FETAL MEDICINE:

Basic Science and Clinical Practice

For Elsevier

Commissioning Editor: Pauline Graham
Development Editor: Ailsa Laing
Project Manager: Kerrie-Anne Jarvis
Senior Designer: Sarah Russell
Illustration Manager: Kirsteen Wright
Illustrator: Richard Prime, Chartwell

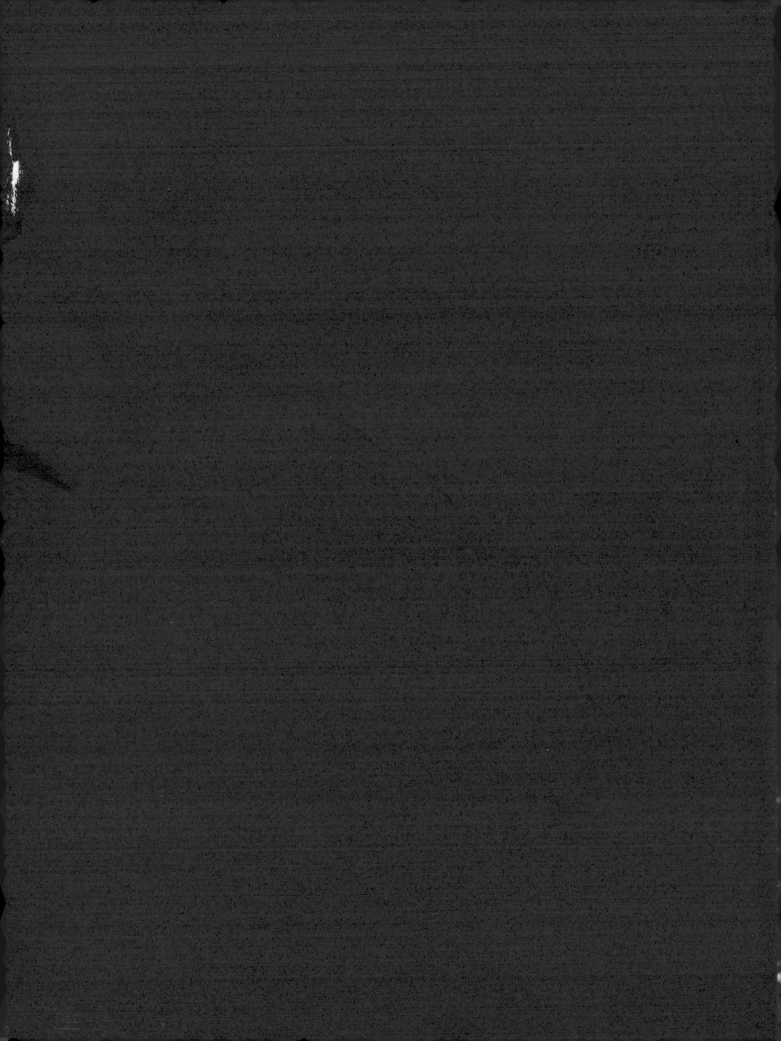

SECOND EDITION

FETAL MEDICINE:

Basic Science and Clinical Practice

Edited by

Charles H Rodeck MB BS BSc DSc FRCOG FRCPath FMedSci

Emeritus Professor, Institute for Women's Health, Obstetrics and Gynaecology, University College London, London, UK

and

Martin J Whittle MD FRCOG FRCP(Glas)

Emeritus Professor of Fetal Medicine, University of Birmingham, Edgbaston, Birmingham, UK

Foreword by

John Queenan

CHURCHILL LIVINGSTONE

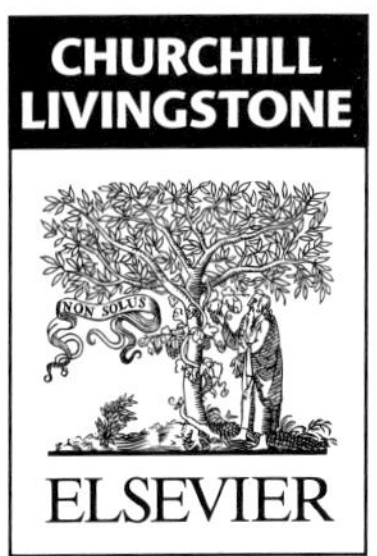

LONDON EDINBURGH NEW YORK PHILADELPHIA SYDNEY TORONTO 2009

CHURCHILL
LIVINGSTONE
ELSEVIER

First Edition 1999
Second Edition 2009
Reprinted 2009

ISBN: 978-0-443-10408-4

British Library Cataloguing in Publication Data
A catalogue record for this book is available from the British Library

Library of Congress Cataloging in Publication Data
A catalog record for this book is available from the Library of Congress

Notice
Knowledge and best practice in this field are constantly changing. As new research and experience broaden our knowledge, changes in practice, treatment and drug therapy may become necessary or appropriate. Readers are advised to check the most current information provided (i) on procedures featured or (ii) by the manufacturer of each product to be administered, to verify the recommended dose or formula, the method and duration of administration, and contraindications. It is the responsibility of the practitioner, relying on their own experience and knowledge of the patient, to make diagnoses, to determine dosages and the best treatment for each individual patient, and to take all appropriate safety precautions. To the fullest extent of the law, neither the Publisher nor the Editors assumes any liability for any injury and/or damage to persons or property arising out of or related to any use of the material contained in this book.

The Publisher

The Publisher's policy is to use paper manufactured from sustainable forests

Printed in China

Contents

Foreword vii
Preface viii
Contributors ix

SECTION 1 **Early fetal development** 1

1 Early concepts and terminology 3
Patricia Collins

2 Cellular mechanisms and embryonic tissues 6
Patricia Collins

3 Staging embryos in development and the embryonic body plan 24
Patricia Collins

4 Development of the head 33
Patricia Collins

5 Development of the heart 47
Roelof-Jan Oostra and Antoon FM Moorman

SECTION 2 **The placenta** 61

6 The immunology of implantation 63
Ashley Moffett and YW Loke

7 Development of the placenta and its circulation 69
Caroline Dunk, Berthold Huppertz and John Kingdom

8 Placental function in maternofetal exchange 97
Thomas Jansson and Theresa L Powell

9 Maternofetal trafficking 110
Diana W Bianchi

SECTION 3 **Fetal physiology and pathology** 117

10 Development of the cardiovascular system 119
Kent L Thornburg and Carley AE Shaut

11 Lung growth and maturation 133
Richard Harding and Stuart B Hooper

12 Development of the kidneys and urinary tract 147
Karen M Moritz, Georgina Caruana and E Marelyn Wintour

13 Maternal medicines and the fetus 158
David Williams and Lila Mayahi

14 The perinatal postmortem 181
Phil Cox

SECTION 4 **Epidemiology** 195

15 Epidemiological techniques in fetal medicine 197
James P Neilson and Zarko Alfirevic

SECTION 5 **Ethics** 205

16 Ethical issues in maternal–fetal medicine 207
Susan Bewley

SECTION 6 **Prenatal screening and diagnosis** 223

17 Conveying information about screening 225
Louise Bryant, Shenaz Ahmed and Jenny Hewison

18 Parental reaction to prenatal diagnosis and subsequent bereavement 234
Jane Fisher and Helen Statham

19 Prenatal screening for open neural tube defects and Down's syndrome 243
James E Haddow, Glenn E Palomaki, Jacob A Canick and George J Knight

20 Ultrasound screening for fetal abnormalities and aneuploidies in the first and second trimesters 265
Fionnuala M Breathnach and Fergal D Malone

21 Non-invasive screening and diagnosis from maternal blood 282
Olav Lapaire, Sinuhe Hahn and Wolfgang Holzgreve

22 Invasive diagnostic procedures 292
Boaz Weisz and Charles Rodeck

23 Cytogenetics 305
Caroline M Ogilvie

24 Mendelian genetics – the old and the new 318
J Michael Connor

25 Preimplantation genetic diagnosis 323
Joyce C Harper and Joy DA Delhanty

26 Hemoglobinopathies 331
John M Old

27 Prenatal screening for thalassemias 344
Mary Tang and Kwok-Yin Leung

28 Cystic fibrosis 349
Mary Porteous and Jon Warner

29 Inborn errors of metabolism 357
Wim J Kleijer and Frans W Verheijen

SECTION 7 **Diagnosis and management of fetal malformations** 377

30 Sonography of the fetal central nervous system 379
Gustavo Malinger and Gianluigi Pilu

31 The heart 412
Helena M Gardiner

32 Fetal lung lesions 429
N Scott Adzick

33 Congenital diaphragmatic hernia 437
Alan W Flake and Holly L Hedrick

34 Abdomen 447
Martin J Whittle

35 Kidney and urinary tract disorders 459
Marc Dommergues, Farida Daïkha-Dahmane, Françoise Muller, Marie Cécile Aubry, Stephen Lortat-Jacob, Claire Nihoul-Fékété, Yves Dumez – updated for the 2nd edition by Mark D Kilby

36 Fetal skeletal abnormalities 478
Lyn S Chitty, Louise Wilson and David R Griffin

37 Fetal hydrops 514
Jon Hyett

38 Fetal tumors 528
Mark P Johnson and Stephanie Mann

SECTION 8 **Diagnosis and management of other fetal conditions** 539

39 Fetal growth and growth restriction 541
Elisabeth Peregrine and Donald Peebles

40 Red cell alloimmunization 559
Charles H Rodeck and Anne Deans

41 Fetal platelet disorders 578
Leendert Porcelijn, Eline SA van den Akker and Humphrey HH Kanhai

42 Treatable fetal endocrine and metabolic disorders 592
Guy Rosner, Shai Ben Shahar, Yuval Yaron and Mark I Evans

43 Early pregnancy failure 602
Jemma Johns and Eric Jauniaux

44 Fetal infections 620
Guillaume Benoist and Yves Ville

45 Amniotic fluid 642
Pamela A Mahon and Karim D Kalache

46 Multiple pregnancy 649
Neelam Engineer and Nicholas Fisk

47 In utero stem cell transplantation 678
Sicco Scherjon and Elles in't Anker

48 Fetal gene therapy 689
Anna David and Charles H Rodeck

SECTION 9 **The neonate** 701

49 Interface of fetal and neonatal medicine 703
Malcolm Chiswick

Self-assessment scenarios 711
Pranav Pandya

Appendix: Charts of fetal measurements 721
LS Chitty and Douglas G Altman

Index 767

Foreword

The last half-century has been an extraordinary time for Fetal Medicine. At the outset, the ravages of prematurity, preeclampsia, Rhesus disease, diabetes mellitus, and even rubella took a large toll on perinatal survival. Modalities such as amniocentesis, ultrasonography, and cardiotocography were not yet available to aid the physicians and nurses caring for high-risk pregnancies. Little was known of fetal physiology or the pathophysiology of fetal disease. In the last 50 years, the inner sanctum of the fetus was probed and tested with medicines, needles, scalpels, and imaging. The secrets of the fetus were systematically explored, and new tests and treatments were developed. This exciting era brought major advances in diagnosis, treatment, and prophylaxis for the fetus.

The fetal medicine scene is quite different today. Perinatal mortality and morbidity have decreased remarkably. Through active immunization, rubella has almost disappeared. Through passive immunization, Rhesus disease is markedly decreased. Fetal aneuploidy can effectively be detected by prenatal genetics, even in the first trimester. Diabetic pregnancies, when appropriately managed, lead to outcomes similar to non-diabetics. Preeclampsia is still common, but the management has lowered the morbidity and mortality for both mother and infant. Unexpected iatrogenic prematurity has almost disappeared because of accurate dating of gestations. Neonatal intensive care nursery skills and equipment have made it possible to save babies born at 23–24 weeks of gestation, while 50 years ago survival rates were low before 34–35 weeks. Now, with fetal surveillance, corticosteroids to promote fetal pulmonary maturity, tocolysis to permit administration of such, and transfer to an appropriate facility for delivery, the prospects for the premature infant are greatly improved.

The two editors of this book were central to the many improvements of Fetal Medicine. As perinatal pioneers, they contributed enormously to the development of new knowledge. Professor Rodeck unlocked the secrets of in-utero health and disease with his fetoscopy, developing diagnostic and therapeutic modalities for the fetus. Professor Whittle has made important contributions in genetics, fetal evaluation, and treatment. What better experts could take on the arduous task of creating a definitive second edition of this textbook?

Unlike most books on high-risk pregnancies, which cover the maternal and fetal aspects, this textbook concentrates on the fetus. They present a comprehensive opus that is truly international, selecting qualified authors who can discuss the basic science as well as the clinical aspects of perinatal problems. This is an essential resource with extraordinary information on embryology, physiology and genetics, and clinical management. It will serve all who care for high-risk pregnancies in the future as we try to conquer the remaining problems causing compromised pregnancy outcome, and to make the next half century of Fetal Medicine even more revolutionary than the last.

John T Queenan, MD
Professor and Chair Emeritus of Obstetrics and Gynecology
Georgetown University School of Medicine
Washington, DC, USA
Deputy Editor, *Obstetrics & Gynecology*

Prefaces

Preface to the second edition

The response to the First Edition was extremely positive but when a Second Edition was suggested, we thought long and hard. The many innovations that have occurred since the publication of the First Edition in 1999 made a revision imperative and rather to our surprise we agreed to the enterprise! We have kept to the Principles outlined in the Preface to the First Edition. We were determined to keep the basic science and to combine it with practical guidance in a variety of clinical circumstances. But there have been many changes. Some chapters are new and others have been completely updated. A self-assessment section with clinical scenarios has been added. We hope that this and the retention of the Appendix with charts of fetal measurements will both assist trainees with learning and continue to add to the value of the book in daily practice. Most sections have been pruned and this Edition is leaner, slimmer, and we believe, fitter.

We have been fortunate that such a constellation of international experts has so generously given their time to share their expertise and we are deeply indebted to them. They have delivered the most up-to-date information possible and balanced the flavour of local practice and experience with a global view. This is a strength which provides individual clinicians, faced with a particular problem, a broader perspective to guide management.

We are also most grateful to our publisher and in particular to Ailsa Laing and Kerrie-Anne Jarvis for their unfailing and patient support and to the commissioning editors, initially Ellen Green and subsequently Pauline Graham. We would also like to thank John Queenan for his constructive comments and kind words.

CHARLES H. RODECK
MARTIN J. WHITTLE

Preface to the first edition

The demise of the large textbook has been repeatedly announced, yet it has failed to happen – why? Perhaps because they provide a summation of knowledge and define a discipline. We believe that this book, the first devoted to Fetal Medicine, fulfils these functions. We thought it essential to include the relevant basic science because the rate of increase in information is outstripping the ability of clinicians to keep up. New scientific terminology and language pose barriers to understanding which we hope that this book will help to overcome.

In such a multidisciplinary field it has been impossible to be all-inclusive: we have preferred to be selective, including only core subjects. In embryology, topics were chosen to illustrate scientific principles, and in neonatology, for their immediate relevance to the fetus. After some initial reluctance, maternal medicine was excluded. Although currently most feto-maternal subspecialists work in both fields, it is likely that a separation will occur in the near future and there are numerous excellent texts dealing with maternal medicine.

We make no apology for some overlap and repetition in a number of the chapters. This has given authors the freedom to express differing views and to develop their own themes, thus maintaining the internal consistency of their chapters. Neither do we apologise for not imposing either cis- or trans-atlantic spelling. That would seem parochial in comparison to the theme of the book and its global authorship and readership.

The development of this book has taken over 10 years, partly due to a series of upheavals in the publishing world. Much credit for its conception must go to the persuasive and persistent charm of Sylvia Hull. Others who have helped to nurture it include Lucy Gardner, Antonia Seymour, Prudence Daniels, Deborah Russell, and most recently Miranda Bromage and Rachel Robson, and they deserve our gratitude. Most of all, we thank our contributors. Their time (much of it doubtless after midnight), expertise and perseverence have provided us with superb chapters.

CHARLES H. RODECK
MARTIN J. WHITTLE

Contributors

N Scott Adzick MD MMM
Surgeon-in-Chief, C Everett Koop Professor of Pediatrics, Department of Surgery, Center for Fetal Diagnosis and Treatment, Children's Hospital of Philadelphia, USA

Shenaz Ahmed BSc(Hons) PhD
Lecturer, Leeds Institute of Health Sciences, Academic Unit of Public Health , The University of Leeds, UK

Zarko Alfirevic MD MRCOG
Professor of Fetal and Maternal Medicine, University Department of Obstetrics and Gynaecology, Liverpool Women's Hospital, Liverpool, UK

Douglas G Altman BSc DSc
Professor of Statistics in Medicine, Centre for Statistics in Medicine, University of Oxford, UK

Marie Cécile Aubry MD
Maternité, Hôpital Necker Enfants Malade, Paris, France

Guillaum Benoist MD
Service de Gynecologie Obstetrique, Centre Hospitalier Intercommunal de Poissy-St Germain, Poissy, France

Susan Bewley MA MD FRCOG
Consultant Obstetrics/Maternal-Fetal Medicine, Women's Services, Guy's and St Thomas's Hospitals, London, UK

Diana W Bianchi MD
Natalie V Zucker Professor of Pediatrics, Obstetrics and Gynaecology, Vice-Chair for Research, Floating Hospital for Children at Tufts Medical Center, Boston, USA

Fionnuala M Breathnach MRCOG MRCPI DCH DipGUMed
Department of Obstetrics and Gynaecology, Royal College of Surgeons in Ireland, The Rotunda Hospital, Dublin, Ireland

Louise Bryant BSc(Hons) Psych PhD
Senior Research Fellow, Leeds Institute of Health Sciences, University of Leeds, UK

Jacob A Canick PhD
Professor, Department of Pathology, The Warren Alpert Medical School of Brown University, Providence; Director, Division of Prenatal and Special Testing, Department of Pathology, Women and Infants Hospital, Providence, USA

Georgina Caruana BSc(Hons) PhD
Research Fellow, Department of Anatomy and Developmental Biology, Monash University, Clayton, Australia

Malcolm L Chiswick MD FRCP(Lond) FRCPCH DCH
Professor of Child Health and Paediatrics, University of Manchester; Honorary Consultant Paediatrician, St Mary's Hospital for Women and Children, Manchester, UK

Lyn S Chitty BSc PhD MBBS MRCOG
Reader and Consultant in Genetics and Fetal Medicine, Institute of Child Health and University College London Hospitals NHS Foundation Trust, London, UK

Patricia Collins BSc PhD
Associate Professor of Anatomy, Anglo-European College of Chiropractic, Bournmouth, Dorset, UK

J Michael Connor MD DSc FRCP
Head of Department and Honorary Consultant, Duncan Guthrie Institute of Medical Genetics, University of Glasgow, Yorkhill Academic Campus, Yorkhill Hospitals, Glasgow, UK

Phil Cox MBBS PhD FRCPath
Consultant Perinatal Pathologist, Department of Histopathology, Birmingham Women's Hospital, Birmingham, UK

Farida Daïkha-Dahmane MD PhD
Praticien Hospitalier, Laboratoire de Biologie du Dévelopement, Hôpital Robert Debré, Paris, France

Anna David BSc(Hons) MB ChB MRCOG PhD
Senior Lecturer and Honorary Consultant in Obstetrics and Fetal Medicine, Institute for Women's Health, University College London, UK

Anne Deans DCH MFFP MRCGP FRCOG
Consultant Obstetrician and Gynaecologist, Frimley Park Hospital and University College Hospital, London, UK

Joy DA Delhanty BSc PhD
Emeritus Professor of Human Genetics, Institute for Women's Health, University College London, UK

Marc Dommergues MD
Praticien Hospitalier, Maternité, Hôpital Antoine Béclère, Clamart, France

Yves Dumez MD
Professor, Maternité Hôpital Necker Enfants-Malades, Paris, France

Caroline Dunk
Research Associate, Women's and Infants' Health, The Samuel Lunerfield Research Institute, Mount Sinai Hospital, Toronto, Canada

Neelam Engineer MBBS MRCOG
Subspecialty Specialist Registrar, Maternal and Fetal Medicine, Centre for Fetal Care, Queen Charlotte's and Chelsea Hospitals, London, UK

Mark I Evans MD
Charlotte B Failing Professor, Acting Chairman and Specialist-in-Chief of Obstetrics and Gynecology; Professor of Molecular

Medicine and Genetics; Professor of Pathology; Director, Division of Reproductive Genetics; Director, Center for Fetal Diagnosis and Therapy; Director, Human Genetics Program, Department of Obs/Gyn, Hutzel Hospital, Detroit, Michigan, USA

Jane Fisher BA MA
Director, Antenatal Results and Choices (ARC), London, UK

Nicholas Fisk PhD MBA FRCOG DDU
Director, University of Queensland Centre for Clinical Research; Specialist in Maternal and Fetal Medicine, Royal Brisbane & Women's Hospital, Herston, Queensland, Australia

Alan W Flake MD
Professor of Pediatric Surgery and Director, Department of Surgery, Children's Hospital of Philadelphia, USA

Helena M Gardiner MD PhD FRCP DCH FRCPCH
Director and Senior Lecturer in Perinatal Cardiology, Institute of Reproductive and Developmental Biology, Faculty of Medicine, Imperial College London, Queen Charlotte's and Chelsea and Royal Brompton Hospitals, London, UK

David R Griffin MB ChB FRCOG
Consultant and Fetal Medicine Lead, West Herts Hospitals NHS Trust, Watford, UK

James E Haddow MD
Director, Division of Medical Screening, Department of Pathology and Laboratory Medicine, Women and Infants Hospital, Providence; Professor of Pathology and Laboratory Medicine (Research), The Warren Alpert Medical School of Brown University, Providence, USA

Sinuhe Hahn MD
Professor, Department of Research, Laboratory for Prenatal Medicine and Gynaecological Oncology, Women's Hospital, Basel, Switzerland

Richard Harding PhD DSc
Department of Anatomy and Developmental Biology, Monash University, Clayton, Victoria, Australia

Joyce C Harper PhD
Reader in Preimplantation Genetics, Institute for Women's Health, University College London, UK

Holly L Hedrick MD
Assistant Professor of Surgery and Obstetrics, Department of Surgery, Children's Hospital of Philadelphia, USA

Jenny Hewison BA MSc PhD
Professor of the Psychology of Healthcare, Leeds Institute of Health Sciences, Academic Unit of Psychiatry and Behavioural Sciences, University of Leeds, UK

Wolfgang Holzgreve Prof. Dr. Med Dr. Lcmulk MS FACOG FRCOG MBA
Professor and Chairman, Department of Obstetrics and Gynaecology, University of Basel, Switzerland

Stuart B Hooper PhD
Associate Professor, Department of Physiology, Monash University, Clayton, Victoria, Australia

Berthold Huppertz
University Professor of Cell Biology, Institute of Cell Biology, Histology and Embryology, Center of Molecular Medicine, Medical University of Graz, Austria

Jon Hyett MBBS MD MRCOG FRANZCOG
Staff Specialist in Maternal and Fetal Medicine, Royal Prince Alfred Hospital, Sydney, Australia

Elles in't Anker MD PhD
Department of Obstetrics, Leiden University Medical Center, Leiden, The Netherlands

Thomas Jansson MD PhD
Associate Professor, Department of Obstetrics and Gynecology, University of Cincinnati Medical Center, Cincinnati, Ohio, USA

Eric Jauniaux MD PhD
Professor of Obstetrics and Fetal Medicine, Institute for Women's Health, University College London, UK

Jemma Johns MBBS MD MRCOG
Honorary Clinical Research Fellow, Institute for Women's Health, University College London, UK

Mark P Johnson MD
Director of Obstetrical Services, Center for Fetal Diagnosis and Treatment, The Children's Hospital of Philadelphia
Associate Professor, Departments of Obstetrics and Gynaecology, Surgery and Pediatrics, the University of Pennsylvania School of Medicine, Philadelphia, USA

Karim D Kalache PrivDoz DrMed
Professor of Obstetrics, Department of Obstetrics, Charité Campus Mitte, Universitätsmedizine Berlin, Germany

Humphrey HH Kanhai MD PhD
Professor of Maternal/Fetal Medicine, Head, Department of Obstetrics, Leiden University Medical Centre, Leiden, The Netherlands

Mark D Kilby MD MBBS MRCOG
Dame Hilda Lloyd Professor in Maternal & Fetal Medicine, Fetal Medicine Centre, Academic Department of Obstetrics & Gynaecology, Birmingham Women's Hospital, Birmingham, UK

John Kingdom MD FRCOG FRCSC MRCP(UK)
Rose Torno Chair, Department of Obstetrics and Gynecology, Medical Imaging and Pathology, University of Toronto; Maternal-Fetal Medicine Specialist, Mount Sinai Hospital, Toronto, Canada

Wim J Kleijer PhD
Clinical Biochemical Geneticist, Department of Clinical Genetics, Erasmus Medical Centre, Rotterdam, The Netherlands

George J Knight PhD
Associate Director, Laboratory Science, Department of Pathology and Laboratory Medicine, Women and Infants Hospital, Providence; Assistant Professor of Pathology and Laboratory Medicine (Research), The Warren Alpert Medical School of Brown University, Providence, USA

Olav Lapaire MD
University Women's Hospital, Basel, Switzerland

Kwok-Yin Leung MBBS MSc FRCOG FHKAM(O&G) DipEpidApplStat
Consultant and Honorary Professor, Department of Obstetrics and Gynaecology, The University of Hong Kong, Queen Mary Hospital, Hong Kong

YW Loke MA MD ScD FRCOG
Professor of Reproductive Immunology, King's College, Cambridge, UK

Stephen Lortat-Jacob MD
Praticien Hospitalier, Service de Chirurgie Infantile, Hôpital Necker Enfants-Malades, Paris, France

Pamela A Mahon DCR(R) DMU MA PhD
Superintendant Sonographer, Southampton Women's Survey Ultrasound Unit, MRC Resource Centre, University of Southampton, Princess Anne Hospital, Southampton, UK

Gustavo Malinger MD
Director, Prenatal Diagnosis Unit, Edith Wolfson Medical Center, Sackler School of Medicine, Tel-Aviv University, Holon, Israel

Fergal D Malone MD
Professor and Chairman, Department of Obstetrics and Gynaecology, Royal College of Surgeons in Ireland, The Rotunda Hospital, Dublin, Ireland

Stephanie Mann MD
Assistant Professor of Surgery, University of Pennsylvania School of Medicine, Center for Fetal Diagnosis and Therapy, Children's Hospital of Philadelphia, USA

Lila Mayahi BSc PhD MRCP
Centre for Clinical Pharmacology, University College London, UK

Ashley Moffett MD MRCP MRCPath
Fellow in Medical Sciences and Director of Clinical Studies, King's College, Cambridge, Reader in Reproductive Immunology, University of Cambridge, UK

Antoon FM Moorman PhD
Professor of Embryology and Molecular Biology of Cardiovascular Diseases, Department of Anatomy and Embryology, Academic Medical Center, Amsterdam, The Netherlands

Karen M Moritz PhD
Research Fellow, School of Biomedical Sciences, University of Queensland, Brisbane, Australia

Françoise Muller MD PhD
Maître de Conférence des Universités, Hôpital Ambroise Paré, Boulogne, France

James P Neilson BSc MD FRCOG
Deputy Dean & Professor of Obstetrics & Gynaecology; Head of School of Reproductive & Developmental Medicine, University of Liverpool; Co-ordinating Editor, Cochrane Pregnancy & Childbirth Group, Liverpool Women's Hospital, Liverpool, UK

Claire Nihoul-Fékété MD
Professor, Service de Chirurgie Infantile, Hôpital Necker Enfants-Malades, Paris, France

Caroline M Ogilvie BSc DPhil
Cytogenetics Department, Guy's & St Thomas' Hospital Foundation Trust; Division of Medical and Molecular Genetics, Guy's, King's & St Thomas' School of Medicine, King's College, London, UK

John M Old PhD FRCPath
Head of Laboratory, National Haemoglobinopathy Reference Service, Churchill Hospital, Headington, Oxford, UK

Roelof-Jan Oostra MD PhD
Lecturer, Department of Anatomy and Embryology, Academic Medical Center, University of Amsterdam, The Netherlands

Glenn E Palomaki BA BS
Associate Director, Division of Medical Screening, Department of Pathology and Laboratory Medicine, Women and Infants Hospital, Providence; Senior Research Associate in Pathology and Laboratory Medicine, The Warren Alpert Medical School of Brown University, Providence, USA

Pranav Pandya BSc MBBS MRCOG MD
Consultant in Fetal Medicine and Obstetrics, Honorary Senior Lecturer, University College London Hospital, UK

Donald M Peebles MA MD MRCOG
Professor of Obstetrics, Institute for Women's Health, University College London, UK

Elisabeth Peregrine MBBS BSc MRCOG MD
Subspecialty Trainee in Materno-Fetal Medicine, Fetal Medicine Unit, Elizabeth Garret Anderson Obstetric Hospital, London, UK

Gianluigi Pilu MD
Consultant in Obstetrics and Gynaecology, Department of Obstetrics and Gynaecology, University of Bologna, Italy

Leendert Porcelijn MD
Head of the Platelet/Leukocyte Serology Department, Sanquin Diagnostic Services, Amsterdam, The Netherlands

Mary Porteous MB ChB MSc MD FRCP(Ed)
Consultant Clinical Geneticist, Director South East of Scotland Genetic Service, Molecular Medicine Centre, Department Clinical Genetics, Western General Hospital, Edinburgh, UK

Theresa L Powell BSc PhD
Department of Obstetrics and Gynecology, University of Cincinnati College of Medicine, Cincinnati, Ohio, USA

Charles H Rodeck MBBS BSc DSc(Med) FRCOG FRCPath FMedSci
Professor Emeritus of Obstetrics and Gynaecology, University College London, UK

Guy Rosner MD
Specialist in Internal Medicine and Medical Genetics, Senior Physician, Tel-Aviv Sourasky Medical Center, Tel-Aviv, Israel

Sicco Scherjon MD PhD
Consultant in Obstetrics, Department of Obstetrics, Leiden University Medical Center, Leiden, The Netherlands

Shai Ben Shachar MD
Specialist in Pediatrics and Medical Genetics, Tel-Aviv Sourasky Medical Center, Tel-Aviv, Israel

Carley A E Shaut PhD
Postdoctoral Fellow, Heart Research Center, Oregon Health and Science University, Portland, Oregon, USA

Helen Statham BSc PhD
Senior Research Associate, Faculty of Social and Political Sciences, University of Cambridge, UK

Mary Tang MBBS FRCOG
Consultant, Prenatal Diagnostic and Counseling Department, Tsan Yuk Hospital, Hong Kong

Kent L Thornburg PhD
M. Lowell Edwards Chair for Research, Professor and Associate Chief for Research, Division of Cardiovascular Medicine; Director, Heart Research Center, Oregon Health & Science University, Portland, Oregon, USA

Eline S A van den Akker MD
Department of Obstetrics, Leiden University Medical Centre, Leiden, The Netherlands

Frans W Verheijen PhD
Clinical Biochemical Geneticist, Department of Clinical Genetics, Erasmus Medical Centre, Rotterdam, The Netherlands

Yves Ville
Professor of Obstetrics and Gynaecology, Service de Gynecologie Obstetrique, Centre Hospitalier Intercommunal, Poissy, France

Jon Warner BSc PhD
Director of Molecular Genetics Service, Human Genetics Unit, Western General Hospital, Edinburgh, UK

Boaz Weisz MD
Senior consultant, Fetal Medicine Unit, Department of Obstetrics and Gynecology, Sheba Medical Center, Israel

Martin J Whittle MD FRCOG FRCP(Glas)
Emeritus Professor of Fetal Medicine, University of Birmingham, Edgbaston, Birmingham, UK

David Williams MBBS PhD FRCP
Consultant Obstetric Physician, Institute for Women's Health, University College London Hospitals, UK

Louise C Wilson BSc MBChB
Consultant in Clinical Genetics, Great Ormond Street Hospital for Children, London, UK

E Marelyn Wintour PhD DSc
Honorary Professor, School of Biomedical Sciences, University of Queensland, Brisbane, Australia

Yuval Yaron MD
Director, Prenatal Genetic Diagnosis Unit, Genetic Institute, Tel-Aviv Sourasky Medical Center, Tel-Aviv; Associate Professor, Department of Obstetrics and Gynaecology, Sackler Faculty of Medicine, Tel-Aviv University, Israel

SECTION 1

Early fetal development

1 Early concepts and terminology 3
Patricia Collins

2 Cellular mechanisms and embryonic tissues 6
Patricia Collins

3 Staging embryos in development and the embryonic body plan 24
Patricia Collins

4 Development of the head 33
Patricia Collins

5 Development of the heart 47
Roelof-Jan Oostra and Antoon FM Moorman

CHAPTER 1

Early concepts and terminology

Patricia Collins

KEY POINTS

- A revision of the 19th century terminology still used to describe early embryos, particularly the outdated term 'germ layers'
- Review of the terms now used for specific embryonic cell populations and the usefulness of histological terms
- Reviews the axes of the early embryo and the terminology used to describe animal and human bodies

Traditional accounts of embryology rely on familiarity with the germ layer concept developed in the latter years of the 19th century. All students are acquainted with ectoderm, endoderm and mesoderm layers and accept the grouping of mature tissues and systems with these layers. However, it is apposite, in the early years of the 21st century, to review and question the usage of our old terminology, and the assumptions which have developed as a consequence, and move forward stating our present knowledge base using the most appropriate language with which to express our existing concepts and hypotheses.

The transitory nature of our conceptual frameworks is acknowledged. We know that the 'snapshots' of knowledge in textbooks may be outdated by the time of publication and are now more likely to turn to the Internet to find the latest publications on a topic. However, the language we use to describe even the most recent findings is still rooted in the past and in many ways hinders our ability to explain developmental processes.

The rapid advances in developmental biology which have increased our understanding of embryological processes have elucidated many cell lines, each of which gives rise to parts of the embryo, each cell type being important in different stages of development. The relatively new methods of cell study, e.g. inter alia, cloning cells taken from early and later stages of development, and production of chimeric embryos where cells from, for example, quail embryos are substituted for cells in chick embryos, have compounded the problem of how to describe cell populations in early embryos so as to marry the older embryological terminology everyone is familiar with to the newer, more specialized, vocabulary of developmental biology.

It has been suggested that to cope with the complex and often conflicting terminologies in embryology, nomenclature relating to the histological appearance of cells is more helpful than the older traditional concepts[1–3]. Indeed, the advances in embryology now make it increasingly difficult to relate older and newer language. This first chapter will give a brief account of the way the older terminology developed and move on to explain the usage of the more recent terminologies.

THE ORIGIN OF THE TRADITIONAL LANGUAGE OF EMBRYOLOGY

The traditional language of embryology comes from work and concepts generated between 1830 and 1900 when, in the mid-1800s, the theory of evolution was being formulated. Ernst Haeckel[4], particularly, promoted a concept which stated that embryos would pass through all the previous evolutionary stages, resembling a series of extant or extinct adult animals as they recapitulated evolution during development. Thus, Haeckel designated a *blastula* stage of development, where a sphere or bilaminar layer of embryonic cells was present, and a later *gastrula* stage achieved after the blastula cells had invaginated to produce more than one or two layers. It is from Haeckel we have the term *gastrulation* to describe the process where cells initially on the embryonic surface move inside the embryo to produce intraembryonic cell populations.

At this time, the instruments for examining embryos were rudimentary and the cell theory was still relatively young. Scientists of the day saw layers of tissue rather than the individual cells composing the layers. Even in those studies where it is clear from the publications that cells could be seen, distinctions between early embryonic cell types probably could not be made with the instruments available. The concepts thus generated by these early embryologists were products of their time, dependent on the methods of experiment and observation customary when they were formulated.

During the process of gastrulation, cells from the outside of the embryo move to the interior and become organized in specific sites. The concept of three main or *germ layers* was formulated by Von Baer[5] and promoted by the Hertwig brothers[6] who supported the doctrine that three germ layers were found in all animal embryos. The layers of adult two-layered creatures had been named *ectoderm* and *endoderm* by Allman[7] and, later, the term *mesoderm* was introduced to describe both the structure that intervened between the ectoderm (exoderm) and endoderm (entoderm) of triploblastic animals and the corresponding embryonic middle layer[4]. At the same time, the more specific embryological terms *epiblast*, *mesoblast* and *hypoblast* were used by Balfour[8] in his studies on chick embryos. Thus, for most of the 20th century, textbooks supported the notion that the tissues of the developed body were derived from one of the three germ layers. While this is not untrue in simplistic terms, the accent on three layers has obfuscated the dynamic differentiation processes occurring in embryos and hindered much description of what can be seen histologically.

A similar process occurred with the description of external embryonic form. Von Baer noted that all vertebrate embryos pass through externally similar stages and Haeckel published a series of drawings demonstrating remarkable similarity between embryos which go on to become very dissimilar adults. This latter concept remained unchallenged for over a century. Recent examination of Haeckel's pictures, together with a clear analysis of the developmental stages of various organs in each embryo revealed a story much closer to the Emperor's new clothes. Richardson[9] noted that drawings by contemporaries of Haeckel show much more accurate interpretations of mammalian embryos of the same developmental stage with clear differences between them. He noted that Haeckel's drawings had given a misleading view of embryonic development. Thus, the idea of one stage of development where all vertebrates are the same, promoted extensively at the turn of the 20th century and repeated unchallenged, obfuscated what really occurs in a number of vertebrate embryos and hindered the search for what is actually present in embryos by limiting our language and expectations.

A description of the developmentally based terminology which recent textbooks of embryology embrace follows, outlining the initial derivation and fate of the early cell lines. As can be seen, the complexities of development now require a redefining of the older terminologies and the introduction of new ones to describe the changes taking place and the cell types involved.

RECENT NOMENCLATURE OF EARLY DEVELOPMENT AND SPECIFICATION OF CELL ORIGIN

The initial zygote cleaves into a number of cells which, because of their position and experiences, have different fates. The earliest positions of cells in the morula will influence the first decision between trophoblastic cells, which will give rise to the placenta and membranes, or embryonic cells. The initial embryonic cells, which are arranged as a disk, are collectively termed *epiblast*. These cells will produce all of the embryonic cell lines and some extraembryonic cell lines. The epiblast cells are supported by an underlying *hypoblast* layer of extraembryonic cells which will later become sequestered into the yolk sac wall. An interaction between epiblast and hypoblast gives rise to the *primitive streak*, a region of cell proliferation and movement, that defines the craniocaudal axis of the embryo. Passage through the primitive streak will confer a fate onto cells specified by the position of invagination or the time of invagination[10]. Predictive fate maps of the epiblast have been constructed from data on the differentiative fate of cells taken from different regions of the embryonic disc and cloned (Fig. 1.1).

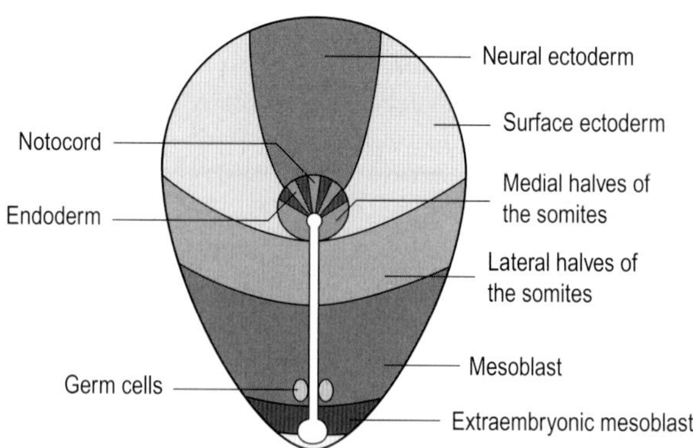

Fig. 1.1 Predictive fates of the epiblast cell population at the time the primitive streak is present. (From *Gray's Anatomy*, 39th edn. Edinburgh: Churchill Livingstone, 2005.)

The primitive streak extends from near the center of the embryonic disk, where it forms the *primitive node*, a curved ridge of cells, to the edge of the disk close to the early connection of the embryo to the developing placenta. Passage of proliferating cells through the primitive node gives rise to the axial cell populations, the *notochord* and the *medial halves of the somites*, and also to the *endoderm* which spreads out beneath the epiblast displacing the hypoblast laterally into the yolk sac wall. Passage through the rostral portion of the primitive streak, however, produces the *lateral halves of the somites* and the middle portion of the streak produces the *lateral plate cells*[11,12]. The next caudal portion of the primitive streak gives rise to the *primordial germ cells*. These are sequestered in the extraembryonic tissues very early on in development and do not return to the embryo until the early gonads have formed. The most caudal portion of the streak contributes cells to the *extraembryonic tissue*.

Once these cells have passed through the primitive streak, the remaining epiblast contains cells populations which will become the surface epithelium of the embryo (this still retains the term 'ectoderm') and the neuroepithelium of the embryo which will form the central, peripheral and autonomic nervous systems. This population is termed 'neurectoderm' prior to neurulation; it is found in front of the primitive node.

The cells within the epiblast are epithelial, when they pass through the primitive streak they undergo a change in morphology allowing them to migrate. This new migratory population is initially termed *mesoblast*[3,13]. All of the early migratory cells derived from ingression through the primitive streak revert to epithelia when they arrive at their final destinations and subsequently form proliferative centers. Cells produced from these early germinal epithelia form populations described as *mesenchyme*, further subdivided according to their position in the embryo. Special populations of mesenchyme also develop from the neural epithelium. At the margins of the neural plate are clusters of neuroepithelial cells termed *neural crest cells*. These cells will form the peripheral nervous system in the trunk and head and an extensive mesenchymal population in the head, often termed 'ectomesenchyme'. The neural crest is found only in vertebrates; it is considered to be an evolutionary advance associated with the development of special sense organs within complex facial structures.

The production of migrating cells from the primitive streak and the development of the neurectoderm which undergoes neurulation (see p. 36) forming the central nervous system, dramatically changes the shape of the embryonic disk causing reflection of the edge of the disk which is displaced to a ventral position with the newly formed neural tube being dorsal.

The early head and tail flexion with corresponding lateral flexion produces the body plan or *Bauplan* and thus a recognizable embryo. Of the developmental studies which have been undertaken over the years in a range of vertebrate species, very few correlate the developmental state of internal organs with external characteristics. Richardson[9], in a study of heterochrony, a change in developmental timing during evolution, has correlated the time of appearance of a number of features to somite number, which is seen as an arbitrary way of expressing developmental age of embryos. This method of investigation allows comparison of the order of development of internal features between a number of embryos and greatly aids our thinking of evolution and development.

ANIMAL MODELS OF DEVELOPMENT

Embryological studies have concentrated on a relatively few species which are easily accessible. Thus chick and quail development has been extensively researched as has *Xenopus* and other amphibians. Mammalian embryos are more difficult to access and difficult to culture for long periods of time, however, the development of the mouse and rat has been closely studied. Although human material has been used for study of very early embryonic development, work is not permitted after 14 days when the primitive streak is formed. Identification of common DNA sequences in vertebrates and invertebrates has meant that embryological processes are now being followed in many species and the findings are equally relevant to human embryos. Avian–mouse chimeras have permitted aspects of mouse neural tube development to be studied in ovo.

The use of diverse species for research means that knowledge about the differences in early development between these species is important. All avian embryos develop from a blastoderm or flattened layer of epiblast above a vast yolk. Mice and rats have folded embryonic regions with the epiblast on the inner surface and the hypoblast on the outer convex surface. During head and tail folding in the mouse, morphological movements alter the embryonic body from a position where the head and tail are in close proximity with the dorsal region fully extended to one where the dorsal region is fully flexed. In human embryos, the embryonic area is disk shaped similar to avia and, although a degree of extension occurs as neurulation proceeds, the extreme extension, as in the mouse, does not occur.

Much confusion in the literature arises because of the difference in nomenclature of axes in animal and human studies. In animals, the axes are described as dorsal/ventral (back to front), lateral/lateral (side to side) and anterior/posterior (nose to tail), and these descriptions are used for embryos. In adult humans, however, the convention for these same axes is posterior/anterior, lateral/lateral and cranial/caudal and this terminology is used variably for human embryos. Much disorientation results from moving from descriptions of human embryos to animal embryos without bearing these terminological differences in mind. For human development in this section the terms dorsal/ventral, lateral/lateral and cranio/caudal, will be used.

REFERENCES

1. Løvtrup S. Epigenetic mechanisms in the early amphibian embryo: cell differentiation and morphogenetic elements. *Biol Rev* **38**:91–130, 1983.
2. Løvtrup S. An introduction to the new evolutionary paradigm. In *Beyond Neo-Darwinism*, Ho Ma-Wan, PT Saunders (eds). London: Academic Press, 1984.
3. Collins P, Billett ES. The terminology of early development: history, concepts and current usage. *Clin Anat* **8**:418–425, 1995.
4. Haeckel E. The gastrea theory, phylogenetic classification of the animal kingdom and the homology of the germ lamellae (trans. EO Wright). *Quart J Micr Sci* **14**:142–165, 223–247, 1874.
5. Von Baer KE. *Entwicklingsgeschichte der Tiere: Beobachtung und Reflexion.* Konigsberg: Bontrager, 1828.
6. Hertwig WAO, Hertwig R. Studies on the germ layers. In *Naturwissenschaften*, pp. 13–16. Jena: Zeit, 1879–1883.
7. Allman GJ. On the structure and development of *Myriothela*. *Phil Trans Roy Soc London* **165**(2):549–575, 1855.
8. Balfour FM. The development and growth of the layers of the blastoderm. *Quart J Micr Sci* **13**:266–276, 1873.
9. Richardson MK. Heterochrony and the phylotypic period. *Develop Biol* **172**:412–421, 1995.
10. Lawson KA, Meneses JJ, Pederson RA. Clonal analysis of epiblast fate during germ layer formation in the mouse embryo. *Development* **113**:891–911, 1991.
11. Selleck MA, Stern CD. Fate mapping and cell lineage analysis of Hensen's node in the chick embryo. *Development* **112**:615–626, 1991.
12. Selleck MA, Stern CD. Commitment of mesoderm cells in Hensen's node of the chick embryo to notochord and somite. *Development* **114**:403–415, 1992.
13. Nakatsuji N. Development of postimplantation mouse embryos: unexplored field rich in unanswered questions. *Devel Growth Differ* **35**:489–499, 1992.

CHAPTER

2 Cellular mechanisms and embryonic tissues

Patricia Collins

KEY POINTS

- This chapter describes the tissue types present in early embryos and the interactions between these tissues
- The membrane systems and cytoskeletal elements within a typical cell are reviewed
- Early embryos contain only epithelial and mesenchymal populations
- Each tissue type produces specialized extracellular matrix molecules and proteins which permit and encourage tissue interactions
- Specific interactions between developing epithelia and mesenchyme are presented and the common cytokines and growth factors discussed

GENERAL CHARACTERISTICS OF ALL CELLS

All cell types have a plasma membrane and internal organelles and all are supported by a range of cytoskeletal structures. The details and arrangement of proteins within cells and within the matrices they synthesize encompass a vast region of research beyond the scope of this text. Only the main proteins and structures necessary for the appreciation of developmental processes are presented. Readers are recommented to consult Alberts et al[1] for further details.

Plasma membrane

The plasma membrane of cells is composed of phospholipid molecules arranged in a bilayer. Within this layer are vast numbers of proteins which may reside entirely within the bilipid layer or protrude intracellularly and/or extracelluarly. Those proteins which project exteriorly are covered with carbohydrates as glycoproteins or proteoglycans and contribute to the *glycocalyx* of the cell (Fig. 2.1). The glycocalyx also contains glycoproteins and proteoglycans which have been secreted into the extracellular space around the cells and then absorbed onto the cell surface. Thus it is difficult to specify exactly where a cell plasma membrane ends and the surrounding extracellular matrix begins. The glycocalyx is fundamental in cell–cell and cell–matrix communication. Cells place specific protein and carbohydrate groups into the glycocalyx when touching and adhering to other cells, when displaying cell markers to other cells, in blood clotting cascades and in inflammatory responses.

The membrane systems (organelles) within the embryonic cells, i.e. nucleus, mitochondria, endoplasmic reticulum, Golgi apparatus, lysosomes and secretory vesicles, are also made of the plasma membrane; secretory vesicles can become incorporated into the external plasma membrane to release contained contents. Intracellular membrane systems are supported within the cytoplasm by a range of cytoskeletal eleme nts which also allow cells to maintain surface specializations (microvilli), to change shape (as in the movements of endocytosis and exocytosis), to move in specific directions and (with the glycocalyx molecules) to adhere strongly to a substrate when movement ceases.

The cytoskeleton

The cytoskeleton is a highly dynamic network of protein filaments that extends throughout the cell. As it also allows the cell to move or move portions of its plasma membrane, the cytoskeleton is less like a bony framework and more like a moveable muscular system. Three types of protein filaments produce a diverse range of cytoskeletal elements including *actin filaments*, *microtubules* and *intermediate filaments* (Fig. 2.2); these are synthesized from actin, tubulin and a range of fibrous proteins, e.g. vimentin, laminin, respectively.

Actin filaments

Actin filaments are polar structures composed of globular molecules of actin arranged as a helix. They work in networks and bundles, often found just beneath the plasma membrane where they crosslink to form the cell cortex. Actin filaments are used to change the shape of the plasma membrane, moving it outwards in projections or inwards in invaginations. Discrete

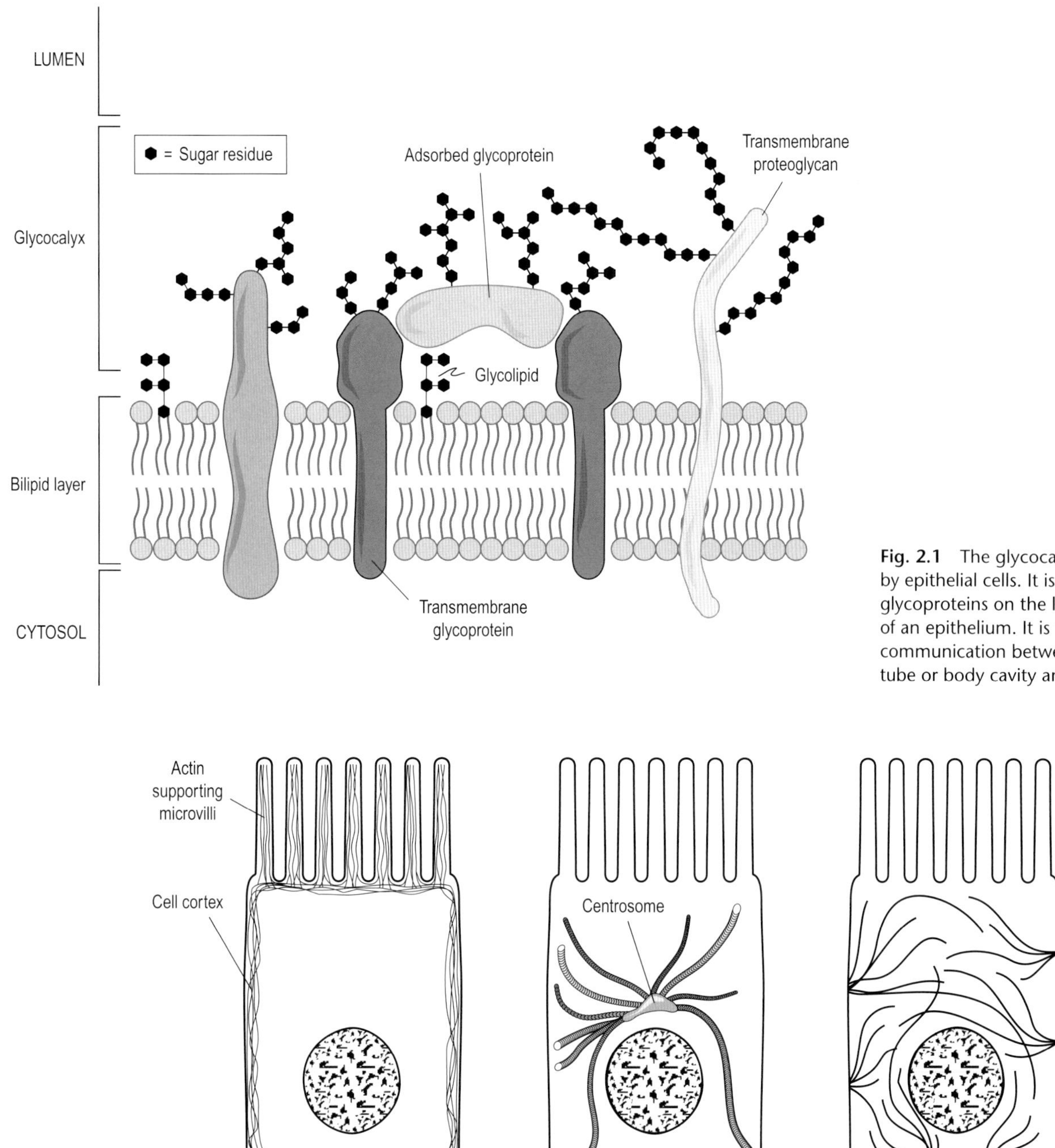

Fig. 2.1 The glycocalyx is synthesized by epithelial cells. It is a feltwork of glycoproteins on the luminal aspect of an epithelium. It is the interface for communication between the lumen of a tube or body cavity and the cells.

Fig. 2.2 Three types of cytoskeletal elements within a cell allow the cell to maintain a shape or move it.

bundles of actin, anchored into the cortex, can produce thin spiky protrusions of the plasma membrane, microvilli, whereas sheet-like extensions of the membrane (lamellipodia) are supported by continuous flattened bundles of actin similarly anchored. Conversely, actin filaments can pull portions of the membrane inwards in the formation of endocytotic vesicles or in cell division. Here, contractile bundles of actin associated with the motor protein myosin form. Although myosin is most familiar in muscle fibers, non-muscle cells contain various myosin proteins. Contractile bundles of actin filaments and myosin filaments are synthesized for specific functions and then disassembled, e.g. during cell division after chromosomal separation, the plasma membrane constricts to the middle of the cell allowing two daughter cells to separate. Such assemblies of actin and myosin are also found in development, near the apical surface of epithelial cells where they play a role in folding of epithelial sheets, and in mesenchyme where they can form stress fibers which allow the cells to exert tension on the extracellular matrix.

Microtubules

Microtubules are long, hollow cylinders composed of the globular protein tubulin. They are much more rigid than actin filaments. Microtubules emanate from the center of the cell in a region termed the centrosome. They lengthen by adding tubulin to the proximal end of each microtubule while subunits are lost from the distal end. The centrosome offers a focus and region of stabilization for the proximal ends of the hundreds of microtubules in a cell; it also contains the two centrioles which are used by the cell when dividing. Vast numbers of microtubules extend in all directions to the plasma membrane and seem to ensure that the centrosome is at the center of the cell. From this position, the microtubule array sites the other cellular organelles and holds them in place using a range of contact proteins. Should the cell touch another cell, there may be internal movements of the organelles driven by the microtubules resulting in repositioning of the centrosome. Microtubules display a dynamic instability, with new subgroups being added or subtracted very rapidly. The turnover of distal units can be slowed by contact with proteins close to the plasma membrane; this allows cells to maintain a particular shape and polarity. Microtubules are also used in cell-surface specializations where they form the basis of cilia in the familiar 9 + 2 arrangement of nine microtubule doublets around a pair of single microtubules.

Intermediate filaments

Intermediate filaments are made of a variety of proteins, all formed from highly elongated fibrous molecules. They are arranged as rope-like fibers which span each cell often from one cell junction to another. They are termed intermediate filaments because their apparent diameter on electron microscopy is between that of actin filaments and thick myosin filaments. Specific varieties of intermediate filaments are present in epithelial and mesenchymal cells. Epithelial cells contain keratin filaments whereas mesenchymal cells have vimentin and vimentin-related filaments and, in those cells which will develop a myogenic lineage, desmin filaments are seen. Neuroepithelial cells develop neurofilaments and glial fibrillary acidic protein filaments are seen in astrocytes.

EMBRYONIC TISSUES

Two early tissue arrangements can be seen in embryos – epithelia and mesenchyme. Individual cells within each arrangement secrete extracellular proteins which form the extracellular matrix. This structures the space around and within cell populations and provides the appriopriate conditions for development.

Epithelia

Cells composing epithelia are polarized with apical and basal surfaces. The apical surface commonly displays specialized features, such as microvilli, whereas the basal surface is the site of extracellular protein deposition in the form of a basal lamina. Laterally, the cells contact their neighbors via varieties of juxtaluminal junctional complexes which bridge the narrow intercellular clefts.

Basal lamina

Basal laminae are thin flexible sheets of extracellular matrix which are made by and underlie epithelial cells (Fig. 2.3). Basal laminae are also found surrounding individual skeletal muscle fibers, fat cells and Schwann cells. The presence or absence of a basal lamina beneath an epithelium during development is of consequence. Basal laminae organize the proteins in adjacent cell membranes, they induce cell differentiation and cell metabolism, they serve as routes for cell migration and can influence cell polarity in those cells that touch them; they can change with time during development and thus can maintain a developmental impetus.

The basal lamina is described in electron microscopic studies as having an electron-lucent layer, the *lamina lucida* or *rara*, closest to the basal surface of the cell and an electron-dense layer, the *lamina densa* below. If the epithelial layer rests on underlying mesenchyme, a layer of collagen fibrils connects the basal lamina to the underlying tissue, sometimes with specialized anchoring collagen fibrils. The strength of this connection is important for development and growth. Many textbooks do not distinguish between the basal lamina as described above and the *basement membrane*, a thicker layer which includes the basal lamina and extracellular components of the underlying connective-tissue matrix.

Embryonic basal laminae are composed chiefly of *laminin*. Later, other extracellular molecules such as *type IV collagen*, *perlecan* and *entactin* (see below) contribute to the feltwork of the layer (see Fig. 2.3). In some regions of the body, basal laminae form specialized structures or units which have a specific function during development or in adult life. An example of this arrangement is seen in tooth development, where initially ameloblasts and odontoblasts are separated by a basal lamina. The ameloblasts deposit enamel directly onto one side of this basal lamina and the odontoblasts deposit dentine onto the other (see Fig. 2.12); in this way, the tooth is formed. In both the kidney and the lung, the basal lamina from the specialized cells of the organ abuts directly onto the endothelial basal lamina producing a selectively permeable barrier. In the kidney, this is the glomerular basement membrane.

In development, the basal lamina acts as a selective barrier to the movement of cells and migrating cells will move along basal laminae but not through them. Cells beneath an epithelial layer see only the basal lamina which the overlying cells produce. Changes in the local basal laminal composition is one way by which the epithelial cells can communicate with the cells migrating beneath them. In adult tissues, the basal lamina permits the movement of macrophages, lymphocytes and nerve processes and plays an important part in tissue regeneration after injury.

Cell–cell junctions

Juxtaposed cells usually do not touch. For contact to be established, the cells produce specific molecules which promote the development of a *cell–cell junction* between them (Fig. 2.4). Junctional complexes allow sheets of epithelial cells to act in concert in maintaining a barrier, or in producing alterations in the overall epithelial morphology; they also permit cell–cell communication and are, in this respect, especially important in development. Cell junctions are classified into three main groups: (i) *tight junctions*, which prevent leakage of molecules between cells from one side of a sheet of cells to the other; (ii) *anchoring junctions*, where the neighboring cell membranes attach and are supported by cytoskeletal elements within the cells, either actin or intermediate filaments – this type of

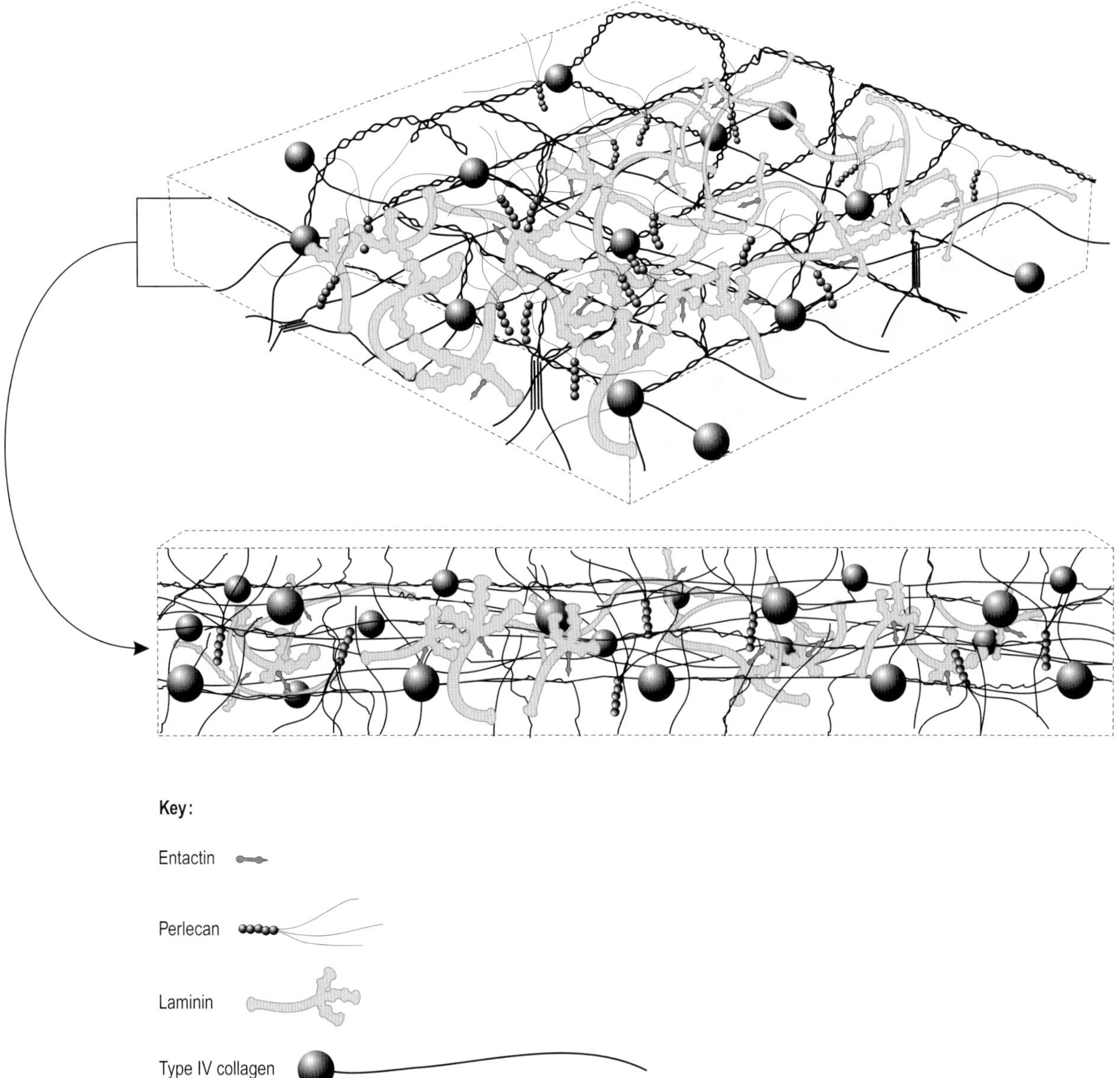

Fig. 2.3 A basal lamina is synthesized by epithelial cells. It is a feltwork of proteins which attach to the epithelial cells and provide an attachment for underlying cells. It is the interface for communication between the extracellular space and the cells.

junction also anchors epithelial cells to the extracellular matrix; (iii) *communicating junctions* mediate the passage of electrical or chemical signals from one cell to another.

The formation of these junctional complexes is dependent on a range of cell adhesion molecules (see Fig. 2.4). In cell–cell anchoring junctions (adhesion belts and desmosomes), the cell adhesion molecules (CAMs) involved are termed *cadherins*; they are attached intracellularly to intermediate or actin filaments in the cell cortex. The latter run parallel to the plasma membrane; thus the actin bundles of adjacent cells are linked. Concomitant contraction of the actin bundles will result in narrowing of the apices of the epithelial cells and rolling of the epithelial layer into a deep groove or a tube.

Epithelial cells contact the underlying basal lamina by different types of anchoring junctions (hemidesomosomes and focal contacts). In these cases, the transmembrane linker proteins belong to the *integrin* family of extracellular matrix receptors. Cytoskeletal filaments support the connection of the integrin within the cell membrane to the matrix.

Communication between adjacent epithelial cells is mediated by *gap junctions*. In forming a gap junction, each cell contributes six identical protein subunits (called connexins) which form a structure, similar to an old-fashioned cotton reel, termed a *connexon*. This is situated across the bilaminar membrane with the thicker rims extending into the extracellular and intracellular spaces. Each connexon is capable of opening and closing, thus controlling the gap. When two connexons from adjacent cells are aligned, a tubular connection is made between the cells. Each gap junction is really a cluster of apposed connexons which each permit molecules smaller than 1000 daltons to pass through them. In early embryos, most cells are electrically coupled to one another by gap junctions. Later in development, epithelial cells synthesize gap junctions at particular stages when it is inferred that information is passing from cell to cell.

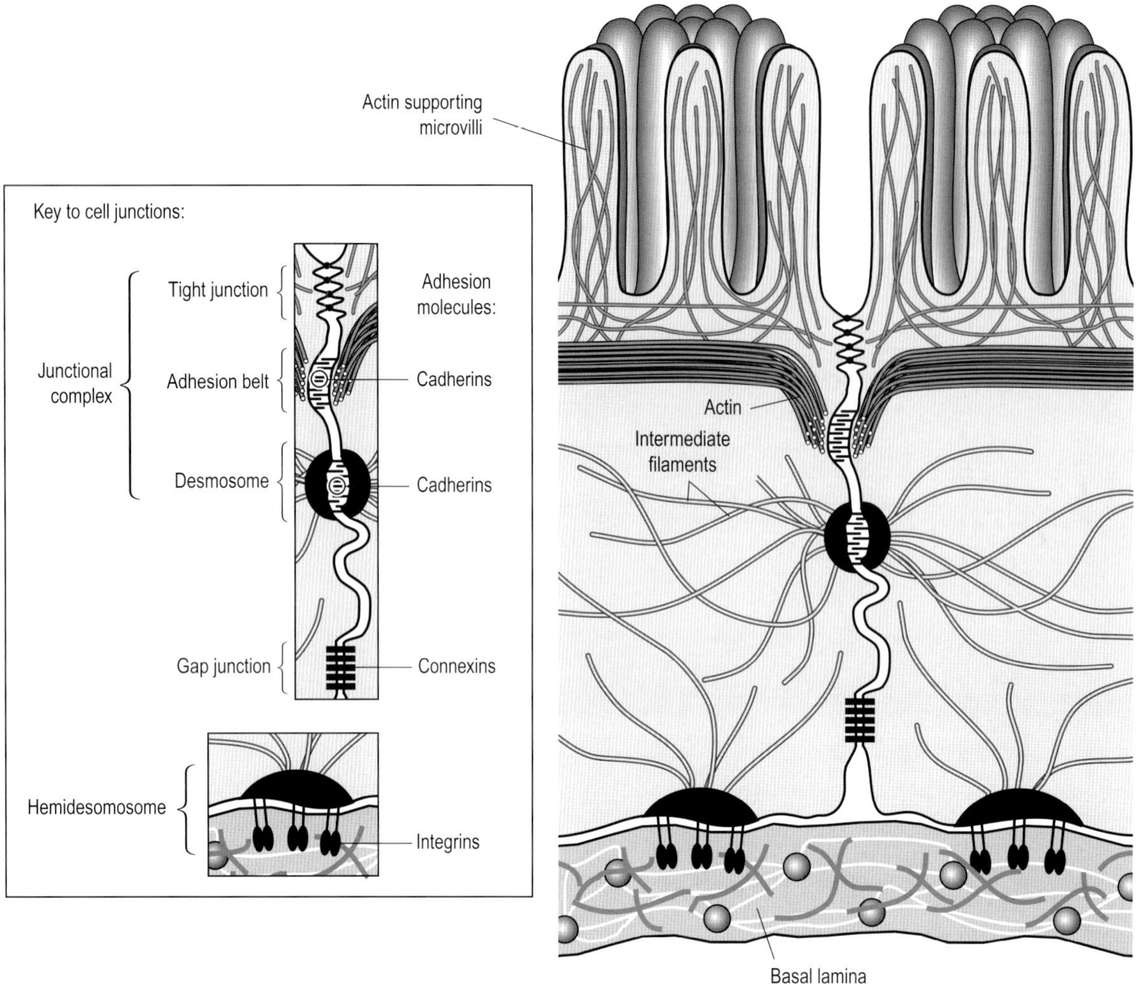

Fig. 2.4 Junction complexes form between epithelial cells preventing passage between cells, permitting communication between cells, and joining cells to each other and to the basal lamina. Junctions are supported by adhesion molecules and the cytoskeletal elements within the cells.

When gap junctions are removed, there is often a difference in differentiation in the cellular progeny. Gap junctions are seen in adult tissues, e.g. connecting cardiac myocytes to permit transmission of the electrical signals of the cardiac cycle. (For further information on cell adhesion molecules see Alberts et al.[1].)

Mesenchymal cells

Mesenchymal cells, in contrast to epithelial cells, have no polarity, thus no directional surface specializations. They have junctional complexes which are not juxtaluminal and they produce extensive extracellular matrix molecules and fibers from the whole cell surface (Fig. 2.5). As development proceeds, proliferating mesenchymal populations begin to differentiate. This is often first seen by the upregulation of specific mRNA in the cell or in the production of different extracellular matrix molecules by selected progeny.

Extracellular matrix

A substantial part of the developing embryo is made up of extracellular matrix. This name is given to the vast array of complex molecules which are secreted locally by mesenchymal cells and assembled into networks which structure the spaces between the embryonic cells. In early development, mesenchymal populations are composed of migrating epithelial cells and mesenchymal cells generated from germinal (proliferative) epithelia. It is the latter group which will give rise to the range of connective tissues seen in the adult. Connective tissues form the architectural framework of the body and it is the matrices which determine the tissue's physical properties, i.e. in bone, cartilage or fascia. It is variation in the constituents and amount of the matrix molecules which gives the diversity of connective tissues (Fig. 2.6).

There are two main classes of extracellular matrix molecules, *glycosaminoglycans* (GAGs), which may be linked covalently to proteins as *proteoglycans* and *fibrous proteins*, e.g. *collagen*, *elastin*, *laminin* and *fibronectin*. The glycosaminoglycan and proteoglycan molecules form a highly hydrated gel-like ground substance into which the fibrous proteins are embedded.

Four main groups of GAGs have been described: (i) hyaluronic acid; (ii) chondroitin sulfate and dermatan sulfate; (iii) heparan sulfate and heparin; (iv) keratan sulfate. Hyaluronic acid is the most simple GAG. It is especially abundant in embryos where it fills the spaces between cells and, because of its level of hydration, becomes turgid and generally resists compression. By synthesizing hyaluronic acid, cells can

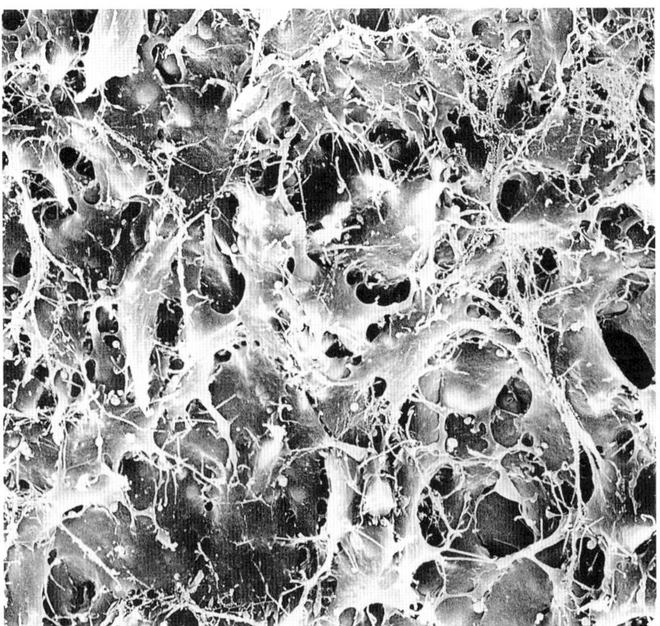

Fig. 2.5 SEM of mesenchyme cells. Mesenchyme cells have no polarity. They control the space around them by their synthesis of extracellular matrix. (Photograph by Dr P Collins.)

open up migration pathways or support epithelia which are undergoing morphological change. The other GAGs, which are more complex than hyaluronic acid, have much shorter disaccharide chains, contain sulfated sugars and are usually bound to a protein core forming proteoglycans. Aggregates of hyaluronate and proteoglycans can make huge molecules which occupy a volume equivalent to a bacterium.

Within tissues, GAGs can form gels of varying pore size and thus act as filters regulating the movement of molecules according to their size or charge. The heparan sulfate proteoglycan *perlecan* is found in the basal lamina of the kidney glomerulus and functions as a filter in the glomerular basement membrane. Proteoglycans which bind various growth factors act as reservoirs for messages which can be positioned in the matrix by cells at one stage to be read by cells developing later. GAGs and proteoglycans associate with the fibrous proteins in the matrix and provide support between the fibers.

Collagens form the major fibrous proteins in the matrix. Several families or groups of collagens are described, each made from a range of basic α-chains and each encoded by a separate gene. Each collagen molecule is made from three α-chains wound around one another like a rope. The main types of fibrillar collagen found in connective tissue are types I, II, III, V and XI. These types aggregate into the huge hawser-like

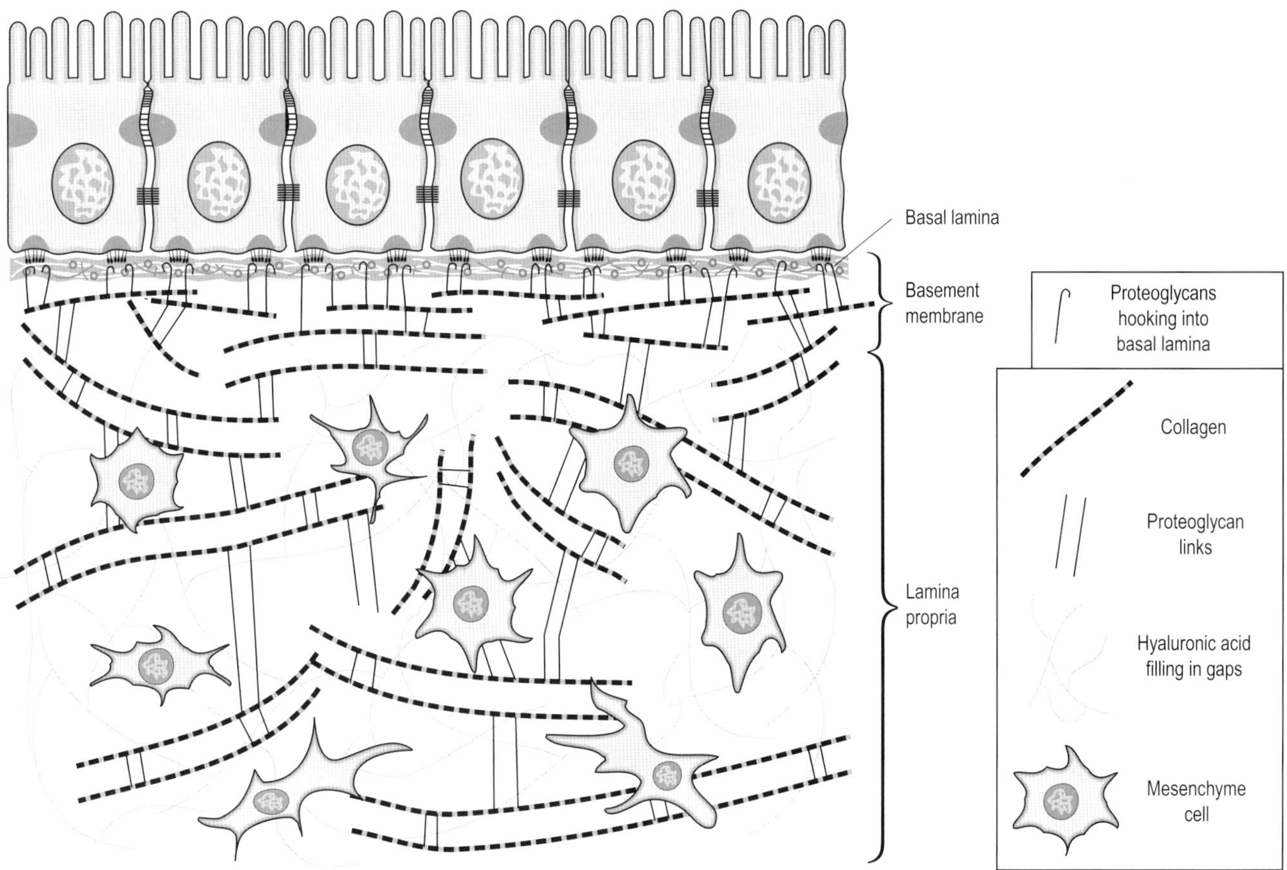

Fig. 2.6 Mesenchyme cells and extracellular matrix forming a lamina propria beneath an epithelium. The mesenchyme cells synthesize collagens, proteoglycans and glycosaminoglycans as a framework and add other proteins, e.g. fibronectin, as necessary. Extracellular matrix is attached to a basal lamina forming a basement membrane.

bundles which can be seen on electron microscopy. Collagen types IX and XII are smaller and link the larger fibers to one another and to other matrix molecules. Types IV and VII are found in the basal laminae where type IV forms the feltwork of the mature basal lamina and VII forms the anchoring structures which attach the basal lamina to the underlying matrix. Collagen is used to provide the initial matrices for cartilage and bone and is particularly seen in tendons and ligaments. In these cases, the amount of GAGs is reduced and the collagen fibers are aligned by the fibroblasts in response to the direction of the stresses acting on the collagen. In this way, the connective tissues of the body are responsive to the physical demands placed upon them. Anomalies of collagen synthesis can give rise to diseases in life, e.g. the condition osteogenesis imperfecta is caused by mutations in type I collagen production, leading to bones which are brittle and fracture with little stress; mutations in type II collagen lead to disorders of cartilage.

Elastin is composed of short elastin proteins which are crosslinked so that when relaxed, the fibers are randomly coiled but, when stretched, each elastin molecule can expand so contributing to the overall effect. Elastic fibers are at least five times more extensible than a rubber band of the same cross-sectional area. Usually collagen fibers are interwoven with elastic fibers to prevent overstretching and damage.

Laminin is one of the first extracellular proteins synthesized in the embryo, forming most of the early basal laminae. Each molecule is shaped like an asymmetric cross. Molecules join together to form a feltwork often supported by smaller entactin molecules.

Fibronectin are high molecular weight glycoproteins found in extracellular matrices and in blood plasma. Within the extracellular matrix fibronectins promote cells adhesion. Generally, contact with fibronectin causes cells to move. It has been shown in culture that neural crest cells will preferentially migrate along fibronectin-rich substrates and, within three-dimensional cultures, migrating cells can achieve their greatest speeds migrating along fibronectin pathways. It is interesting to note that bonding with fibronectin does not necessarily fix a cell to one position within the matrix so contacts with this protein are made and then released with ease.

Cell–matrix junctions

Cells interact with the extracellular matrix molecules via protein receptors or co-receptors in the plasma membrane. *Syndecans* are proteoglycan co-receptors which span the plasma membrane. The extracellular part carries chondroitin sulfate and heparan sulfate chains while the intracellular domain interacts with the cell cortex actin filaments. *Integrins* are receptor proteins which bind to and respond to the extracellular matrix information. An extracellular receptor site binds with matrix molecules, especially fibronectin and laminin; intracellularly, the integrin binds to the actin or intermediate filaments. When the integrins in the cell membrane contact a matrix molecule, e.g. fibronectin, the orientation of the fibronectin will cause alignment of the actin cytoskeleton and a reorientation of the cell itself. Later, when the cells are depositing extracellular matrix molecules, the actin cytoskeleton will exert forces to orient the matrix molecules in a similar configuration. Thus, the interaction between matrix molecules and cells and then cells and matrix can drive development and propagate order from cell to cell.

The cell–matrix junctions permit communications within the embryo just as gap junctions permit communications between cells. However, the cell–matrix mechanisms allow messages to be left in the matrix which may indicate migration routes or halt migrating cells and suggest a differentiation pathway. The matrix information system can thus control the temporal pattern of development.

TRANSFORMATION FROM EPITHELIUM TO MESENCHYME

The two embryonic states of epithelial tissue and mesenchyme are not necessarily immutable and transition from epithelia to mesenchyme and vice versa occurs during development. However, such a change requires a temporal or external inductive agent and causes dramatic upregulation and synthesis of a whole variety of special intra- and extracellular molecules as described above. Generally, in the embryo, epithelial cells seem to derive from existing epithelial populations whereas mesenchymal cells are produced initially from proliferative (germinal) epithelia and then later by amplifying mitoses within the mesenchymal population (see p. 29). Changes from one cell state to another are considered important in development.

The early migrating cells derived from the primitive streak have a mesenchymal morphology yet will become epithelial when they reach their destinations, forming the somites, the somatopleuric and splanchnopleuric epithelia lining the intraembryonic celom, including the lining of the pericardial cavity. All of these epithelia become germinal centers which produce further mesenchymal populations. However, an additional group of mesenchymal cells derived from the neural crest never revert to epithelia. Angiogenic mesenchyme, which is believed to arise from extraembryonic sources initially, is especially proliferative and capable of great migration within the embryo; it differentiates into endothelium throughout early development. A small subset of endothelial cells in the heart are induced to transform back to mesenchyme at the atrioventricular canal and the proximal outflow tract. This may be the only example of a mesenchymal population derived from an endothelial lineage[2]; the cells retain expression of an endothelial marker.

EMBRYONIC INDUCTION AND CELL DIVISION

The earliest cells of the embryo are described as 'totipotent' indicating that they have the capacity to differentiate into any cell type in the body. The pathways cells take to differentiation depend on the regulation of the genes within the cell and the interaction of the cell with its environment and neighbors. Information from these other sources will cause shifts in the differentiative fate of the cell's progeny.

All embryonic cell populations are initially receptive to inductive signals. They respond by becoming '*committed*' to a particular pathway of development which thus restricts their ability to respond to further inductive influences, i.e. they become '*restricted*'. After a series of restrictions cells are said to become '*determined*'. Determined cells are programmed to complete a process of development which will lead to differentiation. The determined state is a heritable characteristic of cells and can be passed on to progeny, it is stable and not dependent on environmental factors; the differentiated state is usually not heritable, it is often dependent on environmental conditions and it may prevent further cell division.

The state of determination or differentiation may be assessed by studying cells in culture. For example, melanocytes display the black pigment melanin. If melanocytes are cultured without the tyrosine needed to synthesize melanin, the cells will become pale and no longer appear differentiated. When the tyrosine is replaced into the culture medium, the cells will once more synthesize melanin and return to their differentiated state, illustrating that they maintained their determination despite not being able to display their differentiation. Similar cultures of cells taken from embryos at different stages of development will reveal which types of protein the cells are capable of synthesizing and thus their level of determination or differentiation. Cell proteins have been classified as 'basic', or 'housekeeping proteins', if they are considered essential for cellular metabolism, and are termed 'primary', as are the genes which regulate them. As cells become determined, they synthesize proteins appropriate to their cell group, e.g. liver and kidney cells, but not myocytes, produce arginase; this class of protein is termed 'secondary'. Finally, at the most differentiated state cells produce 'tertiary' proteins (also called 'luxury proteins') specific to their needs, e.g. hemoglobin in erythrocytes. This range of proteins, primary, secondary and tertiary, is an expression of stages of determination and differentiation and are coded by a range of genes.

Proliferative and quantal mitoses

Within a mesenchymal population, cell divisions will both increase the total numbers of cells but also provide the foci for changes in determination. In normal cell division, sometimes described as proliferative, transient amplifying, or multiplicative mitoses, progeny similar to the parents are produced. In some situations, e.g. as a response to a local inductive influence, the cells will enter a *quantal cell cycle* where the outcome is a *quantal mitosis* which increases the restriction of their progeny. The progeny then continue in amplifying mitoses at the progressive level of determination. It is at these quantal mitoses that binary choices are made in the embryo.

Stem cells and progenitor cells

Within a proliferating cell population, instead of a division producing two progeny with increased determination, the mitosis may produce one determined progeny and another cell with the same state of determination as the parent. This latter cell can reproduce again passing on an increased state of determination to only one offspring. This type of division has been termed 'asymmetric' in contrast to the 'symmetrical' proliferating mitoses. Stem cells are seen in development and in adult life, for example in the bone marrow or in the gut epithelium.

Progenitor cells are those which are already determined to some extent. They may individually follow their differentiation pathway or may proliferate producing more similarly determined progenitor cells. In this case, no stem cell can be identified; all cells seem capable of either differentiation or continued mitosis. An example would be populations of migrating myoblasts in the embryonic limb bud.

Terminal differentiation

The differentiative fates of cells within embryos may be to become long-living lymphoblasts or neuroblasts, but may just as well be to undergo 'apoptosis' also called programmed cell death. Apoptosis is a mechanism whereby cells bequeath their organelles to neighboring cells without releasing any cellular fragments which might stimulate an inflammatory response. Apoptosis occurs in the adult state as well as in embryos. In organogenesis, apoptosis allows for some slack in the system. More cells than may be needed are produced by amplifying mitosis, later the cells are supported by the local extracellular matrix or by innervation or blood supply. Those cells which are in excess and cannot be supported by these means will undergo apoptosis. This proposition has been supported by study of the nematode *Caenorhabditis elegans* which suggests that a cell death program is normally 'on' in all cells and that cell death is prevented by an overriding 'survival' program (reviewed by Raff[3]). As different tissues might be expected to produce different sets of survival factors, a cell in an abnormal location deprived of its specific signals required for survival would die.

The times at which cells cease proliferative mitoses and become differentiated is different for different tissues (Fig. 2.7). Although some tissues will all enter determined pathways and differentiation before birth, other cells retain the ability to divide, e.g. as stem cells, or if environmental conditions changes, as in a wound, are able to revert temporarily to the determined state, affect a repair and then differentiate once again.

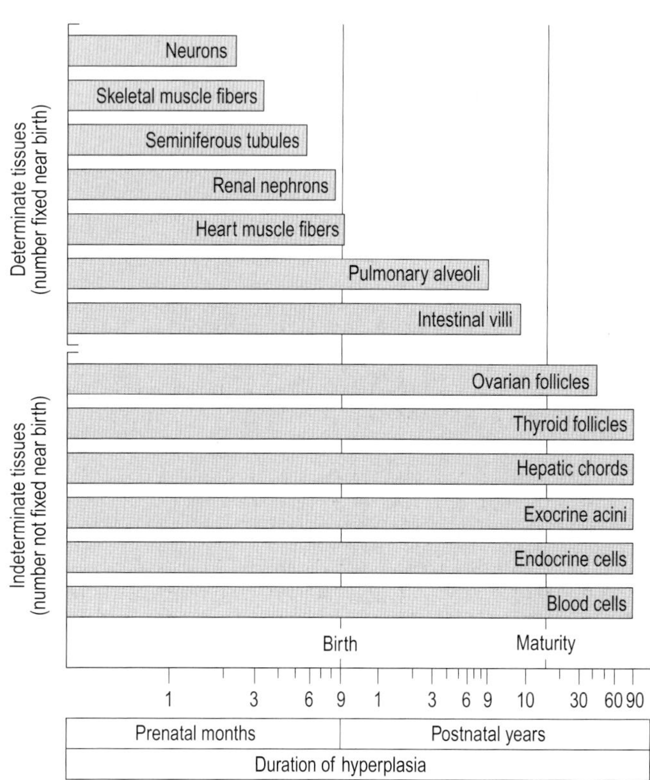

Fig. 2.7 The duration of multiplicative growth for various human tissues. (After Gilbert SF. *Developmental biology*, Sinauer Associates, MA, 1992.)

THE CELL CYCLE

Determination, differentiation and development, in general, all result from a series of interactions in which information from one cell is presented to another and, as a consequence, the behavior of one or both cells is changed. Earlier embryonic studies described the changes in shape which were seen in development and then how these might be modified by experimentation. In these cases, cell populations and morphogenetic movements were observed. Recently, the cues which cause such changes and movements have been investigated as molecular biology has allowed identification of proteins within the cell, the mRNA which indicates the synthesis of such proteins, and latterly isolation and synthesis of individual genes. Through such studies, some of the drivers and checks of development can be studied.

An increase in cell restriction begins with a quantal cell division, thus the mechanisms of mitosis need to be examined. Cells which are undergoing amplifying mitoses pass through a cell cycle which lasts for 12 hours or more. The cell cycle is traditionally divided into four phases, of which the most dramatic is mitosis and cell division (Fig. 2.8). The phases of the cell cycle are noted by the letters M for mitosis and G_1, S and G_2 for the interphase. During mitosis, the cell packs up most of its organelles, the centrioles duplicate and move to each end of the cell and begin synthesis of microtubules which are arranged as the mitotic spindle, and the chromatin in the nucleus condenses into the chromosomes. As the cell has already replicated its DNA, the chromosomes which become visible at metaphase are duplicated but held together at the centromere. The nuclear membrane breaks down, the chromosomes gather at the equator of the cell and are drawn apart towards the poles of the spindle, where they decondense and re-form intact nuclei. The cell cytoplasm divides by cytokinesis, an event which is viewed as the end of the M phase.

G_1 is the time period during which the cell grows until it is large enough to begin DNA synthesis. It may move along to S phase (synthesis) once it has reached an appropriate size and if the environmental conditions are favorable. If the cell is not yet committed to DNA replication, or is going to follow a differentiation pathway, the cell can step out of the cycle into G_0 for days, weeks or longer before resuming proliferation. The majority of cells in the adult are in G_0. The S phase marks replication of the nuclear DNA and is followed by G_2 which is the time taken for further growth. At the end of G_2, the cell must be of sufficient size, have replicated all its DNA, and be in a suitable environment before it can continue into mitosis. Signals from the cells or from the environment can prevent the cell moving from one phase to another.

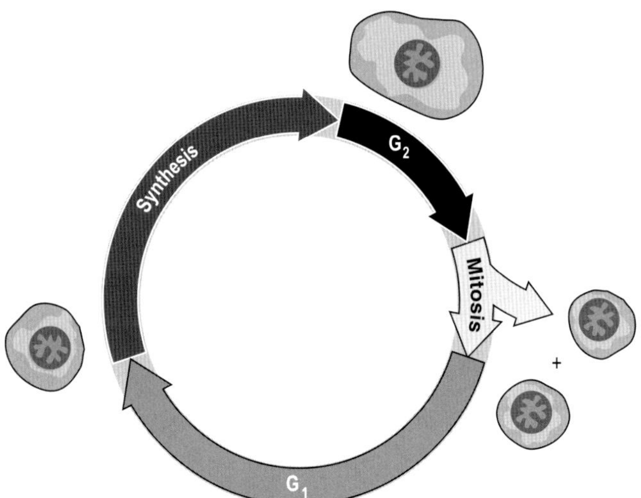

Fig. 2.8 The four stages of the cell cycle. After cell division (mitosis), the cell grows continuously until the next mitosis. The phases G_1, G_2 and S are parts of interphase. (If the cell is not dividing it enters G_0.)

The cycle itself is driven by complexes of cyclins, so called because they undergo synthesis and degradation in each division cycle of the cell. The cyclins bind to cyclin-dependent protein kinases (Cdk) to trigger mitosis and to trigger DNA replication. They thus provide a checkpoint for exit from G_1 and entry into S phase and exit from G_2 and entry into M phase.

In early embryonic cell divisions, the zygote and blastomeres are very large. Growth is not required at this time and the cleavage divisions operate to restore the nuclear to cytoplasm ratio producing cells of typical size. Under these conditions, cells pass through M phase and S phase in quick succession. After each division, the cell progeny are half the size of the parent. Later, the cycle lengthens and various control systems come into operation. It is important that the rate of passage through the S phase allows completion of DNA replication. Should a cell enter M phase before replication is complete, it will die. The cell cycle control system receives a feedback signal from incompletely replicated DNA which will prevent movement to the G_2 phase. Similar protective mechanisms ensure that DNA is only replicated once during S phase.

TISSUE INTERACTIONS

In order for the information carried in the genome of an embryo to be expressed, the cells produced by mitotic division must be able to contact and respond to each other; this process occurs locally by the construction of gap junctions. However, as an embryo grows, it is composed of more and more cell populations which become differentiated into *tissues* and separated by the matrix molecules they produce. In these more complex situations, the tissues have a repertoire of communication methods which require both epithelial and mesenchymal arrangements and their matrices working in concert. From a starting point of an early embryo at the body plan stage, all of the basic organs arise through interactions between close epithelial populations (plus their basal laminae), epithelia and mesenchyme (with the extracellular matrix), and between differentiating mesechymal populations. The basic interactions are the same. Such sequential spatial and temporal reciprocal interactions have been termed *epigenetic cascades*.[4]

Permissive interactions

It has been shown by experimental study that neither epithelia nor mesenchyme will grow alone – each needs the other for DNA synthesis and mitosis to occur. However, in many cases, it is not the cell bodies that are required. Epithelial cells will grow in culture as long as there is some sort of mesenchymal extract in the medium, and mesenchymal cells will grow in culture as long as they can contact a basal lamina. Thus, in both cases, factors in the matrix which have arisen from the cell population are enough to support growth. These basic requirements of development are termed *permissive interactions*. The supporting tissue may not be that usually present in development and, indeed, much research time has been spent in investigating which mesenchymal tissues would support growth of specific epithelia and vice versa. However, in many cases, although growth was maintained in these experiments, development would not proceed at all or in the normal manner. For such development more information is needed from the reciprocating tissues, and such information could enable both tissues to change in a manner that neither of them could do without the information. This is the basis of *instructive interactions*.

Instructive interactions

Wessells[5] proposed four general principles which can be seen in most instructive interactions:

- In the presence of tissue A, responding tissue B develops in a certain way.
- In the absence of tissue A, responding tissue B does not develop in that way.
- In the absence of tissue A, but in the presence of tissue C, tissue B does not develop in that way.
- In the presence of tissue A, a tissue D, which would normally develop differently, is changed to develop like B.

Thus, in an instructive interaction, one tissue induces another to respond in a specific way. If the target tissue can respond to the inductive signal it is called *competent*. If the target tissue does not respond it is described as *non-competent*. Non-competence may be because the tissue has previously responded to an earlier inductive signal which has restricted its repertoire of possible responses. As development proceeds, more and more cell populations will become non-competent as they differentiate.

Inductive interactions may be more or less complicated: only the induced tissue may change or both tissues may change and participate, as in morphogenesis or, more commonly, several reciprocal inductive interactions may be required over a prolonged period of developmental time before a specific organ or tissue will form.

EPITHELIAL–MESENCHYMAL INTERACTIONS

The instructive interactions between epithelia and mesenchyme produce the general morphological changes which are seen in every system throughout embryogenesis. They are a subset of embryonic tissue interactions occurring between epithelial tissue and specific subdivisions of mesenchymal tissue which arise during differentiation. These interactions provide a mechanism for coordinating and fine tuning the mitotic rates and differentiative abilities of the two tissues. A range of interactions occurring in different systems of the embryo are described.

Branching morphogenesis

Most organs, from lungs to kidneys, initially develop a main duct from which branches arise often dichotomously; later these mature into typical patterns seen in the fully formed organ. The mechanism of branching morphogenesis is therefore similar in a variety of systems. Although the early descriptions of this process described only the morphogenesis, now the specific matrix molecules involved during the interaction have been identified (Fig. 2.9).

At the tip of a proliferating duct, the epithelium and its basal lamina is in contact with the underlying mesenchymal cells and their extracellular matrix molecules. Local production of hyaluronidase by the mesenchyme breaks down the basal lamina and promotes proliferation of the epithelium. Cleft production is initiated by the mesenchyme which produces type III collagen fibrils within putative clefts. The collagen acts to protect the basal lamina from the effects of the hyaluronidase and the overlying epithelia have a locally reduced mitotic rate. The region of rapid mitoses at the tip of the acinus is thus split into two and two branches develop from this point. If the type III

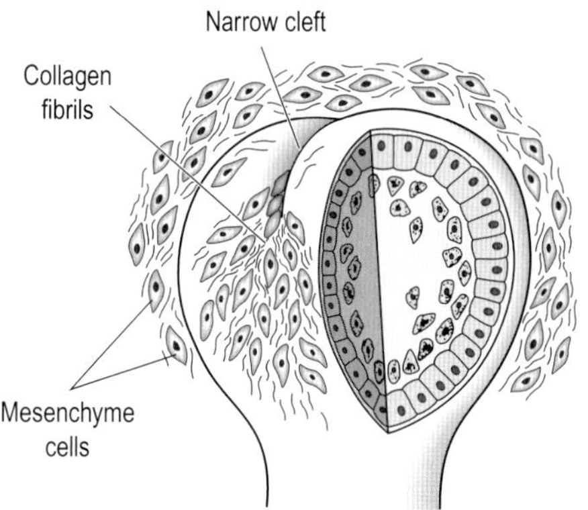

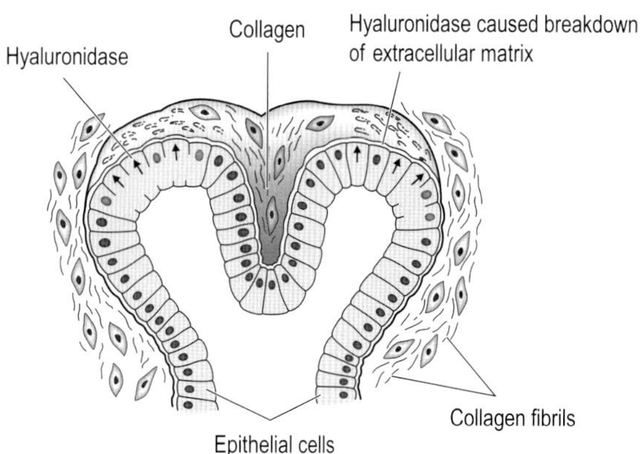

Fig. 2.9 Branching of a tubular duct may occur as a result of an interaction between the proliferating epithelium of the duct and its surrounding mesenchyme and extracellular matrix. Mesenchymal cells initiate cleft formation by producing collagen III fibrils locally within the development clefts and hyaluronidase over other parts of the epithelium. Collagen III prevents local degradation of the epithelial basal lamina by hyaluronidase and slows the rate of mitosis of the overlying epithelial cells. In regions where no collagen III is produced, hyaluronidase breaks down the epithelial basal lamina and locally increases epithelial mitoses forming an expanded acinus. (From *Gray's Anatomy*, 38th edn. Edinburgh: Churchill Livingstone, 1995, p. 114.)

collagen is removed from the cleft, branching does not occur; if excess collagen is not removed, supernumerary clefts appear. Note that this interaction may occur with any epithelial type and any subpopulation of mesenchyme.

Neural ectoderm and surface ectoderm interactions

The above interactions are clearly seen in formation of the lens of the eye. The optic cup is an outgrowth of the diencephalon of the brain. As the cup approaches the overlying surface ectoderm, it induces a local change. The ectoderm cells become narrower at the apical region causing the sheet of cells to curve and move towards the optic cup. Ultimately, a small lens vesicle invaginates and the unaffected surface ectoderm becomes confluent over the structure. If the optic cup is removed no lens vesicle develops. If the optic cup is removed and placed beneath a different portion of surface ectoderm a similar lens vesicle is induced (Fig. 2.10).

Neural ectoderm and neural crest mesenchyme interactions: the 'fly-paper model' of skull development

The subtle interplay between the mesenchyme and the epithelial basal lamina is demonstrated in the fly-paper model of skull development[6]. Here, an interaction occurs between the neuroectoderm of the neural tube and the surrounding neural crest mesenchyme. The neuroepithelium will display fibronectin among other fibrous proteins in the basal lamina. This will ensure the migration of the neural crest over the neural tube and into the developing face. As development proceeds, the neuroepithelium transiently expresses type II collagen in the basal lamina on the basal aspect of the neural tube, around the olfactory regions, around the optic cups prior to and during lens invagination, around the otic vesicles which will form the inner ear, and on the basal and lateral surfaces of the diencephalon, mesencephalon and rhombencephalon. The notochord also expresses type II collagen in its basal lamina. Some time after the type II collagen has been removed from the basal laminae, neural crest mesenchyme adjacent to the regions listed commence synthesis of type II collagen and ultimately differentiate along a chondrogenic pathway. It seems as if the type II collagen in the basal lamina affects those cells which contact it and cause their upregulation of type II collagen. The pattern of the expression of type II collagen in the basal laminae determines the form of the chondrocranium (Fig. 2.11). Slight alterations in the pattern of expression could have profound effects on the shape and form of the chondrocranium, perhaps producing the diversity of skull shapes seen in vertebrates.

Surface ectoderm and neural crest interactions

A further example of a reciprocal tissue interaction can be seen in mammalian tooth development summarized in Fig. 2.12 (from Lumsden[7]). Tooth development begins along the *dental lamina* of the premaxilla, maxilla and mandible. The epithelium proliferates to form an *enamel organ* under the influence of the neural crest mesenchyme which forms a *dental papilla*; together this unit is a tooth bud or germ. The enamel organ induces the dental papilla mesenchyme to become *odontoblasts*; these cells

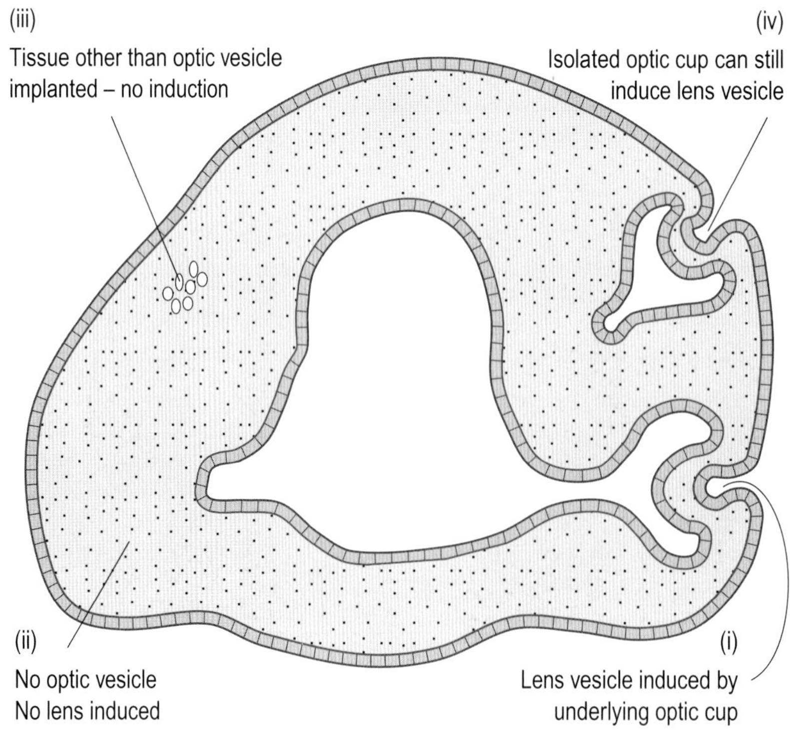
(iii)
Tissue other than optic vesicle
implanted – no induction
(iv)
Isolated optic cup can still
induce lens vesicle
(ii)
No optic vesicle
No lens induced
(i)
Lens vesicle induced by
underlying optic cup

Fig. 2.10 Induction of the lens vesicle by the optic cup. This illustrates clearly the four general principles of an instructive interaction. (After Wessells[5].)

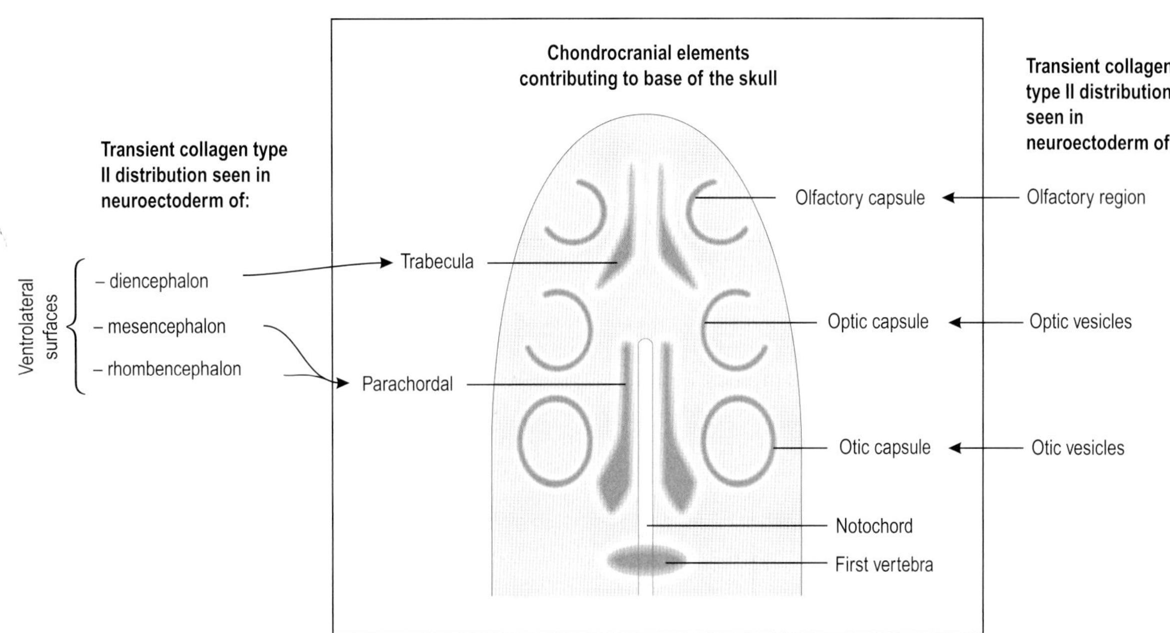

Fig. 2.11 Transient expression of type II collagen in the basal lamina of the neuroepithelium causes mesenchyme cells which touch it to upregulate their own synthesis of type II collagen and differentiate along a chondrogenic pathway. The pattern of expression in the neuroectoderm determines the form of the chondrocranium. (From Thorogood[6] with permission.)

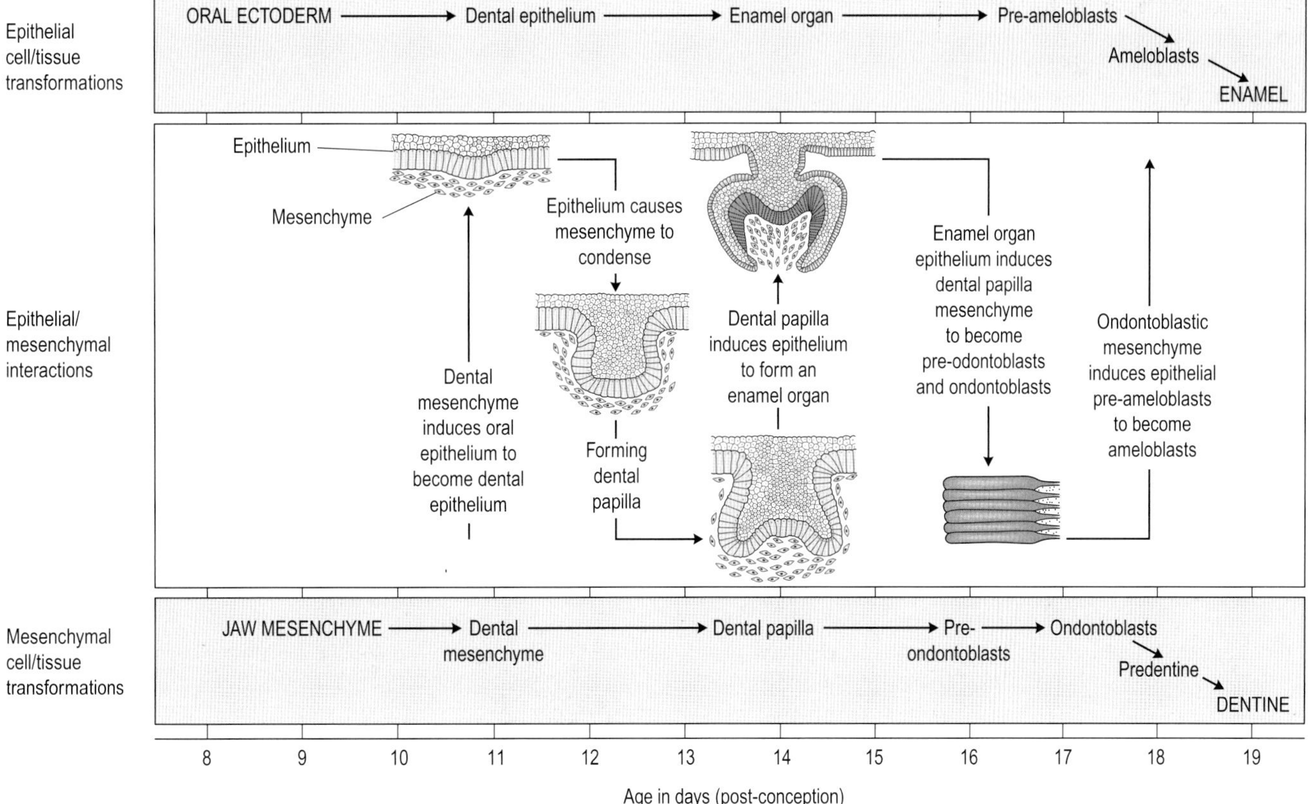

Fig. 2.12 An example of reciprocal tissue interaction in mammalian tooth development. The sequence of epithelial–mesenchymal interactions involved in the development of teeth in the embryonic mouse. E8–19 represent age in days after conception. (From *Gray's Anatomy*, 38th edn. Edinburgh: Churchill Livingstone, 1995, p. 111. After Lumsden[7].)

then induce the epithelial cells to differentiate into *ameloblasts*. The tooth is formed by matrix deposition each side of the epithelial basal lamina, enamel one side and dentine the other.

The neural crest mesenchyme is responsible for patterning development of the pharyngeal arches including tooth formation. Dental papilla mesenchyme is able to induce the formation of teeth in non-oral epithelium, and can specify the type of tooth produced, i.e. incisor or molar. If cranial neural crest is cultured alone it will differentiate into cartilage. When it is recombined with limb epithelium then cartilage and bone will form. However, if cranial neural crest is recombined with mandibular epithelium, salivary islands, hair and teeth form as well as cartilage and bone, indicating that the mandibular epithelium is essential and specific for the development of teeth.

Early recombination (9–11.5 days of development) of mouse mandibular epithelium (first arch) and hyoid mesenchyme (second arch) results in teeth in 90% of cases, this shows that the dental lamina epithelium can induce tooth development in the head neural crest mesenchyme. The reverse recombination, early second arch epithelium and mandibular arch mesenchyme does not produce teeth, indicating that it is only the first arch epithelium which has this property. However, later recombination experiments (11.5–12 days of development), with second arch epithelium and first arch mesenchyme, will produce teeth. In this case, the neural crest mesenchyme has already been induced along a dental lineage[8].

The local specification of particular teeth can be changed experimentally. If presumptive incisor region of the mandibular epithelium is recombined with predetermined molar papillae from post-day 12 tooth germs, the shape of the teeth can be redefined by the epithelium and incisiform teeth develop.

The interaction between oral epithelium and neural crest mesenchyme will operate across species, thus recombination of dental mesenchyme from 16–18-day mouse with oral epithelium from the mandibular epithelium of the chick resulted in tooth formation[9]. This is the more surprising as chicks do not normally develop teeth.

Surface ectoderm and somatopleuric mesenchymal interactions in the limb

The tissues involved in limb development arise from a ridge along the flank of the embryo. Interaction of specialized regions of the *somatopleuric mesenchyme* with the overlying ectoderm gives rise to local, thickened regions of surface ectoderm and proliferation of the underlying mesenchyme. At these sites, the ectoderm forms a longitudinal ridge of high columnar cells, the *apical ectodermal ridge (AER)* and the specialized somatopleuric mesenchyme maintains its growth. The AER and underlying mesenchyme together are termed the *progress zone* and the limb grows meristematically from this point, i.e. proliferation produces the next distal portion of limb. These two populations require each other. Only the apical ectodermal ridge can promote limb outgrowth and only limb mesenchyme will result in limb development. Positional values are assigned to the proliferating epithelial and mesenchymal populations by the progress zone, thus, first the humerus is developed, then the radius and ulna, then the carpals and so on (Fig. 2.13).

Within the portion of the limb which has received its positional value the mesenchyme instructs the overlying ectoderm about the appropriate epidermal structure to develop. Parts of a chick hind limb develop different characteristics with feathers on the thigh and scales on the leg. If mesenchyme from the thigh is transplanted beneath the leg, feathers will develop instead of the normal scales. This type of experiment has been repeated recombining neck ectoderm which will not normally develop feathers with thigh mesenchyme, in this case the epidermis will develop feathers.

If thigh mesenchyme is inserted beneath the apical ectodermal ridge of a developing wing which is at the stage to assign radius and ulna, two things occur. First, information from the apical ectodermal ridge about the age of the limb will override the ‘thighness’ of the mesenchyme and it will express leg characteristics appropriate to the developmental time of the wing. Thus, the proximal limb characteristics are replaced by distal ones. Secondly, the wing epithelium is reassigned to develop leg characteristics by the mesenchyme. Thus the limb develops a fibula and tibia and the epidermis displays scales. This latter experiment show the reciprocal nature of inductive interactions with both tissues giving and responding to information.

Positional information which causes the development of the axes of the limb are controlled by both mesenchyme and epithelium. A subset of mesenchyme situated at the postaxial border of the limb bud termed the *zone of polarizing activity (ZPA)* controls the craniocaudal axis of the limb, i.e. where the thumb develops. Active substances released at this region will cause a number five digit to form, the little finger (see Fig. 2.13). The reducing influence of this substance allows development of digits four, three, two and then the thumb to develop. However, even if this system is disrupted by mixing the mesenchyme up within the limb producing five equally structured digits, the limb still displays dorsal and ventral surfaces. The inductive influence for dorsal/ventral patterning is specified by the ectodermal epithelium.

Endoderm and splanchnopleuric mesenchyme interactions in the lung

The respiratory tree derives from interactions between endodermal epithelium and surrounding splanchnopleuric mesenchyme. The trachea arises from the pharynx as a midline, ventral diverticulum which grows caudally then bifurcates into the primary bronchi which expand dorsally on each side of the esophagus. Originally splanchnopleuric mesenchyme surrounding the pharynx envelopes both the esophagus and the trachea; however, the proximity of the lung buds to the pericardio-peritoneal canals, which will later give rise to the pleural cavities, provides a different mesenchymal population. Proliferation of the adjacent *splanchnopleuric celomic epithelium* (of the primary pleural cavities) provides *investing mesenchyme* around the developing trachea and lung buds from stage 13 of development. The proliferative activity decreases in stage 14 and the mesenchyme becomes arranged in zones around the developing endoderm. This investing mesenchyme contains a mixed population of cells, that which will pattern the endodermal epithelium, a subpopulation of angiogenic mesenchyme which may migrate in to form the endothelial networks surrounding the air sacs, and splanchnopleuric mesenchyme which will give rise to the smooth muscle cells which surround both the respiratory tubes and the blood vessels. The splanchnopleuric celomic epithelium will after its proliferative phase give rise to the visceral pleura.

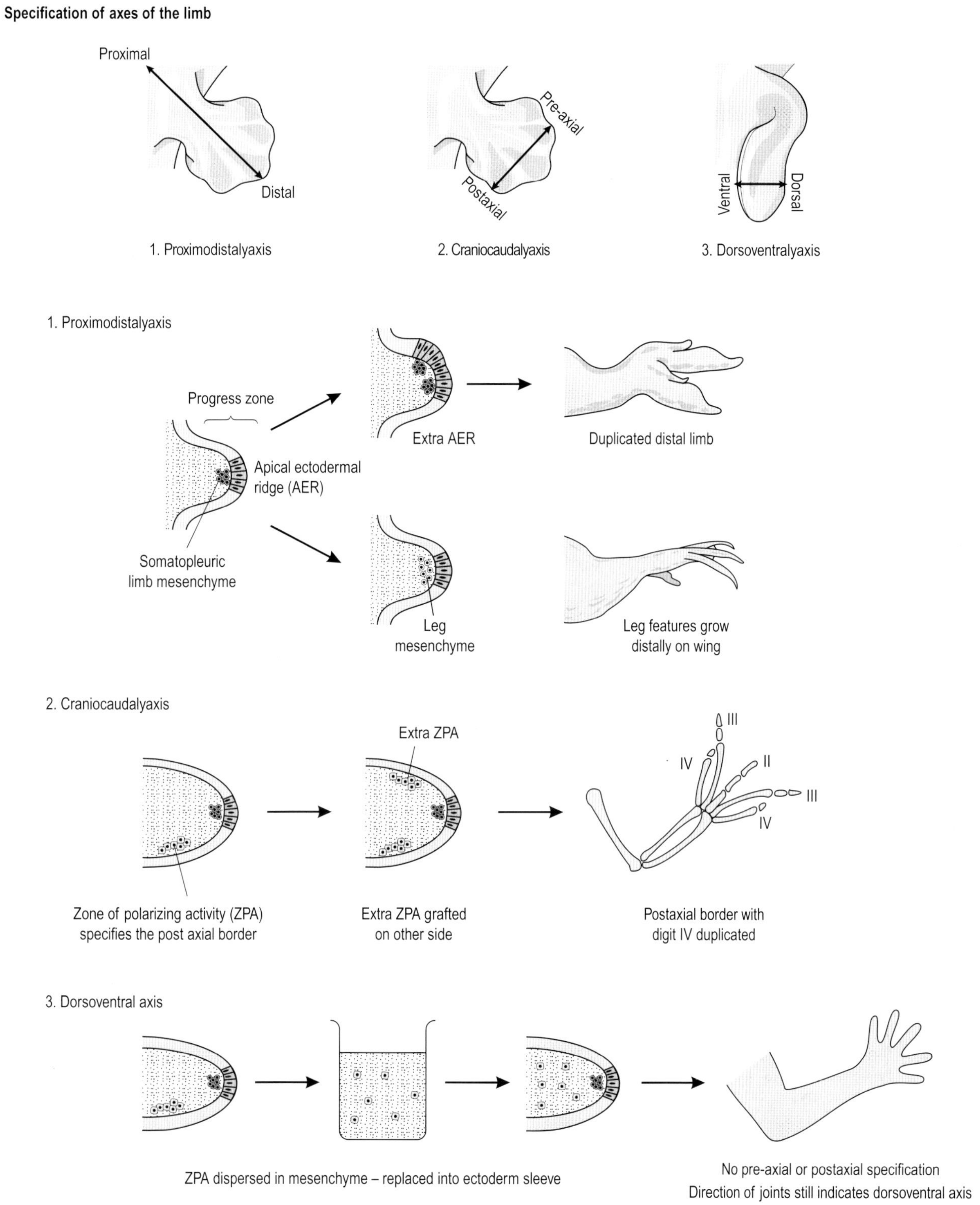

Fig. 2.13 The three axes of the limb are specified by different interactions. The proximodistal axis is specified by the progress zone, the craniocaudal axis by the zone of polarizing activity (ZPA), and the dorsoventral axis by the ectoderm of the limb. The pattern of development within the limb and the ectodermal specializations are controlled by the limb mesenchyme.

The control of the branching pattern of the respiratory tree resides with the *splanchnopleuric mesenchyme*. Recombination of tracheal mesenchyme with bronchial respiratory endoderm causes an inhibition of bronchial branching, whereas recombination of bronchial mesenchyme with tracheal epithelium will induce bronchial outgrowths from the trachea[5,10]. Initially, the tracheal mesenchyme is continuous with that surrounding the ventral wall of the esophagus, but with lengthening and division of the tracheal bud and deviation of the lung buds dorsally, each bud becomes surrounded by its own specific mesenchyme thus permitting regional differences between the lungs, i.e. the number of lobes, or the degree of growth and maturity of a particular lung. Each lung develops by a process of dichotomous branching as described in branching morphogenesis. *Tenascin*, an extracellular matrix molecule (also known as hexabrachion or cytotactin), is present in the budding and distal tip regions, but absent in the clefts. Conversely, fibronectin is found in the clefts and along the sides of the developing bronchi, but not on the budding and distal tips[11].

Endoderm and splanchnopleuric mesenchyme interactions in the gastrointestinal tract

Liver

The liver is a very precocious embryonic organ, functioning as the main center for hemopoiesis in the fetus. It develops from an endodermal evagination of the foregut and from the septum transversum mesenchyme, a region of unsplit lateral plate mesenchyme at the very rostral edge of the disk prior to head folding. The development of the liver is intimately related to the development of the heart as the vitelline, followed by the umbilical veins, are disrupted by the septum transversum to form a hepatic plexus, the forerunner of the hepatic sinusoids.

Endodermal epithelial cells from the foregut proliferate and extend as lines of epithelial cells into the septum transversum mesenchyme. Contact of endodermal epithelium with the mesenchymal cells induces them to form blood islands and endothelium. The advance of the endodermal epithelial cells promotes the conversion of more and more septum transversum mesenchyme into endothelium and blood cells with only a little remaining to form the scanty (human) liver capsule and interlobular connective tissue.

The morphogenesis of the liver lobes are patterned by the septum transversum mesenchyme and both endoderm and septum transversum mesenchyme are required for normal liver development. If a mechanical barrier is inserted across the mesenchymal hepatic area just caudal to the endodermal outgrowth, liver tissue will develop normally cranial to the barrier where it is in contact with the endoderm. However, caudal to the barrier, the mesenchyme will form endothelial cells and hepatic lobes, but there will be no hepatocytes present.

Experiments in which either the epithelium or the mesenchyme is changed will not result in liver development, e.g. cephalic and somitic mesenchyme do not promote the differentiation of hepatic endoderm, and intestinal endoderm cells combined with hepatic mesenchyme will not differentiate into hepatocytes. However, all derivatives of the lateral plate mesenchyme, both somatopleuric and splanchnopleuric mesenchyme can promote the differentiation of hepatic endoderm, although not so strongly as hepatic mesenchyme, and lateral plate mesenchyme will form blood sinusoids under these conditions. It is inferred that matrix or cell surface properties are common throughout the lateral plate mesenchyme but are different from axial mesenchymal cells[12].

Gastric mucosa

Within the gastrointestinal tract, the local organization of the mucosa and smooth muscle layers is under the control of the local splanchnopleuric mesenchyme. Recombination experiments of chick gut epithelium and mouse mesenchyme and vice versa show that the patterning of the intestinal villi will be determined by the underlying mesenchyme. However, the epithelial cells will produce enzymes associated with the relevant species, i.e. mouse epithelium will produce lactase and chick epithelium sucrase, regardless of the origin of the underlying mesenchyme[13].

Intraembryonic mesoderm and intermediate mesenchyme interactions

The metanephric kidney develops from three sources, an evagination of the mesonephric duct, the *ureteric bud*, a local condensation of mesenchyme termed the *metanephric blastema*, and *angiogenic mesenchyme* which migrates into the metanephric blastema slightly later to produce the glomeruli and vasa recta[14–16]. It may also be the case that innervation is necessary for metanephric kidney induction.

During embryonic development, functional mesonephric kidneys develop but are remodeled in male embryos as parts of the reproductive tracts. The mesonephric kidneys develop on the posterior abdominal wall and extend ultimately from the pleural region to the lumbar, with both development and regression proceeding in a craniocaudal progression. However, in the metanephric kidney, a proportion of the mesenchyme remains as stem cells which continue to divide and enter the nephrogenic pathway later as individual collecting ducts lengthen. Thus the temporal development of the metanephric kidney is patterned radially with the outer cortex being the last part to be formed.

In each kidney, a ureteric bud arises as a diverticulum from the mesonephric duct and grows dorsally to enter the metanephric mesenchymal population. The bud bifurcates when it comes into contact with the metanephric blastema as a result of local extracellular matrix molecule synthesis by the mesenchyme. Both chondroitin sulfate proteoglycan synthesis and chondroitin sulfate glycosaminoglycan processing are necessary for this and consequent branching of the ureteric bud[17]. Subsequent divisions of the ureteric bud and the mesenchyme form the gross structure of the kidney with *major* and *minor calyces*; the distal branches of the ureteric ducts will form the *collecting ducts* of the kidney. As the collecting ducts elongate, the metanephric mesenchyme condenses around them. The ureteric bud undergoes a further series of bifurcations within the surrounding metanephric mesenchyme, forming smaller *ureteric ducts*. The metanephric mesenchyme condenses around the dividing ducts into smaller condensations which then undergo a mesenchyme to epithelium transformation forming vesicles. To initiate this transformation, the cells cease production of mesenchymal matrix molecules and commence production of epithelial ones. This has been demonstrated in tissue culture.

Initially, syndecan can be detected between the mesenchymal cells in the condensate. The cells cease expression of the cadherin N-CAM, fibronectin and collagen I and commence production of the cadherin L-CAM (also called uvomorulin) and the basal laminal constituents laminin and collagen IV. The mesenchymal clusters thus convert to small groups of epithelial cells which undergo complex morphogenetic changes (Fig. 2.14). Each epithelial group elongates, forms a comma-shaped, then an S-shaped body, which elongates further. It then fuses to a branch of the ureteric duct at its distal end while expanding as a dilated sac at the proximal end. The sac involutes with

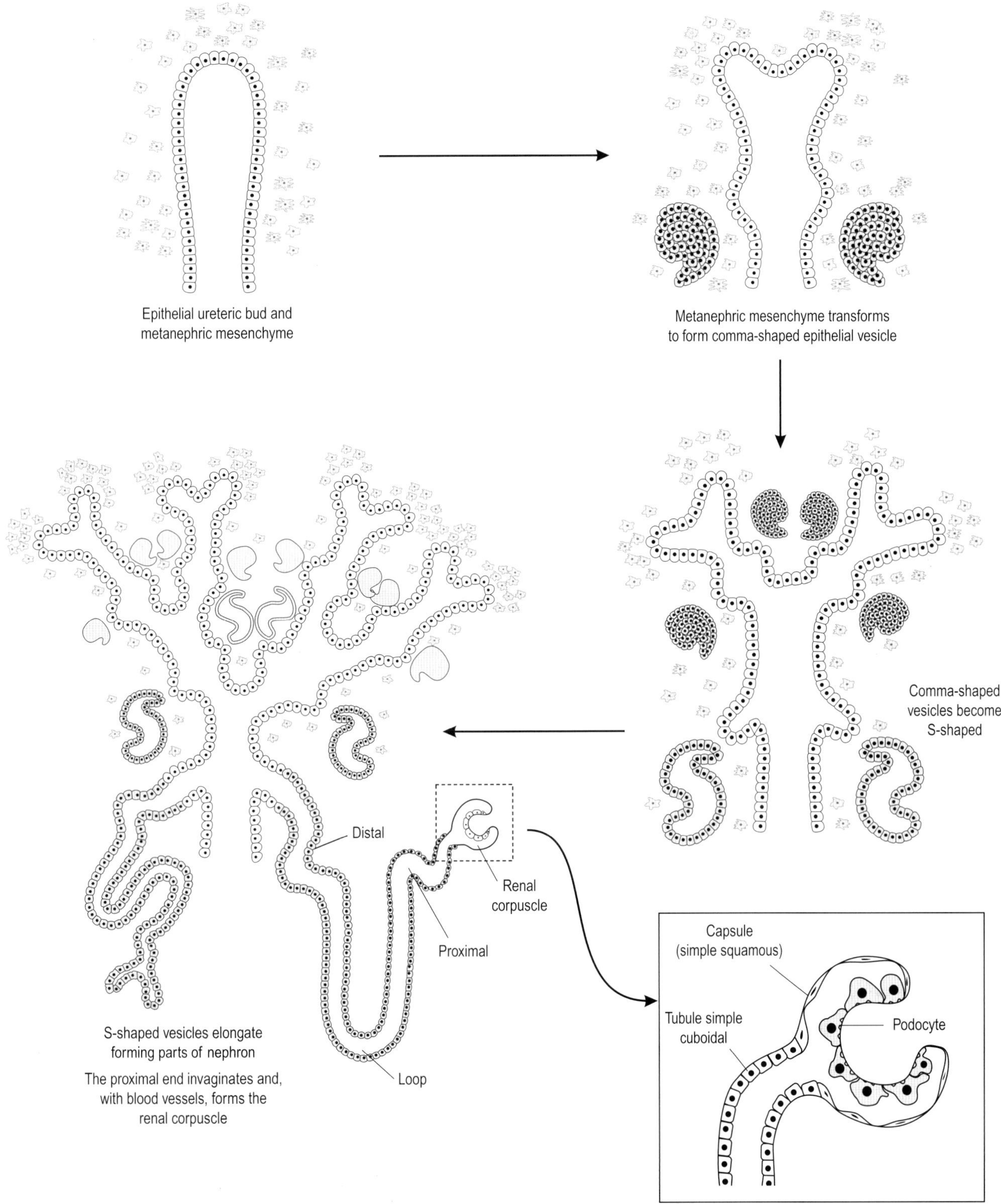

Fig. 2.14 In the developing kidney, there is a mesenchyme-to-epithelial transformation. The epithelial ureteric bud forms the collecting ducts in the kidney. It induces the metanephric mesenchyme to transform into local epithelial vesicles which develop into the nephrons.

local cellular differentiation such that the outer cells become the *parietal glomerular cells*, while the inner ones become *visceral epithelial podocytes*. The podocytes develop in close proximity to invading capillaries which derive from local angiogenic mesenchyme[18]; this third source of mesenchyme produces the endothelial and mesangial cells within the glomerulus. Both the metanephric-derived podocytes and the angiogenic mesenchyme produce fibronectin and other components of the glomerular basal lamina. The isoforms of type IV collagen within this layer follow a specific program of maturation which occurs as the filtration of macromolecules from the plasma becomes restricted[19].

Interestingly, although the interactions in kidney development were usually focused on the induction of metanephric mesenchyme by the ureteric bud epithelium, it had been noted that, when cultured across a filter, the inductive stimulus was quite weak. In contrast, fragments of spinal cord were found to be very potent inducers of metanephric mesenchyme, initiating epithelialization. This suggested that perhaps nerves arriving at the interaction site during development were of some importance. Indeed, it has been shown that blocking nerve growth factor receptor mRNA in the developing kidney not only prevents receptor synthesis, but that nephrogenesis is also completely halted[20].

Other cells types affecting or affected by local interactions

It seems that the basic epithelial–mesenchymal interaction may not be so basic or simple after all. Whereas initial observations were made on cultured embryos, later studies were made on cultured embryonic explants which could be perturbed in some manner. The range of inductive tissues was ascertained, using other mesenchymes or epithelia from the same embryo, from different embryos of the same species and even from different species. Now it seems that the homogeneity of the mesenchymes under examination may have been assumed. The presence of angiogenic mesenchyme may be fundamental for some interactions. Early in development it arises extra-embryonically from the parietal hypoblast. Later, angiogenic mesenchyme is seen close to endodermal epithelia but not ectodermal. It is not clear whether the majority of angiogenic mesenchyme arises close to endodermal populations as it has now been shown to arise from somite-derived mesenchyme[21]. Early embryonic angioblasts are highly invasive, moving in every direction throughout embryonic mesenchymal tissue. It is likely that these cells make a contribution to interactive processes, especially in those organs where close proximity of endothelia to specialized cells is a feature.

Similarly, the innervation of blood vessels, glandular cells and myoepthelial cells may need to be achieved early in development, at the time of the early interactions. Indeed, the condition Hirschsprung's disease which results in a failure of neural crest cells to colonize the gut appropriately and form local constituents of the enteric nervous system, is thought to occur because of disordered basal laminal molecules. The enteric nervous system arises from neural crest cells at somite levels 1–7 and from 28 onwards. Normally, the crest cells invade the splanchnopleuric mesenchyme around the endoderm and site themselves in the putative submucosal and myogenic layers. The splanchnopleuric mesenchyme will develop into both the lamina propria connective tissue lineages and the smooth muscle cells of the muscularis mucosa and the muscularis propria. Hirschsprung's disease is characterized by a dilated segment of colon proximally and lack of peristalsis in the segment distal to the dilation. Infants with this condition show delay in the passage of meconium, constipation, vomiting and abdominal distension. A mouse model has been investigated which demonstrates the same pathology and symptoms[22]. In the normal mouse, laminin and type IV collagen are found beneath the mucosal and serosal epithelia and around the blood vessels. In the mutant mouse, there is a broad zone of these basal laminal proteins around the entire outer gut mesenchyme with increase in the amount of laminin, type IV collagen and heparan sulfate, specifically in the aganglionic portion of bowel. It is suggested that the overabundance of basal laminal components prevents the neural crest cells from penetrating the gut wall; their new position outside the gut does not confer on them the environmental stimuli for enteric nerve differentiation. Consequently, these crest cells differentiate into autonomic ganglia and nerves similar to the parasympathetic nerves which normally modulate enteric nervous system activity. This system demonstrates the importance of local mesenchymal and extracellular matrix activity for the normal induction of neurons as well as epithelial cells.

CYTOKINES AND GROWTH FACTORS

As a result of experiments to find the most appropriate media for maintaining the proliferation of cells in culture, two families of 'factors' were identified, arising initially from lymphocytes and from platelets. Culture of lymphocytes and macrophages revealed a family of factors within the supernatant which was able to facilitate cell–cell communication and proliferation. These soluble factors were isolated and collectively termed *cytokines*. The cytokines include: subtypes of *interleukin (IL)* which cause in the main T- and B-cell proliferation; types of *interferon (IFN)* which are mainly antiviral in nature; *tumour necrosis factor (TNF)* α and β which are cytotoxic; *transforming growth factor β (TGFβ)* which inhibits T- and B-cell proliferation; and *granulocyte-macrophage colony-stimulating factor (GM-CSF)* with factors for granulocytes and macrophages individually, which promote growth. The proliferative actions of cytokines are mediated by specific cell receptors on the surface of target cells.

Culture of mammalian cells was found to be more successful with blood serum added to the medium rather than plasma. Serum is the fluid which remains after blood has clotted whereas plasma is obtained by removing the cells without permitting clotting to occur. The difference between these two fluids was the presence of factors released from platelets as the blood clotted. Experiment showed that an extract of platelets alone added to the medium would support cell-culture proliferation, and the extract was termed a *growth factor*. The particular growth factor from the platelets was shown to be a protein and named *platelet-derived growth factor* or *PDGF*. For PDGF to have an effect on a target cell, the cell must display an appropriate receptor protein on its surface as in the action of cytokines. Receptor proteins for cytokines and growth factors are part of the cell glycocalyx along with, inter alia, cell adhesion molecules and integrins.

Large families of growth factors have now been identified, not all of them proteins; steroid hormones which act on intracellular receptor protein are an example. Growth factors have been divided into broad- and narrow-specificity classes or families. PDGF is a broad-specificity factor as is *epidermal growth factor (EGF)*. PDGF acts on fibroblasts, smooth-muscle cells and neuroglial cells, while EGF acts on epidermal cells and on many embryonic epithelia. Other broad-specificity growth factors are: the *insulin-like growth factors (IGFI, IGFII)* (previously termed 'somatomedins'), stimulating cell metabolism and with other growth factors stimulating cell proliferation; *fibroblast growth factor (FGF)* with subgroups, again being inductive in embryos; and *transforming growth factor β (TGFβ)* having been identified in lymphocytes and also grouped as a cytokine, yet being produced widely by many cell types. The TGFβ family also includes activins and bone morphogenetic proteins (BMPs), which similar to TGFβ, may suppress growth as well as stimulate it.

Of the narrow-specificity factors, *nerve growth factor (NGF)* and related *brain-derived neurotrophic factor (BDNF)*, and neurotrophins 3 and 4 promote survival of neurons; *erythropoietin* promotes proliferation and differentiation of erythrocytes; and *interleukin-3 (IL-3)* and related *hemopoietic colony-stimulating factors (CSFs)*, which are also classed as cytokines, stimulate proliferation of blood cell precursors.

Cytokines and growth factors can signal a wide variety of cellular effects including stimulation or inhibition of growth, differentiation, migration etc[23]. Because each family is so large, and because there are a similarly extensive number of receptors, the possible signaling combinations are considerable. Often, a single growth factor can bind with varying affinities to individual receptor family members. Some of these receptors are monogamous, recognizing only one isoform of the growth factor, whereas others are polygamous, recognizing all isoforms. The effects of any individual growth factor may therefore depend on which receptor isoform, or ratio of isoform receptors, are displayed on the cell surface. It is now clear that developmental information resides, not in any single molecule, but rather in the combination of molecules, to which a cell is exposed. Thus, varying combinations of growth factors, in varying concentrations, can elicit quite different effects on similar cells[24].

As well as an expansion in the range of growth factors identified within development, knowledge of the genes which code for them and ways of demonstrating them has also contributed to the complexity of understanding embryological processes. Many genes have been shown to be ubiquitous throughout embryos and conserved through evolution, making viable transfer of tissues between animal groups possible. Responses to deletion of specific gene action, or application of cytokines and growth factors at inappropriate times and places in the embryo add to the body of knowledge but, because interactions are driven by complex cascades of many growth factors, each study can only add a small piece to the jigsaw. Stern[25] noted that embryos generate complexity with only a few extracellular signals, each of which has multiple roles at different developmental times. Thus, each time we appear to understand a developmental process and declare a 'default' pathway of development that is understood, more complexity is uncovered.

REFERENCES

1. Alberts B, Johnson A, Lewis J, Raff M, Roberts K, Walter P. *Molecular biology of the cell*, 4th edn. New York: Garland Press, 2002.
2. Markwald RR, Mjaatvedt CH, Krug EL, Sinning AR. Interactions in heart development. Role of cardiac edherons in cushion tissue formation. *Ann NY Acad Sci* **588**:13–25, 1990.
3. Raff RA. Evolution of development decisions and morphogenesis: the view from two camps. *Development* (Suppl):15–22, 1992.
4. Hall BK. *Evolutionary developmental biology*. London: Chapman and Hall, 1992.
5. Wessells NK. *Tissue interactions and development*. Menlo Park, CA: Benjamin/Cummings, 1977.
6. Thorogood P. The developmental specification of the vertebrate skull. *Development* **103**(Suppl):141–153, 1988.
7. Lumsden AGS. Neural crest contribution to tooth development in the mammalian embryo. In *Developmental and evolutionary aspects of the neural crest*, PFA Maderson (ed.), pp. 261–300. New York: Wiley, 1987.
8. Kollar EJ, Mina M. Role of the early epithelium in the patterning of the teeth and Meckel's cartilage. *J Craniofac Genet Dev Biol* **11**:223–228, 1991.
9. Kollar EJ, Fisher C. Tooth induction in chick epithelium: expression of quiescent genes for enamel synthesis. *Science* **207**:993–995, 1980.
10. Hilfer SR, Rayner RM, Brown JW. Mesenchymal control of branching pattern in the fetal mouse lung. *Tissue Cell* **127**:523–538, 1985.
11. Abbott LA, Lester SM, Erickson CA. Changes in mesenchymal cell-shape, matrix collagen and tenascin accompany bud formation in the early chick embryo. *Anat Embryol* **183**:299–311, 1992.
12. Le Douarin N. An experimental analysis of liver development. *Med Biol* **53**:427–455, 1975.
13. Haffen K, Kedinger M, Simon-Assmann P. Cell contact dependent regulation of enterocyte differentiation. In *Human gastrointestinal development*, E Lebenthal (ed.). New York: Raven Press, 1989.
14. Grobstein C. Inductive interaction in the development of the mouse metanephros. *J Exp Zool* **130**:319–340, 1955.
15. Saxen L, Koskimies O, Lahti A, Miettinen H, Rapola J, Wartiovarra J. Differentiation of kidney mesenchyme in an experimental model system. *J Adv Morphogen* **7**:251–293, 1968.
16. Saxen L. Failure to demonstrate tubule induction in a heterologous mesenchyme. *Dev Biol* **23**:511–523, 1970.
17. Fouser L, Avner ED. Normal and abnormal nephrogenesis. *Am J Kidney Dis* **21**:64–70, 1993.
18. Ekblom P, Sariola H, Karkinen-Jaaskelainen M, Saxen L. The origin of the glomerular endothelium. *Cell Differentiation* **11**:35–39, 1982.
19. Bard JBL, Woolf AS. Nephrogenesis and the development of renal disease. *Neurol Dial Transplant* **7**:563–572, 1992.
20. Sariola H, Saarma M, Sainio K et al. Dependence of kidney morphogenesis on the expression of nerve growth factor receptor. *Science* **254**:571–573, 1991.
21. Christ B, Huang R, Scaal M. Formation and differentiation of the avian sclerotome. *Anat Embryol* **208**:333–350, 2004.
22. Gershon MD. Phenotypic expression by neural crest-derived precursors of enteric neurons and glia. In *Developmental and evolutionary aspects of the neural crest*, PFA Maderson (ed.). New York: John Wiley, 1987.
23. Sporn MB, Roberts AS. *Peptide growth factors and their receptors*, Vols 1 and 2. Berlin: Springer-Verlag, 1990.
24. Jessell TM, Melton DA. Diffusable factors in vertebrate embryonic induction. *Cell* **68**:257–270, 1992.
25. Stern C. Neural induction: old problem, new findings, yet more questions. *Development* **132**:2007–2021, 2005.

CHAPTER 3

Staging embryos in development and the embryonic body plan

Patricia Collins

KEY POINTS

- This chapter presents the concepts and timing of embryonic development
- The problems of using staging systems to describe a continuous process are discussed
- The method behind staging of chick and human development is presented
- A revision of the timing of early human development is presented
- The problems of equating aspects of animal development directly to human development is discussed
- Embryonic and obstetric stages of development are presented
- The main embryological stages and their approximate times are presented

INTRODUCTION

Estimations concerning the length of time an embryo or fetus has been in utero are based initially on information from the mother on the date of her last menstrual period and subsequently on observation of the embryo or fetus in utero by means of ultrasonography. Knowledge about what external and internal structures would normally be developing at a particular time during early gestation has been generated over the years from study of miscarried or aborted embryos, studies of animal embryos of known gestational age, and now more recently, from ultrasonographic data. Decisions about the health or ill health of the embryo or fetus may be based on comparison of its developmental status with examples found in embryonic staging series.

A variety of staging systems for human embryos were devised in the early years of the last century. To enhance this information, studies on other animals were also performed and externally similar stages compared. However, devising a staging system is very different from describing a day-by-day account of development. It will be clearer to explain how developmental stages for animal embryos have been constructed and then compare this to the ways staging schemes for human embryos were derived.

CHICK STAGE SERIES

Chick development was described by Hamburger and Hamilton[1] (republished by Sanes[2] and Hamilton[3]) as a series of 46 stages. In this series, fertilized eggs were maintained at 39.4°C and embryos were examined over the 20-day incubation. Because development is continuous, dividing it up into stages is a very arbitrary process. It is like seeing the action in a movie only by viewing a succession of freeze-frame images; to show others the story a representative number of images must be selected, but which ones? For the chick series, the major factors were that stages could be identified unequivocally by one or more external morphological features and that successive stages were spaced as closely as possible. Dozens of embryos of the same chronological age were examined to look for the slightest differences in a range of external features. The features under consideration changed as development proceeded and the speed of change varied during the incubation. In the first weeks, the changes in the embryos were so rapid that the stages are only hours apart, whereas in the second half of the incubation, the stages are a day apart. Thus, stages one to seven occur during the first 24 hours of incubation; the somites appear and are used as external features between 23 hours (stage 7) and 53 hours (stage 14). After this time, limb buds and pharyngeal arches are used especially.

The internal characteristics of the chick embryos were not described, so development of particular organs was not initially related to the external features. However, the Hamburger and Hamilton series of stages is supported by extensive photographs of each stage, so that correlation of external features with internal structures identified in subsequent studies is possible.

Hamburger produced similar staging series for *Ambystoma*, *Triturus taeniatus* and *T. cristatus*, species of salamander. Since that time, series have been produced for many reptiles and amphibians. These studies are arduous and time consuming but provide the most valuable hard data on the timing of embryonic development. All of the early series were on amphibian, avian or reptile embryos which are easily accessible throughout incubation. However, the incubation temperature will affect the speed of gestation and, in the case of reptile embryos, will have an effect on the sex of the offspring. In turtles, male embryos result from cool incubations, whereas females arise from warmer temperatures; the opposite occurs in the gecko. In most reptiles, intermediate temperature incubations result in development of both males and females. Mammalian embryos have proved much more inaccessible for study. In laboratory species, gestation in days is universally used as a guide to developmental status, thus the staging is based on chronology rather than external features, although descriptive terms are often also used to indicate the stage.

HUMAN STAGE SERIES

Human embryonic stages are, like the chick stages, universally based on the apparent morphological state of development of the embryo, not on either chronological age or on size. The supposed age of a human embryo is only dubiously estimated from the menstrual history. There is considerable variability in both premenstrual and postmenstrual phases of the menstrual cycle, on top of which there are great possibilities for error in correctly identifying menstruation or erroneously interpreting its absence. The concept of 'postovulatory age' has been used[4], referring to the length of time since the last ovulation before pregnancy began. This is predicated on the very close interval between the time of ovulation and the time of fertilization.

The first comparative description of human embryos is attributed to Wilhelm His (Snr) who, with the use of fixation, sectioning and reconstruction of sections, provided the first insights into internal morphology at different ages. Human embryos were first placed in a staged series by Mall[5], founder of the Department of Embryology of the Carnegie Institution of Washington. Mall arranged 266 human embryos into a series of 14 stages on the basis of their external form. The embryos ranged from 2 to 25 mm in length. His work was continued by George Streeter[6–9] who concentrated on embryos initially up to 32 mm greatest length.

Embryos in the Carnegie Collection were received already in fixative. The greatest length of the embryos, measured with callipers without any attempt to straighten the natural curvature, was recorded usually after 2 weeks in 10% formalin; this was to standardize any shrinkage caused by fixation. Tables of embryonic length correlated to stage and predicted age were produced. These were based on fixed embryos graded as excellent. In each stage, the greatest length may vary by 4 mm within the embryonic period.

All of the embryos were photographed, wax embedded and serially sectioned, the sections were examined and drawings and reconstructions made. Observations were made about the degree of development of a range of internal organs and these were correlated with the external characteristics. No one criterion could place a particular embryo within one stage or another. The stage was estimated from examination of a number of key structures throughout the body. Where human embryos of particular stages were not available, comparison to the development of macaque embryos was made. Now it is known that such comparisons are not warranted. Embryos were assigned to 'horizons' based on these examinations and their ages were thus estimated. Streeter believed such estimations could be ±1 day for any given stage. So, whereas in the chick stage series, the investigators knew the time of incubation and made decisions about whether an embryo demonstrated sufficient external characteristics to warrant inclusion in a particular stage, human embryos were grouped according to similar characteristics and the series was used to infer age. This becomes increasingly difficult as development proceeds and variation in the rate of development or in the size of different embryos becomes more marked.

The strength of Streeter's studies is that portions of embryonic material can often be staged by reference to his work, e.g. he correlated the development of the semi-circular canals to the length of the Müllerian or paramesonephric ducts, such that when the Müllerian duct is up to one-third of the way to the cloaca, one semi-circular canal is present, when the duct is two-thirds of the way to the cloaca, two ducts are present and, when the duct reaches the cloaca, all the semi-circular ducts are present. Thus, a particular stage is not an alternative way of indicating the developmental age of an embryo; a stage conveys the developmental status of many of the systems in concert.

Streeter originally designated the time periods 'horizons'; however, this has now been superseded by 'stage' which is common for other developmental description. His system of stages (now the basis for the Carnegie staging system) range from 1 to 23 over a developmental period from fertilization to 8 postovulatory weeks. Streeter ended the series at stage 23 using the onset of marrow formation in the humerus as the marker for the end of the embryonic and the beginning of the fetal period of development. Embryos at stage 23 are approximately 30 mm long (range 27–31 mm) and 56 postovulatory days.

Streeter's work was continued by Ronan O'Rahilly who has published extensively on human development. The monograph, *Developmental Stages in Human Embryos*, with Fabiola Müller[4] has been a mainstay of embryonic developmental staging for many years and most descriptive research papers on human embryos base the stage and age of development of the specimens they study on this system. O'Rahilly and Müller have always emphasized that the staging system for human embryos is based on internal and external morphological criteria and not founded on length or age[10]. However, recently, ultrasonic examination of embryos in vivo has prompted the revision of some of the ages previously assigned to early embryonic stages. O'Rahilly and Müller also note that inter-embryonic variation may be greater than was thought and some of the ages linked to stages may have been underestimated[11]. Embryos of stages 6–16 are now thought to be up to 3–5 days older than the previously used embryological estimates. For those embryos measuring between 3 and 30 mm, the age of the embryo can be estimated from its embryonic length, by adding number 27 to the length. The resultant figure is an estimation of age. So, for an embryo of greatest length 9 mm, the age estimate would be 36 days. This revision will take some years to percolate through newer embryological studies and it may be some time before the age of neurulation is happily given as 29 days rather than 22 days. O'Rahilly and Müller recommend associating stages to weeks or half weeks of development as more appropriate and note that correlation of a stage of development to a specific age in days may be unreliable.

WHAT IS CONSIDERED 'NORMAL' IN HUMAN EMBRYOS?

A note of caution about existing human stage series must be made. Six hundred embryos were sectioned and examined to arrive at the Carnegie staging system, yet the majority of those were listed as normal. Collections of miscarriages usually contain a large incidence of chromosomally abnormal embryos. The very young embryos in the Carnegie Collection were obtained from hysterectomies and later ones were often received with a scanty background history. Variations and anomalies in individual organs were noted in some embryos. However, the techniques were not available at the time this series was developed, the early 1900s, to check for chromosomal or gene abnormalities. It is suggested that at least 15% of all recognized pregnancies will abort before 12 weeks' gestation (see below for explanation of the timescale referred to) and, of these, 40% will be due to chromosome abnormalities. Thus, collections of miscarried pregnancies can be inferred to contain many abnormal embryos. It should also be noted that estimations of embryonic length may be 1–5 mm less than equivalent in vivo estimates, reflecting the shrinkage of specimens caused by the fixative used to store them.

Similar problems of examining early embryos and predicting what their status would have been at term occur in embryo studies when investigating teratogenic insult. Low level teratogens may affect some developing systems and not others in individual embryos. When examining a mammalian embryo removed during development, the final outcome of the teratogen on that embryo cannot be predicted with certainty. On the one hand, the embryo might have developed to term with sufficient catch up growth to reduce the apparent severity of the condition; on the other hand, the embryo might not have sufficient cell populations to recover from the insult and might have died the following week had the experiment continued. The younger the embryos in such studies, the harder it is to make these predictions.

MOLECULAR MARKERS AND STAGING SYSTEMS

The importance of correlating internal features with external characteristics in embryo series cannot be underestimated, and we should be grateful to the early human embryologists for providing such detailed data. It is now realized that similar external embryonic features of different vertebrate species do not indicate similar internal stages of development[12]. Correlating chick embryos of stage 21 with rat embryos of day 12 and human embryos of stage 14 because the external characteristics look similar does not mean that, for example, the lungs are at the same stage of development in these embryos. This latter consideration has become increasingly important with the advent of molecular biology. Stages of development can now be reinterpreted as the time at which specific gene expression is seen in certain tissues. Because many genes are conserved between vertebrates and because deletion of some genes can cause morphological or developmental anomalies, the effects of gene deletion in mouse embryos are now being studied and correlated with known human conditions displaying the similar gene defects and resulting signs and symptoms. Indeed, many genes are being experimentally removed from the mouse genome in the hope of mimicking a human anomalous condition. However, this approach assumes that the development of any one system either operates in isolation from other systems such that inducers of one population do not have any effect on a distant one, or that all systems in mouse and human are developing along the same timescale.

To correlate gene expression with morphology seems to be the next step forward and accurate staging systems are fundamental to this approach. The leap from species to species is more problematical. The observation that internal and external development is not in any synchronization between vertebrate groups has led to the investigation of heterochrony, a change in developmental timing during evolution[12]. If the time at which a range of developmental events occur in *Homo sapiens* during the somite period is plotted against these same events in other species, it can be seen that although, for example, the heart primordia in many species arise early, the appearance of the nasal placodes may be earlier or later than in *Homo sapiens*. It is not yet clear whether the development of any one system also requires background feedback about the stage of development of other systems for its successful completion.

OBSTETRIC STAGING SCHEMES

Use of the Carnegie staging scheme with reference to individual stages presupposes the adoption of that timescale of development. So, suggesting an embryo is at stage 17, implies that it is six weeks postovulation. In this scale, development averages 266 days, or 9.5 months.

The obstetric timescale is involved in estimating a day of delivery and then assessing the fetus to see if it seems appropriately aged to deliver at that time. The commencement of gestation is determined *clinically* by counting from the date of the last menstrual period. Estimated in this manner, a pregnancy averages 280 days, or 10 lunar months (40 weeks). Examination of Figure 3.1 where both scales are depicted shows the two-week discrepancy between these scales. Generally, books written for obstetricians or fetal physicians will use the lower, obstetric scale, whereas embryology books will use the upper, embryological scale.

There is little information about the growth of the fetus from weeks 9 to 20 (embryonic timescale) and the interaction between developing systems at this time. Yet, today, it is not uncommon for fetuses to be born at ages equivalent to 19 or 20 embryonic weeks and survive. At these stages, estimations of fetal age become less important than estimations of fetal maturity. There are a number of tables showing the expected range of length and weight correlated to obstetric gestation weeks. O'Rahilly and Müller recommend that the words, 'gestational age', 'gestation' and 'gestational weeks' are ambiguous and should be avoided. Fetal staging is fraught with the same errors as embryonic staging. O'Rahilly and Müller note that estimations of embryonic and early fetal age by measuring crown–rump length is unsatisfactory because the two points used for this measurement may not exist or may not be evident in young embryos, and their relative positions may change during development. They recommend the use of greatest length, exclusive of lower limbs, as this measurement is similar to that routinely taken in ultrasound examination. O'Rahilly and Müller also recommend that the term 'crown–rump length' should be replaced by greatest length in ultrasound examination[10].

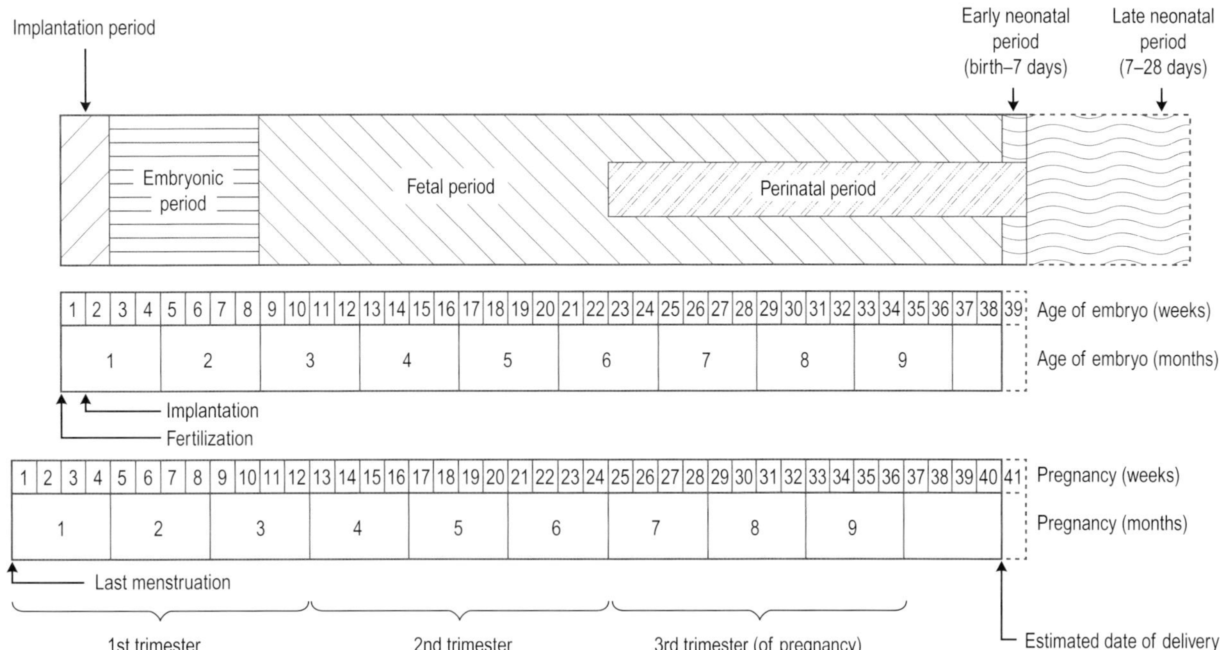

Fig. 3.1 The two time scales used to depict human development. Embryonic development, in the upper scale, is counted from fertilization (or from ovulation, i.e. in postovulatory days).[3] The clinical estimation of pregnancy is counted from the last menstrual period and is shown on the lower scale. Note that there is a two-week discrepancy between these scales. The perinatal period is very long as it includes all of the preterm deliveries. (From *Gray's Anatomy*, 39th edn. Edinburgh: Churchill Livingstone, 2005.)

A number of biometric indices used to determine fetal age in utero have been evaluated in ultrasound studies for accuracy. Charts of first-trimester growth based on biparietal diameter, head circumference and abdominal circumference of normal singleton fetuses, correlated against crown–rump length (from 45 to 84mm) are considered to be more accurate than gestational age by menstrual dates[13]. It is suggested that the femur length/head circumference ratio may be a more robust ratio to characterize fetal proportions than femur length/biparietal diameter[14,15], and combining kidney length, biparietal diameter, head circumference and femur length also increases the precision of dating[16]. Johnsen et al., reported that analysis of measurements of biparietal diameter and head circumference at 10–24 weeks' gestation gave a gestational age assessment of 3–8 days greater than charts in use at that time[14].

MAIN STAGES IN THE EMBRYONIC PERIOD

Embryonic development is not apparent before stage 6. Stages 1–5 are concerned with setting up the cell populations for implantation; most of the cell lines generated are extraembryonic and involved in establishing the placenta and fetal membranes. In stage 6a, the primordial germ cells are sequestered into the extraembryonic mesoblast and, in stage 6b, the primitive streak appears. From this time, intraembryonic cell populations are generated and it is the morphological movements of these populations which produces a recognizable embryo. Figure 3.2 shows stages 1–11 matched to estimated age. The proliferation of cells at the primitive streak occurs through stages 7 and 8, when the notochord is first evident, and provides cell populations which pass within the embryo. By stage 9, the neural populations are becoming defined and result in neurulation and the beginning of somite formation, more clearly seen in stage 10 which typically has 7–12 pairs of somites. The formation of the neural plate and the beginnings of its rostral fusion contribute to the morphological movements of head folding, where the cardiac area, which was rostral to the neural epithelium, becomes ventral and forms a boundary of the cranial intestinal portal. Stages 6b–10 are concerned with embryogenesis when morphogenetic movements affecting the whole embryo move widely dispersed cell populations closer and into their relevant positions for local interactive processes to commence. The stage 11 embryo is at the gateway of organogenesis and all body systems can be seen to originate from this point.

THE STAGE 11 EMBRYO, THE BODY PLAN

The criterion for stage 11 is the presence of 13–20 pairs of somites (Fig. 3.3); during this stage the rostral neuropore will close. Fusion occurs from the rhombencephalon rostrally towards the mesencephalon and from the region of the future optic chiasma towards the mesencephalic roof. The optic primordia have begun evagination towards the surface ectoderm. The otic vesicle, which will invaginate and give rise to the inner ear (cochlea and

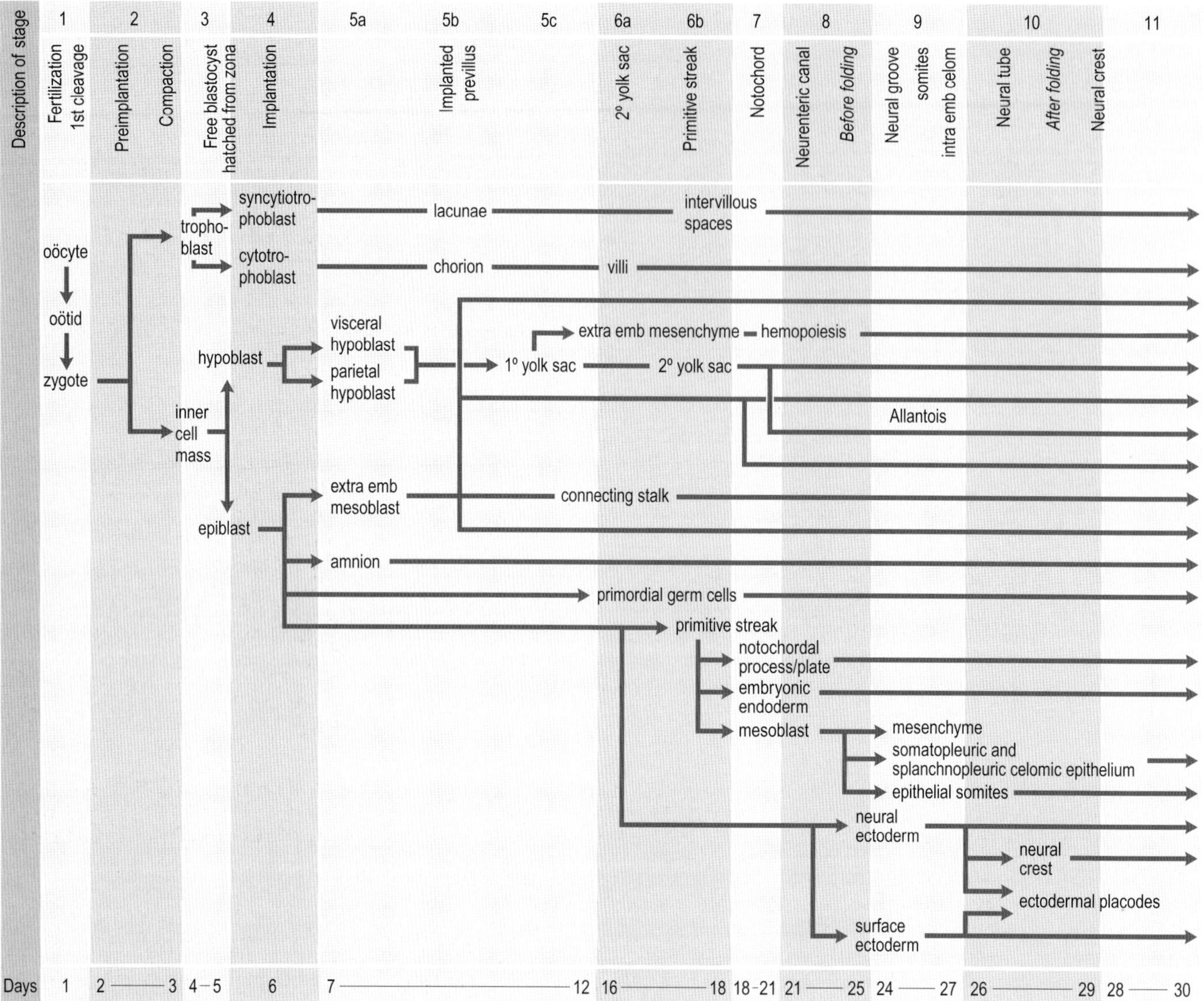

Fig. 3.2 Development processes occurring during the first 10 stages of development. In the early stages a series of binary choices determine the cell lineages. Generally, the earliest stages are concerned with formation of the extraembryonic tissues, whereas the later stages see the formation of embryonic tissues. (Modified from *Gray's Anatomy*, 39th edn. Edinburgh: Churchill Livingstone, 2005.)

semi-circular ducts), has not yet formed, but the surface epithelium has thickened and begun to invaginate. Around the developing pharynx the mandibular processes are present but the maxillary processes have yet to arise. The second pharyngeal arch, the hyoid, is present but not the third. Ventral to the foregut is the heart, this develops very precociously and is seen in stage 9 embryos as tube-like with a united ventricular portion but still separate atrial components. The specialized cells of the celom, which will give rise to the myocardium, can be identified as can the matrix produced locally between the endocardium and the myocardium. Cardiac contractions commence at the beginning of stage 10 when the heart has a recognizable ventricle, bulbus cordis and arterial trunk, and a cardiac loop can be distinguished; the organ is already asymmetrical. By stage 11, the sinus venosus, atria, left and right ventricles, truncus arteriosus and substantial dorsal aortae can be identified. The heart is connected to a range of endothelial vessels and plexuses which are most mature cranially and still forming caudally. The fluid in the vascular system contains relatively few cells. It ebbs and flows because of the pulsations of the myocardium which also cause movement of fluid in the intraembryonic celom. These combined circulations are sufficient to provide nutrient supply to the embryonic tissues.

The intraembryonic celom is especially important at this stage of development. The celom arises from confluent spaces which appear in the embryo from stage 9. As head folding occurs, these spaces coalesce to form a horseshoe-shaped cavity within the embryonic body, which passes between the endoderm of the gut and the ectoderm of the body wall on each side of the developing fore- and midgut, and meets in the midline beneath the rostral neuropore as the future pericardial cavity. The ends of the horseshoe are in wide communication with the

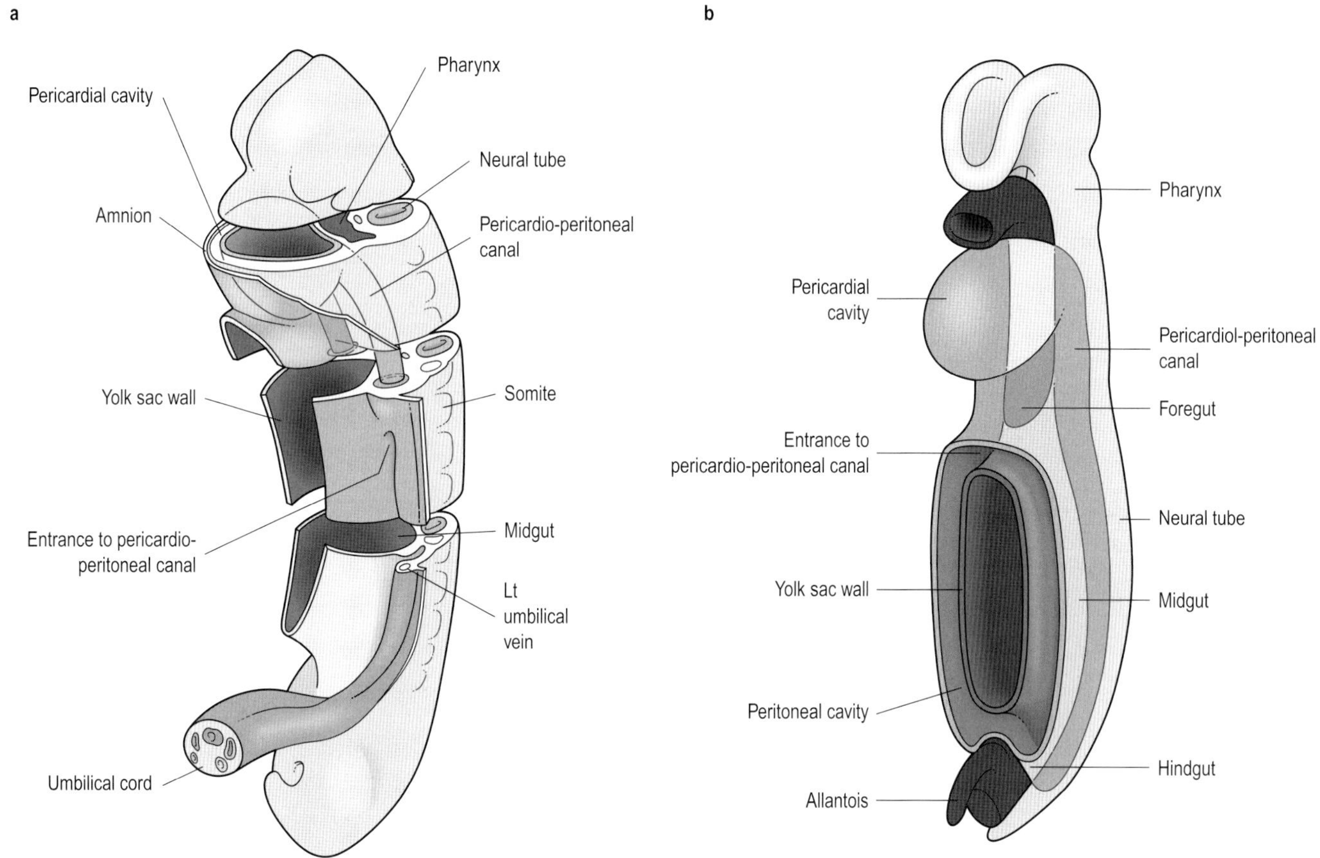

Fig. 3.3 (a) Diagram of a stage-10 embryo with the position of the intraembryonic celom indicated (after Streeter). (b) Diagram of three major epithelial populations within a stage-10 embryo, viewed from a ventrolateral position. The neural tube lies dorsal to the gut; ventrally the intraembryonic celom crosses the midline at the level of the foregut and hindgut, but is lateral to the midgut and a portion of the foregut. (From *Gray's Anatomy*, 39th edn. Edinburgh: Churchill Livingstone, 2005.)

extraembryonic celom around the embryo and within the chorion. The walls of the celom are composed of germinal epithelia which provide mesenchymal cell populations for the connective tissues and smooth muscle of the respiratory and gastrointestinal tracts, the body wall and especially the heart. The myocardium arises directly from the dorsal pericardial wall in the folded embryo. The ventral pericardial wall will give rise to the serous, parietal pericardial layer.

The foregut develops as the head fold elevates and the pericardial cavity swings ventrally. It is flattened dorsoventrally, extending laterally to form the pharyngeal pouches. The buccopharyngeal membrane is present at this stage and may begin to rupture. There is only a small indication of the future respiratory primordium. The liver is represented by the septum transversum mesenchyme and underlying endoderm but the latter is still widely connected to the yolk sac. The nephric system consists of a solid nephrogenic cord lateral to somites 8–13. The cloacal membrane is situated ventrally after tail folding just caudal to the connecting stalk which passes to the developing placenta. The primordial germ cells can be identified in the embryo at stage 11. They are initially in the mesenchyme around the yolk sac and allantoic walls. With tail folding they are brought into the body cavity with the hindgut epithelium and surrounding mesenchyme and then by amoeboid movement and by growth displacement they migrate dorsocranially. They do not reach the gonads until stage 15, some 9 days later, when the local cell population are developed sufficiently to receive them.

During stage 11, the most important epithelial layers attain their position, i.e. surface epithelium, notochord, neural epithelium, somites, gut epithelium and the lining of the celomic cavity (see Fig. 3.3). The germinal epithelia of the somites and the celomic cavity then generate extensive mesenchymal populations at the same time that the neural crest mesenchyme cells are migrating within the head and neck. Finally, each epithelium is surrounded and supported by different mesenchymal populations, i.e. the neural tube and notochord are surrounded by neural crest mesenchyme in the head and somatopleuric mesenchyme in the trunk. The gut epithelium is surrounded by splanchnopleuric mesenchyme which becomes specialized, particularly around the respiratory diverticulum. The surface ectoderm is supported by somatopleuric mesenchyme in the trunk and by neural crest mesenchyme in the head. The celomic epithelia themselves produce specialized epithelial populations which give rise to the gonads, adrenal medulla and the lining of the uterine tubes; these epithelia are all supported by local mesenchyme. Angiogenic mesenchyme is found throughout the embryo from stage 9. It is capable of extensive migration

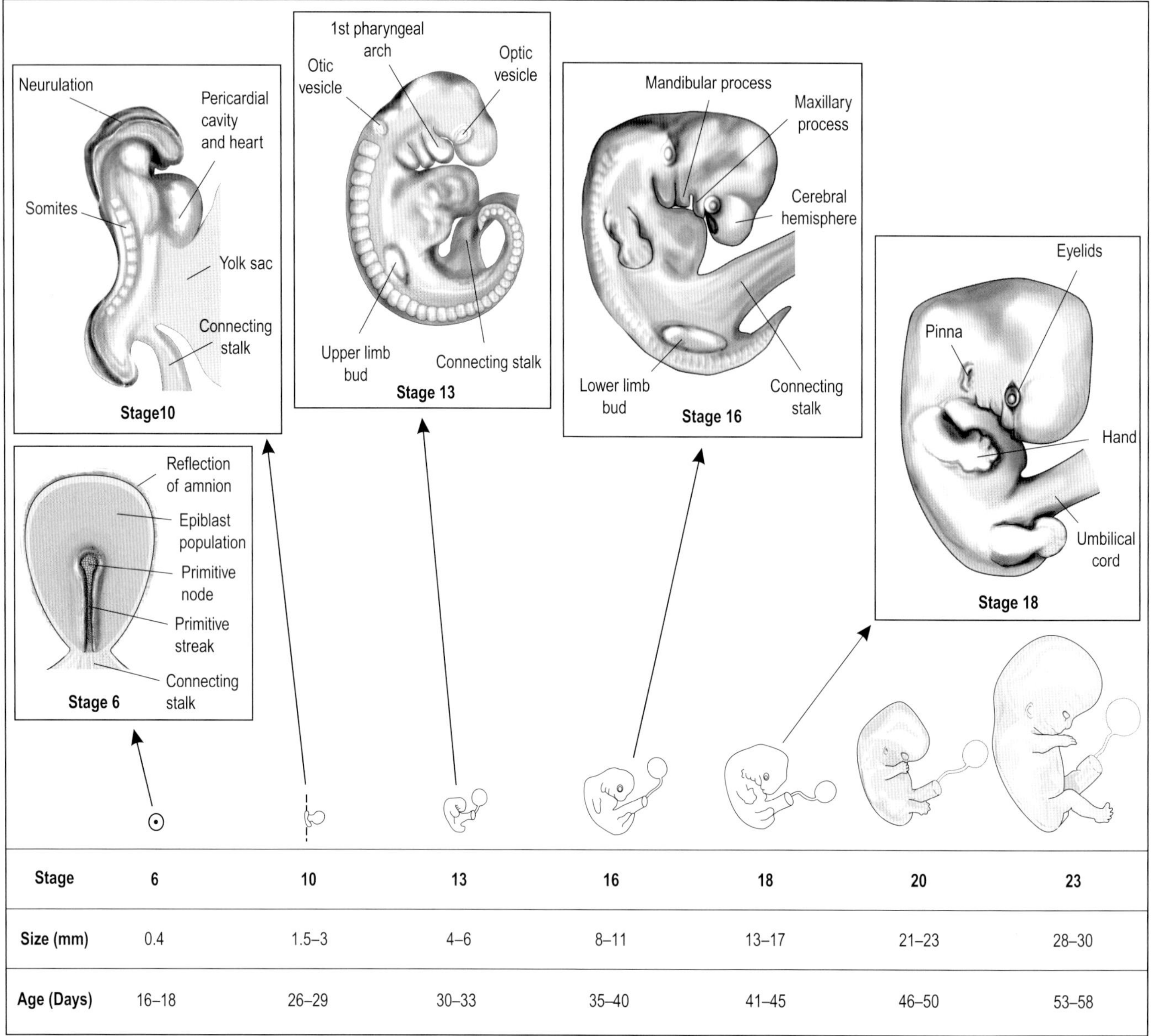

Stage	6	10	13	16	18	20	23
Size (mm)	0.4	1.5–3	4–6	8–11	13–17	21–23	28–30
Age (Days)	16–18	26–29	30–33	35–40	41–45	46–50	53–58

Fig. 3.4 Diagram showing the external appearance and size of embryos between stages 6 and 23. Early in development external features are used to describe the stage, e.g. somites, pharyngeal arches or limb buds. (Modified from *Gray's Anatomy*, 39th edn. Edinburgh: Churchill Livingstone, 2005.)

and differentiates into endothelium or blood cells throughout the embryo. Angiogenic mesenchyme is found within the endodermal and splanchnopleuric layers but never within ectoderm derived tissues.

Stage 11 may be considered to be the body plan stage. To achieve it, genes functioning across the whole embryo are in operation. As stage 11 fades into stage 12, organogenesis is underway and the epithelial/mesenchymal interactions which result in all development are now operating along local lines. Diversity of differentiative outcomes is now possible by upregulation of specific genes in specific regions of the embryo.

Between stage 11 and stage 23, a period of about 32 days, the embryo grows in length from 3 mm to 30 mm. It passes from a general vertebrate embryo to a fully formed but immature human. Figure 3.4 illustrates the dramatic increase in size and developmental status during this time. Figure 3.5 shows the progress in individual systems across the timescale. Although Streeter closed the embryonic period at 56.5 days, the time cut-off is arbitrary, the processes established at that time continue into fetal life and where further growth and maturation proceeds to term and beyond into childhood. Figure 3.6 correlates the stage and age of embryos to length throughout the embryonic period.

Week	1	2	3	4	5	6	7	8	9	10	11	12
Crown-rump length: mm			2	4	10	13	18	30				55
External appearance			Head and tail folding	Pharyngeal arches		Upper lip palate		Digits on hand External ear		Eyelids fuse		
Nervous system			Neurulation First neural crest cells		Otic vesicle Otic cup	Anterior lobe pituitary	Posterior lobe pituitary Membranous labyrinth					
Respiratory				Trachea Lung buds	Primary bronchi			Further division of bronchi				
Gut			Fore-mid hindgut	Thyroid Liver Urorectal septum		Pharyngeal pouches Dorsal and ventral pancreas Rotation of stomach		Midgut loop rotating				Midgut loop returns to abdomen
Kidney				Mesonephros Mesonephric duct	Ureteric bud	Major calyces	Metanephric nephrons	Minor calyces	Kidneys ascend			
Genital				Germ cells in allantoic wall	Indifferent gonad	Mullerian ducts Testis differentiating External genitalia indifferent			Uterus & uterine tubes Vagina		Testis at inguinal canal Prostate External genitalia differentiating	
Cardiovascular			Primitive vascular system Heart tube	Septum primum Heart beats		Septation of ventricles Spleen		Septum secundum				
Musculoskelatal			Somite period 20 days .... 30 days	Forelimb bud		Forelimb digit rays Hindlimb bud	Cartilaginous part of skull		Membranous part of skull			

Fig. 3.5 Timetable of development. The development of individual systems can be seen progressing from left to right. The relative status of different systems can be seen by looking from top to bottom at a particular time. (From *Gray's Anatomy*, 39th edn. Edinburgh: Churchill Livingstone, 2005.)

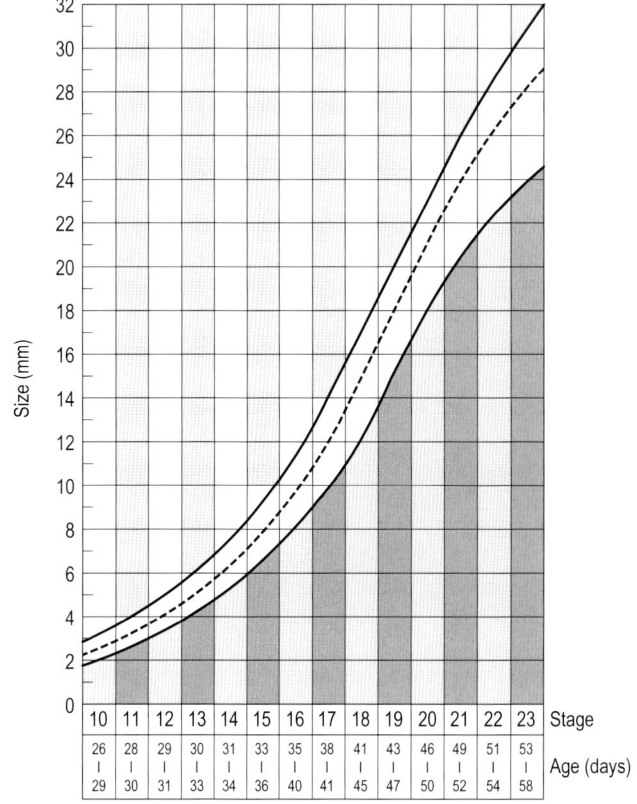

Fig. 3.6 Chart of development stages 10–23 illustrating the range of size embryos attain within the two-day period of a 'stage'[3,7]. (From *Gray's Anatomy*, 39th edn. Edinburgh: Churchill Livingstone, 2005.)

REFERENCES

1. Hamburger V, Hamilton HL. A series of normal stages in the development of the chick embryo. *J Morphol* **88**:49–92, 1951, and *Develop Dynamics* **195**:231–272, 1992.
2. Sanes JR. On the republication of the Hamburger–Hamilton stage series. *Develop Dynamics* **195**:229–230, 1992.
3. Hamilton V. Afterword: The stage series in the chick embryo. *Develop Dynamics* **195**:273–275, 1992.
4. O'Rahilly R, Müller F. *Developmental stages in human embryos*. Publication 637. Carnegie Institution of Washington, 1987.
5. Mall FP. On stages in the development of human embryos from 2 to 25 mm long. *Anat Anz* **46**:78–84, 1914.
6. Streeter GL. Developmental horizons in human embryos. Description of age group XIII, embryos about 4 or 5 millimeters long, and age group XIV, period of indentation of the lens vesicle. Carnegie Institution of Washington Publication 557. *Contrib Embryol* **31**:27–63, 1945.
7. Streeter GL. Developmental horizons in human embryos. Description of age groups XV, XVI, XVII, and XVIII, being the third issue of a survey of the Carnegie Collection. Carnegie Institution of Washington Publication 575. *Contrib Embryol* **32**:133–203, 1948.
8. Streeter GL. Developmental horizons in human embryos. Description of age groups XIX, XX, XXI, XXII, and XXIII, being the fifth issue of a survey of the Carnegie Collection (prepared for publication by CH. Heuser & GW Corner). Carnegie Institution of Washington Publication 592. *Contrib Embryol* **34**:165–196, 1951.
9. Streeter GL. Developmental horizons in human embryos. Description of age group XI, 13 to 20 somites, and age group XII, 21 to 29 somites. Carnegie Institution of Washington. Publication 541. *Contrib Embryol* **30**:211–245, 1942.
10. O'Rahilly R, Müller F. Mini-Review: Prenatal ages and stages – measures and errors. *Teratology* **61**:382–384, 2000.
11. O'Rahilly R, Müller F. *The embryonic human brain. An atlas of developmental stages*, 2nd edn. New York: Wiley-Liss, 1999.
12. Richardson MK. Heterochrony and the phylotypic period. *Develop Biol* **172**:412–421, 1995.
13. Salomon LJ, Bernard JP, Duyme M, Dorion A, Ville Y. Revisiting first-trimester fetal biometry. *Ultrasound Obstet Gynecol* **22**:63–66, 2003.
14. Johnsen SL, Rasmussen S, Sollien R, Kiserud T. Fetal age assessment based on ultrasound head biometry and the effect of maternal and fetal factors. *Acta Obstet Gynecol Scand* **83**:716–723, 2004.
15. Johnsen SL, Rasmussen S, Sollien R. Kiserud T. Fetal age assessment based on femur length at 10–25 weeks of gestation, and reference ranges for femur length to head circumference ratios. *Acta Obstet Gynecol Scand* **84**:725–733, 2005.
16. Konje JC, Abrams KR, Bell SC, Talyor DJ. Determination of gestational age after the 24th week of gestation from fetal kidney length measurements. *Ultrasound Obstet Gynecol* **19**:592–597, 2002.

CHAPTER

4

Development of the head

Patricia Collins

KEY POINTS

- The interactions between different tissue populations occurring in the developing head region are presented
- The following processes are reviewed: early head folding, neurulation, formation of the skull, formation of pharyngeal arches, face and palate, and anomalies of head and neck development
- Nervous tissues arise from the neural plate, neural crest cells and ectodermal placodes
- Each pharyngeal arch is patterned by the neural crest which migrates into it and gives rise to all of the connective tissue elements within the arch. The role of neural crest in the attachment of pharyngeal arch skeletal muscle is presented
- Skeletal muscle within the arches derives from the most rostral unsegmented paraxial mesenchyme. Special populations of preaxial mesenchyme invaginating through the primitive streak ahead of the notochord form the extraocular muscles
- The evolution of the head is discussed

INTRODUCTION

The human head contains the neural tissue necessary for our cognition, coupled with a complex grouping of special sense organs for our perception. There is a vast array of touch and temperature receptors which allow the examination of the local environment with great discrimination and a range of small muscles in the face and the tongue which can be used with exquisite control. Movements of the facial and oral musculature form part of our rich non-verbal communication repertoire, and integration of the skeletal and visceral functions in this region permits the range of reflexes which keep us alive and able to interact in our prescribed social contexts. Complex control of this region occurs in the newborn. Indeed, the sucking and swallowing reflexes seen in the neonate and preterm infant require the coordination of most of the twelve cranial nerves. Within the first couple of feeds, the full-term neonate can suck at a rate of once per second, swallow after five or six sucks, and breathe during every second or third suck. Milk crosses the pharynx en route to the esophagus, and air passes in and out of the nasopharynx and lungs without apparent interruption of breathing and swallowing. Throughout this operation there is little significant misdirection of fluids into the trachea or air into the stomach[1].

The ease with which suckling is established in the neonate is a reflection of the match between the skull shape and palatal development at birth, and the mammary apparatus of the mother. Generally, vertebrate neonates have rounded skulls which assist passage along the birth canal, and relatively short faces which facilitate ease of suckling. It is only after weaning that the range of vertebrate skulls are expressed as in the elongated snouts of the ant eater and the tapir. The ability of the vertebrate skull to produce such a range of variation from what appears to be a basic plan is due to the recruitment of a novel mesenchymal population in the vertebrates alone, the neural crest.

The successful development of the head with all its component parts is due to the accurate expression of genes throughout all of the tissues of the head, from the neuroepithelia, surface ectoderm and endodermal epithelia, to the neural crest, somitic and angiogenic mesenchymal populations.

Development of the head is often dealt with by linear descriptions of individual systems, e.g. nervous system, gastrointestial system, etc. While this approach is helpful for understanding the cranial portions of these systems, it does not convey the interaction and complexity which is seen in head development. This chapter is an attempt to bring together all these aspects so that the integration of the systems in this region can be appreciated. The range of interrelated structures developing in concert in the head can be seen in Figure 4.1.

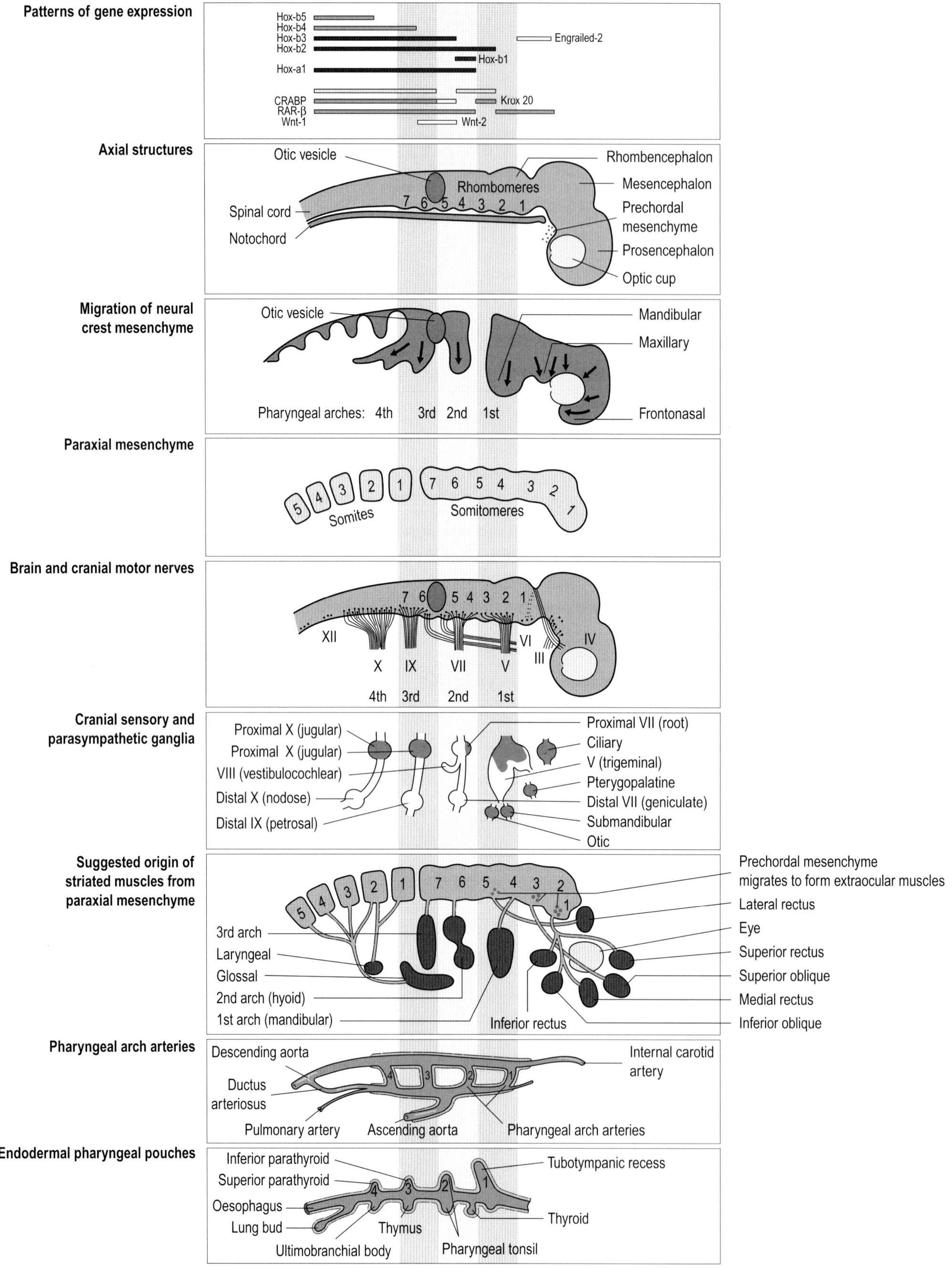

Fig. 4.1 Schema illustrating the organization of the head and pharynx in an embryo at about stage 14. The individual tissue components have been separated but are aligned in register through the numbered zones. (From *Gray's Anatomy*, 38th edn. Edinburgh: Churchill Livingstone, 1995.)

FORMATION OF THE NEURAL POPULATION

Specification of the neural population begins at gastrulation when the primitive streak forms[2]. Cells which proliferate and invaginate at the most rostral end of the streak, the *primitive node* (Hensen's node) form the *notochordal process*, also termed the 'head process' (rather misleadingly), chordamesoderm, or chorda. From this same position, a surface population of neural ectodermal cells proliferate in concert with the notochordal cells. Both populations are suggested to arise from a common progenitor cell[3]. Forward migration of the notochordal cells and the overlying midline neural ectodermal cells is matched and continues rostrally until the cells contact the prechordal plate, a localized thickening of the first endodermal population to ingress at the primitive node. The prechordal plate can be thought of as the site of the future buccopharyngeal membrane, but has other characteristics (see below).

At the onset of primitive streak formation, the putative neural population occupies a zone at the rostral end of the embryonic disk (see Fig. 1.1). After streak formation and the invagination of the notochordal process and the prechordal plate, the neural ectoderm forms a neural plate which is widest at its rostral end, tapering caudally to a narrower zone. The neural plate does not extend to the edges of the embryonic disk, it is surrounded by surface ectoderm. The midline cells of the neural plate match the length of, and are in contact with, the notochordal process. The edges of the plate are raised as folds and distinct from the surface ectoderm. Prior to neurulation, only the brain and cervical regions of the nervous system are represented within the neural plate. As the embryo grows, cells are added to the caudal end of the neural plate matching the increase in notochordal length. The most caudal region of the neural tube develops by a different mechanism (see below).

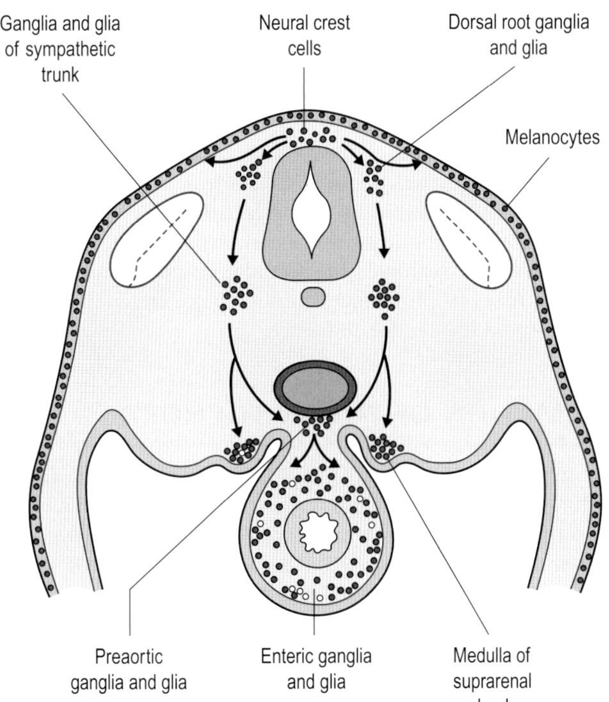

Fig. 4.2 Diagram showing the migration routes taken by neural crest cells in the trunk. (From *Gray's Anatomy*, 39th edn. Edinburgh: Churchill Livingstone, 2005.)

Three distinct neural populations arise from this early arrangement of neural ectoderm:

- The precursors of the central nervous system
- The precursors of the peripheral nervous system
- The ectodermal placodes.

The precursors of the central nervous system arise from the neural plate excluding the edges. The cells produce populations of neurons and glia. The peripheral nervous system arises from populations of cells in the neural folds at the edges of the neural plate, the so-called neural crest. Neural crest cells give rise to all the peripheral ganglia, somatic sensory and autonomic, and their supporting glia, including the neurons and glia of the enteric nervous system (Fig. 4.2). They further produce the cells of the adrenal medulla and melanocytes which later invade the developing epidermis. The ectodermal placodes are neural cells which remain within the surface ectoderm of the head after neurulation to invaginate later. They contribute to the sensory ganglia of the cranial nerves and the epithelium of the inner ear (Fig. 4.3). Some placodal cells, e.g. those forming the olfactory mucosa, are found in the neural folds in local regions where typical crest cells are absent.

CONTRIBUTION OF THE EARLY NEURAL CREST TO THE HEAD

At the time of neurulation, the neural crest cells occupy a zone at the outermost edges of the neural plate, adjacent to the surface ectoderm. When neural epithelial fusion occurs, the crest cells invaginate deep to the surface ectoderm and begin their migration around the forming neural tube. Non-neuronal migratory neural crest cells are produced along the neural axis rostrally as far as the diencephalon, a position corresponding to the extent of the neural floor plate and notochord. Cells arising from the neural fold rostral to this level give rise to the

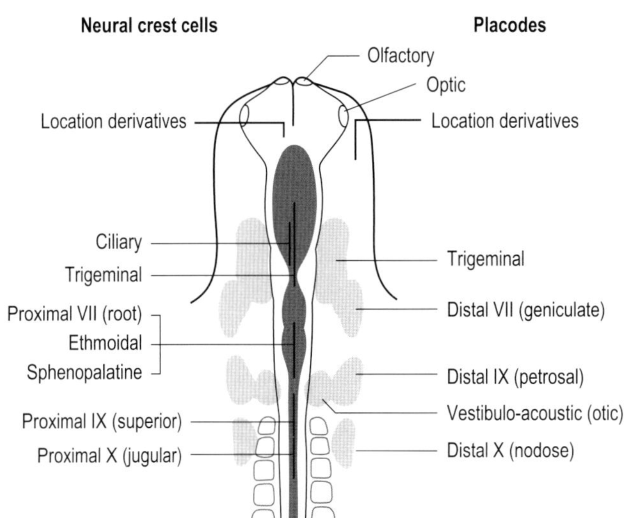

Fig. 4.3 Diagram indicating the contribution of neural crest cells and placodal cells to the ganglia in the head. (From *Gray's Anatomy*, 39th edn. Edinburgh: Churchill Livingstone, 2005.)

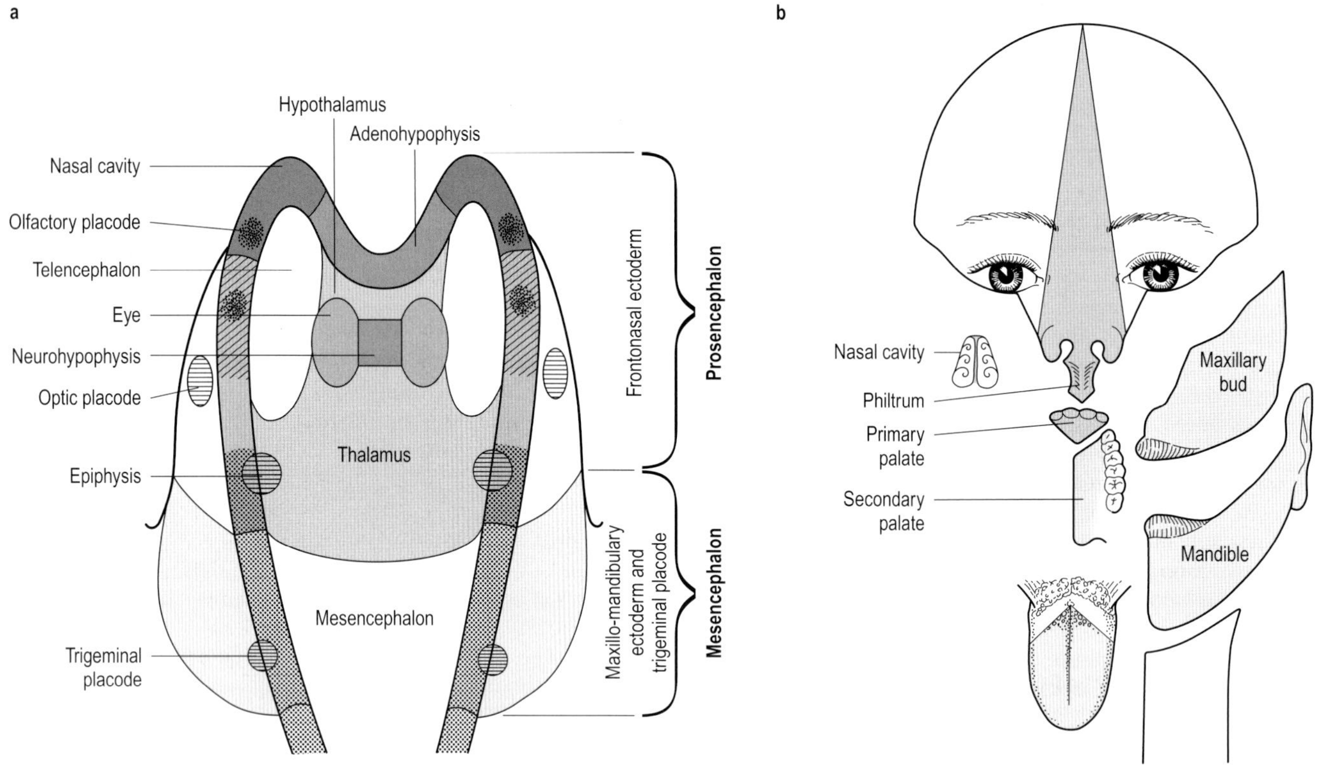

Fig. 4.4 Fate map of the rostral region of the neural primordium as established by the quail–chick chimera system. (a) The various territories yielding rostral head are indicated on the neural plate and neural fold of a 1–3 somite embryo. (b) The results obtained in the avian embryo have been extrapolated to the human head. Thus, the rostral neural fold area yields the epithelium of the rostral roof of the mouth, the nasal cavities and part of the frontal area. (From *Gray's Anatomy*, 39th edn. Edinburgh: Churchill Livingstone, 2005.)

hypophyseal placode, i.e. the future Rathke's pouch, the olfactory placodes and associated nasal epithelium, including the roof of the nasopharynx and the skin of the frontonasal area (Fig. 4.4). The non-neuronal neural crest provides a significant mesenchymal population in the head and neck.

PARAXIAL MESENCHYME AND THE NEURAL TUBE

The neural plate is supported by underlying mesoblast populations which are invaginating through the primitive streak. When neurulation begins, the underlying paraxial mesenchymal population undergoes segmentation to form somites (see below). The process of somitogenesis occurs in concert with neural tube closure. Failure of neurulation will result in incomplete development of the somites and anomalous development of the vertebrae at that level, e.g. spina bifida.

NEURULATION

The neural plate extends much further laterally in the head region than in the trunk. The rapid growth of the plate and underlying mesoblast promotes the ventral movement of the edges of the embryonic disk and neurulation. Neurulation begins at stage 9 (now considered to equate to about 26 post-fertilizational days) when the neural epithelial cells become elongated and then wedge shaped as a result of changes in the conformation of their cytoskeletal elements. The underlying mesoblast and extracellular matrix provide support for the elevating folds and surface ectoderm and assist the alignment of the neural layers as they approach and fuse. Neural tube fusion begins in the hindbrain or upper cervical region at stage 10 (approximately 29 post-fertilizational days). This is primary neurulation. It extends both rostrally and caudally until only small neuropores remain open at each end. The rostral neuropore closes in the middle of the fourth week and the caudal neuropore closes slightly later. Secondary neurulation occurs in the lumbosacral region of the spinal cord and involves cavitation of a mass of pluripotent mesenchyme covered with ectoderm, termed the caudal eminence.

FORMATION OF THE NOTOCHORD

The first cell lines which invaginate through the rostral end of the primitive streak form a *notochordal process*. This is a flat plate of epithelial cells which form the roof of the secondary yolk sac, the notochordal cells being in contact with laterally placed endodermal cells which are invaginating contemporaneously. The notochord separates from the endoderm by a mechanism similar to neurulation, i.e. the cells become wedge shaped and the population forms a groove followed by a tube with the edges opposing and fusing.

The notochord separates from the alimentary tract early in development. However, the last region to contain a notochordal process is the pharynx. Here the notochordal process remains within the endodermal layer until stage 11. It may be that this arrangement facilitates interactions in this region as, whereas in the cervical and more caudal regions, the notochord is involved in sclerotome formation, rostrally the unsegmented paraxial mesenchyme overlying the pharyngeal region may receive different inductive information to initiate its differentiation into skull components; perhaps the later retention of the notochordal process in the pharynx promotes this.

Earlier works identified a mesenchymal population referred to as *prechordal mesenchyme* which was suggested to be part of the prechordal plate (see below). However, more recent experimental studies have shown that, immediately after its formation, the notochordal process is composed of determined myogenic cells[4]; later, myogenic cells are not present. As development proceeds, the posterior portion of the notochordal process becomes transformed into the notochord proper, whereas the prechordal cells retain a mesenchymal morphology and myogenic fate. Orthotopic grafting has demonstrated that these cells later join the more laterally placed paraxial mesenchyme and finally migrate to become the oculomotor musculature of the eyes (see below).

EARLY DEVELOPMENT OF THE BRAIN

Even prior to closure of the neural tube, the neural plate is much more extensive at its rostral end. Here, elevation of the neural folds produces three deep, slit-like early brain regions. The *prosencephalon* or forebrain, the *mesencephalon* or midbrain and the *rhombencephalon* or hindbrain, continuous caudally with the spinal cord. Later, the roof of the rhombencephalon thins and becomes covered with non-neural tissue. As a result of relatively unequal growth occurring in each of these brain regions, three flexures appear in the brain; two flexures are concave ventrally with corresponding flexures of the head, e.g. the mesencephalic flexure at the rostral end of the notochord and the cephalic flexure at the junction of the hindbrain and spinal cord. The third flexure has its convexity directed ventrally at the level of the future pons.

NEUROMERES

With the development of the flexures, the early brain regions are now reassigned into five regions which are used descriptively in the later developing and adult brain. They correspond to segmental regions termed neuromeres, identifiable by transverse subdivisions perpendicular to the longitudinal axis of the developing brain. The prosencephalon will become divided into two parts, the telencephalon, from which paired, lateral evagination will develop into the cerebral hemispheres, and the diencephalon which will form the lateral walls of the IIIrd ventricle (Fig. 4.5). The mesencephalon remains undivided and forms the wall of the cerebral aqueduct. The region of the isthmus rhombencephali is noted as an important landmark between the mesencephalon and rhombencephalon. The rhombencephalon is subdivided by the pontine flexure into the metencephalon rostrally which will give rise to the pons and cerebellum, and the myelencephalon caudally which will give rise to the medulla oblongata.

A series of eight bulges can be seen in the walls of the rhombencephalon, these are termed *rhombomeres*. They constitute the primary patterning units in this region. Single-cell labeling experiments have shown that cells within rhombomeres form segregated non-mixing populations. Rhombomeres can be seen for only a short period of time in early development. However, it is thought that during this period, morphogenetic specification of the neural crest arising from the rhombencephalon occurs (Fig. 4.6). Neural crest cells from rhombomeres 1 and 2 contribute to the trigeminal ganglion, crest cells from rhombomere 4 contribute to the facial and vestibuloacoustic ganglion, while crest cells from rhombomere 6 contribute to the superior petrosal ganglion. There are no contributions to the ganglia from rhombomeres 3 and 5. As well as contributing to the somatic sensory ganglia, the neural crest cells also give rise to the parasympathetic ganglia in the head, the ciliary and pterygopalatine ganglia in the frontonasal region, and the otic and submandibular ganglia within the first arch (see Fig. 4.1). Within the neck, neural crest cells give rise to the cervical ganglia of the sympathetic trunk.

Expression of genes in the Hox a, b, c and d clusters have been studied in a number of vertebrates. Hox genes are expressed in the rhombomeres and also in neural crest arising at the same level. When neural crest migration is complete, the same set of Hox genes is activated in the surface ectoderm[5].

PATTERNING IN THE EARLY NEURAL TUBE

The close relationship between the notochord and neural floor plate is maintained during neurulation and is necessary for the correct specification of the motor and sensory neurons in the spinal cord. Motor neurons differentiate ventrally very close to the floor plate whereas sensory neurons differentiate close to the roof plate. Experiments in the chick have shown that if the notochord is removed the neural floor plate is eliminated and normally dorsally placed sensory neurons are produced, whereas if a notochord or a floor plate is grafted to the dorsal midline of the neural tube ectopic motor neurons are induced (Fig. 4.7).

Within the mesencephalon and rhombencephalon, the same organization of cranial nerves is generally seen, the motor nerves being placed ventrally and the sensory inputs dorsally. With the widening of the rhombencephalic vesicle, the future IVth ventricle, this arrangement is more linear with the motor nerves arising medially and the sensory ones laterally. Thus the motor cranial nerves III, IV, VI and XII broadly parallel the organization of the somatic motor neurons in the spinal cord. However, the mixed cranial nerves V, VII, IX and X, which supply the pharyngeal arches, exit more dorsally than the somatic motor nerves. This is suggested to be because of the effect of the locally migrating neural crest cells.

PREDICTIVE FATE MAPS OF THE NEURAL PLATE AND NEURAL CREST

The close proximity of the neural plate and neural crest populations in the rostral end of the neural plate contribute, in many cases jointly, to structures of the special senses and face. Mapping the fate of cells in this region using chick–quail chimera experimentation has revealed what each part of the floor

Fig. 4.5 (a) The right side of the brain of a human embryo, 9 mm long. (Drawn from a model by His.) (b) The brain of a human embryo about 10.2 mm long: right lateral surface. (From a model by His.) (c) The right side of the brain of a human embryo, 13.6 mm long. The roof of the hindbrain has been removed. (From a model by His.) (Modified from *Gray's Anatomy*, 39th edn. Edinburgh: Churchill Livingstone, 2005.)

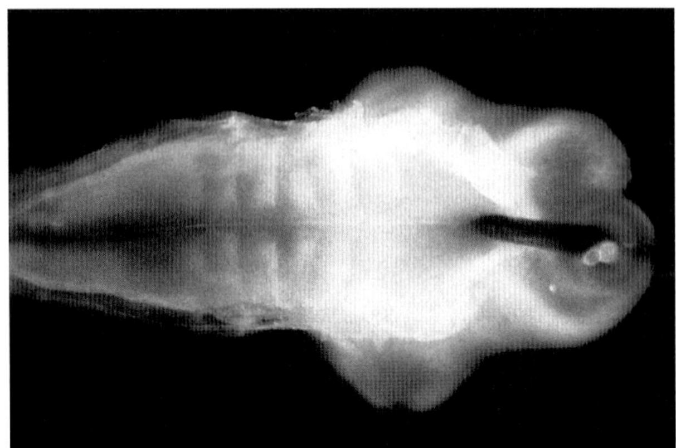

Fig. 4.6 Photograph showing rhombomeric segmentation. (Photograph supplied by Professor A Lumsden, from *Gray's Anatomy*, 39th edn. Edinburgh: Churchill Livingstone, 2005.)

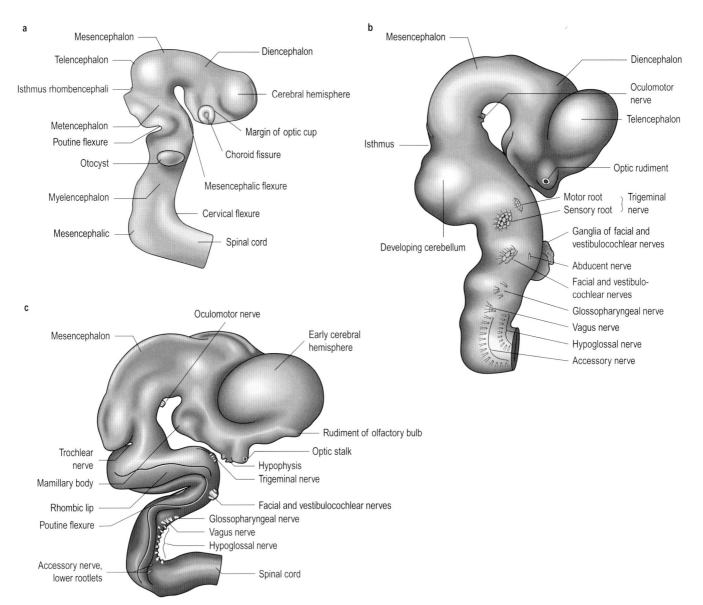

and adjacent neural folds become (see Fig. 4.4). From these studies, the elegant complexity of development can be appreciated. For example, the parts of the hypophysis develop adjacent to each other in the early neural epithelium. The part destined to be the neurohypophysis is found in the floor of the neural plate separated from the adenohypophysis by the hypothalamus. The adenohypophysis, in the rostral neural fold, will remain as an ectodermal placode after neurulation invaginating later as Rathke's pouch to join the neurohypophysis as it evaginates from the diencephalon. The nasal epithelium also arises from the rostral neural folds along with the special epithelium which will give rise to the olfactory placodes. These will form the sensory neurons of the Ist cranial nerve. Much of the frontonasal portion of the face also arises from the neural folds, which contribute both ectodermal and mesenchymal cells to this area.

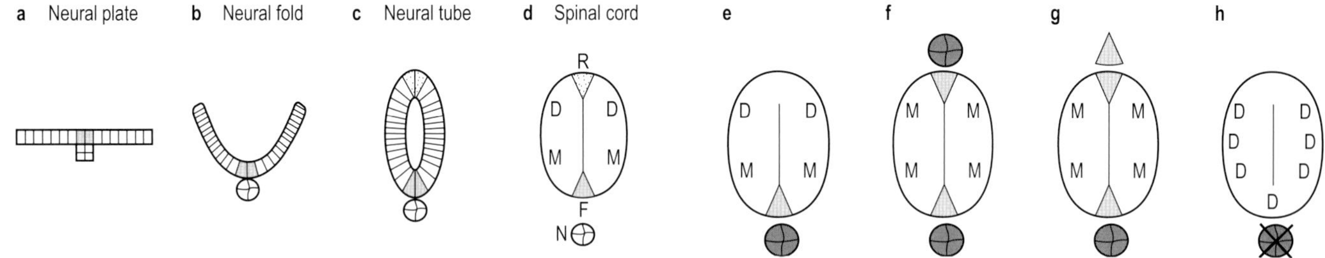

Fig. 4.7 (a–d) Diagrams to show successive stages in the development of the neural tube and spinal cord. (a) The neural plate consists of epithelial cells. Cells at the midline of the neural plate are contacted directly by the notochord. More lateral regions of the neural plate overlie the paraxial mesenchyme (not shown). (b) During neurulation, the neural plate bends at its midline elevating the lateral edges of the plate as the neural folds. Contact between the midline of the neural plate and the notochord is maintained at this stage. (c) The neural tube is formed when the dorsal tips of the neural folds fuse. Cells in the region of fusion form a specialized group of dorsal midline cells, the *roof plate*. (d) Cells at the ventral midline of the neural tube retain proximity to the notochord and differentiate into the *floor plate*. After neural tube closure neuroepithelial cells continue to proliferate and eventually differentiate into defined classes of neurons at different dorsoventral positions within the spinal cord. For example, sensory relay, commissural and other classes of dorsal neurons (D) differentiate near to the roof plate (R), and motor (M) neurons differentiate ventrally near to the floor plate (F), which by this time is no longer in contact with the notochord (N). (e–h) These figures summarize the results obtained from experiments in chick embryos in which a notochord or floor plate is grafted to the dorsal midline of the neural tube and in which the notochord is removed before neural tube closure. (e) The normal condition, showing the ventral location of motor neurons (M) and the dorsal location of sensory relay neurons (D). (f) Dorsal grafts of a notochord result in the induction of a floor plate at the dorsal midline and in the induction of ectopic dorsal motor neurons. (g) Dorsal grafts of a floor plate also result in the induction of a new floor plate at the dorsal midline and in the induction of ectopic dorsal motor neurons. (h) Removal of the notochord results in the elimination of the floor plate and the motor neurons and the expression of dorsal cells types (D) in the ventral region of the spinal cord. (After Jessell & Dodd[6] with permission of WB Saunders.)

DEVELOPMENT OF THE SKULL

The skull has two distinct portions, the *neurocranium* which surrounds the brain and special sense organs, and the *viscerocranium* which includes the lower face and jaws, the palate, hyoid, epiglottis and larynx. The neurocranium is formed from paraxial mesenchyme from the first five somites, the unsegmented paraxial mesenchyme rostral to the first somite, and from neural crest. The viscerocranium is derived exclusively from neural crest mesenchyme.

FORMATION OF SOMITES FROM PARAXIAL MESENCHYME

Paraxial mesenchyme is derived from the early invagination of cells through the primitive node and streak. Cells ingressing through the primitive node form the medial portion of the paraxial mesenchyme, while cells ingressing through the rostral part of the streak form the lateral portion[7]. The paraxial mesenchyme extends rostrally to lie lateral to the notochord. From the lateral sides of the rhombencephalon, caudal to the otic vesicle, the paraxial mesenchyme undergoes segmentation to form the somites. Each somite is formed by the compaction of a cluster of paraxial mesenchymal cells and their transformation into an epithelial cuboid. The cells become polarized with respect to a central lumen, developing cilia on their apical surface. The cells are joined by tight junctions and produce a basal lamina. Processes from the somite cells pass through the basal lamina to contact the basal laminae of the neural tube and notochord. Some cells which do not become part of the epithelial somite remain contained in it, they are termed somitocele cells.

Figure 4.8 summarizes the development of the somites which proceeds in a craniocaudal direction. The cells of the ventromedial wall of the somite undergo an epithelial to mesenchyme transformation and form a proliferating population termed the *sclerotome*. Sclerotomal proliferation fills the spaces between the neural tube and notochord ventrally and also extends dorsally to the midline. Although migration of the sclerotomal cells is often described, it is apparent that proliferation of all cell lines and the general changes in morphology brought about by lateral flexion will result in the sclerotomal cells surrounding the neural tube. Sclerotomal cells and somitocele cells give rise to the bones, joints and ligaments of the vertebral column, the ribs, the local surrounding meninges and some angiogenic mesenchyme. There is a resegmentation of the sclerotomic mesenchyme with the caudal half of one pair of sclerotomes fusing with the cranial half of the pair of sclerotomes below to make a vertebral body initially, then the components of the neural arch and spine later. The spinal nerves preferentially grow through the cranial half of the sclerotomes and the position of the spinal nerves specifies the location of the intervertebral disks.

The remaining cells of the somite are now termed the epithelial plate of the somite or *dermomyotome*. They form a proliferative epithelium which produces skeletal muscle. Proliferation of the dorsomedial, cranial and caudal borders of the dermomyotome give rise to the epaxial myotomes which extend from the cranial to the caudal borders of individual dermomyotomes. The myoblasts remain attached to each end of their original somite and so are finally attached to adjacent vertebrae after sclerotomal resegmentation. The epaxial muscle mass forms the muscles dorsal to the vertebrae, mainly the erector spinae group. Myoblast populations also arise from proliferation of the ventrolateral border of the dermomyotome of specific somites; the occipital somites produce cells which migrate to the tongue and somites opposite the limb buds give rise to limb myoblasts. Both of these origins produce premitotic populations which proliferate as they migrate to their destinations. Finally, the remainder of the dermomyotomes extend into the flank of the body where they fuse to form a premuscular mass which gives rise to the ventrolateral muscles of the body wall, the hypaxial muscles[8].

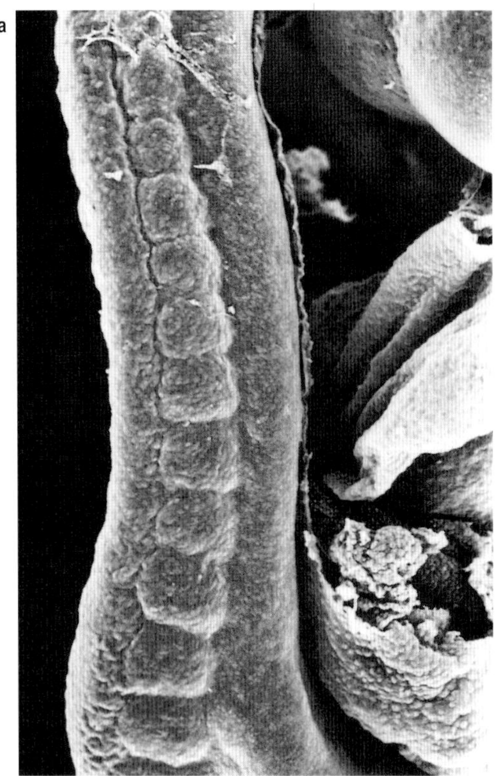

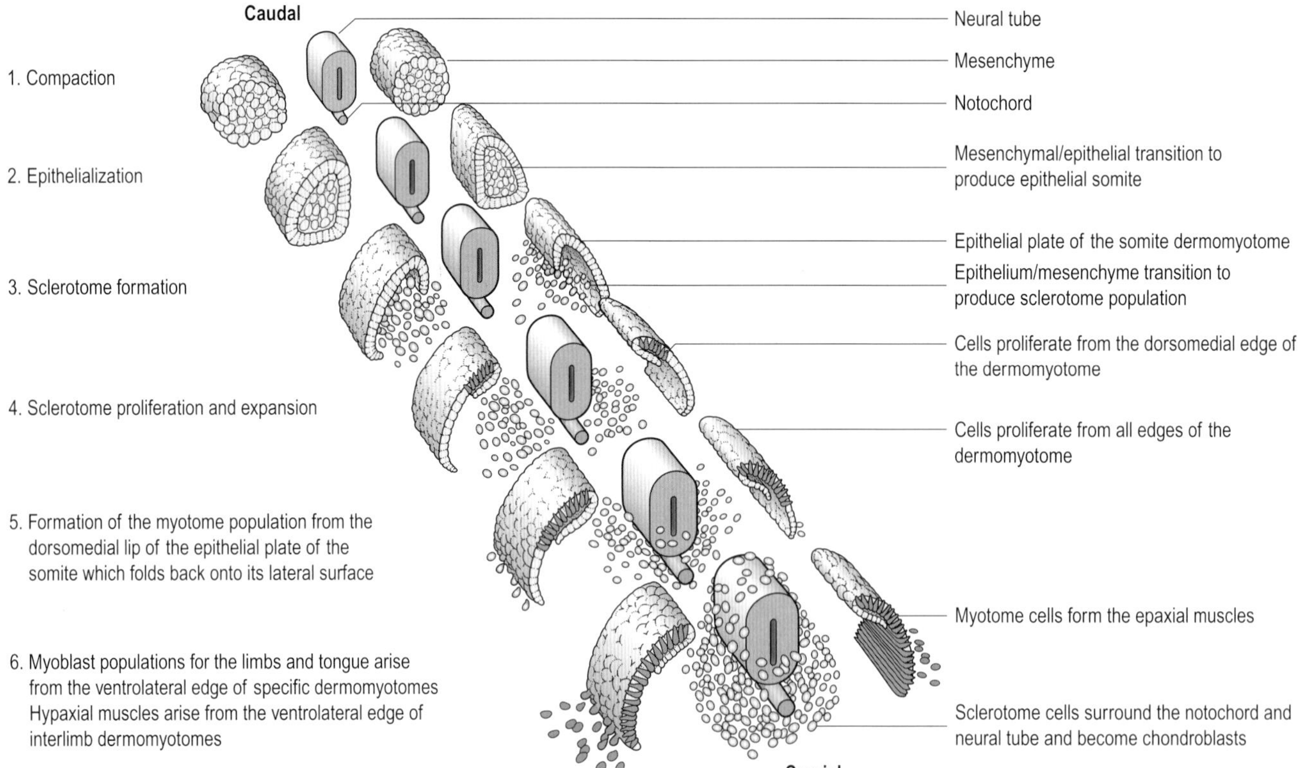

Fig. 4.8 (a) Scanning electron micrograph of a lateral view of an embryo showing the somites. The cranial somites are at the lower border and the more caudal somites are at the upper border. A change in size of the cranially more advanced somites is apparent. (Photograph by P Collins.) (b) The stages of somitogenesis. Development proceeds in a craniocaudal progression. The more cranially placed somites (at the lower right of the figure) are further developed than those caudally placed (at the upper left of the figure). The stages in somitogenesis are given on the left of the figure; more detailed information is given on the right.

The occipitocervical junction is placed at the boundary between somites 4 and 5; this corresponds to occipital somite 4 and cervical somite 1. The paired sclerotomes of occipital somite 4 form the rim of the foramen magnum and the occipital condyles arise from the 1st cervical somite.

Skull base

The basal region of the skull develops from the rostralmost occipital somites and unsegmented paraxial mesenchyme which condenses each side of the notochord and forms most of the clivus. This abuts the hypophyseal cartilage which ossifies to form the postsphenoid part of the sphenoid bone. The region of fusion of these elements corresponds to the spheno-occipital synchondrosis, which is the site of growth up to 20 years of age. Laterally, the otic capsules form the petrous temporal bones and rostrally cartilaginous elements form the nasal capsules and portions of the orbits. The skull base is formed by neural crest rostral to the tip of the notochord.

Skull vault

The skull vault is formed by paired frontal and parietal bones and the squamous parts of the temporal and occipital bones. All of these latter bones develop from membranous ossification via interactions with the meninges. It was thought that all dermal bones derived from neural crest mesenchyme, although evidence now suggests that the frontal and squamous temporal bones, but not the parietal bones, are of neural crest origin. A small line of neural-crest-derived mesenchyme remains between the two parietal bones and contributes to the signaling system that governs growth of the skull vault at the sutures and to the development of the underlying meninges[9]. It should be noted that the conceptual, 'ossification model', which has been the basis of bone and muscle development, i.e. that neural crest is able to produce dermal and endochondral bone whereas mesenchyme populations from paraxial and other early sources form endochondral skeletal elements in the post-otic region, has recently been challenged[10] (see also below).

DEVELOPMENT OF THE PHARYNX

Ventral to the brain and notochord are the foregut and the heart. In the unfolded embryo, the putative foregut region, which includes the prechordal plate, underlies the widest part of the neural plate, the region of the buccopharyngeal membrane, and the surface ectoderm to the rostral edge of the disk. Although head folding is usually described as a movement of the edge of the embryonic disk to a ventral position, the significant proliferation of the neural tissue means that the expansion of the medial (now dorsal) portion of the embryonic disk promotes this morphological change. During this time, the endoderm forms an elongating tube with the proliferating prechordal region at the base.

After head folding, the early foregut is a cul-de-sac with one end open to the midgut and the cranial intestinal portal, and the other closed at the buccopharyngeal membrane. The roof or dorsal wall of the foregut contains the notochordal plate (the notochord proper forms after stage 11), and the floor or ventral wall of the foregut is in close contact with the developing heart, i.e. the angiogenic mesenchyme and celomic epithelium which will form the endocardium, myocardium and pericardial cavity. The caudal portion of the foregut will give rise to the respiratory primordia and the esophagus, while the rostral portion will provide the lining and special glands of the pharynx.

The buccopharyngeal membrane marks the division between the endoderm internally and ectoderm externally. As facial development proceeds, the ectodermal surface of the buccopharyngeal membrane is found at the base of a hollow, the stomodeum. The structures of the face derive from the stomodeal walls and so are covered with epithelia entirely of ectodermal origin. The buccopharyngeal membrane breaks down during stage 12 and subsequent development blurs its original position, which is best thought of as a zone passing from behind the eyes (the adenohypophysis invaginates just in front of the buccopharyngeal membrane) to the posterior part of the anterior two-thirds of the tongue.

With development of the pharyngeal arches (see below), the primitive rostral foregut becomes widened at the putative mouth, narrowing caudally. The foregut is compressed dorsoventrally and there is virtually no lateral wall. Between the arches, the endoderm transiently contacts the overlying ectoderm forming inner and outer depressions where contact is established. Externally, these depressions are termed pharyngeal clefts, internally pharyngeal pouches. The connection remains between the first cleft and pouch, as the tympanic membrane, but more caudal connections are lost. In some cases, the lower pouches develop dorsal and ventral portions with different fates. Thus, the second pouch forms the palatine tonsil, the third pouch forms the thymus ventrally and the parathyroid III dorsally. The fourth pouch forms the parathyroid IV and an ultimobranchial body.

The pharyngeal endoderm is in contact with mesenchyme and epithelia from many sources and may itself be reciprocating in their development. It is intimately involved with neural crest mesenchyme, paraxial mesenchyme – both unsegmented and somitic – lateral plate mesenchyme (of the septum transversum just caudal to the heart) and angiogenic mesenchyme which forms the endocardium and endothelium; it is also associated with notochordal epithelium and cleft ectoderm. The development of the pharyngeal arches is thus likely to involve interactions with all of these sources.

PHARYNGEAL ARCHES

The face, pharynx and larynx develop from mesenchymal and epithelial populations arising from the rostral neural folds and especially from modification of a number of pharyngeal arches which encircle the early foregut. These structures were termed visceral or branchial arches (to note their derivation from gill arches of fish) but are now, in mammalian embryos, most often called pharyngeal arches (Fig. 4.9).

Five pharyngeal arches are seen in mammalian embryos classically numbered I, II, III, IV and VI; there is extensive evidence for not including arch V in the series. Each pharyngeal arch consists of an epithelial covering exteriorly and a mesenchymal core (Fig. 4.10). The epithelium is ectoderm externally and endoderm internally for arches II–VI, and ectoderm entirely for the first arch which is considered atypical. The mesenchyme within each arch arises from specific neural crest

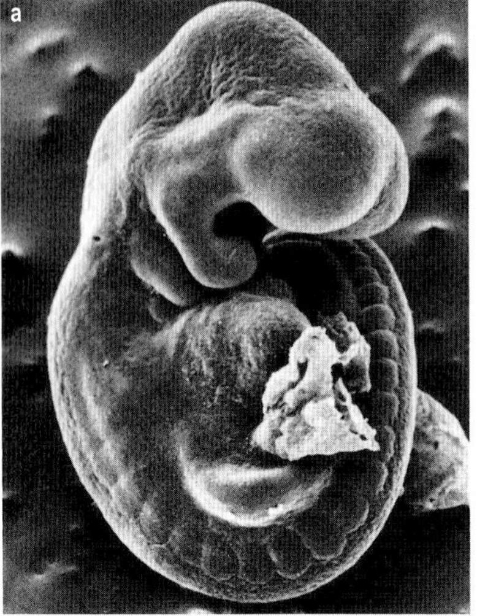

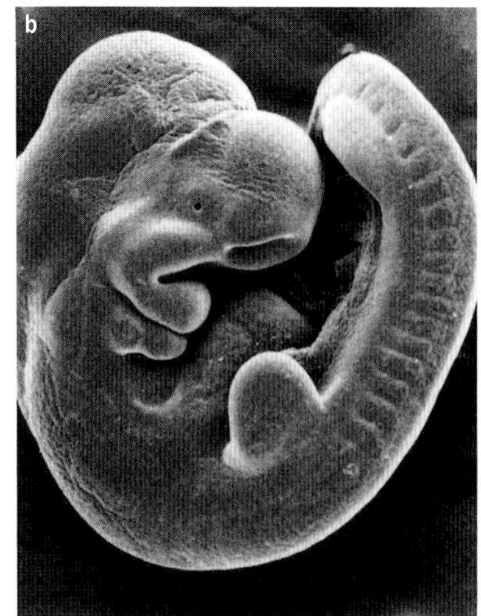

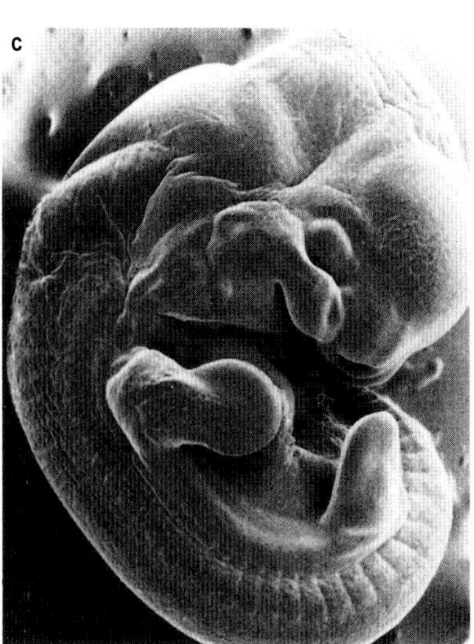

Fig. 4.9 Series of scanning electron micrographs of rat embryos at days 11, 12 and 13: lateral view. (a) Day 11, the pharyngula stage; the otic vesicle is still open but the lens vesicle has yet to invaginate; the first, second and third pharyngeal arches are present; an upper limb bud is present dorsal to the heart. (b) Day 12, the lens vesicle has invaginated but is still open; the maxillary prominence has developed and is beneath the eye; the upper limb is becoming paddle shaped and the lower limb is present. (c) Day 13, the eyelids are beginning to develop; the maxillary prominence is merging with the lateral nasal prominence; both limb buds are well developed. The relative size and number of somites can be seen at each age. (Photographs by P Collins.) (From *Gray's Anatomy*, 39th edn. Edinburgh: Churchill Livingstone, 2005.)

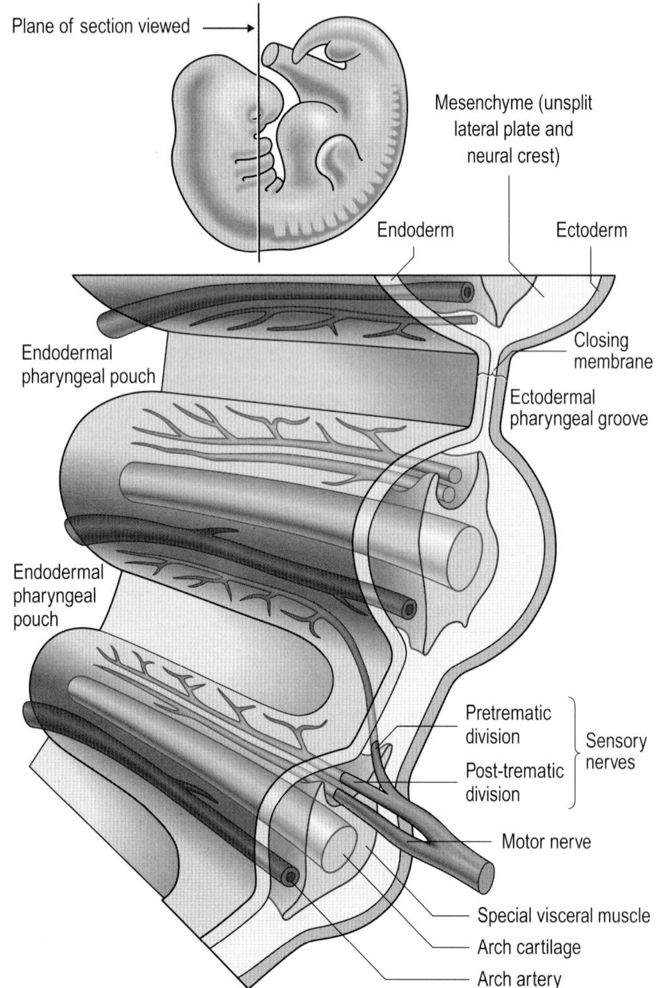

Fig. 4.10 Schema of developing pharyngeal region showing details of generalized pharyngeal constituents, including arches, endodermal pouches and ectodermal grooves. (From *Gray's Anatomy*, 39th edn. Edinburgh: Churchill Livingstone, 2005.)

and paraxial populations. Angiogenic mesenchyme is found throughout the arches especially associated with the endoderm. Motor and sensory cranial nerves are associated with the epithelia and mesenchyme.

Each arch contains:

- specific epithelial structures from ectoderm or endoderm
- skeletal and connective tissue elements from neural crest mesenchyme
- striated muscle from paraxial mesenchyme
- an arch artery from angiogenic mesenchyme
- motor and sensory nerves innervating the arch.

The final topographical arrangement of the tissues within each arch is patterned by Hox gene expression passed from the rhombomeres to the neural crest mesenchyme which migrates to the arches and to the ectoderm.

The developmental pattern of each arch depends on the origin of the neural crest it contains. Neural crest cells migrate from the neural folds of the diencephalon caudally. They do not arise from the prosencephalic folds. The most rostral fold produces epithelium of the nasal cavities, the diencephalic folds give rise to frontonasal mesenchymal populations, while that from the mesencephalic folds, along with the upper rhombomeres, produce mesenchyme for the first arch. Crest cells from rhombomeres 1 and 2 contribute to the first arch mesenchyme, crest cells from rhombomere 4 produce second arch mesenchyme, while crest cells from rhombomere 6 produce third arch mesenchyme. All rhombomeres apart from 3 and 5 contribute migratory neural crest.

The specification of the neural crest, concerning its function within the arches, occurs before it migrates from the neural folds. In grafting experiments, if first arch crest is grafted into the second arch, mandibular structures form suggesting that the differentiation pattern of the second arch surface ectoderm and paraxial mesenchyme is redefined by the new crest mesenchyme[11]. Similar findings are seen in the development of teeth which arise as an interaction between surface ectoderm and crest mesenchyme (see p. 16 and Fig. 2.12).

The axial homeobox genes Hox-a and Hox-b are initially expressed in the rhombomeres then subsequently in the neural crest from the point of origin, during migration and after migration has ceased. Each pharyngeal arch expresses a different combination of Hox genes in the segment restricted manner[12]. Disruption of Hox genes causes failure of neural crest cell proliferation and migration, producing anomalies similar to those seen in human neonates, e.g. DiGeorge's syndrome.

SKELETAL ELEMENTS IN THE PHARYNGEAL ARCHES

The earliest skeletal elements in each arch are cartilage precursors which, in some cases, are replaced by membranous bone. Thus, Meckel's cartilage in the first arch becomes mainly ligamentous or absorbed into the mandible and the second arch cartilage, Reichert's, similarly is reduced for much of its length to a ligament (stylohyoid). The auditory ossicles are initially formed in cartilage but later become ossified. The cartilaginous elements in arches four and six remain as cartilage. That in arch three combines with the second arch and ossifies as the hyoid bone.

Less is known about the origin of the epiglottic cartilage, despite its obvious importance in the functioning of the larynx. The epiglottis arises in the midline ventral to the larynx, in a region termed the hypobranchial eminence. Lateral to the laryngeal inlet are the ventral ends of the sixth arches in which arytenoid swellings appear; these later differentiate into the arytenoid and corniculate cartilages. Together, the arytenoid swellings and the epiglottis reduce the opening into the larynx from a vertical slit to a T-shaped cleft. Later, the cuneiform cartilages differentiate from the epiglottic mesenchyme. It is likely that the epiglottis arises from neural crest mesenchyme, perhaps from fused ventral portions of the sixth arches which later separate from it. However, it has not been established that this is the case.

FACE

The face is formed from the first arch and the frontonasal process which does not contain any cartilage elements. The prosencephalic neural fold produces the frontonasal epithelium and that of the forehead while the most rostral neural fold gives rise to the epithelium of the nasal cavity. The lower portion of the 'C'-shaped first pharyngeal arch containing Meckel's cartilage is termed a mandibular process. Each mandibular process grows first caudally then ventrally to meet and fuse with the process from the other side. (The term 'prominence' is also used to describe these mesenchymal and epithelial structures.) The mandible arises from these merged mesenchymal populations by intramembranous ossification. Rostrally, mesenchyme from the diencephalic neural folds migrates around the olfactory placodes producing surface elevations on each side of the head termed the medial and lateral nasal swellings. The olfactory placodes are originally widely separated and coplanar with the surface ectoderm but, as the nasal swellings develop, they become depressed at the base of olfactory pits. The medial nasal swellings approach each other and extend caudally beyond the lateral nasal swellings. Extensions from the medial swellings into the roof of the stomodeum proliferate to form the premaxillary fields. The upper portion of the first arch, which contains the quadrate cartilage, is termed the maxillary process. Each maxillary process extends beneath the eye in a ventral direction and fuses with the lateral nasal swelling, the two being at first separated by a nasomaxillary groove (naso-optic furrow). The ectoderm between them gives rise to a solid cellular rod, which sinks into the mesenchyme. Its caudal end proliferates to contact the caudal part of the nasal wall, while its cranial end connects with the developing conjunctival sac. The epithelial rod becomes canalized to form the nasolacrimal duct. The epithelium of the upper eyelid and cornea arises from the ectoderm covering the frontonasal process.

The epithelia covering the first, second, third and fourth arches arise from the ectoderm on the lateral side of the head overlying the mesencephalon and rhomebcephalon. The epithelium covering the second arch grows over the caudal arches giving the smooth surface of the neck. Platysma is pulled down with this portion of the arch and thus has superficial fascia both superficial and deep to the muscle.

PALATE

The maxillary processes extend medially during stage 17 (41 days) to produce palatine processes or shelves, which grow towards the midline and downwards, being separated by the developing tongue in the floor of the mouth. At this stage, the tip of the developing tongue is in contact with the cranial surface of the primitive palate, i.e. the stomodeal roof. During stage 23 (56–57 days), the palatine processes rapidly elevate, assuming a horizontal position which allows them to grow towards each other and fuse. The change in position occurs very rapidly caused by matrix changes. Hyaluronic acid is synthesized and accumulates causing swelling and expansion of the mesenchyme, and collagen fibrils are aligned with the mesenchymal cells. The epithelial populations each side of the palatal shelves restrain the swelling. In response to locally released acetylcholine and serotonin, the collagen fibrils and mesenchyme contract causing elevation of the shelves. Other factors also promote palatal elevation. At this time, there is extensive growth in head height rather than head width, there is growth of Meckel's cartilage which allows the tongue to lower into the developing mandible, and also mouth opening, tongue protrusion and hiccup movements have been noted.

The palatal shelves fuse with the premaxilla and with each other from front to back and, at the same time, fuse with the free border of the nasal septum. The mesenchyme within the maxilla, premaxilla and palatal shelves forms bone by intramembranous ossification. Interestingly, the patterning of the neural crest in the palate supports respiratory epithelium (pseudostratified, ciliated columnar epithelium) on the upper, nasal surface and stratified squamous non-keratinizing epithelium on the lower, oral surface.

Generally, male palatal shelf elevation occurs 7 days before females, making congenital cleft palate more likely in female embryos. Such defects may be manifest as cleft lip when a maxillary process and lateral nasal process fail to fuse, or cleft palate if the maxillary processes do not fuse together. More severe conditions result from complete failure of fusion, with facial clefts resulting where the nasolacrimal duct persists as an open furrow. On the other hand, the philtrum (formed from the frontonasal process) may be a separate entity, continuous dorsally with the nasal septum but unattached to the palatine processes; in such cases the floor of the nasal cavity is deficient throughout its extent.

PARAXIAL MESENCHYME IN THE ARCHES – MUSCLES IN THE HEAD AND NECK

The fate of the unsegmented paraxial mesenchyme in the head mirrors that of the somites. The medial mesenchyme forms bony and connective tissue and contributes to elements of the base of the skull, whereas the lateral mesenchyme gives rise to muscle producing the myoblastic lineages which migrate into the pharyngeal arches (see Fig. 4.1). Figure 4.1 shows the developing tissues of the head and neck in register with subdivisions of the paraxial mesenchyme, somitomeres, 4, 6 and 7 supplying the first second and third arches respectively. Studies in the mouse[13] suggests that somitomeres 2 and 3 give rise to the first arch muscle mass which forms the tensor tympani, tensor veli palatini, the masticatory muscles, including mylohyoid and the anterior belly of digastric. Somitomeres 4 and 5 give rise to the second arch muscle mass. The muscles derived from the second arch migrate extensively; stylohyoid, stapedius and the posterior belly of digastric remain attached to the hyoid skeleton, whereas the muscles of facial expression, platysma, the auricular muscles and epicranius all lose connection with it. The paraxial mesenchyme of somitomeres 6 and 7 migrate to the third arch forming stylopharyngeus, and somitomere 7 alone migrates to the fourth arch[13] forming cricothyroid.

The origin of the general musculature of the pharynx, soft palate and larynx has not yet been identified by immunological or chimeric studies. It is thought that myogenic mesenchyme from the third arch migrates into the palate, around the caudal margin of the auditory tube and into the palatopharyngeal arches. However, it is the case that animal studies of the development of this region may not give appropriate information as, in the human, the pharyngeal and laryngeal muscles are developed extensively for vocalization.

Origin of the extraocular muscles

The oculomotor muscles of the eye were described as being derived from 'pre-otic somites', and they are usually indicated close to the developing eye. The pre-otic somites are cavities seen in the developing head which were compared to the somites at their epithelial stage, just after compaction. Although a very early study described the development of oculomotor muscles arising from the prechordal mesenchyme, i.e. that migrating through the primitive streak just ahead of the notochord[14], it was not until chimeric experiments could be performed that this view was confirmed. It has now been demonstrated that the prechordal mesenchyme is displaced laterally at the time of head flexion and that the cells become associated with the more laterally placed paraxial mesenchymal cells[4,15]. Some time later, this mesenchyme migrates and differentiates into the premyoblastic populations for all the extrinsic ocular muscles. In Figure 4.1, the prechordal mesenchyme is indicated with the axial structures and also with the somitomeric mesenchyme which will give rise to the pharyngeal arch musculature. The precursor myoblasts have been grouped with different somitomeres to correspond to the level from which their innervation arises.

INNERVATION OF THE HEAD AND ARCHES

The pharyngeal arches received motor and sensory axons from the cranial nerves. Nerves I, II, VII and VIII are associated with special senses, and there are special sense contributions from IX and X. Nerves III, IV and VI are motor and associated with the eye musculature. The arches are innervated by nerves V, VII, IX and X which supply arches I, II, III and IV respectively; branches of X supply arch VI. In each case the motor nerves are derived from the basal plate of the central nervous system and the sensory nerves from the neural crest cells located in the various somatic ganglia.

Neural crest cells migrate from the mesencephalon and rhombencephalon when 4–10 somites are present, i.e. corresponding to early neurulation[16,17]. These cells provide neural and glial cells for the cranial sensory nerves and for the autonomic ganglia. Throughout the body, four major groups of crest cells have been identified as providing populations for the autonomic system. They are the cranial, vagal, trunk and lumbosacral crest. Within the head region, cranial crest gives rise to the cranial parasympathetic ganglia, whereas vagal crest gives rise to the thoracic parasympathetic ganglia. The vagal crest region also provides neurons and glia for the enteric nervous system.

The ciliary ganglion is formed by crest cells from the caudal third of the mesencephalon and the rostral metencephalon which migrate close to the ophthalmic branch of the trigeminal nerve. The pterygopalatine ganglion arises from pre otic myelencephalic crest and may receive contributions from the ganglia of the trigeminal and facial nerves. The submandibular ganglia and otic ganglia also derive from myelencephalic crest and may have contributions from the facial and glossopharyngeal cranial nerves respectively.

Vagal neural crest from the level of somites 1–7 migrate to the proximal and middle portions of the gut, with sacral neural crest cells supplying the distal gut. It is worth noting that the number of enteric neurons is believed to be of the same magnitude as the number of neurons in the spinal cord[18]. Much fewer preganglionic fibers modulate this system which can mediate its own reflex activity independent of control by the brain and spinal cord. The crest cells destined to become enteric neurons attain their axial value as they leave the neuraxis. If quail crest cells from the trunk are transplanted to the vagal regions of chick hosts they will produce embryos with entirely quail enteric nerves showing that the premigratory neural crest cells are not pre-patterned for specific axial levels. Once these cells reach their destination, they are thought to be regionally patterned by the local splanchnopleuric mesenchyme.

Some neural crest cells arising from a region between the midotic placode and the caudal limit of somite 3 have been termed cardiac neural crest cells. These cells migrate to pharyngeal arches III, IV and VI where they provide support for the embryonic arch arteries and especially contribute to the aorticopulmonary septum and truncus arteriosus.

ANGIOGENIC MESENCHYME IN THE ARCHES

The embryonic aortic arch arteries arise as paired bilateral vessels from a dilated aortic sac (the fused ventral aortae of lower animals), pass laterally around the pharynx within a pharyngeal arch, and join the right or left dorsal aorta as appropriate. As the embryo enlarges, blood flow is directed into a succession of newer and comparatively larger vessels until finally the third, fourth and sixth aortic arch arteries are maintained. Each sixth arch artery is, from its inception, associated with a developing lung bud. When the aorticopulmonary septum divides the truncus arteriosus into pulmonary trunk and ascending aorta, the sixth arch artery retains continuity with the former.

The sixth arch artery, which becomes the ductus arteriosus on the left retains a muscular media and is not elastic like the other arch arteries[19]. Fetal and neonatal ductal tissue produce prostaglandin E_2 (PGE_2), prostaglandin I_2 (PGI_2) and prostaglandin $F_{2\alpha}$ ($PGF_{2\alpha}$) which inhibit the ability of the ductus to contract in response to oxygen. The increased oxygen tension after birth is thus one of the factors involved in ductal closure. Coarctation of the aorta is a condition in which the aorta is constricted just above (preductal) or below (postductal) the entrance of the ductus arteriosus. An abnormal disposition of a smooth muscle media around the aorta at this point could result from an imperfect migration of the cardiac neural crest to establish the usual elastogenic media. The result would be an abnormal constriction of the aorta after birth.

CONNECTIVE TISSUE ELEMENTS IN THE HEAD AND NECK

As previously noted, the neural crest patterns and supports the development of all of the epithelia in the head and neck giving rise to the connective tissue support of the ectodermal and endodermal glands. The ectoderm gives rise to the teeth (see p. 16 and Fig. 2.12), salivary glands and sweat glands, whereas the endoderm with neural crest patterning produces the palatine and pharyngeal tonsils, the thyroid gland, the parathyroid glands and the thymus. In all of the latter cases, the pharyngeal endoderm provides the epithelial cell line which will produce appropriate cytodifferentiation. However, in the absence of neural crest, the endoderm epithelium is not supported or patterned correctly and only limited cytological differentiation of the epithelium occurs. Congenital lack of neural crest, as in DiGeorge's syndrome, is characterized by the absence (or near absence) of the thymus, parathyroids and thyroid glands.

In addition to patterning the development of the glands, interactions between the mesenchyme and surface epithelia persist which continue the maintenance of the differentiated epidermis. Thus, the mucous membrane of the oral cavity differentiates and is maintained as stratified squamous non-keratinizing epithelium, whereas the outer aspect of the face has stratified squamous keratizing epithelium; the special epithelia of the lips delineates the junction between the two.

It is now thought that neural crest mesenchyme also has a role in the development of the attachment points of all pharyngeal arch muscle, regardless of how far that migration may be from the early arches. A 'muscle scaffold model' has been suggested to challenge the 'ossification model' to explain the types of ossification seen especially in the pectoral girdle which, with the disposition and innervation of trapezius and sternocleidomastoid, can be seen to be pharyngeal-arch-derived structures[10]. The neck and shoulder girdle are an interface between spinal nerve innervated trunk muscles, derived from the segementally arranged dermomyotomes, and the cranial nerve innervated pharyngeal arch muscles derived from unsegmented paraxial mesenchyme. Matsuoka et al. (2005) have demonstrated that the connections of the trapezius muscle are formed from post-otic neural crest at the cranial attachment to the nuchal line of the occipital bone proximally and also at the attachment to the scapular spine distally[10]. They noted that the post-otic neural crest generates areas of endochondral ossification in the cervical vertebral column and in the pectoral girdle associated with these distal attachment sites. They view a number of syndromes including, Klippel-Feil disease, Sprengel's deformity, cleidocranial dysplasia and Arnold-Chiari I/II malformation, all of which have pharyngeal/laryngeal, occipital, cervical and shoulder dysmorphologies and co-occurrence of swallowing problems, as defects in the final fate of the post-otic neural crest cells. They note that defects in the fate choices of the neural crest could result in ectopic ossifications of trapezius connective tissue around the neck vertebrae and ectopic ossification of the pre-vertebral ligaments of pharyngeal muscles, and promote this as a reason for Klippel-Feil disease, rather than the previous interpretation of the condition as an aberration of cervical somite segmentation.

EXTERNAL FEATURES OF HEAD DEVELOPMENT

Structures composing the head can be first discerned in embryos of 29 post-fertilizational (p.f.) days[20] (stage 10). Although little is obvious externally, all the development described in this chapter is progressing. Neurulation begins at this stage and 4–12 pairs of somites are present. Facial development begins with the mandibular and hyoid arches becoming visible. However, the proximity of the rostral neural fold, the buccopharyngeal membrane and the heart primordium makes identification of these structures difficult. By 30 p.f. days (stage 11[20]), the neural tube has formed and brain vesicles are present. During this stage, the rostral neuropore will close. The mandibular and hyoid arches are enlarging as neural crest cells stream into them. This increase in mesenchymal population facilitates the invagination of the otic placode which commences.

By 31 p.f. days, three pharyngeal arches can be seen with deepening clefts between them where the surface ectoderm and pharyngeal endoderm are in contact. Dorsal and ventral portions of the arches can be discerned. The otic vesicle has invaginated and only a small opening is now present. The optic vesicle is evaginated from the diencephalon and approaching the surface ectoderm.

During stage 14 (33 p.f. days), the maxillary process can be seen, the lens has invaginated from the surface ectoderm and a small hole may remain on the surface. Stage 15 sees the cerebral evaginations. During stage 16 (37 p.f. days), the mandibular processes fuse across the midline and the maxillary processes meet with the lateral nasal swellings. In stage 17 (40 p.f. days), the medial nasal swellings move closer and extend caudal to the lateral nasal swellings, thus producing the premaxilla. They meet the medially moving maxillary processes during this period. Auricular hillocks can be identified at this stage and their development continues in stage 18 (42 p.f. days) forming the auricular pinna. The eyes are pigmented at this time and the edges of the eyelids can be identified at the edges of the globe. By stage 19 (44 p.f. days), the lower border of arch two has fused with the ectoderm on the cranial aspect of the pericardial region and the neck appears smooth. During stage 20 (47 p.f. days), the pinna is recognizable, the nostrils face anteriorly and the eyelids are covering the edges of the eyes. There is still a significant neck flexion and the mouth is in contact with the pericardial bulge. From this time to stage 23 (56–57 p.f. days), the embryo shows less cervical flexion and the lower border of the mandible gains contact with the pericardial bulge. By this stage, the eyelids have still not yet met and fused.

EVOLUTION OF THE HEAD

It is suggested that the evolution of the head has occurred because of the recruitment, by vertebrates, of a novel mesenchymal population in the head, the neural crest. Creatures such as the cephalocaudate *Amphioxus*, which do not have neural crest, develop via similar mechanisms throughout the cephalic end of their body and along the trunk. The developmental mechanisms which are seen in the vertebrate head are different from those in the trunk. This observation can be used to deduce that the vertebrate head evolved by a different route from the other axial structures, using different cell populations which do not respond to the usual inducers produced in the trunk.

The hypothesis of head evolution put forward by Gans and Northcutt[21] and Northcutt and Gans[22] proposes that the rostral portion of the head, including the sense organs, prosencephalon, mesencephalon and surrounding skull is derived from the neuroectoderm. Certainly, the neuroectoderm gives rise to the sense organs via a series of ectodermal placodes, often situated initially in the edges of the neural plate. This same region also gives rise to a unique migratory mesenchyme population, the neural crest, which forms the 'prechordal' skull, i.e. that part rostral to the notochord[23].

The neural crest in the head appears to fulfil a role similar to that of the somatic and splanchnopleuric mesenchymes within the trunk, i.e. it patterns the adjacent epithelia and intrinsic mesenchymal tissue. It is able to differentiate along a chondrogenic lineage in the head, a fate which cannot occur in the trunk, and can thus contribute to the base plan of the skull, which provides a template for the wide range of vertebrate head shapes, and to the modification of the pharyngeal arches into oral structures. The concept that the neural crest was preprogrammed prior to emigration from the neural tube, and that the specific Hox codes, derived from the rhombencephalon, were taken into the pharyngeal arches supported this notion. More recent studies now support a 'neural crest plasticity and independent gene regulation model'[24]. This suggests that the extracellular environment into which neural crest cells migrate also plays a role in the differentiation pathways the crest cells follow. The notion that neural crest cells are pre-programmed may thus be more limiting than the idea that crest cells have more plasticity and that, as they migrate, their gene expression is regulated, independently, in the different tissues of the head. This latter concept could provide more understanding of the development of diversity of head shape and successful adaptation to the environment seen in vertebrates.

REFERENCES

1. Herbst JJ. Development of suck and swallow. In *Human gastrointestinal development*, E Lebethal (ed.), pp. 229–239. New York: Raven Press, 1989.
2. Selleck MAJ, Stern CD. Commitment of mesoderm cells in Hensen's node of the chick embryo to notochord and somite. *Development* **114**:403–415, 1992.
3. Jessel TM, Bovolenta P, Placzek M, Tessier-Lavigne M, Dodd J. Polarity and patterning the neural tube: the origin and function of the floor plate. In *Cellular basis of morphogenesis CIBA Foundation Symposium 144*, L. Wolpert (ed.), pp. 255–280. Chichester: John Wiley, 1989.
4. Wachtler F, Jacob M. Origin and development of the cranial skeletal muscles. *Bibl Anat* **29**:24–46, 1986.
5. Couly GF, Le Douarin NM. Head morphogenesis in embryonic avian chimeras: evidence for a segmental pattern in the ectoderm corresponding to the neuromeres. *Development* **108**:543–558, 1990.
6. Jessell TM, Dodd J. Floor-plate-derived signals and the control of neural cell pattern in vertebrates. *Harrey Lect* **86**:645–659, 1992.
7. Selleck MAJ, Stern CD. Fate mapping and cell lineage analysis of Hensen's node in the chick embryo. *Development* **112**:615–626, 1991.
8. Christ B, Huang R, Scaal M. Formation and differentiation of the avian sclerotome. *Anat Embryol* **208**:333–350, 2002.
9. Jiang X, Iseki S, Maxson RE, Sucov HM, Morris-Kay GM. Tissue origins and interactions in the mammalian skull vault. *Dev Biol* **241**:106–116, 2002.
10. Matsuoka T, Ahlberg PE, Kessaris N et al. Neural crest origins of the neck and shoulders. *Nature* **436**:347–355, 2005.
11. Noden DM. Interactions and fates of avian craniofacial mesenchyme. *Development* **103**(suppl):121–140, 1988.
12. Hunt P, Gulisano M, Cook M et al. A distinct Hox code for the branchial region of the head. *Nature* **353**:861–864, 1991.
13. Trainor PA, Tan S, Tam PPL. Cranial paraxial mesoderm: regionalisation of cell fate and impact on craniofacial development in mouse embryos. *Development* **120**:2397–2408, 1994.
14. Adelmann HB. The development of the eye muscles in the chick. *J Morphol* **44**:29–87, 1927.
15. Christ B, Jacob M, Jacob HJ, Brand B, Wachtler F. Myogenesis: a problem of cell distribution and cell interactions. In *Somites in developing embryos. NATO ASI Series. Series A: Life Sciences*, R Bellairs, DA Ede, JW Lash (eds), pp. 261–275. New York: Plenum Press, 1986.
16. Nichols DH. Ultrastructure of neural crest formation in the midbrain/rostral hindbrain and preotic hindbrain regions of the mouse embryo. *Am J Anat* **179**:148–154, 1987.
17. Chan WY, Tam PPL. A morphological and experimental study of the mesencephalic neural crest cells in the mouse embryo using wheat germ agglutinin–gold conjugate as the cell marker. *Development* **102**:427–442, 1988.
18. Furness JB, Costa M. Types of nerves in the enteric nervous system. *Neuroscience* **5**:1–20, 1980.
19. Ruiter DJ, Schlingermann RO, Reitveld FJR, de Wall MW. Monoclonal antibody-defined human endothelial antigens as vascular markers. *J Invest Dermatol* **93**:25S–32S, 1989.
20. O'Rahilly R, Müller F. *The embryonic human brain. An atlas of developmental stages*, 2nd edn. New York: Wiley-Liss,, 1999.
21. Gans C, Northcutt RG. Neural crest and the origin of vertebrates: a new head. *Science* **220**:268–274, 1983.
22. Northcutt RG, Gans C. The genesis of neural crest and epidermal placodes: a reinterpretation of vertebrate origins. *Q Rev Biol* **58**:1–28, 1983.
23. Couly GF, Coltey PM, Le Douarin NM. The developmental fate of the cephalic mesoderm in quail–chick chimeras. *Development* **114**:1–15, 1992.
24. Trainor PA, Melton KR, Manzanares M. Origins and plasticity of neural crest cells and their roles in jaw and craniofacial evolution. *Int J Dev Biol* **47**:541–553, 2003.

CHAPTER

5

Development of the heart

Roelof-Jan Oostra and Antoon FM Moorman

KEY POINTS

- The primary heart tube originates from the lateral plate mesoderm of the cardiogenic crescent but contributes to little more than the left ventricle. While the heart tube is elongating and looping, myocardium is still added on both ends, which will contribute to the other cardiac compartments
- The atria and ventricles should not be considered as segments of the primary heart tube. Instead, their primordia result from distension (ballooning) of the outer curvature wall of the heart tube, consisting of fast-conducting, synchronously contracting functional myocardium
- The heart tube functions as a peristaltic pump and consists of primary myocardium which is slow in conduction and contraction but high in automaticity
- The parts of the heart tube flanking the ballooning compartments, i.e. the inflow tract, the atrioventricular canal, the interventricular ring and the outflow tract, as well as the interconnecting heart tube's inner curvature, retain the original primary myocardial characteristics. Later on, they will give rise to the central conduction system of the heart
- In the ballooning but still valve-less heart, the slowly contracting and relaxing primary myocardium of the inflow tract, the atrioventricular canal and the outflow tract act as sphincters that prevent blood regurgitation during alternating atrial and ventricular contractions
- The coronary vessels originate from mesenchymal cells generated by the epicardium which, in contrast to the endocardium and myocardium, has an extracardiac origin. Subsequently, the coronary arteries penetrate the aortic root instead of sprouting from it

INTRODUCTION

In the developing vertebrate organism, the circulatory system is the first functioning organ to appear. In the earliest stages of embryonic development, diffusion from and to surrounding tissues is the only mechanism by which nutrients are distributed. This soon becomes insufficient in the exponentially growing embryo, which raises the need for a proper transportation system for nutrients and waste products. Already in the fourth week of human embryonic development, a closed blood circulation is achieved, driven by a simple but adequate cardiac pump. In the next five weeks, while functioning and responding to the ever increasing demands of the developing embryonic body, it transforms from a single peristaltic pump into a double-circuited, four-chambered, synchronously contracting heart, equipped with septa, valves, a conduction system and its own blood supply. Needless to see that this requires profound and complex remodeling processes which have intrigued and puzzled scientists for decades. Understanding these processes is now coming within reach, thanks to the exponentially growing knowledge with respect to the molecular mechanisms involved in developmental biology. An outline of the state of the art concerning cardiac embryology is presented here.

THE EARLIEST STAGES OF HEART DEVELOPMENT

The heart primordium is formed during the process known as gastrulation, which gives rise to a three-layered embryo. During stage 7 of human embryonic development (16 days post coitum (dpc)), ingression of epiblast cells gives rise to a third embryonic disk layer in between the already formed endoderm layer and the remaining epiblast (which will become the ectoderm). This third layer is the intraembryonic mesoderm. It consists of four component parts, one of which is horseshoe shaped and situated in the anterior part of the embryonic disk: the lateral plate mesoderm. During stage 8 (17–19 dpc), small cavities appear in this arch-shaped band of mesoderm which coalesces to give rise to a structure that is typical to all vertebrates and other chordates: the intraembryonic celom. This space separates the lateral plate mesoderm into two epithelial layers, i.e. one facing the ectoderm (the parietal or somatic mesoderm), and one that is apposed to the endoderm (the visceral or splanchnic mesoderm). The anlage of the heart is formed in the median part of the visceral mesoderm and the intraembryonic celom at this level will become the pericardial cavity. The whole area is known as the cardiogenic crescent (heart-forming region). The extremities of intraembryonic celom form the pleuro-peritoneal ducts (celomic ducts), which connect to the peritoneal cavity.

The first signs of blood vessel formation (vasculogenesis) are seen in the extraembryonic mesoderm of the yolk sac and later on also at various sites in the lateral plate mesoderm of the embryo itself. Mesenchymal cells give rise to vacuolated cords of endothelial cells and, at least in the extraembryonic mesoderm, to islands of blood cells[1]. In recent years, much has become known about the characteristics of these endothelial precursor cells (which in postnatal life play important roles in e.g. tumor development) and their response to various growth factors[2]. Subsequently, these primitive vessels are remodeled to give rise to a mature system of capillaries, arteries and veins, a process known as angiogenesis[3]. In the visceral plate of the cardiogenic crescent, these angioblasts give rise to the endocardial plexus[4]. This plexus, situated in the midline, connects anteriorly (and peripherally) with the central venous system formed in the lateral parts of the embryonic disk and posteriorly (and centrally) with the dorsal aortae that are located on either side of the notochord. In most species, two endothelial tubes form from the endocardial plexus which fuse in the midline to form the primitive endocardial tube, whereas in human embryos, around stage 10 (21–23 dpc), an unpaired endocardial tube seems to be formed directly from the plexus (Steding, personal communications). The endocardial tube is surrounded by a mantle of primary myocardium, another derivative of the visceral mesoderm, which generates a glycosamine-rich extracellular layer in between the endocardial tube and the myocardial mantle. This material is known as cardiac jelly, which at this stage is acellular. Shortly after the primitive heart tube has been formed, the first cardiac contractions can be noticed even before the circulation is completely closed. In spite of what has been assumed for a long time, the initial heart tube that forms from the fusing endocardial plexus only contributes to the formation of little more than the future left ventricle,[5] which means that those parts of the heart tube that contribute to all other cardiac compartments have yet to be formed. Indeed, as development proceeds, cardiac progenitor cells are recruited from the flanking visceral mesoderm, at both the anterior[6–8] and posterior[9,10] ends of the elongating heart tube.

LOOPING OF THE HEART TUBE AND INITIATION OF CHAMBER FORMATION

Two processes, more or less occurring simultaneously, accompany the formation of the primitive heart tube. First, around stage 9 (19–21 dpc), the embryonic disk starts to flex and folds along both its transverse and longitudinal axes, probably in response to the proliferation of neurectoderm. As a result of the thus formed anterior (head) fold, the most anteriorly positioned structures of the embryonic disk, including the developing heart, curve ventrally at an angle of more than 180° and acquire their definite position ventral to the foregut. Secondly, prior to complete coalescence of the cardiac plexus, parts of the heart tube start to bend in different directions from the beginning of stage 10 onward, a process known as cardiac looping. The first loop to appear is found at the coalescence site of the endocardial plexus, i.e. where the left ventricle will develop later on, and locally causes the tube to curve in a dextroventral direction. As elongation of the heart tube proceeds, a second loop occurs in the region of the future atria and the atrioventricular connection, causing this part of the tube to curve in a levodorsal direction. The heart tube thus attains an S-like shape when seen from both its ventral and lateral sides. Subsequently, the first (ventricular) loop bulges over the second (atrial) loop and twists to the right. As a result, the initial left-sided part of the ventricular loop presents in a ventral position, whereas the right side is now positioned dorsally. In the past, several studies have been performed (mostly in chicken embryos) to analyze the extent of extrinsic factors being involved in the process of cardiac looping. Evidently, this process is intrinsically dictated[11–13] but experimental manipulation of the developing embryo during looping may have profound effects on the eventual morphological outcome[14–17]. The loops of the expanding and elongating heart tube protrude into the pericardial cavity, i.e. the heart tube becomes entirely enclosed by the pericardial cavity except for its dorsal-most aspect. Here the heart tube remains connected over its entire length to the dorsal body wall by means of a tissue suspension known as the dorsal mesocardium, which becomes very thin and disappears almost completely, leaving a communication between either side of the pericardial cavity. In the mature heart, this passage is known as the transverse pericardial sinus. Up to the moment of breakthrough, the dorsal mesocardium can be considered as a source of myocardial recruitment, in addition to the anterior and posterior ends of the heart tube. With the anterior end (arterial pole) of the heart tube connected to the aortae and the posterior end (venous pole) to the venous collecting system, the only other connection of the heart tube with the dorsal body wall that remains is situated immediately downstream of the venous pole. This connection, known as the heart stalk or persistent dorsal mesocardium[18] will play an important role in the development of the pulmonary veins.

Compared to the working myocardium of mature hearts, the muscular tissue of the heart tube is much lower in conduction velocity, contractility and sarcoplasmatic reticular activity but its ability for spontaneous depolarization (automaticity) is much higher. In fact, this primary myocardium functionally resembles the myocardium of the mature sinu-atrial and atrioventricular nodes in many aspects. The first signs of pacemaker activity and impulse propagation in the tubular heart are soon to be followed by myocardial contractions and initiation of blood propulsion. Although the first contractions in this primary myocardium are seen in the ventricular loop, dominant pacemaker activity is always and exclusively found at the posterior-most (i.e. inflow) end of the heart tube[19,20]. Since myocardium is still added at both sides of the heart tube during early development, this would imply that pacemaker dominance is constantly shifted posteriorly. Indeed, this seems to be in line with the results of gene expression studies performed in mouse embryos which show that the expression of Nkx 2.5 (a quintessential gene in cardiac development) relegates pacemaker activity to the most recently added cells at the posterior end of the heart tube[21]. These Nkx2.5-negative cells express Hcn4 which is required for pacemaker activity[22]. In the tubular heart, impulse propagation and circular contraction of the primary myocardium follow a peristaltic pattern running from the posterior to the anterior end. Optimal constriction of the tubular lumen required for blood propulsion is achieved by the layer of cardiac jelly in between the endocardium and myocardium. Although the heart at this stage has a single tubular lumen, separate preferential flow patterns have been observed in the early looped heart of chicken embryos by various observers. Thus far, it has remained inconclusive whether these blood streams are of influence on the eventual outcome of cardiogenesis[23].

A direct result of the cardiac looping process is that the looped parts of the heart tube have a convex outer curvature and a concave inner curvature which initially present in a sagittal plane. In the atrial loop this will remain unchanged, whereas in the ventricular loop, due to the local rightward twisting, the curvatures end up in a more or less coronal plane. The first signs of cardiac chamber formation are seen in the ventricular area during stage 11 (24 dpc) Here the outer curvature wall of the heart tube starts to distend to give rise to the ballooning primordia of the left ventricle and, from stage 12 (26 dpc) onward, of the right ventricle (Fig. 5.1). The left and right ventricular primordia are positioned anteroposteriorly along the outer curvature which results in a left-right positioning as a consequence of the rightward twist of the ventricular loop. The ballooning of the atrial primordia, which initiates during stage 12, is comparable to what occurs in the ventricular area, albeit that the atria develop on either side of the outer curvature midline. This difference can be visualized by staining for the expression of genes involved in left-right patterning. Expression of Pitx-2, which is a mediator of left-sided signaling, is confined to the derivatives of the left half of the cardiogenic crescent[24]. These include the complete left atrial primordium and the original left half of both the right and the left ventricular primordia which, after rightward twisting of the ventricular loop, become the ventral side of both ventricles[25]. It should therefore be borne in mind that the designation of 'left' and 'right' ventricle does not refer to the molecular patterning of the left-right body axis, but merely reflects the mutual position of the ventricles after completion of cardiac looping. Since ballooning of compartments occurs only at the outer curvature of the atrial and ventricular loops, the remaining parts of the heart tube retain their original morphology. These are the inflow and outflow tracts at the posterior and anterior ends and the atrioventricular canal in between the atrial and ventricular loops. Notably, the inner curvature and the lumen of the tube, which are not involved in the ballooning of compartments[26], interconnect the non-ballooning parts of the heart. Therefore, the atrial and ventricular primordia are not parts or segments of the heart tube but merely appendages. Molecularly, the development of cardiac chambers is characterized by the initiation of a chamber-specific expression program of genes, including Chisel, atrial natriuretic factor (ANF), connexin 40 and 43 and Irx5[27,28]. In fact, the expression of these genes precedes the visible formation of chamber primordia. The primary myocardium has its own specific set of expressed genes. Two of these are transcription factors called Tbx2 and Tbx3, which are capable of suppressing the expression of chamber-specific genes, thereby maintaining primary myocardial properties[29,30] (Fig. 5.2).

The molecular profile reflects the specific phenotype of chamber myocardium which consists of synchronously contracting muscle fibers that show abundant gap junctions and high-voltaged depolarizations with fast conduction velocities. The initially homogeneous pattern of primary myocardium, with its low-voltaged, slowly propagating discharges, circular contraction and peristaltoid propulsion, will be disrupted with the localized appearance of chamber myocardium. Hemodynamically, the early chambered heart is characterized by the filling and emptying of atria and ventricles in an alternated fashion, thus resembling the situation in the mature heart. However, the persistent presence of the slowly contracting and relaxating primary myocardium at the inflow and outflow ends of the heart tube and at the atrioventricular canal (AVC) is of crucial importance for the blood to be propelled exclusively in an anterior direction since the heart at this stage has neither atrioventricular nor ventriculo-arterial valves. When a pulse generated at the inflow end arrives at the atrial chamber myocardium, contraction will propel the blood through the AVC into the ventricles since the primary myocardium at the inflow end is still contracted, thus preventing regurgitation into the venous system. Similarly, blood is exclusively propelled into the arterial system when the ventricles contract because the primary myocardium of the AVC, activated by the atrial myocardium, is still contracted at that time. The primary myocardium of the outflow tract is still contracted when the ventricles relax, again to prevent regurgitation. In this respect, the remaining tubular parts of primary myocardium act as a set of sphincters to guarantee unidirectional blood propulsion[31]. The sequence of alternating slowly and rapidly impulse propagation in the early chambered heart creates an electrocardiogram which is remarkably reminiscent to that of a mature heart[20] and forecasts the eventual transformation of primary myocardial elements into the mature conduction system.

DEVELOPMENT AND SEPTATION OF THE ATRIA AND INFLOW TRACT

Venous blood enters the heart tube at the posterior or inflow end. The two major vessels that drain here, commonly known as the right and left sinus horns, receive blood from the vitelline, umbilical and common cardinal veins. Their connection with the heart tube is known as the sinu-atrial foramen[32], which implies that they join to form a common draining structure, the sinus venosus. However, as is apparent from expression studies in mouse embryos, both these so-called sinus horns connect separately to the heart tube and remain so throughout cardiac development, without forming a single structure[33]. In fact, with the elongation of the primary heart tube by means of recruiting visceral mesoderm (see above), these draining channels become incorporated and contribute to the formation of the atrial chambers[34]. As soon as ballooning is initiated in human embryonic hearts (stage 12), a slight asymmetry can be noted with respect to the size of the systemic venous conduits, favoring the right- over the left-sided parts. As development proceeds, the opening of the left venous channel gradually shifts towards the right[35]. Eventually, both the right- and the left-sided channels will drain into the right atrium. The area in between these openings is known as the sinus septum[32,36], which appears as the crotch in a pair of trousers when seen from the luminal side[18]. Subsequently, the right venous valve

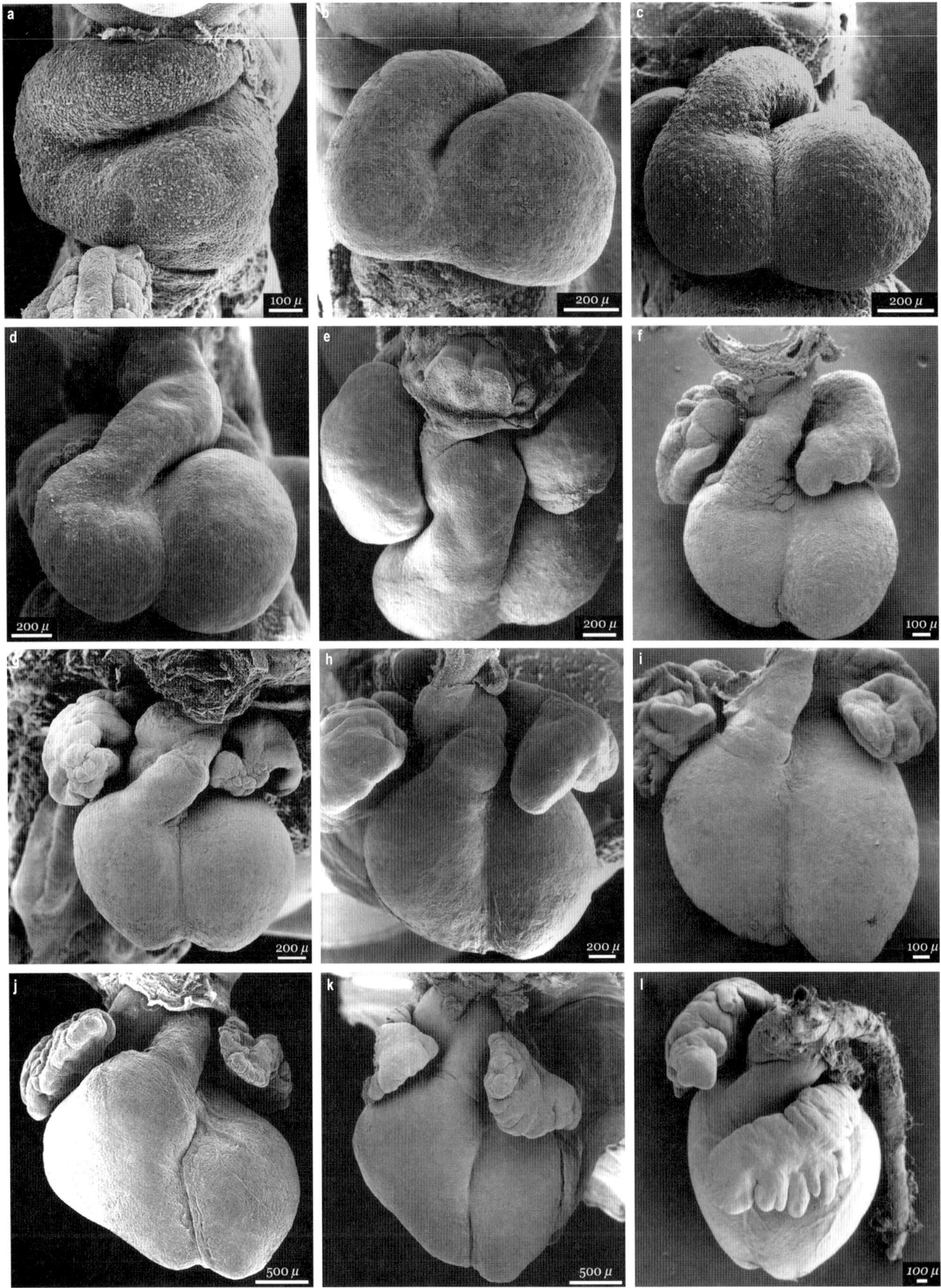

Fig. 5.1 Scanning electron microscopy photographs showing the exterior view of embryonic human hearts in various stages of development. (a) Stage 12 (26 days post coitum (dpc), crown–rump length (CRL): 3–5 mm), (b) stage 13 (28 dpc, CRL: 4–6 mm), (c) stage 14 (32 dpc, CRL: 5–7 mm), (d): stage 15 (33 dpc, CRL: 7–9 mm), (e) stage 16 (37dpc, CRL: 8–11 mm), (f) stage 17 (41 dpc, CRL: 11–14 mm), (g) stage 18 (44 dpc, CRL: 13–17 mm), (h) stage 19 (47 dpc, 16–18 mm), (i) stage 20 (50 dpc, CRL: 18–22 mm), (j) stage 22 (54 dpc, CRL: 23–28 mm), (k) 9 weeks pc (CRL: 25–35 mm), (l) 10 weeks pc (CRL: 35–40 mm). (Reproduced from Oostra et al.[23] with permission of Springer.)

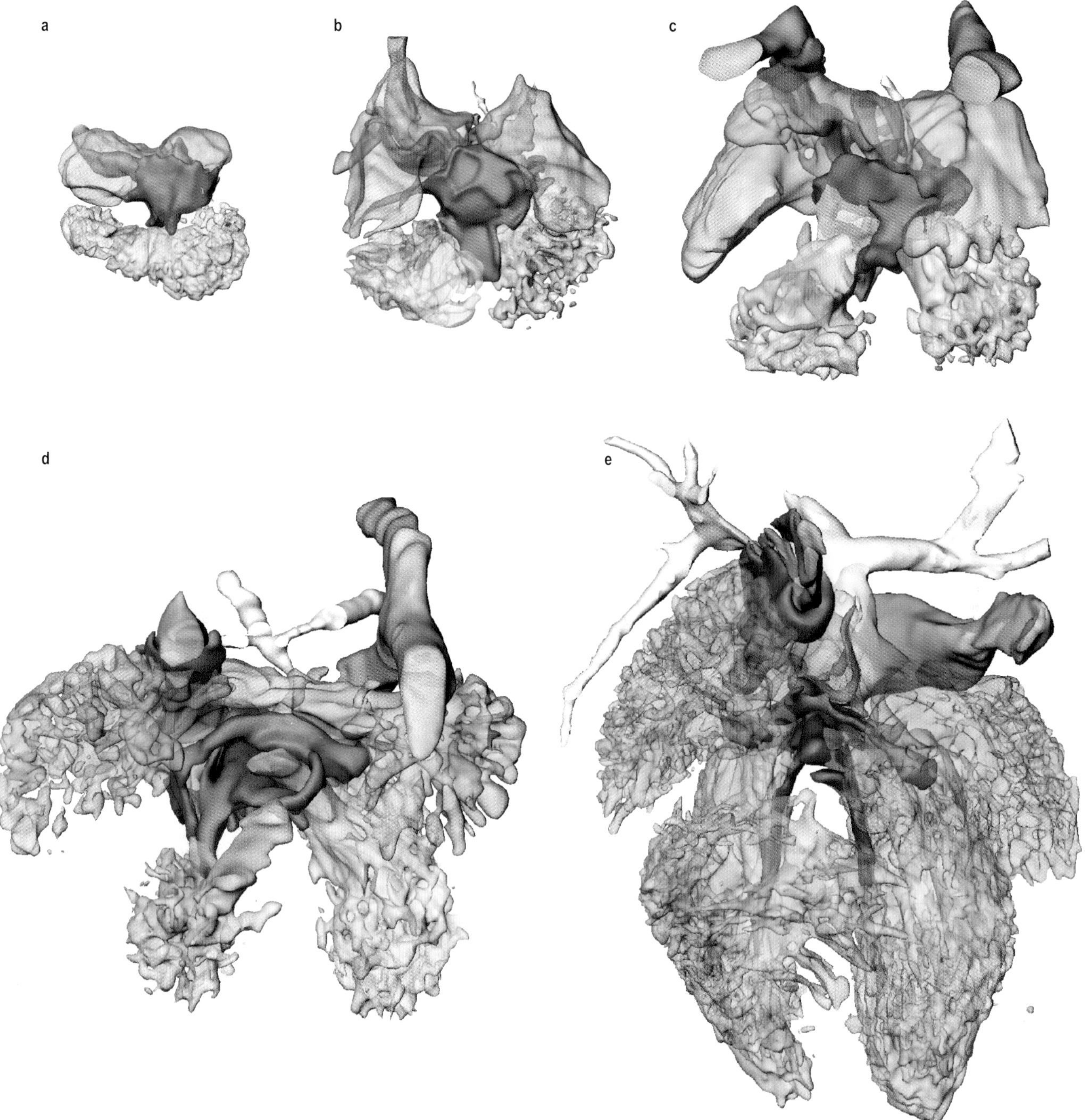

Fig. 5.2 Reconstructions of sectioned embryonic mouse hearts at embryonic day (ED) 9.5 (a), ED 10.5 (b), ED 12.5 (c), ED 14.5 (d) and ED 17.5 (e), ventral view, showing the Tbx3 expression (red) of the primary myocardium and its derivatives. The remaining myocardium has been removed, revealing the lumen. (Reproduced from Hoogaars WM et al. 2004 The transcriptional repressor Tbx3 delineates the developing central conduction system of the heart. *Cardiovasc Res* **62**:489–499, with permission.)

appears, which is an infolding of the right atrial wall at the side of its junction with the venous channels, which will give rise to the Eustachian and Thebesian valves. Later on, a strand of fibrous tissue (the tendon of Todaro) will run from where the valves remain connected towards the endocardial cushions in the atrioventricular canal[37]. The left venous valve, by contrast, is formed from an ingrowing myocardial protrusion[38], the superior edge of which fuses with the edge of the right venous valve to form the spurious septum, flanking the opening of the superior caval vein. Eventually, it will become part of the terminal crest, which separates the pectinated from the smooth-walled parts of the right atrium. The other end of the spurious septum fuses with the primary interatrial septum.

As stated above, the dorsal mesocardium, which initially connects the heart tube over its entire length with the dorsal body wall, disappears almost completely with exception of the area directly anterior to the left and right openings of the system venous tributaries. This persisting dorsal mesocardium is the site where the pulmonary veins will enter the inflow end of the developing heart. From the luminal side, this area appears as a dimple, known as the pulmonary pit[18]. This dimple is surrounded by a horseshoe-shaped myocardial elevation, the legs of which are the right and left pulmonary ridges, whereas the arch is continuous with the primary interatrial septum (see below). Development of the pulmonary veins initiates at stage 12, although it takes to stage 20 (50 dpc) before more than one vein has developed[39]. It was previously considered to involve budding from the atrial wall[40,41], but it appears that these veins canalize from endothelial strands in the midpharyngeal mesenchyme[38,42,43]. Since the primary myocardium surrounding the posterior end of the forming and elongating heart tube, commonly but erroneously known as the sinus venosus, contributes to the formation of the atria (see above), it is no surprise that some investigators consider the myocardium surrounding the pulmonary venous entrance to have the same origin[42]. However, it appears that this myocardium, from its first appearance onward, has a molecular expression profile distinctive of both primary and working myocardium, in that it expresses connexin 40 (which makes it fast-conducting myocardium) but no ANF. Because of this clear molecular distinction, the myocardium surrounding the pulmonary venous entrance, which expands profoundly soon after its first appearance and contributes substantially to the smooth-walled parts of both atria, has been dubbed the dorsal or mediastinal myocardium[33,44]. Therefore, the pulmonary venous entrance should not be considered to originate from the sinus venous, which never exists in mammalian cardiac development[34].

The atrial loop of the primary heart tube, together with its ballooning parts, initially enclose a single cavity with symmetrical systemic venous entrance and midline presentation of the sinus septum and the dorsal mesocardium (see above). This all changes from stage 11 onward, with the systemic venous entrances moving to the right and the dorsal mesocardium to the left. This coincides with the initiation of atrial septation. The primary interatrial septum commences as a myocardial protrusion that appears in the midline of the dorsal cranial wall of the atrial cavity, its dorsal rim being in continuity with the cranial aspect of the pulmonary ridges (see above). While the septum proliferates and approaches the atrioventricular transition, the space that separates the free rim of the septum from the atrioventricular cushions (the primary interatrial foramen) is diminishing steadily until it disappears when the epithelially lined mesenchymal cells that cover both the septal rim and the cushions fuse by the time development enters stage 17 (41 dpc)[37]. It was recently shown that this mesenchyme is entirely endocardially derived except for a molecularly distinct population of cells that are contiguous with the mesenchyme inside the dorsal mesocardium and therefore considered to be of extracardiac origin[45]. During its formation, the primary septum starts to show perforations in its dorsal cranial part that merge to form the secondary interatrial foramen. By the time the primary foramen obliterates, an inward folding of the ventral cranial wall of the atrium appears immediately to the right of the primary interatrial septum. This fold, known as the secondary interatrial septum, eventually covers the secondary foramen, although it takes to stage 21 (52 dpc) before this process becomes clearly distinguishable[46]. The oval foramen, which is the space encircled by the free rim (the limbus) of the secondary septum, is covered by the primary septum, thus presenting as the oval fossa. Prenatally, the oxygenated blood returning from the placenta enters the right atrium through the umbilical and inferior caval veins, crosses the oval foramen, and is shunted to the left side of the heart. From there it mainly enters the aortic arch branches (subclavian and carotid arteries) to comply with the high energy demand of the developing brain. The remainder mixes with blood that returns from the body through the superior caval vein, passes the right side of the heart, the pulmonary trunk and the arterial duct, and enters the descending aorta. After birth, with the pulmonary circulation functional, pressure differences between the right and left atria change and the shunt is closed. This functional closure is usually followed by a fusion of the primary septum with the limbus of the secondary septum within the first two years of life but it remains patent in 25% of the population[47].

As mentioned above, the definitive atria receive contributions from various tissue sources, all having a specific molecular expression pattern[33,44]. These sources include the primary myocardium of the atrial loop and inflow end recruited from the visceral mesoderm, the working myocardium of the ballooning parts, and the dorsal or mediastinal myocardium. A fourth component is the primary myocardium surrounding the atrioventricular canal. The definitive atria consist of smooth-walled parts that are mainly derived from the dorsal myocardium, and the trabeculated auricles which are the remnants of the ballooning parts of working myocardium[33]. In fact, the myocardium of the ballooning parts is initially smooth walled too, until stage 16 (37 dpc) when the typical pectinate muscles or carneous trabeculae start to appear (see Fig. 5.1). The auricles will lose their function in blood propulsion from stage 14 (32 dpc) onward, whereas the differences with respect to their specific morphology[48] start to appear during stage 17[23]. The role of the auricles and their trabeculae in the functioning of the mature heart is unknown. Most of the primary myocardial components of the atria will either disappear or transform into fast-conducting myocardium, with exception of the parts that will give rise to the central conduction system (see below)[30]. This raises the need for electrical isolation of the atria from the ventricles in order to maintain sequential depolarization and contraction. This process starts off during stage 14 with the proliferation of epicardially derived extracardiac mesenchyme in the atrioventricular sulcus, which subsequently becomes enclosed by the bulging lateral ventricular wall[38]. Interruption of the atrioventricular myocardial continuity by fusion of the extracardiac mesenchyme with the endocardial mesenchyme of the atrioventricular cushions commences during stage 20 but is not completed before the end of the 3rd gestational month, the atrioventricular node and bundle being the only remaining sites of electrical permeability[38]. These structures are derivatives of the primary myocardium, i.e. the atrioventricular canal, the interventricular ring (see below) and the interconnecting part of the inner curvature, and have retained the corresponding properties including slow conduction and high automaticity[30,49].

DEVELOPMENT AND SEPTATION OF THE VENTRICLES AND OUTFLOW TRACT

Despite its resemblance with atrial ballooning, formation of the ventricles is different in many ways. Both processes are characterized by expression of a chamber-specific set of genes but, whereas the atria are formed on both sides of the heart tube's outer curvature, the ventricular compartments balloon from the midline of the outer curvature with the right ventricle being formed anteriorly from the left ventricle. This requires extensive remodeling of the whole area downstream of the atria to obtain proper inlet and outlet connections. Moreover, in contrast to the initially smooth-walled ballooning atria (which afterwards become trabeculated), myocardial trabeculation accompanies the ventricular formation from the beginning onward. These trabeculae, which enhance contractility[50] and coordinate intraventricular conduction[31], enable the ventricles to grow without needing a yet to be formed coronary circulation[51]. Tissue proliferation in the outermost layer of the ventricles, which consists of compact myocardium, causes the ventricles to grow[52–54]. Provided that the inner layers and the endocardium do not participate (to the same degree) in the proliferation, one could imagine that the ballooning process[55], perhaps facilitated by the contraction activity[56], causes these layers to tear and perforate. The tissue strands thus formed would become, after recoating with endocardium, the first generation of trabeculae. Continuous repetition of this process would create a radially expanding spongy layer of trabeculated myocardium[57,58]. It has been established recently that the interaction between myocardium and endocardium, leading to the differentiation of trabeculated and compact myocardial layers is controlled by Notch signaling[59]. Meanwhile, the proliferative outer layer, which retains its compaction, is able to expand considerably once a coronary circulation is established, thus exceeding the trabeculated layer in mass contribution by far[60]. Aggregation and compression of the basal trabeculae contributes to the increasing thickness of the compact layer[61] and is more pronounced in the left ventricle. This mechanism seems to be also responsible for the formation of the interventricular septum[62], which is a gradually thickening and rising muscular ridge in between the ventricles. The cause of differences between left and right ventricles concerning their trabeculation patterns[48], which become clearly distinguishable in the early fetal period, is unknown. Although the left ventricle is somewhat larger than the right from their first appearance onward, it is not before stage 17 that the apex of the left ventricle reaches beyond that of the right one (see Fig. 5.1). By that time, the interventricular groove has flattened and the ventricles attain their mature shape, being cylindrical for the left and tetrahedrical for the right.

According to the classical concept, the region of the heart downstream of the atria is considered to consist of four serial segments, these being the atrioventricular canal, the left ventricle, the right ventricle and the outflow tract, which implies that blood coming from the atria would successively pass each of these segments before entering the arterial system. In this model, therefore, the right ventricle would not have a separate inlet other than the left ventricle, nor would the left ventricle have its own outlet except for the right ventricle. Quintessential to this erroneous concept is the assumption that the supposedly formed segments of the heart tube become exclusively committed to the ventricles that balloon from their outer curvature. In fact, however, the heart tube, except for its outer curvature, is not involved in the formation of the ventricles. Instead, its derivatives remain to serve as parallel inlets and outlets of both the right and the left ventricle throughout development. This is most vividly illustrated at the site of the so-called interventricular foramen, which is merely a cross section through the heart tube in between the ballooning ventricles, the outer curvature part of which is the free edge of the interventricular septum. The interventricular foramen therefore hardly qualifies as a foramen but, more importantly, it is not positioned interventricularly. Blood coming from the atrioventricular canal during diastole runs to both ventricles, directly to the left ventricle but, by crossing the interventricular foramen, to the right ventricle. Likewise, during systole the right ventricle empties directly into the outflow tract, but blood from the left ventricle first crosses the interventricular foramen. Hence, the interventricular foramen acts as right ventricular inlet (during diastole) and as left ventricular outlet (during systole), but never during normal cardiac development does blood pass from one ventricle to another through this foramen.

The primary myocardium surrounding the interventricular foramen specifically expresses a gene called GlN2, which makes it a discernable structure, the fate of which can be traced in the course of subsequent development[49,63]. Differential growth patterns cause the atrioventricular canal and the outflow tract to expand preferentially in rightward and leftward directions respectively, thereby facilitating right ventricular inflow and left ventricular outflow. As a result, the upper dorsal third of the tissue ring that encircles the interventricular foramen shifts to the right to enclose the right atrioventricular (tricuspid) orifice, whereas the upper ventral third moves to the left and encloses the left outflow tract (aortic) orifice. The remainder of the tissue ring, being the lower (dorsal and ventral) third, retains its position on top of the interventricular septum and is not involved in any blood passage, either to or from the ventricles. Nevertheless, it is the only part of the ring, and therefore of the foramen, that could rightly be named interventricular, since it has to be closed to prevent blood shunting from one ventricle to the other after birth. The closure of this part of the foramen is one of the goals to achieve during septation of the ventricles and outflow tract (see below). Since the interventricular ring consists of primary myocardium all parts, including those encircling the tricuspid and aortic orifices, initially have corresponding physiological properties and express specific genes, including Tbx3, as has been demonstrated in chicken and mouse embryos[30,49] (see Fig. 5.2). Only the part on top of the dorsal free edge of the interventricular septum will retain these properties throughout development. This is to become the atrioventricular bundle. On each side of the interventricular septum, a sprout becomes apparent from this bundle that ramifies into the septal myocardium. These are the bundle branches, the proximal parts of which initially express Tbx3, whereas the distal parts, and later on (during the fetal period) the proximal parts as well, express chamber-specific genes[30]. In line with this, the myocytes of the bundle branches, especially the distal parts, are fast conducting.

Proper cardiac blood flow patterns do not require septation of compartments, despite what might be assumed. As stated before, separate parallel blood streams are already present in the looping heart tube stages, i.e. long before septation commences. Rather than separating blood flows, the main purpose of cardiac septation is to separate the different hemodynamic pressures between the systemic and pulmonary circulations, which will occur once the fetus is born. Septation of the region downstream of the atria mainly concerns the derivatives of the primary heart tube, i.e. the atrioventricular canal, the interventricular foramen and the outflow tract (Fig. 5.3). Since peristaltic

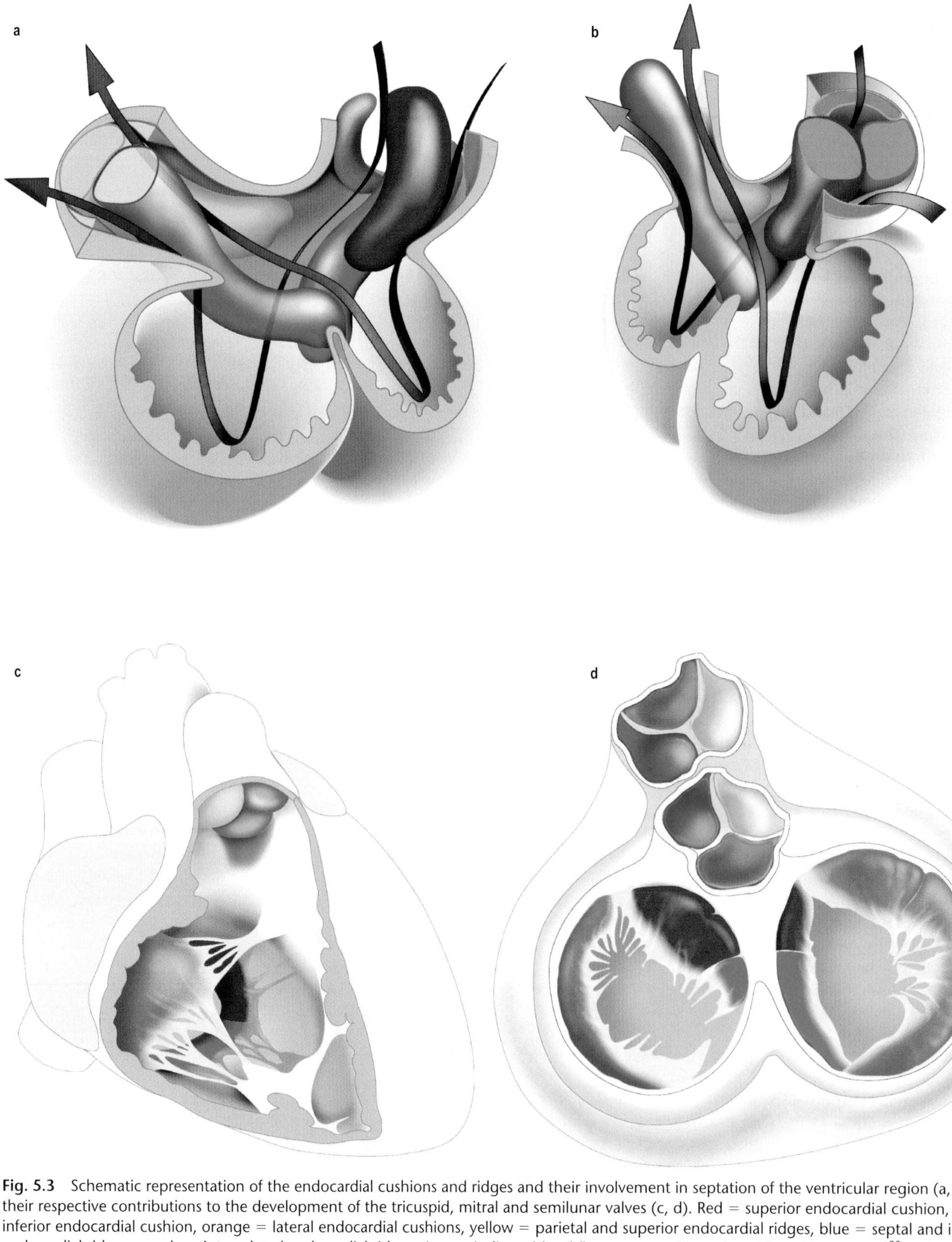

a

b

c

d

Fig. 5.3 Schematic representation of the endocardial cushions and ridges and their involvement in septation of the ventricular region (a, b) and their respective contributions to the development of the tricuspid, mitral and semilunar valves (c, d). Red = superior endocardial cushion, green = inferior endocardial cushion, orange = lateral endocardial cushions, yellow = parietal and superior endocardial ridges, blue = septal and inferior endocardial ridges, purple = intercalated endocardial ridges. Arrows indicate blood flow patterns. Reproduced from Oostra et al.[23] with permission of Springer.)

propulsion of blood is the primordial function of the heart tube, the acellular cardiac jelly is initially regularly deposited in between the myocardial and endocardial layers. At the site of the ballooning compartments, the cardiac jelly disappears whereas it persists and accumulates in two opposing proliferations at the atrioventricular canal and the outflow tract. During subsequent development, these endocardial cushions (in the atrioventricular canal) and ridges (in the outflow tract) become invested with mesenchymal cells originating from the endocardium[64,65] and will mutually fuse to create physically separated right and left blood streams (Figs. 5.3 and 5.4). In the atrioventricular canal, these passages become the tricuspid and mitral orifices at the right and left sides of the fused cushions respectively. Upstream, the endocardial mesenchyme of the fusing cushions is in continuity with the tissue covering the free rim of the primary interatrial septum that encircles the primary foramen (see above). The moment of actual fusion of the atrioventricular cushions is highly variable and takes place somewhere between stage 16 and stage 19 (47 dpc)[23].

Apart from these two cushions (usually dubbed superior and inferior), two other cardiac jelly proliferations are formed in the atrioventricular canal, which flank the tricuspid and mitral orifices at their lateral sides. Both these lateral cushions, which are not involved in septation, as well as the fused superior and inferior cushions start to proliferate at the beginning of stage 18 (44 dpc) and grow over the ventricular walls, including both sides of the interventricular septum, in the direction of the ventricular apex[66]. Concomitantly, confluent spaces appear in the myocardium of the ventricular walls that are covered by the proliferating cushions[67]. The spaces formed by this process of undermining become part of the lumen, thus enhancing the ventricular capacity. As a result, the cushion proliferations, together with the reducing myocardial layer that they cover, form movable leaflets, the free edges of which form the tendineous chordae that remain connected with the future papillary musculature. The septal leaflets of both valves are thus formed from the fused superior and inferior cushions while the mural leaflets originate from the lateral cushions. The central part of the septal leaflet of the mitral valve is formed slightly differently, in that it is flanked by the aortic outlet and therefore has no myocardial layer[66]. The forming leaflets appear not to receive any contribution from the extracardiac mesenchyme[38,68,69]. Eventually, the myocardial layer of the leaflets will disappear although it will take up to the early fetal period before this process is completed[66,68]. Therefore, the definitive leaflets are entirely endocardially derived[69] (see Fig. 5.3).

To a certain extent, the septation process in the atrioventricular canal is comparable to what will happen in the outflow tract, which connects the ventricles with the aortic sac and its derivatives. From stage 13 (28 dpc) onward, a proximal and a distal part can be appreciated with a clearly distinguishable bend in between. In both parts, two opposing cardiac jelly proliferations appear, being the parietal (or right) and septal (or left) ridges in the proximal part and the superior and inferior ridges in the distal part. The ridges are named after the position of their most proximal ends, with the parietal and superior ridges being in line with each other as well as the septal and inferior ridges, but they both have a clockwise spiraling course which, in total, covers about 180 degrees. Both sets of ridges fuse in distal to proximal direction, starting with the ridges in the distal part (see Fig. 5.4). The timing of these processes is quite variable and ranges from stage 15 (33 dpc) to stage 20[23]. Formation and fusion of the ridges can be noticed from the exterior aspect from stage 15 onward with the appearance of a spiraling longitudinal flattening that disrupts the regular contour of the outflow tract. Distally, the superior and inferior ridges connect respectively with the ventral and dorsal legs of the aorticopulmonary septum in the aortic sac, which separates the systemic parts of the pharyngeal arch arteries from the pulmonary parts. The formation of this septum is supposed to be achieved by ingrowth of migrating neural crest cells[8]. The externally visible bend in the outflow tract is where the two sets of fused ridges meet each other and give rise to the facing cusps and sinuses of the semilunar valves of the aorta and pulmonary trunk[57,70–72]. At this level, two additional cardiac jelly proliferations (the intercalated ridges) appear in a plane perpendicular to that of the fused ridges, which will form the non-facing cusps and sinuses. For a long time, the coronary arteries have been considered to sprout from the two facing sinuses of the aortic valve by means of angiogenesis. However, this assumption is in contradiction with two important observations. First of all, coronary vessels are already developing before the coronary orifices have formed[73]. Secondly, vessel formation by angiogenesis cannot initiate from non-capillary vessels. This implies that coronary arteries must penetrate the aortic sinuses rather than originate from them[74]. In fact, vasculogenesis causes angioblasts to be formed from pluripotent mesenchymal cells in the subepicardial space which, in turn, create a capillary network (angiogenesis) that invades the myocardium and finally penetrate the aortic sinuses by means of apoptosis[75]. The mesenchymal cells in the subepicardial space are derived from the overlying epicardium[76] which, in contrast to the myocardium and endocardium, has an extracardiac origin. It is generated by the pro-epicardial organ, a mesenchymal cell mass originating from the mesothelium at the transition of the inflow end of the heart tube and the transverse septum during the looping stages[77], and subsequently creates a covering of the myocardial surface[78].

Since myocardium is still added at both ends of the primary heart tube during the looping stages (see above) it takes, in human embryos, probably up to stage 13 before the myocardium of the outflow tract, being the anterior most part of the heart tube, is completely recruited from the pharyngeal mesenchyme[72]. In line with this, experiments in mice and chicken embryos have shown that myocardium in the anterior parts of the looping heart tube, initially appearing as (proximal) outflow tract, eventually end up in the wall and infundibulum of the right ventricle[79–82]. At the end of the looping stages the myocardium in the distal part of the outflow tract starts to disappear which, in human embryos, is visible form stage 15 onward, and proceeds in proximal direction (see Fig. 5.1). In chicken embryos, this already occurs before the outflow tract has reached its maximum length, with the non-myocardial component being derived from pharyngeal mesoderm and neural crest cells[82]. Subsequently, the myocardial component, concerning the proximal part of the outflow tract, regresses progressively, while the non-myocardial or distal part increases. In chicken embryos, this does not result from transdifferentation or apoptosis but from migration of myocardial cells in the direction of the right ventricle[82]. The fused superior and inferior ridges in the distal, non-myocardial segment of the outflow tract create the lumina that, after apoptosis-mediated separation[83,84], will form the intrapericardial parts of the aorta

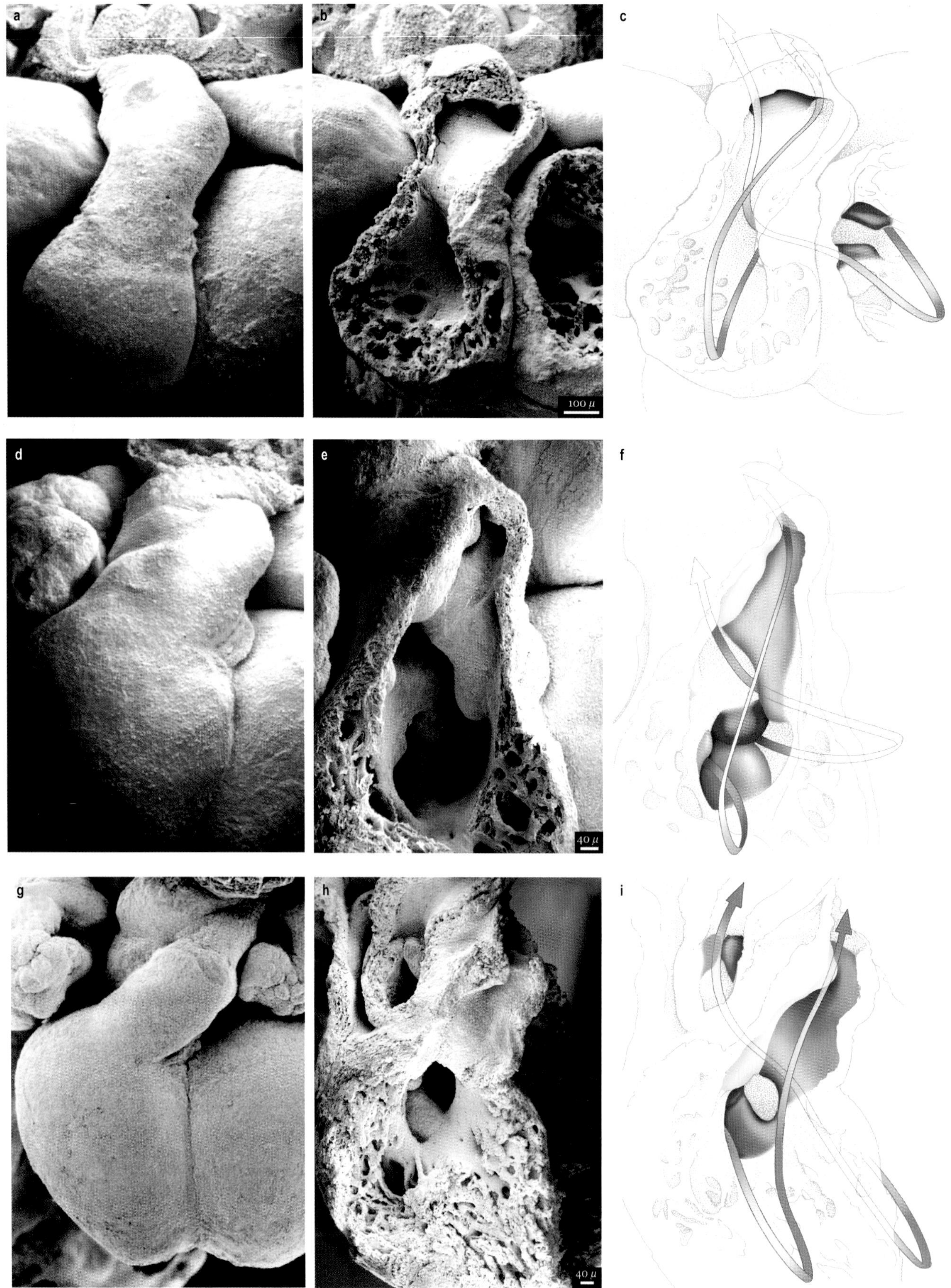

Fig. 5.4 Scanning electron microscopy photographs showing the exterior and interior views of the ventricular region of embryonic human hearts in stage 15 (a, b, c), stage 17 (d, e, f) and stage 18 (g, h, i). See Fig. 5.3 for color coding. Arrows indicate blood flow patterns. (Reproduced from Oostra et al.[23] with permission of Springer.)

and pulmonary trunk. The initially spiraling course of the outflow tract ridges seems to cause the twisting of the aorta and pulmonary trunk[57,72], although it remains elusive as to what extent rotation of the outflow tract myocardium[85] is involved in this process. The ridges in the proximal part of the outflow tract, which mainly contributes to the infundibuli of the aorta and pulmonary trunk, play a crucial role in the physical septation of the right and left ventricular blood streams (see Fig. 5.4). Initially, fusion of these ridges will not be completed up to their proximal extremities for this would leave the right ventricle deprived of an inlet. Instead the septal ridge will grow in the direction of the atrioventricular canal thereby approaching the interventricular foramen from its ventral side. Arriving at the free edge of the interventricular septum, it meets the inferior atrioventricular cushion that is approaching from the dorsal side. The superior cushion will not contact the free rim of the interventricular septum but, instead, encircles the dorsal side of the interventricular foramen. When seen from the left ventricular lumen, the fused cushions are dome shaped and form the roof of the left ventricular outlet. Later on, it will give rise to the aortic leaflet of the mitral valve (see above). By now, a more or less triangular space remains bordered by the inferior atrioventricular cushions and the non-fused parts of the outflow tract ridges. This space, which is the floor of the left ventricular outlet and a potential communication with the right ventricular inlet, is the remainder of the interventricular foramen. Closure is achieved at the end of the embryonic period and completes the septation process. In contrast to the already fused parts of the proximal outflow tract ridges, which subsequently become muscularized[68,86], this area remains void of myocytes and can be recognized in the mature heart as the membranous interventricular and atrioventricular septum.

REFERENCES

1. Noden DM. Embryonic origins and assembly of blood vessels. *Am Rev Respir Dis* **140**:1097–1103, 1989.
2. Ribatti D. The discovery of endothelial progenitor cells: an historical review. *Leuk Res* [Epub ahead of print] 2006.
3. Poole TJ, Coffin JD. Vasculogenesis and angiogenesis: two distinct morphogenetic mechanisms establish embryonic vascular pattern. *J Exp Zool* **251**:224–231, 1989.
4. Viragh S, Szabo E, Challice CE. Formation of the primitive myo- and endocardial tubes in the chicken embryo. *J Mol Cell Cardiol* **21**:123–137, 1989.
5. Buckingham M, Meilhac S, Zaffran S. Building the mammalian heart from two sources of myocardial cells. *Nat Rev Genet* **6**:826–835, 2005.
6. Kelly RG, Brown NA, Buckingham ME. The arterial pole of the mouse heart forms from Fgf10-expressing cells in pharyngeal mesoderm. *Dev Cell* **1**:435–440, 2001.
7. Mjaatvedt CH, Nakaoka T, Moreno-Rodriguez R et al. The outflow tract of the heart is recruited from a novel heart-forming field. *Dev Biol* **238**:97–109, 2001.
8. Waldo KL, Kumiski DH, Wallis KT et al. Conotruncal myocardium arises from a secondary heart field. *Development* **128**:3179–3188, 2001.
9. Van den Hoff MJ, Kruithof BP, Moorman AF. Making more heart muscle. *Bioessays* **26**:248–261, 2004.
10. Christoffels VM, Mommersteeg MT, Trowe MO et al. Formation of the venous pole of the heart from an Nkx2-5-negative precursor population requires Tbx18. *Circ Res* **98**:1555–1563, 2006.
11. Manasek FJ, Monroe RG. Early cardiac morphogenesis is independent of function. *Dev Biol* **27**:584–588, 1972.
12. Manning A, McLachlan JC. Looping of chick embryo hearts in vitro. *J Anat* **168**:257–263, 1990.
13. De la Cruz MV, Sanchez-Gomes C. Straight heart tube. Primitive cardiac cavities vs. primitive cardiac segments. In *Living Morphogenesis of the Heart*, MV De la Cruz, RR Markwald (eds), pp. 85–98. Boston: Birkhäuser, 1999.
14. Männer J, Seidl W, Steding G. Correlation between the embryonic head flexures and cardiac development: an experimental study in chick embryos. *Anat Embryol* **188**:269–285, 1993.
15. Kosaki K, Mendoza A, Jones KL. Cervical flexion: its contribution to normal and abnormal cardiac morphogenesis. *Teratology* **54**:135–144, 1996.
16. Hogers B, De Ruiter MC, Gittenberger-de Groot AC, Poelmann RE. Unilateral vein ligation alters intracardiac blood flow patterns and morphogenesis in the chick embryo. *Circ Res* **80**:473–481, 1997.
17. Hogers B, De Ruiter M, Gittenberger-de Groot AC, Poelmann RE. Extraembryonic venous obstructions lead to cardiovascular malformations and can be embryolethal. *Cardiovasc Res* **41**:87–99, 1999.
18. Webb S, Brown NA, Wessels A, Anderson RH. Development of the murine pulmonary vein and its relationship to the embryonic venous sinus. *Anat Rec* **250**:325–334, 1998.
19. Patten BM. Initiation and early changes in the character of the heartbeat in vertebrate embryos. *Physiol Rev* **29**:31–47, 1949.
20. Van Mierop LHS. Localization of pacemaker in chick embryo heart at the time of initiation of heartbeat. *Am J Physiol* **212**:407–415, 1967.
21. Mommersteeg MT, Hoogaars WM, Prall OW et al. Molecular pathway for the localized formation of the sinoatrial node. *Circ Res* **100**:354–362, 2007.
22. Stieber J, Herrmann S, Feil S et al. The hyperpolarization-activated channel HCN4 is required for the generation of pacemaker action potentials in the embryonic heart. *Proc Natl Acad Sci USA* **100**:15235–15240, 2003.
23. Oostra RJ, Steding G, Lamers WH, Moorman AFM. *Steding's and Virágh's scanning electron microscopy atlas of the developing human heart*. New York: Springer, 2007.
24. Ryan AK, Blumberg B, Rodriguez-Esteban C et al. Pitx2 determines left-right asymmetry of internal organs in vertebrates. *Nature* **394**:545–551, 1998.
25. Campione M, Ros MA, Icardo JM et al. Pitx2 expression defines a left cardiac lineage of cells: evidence for atrial and ventricular molecular isomerism in the iv/iv mice. *Dev Biol* **231**:252–264, 2001.
26. Moorman AF, Christoffels VM. Cardiac chamber formation: development, genes, and evolution. *Physiol Rev* **83**:1223–1267, 2003.
27. Moorman AF, Schumacher CA, de Boer PA et al. Presence of functional sarcoplasmic reticulum in the developing heart and its confinement to chamber myocardium. *Dev Biol* **223**:279–290, 2000.
28. Christoffels VM, Habets PE, Franco D et al. Chamber formation and morphogenesis in the developing mammalian heart. *Dev Biol* **223**:266–278, 2000.
29. Christoffels VM, Hoogaars WM, Tessari A, Clout DE, Moorman AF, Campione M. T-box transcription factor Tbx2 represses differentiation and formation of the cardiac chambers. *Dev Dyn* **229**:763–770, 2004.
30. Hoogaars WM, Tessari A, Moorman AF et al. The transcriptional repressor Tbx3 delineates the developing central conduction system of the heart. *Cardiovasc Res* **62**:489–499, 2004.
31. De Jong F, Opthof T, Wilde AA et al. Persisting zones of slow impulse conduction in developing chicken hearts. *Circ Res* **71**:240–250, 1992.
32. Steding G, Xu JW, Seidl W, Manner J, Xia H. Developmental aspects of the sinus valves and the sinus venosus septum of

the right atrium in human embryos. *Anat Embryol (Berl)* **181**:469–475, 1990.
33. Soufan AT, van den Hoff MJ, Ruijter JM et al. Reconstruction of the patterns of gene expression in the developing mouse heart reveals an architectural arrangement that facilitates the understanding of atrial malformations and arrhythmias. *Circ Res* **95**:1207–1215, 2004.
34. Anderson RH, Brown NA, Moorman AF. Development and structures of the venous pole of the heart. *Dev Dyn* **235**:2–9, 2006.
35. Knauth A, McCarthy KP, Webb S et al. Interatrial communication through the mouth of the coronary sinus. *Cardiol Young* **12**:364–372, 2002.
36. Vernall DG. The human embryonic heart in the seventh week. *Am J Anat* **111**:17–24, 1962.
37. Webb S, Brown NA, Anderson RH. Formation of the atrioventricular septal structures in the normal mouse. *Circ Res* **82**:645–656, 1998.
38. Wessels A, Markman MW, Vermeulen JL, Anderson RH, Moorman AF, Lamers WH. The development of the atrioventricular junction in the human heart. *Circ Res* **78**:110–117, 1996.
39. Bliss DF, Hutchins GM. The dorsal mesocardium and development of the pulmonary veins in human embryos. *Am J Cardiovasc Pathol* **5**:55–67, 1994.
40. Neill CA. Development of the pulmonary veins. *Pediatrics* **18**:880–887, 1956.
41. Los JA. De embryonale ontwikkeling van de venae pulmonales en de sinus coronarius bij de mens. Thesis. Leiden: University of Leiden, p. 131, 1958.
42. De Ruiter MC, Gittenberger-de Groot AC, Wenink AC, Poelmann RE, Mentink MM. In normal development pulmonary veins are connected to the sinus venosus segment in the left atrium. *Anat Rec* **243**:84–92, 1995.
43. Blom NA, Gittenberger-de Groot AC, Jongeneel TH, DeRuiter MC, Poelmann RE, Ottenkamp J. Normal development of the pulmonary veins in human embryos and formulation of a morphogenetic concept for sinus venosus defects. *Am J Cardiol* **87**:305–309, 2001.
44. Franco D, Campione M, Kelly R et al. Multiple transcriptional domains, with distinct left and right components, in the atrial chambers of the developing heart. *Circ Res* **87**:984–991, 2000.
45. Mommersteeg MT, Soufan AT, de Lange FJ et al. Two distinct pools of mesenchyme contribute to the development of the atrial septum. *Circ Res* **99**:351–353, 2006.
46. Anderson RH, Brown NA, Webb S. Development and structure of the atrial septum. *Heart* **88**:104–110, 2002.
47. Hagen PT, Scholz DG, Edwards WD. Incidence and size of patent foramen ovale during the first 10 decades of life: an autopsy study of 965 normal hearts. *Mayo Clin Proc* **59**:17–20, 1984.
48. Anderson RH, Becker RA. *Cardiac anatomy: an integrated text and colour atlas*. London: Gower Medical Publishing, Churchill Livingstone, 1980.
49. Moorman AF, de Jong F, Denyn MM, Lamers WH. Development of the cardiac conduction system. *Circ Res* **82**:629–644, 1998.
50. Challice CE, Viragh S. The architectural development of the early mammalian heart. *Tissue Cell* **6**:447–462, 1973.
51. Van Mierop LHS, Kutsche LM. Comparative anatomy and embryology of the ventricles and arterial pole of the vertebrate heart. In *Congenital heart disease: causes and processes*, JJ Nora, A Takao (eds), pp. 459–479. New York: Futura, 1984.
52. Rumyantsev PP. Interrelations of the proliferation and differentiation processes during cardiac myogenesis and regeneration. *Int Rev Cytol* **51**:186–273, 1977.
53. Thompson RP, Kanai T, Germroth PG et al. Organization and function of early specialized myocardium. In *Developmental mechanisms of heart disease*, EB Clark, RR Markwald, A Takao (eds), pp. 269–279. Armonk: Futura Publishing Co Inc, 1995.
54. Henderson DJ, Copp AJ. Versican expression is associated with chamber specification, septation, and valvulogenesis in the developing mouse heart. *Circ Res* **83**:523–532, 1998.
55. Sedmera D, Pexieder T, Vuillemin M, Thompson RP, Anderson RH. Developmental patterning of the myocardium. *Anat Rec* **258**:319–337, 2000.
56. Thompson RP, Soles-Rosenthal P, Cheng G. Origin and fate of cardiac conduction tissue. In *Fifth International Symposium on Etiology and Morphogenesis of Congenital Heart Disease*, EB Clark, A Takao (eds). New York: Futura, 2000.
57. Steding G, Seidl W. Contribution to the development of the heart. Part 1: normal development. *Thorac Cardiovasc Surg* **28**:386–409, 1980.
58. Mikawa T, Borisov A, Brown AM, Fischman DA. Clonal analysis of cardiac morphogenesis in the chicken embryo using a replication-defective retrovirus: I. Formation of the ventricular myocardium. *Dev Dyn* **193**:11–23, 1992.
59. Grego-Bessa J, Luna-Zurita L, del Monte G et al. Notch signaling is essential for ventricular chamber development. *Dev Cell* **12**:415–429, 2007.
60. Blausen BE, Johannes RS, Hutchins GM. Computer-based reconstructions of the cardiac ventricles of human embryos. *Am J Cardiovasc Pathol* **3**:37–43, 1990.
61. Rychterova V. Principle of growth in thickness of the heart ventricular wall in the chick embryo. *Folia Morphol Praha* **19**:262–272, 1971.
62. Harh JY, Paul MH. Experimental cardiac morphogenesis. I. Development of the ventricular septum in the chick. *J Embryol Exp Morphol* **33**:13–28, 1975.
63. Wessels A, Vermeulen JL, Verbeek FJ et al. Spatial distribution of 'tissue-specific' antigens in the developing human heart and skeletal muscle. III. An immunohistochemical analysis of the distribution of the neural tissue antigen G1N2 in the embryonic heart; implications for the development of the atrioventricular conduction system. *Anat Rec* **232**:97–111, 1992.
64. Markwald RR, Fitzharris TP, Adams-Smith WN. Structural analysis of endocardial cytodifferentiation. *Dev Biol* **42**:160–180, 1975.
65. Markwald RR, Fitzharris TP, Manasek FJ. Structural development of endocardial cushions. *Amer J Anat* **148**:85–120, 1977.
66. Oosthoek PW, Wenink AC, Vrolijk BC et al. Development of the atrioventricular valve tension apparatus in the human heart. *Anat Embryol (Berl)* **198**:317–329, 1998.
67. Van Mierop LHS, Alley RD, Kausel HW, Stranahan A. The anatomy and embryology of endocardial cushion defects. *J Thorac Cardiovasc Surg* **43**:71–83, 1962.
68. Lamers WH, Viragh S, Wessels A, Moorman AF, Anderson RH. Formation of the tricuspid valve in the human heart. *Circulation* **91**:111–121, 1995.
69. De Lange FJ, Moorman AF, Anderson RH et al. Lineage and morphogenetic analysis of the cardiac valves. *Circ Res* **95**:645–654, 2004.
70. Ya J, Van Den Hoff MJB, De Boer PAJ, Tesink-Taekema Franco D, Moorman AFM, Lamers WH. Normal development of the outflow tract in the rat. *Circ Res* **82**:464–472, 1998.
71. Qayyum SR, Webb S, Anderson RH, Verbeek FJ, Brown NA, Richardson MK. Septation and valvar formation in the outflow tract of the embryonic chick heart. *Anat Rec* **264**:273–283, 2001.
72. Webb S, Qayyum SR, Anderson RH, Lamers WH, Richardson MK. Septation and separation within the outflow tract of the developing heart. *J Anat* **202**:327–342, 2003.
73. Bogers AJJC, Gittenberger-de Groot AC, Dubbeldam JA, Huysmans HA. The inadequacy of existing theories on development of the proximal coronary arteries and their connexions with the arterial trunks. *Int J Cardiol* **20**:117–123, 1988.
74. Waldo KL, Willner W, Kirby ML. Origin of the proximal coronary artery stems and a review of ventricular vascularization in the chick embryo. *Am J Anat* **188**:109–120, 1990.
75. Bernanke DH, Velkey JM. Development of the coronary blood supply: changing concepts and current ideas. *Anat Rec* **269**:198–208, 2002.
76. Perez-Pomares JM, Macias D, Garcia-Garrido L, Munoz-Chapuli R.

Contribution of the primitive epicardium to the subepicardial mesenchyme in hamster and chick embryos. *Dev Dyn* **210**:96–105, 1997.

77. Viragh S, Gittenberger-de Groot AC, Poelman RE, Kalman F. Early development of the quail heart epicardium and associated vascular and glandular structures. *Anat Embryol* **188**:381–393, 1993.
78. Männer J, Perez-Pomares JM, Macias D, Munoz-Chapuli R. The origin, formation and developmental significance of the epicardium: a review. *Cells Tissues Organs* **169**:89–103, 2001.
79. Cai CL, Liang X, Shi Y et al. Isl1 identifies a cardiac progenitor population that proliferates prior to differentiation and contributes a majority of cells to the heart. *Dev Cell* **5**:877–889, 2003.
80. Meilhac SM, Esner M, Kelly RG, Nicolas JF, Buckingham ME. The clonal origin of myocardial cells in different regions of the embryonic mouse heart. *Dev Cell* **6**:685–698, 2004.
81. Verzi MP, McCulley DJ, De VS, Dodou E, Black BL. The right ventricle, outflow tract, and ventricular septum comprise a restricted expression domain within the secondary/anterior heart field. *Dev Biol* **287**:134–145, 2005.
82. Rana MS, Horsten NC, Tesink-Taekema S, Lamers WH, Moorman AF, van den Hoff MJ. Trabeculated right ventricular free wall in the chicken heart forms by ventricularization of the myocardium initially forming the outflow tract. *Circ Res* **100**:1000–1007, 2007.
83. Watanabe M, Choudry A, Berlan M et al. Developmental remodeling and shortening of the cardiac outflow tract involves programmed cell death. *Development* **125**:3809–3820, 1998.
84. Schaefer KS, Doughman YQ, Fisher SA, Watanabe M. Dynamic patterns of apoptosis in the developing chicken heart. *Dev Dyn* **229**:489–499, 2004.
85. Bajolle F, Zaffran S, Kelly RG et al. Rotation of the myocardial wall of the outflow tract is implicated in the normal positioning of the great arteries. *Circ Res* **98**:421–428, 2006.
86. Van Den Hoff MJB, Moorman AFM, Ruijter JM et al. Myocardialisation of the cardiac outflow tract. *Dev Biol* **212**:477–490, 1999.

SECTION 2

The placenta

6 The immunology of implantation 63
Ashley Moffett and YW Loke

7 Development of the placenta and its circulation 69
Caroline Dunk, Berthold Huppertz and John Kingdom

8 Placental function in maternofetal exchange 97
Thomas Jansson and Theresa L Powell

9 Maternofetal trafficking 110
Diana W Bianchi

CHAPTER 6

The immunology of implantation

Ashley Moffett and YW Loke

KEY POINTS

- The extravillous pathway of trophoblast differentiation is essential for the development of the fetoplacental blood supply
- Extravillous trophoblast cells express a unique array of human leukocyte antigen (HLA) class I molecules, HLA-G, HLA-E and HLA-C
- The main population of maternal immune cells in the decidua during placentation are uterine natural killer (NK) cells
- Interaction between receptors on maternal NK cells and their HLA ligands on fetal trophoblast cells may regulate the depth and extent of vascular modification by trophoblast

INTRODUCTION

The traditional way to study pregnancy immunology follows the classical transplantation model, which views the fetus as an allograft. A more recent approach focuses on the unique, local uterine immune response to the implanting placenta. This approach requires knowledge of implantation and placental structure, as this impacts greatly on the type of immune response produced by the mother. At the implantation site, cells from the mother and the fetus intermingle during pregnancy. Unravelling what happens here is crucial to our understanding of why some human pregnancies are successful while others are not.

NIDATION

The initial event in implantation is achieved by contact and adhesion between the embryonic trophectoderm of the blastocyst and the uterine surface epithelium[1]. The polarity of the surface epithelial cells is essential as it is the apical surface that will interact with the apical surface of the trophectoderm. Because material from this early phase of the process is not readily available for study in humans, the mechanisms involved are still not clearly understood. The apical surface of the epithelium is generally considered to be repellent to cellular attachment most of the time and only becomes receptive at a specific period under the appropriate hormonal stimulus. This period of receptivity or 'implantation window' is estimated to last approximately 6–10 days after the luteinizing hormone (LH) surge in humans. The stage of embryonic development must also coincide with this 'window' for implantation to occur. The small number of successful pregnancies achieved by in vitro fertilization (IVF) relative to the high rate of successful fertilization could be due to failure to synchronize the state of development of the blastocyst with this 'implantation window'.

Blastocysts will attach readily to uterine stromal cells at all times of the menstrual cycle indicating that the surface epithelium is responsible for the tight window of receptivity. There have been many attempts to identify the structural or phenotypic features of these epithelial cells which may characterize the period of the 'window'[2]. Ultrastructural changes, such as loss of microvilli, alteration of tight junctions and modification of the glycocalyx have been reported. Characteristic structures known as 'pinopods', which are visualized by scanning electron microscopy of the uterine epithelium, have been described to correlate with the time of implantation[3]. Production of the mucin-type secretory glycoprotein, MUC-1, is observed to increase markedly in the secretory phase of the cycle at the apical epithelial surface. Since similar glycosaminoglycans can facilitate attachment and spreading of mouse blastocysts in vitro, this glycoprotein could play an important role in human implantation. Initial blastocyst attachment results in loss of MUC-1 from subjacent cells allowing subsequent high affinity interactions of adhesion molecules between epithelial cells and trophectoderm. The embryo can mediate its own attachment by secretion of proteins such as human chorionic gonadotrophin (hCG) or pregnancy-specific glycoproteins (PSG). Additional adhesion molecules include the integrin subunits, CD9, trophinin and osteopontin. Soon after the initial attachment to the apical surface, the spaces between the surface epithelial cells alter as the trophoblast insinuates itself to move to the stroma beneath[2].

TROPHOBLAST POPULATIONS

At the time when the blastocyst adheres to the epithelial lining of the uterine mucosa, it is surrounded by a layer of cells derived from the trophectoderm. As the blastocyst penetrates through the surface epithelium into the uterine mucosa, this layer differentiates into an outer multinucleated syncytiotrophoblast (primitive syncytium) and an inner layer of primitive mononuclear cytotrophoblast. Lacunae soon appear in the syncytium and these rapidly enlarge by fusing with each other. The uteroplacental circulation is potentially established when this lacuna system erodes through the uterine capillaries. The intervillous space of the definitive placenta is a derivation of these lacunae.

The subsequent differentiation of trophoblast occurs along two main pathways – villous and extravillous (Fig. 6.1). Villous trophoblast is in contact with maternal blood and its main functions are transport of nutrients and oxygen to the fetus and secretion of hormones and other proteins. Extravillous trophoblast is involved in the establishment of the placental blood supply and these are the trophoblast cells that directly contact maternal uterine tissues[4]. At the tips of some chorionic villi, cytotrophoblast cells proliferate into solid masses of tissue known as cytotrophoblast columns that anchor these villi to the underlying decidua. From these columns individual trophoblast cells break off to invade the decidua. These interstitial trophoblast cells appear to move towards the decidual spiral arteries, encircling these vessel s which then show endothelial swelling and a characteristic 'fibrinoid' destruction of the smooth muscle of the media. How trophoblast cells induce these changes in the vessel wall is presently unknown. When the trophoblast cells reach the decidual–myometrial junction, many of them become multinucleated and are now known as placental bed giant cells. These can be regarded as the endpoint of the extravillous pathway of trophoblast differentiation.

Cytotrophoblast cells from the cell columns that lie over the openings of the decidual spiral arteries form a plug of cells that are known as endovascular trophoblast. Early in gestation, these plugs appear partially to occlude the lumen of the vessels[5]. These plugs limit the influx of blood into the intervillous space in the first trimester so that there is only a seepage of serum into the intervillous space. This means that the embryo in the first trimester exists in a low oxygen environment. From these plugs, trophoblast cells extend in a retrograde manner along the inner wall of the blood vessel rather like 'wax dripping down a candle', replacing the endothelial lining. Eventually, trophoblast cells become incorporated into the fibrinoid material of the vessel wall, both from endovascular trophoblast invading outwards through the wall and from interstitial trophoblast coming in from the decidua outside.

Transformation of the spiral arteries by trophoblast is crucial to successful implantation because these changes convert the arteries from muscular vessels into flaccid sacs capable of transmitting the increased blood flow required for the developing fetoplacental unit. Failure of this arterial transformation will result in reduced conductance and poor perfusion of the placenta, which will affect the growth and development of the villous tree. This in turn will lead to clinical conditions such as miscarriage, stillbirth, unexplained intrauterine growth retardation (IUGR) and pre-eclampsia (Fig. 6.2)[6].

DECIDUALIZATION

The uterine endometrial mucosa is transformed into decidua during pregnancy[7]. Morphologically, the most obvious changes are seen in the stromal cells which become rounded and glycogen-rich. There is also infiltration by large numbers of bone-marrow-derived cells. These changes begin during the luteal phase of the menstrual cycle (pre-decidual change) but, if pregnancy occurs, the decidualization process continues. This is unlike the situation in most other species where decidualization only begins at implantation. Decidualization is under the control of sex hormones, estrogen and progesterone and sequential expression of their receptors is seen in the menstrual cycle. Both glandular and stromal cells of the endometrium

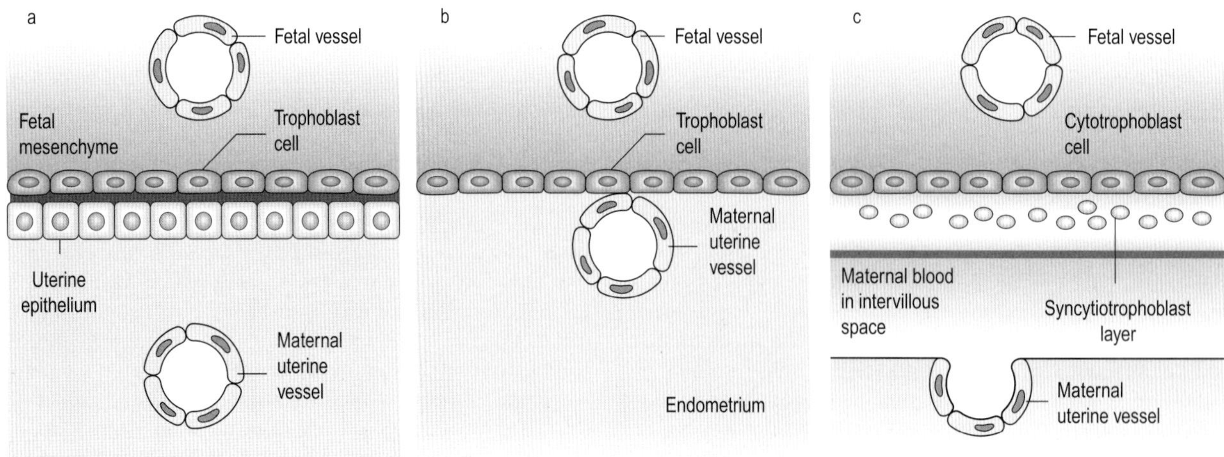

Fig. 6.1 Villous and extravillous pathways of trophoblast differentiation. (From Loke and King, *Human Implantation: Cell Biology and Immunology*, Cambridge University Press.)

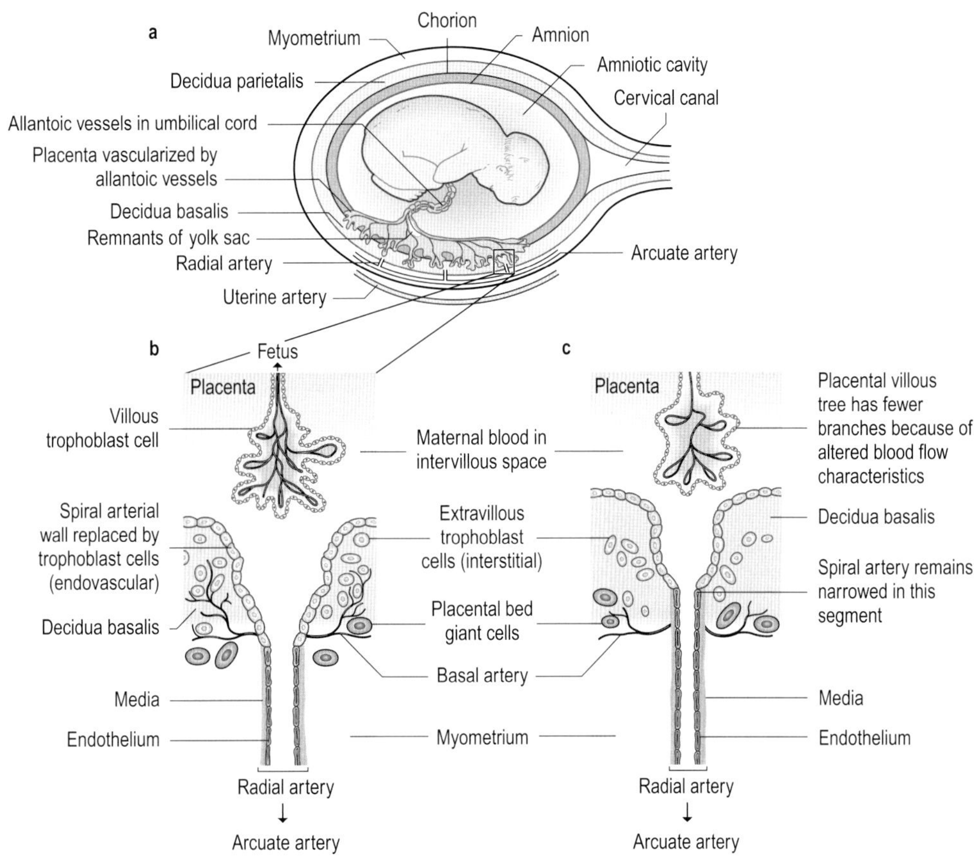

Fig. 6.2 Disorders of human pregnancy resulting from abnormal placentation. (a) The blood supply to the human pregnant uterus is shown. (b) Normal pregnancy. The spiral arteries of the placental bed are converted to uteroplacental arteries by the action of migratory extravillous trophoblast cells. Both the arterial media and the endothelium are disrupted by trophoblast cells, converting the artery into a wide caliber vessel that can deliver blood to the intervillous space at low pressure. The small basal arteries are not involved and remain as nutritive vessels to the inner myometrium and decidua basalis. (c) Pre-eclampsia and fetal growth restriction. When trophoblast cell invasion is inadequate, there is deficient transformation of the spiral arteries. The disturbed pattern of blood flow leads to reduced growth of the branches of the placentalvillous tree, which results in poor fetal growth.

increasingly express estrogen receptors and progesterone receptors until the time of ovulation and expression then declines in the glands. Meanwhile, in the stroma, expression of progesterone receptors continues throughout the secretory phase and in early decidua. Prolonged exposure to progesterone results in large, rounded cells that secrete high levels of prolactin and insulin growth-factor binding protein-1 (IGFBP-1). Other changes include secretion of interleukin-15 (IL-15), metalloproteinases and chemokines and the laying down of a peri-cellular rim of matrix proteins, particularly fibronectin.

Regarding the function of decidua, popular opinion favors the view that it facilitates implantation by providing an appropriate substrate for trophoblast migration and a fertile soil for nourishment of the developing fetus throughout gestation. However, it is also possible that decidua provides a restraining influence against over-invasion by trophoblast[6]. This view is in accord with observations that, in situations where decidualization is inadequate, such as in ectopic pregnancies or implantation over a previous cesarean section scar tissue, trophoblast invasion is unrestrained. It is likely that decidua provides a balance allowing migration of trophoblast but only to a certain depth. Thus, mammalian reproduction may be considered as a parental tug-of-war between the requirements of the fetus to derive as much nourishment as possible from the mother, and the defense of the mother to reduce this nutritional burden for the sake of her own health and for future pregnancies.

TROPHOBLAST INTERACTION WITH EXTRACELLULAR MATRIX

Cell migration is dependent on the expression of adhesion molecules which bind to matrix proteins in the extracellular environment. For example, the physiological migration of epithelial cells in wound healing and the pathological invasion of cancer cells require cell–matrix interaction. Trophoblast migration into decidua appears to utilize a similar mechanism. There are four families of adhesion molecules, of which the most important for adhesion to the extracellular matrix (ECM) is the family of integrins. These are transmembrane glycoproteins consisting of non-covalently associated α and β subunits. Different α and β subunits exist and the way they combine determines the ligand specificity of the integrin. For example, the heterodimers $\alpha1\beta1$ and $\alpha6\beta4$ are receptors for the ECM protein, laminin, while $\alpha5\beta1$, $\alpha4\beta1$ and $\alpha4\beta7$ bind fibronectin.

Using monoclonal antibodies specific for various subunits, the pattern of expression of integrins by different trophoblast populations at the implantation site is now well documented. The $\alpha6\beta4$ integrin is seen on the layer of villous cytotrophoblast cells and continues to be expressed by those cytotrophoblast cells of the cell columns nearest the villous core. This integrin disappears further out in the cell columns to be replaced by the heterodimers $\alpha5\beta1$ that continue to be expressed by the interstitial trophoblast invading into decidua. Thus, there appears to be a downregulation of the $\alpha6\beta4$ laminin receptor with a concomitant upregulation of the $\alpha5\beta1$ fibronectin receptor as trophoblast invades the decidua. This observation is very similar to that seen during the healing of a skin wound where the sessile keratinocytes that form the normal epidermis express $\alpha6\beta4$ while those keratinocytes which migrate over to close the wound express $\alpha5\beta1$. Binding of trophoblast to fibronectin seems to be of particular importance and can result in signaling through integrins to the trophoblast cell with changes in gene expression that will affect trophoblast function[1]. In pre-eclampsia, trophoblast fails to downregulate $\beta4$ and to upregulate $\alpha1$ subunits as seen in normal pregnancy, indicating that disregulation of these integrins could be responsible for the inadequate trophoblast invasion of decidua associated with this pathological condition. What factors determine this switch from one integrin to another, however, are not known.

MATRIX DEGRADATION BY TROPHOBLAST

Besides adhesion to ECM proteins via integrins, cellular migration also requires degradation of the matrix. This process involves the production of proteolytic enzymes by the migrating cell[8]. The two main groups of enzymes are members of the plasminogen activator (PA) system of serine proteases and the family of matrix metalloproteinases (MMP). The MMP family is divided into three main classes based on their substrate specificities: the collagenases, the gelatinases and the stromelysins. There is an intricate interaction between the PA and MMP systems, and together they can break down the major components of ECM. The activity of these proteases is subjected to close control by specific inhibitors. There are two inhibitors for PA (PAI) designated as PAI-1 and PAI-2, and two tissue inhibitors for MMP (TIMP) designated as TIMP-1 and TIMP-2.

Trophoblast cells possess proteolytic activity which can be demonstrated in vitro by their digestion of the surrounding matrix on which the cells are seeded. Zymogram studies have shown that trophoblast cells produce a wide array of proteases, this production being greater in first-trimester trophoblast compared to trophoblast later in gestation which, therefore, mirrors the invasive capacity of early trophoblast. These observations have led to the conclusion that PA, MMP, PAI and TIMP together provide an intricate network that controls matrix degradation during trophoblast invasion.

ENDOVASCULAR TROPHOBLAST MIGRATION

Endovascular trophoblast cells move down the spiral artery against the flow of blood and become incorporated into the vessel wall replacing the endothelial cells. This process has parallels with emigration of leukocytes during inflammation and it is not surprising that members of the selectin family may be involved[9]. Endovascular trophoblast cells also express high levels of CD56 – otherwise known as NCAM. NCAM forms homotypic interactions and these may be important in formation of the loose plug of trophoblast cells in the first trimester. Secretion of angiogenic factors such as Vascular Endothelial growth factor-C (VEGF-C) and Angiopoietin2 (Ang2) that may influence the maternal arteries directly is also a feature of these cells.

TROPHOBLAST EXPRESSION OF MAJOR HISTOCOMPATIBILITY COMPLEX (MHC) ANTIGENS

Major histocompatibility complex (MHC) class I and class II antigens serve as important recognition molecules for immune cells. In humans, these antigens are also known as human leukocyte antigens (HLA). HLA class I antigens are expressed on nearly all nucleated cells and class II antigens on specialized cells involved in antigen presentation such as dendritic cells, macrophages and B cells. Both HLA class I and class II antigens are highly polymorphic and incompatibility for these antigens between donor and recipient is the basis of graft rejection.

None of the trophoblast cell populations described above express HLA class II antigens and villous trophoblast is also negative for HLA class I. However, extravillous trophoblast cells that invade decidua and interact with uterine tissues do express an unusual and unique array of HLA class I antigens. Presently, there are six HLA class I loci that code for an expressed protein: three classical loci (HLA-A, -B and -C) and three non-classical loci (HLA-E, -F and -G). Normal somatic cells express HLA-A, -B and -C, while the antigens expressed by extravillous trophoblast are HLA-C, HLA-E and HLA-G[6]. In healthy individuals, the expression of HLA-G appears to be restricted to extravillous trophoblast and this suggests that it might have an important role to play in implantation.

LEUKOCYTE POPULATIONS IN DECIDUA

Analysis of the leukocyte populations in decidua has shown that the predominant cell type is natural killer (NK) cells rather than classical lymphocytes, T or B cells[10]. The NK cells have prominent granules in their cytoplasm and hence were originally referred to as large granular lymphocytes (LGL). They have the unusual phenotype of $CD56^{bright}$ $CD16^{-}$ and this differentiates them from the classical NK cells in peripheral blood which are $CD56^{dim}$ $CD16^{+}$. The number of these NK cells in the uterine mucosa varies throughout the menstrual cycle. They are sparse during the proliferative phase, increase significantly by the secretory phase and remain in high numbers in decidua during the early part of gestation. This suggests that their recruitment is hormonally controlled. The numbers then decline as pregnancy progresses and only very few cells remain by term. During the first trimester, these NK cells are particularly abundant in the decidua basalis in close contact with invading trophoblast cells. This temporal and spatial association with the implanting placenta has led to the proposal that these decidual NK cells might play an important role in the control of trophoblast migration and differentiation.

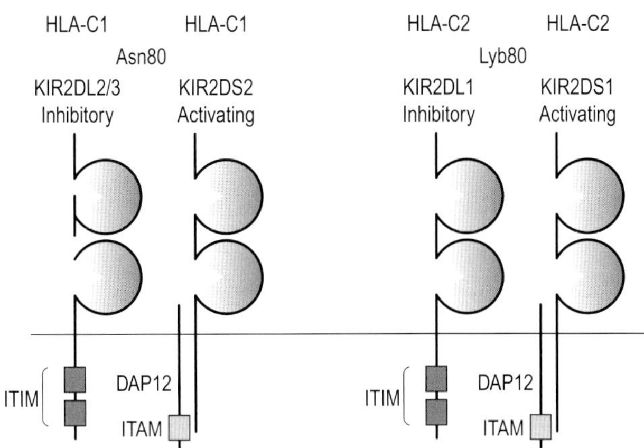

Fig. 6.3 KIR receptors and their HLA-C ligands. Both HLA-C1 and HLA-C2 groups have corresponding inhibitory and activating KIR receptors. Inhibitory receptors signal through intercellular ITIM motifs and activating receptors on association with the adaptor molecule DAP-12 which has ITAM motifs.

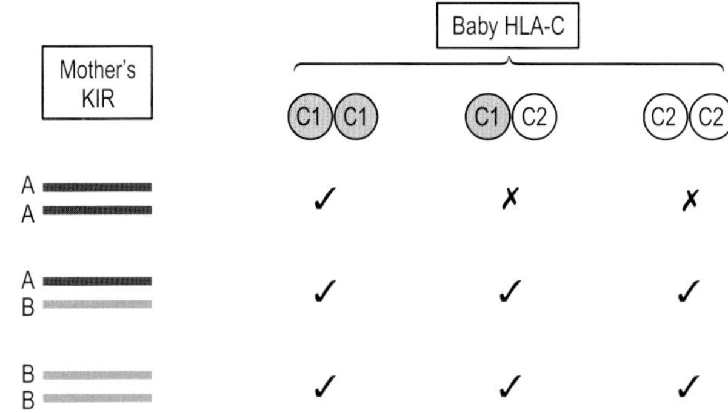

Fig. 6.4 Certain combinations of maternal KIR and fetal HLA-C genotypes increase susceptibility to pre-eclampsia. A cross (x) indicates the increased risk of a poor clinical outcome.

UTERINE NK CELL RECOGNITION OF TROPHOBLAST

Uterine NK cells express an array of receptors, some of which are known to bind to the HLA class I molecules expressed by extravillous trophoblast[10] (Fig. 6.3). Unlike blood NK cells, all uterine NK (uNK) cells express high levels of the C-type lectin family member CD94/NKG2A, which binds to HLA-E resulting in inhibition of NK-cell cytotoxicity. This is likely to be the signal that stops uNK cells from killing trophoblast and the maternal cells in the decidua. uNK cells also express members of the killer immunoglobulin-like receptors (KIR) family of receptors[11]. These differ in the number of extracellular immunoglobulin-like domains and this will determine their binding specificity. They also differ in the length of their cytoplasmic tail that either results in an inhibitory or an activating signal to the NK cell. Those that have a short tail (S) are activating (KIR2DS) and those that are long (L) are inhibitory (KIR2DL) receptors. In all populations, there are two main KIR haplotypes, A and B, these differ in the presence of additional activating receptors in the B haplotype. HLA-C, which is the only polymorphic MHC class I molecule expressed by extravillous trophoblast, is the dominant ligand for these KIR receptors. These HLA-C ligands also belong to two groups, HLA-C1 and HLA-C2. The maternal–fetal immunological interaction that occurs at the site of implantation between uNK and trophoblast, therefore, involves two gene systems, maternal KIR and fetal HLA-C molecules. Because these are both polymorphic, the exact KIR/HLA-C interaction will differ in each pregnancy. Some KIR/HLA-C combinations might be more favorable to trophoblast invasion than others thus affecting reproductive outcome. This has now been shown to be the case and three major conditions of pregnancy, recurrent miscarriage, fetal growth restriction (FGR) and pre-eclampsia all show the same association. When the fetus has an HLA-C2 group and the mother lacks the activating receptor for C2 (known as KIR2DS1), then trophoblast invasion fails to some degree (Fig. 6.4)[11].

Trophoblast HLA-G is a ligand for the KIR family member, KIR2DL4, the interaction of which results in upregulation of pro-inflammatory and pro-angiogenic cytokines, indicating a mechanism by which the placenta can increase its own blood supply. In addition, HLA-G binds with high affinity to leukocyte immunoglobulin-like receptors (LILR) expressed by myelomonocytic cells. This interaction results in the induction of 'tolerogenic' population of dendritic cells (DC) which, in a transplantation setting, leads to tolerance. The idea that the placenta itself (via HLA-G) is modifying the maternal immune reactivity locally in the uterus to downregulate damaging alloreactive T-cell responses during pregnancy is attractive. Thus, HLA-G could signal to the decidual innate immune system through both KIR2DL4 on uNK cells and LILRB1 on myelomonocytic cells. By alerting two different cell types, HLA-G might be acting as a 'placental' signal that induces pregnancy-specific immune functions in the uterus[6].

CONCLUSION

Elucidation of the molecular and cellular interactions occurring during placental implantation is essential for a clear understanding of what happens in the early stages of gestation. Correct implantation is required for proper placental and fetal growth. In addition, epidemiological data have shown that growth retardation in utero is associated with an increase in incidence of diseases in adult life. Thus, any disregulation of this process will have far-reaching consequences. The role of NK cells is uncertain although, in humans, there is an indication that NK-cell KIR/trophoblast HLA-C interactions do regulate the depth of invasion. A direct effect of uterine NK cells on spiral artery structure and function (possibly modified by soluble trophoblast-derived factors) is also likely. The relative importance of interactions between the three components – uterine NK cells, trophoblast and arteries – probably varies in different species. Whatever mechanisms are involved, the maternal immune system must provide a balance between the need for fetal intrusion into the mother's resources and the need to protect the mother from excessive fetal greed. In studying this, the view of the uterus as a 'privileged site' is no longer valid as all anatomical sites have unique immune features and this applies particularly to mucosal surfaces. The comparison of the uterine mucosa to the gut or the nose (which CD56^{bright} NK-like cells also frequent) would seem far more informative than to the traditional sites of immune privilege, the eye, brain or testis.

REFERENCES

1. Armant DR. Blastocysts don't go it alone. Extrinsic signals fine-tune the intrinsic developmental program of trophoblast cells. *Dev Biol* **280**:260–280, 2005.
2. Aplin JD. Embryo implantation: the molecular mechanism remains elusive. *Reprod BioMed Online* **13**:833–839, 2006.
3. Lopota A, Bentin-Ley U, Enders A. 'Pinopodes' and implantation. *Rev Endocrine Metabol Dis* **3**:77–86, 2002.
4. Pijnenborg R, Vercruysse L, Hanssens M. The uterine spiral arteries in human pregnancy: facts and controversies. *Placenta* **27**:939–958, 2006.
5. Burton GJ, Jauniaux E, Watson AL. Maternal arterial connections to the placental intervillous space during the first trimester of human pregnancy: the Boyd collection revisited. *Am J Obstet Gynecol* **181**:718–724, 1999.
6. Moffett-King A. Natural killer cells and pregnancy. *Nat Rev Immunol* **2**:656–663, 2002.
7. Dunn CL, Kelly RW, Critchley HO. Decidualization of the human endometrial stromal cell: an enigmatic transformation. *Reprod Biomed Online* **7**:151–161, 2003.
8. Cohen M, Meisser A, Bischof P. Metalloproteinases and human placental invasiveness. *Placenta* **27**:783–793, 2006.
9. Red-Horse K, Zhou Y, Genbacev O et al. Trophoblast differentiation during embryo implantation and formation of the maternal-fetal interface. *J Clin Invest* **114**:744–754, 2004.
10. Moffett A, Loke C. Immunology of placentation in eutherian mammals. *Nat Rev Immunol* **6**:584–594, 2006.
11. Moffett A, Hiby SE. How does the maternal immune system contribute to the development of pre-eclampsia?. *Placenta* (Suppl A):S51–S56, 2007.

CHAPTER

7

Development of the placenta and its circulation

Caroline Dunk, Berthold Huppertz and John Kingdom

KEY POINTS

- The development and structure of the human hemochorial placenta, describing in detail the development of the uteroplacental and fetoplacental circulations
- Recent developments in our understanding of the development and prenatal diagnosis of the placental pathologies in pre-eclampsia and intrauterine growth restriction
- A review of some of molecular mediators of human placental development including the basic helix loop helix transcription factors and the HGF, TGF, IGF, EGF, VEGF and angiopoietin growth factors and their dysregulation in placental pathology

INTRODUCTION

In this chapter, we intend to draw the reader into areas in which placental biology and pathology directly impinge on their practice. Pregnancies complicated by stillbirth, severe pre-eclampsia and/or intrauterine growth restriction (IUGR), especially those that deliver before 34 weeks, are associated with significant gross and microscopic placental pathology. Prenatal diagnosis of pregnancies at risk of these severe complications is now possible because we can recognize these features of 'placental insufficiency' at the 20 week stage[1–3]. Furthermore, new biomarkers analyzed from maternal blood samples show increasing power of prediction in the second trimester[4] with some of them showing predictive value as early as the first trimester of pregnancy[5,6]. These advances underscore the need for a greater understanding of placental development and pathology. More detailed information can be found in the following references[7,8].

THE PLACENTA AT DELIVERY

The full-term human placenta is a disk-like circular organ commonly inspected in its 'inverted' state from the fetal, or chorionic plate, surface. The chorionic plate is a fibrous disk into which the umbilical arteries ramify as chorionic plate vessels in a dichotomous fashion, each penetrating the plate to enter the stem (truncus) of a villous tree, and accompanied by a vein draining oxygenated blood back towards the umbilical vein. The chorionic plate vessels are covered by the amniotic membrane, which is normally glossy and can easily be peeled off. At the placental margin, the chorionic plate thickens to form a ring and continues and fuses with the basal plate to form the chorion laeve, the fetal membranes. The gross structure of the full-term placenta is illustrated in cross-section in Figure 7.1.

Macroscopic abnormalities, such as succenturiate lobes, velamentous cord insertion, or circumvallate margin, where the ring is undergrown by villous trees and the intervillous space and the membranes insert medial to the edge of the chorionic plate, are identified from this aspect and occur in approximately 10% of cases at full-term[9]. In isolation, these abnormalities have weak associations with low birth weight or pre-eclampsia[10] and may therefore be ignored if other aspects of placentation are normal. Nevertheless, experience in second-trimester ultrasonographic examination of the placenta is increasing[2], with rare but clinically relevant problems, such as vasa previa, being identified by ultrasound resulting in dramatic improvements in perinatal survival[11,12].

The fetal surface of the placenta may also be inspected at delivery for evidence of intra-amniotic infection, such as cloudy yellow malodorous discoloration, or chronic staining by meconium, when clinically relevant. Successful diagnosis of chorioamnionitis at delivery is facilitated by collection of fluid/pus (for gas chromatography), a membrane roll (from rupture point to edge of placenta) and a sample of umbilical cord into sterile containers, prior to transport of the placenta to the pathology department. Cloudy nodular discolorations of the amnion, termed amnion nodosum, are indicative of prolonged rupture of the membranes and oligohydramnios[7].

The maternal surface of the placenta (referred to as the basal plate) is an artificial surface in that delivery of the 'placenta' requires the organ to be cleaved through the basal plate (see Fig. 7.1). In this sense, part of the trophoblast remains undelivered in the placental bed, normally regressing over the

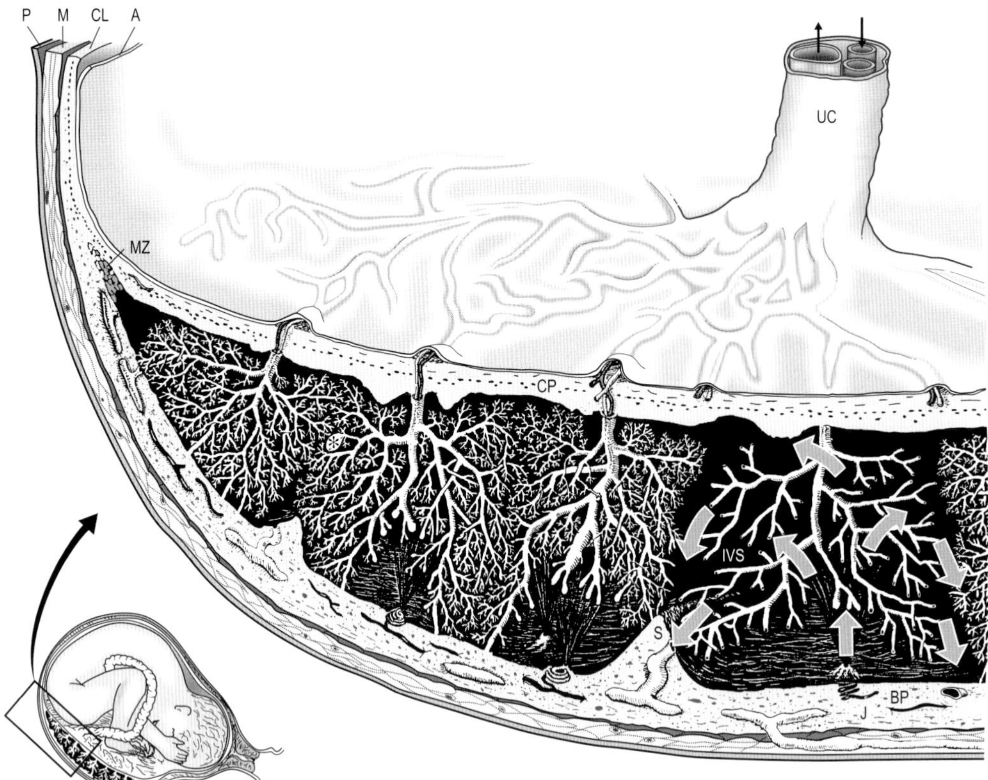

Fig. 7.1 The mature human placenta. Nearly mature human placenta in situ. On the fetal side, the amnion covers the chorionic plate, from which the umbilical cord continues towards the fetus. From the chorionic plate the villous trees extend into the intervillous space, which is filled with maternal blood. On the maternal side, the basal plate demarcates the placenta from the placental bed, which defines that part of the uterine wall directly underneath the placenta. Within the placental bed trophoblast invasion takes place and transformation of spiral arteries can be found. At the margin of the placenta, chorionic plate and basal plate fuse to circumvent the intervillous space and to generate the fetal membranes. CP = chorionic plate; IVS = intervillous space; P = serosa; M = myometrium; CL = chorion laeve; A = amnion; MZ = marginal zone between placenta and fetal membranes, with obliterated intervillous space and ghost villi; S = septum; J = junctional zone; BP = basal plate; UC = umblical cord. From Kaufmann and Scheffen[290] with permission.

ensuing weeks. The basal plate is a heterogeneous mixture of trophoblastic and decidual cells, embedded in large amounts of extracellular debris, fibrinoid and blood clot. The basal surface is divided by a system of grooves into 10–40 elevated areas referred to as the maternal lobes of the placenta. These correspond approximately to the underlying arrangement of villous trees with three or four trees per lobe in the center; small lobes at the periphery of the placenta are generally occupied only by a single villous tree. Only the latter correspond to what Schuhmann[13] described as a placentone: a villous tree together with its surrounding part of the intervillous space and its corresponding uteroplacental vessels. Terms such as 'fetal placenta' for the chorionic plate (including villous trees) and 'maternal placenta' for the basal plate (including uteroplacental vessels invaded by trophoblast) are tempting from a clinical perspective, as will be discussed in relation to Doppler studies[14]. However, since it is impossible to separate physically the fetal and maternal cellular constituents, this concept must be viewed with caution.

Many academic departments take an active interest in placental genetics, structure and function, as they relate to development, pathology and the new science of perinatal programming. Sampling of the placenta at delivery is thus an increasingly important task. Since the organ is inherently heterogeneous, a strategy of systematic random block sampling, employed in studies that use stereology methods[15], is preferred. When the focus is on vascular structure and villous development, the best approach is immediately to clamp the cord root (to prevent fetoplacental vascular collapse) and allow the organ to fix for several days in formaldehyde[16]. However, since both mRNAs and proteins are rapidly degraded following delivery, especially in the metabolically active villous trophoblast, when studies at a protein, molecular, or ultra-structural level are undertaken, a better approach is to open the placenta at random sites from the basal plate to excise samples of villous tissue that can be divided and rapidly frozen (for protein extraction) or placed into RNA fixative.

Sampling of the placental bed is far more challenging than that of the delivered placenta. Nevertheless, several groups have advanced the field of placental bed pathologies as it relates to abnormal uterine artery Doppler[17,18]. The introduction of punch biopsy of the placental bed now permits several samples to be taken[19], including samples from women following vaginal deliveries and earlier miscarriages[20].

HEMOCHORIAL PLACENTAL BLOOD FLOW

The human placenta is termed hemochorial because it provides direct contact between maternal blood and the chorionic (fetal) villi in the intervillous space (see Fig. 7.1). Maternal blood leaves the openings of the transformed spiral arteries and circulates around the villi. Some villi anchor the villous trees to the basal plate whereas the bulk of the placenta comprises trees of gas-exchanging terminal villi floating in maternal blood. The classic injection studies of spiral arteries by Wigglesworth indicated that a majority of the 60–70 villous trees at term, branching from the chorionic plate, are maternally perfused from their centers thus creating hollow-centered structures[21]. His concept was substantiated by Schuhmann's description of the 50–100 maternal arterial inlets as being located near the centers of the villous trees[13,22]. The 50–200 maternal venous outlets per placenta at term are thought to be arranged around the periphery of the villous trees such that each villous tree is perfused in a centrifugal manner. The radioangiographic studies conducted in the rhesus monkey[23] and the human[24] support the placentone concept; color flow Doppler imaging can now be used to study intraplacental blood flow relationships[25]. The maternal arterial jet flows rapidly upwards through the central cavity, dispersing in a centrifugal manner to perfuse the surrounding well-developed and more densely packed villi of mature intermediate and terminal type (see below)[26]. Reduced intervillous perfusion of a placentone results in villous placental hypoxia since fetal perfusion continues to remove oxygen bound to fetal hemoglobin. In response, the stem villous arterioles will constrict to reduce the rate of removal of oxygen until intervillous oxygen tension equilibrates again. In this way, the individual placentones self-regulate to maximize maternal–fetal exchange. Persistent lack of intervillous perfusion can cause stem villous arterial thrombosis[27]. However, the central portions of the placenta have the largest placentones and the most-transformed spiral arteries, so central vascular pathology is therefore rare in normal pregnancy. By contrast, spiral artery thrombosis and villous infarction is often found at the margins of the placental disk after a term delivery, with no apparent ill-effects.

It is the uniquely invasive properties of the extravillous trophoblast that transform the uterine spiral arteries, which result in the hemochorial arrangement that characterizes human placentation. The process of invasion is precisely controlled and it is thought that the disordered extravillous trophoblast proliferation/migration, in combination with the placental vascular pathology which relates to major clinical conditions such as pre-eclampsia and IUGR (inadequate invasion) or placenta percreta (excessive invasion) and is discussed in detail later in this chapter.

EARLY STAGES OF PLACENTAL DEVELOPMENT

Placental development begins with blastocyst attachment to the uterine wall. At this stage the first extraembryonic cell lineage differentiates and is termed the trophoblast[28]. Signals from the embryo (inner cell mass), including fibroblast growth factor 4 (FGF4) expand the population of trophoblast stem (TS) cells that are capable of differentiating along both the extravillous and villous pathways of development. Considerable knowledge of trophoblast differentiation has been obtained using transgenic mice and mouse TS cells and is summarized in recent reviews[29,30]. Blastocyst symmetry is directed by the inner cell mass since only those trophoblast cells overlying the inner cell mass make direct contact with the uterine epithelium (Fig. 7.2a). Abnormal orientation of these structures likely causes abnormalities in the site of umbilical cord insertion into the placental disk[31]. It is of interest that these gross abnormalities of placental development are more common in pregnancies arising from in vitro fertilization (IVF)[32].

The *prelacunar stage* of development (Fig. 7.2b) is characterized by the formation of an outer shell of syncytiotrophoblast that is distinct from the later villous syncytiotrophoblast by being able to penetrate the uterine epithelium and embed the conceptus in the uterine stroma[33]. The more proximal trophoblast cell population is referred to as cytotrophoblast and is positioned between the syncytiotrophoblast and embryoblast. The cytotrophoblast layer is assumed to be a multipotent stem cell population capable of subsequently producing each type of trophoblast, as in the mouse[34]. Around day 14 post conception (pc), the conceptus is fully embedded within uterine tissues and the syncytiotrophoblast starts to develop fluid-filled spaces termed lacunae (Fig. 7.2c). The lacunae gradually coalesce to form one large intervillous space of the placenta. This *lacunar stage* results in the formation of syncytiotrophoblast columns, referred to as trabeculae, which reach from the embryonic side of the placenta to the maternal decidual tissues. The development of the lacunae and the establishment of the intervillous space compartmentalize the growing placenta as follows:

- the site of attachment, comprising anchoring villi and the basal plate
- the lacunar spaces, forming the intervillous space
- branches that derive from the trabeculae develop into floating villi
- the embryonic side develops into the chorionic plate.

Further invasion of the maternal tissues by the placenta is necessary so as to transform the spiral arteries of the uteroplacental circulation. The first step is the streaming of cytotrophoblast cells down the center of the syncytiotrophoblast trabeculae, creating a new lineage of extravillous cytotrophoblast that is in direct into contact with maternal tissues beyond the initial wave of syncytiotrophoblast invasion (Fig. 7.2d–f). Cytotrophoblasts at the tips of the trabeculae, their maternal ends now referred to as anchoring villi, form trophoblast cell columns. The proximal cells proliferate as the source of all subsequent subtypes of invasive extravillous trophoblast cells. Initially, the invasion of maternal decidual tissues by cytotrophoblasts begins in the connective tissue (interstitial extravillous trophoblast) followed by the walls of the spiral arteries (endovascular trophoblast cells)[35,36].

Trophoblast invasion into maternal tissues is not restricted to the process of implantation and early placentation, but is a continuous process throughout pregnancy serving a number of purposes. The trophoblastic cell columns at the base of the anchoring villi provide the cellular sources for this invasive process. The cell columns do not contain stroma since they were not excavated by mesenchyme during formation of the villous trees. The cytotrophoblast cells composing these cell

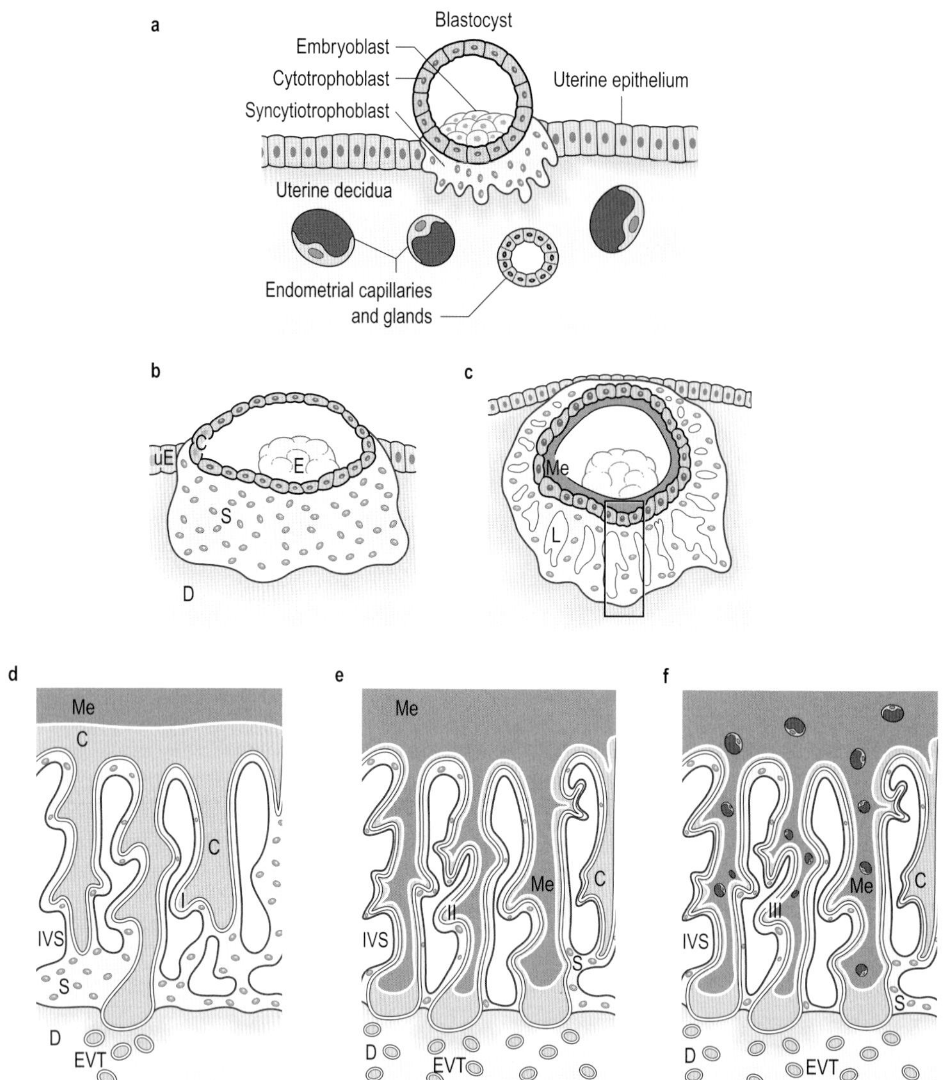

Fig. 7.2 Early placental development. (a) The blastocyst is covered by a monolayer of trophoblast cells that encircle a fluid-filled cavity, the blastocele, and the developing embryoblast. A crucial developmental prerequisite for implantation is a next differentiation step of those trophoblast cells in direct contact to the uterine epithelium. Only syncytial fusion of those cells to develop a first syncytiotrophoblast enables the blastocyst to penetrate the uterine epithelium and to further implant into the maternal uterine tissues. (b) During the *prelacunar stage*, the syncytiotrophoblast (S) has penetrated the uterine epithelium (uE) and has reached the decidua (D), continuing the direct contact to maternal cells. The layer of cytotrophoblast cells (C) does not have direct contact to maternal cells but lies in second row between syncytiotrophoblast and embryo (E). (c) During the *lacunar stage*, first, fluid-filled spaces, lacunae (L), appear within the mass of the syncytiotrophoblast, grow and flow together finally to generate one large fluid-filled space, the intervillous space. Between embryo and cytotrophoblast extraembryonic mesenchyme (Me) has spread out. (d–f) *Villous stages*: the further development of the placenta is shown using the black rectangle in (c). The cytotrophoblast (C) begins to penetrate into the syncytiotrophoblast (S) and reaches the opposite side of the placenta and thus reaches maternal tissues of the decidua (D). Cytotrophoblast cells that leave the proper placenta are termed extravillous trophoblast (EVT). Within the placenta first sprouting of the syncytiotrophoblast can be found (d), protruding towards the intervillous space (IVS). This is the development of the first primary villi (I). A few days later the extraembryonic mesenchyme (Me) starts to penetrate the syncytiotrophoblast as well and displaces the cytotrophoblast from the core of the trabeculae and primary villi. This leads to the development of the secondary villi (II) (e). Slightly later first blood vessels develop within the placental mesenchyme and lead to the formation of tertiary villi (III).

columns, together with trophoblast cells in the placental bed, basal plate, chorionic plate and membranes, are collectively described as extravillous trophoblast[37].

The trophoblastic cell columns resting on the basal plate should be viewed as a rapidly proliferating zone from which extravillous trophoblast cells migrate continuously into maternal tissues (Fig. 7.3). However, as soon as the extravillous trophoblast cells leave this proliferative zone, they leave the cell division cycle and change to an invasive phenotype. Their pattern of integrin expression, secretion of proteolytic enzymes and production of extracellular matrix proteins is strikingly similar to that of malignant tumor cells[37]. Fortunately, they differ in one fundamental aspect – they have lost their ability to proliferate during invasion. This is one of the reasons why the depth of invasion into maternal tissues is limited, due to their individual life span. If deportation into the maternal circulation

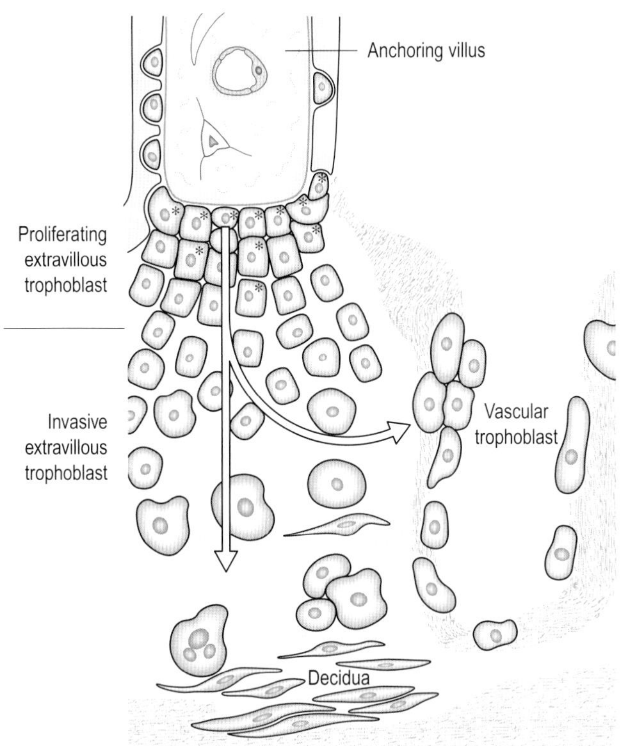

Fig. 7.3 Trophoblastic cell column. Schematic drawing of a trophoblastic cell column connecting a villous stem (above) to the basal plate (below). Proliferating stem cells (*) of the extravillous trophoblast. The arrow symbolizes the invasive pathway. Fibrin-type fibrinoid (line shading). Extracellular matrix (light point shading).

occurs, metastatic growth is impossible since these cells have lost their generative potency.

Invasion by extravillous trophoblast serves two very different purposes, namely adhesion of the placenta to the uterine wall and adaptation of uteroplacental arteries to the fetal requirements.

PHENOTYPES OF EXTRAVILLOUS TROPHOBLAST

Among the invasive trophoblast cells, a subset of cells secretes huge amounts of extracellular matrix (composed of laminins, collagen IV, fibronectins, vitronectin and heparan sulfate) known as matrix-type fibrinoid[38] into which they are embedded. The extravillous trophoblast cells adhere to the extracellular matrix via the surface expression of molecules known as integrins. Likewise, the endometrial stromal cells adhere via similar mechanisms; root-like projections of extravillous trophoblast, together with its associated matrix, penetrate deep into the myometrium, thereby ensuring perfect anchoring of the placenta. Adhesion of the placenta by the glue-like extracellular matrix[39] depends on the viability of the extravillous trophoblast cells expressing integrins; in this sense, it is reversible at delivery. This anchoring process is essential; otherwise entry of maternal blood into the intervillous space at high velocity would shear off the chorionic plate.

Along the invasive pathway through the decidual interstitium extravillous trophoblast cells show morphologically and functionally different phenotypes. These different phenotypes display a varying behavior regarding contact to maternal cells, secretion of matrix and invasiveness. At present, the molecular basis of these different phenotypes is not known, though has recently been described in the related mouse placenta[40]. Such knowledge may in future help us to understand the pathways that prevent this physiologic process from occurring in certain specific diseases, such as abruption (premature separation), pre-eclampsia and IUGR.

In a normal intrauterine pregnancy, extravillous trophoblast cells that are invading the decidual interstitium can be subdivided into three morphologically and functionally different subtypes.

Large polygonal cells

This subtype of large polygonal extravillous trophoblast cells corresponds to the well-described former X-cells[7]. Compared to the subset of small spindle-shaped cells, the relative number of this subtype increases from 45% at weeks 9–12 to 69% at weeks 16–24 and makes up about 89% in weeks 31–39[41]. Hence this subtype is the prevailing phenotype of extravillous trophoblast at the time of delivery. These cells are evenly distributed throughout the basal plate as well as along the route of invasion reaching the upper third of the myometrium. Morphologically, these cells are large, polygonal, uninucleated extravillous trophoblast cells displaying big, irregularly shaped and intensely staining nuclei. No other subtype of all trophoblast cells displays a stronger immunoreactivity for cytokeratin 7 than these large polygonal cells. At the same time, they are always immunonegative for proliferation markers such as anti-Ki67.

These cells secrete the typical extracellular matrix of extravillous trophoblast, the matrix-type fibrinoid[38,42]. This basement membrane-like extracellular matrix comprises three different patches of matrix molecules, collagen IV and laminin, an amorphous ground substance containing heparan sulfate and vitronectin, and fibronectins and fibrillin embedded in the same amorphous ground substance[42–45]. The large cells fix themselves within their self-secreted matrix by expression and exposition of the respective integrins, such as $\alpha5/\beta1$, $\alpha1/\beta1$ and α-v/$\beta3/5$ integrins[46–48]. These cells organize themselves in clusters, which are usually void of maternal tissue components but filled with matrix-type fibrinoid. The above features do not support the classical thinking that the large polygonal cells ('X-cells') are highly invasive cells. Rather, it appears as if this subtype of interstitial extravillous trophoblast may have a function in fixing and adhering the placenta to the uterine wall by secreting matrix-type fibrinoid, which has been termed the 'trophoblast glue'[39].

Small spindle-shaped extravillous trophoblast cells

This subtype of the interstitial trophoblast is also negative for proliferation markers and only moderately immunoreactive for cytokeratin 7 and can be found from the transitional zone of trophoblastic cell columns reaching the upper third of the myometrium. Hence this subtype shares the spatial distribution pattern with the subtype of the large polygonal cells. Opposing the large polygonal subtype, this small subtype displays a decrease in numbers towards term from 55% in the first trimester to 31% in the second trimester reaching only about 11% at term[41]. Structurally, this subtype is characterized by elongated, partly filiform cell bodies mostly oriented radially to the uterine wall containing small ovoid nuclei. This small subtype usually forms loosely arranged arrays of cells, surrounded by only very little matrix.

There are only a few descriptions of these small spindle-shaped trophoblast cells so far[41], which may be due to the fact that these small, usually filiform cells easily escape the investigators' attention, the reason being that they are rarely represented in one section in full length. The small cells only secrete little amounts of self-secreted matrix, which is mostly composed of cellular and oncofetal isoforms of fibronectin[42–44,49]. At the same time, these cells only express 'interstitial' integrins such as $\alpha 5/\beta 1$ and α-v-integrins. The predominant expression of 'interstitial' integrins in combination with the expression of oncofetal fibronectins is an essential mechanism of trophoblast invasiveness[42,50,51]. Aplin and coworkers have elegantly shown that interactions between $\alpha 5/\beta 1$ integrins and fibronectins are crucial for trophoblast invasion[52].

In the last decade, an integrin switch has been described during the course of trophoblast invasion[47,53]. In the light of the data presented above, this phenomenon could be explained as follows: the small subtype of cells expresses only 'interstitial' integrins and prevails in deeper zones of the invasive pathway since this phenotype is really invasive. The large subtype additionally expresses 'epithelial' integrins. Therefore, the integrin switch may relate to the terminal differentiation of the motile spindle shaped to the non-motile polygonal trophoblast cells, this process occurs over the course of gestation and may account for the increasing percentage of polygonal trophoblast cells and corresponding decrease in spindle-shaped trophoblast cells.

Multinucleated giant cells

This subtype prevails in the depth of the placental bed, at the border between decidua and myometrium and does not show any proliferative activity. A distinct difference to the above mentioned subtypes is that these cells contain more than one and up to 10 irregularly shaped nuclei of varying size, leading to a much larger volume with a diameter ranging between 50 and 100 μm[41]. These multinucleated cells are either immunonegative for cytokeratin 7 or show few spots of reactivity – and thus may easily be missed during superficial inspection of immunohistochemical sections of the placental bed. Although a fusion event of such cells has never been observed, it is generally accepted that fusion of interstitial extravillous trophoblast cells does occur.

REGULATION OF TROPHOBLAST INVASION

The invasive extravillous trophoblast cells finally reach the upper third of the myometrium where they can be found between the layers of smooth muscle cells. Arrest at this stage is crucial so that pathological placental invasion does not occur. Some insight into the mechanisms that permit further trophoblast invasion into the uterus has come from studies in placenta accreta specimens[54].

Hypotheses favoring extrinsic factors

- Trigger gradient: extravillous trophoblast cells need a trigger to be invasive. This trigger is derived from the mesenchymal stroma of anchoring villi[55]. Cell invasion is therefore limited by a requirement for this diffusible factor.
- Cellular interaction: cells within the myometrium (smooth muscle cells, specific immune cells) or endometrium may arrest invasion.

Hypotheses favoring intrinsic factors and programs

- Apoptosis: programmed cell death occurs in extravillous trophoblast cells[56–60]. The rates of apoptosis differ significantly between studies, due to technical and sampling limitations. Therefore, at present, the role of apoptosis as a critical regulator of trophoblast invasion is uncertain.
- Polyploidization: the subtype of large polygonal trophoblast cells is most probably differentiated from the small spindle-shaped cells by polyploidization[61]. This leads to a non-invasive phenotype that secretes ample matrix that acts as a trophoblast–decidual glue[39] to anchor the placenta to its implantation site.
- Syncytial fusion: it is generally accepted that the multinucleated giant cells derive from syncytial fusion of their mononucleated counterparts[7]. The non-invasive multinucleated cells accumulate close to the border between decidua and myometrium and may act as a trap for those trophoblast cells that try to trespass into deeper layers. Cell–cell fusion likely occurs via expression of the fusogenic protein syncytin[62]. These terminally differentiated multinucleated structures may participate in the maternal recognition and adaptation to pregnancy.

The invasive nature of hemochorial placentation is precisely regulated under normal circumstances; when it occurs to excess, extravillous trophoblast cells may invade deeply into (accreta) or through (percreta) the uterine wall, such that physiological separation of the placenta can no longer occur. Invasive placentation is more common in a scarred uterus from multiple previous cesarean sections[63] and in pregnancies following successful endoscopic surgery for Asherman's syndrome (uterine adhesion from patchy loss of endometrium)[64].

Conversely, a failure of this invasive anchoring process predisposes to premature placental separation (abruption), either during the antepartum period or during labor. These important conditions underscore the importance of understanding how extravillous trophoblast invasion and production of an adhesive matrix is disturbed in these conditions.

PLACENTAL PERFUSION DURING EMBRYOGENESIS

During implantation, the expanding and invading early syncytiotrophoblast initially comes into contact with the superficial capillary system of the decidua underneath the uterine epithelium. Capillaries may leak maternal erythrocytes into the lacunar spaces of the placenta[65,66], but the predominating observation is that the stromal capillaries are blocked by extravillous trophoblast and no arterial connections are made between the maternal circulation and the primitive intervillous space[67,68]. Maternal erythrocytes are not consistently identified within the intervillous space prior to week 10 of gestation[69]. This apparent lack of intervillous blood perfusion has been shown by transcervical endoscopic observations of the intervillous space[70], Doppler ultrasound[71] and by elegant studies which demonstrate an oxygen gradient between maternal stroma and villous placenta in the first trimester[72]. During embryogenesis, the intervillous space is filled with a clear fluid[73] comprising filtered maternal plasma and uterine gland secretion products rich in nutrients and growth factors crucial for placental and embryonic development[74]. The glandular secretion has a high lipid content termed 'uterine milk'[73,75].

Occlusion of maternal vessels during implantation is designed to facilitate embryogenesis in a low oxygen environment below 20 mmHg until week 10 of gestation[76] and has the following advantages:

- Reduction of the amount of free radicals to protect the embryo from teratogenesis during this critical phase of tissue and organ development[76,77].
- Mammalian cells grow much faster under low oxygen as compared to higher oxygen tensions. Embryo development is characterized by rapid cell division and thus a low oxygen is ideal to generate an environment to achieve and maintain a high level of cell divisions.
- Connection between placental and embryonic vessels is not fully established before week 7 of gestation. Hence there is no need to perfuse the placenta with maternal blood to feed the embryo before this time.
- Perfusion of maternal plasma without blood cells may protect the early villous syncytiotrophoblast from direct contact with circulating maternal immune cells.

TRANSFORMATION OF THE UTEROPLACENTAL ARTERIES

Starting from the interstitial route of invasion, a subset of extravillous trophoblast cells penetrate the walls of uterine spiral arteries[7,35]. This subset of invasive extravillous trophoblast cells is termed endovascular trophoblast[35,78]. The endovascular trophoblast cells intravasate from the interstitium and may migrate inside the arterial lumen along the arterial wall and later may even extravasate focally to re-enter the walls of the spiral arteries.

The major role of endovascular trophoblast is to transform the distal spiral arteries into dilated segments that facilitate increased uteroplacental blood flow. The transformation of spiral arteries is divided into three stages (Fig. 7.4).

1. Maternal signals such as the local decidual artery renin–angiotensin systems[79] induce the first changes of uterine spiral arteries very early during pregnancy, still in the absence of any invading trophoblast in their vicinity (Fig. 7.4a). The vessels begin to dilate via a disorganization of vascular smooth muscle cells and altered endothelial cell morphology[79].
2. Before penetrating the spiral artery walls, extravillous trophoblast cells remodel the vessel walls (Fig. 7.4b). This has been demonstrated in the guinea pig[80–82], where smooth muscle cell depletion and fibrinoid deposition

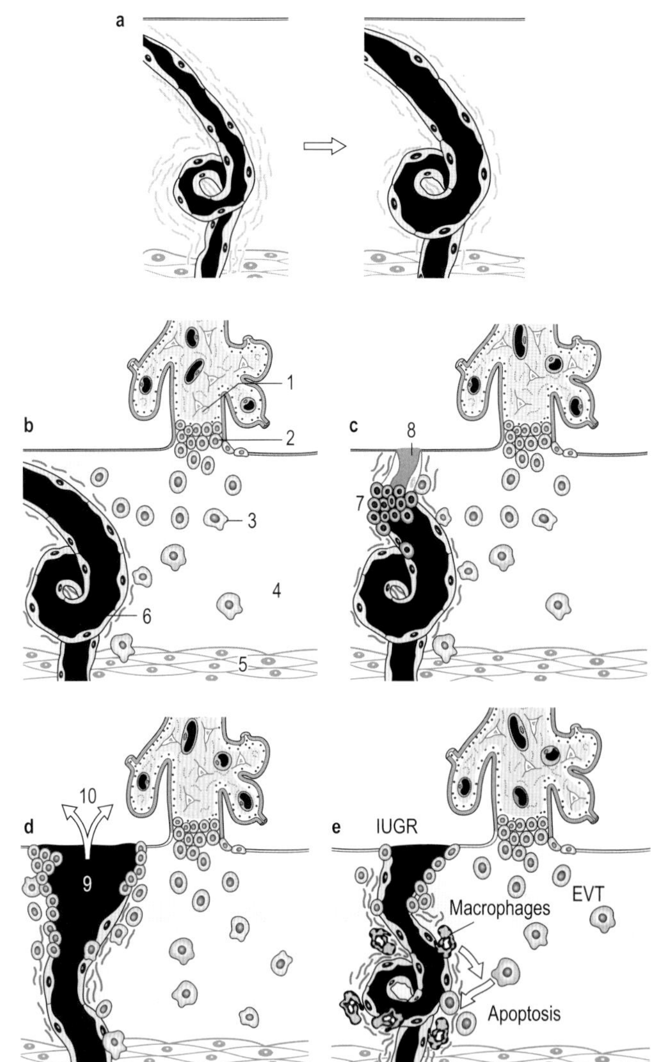

Fig. 7.4 Transformation of spiral arteries. (a) First transformation of spiral arteries early during pregnancy in the absence of trophoblast invasion. Already during early implantation the spiral arteries are altered by signals from the mother. The muscle within the arterial wall is reduced and a first widening of the lumen can be seen. These events are supposed to be preparative steps towards trophoblast infiltration of the arterial walls. (b) Beginning during the third week of pregnancy, invasion of extravillous trophoblast cells starts. At the lower tip of anchoring villi (1) trophoblastic cell columns form (2). These columns are the source of interstitial trophoblast cells (3) that migrate into the connective tissues of the decidua (4). Some trophoblast cells reach the upper third of the myometrium (5), while others take a side route and penetrate the spiral arteries (6). (c) The trophoblast cells that have reached the spiral arteries are termed endovascular trophoblast (EVT) (7), which can be found in the wall as well as in the lumen of spiral arteries. Within the lumen they build plugs (8) that during the first trimester hinder maternal blood cells to flow into the intervillous space. (d) Only around the end of the first trimester the trophoblastic plugs disintegrate. Now maternal blood containing blood cells flow through the maximally enlarged uteroplacental arteries (9) and reach the intervillous space (10) of the placenta. (e) In intrauterine growth restriction (IUGR), invasion of spiral arteries does not take place in a normal manner. Reduced depth of invasion in combination in a decreased number of invaded spiral arteries leads to malperfusion of the placenta. Maternal macrophages may play a role in hindering endovascular trophoblast invasion by induction of trophoblast apoptosis.

are seen before the extravillous trophoblast cells invade into the vessel media. The human trophoblast-decidua co-culture model has been used to demonstrate the same phenomenon[83].

3. Endovascular trophoblast infiltrates the arterial walls resulting in remodeling of the uteroplacental arteries (Fig. 7.4c,d). The further dilation of the arteries results in lumen diameters several times greater than the original diameter[7,84]. The reduced activity of smooth muscle cells[82,85] and the loss of elastic fibers[86] are clear indications of the disruptive properties of the endovascular trophoblast in the vessel media.

The number of uteroplacental spiral arteries supplying the intervillous space reduces as pregnancy advances due to vascular obliteration, such that, by term, the intervillous space is perfused by approximately one hundred spiral arteries[33]. However, intervillous blood flow increases considerably due to these physiological changes in the uteroplacental arteries including loss of autonomic innervation[87]. The dilated and denervated uteroplacental arteries are released from autonomic and local vasomotor influences such that intervillous perfusion is regulated by systemic arterial pressure. Differential regulation of uteroplacental blood flow by the mother is no longer possible so hypotension, such as following the insertion of an epidural anesthetic during labor may cause temporary fetal distress due to a fall in uteroplacental perfusion, which is then corrected by intravenous crystalloid volume expansion and ephedrine.

The virtual absence of endovascular trophoblast invasion characterizes the placental bed in chromosomally normal late first-trimester miscarriages[20]. Focal inadequate occlusion of invaded endometrial stromal vessels by extravillous trophoblast results in a premature entry of oxygenated maternal blood into the intervillous space, arresting trophoblast proliferation, villous angiogenesis and therefore overall development of the chorio-allantoic placenta[88]. This is recognized clinically by transvaginal ultrasound[89] and by low levels of trophoblast-derived pregnancy-associated placental protein A (PAPP-A) in maternal blood[90]. By contrast, no abnormalities of trophoblast invasion are found in early first-trimester losses[91]. Less severe reductions in trophoblast invasion characterize IUGR and early onset pre-eclamptic pregnancies[58,92,93] and are discussed in detail later.

FLOW OF MATERNAL BLOOD INTO THE INTERVILLOUS SPACE

During the course of the first trimester, extravillous trophoblast cells generated from the anchoring cell columns penetrate the decidua and come into contact with the uterine spiral arteries to begin the process of physiological transformation of these vessels. The extravillous trophoblast cells reorganize the vessel walls and also aggregate in the lumen of these vessels resulting in the plugging of the distal portions of the vessels (see Fig. 7.4c)[94,95]. Hence, there is no free communication of maternal blood cells between these eroded vessels and the intervillous space of the placenta until the end of the first trimester. Only then do the intra-arterial plugs of trophoblast cells become permeable and begin to dislocate. This finally enables maternal blood cells to enter the intervillous space of the placenta (see Fig. 7.4d)[77,96].

As detailed above, there is a gradient in trophoblast development during the first trimester of pregnancy with the most advanced stages in the center below the embryo and the less advanced stages in the periphery underlying the uterine epithelium (Fig. 7.5). Similarly, the plugging of the spiral arteries follows this gradient with the deepest invasion and the highest number of extravillous trophoblast plugs found in the center of the placental bed[97]. The low number of invading cells in the peripheral part of the placenta, together with the superficial invasion of spiral arteries, enables maternal blood cells to override the outer trophoblastic plugs first, even well before 10 weeks of gestation[98]. The inflow of maternal blood and blood cells at this time results in enormous oxidative stress in these peripheral parts of the placenta leading to damage of villous trophoblast[98]. Subsequently, degeneration of villi can be observed at these sites. Thus, in the peripheral parts of the

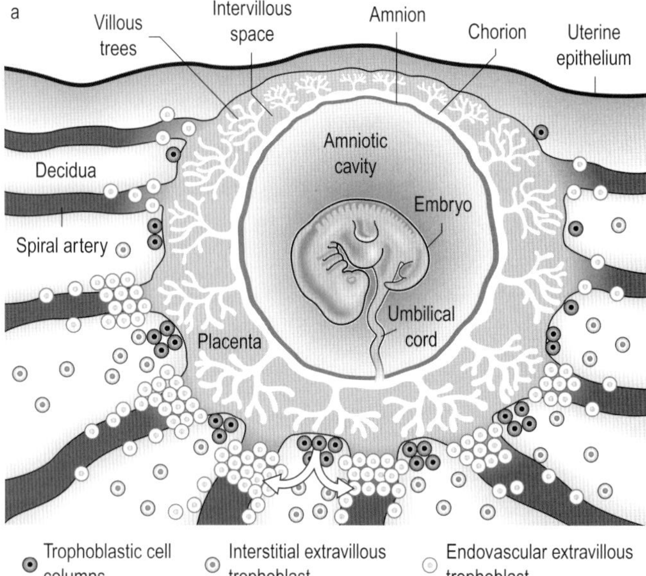

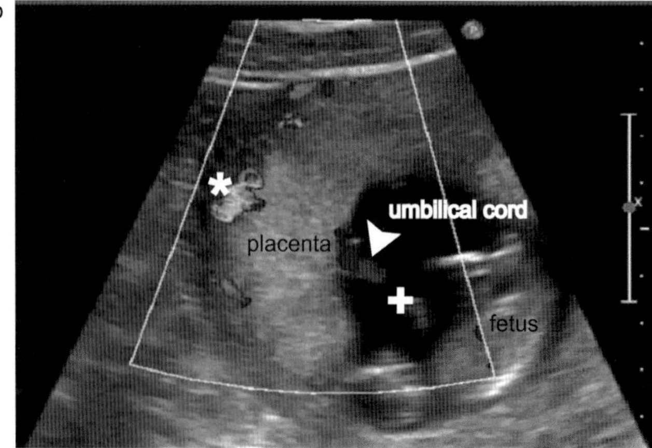

Fig. 7.5 Onset of placental perfusion. Placental blood flow in the first trimester. At this time, the spiral arterioles beneath the definitive placenta are occluded by endovascular trophoblast (a). As a result, maternal blood bypasses the intervillous space, but can be seen to flow in the myometrium using color Doppler ultrasound (*). (b) Note that the fetoplacental circulation is established at this time and is detected by color flow in the umbilical cord (+).

placenta below the uterine epithelium villi regress resulting in a secondary smoothing of the chorion and hence the development of the chorion laeve, the fetal membranes.

The removal of the centrally located plugs within the spiral arteries is achieved only after the flow of maternal blood in the peripheral parts of the placenta has been established[98]. With the onset of maternal blood flow into the placenta, a direct contact between maternal blood cells and the fetal syncytiotrophoblast is established resulting in a more than threefold increase in intraplacental oxygen concentrations, from less than 20 mmHg to about 60 mmHg[77,96]. The reorganization of villous tissues within the placenta at the end of the first trimester results in the definitive disk-shaped placenta with the central and remaining part of the villous tissues developing into the chorion frondosum. The temporal difference between the two onsets of blood flow into the different parts of the placenta may play an essential role in the generation of the decisive shape of the human placenta. Before 10 weeks of gestation, villi regress with increasing oxygen concentrations, while the same phenomenon between weeks 10 and 12 (increasing oxygen concentrations) provides a stimulus for trophoblast differentiation. It has to be stressed though that also at that time oxidative stress within the placenta occurs, partly resulting in damage of the syncytiotrophoblast[77,99].

In the human, the process of uteroplacental dilatation and invasion begins in the central part of the placenta and spreads towards the periphery[92]. When the placenta is predominantly located on one side of the uterus, Doppler examination of the ipsilateral uteroplacental artery during the second trimester indicates lower impedance than the opposite side. Persistent high-impedance waveforms with preservation of the early diastolic notch on the placental side of the uterus is associated with placental complications of pregnancy such as intrauterine growth restriction and abruption[3,100]. The non-invasive Doppler studies are supported by earlier histological studies demonstrating incomplete trophoblast invasion of spiral arteries in these conditions[92,93,101,102].

The uteroplacental veins, approximately 50–200 in number, drain the intervillous space from the margins of the fetal cotyledons, thus surrounding the basal parts of the villous trees[7]. In contrast to the arteries, the veins are only poorly invaded by extravillous trophoblast and obviously are not involved in the regulation of the intervillous blood flow.

DEVELOPMENT OF PLACENTAL VILLI

At about day 14 pc, cytotrophoblast cells within the syncytial trabeculae begin to proliferate and push the syncytial layer to generate protrusions that bulge into the intervillous space. These pure trophoblastic structures are termed primary villi, which are composed of an outer syncytial layer and a core filled with mononucleated cytotrophoblast cells (see Fig. 7.2d). Shortly after, the mesenchymal cells from the extraembryonic mesoderm follow the cytotrophoblast cells and migrate into the syncytial trabeculae, this time displacing the cytotrophoblast cells from the core of the trabeculae. The mesenchymal cells follow the cytotrophoblast into the primary villi, fill them with a first connective tissue and hence generate secondary villi (see Fig. 7.2e). At around day 20 pc, first primitive blood vessels and hemangioblastic stem cells[103] develop within the mesenchyme, generating tertiary villi (see Fig. 7.2f)[72,104]. The development of the placental vascular bed is independent of that of the embryo and both vessel beds only connect to each other to establish a fully embryo–placental circulation at day 35 pc[105]. During the first trimester, hematopoiesis can be observed within newly formed placental capillaries, thereafter the fetal liver takes over. By 12–13 weeks, most villi have transformed to tertiary vascularized villi, through an intense period of branching angiogenesis. This is driven in part by the intraplacental low oxygen tension due to effective occlusion of the decidual stromal blood vessels over an area of the uterine wall that is destined to become the definitive placenta (see Fig. 7.5).

Premature entry of maternal blood into the intervillous space can be detected by color Doppler ultrasound, and is observed in non-viable pregnancies destined for miscarriage[105]. While many miscarriages are aneuploid, this phenomenon is seen in euploid miscarriages, and may therefore represent early pregnancy failure due to lack of adequate initial endovascular occlusion of stromal blood vessels. Non-lethal variants of this may result in villous obliteration and 'chorion regression syndrome' whereby most severe preterm IUGR placentas are <10th centile for weight and have eccentric cord insertions[3,106]. This pathology of pregnancy is discussed in detail below.

ARCHITECTURE OF THE VILLOUS TREES

Placental villi are composed of two compartments, a superficial layer of trophoblast comprising cytotrophoblasts covered by a continuous syncytiotrophoblast, and the villous core, comprising stroma and fetally derived blood vessels[7]. Syncytiotrophoblast is generated by syncytial fusion of a subset of villous cytotrophoblasts (Langhans cells). Cytotrophoblast numbers remain fairly constant throughout the second and third trimesters[107], while the volume of syncytiotrophoblast increases to cover the exponentially growing specialized villi. Consequently, the cytotrophoblast population becomes dispersed[108]. Mitosis is confined to the cytotrophoblast layer and these cells are analyzed for the preliminary karyotype by chorionic villous sampling. Determination of fetal karyotype by culture of villous explants depends upon the slower multiplication of villous stromal cells; since these are derived from embryonic (allantoic) tissues, they more accurately reflect the karyotype in fetal tissues[109].

From a functional perspective, fusion of newly formed cytotrophoblast into the outer syncytium results in the transfer of fresh organelles, enzyme systems and messenger RNA transcripts into the syncytium. Aged syncytial nuclei cluster together, known as 'syncytial knots', and protrude into the intervillous space, prior to release into the maternal circulation[110,111]. Continued rejuvenation of the syncytial layer is essential in order to sustain the intense metabolic activity required for maternofetal transfer processes, secretory and endocrine functions. As gestation advances, this process of rejuvenation appears to slow down, since the ratio of cytotrophoblast to syncytial nuclei within individual terminal villi decreases as syncytial knots become more common[112]. However, stereological analysis of the total trophoblast number shows that the ratio between cytotrophoblast nuclei and syncytiotrophoblast nuclei remains mostly constant throughout gestation with a value of 9 at 13–16 weeks and again a value of 9 at 37–41 weeks of gestation[113].

Groups of degenerating syncytial nuclei protrude into the intervillous space as syncytial knots (Fig. 7.6) and may break

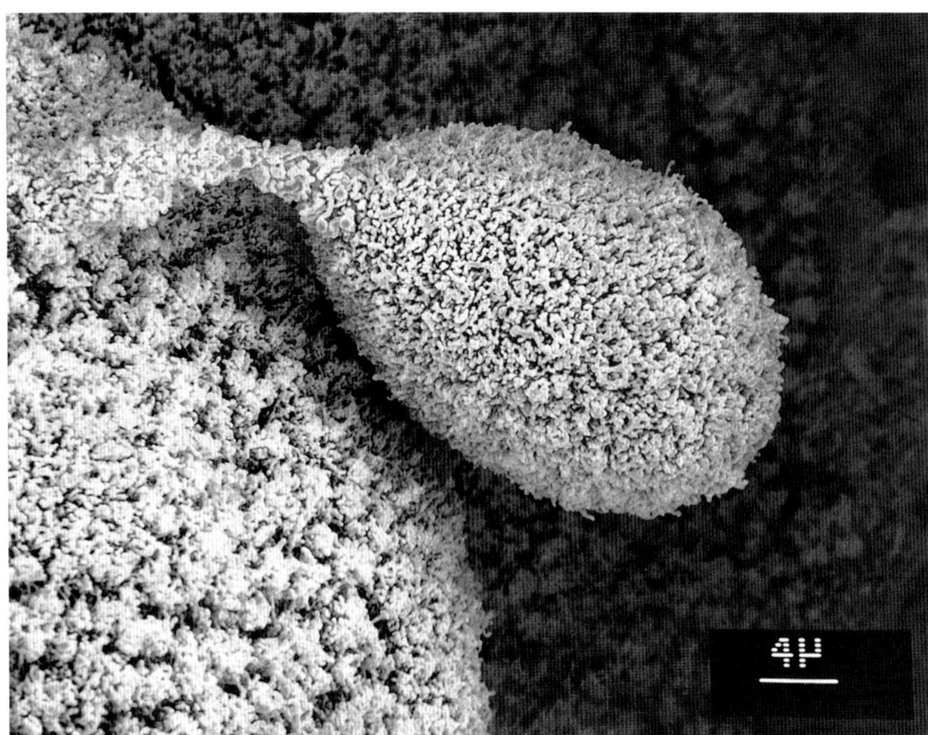

Fig. 7.6 Term placenta with syncytial knot. A syncytial knot (center) is connected to a terminal villus (left) by a thin stalk and protrudes into the intervillous space (right). This type of sprout may detach and enter the maternal circulation. Scanning electron micrograph, ×2500.

away; the resulting syncytial globules are deported in the maternal blood, most becoming lodged in the pulmonary capillary bed. It has been estimated that up to 150000 such globules enter the maternal circulation each day[114], a mechanism by which aged syncytial nuclei can be shed. This phenomenon may play a role in modifying the maternal immune system, although how this is achieved by tissue devoid of major histocompatibility complex (MHC) antigens remains uncertain.

The syncytial knots that are released into maternal blood are characterized by a tightly sealed membrane surrounding a corpuscular structure containing numerous nuclei. Recent calculations[115,116] including cytotrophoblast proliferation, syncytial fusion and villous growth over gestation have revealed that at term several grams of apoptotic syncytial knots per day are deported into the maternal circulation[7,114,115].

Deported syncytial knots have been detected in uterine vein blood behind the placenta[117] and in lung vessels[118,119], where they infrequently lead to a lung embolism[120–122]. Since syncytial knots are engulfed by lung macrophages[118,123], they are found in uterine venous, but not arterial, blood of pregnant women[117,124]. Syncytial shedding and villous trophoblast morphology are abnormal in severe forms of IUGR and preeclampsia and will be discussed in the pathology section.

The fetal vessels within the stem villi comprise muscularized arteries and veins[125]. These lead into the elongated capillaries of the mature intermediate and terminal villi, the latter providing a surface for gas exchange thought to exceed $10\,m^2$[27]. The endothelium of the fetal capillaries acts as a passive filter, limiting macromolecular transfer across the vessel wall to molecules below 20000 Da[126,127], depending upon molecular charge[127,128]. The contractile cells that surround the walls of the arteries and arterioles of the stem villi are of great interest clinically since reduced fetoplacental perfusion, detected by Doppler ultrasound examination of the umbilical arteries in vivo, is associated with poor fetal growth, fetal death and perinatal loss[129]. Since these vessels have no autonomic innervation[130], blood flow must be regulated by local and systemic vasomotor factors, together with the anatomical arrangements and fetal cardiac output[131].

Connective tissue cells within the stroma are heterogeneous in nature, producing various connective-tissue fibers, which increase the mechanical stability of the villous core. In addition, the villous core contains macrophages (Hofbauer cells) that are capable of producing a variety of growth factors regulating growth and differentiation of all villous components[132]. Moreover, they express the CD4 antigen[133] which functions as the membrane receptor for infection by human immunodeficiency virus. Virus accumulation within the Hofbauer cells has been described[134], and it has been proposed that HIV vertical transmission across the placenta may occur through direct cell–cell contacts between CD4 positive leukocytes such as T cells and Hofbauer cells and the placental trophoblast[135].

VILLOUS DEVELOPMENT

The importance of appreciating villous development is underscored by the significant alterations of the fetoplacental blood vessels, and villi, in the various forms of intrauterine growth restriction (IUGR) resulting from placental insufficiency. For a detailed review of placental villous and vascular development see Kaufmann et al.[136]. Five types of villi have been distinguished on the basis of their caliber, stromal characteristics and vessel structure (Fig. 7.7)[33,137–139].

1. *Stem villi*[33,138] represent the first 5–30 generations of unequal dichotomous branchings and serve to give mechanical support to the villous trees. They range from about 100 μm to several millimeters in diameter and are characterized

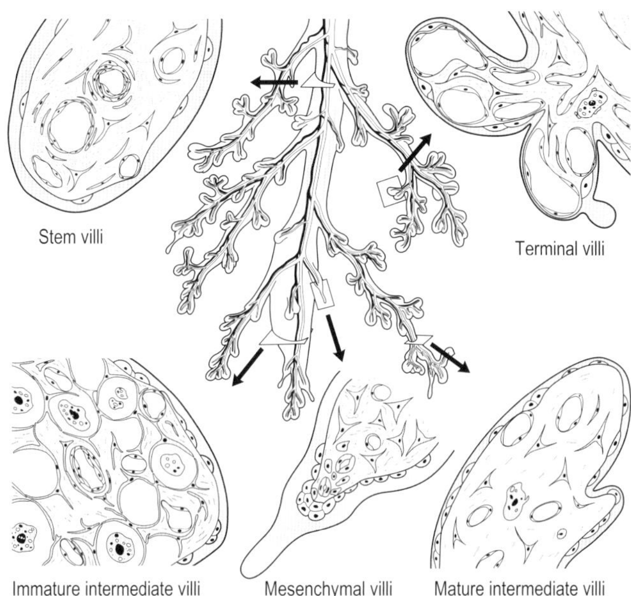

Fig. 7.7 Villous types. Simplified representation of a peripheral part of a mature placental villous tree, together with typical cross-sections of the various villous types. For details, see text. From Kaufmann[291], with permission.

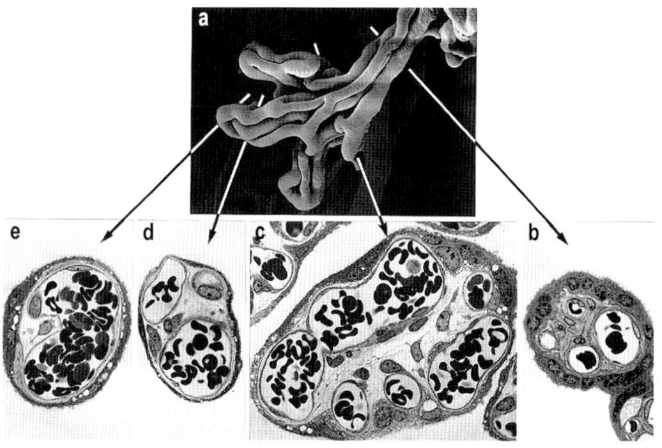

Fig. 7.8 Fetal vascularization of terminal villi. (a) Cast of vessels from a group of terminal villi. Corresponding semi-thin sections of the transition to a mature intermediate villus (b), the basis of the branching terminal villi (c), a single terminal villus near its tip (d), and a flat section of the terminal villous tip (e). These pictures demonstrate the structural variability of terminal villi; they all have in common that fetal capillaries and the highly dilated sinusoids amount to more than 50% of the stromal volume as long as postpartal collapse can be avoided by early fixation. ×300. From Kaufmann et al.[146], with permission.

by a compact fibrous stroma containing centrally located arteries or larger arterioles, and veins or venules.

2. *Mature intermediate villi*[138], ranging from 80 to 120 μm in diameter, arise from the ends of the last generation of stem villi. These are often gently curving and terminal villi arise at intervals from the convex aspects of their surface. Internally, they consist of a loose stromal core and, embedded within this, are narrow arterioles, characterized by a single layer of contractile cells leading into long capillaries.
3. *Terminal villi*[33,138] are the final branches of the villous tree and, from a physiological viewpoint, are the most important component. They are short stubby protuberances, up to 200 μm in length with a diameter of 50–100 μm, arising from the surface of mature intermediate villi. Their characterizing feature is the high degree of capillarization – more than 50% of terminal villous volume is represented by capillaries (Fig. 7.8).The thickness of the syncytiotrophoblast is not uniform over the terminal villous surface, rather, there are areas where the trophoblast is extremely attenuated, devoid of syncytial nuclei (Fig. 7.9), known as the 'vasculosyncytial membrane' (VSM). Underlying such areas are dilated segments of fetal capillaries, referred to as 'sinusoids', where the diffusional distance between maternal and fetal plasma is reduced to as little as 0.5–2.0 μm. The proportion of villous surface area occupied by VSM increases as gestational age advances towards term[139]. At other points on the villous surface, the syncytiotrophoblast is relatively thick containing clusters of syncytial nuclei. These are the most important sites of metabolic and endocrine activity.
4. *Immature intermediate villi*[138] represent peripheral continuations of stem villi that are in the process of development. Thus, while common in immature placentas, their distribution in the mature organ is generally limited to the central regions of the lobules, surrounding the central cavities, characteristically lacking terminal villi. These villi are recognized by the characteristically loose reticular meshwork in the stroma, in which numerous macrophages (Hofbauer cells) are found. Embedded among the stromal cells are arterioles and venules, confirming that these villi are the forerunners of stem villi. It is important that their presence in normal term pregnancy is recognized and that they are not incorrectly interpreted as edematous villi.

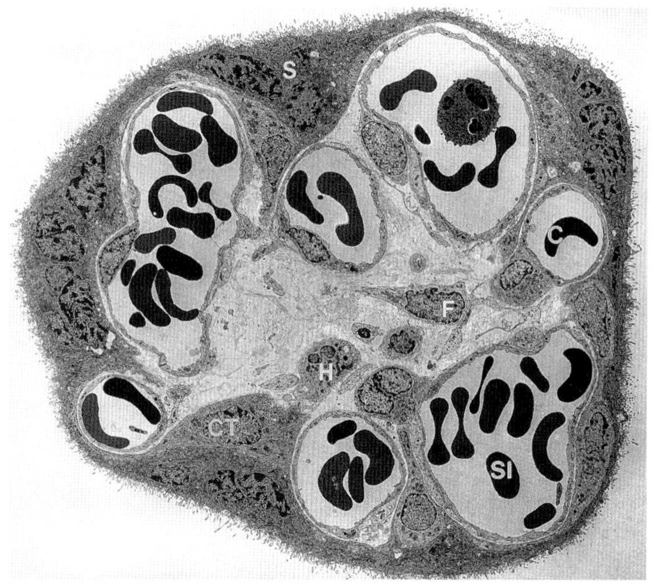

Fig. 7.9 Ultrastructure of the terminal villi. Electron micrograph of a terminal villus from a fully mature placenta showing capillaries (C) and sinusoids (SI). The sparse connective tissue is composed of macrophages (H) and fibroblasts (F). S = syncytiotrophoblast; CT = cytotrophoblastic cell. ×1400. From Becker et al.[292], with permission.

5. *Mesenchymal villi*[140]. This is again a transient population, seen predominantly in the earliest stages of pregnancy where these villi are the precursors of immature intermediate villi. In the more mature placenta, they are inconspicuous, usually situated at the surfaces of immature intermediate villi where they represent the points of villous sprouting and development.

The development of the villous tree starts by the formation of syncytial or trophoblastic sprouts; in early gestation these are seen arising in an apparently random pattern from the surfaces of mesenchymal and immature intermediate villi (IIV)[140,141]. These primary syncytiotrophoblastic sprouts are invaded centrally by cytotrophoblast, followed by a second central invasion by mesenchyme, to form secondary villi; the latter differentiates into stroma and capillaries resulting in tertiary (mesenchymal) villi. Most villi at the end of the first trimester are of this type. As development proceeds into the second trimester, mesenchymal villi transform into IIV[140]. New syncytial sprouts continue to form from the IIV until they themselves are transformed into terminally differentiated stem villi. Thus, growth of the placental villous trees is controlled by the activity of the IIV. This concept is important to appreciate because the clinical literature[142–144] erroneously refers to primary, secondary and tertiary stem villi; in truth, the number of generations of stem villi is variable, ranging from 5 to 30 generations, due to the local activity of the immature intermediate villi. This mechanism of placental villous growth is illustrated in Figure 7.10. By the onset of the third trimester, the immature villous types (mesenchymal and immature intermediate villi) have transformed into their mature counterparts (mature intermediate villi (MIV) and stem villi, respectively). The MIV are, by definition, the structure that makes the terminal villi, where gas exchange and nutrient transfer takes place, primarily across the 'vasculosyncytial membrane' – the functional structure of the placenta.

Formation of terminal villi is thought to be the result of stimulated capillary growth (Fig. 7.11)[145,146]. Within mature intermediate villi, arterioles give way to long slender capillaries. Under normal conditions, elongation of these capillaries is increased during the third trimester and exceeds that of the containing villi. As a result, capillary coils are formed, which protrude from the surface, raising an attenuated blister of trophoblast before them. In this way, terminal villi are formed, and the same capillary may run through several terminal villi in series before communicating with a venule. The degree of capillarization and formation of terminal villi is regulated by angiogenesis, and therefore indirectly by local oxygen partial pressure[146–149] and is summarized in Kingdom & Kaufmann[150]. The switch in differentiation pathways at the start of the third trimester is of key importance in placental development[137,140]. If this takes place too early, or is arrested, terminal villi will

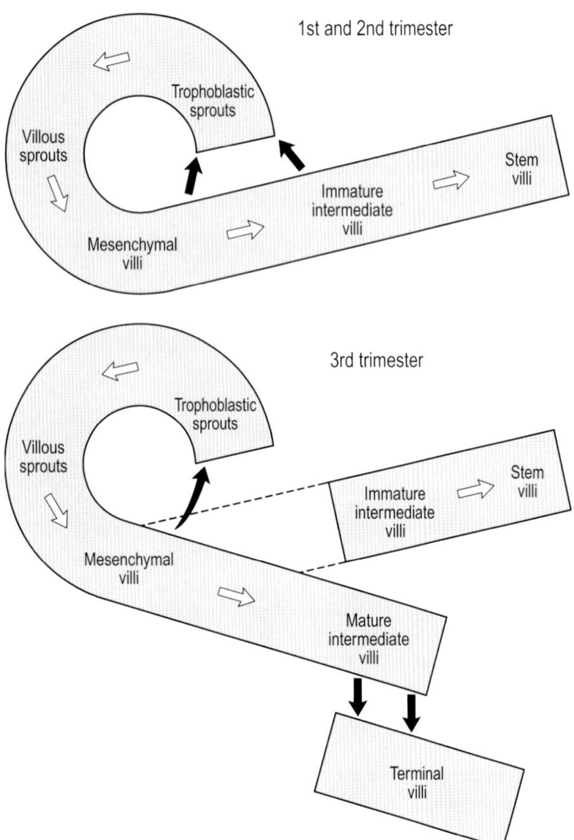

Fig. 7.10 Routes of villous development during early and late pregnancy. White arrows = transformation of one villous type into another. Black arrows = new production of villi or sprouts along the surface of other villi. Slightly modified from Castellucci et al.[140], with permission.

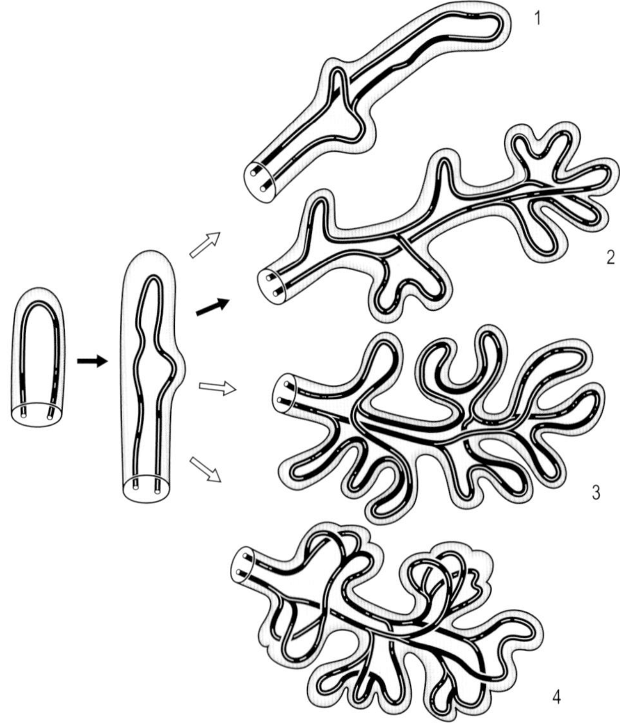

Fig. 7.11 Simplified diagram of the terminal villous development in relation to capillary growth. Varying degrees of imbalance between villous and capillary growth result in different types of terminal villous development, such as terminal villi deficiency (1), normal mature placenta (2), hypermaturity (3), and hypoxic hypervascularization, e.g. pre-eclampsia or maternal anemia (4), the conditions 1 and 3 are found e.g. in intrauterine growth restriction (IUGR) combined with absent end-diastolic flow velocities (AEDFV). From Kaufmann et al.[146], with permission.

not form in normal amounts[151], while overgrowth, as seen in chronic fetal anemia, will result in an excessively thick placenta, excessive trophoblast shedding and the mirror-syndrome form of pre-eclampsia[152]. These changes are discussed in the pathology section[7,150].

THE PLACENTAL BARRIER

Maternal and fetal blood are separated by the following layers (see Fig. 7.9):

1. *Syncytiotrophoblast*. This continuous layer of villous trophoblast does not possess any lateral cell borders and thus represents a single layer containing millions of nuclei and covering all villi of a single placenta. The syncytiotrophoblast represents the outermost layer of the placental villi and is the fetal layer in direct contact to maternal blood and blood cells.
2. *Cytotrophoblast*. The initially complete layer of mononucleated cytotrophoblast cells (first trimester) becomes discontinuous later during pregnancy (second and third trimester).
3. *Basement membrane*. The epithelial-like villous trophoblast rests on a basement membrane that is typically composed of laminins and collagen IV. This trophoblastic basement membrane may fuse with the basement membrane of the endothelium of the placental capillaries and sinusoids in the last trimester due to thinning of the stroma.
4. *Stromal connective tissue*. The basement membranes of trophoblast and capillaries are separated by connective tissue derived from the extraembryonic mesoderm.
5. *Fetal endothelium*. The cytoplasm of the endothelium becomes thinner in the third trimester, due to capillary loop sinusoid formation at the apex of terminal villi.

These changes gradually increase the conductance of the placenta to oxygen and permit exponential growth of the fetus in the third trimester[153]. The maternofetal diffusion distance, which is 50–100 μm in the first trimester, is eventually reduced to 4–5 μm at term by the following mechanisms[7]:

- The thickness of the villous trophoblast is reduced from 20 μm in early pregnancy to about 3.5 μm at term[7]. The vasculosyncytial membrane reduces this to 0.5–2.0 μm.
- At sites of the vasculosyncytial membrane cytotrophoblasts disappear and are found in niches where they do not disturb the diffusion and transport between the maternal and fetal blood system.
- Mean villous diameter decreases as the villi differentiate. In addition, the blood vessels inside the villi become demuscularized and reside directly under the trophoblast basement membrane.

INTEGRITY OF THE PLACENTAL BARRIER

Alpha-fetoprotein (AFP) is produced by the fetal liver. Its concentration in the fetal blood is 50 000 times higher than in the maternal blood due to the fact that the trophoblastic barrier is generally not permeable to proteins[137]. The introduction of mid-trimester maternal serum AFP screening programs for the detection of fetal spina bifida led to the observation that elevated levels of AFP (>2 multiples[163] of the median (MOM) value for gestation) with no associated fetal malformation had an increased risk of adverse outcomes such as pre-eclampsia, intrauterine growth restriction and antepartum fetal death[154]. The implication is that increased placental permeability may lead to impaired pregnancy outcome. Abnormal Doppler values[155] and/or abnormal placental shape[156] identify those at greatest risk of perinatal death and preterm delivery from placental damage. Villous repair following loss of trophoblast involves deposition of fibrin, and in vitro studies using horseradish peroxidase confirm these as sites of increased permeability, and so are responsible for the increased release of AFP into the maternal circulation[157]. In the normal term placenta, fibrin deposits that may be responsible for the passage of macromolecules cover approximately 7% of the villous surface.

Another paratrophoblastic transfer route for smaller molecules is provided by the transtrophoblastic channels, approximately 20 nm in diameter and seen only by electron microscopy[158–161]. These exist to allow transfer of water-soluble, lipophobic molecules with an effective molecular diameter <1.5 nm[160,161] and may be important for the regulation of fluid balance[137,162]. Under certain circumstances, such as fetal hydrops, increased fetal venous pressure, or reduced fetal oncotic pressure, these channels dilate such that not only water, but also fetal proteins, may pass into the maternal circulation[137,159].

PHYSIOLOGY OF FETOPLACENTAL BLOOD FLOW

Fetal size, and thus oxygen and nutritional demands, rapidly outstrip growth of the placenta such that by term, 1 g of placenta supports 6 g of fetus. In order to meet these demands, the peripheral villous placenta differentiates such that, by term, the proportion of descending aortic blood flow entering the umbilical arteries is increased to 40%[163] and the diffusive capacity is increased 10-fold[98]. These alterations are almost wholly dependent upon the exponential elaboration of terminal villi in the second half of pregnancy[110]. As in the uteroplacental circulation, which becomes 'denervated' by trophoblast, so the villous tree remains free of fetal autonomic influences and is dependent upon fetal cardiac output since it is devoid of nerves[130]. The fetoplacental circulation competes with the lower fetal body for aortic blood. The umbilical arteries receive this large proportion of descending aortic blood flow due to low impedance.

Doppler studies of the umbilical arteries indicate a progressive fall in fetoplacental vascular impedance, reflected by increasing end-diastolic flow velocity[164]. During the first trimester, end-diastolic velocities are absent[165], becoming consistently present by 14 weeks of gestation[166]. Thereafter, the steady rise in end-diastolic velocity parallels differentiation of the villous tree into its mature form[71]. The dramatic changes in peripheral capillarization of villi throughout pregnancy (see Fig 7.11), contribute to changes in umbilical artery blood flow, in addition to the local vasomotor regulatory process in muscularized stem villous arterioles[131].

Systemic vascular beds have a relatively short distance between arterioles and venules and these are bridged by many parallel capillaries, so that impedance/flow is regulated by autonomically innervated precapillary sphincters; these structures regulate blood flow across a wide range, for example in muscle that may exercise or rest. By contrast, fetoplacental blood flow must be constant, and ever increasing; the capillary bed of the peripheral villi is much longer than in muscle (2000–4000 μm), less richly branched, and is focally dilated into sinusoids within terminal villi (see Figs 7.8 and 7.11).

PLACENTAL PATHOLOGY OF IUGR AND PRE-ECLAMPSIA

The increasing use of Doppler studies as part of the fetal monitoring strategy in pregnancies affected by intrauterine growth restriction (IUGR) has contributed significantly to our understanding of the placental basis of this disease, stillbirth and pre-eclampsia. Severe early-onset IUGR may cause stillbirth, and is often associated with pre-eclampsia. The pathology of this condition, resulting in death or delivery before 32 weeks of gestation, is summarized in Figures 7.12 and 7.13[167].

Placental bed disease in IUGR and early onset pre-eclampsia

In our experience, around 85% of severe IUGR pregnancies with absent/reversed end-diastolic velocities in the umbilical arteries (AEDF) have bilateral abnormal uterine artery Doppler waveforms[3]. Similar abnormalities in uterine artery Doppler are found in early-onset severe pre-eclampsia, but not with mild disease near term[168]. Several investigators have performed direct-vision placental bed biopsies at cesarean section in severe IUGR/hypertensive patients, demonstrating an association between abnormal uterine artery Doppler and non-transformation of myometrial spiral artery segments[169,170]. The risk and severity of IUGR[171] and the severity of the uterine artery Doppler changes[172,173] correlate with the depth of interstitial extravascular trophoblast invasion. Clinicians use the term 'uteroplacental vascular insufficiency' to describe severe bilateral abnormal uterine Doppler, and the histologic findings represent varying combinations of the following features on H&E sections:

- Persistent muscularization of the spiral artery segments
- Lack of endovascular trophoblast
- Apoptosis of endovascular extravillous trophoblast
- A maternal leukocyte infiltrate, capable of inducing trophoblast apoptosis
- Atherosis and further narrowing of the vessel lumens
- Thrombosis in the spiral artery.

Collectively, these features are termed decidual vasculopathy by pathologists and are illustrated in Figure 7.13.

More recently, investigators have attempted to determine why the decidual penetration and transformation of muscularized spiral arteries by both interstitial and endovascular trophoblast is impaired. These pathways are summarized in Figure 7.4 and include:

- Interstitial trophoblast invasion occurs, but the cells surround non-transformed muscularized spiral artery segments – so-called 'peri-arterial' trophoblast[59]
- Interstital trophoblast may be unable to invade the arterial wall due to suppression of the required matrix-metalloproteinase (MMP3 & 7) enzymes[174]
- Endovascular trophoblast is patchy or absent within the lumen of spiral artery segments[35]
- Apoptosis events are increased in the endovascular trophoblast[56]
- Maternal leukocyte subpopulations infiltrate the placental bed and spiral arteries, where they inhibit trophoblast invasion via several mechanisms including:
  - Leukemia inhibitory factor (LIF)-mediated suppression of MMP3 & 7 expression via natural killer cells[174]
  - Macrophage-mediated trophoblast apoptosis via tryptophan depletion and tumor-necrosis factor alpha (TNFα)[60].

Though placental bed biopsy specimens can now be obtained following vaginal delivery using ultrasound-guided forceps[19], they remain in the research domain. Nevertheless, information regarding likely placental bed disease can be inferred from analysis of decidual spiral artery segments located in membrane rolls of decidua capsularis at delivery, or from samples of the decidua basalis, the base of the delivered placenta[175]. In an impressive study of 350 placentas from hypertensive women, vasculopathy changes were seen in 21%, more commonly in the decidua capsularis than parietalis[176]. Neither study related these pathologic findings to in-vivo uterine artery Doppler. A smaller cohort study of severe IUGR, in which 86% of pregnancies had abnormal uterine artery Doppler prior to delivery, this Doppler observation had a 51% positive predictive value for decidual vasculopathy in a membrane roll[3].

Pathology of the villous placenta in IUGR and pre-eclampsia

Consensus on the types of pathologic findings in the placenta from pregnancies complicated by pre-eclampsia and IUGR is gradually being achieved. First, this is due to better clinical methodology (distinguishing preterm from term disease and integrating uterine and umbilical artery Doppler in the clinical phenotype analysis[3,151] and second to the wider adoption of systematic random-block sampling that is a prerequisite for stereologic analysis of this notoriously heterogeneous organ[15]. Recent stereologic studies have established that there are no discernible alterations to villous morphology in the placenta from term deliveries of pre-eclamptic women[177] but that villous volume and structure are altered in IUGR pregnancies across gestation, even in the presence of pre-eclampsia[178]. The delivered portion of the placenta is affected by several factors including the host environment such as high altitude[179], maternal anemia[180] and from a reduced uteroplacental blood supply.

In severe IUGR cases with abnormal umbilical artery Doppler, stereologic studies demonstrate a significant reduction in gas-exchanging terminal villi[165], which can be seen using 3-dimensional scanning electron microscopy[151]. Therefore, severe forms of IUGR resulting in preterm delivery are associated with defective formation of the placental villi and a high perinatal loss rate[181] (see Fig. 7.12). A number of molecular pathways are known to regulate branching morphogenesis in the mammalian placenta and will become the focus of future research in human pathology as discussed below[182].

Uteroplacental vascular insufficiency is predicted to increase placental weight due to enhanced hypoxic angiogenesis[183]. This so-called 'chorio-angiosis' in placental villi is found in IUGR

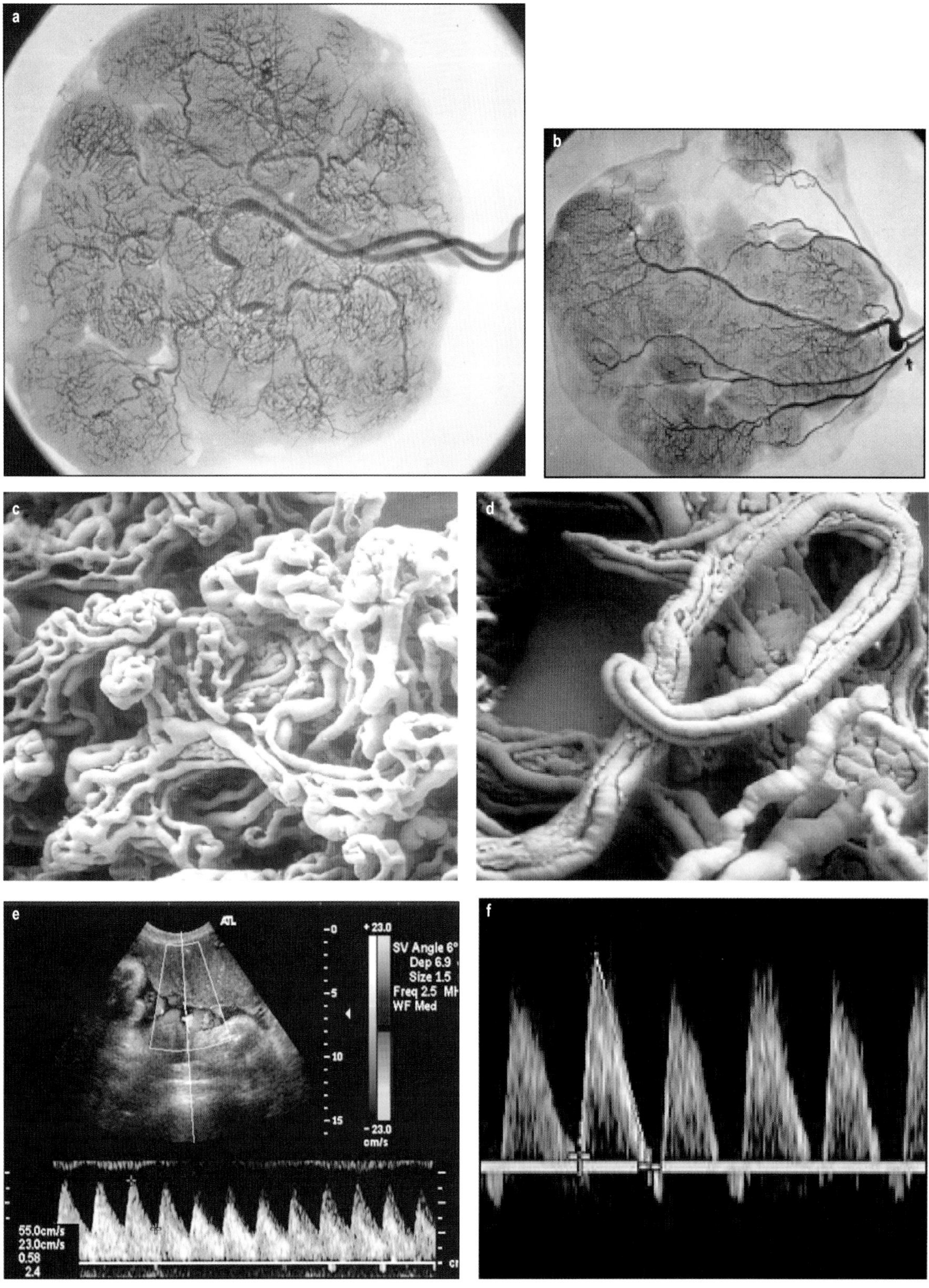

Fig 7.12 Abnormal terminal villus development and abnormal umbilical blood flows are characteristic of severe IUGR. (a) Radio-angiogram of a normal term placenta and (b) a severely growth restricted placenta showing chorionic villus regression resulting in an eccentric cord insertion in a small placental disk. (c) Scanning electron microscopy of casts from placental terminal capillaries, normal placenta show B a richly branched and looping capillary network, while IUGR placenta show B reduced numbers of long narrow straight capillaries (d). Umbilical artery Doppler waveforms from normal (e) and severely growth-restricted (f) pregnancies corresponding to (c) and (d) respectively. Note absent/reversed end-diastolic flow velocity in severe IUGR. (a) From Nordenvall M et al. 1991 Placental morphology in relation to umbilical artery blood velocity waveforms. *Eur J Obstet Gynecol Reprod Biol* **40**: 79–190. (b) from Viero S et al. 2004 Prognostic value of placental ultrasound in pregnancies complicated by absent end-diastolic flow velocity in the umbilical arteries. *Placenta* **25**:735–74, and (c) and (d) from Krebs C et al. 1996 Intrauterine growth restriction with absent end-diastolic flow velocity in the umbilical artery is associated with maldevelopment of the placental terminal villous tree. *Am J Obstet Gynecol* **175**:1534–1542, with permission.

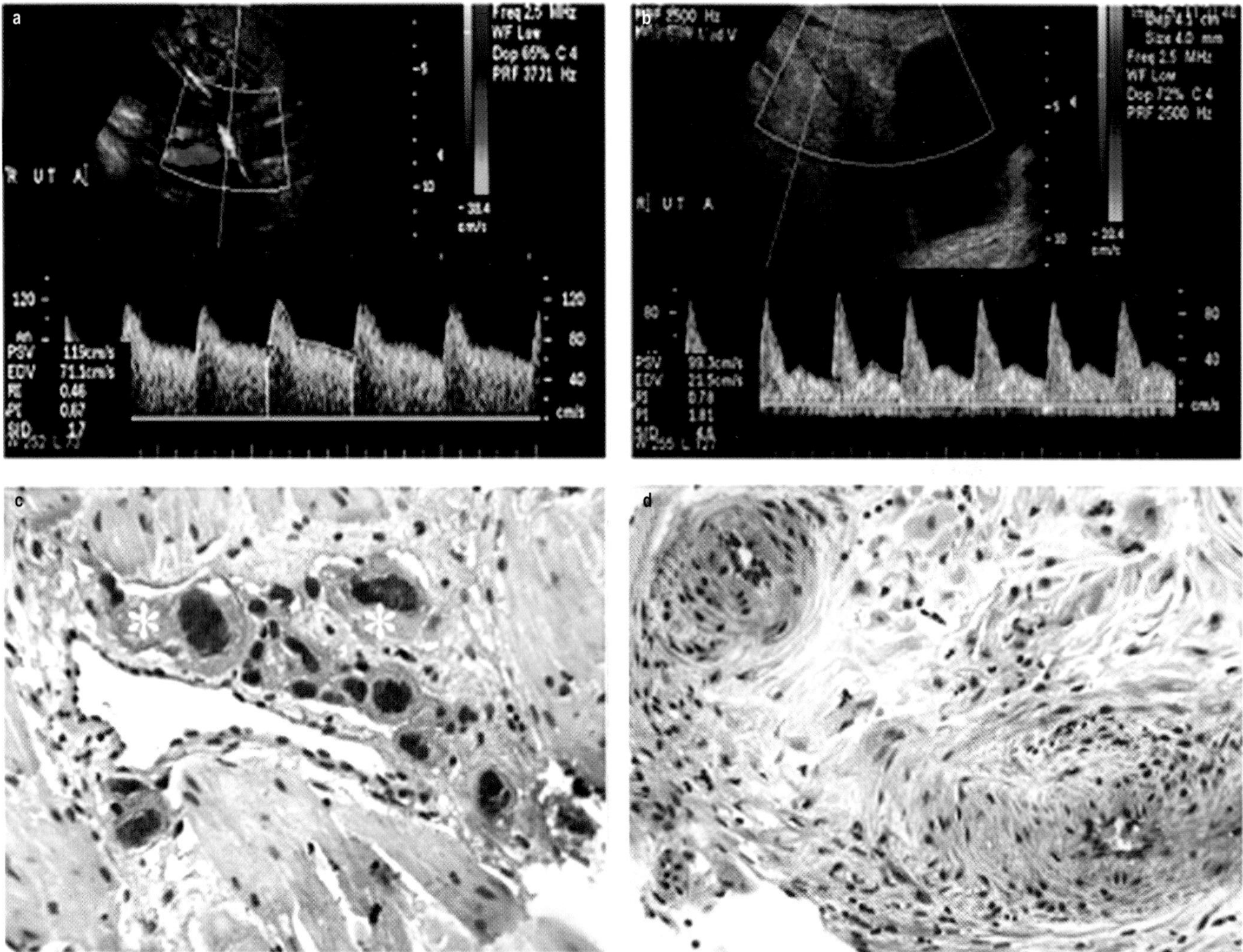

Fig 7.13 Normal and abnormal uterine Doppler waveforms and immunocytochemistry (ICC) of placental bed vessel. Uteroplacental vascular insufficiency correlates with failure of extra-villous trophoblast (EVT) to transform uterine vessels. (a) Normal uterine artery Doppler at 22 weeks' gestation (pulsatility index (PI) = 0.67). (b) Abnormal waveform (pulsatility index (PI) = 1.87) with early diastolic notching indicating uteroplacental vascular insufficiency. (c) Cytokeratin staining of multinucleated (*) EVT associated with a transformed spiral artery from a placental bed biopsy from a normal term. (d) H&E staining of a pathological placental bed biopsy showing a non-transformed spiral artery. With thanks to Dr Sarah Keating, Dept of Pathology, Mt Sinai Hospital, Toronto, Canada.

pregnancies[184] that have persistent end-diastolic velocities in the umbilical arteries up until delivery[184]. This mechanism of adaptive villous angiogenesis appears to fail in high-risk pregnancies with abnormal uterine artery Doppler. In a prospective cohort study of placentas from pregnancies with abnormal uterine artery Doppler, 74% weighed <10th centile for gestation[106]. One explanation for this excess risk of a small-for-dates placenta may be regression of parts of the chorion frondosum that develops into the definitive placenta, leaving an eccentric or velamentous cord insertion[3,185].

In pre-eclamptic pregnancies, the apoptotic release of syncytiotrophoblast material into the maternal circulation is altered in that the release shifts from apoptosis towards non-apoptotic mechanisms[116,186], including necrosis and aponecrosis[187]. It is hypothesized that the release of necrotic and/or aponecrotic syncytial material triggers the endothelial damage and activation typically found in pre-eclampsia[188]. In this situation, no longer sealed membrane fragments releasing cell-free molecules may circulate freely and pass the capillaries of the lung[124] thereby inducing a systemic inflammatory response of the mother.

Placentas from women with early-onset pre-eclampsia being affected by IUGR as well also have increased rates of ischemic-thrombotic disease, such as villous infarction[189]. In this mixture of syndromes, the extent of the pathologies correlates with prior documentation of abnormal uterine artery Doppler[190,191]. Other lesions compromising gas exchange across villi, such as intervillous thrombosis[176] and perivillous fibrin deposition[106] are also prevalent in underperfused placentas, as areas of chorio-angiosis (excessive villous vascularization in response to local hypoxia)[176] that are an attempt to improve gas exchange. The severity of the placental pathology of severe IUGR is thus variable and comprises a spectrum of developmental defects and progressive ischemic-thrombotic vascular damage to the remaining villous tissues[167].

A final pathologic process that mediates abnormal umbilical artery blood flow is damage to the fetoplacental vascular endothelium since local endocrine, paracrine and flow-dependent vasodilator mechanisms operate in the fetoplacental vasculature[131]. Many of these systems are abnormal in severe IUGR and appear to be intrinsically abnormal, as opposed to being influenced by factors in maternal blood[192]. Recent data suggest that growth factors, such as trophoblast-derived vascular endothelial growth factor (VEGF), induce local fetoplacental vasodilation and that this effect is reduced by 50% in IUGR pregnancies[193]. Selective extraction of microvascular endothelium from the IUGR placenta reveals increased expression of the following that indicate endothelial injury: intercellular adhesion molecule-1 and platelet endothelial cell adhesion molecule-1[194], fibroblast growth factor receptor-1 (FGFR-1) and its transcription factor early growth response factor-1 (Egr-1) expression[195]. When each of these pathologic processes acts in concert, the reduction in fetoplacental blood flow is manifested as absent/reversed end-diastolic flow velocity (ARED) in the umbilical arteries. An appreciation of the pathology helps to understand why umbilical artery Doppler surveillance is so important in high-risk, IUGR and pre-eclamptic pregnancies since perinatal mortality will be reduced as a result of selective intensive monitoring of the subset identified with ARED in the umbilical arteries[196]. The prospective risk of ARED occurring in high-risk women with abnormal uterine artery Doppler is significant (30%)[106].

PRENATAL DIAGNOSIS OF PLACENTAL INSUFFICIENCY

The possibility of making a useful diagnosis of placental insufficiency, as opposed to merely IUGR in the fetus and/or pre-eclampsia in the mother, arises as a result of appreciating the developmental and vascular pathology found in these overlapping conditions. Interest in placental imaging has grown rapidly in the past decade and is recently reviewed[197].

As a single screening test for adverse perinatal outcomes, uterine artery Doppler performs poorly in low-risk[198] and in unselected women[199]. The screening test characteristics for pre-eclampsia are improved by the incorporation of maternal characteristics[200]. More recently, the wider implications of abnormal uterine artery Doppler, such as the potential for preventing preterm stillbirth[201] underscores the broader concept of making a prenatal diagnosis of placental insufficiency, as opposed to individual placenta-specific diseases. Useful adjuncts to uterine artery Doppler include maternal serum biochemistry tests for Down's syndrome and spina bifida[167] and a simple description of placental morphology[156]. Significant reassurance can be given to apparently high-risk women when all 3 tests (biochemistry, morphology and uterine artery Doppler) are normal in the window 19–23 weeks[2]. In the last few years, testing maternal blood using biochemical markers has led to an increased power of prediction for pregnancies at risk[4–6].

Sceptics of the rationale of placental function testing cite either the lack of any treatment modalities to improve perinatal outcome, or the possibility that the program identifies pregnancies with such severe disease that the most important intervention (timed delivery by cesarean section or induction of labor in the fetal interest) is inappropriate. At present, no study of anticoagulant drugs, to prevent secondary thrombotic injury to ischemic villi, has shown any benefit. In a large randomized controlled trial of 19950 unselected women, the selective prescription of low-dose aspirin to those with abnormal uterine artery Doppler conferred no benefit[202]. The more potent drug heparin has to date been very poorly researched, with only 2 small cohort studies and one small pilot randomized controlled trial meeting basic methodology to date[203]. However, in vitro studies have shown a beneficial effect of heparin on placental viability[203–205].

Further studies of heparin in women with multiparameter placental dysfunction are in progress to meet the challenge that we need a therapeutic option for such women. In the meantime, several clinical options, including selective involvement of a high-risk obstetrician, education about pre-eclampsia, increased ultrasound-based fetal monitoring and selective use of corticosteroids to enhance fetal lung maturation, are legitimate activities that can improve maternal–fetal outcome.

MOLECULAR CONTROL OF TROPHOBLAST AND ENDOTHELIAL DIFFERENTIATION

As discussed in the sections above, successful placental development is largely dependent on the tightly coordinated proliferation and differentiation of both trophoblast and endothelial cells to establish the richly branched and specialized structures of the mature villous tree and the uteroplacental circulation. Over the past two decades, our understanding of the underlying molecular mechanisms that control these events has improved, largely due to data from mouse knock out studies[206]. Increasing evidence suggests that the effects may converge upon placental villous development via oxygen-sensitive factors such as hypoxia-inducible factor-1 (HIF-1)[207]. Other molecular mediators including basic helix loop helix transcription factors and growth factors have been shown to play an important role in placental development and their deregulation is associated with the placental pathologies. Good molecular evidence now exists to support the concept of dysregulation of oxygen-sensing molecules such as HIF1α[208]; that in turn not only enhance villous angiogenesis[150] but upregulate the production of soluble Flt-1 leading to endothelial cell damage[207]. In the following sections we will give a brief overview of some of these factors.

Transcription factors in trophoblast differentiation

The basic helix loop helix (bHLH) transcription factors (including, mammalian achaete-scute homologue 2 (Mash-2)/Hash-2, Glial cell missing-1 (Gcm-1), Stra13, E-factor, NeuroD1/NeuroD2 and Id genes) are expressed in the human placenta and, as in the mouse placenta, are dynamically regulated during differentiation of trophoblast cells[209–212]. For example, in the mouse, Gcm-1 is specifically expressed at the time of chorionic fusion and early labyrinth development and knock out of Gcm-1 leads to embryonic death by day 10.5[210,213]. We have similarly shown in the human placenta that Gcm-1 is expressed in the daughter cytotrophoblasts that are committed to syncytial fusion and that inhibition of Gcm-1 prevents trophoblast cell–cell fusion[209,214]. We have also shown that Gcm-1 is implicated in the differentiation of cytotrophoblast to invasive extravillous trophoblast suggesting that it is a key molecular mediator of trophoblast cell cycle arrest in both pathways of differentiation[214]. Interestingly, Gcm-1 levels are decreased in placentas from pre-eclamptic patients[215] and in severe IUGR[216], and we have suggested that this decrease may account for the disturbances in the trophoblast turnover, increased syncytial shedding and uteroplacental placental pathology seen in these cases[217]. Furthermore, a recent study has implicated another transcription factor, namely STOX1, a winged helix domain protein, in the development of pre-eclampsia and has shown that missense mutations in STOX1 cosegregate with pre-eclampsia and follow matrilineal inheritance in a Dutch population[218]. These authors also showed that STOX1A is restricted to the polyploid extravillous trophoblast and suggest a defect in extravillous trophoblast polyploidization and differentiation may account for the failure of the extravillous trophoblast to remodel the uterine vasculature in these cases[218].

Role of the growth factors in placental development

Many growth factors and cytokines have been shown to play a biological role in placental development. Some of those that play a dual role in cytotrophoblast cell fusion, trophoblast invasion and/or placental angiogenesis and whose expression levels have been shown to be altered in pathological pregnancies are detailed below.

Hepatocyte growth factor

The hepatocyte growth factor (HGF) is a potent mitogen and has been shown to stimulate dissociation and mobility of epithelial cells[219]. In the placenta, HGF promotes trophoblast migration and invasion but does not effect cellular proliferation[220,221]. HGF is produced by the chorionic mesenchyme and acts in a paracrine fashion through its receptor, c-met, which is expressed by cytotrophoblast[222,223]. HGF effects extravillous trophoblast cell mobility by stimulating an increase in nitric oxide (NO) production[220] through the induction of inducible nitric oxide synthase (iNOS) via both PI 3-k Kinase and MAPK pathways[224]. Extravillous trophoblast express two isoforms of nitric oxide sythase, iNOS[225] and the constitutively expressed endothelial NOS (eNOS)[226]; both have been shown to be involved in the migration of extravillous trophoblast, though at present the mechanism for this effect is not known. A potential deregulation of the HGF system is suggested in severe IUGR with reports of the HGF expression in the villous mesenchyme of the placenta being decreased in IUGR[227] while its cmet receptor is increased[228].

Insulin-like growth factor (IGF) family

The majority of studies into the effect of IGF family members on trophoblast phentoype support their role in promoting trophoblast invasion and not proliferation. IGF-II induces trophoblast invasion by stimulating trophoblast migration through the direct binding to the type-2 IGF receptor (IGF-R2), also called the mannose-6-phosphate receptor, and subsequent signaling through the MAPK pathway. This effect was achieved independently of insulin-like growth factor binding protein (IGFBP) binding[229,230]. Members of the insulin-like growth factor family have been identified throughout the tissues at the maternal/fetal interface. Studies have shown that the placenta produces the IGF proteins while the binding proteins are secreted by the decidua. While both IGF-1 and IGF-II localize to trophoblast cells, only IGF-II exhibits a differential pattern of expression with higher levels detected in extravillous trophoblast at the invading front of the cell column[231].

Similarly, all IGFBPs are expressed in the decidua, but IGFBP-1 is expressed most abundantly and at sites adjacent to the invading extravillous trophoblast, which express IGF-II. In early pregnancy, epithelial cells of the endometrial glands and some early decidual stromal cells first express IGFBP-1; within a few weeks following the establishment of pregnancy, all decidual stromal cells secrete IGFBP-1[232]. While both IGF-II and IGFBP-1 were shown to affect trophoblast invasiveness, several studies have established that they accomplish this independently of each other[229,233]. Interestingly, IGFBP-1 levels in maternal plasma were observed to be lower during early pregnancy in women destined to become pre-eclamptic than normal controls[234]. The lower levels of IGFBP-1 during the period of early placentation may result in a decreased migration stimulus to extravillous trophoblast and consequently to hypoinvasion of the uterine tissues and a failed uteroplacental vascular transformation.

Transforming growth factor β family

The transforming growth factor (TGF)-β family is comprised of three related proteins, TGF-β1, -2 and -3. Many studies have demonstrated that these proteins exert anti-proliferative, anti-migratory and anti-invasive effects on extravillous trophoblast by restricting their differentiation along the invasive pathway. At the maternal/fetal interface, TGF-β proteins are produced predominantly by the decidua and localize to the decidual ECM[235], however they exhibit an intriguing pattern of expression in extravillous trophoblast. Here, TGF-β1 and TGF-β2 mRNA are expressed at constant levels throughout the first trimester but, TGF-β3 levels, which are expressed at very low levels during the 5th–6th weeks of gestation, increase between the 7th and 8th weeks of gestation before dropping off at 9 weeks, corresponding to the increase in placental pO_2 at this time[236]. Pre-eclampsia is associated with a failure to downregulate TGF-β3 and this may in part account for the insufficient uterine invasion characteristic of the disease[236]. Several mechanisms have been elaborated to account for TGF-β–mediated suppression of extravillous trophoblast invasion:

- TGF-β inhibits the total gelatinolytic activity and MMP-9 activity of trophoblast cells[237] upregulates TIMP-1[238,239] and plasminogen activator inhibitor (PAI)-1, and downregulates uPA[240,241], thus decreasing the invasive capacity of the extravillous trophoblast.
- TGF-β2 upregulates α_1, α_3, α_5, α_v integrin expression on trophoblast leading to increased adhesiveness and decreased extravillous trophoblast migration[48].
- TGF-β1 enhances differentiation of invasive extravillous trophoblast into multinucleated, non-migratory cells[242].
- TGF-β3 inhibits trophoblast invasion along the invasive pathway and prevents expression of invasive-extravillous trophoblast markers[236,243].
- TGF-β1 inhibits the invasion-promoting effects of HGF (discussed above) by preventing HGF-induction of iNOS[244].

The effects of TGF-β on trophoblast differentiation are mediated through the oxygen-regulated transcription factor, HIF-1α. This regulatory mechanism seems to ensure that trophoblast proliferation is maximal while invasion is restricted until the oxygen level in the intervillous space rises at approximately 9 weeks' gestation[243]. In addition, the inhibitory effects of TGF-β1 and –β2 require co-expression with their co-receptor protein endoglin[245]. Interestingly, a recent publication has described the identification of a soluble isoform of endoglin and shown that its levels are increased in the maternal serum of pre-eclamptic patients[246]. These authors further showed that treatment of pregnant rats with sol-endoglin induced vascular permeability and hypertension similar to the changes seen in the maternal vasculature of pre-eclamptic patients[246]. A further study has shown elevated sol-endoglin as early as 17 weeks' gestation in pre-eclamptic patients making this a potential biomarker for early diagnosis of this disease[247].

Epidermal growth factor family

The epidermal growth factor (EGF) family includes more than 10 proteins that bind the EGF receptor (HER) group of tyrosine kinase receptors including EGF, heparin-binding (HB)-EGF, transforming growth factor (TGF)α, amphiregulin (AR), epiregulin (EPR) and betacellulin (BTC)[248]. Many of these EGF ligands are expressed in the placental and decidual tissues and the HER isoforms have been detected on trophoblast cells indicating that they are capable of responding to stimulation by EGF family ligands. The following sections review the research that has established a role for EGF family ligands in trophoblast differentiation and invasion.

HER expression in trophoblast

EGF family ligands have been shown to have different effects on different trophoblast populations[249]. This has been attributed to the differential expression of their receptors, the HER proteins, on trophoblast cells. Many studies have demonstrated that the HER proteins are expressed by every trophoblast subtype, for example, the cytotrophoblast express high levels of HER-1[249,250]. Within the extravillous trophoblast lineage, HER-1 protein is expressed by proliferative extravillous trophoblast of the proximal cell column and not by invasive extravillous trophoblast. However, as extravillous trophoblast differentiate to the invasive phenotype, there is a switch in HER expression such that the HER-2 protein is expressed by the non-proliferative invasive extravillous trophoblast in the distal portion of the cell columns and the interstitial extravillous trophoblast, while HER-1 expression disappears. The precise spatial segregation of HER proteins suggests that HER-1 may be important for cellular proliferation, while HER-2 may be involved in extravillous trophoblast invasion into the maternal decidua[250,251]. Interestingly, amplification of HER-2 occurs in many adenocarcinomas and studies have demonstrated that it induces a higher metastatic potential by promoting adhesion and invasion steps in the metastatic cascade[250,252].

Epidermal growth factor

EGF has been shown to mediate many activities in trophoblast cells from differentiation of cytotrophoblast to syncytiotrophoblast[253,254] to proliferation of cytotrophoblast[255]. Within the extravillous trophoblast cell lineage, EGF does not stimulate cell division[256], but has been implicated in the process of differentiation from the proliferative to invasive phenotype[254,256]. The means by which EGF induces extravillous trophoblast differentiation remain unclarified, although it is likely to involve the induction of genes for MMPs[257], the deterioration of adhesive cell surface molecules and activation of integrin-dependent cell migration[258,259]. Indeed, we have shown that EGF down regulates Cx40, a marker of the proliferative extravillous trophoblast and we suggest that this is a prerequisite for the initiation of extravillous trophoblast invasion[260].

Transforming growth factor-α

TGF-α, previously referred to as sarcoma growth factor, shares a 30% sequence homology to EGF and binds and activates the same complement of HERs[261,262], however, there are distinguishable differences in their biological activities[263–265] which have been attributed to their binding different sites on the HER-1 ectodomain[265]. TGF-α treatment of cultured first-trimester trophoblast stimulated the proliferation and growth of these cells[249,266].

Heparin-binding epidermal growth factor

HB-EGF is a member of the EGF family that can bind both HER-1 and HER-4 and therefore can activate a broader spectrum of HER dimers than either EGF or TGF-α[248,267]. In the placenta, HB-EGF has been shown to maintain the invasive phenotype of extravillous trophoblast; furthermore, it may also play a role in uterine vascular remodeling[268] and the differentiation to the non-invasive vascular phenotype of endovascular extravillous trophoblast[269]. Direct evidence from placental explant studies has confirmed that HB-EGF treatment enhances extravillous trophoblast differentiation along the invasive pathway while treatment of the trophoblast cell line HTR-8/SVneo did not effect cellular proliferation but, rather, initiated integrin switching characteristic of extravillous trophoblast differentiation[270]. HB-EGF is expressed during early pregnancy by the decidua (stromal cells and blood vessel endothelium), cytotrophoblast and extravillous trophoblast[269]. Interestingly, expression of HB-EGF was highest during the first 8 weeks of pregnancy suggesting that its expression may be induced by hypoxia[269]. This observation coupled with evidence that HB-EGF exerts cytoprotective effects on organs and prevents low oxygen-induced cell death in a kidney-ischemia reperfusion model[271] indicate that it may also protect trophoblast from low oxygen damage during the first trimester of pregnancy[269]. Moreover, reports have recently emerged indicating HB-EGF expression is fivefold lower in pre-eclamptic patients compared with controls[272,273] suggesting impaired trophoblast invasion, accelerated cell death and failed arterial remodeling may be caused by HB-EGF deficiency in some cases of pre-eclampsia.

Vascular endothelial and angiopoietin growth factor families

Recently, much placental research has focused on the roles and regulation of the angiogenic growth factors vascular endothelial growth factor (VEGF), placenta growth factor (PlGF) and the angiopoietins 1 and 2 during human placental development[274]. The diametric expression of these factors in the human trophoblast, together with the demonstration that their functional receptors (VEGFR1 (flt-1) and 2 (KDR) and Tie-2) are expressed by both trophoblast and endothelial cells support a key role for these factors during placental development[275–278]. In addition to their potent angiogenic effects VEGF, PlGF and angiopoietin 2, have all been demonstrated to affect trophoblast function by promoting the proliferation of cytotrophoblast cells and extravillous trophoblast[277,279–281] while angiopoietin 1 was shown to increase extravillous trophoblast migration[277]. Moreover, VEGF expression is upregulated by hypoxic induction of HIF1α[282], thus supporting an important role for this growth factor for promoting trophoblast proliferation in the first weeks of pregnancy. The high expression levels of VEGF and angiopoetin-1 during early placental development characterized by high levels of trophoblast and endothelial cell proliferation, proposes that these factors play a fundamental role stimulating the rapid proliferation and differentiation of trophoblast and endothelial cells during the formation of the richly branched mesenchymal and immature intermediate villi.

PlGF and angiopoietin-2 expression levels increase as gestation progresses to term correlating with the increase in placental pO_2 at this time and the observed effects of hypoxia on PlGF expression in term trophoblast[281]. During the second and third trimester of placental development, the mesenchymal villous differentiation changes to form the mature intermediate and terminal villi. Thus, it has been suggested that the increase in these factors during later gestation may play a definitive role in modulating the change from branching to non-branching angiogenesis.

The first molecular evidence for the hypothesis of 'placental hyperoxia' in severe IUGR[150] was provided by the observation that levels of placental PlGF increase in severe IUGR placentas[281]. Moreover, it has been reported that the pO_2 of uterine venous blood behind the placenta is higher in cases of severe IUGR compared with control cases[283]. Levels of angiopoietin-2 are also reported to decrease in severe IUGR, suggesting that these factors may contribute to the accelerated maturation of the fetal vasculature, poor terminal villous development and disturbances in rate of cytotrophoblast proliferation and syncytial formation associated with severe IUGR[277].

More recently, many groups have documented the hypoxic mediated upregulation of an alternatively spliced soluble form of flt1 (sol-Flt1)[207] and a corresponding decrease in PlGF in the maternal plasma of severe pre-eclamptic pregnancies[284–286]. These authors suggest that this naturally occurring antagonist of VEGF and PlGF function may cause the maternal endothelial cell damage seen in these cases[287]. A systematic review of the literature to date has concluded that, while these data from patients later than 25 weeks provide evidence for the etiology of the syndrome, its use as a screening tool in the first and second trimesters is unproven[286], although a recent study has suggested that in combination with sol-endoglin it may perform better[247]. More recently, a similar increase in sol-Flt1 has been reported in severe IUGR placentas[288], though to date inconsistent results in maternal serum have been reported[284,289] possibly due to the heterogeneity and severity of the condition of IUGR in these cases.

CONCLUDING REMARKS

We hope the reader has appreciated the clinical relevance of human placental development. A wide range of important clinical problems such as adult cardiac disease, have their origins in placental maldevelopment and pathology. Increasing interest in placental research and important contributions by clinicians, especially collaboration to obtain Doppler and real-time ultrasound information of the placenta just prior to delivery, has led to important advances in our understanding of the pathological basis of placental insufficiency syndromes that cause stillbirth and premature death. In the near future, we predict a more widespread acceptance among maternal–fetal medicine clinicians of the value of making a prenatal diagnosis of placental insufficiency, and as a direct consequence, advances in the therapeutic options for at risk women.

REFERENCES

1. Alkazaleh F, Viero S, Simchen M et al. Ultrasound diagnosis of severe thrombotic placental damage in the second trimester: an observational study. *Ultrasound Obstet Gynecol* **23**:472–476, 2004.
2. Toal M, Chan C, Fallah S et al. Usefulness of a placental profile in high-risk pregnancies. *Am J Obstet Gynecol* **196**:363 e1–7, 2007.
3. Viero S, Chaddha V, Alkazaleh F et al. Prognostic value of placental ultrasound in pregnancies complicated by absent end-diastolic flow velocity in the umbilical arteries. *Placenta* **25**:735–741, 2004.
4. Spencer K, Cowans NJ, Chefetz I, Tal J, Kuhnreich I, Meiri H. Second-trimester uterine artery Doppler pulsatility index and maternal serum PP13 as markers of pre-eclampsia. *Prenat Diagn* **27**:258–263, 2007.
5. Cowans NJ, Spencer K. First-trimester ADAM12 and PAPP-A as markers for intrauterine fetal growth restriction through their roles in the insulin-like growth factor system. *Prenat Diagn* **27**:264–271, 2007.
6. Spencer K, Cowans NJ, Chefetz I, Tal J, Meiri H. First-trimester maternal serum PP-13, PAPP-A and second-trimester uterine artery Doppler pulsatility index as markers of pre-eclampsia. *Ultrasound Obstet Gynecol* **29**:128–134, 2007.
7. Benirschke K, Kaufmann P. *Pathology of the Human Placenta*. New York: Springer-Verlag, 2006.
8. Knobil E, Neill J. *Knobil and Neill's Physiology of Reproduction*. London: Elsevier Science & Technology, 2005.
9. Torpin R. *The Human Placenta*. Springfield, Il: Charles C Thomas, 1969.
10. Liu CC, Pretorius DH, Scioscia AL, Hull AD. Sonographic prenatal diagnosis of marginal placental cord insertion: clinical importance. *J Ultrasound Med* **21**:627–632, 2002.
11. Jauniaux E, Ramsay B, Campbell S. Ultrasonographic investigation of placental morphologic characteristics and size during the second trimester of pregnancy. *Am J Obstet Gynecol* **170**:130–137, 1994.
12. Oyelese Y, Smulian JC. Placenta previa, placenta accreta, and vasa previa. *Obstet Gynecol* **107**:927–941, 2006.
13. Schuhmann K. Plazenton: Begriff, Entstehung, funktionelle Anatomie. In *Die Plazenta des Menschen*, V Becker, TH Schiebler, F Kubli (eds), pp. 199–207. Stuttgart: Thieme Verlag, 1981.
14. Zimmermann P, Eirio V, Koskinen J, Kujansuu E, Ranta T. Doppler assessment of the uterine and uteroplacental circulation in the second trimester in pregnancies at high risk for pre-eclampsia and/or intrauterine growth retardation: comparison and correlation between different Doppler parameters. *Ultrasound Obstet Gynecol* **9**:330–338, 1997.
15. Mayhew TM. Stereology and the placenta: where's the point? – a review. *Placenta* **27**(Suppl A): S17–25, 2006.
16. Egbor M, Ansari T, Morris N, Green CJ, Sibbons PD. Morphometric placental villous and vascular abnormalities in early- and late-onset pre-eclampsia with and without fetal growth restriction. *Br J Obstet Gynaecol* **113**:580–589, 2006.
17. Kim YM, Chaiworapongsa T, Gomez R et al. Failure of physiologic transformation of the spiral arteries in the placental bed in preterm premature rupture of

membranes. *Am J Obstet Gynecol* **187**:1137–1142, 2002.

18. Lyall F. The human placental bed revisited. *Placenta* **23**:555–562, 2002.
19. Robson SC, Simpson H, Ball E, Lyall F, Bulmer JN. Punch biopsy of the human placental bed. *Am J Obstet Gynecol* **187**:1349–1355, 2002.
20. Ball E, Bulmer JN, Ayis S, Lyall F, Robson SC. Late sporadic miscarriage is associated with abnormalities in spiral artery transformation and trophoblast invasion. *J Pathol* **208**:535–542, 2006.
21. Wigglesworth JS. Vascular organization of the human placenta. *Nature* **216**:1120–1121, 1967.
22. Schuhmann R, Wehler V. Histological differences of placental villi within materno-fetal circulation units. Contribution to the functional morphology of the placenta. *Arch Gynakol* **210**:425–439, 1971.
23. Ramsey EM, Corner GW Jr, Donner MW. Serial and cineradioangiographic visualization of maternal circulation in the primate (hemochorial) placenta. *Am J Obstet Gynecol* **86**:213–225, 1963.
24. Borell U, Fernstrom I, Westman A. Eine arteriographische Studie des Plazentarkreilaufs. *Geburtshilfe Frauenheilhd* **18**:1–9, 1958.
25. Konje JC, Huppertz B, Bell SC, Taylor DJ, Kaufmann P. 3-dimensional colour power angiography for staging human placental development. *Lancet* **362**:199–1201, 2003.
26. Moll W. Physiologie der maternen plazentaren Durchblutung. In *Die Plazenta des Menschen*, V Becker, TH Schiebler, F Kubli (eds), pp. 172–194. Stuttgart: Thiem, 1981.
27. McDermott M, Gillan JE. Chronic reduction in fetal blood flow is associated with placental infarction. *Placenta* **16**:165–170, 1995.
28. Kunath T, Strumpf D, Rossant J. Early trophoblast determination and stem cell maintenance in the mouse – a review. *Placenta* **25** Suppl A:S32-38, 2004.
29. Quinn J, Kunath T, Rossant J. Mouse trophoblast stem cells. *Methods Mol Med* **121**:125–148, 2006.
30. Simmons DG, Cross JC. Determinants of trophoblast lineage and cell subtype specification in the mouse placenta. *Dev Biol* **284**:12–24, 2005.
31. McLennan JE. Implications of the eccentricity of the human umbilical cord. *Am J Obstet Gynecol* **101**:1124–1130, 1968.
32. Jauniaux E, Englert Y, Vanesse M, Hiden M, Wilkin P. Pathologic features of placentas from singleton pregnancies obtained by in vitro fertilization and embryo transfer. *Obstet Gynecol* **76**:61–64, 1990.
33. Boyd JD, Hamilton WJ. *The Human Placenta*. Cambridge: Heffer, 1970.
34. Potgens AJ, Schmitz U, Bose P, Versmold A, Kaufmann P, Frank HG. Mechanisms of syncytial fusion: a review. *Placenta* **23** Suppl A:S107–113, 2002.
35. Kaufmann P, Black S, Huppertz B. Endovascular trophoblast invasion: implications for the pathogenesis of intrauterine growth retardation and preeclampsia. *Biol Reprod* **69**:1–7, 2003.
36. Pijnenborg R, Bland JM, Robertson WB, Brosens I. Uteroplacental arterial changes related to interstitial trophoblast migration in early human pregnancy. *Placenta* **4**:397–413, 1983.
37. Kaufmann P, Castellucci M. Extravillous trophoblast in the human placenta. *Trophoblast Res* **10**:21–65, 1997.
38. Frank HG, Malekzadeh F, Kertschanska S et al. Immunohistochemistry of two different types of placental fibrinoid. *Acta Anat (Basel)* **150**:55–68, 1994.
39. Feinberg RF, Kliman HJ, Lockwood CJ. Is oncofetal fibronectin a trophoblast glue for human implantation? *Am J Pathol* **138**:537–543, 1991.
40. Simmons DG, Fortier AL, Cross JC. Diverse subtypes and developmental origins of trophoblast giant cells in the mouse placenta. *Dev Biol* **304**:567–578, 2007.
41. Kemp B, Kertschanska S, Kadyrov M, Rath W, Kaufmann P, Huppertz B. Invasive depth of extravillous trophoblast correlates with cellular phenotype: a comparison of intra- and extrauterine implantation sites. *Histochem Cell Biol* **117**:401–414, 2002.
42. Huppertz B, Kertschanska S, Frank HG, Gaus G, Funayama H, Kaufmann P. Extracellular matrix components of the placental extravillous trophoblast: immunocytochemistry and ultrastructural distribution. *Histochem Cell Biol* **106**:291–301, 1996.
43. Frank HG, Huppertz B, Kertschanska S, Blanchard D, Roelcke D, Kaufmann P. Anti-adhesive glycosylation of fibronectin-like molecules in human placental matrix-type fibrinoid. *Histochem Cell Biol* **104**:317–329, 1995.
44. Huppertz B, Kertschanska S, Demir AY, Frank HG, Kaufmann P. Immunohistochemistry of matrix metalloproteinases (MMP), their substrates, and their inhibitors (TIMP) during trophoblast invasion in the human placenta. *Cell Tissue Res* **291**:133–148, 1998.
45. King BF, Blankenship TN. Immunohistochemical localization of fibrillin in developing macaque and term human placentas and fetal membranes. *Microsc Res Tech* **38**:42–51, 1997.
46. Damsky CH, Fitzgerald ML, Fisher SJ. Distribution patterns of extracellular matrix components and adhesion receptors are intricately modulated during first trimester cytotrophoblast differentiation along the invasive pathway, in vivo. *J Clin Invest* **89**:210–222, 1992.
47. Damsky CH, Librach C, Lim KH et al. Integrin switching regulates normal trophoblast invasion. *Development* **120**:3657–3666, 1994.
48. Irving JA, Lala PK. Functional role of cell surface integrins on human trophoblast cell migration: regulation by TGF-beta, IGF-II, and IGFBP-1. *Exp Cell Res* **217**:419–427, 1995.
49. Feinberg RF, Kliman HJ. Fetal fibronectin and preterm labor. *N Engl J Med* **326**:708; author reply 709, 1992.
50. Fisher SJ, Damsky CH. Human cytotrophoblast invasion. *Semin Cell Biol* **4**:183–188, 1993.
51. Menzin AW, Loret de Mola JR, Bilker WB, Wheeler JE, Rubin SC, Feinberg RF. Identification of oncofetal fibronectin in patients with advanced epithelial ovarian cancer: detection in ascitic fluid and localization to primary sites and metastatic implants. *Cancer* **82**:152–158, 1998.
52. Aplin JD, Haigh T, Jones CJ, Church HJ, Vicovac L. Development of cytotrophoblast columns from explanted first-trimester human placental villi: role of fibronectin and integrin alpha5beta1. *Biol Reprod* **60**:828–838, 1999.
53. Zhou Y, Fisher SJ, Janatpour M et al. Human cytotrophoblasts adopt a vascular phenotype as they differentiate. A strategy for successful endovascular invasion? *J Clin Invest* **99**:2139–2151, 1997.
54. Tseng JJ, Chou MM. Differential expression of growth-, angiogenesis- and invasion-related factors in the development of placenta accreta. *Taiwan J Obstet Gynecol* **45**:100–106, 2006.
55. Aplin JD, Lacey H, Haigh T, Jones CJ, Chen CP, Westwood M. Growth factor-extracellular matrix synergy in the control of trophoblast invasion. *Biochem Soc Trans* **28**:199–202, 2000.
56. DiFederico E, Genbacev O, Fisher SJ. Preeclampsia is associated with widespread apoptosis of placental cytotrophoblasts within the uterine wall. *Am J Pathol* **155**:293–301, 1999.
57. Kadyrov M, Kingdom JC, Huppertz B. Divergent trophoblast invasion and apoptosis in placental bed spiral arteries from pregnancies complicated by maternal anemia and early-onset preeclampsia/intrauterine growth restriction. *Am J Obstet Gynecol* **194**:557–563, 2006.
58. Kadyrov M, Schmitz C, Black S, Kaufmann P, Huppertz B. Pre-eclampsia and maternal anaemia display reduced apoptosis and opposite invasive phenotypes of extravillous trophoblast. *Placenta* **24**:540–548, 2003.
59. Reister F, Frank HG, Heyl W et al. The distribution of macrophages in spiral arteries of the placental bed in pre-eclampsia differs from that in healthy patients. *Placenta* **20**:229–233, 1999.

60. Reister F, Frank HG, Kingdom JC et al. Macrophage-induced apoptosis limits endovascular trophoblast invasion in the uterine wall of preeclamptic women. *Lab Invest* **81**:1143–1152, 2001.
61. Zybina TG, Frank HG, Biesterfeld S, Kaufmann P. Genome multiplication of extravillous trophoblast cells in human placenta in the course of differentiation and invasion into endometrium and myometrium. II. Mechanisms of polyploidization. *Tsitologiia* **46**:640–648, 2004.
62. Malassine A, Handschuh K, Tsatsaris V et al. Expression of HERV-W Env glycoprotein (syncytin) in the extravillous trophoblast of first trimester human placenta. *Placenta* **26**:556–562, 2005.
63. Silver RM, Landon MB, Rouse DJ et al. Maternal morbidity associated with multiple repeat cesarean deliveries. *Obstet Gynecol* **107**:1226–1232, 2006.
64. Fernandez H, Al-Najjar F, Chauveaud-Lambling A, Frydman R, Gervaise A. Fertility after treatment of Asherman's syndrome stage 3 and 4. *J Minim Invasive Gynecol* **13**:398–402, 2006.
65. Adams EC, Hertig AT, Rock J. A description of 34 human ova within the first 17 days of development. *Am J Anat* **98**:435–493, 1956.
66. Carter AM. When is the maternal placental circulation established in man? *Placenta* **18**:83–87, 1997.
67. Burton GJ, Jauniaux E, Watson AL. Maternal arterial connections to the placental intervillous space during the first trimester of human pregnancy: the Boyd collection revisited. *Am J Obstet Gynecol* **181**:718–724, 1999.
68. Hamilton WJ, Boyd JD. Development of the human placenta in the first three months of gestation. *J Anat* **94**:297–328, 1960.
69. Hustin J, Schaaps JP, Lambotte R. Anatomical studies of the utero-placental vascularization in the first trimester of pregnancy. 1988.
70. Schaaps JP, Hustin J. In vivo aspect of the maternal-trophoblastic border during the first trimester of gestation. *Trophoblast Res* **3**:39–48, 1988.
71. Jauniaux E, Jurkovic D, Campbell S, Kurjak A, Hustin J. Investigation of placental circulations by color Doppler ultrasonography. *Am J Obstet Gynecol* **164**:486–488, 1991.
72. Rodesch F, Simon P, Donner C, Jauniaux E. Oxygen measurements in endometrial and trophoblastic tissues during early pregnancy. *Obstet Gynecol* **80**:283–285, 1992.
73. Jauniaux E, Gulbis B, Burton GJ. The human first trimester gestational sac limits rather than facilitates oxygen transfer to the foetus – a review. *Placenta* **24** Suppl A:S86–93, 2003.
74. Lennard SN, Gerstenberg C, Allen WR, Stewart F. Expression of epidermal growth factor and its receptor in equine placental tissues. *J Reprod Fertil* **112**:49–57, 1998.
75. Gray CA, Taylor KM, Ramsey WS et al. Endometrial glands are required for preimplantation conceptus elongation and survival. *Biol Reprod* **64**:1608–1613, 2001.
76. Burton GJ, Jauniaux E. Maternal vascularisation of the human placenta: does the embryo develop in a hypoxic environment? *Gynecol Obstet Fertil* **29**:503–508, 2001.
77. Jauniaux E, Watson A, Burton G. Evaluation of respiratory gases and acid-base gradients in human fetal fluids and uteroplacental tissue between 7 and 16 weeks' gestation. *Am J Obstet Gynecol* **184**:998–1003, 2001.
78. Pijnenborg R. Trophoblast invasion and placentation in the human: morphological aspects. *Trophoblast Res* **4**:33–47, 1990.
79. Craven CM, Morgan T, Ward K. Decidual spiral artery remodelling begins before cellular interaction with cytotrophoblasts. *Placenta* **19**:241–252, 1998.
80. Hees H, Moll W, Wrobel KH, Hees I. Pregnancy-induced structural changes and trophoblastic invasion in the segmental mesometrial arteries of the guinea pig (Cavia porcellus L.). *Placenta* **8**:609–626, 1987.
81. Moll W, Nienartowicz A, Hees H, Wrobel KH, Lenz A. Blood flow regulation in the uteroplacental arteries. *Trophoblast Res* **3**, 1988.
82. Nanaev A, Chwalisz K, Frank HG, Kohnen G, Hegele-Hartung C, Kaufmann P. Physiological dilation of uteroplacental arteries in the guinea pig depends on nitric oxide synthase activity of extravillous trophoblast. *Cell Tissue Res* **282**:407–421, 1995.
83. Dunk C, Petkovic L, Baczyk D, Rossant J, Winterhager E, Lye S. A novel in vitro model of trophoblast-mediated decidual blood vessel remodeling. *Lab Invest* **83**:1821–1828, 2003.
84. Hirano H, Imai Y, Ito H. Spiral artery of placenta: development and pathology-immunohistochemical, microscopical, and electron-microscopic study. *Kobe J Med Sci* **48**:13–23, 2002.
85. De Wolf F, De Wolf-Peeters C, Brosens I. Ultrastructure of the spiral arteries in the human placental bed at the end of normal pregnancy. *Am J Obstet Gynecol* **117**:833–848, 1973.
86. Robertson WB. Uteroplacental vasculature. *J Clin Pathol Suppl (R Coll Pathol)* **10**:9–17, 1976.
87. Brosens I, Robertson WB, Dixon HG. The physiological response of the vessels of the placental bed to normal pregnancy. *J Pathol Bacteriol* **93**:569–579, 1967.
88. Hustin J, Jauniaux E, Schaaps JP. Histological study of the materno-embryonic interface in spontaneous abortion. *Placenta* **11**:477–486, 1990.
89. Jauniaux E, Greenwold N, Hempstock J, Burton GJ. Comparison of ultrasonographic and Doppler mapping of the intervillous circulation in normal and abnormal early pregnancies. *Fertil Steril* **79**:100–106, 2003.
90. Tong S, Marjono B, Mulvey S, Wallace EM. Low levels of pregnancy-associated plasma protein-A in asymptomatic women destined for miscarriage. *Fertil Steril* **82**:1468–1470, 2004.
91. Ball E, Robson SC, Ayis S, Lyall F, Bulmer JN. Early embryonic demise: no evidence of abnormal spiral artery transformation or trophoblast invasion. *J Pathol* **208**:528–534, 2006.
92. Brosens I. The uteroplacental vessels at term – the distribution and extent of physiological changes. *Trophoblast Res* **3**:61–67, 1988.
93. Sheppard BL, Bonnar J. The maternal blood supply to the placenta in pregnancy complicated by intrauterine fetal growth retardation. *Trophoblast Res* **3**:69–82, 1988.
94. Burton GJ, Hempstock J, Jauniaux E. Oxygen, early embryonic metabolism and free radical-mediated embryopathies. *Reprod Biomed Online* **6**:84–96, 2003.
95. Nicol CJ, Zielenski J, Tsui LC, Wells PG. An embryoprotective role for glucose-6-phosphate dehydrogenase in developmental oxidative stress and chemical teratogenesis. *Faseb J* **14**:111–127, 2000.
96. Watson AL, Skepper JN, Jauniaux E, Burton GJ. Susceptibility of human placental syncytiotrophoblastic mitochondria to oxygen-mediated damage in relation to gestational age. *J Clin Endocrinol Metab* **83**:1697–1705, 1998.
97. Corner GW. A well-preserved human embryo of 10 somites. *Carnegie Contrib Embryol* **20**:81–102, 1929.
98. Jackson MR, Mayhew TM, Boyd PA. Quantitative description of the elaboration and maturation of villi from 10 weeks of gestation to term. *Placenta* **13**:357–370, 1992.
99. Kaufmann P, Huppertz B, Frank HG. The fibrinoids of the human placenta: origin, composition and functional relevance. *Ann Anat* **178**:485–501, 1996.
100. Bewley S, Cooper D, Campbell S. Doppler investigation of uteroplacental blood flow resistance in the second trimester: a screening study for pre-eclampsia and intrauterine growth retardation. *Br J Obstet Gynaecol* **98**:871–879, 1991.
101. Brosens IA, Robertson WB, Dixon HG. The role of the spiral arteries in the pathogenesis of pre-eclampsia. *J Pathol* **101**:vi, 1970.

102. Khong TY, De Wolf F, Robertson WB, Brosens I. Inadequate maternal vascular response to placentation in pregnancies complicated by pre-eclampsia and by small-for-gestational age infants. *Br J Obstet Gynaecol* **93**:1049–1059, 1986.
103. Demir R, Kaufmann P, Castellucci M, Erbengi T, Kotowski A. Fetal vasculogenesis and angiogenesis in human placental villi. *Acta Anat (Basel)* **136**:190–203, 1989.
104. Burton GJ, Watson AL, Hempstock J, Skepper JN, Jauniaux E. Uterine glands provide histiotrophic nutrition for the human fetus during the first trimester of pregnancy. *J Clin Endocrinol Metab* **87**:2954–2959, 2002.
105. Jauniaux E, Watson AL, Hempstock J, Bao YP, Skepper JN, Burton GJ. Onset of maternal arterial blood flow and placental oxidative stress. A possible factor in human early pregnancy failure. *Am J Pathol* **157**:2111–2122, 2000.
106. Toal M, Keating S, Machin G et al. Determinants of adverse perinatal outcome in high-risk women with abnormal uterine artery doppler. *Am J Obstet Gynecol* **198**:330 e1–7, 2008.
107. Mayhew TM. Villous trophoblast of human placenta: a coherent view of its turnover, repair and contributions to villous development and maturation. *Histol Histopathol* **16**:1213–1224, 2001.
108. Simpson RA, Mayhew TM, Barnes PR. From 13 weeks to term, the trophoblast of human placenta grows by the continuous recruitment of new proliferative units: a study of nuclear number using the disector. *Placenta* **13**:501–512, 1992.
109. Wilkins-Haug L, Roberts DJ, Morton CC. Confined placental mosaicism and intrauterine growth retardation: a case-control analysis of placentas at delivery. *Am J Obstet Gynecol* **172**:44–50, 1995.
110. Benirschke K, Kaufmann P. *Pathology of the Human Placenta*. New York: Springer-Verlag, 1995.
111. Huppertz B, Kingdom J, Caniggia I et al. Hypoxia favours necrotic versus apoptotic shedding of placental syncytiotrophoblast into the maternal circulation. *Placenta* **24**:181–190, 2003.
112. Macara L, Kingdom JC, Kaufmann P et al. Structural analysis of placental terminal villi from growth-restricted pregnancies with abnormal umbilical artery Doppler waveforms. *Placenta* **17**:37–48, 1996.
113. Mayhew TM, Leach L, McGee R, Ismail WW, Myklebust R, Lammiman MJ. Proliferation, differentiation and apoptosis in villous trophoblast at 13–41 weeks of gestation (including observations on annulate lamellae and nuclear pore complexes). *Placenta* **20**:407–422, 1999.
114. Ikle A. Trophoblast cells in the circulating blood. *Schweiz Med Wochenschr* **91**:943–945, 1961.
115. Huppertz B, Frank HG, Kingdom JC, Reister F, Kaufmann P. Villous cytotrophoblast regulation of the syncytial apoptotic cascade in the human placenta. *Histochem Cell Biol* **110**:495–508, 1998.
116. Huppertz B, Kaufmann P, Kingdom J. Trophoblast turnover in health and disease. *Fetal Maternal Med Rev* **13**:103–118, 2002.
117. Johansen M, Redman CW, Wilkins T, Sargent IL. Trophoblast deportation in human pregnancy – its relevance for pre-eclampsia. *Placenta* **20**:531–539, 1999.
118. Ikle FA. Dissemination of syncytial trophoblastic cells in the maternal blood stream during pregnancy. *Bull Schweiz Akad Med Wiss* **20**:62–72, 1964.
119. Lunetta P, Penttila A. Immunohistochemical identification of syncytiotrophoblastic cells and megakaryocytes in pulmonary vessels in a fatal case of amniotic fluid embolism. *Int J Legal Med* **108**:210–214, 1996.
120. Cohle SD, Petty CS. Sudden death caused by embolization of trophoblast from hydatidiform mole. *J Forensic Sci* **30**:1279–1283, 1985.
121. Delmis J, Pfeifer D, Ivanisevic M, Forko JI, Hlupic L. Sudden death from trophoblastic embolism in pregnancy. *Eur J Obstet Gynecol Reprod Biol* **92**:225–227, 2000.
122. Kamoi S, Ohaki Y, Mori O et al. Placental villotrophoblastic pulmonary emboli after elective abortion: immunohistochemical diagnosis and comparison with ten control cases. *Int J Gynecol Pathol* **22**:303–309, 2003.
123. Lee W, Ginsburg KA, Cotton DB, Kaufman RH. Squamous and trophoblastic cells in the maternal pulmonary circulation identified by invasive hemodynamic monitoring during the peripartum period. *Am J Obstet Gynecol* **155**:999–1001, 1986.
124. Knight M, Redman CW, Linton EA, Sargent IL. Shedding of syncytiotrophoblast microvilli into the maternal circulation in pre-eclamptic pregnancies. *Br J Obstet Gynaecol* **105**:632–640, 1998.
125. Macara L, Kingdom JC, Kohnen G, Bowman AW, Greer IA, Kaufmann P. Elaboration of stem villous vessels in growth restricted pregnancies with abnormal umbilical artery Doppler waveforms. *Br J Obstet Gynaecol* **102**:807–812, 1995.
126. Sibley CP, Bauman KF, Firth JA. Permeability of the foetal capillary endothelium of the guinea-pig placenta to haem proteins of various molecular sizes. *Cell Tissue Res* **223**:165–178, 1982.
127. Sibley CP, Bauman KF, Firth JA. Molecular charge as a determinant of macromolecule permeability across the fetal capillary endothelium of the guinea-pig placenta. *Cell Tissue Res* **229**:365–377, 1983.
128. Firth JA, Bauman KF, Sibley CP. Permeability pathways in fetal placental capillaries. *Trophoblast Res* **3**:163–177, 1988.
129. Alfirevic Z, Neilson JP. Doppler ultrasonography in high-risk pregnancies: systematic review with meta-analysis. *Am J Obstet Gynecol* **172**:379–1387, 1995.
130. Reilly RD, Russell PT. Neurohistochemical evidence supporting an absence of adrenergic and cholinergic innervation in the human placenta and umbilical cord. *Anat Rec* **188**:277–286, 1977.
131. Kingdom JC, Burrell SJ, Kaufmann P. Pathology and clinical implications of abnormal umbilical artery Doppler waveforms. *Ultrasound Obstet Gynecol* **9**:271–286, 1997.
132. Castellucci M, Muhlhauser J, Zaccheo D. The Hofbauer cell: the macrophage of the human placenta. In *Immunobiology of normal and diabetic pregnancy*, D Andreani, GD Bompiani, U Di Mario, WP Faulk, A Galluzzo (eds), pp. 135–144. New York: John Wiley, 1990.
133. Goldstein J, Braverman M, Salafia C, Buckley P. The phenotype of human placental macrophages and its variation with gestational age. *Am J Pathol* **133**:648–659, 1988.
134. Backe E, Jimenez E, Unger M, Schafer A, Jauniaux E, Vogel M. Demonstration of HIV-1 infected cells in human placenta by in situ hybridisation and immunostaining. *J Clin Pathol* **45**:871–874, 1992.
135. Arias RA, Munoz LD, Munoz-Fernandez MA. Transmission of HIV-1 infection between trophoblast placental cells and T-cells take place via an LFA-1-mediated cell to cell contact. *Virology* **307**:266–277, 2003.
136. Kaufmann P, Mayhew TM, Charnock-Jones DS. Aspects of human fetoplacental vasculogenesis and angiogenesis. II. Changes during normal pregnancy. *Placenta* **25**:114–126, 2004.
137. Kaufmann P, Schroder H, Leichtweiss HP. Fluid shift across the placenta: II. Fetomaternal transfer of horseradish peroxidase in the guinea pig. *Placenta* **3**:339–348, 1982.
138. Kaufmann P, Sen DK, Schweikhart G. Classification of human placental villi. I. Histology. *Cell Tissue Res* **200**:409–423, 1979.
139. Sen DK, Kaufmann P, Schweikhart G. Classification of human placental villi. II. Morphometry. *Cell Tissue Res* **200**:425–434, 1979.
140. Castellucci M, Scheper M, Scheffen I, Celona A, Kaufmann P. The development of the human placental villous tree. *Anat Embryol (Berl)* **181**:117–128, 1990.

141. Burton GJ. The fine structure of the human placental villus as revealed by scanning electron microscopy. *Scanning Microsc* **1**:1811–1828, 1987.
142. Bracero LA, Beneck D, Kirshenbaum N, Peiffer M, Stalter P, Schulman H. Doppler velocimetry and placental disease. *Am J Obstet Gynecol* **161**:388–393, 1989.
143. Giles WB, Trudinger BJ, Baird PJ. Fetal umbilical artery flow velocity waveforms and placental resistance: pathological correlation. *Br J Obstet Gynaecol* **92**:31–38, 1985.
144. McCowan LM, Mullen BM, Ritchie K. Umbilical artery flow velocity waveforms and the placental vascular bed. *Am J Obstet Gynecol* **157**:900–902, 1987.
145. Kaufmann P, Bruns U, Leiser R, Luckhardt M, Winterhager E. The fetal vascularisation of term human placental villi. II. Intermediate and terminal villi. *Anat Embryol (Berl)* **173**:203–214, 1985.
146. Kaufmann P, Luckhardt M, Leiser R. Three-dimensional representation of the fetal vessel system in the human placenta. *Trophoblast Res* **3**, 1988.
147. Bacon BJ, Gilbert RD, Kaufmann P, Smith AD, Trevino FT, Longo LD. Placental anatomy and diffusing capacity in guinea pigs following long-term maternal hypoxia. *Placenta* **5**:475–487, 1984.
148. Jackson MR, Mayhew TM, Haas JD. Morphometric studies on villi in human term placentae and the effects of altitude, ethnic grouping and sex of newborn. *Placenta* **8**:487–495, 1987.
149. Scheffen I, Kaufmann P, Philippens L, Leiser R, Geisen C, Mottaghy K. Alterations of the fetal capillary bed in guinea pig placenta following long-term hypoxia. In *Oxygen transfer to tissue, pp*, J Piiper, TK Goldstick (eds), pp. 779–790. New York: Plenum Press, 1990.
150. Kingdom JC, Kaufmann P. Oxygen and placental villous development: origins of fetal hypoxia. *Placenta* **18**:613-621; discussion 623–616, 1997.
151. Krebs C, Macara LM, Leiser R, Bowman AW, Greer IA, Kingdom JC. Intrauterine growth restriction with absent end-diastolic flow velocity in the umbilical artery is associated with maldevelopment of the placental terminal villous tree. *Am J Obstet Gynecol* **175**:1534–1542, 1996.
152. Espinoza J, Romero R, Nien JK et al. A role of the anti-angiogenic factor sVEGFR-1 in the 'mirror syndrome' (Ballantyne's syndrome). *J Matern Fetal Neonatal Med* **19**:607–613, 2006.
153. Mayhew TM. Allometric studies on growth and development of the human placenta: growth of tissue compartments and diffusive conductances in relation to placental volume and fetal mass. *J Anat* **208**:785–794, 2006.
154. Alkazaleh F, Chaddha V, Viero S et al. Second-trimester prediction of severe placental complications in women with combined elevations in alpha-fetoprotein and human chorionic gonadotrophin. *Am J Obstet Gynecol* **194**:821–827, 2006.
155. Konchak PS, Bernstein IM, Capeless EL. Uterine artery Doppler velocimetry in the detection of adverse obstetric outcomes in women with unexplained elevated maternal serum alpha-fetoprotein levels. *Am J Obstet Gynecol* **173**:1115–1119, 1995.
156. Williams MA, Hickok DE, Zingheim RW et al. Elevated maternal serum alpha-fetoprotein levels and midtrimester placental abnormalities in relation to subsequent adverse pregnancy outcomes. *Am J Obstet Gynecol* **167**:1032–1037, 1992.
157. Brownbill P, Edwards D, Jones C et al. Mechanisms of alphafetoprotein transfer in the perfused human placental cotyledon from uncomplicated pregnancy. *J Clin Invest* **96**:2220–2226, 1995.
158. Kaufmann P. Development and differentiation of the human placental villous tree. *Bibl Anat* 29–39, 1982.
159. Kertschanska S, Kosanke G, Kaufmann P. Is there morphological evidence for the existence of transtrophoblastic channels in the human placental villi? *Trophoblast Res* **8**:581–596, 1994.
160. Stulc J, Friedrich R, Jiricka Z. Estimation of the equivalent pore dimensions in the rabbit placenta. *Life Sci* **8**:167–180, 1969.
161. Thornburg KL, Faber JJ. Transfer of hydrophilic molecules by placenta and yolk sac of the guinea pig. *Am J Physiol* **233**:C111–124, 1977.
162. Nelson DL, Thompson G, Moore JA. Identification of factors of affective meaning in four selected activities. *Am J Occup Ther* **36**:381–387, 1982.
163. Eik-Nes SH, Marsal K, Brubakk AO, Kristofferson K, Ulstein M. Ultrasonic measurement of human fetal blood flow. *J Biomed Eng* **4**:28–36, 1982.
164. Hendricks SK, Sorensen TK, Wang KY, Bushnell JM, Seguin EM, Zingheim RW. Doppler umbilical artery waveform indices – normal values from fourteen to forty-two weeks. *Am J Obstet Gynecol* **161**:761–765, 1989.
165. Jackson MR, Walsh AJ, Morrow RJ, Mullen JB, Lye SJ, Ritchie JW. Reduced placental villous tree elaboration in small-for-gestational-age pregnancies: relationship with umbilical artery Doppler waveforms. *Am J Obstet Gynecol* **172**:518–525, 1995.
166. Fisk NM, MacLachlan N, Ellis C, Tannirandorn Y, Tonge HM, Rodeck CH. Absent end-diastolic flow in first trimester umbilical artery. *Lancet* **2**:1256–1257, 1988.
167. Whittle W, Chaddha V, Wyatt P, Huppertz B, Kingdom J. Ultrasound detection of placental insufficiency in women with 'unexplained' abnormal maternal serum screening results. *Clin Genet* **69**:97–104, 2006.
168. Crispi F, Dominguez C, Llurba E, Martin-Gallan P, Cabero L, Gratacos E. Placental angiogenic growth factors and uterine artery Doppler findings for characterization of different subsets in preeclampsia and in isolated intrauterine growth restriction. *Am J Obstet Gynecol* **195**:201–207, 2006.
169. Olofsson P, Laurini RN, Marsal K. A high uterine artery pulsatility index reflects a defective development of placental bed spiral arteries in pregnancies complicated by hypertension and fetal growth retardation. *Eur J Obstet Gynecol Reprod Biol* **49**:161–168, 1993.
170. Voigt HJ, Becker V. Doppler flow measurements and histomorphology of the placental bed in uteroplacental insufficiency. *J Perinat Med* **20**:139–147, 1992.
171. Lin S, Shimizu I, Suehara N, Nakayama M, Aono T. Uterine artery Doppler velocimetry in relation to trophoblast migration into the myometrium of the placental bed. *Obstet Gynecol* **85**:760–765, 1995.
172. Espinoza J, Romero R, Mee Kim Y et al. Normal and abnormal transformation of the spiral arteries during pregnancy. *J Perinat Med* **34**:447–458, 2006.
173. Sagol S, Ozkinay E, Oztekin K, Ozdemir N. The comparison of uterine artery Doppler velocimetry with the histopathology of the placental bed. *Aust NZ J Obstet Gynaecol* **39**:324–329, 1999.
174. Reister F, Kingdom JC, Ruck P et al. Altered protease expression by periarterial trophoblast cells in severe early-onset preeclampsia with IUGR. *J Perinat Med* **34**:272–279, 2006.
175. Walford N, Htun K, Akhilesh M. Detection of atherosis in preeclamptic placentas: comparison of two gross sampling protocols. *Pediatr Dev Pathol* **8**:61–65, 2005.
176. Zhang P, Schmidt M, Cook L. Maternal vasculopathy and histologic diagnosis of preeclampsia: poor correlation of histologic changes and clinical manifestation. *Am J Obstet Gynecol* **194**:1050–1056, 2006.
177. Mayhew TM, Wijesekara J, Baker PN, Ong SS. Morphometric evidence that villous development and fetoplacental angiogenesis are compromised by intrauterine growth restriction but not by pre-eclampsia. *Placenta* **25**:829–833, 2004.
178. Mayhew TM, Manwani R, Ohadike C, Wijesekara J, Baker PN. The placenta in pre-eclampsia and intrauterine growth

restriction: studies on exchange surface areas, diffusion distances and villous membrane diffusive conductances. *Placenta* **28**:233–238, 2007.

179. Zamudio S. The placenta at high altitude. *High Alt Med Biol* **4**:171–191, 2003.
180. Hindmarsh PC, Geary MP, Rodeck CH, Jackson MR, Kingdom JC. Effect of early maternal iron stores on placental weight and structure. *Lancet* **356**:719–723, 2000.
181. Karsdorp VH, van Vugt JM, van Geijn HP et al. Clinical significance of absent or reversed end diastolic velocity waveforms in umbilical artery. *Lancet* **344**:1664–1668, 1994.
182. Cross JC, Nakano H, Natale DR, Simmons DG, Watson ED. Branching morphogenesis during development of placental villi. *Differentiation* **74**:393–401, 2006.
183. Soleymanlou N, Jurisica I, Nevo O et al. Molecular evidence of placental hypoxia in preeclampsia. *J Clin Endocrinol Metab* **90**:4299–4308, 2005.
184. Todros T, Sciarrone A, Piccoli E, Guiot C, Kaufmann P, Kingdom J. Umbilical Doppler waveforms and placental villous angiogenesis in pregnancies complicated by fetal growth restriction. *Obstet Gynecol* **93**:499–503, 1999.
185. Nordenvall M, Ullberg U, Laurin J, Lingman G, Sandstedt B, Ulmsten U. Placental morphology in relation to umbilical artery blood velocity waveforms. *Eur J Obstet Gynecol Reprod Biol* **40**:179–190, 1991.
186. Huppertz B, Kingdom JC. Apoptosis in the trophoblast – role of apoptosis in placental morphogenesis. *J Soc Gynecol Investig* **11**:353–362, 2004.
187. Formigli L, Papucci L, Tani A, Schiavone N et al. Aponecrosis: morphological and biochemical exploration of a syncretic process of cell death sharing apoptosis and necrosis. *J Cell Physiol* **182**:41–44, 2000.
188. Goswami D, Tannetta DS, Magee LA et al. Excess syncytiotrophoblast microparticle shedding is a feature of early-onset pre-eclampsia, but not normotensive intrauterine growth restriction. *Placenta* **27**:56–61, 2006.
189. Moldenhauer JS, Stanek J, Warshak C, Khoury J, Sibai B. The frequency and severity of placental findings in women with preeclampsia are gestational age dependent. *Am J Obstet Gynecol* **189**:1173–1177, 2003.
190. Aardema MW, Oosterhof H, Timmer A, van Rooy I, Aarnoudse JG. Uterine artery Doppler flow and uteroplacental vascular pathology in normal pregnancies and pregnancies complicated by pre-eclampsia and small for gestational age fetuses. *Placenta* **22**:405–411, 2001.
191. Ferrazzi E, Bulfamante G, Mezzopane R, Barbera A, Ghidini A, Pardi G. Uterine Doppler velocimetry and placental hypoxic-ischemic lesion in pregnancies with fetal intrauterine growth restriction. *Placenta* **20**:389–394, 1999.
192. Wang X, Athayde N, Trudinger B. Maternal plasma from pregnant women with umbilical placental vascular disease does not affect endothelial cell mRNA expression of nitric oxide synthase. *J Soc Gynecol Investig* **11**:149–153, 2004.
193. Szukiewicz D, Szewczyk G, Watroba M, Kurowska E, Maslinski S. Isolated placental vessel response to vascular endothelial growth factor and placenta growth factor in normal and growth-restricted pregnancy. *Gynecol Obstet Invest* **59**:02–107, 2005.
194. Wang X, Athayde N, Trudinger B. Microvascular endothelial cell activation is present in the umbilical placental microcirculation in fetal placental vascular disease. *Am J Obstet Gynecol* **190**:596–601, 2004.
195. Wang X, Athayde N, Trudinger B. Egr-1 transcription activation exists in placental endothelium when vascular disease is present. *Br J Obstet Gynaecol* **113**:683–687, 2006.
196. Westergaard HB, Langhoff-Roos J, Lingman G, Marsal K, Kreiner S. A critical appraisal of the use of umbilical artery Doppler ultrasound in high-risk pregnancies: use of meta-analyses in evidence-based obstetrics. *Ultrasound Obstet Gynecol* **17**:466–476, 2001.
197. Abramowicz JS, Sheiner E. In utero imaging of the placenta: importance for diseases of pregnancy. *Placenta* **28** Suppl A:S14–22, 2007.
198. Audibert F, Benchimol Y, Benattar C, Champagne C, Frydman R. Prediction of preeclampsia or intrauterine growth restriction by second trimester serum screening and uterine Doppler velocimetry. *Fetal Diagn Ther* **20**:48–53, 2005.
199. Papageorghiou AT, Yu CK, Bindra R, Pandis G, Nicolaides KH. Multicenter screening for pre-eclampsia and fetal growth restriction by transvaginal uterine artery Doppler at 23 weeks of gestation. *Ultrasound Obstet Gynecol* **18**:441–449, 2001.
200. Yu CK, Smith GC, Papageorghiou AT, Cacho AM, Nicolaides KH. An integrated model for the prediction of preeclampsia using maternal factors and uterine artery Doppler velocimetry in unselected low-risk women. *Am J Obstet Gynecol* **193**:429–436, 2005.
201. Smith GC, Yu CK, Papageorghiou AT, Cacho AM, Nicolaides KH. Maternal uterine artery Doppler flow velocimetry and the risk of stillbirth. *Obstet Gynecol* **109**:144–151, 2007.
202. Yu CK, Papageorghiou AT, Parra M, Palma Dias R, Nicolaides KH. Randomized controlled trial using low-dose aspirin in the prevention of pre-eclampsia in women with abnormal uterine artery Doppler at 23 weeks' gestation. *Ultrasound Obstet Gynecol* **22**:233–239, 2003.
203. Dodd J, Sahi K, Kingdom J, Windrim R. A systematic review of anticoagulation to prevent placental insufficiency symdromes. *Acta Obstet Gynecol Scand* (in press).
204. Bose P, Black S, Kadyrov M, et al. Adverse effects of lupus anticoagulant positive blood sera on placental viability can be prevented by heparin in vitro. *Am J Obstet Gynecol* **191**:2125–213, 12004.
205. Bose P, Black S, Kadyrov M et al. Heparin and aspirin attenuate placental apoptosis in vitro: implications for early pregnancy failure. *Am J Obstet Gynecol* **192**:23–30, 2005.
206. Rossant J, Cross JC. Placental development: lessons from mouse mutants. *Nat Rev Genet* **2**:538–548, 2001.
207. Nevo O, Soleymanlou N, Wu Y et al. Increased expression of sFlt-1 in in vivo and in vitro models of human placental hypoxia is mediated by HIF-1. *Am J Physiol Regul Integr Comp Physiol* **291**: R1085-1093, 2006.
208. Many A, Todros T, Wu Y et al. Mechanisms of oxygen sensing in intra uterine growth restriction placentae. *J Soc Gynecol Invest* **13**:214A, 2006.
209. Baczyk D, Radulovich N, Dunk C, Kingdom J. siRNA-Mediated GCM1 Gene Silencing *in vitro*. *Placenta* **25**:A50, 2004.
210. Cross JC, Baczyk D, Dobric N et al. Genes, development and evolution of the placenta. *Placenta* **24**:123–130, 2003.
211. Janatpour MJ, Utset MF, Cross JC et al. A repertoire of differentially expressed transcription factors that offers insight into mechanisms of human cytotrophoblast differentiation. *Dev Genet* **25**:46–157, 1999.
212. Westerman BA, Poutsma A, Maruyama K, Schrijnemakers HF, van Wijk IJ, Oudejans CB. The proneural genes NEUROD1 and NEUROD2 are expressed during human trophoblast invasion. *Mech Dev* **113**:85–90, 2002.
213. Anson-Cartwright L, Dawson K, Holmyard D, Fisher SJ, Lazzarini RA, Cross JC. The glial cell missing-1 protein is essential for branching morphogenesis in the chorioallantoic placenta. *Nat Genet* **25**:11–314, 2000.
214. Baczyk D, Dunk C, Huppertz B et al. Bi-potential behaviour of cytotrophoblasts in first trimester chorionic villi. *Placenta* **27**:367–374, 2006.
215. Chen CP, Chen CY, Yang YC, Su TH, Chen H. Decreased placental GCM1 (glial cell missing) gene expression in pre-eclampsia. *Placenta* **25**:413–421, 2004.
216. Keunen J, Baczyk D, Dunk C et al. The molecular placental phenotype in severe

IUGR and preeclampsia is consistent with a precise (siRNA mediated inhibition of glial cell missing-1) alteration in BeWo cytotrophoblast behaviour. In *Society for Gynecologic Investigation*, p. 216A. Toronto, Canada, 2006.

217. Baczyk D, Drewlo S, Dunk C, et al. Glial cell missing-1 transcription factor is required for the differentiation of the human trophoblast. Cell Death and Diff (submitted) 2008.
218. van Dijk M, Mulders J, Poutsma A et al. Maternal segregation of the Dutch preeclampsia locus at 10q22 with a new member of the winged helix gene family. *Nat Genet* **37**:514–519, 2005.
219. Jiang WG, Hiscox S. Hepatocyte growth factor/scatter factor, a cytokine playing multiple and converse roles. *Histol Histopathol* **12**:537–555, 1997.
220. Cartwright JE, Holden DP, Whitley GS. Hepatocyte growth factor regulates human trophoblast motility and invasion: a role for nitric oxide. *Br J Pharmacol* **128**:181–189, 1999.
221. Nasu K, Zhou Y, McMaster MT, Fisher SJ. Upregulation of human cytotrophoblast invasion by hepatocyte growth factor. *J Reprod Fertil Suppl* **55**:73–80, 2000.
222. Furugori K, Kurauchi O, Itakura A et al. Levels of hepatocyte growth factor and its messenger ribonucleic acid in uncomplicated pregnancies and those complicated by preeclampsia. *J Clin Endocrinol Metab* **82**:2726–2730, 1997.
223. Kauma S, Hayes N, Weatherford S. The differential expression of hepatocyte growth factor and met in human placenta. *J Clin Endocrinol Metab* **82**:949–954, 1997.
224. Cartwright JE, Tse WK, Whitley GS. Hepatocyte growth factor induced human trophoblast motility involves phosphatidylinositol-3-kinase, mitogen-activated protein kinase, and inducible nitric oxide synthase. *Exp Cell Res* **279**:219–226, 2002.
225. Lyall F, Jablonka-Shariff A, Johnson RD, Olson LM, Nelson DM. Gene expression of nitric oxide synthase in cultured human term placental trophoblast during in vitro differentiation. *Placenta* **19**:253–260, 1998.
226. Martin D, Conrad KP. Expression of endothelial nitric oxide synthase by extravillous trophoblast cells in the human placenta. *Placenta* **21**:23–31, 2000.
227. Somerset DA, Li XF, Afford S et al. Ontogeny of hepatocyte growth factor (HGF) and its receptor (c-met) in human placenta: reduced HGF expression in intrauterine growth restriction. *Am J Pathol* **153**:1139–1147, 1998.
228. Baykal C, Guler G, Al A et al. Expression of hepatocyte growth factor/scatter factor receptor in IUGR fetuses' placentas: an immunohistochemical analysis. *Fetal Diagn Ther* **20**:249–253, 2005.
229. Gleeson LM, Chakraborty C, McKinnon T, Lala PK. Insulin-like growth factor-binding protein 1 stimulates human trophoblast migration by signaling through alpha 5 beta 1 integrin via mitogen-activated protein Kinase pathway. *J Clin Endocrinol Metab* **86**:2484–2493, 2001.
230. Hamilton GS, Lysiak JJ, Han VK, Lala PK. Autocrine-paracrine regulation of human trophoblast invasiveness by insulin-like growth factor (IGF)-II and IGF-binding protein (IGFBP)-1. *Exp Cell Res* **244**:147–156, 1998.
231. Han VK, Bassett N, Walton J, Challis JR. The expression of insulin-like growth factor (IGF) and IGF-binding protein (IGFBP) genes in the human placenta and membranes: evidence for IGF-IGFBP interactions at the feto-maternal interface. *J Clin Endocrinol Metab* **81**:2680–2693, 1996.
232. Han VK, Matsell DG, Delhanty PJ, Hill DJ, Shimasaki S, Nygard K. IGF-binding protein mRNAs in the human fetus: tissue and cellular distribution of developmental expression. *Horm Res* **45**:60–166, 1996.
233. Chakraborty C, Gleeson LM, McKinnon T, Lala PK. Regulation of human trophoblast migration and invasiveness. *Can J Physiol Pharmacol* **80**:116–124, 2002.
234. Anim-Nyame N, Hills FA, Sooranna SR, Steer PJ, Johnson MR. A longitudinal study of maternal plasma insulin-like growth factor binding protein-1 concentrations during normal pregnancy and pregnancies complicated by pre-eclampsia. *Hum Reprod* **15**:2215–2219, 2000.
235. Lysiak JJ, Hunt J, Pringle GA, Lala PK. Localization of transforming growth factor beta and its natural inhibitor decorin in the human placenta and decidua throughout gestation. *Placenta* **16**:221–231, 1995.
236. Caniggia I, Grisaru-Gravnosky S, Kuliszewsky M, Post M, Lye SJ. Inhibition of TGF-beta 3 restores the invasive capability of extravillous trophoblasts in preeclamptic pregnancies. *J Clin Invest* **103**:1641–1650, 1999.
237. Meisser A, Chardonnens D, Campana A, Bischof P. Effects of tumour necrosis factor-alpha, interleukin-1 alpha, macrophage colony stimulating factor and transforming growth factor beta on trophoblastic matrix metalloproteinases. *Mol Hum Reprod* **5**:252–260, 1999.
238. Graham CH, Lala PK. Mechanism of control of trophoblast invasion in situ. *J Cell Physiol* **148**:228–234, 1991.
239. Khoo NK, Bechberger JF, Shepherd T et al. SV40 Tag transformation of the normal invasive trophoblast results in a premalignant phenotype. I. Mechanisms responsible for hyperinvasiveness and resistance to anti-invasive action of TGFbeta. *Int J Cancer* **77**:429–439, 1998.
240. Graham CH. Effect of transforming growth factor-beta on the plasminogen activator system in cultured first trimester human cytotrophoblasts. *Placenta* **18**:37–143, 1997.
241. Graham CH, Hawley TS, Hawley RG et al. Establishment and characterization of first trimester human trophoblast cells with extended lifespan. *Exp Cell Res* **206**:204–211, 1993.
242. Graham CH, Lysiak JJ, McCrae KR, Lala PK. Localization of transforming growth factor-beta at the human fetal-maternal interface: role in trophoblast growth and differentiation. *Biol Reprod* **46**:561–572, 1992.
243. Caniggia I, Mostachfi H, Winter J et al. Hypoxia-inducible factor-1 mediates the biological effects of oxygen on human trophoblast differentiation through TGFbeta(3). *J Clin Invest* **105**:577–587, 2000.
244. Tse WK, Whitley GS, Cartwright JE. Transforming growth factor-beta1 regulates hepatocyte growth factor-induced trophoblast motility and invasion. *Placenta* **23**:699–705, 2002.
245. Caniggia I, Taylor CV, Ritchie JW, Lye SJ, Letarte M. Endoglin regulates trophoblast differentiation along the invasive pathway in human placental villous explants. *Endocrinology* **138**:4977–4988, 1997.
246. Venkatesha S, Toporsian M, Lam C et al. Soluble endoglin contributes to the pathogenesis of preeclampsia. *Nat Med* **12**:642–649, 2006.
247. Levine RJ, Lam C, Qian C et al. Soluble endoglin and other circulating antiangiogenic factors in preeclampsia. *N Engl J Med* **355**:992–1005, 2006.
248. Riese DJ, 2nd, Stern DF. Specificity within the EGF family/ErbB receptor family signaling network. *Bioessays* **20**:41–48, 1998.
249. Lala PK, Hamilton GS. Growth factors, proteases and protease inhibitors in the maternal-fetal dialogue. *Placenta* **17**:545–555, 1996.
250. Jokhi PP, King A, Loke YW. Reciprocal expression of epidermal growth factor receptor (EGF-R) and c-erbB2 by non-invasive and invasive human trophoblast populations. *Cytokine* **6**:433–442, 1994.
251. Muhlhauser J, Crescimanno C, Kaufmann P, Hofler H, Zaccheo D, Castellucci M. Differentiation and proliferation patterns in human trophoblast revealed by c-erbB-2 oncogene product and EGF-R. *J Histochem Cytochem* **41**:165–173, 1993.
252. Yu D, Hamada J, Zhang H, Nicolson GL, Hung MC. Mechanisms of c-erbB2/neu oncogene-induced metastasis and

repression of metastatic properties by adenovirus 5 E1A gene products. *Oncogene* **7**:2263–2270, 1992.

253. Brice EC, Wu JX, Muraro R, Adamson ED, Wiley LM. Modulation of mouse preimplantation development by epidermal growth factor receptor antibodies, antisense RNA, and deoxyoligonucleotides. *Dev Genet* **14**:74–184, 1993.
254. Morrish DW, Dakour J, Li H. Functional regulation of human trophoblast differentiation. *J Reprod Immunol* **39**:179–195, 1998.
255. Haimovici F, Anderson DJ. Effects of growth factors and growth factor-extracellular matrix interactions on mouse trophoblast outgrowth in vitro. *Biol Reprod* **49**:124–130, 1993.
256. Bass KE, Morrish D, Roth I et al. Human cytotrophoblast invasion is up-regulated by epidermal growth factor: evidence that paracrine factors modify this process. *Dev Biol* **164**:550–561, 1994.
257. Delany AM, Brinckerhoff CE. Post-transcriptional regulation of collagenase and stromelysin gene expression by epidermal growth factor and dexamethasone in cultured human fibroblasts. *J Cell Biochem* **50**:400–410, 1992.
258. Mainiero F, Pepe A, Yeon M, Ren Y, Giancotti FG. The intracellular functions of alpha6beta4 integrin are regulated by EGF. *J Cell Biol* **134**:241–253, 1996.
259. Pollheimer J, Knofler M. Signalling pathways regulating the invasive differentiation of human trophoblasts: a review. *Placenta* **26** Suppl A:S21–30, 2005.
260. Wright JK, Dunk CE, Perkins JE, Winterhager E, Kingdom JCP, Lye SJ. EGF modulates trophoblast migration through regulation of connexin 40. *Placenta* (in press), 2006.
261. Carpenter G, Stoscheck CM, Preston YA, DeLarco JE. Antibodies to the epidermal growth factor receptor block the biological activities of sarcoma growth factor. *Proc Natl Acad Sci USA* **80**:5627–5630, 1983.
262. Ullrich A, Coussens L, Hayflick JS et al. Human epidermal growth factor receptor cDNA sequence and aberrant expression of the amplified gene in A431 epidermoid carcinoma cells. *Nature* **309**:418–425, 1984.
263. Reynolds RK, Hu C, Baker VV. Transforming growth factor-alpha and insulin-like growth factor-I, but not epidermal growth factor, elicit autocrine stimulation of mitogenesis in endometrial cancer cell lines. *Gynecol Oncol* **70**:202–209, 1998.
264. Schreiber AB, Winkler ME, Derynck R. Transforming growth factor-alpha: a more potent angiogenic mediator than epidermal growth factor. *Science* **232**:1250–1253, 1986.
265. Winkler ME, O'Connor L, Winget M, Fendly B. Epidermal growth factor and transforming growth factor alpha bind differently to the epidermal growth factor receptor. *Biochemistry* **28**:6373–6378, 1989.
266. Lysiak JJ, Han VK, Lala PK. Localization of transforming growth factor alpha in the human placenta and decidua: role in trophoblast growth. *Biol Reprod* **49**:885–894, 1993.
267. Carpenter G. ErbB-4: mechanism of action and biology. *Exp Cell Res* **284**:66–77, 2003.
268. Arkonac BM, Foster LC, Sibinga NE et al. Vascular endothelial growth factor induces heparin-binding epidermal growth factor-like growth factor in vascular endothelial cells. *J Biol Chem* **273**:4400–4405, 1998.
269. Leach RE, Khalifa R, Ramirez ND et al. Multiple roles for heparin-binding epidermal growth factor-like growth factor are suggested by its cell-specific expression during the human endometrial cycle and early placentation. *J Clin Endocrinol Metab* **84**:3355–3363, 1999.
270. Leach RE, Kilburn B, Wang J, Liu Z, Romero R, Armant DR. Heparin-binding EGF-like growth factor regulates human extravillous cytotrophoblast development during conversion to the invasive phenotype. *Dev Biol* **266**:223–237, 2004.
271. Homma T, Sakai M, Cheng HF, Yasuda T, Coffey RJ Jr., Harris RC. Induction of heparin-binding epidermal growth factor-like growth factor mRNA in rat kidney after acute injury. *J Clin Invest* **96**:1018–1025, 1995.
272. Lala PK, Chakraborty C. Factors regulating trophoblast migration and invasiveness: possible derangements contributing to pre-eclampsia and fetal injury. *Placenta* **24**:575–587, 2003.
273. Leach RE, Romero R, Kim YM et al. Pre-eclampsia and expression of heparin-binding EGF-like growth factor. *Lancet* **360**:1215–1219, 2002.
274. Charnock-Jones DS, Kaufmann P, Mayhew TM. Aspects of human fetoplacental vasculogenesis and angiogenesis. I. Molecular regulation. *Placenta* **25**:03–113, 2004.
275. Ahmed A, Dunk C, Ahmad S, Khaliq A. Regulation of placental vascular endothelial growth factor (VEGF) and placenta growth factor (PIGF) and soluble Flt-1 by oxygen--a review. *Placenta* **21**(Suppl A):S16-24, 2000.
276. Dunk C, Ahmed A. Expression of VEGF-C and activation of its receptors VEGFR-2 and VEGFR-3 in trophoblast. *Histol Histopathol* **16**:359–375, 2001.
277. Dunk C, Shams M, Nijjar S, Rhaman M, Qiu Y, Bussolati B, Ahmed A. Angiopoietin-1 and angiopoietin-2 activate trophoblast Tie-2 to promote growth and migration during placental development. *Am J Pathol* **156**:2185–2199, 2000.
278. Li XF, Ferriani RA, Michell RH, Ahmed A. Localisation of bradykinin-like immunoreactivity and modulation of bradykinin-evoked phospholipase D activity by 17 beta-oestradiol in human endometrium. *Growth Factors* **12**:203–209, 1995.
279. Athanassiades A, Hamilton GS, Lala PK. Vascular endothelial growth factor stimulates proliferation but not migration or invasiveness in human extravillous trophoblast. *Biol Reprod* **59**:643–654, 1998.
280. Athanassiades A, Lala PK. Role of placenta growth factor (PIGF) in human extravillous trophoblast proliferation, migration and invasiveness. *Placenta* **19**:465–473, 1998.
281. Khaliq A, Dunk C, Jiang J et al. Hypoxia down-regulates placenta growth factor, whereas fetal growth restriction up-regulates placenta growth factor expression: molecular evidence for 'placental hyperoxia' in intrauterine growth restriction. *Lab Invest* **79**:151–170, 1999.
282. Shweiki D, Itin A, Soffer D, Keshet E. Vascular endothelial growth factor induced by hypoxia may mediate hypoxia-initiated angiogenesis. *Nature* **359**:843–845, 1992.
283. Radaelli T, Cetin I, Ayuk PT, Glazier JD, Pardi G, Sibley CP. Cationic amino acid transporter activity in the syncytiotrophoblast microvillous plasma membrane and oxygenation of the uteroplacental unit. *Placenta* **23**(Suppl A): S69–74, 2002.
284. Shibata E, Rajakumar A, Powers RW et al. Soluble fms-like tyrosine kinase 1 is increased in preeclampsia but not in normotensive pregnancies with small-for-gestational-age neonates: relationship to circulating placental growth factor. *J Clin Endocrinol Metab* **90**:4895–4903, 2005.
285. Thadhani R, Mutter WP, Wolf M et al. First trimester placental growth factor and soluble fms-like tyrosine kinase 1 and risk for preeclampsia. *J Clin Endocrinol Metab* **89**:770–775, 2004.
286. Widmer M, Villar J, Benigni A, Conde-Agudelo A, Karumanchi SA, Lindheimer M. Mapping the theories of preeclampsia and the role of angiogenic factors: a systematic review. *Obstet Gynecol* **109**:168–180, 2007.
287. Maynard SE, Min JY, Merchan J et al. Excess placental soluble fms-like tyrosine kinase 1 (sFlt1) may contribute to endothelial dysfunction, hypertension, and proteinuria in preeclampsia. *J Clin Invest* **111**:649–658, 2003.

288. Nevo O, Xu J, Many A et al. sFlt-1 expression is increased in placentae fom IUGR pregnancies. In *Society for gynecologic investigation*, p. 285A, Toronto, Canada, 2006.
289. Wallner W, Sengenberger R, Strick R et al. Angiogenic growth factors in maternal and fetal serum in pregnancies complicated by intrauterine growth restriction. *Clin Sci (Lond)* **112**:51–57, 2007.
290. Kaufmann P, Scheffen I. Placental development. In *Neonatal and fetal medicine – physiology and pathophysiology*, R Pollin, W Fox (eds). Orlando: WB Saunders, 1992.
291. Kaufmann P. Basic morphology of the fetal and maternal circuits in the human placenta. *Contrib Gynecol Obstet* **13**:5–17, 1985.
292. Becker V, Schiebler TH, Kubli F. *Die Plazenta des Menschen*. Stuttgart: Georg Thieme, 1981.

CHAPTER

8

Placental function in maternofetal exchange

Thomas Jansson and Theresa L Powell

KEY POINTS

- The primary determinant of fetal growth is oxygen and nutrient supply, which is directly dependent on placental transport functions
- Oxygen diffuses readily across the placental barrier and oxygen transfer is markedly affected by changes in blood flow
- The transfer of nutrients and most ions is dependent on the presence of transport proteins in the plasma membranes of the syncytiotrophoblast, the transporting epithelium of the human placenta, and is not significantly affected by acute changes in blood flow
- The placenta has a very high capacity for glucose transport, which is facilitated by the expression of glucose transporter 1 in the placental barrier. Net glucose transport is strongly influenced by the concentration gradient
- Placental amino acid uptake into the syncytiotrophoblast is an active process, in many cases energized by the gradient for sodium ions
- Free fatty acids bound to albumin or released from maternal lipoproteins by placental lipases are transferred across the microvillous plasma membrane of the syncytiotrophoblast, possibly mediated by specific proteins. Inside the cell, free fatty acids are bound to cytosolic fatty acid binding proteins and delivered to the fetal side of the barrier
- Regulation of placental transporters is not well established. Amino acid transporters are regulated by oxygen, growth factors and hormones such as insulin, leptin and IGF-I
- Placental nutrient and ion transporters are specifically altered in intrauterine growth restriction and fetal overgrowth, respectively. In intrauterine growth restriction, placental amino acid transporters are downregulated and, in fetal overgrowth, the activity of placental glucose and amino acid transporters is increased
- It has been proposed that changes in placental nutrient transport directly contribute to pathological fetal growth and that targeting placental transporters may provide a novel avenue for intervention in these pregnancy complications

INTRODUCTION

The mammalian placenta is a unique biological structure constituting the interface between maternal and fetal blood circulations. From the fetal perspective, the placenta has functions that are similar to those of the lung, kidney and digestive tract in postnatal life. These primary functions include:

- providing an immunological barrier between mother and fetus
- hormone production that alters the metabolic status of the mother
- transport of nutrients, respiratory gases, ions and water to the fetus
- transport of waste products away from the fetus.

Normal fetal growth and development are critically dependent on the maternofetal exchange functions of the placenta and recent advances in placental research suggest that changes in placental transport functions are directly involved in the pathophysiology of intrauterine growth restriction and fetal overgrowth[1,2]. Therefore, a basic knowledge of the mechanisms involved in placental transport is essential to understand the factors governing normal fetal growth as well as fully appreciate how important pregnancy complications develop. There are several excellent reviews on placental transport mechanisms[3–9], albeit none of these are very recent.

In this chapter, we will describe the functions of the syncytiotrophoblast, the transporting epithelium of the human placenta, using information obtained in various in vitro preparations of the human placenta, including isolated syncytiotrophoblast plasma membranes, primary villous fragments and cultured trophoblast cells, as well as studies in the pregnant woman. We will not discuss the well-established in vitro techniques with which to study human placental transport functions, but the reader is referred to some excellent and recent reviews for this information[10–14]. Animal experimental studies will be discussed only where data from the human are unavailable. We will discuss the mechanisms whereby molecules are transported, how these processes are regulated and in what context these placental functions in maternofetal exchange may be clinically relevant.

THE PLACENTAL BARRIER

Maternofetal exchange can be affected by numerous factors including placental and umbilical blood flows, concentration gradients, placental metabolism and transporter expression/activity in the placental barrier. Of these factors, the transport capacity of the placental barrier, as represented by the activity of numerous, specific transporter proteins, is of particular importance since this appears to be the primary factor that is subjected to regulation.

The maternal and fetal blood supplies, while kept separate at all times, must come into close proximity to allow for efficient transfer of respiratory gases, ions and nutrients. The human placenta is of the hemochorial type, i.e. maternal blood delivered by the spiral arteries into the intervillous space comes in direct contact with the trophoblast villi containing the fetal capillaries. There are only two cell layers separating the fetal and maternal circulations in the term human placenta; the *fetal capillary endothelium* and *the syncytiotrophoblast*[15] (Fig. 8.1). Fetal placental capillaries are of the continuous type, allowing the unrestricted passage of molecules of the size of glucose and amino acids between cells through intercellular spaces but restricting the transfer of large molecules such as immunoglobulins[16]. The syncytiotrophoblast cell layer is supported by an underlying *basement membrane* (see Fig. 8.1). These three structures collectively constitute the 'placental barrier'. The syncytiotrophoblast is the transporting epithelium of the human placenta and is a true syncytium generated by fusion of underlying cytotrophoblast cells. In early pregnancy, cytotrophoblast cells are highly abundant creating a continuous cell layer between the syncytium and the fetal capillary. In late pregnancy, however, cytotrophoblast cells are less abundant. The syncytiotrophoblast has two polarized plasma membranes, the microvillous plasma membrane (MVM) directed towards the maternal blood in the intervillous space and the basal plasma membrane (BM) facing the fetal capillary (see Fig. 8.1). The syncytial nature of the syncytiotrophoblast allows for a relatively tight barrier function since no intercellular spaces are available for transport of large molecules or large volumes of fluid. However, there is ample evidence to suggest the presence of so-called paracellular or transtrophoblastic channels that constitute a conduit across the barrier for larger molecules such as alpha-fetoprotein[17–20]. Furthermore, temporary breaks are likely to occur occasionally in the barrier, which can explain the presence of small amounts of fetal blood cells in the maternal circulation.

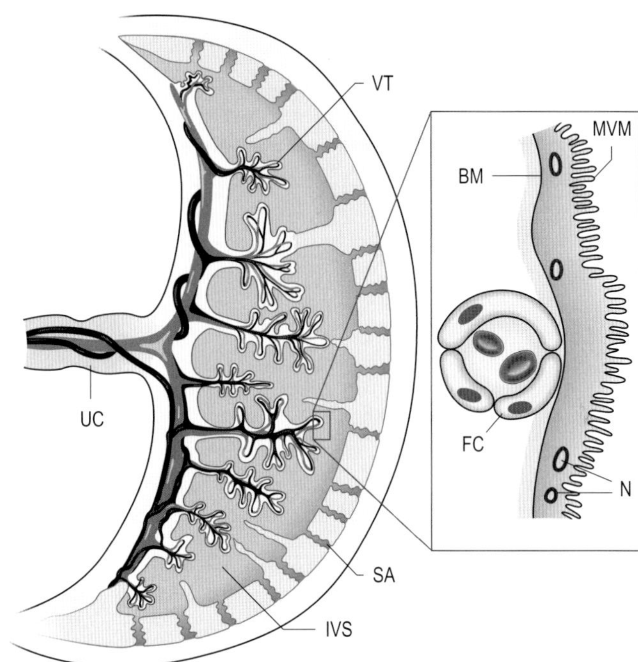

Fig. 8.1 The placental barrier primarily consists of the syncytiotrophoblast cell and the fetal capillary (FC) endothelial cell. Of these structures, it is primarily the two polarized plasma membranes, the microvillous (MVM) and the basal plasma membrane (BM) of the syncytiotrophoblast that restrict the transfer of molecules like glucose and amino acids. N = nucleus of syncytiotrophoblast cell, IVS = intervillous space, SA = spiral artery, VT = villous tree, UC = umbilical cord.

For many molecules, the transport characteristics of MVM and BM are the most important limiting factors for transplacental transport, providing the rationale for isolating these plasma membranes separately and studying their transport properties in vitro. Thus, studies of the transport properties of isolated syncytiotrophoblast plasma membranes may provide important information on transplacental transport in normal and pathological pregnancies. The presence of microvilli on the apical plasma membranes considerably increases the placental surface area exposed to maternal blood[21], which is estimated to be approximately 50 m^2. This, together with the high rates of placental and umbilical blood flow and the short diffusion distance between the maternal and fetal circulation (as little as a few micrometers in some regions of the barrier)[22], is critical to ensuring an efficient exchange between the mother and her fetus.

TYPES OF TRANSPORT INVOLVED IN MATERNOFETAL EXCHANGE

The transport of a molecule across a barrier can be limited by the blood flow transporting the molecule to and from the barrier ('flow-limited' transport) and/or by diffusion across the barrier itself ('diffusion-limited' transport). An example of a molecule with blood flow-limited transport across the placental barrier is oxygen, which is a small molecule with high lipid solubility, allowing rapid diffusion across the syncytiotrophoblast and fetal capillary endothelium. Even brief reductions in blood flow may therefore affect fetal oxygenation. In contrast, the transport of nutrients, such as glucose and amino acids, is primarily limited by the transport characteristics of the barrier itself. For molecules with a flow-limited transport there are no specific mechanisms or transporters in the barrier and the transport is characterized as 'non-mediated'. For many molecules with diffusion-limited transport there are transporters, binding proteins or receptors expressed in the syncytiotrophoblast plasma membranes or cytosol which increase the rate of transfer ('mediated transport').

Non-mediated transport

The rate of transplacental transport of molecules which lack specific transport mechanisms in the placental barrier is dependent on the physical and chemical properties of the molecules, in particular their charge, size, lipid solubility and degree of protein binding. Thus, a molecule with high lipid solubility, no charge or protein binding and with a low molecular weight diffuses rapidly between the two blood circulations. In general, the same physicochemical properties govern the non-mediated transfer of pharmaceutical drugs across the placental barrier. Indeed, oral anticoagulants such as dicumarol have a relatively low molecular weight and cross the placental barrier readily, whereas heparin, which is a charged molecule with a high molecular weight, crosses the barrier only with great difficulty[23]. However, a significant number of drugs are subjected to mediated uptake, metabolism by cytochrome 450 enzymes and/or extrusion from the syncytiotrophoblast by efflux pumps such as P-glycoprotein, limiting the value of generalized statements about placental drug transfer. This subject is covered comprehensively by recent reviews[24,25].

Mediated transport

The transplacental transfer of most nutrients and ions is mediated, i.e. there are specific transport mechanisms present in the placental barrier. When mediated transport is achieved without energy expenditure the transport is termed 'facilitated'. The term 'active' transport is used when energy is consumed, either directly (primary active transport) or indirectly (secondary active transport). The most common mechanism for mediated transport in the placental barrier is the presence of transporter proteins in the syncytiotrophoblast plasma membranes. Glucose transport is an example of facilitated transport across the placental barrier, achieved by the presence of facilitative glucose transporters in the MVM and BM. Calcium transport across the BM mediated by Ca^{2+}-ATPase is an example of primary active transport, and Na^{+}-dependent transport systems for amino acids, such as System A, represent an example of a secondary active transport mechanism. Transplacental transport may also be facilitated by the expression of receptors in the MVM (e.g. the transferrin receptor, which binds transferrin-iron complex in maternal blood thereby facilitating the placental uptake of iron) or binding proteins in syncytiotrophoblast plasma membranes or cytosol (such as fatty acid binding proteins). These transport mechanisms will be discussed in detail below.

Endocytosis/transcytosis

Endocytosis/transcytosis constitutes a special form of transport involving vesicle formation on one side of the syncytiotrophoblast by invagination of the plasma membrane and, on the opposite side of the cell, fusion of vesicles with the plasma membrane, resulting in the release of vesicle content into the extracellular space. Endocytosis/transcytosis can be non-mediated in that vesicles are formed at the plasma membrane incorporating fluid and any dissolved solute (fluid-phase endocytosis) and vesicles can be transferred across the syncytium mediated only by Brownian movements. Mediated endocytosis involves binding of a specific ligand to a receptor in the plasma membrane, which causes endocytosis and transcytosis can be mediated by components of the cytoskeleton. Endocytosis/transcytosis plays an important role in the transplacental transfer of IgG, iron and lipoproteins[26], which is discussed further below.

OXYGEN EXCHANGE

Transfer of oxygen from maternal to fetal blood occurs rapidly due to the high permeability of the placental barrier to respiratory gases. Furthermore, net transfer in the maternofetal direction is facilitated by a marked difference in pO_2 between maternal and fetal blood. This difference is large when comparing pO_2 in maternal arterial blood (100 mmHg) and pO_2 in the umbilical vein (approximately 34–41 mmHg at the end of pregnancy). This large pO_2 gradient cannot be attributed to restriction of oxygen diffusion across the placental barrier, but is likely to be due to (1) a high oxygen consumption by the placenta itself and (2) the mixing of 'arterial' and 'venous' blood in the intervillous space resulting in a pO_2 significantly lower than in maternal arterial blood. Other factors facilitating movement of oxygen in the maternofetal direction are higher hemoglobin concentrations in fetal blood, resulting in a significantly higher oxygen carrying capacity of fetal blood, and a higher affinity of fetal (HbF) hemoglobin for oxygen as compared to maternal hemoglobin (HbA). The higher oxygen affinity of HbF is due to its lower affinity to bind 2,3-diphosphoglycerate[27], which shifts the oxygen–hemoglobin dissociation curve to the left in fetal blood.

The effect of reductions in uteroplacental or umbilical blood flow on fetal pO_2 and fetal oxygen uptake has been studied in detail in fetal sheep, and it is likely that the principal findings in these studies can be extrapolated to the human fetus. Indeed, fetal O_2 uptake is maintained remarkably constant via compensatory changes in fractional O_2 extraction, i.e. subsequent to the decrease in umbilical vein pO_2, umbilical artery pO_2 decreases in parallel[28,29]. Therefore, in response to an acute reduction in placental blood flow, umbilical artery pO_2 will decrease, resulting in hypoxemia. However, the increase in fractional oxygen extraction will maintain fetal oxygen uptake, thereby counteracting the development of tissue hypoxia and acidosis. While responses to short-term hypoxemia are observed in clinical situations such as cord compression, maternal exercise, fetal activity or uterine contractions, no effect on long-term outcome has been demonstrated. However, fetal sheep subjected to long-term hypoxemia show altered metabolism and reduced growth[30,31].

SODIUM TRANSPORT

Uptake of sodium by the fetus is critical for growth and development but must be carefully controlled to maintain correct osmotic and fluid balance in the fetal compartment. The inwardly directed sodium gradient in the syncytiotrophoblast cell is maintained by Na^+K^+-ATPase in the plasma membrane and is used to transport a large number of nutrients and other ions (i.e. amino acids, phosphorus, magnesium and calcium) to the syncytial cytoplasm. Sodium is transported to the fetus against its electrochemical gradient across the BM by the Na^+K^+-ATPase[32] but, interestingly, we have also found Na^+K^+-ATPase in the MVM[33], which would seem counterintuitive for net sodium transport in the direction of the fetus. We have proposed that unidirectional transport of sodium toward the fetus would result in rapid overhydration of the closed fetal compartment resulting in elevated blood pressure and polyhydramnios[33]. Therefore, in order to use the sodium gradient to drive nutrient and ion uptake and waste removal, an efficient mechanism to return sodium to the maternal compartment and maintain the gradient must be localized to the MVM. The presence of the Na^+K^+-ATPase in the MVM would provide such a mechanism.

WATER

Close to term, the human fetus has a daily water requirement of 22 ml[34]. Since only approximately 20% of the fetal water accumulation can be accounted for by water produced by fetal metabolism[35], most of the water must be obtained from the mother, which is primarily transferred across the placenta[36]. The driving forces for net maternofetal water movement and the pathways for water and solute transfer across the human placenta remain poorly defined. However, values for pressure in the umbilical circulation and intervillous space, obtained by transabdominal techniques[37–41], clearly suggest that hydrostatic pressure differences across the human placenta promote transfer of water from the fetus to the mother. Since colloidal osmotic pressure differences[35,42,43] also cause water to move in the maternal direction, net transplacental movement of water must be driven by a gradient of solutes. However, no significant gradient has been clearly demonstrated when maternal and fetal osmotic pressures have been measured[44]. This apparent contradiction has been resolved by studies demonstrating that the water permeability of the syncytiotrophoblast plasma membranes is significant[45,46] suggesting that water accumulation by the human fetus could be driven by a solute gradient across the placental barrier small enough to be within the error of standard osmolarity measurements[46]. In an analogous situation described for the rat placenta[36,47,48], available data for the human placenta suggest that solute is actively transported into the fetal compartment and water follows osmotically via a transcellular pathway. Subsequently, water recirculates back to the maternal compartment through transtrophoblast channels driven by the hydrostatic and colloid osmotic pressure gradients. Isoforms 3, 8 and 9 of aquaporin water channels have been shown to be expressed at the RNA and protein level in the human syncytiotrophoblast[49–51]. However, the functional role of these aquaporins in the syncytiotrophoblast remains to be fully established since there is currently no evidence to suggest significant aquaporin mediated water permeation across isolated microvillous and basal plasma membranes[46]. Aquaporin 3 and 9 mediate the transport of small solutes such as urea in addition to water[52] and it has been suggested that placental aquaporins are involved in solute transport[49].

ACID–BASE BALANCE, CARBON DIOXIDE AND PROTONS

The fetus is dependent on the placenta for regulation of its acid–base balance. Large amounts of carbon dioxide are continuously produced by the fetus and the placenta as a result of oxidative metabolism. In postnatal life, CO_2 is rapidly eliminated via the lungs but is also in equilibrium with carbonic acid, which can rapidly produce protons. In the context of fetal acid–base balance, CO_2 is therefore characterized as a 'respiratory acid'. Carbon dioxide produced in the fetus readily crosses the placental barrier via non-mediated transfer and is eliminated by the mother. Due to hyperventilation, arterial pCO_2 is lower in the pregnant woman (between 26 and 34 mmHg)[53] as compared to the non-pregnant woman. Umbilical vein pCO_2 at term is between 38 and 45 mmHg[54], providing a substantial diffusion gradient promoting fetal–maternal CO_2 transfer. Due to its high lipid solubility, transplacental transfer of CO_2 is blood flow limited. Catalyzed by carbonic anhydrase in erythrocytes, the majority of the CO_2 in blood is present as H^+ and bicarbonate ions. Some CO_2 is associated with deoxygenated Hb, as carbamino-Hb, and only a small amount is dissolved. In order to be readily transferred across the placenta, CO_2 is produced from H^+ and HCO_3^- at the placental barrier, a reaction facilitated by the action of carbonic anhydrase expressed in endothelial and trophoblast cells[55]. If placental and/or umbilical blood flows are reduced, respiratory acidosis may develop quickly, which is normalized following re-establishment of adequate blood flows.

Acid equivalents produced metabolically by the fetus cannot be eliminated across the placental barrier by the movement of CO_2, but require transport of protons from the fetal to the maternal circulations or, alternatively, bicarbonate in the reverse direction. This is achieved by specific transporters expressed in the MVM and BM. The most important placental transporter involved in acid–base regulation is the sodium–proton exchanger (NHE), which is highly active in the MVM[56]. Several NHE isoforms have been identified in the human placenta and all utilize the inwardly directed Na^+ gradient to exchange sodium moving in with protons moving out of the syncytiotrophoblast cells into the intervillous space[57]. In intrauterine growth restriction (IUGR), the protein expression and activity of MVM NHE is decreased, which has been proposed to contribute to the in utero acidosis that some IUGR fetuses develop[58].

During fetal life, lactate is an important energy source in the heart, brain and skeletal muscle and fetal levels of lactate are higher than maternal levels. The placenta may be a source of lactate even when oxygen supplies are adequate[59]. However, the placenta is also an important site for clearance of fetally produced lactate, especially in cases of fetal hypoxia[60]. Studies in human placenta indicate that lactate is taken up by both syncytiotrophoblast plasma membranes by a lactate/H^+ co-transporter also known as monocarboxylate transporter (MCT) isoforms 1 and 4[61]. The capacity to take up lactate is reduced in the BM from placentas of IUGR pregnancies but not in the MVM[62]. This decrease in activity may contribute to the lactacidemia often associated with this pregnancy complication.

CALCIUM TRANSPORT

The fetus requires approximately 30 g of calcium to develop normally, and much of this accumulation takes place in the third trimester when fetal bone mineralization occurs. As in other cells, the intracellular calcium concentration in the syncytiotrophoblast is approximately one million times lower than extracellular concentrations, allowing intracellular calcium to participate in critical signal transduction pathways. Calcium entry across the MVM is therefore primarily mediated by calcium channels which allow for diffusion of calcium down its electrochemical gradient. Several types of non-selective cation channels have been localized in the MVM that would allow for calcium entry from the maternal plasma[63–65]. Once calcium enters the cytoplasm, it is quickly sequestered into intracellular compartments or bound to calcium-binding proteins such as calmodulin or calbindin. Sequestration into endoplasmic reticulum allows for regulation of intracellular calcium concentrations and release of calcium in response to signaling through a DAG-PKC-IP3 pathway. Cytoplasmic calcium binding proteins transport calcium through the cytoplasm and help to buffer intracellular calcium. In the rat placenta, calbindin-9k has been found to be highly expressed in late gestation and to be the rate-limiting step in transplacental transport[66]. However, the role of calbindin-9k is less clear in humans[67]. The calcium pump (or Ca^{2+}-ATPase) is highly expressed in the basal plasma membrane and this transporter pumps calcium out of the syncytiotrophoblast in the fetal direction against a formidable concentration gradient. As a result of this primary active transport, fetal blood Ca^{2+} concentrations are higher than maternal. The activity of the basal membrane calcium pump was found to increase significantly from gestational week 32 to 37 suggesting an increased transport capacity during fetal skeletal mineralization[68]. Interestingly, BM Ca^{2+}-ATPase activity was found to be increased in both IUGR and in fetal overgrowth in association to maternal diabetes, possibly to meet fetal calcium needs that, in relation to placental and fetal weight, are in fact increased in these pregnancy complications[69].

Human placental Ca^{2+}-ATPase has been shown to be regulated by PTHrP (38-94), a mid-molecule fragment of parathyroid hormone-related peptide, and increased fetal concentrations of PTHrP (38-94) may provide a mechanisms for the increased placental Ca^{2+}-ATPase activity in IUGR[70]. In studies of mice homozygous for the deletion of the PTHrP gene, the normally occurring maternal to fetal calcium gradient was absent as was the transfer of maternally administered isotope-labeled calcium. Treating the fetuses with various PTH and PTHrP fragments defined the mid-molecule fragment of PTHrP as the portion responsible for the regulation of placental calcium transport[71].

IRON

During pregnancy, diferric (Fe^{3+}) transferrin in maternal plasma binds to the transferrin receptor in the MVM of the syncytiotrophoblast[72,73] and is internalized in a clathrin-mediated endocytosis. The iron is reduced (Fe^{2+}) and released in the acidic endosome and the maternal apotransferrin is returned to the plasma membrane for release. No maternal transferrin enters the fetal circulation. Efflux of iron from the endosome is likely mediated by the divalent metal transporter protein (DMT1)[74]. Once in the cytoplasm, the iron is used in biosynthetic pathways, stored (bound to ferritin or as free iron pool), or transported across the basal membrane to the fetus. Once released in the syncytiotrophoblast cytoplasm, the iron is believed to be oxidized by endogenous ferroxidase, a ceruloplasmin homologue[75,76], before being transported by ferroportin, also known as iron regulated gene (IREG1) or metal transport protein (MTP1), across the basal membrane to the fetus. In iron deficiency states, the fetus has the capacity to upregulate the transferrin receptor on the maternal facing membrane and DMT1 in the cytoplasm to ensure adequate transport to the fetus while leading to further deficiency in the mother.

IMMUNOGLOBULINS

Maternal antibodies, primarily IgG, are transported by the human placenta and mediate passive immunity to the fetus and neonate[77]. Placental IgG transport becomes significant in mid pregnancy[78] and increases in the third trimester[79]. IgG1 appears to be preferentially transported as compared to the other IgG subclasses[78]. At term, fetal IgG levels exceed those in the maternal circulation suggesting an active transport against a concentration gradient[80]. The mechanisms by which IgG is transferred across the placental barrier in the human are not well established. Uptake across the microvillous plasma membrane is proposed to be mediated by fluid-phase endocytosis into acidic early endosomes, rather than by receptor-mediated endocytosis mediated by the human Fc receptor isoform FcRIII[26,81]. There is strong evidence to suggest that another Fc receptor, the human neonatal Fcg receptor (hFcRn) with a pH optimum for IgG binding at pH 6, plays a crucial role in the transfer across the syncytiotrophoblast in acidic vesicles[26,82]. The IgG transfer across BM is less clear, however, it is assumed that acidic vesicles containing IgG bound to hFcRn are targeted to the basal plasma membrane[26]. Once IgG reaches the interstitial space on the fetal side of the syncytiotrophoblast, it has to traverse the basement membrane and fetal capillary endothelium. Although the former does not appear to present a significant barrier[83,84], the latter does; the available data suggest that transcytosis in vesicles is a more likely route of transfer across the endothelium than is diffusion through the lateral intercellular spaces between endothelial cells[83,85,86].

GLUCOSE

Glucose is the primary substrate for energy metabolism in the placenta and fetus. Of the total amount of glucose taken up by the placenta from the uterine circulation, 30–40% is consumed by the placenta itself. Transplacental glucose transport is Na^+-independent and facilitated by glucose transporters (GLUTs) expressed in the two polarized syncytiotrophoblast plasma membranes[3,87–92] and as reviewed in[93–96] (Fig. 8.2). In the first trimester, at least four different GLUT isoforms are expressed in the syncytiotrophoblast: GLUT 1, 3, 4 and 12[97,98] of which GLUT 4 and 12 are sensitive to regulation by insulin.

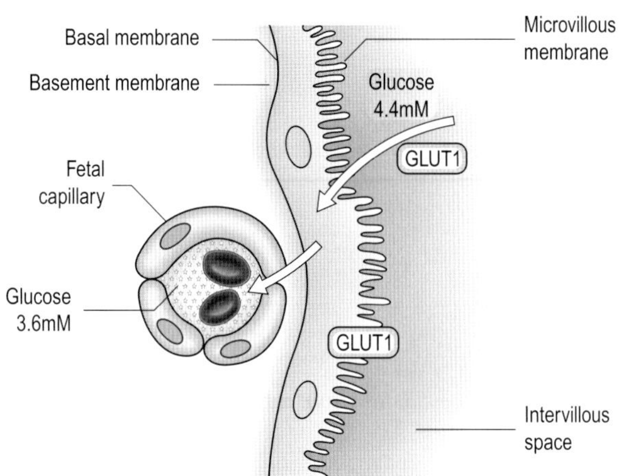

Fig. 8.2 Principles for placental glucose transport. Glucose transport across the placental barrier is primarily mediated by glucose transporter 1 (GLUT1), an isoform of the family of facilitated glucose transporters. Despite the high glucose consumption of the placenta itself, the glucose concentrations in the umbilical vein are only approximately 1 mM lower than in the intervillous space, indicating a large transport capacity for glucose. Due to the facilitated nature of glucose transport net transfer is sensitive to changes in the concentration gradient (see text). MVM = microvillous plasma membrane, BM = basal plasma membrane.

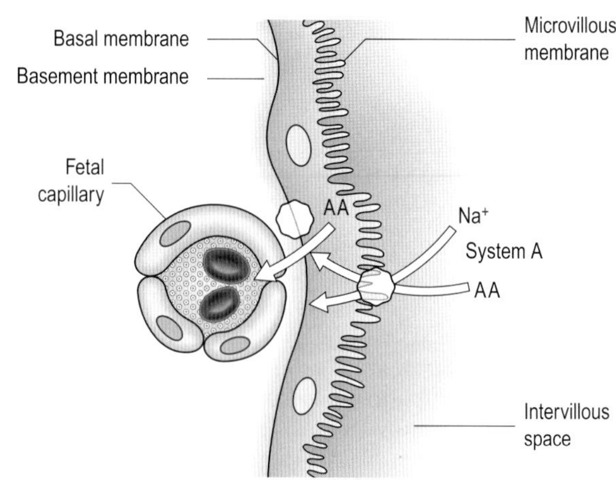

Fig. 8.3 Principles for placental amino acid transport. Amino acid (AA) transport across the placenta is an active transport resulting in higher concentrations of AA in fetal blood as compared to the maternal circulation. The transport across the syncytiotrophoblast microvillous plasma membrane (MVM) constitutes the active step, often energized by the inwardly directed Na^+-gradient. As a consequence, AA concentrations in the syncytiotrophoblast cytoplasm are much higher than in maternal and fetal blood. The transport across the basal plasma membrane (BM) is facilitated by specific transporters and driven by the outwardly directed concentrations gradient for AA.

In late pregnancy, however, GLUT1 is the primary GLUT isoform mediating glucose transport across the placental barrier in the human[92,97]. This marked difference between early and late pregnancy in the expression of glucose transporters in the syncytium may explain experimental findings that insulin stimulates placental glucose uptake primarily in the first trimester[97]. Both first-trimester and term human placenta showed greater GLUT1 immunoreactivity on the microvillous plasma membrane compared with the basal plasma membrane[91,92]. This asymmetry in GLUT1 distribution together with the much greater surface area of the microvillous membrane may well result in syncytial intracellular glucose concentrations approaching maternal levels, providing a maximal gradient for transfer to the fetus[92]. Based on these findings, it has been suggested that it is the transport across the basal plasma membrane that constitutes the rate-limiting step of transplacental glucose transport[92], and some recent studies in polarized BeWo cells have provided some support for this hypothesis[99].

The driving force for transfer of glucose in the maternofetal direction is the higher glucose concentration in maternal as compared to fetal blood[100]. An important consequence of the facilitated nature of placental glucose transport and the fact that the glucose concentration in the maternal and fetal blood circulations are much lower[100] than the affinity of the GLUT transporters[87,89], is that net transfer is critically dependent on the glucose concentration difference between maternal and fetal blood. Maternal hyperglycemia in diabetes with suboptimal metabolic control will therefore result in an increased glucose transfer, which will increase fetal insulin secretion and consequently fetal growth. Paradoxically, placental glucose transporters are upregulated in type 1 diabetes[101], which could increase placental glucose transport even during normoglycemia. Indeed, these changes have been proposed to explain fetal overgrowth in type-1 diabetes with apparent optimal glucose control[101]. Fetal hypoglycemia in IUGR is unlikely to be due to changes in placental glucose transporters since both GLUT1 protein expression and glucose transport activity in syncytiotrophoblast plasma membranes have been reported to be unaltered in IUGR[92,102].

AMINO ACIDS

Amino acids constitute building blocks for fetal protein synthesis and non-essential amino acids are also used as energy substrates. The transfer of amino acids across the placental barrier is an active process resulting in concentrations for most amino acids that are higher or much higher in the umbilical vein as compared to the uterine artery[103,104]. Placental amino acid transport is complex and the syncytiotrophoblast expresses at least 15 different amino acid transporters, each transporter mediating the uptake of several different amino acids, and one specific amino acid can be transported by multiple transport systems, as discussed in detail in previously published reviews[105–108]. The uptake across the MVM represents the active step in transplacental amino acid transfer by concentrating amino acids in the cytosol of the syncytiotrophoblast by means of secondary active transport[106] (Fig. 8.3). The driving force for the amino acid uptake across the MVM is, in many cases, the inwardly directed Na^+-gradient (e.g. the System A transporter and the taurine transporter), but can also be a result of the electrical potential difference with the inside of the cell negative (the driving force for the uptake of the cationic amino acids arginine and lysine). Some amino acid transporters are exchangers, i.e. one amino acid is exchanged for another one across the plasma membrane[107]. The L-amino acid transporter system is one example of an exchanger, which uses the steep outwardly directed concentration gradient of some non-essential amino acids such as glycine to drive uptake of leucine, an essential amino acid, against its concentration gradient[109]. In all these cases, the energy for the uphill transport is ultimately generated by the Na^+K^+-ATPase which extrudes sodium in exchange for potassium thereby maintaining a low intracellular Na^+ concentration and creating a potential difference across the plasma membrane[33]. After being concentrated in the cytosol of the syncytiotrophoblast, amino acids cross the syncytiotrophoblast basal plasma membrane into the fetal circulation by facilitated transport using the large outwardly directed concentration gradient for most amino acids[106] (see Fig. 8.3). Thus, the concentrations of amino acids in the cytosol of the syncytiotrophoblast are much higher than those in both maternal and fetal blood[110,111]. The asymmetric distribution of amino acid transporters between the two syncytiotrophoblast plasma membranes, with secondary active transport systems primarily expressed in the MVM, is critical in order to generate a net flux of amino acids from mother to fetus.

The activity of amino acid transporters in the human placenta is reduced in association with IUGR and increased in fetal overgrowth suggesting that changes in placental nutrient transporters may contribute to pathological fetal growth (reviewed in[1,2]). The activity of System A, a Na^+-dependent transporter mediating the uptake of non-essential neutral amino acids, is markedly reduced in the MVM in IUGR[112,113], in particular in severely compromised IUGR babies delivered prematurely[102]. In addition, the activity of a number of placental transport systems for essential amino acids, such as lysine and leucine[109] and taurine[114], are reduced in MVM and/or BM isolated from IUGR placentas. These in vitro findings are compatible with a study in pregnant women in which Paolini and coworkers demonstrated, using stable isotope techniques, that placental transfer of the essential amino acids leucine and phenylalanine is reduced in IUGR[115]. The downregulation of placental amino acid transporters in IUGR results in a decreased delivery of amino acids to the fetus and is likely to be an important factor causing the low fetal plasma concentrations of certain amino acids in this pregnancy complication[116–118]. Amino acids are, together with glucose, the primary stimuli for secretion of fetal insulin, probably the most important growth-promoting hormone in utero. Therefore, it appears that there is a direct link between downregulation of placental amino acid transporters and restricted fetal growth in IUGR. Currently, there is no unequivocal evidence demonstrating that downregulation of placental amino acid transporters causes IUGR. However, recent experimental data demonstrate that downregulation of placental amino acid transporters precedes reduced fetal growth in animal models of IUGR[119].

LIPIDS

While lipids are relatively soluble in plasma membranes, a number of mechanisms ensure adequate transport of free fatty acids (FFA) to the fetus. The source of fatty acids to be transported to the fetus is either triglyceride (TG)-rich maternal lipoproteins, such as chylomicrons and very low density lipoprotein (VLDL), or FFA bound to albumin. Maternal lipid metabolism changes during pregnancy and plasma FFA concentrations increase rapidly during the third trimester and represent the main class of lipids crossing the placenta[120–122]. Most essential fatty acids (EFA) and long-chain polyunsaturated fatty acids (LCPUFA) are delivered to the placenta incorporated into TGs in lipoproteins[123]. Net transfer of FFA to the fetus is thought to be driven by the maternal–fetal gradient[124]. TGs cannot be transported intact over the syncytiotrophoblast but must first be hydrolyzed into FFA by lipase enzymes in the microvillous membrane or endocytosed as intact lipoprotein particles (Fig. 8.4). Both processes are initiated by lipoprotein binding to lipoprotein receptors (VLDL and low density lipoprotein (LDL) receptors) in the MVM[125,126].

Lipoprotein lipase (LPL) is bound to heparin sulfate proteoglycans in the MVM[127] and hydrolyzes TG from lipoproteins to FFA. Other lipases are also present including endothelial lipase[128] and possibly a placental specific lipase[129]. The FFA are thought to reach the intracellular compartment by simple diffusion[130] or by the action of the membrane-bound fatty acid binding proteins (FABPs) which facilitate FFA transfer across membranes and provide a mechanism for intracellular channeling of fatty acids[131]. The FABP found in placental membranes include a placenta-specific FABP[132] which acts as an extracellular fatty acid acceptor and fatty acid transfer proteins (FAT/CD36 and FATP) which span the lipid bilayer and function as fatty acid transporters/translocases. The plasma membrane FABP has been found only in the MVM, whereas FAT/CD36 and FATP are found both in MVM and BM[133]. Several studies have shown a preferential uptake of LCPUFAs by the placenta[121]. Further, fetal blood docosahexaenoic acid, as a percent of total fatty acids, is increasing exponentially after 20 weeks of gestation[134]. No preference in LCPUFA

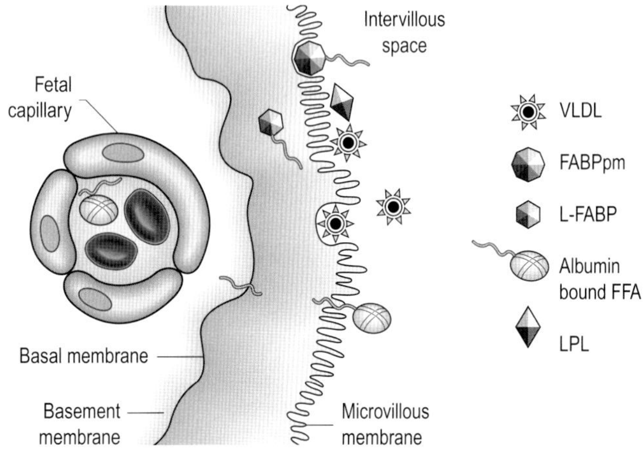

Fig. 8.4 Principles for placental lipid transport. In the maternal blood there are two major sources for free fatty acids (FFA) that can be transported to the fetus: 1. FFA bound to albumin in an albumin–FFA complex, which can interact with fatty acid binding protein proteins in MVM, resulting in transfer of FFA across the MVM. 2. Triglycerides in maternal lipoproteins, in particular very low density lipoproteins (VLDL), which are hydrolyzed into FFA by lipoprotein lipase (LPL) expressed in the MVM. FFA is subsequently transferred across the MVM. Alternatively, maternal lipoproteins interact with LDL/VLDL receptors in MVM resulting in endocytosis and intracellular hydrolysis, which releases FFA. Intracellularly, FFA are transported bound to fatty acid binding proteins. The mechanisms for FFA transfer across the basal plasma membrane (BM) are not well established.

uptake has been observed for FAT/CD36 or FATP, indicating that these transporters, present in both MVM and BM, allow for the non-selective transfer of fatty acids across both membranes. Therefore, most of the selective uptake is taking place in the MVM and ensures the enrichment of LCPUFAs in the syncytiotrophoblast[135].

Internalization of lipoproteins is through clathrin-mediated endocytosis. The vesicles are acidified and the receptors release the lipoprotein particle and are returned to the apical membrane. The lipoproteins are processed in endosomes and lysosomes and eventually the TG is hydrolyzed by intracellular lipases such as hormone-sensitive lipase (for review see[26]). FFA in the syncytial cytoplasm bind to cytoplasmic FABP and are directed to different sites for esterification, beta-oxidation or for transport over to the fetus across the BM. Two types of FABPs have been detected in syncytiotrophoblast cytoplasm; the liver-FABP (L-FABP) and cardiac-FABP (C-FABP)[132]. The transport of fatty acids over the BM is thought to be either through diffusion or by assistance by the FATPs. However, recent data suggest that the placenta produces and secretes ApoB particles, but whether these are released to the maternal or fetal compartment remains unclear[136].

REGULATION OF PLACENTAL NUTRIENT TRANSPORTERS

Fetal growth is primarily determined by nutrient availability, which is intimately related to placental nutrient transport. The findings reviewed above, demonstrating that both IUGR and fetal overgrowth are conditions associated with specific changes in placental nutrient transporters, have stimulated inquiries into the factors which maybe responsible for the changes in placental transport function. Indeed, detailed information on the regulation of placental nutrient transporters is critical in order to understand the mechanisms underlying altered fetal growth, and may also provide novel avenues for intervention. Placental transport is determined by numerous factors including concentration gradients, placental metabolism and blood flow. For glucose and amino acids, the expression and activity of plasma membrane transport proteins are particularly important in maintaining the nutrient supply to the developing fetus. In addition, the transfer of lipids across the placenta is dependent on lipases, lipoprotein receptors and membrane-bound and cytosolic fatty acid binding proteins.

Glucocorticoids decrease the expression of placental glucose transporters[137]. Some in vitro studies[138,139] have shown that insulin does not affect placental glucose uptake at term, whereas other investigators have demonstrated a modest stimulating effect of insulin on placental glucose uptake[140,141]. In a first-trimester trophoblast cell line, glucose transport activity was increased after 1 hour of incubation with insulin, insulin-like growth factors (IGF-I or IGF-II)[142,143]. Using primary villous fragments from human placenta, it was demonstrated that placental glucose transporter activity was not affected by hormones such as leptin, GH, IGF-I, insulin and cortisol, at term[139]. However, in the first trimester, insulin markedly stimulated glucose uptake at 6–8 weeks of gestation[97], which may be related to the findings of expression of the insulin-sensitive glucose transporter GLUT 4 in the cytosol and microvillous plasma membranes of the syncytiotrophoblast in first trimester[97].

With regard to the regulation of placental amino acid transporters, system A, a key transporter for neutral amino acids, has been the focus of most studies. Using cultured trophoblast cells, placental system A transporter activity has been shown to be stimulated by insulin, IGF-I and epidermal growth factor (EGF) and by decreased substrate concentrations[144,145]. A 1-hour incubation with leptin and insulin stimulated System A activity uptake by 50–60% in primary villous fragments at term[146]. Furthermore, in cultured trophoblast cells, hypoxia decreased system A activity, which could be explained by a decreased protein expression of the two System A transporter isoforms SNAT 1 and 2[147]. Recently, it was shown that inhibition of the mammalian target of rapamycin signaling system in primary villous fragments of human placenta, markedly reduced the transport of the essential amino acid leucine, and that placental mTOR signaling activity was downregulated in IUGR[148]. These findings implicate placental mTOR signaling as a regulator of placental amino acid transporters.

The factors regulating lipid and ion transport in the human placenta are largely unknown. Placental LPL activity has been shown to be inhibited by high substrate concentrations[149] and stimulated by estradiol and the combination of hyperinsulinemia and hyperglycemia[150]. The activity of BM Ca^{2+}-ATPase has been shown to be under the regulation of a fetal hormone, an active fragment of parathyroid hormone-related peptide (PTHrp 38-94)[70].

CLINICAL IMPLICATIONS

A large body of data suggests that specific changes in placental transport of nutrient and ions directly contribute to pathological fetal growth[1,2]. Thus, the restricted nutrient delivery in 'placental insufficiency' is not only a matter of decreased blood flow or a smaller placenta but also a downregulation of placental nutrient transporters. Similarly, the increased fetal nutrient delivery in fetal overgrowth in association with maternal diabetes is due to an upregulation of placental nutrient transporters in addition to elevated maternal nutrient levels. It has been discussed in the literature that mechanisms for maternofetal exchange may adapt in order to increase nutrient transport capacity in IUGR and to downregulate placental nutrient transport in fetal overgrowth in diabetes, thereby 'protecting' the fetus from high glucose levels. However, the data discussed in this chapter indicate the opposite, although it cannot be excluded that compensatory changes in placental transport may be present earlier in pregnancy.

In order to understand the pathophysiology of altered fetal growth, information on the factors that regulate placental transporters is critical. As discussed previously, studies in different in vitro preparations of the human placenta have demonstrated that placental transporters are under the regulation of hormones and growth factors including IGF-I, insulin and leptin. The receptors in the placenta for these factors are primarily localized in the microvillous plasma membrane of the syncytiotrophoblast[151–153] and, therefore, directly exposed to maternal blood. Furthermore, the placenta produces many hormones, including IGF-I and leptin[154,155], which are secreted into the intervillous space where they can interact with the receptors on the microvillous plasma membrane, constituting an autocrine/paracrine regulation. Thus it appears that placental transporters are under the regulation of maternal and placental hormones and growth factors. It is interesting to note that in IUGR and fetal overgrowth, the maternal serum concentrations and placental production of these factors, as well as receptor number or activity in the placenta for these growth factors and hormones, are changed in a direction compatible with the possibility that these factors play a critical role in regulating placental transport and fetal growth in clinically important pregnancy complications. In IUGR, for example, maternal serum concentrations of IGF-I are decreased[156] and some studies indicate that maternal serum leptin concentrations are reduced[157]. Furthermore, placental insulin receptor number[158], placental IGF-I signaling activity[159] and placental leptin production[160] are reduced in IUGR. In contrast, circulating maternal IGF-I is increased in pregnancies with diabetes and accelerated fetal growth[161], placental insulin receptor binding and insulin receptor kinase activity are increased in gestational diabetes with accelerated fetal growth[162], and placental leptin production is elevated in maternal diabetes[160].

In animal models of IUGR, changes in placental transport functions are observed before fetal growth rate is affected[119], suggesting that targeting placental transport functions may be advantageous both in early diagnosis and treatment of pathological fetal growth. Currently, there are no non-invasive simple techniques to assess placental transport function in the pregnant woman. However, a change in placental nutrient transport is likely to affect placental growth before altering fetal growth, compatible with the idea that decreased placental growth constitutes an early sign of developing IUGR. Indeed, 3D ultrasound measurement of placental volume in the second trimester correlates significantly with birth weight[163–165]. Placental volume measurements may therefore provide a predictor of subsequent decreases in fetal growth rate.

The development of specific strategies for treatment and intervention in cases of altered fetal growth has been hampered by our limited understanding of the underlying pathophysiology. However, significant progress has been made recently in elucidating the key mechanisms involved in pathological growth and this knowledge will provide the necessary foundation for designing novel intervention strategies in the near future. For example, maternal IGF-I administration stimulates fetal growth in animal experiments and has been proposed as a possible therapy in cases of IUGR[166,167]. The mechanisms involved have been suggested to be effects on placental function and possibly the transfer of nutrients across the placenta[166,167], compatible with in vitro studies demonstrating that IGF-I stimulates trophoblast glucose and amino acid uptake[143,168]. Thus, maternal IGF-I administration is an example of an intervention targeting placental transport function that may be of value in order to alleviate restricted fetal growth.

REFERENCES

1. Jansson T, Powell TL. Human placental transport in altered fetal growth: does the placenta function as a nutrient sensor? A review. *Placenta* **27**(Suppl):91–97, 2006.
2. Sibley CP, Turner MA, Cetin I et al. Placental phenotypes of intrauterine growth. *Pediatr Res* **58**:827–832, 2005.
3. Sibley CP, Boyd RDH. Control of transfer across the mature placenta. In *Oxford reviews of reproductive biology*, JR Clarke (ed.), Vol. 10. Oxford: OUP, 1988.
4. Smith CH, Moe AJ. Nutrient transport pathways across the epithelium of the placenta. *Annu Rev Nutr* **12**:183–206, 1992.
5. Sibley CP, Boyd RDH. Mechanisms of transfer across the human placenta. In *Fetal and neonatal physiology*, RA Polin, WW Fox (eds). Philadelphia: WB Saunders Co, 1998.
6. Sibley C, D´Souza S, Glazier J et al. Mechanisms of solute transfer across the human placenta: effects of intrauterine growth restriction. *Fetal Maternal Med Rev* **10**:197–206, 1998.
7. Faber JJ, Thornburg KL. *Placental physiology: structure and function of fetomaternal exchange*. New York: Raven Press, 1983.
8. Morriss FH, Boyd RDH, Mahendran D. Placental transport. In *The physiology of reproduction*, E Knobil, JD Neill (eds). New York: Raven Press Limited, 1994.
9. Page K. *The physiology of the human placenta*. London: University College London Press, 1993.
10. Ganapathy V, Fei YJ, Prasad PD. Heterologous expression systems for studying placental transporters. *Methods Mol Med* **122**:285–300, 2006.
11. Xu Y, Cook TJ, Knipp GT. Methods for investigating placental fatty acid transport. *Methods Mol Med* **122**:265–284, 2006.
12. Glazier JD, Sibley CP. In vitro methods for studying human placental amino acid transport: placental plasma membrane vesicles. *Methods Mol Med* **122**:241–252, 2006.
13. Greenwood SL, Sibley CP. In vitro methods for studying human placental amino acid transport: placental villous fragments. *Methods Mol Med* **122**:253–264, 2006.
14. Trundley A, Gardner L, Northfield J et al. Methods for isolation of cells from the human fetal–maternal interface. *Methods Mol Med* **122**:109–122, 2006.
15. Kaufmann P, Burton GJ. Anatomy and genesis of the placenta. In *The physiology of reproduction*, E Knobil, JD Neill (eds). New York: Raven Press, 1994.
16. Firth JA, Leach L. Not trophoblast alone: a review of the contribution of the fetal microvasculature to transplacental exchange. *Placenta* **17**:89–96, 1996.
17. Edwards D, Jones CJP, Sibley CP et al. Paracellular permeability pathways in the human placenta: a quantitative and morphological study of maternal–fetal transfer of horseradish peroxidase. *Placenta* **14**:63–73, 1993.
18. Brownbill PD, Edwards D, Jones C et al. Mechanisms of alphafetoprotein transfer in the perfused human placental cotyledon from uncomplicated pregnancy. *J Clin Invest* **96**:2220–2226, 1995.
19. Kertschanska S, Kosanke G, Kaufmann P. Is there morphological evidence for the existence of transtrophoblastic channels in human placental villi? *Trophoblast Res* **8**:581–596, 1995.
20. Brownbill PD, Mahendran D, Owen D et al. Denudations as paracellular routes for alphafetoprotein and creatinine across the human syncytiotrophoblast. *Am J Physiol Regul Integr Com Physiol* **278**:R677–R683, 2000.
21. Teasdale F, Jean-Jacques G. Intrauterine growth retardation: morphometry of the microvillous membrane of the human placenta. *Placenta* **9**:47–55, 1988.
22. Feneley MR, Burton GJ. Villous composition and membrane thickness in the human placenta at term: a stereological study using unbiased estimators and optimal fixation techniques. *Placenta* **12**:131–142, 1991.
23. Bajoria R, Contractor SF. Transfer of heparin across the human placenta. *J Pharm Pharmacol* **44**:952–959, 1992.
24. Marin JJG, Briz O, Serrano MA. A review on the molecular mechanisms involved in the placental barrier for drugs. *Curr Drug Deliv* **1**:275–289, 2004.
25. Syme MR, Paxton JW, Keelan JA. Drug transfer and metabolism by the human

placenta. *Clin Pharmacokinet* **43**:487–514, 2004.
26. Fuchs R, Ellinger I. Endocytic and transcytotic processes in villous syncytiotrophoblast: role in nutrient transport to the human fetus. *Traffic* **5**:725–738, 2004.
27. Banner CH, Ludwig I, Ludwig M. Different effects of 2,3-diphosphoglycerate and adenosine triphosphate on the oxygen affinity of adult and foetal haemoglobin. *Life Sci* **7**:1339–1343, 1968.
28. Edelstone DI, Peticca BB, Goldblum LJ. Effects of maternal oxygen administration on fetal oxygenation during reductions in umbilical blood flow in fetal lambs. *Am J Obstet Gynecol* **152**:351–358, 1989.
29. Wilkening RB, Meschia G. Fetal oxygen uptake, oxygenation and acid–base balance as a function of uterine blood flow. *Am J Physiol* **244**:H749–H755, 1983.
30. Anderson DF, Parks CM, Faber JJ. Fetal O2 consumption in sheep during controlled long-term reductions in umbilical blood flow. *Am J Physiol* **250**:H1037–H1042, 1986.
31. Jacobs R, Robinson JS, Owens JA et al. The effect of prolonged hypobaric hypoxia on growth of fetal sheep. *J Dev Physiol* **10**:97–112, 1988.
32. Whitsett J, Wallick E. (^{3}H)–ouabain binding and Na^+/K^+ ATPase activity in human placenta. *Am J Physiol* **238**:E38–E45, 1980.
33. Johansson M, Jansson T, Powell TL. Na^+/K^+-ATPase is distributed to microvillous and basal membrane of the syncytiotrophoblast in the human placenta. *Am J Physiol* **279**:R287–R294, 2000.
34. Hytten FE. Water transfer. In *Placental transfer*, G Chamberlain, A Wilkinson (eds). Tunbridge Wells: Pitman Medical Publishing Co Ltd, 1979.
35. Power GG, Roos PJ, Longo LD. Water transfer across the placenta: hydrostatic and osmotic forces and the control of fetal cardiac output. In *Fetal and newborn cardiovascular physiology*, L Longo, D Reneau (eds), Vol. 1. New York: Garland STPM Press, 1978.
36. Stulc J. Placental transfer of inorganic ions and water. *Physiol Rev* **77**:805–836, 1997.
37. Nicolini U, Fisk NM, Talbert DG et al. Intrauterine manometry: technique and application to fetal pathology. *Prenatal Diagnosis* **9**:243–254, 1989.
38. Weiner CP, Pelzer GD, Heilskov J et al. The effect of intravascular transfusion on umbilical venous pressure in anemic fetuses with and without hydrops. *Am J Obstet Gynecol* **161**:1498–1501, 1989.
39. Weiner CP, Heilskov J, Pelzer G et al. Normal values for human umbilical venous and amniotic fluid pressures and their alteration by fetal disease. *Am J Obstet Gynecol* **161**:714–717, 1989.
40. Moise KJ, Mari G, Fischer DJ et al. Acute fetal hemodynamic alterations after intrauterine transfusion for treatment of severe red blood cell alloimmunization. *Am J Obstet Gynecol* **163**:776–784, 1990.
41. Weiner CP, Spies SL, Wenstrom K. The effect of fetal age upon normal fetal laboratory values and venous pressure. *Obstet Gynecol* **79**:713–718, 1992.
42. Hinkley CM, Blechner JN. Colloidal osmotic pressures of human maternal and fetal blood plasma. *Am J Obstet Gynecol* **103**:71–72, 1969.
43. Delivoria-Papadopoulos M, Battaglia FC, Meschia G. A comparison of fetal versus maternal plasma colloidal osmotic pressure in man. *Proc Soc Expr Biol Med* **131**:84–87, 1969.
44. Battaglia F, Prystowsky H, Smisson V et al. Fetal blood studies. XIII. The effect of the administration of fluids intravenously to mothers upon the concentrations of water and electrolytes in plasma of human fetuses. *Pediatrics* **25**:2–10, 1960.
45. Illsley N, Verkman A. Serial permeability barriers to water transport in human placental vesicles. *J Membrane Biol* **94**:267–278, 1986.
46. Jansson T, Illsley NP. Osmotic water permeabilities of human placental microvillous and basal membranes. *J Membrane Biol* **132**:147–155, 1993.
47. Stulc J, Stulcova B. Asymmetrical transfer of inert hydrophilic solutes across rat placenta. *Am J Physiol* **265**:R670–R675, 1993.
48. Stulc J, Stulcova B. Effect of NaCl load administered to the fetus on the bidirectional movement of ^{51}Cr-EDTA across the rat placenta. *Am J Physiol* **270**:R984–R989, 1996.
49. Damiano A, Zotta E, Goldstein J et al. Water channel proteins AQP3 and AQP9 are present in the syncytiotrophoblast of human term placenta. *Placenta* **22**:776–781, 2001.
50. Wang S, Chen J, Beall M et al. Expression of aquaporin 9 in human chorioamniotic membranes and placenta. *Am J Obstet Gynecol* **191**:2160–2167, 2004.
51. Wang S, Kallichanda N, Song W et al. Expression of aquaporin–8 in human placenta and chorioamniotic membranes: evidence of molecular mechanism for intramembraneous amniotic fluid resorption. *Am J Obstet Gynecol* **185**:1226–1231, 2001.
52. King LS, Kozono D, Agre P. From structure to disease: the evolving tale of aquaporin biology. *Nature Rev Mol Cell Biol* **5**:687–698, 2004.
53. Robson SC. Maternal respiratory and cardiovascular changes during pregnancy. In *Scientific essentials of reproductive medicine*, SG Hiller, HC Kitchener, JP Neilson (eds). London: WB Saunders, 1996.
54. Economides DL. Acid–base balance in the fetus. In *Scientific essentials of reproductive medicine*, SG Hiller, HC Kitchener, JP Neilson (eds). London: WB Saunders, 1996.
55. Muhlhauser J, Crescimanno C, Rajaniemi H et al. Immunohistochemistry of carbonic anhydrase in human placenta and fetal membranes. *Histochemistry* **101**:91–98, 1994.
56. Sibley CP, Glazier JD, Greenwood SL et al. Regulation of placental transfer: the Na^+/H^+ exchanger. *Placenta* **23**(Suppl A):S39–sS46, 2002.
57. Speake PF, Mynett KJ, Glazier JD et al. Actiivity and expression of Na+/H+ exchanger isoforms in the syncytiotrophoblast of the human placenta. *Pflugers Arch* **450**:123–130, 2005.
58. Johansson M, Karlsson L, Wennergren M et al. Activity and protein expression of Na^+K^+ ATPase are reduced in microvillous syncytiotrophoblast plasma membranes isolated from pregnancies complicated by intrauterine growth restriction. *J Clin Endocrinol Metab* **88**:2831–2837, 2003.
59. Burd LI, Jones MDJ, Simmons MA et al. Placental production and foetal utilisation of lactate and pyruvate. *Nature* **254**:710–711, 1975.
60. Hooper SB, Walker DW, Harding R. Oxygen, glucose, and lactate uptake by fetus and placenta during prolonged hypoxemia. *Am J Physiol* **268**:R303–R309, 1995.
61. Settle P, Mynett KJ, Speake PF et al. Polarized lactate transporter activity and expression in the syncytiotrophoblast of the term human placenta. *Placenta* **25**:496–504, 2004.
62. Settle P, Sibley CP, Doughty IM et al. Placental lactate transporter activity and expression in intrauterine growth restriction. *J Soc Gynecol Invest* **13**:357–363, 2006.
63. Clarson LH, Roberts VH, Hamark B et al. Store-operated Ca2+ entry in the first trimester and term human placenta. *J Physiol* **15**:515–528, 2003.
64. Roberts VH, Waters LH, Powell TL. Purinergic receptor expression and activation in first trimester and term human placenta. *Placenta* **28**:339–347, 2007.
65. Belkacemi L, Bedard I, Simoneau L et al. Calcium channels, transporters and exchangers in placenta: a review. *Cell Calcium* **37**:1–8, 2005.
66. Glazier JD, Atkinson DE, Thornburg KL et al. Gestational changes in Ca2+ transport across rat placenta and mRNA for calbindin9 K and Ca2+ -ATPase. *Am J Physiol* **263**:R930–rR935, 1992.
67. Belkacemi L, Gariepy G, Mounier C et al. Calbindin–D9k (CaBP9k) localization and levels of expression in trophoblast cells from human term placenta. *Cell Tissue Res* **315**:107–117, 2004.
68. Strid H, Powell TL. ATP dependent Ca^{2+} transport is upregulated during third

trimester in human syncytiotrophoblast basal membrane. *Pediatr Res* **48**:58–63, 2000.
69. Strid H, Bucht E, Jansson T et al. ATP-dependent Ca2+ transport across basal membrane of human syncytiotrophoblast in pregnancies complicated by diabetes or intrauterine growth restriction. *Placenta* **24**:445–452, 2003.
70. Strid H, Care AD, Jansson T et al. PTHrp midmolecule stimulates Ca^{2+} ATPase in human syncytiotrophoblast basal membrane. *J Endocrinol* **175**:517–524, 2002.
71. Kovacs CS, Lanske B, Hunzelman JL et al. Parathyroid hormone-related peptide (PTHrP) regulates fetal–placental calcium transport through a receptor distinct from the PTH/PTHrP receptor. *Proc Natl Acad Sci USA* **93**:15233–15238, 1996.
72. Morris Buus R, Boockfor FR. Transferrin expression by placental trophoblastic cells. *Placenta* **25**:45–52, 2004.
73. Bastin J, Drakesmith H, Rees M et al. Localisation of proteins of iron metabolism in the human placenta and liver. *Br J Haematol* **134**:532–543, 2006.
74. Georgieff MK, Wobken JK, Welle J et al. Identification and localization of divalent metal transporter-1 (DMT-1) in term human placenta. *Placenta* **21**:799–804, 2000.
75. Srai SKS, Bomford A, McArdle HJ. Iron transport across cell membranes: molecular understanding of duodenal and placental iron uptake. *Best Pract Res Clin Haematol* **15**:243–259, 2002.
76. McKie AT, Barlow DJ. The SLC40 basolateral iron transporter family (IREG1/ ferroprotein/ MTP1). *Pflugers Arch* **447**:801–806, 2004.
77. Simister NE. Placental transport of immunoglobulin G. *Vaccine* **21**:3365–3369, 2003.
78. Malek A, Sager R, Kuhn P et al. Evolution of maternofetal transport of immunoglobulins during human pregnancy. *Am J Reprod Immunol* **36**:248–255, 1996.
79. Malek A, Sager R, Schneider H. Maternal–fetal transport of immunoglobulin G and its subclasses during the third trimester of human pregnancy. *Am J Reprod Immunol* **32**:8–14, 1994.
80. Kohler PF, Farr RS. Elevation of cord blood over maternal IgG immunoglobulin: evidence for active placental IgG transport. *Nature* **210**:1070–1071, 1966.
81. Kristoffersen EK. Placental Fc receptors and the transfer of maternal IgG. *Transfus Med Rev* **14**:234–243, 2000.
82. Firan M, Bawdon R, Radu C et al. The MHC class I-related receptor, FcRn, plays an essential role in the maternofetal transfer of gamma-globulins in humans. *Int Immunol* **13**:993–1002, 2001.
83. King BF. Absorption of peroxidase conjugated immunoglobulin G by human placenta: an in vitro study. *Placenta* **3**:395–406, 1982.
84. Lin CT. Immunoelectron microscopic localization of immunoglobulin G in human placenta. *J Histochem Cytochem* **28**:339–346, 1980.
85. Leach L, Eaton BM, Firth JA et al. Immunogold localisation of endogenous immunoglobulin-G in ultrathin frozen sections of the human placenta. *Cell Tissue Res* **257**:603–607, 1989.
86. Leach L, Eaton BM, Firth JA et al. Immunocytochemical and labelled tracer approaches to uptake and intracellular routing of immunoglobulin G (IgG) in the human placenta. *Histochem J* **23**:444–449, 1991.
87. Johnson LW, Smith CH. Monosaccharide transport across microvillous membrane of human placenta. *Am J Physiol* **238**:C160–C168, 1980.
88. Bissonette J, Black J, Wickham W et al. Glucose uptake into plasma membrane vesicles from the maternal surface of human placenta. *J Membrane Biol* **58**:75–80, 1981.
89. Johnson L, Smith C. Glucose transport across basal plasma membrane of human placental syncytiotrophoblast. *Biochem Biophys Acta* **815**:44–50, 1985.
90. Takata K, Kasahara T, Kasahara M et al. Localization of erythrocyte/Hep G2-type glucose transporter (GLUT 1) in human placental villi. *Cell Tissue Res* **267**:407–412, 1992.
91. Barros L, Baldwin S, Jarvis S et al. In human placenta the erythroid glucose transporter GLUT1 is abundant in the brush border and basal membranes of the trophoblast but the insulin-dependent isoform GLUT4 is absent: neither transporter is detectable in endothelial cells. *J Physiol* **446**:345P (Abstr.) 1992.
92. Jansson T, Wennergren M, Illsley NP. Glucose transporter protein expression in human placenta throughout gestation and in intrauterine growth retardation. *J Clin Endocrinol Metab* **77**:1554–1562, 1993.
93. Bissonnette JM, Ingermann RL, Thornburg KL. Placental sugar transport. In *Carrier mediated transport of solutes from blood to tissue*, DL Yudilevich, DL Mann (eds). London: Longman, 1985.
94. Ingermann RL. Control of placental glucose transfer. *Placenta* **8**:557–571, 1987.
95. Hahn T, Desoye G. Ontogeny of glucose transport systems in the placenta and its progenitor tissues. *Early Pregnancy: Biol Med* **2**:168–182, 1996.
96. Illsley NP. Glucose tranporters in the human placenta. *Placenta* **21**:14–22, 2000.
97. Ericsson A, Hamark B, Powell TL et al. Glucose transporter isoform 4 is expressed in the syncytiotrophoblast of first trimester human placenta. *Hum Reprod* **20**:521–530, 2005.
98. Gude NM, Stevenson JL, Rogers S et al. GLUT12 expression in human placenta in first trimester and term. *Placenta* **24**:566–570, 2003.
99. Vardhana PA, Illsley NP. Transepithelial glucose transport and metabolism in BeWo choriocarcinoma cells. *Placenta* **23**:653–660, 2002.
100. Economides DL, Nicolaides KH, Campbell S. Relation between maternal-to-fetal blood glucose gradient and uterine and umbilical Doppler blood flow measurements. *Br J Obstet Gynaecol* **97**:543–544, 1990.
101. Jansson T, Wennergren M, Powell TL. Placental glucose transport and GLUT 1 expression in insulin dependent diabetes. *Am J Obstet Gynecol* **180**:163–168, 1999.
102. Jansson T, Ylvén K, Wennergren M et al. Glucose transport and system A activity in syncytiotrophoblast microvillous and basal membranes in intrauterine growth restriction. *Placenta* **23**:386–391, 2002.
103. Cetin I, Marconi AM, Corbetta C et al. Fetal amino acids in normal pregnancies and in pregnancies complicated by intrauterine growth retardation. *Early Hum Dev* **29**:183–186, 1992.
104. Young M, Prenton MA. Maternal and fetal plasma amino acid concentrations during gestation and in retarded fetal growth. *Br J Obstet Gynaecol* **76**:333–334, 1969.
105. Moe AJ. Placental amino acid transport. *Am J Physiol* **268**:C1321–C1331, 1995.
106. Jansson T. Amino acid transporters in the human placenta. *Pediatr Res* **49**:141–147, 2001.
107. Kudo Y, Boyd CA. Human placental amino acid transporter genes: expression and function. *Reproduction* **124**:593–600, 2002.
108. Cariappa R, Heath-Moning E, Smith CH. Isoforms of amino acid transporters in placental syncytiotrophoblast; plasma membrane localisation and potential role in maternal/fetal transport. *Placenta,* **24**:713–726, 2003.
109. Jansson T, Scholtbach V, Powell TL. Placental transport of leucine and lysine is reduced in intrauterine growth restriction. *Pediatr Res* **44**:532–537, 1998.
110. Sooranna S, Burston D, Ramsey B et al. Free amino acid concentrations in human first and third trimester placental villi. *Placenta* **15**:747–751, 1994.
111. Pearse W, Sornson H. Free amino acids of normal and abnormal human placenta. *Am J Obstet Gynecol* **105**:696–701, 1969.
112. Mahendran D, Donnai P, Glazier JD et al. Amino acid (System A) transporter activity in microvillous membrane vesicles from the placentas of appropriate and small for gestational age babies. *Pediatr Res* **34**:661–665, 1993.
113. Glazier JD, Cetin I, Perugino G et al. Association between the activity of the system A amino acid transporter in the microvillous plasma membrane of the human placenta and severity of fetal

compromise in intrauterine growth restriction. *Pediatr Res* **42**:514–519, 1997.
114. Norberg S, Powell TL, Jansson T. Intrauterine growth restriction is associated with a reduced activity of placental taurine transporters. *Pediatr Res* **44**:233–238, 1998.
115. Paolini CL, Marconi AM, Ronzoni S et al. Placental transport of leucine, phenylalanine, glycine, and proline in intrauterine growth-restricted pregnancies. *J Clin Endocrinol Metab* **86**:5427–5543, 2001.
116. Cetin I, Corbetta C, Sereni LP et al. Umbilical amino acid concentrations in normal and growth-retarded fetuses sampled in utero by cordocentesis. *Am J Obstet Gynecol* **162**:253–261, 1990.
117. Cetin I, Marconi AM, Bozzetti P et al. Umbilical amino acid concentrations in appropriate and small for gestational age infants: a biochemical difference present in utero. *Am J Obstet Gynecol* **158**:120–126, 1988.
118. Economides DL, Nicolaides KH, Gahl WA et al. Plasma amino acids in appropriate- and small-for-gestational-age fetuses. *Am J Obstet Gynecol* **161**:1219–1227, 1989.
119. Jansson N, Pettersson J, Haafiz A et al. Down-regulation of placental transport of amino acids precedes the development of intrauterine growth restriction in rats fed a low protein diet. *J Physiol (Lond)* **576**:935–946, 2006.
120. Herrera E, Amusquivar E, Lopez-Soldado I et al. Maternal lipid metabolism and placental lipid transfer. *Horm Res* **65**(Suppl 3):59–64, 2006.
121. Benassayag C, Mignot TM, Haourigui M et al. High polyunsaturated fatty acid, thromboxane A2, and alpha–fetoprotein concentrations at the human feto–maternal interface. *J Lipid Res* **38**:276–286, 1997.
122. Burt RL. Plasma nonesterfied fatty acids in normal pregnancy and puerperium. *Obstet Gynecol* **15**:460–464, 1960.
123. Herrera E. Implications of dietary fatty acids during pregnancy on placental, fetal and postnatal development – a review. *Placenta* **23**(Suppl A):S9–S19, 2002.
124. Knopp RH, Warth MR, Charles D et al. Lipoprotein metabolism in pregnancy, fat transport to the fetus, and the effects of diabetes. *Biol Neonate* **50**:297–317, 1986.
125. Furuhashi M, Seo H, Mizutani S et al. Expression of low density lipoprotein receptor gene in human placenta during pregnancy. *Mol Endocrinol* **3**:1252–1256, 1989.
126. Wittmaack FM, Gafvels ME, Bronner M et al. Localization and regulation of the human very low density lipoprotein/apolipoprotein-E receptor: trophoblast expression predicts a role for the receptor in placental lipid transport. *Endocrinology* **136**:340–348, 1995.
127. Waterman I, Emmison N, Dutta-Roy A. Characterisation of triacylglycerol hydrolase activities in human placenta. *Biochim Biophys Acta* **1394**:169–176, 1998.
128. Lindegaard ML, Olivecrona G, Christoffersen C et al. Endothelial and lipoprotein lipases in human and mouse placenta. *J Lipid Res* **46**:2339–2346, 2005.
129. Waterman IJ, Emmison N, Sattar N et al. Further characterization of a novel triacylglycerol hydrolase activity (pH 6.0 optimum) from microvillous membranes from human term placenta. *Placenta* **21**:813–823, 2000.
130. Kamp F, Zakim D, Zhang F et al. Fatty acid flip-flop in phospholipid bilayers is extremely fast. *Biochemistry* **34**:11928–11937, 1995.
131. Veerkamp JH, Peeters RA, Maatman RG. Structural and functional features of different types of cytoplasmic fatty acid-binding proteins. *Biochim Biophys Acta* **1081**:1–24, 1991.
132. Campell FM, Gordon MJ, Dutta-Roy AK. Placental membrane fatty acid-binding protein preferentially binds arachidonic and docosahexaenoic acids. *Life Sci* **63**:235–240, 1998.
133. Dutta-Roy AK. Cellular uptake of long-chain fatty acids: role of membrane–associated fatty-acid-binding/transport proteins. *Cell Mol Life Sci* **57**:1360–1372, 2000.
134. Al MD, van Houwelingen AC, Kester AD et al. Maternal essential fatty acid patterns during normal pregnancy and their relationship to the neonatal essential fatty acid status. *Br J Nutr* **74**:55–68, 1995.
135. Haggarty P. Effect of placental function on fatty acid requirements during pregnancy. *Eur J Clin Nutr* **58**:1559–1570, 2004.
136. Madsen EM, Lindegaard ML, Andersen CB et al. Human placenta secretes apolipoprotein B-100-containing lipoproteins. *J Biol Chem* **279**:55271–55276, 2004.
137. Hahn T, Barth S, Graf R et al. Placental glucose transporter expression is regulated by glucocorticoids. *J Clin Endocrinol Metab* **84**:1445–1452, 1999.
138. Challier JC, Hauguel S, Desmaizieres V. Effect of insulin on glucose uptake and metabolism in the human placenta. *J Clin Endocrinol Metab* **62**:803–807, 1986.
139. Ericsson A, Hamark B, Jansson N et al. Hormonal regulation of glucose and system A amino acid transport in first trimester placental villous fragments. *Am J Physiol Regul Integr Comp Physiol* **288**:R656–R662, 2005.
140. Brunette M, Lajeunesse D, Leclerc M et al. Effect of insulin on D-glucose transport by human placental brush border membranes. *Mol Cell Endocrin* **69**:59–68, 1990.
141. Acevedo CG, Marquez JL, Rojas S et al. Insulin and nitric oxide stimulates glucose transport in human placenta. *Life Sci* **76**:2643–2653, 2005.
142. Gordon MC, Zimmerman PD, Landon MB et al. Insulin and glucose modulate glucose transporter messenger ribonucleic acid expression and glucose uptake in trophoblasts isolated from first-trimester chorionic villi. *Am J Obstet Gynecol* **173**:1089–1097, 1995.
143. Kniss DA, Shubert PJ, Zimmerman PD et al. Insulin growth factors: their regulation of glucose and amino acid transport in placental trophoblasts isolated from first-trimester chorionic villi. *J Reprod Med* **39**:249–256, 1994.
144. Karl PI, Alpy KL, Fischer SE. Amino acid transport by the cultured human placental trophoblast: effect of insulin on AIB transport. *Am J Physiol* **262**:C834–C839, 1992.
145. Bloxam DL, Bax BE, Bax CMR. Epidermal growth factor and insulin-like growth factor I differentially influence the directional accumulation and transfer of 2-aminoisobutyrate (AIB) by human placental trophoblast in two-sided culture. *Biochim Biophys Res Commun* **199**:922–929, 1994.
146. Jansson N, Greenwood S, Johansson BR et al. Leptin stimulates system A activity in human placental villous fragments. *J Clin Endocrinol Metab* **88**:1205–1211, 2003.
147. Nelson DM, Smith SD, Furesz TC et al. Hypoxia reduces expression and function of system A amino acid transporters in cultured term human trophoblasts. *Am J Physiol* **284**:C310–C315, 2003.
148. Roos S, Jansson N, Palmberg I, et al. Mammalian target of rapamycin in the human placenta regulates leucine transport and is down-regulated in restricted fetal growth. *J Physiol* **582**:449–459, 2007.
149. Magnusson-Olsson AL, Lager S, Jacobsson B, et al. The effect of maternal lipids on placental lipoprotein lipase in cultured primary trophoblast cells and in a case of maternal LPL deficiency. *Am J Physiol* **293**:E24–E30, 2007.
150. Magnusson-Olsson AL, Hamark B, Ericsson A et al. Gestational and hormonal regulation of human placental lipoprotein lipase. *J Lipid Res* **47**:2551–2561, 2006.
151. Desoye G, Hartmann M, Blaschitz A et al. Insulin receptors in syncytiotrophoblast and fetal endothelium of human placenta. *Immunohistochemical evidence for developmental changes in distribution pattern. Histochemistry,* **101**:277–285, 1994.
152. Ebenbichler CF, Kasser S, Laimer M et al. Polar expression and phosphorylation of human leptin

receptor isoforms in paired syncytial, microvillous and basal membranes from human term placenta. *Placenta* **23**:516–521, 2002.
153. Fang J, Furesz TC, Lurent RS et al. Spatial polarization of insulin-like growth factor receptors on the human syncytiotrophoblast. *Pediatr Res* **41**:258–265, 1997.
154. Masuzaki H, Ogawa Y, Sagawa N et al. Nonadipose tissue production of leptin: leptin as a novel placenta-derived hormone in humans. *Nature Med* **3**:1029–1033, 1997.
155. Reis FM, Florio P, Cobellis L et al. Human placenta as a source of neuroendocrine factors. *Biol Neonate* **79**:150–156, 2001.
156. Holmes R, Montemagno R, Jones J et al. Fetal and maternal plasma insulin-like growth factors in pregnancies with appropriate or retarded fetal growth. *Early Hum Dev* **49**:7–17, 1997.
157. Yildiz L, Avci B, Ingec M. Umbilical cord and maternal blood leptin concentrations in intrauterine growth retardation. *Clin Chem Lab Med* **40**:1114–1117, 2002.
158. Potau N, Riudor E, Ballabriga A. Insulin receptors in human placenta in relation to fetal weight and gestational age. *Pediatr Res* **15**:798–802, 1981.
159. Laviola L, Perrini S, Belsanti G et al. Intrauterine growth restriction in humans is associated with abnormalities in placental insulin-like growth factor signaling. *Endocrinology* **146**:1498–1505, 2005.
160. Lea RG, Howe D, Hannah LT et al. Placental leptin in normal diabetic and fetal growth-retarded pregnancies. *Mol Hum Reprod* **6**:763–769, 2000.
161. Lauszus FF, Klebe JG, Flyvbjerg A. Macrosomia associated with maternal serum insulin-like growth factor-I and -II in diabeteic pregnancy. *Obstet Gynecol* **97**:734–741, 2001.
162. Takayama–Hasumi S, Yoshino H, Shimisu M et al. Insulin-receptor kinase is enhanced in placentas from non-insulin-dependent diabetic women with large-for-gestational age babies. *Diabetes Res Clin Pract* **22**:107–116, 1994.
163. Hafner E, Philipp T, Schuchter K et al. Second trimester measurements of placental volume by 3D ultrasound to predict SGA-infants. *Ultrasound Obstet Gynecol* **12**:97–102, 1998.
164. Hafner E, Metzenbauer M, Höfinger D et al. Placental growth from the first to the second trimester of pregnancy in SGA-fetuses and pre-eclamptic pregnancies compared to normal foetuses. *Placenta* **24**:336–342, 2003.
165. Kinare AS, Naetkar AS, Chinchwadkar MC et al. Low midpregnancy placental volume in rural Indian women: a cause for low birth weight. *Am J Obstet Gynecol* **182**:443–448, 2000.
166. Gluckman PD, Harding JE. The pathophysiology of intrauterine growth retardation. *Horm Res* **48**(Suppl 1):11–16, 1997.
167. Harding JE, Bauer MK, Kimble RM. Antenatal therapy for intrauterine growth retardation. *Acta Paediatr Suppl* **423**:196–997, 2001.
168. Karl PI. Insulin-like growth factor-1 stimulates amino acid uptake by the cultured human placental trophoblast. *J Cell Physiol* **165**:83–88, 1995.

CHAPTER

9

Maternofetal trafficking

Diana W Bianchi

KEY POINTS

- Bidirectional maternofetal cell trafficking occurs in rodents and humans
- Fetal cells in the mother may play a role in the 'cause' or 'cure' of diseases
- Fetal cells have characteristics that are between adult and embryonic stem cells
- Adult stem cell researchers (to date) have not considered the role of pregnancy in a donor or recipient when evaluating transdifferentiation or clinical impact
- Maternal cells in a newborn or child may also play a role in the etiology or treatment of disease

INTRODUCTION

Georg Schmorl, in his 1896 treatise on pre-eclampsia, painstakingly documented the transfer of (fetal) syncytiotrophoblasts into the lungs of women who died of eclampsia[1]. He was arguably the first physician-scientist to recognize that fetomaternal trafficking occurred, and that this was possibly associated with disease. Yet, despite his seminal paper (published in German), during the 19th and 20th centuries, most medical students were taught that the fetal and maternal circulations were largely separate. Today, we know that they are not. This fact has implications for both non-invasive prenatal diagnosis (discussed in Chapter 21) and for the long-term health of the mother and child. In this chapter, I will discuss the evidence demonstrating that bidirectional maternofetal trafficking occurs in both rodents and humans, and focus on the potential consequences of this trafficking with reference to maternal and child health.

FETOMATERNAL TRAFFICKING IN THE MOUSE MODEL

Fetomaternal cellular trafficking was first described in the mouse in France in the late 1970s. Gaillard et al.[2] studied mouse matings in which a wild-type female was bred to a male that carried a unique cytogenetic marker known as the T6 chromosome. During the pregnancies that followed from these matings, fetal cells carrying the T6 marker accumulated in the maternal spleen. The fetal T6 positive cells in the mother were shown to be capable of mitotic division, survived post partum, and increased in number during a second pregnancy. Subsequently, Liégeois et al.[3] demonstrated that the T6 positive cells could be found in maternal spleen and bone marrow even when the later pregnancies resulted from matings with males that did not carry this marker. Thus, in the mouse, fetal cells were shown to persist from prior pregnancies. This group coined the term 'microchimerism' to describe the apparently stable long-term survival and proliferation of allogenic fetal cells in the maternal mouse without the induction of obvious graft-versus-host disease.

Many years later, in our laboratory, we were able to use real-time polymerase chain reaction (PCR) amplification of unique fetal transgenes to study the natural history of fetal cell microchimerism during and following murine pregnancy[4]. We bred 8-week-old C57B1/6J (H-2^b) virgin females to congenic males that carried a green fluorescent protein (GFP) transgene. Mice were sacrificed during pregnancy and one, two, or three weeks after a first, second, or third delivery. Liver, spleen, kidney, heart, lung, brain and skin were obtained. Genomic DNA was extracted and amplified for a 75 base pair region of the transgene. The mean number of fetal cells per million maternal cells was higher in lungs compared to other tissues. One week after a first delivery only 40% of the mice had detectable fetal cells. None of the mice had detectable fetal cells by two to three weeks after a first delivery. However, by a third delivery 40% of the mice had evidence of long-term persistence of fetal cells. These data suggested that reproductive history played a role in the development and persistence of fetomaternal trafficking.

Other factors that influence the numbers of fetal cells in the maternal mouse include whether or not the fetus is syngenic (i.e. identical for histocompatibility alleles at the H-2 locus). Bonney and Matzinger[5] showed that female mice carrying a syngenic fetus had higher numbers of microchimeric cells in their hematopoietic tissues compared with female mice with allogenic fetuses. Khosrotehrani et al.[4] also showed that the level of microchimerism was higher in congenic versus allogenic pregnancies.

More recently, the timing of bidirectional trafficking of GFP+ cells was elegantly demonstrated in the murine placenta[6]. Placental implantation sites were harvested between days 6 and 19 post-coitum (pc), cryosectioned, and analyzed after nuclear (Hoechst) staining. The precise juxtaposition between maternal and fetal tissues could be studied under the microscope, as either the mother or fetus expressed the GFP transgene. In this study, no exchanges of cells between mother and fetuses occurred before day 10 pc. Starting at days 10–12 pc, fetal cells began to be organized in maternal blood. After day 13, the fetomaternal interface became significantly modified; about one-third of the decidua was invaded by fetal cells. The number of fetal cells in the decidua regularly increased between days 13 and 16 and remained constant thereafter throughout pregnancy. The mean number of fetal cells observed in each 600 μm × 400 μm area of the decidua was comparable in syngenic and allogenic matings, but significantly decreased in outbred crosses. Using a nested PCR assay for the *gfp* transgene, this group did not detect any fetal cells in maternal blood before day 10 pc, but thereafter frequently found them at days 10–19 pc[6].

In the healthy pregnant mouse, therefore, fetal cell trafficking occurs after day 10. There are predictable patterns of migration through the decidua. During pregnancy fetal cells are found with different frequencies in different organs. The lung contains the most fetal cells. Trafficking and microchimerism are affected by reproductive history and immunogenetic relationships between the mother and fetus.

FETOMATERNAL TRAFFICKING IN HUMANS

In 1996, while searching for novel antibodies to isolate fetal nucleated erythrocytes for non-invasive prenatal diagnosis, we made the novel observation that, in 75% of women with sons, fetal hematopoietic stem cells, expressing the CD34 antigen, and lymphoid precursors, expressing CD34 and CD38, could be isolated from the circulation of healthy, non-transfused mothers[7]. This finding has been validated and extended by others. Guetta et al.[8] calculated that there were 0–2 fetal progenitor cells per ml of blood in pregnant women. Following growth factor mobilization of hematopoietic stem cells, 50% of postpartum women have fetal cells in the CD34+ enriched fraction of their apheresis products[9]. Fetal mesenchymal stem cells (MSC) were isolated from the peripheral blood of an adult woman who underwent termination of pregnancy[10].

Factors that affect the extent of fetomaternal trafficking in humans include the following: abnormal placentation (such as with pre-eclampsia), fetal aneuploidy, the presence of specific tissue-type antigens such as HLA-DQAI*0501[11], and the amount of time that has elapsed since pregnancy and delivery[7,12]. Fetal cells are not detected in women with young sons; it may take time to establish a microchimeric population of cells.

A key element in the development of microchimerism is a woman's reproductive history. Using quantitative PCR amplification of a Y-chromosome sequence, we showed that women who undergo elective termination of pregnancy receive as many as 500 000 nucleated cells from their fetuses as a result of the procedure[13]. A significant percentage of these first- and second-trimester cells are likely to be stem or progenitor cells. The biologic consequences of termination-associated trafficking are largely unknown. By systematically analyzing all published cases of microchimerism that reported the study subjects' individual pregnancy histories, we observed that a prior history of fetal loss (through miscarriage or termination) significantly increases the chance that fetal cells can be detected in the woman's blood or organs[14]. In our study, women with a history of fetal loss had 2.4 fold (95% confidence interval: 1.2–6.0) increased chance of having microchimerism compared to women with no history of fetal loss. Our meta-analysis was unable to ascertain differences between miscarriage and termination because the primary references did not record that information. There may be significant differences in the incidence or quantity of microchimerism in each of these reproductive scenarios. In another study, however, blood microchimerism was shown to be more frequent and occurred at greater levels in women with a history of elective termination compared with women who had other pregnancy histories[15].

Some researchers are beginning to analyze baseline autopsy data to determine the incidence and frequency of fetal cell microchimerism in parous women. In one paper, 75 autopsied women with known transfusion status and gender of living children had their organs studied by fluorescence in situ hybridization (FISH) using X- and Y-chromosome specific probes[16]. Cells containing a Y chromosome were found in 13/51 kidneys, 10/51 livers and 4/69 hearts, thus indicating widespread tissue microchimerism. This study, however, had limitations in that the reproductive histories were not obtained from the subjects themselves (as they were deceased) but rather from their general physicians. There were no records of miscarriage or abortion, which could explain why some women without sons had male cells detected. In addition, 45/75 women had a history of at least one blood transfusion, which could be another source of male cells. Nonetheless, the study demonstrated that fetal cell microchimerism occurs in the healthy organs of parous women[16].

It is important to recognize that fetomaternal cell trafficking occurs independent of fetal gender. Although many studies document fetal microchimerism using the presence of the Y chromosome, this is only because it is a universal non-maternal marker. Female fetal cell trafficking occurs with equal frequency, and has the same biologic significance as male fetal cell trafficking. Note that in rodent studies, non-gender dependent paternally inherited transgenes such as *gfp*, are used to document fetal cells in the mother.

FETOMATERNAL TRAFFICKING AND DISEASE

Humans

In 1996, Nelson put forth the hypothesis that some autoimmune diseases that preferentially occur in middle-aged women following their reproductive years, and that have clinical and pathological similarities with graft-versus-host disease, may in fact be a form of alloimmune disease[17]. This hypothesis has been tested in surgical and autopsy tissues obtained from women with a variety of autoimmune diseases, including systemic sclerosis, systemic lupus erythematosus (SLE), primary biliary cirrhosis (PBC), Sjögren syndrome, Hashimoto's and Graves' diseases and cutaneous lichen planus (data reviewed in reference[18]). In several studies, the number of fetal cells present in blood and organs of women affected with systemic sclerosis was significantly higher than in controls[19–25]. Chimeric cells in localized scleroderma are more likely to carry dendritic cell and/or B lymphocyte cell surface markers[25]. Similarly, women with autoimmune thyroid disease and Hashimoto's disease in particular, have consistently shown increased fetal cell microchimerism[26–28]. The data on women with lupus is less consistent. Some women with mild cutaneous lupus do not appear to have increased fetal cell microchimerism[29]. In one study, Y-chromosome sequences were detected in the blood of 68% of women with SLE, as compared with 33% of controls[12]. It appears that fetal cell microchimerism is more likely to be found in women with SLE if their tissues are severely clinically affected, such as in lupus nephritis[30]. Johnson et al.[31] demonstrated that, in a woman with SLE who died due to a severe intestinal vasculitis, diseased tissues had more fetal cells present than did healthy tissues.

Other conditions, such as PBC, are inconsistently associated with fetomaternal trafficking. This is somewhat surprising as this disease presents almost exclusively in women. Studies of peripheral blood and salivary glands of women with Sjögren syndrome do not show an increase in microchimerism, although when either PBC or Sjögren syndrome presents in association with systemic sclerosis, significantly increased fetal cell microchimerism has been demonstrated[32,33].

To date, there has been no evidence, either in vivo or in vitro, that fetal cells cause autoimmune disease. Other variables may play a key role in the pathogenesis of disease, such as the class II HLA (human leukocyte antigen) relationships between mother and fetus, grandmother and mother, or grandmother and fetus. Furthermore, the presence of fetal cell microchimerism in affected tissues from women with non-autoimmune diseases such as hepatitis C,[34] cervical cancer[35] and cardiomyopathy[36] has been shown.

In a study of thyroid biopsy material from 29 women with a variety of thyroid conditions, we unexpectedly found large numbers of male fetal cells in an otherwise healthy woman with benign thyroid adenoma. Via FISH analysis using X and Y probes, we showed that mature follicles from the woman's thyroid specimen were partly male and partly female[26]. She had no other potential sources of microchimeric cells. She had never received a blood transfusion or organ transplant, and she was not a twin. This observation prompted us to hypothesize that fetal cells from this woman's son, transferred during pregnancy or delivery, had persisted within the body, and eventually developed into part of her thyroid.

Another case helped us to refine the hypothesis and ask the question as to whether fetal cells, transferred into the mother during pregnancy or delivery, were actually stem or progenitor cells with the capacity to repair maternal disease or injury. In this second case, we analyzed a liver biopsy from an intravenous drug abuser with hepatitis C. Her reproductive history included one son, two miscarriages and two elective terminations[34]. This woman had a high viral load, but was inconsistently taking her medication and ultimately stopped treatment against medical advice. Despite this, she clinically improved. Her liver biopsy specimen showed the presence of thousands of male cells, again using FISH with probes for the X and Y chromosome. She had never received a blood transfusion and was not a twin. Because so many male cells were present, it was technically feasible to perform additional studies using single nucleotide polymorphism (SNP) analysis. We obtained peripheral blood from the woman, her son, and the fathers for her miscarriages and one termination. The results suggested that the likely source of the male cells in her liver was a pregnancy that she had terminated between 17 and 19 years earlier. In this case, the male cells in the liver were morphologically indistinguishable from surrounding liver tissue, suggesting that they were hepatocytes.

An intriguing question is whether women develop fetal cell microchimerism from every pregnancy, or whether it is from the first pregnancy, or from a specific later pregnancy. In the thyroid case described above, her son was her first pregnancy. In the liver case, the microchimerism developed from either the first or second pregnancy. Further elucidation of this issue will require additional study of women whose children are all available for polymorphism analysis.

The liver and thyroid studies did not identify the male (fetal) cell type. To address this issue we combined FISH and immunochemical analysis in new slides from 10 women with sons who were previously found to have significant levels of microchimerism. Immunolabeling was performed using anti-cytokeratin (AE1/AE3) to mark epithelial cells, anti-CD45 to mark leukocytes, and heppar-1 as a hepatocyte marker[37]. In epithelial tissues such as thyroid, intestine, gall bladder or cervix, 14–60% of fetal cells expressed cytokeratin. In the liver, 4% of male cells expressed heppar-1. In spleen and lymph nodes, 90% of male cells expressed CD45. Histologic and immunochemical evidence of differentiation was highly concordant. In addition, the differentiation pattern of XY+ cells, according to their physical location within a diseased or healthy area, was studied. Fetal cells were shown more frequently to express cytokeratin, as opposed to CD45, if they were in the diseased area.

Simlarly, Stevens and colleagues[38] studied liver biopsy samples from 14 women with PBC, 8 with hepatitis C and 6 with other diseases such as steatosis. All women studied had sons. Male cells were found in 43% of women with PBC, 25% with hepatitis C and 33% of others. No male cells expressed CD45 or von Willebrand factor, an endothelial cell marker. A fourth of the male cells with hepatocyte morphology expressed the hepatocyte cytokeratin marker CAM 5.2.

These two studies imply that fetal cells, possibly of hematopoietic origin, home to the site of injury or disease and adopt the local maternal tissue phenotype. Whether the fetal cells transdifferentiate or fuse with maternal cells is unknown. However, in our FISH analyses we never observed tetraploid signals that would suggest fusion as the underlying basis for the results.

Animals

As shown above in humans, parallel data demonstrate that fetal cell microchimerism is increased above baseline in the diseased or injured maternal mouse. Furthermore, more recent studies show that fetal cells can acquire the maternal mature tissue phenotype. As examples, Christner and Jimenez[39] increased the number of fetal cells present by 48-fold in the peripheral blood of maternal mice by injection of vinyl chloride, which is associated with the development of dermal fibrosis and is a model for studies of systemic sclerosis. Imaizumi et al.[40] showed that fetal cells accumulate in the thyroid glands of mice with peripartum autoimmune thyroiditis. In a rat model, transgenic cells that expressed GFP migrated to kidneys damaged by gentamicin; fetal cells resembled renal tubular epithelium[41]. Remarkably, Tan et al.[42] demonstrated that fetal GFP+ cells could cross the blood–brain barrier. In an induced central nervous system lesion, the fetal cells migrated to the site of injury and expressed neural markers. In a study of the ability of maternal inflammation to recruit fetal cells, a contact hypersensitivity skin reaction was induced in wild-type pregnant mice that were mated to transgenic males[43]. Fetal cells were identified using real-time PCR of the transgene, FISH using the Y chromosome, immunohistochemical studies and in vivo imaging. Fetal cells were found in the inflamed areas of all mice (17/17), with higher frequency and amounts in the inflamed compared with control areas ($P = 0.01$). Double labeling showed that the GFP+ cells also expressed CD31 and organized as blood vessels, implying that pregnant mice acquire fetal endothelial cells that participate in maternal angiogenesis.

Pregnancy-associated progenitor cells

The identification of fetal cells transferred to the human and murine female during pregnancy, with the subsequent demonstration of their capacity to develop multiple lineages, has led to the concept of a pregnancy-associated progenitor cell (PAPC)[37]. The origin of PAPCs is currently under study. Candidate cell types include hematopoietic stem cells that express CD34, endothelial cells that express CD31, placenta-derived stem cells (either hematopoietic or fibroblast-like) or cytotrophoblasts.

An excellent candidate for the origin of the PAPC is the mesenchymal stem cell (MSC), based on the data of O'Donoghue et al.[44]. This group cultured male MSCs from the rib marrow of parous women who were undergoing clinically indicated thoracotomies. Male MSCs were found in every woman who had giving birth to a son 13–51 years previously. They were able to induce the MSCs to differentiate into fat and bone. This important study proved that an actual population of fetal stem cells persisted in the parous women for decades.

FETOMATERNAL TRAFFICKING: RELEVANCE FOR THE STEM CELL DEBATE

The fact that women become chimeras following pregnancy has relevance for the debate that occurs over the relative benefits and limitations of adult and embryonic stem cells. Whereas, in general, adult stem cells are thought to have low plasticity, conflicting reports exist of transdifferentiation outside traditional lineage boundaries. Perhaps this transdifferentiation is due to the transfusion or transplant of a population of cells from women that also contain their fetal cells from prior pregnancies. Surprisingly, the reproductive history of adult stem cell donors and/or recipients has been excluded from most studies of sex-mismatched transplants[45]. This is important because many articles conclude that gender-discordant cells, such as XY+ cells in a woman following a bone marrow transplant, are the result of transdifferentiation of the transplanted cells. An alternate explanation is that male cells in a woman's body could derive from her male fetuses. Bianchi and Fisk recommend that all studies of adult stem cells that examine their subsequent fate after transplantation should include the complete reproductive history of the donor and/or the recipient, as appropriate[45]. This is particularly important in the evaluation of clinical outcomes of human stem cell trials.

MATERNOFETAL TRAFFICKING

Human

Thus far, this chapter has focused on transfer of cells from fetus to mother. The reverse also occurs. Maternal cell microchimerism was first appreciated as early as the 1960s, when large-scale karyotyping of newborn male infants revealed the presence of maternal cells[46,47]. Decades later, using more sensitive molecular techniques such as FISH and PCR, investigators showed that 40–50% of male newborn umbilical cord blood samples contained uniquely maternal gene sequences[48–50]. Because this finding could reflect a delivery-associated mixing of the fetal and maternal circulations, subsequent studies were performed using cordocentesis samples from second- and third-trimester fetuses[51,52]. Again, maternofetal trafficking was demonstrated even as early as 13 weeks of gestation. Remarkably, maternal cells persist in immunocompetent children well into adult life[53]. Maloney and colleagues developed a sensitive human leukocyte antigen (HLA)-specific PCR, and used non-shared maternal HLA sequences as a target to detect persistent maternal microchimerism in healthy subjects and subjects with scleroderma. Uniquely maternal DNA was detected in 17/31 (55%) study subjects, at a mean age of 34 years for the scleroderma patients, and 25 years for the normal controls. There were no differences between scleroderma patients and normal controls in number or frequency of maternal cell chimerism. In a subsequent study by the same laboratory, maternal cell microchimerism was shown to be more frequent among women with scleroderma (72%) than among healthy women (22%) ($P = 0.001$), but the numbers of maternal cells, expressed as genome equivalents of maternal cells per million child cells, did not significantly differ among the two groups[54].

In 2000, in parallel to studies mentioned earlier in the chapter that explored the relationship between fetal cell microchimerism and autoimmune disease, two different groups reported that maternal cell microchimerism was more common in children affected by dermatomyositis than in their healthy siblings[55,56]. Juvenile dematomyositis has clinical similarities with graft-versus-host disease. In both of these studies, the affected child was several years old and it was unclear whether maternal cells were always present in affected tissues or whether they migrated there as a result of the disease process. In 2003, we performed a study to determine if maternal cells could be detected in autopsy tissues from non-transfused male infants who died within the first week of life[57]. Female cells, as defined by the presence of intact nuclei with two X-chromosome signals, were found in multiple tissue types in all 4 neonates studied. The number of female cells varied from 3 to 45 per slide. More recent studies also suggest that maternal cell microchimerism develops during fetal life[58,59]. In one second-trimester fetus that was terminated for the presence of malformations, CD3+, CD19+, CD34+ and CD45+ cells of maternal origin were demonstrated in fetal liver, lung, heart, thymus, spleen, adrenal gland, kidney and placenta[58].

The biologic effects of maternal cell microchimerism are not known for sure, but three studies involving very different diseases have shown that maternal cells are present in affected organs in statistically significantly higher amounts than in control tissue sections[60–62]. Furthermore, immunohistochemical staining suggests that maternal cells are capable of exhibiting tissue-specific differentiation in the diseased organ. In the first study, myocardial and atrioventricular nodal tissue from 4 male fetuses or newborns that died of congenital heart block due to maternal lupus were studied by FISH and monoclonal antibody to CD45, a leukocyte marker, and sarcomeric alpha-actin, a cardiac myocyte marker[60]. Maternal cells were found in all tissue sections obtained from subjects affected with neonatal lupus. Most of these cells expressed sarcomeric alpha-actin and not CD45. The authors speculated that maternofetal transfer of cells could contribute to the pathogenesis, or alternatively, the repair of cardiac injury in neonatal lupus. Similarly, archived skin biopsy specimens from young males with pityriasis lichenoides, a T-cell mediated condition, were analyzed for the presence of maternal microchimerism. The numbers of maternal cells were higher than in skin biopsies obtained from controls[61]. Furthermore, all maternal cells expressed cytokeratin, and not hematopoietic markers. Lastly, PCR assays targeting non-transmitted, non-shared, maternal-specific HLA alleles were used to show that levels of maternal microchimerism were higher in male children with type 1 diabetes mellitus than in their healthy siblings[62]. In pancreatic tissue, the female cells were shown by immunohistochemistry to make insulin, implying that maternal microchimerism contributes to islet β cells.

Overall, as in fetal cell microchimerism, many different studies have shown that low levels of maternal cell microchimerism are present in healthy tissue, but it increases in a diseased or injured organ. Maternal cells also appear capable of transdifferentiation. At present, it is not known whether maternal cells benefit the fetus or newborn by 'educating' the immune system or by providing missing material, such as insulin, or cells for tissue repair.

Mouse

The mouse model has also been used to demonstrate the presence of maternofetal trafficking. Using GFP+ mothers mated to wild-type males, Vernochet et al.[6] studied maternofetal cellular exchange between days 10 and 19 post conception. As early as day 10, maternal cells were detected in very small numbers in the spongiotrophoblast. After day 13, they were found in the labyrinth zone.

A variety of mutant and transgenic mice have been used to document that maternal cells traffic into neonatal blood, bone marrow, liver, thymus, lung, heart and brain[63–65]. The presence of maternal cells within primary lymphoid organs of fetuses was hypothesized to influence the repertoire of the developing fetal immune system. As in the Maloney study performed in humans, Marleau et al.[66] showed that murine maternal cells persisted into adulthood in their offspring.

Another source of maternal cell microchimerism is postnatal transfer through milk[67,68]. GFP negative neonates nursed by GFP+ mothers show the presence of GFP+ cells in the digestive tract and liver.

To date, there have not yet been studies of specific neonatal disease processes to evaluate the role of maternal cells in repair or pathogenesis.

SUMMARY

Multiple lines of evidence demonstrate that low levels of chimeric cells are present in healthy mothers and children as a result of bi-directional maternofetal trafficking. Higher numbers of chimeric cells are present in diseased or injured tissues. These chimeric cells express differentiation markers characteristic of the surrounding tissue. Bi-directional cellular trafficking between the pregnant woman and her fetus may have long-term consequences for the health status of each individual. Animal models, such as the rodent, will allow us to understand better the therapeutic capabilities of these cells.

REFERENCES

1. Lapaire O, Holzgreve W, Oosterwijk JC, Brinkhaus R, Bianchi DW. Georg Schmorl on trophoblasts in the maternal circulation. *Placenta* **28**:1–5, 2007. Epub 2006 Apr 18
2. Gaillard MC, Ouvre E, Liégeois A, Lewin D. The concentration of fetal cells in maternal haematopoietic organs during pregnancy. An experimental study in mice. *J Gynecol Obstet Biol Reprod* **7**:1043–1050, 1978.
3. Liégeois A, Gaillard MC, Ouvre E, Lewin D. Microchimerism in pregnant mice. *Transplant Proc* **13**:1250–1252, 1981.
4. Khosrotehrani K, Johnson KL, Guegan S, Stroh H, Bianchi DW. Natural history of fetal cell microchimerism during and following murine pregnancy. *J Reprod Immunol* **66**:1–12, 2005.
5. Bonney EA, Matzinger P. The maternal immune system's interaction with circulating fetal cells. *J Immunol* **158**:40–47, 1997.
6. Vernochet C, Caucheteux SM, Kanellopoulos-Langevin C. Bi-directional cell trafficking between mother and fetus in mouse placenta. *Placenta* **28**:639–649, 2007. Epub 2006 Nov 20.
7. Bianchi DW, Zickwolf GK, Weil GJ, Sylvester S, DeMaria MA. Male fetal progenitor cells persist in maternal blood for as long as 27 years postpartum. *Proc Natl Acad Sci USA* **93**:705–708, 1996.
8. Guetta E, Gordon D, Simchen MJ, Goldman B, Barkai G. Hematopoietic progenitor cells as targets for non-invasive prenatal diagnosis: detection of fetal CD34+ cells and assessment of post-delivery persistence in the maternal circulation. *Blood Cells Mol Dis* **30**:13–21, 2003.
9. Adams KM, Lambert NC, Heimfeld S et al. Male DNA in female donor apheresis and CD34-enriched products. *Blood* **102**:3845–3847, 2003. Epub Jul 17, 2003.
10. O'Donoghue K, Choolani M, Chan J et al. Identification of fetal mesenchymal stem cells in maternal blood: implications for non-invasive prenatal diagnosis. *Mol Hum Reprod* **9**:497–502, 2003.
11. Lambert NC, Evans PC, Hashizumi TL, et al. Cutting edge: persistent fetal microchimerism in T lymphocytes is associated with HLA-DQA1*0501: implications in autoimmunity. *J Immunol* **164**:5545–5548, 2000.
12. Abbud Filho M, Pavarino-Bertelli EC, Alvarenga MP et al. Systemic lupus erythematosus and microchimerism in autoimmunity. *Transplant Proc* **34**:2951–2952, 2002.
13. Bianchi DW, Farina A, Weber W et al. Significant fetal-maternal hemorrhage after termination of pregnancy: implications for development of fetal cell microchimerism. *Am J Obstet Gynecol* **184**:703–706, 2001.
14. Khosrotehrani K, Johnson KL, Lau J, Dupuy A, Cha DH, Bianchi DW. The influence of fetal loss on the presence of fetal cell microchimerism: a systematic review. *Arthritis Rheum* **48**:3237–3241, 2003.
15. Yan Z, Lambert NC, Guthrie KA, Porter AJ, Loubiere LS, Madeleine MM et al.

Male microchimerism in women without sons: quantitative assessment and correlation with pregnancy history. *Am J Med* **118**:899–906, 2005.
16. Koopmans M, Kremer Hovinga IC, Baelde HJ et al. Chimerism in kidneys, livers and hearts of normal women: implications for transplantation studies. *Am J Transplant* **5**:1495–1502, 2005.
17. Nelson JL. Maternal-fetal immunology and autoimmune disease: is some autoimmune disease auto-alloimmune or allo-autoimmune? *Arthritis Rheum* **39**:191–194, 1996.
18. Khosrotehrani K, Bianchi DW. Multi-lineage potential of fetal cells in maternal tissue: a legacy in reverse. *J Cell Sci* **118**:1559–1563, 2005.
19. Nelson JL, Furst DE, Maloney S et al. Microchimerism and HLA-compatible relationships of pregnancy in scleroderma. *Lancet* **351**:559–562, 1998.
20. Artlett CM, Smith JB, Jimenez SA. Identification of fetal DNA and cells in skin lesions from women with systemic sclerosis. *N Engl J Med* **338**:1186–1191, 1998.
21. Evans PC, Lambert N, Maloney S, Furst DE, Moore JM, Nelson JL. Long-term fetal microchimerism in peripheral blood mononuclear cell subsets in healthy women and women with scleroderma. *Blood* **93**:2033–2037, 1999.
22. Ohtsuka T, Miyamoto Y, Yamakage A, Yamazaki S. Quantitative analysis of microchimerism in systemic sclerosis skin tissue. *Arch Dermatol Res* **293**:387–391, 2001.
23. Johnson KL, Nelson JL, Furst DE et al. Fetal cell microchimerism in tissue from multiple sites in women with systemic sclerosis. *Arthritis Rheum* **44**:1848–1854, 2001.
24. Artlett CM, Cox LA, Ramos RC et al. Increased microchimeric CD4+ T lymphocytes in peripheral blood from women with systemic sclerosis. *Clin Immunol* **103**:303–308, 2002.
25. McNallan KT, Aponte C, el-Azhary et al. Immunophenotyping of chimeric cells in localized scleroderma. *Rheumatology* **46**:398–402, 2007.
26. Srivatsa B, Srivatsa S, Johnson KL, Samura O, Lee SL, Bianchi DW. Microchimerism of presumed fetal origin in thyroid specimens from women: a case-control study. *Lancet* **358**:2034–2038, 2001.
27. Renne C, Ramos Lopez E, Steimle-Grauer SA et al. Thyroid fetal male microchimerisms in mothers with thyroid disorders: presence of Y-chromosomal immunofluorescence in thyroid-infiltrating lymphocytes is more prevalent in Hashimoto's thyroiditis and Graves' disease than in follicular adenomas. *J Clin Endocrinol Metab* **89**:5810–5814, 2004.
28. Klintschar M, Immel UD, Kehlen A et al. Fetal microchimerism in Hashimoto's thyroiditis: a quantitative approach. *Eur J Endocrinol* **154**:237–241, 2006.
29. Khosrotehrani K, Mery L, Aractingi S, Bianchi DW, Johnson KL. Absence of fetal cell microchimerism in cutaneous lesions of lupus erythematosus. *Ann Rheum Dis* **64**:159–160, 2005.
30. Mosca M, Curcio M, Lapi S et al. Correlations of Y chromosome microchimerism with disease activity in patients with SLE: analysis of preliminary data. *Ann Rheum Dis* **62**:651–654, 2003.
31. Johnson KL, McAlindon TE, Mulcahy E, Bianchi DW. Microchimerism in a female patient with systemic lupus erythematosus. *Arthritis Rheum* **44**:2107–2111, 2001.
32. Corpechot C, Barbu V, Chazouilleres O, Poupon R. Fetal microchimerism in primary biliary cirrhosis. *J Hepatol* **33**:696–700, 2000.
33. Aractingi S, Sibilia J, Meignin V et al. Presence of microchimerism in labial salivary glands in systemic sclerosis but not in Sjögren's syndrome. *Arthritis Rheum* **46**:1039–1043, 2002.
34. Johnson KL, Samura O, Nelson JL, McDonnell M d WM, Bianchi DW. Significant fetal cell microchimerism in a nontransfused woman with hepatitis C: Evidence of long-term survival and expansion. *Hepatology* **36**:1295–1297, 2002.
35. Cha D, Khosrotehrani K, Kim Y, Stroh H, Bianchi DW, Johnson KL. Cervical cancer and microchimerism. *Obstet Gynecol* **102**:774–781, 2003.
36. Bayes-Genis A, Bellosillo B, de la Calle O et al. Identification of male cardiomyocytes of extracardiac origin in the hearts of women with male progeny: male fetal cell microchimerism of the heart. *J Heart Lung Transplant* **24**:2179–2183, 2005.
37. Khosrotehrani K, Johnson KL, Cha DH, Salomon RN, Bianchi DW. Transfer of fetal cells with multilineage potential to maternal tissue. *J Am Med Assoc* **292**:75–80, 2004.
38. Stevens AM, McDonnell WM, Mullarkey ME, Pang JM, Leisenring W, Nelson JL. Liver biopsies from human females contain male hepatocytes in the absence of transplantation. *Lab Invest* **84**:1603–1609, 2004.
39. Christner PJ, Jimenez SA. Animal models of systemic sclerosis: insights into systemic sclerosis pathogenesis and potential therapeutic approaches. *Curr Opin Rheumatol* **16**:746–752, 2004.
40. Imaizumi M, Pritsker A, Unger P, Davies TF. Intrathyroidal fetal microchimerism in pregnancy and postpartum. *Endocrinology* **143**:247–253, 2002.
41. Wang Y, Iwatani H, Ito T et al. Fetal cells in mother rats contribute to the remodeling of liver and kidney after injury. *Biochem Biophys Res Commun* **325**:961–967, 2004.
42. Tan XW, Liao H, Sun L, Okabe M, Xiao ZC, Dawe GS. Fetal microchimerism in the maternal mouse brain: a novel population of fetal progenitor or stem cells able to cross the blood-brain barrier? *Stem Cells* **23**:1443–1452, 2005. Epub Aug 9, 2005.
43. Huu SN, Oster M, Uzan S, Chareyre F, Aractingi S, Khosrotehrani K. Maternal neoangiogenesis during pregnancy partly derives from fetal endothelial progenitor cells. *Proc Natl Acad Sci USA* **104**:1871–1876, 2007. Epub Jan 31, 2007.
44. O'Donoghue K, Chan J, de la Fuente J et al. Microchimerism in female bone marrow and bone decades after fetal mesenchymal stem-cell trafficking in pregnancy. *Lancet* **364**:179–182, 2004.
45. Bianchi DW, Fisk NM. Fetomaternal cell trafficking and the stem cell debate: gender matters. *J Am Med Assoc* **297**:1489–1491, 2007.
46. Turner JH, Wald N, Quinlivan WL. Cytogenetic evidence concerning possible transplacental transfer of leukocytes in pregnant women. *Am J Obstet Gynecol* **95**:831–833, 1966.
47. el-Alfi OS, Hathout H. Maternofetal transfusion: immunologic and cytogenetic evidence. *Am J Obstet Gynecol* **103**:599–600, 1969.
48. Socie G, Gluckman E, Carosella E, Brossard Y, Lafon C, Brison O. Search for maternal cells in human umbilical cord blood by polymerase chain reaction amplification of two minisatellite sequences. *Blood* **83**:340–344, 1994.
49. Petit T, Gluckman E, Carosella E, Brossard Y, Brison O, Socie G. A highly sensitive polymerase chain reaction method reveals the ubiquitous presence of maternal cells in human umbilical cord blood. *Exp Hematol* **23**:1601–1605, 1995.
50. Hall JM, Lingenfelter P, Adams SL, Lasser D, Hansen JA, Bean MA. Detection of maternal cells in human umbilical cord blood using fluorescence in situ hybridization. *Blood* **86**:2829–2832, 1995.
51. Petit T, Dommergues M, Socie G, Dumez Y, Gluckman E, Brison O. Detection of maternal cells in human fetal blood during the third trimester of pregnancy using allele-specific PCR amplification. *Br J Haematol* **98**:767–771, 1997.
52. Lo ES, Lo YM, Hjelm NM, Thilaganathan B. Transfer of nucleated maternal cells into fetal circulation during the second trimester of pregnancy. *Br J Haematol* **100**:605–606, 1998.
53. Maloney S, Smith A, Furst DE et al. Microchimerism of maternal origin persists into adult life. *J Clin Invest* **104**:41–47, 1999.
54. Lambert NC, Erickson TD, Yan Z et al. Quantification of maternal microchimerism by HLA-specific

real-time polymerase chain reaction: studies of healthy women and women with scleroderma. *Arthritis Rheum* **50**:906–914, 2004.

55. Reed AM, Picornell YJ, Harwood A, Kredich DW. Chimerism in children with juvenile dermatomyositis. *Lancet* **356**:2156–2157, 2000.
56. Artlett CM, Ramos R, Jiminez SA, Patterson K, Miller FW, Rider LG. Chimeric cells of maternal origin in juvenile idiopathic inflammatory myopathies. *Lancet* **356**:2155–2156, 2000.
57. Srivatsa B, Srivatsa S, Johnson KL, Bianchi DW. Maternal cell microchimerism in newborn tissues. *J Pediatr* **142**:31–35, 2003.
58. Gotherstrom C, Johnsson AM, Mattsson J, Papadogiannakis N, Westgren M. Identification of maternal hematopoietic cells in a 2nd-trimester fetus. *Fetal Diagn Ther* **20**:355–358, 2005.
59. Berry SM, Hassan SS, Russell E, Kukuruga D, Land S, Kaplan J. Association of maternal histocompatibility at class II HLA loci with maternal microchimerism in the fetus. *Pediatr Res* **56**:73–78, 2004.
60. Stevens AM, Hermes HM, Rutledge JC, Buyon JP, Nelson JL. Myocardial-tissue-specific phenotype of maternal microchimerism in neonatal lupus congenital heart block. *Lancet* **362**:1617–1623, 2003.
61. Khosrotehrani K, Guegan S, Fraitag S et al. Presence of chimeric maternally derived keratinocytes in cutaneous inflammatory diseases of children: the example of pityriasis lichenoides. *J Invest Dermatol* **126**:345–348, 2006.
62. Nelson JL, Gillespie KM, Lambert NC et al. Maternal microchimerism in peripheral blood in type 1 diabetes and pancreatic islet beta cell microchimerism. *Proc Natl Acad Sci USA* **104**:1637–1642, 2007.
63. Shimamura M, Ohta S, Suzuki R, Yamazaki K. Transmission of maternal blood cells to the fetus during pregnancy: detection in mouse neonatal spleen by immunofluorescence flow cytometry and polymerase chain reaction. *Blood* **83**:926–930, 1994.
64. Piotrowski P, Croy BA. Maternal cells are widely distributed in murine fetuses in utero. *Biol Reprod* **54**:1103–1110, 1996.
65. Kaplan J, Land S. Influence of maternal-fetal histocompatibility and MHC zygosity on maternal microchimerism. *J Immunol* **174**:7123–7128, 2005.
66. Marleau AM, Greenwood JD, Wei Q, Singh B, Croy BA. Chimerism of murine fetal bone marrow by maternal cells occurs in late gestation and persists into adulthood. *Lab Invest* **83**:673–681, 2003.
67. Zhou L, Yoshimura Y, Huang Y et al. Two independent pathways of maternal cell transmission to offspring: through placenta during pregnancy and by breast-feeding after birth. *Immunology* **101**:570–580, 2000.
68. Arvola M, Gustafsson E, Svensson L et al. Immunoglobulin-secreting cells of maternal origin can be detected in B cell-deficient mice. *Biol Reprod* **63**:1817–1824, 2000.

SECTION 3

Fetal physiology and pathology

10 Development of the cardiovascular system 119
Kent L Thornburg and Carley AE Shaut

11 Lung growth and maturation 133
Richard Harding and Stuart B Hooper

12 Development of the kidneys and urinary tract 147
Karen M Moritz, Georgina Caruana and E Marelyn Wintour-Coghlan

13 Maternal medicines and the fetus 158
David Williams and Lila Mayahi

14 The perinatal postmortem 181
Phil Cox

CHAPTER 10

Development of the cardiovascular system

Kent L Thornburg and Carley AE Shaut

KEY POINTS

- The heart is the first organ to develop within the fetus, and it follows several key morphological stages to become a four-chambered heart: fusion, looping and septation
- Cardiomyocytes must be functional while they are still differentiating, and so they have several modifications to allow adequate cardiac physiology and function
- In large mammals, cardiomyocytes grow by proliferation until late gestation, whereupon they undergo terminal differentiation and cease to divide
- During fetal life, the right ventricle is larger and at a mechanical disadvantage compared to the left ventricle
- The fetal coronary circulation is characterized by the ability to dilate dramatically in response to hypoxemia and to remodel extensively in response to increase shear forces
- The risk of acquiring adult-onset ischemic heart disease is set, in large part, during fetal life

INTRODUCTION

The formation of a properly working heart is an extremely complex process. The developing heart must coordinate and respond to multiple transformative signals: the genetic program that specifies the heart field, chambers and cell types; hemodynamic forces from circulating blood cells against the inner heart wall influence gene activation, extracellular and intracellular structural proteins and signaling machinery; and continued differentiation, growth and morphological changes of the heart (i.e. fusion, looping, septation). Moreover, since the developing heart must be functional while it is still forming, great physiological changes are occurring in regulating circulation and cardiac output, especially when we compare the fetal heart to the better understood adult heart physiology. Finally, due to the complexity of signals and morphological changes, it is no wonder that even small variations in the normal heart development (such as cell migrations, altered gene expression, fetal blood pressure and cardiac output) can lead to a wide breadth of defects, from severe congenital cardiovascular defects to greater prevalence of cardiovascular disease in adults.

CARDIAC DEVELOPMENT

Immediately following gastrulation, two specific areas of splanchnic mesoderm in the mammalian embryo become cardiac precursor cells[1]. As development proceeds, these areas fold beneath the embryo within the 'wings' of lateral tissue that enclose the space that will become primitive foregut (Fig. 10.1). During the folding process, these areas form bilateral heart tubes that become the cardiac crescent. Each has the potential to become a complete heart but instead, the two heart tubes come together on the ventral side of the embryo and fuse to make a complete single tube, marking the *fusion stage* (see Fig. 10.1). This takes place on about day 21–22 postovulation in the human and represents the stage that cardiomyocytes become capable of beating.

As the tube matures, it becomes composed of three layers (inside to outside): endocardium, cardiac jelly and myocardium. The inner lumen containing blood is lined by endocardium which is surrounded by gelatinous cardiac jelly. The physiological role of cardiac jelly is unknown. The outside layer is muscle composed of primitive but already specialized working myocardium. At this stage, the tube contains regions destined to become structures of the mature heart (see Fig. 10.1). These regions include, from anterior to posterior, truncus arteriosus, bulbus, ventricle, atrium and sinus venosus. As soon as the vascular tree has formed a complete circuit, the heart begins to perform as a beating pump. Thus the heart, though primitive, is the first functioning organ of the body. The sequential segmental contraction of the heart tube at discrete points along the tube allows the wall thickenings to function as valves so that the heart operates as an efficient forward motion pump. The heart tube then grows in a fashion that causes the bulboventricular region to bulge rightward to form a right-handed loop as the heart forms an S-shaped structure (see Fig. 10.1) – the *looping stage* – and is found in the 25–27-day human embryo. The rightward looping of the heart marks the first physical left-right asymmetry within the developing embryo, and this process is controlled by key signaling and transcription factors such as Shh, Nodal, BMPs and Pitx2, among others[4]. At present, the physical and biological mechanisms that underlie the looping process are unknown.

The most complex part of heart formation is the *septation stage* in which all heart chambers and outflow tracts are

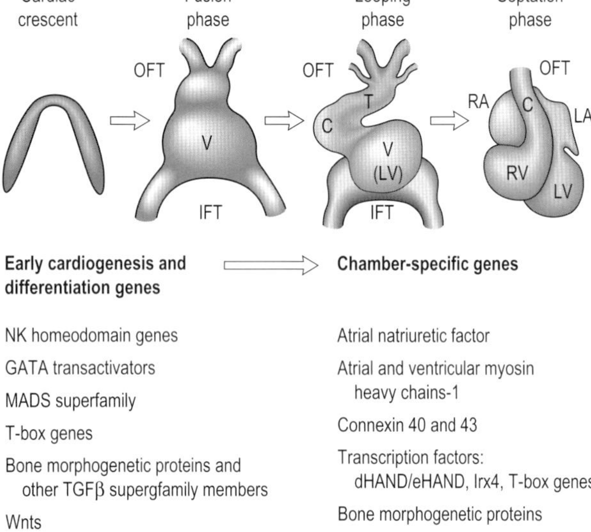

Fig. 10.1 Diagrams of the developing heart. Fusion of the paired endocardial and myoepicardial tubes, cardiac crescent, results in a single straight cardiac tube. These early heart stages are associated with activation of early cardiogenesis gene families. Heart development progresses as the heart loops to the left and the chambers are specified, as observed by the morphological changes and the chamber-specific gene expression. IFT, inflow tract; OFT, outflow tract; T, truncus; C, conus; RV, right ventricle; LV, left ventricle; RA, right atrium; LA, left atrium; V, ventricles. After van Wijk et al.[2] and Bruneau.[3]

formed. It is likely that many structural heart defects arise at this stage. The interatrial septum is formed by two migrating membranous tissue walls that form in succession between the right and left atria (Fig. 10.2). The first (septum primum) grows from the roof of the atrium down to the floor, making a complete wall. This would prevent the necessary flow of blood from the right atrium to the left atrium, if it were not that a hole forms in the wall as it grows. A second wall (septum secundum) then grows from the roof alongside the first septum but it does not grow completely to the floor. The combination of these two membranes form the foramen ovale and provide its flap valve properties.

The interventricular septum is formed internally from a trabecular ridge that originates at the point where the primitive ventricle and bulbus cordis join. Septal tissue forms from a compaction of trabecular tissue. The latter arises from endocardium that invades the cardiac jelly and grows toward the outer myocardial layer in the looping stage. As the jelly disappears, a complex network of spongy pockets (lacunae) and trabeculae are formed. The coalescence of the inner spongy layer gives rise to the interventricular ridge that eventually forms the muscular septum and the papillary muscles. During the septation stage, the interventricular septum slowly migrates in an upward direction toward the atria, leaving an open channel between the ventricles. As the heart matures and twists in shape, this interventricular channel is closed by a downward-growing membranous septum that arises from bulbar ridges and cushion tissue. A persistent 'hole' between the ventricles is the most common type of congenital heart defect, a ventricular septal defect (VSD).

The truncus arteriosus is the outflow vessel of the embryonic heart tube. It divides longitudinally to become the aorta that serves the body and the pulmonary artery that serves the lungs. The septation of the truncus into its component arteries is complicated because the two great vessels must twist upon themselves to match their proper circuits. A spiral septum is derived from two longitudinal ridges that spiral down the inside of the truncus and fuse within the bulbotruncal region of the heart[1] (Fig. 10.3). The ridges gradually fuse along the entire outflow tract and form the two intertwining vessels. Truncal septation cannot occur unless the spiral septum is 'seeded' by

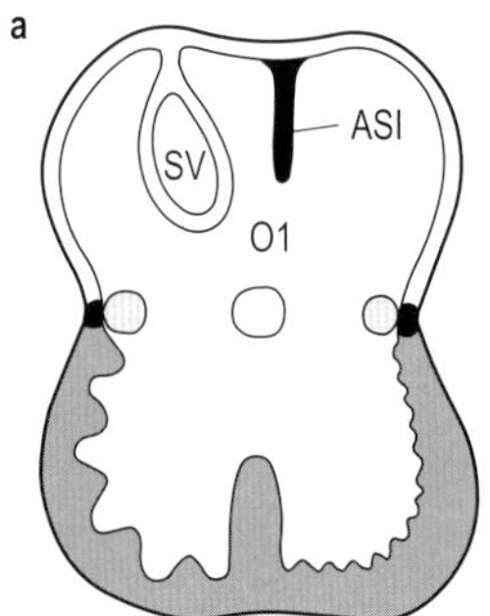

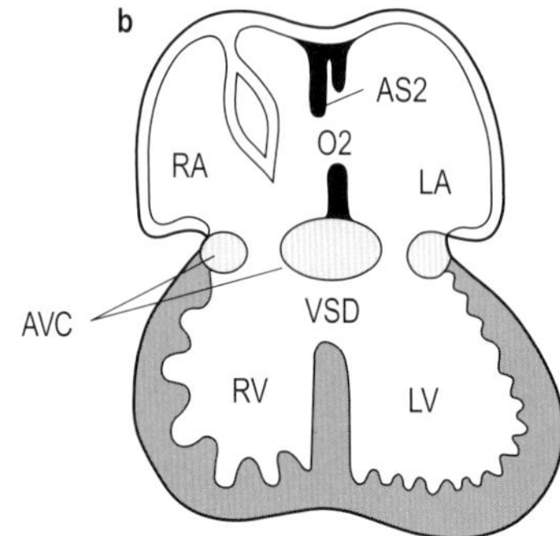

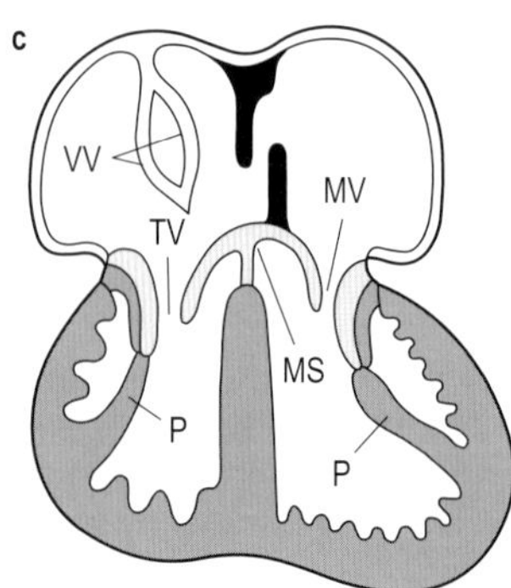

Fig. 10.2 Stages in cardiac chamber septation; the diagrams represent coronal sections of the heart. (a) Early stage – commencing atrial and ventricular septation. (b) Atrial ostium primum closed and ostium secundum forming; ventricular septation incomplete. (c) Septation complete and membranous septum formed. The atrioventricular valves have been formed by cushion tissue and delamination of myocardium. AS1, Atrial septum primum; AS2, atrial septum secundum; AVC, atrioventricular cushion; LA, left atrium; LV, left ventricle; MS, membranous septum; MV, mitral valve; O1, atrial ostium primum; O2, atrial ostium secundum; P, papillary muscles; RA, right atrium; RV, right ventricle; SV, sinus venosus; TV, tricuspid valve; VSD, ventricular septal defect; VV, venous valves. After Reller et al.[1].

neural crest cells that migrate from the neural tube, travel along the branchial clefts down to the truncus arteriosus and invade the regions of the spiral septum and the heart proper. When migration is impeded, a non-septated truncus arteriosus results (called persistent truncus arteriosus), a defect often seen as part of the spectrum of cardiovascular congenital anomalies.

Many genes essential for heart development have been investigated using animal models such as fruit fly, zebrafish, chick and mouse. Genetic screens, expression analysis, transgenic and knockout mouse models and transplantation/ablation studies have helped identify the precise requirement for specific 'heart' genes during each stage of its development. Many transcriptional regulators, signaling molecules and structural molecules are essential for proper heart formation[2,3] (see Fig. 10.1). Transcriptional regulators (i.e. transcription factors, cofactors) set precursor cells down cardiac pathways, activating cardiogenic markers that direct heart morphogenesis. Also, signaling molecules such as growth factors, cell receptors and intracellular signaling molecules, help cardiomyocytes interact with each other and specify the positional cues (i.e. anteroposterior). Many genes are initially expressed throughout the looping heart, followed by restriction of their expression to specific heart chambers or cells.

Some human cardiovascular defects are linked to specific genes and they can be studied by recreating similar mutations or knockout mouse models. For example, point mutations in the T-box transcription factor gene *Tbx5* is associated with Holt-Oram syndrome in humans, which presents with many cardiovascular defects[6]. Tbx5 is expressed within discrete regions of the developing heart. Mice heterozygous for Tbx5 mutant allele partially phenocopy the heart defects seen in Holt-Oram syndrome (defects in septation, pacemaking and conduction)[7]. Overall, more research is needed to combine all the genetic cues to the biological, morphological and physiological aspects of heart development. There is a fuller description of cardiac development in Chapter 5.

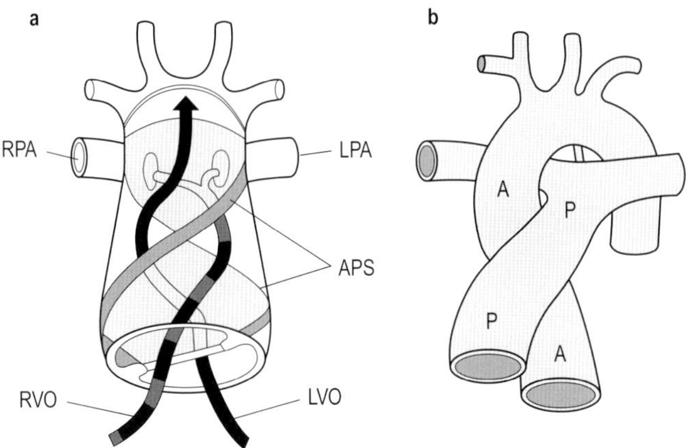

Fig. 10.3 Septation of the truncus arteriosus. (a) Diagram showing the spiral aorticopulmonary septum, which separates the systemic arterial flow (*solid dark line*) from the pulmonary arterial flow (*broken line*). (b) The mature pulmonary artery and aorta, after septation and separation, showing the persisting spiral relationship. A, Aorta; APS, aorticopulmonary septum; LPA, left pulmonary artery; LVO, left ventricular outflow pathway; P, pulmonary trunk; RPA, right pulmonary artery; RVO, right ventricular outflow pathway. After Reller et al.[1].

Mature myocyte

The histological arrangement within the mature cardiac myocyte is common to all mammals. The cell membrane of the cardiomyocyte, known as the sarcolemma, contains the proteins that propagate the action potential and other crucial homeostatic transport proteins[8]. As the myocyte matures, the sarcolemma invaginates at regular intervals and forms tubules that reach the interior of the cell. These transverse tubules or T-tubules carry the action potential to the cell interior. The most striking feature of the mature cell is its striated muscle pattern derived from the registry of contractile proteins that compose the muscle strands known as myofibrils. Myofibrils are composed of a series of sarcomeres, the individual contractile units of striated muscle (Fig. 10.4). The most easily visible protein strand is myosin, which composes the heavy strands (thick filaments) that run from the darkly stained Z-line toward the center of the sarcomere. Thin actin filaments are found in the center of the sarcomere reaching between the thick filaments with which they overlap. Another important structural protein is titin, the largest protein in the body. It traverses the sarcomere from the Z-line to the M-line. It is important because different isoforms may be expressed over development and upon changes in loading conditions. It also has a kinase domain that is important in cell signaling.

The mature cell is characterized by alternating layers of myofibrils and mitochondria. There hardly seems to be room for necessary organelles. Every mature cell has one or more nuclei and contains a complex inner network, the sarcoplasmic reticulum (SR). SR forms special couplings near the sarcolemma (SL). Small fluxes of Ca^{2+} traverse the SL in response to an action potential via voltage-gated Ca^{2+} channels (dihydropyridine receptor). In response to stimulation, Ca^{2+} is released into the cytosol from SR stores via ryanodine-sensitive release channels. Contraction proceeds as myosin and actin interact in the presence of activator Ca^{2+}.

Embryonic hearts have many attributes similar to mature hearts. They are capable of circulating blood even before the

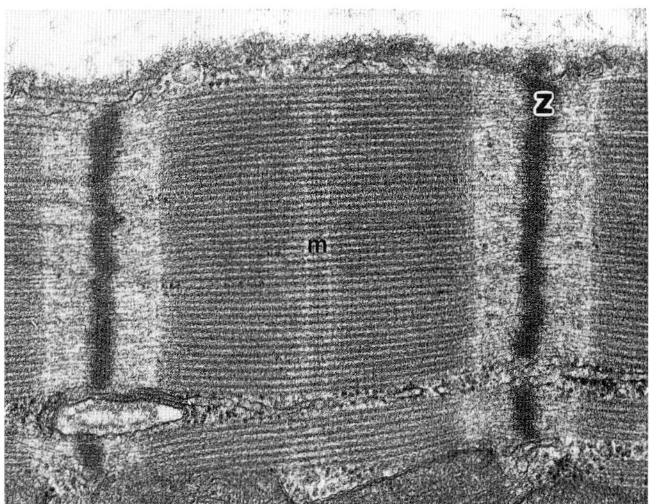

Fig. 10.4 Showing electron micrograph of a single sarcomere of a near-term sheep heart. Note the Z-line (Z) and M-line (m). The heavy electron-dense line between Z-lines is the contractile protein, myosin. Courtesy KL Thornburg.

working cells have a distinct myocyte appearance. Embryonic hearts carry out the basic pump functions as expected from a mature heart in that they generate pressures (very low) with characteristic pressure waves (Fig. 10.5), they respond to preload and afterload and they control output via changes in venous flow, stroke volume and heart rate[10,11]. However, after looking at the ultrastructural features of the early cardiomyocyte, one is surprised by its functional capability. The immature contractile units (sarcomeres) are scarce, disorganized and sometimes seen at odd angles with respect to the SL (Fig. 10.6). The amazing feature among vertebrate hearts is the gradual increasing complexity of the cardiomyocyte, while continually providing kinetic energy to circulating blood.

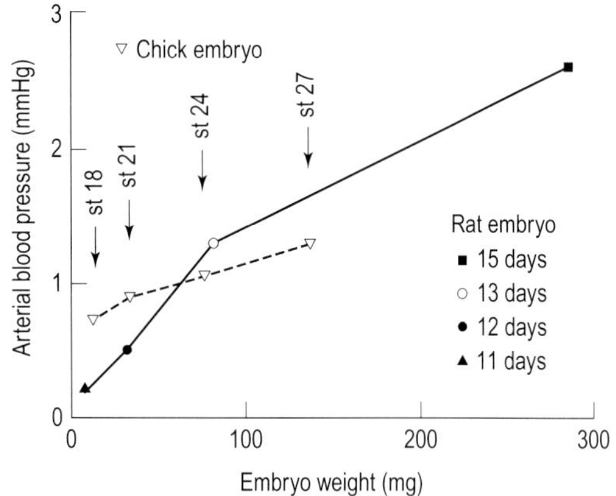

Fig. 10.5 Changes in blood pressure in chick and rat embryos with respect to wet weight of embryo. Stage (st) 18 is equivalent to 3 days; stage 21, 3.5 days; stage 24, 4.5 days; and stage 27, 5.5 days. After Nakazawa et al.[9].

Altricial animals are born in a very immature, dependent state at which time they often have their eyes closed and may have little fur. Rats and rabbits are examples. In contrast, precocial animals are born in a mature state. They are often on their feet within minutes of birth and some are even able to eat solid food within hours. Guinea pigs and most large mammals are examples. In general, altricial mammals are born with hearts that are histologically and functionally immature and most precocial animals have hearts that are rather mature by comparison. The immature fetal cell of either type of animal is characterized by its small size and histological arrangement where myofibrils are located only at the periphery of the cell; the central portion of the myocyte contains large fluid filled 'spaces' that contain mitochondria, Golgi apparatus, glycogen and polyribosomes. Figure 10.7 compares the ultrastructure of the immature cat heart with the adult cat heart.

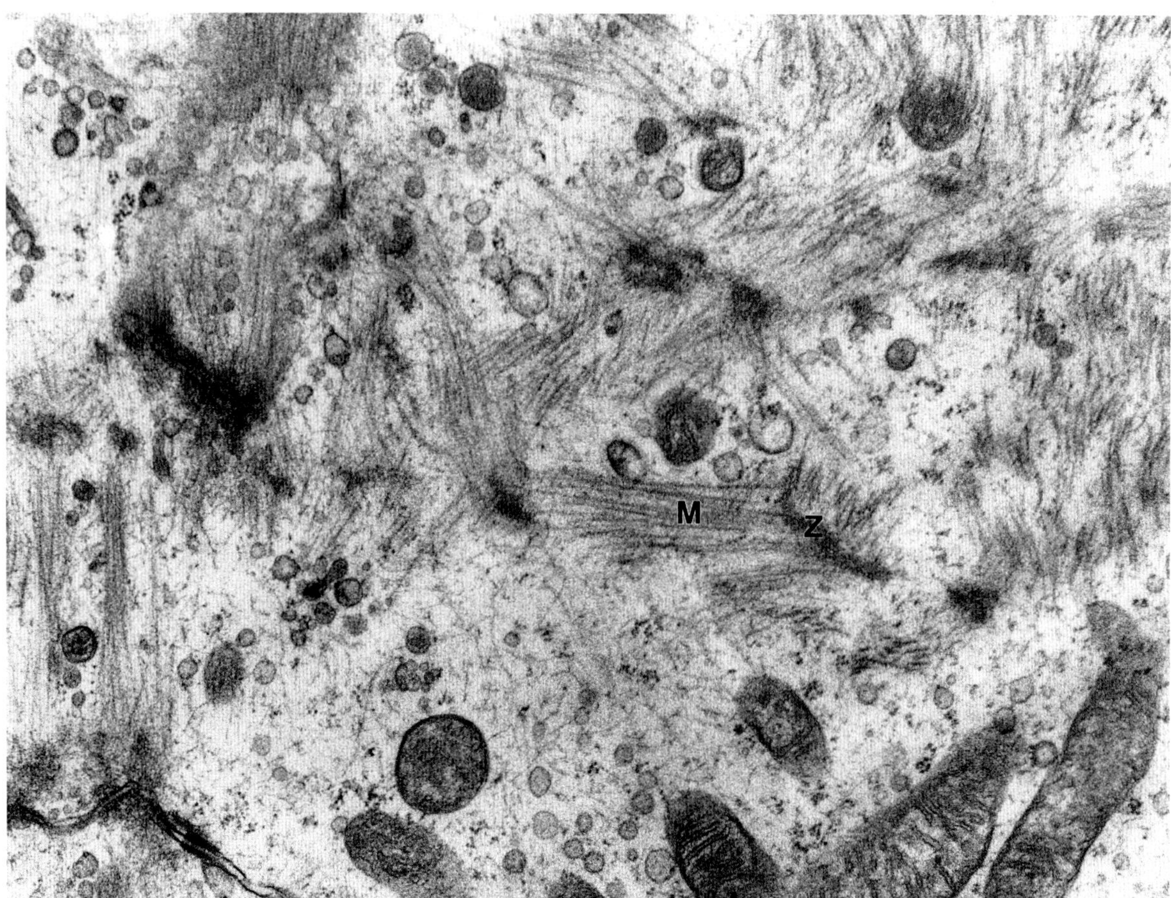

Fig. 10.6 Showing electron micrograph of an embryonic chick heart cell from postfusion stage. This cell is in early stages of sarcomerogenesis but is capable of contraction. Z, Z-line; M, contractile protein forming a myofibril. Courtesy KL Thornburg.

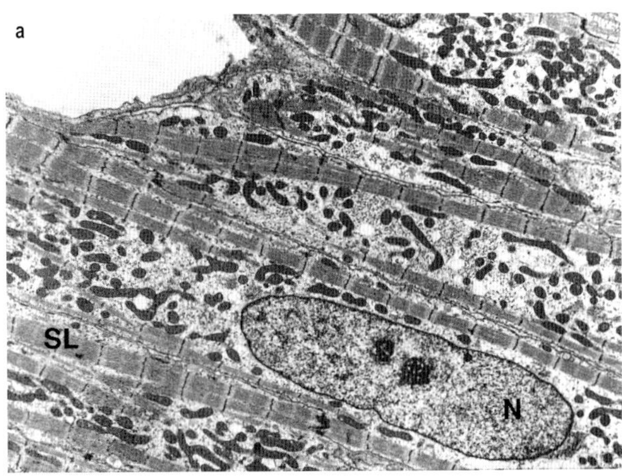

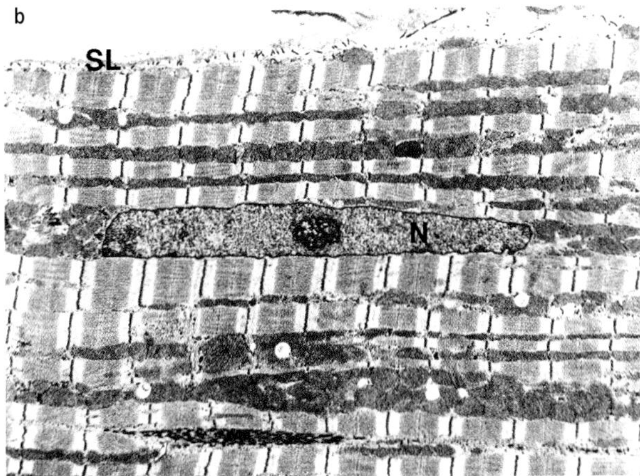

Fig. 10.7 Electron micrographs of heart muscle from immature cat. (a) In the neonatal cat five cells are seen separated by sarcolemma (SL). (b) In the adult heart, one cell is seen. Contractile material is found at the periphery in neonate cells but throughout the cytoplasm in the adult cell. The nucleus (N) in the neonate is centered within the cell and mitochondria are scattered throughout the central cytoplasm. In the adult, mitochondria are sandwiched between the layers of myofibrilla material. ×2 After Maylie[12].

Myocyte size

Embryonic hearts grow by myocyte hyperplasia (cell division) in all species. In altricial species, this growth pattern continues over the life of the fetus. In rats, myocytes do not increase much in size throughout gestation after the early embryonic period. After birth, rat myocytes undergo a terminal maturation process by which they become binucleate and cease to divide. Clubb and Bishop[13] have shown that the binucleation stage takes place during postnatal life so that about 50% of the cells are binucleate at 9 postnatal days. A similar process is found in all mammalian hearts[14]. The number of cells present in the heart at the stage of terminal maturation is the number that will be present in the heart for the life of the individual. The entire heart organ must grow considerably to keep up with the growth of the animal. For this growth, the chambers enlarge by increasing the dimensions and volume of the individual myocytes and by architectural rearrangement of the matrix scaffold.

Table 10.1 Cardiac contraction in the rabbit*

Gestation (days)	*Maximal developed tension (g/g cardiac muscle)*	*Percentage of cardiac muscle that is myofibril*	*Maximal developed tension (g/g cardiac muscle)*
18	18	13	1.4
21	22	15.3	1.4
28	40	24.3	1.6
New-born	68	39	1.7
Adult	78	50	1.6

*Adapted from Nakanishi et al.[15]

Functional maturity of the myocyte

As mentioned above, cardiomyocytes are able to contract as soon as functioning myofibrils are present while their morphology and biochemical development is primitive. One of the most important physiological features is the maturation of the Ca^{2+} transport and sequestration systems. The primitive myocyte has virtually no SR. The rate at which functional SR will be integrated into the cell is species dependent – the sheep has abundant SR at birth, the cat has almost none. Because SR is the storage site for most intracellular Ca^{2+}, the immature myocyte must acquire and extrude Ca^{2+} across the SL during systole and diastole, respectively, each and every beat. In the immature myocyte, it appears that Ca^{2+} enters the myocyte through voltage-gated Ca^{2+} channels, in response to an action potential, in sufficient quantity to provide *activator* Ca^{2+} for each beat. The lack of internal Ca^{2+} storage places limitations on myocyte growth because the myocyte must not get so large that diffusion distances are rate limiting at fetal heart rates. Fetal cardiac myocytes are designed with small diameters in early fetal life and they grow only as SR is developed. The myocytes have important adaptations. Myofibrillar material is found only at the periphery of the cell in immature cells with direct access to Ca^{2+} fluxes crossing the SL each beat. As these cells mature, and SR and T tubules are manufactured by the cell, the myofibrillar material is placed more deeply within the cell. Table 10.1 shows the relative importance of SR and SL contributions to the rate of tension generation in developing myocardium of rabbits[15].

ADULT CIRCULATION

Most physiology textbooks contain information only on adult organ function. However, the fetal cardiovascular system functions so differently from the adult that one cannot extrapolate directly from these textbooks. The differences are explained by differing anatomical, cytomorphological and biochemical characteristics. In the adult heart, the right and left ventricles beat in series with almost exactly the same stroke volume per beat, with small short-term differences being compensated by the Frank–Starling mechanism (discussed below). The adult right ventricle is designed to be a low pressure–volume pump that ejects blood through the inflated lungs with their vascular resistance some tenfold lower than that of the systemic circulation. The left ventricle, on the other hand, is designed to be a high-pressure pump for perfusing the systemic circulation. Further, because the adult circulation is in series, virtually all blood that returns to the heart is passed through the lung before returning to the systemic circuit.

THE FETAL CIRCULATION

Figure 10.8 shows the fetal circulatory arrangement that is quite different from that of the adult arrangement[16]. The fetal circulation is characterized by four shunts:

1. the umbilical circulation
2. the ductus venosus
3. the foramen ovale and
4. the ductus arteriosus.

The *umbilical circulation* is a special vascular configuration that carries 40% of the fetal cardiac output to the placenta for gas exchange. The umbilical arteries arise at the caudal end of the dorsal aorta. Just beyond the branching of the external iliac arteries, the dorsal aorta becomes the common umbilical artery that serves mostly the umbilical arteries except for small branches to the legs. In normal fetuses, the umbilical circulation is a low-resistance circuit. However, several pathological conditions are characterized by an increase in placental vascular resistance and the fetal heart must increase its workload substantially just to perfuse the placenta. The hemoglobin in blood returning to the fetus from the placental circulation is some 80% saturated with oxygen. Placental blood flows through the umbilical vein to the liver where a small portion oxygenates the liver but most flows through the second shunt, the *ductus venosus*, and joins desaturated blood from the lower body inferior vena cava (IVC). The ductus venosus is not found in the guinea pig[17]. The IVC courses through the diaphragm and bifurcates in the chest near the heart. Some 30–90% of the IVC flow (depending on species) is directed across the *foramen ovale* into the left atrium[17,18]. The foramen ovale is usually described in textbooks as a one-way flap valve between the atria that allows only right to left flow. In sheep, the foramen is a rather long wind-sock-shaped membrane containing muscle fibers that originates as a branch of the IVC at the bifurcation, the crista terminalis. There is evidence that oxygenated blood from the placenta is preferentially directed to the left atrium via the foramen ovale[19] and that the flow through the foramen is highly dependent on the kinetic energy of the blood in the IVC[20]. The oxygenated blood entering the left heart via the foramen ovale is primarily delivered to heart and brain. Blood returning from the head and the lower body flows through the right atrium and ventricle and is ejected into the main pulmonary artery. Most of the pulmonary arterial flow is directed across the *ductus arteriosus*, a shunt that connects the pulmonary artery with the descending aorta. Because the lungs are not inflated in utero, their vascular resistance is high and their oxygen flow needs low. In the fetus, desaturated blood flowing through the pulmonary artery joins blood from the aortic isthmus and travels down the descending aorta to the placenta for reoxygenation. The fetal shunts are crucial for survival of the fetus but, after the placental circulation is abruptly disrupted at birth, they are no longer needed. All disappear shortly after birth. It is not uncommon in humans for the ductus arteriosus to remain open longer than desired and it is sometimes closed via a catheter-placed obstruction device or by surgical ligation.

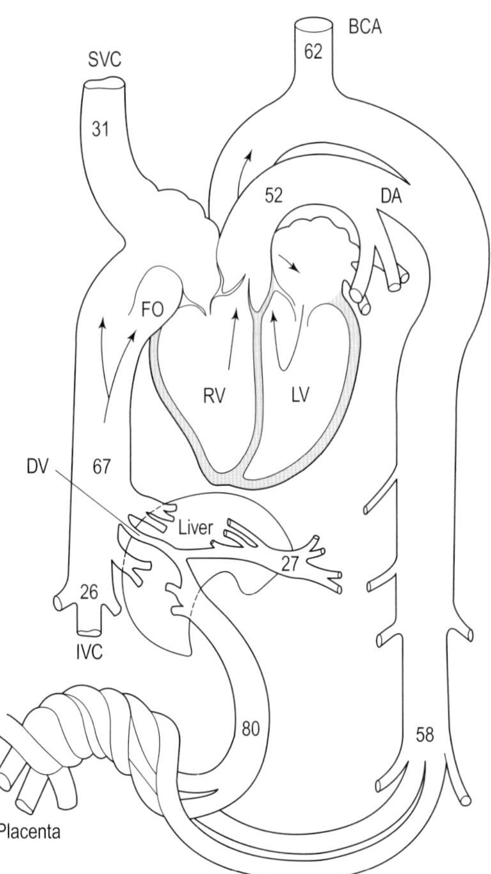

Fig. 10.8 Circulation of the mature fetal lamb. Numbers indicate mean oxygen saturation (%). RV, right ventricle; LV, left ventricle; SVC, superior vena cava; BCA, brachiocephalic artery; FO, foramen ovale; DA, ductus arteriosus; DV, ductus venosus, IVC, inferior vena cava. After Dawes[16].

FETAL HAEMODYNAMICS

Flow through blood vessels is often described by the hemodynamic equivalent of Ohm's law:

$$\dot{Q} = \Delta P/R \quad (10.1)$$

where $\dot{Q}$ is blood flow, ΔP the driving pressure ($P_{art} - P_{ven}$) and R the resistance to flow. This simple concept is mostly adequate for understanding the physics of the circulation in the fetus. However, it does not take into account the complex resistance forces that occur as a result of pulsatile flow and reflections of pulse waves from distant bifurcations. To take these factors into account, one can estimate the total impedance of the vascular tree using high-fidelity measurements of pressure and flow at the pulmonary and aortic roots. The impedance is the total hindrance to the ejection of blood by the ventricle due to both vascular resistance and pulsatile flow[21]. There are recent studies examining impedance within the fetal circulation[22].

Table 10.2 **Fetal organ blood flows in near-term animals (ml/min/100 g)**

Organ	*Llama****	*Guinea pig**	*Sheep***	*(Percentage biventricular output)*
Brain	85		150	4
Heart	165	165	265	3
Lung	–	–	160	6
Adrenals	330	385	395	0.1
Kidney	95	110	245	3
Placenta		125	140	40
Carcass	8	20	15	35

Modified from *Carter (1984)[17], **Teitel (1988)[24] and ***Llanos (1995)[25]

The regulation of blood flow in the fetus has been studied extensively. The advent of several techniques was prerequisite to the feasibility of performing these studies. Foremost was the chronic catheterization of the sheep fetus[23]. Most of what we know about fetal cardiovascular physiology has been learned from this model. The microsphere technique has also been a very valuable tool because it allows the measurement of organ flows (e.g. Table 10.2). Electromagnetic flow sensors and later transonic and Doppler methods have greatly expanded our capability to measure flows and flow velocities continuously within specific beds. Ultrasonic sonomicrometer piezoelectric crystals have been used extensively to obtain instantaneous dimensions of the heart[26,27], ductus arteriosus and other structures. Using sonomicrometry, pressure–dimension relation of the fetal heart can be determined under a variety of physiological conditions.

The hemodynamic features of the fetal circulation are also very different from those of the adult. The mean arterial pressure increases gradually over gestation and reaches ≈50 mmHg in the mature fetus. Because of the unique fetal shunt system, the fetal ventricles eject against similar mean arterial pressures and are filled by similar filling pressures (3–5 mmHg) throughout fetal life. The arrangement of the arterial tree in the fetus may affect heart function. The right ventricle ejects into the pulmonary artery that feeds the low-resistance placental circulation. One might guess, therefore, that the impedance to ejection is less for the right ventricle than for the left ventricle which ejects into the circuit that perfuses the head and the smaller aortic isthmus (the segment between the brachiocephalic artery and ductus arteriosus).

Fetal cardiac output

Because the two fetal ventricles pump in parallel rather than in series, the output of the heart is best expressed as the combined ventricular output. The biventricular output of the 'resting' sheep fetus is about 500 ml/min/kg and represents a flow that cares for the total oxygen needs of the fetal body. In contrast, an adult sheep has a cardiac output of about 150 ml/min/kg[28]. A near-term sheep fetus of 4 kg pumps about 21 ml/min. The output of the human fetus at 38 weeks is also about 21 ml/min as estimated from Doppler flow velocities and estimates of tricuspid and mitral valve cross-sectional areas[29]. In the sheep fetus, the right ventricle contributes about 60–70% of the cardiac output[18,30]. In the human fetus, the estimated contribution of the total cardiac output from the right ventricle is 55–60% near term[31].

It seems obvious that the heart cannot pump more than is returned to it through the veins. Indeed, the fetal heart and circulation are precisely coupled through mean atrial pressure so that venous return and cardiac output are equal. This coupling is complex because it involves regulating the fetal blood volume. The equilibrated pressure in the fetal circulation when the heart is at rest has been estimated[32] and is thought to be two times higher (≈14 mmHg) than for adults. This may indicate that the fetal circulation is relatively 'over-filled' compared to the adult circulation. The difference between the mean systemic pressure and mean right atrial pressure is thought to estimate a driving pressure for venous flow back to the heart[33]. Therefore, the downstream pressure of venous return is also the filling pressure of the heart that operates on the Frank–Starling principle (see below).

Distribution of cardiac output

Blood flow is distributed to the organs of the fetal body according to the inherent vascular resistance of the organ in question and autoregulatory needs of the organ. It is not known how an organ acquires its unique autoregulatory capability. Table 10.2 shows weight specific flows for different organs under normoxemic conditions.

It is generally accepted that there is autoregulatory capability at the organ level in the fetus and that this is an important component of the blood-pressure regulation system[18]. Autoregulation, the tendency of an organ to keep its blood flow constant over a range of driving pressures, is thought to be the result of local metabolic control of vascular resistance at the arteriolar level to maintain oxygen delivery at an appropriate level. Nevertheless, there is considerable variation among organs in the direction and magnitude of blood-flow change with fluctuations in arterial oxygen content. The lungs vasodilate in the presence of increased oxygen content[34]. Other organs vasoconstrict. There are powerful organ-specific blood flow reallocations within the fetus during episodes of hypoxemia.

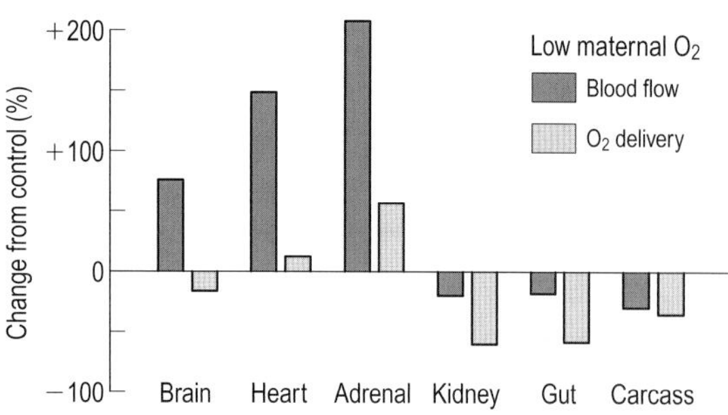

Fig. 10.9 Changes in blood flow and estimated oxygen deliveries to selected sheep fetal organs during an acute fetal hypoxemic episode induced by allowing the ewe to breathe air containing a reduced fraction of oxygen (Cohn et al.[61]). Oxygen deliveries were estimated from published relationships between organ flows and blood oxygen contents for various organs and the estimated contents from similar experiments in other laboratories (Longo et al.[35,36], Peeters et al.[37]; oxygen deliveries are only rough approximations). After Thornburg[38].

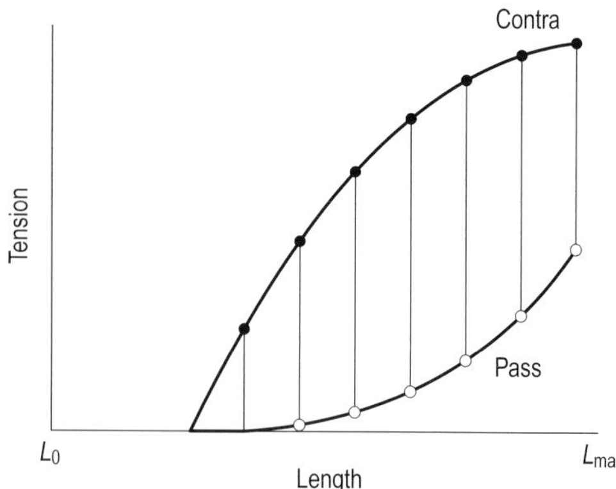

Fig. 10.10 The relationship of length to tension for passive (open circles) and contracting (closed circles) cardiac muscle strips is shown schematically. The vertical lines connect the diastolic length–tension point to the systolic length–tension point for an isometric contraction. L_0 is the unstressed muscle length and L_{max} is the muscle length that produces the maximum tension during isometric contraction. The rapid increase in active tension at muscle lengths above L_0 is the basis for the Frank–Starling mechanism. After Thornburg and Morton[40].

Blood flow to the heart, brain and adrenal glands is increased dramatically as flow to the fetus is diminished (Fig. 10.9).

Determinants of cardiac output

Heart rate

Cardiac output is defined as the product of heart rate and stroke volume and each is regulated. The fetal heart normally beats at a rate set by the pacemaker in the sinoatrial node. The inherent beating rate of the heart increases during early embryonic life and then decreases over the life of the fetus, being about 200/min by mid gestation in sheep and 150/min at birth. Interestingly, fetuses of mammals of all sizes have about the same inherent heart rate. The decrease in rate with fetal age is largely due to increasing cholinergic parasympathetic tone as vagal innervation becomes established at the sinus node. Antagonism of the cholinergic muscarinic receptors by atropine returns the fetal heart to its inherent ($\approx$200/min) rate. Rapid pacing of the fetal heart decreases stroke volume as filling time decreases, but with output being different depending on which ventricle is being paced. There has been debate about whether heart rate or stroke volume holds the prominent place in the regulation of cardiac output in vivo. The issue is moot since both affect output and both depend on cooperation with the circulation via venous return.

Stroke volume

In the adult mammalian heart, there are three primary determinants of stroke volume: preload, afterload and contractility. In the immature heart, one must also consider chamber growth because over gestation it affects stroke volume more than is possible by the other three determinants. Our knowledge about how each affects the volume of blood ejected from the ventricle is derived from nearly a century of research on striated muscle and its application to the odd-shaped ventricles of the heart by Braunwald et al.[39].

Preload

In the heart, the force per unit cross-sectional area present within the ventricular wall just before it contracts (end diastole) is called preload. End-diastolic pressure (EDP) or end-diastolic volume (EDV) are often used as surrogates for preload when force per unit cross-sectional area is unknown. From Figure 10.10, one could predict that as preload increases and muscle fibers are lengthened, they would generate more tension. Thus, it follows that the fraction of the end-diastolic volume that is actually ejected each beat (ejection fraction) is a function of the transmural pressure across the ventricular wall that determines wall tension preceding that beat (preload). As end-diastolic volume increases, stroke volume increases. This has long been known as the Frank–Starling relation or as the Starling's law of the heart which was originally stated as, 'The mechanical energy set free on passage from the resting to the contracted state is a function of the length of the muscle fiber, i.e. of the area of chemically active surfaces'[41].

Afterload

A second determinant of stroke volume is afterload, the force per cross-sectional area within the myocardium (wall stress) during contraction. Ventricular wall stress can be estimated using a simplified form of Laplace's law which states:

$$S_w = \frac{1}{2} P_t (r/h) \qquad (10.2)$$

where S_w is wall stress (force per unit cross sectional area), P_t is transmural pressure, r is radius of curvature, h is wall thickness. From this relationship, one can see that the wall stress will increase in direct proportion to the radius of curvature (r) if wall thickness (h) is constant. From this equation, one can appreciate the physiological benefit of increasing wall thickness in response to pressure load (compensatory hypertrophy) because S_w decreases as wall thickness increases, making ejection easier (Fig. 10.11).

Decreases in stroke volume with increased wall stress are explained by the force–velocity relationship of striated muscle. One can see that as arterial blood pressure goes up, the heart has an increasing load against which it must eject its stroke volume. Pressure is the largest component of afterload. However, a more accurate estimate of afterload is the total impedance

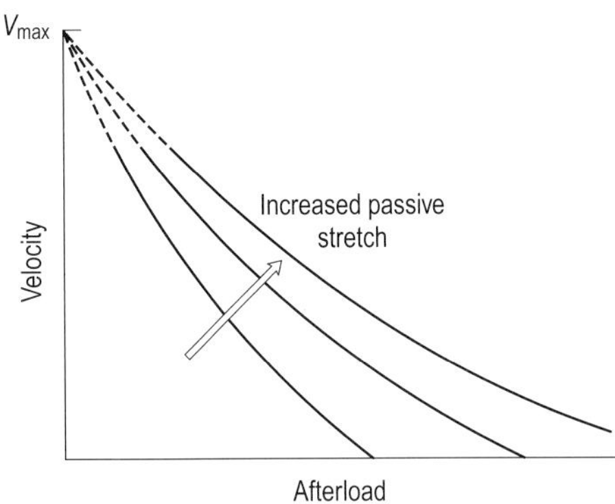

Fig. 10.11 The relationship of velocity of contraction to systolic tension or afterload is shown schematically for isotonically contracting cardiac muscle strips. Velocity and extent of contraction are inversely related to afterload. Increased preload or passive stretch and increased contractility increase velocity of shortening at any given afterload. V_{max} is the extrapolated intercept velocity at zero afterload and is relatively constant at different preloads allowing it to be used as an index of contractility. The reciprocal relationship between extent of shortening and afterload is the basis for the reciprocal relationship between arterial pressure and stroke volume. After Thornburg and Morton[40].

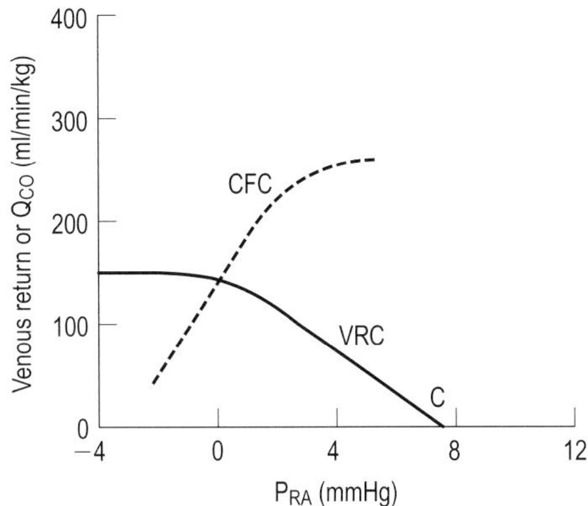

Fig. 10.12 Theoretical venous return curve (VRC) and cardiac function curve (CFC) for normal adults. Modified from Gilbert[32].

of the vascular tree. As mentioned above, the vascular impedance is the additive resistive forces of mean and pulsatile flow components.

Contractility

When preload and afterload are kept constant, a ventricle can increase or decrease its ejection fraction through changes in contractility. Contractility (intropy) is the relative contractile state (strength) of the myocardium. Increases in contractility are usually the result of greater cytosolic Ca^{2+} concentrations during systole. However, the sensitivity of the contractile elements to Ca^{2+} ion and the ATPase activity of the myosin isoforms are also factors that affect contractility. Drugs that increase contractility are inotropic agents. Increases in heart rate affect myocyte intracellular Ca^{2+} concentration and therefore alter contractility.

There are important differences between immature myocardium and adult myocardium with regard to contractile capability. Friedman[42] showed that fetal myocardium generates less tension per gram than does adult myocardium. Similarly, Nakanishi et al.[15] reported that the 18-day rabbit heart could generate about 18 g of tension for each gram of cardiac muscle, whereas the adult could generate nearly 78 g (see Table 10.1). Such changes have been assumed to be largely due to the reduced proportion of the myocyte volume containing contractile material[42]. Contraction velocities of unloaded muscle from fetal and adult myocardium are about equal, suggesting that mature and immature sarcomeres behave similarly. However, this is now known to be more complex than originally thought and there may be genuine contractility increases with maturity.

There are differences in contraction velocity of cardiac muscle depending on which of several types of myosin is present. For example, alpha-myosin (V_1) has high ATPase activity whereas beta-myosin (V_3) has low ATPase activity. The ventricular myocardium of the rat switches from V_3 to V_1 in the postnatal period and again to V_3 in old age. V_3 is the prominent isoform in adult humans over the life of the individual. Therefore, it has not been possible to interpret changes in the contractile state with isoenzyme activity in humans.

To what extent do preload, afterload and contractility determine stroke volume in the intact fetus? This question is often raised among physiologists and answers have come in various forms. The cardiac function curve is often used to investigate preload. The function curve is a plot of cardiac output, stroke volume or stroke work (stroke volume × driving pressure) against an index of ventricular filling (mean atrial pressure, end-diastolic pressure or end-diastolic volume)[43]. Function curves have been constructed for the whole heart of the fetus[32]. Figure 10.12 shows that as mean atrial pressure (above amniotic pressure) increases from a low level, cardiac output increases proportionately up the ascending limb until the plateau limb is reached, above which no further increases can be generated. The conclusion is that the fetus operates near the top of the curve and that there is very little 'preload reserve' on the plateau. When the fetal ventricles were studied independently, the same conclusion was reached for each ventricle[44,45]. Interestingly, the function curve of the right ventricle is situated well above the curve of the left ventricle. This indicates that for the same filling pressure and ejection fraction, the stroke volume is greater for the right ventricle than for the left.

The shape of the function curve is important. When mean atrial pressure is referenced to amniotic fluid pressure, true ventricular filling pressure is not being measured. The transmural pressure difference across the ventricular wall is the best measure of filling pressure. Transmural pressure can be estimated by referring intraventricular pressure to pressure in the pericardial space, especially since the physical behavior of the catheter in that space is known[46]. Surprisingly, the placement of a pericardial catheter does not much alter the shape of the function curve. However, it is known that augmentation of end-diastolic volume inevitably leads to increases in stroke volume. Thus, while increasing pressures on the plateau of the function curve represents measurments in vivo, it does not appear to represent true increases in end-diastolic volume. This points to the difficulty of measuring local transmural pressures at the freewall of the ventricle in vivo.

It has long been known in adults that increased afterload reduces ventricular shortening velocity and thus, ejection fraction. When afterload was increased in the fetus, it was found that the two ventricles responded very differently. Figure 10.13 shows the relationship between stroke volume and arterial pressure for each ventricle[47] as arterial pressure is increased by inflating an occluder around the descending aorta just beyond the ductus arteriosus. The right ventricular stroke volume decreases rapidly with increasing pressure while the left

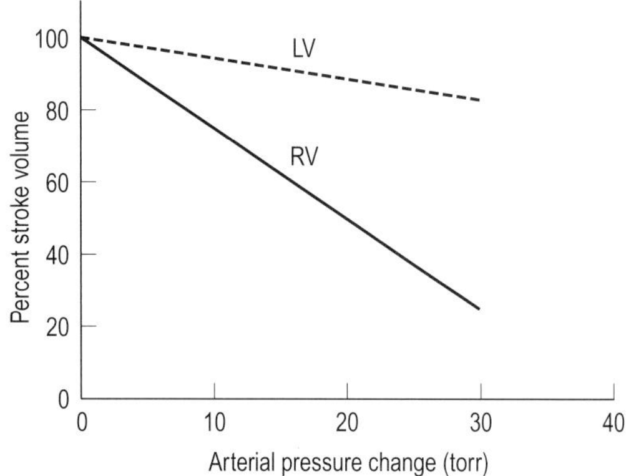

Fig. 10.13 The simultaneous average responses of the right and left ventricles to increased arterial pressure are shown for nine fetuses. Stroke volume is expressed as a percent of control value and arterial pressure as the increment above control. The linear regression coefficient for each ventricle was calculated, the average slope forced through 100% on the Y-axis and the lines extended through the pressure range studied. The right ventricular pressure sensitivity (−2.5 ± 1.4% stroke volume/torr) was more than fivefold the left ventricular pressure sensitivity (−0.5 ± 0.7% stroke volume/torr) ($P < 0.001$). After Reller et al.[47].

ventricular stroke volume decreases hardly at all. This indicates that the right ventricle is inherently unable to maintain its stroke volume in the face of increased arterial pressure compared to the left ventricle. This 'afterload sensitivity' of the right ventricle is physiologically important because it shows that increases in arterial pressure from hypoxemia or placenta growth abnormalities will preferentially affect the right ventricle and will change hemodynamic patterns in the fetus.

There is no convincing evidence that contractility of the fetal heart is significantly regulated on a beat-to-beat basis, though in hypoxemic fetuses, catecholamine concentrations may be high and direct inotropic stimulation of the myocardium is likely.

Ventricular geometry

The fetal ventricles were long thought to be nearly identical in shape and function[48–50]. This impression likely came from the stark contrast between adult and fetal hearts. In adult hearts, the thin-walled right ventricle appears to be a crescent-shaped add-on to the thick-walled cylindrical left ventricle. In contrast, the fetal ventricles have nearly identical wall thicknesses and their cross-sectional views look similar in certain cross-sectional views. Unfortunately, this impression is misleading. The fetal ventricles are sufficiently different in shape and architecture that their physiological function is importantly affected. This interventricular difference in form and function is exaggerated over time during postnatal life (Fig. 10.14). The internal dimensions of

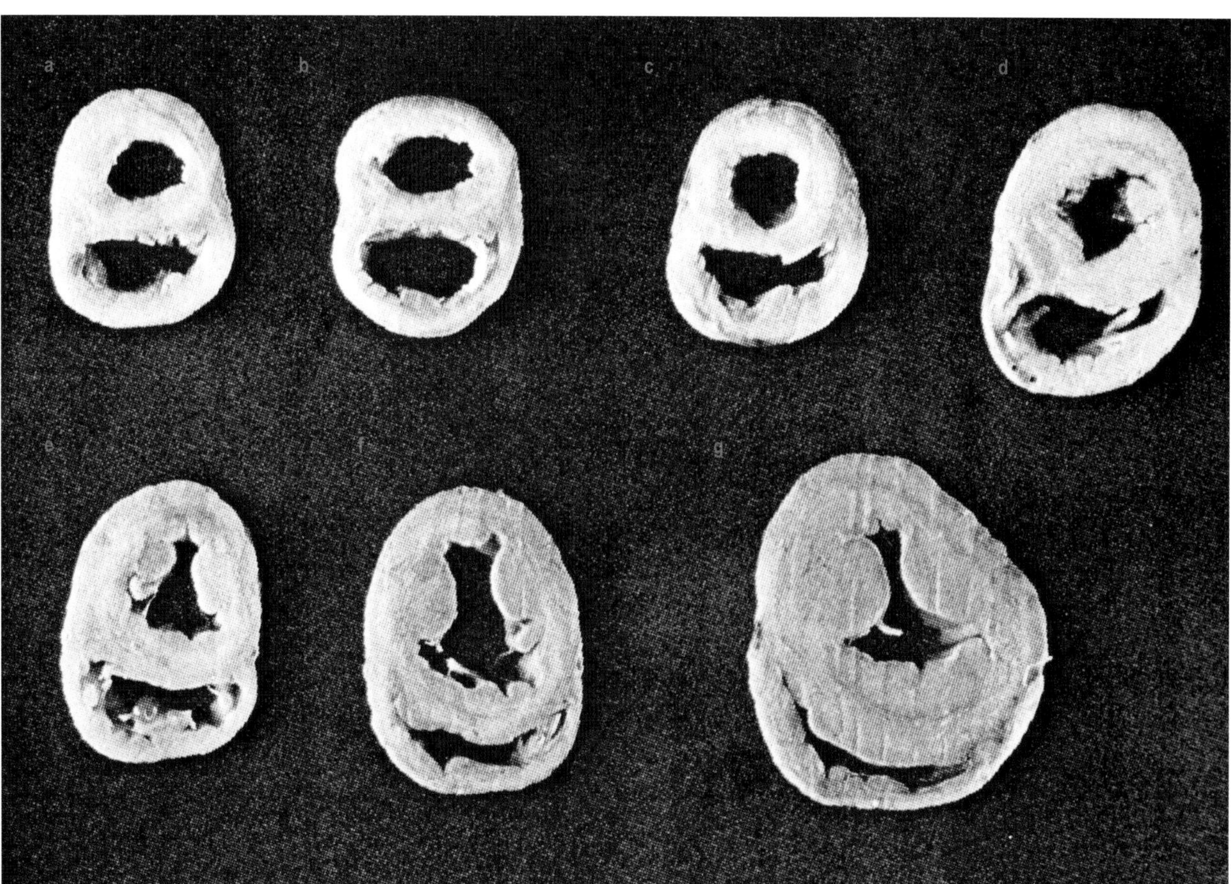

Fig. 10.14 Horizontal sections across the ventricles of pig hearts from 1 day to 9 weeks old with the left ventricle on the top of each slice. a = 1 day; b = 2 days; c = 3 days; d = 9 days; e = 18 days; f = 37 days; g = 9 weeks. After Versprille et al.[51].

the near term fetal ventricles have been determined for sheep[52] from hearts fixed at physiological filling pressures (Fig. 10.15) as have the component weights (Table 10.3). Several key physical features are important in understanding the physiology of the working heart in utero:

- The right ventricular chamber of the sheep is some 30% larger than the left ventricular chamber. The difference between the ventricles is present in the human fetal heart but it is not quite so pronounced. If filling pressures and ejection fractions are about equal, this finding explains the dominant right-ventricular stroke volume in the fetus.
- The meridianal radius to wall thickness ratio is larger for the right ventricle than for the left[52]. For the mid-section of the fetal heart the average radius of curvature (r) for the right ventricle is 12.8 mm versus 10.9 mm for the left ventricle. The wall thicknesses (h) are about 3.0 mm and 4.2 mm respectively. Thus, the r/h of the right ventricle (4.5) compared to the smaller r/h (2.6) indicates that the right ventricle has a higher resting wall stress and is at a mechanical disadvantage compared to the left ventricle.

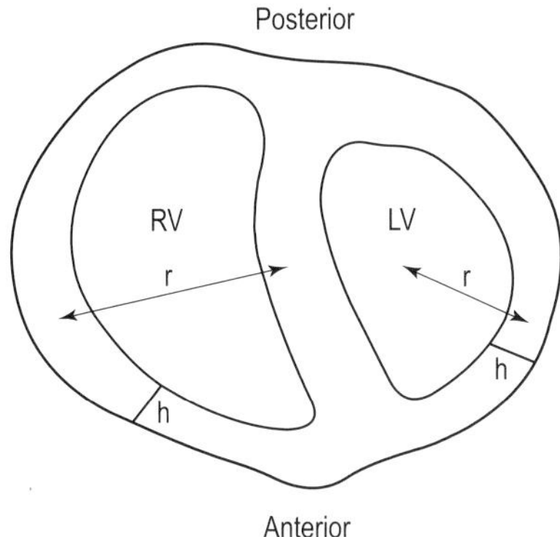

Fig. 10.15 Cross-sectional slice from a near-term fetal heart cut half-way between the apex and annulus. Note that the two ventricles are clearly distinguishable in shape at this stage of gestation. Even by inspection, one could estimate that the right ventricle has a larger radius of curvature than the left ventricle (see Eqn 10.2). After Thornburg et al.[53].

Table 10.3 **Heart mass for the 129-day sheep fetus (*n* = 44)**

	Weight (g)	*SD*
Total atrial	3.1	0.9*
Total ventricular	16.0	4.8
Left ventricle	6.2	1.8
Right ventricle	5.8	1.9
Septum	4.0	1.2
Fetal mass	2.9 (kg)	0.8
Ventricular/fetal mass	5.5 (g/kg)	0.9
Dry/wet heart mass	0.17	0.02**

*n = 34; **n = 21

This provides a physical explanation for ventricular differences in sensitivity to arterial pressure as predicted by Laplace's law (see Eqn 10.2).

There are several pathological conditions where the right ventricle must carry the workload of the systemic circulation. This can be done more easily if the ventricle is conditioned by episodes of moderate pressure loading before being harnessed to the high resistance of the systemic circulation. The fetal sheep right ventricle has been studied to determine whether it is able to compensate for increased pressure load over time by inflation of an occluder around the main pulmonary artery[54]. The mean pressure in the pulmonary artery was increased by about 10 mmHg above the usual 45–50 mmHg for a 10-day period. Right ventricular wall thickness and weight were both increased. The pressure–volume curves of both ventricles were left shifted which means that the chamber volume was smaller for any given filling pressure (Fig. 10.16). Thus, the fetal right ventricle adapts to a pressure load by increasing free wall thickness (a lesson already learned from mature hearts) but at the expense of the chamber volume.

Figure 10.17 shows the change in sensitivity to increasing arterial pressure following pressure loading. Note that the right ventricular stroke volume curve dramatically decreases its slope so that the conditioned ventricle is able to eject a larger volume at any pulmonary arterial pressure than before loading. Also note that r/h (see Eqn 10.2) approaches that of the left ventricle and that the function of the two ventricles is now similar.

Regulation of coronary flow

The flow of blood through the coronary circulation has been studied extensively in the adult but only little in immature hearts[56–58]. The concept of flow reserve has been helpful. When the heart is fully dilated by a pharmacological agent, coronary flow increases linearly with the driving pressure ($P_{art} - P_{cs}$), where P_{art} is the inflow pressure in the coronary artery and

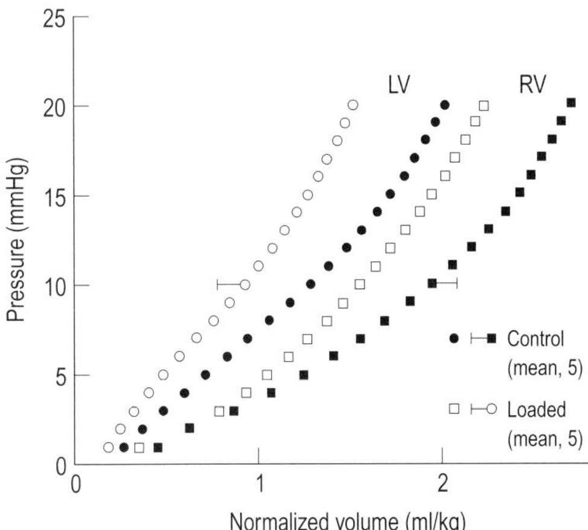

Fig. 10.16 Pressure–volume relations of K$^+$-arrested fetal hearts in vitro. Curves were made by rapidly infusing isotonic saline into left ventricular (LV) and right ventricular (RV) chambers through a plug in the valve annulus while simultaneous pressure measurements were made. Measurements are shown with the contralateral ventricle at 10 mmHg transmural pressure and the pericardium in place. After Pinson et al.[54].

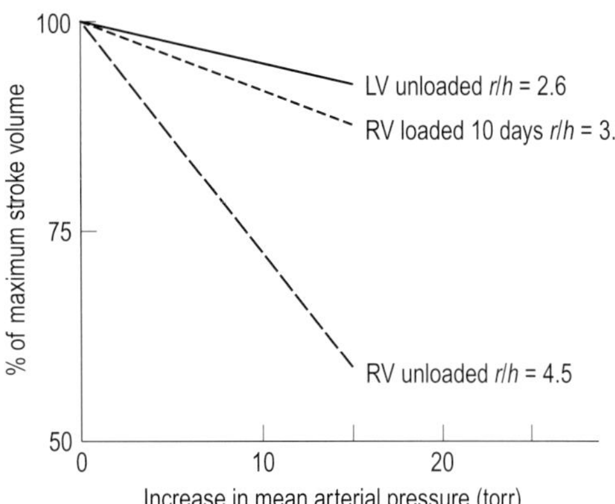

Fig. 10.17 Percentage change in right ventricular stroke volume of fetuses plotted as a function of increase in pulmonary artery pressure. The normal relationships between stroke volume and mean arterial pressure for the unloaded right ventricle (RV unloaded) and the unloaded left ventricle (LV unloaded) are taken from Figure 10.13. The relationship between stroke volume and pulmonary arterial pressure after 10 days of mild pressure loading is shown as 'RV loaded 10 days'. Each curve is shown with its respective radius to wall thickness ratios which affect wall tension as shown in Eqn 10.2. After Thornburg et al.[55].

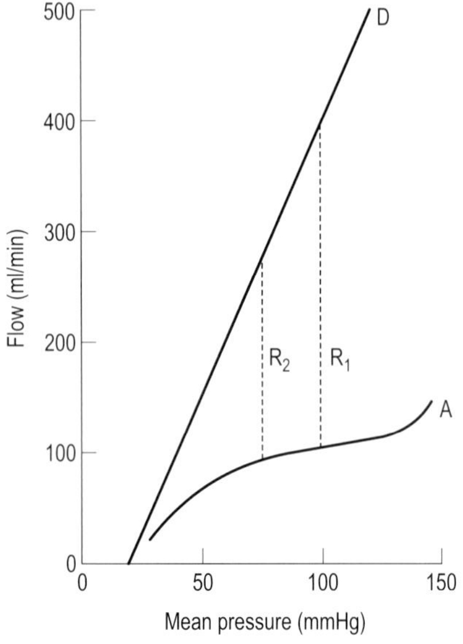

Fig. 10.18 Diagram of pressure–flow relationships in normal left ventricle during autoregulation (A) and maximal vasodilatation (D). R_1 and R_2 are the coronary flow reserves at mean coronary perfusing pressures of 75 and 100 mmHg when aortic pressure and heart rate are constant. After Hoffman[31].

P_{cs} is the outflow pressure in the coronary sinus (Fig. 10.18). However, coronary flow at rest is only a fraction of its potential at any given pressure. In fact, if inflow coronary pressure is increased, flow increases very little over its autoregulatory range (the plateau in Figure 10.18). The difference between the autoregulated flow and the flow at full chemical dilation is the 'flow reserve', a value that clearly depends on the pressure at which the measurement is made.

Coronary flow correlates best with oxygen consumption which in turn is affected by pressure and heart rate. In the sheep fetus, coronary flow has been measured using microspheres[56] and Doppler sensors that indicate flow velocity[59]. The oxygen consumption of the heart is similar on a gram basis to the adult heart[56]. However, the oxygen content of the fetal arterial blood is half that of the adult. Thus, coronary flow in the fetus must be about twice that of the adult. In fetal sheep, the resting coronary flow is about 200–250 ml/min/100 g and coronary flow in adult animals ranges between 80 and 110 ml/min/100 g[28,59].

When the fetal sheep coronary circulation is dilated maximally with increasing doses of adenosine, the maximal right ventricular flow is about 600 ml/min/100 g at resting pressure[59]. The right ventricle was studied during gradual increases in pressure load as an occluder around the pulmonary artery was inflated in a near-term sheep[60]. Fetal coronary flow increased with increases in pressure load until mean pulmonary arterial pressure reached 80 mmHg, the point where the ventricle failed. At this pressure, right ventricular flow was ≈400 ml/min/100 g, a value that was two-thirds less than flow during dilation with adenosine. This indicates that right ventricular work is not able to elicit a flow response to take full advantage of potential flow reserve even when the ventricle is failing. The fetal myocardium, like the adult myocardium, is not able to recruit all of its reserve under physiological conditions. However, the fetal heart appears to be especially equipped to handle hypoxemic episodes in utero. When the fetus is made acutely hypoxemic by the administration of low oxygen gas mixtures to the ewe, coronary flow increases with decreasing arterial oxygen content. At very low oxygen concentrations (<1 mM) flows in the myocardium are dramatic and may reach 1.6 l/min/100 g. Stroke volume is maintained at this level of oxygenation for short periods (≈15 min).

Developmental plasticity and life-long disease

Epidemiological evidence indicates that fetal growth stressors elicit changes in gene expression and growth patterns that predispose the body for life-long disease. These findings have led to a decade of intense research on the roles of hypoxemia, malnutrition and glucocorticoid excess in programming a fetus for adult onset disease risk. Several fetal responses to stress are known to stimulate common responses by the cardiovascular system depending on the window of development in which the stress is applied. Common alterations include:

1. reduced nephron numbers and anatomy
2. endothelial dysfunction
3. altered cardiomyocyte numbers
4. enhanced or reduced cardiac myocardial mass
5. remodeled coronary tree.

Each of these changes confers a predisposition for the fetus at the time of birth. Hormones that regulate cardiomyocyte growth include insulin-like growth factor (IGF)-1, angiotensin II, thyroid hormone and cortisol.

Recent experiments have shown that the fetal coronary vessels are very plastic. A 7-day episode of severe anemia in the near-term fetus stimulates the coronary tree to increase its cross-sectional area at the level of the microcirculation. Flows in the fully dilated coronary tree can increase over three- to fourfold within a few days. The striking finding, however, is that the proportional increase in flow for any perfusion pressure (conductance) remains into adulthood. Thus, the coronary tree is highly plastic during the perinatal period and changes in coronary architecture during that period have life-long consequences.

ACKNOWLEDGMENTS

We would like to thank our colleagues who have been co-investigators, technicians and supporters: George D Giraud, Lowell Davis, J Job Faber, Debra Anderson, Mark J Morton, Mark D Reller, Antonio Barbera, John Bissonnette, James Metcalfe, C Wright Pinson, Deborah Reid, David Wu, Mike Burson, Tom Green, Bob Webber, Pat Renwick, Lisa Rhuman. From these, we have received more than we have given.

REFERENCES

1. Reller MD, McDonald RW, Gerlis LM, Thornburg KL. Cardiac embryology: basic review and clinical correlations (review). *J Am Soc Echocardiogr* **4**(5):519–532, 1991.
2. van Wijk B, Moorman AFM, van den Hoff MJB. Role of bone morphogenetic proteins in cardiac differentiation (review). *Cardiovasc Res* **74**:44–255, 2007.
3. Bruneau BG. Developmental biology: tiny brakes for a growing heart (review). *Nature* **436**:181–182, 2005.
4. Kathiriya IS, Srivastava D. Left-right asymmetry and cardiac looping: implications for cardiac development and congenital heart disease. *Am J Med Genet (Semin Med Genet)* **97**:271–279, 2000.
5. Zaffran S, Frasch M. Early signals in cardiac development (review). *Circ Res* **91**:457–469, 2002.
6. Kirby ML. Molecular embryogenesis of the heart (review). *Pediatr Dev Pathol* **5**:516–543, 2002.
7. Ryan K, Chin AJ. T-Box genes and cardiac development (review). *Birth Defects Res (Part C)* **69**:25–37, 2003.
8. Katz AM. *Physiology of the heart*, 2nd edn. New York: Raven Press, 1992.
9. Nakazawa M, Miyagawa S, Ohno T, Miura S, Takao A. Developmental hemodynamic changes in rat embryos at 11 to 15 days of gestation: normal data of blood pressure and the effect of caffeine compared to data from chick embryo. *Ped Res* **23**(2):200–205, 1988.
10. Faber JJ, Green TJ, Thornburg KL. Embryonic stroke volume and cardiac output in the chick. *Dev Biol* **41**(1):14–21, 1974.
11. Keller BB. Overview: functional maturation and coupling of the embryonic cardiovascular system. In *Developmental mechanisms of heart disease*, EB Clark, RR Markwald, A Takao (eds), pp. 367–385. Armonk NY: Futura, 1995.
12. Maylie JG. Excitation–contraction coupling in neonatal and adult myocardium of cat. *Am J Physiol* **242**(5):H834–H843, 1982.
13. Clubb FJ, Bishop SP. Formation of binucleated myocardial cells in the neonatal rat: an index for growth hypertrophy. *Lab Invest* **50**:571–577, 1984.
14. Rakusan K. Cardiac growth, maturation, and aging. In *Growth of the heart in health and disease*, R Zak (ed.), pp. 131–164. New York: Raven Press, 1984.
15. Nakanishi T, Seguchi M, Takao A. Development of the myocardial contractile system (review). *Experientia* **44**(11–12):936–944, 1988.
16. Dawes GS. *Foetal and neonatal physiology*. Chicago: Year Book Medical Publishers, 1968.
17. Carter AM. The blood supply to the abdominal organs of the fetal guinea-pig. *J Dev Physiol* **6**:407–416, 1984.
18. Anderson DF, Bissonnette JM, Faber JJ, Thornburg KL. Central shunt flows and pressures in the mature fetal lamb. *Am J Physiol* **241**(1):H60–H66, 1981.
19. Reuss ML, Rudolph AM. Distribution and recirculation of umbilical and systemic venous blood flow in fetal lambs during hypoxia. In *Journal of developmental physiology*, CT. Jones (ed.), Vol. 2, pp. 71–84. Oxford: Blackwell Scientific Publications, 1980.
20. Anderson DF, Faber JJ, Morton MJ, Parks CM, Pinson CW, Thornburg KL. Flow through the foramen ovale of the fetal and new-born lamb. *J Physiol (Lond)* **365**:29–40, 1985.
21. Nichols WW, O'Rourke MF. *McDonald's blood flow in arteries: theoretic, experimental and clinical principles*, 3rd edn. Philadelphia: Lea & Febiger, 1990.
22. Langille BL, Adamson SL. Thoracic aortic pressure–flow relationships and vascular impedance in fetal sheep. *Am J Physiol* **263**:H824–H32, 1992.
23. Meschia G, Cotter JR, Breathnach CS, Barron DH. The hemoglobin, oxygen, carbon dioxide and hydrogen ion concentrations in the umbilical bloods of sheep and goats as sampled via indwelling plastic catheters. *Q J Exp Physiol* **50**:185–195, 1965.
24. Teitel DF. Circulatory adjustments of postnatal life. *Sem Perinatol* **12**:96–103, 1988.
25. Llanos AJ, Riquelme RA, Moraga FA, Cabello G, Parer JT. Cardiovascular responses to graded degrees of hypoxaemia in the llama fetus. *Progr Perinatal Physiol Reproduct Fertil Develop* **7**:247–250, 1995.
26. Kirkpatrick SE, Friedman WF. Myocardial determinants of fetal cardiac output. In *Fetal and newborn cardiovascular physiology*, LD Longo, DD Reneau (eds), Vol. 1, pp. 369–389. New York: Garland STPM Press, 1978.
27. Anderson PAW, Glick KI, Manring A, Crenshaw C, Jr. Developmental changes in cardiac contractility in fetal and postnatal sheep: *in vitro* and *in vivo*. *Am J Physiol* **247**:H371–H379, 1984.
28. Jacobson S-L, Eicher AL, Paul MS, Giraud GD, Morton MJ, Thornburg KL. The sequential effects of estrogen administration and hypertension on cardiac function in ewes. *Am J Obstet Gynecol* **179**:610–619, 1998.
29. Rasanen J, Wood DC, Weiner S, Ludomirski A, Huhta JC. Role of the pulmonary circulation in the distribution of human fetal cardiac output during the second half of pregnancy. *Circulation* **94**:1068–1073, 1996.
30. Heymann MA, Creasy RK, Rudolph AM. Quantitation of blood flow patterns in the foetal lamb *in utero*. In *Foetal and neonatal physiology*, KS Combline, KW Cross, GS Dawes, PW Nathanielsz (eds), pp. 129–135. Cambridge: Cambridge University Press, 1973.
31. Hoffmann JIE. Maximal coronary flow and the concept of coronary vascular reserve (review). *Circulation* **70**(2):153–159, 1984.
32. Gilbert RD. Venous return and control of fetal cardiac output. In *Fetal and newborn cardiovascular physiology, vol. 1: developmental aspects*, LD Longo, DD Reneau (eds), pp. 299–316. New York: Garland STPM Press, 1978.
33. Guyton AC, Lindsey AW, Abernathy JB, Richardson T. Venous return at various right atrial pressures and the normal venous return curve. *Am J Physiol* **189**:609–615, 1957.
34. Morin FC, Eagan EA. Pulmonary hemodynamics in fetal lambs during development at normal and increased oxygen tension. *J Appl Physiol* **73**:213–218, 1992.
35. Longo LD, Wyatt JF, Hewitt CW, Gilbert RD. A comparison of circulatory responses to hypoxic hypoxia and carbon monoxide hypoxia in fetal blood flow and oxygenation. In *Fetal and newborn cardiovascular physiology*, LD Longo, DD Reneau (eds), pp. 259–288. New York: Garland STPM Press, 1976.
36. Longo LD, Packianathan S. Hypoxia-ischaemia and the developing brain: hypotheses regarding the pathophysiology of fetal-neonatal brain damage. *Br J Obstet Gynaecol* **104**(6):652–662, 1997.
37. Peeters LLH, Sheldon RE, Jones MD, Jr., Makowski EL, Meschia G. Blood flow to

fetal organs as a function of arterial oxygen content. *Am J Obstet Gynecol* **135**:637–646, 1979.

38. Thornburg KL. Fetal response to intrauterine stress (review). In *Childhood environment and adult disease*, GR Bock, J Whelan (eds), pp. 17–37. (Ciba Foundation Symposium 156) Chichester: John Wiley, 1991.
39. Braunwald E, Ross J, Jr., Sonnenblick EH. *Mechanisms of contraction of the normal and failing heart*. Boston: Little, Brown, 1976.
40. Thornburg KL, Morton MJ. Development of the cardiovascular system. In *Textbook of fetal physiology*, GD Thorburn, R Harding (eds), pp. 95–130. Oxford: Oxford University Press, 1994.
41. Paterson SW, Starling EH. On mechanical factors which determine output of ventricles. *J Physiol (Lond)* **48**:357–379, 1914.
42. Friedman WF. The intrinsic physiologic properties of the developing heart. *Prog Cardiovasc Dis* **15**:87, 1972.
43. Bishop VS, Stone HL, Guyton AC. Cardiac function curves in conscious dogs. *Am J Physiol* **207**:677–682, 1964.
44. Thornburg KL, Morton MJ. Filling and arterial pressures as determinants of RV stroke volume in the sheep fetus. *Am J Physiol* **244**(5):H656–H663, 1983.
45. Thornburg KL, Morton MJ. Filling and arterial pressures as determinants of left ventricular stroke volume in fetal lambs. *Am J Physiol* **251**(5, Pt 2):H961–H968, 1986.
46. Morton MJ, Pinson CW, Thornburg KL. *In utero* ventilation with oxygen augments left ventricular stroke volume in lambs. *J Physiol (Lond.)* **383**:413–424, 1987.
47. Reller MD, Morton MJ, Reid DL, Thornburg KL. Fetal lamb ventricles respond differently to filling and arterial pressures and to *in utero* ventilation. *Pediatr Res* **22**(6):621–626, 1987.
48. Pohlman AG. The course of the blood through the heart of the fetal mammal, with a note on the reptilian and amphibian circulations. *Anat Rec* **3**:75–109, 1909.
49. Cassin S, Dawes GS, Mott JC, Ross BB, Strang LB. The vascular resistance of the fetal and newly ventilated lung of the lamb. *J Physiol (Lond.)* **171**:61–79, 1964.
50. St John-Sutton MG, Gewitz MH, Shah B et al. Quantitative assessment of growth and function in the cardiac chambers in the normal human fetus: a prospective longitudinal echocardiographic study. *Circulation* **69**:645–654, 1984.
51. Pinson CW, Morton MJ, Thornburg KL. An anatomic basis for fetal right ventricular dominance and arterial pressure sensitivity. *J Dev Physiol* **9**(3): 253–269, 1987.
52. Versprille A, Jansen JRC, Harnick E, van Nie CJ, deNeef KJ. Functional interaction of both ventricles at birth and the changes during the neonatal period in relation to the changes of geometry. In *Fetal and newborn cardiovascular physiology*, LD Longo, DD Reneau (eds), vol. 1, pp. 399–413. New York: Garland STPM Press, 1978.
53. Thornburg KL, Morton MJ, Pinson CW, Reller MD, Reid DL. Anatomic and functional distinctions between the fetal heart ventricles. In *Perinatal development of the heart and lung*, J Lipshitz, J Maloney, C Nimrod, G Carson (eds), pp. 49–82. Ithaca, NY: Perinatology Press, 1991.
54. Pinson CW, Morton MJ, Thornburg KL. Mild pressure loading alters right ventricular function in fetal sheep. *Circ Res* **68**(4):947–957, 1991.
55. Thornburg KL, Morton MJ. Growth and development of the heart. In *Fetus and neonate: physiology and clinical applications, vol. 1: the circulation*, MA Hanson, JAD Spencer, CH Rodeck (eds), pp. 137–159. Cambridge: Cambridge University Press, 1993.
56. Fisher DJ, Heymann MA, Rudolph AM. Myocardial oxygen and carbohydrate consumption in fetal lambs and in adult sheep. *Am J Physiol* **238**:H399–H405, 1980.
57. Fisher DJ, Heymann MA, Rudolph AM. Fetal myocardial oxygen and carbohydrate consumption during acutely induced hypoxemia. *Am J Physiol* **242**:H657–H661, 1982.
58. Fisher DJ, Heymann MA, Rudolph AM. Regional myocardial blood flow and oxygen delivery in fetal, newborn, and adult sheep. *Am J Physiol* **243**:H729–H731, 1982.
59. Reller MD, Morton MJ, Giraud GD, Wu DE, Thornburg KL. Maximal myocardial blood flow is enhanced by chronic hypoxemia in late gestation fetal sheep. *Am J Physiol* **263**(4, Pt 2):H1327–H1329, 1992.
60. Reller MD, Morton MJ, Giraud GD, Wu DE, Thornburg KL. Severe right ventricular pressure loading in fetal sheep augments global myocardial blood flow to sub-maximal levels. *Circulation* **86**(2):581–588, 1992.
61. Cohn HE, Sacks EJ, Heyman MA, Rudolph AM. Cardiovascular responses to hypoxemia and academia in fetal lambs. *Am J Obstet Gynecol* **120**:817–824, 1974.

CHAPTER

11

Lung growth and maturation

Richard Harding and Stuart B Hooper

KEY POINTS

- Survival at birth depends upon the lung being well grown and structurally mature during fetal life. This chapter deals with mechanisms underlying normal and impaired lung growth and development
- The fetal lung has a low level of recoil and its lumen is liquid filled; it develops in an expanded state which is necessary for normal growth and maturation
- The level of fetal lung expansion is determined by its physical environment, including amniotic fluid volume, intrathoracic space and fetal breathing movements. Lung tissue stretch stimulates gene networks leading to tissue growth and differentiation. Lung hypoplasia results if the fetal lung is chronically under-expanded
- The secretion of fetal lung liquid by the pulmonary epithelium is an active process that is hormonally regulated; with the onset of labor, secretion slows and is reversed due to increasing levels of adrenaline and cortisol. Remaining lung liquid is absorbed after birth
- The fetal lung has a low blood flow that is appropriate for tissue mass; at birth, constrictor processes must be overcome and dilator processes activated to lower pulmonary vascular resistance to permit adequate gas exchange
- The production of pulmonary surfactant by epithelial type II cells is critical for survival of the newborn. The number of type II cells is related to the level of lung expansion. Surfactant production and maturation of lung parenchyma are stimulated by endogenous and exogenous corticosteroids

INTRODUCTION

At birth, the lungs must immediately take over the role of gas exchange from the placenta. This transition is normally uneventful, which is remarkable given that prior to birth the lungs are liquid filled, have a relatively modest blood supply (i.e. appropriate for tissue mass, but inappropriate for gas exchange) and have never performed this role. In order for the lung to function as an organ of gas exchange it must cease its secretion of lung liquid, secrete surfactant, clear the airways of liquid and greatly reduce pulmonary vascular resistance, allowing it to receive the entire output of the right ventricle. During normal fetal development, the lung becomes progressively prepared for these dramatic changes in physiology at birth. However, if lung growth or maturation in utero is impaired, respiratory insufficiency in the newborn can result, which may contribute to the development of respiratory disorders in later life. This chapter will focus on the processes controlling prenatal lung growth and maturation. Some of the more common respiratory complications in the neonate, and their fetal origins, will be discussed together with strategies for their treatment.

STAGES OF LUNG DEVELOPMENT

Pulmonary morphologists recognize five or six major stages in human lung development[1,2] (Table 11.1).

Embryonic stage (3–7 weeks): the lung first appears as an outgrowth of the primitive foregut (i.e. endodermal tissue) at 22–26 days post-conception. This bud elongates and divides to form the trachea and left and right bronchi; these structures then undergo dichotomous branching to form the major units of the bronchial tree. By 34 days, each of the major bronchopulmonary segments has formed. During early embryonic development, epithelial cells that are endodermal in origin form the developing 'airways' and grow into the surrounding tissue which is derived from splanchnic mesoderm. This mesodermal tissue gives rise to the mesenchymal cells that form the non-epithelial structures of the lung including blood and lymph vessels, airway cartilage and smooth muscle, fibrous tissue and other parenchymal components. The mature lungs contain more than 40 different cell types, all derived from embryonic endodermal and mesenchymal tissue.

Table 11.1 **Stages of lung development in the human**

Stage	*Timing*	*Major events*
Embryonic	4–7 weeks	Appearance of ventral bud in foregut. Epithelial tube branches and grows into surrounding mesenchyme. Vascular connections formed
Pseudoglandular	5–17 weeks	Development of conductive airway tree, paralleled by formation of vascular tree. Lung periphery contains parenchymal precursors
Canalicular	16–26 weeks	Addition of further generations of airways and of vascular tree. Differentiation of type-I and type-II epithelial cells. Formation of thin air–blood barrier. Start of surfactant production
Saccular stage	25–40 weeks (term)	Formation of additional airway generations. Dilation of prospective gas-exchanging airspaces. Maturation of surfactant system
Alveolar stage	36 weeks–18 months	Start of alveolar formation at 36 weeks. Formation of alveoli by outgrowth of secondary septa
Microvascular	Before birth–3 years	Change from double- to single-capillary layer. Reduction in interstitial tissue mass; fusion of endothelial cell and epithelial cell basement membranes. Preferential growth of single-layered capillary network areas

Reproduced in modified form, with permission, from Burri [1]

Pseudoglandular stage (8–16 weeks): during the pseudoglandular stage, the lung resembles a typical exocrine gland. The major bronchi and associated functional units of the lung (i.e. acini) are progressively formed which are paralleled by the formation and growth of pulmonary arterial tree. As a result, each major 'airway' is accompanied by a branch of the pulmonary artery. The formation of acini occurs as a result of repeated branching of distal extremities of blind-ending tubes or 'airways' comprised of epithelial cells (Fig. 11.1). The process of branching, which is critical to the growth of new orders of 'airways', is induced by the interaction between airway epithelial cells and adjacent mesenchymal cells; this process probably depends upon mitogens acting in a paracrine manner. The developing airways are surrounded by mesenchymal tissue which, at this stage, has only a loose network of blood capillaries (see Fig. 11.1), thereby precluding, or at least greatly restricting, pulmonary gas exchange. Airway epithelial cells gradually differentiate (in a centrifugal direction) into ciliated cells (by 11–13 weeks), as well as goblet cells and mucous glands.

Canalicular stage (17–25 weeks): during the canalicular stage of lung development, the airways grow and enlarge (both widen and lengthen – i.e. canalization) and the mesenchymal tissue, surrounding the terminal air ways, attenuates (see Fig. 11.1). This results in a substantial increase in luminal volume of the lung. During the canalicular stage, the functional units of the lung are formed, consisting of terminal bronchioles ending with enlargements that subsequently give rise to terminal sacs (primitive alveoli). A network of blood capillaries develops around the developing terminal airsacs, thereby increasing the proximity of blood capillaries with the epithelial cell layer of the gas-exchange units; this marks the beginnings of the air–blood interface that is required for effective gas exchange (see Fig. 11.1). Thus, the mid-late canalicular stage is the earliest that the lungs can potentially support independent life.

Terminal sac stage (28–35 weeks): this stage of lung development, sometimes called the saccular stage, sees a progressive enlargement of the distal 'airspaces'. This results from further attenuation of peri-saccular mesenchymal tissue and leads to a further increase in luminal volume relative to total lung volume. During the terminal sac stage, the development of secondary septa first begins; these are outgrowths from primary septa and will eventually subdivide the terminal sac into multiple alveoli (see Fig. 11.1). The primary septa are considered primitive in that they are wider than the secondary septa and contain a double capillary network, rather than the single capillary layer of the mature lung. Elastic fibers are formed by myofibroblasts within the secondary septa and are deposited at their tips, thereby contributing to the elastic (recoil) properties of the lung. The epithelial layer becomes thinner and both type I and type II epithelial cells differentiate. As a result of these structural changes, the separation between luminal 'air' and capillary blood becomes smaller, thereby enhancing the ability of the lung to exchange respiratory gases.

Alveolar stage (36 weeks of gestation – 1–2 years): by the time of term birth in human infants, several million definitive pulmonary alveoli are present; estimates vary between 20 and 50 million. In the adult human lung, some 300 million alveoli are present, indicating that most are formed postnatally. The alveolar stage of lung development is thought to continue for at least one or two years after birth. In species born at an earlier stage of development (e.g. rats and mice), the alveolar stage begins after birth and, therefore, at birth, gas exchange occurs across the simpler, more primitive terminal sacs in these species.

During the alveolar stage, terminal sacs are subdivided by the outgrowth of secondary septa, from the primary septa, to form alveoli. Initially, these alveoli resemble shallow cups, but they deepen due to elongation of the secondary septa. Septal walls and epithelial cells lining the alveoli become thinner, leading to the formation of definitive alveoli. The mean alveolar diameter increases greatly, from $\approx 30\,\mu m$ at 30 weeks to $\approx 150\,\mu m$ at 40 weeks. The final stage of alveolar maturation involves the restructuring of the capillary network, such that the more primitive double capillary layer lining the terminal sacs/alveoli is transformed into a single layer of capillaries[3] (see Fig. 11.1); this marks the existence of definitive alveoli.

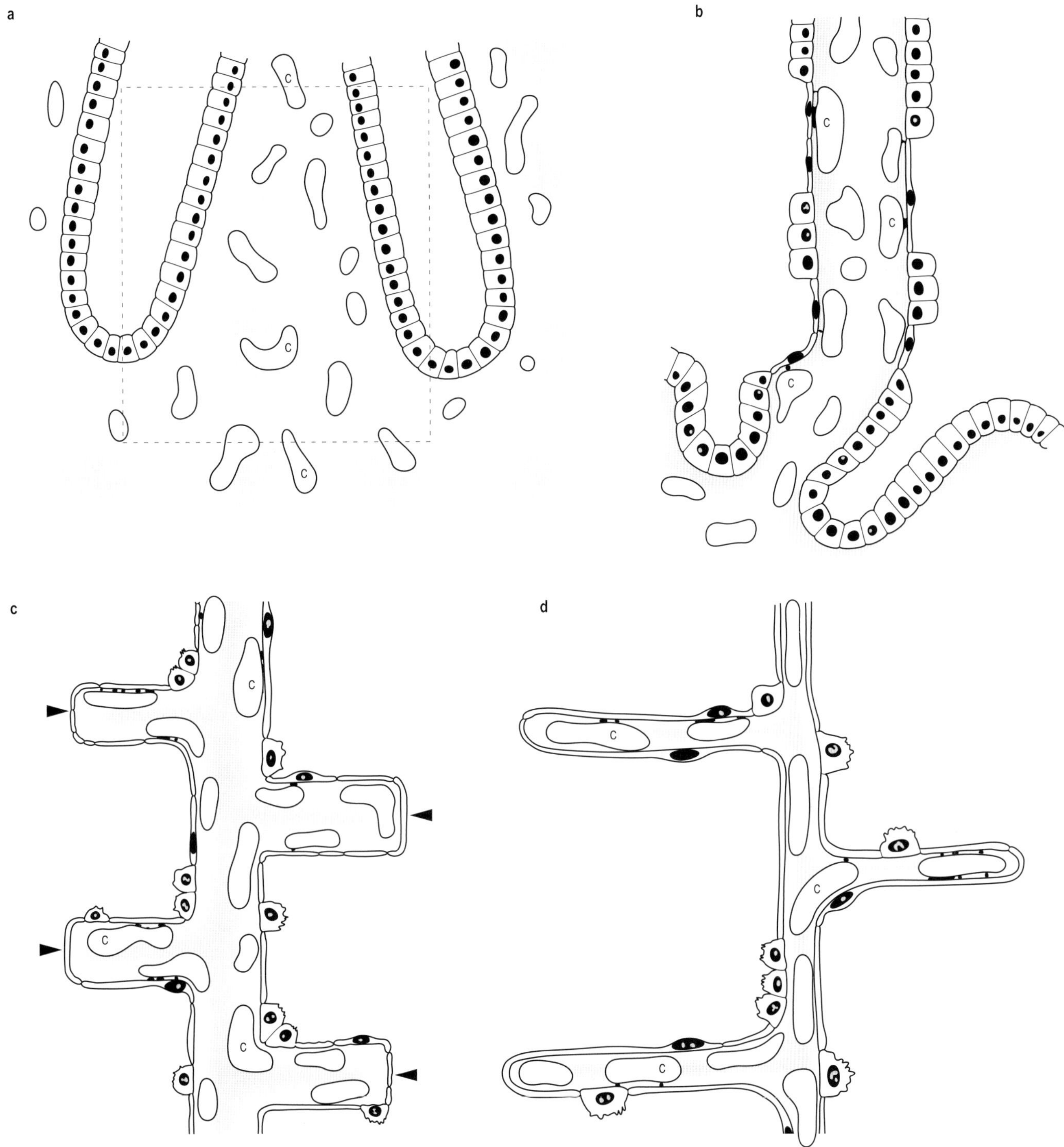

Fig. 11.1 Diagram showing development of lung parenchyma and its microvasculature. (a) Pseudoglandular stage, during which epithelial tubes lined by columnar epithelial cells invade the mesenchyme which contains a loose network of blood capillaries. (C = capillaries.) Remaining panels show further development of structures enclosed by the frame in the upper left panel. (b) Canalicular stage, showing differentiation of 'airspace' epithelium and expansion of airspaces resulting in attenuation of mesenchyme; capillaries are rearranged around the epithelial tubes so that walls between 'airspaces' contain a double layer of capillaries. A thin 'air'–blood interface develops and types-I and II epithelial cells become apparent. (c) Terminal sac/alveolar stages, showing development of secondary septa (arrowheads) from primary septa; septa are primitive in that they contain a double capillary network and a central layer of connective tissue. (d) Mature lung, showing thin interalveolar walls containing a single capillary layer. Reproduced with permission from Burri[2].

PULMONARY CIRCULATION

Structural development

The structural development of the pulmonary vasculature has been recently reviewed[4]. The lung develops with two anatomically and functionally distinct vascular systems: the pulmonary system, which supplies the alveoli, and the bronchial system, which perfuses the non-gas-exchanging regions of the lung. The arteries of the bronchial circulation follow the bronchi but do not extend to the most peripheral parts of the bronchial tree, giving rise to capillaries which supply the walls of the bronchi and bronchioles; venous blood returns via the pulmonary veins due to anastomoses between the bronchiolar and pulmonary circulations. The pulmonary arteries develop with a muscular wall, except near the lung periphery where the arteries are only partially muscularized. Pulmonary veins show a branching pattern similar to that of arteries, but do not follow the arteries and airways, rather they tend to run at right angles in the mesenchyme.

Arterioles are virtually absent in the pulmonary circulation of the adult and, therefore, pulmonary blood flow (PBF) is determined largely by the resistance of the alveolar capillaries. In the fetus and newborn, however, the smooth muscle surrounding the small pulmonary arteries is thicker, relative to total diameter, and extends further down the vascular tree, than in the adult lung. This likely contributes to the high vascular resistance of the fetus. In the first few weeks after birth, the arterial smooth muscle thins, leading to a reduction in wall thickness.

The creation of an efficient gas-exchange surface within the lung depends upon the development of a dense capillary bed in close proximity to the epithelium of the terminal sacs/alveoli. Early in development, capillaries form a loose network adjacent to the immature air spaces, but the two structures are usually separated by other cells and extracellular matrix components. During the canalicular stage, the number of capillaries increases greatly and they come into close contact with the primitive airsacs. By the terminal sac stage, the capillaries form a dense network around the terminal air spaces and, with further attenuation of tissue between adjacent sacs, the basement membrane underlying the capillary endothelial cells fuses with the basement membrane underlying the alveolar epithelial cells (Fig. 11.2). The sites of basement membrane fusion are initially focal, but expand as the lung matures, providing a very thin barrier for gas exchange.

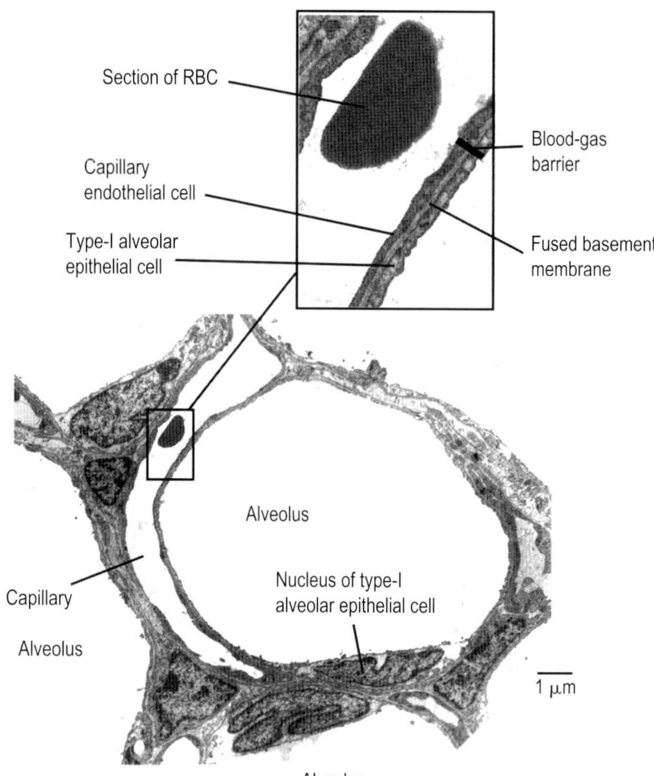

Fig. 11.2 An electron micrograph of an alveolus and an adjacent capillary, demonstrating the very thin barrier that separates the airspace from the capillary lumen (air/blood gas barrier). Note that this barrier consists of the attenuated cytoplasms of an alveolar epithelial cell and a capillary endothelial cell, which are separated by their respective basement membranes that have fused (see insert). In this micrograph, the attenuated cytoplasmic extension of the type-I cell indicated extends around the entire alveolus. RBC = red blood cell.

Functional development

This topic has recently been reviewed[5]. During late fetal life, only 8–10% of total cardiac output flows through the pulmonary vascular bed; at mid-gestation this figure is only 3–4%[5]. In the fetus, most (≈88%) of right ventricular output is diverted away from the lungs to the descending aorta via the ductus arteriosus. Mean pulmonary arterial pressure in the near-term fetus is ≈55 mmHg, which is ≈5 mmHg higher than mean aortic pressure, thereby maintaining flow from the pulmonary to the systemic circulation through the ductus arteriosus. Although pulmonary vascular resistance (PVR) declines progressively during fetal life, due to a large increase in total cross-sectional area of the pulmonary vascular bed, it remains much higher (up to eightfold) just before birth compared to immediately after birth[5].

PVR in the fetus is influenced by a range of factors, including the physical and oxygen environments of pulmonary vessels and the presence of vasoactive agents. Comprehensive reviews of this complex topic have been published recently[5,6] and only a brief outline will be provided here. Studies in fetal sheep have shown that there is a direct relationship between lung liquid volume and PVR[7]. Increasing the volume, and hence pressure, within the terminal airsacs likely compresses the small pulmonary vessels (mainly capillaries), thereby increasing PVR[7]. The low Po_2 of blood perfusing the fetal lungs also contributes to a high PVR. In postnatal lambs, perfusion of the lungs with blood having a Po_2 similar to the fetus causes the normally low PVR to be greatly increased[8]. Studies in fetal sheep have shown that lowering and raising the Po_2 of arterial blood (i.e. hypoxia and hyperoxia) induce, respectively, increases and decreases in PVR[5]. The mechanism by which oxygen tension influences PVR is unknown, but may involve the release of prostacyclin (PGI_2) and endothelium-derived nitric oxide (NO) both of which affect vascular smooth muscle.

Leukotrienes (LT) C_4 and D_4, both of which are potent vasoconstrictors in the pulmonary circulation, may also contribute to the high PVR in the fetus. In fetal sheep, blockade of LT receptors or inhibition of LT synthesis leads to increases in PBF to levels similar to that seen in the newborn[5]. Other vasoactive substances that may be involved in maintaining a high PVR in the fetus include endothelin-1, a potential vasodilator released from endothelial cells, and thromboxane A_2, another product of arachidonic acid[5,6].

Changes at birth

With the clearance of lung liquid at birth, the onset of breathing and the increase in arterial Po_2, PVR greatly diminishes, allowing PBF to increase by eight- to tenfold[5]. The increase in PBF and pulmonary venous return leads to an increase in left (above right) atrial pressure which results in closure of the foramen ovale. This, together with the closure of the ductus arteriosus, results in functional separation of the pulmonary and systemic circulations soon after birth.

The mechanisms underlying the large fall in PVR at birth are complex[9] and probably involve physical factors, the oxygen environment and alterations in the balance between vasodilator and vasoconstrictor substances in the pulmonary vascular bed. Because the alveolar epithelium and capillary endothelium are mechanically coupled, the creation at birth of an air–liquid interface in the alveoli, and the partial recoil of the lungs (see below), are likely to alter the geometry of small pulmonary vessels causing them to dilate (see Fig. 11.2). Rhythmic expansion of the lungs at birth, and increased oxygenation, release vasodilators such as PGI_2, possibly mediated by bradykinin (a potent vasodilator in the fetus) or angiotensin II. Nitric oxide (NO) is now thought to play an important role in pulmonary vasodilation after birth. The inhibition of NO synthesis prior to birth attenuates the birth-induced increase in PBF and results in pulmonary hypertension in the newborn[5]. It is apparent that many factors are involved in the switch from a high PVR in the fetus to a low PVR in the neonate.

FETAL BREATHING MOVEMENTS

Episodes of breathing-like movements occur intermittently throughout much of gestation in healthy mammalian fetuses[10]. These movements, termed 'fetal breathing movements' (FBM), share important features with postnatal breathing and are thought to be an early expression of coordinated, rhythmical activity in brain regions responsible for respiratory control. FBM involve rhythmic 'inspiratory' activation of the diaphragm and dilator muscles of the larynx[11]. Expiratory muscles (e.g. intercostal muscles, upper airway constrictors) are not significantly active during unstimulated FBM. Like postnatal breathing, FBM are stimulated by increased arterial $PaCO_2$ and by decreased pH of the blood or cerebrospinal fluid, probably via stimulation of centrally located chemoreceptors[12]. FBM are also influenced by fetal behavioral states. During late gestation, FBM are inhibited during the fetal state resembling quiet (slow wave or non-rapid-eye movement) sleep and are common during the fetal state resembling rapid-eye-movement (or active, or desynchronized) sleep[10]. Whether the fetus is ever in a state resembling wakefulness is controversial; however, there is some evidence that a fetal awake state does exist which is associated with FBM. The suppression of FBM during fetal quiet sleep is of considerable interest because this suppression must cease after birth when breathing becomes continuous; discontinuous breathing postnatally is of potential relevance to the sudden infant death syndrome.

FBM differ from postnatal breathing in that the 'tidal volume' is very small and each 'breath' is essentially isovolumic; the low tidal volume of the fetus can be attributed to the high viscosity (and inertia) of water relative to air, and the high resistance of the fetal upper respiratory tract to the ingress of liquid[13]. In ovine fetuses, the 'tidal volume' is normally less than 1 ml[14], compared with 40–50 ml (8–10 ml/kg) in newborns[15]; a similar difference exists in humans. That is, the change in lung luminal volume associated with individual FBM in late gestation is normally less than 2% of resting (baseline) luminal volume. Thus, FBM resemble postnatal breathing with an obstructed upper airway; this presumably gives rise to the paradoxical nature of FBM; during 'inspiration' the chest wall retracts and the abdominal wall moves out[16,17].

FBM are readily detected by ultrasound and, as part of the fetal biophysical profile[18], are used to assess fetal health. The incidence of FBM is reduced in fetuses that are subjected to intrauterine stresses such as the impaired delivery of primary nutrients (oxygen and glucose), intrauterine infection, increased levels of prostaglandins or labor[10,19]. FBM may be absent or impaired in fetuses with congenital abnormalities of the nervous system or skeletal muscle. Maternal drug use can also abolish or attenuate FBM; for example alcohol, tobacco smoking as well as common sedatives and narcotics can inhibit FBM.

FBM are now known to be important for normal lung growth and development as their prolonged absence can lead to the development of lung hypoplasia, a condition in which the lungs are small and structurally immature[20,21]. If severe, it can result in respiratory insufficiency or death in the newborn. FBM play a critical role in maintaining the fetal lungs in an expanded state by resisting the tendency of the fetal lung to recoil. Lung expansion during fetal life is known to be necessary for the normal growth and structural maturation of the lungs. The role of FBM in the maintenance of lung expansion and lung growth is discussed in more detail below.

FETAL LUNG LIQUID

Control of fetal lung liquid secretion

During fetal life, the future airspaces of the lungs are filled with a liquid that is secreted by the pulmonary epithelium. This liquid is not inhaled amniotic fluid as it accumulates in the lungs when the trachea is obstructed[11] and it has an ionic composition which is different to that of amniotic fluid[22] (Table 11.2). Measurements of unidirectional ion fluxes in fetal sheep lungs have indicated that lung liquid secretion results from the net movement of chloride and sodium ions across the pulmonary epithelium into the 'airway' lumen[23]. This generates an osmotic gradient across the epithelium which promotes the movement of water towards the lung lumen. It is thought that Na^+, K^+-ATPase, located on the basolateral surface of pulmonary epithelial cells, provides the electrochemical gradient for Na^+ to enter the cell coupled to Cl^-. The Cl^- then exits the cell across its apical membrane and enters the lung lumen down its electrochemical gradient. The net movement of Cl^- into the lung lumen provides an electrical gradient for Na^+ to enter as well, which together create an osmotic gradient for the movement of water in the same direction.[23] Once secreted, fetal lung liquid leaves the lung via the the trachea and pharynx, from where it is either swallowed or enters the amniotic sac[24,25].

Table 11.2 **Composition of fetal lung liquid in comparison to fetal plasma and amniotic fluid in sheep**

Parameter	*Plasma*	*Lung liquid*	*Amniotic fluid*
Na^+ (mmol/l)	150 ± 0.7	150 ± 1.3	113 ± 6.5
K^+ (mmol/l)	4.8 ± 0.2	6.3 ± 0.7	7.6 ± 0.8
Cl^- (mmol/l)	107 ± 1.0	157.1 ± 4.1	87 ± 5
Ca^{2+} (mmol/l)	3.3 ± 0.1	0.8 ± 0.1	1.6 ± 0.1
HCO_3^-(mmol/l)	24 ± 1.2	2.8 ± 0.3	19 ± 3
Urea (mmol/l)	8.2 ± 1.4	7.9 ± 2.7	10.5 ± 2.4
Osmolality (mOsm)	291 ± 2	294 ± 2	265 ± 2
Protein (mg/100 ml)	4090 ± 260	27 ± 2	100 ± 10
pH	7.34 ± 0.04	6.27 ± 0.5	7.02 ± 0.09

Values from Adamson et al.[22]

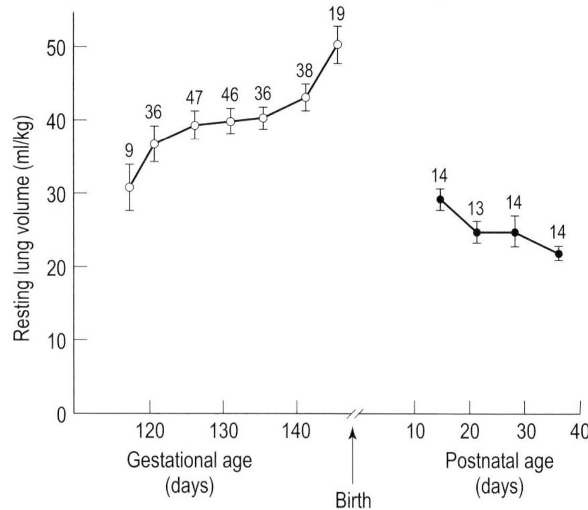

Fig. 11.3 The volume of fetal lung liquid, measured by dye dilution, during the last 40 days of gestation in fetal sheep. Measurements of functional residual capacity (FRC) in postnatal lambs, made using a He-dilution technique, have been included for comparison[15]. Numbers represent the number of animals from which measurements were made at each gestational or postnatal age.

During the last third of gestation, before the onset of labor, healthy fetal sheep secrete lung liquid at a rate of 3–4 ml/kg/h[26]; no data are available for human fetuses. The rate of secretion is controlled by endocrine, metabolic and physical factors. Both adrenaline, acting via β-adrenergic receptors[27,28], and arginine vasopressin[29] are potent inhibitors of lung liquid secretion in vivo, possibly via activation of adenylate cyclase leading to an increase in intracellular cAMP concentrations[30]. Because the inhibitory effect of these hormones increases with gestational age, it is likely that they play an important role in the reabsorption of lung liquid at birth (see below). Other hormones known to affect fetal lung liquid secretion include: cortisol which increases lung liquid secretion in vivo[31,32] but inhibits it in vitro[33]; aldosterone which inhibits lung liquid secretion in vitro[33]; and prolactin which stimulates lung liquid secretion when administered directly into lung liquid in vivo[34].

Hypoxemia is also a potent inhibitor of fetal lung secretion, whether it is acute or chronic[35,36]. Its effect is unlikely to be mediated by an associated stress-related increase in circulating adrenaline and vasopressin concentrations[28,37], but rather from a reduction in oxidative metabolism and/or associated changes in tissue pH[38]. Indeed, the lung liquid secretory process appears to be oxygen dependent[23,39] and acidemia has been shown to enhance the inhibitory effect of hypoxaemia[38]. In this regard, it is of interest that acidemia potentiates the reduction in PBF, and hence pulmonary oxygen delivery, in fetal sheep exposed to hypoxemia.

Physical factors such as the pulmonary luminal pressure can influence the secretion of fetal lung liquid. Experimental manipulations that lead to a reduction in fetal lung expansion, and hence a reduction in luminal pressure, result in an increase in lung liquid secretion rates[40–42]. In contrast, sustained increases in lung expansion, and hence increases in luminal pressure, cause either a reduction[43] or complete cessation of fetal lung liquid secretion[41,44]. The driving force for the net movement of water across the epithelium must be governed by the sum of all forces affecting fluid movement. Under normal conditions, a small hydrostatic pressure exists across the lungs (lung lumen is 1–2 mmHg > amniotic sac pressure[11]), which opposes the osmotic pressure resulting from the movement of chloride ions. The osmotic pressure promoting liquid secretion must exceed the opposing hydrostatic pressure for liquid to cross the epithelium into the lung lumen. Thus, reductions or increases in the intraluminal pressure, resulting from alterations in lung liquid volume, would be expected to increase or reduce net production rates of lung liquid by altering the magnitude of the opposing hydrostatic pressure, i.e. without directly affecting the ionic mechanism of lung liquid secretion.

Control of fetal lung liquid volume

The volume of liquid within the future airways increases markedly over the last half of gestation in most species, but there is likely to be much variability between individuals[45]. Over the last third of gestation in fetal sheep, lung liquid volume typically increases from 25–30 ml/kg to 45–50 ml/kg near term (145–150 days) (Fig. 11.3). In contrast, the corresponding volume of the air-filled lung in newborn lambs (functional residual capacity; FRC) is 20–25 ml/kg[15]. Thus, during late gestation, the fetal lung is hyperexpanded relative to the postnatal air-filled lung (see Fig. 11.3). The reason for the reduction in lung luminal volume (i.e. FRC) at birth is likely to be due to the formation of an air–liquid interface, and hence surface tension, within the lung which constitutes the major part of the postnatal lung's elastic recoil. Although the presence of surfactant greatly reduces these surface forces, it does not eliminate them and, as a consequence, the lung tends to collapse away from the chest wall after birth. This partial recoil of the lung after birth results in the formation of a subatmospheric pressure in the intrapleural space which is not present in the fetus[11].

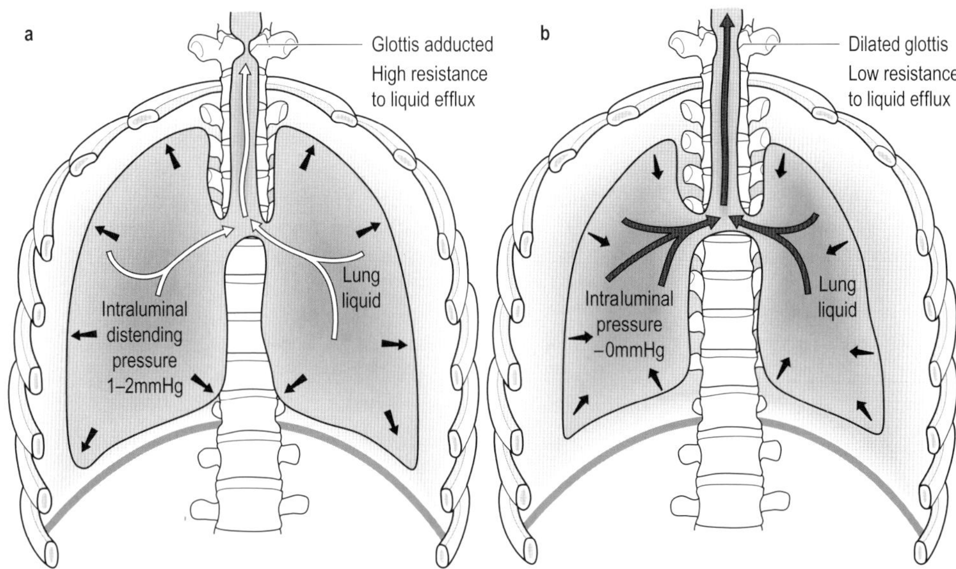

Fig. 11.4 Control of fetal lung liquid volumes during periods of (a) apnea and (b) fetal breathing movements (FBM). During apnea, the glottis is actively adducted which restricts the efflux of lung liquid and promotes its accumulation within the future airways, thereby maintaining an intraluminal distending pressure of 1–2 mmHg above ambient pressure (amniotic sac pressure). During periods of FBM, the glottis phasically dilates which greatly reduces the resistance to lung liquid efflux. As a result, liquid leaves the lungs at a higher rate, causing a reduction in lung liquid volume and the distending pressure (at end-expiration) declines to ambient pressure.

During fetal life, the volume of lung liquid is largely maintained by factors that control transpulmonary pressure and the efflux of liquid from the lungs, rather than by alterations in the rate of secretion[11]. The rate of efflux of lung liquid is controlled by transpulmonary pressure and the resistance of the upper airway, particularly the larynx[13,46]. During 'non-breathing' periods (i.e. during fetal 'apnea'), tonic activity in the laryngeal constrictor muscles imposes a resistance to lung liquid efflux, thereby opposing the tendency of the lungs to collapse as a result of their elastic recoil (Fig. 11.4). During periods of FBM, the laryngeal dilator muscles are phasically active leading to widening of the glottis and a reduction in the resistance to lung liquid efflux. Consequently, due to the combined effect of the elastic recoil of lung tissue and the lowered resistance to lung liquid efflux, liquid loss from the lung accelerates and the lungs partially collapse[24,25]. However, the loss of lung liquid during periods of FBM is opposed by a simultaneous contraction of the diaphragm muscle[40,42]. That is, contraction of the diaphragm muscle during the inspiratory phase of FBM tends to oppose the elastic recoil of lung tissue, thereby limiting the loss of lung liquid[11] (see Fig. 11.4). Thus, the high degree of lung expansion in the fetus is apparently due to (i) the low level of elastic recoil (owing to the absence of an air–liquid interface), (ii) the high resistance to lung liquid efflux offered by the larynx during non-breathing periods and (iii) the contractions of the diaphragm muscle during FBM episodes when the resistance to lung liquid efflux is reduced.

Clearance of lung liquid at birth

Fetal lung liquid must be cleared from the airways at birth so that the newborn can establish effective pulmonary gas exchange. This process begins before birth and continues for some time after birth. Studies in fetal sheep show that lung liquid clearance begins at the start of labor[45] and that, in healthy fetuses with normal amniotic fluid volumes, much of the liquid is cleared during labor. It is now recognized that increased circulating concentrations of adrenaline and arginine vasopressin (AVP) in fetal plasma, released in response to labor[27,29], play an important role in inhibiting secretion and inducing lung liquid reabsorption. These hormones are thought to act via a cAMP-mediated activation of amiloride-blockable sodium channels on the luminal surface of pulmonary epithelial cells[30,47]. Activation of these channels causes an increase in Na^+ and Na^+-linked Cl^- flux away from the lung lumen to the interstitium, thereby reversing the osmotic gradient across the epithelium and leading to lung liquid reabsorption[47]. While this mechanism is likely to be important, any factor that increases transpulmonary pressure can contribute to the loss of liquid during labor. For instance, in unstressed fetal sheep at term, we have observed the loss of large amounts of lung liquid (≈50%) during the early stages of labor before fetal circulating concentrations of adrenaline and AVP increase.[45] This reduction in lung liquid volume is probably caused by compression of the lungs resulting from postural changes imposed on the fetus by the shortening of the uterine muscle during labor; it has been established that fetal trunk flexion causes substantial loss of lung liquid[48].

LUNG GROWTH

Regulation of fetal lung growth

Most research to date indicates that the degree of lung expansion, and hence degree of lung tissue stretch, plays a critical role in normal fetal lung growth and maturation[49,50]. Indeed, it is now apparent that most, if not all, of the many clinical conditions that lead to fetal lung hypoplasia do so by causing a prolonged reduction in lung expansion[11,26]. These include disorders that cause the fetal lung to collapse (e.g. diaphragmatic hernias), that reduce intrathoracic space (e.g. pleural fluid accumulation), that cause compression of the chest (e.g. oligohydramnios) and that impair skeletal muscle activity.

The critical importance of fetal lung expansion with luminal liquid was first demonstrated by experiments showing profound changes in lung growth and maturation following prolonged alterations in lung liquid volume. For example, prolonged drainage of lung liquid via the trachea, which causes the lungs to deflate, results in a total cessation of fetal lung growth[41,51] and severe lung hypoplasia[41,52]. In contrast, increasing the volume of lung liquid (by obstructing the fetal trachea) markedly increases fetal lung growth and enhances alveolarization[51–53]. The lung growth response to tracheal obstruction is rapid and can cause an almost doubling in total lung cell number within 7 days[51]. The growth response, in terms of cell proliferation rates, follows a specific time course, with maximum rates being detected at 1–2 days, which return to control levels by 10 days[44]. Thus, the mechanisms by which increases in fetal lung expansion induce an acceleration in lung growth are only active within a relatively narrow window of time.

Mechanisms relating lung stretch to lung growth

The cellular and molecular mechanisms by which changes in fetal lung expansion affect lung growth are localized to expanded or deflated regions of the lung[53]. This response is not unique to the lung as mechanical forces are well known to affect DNA synthesis as well as the phenotypic expression, via the activation or repression of genes, of many different types of cells[54]. However, the mechanisms by which mechanical forces are translated into cellular responses are not yet fully understood. It is likely that the distortion of lung tissue associated with a change in lung expansion is transmitted via the extracellular matrix and causes changes in cell shape and/or tension within the cytoskeleton. This stimulus may be translated into a cellular response due to direct activation of stretch sensitive ion channels and/or to the direct activation of second messenger systems (e.g. tyrosine kinases and phospholipases) associated with the proteins that interlink extracellular matrix receptors (e.g. integrins) with the cytoskeleton[55]. It is also possible that distortion of a cell may directly activate or inactivate genes and/or DNA synthesis via changes in tension or orientation of cytoskeletal and nuclear structural components[55].

It is possible that alterations in gene expression for a variety of growth factors contribute to the growth response induced by changes in lung expansion, possibly by integrating and propagating the response. Indeed, alterations in fetal lung expansion induce corresponding changes in insulin like growth factor-II (IGF-II) gene expression[40,51]. IGF-II has potent mitogenic and differentiating activities and is thought to play an important role in fetal growth. Similarly, intermittent stretch of pulmonary epithelial cells in culture is a potent stimulus for DNA synthesis[56] and increases platelet-derived growth factor (PDGF) gene expression[56]. As the effect of phasic stretch on DNA synthesis in cultured pulmonary epithelial cells can be blocked by antisense oligonucleotides for PDGF, PDGF must play a crucial role in this response[57]. However, a more recent in vivo study has failed to demonstrate an increase in PDGF and IGF-II expression when cell proliferation rates are high, in response to an increase in fetal lung expansion[58]. Furthermore, a differentiatial gene expression analysis, designed to identify genes activated and repressed by increases in fetal lung expansion, failed to identify a number of other growth factors thought to mediate expansion-induced fetal lung growth[59]. However, numerous other genes were identified which are likely to be activated directly by the mechanical stimulus and play a vital role in this process[59].

Fetal lung hypoplasia

Lung hypoplasia at birth is a graded phenomenon and increases the risk of neonatal morbidity and mortality[60]. In humans, the neonatal lung is considered to be hypoplastic if the lung to body weight ratio is <0.015 at less than 28 weeks of gestation and <0.012 after 28 weeks[61]. Lung hypoplasia occurs in ≈ 1.1 babies per 1000 live births[62], although this value probably underestimates the true incidence due to the many neonates that survive following extensive postnatal treatment. However, of babies born after 35 weeks of gestation and who die in their first postnatal week, almost one-third have severe lung hypoplasia[62]. It is important to recognize that the hypoplastic fetal lung is not simply small, but is also structurally immature. For example, hypoplastic lungs contain reduced numbers of airways and alveoli[61,63], have a reduced proportion of airspace, reduced elastin development, narrower airways and altered vascular development[64]. The maturation of the respiratory epithelium is impaired, as evidenced by the persistence of cuboidal cells, particularly in the peripheral parts of the acinus[65]. This structural immaturity, which results in the reduced size and effectiveness of the gas-exchanging surface, leads to the impaired gas exchange that contributes to neonatal respiratory compromise. Another important factor that limits gas exchange is increased pulmonary vascular resistance in hypoplastic lungs; this is considered to be due to altered structural and functional development of the pulmonary vascular bed[64]. The severity and range of pathological changes in the lungs will depend on the duration and degree of reduced lung expansion[66].

Fetal lung hypoplasia is commonly associated with disorders of the central nervous system and skeletal muscle that affect the thorax, as well as disorders that reduce fetal intrathoracic volume, for example pleural effusions and herniation of the diaphragm[60]. Oligohydramnios is also a common cause of fetal lung hypoplasia, whether the reduction in amniotic fluid results from premature rupture of the membranes or from renal or urinary tract abnormalities[67]. Although it appears that a diverse range of antenatal factors can cause lung hypoplasia, it is likely that they all act via a common final mechanism, namely a prolonged reduction in fetal lung expansion. Thus, the lung hypoplasia most probably results from the absence of a growth stimulus (i.e. tissue stretch), rather than from an active inhibition of growth.

Because fetal lung growth is so sensitive to alterations in lung expansion, tracheal obstruction has been trialed to reverse lung growth deficits in human fetuses. Experimental obstruction of the fetal trachea, which results in intraluminal fluid accumulation and increased lung tissue stress, prevents the pulmonary hypoplasia caused by oligohydramnios[68] and congenital diaphragmatic hernia[69]. As little as 6 days of tracheal obstruction in fetal sheep is sufficient to reverse almost totally an existing, severe lung growth deficit[41]. Although the fetal lungs, subjected to limited periods of accelerated growth by tracheal obstruction, appear functionally normal after birth[70], they may retain ongoing structural deficits, particularly with regard to alveolar development[71]. Furthermore, the available evidence suggests that a number of unwanted side effects need to be considered. In particular, tracheal obstruction alters the distribution of epithelial cell types in the terminal airways resulting in fewer type II cells[52,72,73] and reduced surfactant protein-A, -B, and -C gene expression[74]. Thus, much more information is needed regarding the physiological consequences of altering the degree of fetal lung expansion to avoid complications that may result from this treatment.

LUNG MATURATION

Structural maturation of the lung

The unique architecture of the lung is largely dependent upon its extracellular matrix (ECM) and on cell-to-cell and cell-substrate adhesion properties. Within the lung, the components of the ECM are synthesized by a variety of cell types and provide the structural scaffolding that supports the lung cells[75]. Consequently, the ECM plays an integral role in lung development from the early in utero stages through to its postnatal function of gas exchange. Indeed, different components of the ECM are considered to be critically involved with cell migration, branching morphogenesis, cellular proliferation and cytodifferentiation as well as determining tissue compliance[75]. The ECM of the lungs is comprised of collagen (principally types I, III, V and VI), elastin, glycoproteins (e.g. fibronectin and laminin) and proteoglycans[75]. At the level of the peripheral airway units, these components form the epithelial and endothelial basement membranes and the structural fibers that course through the interstitium located at the interalveolar septa; these connect with axial fibers running in parallel with major conducting airways and blood vessels and are further braced by fibers projecting in from the pleura[76]. A recent study has demonstrated that versican is one of the most abundant proteoglycans located within the peri-saccular parenchyma of the developing lung[77]. The high ionic charge density of versican promotes the retention of water within tissue which contributes to tissue volume and has a major influence on tissue viscoelastic properties. As versican content decreases in parallel with the decrease in distal airway tissue volumes in late gestation, it is possible that a loss of versican from the peri-alveolar tissue compartment contributes to the reduction in tissue volumes and the thinning of interalveolar walls[77]. Thus, major alterations in lung architecture, such as those that occur during development, likely involve remodeling of the ECM.

The increase in fetal plasma cortisol concentrations prior to parturition is thought to play an important role in maturing the lung by influencing its architecture, its tissue compliance, development of the vascular bed, differentiation of epithelial cells and the synthesis of surfactant[78]. These changes lead to an increase in potential airspace volume, a reduction in gas-diffusing distances and an increase in compliance of the air-filled lung. Indeed, over the last third of gestation in fetal sheep, there is a large increase in lung luminal volume (see Fig. 11.3) which is associated with increased alveolar surface area and reduced interalveolar tissue distances[79]. The findings that fetal infusions of corticosteroids accelerate these changes in lung architecture, whereas adrenalectomy or hypophysectomy (which removes or reduces the source of endogenous fetal corticosteroids) retards them[31,32], indicates that corticosteroids are intimately involved in the structural modification of the lung during late gestation. The structural changes caused by adrenalectomy or hypophysectomy are characteristic of immature lungs and are reversed by the reinfusion of either cortisol or adrenocorticotrophin (ACTH)[80]. Furthermore, mice with a targeted disruption of the glucocorticoid receptor gene die at birth due to respiratory failure[81]. The lungs are morphologically immature, hypercellular with abnormal development of the terminal airways[82]; similar effects have been observed in corticotrophin-releasing hormone (CRH)-deficient mice[83]. Collectively, these findings indicate that a progressive increase in circulating concentrations of fetal corticosteroids plays an important role in promoting structural changes within the lung. This concept is consistent with numerous studies demonstrating that antenatal corticosteroid treatment greatly increases lung compliance[78,84] and ventilatory efficiency[85] in prematurely delivered fetuses. The relative involvement of thyroid hormones in the corticosteroid-induced changes in lung structure, however, is still unclear. It is interesting that sustained lung deflation in fetal sheep causes changes in lung structure that are very similar to those reported for corticosteroid withdrawal[52].

The mechanisms by which corticosteroids stimulate the structural maturation of the fetal lungs are not well understood, but most probably include remodeling of the ECM. Over the last third of ovine gestation, the content of collagen in lung parenchyma increases markedly, with most of the increase occurring over the final 25–30 days[86]. Similarly, elastin mRNA levels in ovine fetal lungs increase markedly over the last third of gestation and, in particular, tropoelastin (elastin precursor) production peaks just before birth[87]. This period of gestation coincides with the exponential increase in circulating cortisol concentrations in the fetus and a large increase in the luminal volume of the fetal lungs[26,32]. Thus, because the components of the lung ECM are rapidly turned over, at least in culture[88], it is likely that endocrine factors like cortisol induce remodeling of the ECM by altering the expression of its specific components or via alterations in the activity of metalloproteinases or their specific inhibitors. Whatever the mechanisms, endogenous glucocorticoids apparently play an important role in regulating the ECM of the lung and, therefore, are able to influence its structural development and thus its ability to function as a gas-exchange organ after birth.

Epithelial cell differentiation

The success of pulmonary gas exchange after birth depends on many factors. These include a large surface area for gas exchange, adequate blood flow through alveolar capillaries, a thin barrier between air and blood, and a high degree of lung compliance. Many of these factors are dependent upon the maturation of pulmonary epithelial cells. During early stages of lung development, epithelial cells are either columnar (pseudoglandular stage) or cuboidal (canalicular stage) and are unable to synthesize surfactant, although they do express a number of surfactant proteins. These primitive epithelial cells contain abundant glycogen deposits and form a thick barrier to gas exchange. During the canalicular stage (by 22–24 weeks), epithelial cells begin to differentiate into thinner type I cells (which form the gas-exchange surface) and cuboidal type II cells (which are able to synthesize, store and release pulmonary surfactant) (Fig. 11.5).

The mechanisms that regulate the differentiation of pulmonary epithelial cell are largely unknown. Type I epithelial cells make up >90% of the surface area of the lung and their attenuated cytoplasmic extensions provide a minimal barrier for gas exchange. Type II cells have a much smaller surface area but are the source of surfactant which is critical for lowering surface forces in the lungs[90].

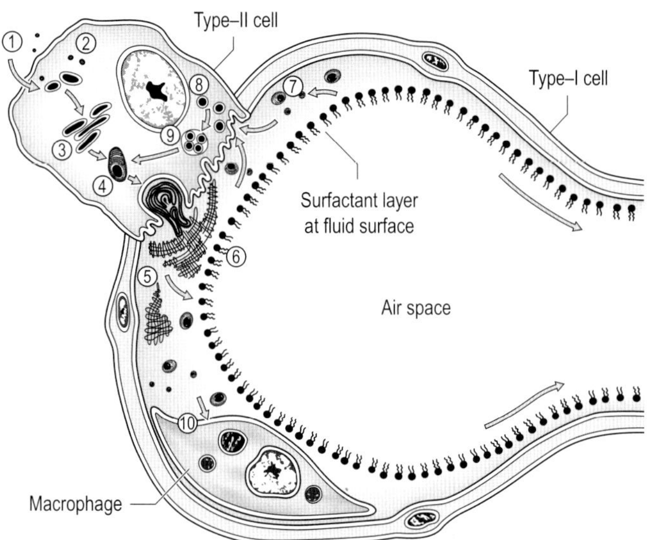

Fig. 11.5 Schematic diagram of a section through a single alveolus, showing the movement of surfactant components through the type-II cell and alveolar liquid (not to scale). 1, Surfactant precursors such as glucose, amino acids and fatty acids; 2, endoplasmic reticulum; 3, Golgi apparatus; 4, lamellar bodies; 5, tubular myelin; 6, surface film with adsorbed phospholipids; 7, vesicular and myelin forms of surfactant, possibly derived from material desorbed from the film; 8 and 9, endocytic compartments including multivesicular bodies; 10, alveolar macrophage. Reproduced with permission from Hawgood and Clements[89].

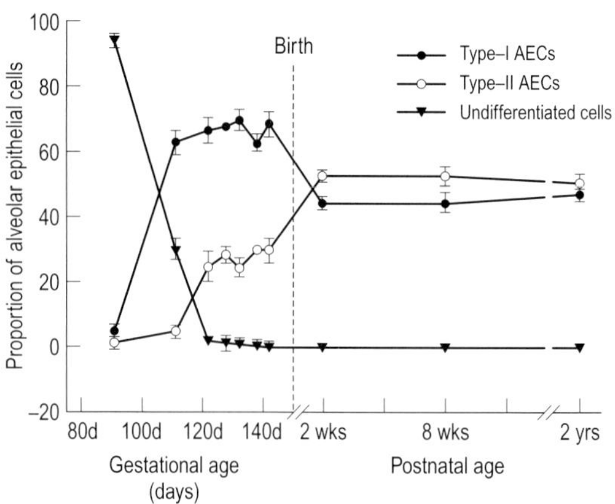

Fig. 11.6 Changes in the relative proportions of undifferentiated (closed triangles), type-I (closed circles) and type-II (open circles) alveolar epithelial cells (AECs) in sheep during the last third of gestation and up to 2 years of age. Redrawn from Flecknoe et al.[91].

During the early stages of lung development, all epithelial cells within the terminal airways are undifferentiated[79,91] and gradually differentiate into both cell types as development progresses (Fig. 11.6); the factors controlling differentiation from the undifferentiated phenotype are unknown. Type-I cells can be identified at an earlier stage of development than type-II cells, indicating that undifferentiated epithelial cells can differentiate directly into type-I cells[79,91]. At this stage of development, the type-I cells quickly become the most numerous epithelial cell phenotype, but a rapid increase in the proportion of type-II cells soon follows[91]. However, in late gestation and at term, when the alveolar epithelium has fully differentiated (undifferentiated epithelial cells are <1%), there are approximately twice as many type-I as type-II cells[80,91]. Although it is widely considered that both types of differentiated epithelial cells arise as daughter cells from proliferating type-II cells, more recent data indicate that this concept may not be correct for the following reasons: (1) in the sheep fetus, type-I cells can be detected at an earlier period in gestation than type-II cells[79,91] and (2) increased fetal lung expansion induces type-II to type-I cell trans-differentiation whereas reductions in fetal lung expansion induce type-I to type-II cell trans-differentiation[73].

Whatever the mechanisms that control epithelial cell differentiation in the developing lungs, this process is influenced by both corticosteroids[80,82] and the degree of fetal lung expansion (i.e. tissue stress)[52,72,73]. Fetal hypophysectomy, which prevents the normal gestational age-related increase in fetal plasma cortisol concentrations and the onset of labor, results in increased type-II cell and reduced type-I cell densities compared to controls[80]; adrenocorticotrophic hormone (ACTH) and cortisol replacement both restore type-I and type-II cell densities[80]. Similarly, ablation of the glucocorticoid receptor in genetically modified mice delays epithelial cell differentiation resulting in a much greater proportion of undifferentiated epithelial cells; the proportion of type-II cells was increased, whereas the proportion of type-I cells was markedly reduced[82]. Similar changes in type-I and type-II cell proportions can be observed following alterations in fetal lung expansion, indicating that there may be a common link between tissue stretch and corticosteroids[72]. Studies in fetal sheep have shown that prolonged reductions in lung expansion increase the density of type-II cells and reduce the proportion of type-I cells[72]. On the other hand, increasing the degree of lung expansion reduces the density of type-II epithelial cells and increases the density of type-I cells[52,72]. Importantly, these studies have also shown that the density of type-II cells is reduced to ≈2% (from ≈30%) of all epithelial cells following a prolonged increase in fetal lung expansion and that a subsequent period of lung deflation gradually restores the proportion of type-II cells to ≈30%[73]. As the increase in type-II proportions did not include an increase in type-II proliferation, the increase must have resulted from type-I to type-II cell trans-differentiation[73].

PULMONARY SURFACTANT

Pulmonary surfactant is essential for postnatal lung function as, without adequate amounts of surfactant, the lungs are difficult to expand, the work of breathing is greatly increased and gas exchange is impaired. Surfactant deficiency is common in preterm infants and can lead to the respiratory distress syndrome (RDS, or hyaline membrane disease); this is characterized by labored breathing and progressive cyanosis due to ineffective respiratory gas exchange[92,93]. In preterm infants, the effects of surfactant deficiency may be exacerbated by structural immaturity of the lungs. Prenatal treatment with glucocorticoids can not only stimulate surfactant synthesis but can enhance structural maturation of the lungs[94], both of which are essential for lung function after birth.

Composition of surfactant

Pulmonary surfactant is a complex mixture of phospholipids and proteins (approximately 90% lipid and 10% protein) and is synthesized within type-II epithelial cells[95]. Once secreted, it forms a monolayer of tightly packed lipid molecules at the air–liquid interface of the internal liquid layer that covers and protects the alveolar epithelial cells (see Fig. 11.5). This monolayer displaces water molecules from the interface, thereby greatly lowering the surface tension. As a result, alveoli can be expanded more easily during inspiration, and during expiration the deflating alveoli are stabilized so that they do not collapse at end-expiration. The bioactive properties of surfactant are primarily attributed to dipalmitoyl phosphatidylcholine (DPPC) which accounts for ≈45% of pulmonary surfactant[96]; other phospholipids with surface active properties include phosphatidylglycerol and phosphatidylinositol.

In addition to lipids, four surfactant-associated proteins (or apoproteins) have been identified; surfactant proteins (SP) A, B, C and D. SP-A is the largest and most abundant of the surfactant proteins, is a water-soluble glycoprotein with a molecular weight of 28–30 kDa and is made up of 18 subunits. In vitro, SP-A, together with SP-B and SP-C, accelerates the formation and spreading of the surface layer[97], although in vivo, SP-A is thought primarily to aid in host defense. SP-B and SP-C are small lipophilic proteins (8 and 5 kDa, respectively) which facilitate the formation of a phosopholipid surface layer; in preterm animals, mixtures of SP-B and phospholipids are able to increase lung compliance and alveolar stability. SP-D is a hydrophilic glycoprotein (43 kDa) and does not appear to be involved in the surface active function of surfactant. As SP-D contains sequences that bind to bacteria, its major role is thought to involve host defense within the lung. Although ablation of the SP-D gene is not lethal at birth, the neonates gradually develop emphysematous-like changes in lung structure, indicating that SP-D plays an important role in maintaining the integrity of alveolar structures.

All lipid and protein components of surfactant are synthesized in alveolar type-II cells[98], although much of this material is recycled following re-uptake by type-II cells via endocytosis. Within the type-II cells, the lipid and surfactant proteins (SP A–C) are incorporated into lamellar bodies which are made up of concentrically arranged layers of phospholipids. Surfactant is released into the alveolar space by exocytosis following fusion of the lamellar body to the type-II cell membrane (see Fig. 11.5). Once outside the cell, surfactant forms a meshwork of tubular myelin made up of long tubules with intersecting lipid bilayers containing SP-A and SP-B[99]. The phospholipids are then incorporated into the monolayer at the air–liquid interface.

Surfactant synthesis and release

In human fetuses, pulmonary concentrations of DPPC begin to increase after 20 weeks, when type-II cells containing lamellar bodies are first detected. By 24 weeks, concentrations reach ≈35% of adult levels, although no surfactant is released until about 30 weeks when it can be first detected in amniotic fluid. After 30 weeks, it is thought that the synthesis and release of surfactant from type-II cells continues to increase until term. The synthesis of DPPC is controlled by the enzyme fatty acid synthetase, the activity of which increases during late fetal life in parallel with increasing DPPC content. Studies on the ontogeny of surfactant proteins show that levels increase during the latter half of gestation. The presence of SP-A in amniotic fluid, like that of DPPC, is detected first around 30 weeks and then progressively increases in parallel with the increases in surfactant protein mRNA levels in lung tissue.

TREATMENTS FOR LUNG IMMATURITY

It is now well established that exogenous glucocorticoids can accelerate maturation of the fetal lung; the resulting functional and structural changes have been well described[93,94]. In particular, antenatal glucocortioids are known to enhance surfactant synthesis as well as structural maturation of the lung, as indicated by an attenuation of mesenchymal tissue, an increase in the proportion of potential airspace and an increase in the synthesis of elastin and collagen. Thus, the effect of glucocorticoids in improving lung distensibility of the preterm neonate is attributable to both enhanced structural maturation and increased surfactant synthesis[97]. In addition, more recent evidence indicates that antenatal glucocorticoids may have a beneficial effect on the pulmonary vascular bed[100,101]. In particular, antenatal glucorticoids were shown to lower PVR in the fetus and to increase pulmonary blood flow after birth, both in normal neonates[100] and in neonates with hypoplastic lungs[101].

Thyroid hormones appear to be important in lung development as fetal thyroidectomy impairs structural maturation and reduces surfactant content in type-II cells and lavage fluid[97]. In vitro and in vivo studies have shown that triiodothyronine (T_3), thyroxine (T_4) and thyrotropin-releasing hormone (TRH) stimulate the synthesis of surfactant phospholipids[102]; T_3 appears to be more potent than T_4 in this regard. It has also been shown that the stimulatory effects of thyroid hormones are potentiated by glucocorticoids; i.e. the effects of these hormones when administered together are greater than when given alone. This potentiation has formed the basis for clinical trials of the stimulation of lung maturation in cases of threatened preterm delivery[103]. In animal studies, a greater degree of potentiation was achieved when catecholamines were administered along with glucocorticoids and thyroid hormones. Catecholamines have been shown to stimulate the reabsorption of lung liquid and surfactant release from type-II cells. Studies in animals have indicated that lung maturation is dependent upon a number of key hormone systems, principally glucocorticoids, thyroid hormones and catecholamines, and it is likely that this is also true in the human.

Preterm birth is the major cause of early postnatal respiratory disease and mortality. Of babies born at 30 weeks, approximately one-half will develop the respiratory distress syndrome (RDS) and chronic lung disease (CLD). Antenatal therapy with glucocorticoids has greatly reduced the incidence of RDS in preterm infants, although, to be effective, they must be administered 1–2 days prior to birth[93,97]. In animal studies, glucocorticoids have been found to increase the activities of antioxidant enzymes in the lungs, as well as increasing surfactant synthesis.

Prenatal prevention of RDS with glucocorticoids alone is not always effective and clinical trials have tested the combined administration of adding TRH[103]; however, the results of such trials have been conflicting. The treatment of RDS by the intrapulmonary administration of replacement surfactant is now widely used with considerable success, often in combination with antenatal glucocorticoid treatment. However, the earliest gestational age at which such treatments can be successful will be determined by the presence of the basic structural requirements for gas exchange, which first appear at approximately 22–24 weeks. Infants born earlier than this have been supported by ECMO (extracorporeal membrane oxygenation) until the lungs have developed sufficiently to support gas exchange.

REFERENCES

1. Burri PH. Structural development of the lung in the fetus and neonate. In *Fetus and neonate. Physiology and clinical implications*, MA Hanson, JAD Spencer, CH Rodeck, DV Walters (eds), pp. 3–19. Cambridge: Cambridge University Press, 1994.
2. Burri PH. Fetal and postnatal development of the lung. *Annu Rev Physiol* **46**:617–628, 1984.
3. Burri PH. Structural aspects of postnatal lung development – alveolar formation and growth. *Biol Neonate* **89**:313–322, 2006.
4. Jones R, Reid LM. Development of the pulmonary vasculature. In *The lung: development, aging and the environment*, R Harding, KE Pinkerton, CG Plopper (eds), p. 81. London: Elsevier Academic Press, 2004.
5. Abman SH. Developmental physiology of the pulmonary circulation. In *The lung: development, aging and the environment*, R Harding, KE Pinkerton, CG Plopper (eds), pp. 105–117. Oxford: Butterworth Heinemann, 2004.
6. Tod ML, Cassin S. Fetal and neonatal pulmonary circulation. In *The lung: scientific foundations*, RG Crystal, DB West, ER Weibel, PJ Barnes (eds), p. 2129. Philadelphia: Lippincott-Raven, 1997.
7. Hooper SB. Role of luminal volume changes in the increase in pulmonary blood flow at birth in sheep. *Exp Physiol* **83**:833–842, 1998.
8. Rudolph AM. Fetal and neonatal pulmonary circulation. *Annu Rev Physiol* **41**:383–395, 1979.
9. Hooper SB, Harding R. Pulmonary transition at birth. In *The lung: development, aging and the environment*, R Harding, KE Pinkerton, CG Plopper (eds), pp. 201–212. Elsevier Academic Press, 2004.
10. Harding R. Fetal breathing movements. In *The lung: scientific foundations*, RG Crystal, JB West, ER Weibel, PJ Barnes (eds), p. 2093. New York: Lippincott-Raven, 1997.
11. Harding R, Hooper SB. Regulation of lung expansion and lung growth before birth. *J Appl Physiol* **81**:209–224, 1996.
12. Moore PJ, Hanson MA. Control of breathing: central influences. In *Fetus and neonate: breathing*, MA Hanson, JAD Spencer, CH Rodeck, DV Walters (eds), p. 109. Cambridge: Cambridge University Press, 1994.
13. Harding R, Bocking AD, Sigger JN. Influence of upper respiratory tract on liquid flow to and from fetal lungs. *J Appl Physiol* **61**:68–74, 1986.
14. Maloney JE, Adamson TM, Brodecky V, Cranage S, Lambert TF, Ritchie BC. Diaphragmatic activity and lung liquid flow in the unanesthetized fetal sheep. *J Appl Physiol* **39**:423–428, 1975.
15. Jakubowska AE, Billings K, Johns DP, Hooper SB, Harding R. Respiratory function in lambs following prolonged oligohydramnios during late gestation. *Pediatr Res* **34**:611–617, 1993.
16. Patrick J, Natale R, Richardson B. Patterns of human fetal breathing activity at 34 to 35 weeks' gestational age. *Am J Obstet Gynecol* **132**:507–513, 1978.
17. Harding R, Liggins GC. Changes in thoracic dimensions induced by breathing movements in fetal sheep. *Reprod Fertil Dev* **8**:117–124, 1996.
18. Bocking AD, Gagnon R. Assessment of fetal health. In *Textbook of fetal physiology*, GD Thorburn, R Harding (eds), p. 186. Oxford: Oxford University Press, 1994.
19. Hooper SB, Harding R. Respiratory system. In *Fetal growth and development*, R Harding, AD Bocking (eds), p. 114. Cambridge: Cambridge University Press, 2001.
20. Wigglesworth JS, Desai R. Effects on lung growth of cervical cord section in the rabbit fetus. *Early Hum Dev* **3**:51–65, 1979.
21. Liggins GC, Vilos GA, Campos GA, Kitterman JA, Lee CH. The effect of spinal cord transection on lung development in fetal sheep. *J Develop Physiol* **3**:267–274, 1981.
22. Adamson TM, Boyd RDH, Platt HS, Strang LB. Composition of alveolar liquid in the foetal lamb. *J Physiol* **204**:159–168, 1969.
23. Olver RE, Strang LB. Ion fluxes across the pulmonary epithelium and the secretion of lung liquid in the foetal lamb. *J Physiol* **241**:327–357, 1974.
24. Harding R, Sigger JN, Wickham PJD, Bocking AD. The regulation of flow of pulmonary fluid in fetal sheep. *Respir Physiol* **57**:47–59, 1984.
25. Brace RA, Wlodek ME, McCrabb GJ, Harding R. Swallowing and urine flow responses of the ovine fetus to 24 h of hypoxia. *Am J Physiol* **266**:R1345–R1352, 1994.
26. Hooper SB, Harding R. Fetal lung liquid: a major determinant of the growth and functional development of the fetal lung. *Clin Exp Pharmacol Physiol* **22**:235–247, 1995.
27. Brown MJ, Olver RE, Ramsden CA, Strang LB, Walters DV. Effects of adrenaline and of spontaneous labour on the secretion and absorption of lung liquid in the fetal lamb. *J Physiol* **344**:137–152, 1983.
28. Hooper SB, Harding R. Effects of b-adrenergic blockade on lung liquid secretion during fetal asphyxia. *Am J Physiol* **257**:R705–R710, 1989.
29. Wallace MJ, Hooper SB, Harding R. Regulation of lung liquid secretion by arginine vasopressin in fetal sheep. *Am J Physiol* **258**:R104–R111, 1990.
30. Walters DV, Ramsden CA, Olver RE. Dibutyryl cAMP induces a gestation-dependent absorption of fetal lung liquid. *J Appl Physiol* **68**:2054–2059, 1990.
31. Wallace MJ, Hooper SB, Harding R. Effects of elevated fetal cortisol concentrations on the volume, secretion and reabsorption of lung liquid. *Am J Physiol* **269**:R881–R887, 1995.
32. Wallace MJ, Hooper SB, Harding R. Role of the adrenal glands in the maturation of lung liquid secretory mechanisms in fetal sheep. *Am J Physiol* **270**:R1–R8, 1996.
33. Kindler PM, Chuang DC, Perks AM. Fluid production by in vitro lungs from near-term fetal guinea pigs: effects of cortisol and aldosterone. *Acta Endocrinologica* **129**:169–177, 1993.
34. Cassin S, Perks AM. Studies of factors which stimulate lung fluid secretion in fetal goats. *J Develop Physiol* **4**:311–325, 1982.
35. Hooper SB, Dickson KA, Harding R. Lung liquid secretion, flow and volume in response to moderate asphyxia in fetal sheep. *J Develop Physiol* **10**:473–485, 1988.
36. Hooper SB, Harding R. Changes in lung liquid dynamics induced by prolonged fetal hypoxemia. *J Appl Physiol* **69**:127–135, 1990.
37. Hooper SB, Wallace MJ, Harding R. Amiloride blocks the inhibition of fetal lung liquid secretion caused by AVP but not by asphyxia. *J Appl Physiol* **74**:111–115, 1993.
38. Wallace MJ, Hooper SB, McCrabb GJ, Harding R. Acidemia enhances the inhibitory effect of hypoxia on fetal lung liquid secretion. *Reprod Fertil Dev* **8**:327–333, 1996.
39. Perks AM, Ruiz T, Chua B, Muhll IV, Kindler PM, Blair W. Reabsorption of lung liquid produced by 2,4-dinitrophenol in *in vitro* lungs from fetal guinea pigs. *Can J Physiol Pharmacol* **71**:1–11, 1993.
40. Harding R, Hooper SB, Han VKM. Abolition of fetal breathing movements by spinal cord transection leads to reductions in fetal lung liquid volume, lung growth and IGF-II gene expression. *Pediatr Res* **34**:148–153, 1993.
41. Nardo L, Hooper SB, Harding R. Lung hypoplasia can be reversed by short-term obstruction of the trachea in fetal sheep. *Pediatr Res* **38**:690–696, 1995.
42. Miller AA, Hooper SB, Harding R. Role of fetal breathing movements in control of fetal lung distension. *J Appl Physiol* **75**:2711–2717, 1993.
43. Perks AM, Cassin S. The rate of production of lung liquid in fetal goats, and the effect of expansion of the lungs. *J Develop Physiol* **7**:149–160, 1985.
44. Nardo L, Hooper SB, Harding R. Stimulation of lung growth by tracheal obstruction in fetal sheep: relation to luminal pressure and lung liquid volume. *Pediatr Res* **43**:184–190, 1998.

45. Lines A, Hooper SB, Harding R. Lung liquid production rates and volumes do not decrease before labor in healthy fetal sheep. *J Appl Physiol* **82**:927–932, 1997.
46. Harding R, Bocking AD, Sigger JN. Upper airway resistances in fetal sheep: the influence of breathing activity. *J Appl Physiol* **60**:160–165, 1986.
47. Olver RE, Ramsden CA, Strang LB, Walters DV. The role of amiloride-blockable sodium transport in adrenaline-induced lung liquid reabsorption in the fetal lamb. *J Physiol* **376**:321–340, 1986.
48. Harding R, Hooper SB, Dickson KA. A mechanism leading to reduced lung expansion and lung hypoplasia in fetal sheep during oligohydramnios. *Am J Obstet Gynecol* **163**:1904–1913, 1990.
49. Hooper SB, Wallace MJ. Physical, endocrine and growth factors in lung development. In *The lung: development, aging and the environment*, R Harding, KE Pinkerton, CG Plopper (eds), pp. 131–148. Elsevier Academic Press, 2004.
50. Hooper SB, Wallace MJ. Role of the physicochemical environment in lung development. *Clin Exp Pharmacol Physiol* **33**:273–279, 2006.
51. Hooper SB, Han VKM, Harding R. Changes in lung expansion alter pulmonary DNA synthesis and IGF-II gene expression in fetal sheep. *Am J Physiol* **265**:L403–lL409, 1993.
52. Alcorn D, Adamson TM, Lambert TF, Maloney JE, Ritchie BC, Robinson PM. Morphological effects of chronic tracheal ligation and drainage in the fetal lamb lung. *J Anat* **123**:649–660, 1977.
53. Moessinger AC, Harding R, Adamson TM, Singh M, Kiu GT. Role of lung fluid volume in growth and maturation of the fetal sheep lung. *J Clin Invest* **86**:1270–1277, 1990.
54. Vandenburgh HH. Mechanical forces and their second messengers in stimulating cell growth in vitro. *Am J Physiol* **262**:R350–R355, 1992.
55. Ingber DE. The riddle of morphogenesis: a question of solution chemistry or molecular cell engineering – minireview. *Cell* **75**:1249–1252, 1993.
56. Liu M, Xu J, Liu J, Kraw ME, Tanswell AK, Post M. Mechanical strain-enchanced fetal lung cell proliferation is mediated by phospholipases C and D and protein kinase C. *Am J Physiol* **268**:L729–L738, 1995.
57. Liu M, Liu J, Buch S, Tanswell AK, Post M. Antisense oligonucleotides against PDGF-B and its receptor inhibit mechanical strain-induced fetal lung cell growth. *Am J Physiol* **269**:L178–L184, 1995.
58. Wallace MJ, Thiel AM, Lines AM, Polglase GR, Sozo F, Hooper SB. Role of platelet-derived growth factor-B, vascular endothelial growth factor, insulin-like growth factor-II, mitogen-activated protein kinase and transforming growth factor-beta 1 in expansion-induced lung growth in fetal sheep. *Reprod Fertil Dev* **18**:655–665, 2006.
59. Sozo F, Wallace MJ, Zahra VA, Filby CE, Hooper SB. Gene expression profiling during increased fetal lung expansion identifies genes likely to regulate development of the distal airways. *Physiol Genomics* **24**:105–113, 2006.
60. Harding R, Albuquerque C. Lung hypoplasia: role of mechanical factors in prenatal lung growth. In *Lung development*, C Gaultier, J Bourbon, M Post (eds), pp. 364–394. Oxford: Oxford University Press, 1999.
61. Askenazi SS, Perlman M. Pulmonary hypoplasia: lung weight and radial alveolar count as criteria of diagnosis. *Arch Dis Child* **54**:614–618, 1979.
62. Moessinger AC, Santiago A, Paneth NS, Rey HR, Blanc WA, Driscoll JM, Jr. Time trends in necropsy prevalence and birth prevalence of lung hypoplasia. *Paediatr Perinat Epidemiol* **3**:421–431, 1989.
63. Thibeault DW, Beatty EC, Hall RT, Bowen SK, O'Neill DH. Neonatal pulmonary hypoplasia with premature rupture of fetal membranes and oligohydramnios. *J Pediatr* **107**:273–277, 1985.
64. Suzuki K, Hooper SB, Cock ML, Harding R. Effect of lung hypoplasia on birth-related changes in the pulmonary circulation in sheep. *Pediatr Res* **57**:530–536, 2005.
65. Wigglesworth JS. Pathology of the lung in the fetus and neonate, with particular reference to problems of growth and maturation. *Histopathology* **11**:671–689, 1987.
66. Moessinger AC, Collins MH, Blanc WA, Rey HR, James LS. Oligohydramnios-induced lung hypoplasia: the influence of timing and duration in gestation. *Pediatr Res* **20**:951–954, 1986.
67. Nimrod C, Varela-Gittings F, Machin G, Campbell D, Wesenberg R. The effect of very prolonged membrane rupture on fetal development. *Am J Obstet Gynecol* **148**:540–543, 1984.
68. Wilson JM, DiFiore JW, Peters CA. Experimental fetal tracheal ligation prevents the pulmonary hypoplasia associated with fetal nephrectomy: possible application for congenital diaphragmatic hernia. *J Pediatr Surg* **28**:1433–1440, 1993.
69. Hedrick MH, Estes JM, Sullivan KM et al. Plug the lung until it grows (PLUG): a new method to treat congenital diaphragmatic hernia in utero. *J Pediatr Surg* **29**:612–617, 1994.
70. Davey MG, Hooper SB, Tester ML, Johns DP, Harding R. Respiratory function in lambs after in utero treatment of lung hypoplasia by tracheal obstruction. *J Appl Physiol* **87**:2296–2304, 1999.
71. Davey MG, Hooper SB, Cock ML, Harding R. Stimulation of lung growth in fetuses with lung hypoplasia leads to altered postnatal lung structure in sheep. *Pediatr Pulmonol* **32**:267–276, 2001.
72. Flecknoe S, Harding R, Maritz G, Hooper SB. Increased lung expansion alters the proportions of type I and type II alveolar epithelial cells in fetal sheep. *Am J Physiol* **278**:L1180–L1185, 2000.
73. Flecknoe SJ, Wallace MJ, Harding R, Hooper SB. Determination of alveolar epithelial cell phenotypes in fetal sheep: evidence for the involvement of basal lung expansion. *J Physiol* **542**:245–253, 2002.
74. Lines A, Nardo L, Phillips ID, Possmayer F, Hooper SB. Alterations in lung expansion affect surfactant protein A, B and C mRNA levels in fetal sheep. *Am J Physiol* **276**:L239–L245, 1999.
75. Schellenberg JC. The development of connective tissue and its role in pulmonary mechanics. In *Respiratory control and lung development in the fetus and newborn*, BM Johnston, PD Gluckman (eds), pp. 3–62. Ithaca: Perinatology Press, 1986.
76. Clark JG, Kuhn C, III, McDonald JA, Mecham RP. Lung connective tissue. *Int Rev Connect Tissue Res* **10**:249–331, 1983.
77. Faggian J, Fosang AJ, Zieba M., Wallace MJ, Hooper SB. Changes in versican and chondroitin sulphate proteoglycans during structural development of the lung. *Am J Physiol* in press, 2007.
78. Liggins GC, Schellenberg J-C, Finberg K, Kitterman JA, Lee CH. The effects of ACTH1-24 or cortisol on pulmonary maturation in the adrenalectomized ovine fetus. *J Develop Physiol* **7**:105–111, 1985.
79. Alcorn DG, Adamson TM, Maloney JE, Robinson PM. A morphologic and morphometric analysis of fetal lung development in the sheep. *Anat Rec* **201**:655–667, 1981.
80. Crone RK, Davies P, Liggins GC, Reid L. The effects of hypophysectomy, thyroidectomy, and postoperative infusion of cortisol or adrenocorticotrophin on the structure of the ovine fetal lung. *J Develop Physiol* **5**:281–288, 1983.
81. Cole TJ, Blendy JA, Monaghan AP et al. Targeted disruption of the glucocorticoid receptor gene blocks adrenergic chromaffin cell development and severely retards lung maturation. *Genes Dev* **9**:1608–1621, 1995.
82. Cole TJ, Solomon NM, Van Driel R et al. Altered epithelial cell proportions in the fetal lung of glucocorticoid receptor null mice. *Am J Respir Cell Mol Biol* **30**:613–619, 2004.
83. Muglia LJ, Bae DS, Brown TT et al. Proliferation and differentiation defects during lung development in corticotropin-releasing hormone-deficient mice. *Am J Respir Cell Mol Biol* **20**:181–188, 1999.
84. Jobe AH, Polk D, Ikegami M et al. Lung responses to ultrasound-guided fetal

treatments with corticosteroids in preterm lambs. *J Appl Physiol* **75**:2099–2105, 1993.
85. Polk DH, Ikegami M, Jobe AH et al. Postnatal lung function in preterm lambs: effects of a single exposure to betamethasone and thyroid hormones. *Am J Obstet Gynecol* **172**:872–881, 1995.
86. Schellenberg J-C, Liggins GC. Elastin and collagen in the fetal sheep lung. I. Ontogenesis. *Pediatr Res* **22**:335–338, 1987.
87. Shibahara S, Davidson JM, Smith K, Crystal RG. Modulation of tropoelastin production and elastin messenger ribonucleic acid activity in developing sheep lung. *Biochem* **20**:6577–6584, 1981.
88. Dunsmore SE, Rannels DE. Turnover of extracellular matrix by type II pulmonary epithelial cells. *Am J Physiol* **268**:L336–L346, 1995.
89. Hawgood S, Clements JA. Pulmonary surfactant and its apoproteins. *J Clin Invest* **86**:1–6, 1990.
90. Possmayer F. The perinatal lung. In *The biochemical development of the fetus and neonate*, CT Jones (ed.), pp. 337–391. Amsterdam: Elsevier, 1982.
91. Flecknoe SJ, Wallace MJ, Cock ML, Harding R, Hooper SB. Changes in alveolar epithelial cell proportions during fetal and postnatal development in sheep. *Am J Physiol Lung Cell Mol Physiol* **285**:L664–L670, 2003.
92. Whitsett JA. Pulmonary surfactant and respiratory distress syndrome in the newborn infant. In *The lung: scientific foundations*, RG Crystal, JB West, ER Weibel, PJ Barnes (eds), p. 2167. Philadelphia: Lippincott-Raven, 1997.
93. Jobe AH, Ikegami M. Lung development and function in preterm infants in the surfactant treatment era. *Annu Rev Physiol* **62**:825–846, 2000.
94. Liggins GC, Schellenberg J-C. Hormones and lung maturation. In *Respiratory control and lung development in the fetus and newborn*, BM Johnston, PD Gluckman (eds), pp. 107–133. Perinatology Press, 1986.
95. Orgeig S, Daniels CB, Sullivan LC. Development of the pulmonary surfactant system. In *The lung: development, aging and the environment*, R Harding, KE Pinkerton, CG Plopper (eds), pp. 149–167. London: Elsevier Academic Press, 2004.
96. Hawgood S. Surfactant: composition, structure, and metabolism. In *The lung: scientific foundations*, RG Crystal, JB West, ER Weibel, PJ Barnes (eds), pp. 557–571. Philadelphia, New York: Lippincott-Raven, 1997.
97. Froh DK, Ballard PL. Fetal lung maturation. In *Textbook of fetal physiology*, GD Thorburn, R Harding (eds), pp. 168–185. Oxford: Oxford University Press, 1994.
98. Mason RJ, Shannon JM. Alveolar type II cells. In *The lung: scientific foundations*, RG Crystal, JB West, ER Weibel, PJ Barnes (eds), pp. 543–555. Philadelphia, New York: Lippincott-Raven, 1997.
99. Williams MC, Hawgood S, Hamilton RL. Changes in lipid structure produced by surfactant proteins Sp-A, Sp-B, and Sp-C. *Am J Respir Cell Mol Biol* **5**:41–50, 1991.
100. Deruelle P, Houfflin-Debarge V, Magnenant E et al. Effects of antenatal glucocorticoids on pulmonary vascular reactivity in the ovine fetus. *Am J Obstet Gynecol* **189**:208–215, 2003.
101. Suzuki K, Hooper SB, Wallace MJ, Probyn ME, Harding R. Effects of antenatal corticosteroid treatment on pulmonary ventilation and circulation in neonatal lambs with hypoplastic lungs. *Pediatr Pulmonol* **41**:844–854, 2006.
102. Liggins GC. Thyrotropin-releasing-hormone (Trh) and lung maturation. *Reprod Fertil Dev* **7**:443–450, 1995.
103. Moya FR, Gross I. Combined hormonal therapy for the prevention of respiratory-distress syndrome and its consequences. *Semin Perinatol* **17**:267–274, 1993.

Development of the kidneys and urinary tract

CHAPTER 12

Karen M Moritz, Georgina Caruana and E Marelyn Wintour

KEY POINTS

- Development of the permanent (metanephric) kidney involves complex interactions between the ureteric bud and the metanephric mesenchyme. Correct temporal and spatial expression of many genes in these compartments is critical for normal renal development
- The fetal kidney produces a large volume of dilute urine (necessary for maintaining amniotic fluid volume) as well as a number of hormones (erythropoietin, angiotensin II)
- Nephron number (endowment) in the human is complete prior to birth and is permanent. Normal nephron endowment in the human ranges from around 200 000 to more than 2 million nephrons per kidney. Estimation of nephron endowment should only be performed using unbiased stereology
- Exposure to a poor intrauterine environment (maternal low-protein diet, maternal glucocorticoid exposure, placental restriction) can deleteriously affect renal development and result in a low nephron endowment
- A low nephron endowment from birth is strongly linked to the development of adult onset diseases such as hypertension and type-2 diabetes
- Alterations in the renal renin–angtiotensin system are associated with abnormal renal development and appear to be an important mechanism through which a poor intrauterine exposure may contribute to adult onset disease

INTRODUCTION

Since the first edition of this book the importance of studying kidney development has taken on increased significance[1]. In that first edition, we alluded to the 'Barker Hypothesis' as one of the reasons for investigating the development of renal structure and function. This hypothesis suggested that factors such as the diet or stress levels of the mother might impact on the development of various organs and systems in the fetus in such a way as to change, permanently, the function of these organs/systems and thus 'program' the propensity of the adult to develop diseases such as hypertension or type-2 diabetes [2–4]. It has now been expanded to include influences occurring before conception and in the neonatal period, and has been termed the developmental origins of health and adult disease (DOHaD) or developmental programming[5]. There is now substantial evidence that the developing kidney is, indeed, very susceptible to a wide variety of alterations in the 'environment', which can alter (reduce) the permanent number of functioning units (nephron endowment), and also the expression of a number of genes involved in the regulation of normal renal and cardiovascular function[6–8]. The current chapter will expand on this concept and discuss the optimum methodology for the determination of nephron number and evaluation of cardiovascular function. The importance of a low nephron endowment has been studied in models of uninephrectomy during the period of metanephric development and results demonstrate significant alterations in structure and function of the remaining kidney with increased risk of adult cardiovascular disease. These data will be discussed, along with such evidence as has been investigated of the consequences of having a single kidney in human newborns.

In the first edition, we discussed the morphological development of the mammalian kidney through the three forms, pro-, meso- and metanephros, and alluded to a relatively small number of genes then known to be essential for normal development. There has been an explosion of information in this area and the discussion of morphological development can now include extensive gene expression data. In addition, the known roles of the renin–angiotensin system and the eicosanoids in the developing kidney that were discussed in the first edition can now be correlated with alterations in gene expression patterns at various stages of development and in models of developmental programming.

RENAL DEVELOPMENT

Pronephros and mesonephros

The final, permanent metanephric kidney can only be formed normally if it is preceded by the development and subsequent regression of two more primitive forms – the pronephros and the mesonephros. The pronephros consists of one to three filtering units (the glomerulus) which filter(s) fluid into a body compartment – the nephrocele. From here fluid is collected by the ciliated nephrostome and some reabsorption takes place into the surrounding blood sinus before excretion of the remainder into the cloaca. The pronephros has its origin in the nephrogenic ridge which forms on either side of the midline in the human embryo some 23–24 days after conception and the pronephros forms at the cranial end[9]. The mesonephros is the second transient kidney. In comparison to the metanephros, the mesonephros has a small number of nephrons, lacks a loop of Henle and macula densa, but is a filtering kidney which produces a dilute urine[10,11]. This fluid is the major contribution to the allantoic compartment in species such as sheep and cow, with a cotyledonary placenta. The influx of fluid helps the expansion of the allantoic membrane which carries the blood vessels to vascularize the cotyledons even in the non-pregnant horn. In addition, the mesonephros secretes renin[12] and erythropoietin[13], is a source of cells which go on to form the adrenals and gonads[14,15], and is the permanent site of erythropoiesis in the fish[16]. Much recent information has shown the aorta-gonadal-mesonephros region (AGM) to be an important site for stem cells for the hemopoietic system[17–20]. The timing of mesonephric development and major functions of the mesonephros are summarized in Tables 12.1 and 12.2, respectively.

Metanephros

The development of the permanent mammalian kidney (metanephros) is initiated with the outgrowth of the ureteric bud (UB) from the caudal end of the Wolffian duct (WD). This occurs at approximately day 30 in human gestation and at embryonic day (E) 10.5 in the mouse. The timing and site at which the UB emerges from the WD is well orchestrated such that it invades a mass of metanephric mesenchyme (MM) which will become the metanephros. Reciprocal inductive signals occur between the UB and MM[21]. The MM induces the UB to grow and repetitively bifurcate to form the ureteric tree via branching morphogenesis. The ureteric tree subsequently forms the collecting ducts, calyces and renal pelvis. The region of the UB that does not enter the MM becomes the ureter. Simultaneously, the epithelial cells of the tips of the ureteric tree induce committed MM cells to condense forming 'caps' and pre-tubular aggregates[22]. The pre-tubular aggregates undergo a mesenchyme-to-epithelial transition to form renal vesicles. The epithelial cells of the renal vesicle develop into nephrons. This occurs through a number of stages as the renal vesicle develops first into a comma-shaped body followed by an S-shaped body. The lower limb of the S-shaped tubule forms the glomerulus after invasion by capillaries. The S-shaped tubule fuses with the ureteric duct (collecting duct). Progressive growth and differentiation occurs, so that the proximal tubule, convoluted and straight, loop of Henle (descending thin limb and ascending thick limb, macula densa, and distal tubule) form. Nephrogenesis always occurs on the outermost rim of the developing kidney and 'the oldest' glomeruli are pushed progressively to the innermost area of the cortex. The loops of these inner cortical nephrons grow into the inner medulla, whereas those of the last-formed outer glomeruli reach only as far as the outer stripe of the outer medulla[23–26].

Molecular regulation of ureteric budding and branching morphogenesis

The outgrowth of the UB from the WD involves the interplay between two major transforming growth factor-β (TGF-β) superfamily signaling pathways, the bone morphogenetic protein 4 (BMP4) and glial cell line-derived neurotrophic factor (GDNF)/Ret pathways. BMP4 is an inhibitor of ureteric budding and branching whereas GDNF/Ret promotes both of these events. BMP4 is expressed in the mesenchymal cells surrounding the WD[27]. GDNF is expressed in the intermediate mesoderm

Table 12.1 **Timing of mesonephric development and regression and the relative period of gestation over which this occurs in a number of species**

Species	*Days of mesonephric development*	*Relative period of gestation*
Human	28–112	12–38%
Sheep	17–57	10–40%
Pig	15–24	9–21%
Mouse	10–13	53–70%
Rat	12–17	57–81%

Table 12.2 **Structural and functional characteristics of the mesonephros**

Structure	No loops of Henle, small number of relatively large glomeruli
Excretory function	Present in some species – produces dilute urine and contributes to allantoic fluid
Hormonal function	Produces erythropoietin, renin and contains receptors for angiotensin II, glucocorticoids and mineralocorticoids, growth hormone
Hemopoiesis	AGM (aorta-gonadal-mesonephros) is site of stem cells with potential capacity to reconstitute multilineage hemopoietic cells
Other possible functions	Cells from mesonephros have been shown to contribute to development of gonads and adrenals

(presumptive metanephric blastema) adjacent to the WD[28]. Both the WD and UB express the c-Ret tyrosine kinase receptor, the receptor for GDNF. The signaling interplay between the BMP4 and GDNF/c-Ret pathways allows the emergence of the UB at precisely the right site from the WD. Upon branching of the ureteric tree, c-Ret becomes restricted to the tips and GDNF to the mesenchyme surrounding the tips allowing continued induction of branching to occur only at the tips. Mice lacking *GDNF* or *c-Ret* display renal agenesis due to lack of budding or blind-ended ureters or small disorganized kidney rudiments[29–32]. Several genes have been shown to promote the expression of GDNF (*Pax2, Eya1, Sall1* and *Hox11* paralogs), regulate the GDNF expression domain (*Foxc1/2* and *Slit2/Robo2*) or the response to GDNF (*sprouty1*) (reviewed in[33,34]).

Several other molecules have been shown to promote branching (e.g. hepatocyte growth factor (HGF), heparan sulfate proteoglycans, integrins α3 and α8, matrix metalloproteinase-9, Erk MAP-kinase), inhibit branching (e.g. activin, TGF-β2, BMP-2, protein kinase A pathway), regulate branch elongation (TGFβ1 and HGF)[35–39], or control branch symmetry (Hoxa11, Hoxd11 and BMP4)[40–42]. Many of these molecules demonstrate a temporal-spatial expression pattern in the MM and/or UB.

Molecular regulation of nephrogenesis

Prior to nephrogenesis, the uninduced MM expresses the zinc-finger transcription factor, Wilms' tumor (WT-1). Inactivation of *WT-1* in mice results in agenesis due to the inability of condensates to form and apoptosis of the MM[43]. The first step of nephrogenesis involves the epithelialization of the uninduced MM through factors secreted by the ureteric bud. These include leukemia inhibitory factor (LIF), transforming growth factor-β2, lipocalin-2, Wnt-6, BMP7 and cytokine receptor-like factor-1 (CRLF-1)[44–48] (reviewed by[22,49]). The cap mesenchyme expresses a number of transcription factors, such as Pax-2, Cited-1, Six1, Sall1 and Eya1 (reviewed in[49,50]). The cells of the pre-tubular aggregate, which develop into the nephron, express Wnt-4, Lim-1 and begin to express epithelial markers[22,45,46,49].

As nephrogenesis proceeds, genes become spatially restricted to various segments of the nephron. These include members of the cadherin family[51], notch signaling pathway[52,53], Robo/Slit family[54] and aquaporins[55] just to name a few. Gene inactivation in mice of podocyte expressed genes such as *Nephrin* and *podocin* result in nephrotic syndromes demonstrating the importance of these cells in the function of the glomerular filtration barrier (reviewed in[56]). Gene inactivation of a number of genes expressed in the renal stroma in the mouse has demonstrated the importance of this renal subcompartment in regulating both branching morphogenesis and nephrogenesis (reviewed by[57]). The renal stroma provides structural support and is involved in nephron maturation.

In this section, we have described the importance of a number of key genes that play a role in the development of the metanephros. In recent years, there has been an explosion in the number of genes known to be temporally and spatially expressed in the developing metanephros through the analysis of global gene expression[48,58–63]. Many of these genes await functional analysis to determine their roles in the development of the metanephros.

NEPHRON ENDOWMENT

What is a normal nephron number?

Until quite recently, it was thought that each human kidney contained approximately one million nephrons with relatively little variance among individuals. Over the last decade, with the use of unbiased stereological methods, it has been demonstrated that there is a huge, almost 10-fold range in nephron endowment in kidneys collected at autopsy from people with no noted medical condition. Table 12.3 shows normal nephron number in the human in four reported studies in which reliable stereological methods have been used[64–67]. Interestingly, Australian Aborigines show a significantly lower nephron number than other racial groups. Data from Hughson et al.[67] can be reanalyzed according to gender to show females have a lower nephron endowment than males.

Table 12.3 **Nephron number in the human**

Nephron number	*Sample size*	*Sex*	*Race*	*Pathology*	*Reference*
617 000 (mean)	37	19M/18F			Nyengaard 1992[65]
1 429 200 (median)	10	9M/1F	White European	Normotensive	Keller 2003[64]
702 379 (median)	10	9M/1F	White European	Hypertensive	Keller 2003[64]
961 840 ± 292 750	21	Mixed	African American	Normotensive	Hughson 2006[67]
867 358 ± 341 958	41	Mixed	African American	Hypertensive	Hughson 2006[67]
923 377 ± 256 291	36	Mixed	White American	Normotensive	Hughson 2006[67]
754 319 ± 329 506	21	Mixed	White American	Hypertensive	Hughson 2006[67]
683 174 (mean)	17	11M/6F	Australian Aboriginal	Not known	Hoy 2006[66]
885 318 (mean)	24	21M/3F	Non-aboriginal Australian	Not known	Hoy 2006[66]

These studies all used the optimal method of unbiased stereology to determine nephron endowment in human kidneys obtained at autopsy

Why is nephron endowment important?

Cardiovascular and renal disease now contribute to more than 40% of all deaths in Western society, a figure expected to increase dramatically in the upcoming decades. Although these diseases have in many instances been considered to be dependent upon genetic and lifestyle factors, studies have indicated that a suboptimal in utero environment may 'program' an individual to be born with an increased risk of developing these diseases. As the kidney is intrinsically linked to the long-term regulation of blood pressure and directly to renal function, it is not surprising that the kidney has been the focus of much study. As discussed below, a low nephron endowment has been strongly associated with the development of hypertension in the human and a variety of animal models, although it is difficult to establish direct cause and effect. Two of the studies in Table 12.3 also separate the groups according to known blood pressure prior to death. This demonstrates that, at least in white populations, a low nephron endowment is associated with hypertension. The low nephron endowment may also contribute the very high rates of renal and cardiovascular disease in Aboriginal Australians compared to white Australians[68,69]. Black Americans also tend to have a higher incidence of these diseases than their white counterparts, but do not appear to have a nephron deficit. It should be noted that nephrons are lost with age and this needs to be taken in account when analyzing nephron number from autopsy samples, as the estimated nephron number at the age of death may not be directly related to the number present at birth.

Links between a congenital nephron deficit and elevated blood pressure form part of the 'Brenner Hypothesis'. Brenner and colleagues proposed, almost 20 years ago, that a congenital nephron deficit was likely to be associated with increased hydrostatic pressure in the glomerular capillaries and glomerular hyperfiltration which would result in glomerular hypertrophy[70]. This would act to maintain overall normal glomerular filtration rate but this 'adaptation' could only suffice for a defined period and eventually glomerulosclerosis would result, further perpetuating nephron loss. Figure 12.1 demonstrates how a low nephron endowment may contribute to adult disease.

The timing of nephrogenesis in the metanephric kidney and the extent to which it occurs in utero/postnatally varies extensively among species and appreciation of these differences is crucial to our understanding of the impact of the in utero environment of future disease outcomes. Table 12.4 shows the great variation among species. Of greatest importance is the fact that humans complete nephrogenesis at 36 weeks of gestation while many animal models (particularly rodents) continue nephron formation for a considerable time after birth. This means that a human kidney in relatively early pregnancy is similar, developmentally, to a rodent kidney in late gestation. This is illustrated in Figure 12.2 which depicts a human kidney at approximately 9 weeks of pregnancy (out of a 39–40 week pregnancy) at an approximately similar stage of development to a rat kidney at day 20 (out of a 22 day) pregnancy.

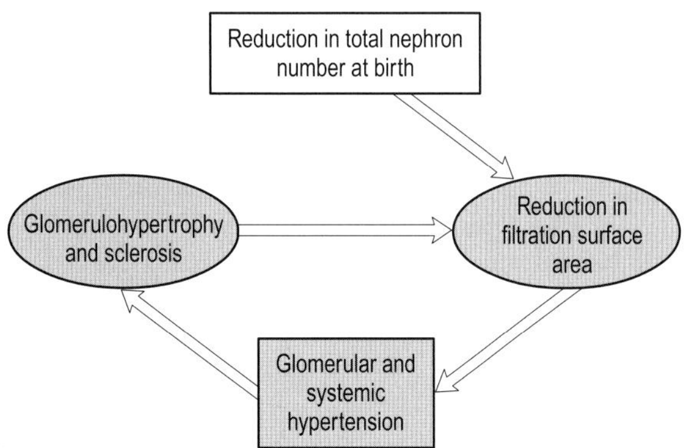

Fig. 12.1 Mechanisms through which a low nephron endowment may lead to hypertension.

How to measure nephron endowment

At present, estimation of nephron number can only be performed on kidneys obtained at autopsy. Estimation of the number of nephrons in the kidney can be performed in a number of ways including acid maceration and morphological/histological techniques. The use of different methodologies to measure nephron number remains a potential source of great variation in findings between studies. Unbiased stereology is the gold standard for measurement of glomerular (nephron) number and its use is recommended by International Nephrology associations[71]. However, it has not been utilized extensively as it is relatively time-consuming. It has the added advantage that glomerular volume is obtained, allowing the degree of glomerular hypertrophy to be determined. Use of methods such as acid maceration may be valid in some cases but not when performed by inexperienced researchers or where there may be high levels of glomerulosclerosis.

In utero factors that influence nephron endowment

Many studies now provide strong evidence that a large number of maternal perturbations can alter normal development and many of these can influence nephron endowment. This chapter

Table 12.4 **Approximate period over which nephrogenesis occurs in a number of species**

Species	*Length of pregnancy*	*Approximate period of nephrogenesis*	*Relative period of gestation*
Human	40 weeks	5–36 weeks	12–90%
Sheep	150 days	30–130 days	20–90%
Guinea pig	63 days	22–55 days	35–90%
Spiny mouse	40 days	19–37 days	50–90%
Mouse	20 days	E11–PN5–7 days	55–125%
Rat	22 days	E12–PN8–10	55–140%
Rabbit	32 days	E12–PN21	35–160%
Pig	112 days	E20–PN21–25	20–120%

Note: the first 4 species complete nephrogenesis prior to birth while the remaining species complete nephrogenesis in the postnatal period. E = embryonic day and PN = postnatal day

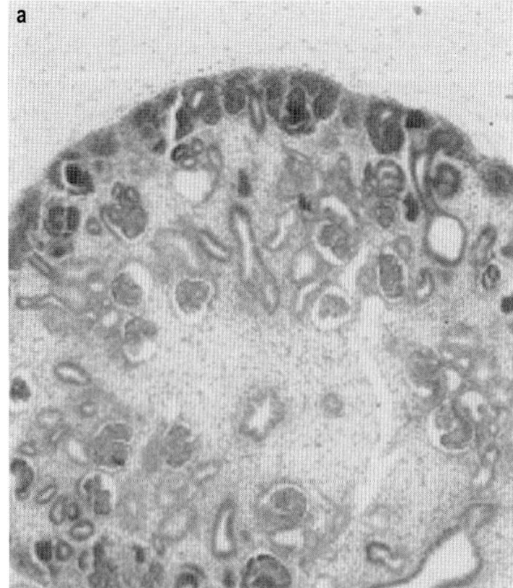

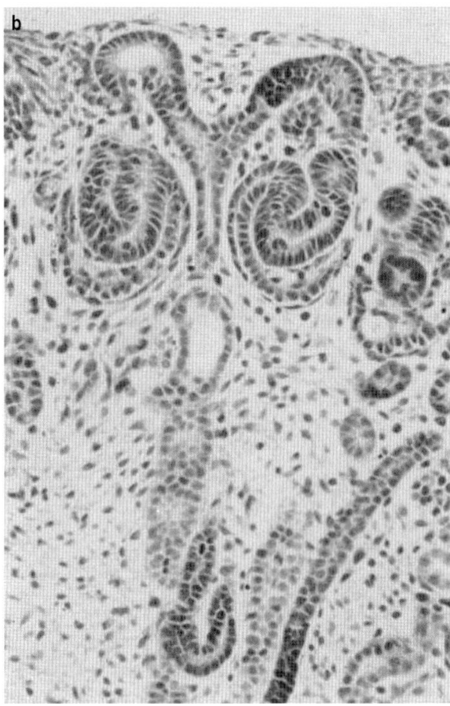

Fig. 12.2 Metanephric development of a human kidney at 9 weeks of pregnancy (a) and a rat kidney at 20 days of gestation (b). In both cases branching of the ureteric bud can be seen along with immature, developing glomeruli. It should be noted this represents the first trimester of human pregnancy (39–40 weeks gestation) but close to birth (a 22-day pregnancy) in the rat, highlightling the different time periods, as a proportion of gestation, over which metanephric development takes place. (NB Pictures at different magnification.)

will not attempt to cover in detail all studies in this field, but refer readers to some recent reviews on this topic[6,72–74]. Here, we shall concentrate on studies in which the optimal methodology of unbiased stereology has been utilized to determine nephron endowment.

Human studies

It is obviously difficult to examine directly the effect of a maternal insult on nephron endowment in the human. One study has demonstrated a strong correlation between low birth weight (used as an indicator of a poor intrauterine exposure) and nephron endowment with a predicted increase of approximately 250000 nephrons per kg increase in birth weight[75]. Other epidemiological studies in humans suggest that maternal diabetes can cause abnormal renal development[76], as may maternal micronutrient deficiencies[77], however, nephron number has not been assessed. Use of particular drugs, including those for medicinal purposes (e.g. angiotensin converting enzyme (ACE) inhibitors) are known to affect fetal renal development and should be avoided in pregnancy[78].

Animal studies

Many maternal manipulations can influence nephron endowment. It should first be acknowledged that the overall outcome of these studies is highly dependent on a number of factors including the type, severity and timing of the insult, the sex of the fetus and the species utilized. Undernutrition, in which mothers (most often rats but also performed in sheep and mice) are placed on diets low in calories, protein or other nutrients for all or part of pregnancy, has been extensively used. This regimen in general produces offspring of low birth weight with a reduced nephron number[79–82]. In many cases (but not always), the offspring develop hypertension as adults. Maternal vitamin A deficiency in rats is also associated with a decreased nephron endowment in offspring[83] as is maternal anemia[84].

Maternal exposure to glucocorticoids has been performed in rats, sheep and spiny mice. These studies are of great interest as maternal stress during pregnancy may be of greater relevance to women in Western society than severe undernutrition. It has been shown that a very short exposure (48–60 hours) to either synthetic glucocorticoids (dexamethasone in the sheep, rat or spiny mouse) or natural ones (cortisol in the sheep and corticosterone in the rat) can result in an ≈30% nephron deficit[85–88]. This model is highly dependent upon timing of the exposure with the period of very early renal development being particularly susceptible. Interestingly, in these models of short exposure to glucocorticoids, the nephron deficit occurs even though the offspring are of normal birth weight. It has been suggested that low-protein diets may work via increased exposure to maternal glucocorticoids, at least in males[89]. However, recently, an argument has been made that dexamethasone programmed hypertension in rat offspring may be due to reduction in food intake[90]. This probably only occurs if the exposure to dexamethasone continues for an extended period (5 days) and results in growth restriction[91]. Also highly relevant to Western obstetric care are results from models of placental ligation which causes reduced placental perfusion. Bilateral uterine vessel ligation in the rat can cause a reduction in nephron endowment in rat offspring[92,93].

Unilateral nephrectomy as a model of reduced nephron endowment

The most direct evidence defining the link between nephron number and adult blood pressure comes from animal models in which a kidney is removed during nephrogenesis thereby decreasing nephron number from early in life. This was first performed in the rat where removal of one kidney on postnatal day 1 resulted in offspring with elevated blood pressure in adulthood[94,95]. In the sheep, which like the human completes nephrogenesis prior to birth, removal of one kidney at 100 days of gestation (where nephrogenesis is complete around 130 days) resulted in female offspring with hypertension[96]. It also caused a reduction in glomerular filtration rate (GFR) by approximately 30% and an inability to excrete a protein load[96,97]. These animals developed elevated plasma creatinine concentrations suggestive of mild renal failure[97]. We have recently shown this treatment also causes a hypertension in male offspring and also results in impaired cardiac function as measured by a reduced cardiac functional reserve (unpublished). Future studies in this model may help elucidate the mechanisms through which a reduced nephron endowment from birth results in altered cardiovascular and renal function. Interestingly, in the sheep, removal of the kidney at 100 days resulted in compensatory nephrogenesis in the remaining kidney[98], resulting in an overall nephron deficit of approximately 30% rather than 50%.

FUNCTIONAL DEVELOPMENT OF THE METANEPHROS

The most important roles of the fetal metanephros are the production of a relatively large volume of dilute urine (from a blood flow equivalent to only 3% of the cardiac output), support of the fetal circulation (by the production of erythropoietin to increase red blood cell production and the secretion of vasoactive factors), and to support growth of the fetus by production of hormones and binding proteins. The production of the large volume of dilute fetal urine (25–35% body weight per day, approximate osmolality of 100–150 mOsmol/kg water) is essential for the maintenance of the amniotic fluid volume, which allows symmetrical normal growth of the fetus and expansion of lungs. The relative inability of the fetal metanephros to produce a concentrated urine is due to the fact that the aquaporin 2 (water channel target of arginine vasopressin) gene expression is less than half that of the adult kidney at term[99]. The ontogeny of the water channel genes in the developing kidney has been discussed extensively in recent reviews[55,100]. As discussed in the previous edition, some hormones (cortisol, atrial natriuretic peptide, angiotensin II) have exaggerated diuretic and natriuretic effects in immature kidneys because they tend to increase glomerular filtration rate while there is a disruption of glomerulo-tubular balance.

Production and biochemical analysis of fetal urine

The healthy fetus produces hypotonic urine. Fetal urine, in the human, is excreted into the amniotic fluid compartment from at least 12 weeks of gestation and, although amniotic fluid differs significantly in composition from fetal urine, a steady input of dilute fetal urine is essential for normal amniotic fluid volume maintenance. At 16 weeks (0.4) of gestation, human fetal urine solutes (obtained from the fetal bladder) showed the following concentrations (mmol/l): sodium 80–150, potassium 3, calcium 0.21, phosphate 0.91, creatinine 0.1 and urea 0.008[101]. Just before birth, there was a decrease in sodium and an increase in urea and creatinine. Elevation in urinary sodium, chloride, calcium and osmolality are good indices of fetal renal injury and may suggest irreversible renal dysplasia. Repeated fetal urine sampling throughout pregnancy has been recommended to improve diagnostic accuracy of fetal renal abnormalities[102]. However, fetal urine electrolyte parameters did not prove always reliable for the prediction of renal dysplasia. Nicolini and colleagues[101] found fetal urinary calcium as a most sensitive marker in predicting renal dysplasia, with a calcium <1.3 mmol/l suggesting normal renal function. β2-microglobulin (molecular weight of 11 800 Da) and α_1-microglobulin (molecular weight of 33 000 Da) have been proposed as more sensitive indices of renal function[103,104]. Mandelbrot and colleagues suggested that the combination of urinary sodium <70 mmol/l and β_2-microglobulin <4 mg/l are the best predictors for normal fetal renal function[105]. Elevation in urinary *N*-acetyl-β-D-glucosaminidase (NAD) correlated well with renal cellular injury in some studies[106,107] but was not useful as a marker of renal maturation[105]. The use of proton nuclear magnetic resonance spectroscopy to measure low-molecular-weight metabolites such as amino acids, amines and sugars may allow clear identification of fetuses with impaired renal function[108]. In addition, medullary osmolytes, taurine, myo-inositol and trimethylamide-*N*-oxide (TMAO) could be potentially used in the evaluation of fetal renal function[109]. In all cases, the value of fetal urine sampling must be weighed against the risk for the fetus[110].

RENIN–ANGIOTENSIN SYSTEM (RAS)

During fetal development, the major action of the RAS appears to be on the kidney where it acts to maintain GFR and ensure a high rate of urine production[111]. Angiotensin II is also important for normal kidney development[9]. Understanding of the fetal RAS is very important as use of angiotensin converting enzyme (ACE) inhibitors is contraindicated in pregnancy. It has been observed in clinical practice that women treated with ACE inhibitors during pregnancy often had oligohydramnios. This was associated with anuria and lung abnormalities after birth[77]. All components of this system – renin, angiotensinogen, angiotensin converting enzyme and the angiotensin receptors – are produced in the fetal meso- and metanephros from very early in gestation allowing for local production and action[12]. Over the last few years, significant alterations in the renal RAS have been documented in the offspring of mothers exposed to a variety of perturbations including protein restriction or glucocorticoid exposure during pregnancy and placental restriction. Together, these data suggest alterations in the renal RAS may be a key mediator of 'programming' effects.

Altered RAS during renal development

Studies of the RAS have been performed in many models of developmental programming. During the period of nephrogenesis, there is supression of the renal RAS in offspring of rat dams exposed to protein restriction during pregnancy[79] and decreased expression of the angiotensin type 1 (AT1) receptor[112]. Glucocorticoid exposure in the rat also alters AT1 receptor expression[87]. Angiotensin II binding to the AT1 receptor has been shown at least in culture systems to mediate the process of branching morphogenesis[113]. Thus, decreased expression of the AT1 receptor may result in less branching of the ureteric bud and thus a reduction in nephron endowment. Increased expression of the angiotensin type II (AT2) receptor has been reported in the fetal kidney following glucorticoid exposure in the rat[87]. The AT2 receptor is thought to be involved in apoptosis[114].

Increased apoptosis has been shown in in the kidneys of embryos from rat dams exposed to a low-protein diet[115,116] and is another potential mechanism through which maternal perturbations lead to a decrease in neprhon endowment.

Compensatory changes in the renal RAS contributing to cardiovascular disease

Interestingly, after completion of nephrogenesis, components of the RAS, particularly the AT1 receptor, appear to present at higher levels in the kidneys of offspring that have been programmed in utero. This has been observed in rats and sheep exposed to glucocorticoids[87,117], rats exposed to low protein[118] and male rats exposed to placental insufficiency[93]. There is now evidence to suggest that increased activation of the renal RAS may cause sodium retention and contribute to sustained elevations in blood pressure[119].

EICOSANOIDS

The eicosanoid family include prostaglandins, thromboxane, leukotrienes, monohydroxylated eicosatetraenoic acids (HETES) and eoxides of arachidonic acid. Vasodilator prostaglandins are produced in large amounts by fetal kidneys and the urinary excretion rate is higher in premature human neonates than in children or adults[120]. These prostaglandins are produced by the action of the enzyme, cyclo-oxygenase (COX), of which there are two isoforms, and can be inhibited by compounds such as aspirin and indomethacin. COX-1 is constitutively expressed, COX-2 is expressed as part of the inflammatory response, but appears to be constitutively expressed in rat kidney[121]. COX-2 gene knockout studies in mice have demonstrated renal defects including retarded development of the mesenchyme, resulting in fewer mature nephrons, suggestive that COX-2 has a role in ureteric bud induction of the metanephric mesenchyme. COX-2 inhibiton during pregnancy and weaning impairs glomerulogenesis and renal cortical development[122]. In human fetal kidneys, temporal expression of the COX-2 isoform in the podocytes of post-vascularized glomeruli has been observed and is suggestive of a potential regulatory role in glomerular hemodynamics. The abundant expression of COX-1 during renal development suggests this isoform is more important in humans than in murine species, with renal impairment resulting from indomethacin treatment during pregnancy thought to relate more to inhibition of this isoform. Treatment with the COX-1 inhibitor indomethacin has been used in women with polyhydramnios to reduce amniotic fluid volume by decreasing urine production[123–125]. COX-2 inhibitors, although originally thought to be useful in preventing preterm labor, have now been shown to reduce renal function in the fetus and impair renal development[126,127]. New agents that specifically target the PGF2α receptor (FP) may prove to be more specific in preventing preterm birth without unwanted side effects in the developing baby[127].

RENAL AGENESIS AND CONGENITAL URINARY TRACT MALFORMATIONS

The increased use of ultrasound in pregnancy has resulted in an increase in the diagnosis of renal malformations of the fetus. Prenatal diagnosis is important and enables either special obstetric management, termination of pregnancy and the possibility of intrauterine intervention. Below, we discuss what is known about human cases of renal agenesis and congenital urinary tract malformations and what can be learnt from experimental models of these abnormalities.

Bilateral renal agenesis (Potter's syndrome)

Renal agenesis may be due to a defect either in the ureteric bud or in the metanephric blastema resulting in a failure of the ureteric bud to induce development in the metanephric blastema, as described earlier. The infant passes no urine and dies within hours of birth from respiratory failure caused by pulmonary hypoplasia[128,129]due at least in part to the absence of amniotic fluid. The lack of amniotic fluid – oligohydramnios – causes compression of the fetus resulting in fetal deformations such as those seen in Potter's syndrome.

What we have learnt from experimental bilateral nephrectomy?

Roles of the fetal kidneys in growth, lung development, regulation of arterial pressure and erythropoietin production have been studied experimentally in nephrectomized ovine fetuses. Removal of both fetal kidneys after mid gestation results in decreases in fetal arterial pressure[130] and in significant decrease in extracellular fluid volume[131]. It also casues a decrease in plasma chloride, without a change in plasma sodium, and doubling of plasma creatinine, phosphate and magnesium[132] and, in some cases, is accompanied by growth retardation, presumably through a decrease in blood flow which leads to fetal tissue hypoxia. In addition, redistribution of fetal blood occurs with shunting to the brain, heart and adrenal glands. These effects of fetal nephrectomy could at least in part be responsible for the fetal growth retardation seen in some models of fetal bilateral nephrectomy[133]. Another possible mechanism that leads to fetal growth retardation is loss of kidney-related growth factors such as epidermal growth factor (EGF), synthesis of which directly stimulates synthesis of insulin-like growth factor-I (IGF-I) in the renal collecting duct[134,135]. Although fetal nephrectomy leads to a transient increase in the plasma concentration of IGF-I, reduced effectiveness may occur because of an increase in IGF-binding proteins[136,137].

Congenital anomalies of the kidney and urinary tract

Congenital anomalies of the kidney and urinary tract (CAKUT) is a clinical description of complex developmental renal and ureteric abnormalities that have been recognized within families. They include renal hypoplasia/dysplasia, multicystic dysplastic or duplex kidney often associated with vesicoureteric reflux (VUR), hydroureter, hydronephrosis or obstruction at the vesicoureteric (VUJ) or ureteropelvic (UPJ) junction. These anomalies occur in various combinations within families suggesting an incomplete or variable genetic penetrance. Severity may vary from incidental clinical findings to chronic ill health and end stage renal failure in childhood[138–140].

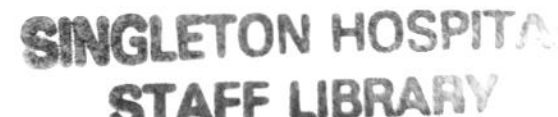

Experimental models of CAKUT

The identification of the key events that are perturbed in patients with CAKUT has come about through the study of mouse models. Mice heterozygous for a null mutation in bone morphogenetic protein 4 ($BMP4^{+/-}$) have been the most extensively studied model. These mice develop renal and ureter abnormalities that mimic those seen in human CAKUT including renal hypo/dysplasia (HK/DK), VUJ obstruction with hydronephrosis and duplex renal systems[141]. Many of these phenotypes can be attributed to abnormalities in the development of the ureter. If the UB (presumptive ureter) fails to bud at the appropriate site along the WD or buds more than once it will not invade the MM appropriately leading to renal dysgenesis (such as renal aplasia, HK/DK kidney, UPJ obstruction, megaureter or duplex collecting system). Inappropriate budding can also lead to ectopic insertion into the bladder resulting in VUJ obstruction and reflux, hydroureter (dilation of the ureter) and hydronephrosis (dilation of the renal pelvis)[138–140]. These conditions arise due to backflow of urine from the bladder into the kidney. In addition, the conditions of hydroureter and hydronephrosis have been associated with smooth muscle cell abnormalities in the ureter and subsequent peristalsis defects[141–143].

Unilateral renal agenesis in the human

Unilateral renal agensis (URA) in the human is a relatively common malformation with an incidence of 1 in every 800–1000 live births. Individuals with URA would be expected to have an overall lower nephron endowment compared to someone with two kidneys and thus may be at risk for hypertension and impaired renal function. Studies have shown modest increases in blood pressure in children with URA[144], although this may be dependent upon what occurs in the remaining kidney. The size of the remaining kidney was inversely correlated to blood pressure in a study including patients with URA, unilateral nephrectomy, unilateral atrophic kidney and controls suggesting the degree of hypertrophy in the remaining kidney was predictive of outcome[145]. Scarring in the remaining kidney in URA patients was also strongly linked to elevated blood pressure[146]. Obesity has also been found to play a role in the development of proteinuria in patients with a single kidney[147]. These studies highlight that compensatory factors and lifestyle can influence disease outcomes in instances of a low nephron endowment.

CONCLUSION

Formation of an adequate nephron endowment during development is essential for the long-term health of an individual. Many factors including maternal stress, protein/calorie restriction and placental insufficiency can impact deleteriously on fetal renal development resulting in a nephron deficit at birth. Future studies examining mechanisms, especially gene pathways contributing to a nephron deficit, will aid our understanding of renal development and hopefully identify potential sites for therapeutic intervention.

REFERENCES

1. Wintour EM, Dodic M, Johnston H, Moritz K, Peers A. Kidney and urinary tract. In *Fetal medicine: basic science and clinical practice*, C Rodeck, W Whittle (eds), pp. 155–171. London: Harcourt, Brace, Abramovich, 1999.
2. Barker DJP, Osmond C, Winter PD, Margetts Bl, Simmonds SJ. Weight in infancy and death from ischaemic heart disease. *Lancet* **2**:577–580, 1989.
3. Barker DJP. *Mothers, babies and diseases in later life*. London: BMJ Publishing Group, 1994.
4. Barker DJP, Eriksson JG, Forsèn T, Osmond C. Fetal origins of adult disease: strength of effects and biological basis. *Int J Epidemiol* **31**:1235–1239, 2002.
5. Gluckman P, Hanson MA. The developmental origins of health and disease: an overview. In *Developmental origins of health and disease*, Gluckman, Hanson (eds), p. 105. Cambridge: Cambridge University Press, 2006.
6. Moriz KM, Dodic M, Wintour EM. Kidney development and the fetal programming of adult disease. *Bioessays* **25**:212–220, 2003.
7. Moritz KM, Boom WM, Wintour EM. Glucocorticoids and fetal programming. *Cell Tissue Res* **322**:81–88, 2005.
8. Moritz MK, Bertram JF. Barker and Brenner: a basis for hypertension? *Curr Hypertens Rep* **2**:179–185, 2006.
9. Wintour EM, Alcorn D, Rockell MD. Development and function of the fetal kidney. In *Fetus and neonate: physiology and clinical applications*, AB Brace, MA Hanson, CH Rodeck (eds), pp. 3–56. Cambridge: Cambridge University Press, 1998.
10. De Martino C, Zamboni L. A morphologic study of the mesonephros of the human embryo. *J Ultrastruct Res* **16**:399–427, 1966.
11. Wintour EM, Alcorn D, Butkus A et al. Ontogeny of hormonal and excretory function of the meso- and meta-nephros in the ovine fetus. *Kidney Int* **50**:1624–1633, 1996.
12. Schutz S, Le Moullec J-M, Corvol P, Gasc J-M. Early expression of all the components of the renin–angiotensin system in human development. *Am J Pathol* **149**:2067–2079, 1996.
13. Wintour EM, Butkus A, Earnest L, Pompolo S. The erythropoietin gene is expressed strongly in the mammalian mesonephros. *Blood* **88**:3349–3353, 1996.
14. Updhyay S, Zamboni L. Preliminary observations on the role of the mesonephros in the development of the adrenal cortex. *Anat Rec* **202**:105–111, 1982.
15. Buehr M, Gu S, McLaren A. Mesonephric contributions to testis differentiation in the fetal mouse. *Development* **117**:273–281, 1993.
16. Esteban MA, Meseguer J, Ayala AG, Agulleiro B. Erythropoiesis and thrombopoiesis in the head-kidney of the sea bass (*Dicentrarchus labrax* L.): an ultrastructural study. *Arch Histol Cytol* **52**:407–419, 1989.
17. Samokhvalov IM, Samokhvalova NI, Nishikawa SI. Call tracing shows the contribution of the yolk sac to adult haematopoiesis. *Nature* **446**:1056–1061, 2007.
18. Zambidis, E, Sinka L, Tavian M et al. Emergence of human angio-haemopoietic cells in normal development and from cultured embryonic stem cells. *Ann NY Acad Sci* (in press), 2007.
19. Yao H, Liu B, Wang X et al. Identification of high proliferative potential precursors with haemangioblastic activity in the mouse AGM region. *Stem Cells* (in press), 2007.
20. Nobihisa I, Ohtsu N, Okada S, Nagata N, Taga T. Identification of a population of cells with haemopoietic stem cell properties in mouse aorta-gonad-mesonephros cultures. *Exp Cell Res* **313**(5):965–974, 2007.

21. Saxen L, Sariola H. Early organogenesis of the kidney. *Pediatr Nephrol* **1**:385–392, 1987.
22. Sariola H. Nephron induction revisited: from caps to condensates. *Curr Opin Nephrol Hypertens* **11**:17–21, 2002.
23. Clark A, Bertram JF. Molecular regulation of nephron endowment. *Am J Physiol* **276**:F485–F97, 1999.
24. Davies JA, Fisher CE. Genes and proteins in renal development. *Exp Nephrol* **10**:102–113, 2002.
25. Carroll TJ, McMahon AP. Overview: the molecular basis of kidney development. In *The kidney: from normal development to congenital disease*, PD Vize, AS Woolf, JBL Bard (eds), pp. 343–376. London: Academic Press, 2003.
26. Yu J, McMahon AP, Valerius MT. Recent genetic studies of mouse kidney development. *Curr Opin Genet Dev* **14**: 550–557, 2004.
27. Miyazaki Y, Oshima K, Fogo A et al. Bone morphogenetic protein 4 regulates the budding site and elongation of the mouse ureter. *J Clin Invest* **105**:863–873, 2000.
28. Hellmich HL, Kos L, Cho ES, Mahon KA, Zimmer A. Embryonic expression of glial cell-line derived neurotrophic factor (GDNF) suggests multiple developmental roles in neural differentiation and epithelial-mesenchymal interactions. *Mech Dev* **54**:95–105, 1996.
29. Pichel J, Shen L, Sheng H et al. Defects in enteric innervation and kidney development in mice lacking GDNF. *Nature* **382**:73–76, 1996.
30. Schuchardt A, D'Agati V, Larsson-Blomberg L, Costantini F, Pachnis V. Defects in the kidney and enteric nervous system of mice lacking the tyrosine kinase receptor Ret. *Nature* **367**:380–383, 1994.
31. Moore MW, Klein RD, Farinas I et al. Renal and neuronal abnormalities in mice lacking GDNF. *Nature* **382**:76–79, 1996.
32. Sanchez MP, Silos-Santiago I, Frisen J, He B, Lira SA, Barbacid M. Renal agenesis and the absence of enteric neurons in mice lacking GDNF. *Nature* **382**:70–73, 1996.
33. Bouchard M. Transcriptional control of kidney development. *Differentiation* **72**:295–306, 2004.
34. Costantini F, Shakya R. GDNF/Ret signaling and the development of the kidney. *Bioessays* **28**:117–127, 2006.
35. Clark AT, Bertram JF. Molecular regulation of nephron endownment. *Am J Physiol Renal Physiol* **276**:485–497, 1999.
36. Clark AT, Young RJ, Bertram JF. In vitro studies on the roles of transforming growth factor-beta 1 in rat metanephric development. *Kidney Int* **59**:1641–1653, 2001.
37. Martinez G, Cullen-McEwen L, Bertram JF. Transforming growth factor-beta superfamily members: roles in branching morphogenesis in the kidney. *Nephrology* **6**:274–284, 2001.
38. Pohl M, Stuart RO, Sakurai H, Nigam SK. Branching morphogenesis during kidney development. *Annu Rev Physiol* **62**:595–620, 2000.
39. Davies J. Intracellular and extracellular regulation of ureteric bud morphogenesis. *J Anat* **198**:257–264, 2001.
40. Patterson LT, Pembaur M, Potter SS. Hoxa11 and Hoxd11 regulate branching morphogenesis of the ureteric bud in the developing kidney. *Development* **128**:2153–2161, 2001.
41. Raatikainen-Ahokas A, Hytonen M, Tenhunen A, Sainio K et al. BMP-4 affects the differentiation of metanephric mesenchyme and reveals an early anterior-posterior axis of the embryonic kidney. *Dev Dyn* **217**:146–158, 2000.
42. Cain JE, Nion T, Jeulin D, Bertram JF. Exogenous BMP-4 amplifies asymmetric ureteric branching in the developing mouse kidney in vitro. *Kidney Int* **67**:420–431, 2005.
43. Kreidberg JA, Sariola H, Loring JM et al. WT-1 is required for early kidney development. *Cell* **74**:679–691, 1993.
44. Perantoni AO, Dove LF, Karavanova I. Basic fibroblast growth factor can mediate the early inductive events in renal development. *Proc Natl Acad Sci USA* **92**:4696–4700, 1995.
45. Barasch J, Yang J, Ware CB et al. Mesenchymal to epithelial conversion in rat metanephros is induced by LIF. *Cell* **99**:377–386, 1999.
46. Plisov SY, Yoshino K et al. TGF beta 2, LIF and FGF2 cooperate to induce nephrogenesis. *Development* **128**:1045–1057, 2001.
47. Itäranta P, Lin Y, Perasaari J, Roel G, Destree O, Vainio S. Wnt-6 is expressed in the ureter bud and induces kidney tubule development in vitro. *Genesis* **32**:259–268, 2002.
48. Schmidt-Ott KM, Yang J, Chen X et al. Novel regulators of kidney development from the tips of the ureteric bud. *J Am Soc Nephrol* **16**:1993–2002, 2005.
49. Schmidt-Ott KM, Lan D, Hirsh BJ, Barasch J. Dissecting stages of mesenchymal-to-epithelial conversion during kidney development. *Nephron Physiol* **104**:56–60, 2006.
50. Boyle S, de Caestecker M. Role of transcriptional networks in coordinating early events during kidney development. *Am J Physiol Renal Physiol* **291**:F1–F8, 2006.
51. Dahl U, Sjodin A, Larue L et al. Genetic dissection of cadherin function during nephrogenesis. *Mol Cell Biol* **22**:1474–1487, 2002.
52. Chen L, Al-Awqati Q. Segmental expression of Notch and Hairy genes in nephrogenesis. *Am J Physiol Renal Physiol* **288**:F939–F952, 2005.
53. Piscione TD, Wu MY, Quaggin SE. Expression of Hairy/Enhancer of Split genes, Hes1 and Hes5, during murine nephron morphogenesis. *Gene Expr Patterns* **4**:707–711, 2004.
54. Piper M, Georgas K, Yamada T, Little M. Expression of the vertebrate slit gene family and their putative receptors, the Robo genes, in the developing murine kidney. *Mech Dev* **94**:213–217, 2000.
55. Liu H, Wintour EM. Aquaporins in development – a review. *Reprod Biol Endocrinol* **3**:18, 2005.
56. Patari-Sampo A, Ihalmo P, Holthofer H. Molecular basis of the glomerular filtration: nephrin and the emerging protein complex at the podocyte slit diaphragm. *Ann Med* **38**:483–492, 2006.
57. Cullen-McEwen LA, Caruana G, Bertram JF. The where, what and why of the developing renal stroma. *Nephron Exp Nephrol* **99**:e1–e8, 2005.
58. Challen GA, Martinez G, Davis MJ et al. Identifying the molecular phenotype of renal progenitor cells. *J Am Soc Nephrol* **15**:2344–2357, 2004.
59. Challen G, Gardiner B, Caruana G et al. Temporal and spatial transcriptional programs in murine kidney development. *Physiol Genomics* **23**:159–171, 2005.
60. Schwab K, Patterson LT, Aronow BJ, Luckas R, Liang HC, Potter SS. A catalogue of gene expression in the developing kidney. *Kidney Int* **64**:1588–1604, 2003.
61. Stuart RO, Bush KT, Nigam SK. Changes in gene expression patterns in the ureteric bud and metanephric mesenchyme in models of kidney development. *Kidney Int* **64**:1997–2008, 2003.
62. Takasato M, Osafune K, Matsumoto Y et al. Identification of kidney mesenchymal genes by a combination of microarray analysis and Sall1-GFP knockin mice. *Mech Dev* **121**:547–557, 2004.
63. Caruana G, Cullen-McEwen L, Nelson AL et al. Spatial gene expression in the T-stage mouse metanephros. *Gene Expr Patterns* **6**:807–825, 2006.
64. Keller G, Zimmer G, Mall G, Ritz E, Amann K. Nephron number in patients with primary hypertension. *N Engl J Med* **348**:101–108, 2003.
65. Nyengaard JR, Bendtsen TF. Glomerular number and size in relation to age, kidney weight, and body surface in normal man. *Anat Rec* **232**:194–204, 1992.
66. Hoy WE, Hughson M, Singh, Douglas-Denton R, Bertram JF. Reduced neprhon number and glomerulomegaly in Australian Aborigines: a group at high risk for renal disease and hypertension. *Kidney Inter* **70**:104-110.
67. Hughson MD, Douglas Denton R, Bertram JF, Hoy WE. Hypertension, glomerular number and birth weight in African Americans and white subjects in the southeastern United States. *Kidney Inter* **69**; 671-678.
68. McDonald SP, Maguire GP, Hoy WE. Renal function and cardiovascular risk markers in a remote Australian Aboriginal community. *Nephrol Dial Transplant* **18**:1555–1561, 2003.

69. Singh GR, Hoy WE. Kidney volume, blood pressure and albuminuria: findings in an Australian Aboriginal community. *Am J Kidney Dis* **43**:254–259, 2004.
70. Brenner BM, Garcia DL, Anderson S. Glomeruli and blood pressure. Less of one, more the other? *Am J Hypertens* **4**:335–347, 1998.
71. Bertram JF, Nurcombe V. Counting cells with the new stereology. *Trends Cell Biol* **2**:177–180, 1992.
72. Kett MM, Bertram JF. Nephron endowment and blood pressure: what do we really know? *Curr Hypertens Rep* **6**:133–139, 2004.
73. McMillan IC, Robinson JS. Developmental origins of the metabolic syndrome: prediction, plasticity and programming. *Physiol Rev* **85**(2):571–633, 2005.
74. Armitage JA, Khan IY, Taylor PD Nathanielsz PW, Poston L. Developmental programming of the metabolic syndrome by maternal nutritional imbalance: how strong is the evidence from experimental models in mammals? *Physiology* **561**:355–377, 2004.
75. Hughson M, Farris AB, 3rd, Douglas-Denton R, Hoy WE, Bertram JF. Glomerular number and size in autopsy kidneys: the relationship to birth weight. *Kidney Int* **63**:2113–2122, 2003.
76. Chugh SS, Wallner EI, Kanwar YS. Renal development in high-glucose ambience and diabetic embryopathy. *Semin Nephrol* **23**:583–592, 2003.
77. Fall CH, Yajnik CS, Rao S, Davies AA, Brown N, Farrant HJ. Micronutrients and fetal growth. *J Nutr* **133**:1747–1756S, 2003.
78. Shotan A, Widerhorn J, Hurst A, Elkayam U. Risks of angiotensin-converting enzyme inhibition during pregnancy: experimental and clinical evidence, potential mechanisms, and recommendations for use. *Am J Med* **96**:451–456, 1994.
79. Woods LL, Weeks DA, Rasch R, Nyengaard JR, Rasch R. Maternal protein restriction suppresses the newborn renin-angiotensin system and programs adult hypertension in rats. *Pediatr Res* **49**:460–467, 2001.
80. Woods LL, Weeks DA, Rasch R. Programming of adult blood pressure by maternal protein restriction: role of nephrogenesis. *Kidney Int* **65**:1339–1348, 2004.
81. Zimanyi MA, Bertram JF, Black MJ. Does a neprhon deficit predispose to sal-sensitive hypertension? *Kidney Blood Press Res* **27**(4):239–247, 2004.
82. Hoppe CC, Evans RG, Moritz KM et al. Combined prenatal and postnatal protein restriction influences adult kidney structure, function, and arterial pressure. *Am J Physiol (Regul Integr Comp Physiol)* **292**(1):R462–R469, 2007.
83. Lelievre-Pegorier M, Vilar J et al. Mild vitamin A deficiency leads to inborn nephron deficit in the rat. *Kidney Int* **54**:1455–1462, 1998.
84. Lisle SJ, Lewis RM, Petry CJ, Ozanne SE, Hales CN, Forhead AJ. Effect of maternal iron restriction during pregnancy on renal morphology in the adult rat offspring. *Br J Nutr* **90**:33–39, 2003.
85. Wintour EM, Moritz KM, Johnson K, Ricardo S, Samuel CS, Dodic M. Reduced nephron number in adult sheep hypertensive as a result of prenatal glucocorticoid treatment. *J Physiol* **549**:929–935, 2003.
86. Dickinson H, Walker DW, Wintour EM, Moritz K. Maternal dexamethasone treatment at midgestation reduces nephron number and alters renal gene expression in the fetal spiny mouse. *Am J Physiol Regul Integr Comp Physiol* **292**:R453–R461, 2007.
87. Singh RR, Cullen-McEwen LA, Kett MM et al. Prenatal corticosterone exposure results in altered AT1/AT2, nephron deficit and hypertension in the rat offspring. *J Physiol* **579**:503–513, 2007.
88. Oritz LA, Quan A, Weinberg A, Baum M. Effect of prenatal dexamethasone on rat renal development. *Kidney Int* **59**:1663–1669, 2001.
89. McMullen S, Langley-Evans SC. Maternal low-protein diet in rat pregnancy programs blood pressure through sex-specific mechanisms. *Am J Physiol Regul–Integr Comp Physiol* **288**:R85–R90, 2005.
90. Woods LL, Weeks DA. Prenatal programming of adult blood pressure: role of maternal corticosteroids. *Am J Physiol Regul Integr Comp Physiol* **289**:R955–R962, 2005.
91. Woods LL. Maternal glucocorticoids and prenatal programming of hypertension. *Am J Physiol Regul Integr Comp Physiol* **291**(4):R1069–R1075, 2006.
92. Schreuder MF, Nyengaard JR, Fodor M, vanWijk JA, Delmarre-van de Waal HA. Glomerular number and function are influenced by spontaneous and induced low birth weight in rats. *J Am Soc Nephrol* **16**(10):2913–2919, 2005.
93. Wlodek ME, Mibus A, Tan A, Siebel AL, Owens JA, Moritz KM. A normal lactational environment restores nephron endowment and prevents hypertension after placental restriction in the rat. *J Am Soc Nephrol* (in press), 2007.
94. Woods LL. Neonatal uninephrectomy causes hypertension in adult rats. *Am J Physiol Regul Integr Comp Physiol* **276**:R974–R978, 1999.
95. Woods LL, Weeks DA, Rasch R. Hypertension after neonatal uninephrectomy in rats precedes glomerular damage. *Hypertension* **38**(3):337–342, 2001.
96. Moritz KM, Wintour EM, Dodic M. Fetal uninephrectomy leads to postnatal hypertension and compromised renal function. *Hypertension* **39**:1071–1076, 2002.
97. Moritz KM, Jefferies A, Wong J, Wintour EM, Dodic M. Reduced renal reserve and increased cardiac output in female sheep uninephrectomised as fetuses. *Kidney Int* **67**:822–828, 2005.
98. Douglas-Denton R, Moritz KM, Bertram JF, Wintour EM. Compensatory renal growth after unilateral nephrectomy in the ovine fetus. *J Am Soc Nephrol* **13**:406–410, 2002.
99. Butkus A, Earnest L, Jeyaseelan K et al. Ovine AQP_2–cDNA cloning, ontogeny and control of renal gene expression. *Pediatr Nephrol* **13**:379–390, 1999.
100. Jeyaseelan K, Sepramaniam S, Armugam A, Wintour EM. Aquaporins: a promising target for drug development. *Expert Opin. Ther Targets* **10**:889–909, 2006.
101. Nicolini U, Fisk NM, Rodeck CH, Beacham J. Fetal urine biochemistry: an index of renal maturation and dysfunction. *Br J Obstet Gynaecol* **99**:46–50, 1992.
102. Nicolini U, Spelzini F. Invasive assessment of fetal renal abnormalities: urinalysis, fetal blood sampling and biopsy. *Prenatal Diagn* **21**(11):964–969, 2001.
103. Konda R, Sakai K, Ota S, Takeda A, Orikasa S. Follow-up study of renal function in children with reflux nephropathy after resolution of vesicoureteral reflux. *J Urol* **157**:975–979, 1997.
104. Oliveira FR, Barros EG, Magalhaes JA. Biochemical profile of amniotic fluid for the assessment of fetal and renal development. *Braz J Med Biol Res* **35**(2):215–222, 2002.
105. Mandelbrot L, Dumez Y, Muller F. Prenatal prediction of renal function in fetal obstructive uropathies. *J Perinat Med* **19**:283–287, 1991.
106. Huland H, Gonnermann D, Werner B, Possin U. A new test to predict reversibility of hydronephrotic atrophy after stable partial unilateral ureteral obstruction. *J Urol* **140**:1591–1594, 1988.
107. Carr MC, Peters CA, Retik AB, Mandell J. Urinary levels of renal tubular enzyme *N*-acetyl-β-D-glucosaminidase in relation to grade of vesicoureteral reflux. *J Urol* **146**:654–656, 1991.
108. Foxall PJD, Bewley S, Neild GH, Rodeck CH, Nicholson JK. Analysis of fetal and neonatal urine using proton nuclear magnetic resonance spectroscopy. *Arch Dis Child* **73**:F153–F157, 1995.
109. Sizeland PCB, Chambers ST, Lever M, Bason LM, Robson RA. Organic osmolytes in human and other mammalian kidneys. *Kidney Int* **43**:448–454, 1993.
110. Miguelez J, Bunduki V, Yoshizaki CT et al. Fetal obstructive uropathy: is urine sampling useful for prenatal counseling. *Prenat Diagn* **26**(1):81–84.

111. Lumbers ER. Functions of the renin–angiotensin system during development. *Clin Exp Pharmacol Physiol* **22**:499–505, 1995.
112. Vehaskari VM, Stewart T, Lafont D, Soyez C, Seth D, Manning J. Kidney angiotensin and angiotensin receptor expression in prenatally programmed hypertension. *Am J Physiol Renal Physiol* **287**:F262–F267, 2004.
113. Yosypiv IV, El-Dahr WE. Role of the renin-angiotensin system in the development of the uteric bud and renal collecting system. *Pediatric Nephrol* **20**:1219–1229, 2005.
114. Tufro-McReddie A, Romano LM, Harris JM, Ferder L, Gomez RA. Angiotensin II regulates nephrogenesis and renal vascular development. *Am J Physiol Renal Physiol* **269**:F110–F115, 1995.
115. Welham SJ, Wade A, Woolf AS. Protein restriction in pregnancy is associated with increased apoptosis of mesenchymal cells at the start of rat metanephrogenesis. *Kidney Int* **61**:1231–1242, 2002.
116. Welham S, Riley PR, Wade A, Hubank M, Woolf AS. Maternal diet programs embryonic kidney gene expression. *Physiol Genomics* **22**:48–56, 2005.
117. Moritz KM, Butkus A, Hantzis V, Peers A, Wintour EM, Dodic M. Prolonged low dose dexamethasone in early gestation has no long term deleterious effect on normal ovine fetuses. *Endocrinology* **143**:1159–1165, 2002.
118. Sahajpal V, Ashton N. Renal function and angiotensin AT1 receptor expression in young rats following intrauterine exposure to a maternal low-protein diet. *Clin Sci* **104**:607–614, 2003.
119. Ichihara A, Kobori U, Nishiyama A, Navar LG. Renal renin-angiotensin system. *Contrib Nephrol* **143**:117–130, 2004.
120. Seikaly MG, Arant BS. Development of renal hemodynamics: glomerular filtration and renal blood flow. *Clin Perinatol* **19**:1–13, 1992.
121. Komhoff M, Hermann-Josef G, Thomas K, Hennsjoerg W, Seyberth HW, Nusing RM. Localization of cyclooxygenase-1 and 2 in adult and fetal human kidney: implications for renal function. *Am J Physiol Renal Physiol* **272**:F460–F468, 1997.
122. Komhoff M, Wang JL et al. Cyclooxygenase-2-selective inhibitors impair glomerulogenesis and renal cortical development. *Kidney Int* **57**:414–422, 2000.
123. Kirshon B, Mari G, Moise KJ. Indomethacin therapy in the treatment of symptomatic polyhydramnios. *Obstet Gynecol* **75**:202–205, 1990.
124. Kirshon B, Moise KJ, Wasserstrum N, Ou C, Huhta JC. Influence of short-term indomethacin therapy on fetal urine output. *Obstet Gynecol* **72**:51–53, 1988.
125. Mamopoulos M, Assimakopoulos E, Reece A, Andreou A, Zheng X, Mantalenakis S. Maternal indomethacin therapy in the treatment of polyhydramnios. *Am J Obstet Gynecol* **162**:1225–1229, 1990.
126. Groom KM, Shennan AH, Jones BA, Seed P, Bennett PR. TOCOX-a randomized, double-blind, placebo-controlled trial of rofecoxib (a COX-2-specific prostaglandin inhibitor) for the prevention of preterm delivery in women at high risk. *Br J Obstet Gynaecol* **112**:725-730.
127. Olson DM, Ammann C. Role of the prostaglandins in labour and prostaglandin receptor inhibitors in the prevention of preterm labour. *Front Biosci* **12**:1329–1343, 2007.
128. Bain AD, Scott JS. Renal agenesis and severe urinary tract dysplasia: a review of 50 cases with a particular reference to the associated abnormalities. *Br Med J* i:841–846, 1960.
129. Potter EL. Bilateral absence of ureters and kidneys. *Obstet Gynecol* **25**:3–12, 1965.
130. Anderson DF, Barbera A, Faber JJ. Substantial reductions in blood pressure after bilateral nephrectomy in fetal sheep. *Am J Physiol* **266**:H17–H20, 1994.
131. Gibson KJ, Lumbers ER. The effects of bilateral nephrectomy on the volume and composition of fetal body fluids. *Proc Austral Soc Med.Res* Abstract 032, 1993.
132. Moritz KM, Macris M, Talbo G, Wintour EM. Foetal fluid balance and hormone status following nephrectomy in the foetal sheep. *Clin Exp Pharmacol Physiol* **26**:857–864, 1999.
133. Karnak I, Adrian F, Tanyel FC et al. The effects of nephrectomy on the developing fetus. *Eur J Pediatr Surg* **6**:270–273, 1996.
134. Rogers SA, Miller SB, Hammerman MR. Growth hormone stimulates *IGF-I* gene expression in isolated rat renal collecting duct. *Am J Physiol Renal Physiol* **259**:F474–F479, 1990.
135. Rogers SA, Miller SB, Hammerman MR. Enhanced renal IGF-I expression following partial kidney infarction. *Am J Physiol Renal Physiol* **264**:F963–F967, 1993.
136. Iwamoto HS, McConnell CJ. Effects of fetal nephrectomy on insulin-like growth factors and their binding proteins in sheep. *Biol Neonate* **71**:92–101, 1997.
137. Beanland C, Browne C, Young R, Owens J, Walton P, Thorburn G. Fetal plasma insulin-like growth factor-binding protein-3 concentrations are elevated following bilateral nephrectomy in fetal sheep. *Reprod. Fertil Dev* **7**:345–349, 1995.
138. Pope J, 4th, Brock J, 3rd, Adams M, Stephens F, Ichikawa I. How they begin and how they end: classic and new theories for the development and deterioration of congenital anomalies of the kidney and urinary tract, CAKUT. *J Am Soc Nephrol* **9**:2018–2028, 1999.
139. Miyazaki Y, Ichikawa I. Ontogeny of congenital anomalies of the kidney and urinary tract, CAKUT. *Pediatr Int* **45**: 598–604, 2003.
140. Woolf AS, Price KL, Scambler PJ, Winyard PJ. Evolving concepts in human renal dysplasia. *J Am Soc Nephrol* **15**:998–1007, 2004.
141. Miyazaki Y, Tsuchida S, Nishimura H et al. Angiotensin induces the urinary peristaltic machinery during the perinatal period. *J Clin Invest* **102**: 1489–1497, 1998.
142. Airik R, Bussen M, Singh MK, Petry M, Kispert A. Tbx18 regulates the development of the ureteral mesenchyme. *J Clin Invest* **116**:663–674, 2006.
143. Mahoney ZX, Sammut B, Xavier RJ et al. Discs-large homolog 1 regulates smooth muscle orientation in the mouse ureter. *Proc Natl Acad Sci USA* **103**:19872–19877, 2006.
144. Mei-Zahav M, Korzets Z, Cohen I et al. Ambulatory blood pressure monitoring in children with a solitary kidney – a comparison between unilateral renal agenesis and uninephrectory. *Blood Press Monit* **6**:263–267, 2001.
145. Dursun H, Bayazit AK, Cengiz N et al. Ambulatory blood pressure monitoring and renal functions in children with a solitary kidney. *Pediatr Nephrol* **22**:559–564, 2007.
146. Seeman T, Patzer L, John U et al. Blood pressure, renal function and proteinuria in children with unilateral renal agenesis. *Kidney Blood Press Res* **29**:210–215, 2006.
147. Gonzalez E, Gutierrez E, Morales E et al. Factors influencing the progression of renal damage in patients with unilateral renal agenesis and remnant kidney. *Kidney Int* **68**:263–270, 2005.

CHAPTER

13 Maternal medicines and the fetus

David Williams and Lila Mayahi

KEY POINTS

- A clinician prescribing medicines in pregnancy often needs to make a unique decision about the potential harm to the fetus of a drug and the potential harm to mother and fetus of leaving the condition untreated
- With few notable exceptions, underlying maternal diseases are more likely to cause fetal malformations than the drug prescribed for treatment
- Very few drugs are known to be teratogenic (see Table 13.1)
- Major congenital malformations affect 3–4% of the general population
- If possible, prescribe the lowest *effective* dose of a drug with a proven record of safety in pregnancy
- Support and guidance for prescribing decisions in pregnancy is most likely to come from medical case series and registries than from the pharmaceutical industry

INTRODUCTION

Drug treatment of maternal disease during pregnancy requires the clinician to make a judgment between potential harm to the fetus from the drug and potential harm to the mother *and* fetus from leaving the maternal condition untreated. The clinician has limited information on which to make this judgment. Pharmaceutical companies rarely support the use of a drug for an otherwise licensed indication in pregnant women. A sentiment reinforced by a strong memory of the consequences that followed those very few drugs that have been shown to be teratogenic.

It is difficult to obtain compelling evidence of 'no harm' to a human fetus. Pregnant women are rarely included in clinical trials. Observational studies that aim to identify birth defects associated with individual drugs need large numbers of treated women in order to identify an effect that is greater than the background prevalence. Yet the cost of not identifying a teratogenic drug before it does harm can be enormous, both in personal terms to the victim and in financial terms to the pharmaceutical company. In this chapter, we review the issues surrounding prescribing in pregnancy and discuss the pharmaceutical management of maternal conditions and their potential impact on the developing fetus.

WHAT IS A TERATOGEN?

A teratogen is a drug, chemical, infectious disease or environmental agent that interferes with the normal development of a fetus and results in pregnancy loss, congenital malformation, growth restriction or behavioral changes in the neonate. For a causal relationship to be confirmed, the teratogen needs reproducibly to cause a specific effect in a dose-dependent manner. These criteria are even more difficult to fulfil because most teratogenic drugs only cause a relatively small increased risk over and above that observed in a western population (Table 13.1)[1].

Background rates of adverse pregnancy outcomes[1] are estimated as follows:

- spontaneous abortion (in recognized pregnancies) 15%
- premature delivery 6–10%
- major congenital malformations 4%
- additional minor malformations 5%.

However, these will vary in different populations and at different maternal ages.

IDENTIFYING A TERATOGEN

Most information on drug-induced congenital anomalies is derived from post-marketing surveillance. Case reports of adverse drug outcomes go to government agencies, e.g. FDA in USA and MHRA in UK. Despite limitations, case reports have led to the identification of teratogenic drugs. Epidemiological studies also provide useful information, but tend towards bias with patient selection and outcome. When concern is raised from repeated case reports or epidemiological studies, registries

Table 13.1 **Drugs with proven teratogenic effects in humans**

Drug	*Teratogenic effects*
Cardiovascular system	
Angiotensin-converting enzyme inhibitors, angiotensin II receptor blockers	Decreased skull ossification, renal tubular dysgenesis, neural and cardiac defects
Warfarin	Fetal warfarin syndrome. Optic atrophy, cataracts, mental retardation, microcephaly, microphthalmia, Dandy–Walker syndrome
Statins	Weak, possible teratogen in first trimester. Limb deformities, neural tube defect including spina bifida
Endocrine	
Methimazole	Care-reports of aplasia cutis only
Androgens such as danazol	Masculinization of female fetus
Diethylstilbestrol	Vaginal carcinoma and other genitourinary defects in female offspring and increased risk of hypospadia in male offspring
Gastrointestinal	
Misoprostol	Moebius sequence
Neurology and psychiatry	
Carbamazepine	Craniofacial abnormalities, growth retardation, neural tube defects, fingernail hypoplasia
Phenytoin	Fetal hydantoin syndrome including heart defect, low nasal bridge, growth retardation, nail hypoplasia, mental retardation
Valproic acid	Spina bifida, facial anomalies, slow development, microcephaly, CNS and cardiac defects
Lithium	Ebstein's anomaly, other cardiac defects
Dermatology	
Retinoids (isotretinoin and etretinate)	Heart defect, spontaneous abortion, microtia, microcephalus, hydrocephalus, deformity of ears, face, limbs, liver, cognitive defects, thymic hypoplasia
Antibacterial	
Aminoglycosides	VIII cranial nerve damage
Tetracyclines	Weakened fetal bone and tooth enamel dysplasia, permanent tooth discoloration
Trimethoprim	Possible neural tube defects in first trimester
Antiretroviral	
Zidovudine	Hypospadia
Vitamins	
Vitamin A (greater than 25 000 IU/day)	Microtia, craniofacial, CNS and cardiac anomalies, bowel atresia, limb reductions, urinary tract defects
Others	
Alcohol	Fetal alcohol syndrome
Antimetabolites	Growth retardation, malformation of ear, eye, nose, cleft palate, malformation of extremities, fingers, brain, skull
Alkylating agents, e.g. busulphan, cyclophosphamide	Growth retardation, cleft palate, microphthalmia, cloudy cornea, agenesis of kidney, cardiac defects
Cocaine	Bowel atresia, defects of genitourinary system, heart, limbs, face
Ergometrine (high doses)	Intestinal atresia, cerebral atrophy and multiple arthrogryposis
Thalidomide	Anomalies of ears, teeth, eyes, intestine, limbs, heart, kidney, deafness

can be set up to document pregnancy outcome for individual drugs or classes of drugs. Further up-to-date information about teratogens can be found on two well-linked websites:

1. Organisation of Teratology Information Specialists (OTIS) http://www.otispregnancy.org/
2. International Birth defects Informations Systems (IBIS) http://www.ibis-birthdefects.org/start/index.htm

HOW COMMON ARE DRUG-INDUCED EFFECTS ON THE FETUS?

Only a small fraction of congenital malformations (0.1–0.2% of live births) can be attributed to maternal drug use. Despite this reassuring epidemiological evidence, there are many well-recognized classes of drugs which can harm the fetus and cause life-long problems for the victim and their family.

PRE-EXISTING MATERNAL DISEASE AND CONGENITAL MALFORMATION

More often the maternal condition for which treatment is given is responsible for fetal harm. Up to 10% of congenital malformations are secondary to maternal disease, for example, diabetes mellitus, the maternal condition most frequently associated with congenital abnormalities, in particular with poor blood glucose control during the first trimester. Congenital heart lesions run in families and now that corrective cardiac surgery allows many women to reach a fertile age and reproduce, there are increasing numbers of affected fetuses and infants. Maternal infections such as rubella, chicken pox and toxoplasmosis are all associated with congenital malformations (see Chapter 44).

Medication for maternal disease may therefore be inappropriately blamed for a major congenital malformation to which the fetus was vulnerable due to a pre-existing or transient maternal condition, an inherited risk or novel mutation.

DRUG METABOLISM DURING PREGNANCY

During pregnancy, major maternal physiological changes alter drug metabolism and have an impact on drug concentration. These changes include reduced bowel motility and protein binding, altered hepatic metabolism, increased plasma volume, cardiac output and renal excretion[2]. Depending on whether the drug is predominantly metabolized, excreted or protein bound will have an effect on how much passes across the placenta from the maternal circulation to the fetus.

THE PLACENTA

The placenta is a mechanical barrier which blocks the passage of cells (e.g. erythrocytes, malaria parasites) and large molecules between mother and fetus, but most drugs eventually pass across its lipid membrane by passive diffusion. Drugs which pass across the placenta most quickly are of high lipid solubility, low molecular weight and have reduced protein binding and slow elimination from the maternal circulation.

There are several other ways in which drugs pass across the placenta. These include passive diffusion, active transfer, facilitated diffusion, phagocytosis and pinocytosis[3]. Placental transporters, e.g. multidrug resistance proteins, P-glycoprotein and breast cancer resistance proteins, have a role in effluxing drugs such as glyburide and protease inhibitors from the fetal circulation[4]. The placenta is also filled with enzymes that degrade drugs and hormones. For example, thyroxine is metabolized by type 3 iodothyronine deiodinase (D3) and reduces uteroplacental passage of maternal thyroxine, whether endogenous or supplemental[5].

TIMING AND DOSING OF DRUG EXPOSURE DURING PREGNANCY

It has been suggested that the toxic effects of fetal exposure to drugs be organized into 5 categories that relate to the timing of drug use:

1. intrauterine death
2. physical malformation
3. growth impairment
4. behavioral teratology
5. neonatal toxicity[6].

Exposure to a teratogen in the 14 days post conception, is likely to result in miscarriage. Drug exposure during days 14–35 is the time when there will be greatest effect on structural and neurochemical development[7]. However, maternal drugs taken throughout pregnancy can have an impact on fetal neurodevelopment that is only evident when the infant is found to have behavioral problems. Maternal medicines taken near delivery can have a direct toxic effect on the neonate, e.g. benzodiazepines at term may cause transient sedation of the neonate and then withdrawal symptoms[8]. Paroxetine has been weakly associated with congenital malformations at the time of organogenesis in the first trimester and with persistent pulmonary hypertension of the neonate in the third trimester (see later).

The risk of a drug-induced effect is also associated with the dose of drug taken. A dose-related teratogenic effect has been observed with sodium valproate[9], warfarin[10] and paroxetine[11] (see later). Furthermore, the concentration or binding of a drug in the fetal circulation may differ from that in the maternal circulation with therapeutic consequences that may have a significant effect on fetal health, e.g. warfarin appears to be more potent in the fetal circulation than in the maternal[12].

The USA Food and Drug Administration (FDA) has developed categories for drug use in pregnancy (Table 13.2).

GENERAL PRINCIPLES OF PRESCRIBING IN PREGNANCY

If a drug needs to be given in pregnancy, the lowest effective dose for the shortest duration of time should be chosen. This does not mean an ineffectively low dose, which is so often prescribed by the uncertain clinician. If possible, multidrug prescribing should be avoided. Accumulating clinical experience about the safety of new drugs in pregnancy takes many years. Prescribing older drugs, for which there is more clinical experience in pregnancy, is preferable to equipotent newer drugs for which there is less knowledge of safety. If newer drugs

Table 13.2 USA Food and Drug Administration (FDA) categories for drug use in pregnancy

Category	*Interpretation*
A	Adequate, well-controlled studies in pregnant women have not shown an increased risk of fetal abnormalities to the fetus in any trimester of pregnancy
B	Animal studies have revealed no evidence of harm to the fetus; however, there are no adequate and well-controlled studies in pregnant women *or* Animal studies have shown an adverse effect, but adequate and well-controlled studies in pregnant women have failed to demonstrate a risk to the fetus in any trimester
C	Animal studies have shown an adverse effect and there are no adequate and well-controlled studies in pregnant women *or* No animal studies have been conducted and there are no adequate and well-controlled studies in pregnant women
D	Adequate well-controlled or observational studies in pregnant women have demonstrated a risk to the fetus. However, the benefits of therapy may outweigh the potential risk. For example, the drug may be acceptable if needed in a life-threatening situation or serious disease for which safer drugs cannot be used or are ineffective
X	Adequate well-controlled or observational studies in animals or pregnant women have demonstrated positive evidence of fetal abnormalities or risks. The use of the product is contraindicated in women who are or may become pregnant

are used, then all adverse outcomes must be reported, whether to government prescribing agencies or established drug registries. Adding to the cumulative knowledge of a drug's potential for harm should be considered part of our clinical responsibility.

HYPERTENSION

Hypertension is one of the most common medical disorders during pregnancy, with an estimated incidence of 6–8% of all pregnancies[13,14].

Hypertension in pregnancy can be divided into three categories:

1. chronic hypertension, pre-dating and continuing through pregnancy
2. gestational hypertension or pregnancy-induced hypertension, i.e. onset of isolated hypertension in the second half of pregnancy
3. pre-eclampsia (new onset hypertension >140/90 mmHg and >300 mg/24 h[15].

Antihypertensive medication

Maternal indication

There is no consensus as to the target level of blood pressure (BP) needed for optimum maternal and fetal outcome. This is due to a 'trade-off' between the lower BP that would protect the mother from cardiovascular end-organ damage, but have a negative effect on fetal growth and a higher BP that allows better uteroplacental perfusion, but increases maternal cardiovascular risk.

Treatment of mild to moderate BP (140–169/90–110 mmHg) halves the risk of progression to severe hypertension[16]. Beta-blockers appear to be more effective than methyldopa in reducing progression to severe hypertension[16]. However, treatment of mild to moderate hypertension has no effect on the prevention of pre-eclampsia, fetal or neonatal death, small-for-gestational-age infants or preterm delivery[16].

Treatment of pregnancy-induced hypertension (PIH) has not prevented development of pre-eclampsia or improved fetal outcome[17]. Given the multisystem nature of pre-eclampsia, these results are not surprising as lowering the blood pressure would not deal with the global pathophysiology of this disease. Most importantly, there is concern that treatment of hypertension to the same target levels as required for long-term cardiovascular protection leads to placental hypoperfusion and fetal growth restriction[18]. Nevertheless, in the setting of severe hypertension, there is a definite role for pharmacological treatment[19].

It is likely that antihypertensive drugs will cause altered fetal and neonatal heart rate, secondary to the level of maternal BP, rather than due to a direct toxic effect on the fetus. Lowering maternal BP too precipitously with any antihypertensive agent can cause fetal bradycardia[20].

Pre-eclampsia

The aim of treatment in cases of pre-eclampsia remote from term (<32 weeks) is to prolong pregnancy without harming the mother. Conservative treatment of early pre-eclampsia can prolong pregnancy by 8–11 days using antihypertensive drugs and steroids for fetal lung maturity[18,21].

Antihypertensive drugs and pregnancy

Methyldopa

There is no single antihypertensive agent that consistently performs better than any other in the management of hypertension in pregnancy. The widespread use of methyldopa has followed proof that it is not harmful to the developing fetus, rather than because of improved efficacy. Indeed, methyldopa has been relegated to a third/fourth line antihypertensive outside of pregnancy due to the emergence of more effective and better tolerated drugs.

Maternal indication

Methyldopa is the most commonly used antihypertensive to treat hypertension in pregnancy. It is a centrally acting antihypertensive that reduces sympathetic discharge.

Maternal and fetal outcome

Short-term treatment with methyldopa in the third trimester does not affect uteroplacental or fetal hemodynamics[22]. In addition, there are no short-term effects on the neonate[23] nor long-term effects during infancy[24] for offspring born to mothers who took methyldopa throughout pregnancy. However, none of the randomized trials has shown superiority in primary end point in lowering BP or prevention of pre-eclampsia, placental abruption or preterm delivery when compared to other antihypertensives, such as labetolol[23]. Methyldopa causes significant side effects in the mother, such as somnolence and lethargy and, therefore, alternative treatments may be preferred. A loading dose of methyldopa aggravates this side effect without speeding up the antihypertensive effect.

Beta-blockers

Beta-blockers are competitive antagonists of beta-adrenoceptors. They are selective for B1 or B2 receptors or non-selective where they work on both types. Examples of selective B1 antagonists include metoprolol and atenolol. While labetolol is a non-selective beta-blocker with partial alpha-blocker activity.

Maternal and fetal outcome

Beta-blockers cross the placenta and are found in breast milk. When beta-blockers are used to treat mild to moderate hypertension in pregnancy, there is a lower risk of severe hypertension or the need for additional antihypertensive agent compared to placebo[16]. Beta-blockers have been associated with an increased risk of small-for-gestational-age infants, but many of these studies used very high doses of beta-blocker, e.g. atenolol 200 mg daily[25]. It is likely that depression of maternal cardiac output with overtreatment of hypertension will reduce uteroplacental blood flow and pressure. More recently, comparison between beta-blockers and methyldopa revealed equal efficacy and safety[26].

The data on specific beta-blocker use in pregnancy are too limited to make any firm conclusions. The selective B1 agonist atenolol (25–100 mg) has been reported to have reduced the incidence of severe hypertension and preterm delivery, but it was the failure to adjust the dose according to BP response that led to an excessive fall in cardiac output that was associated with reduced fetal growth[27]. Maybe for this reason atenolol taken from the time of conception or during the first trimester of pregnancy is associated with a low birth weight, independent of an effect of superimposed pre-eclampsia[28,29].

Parenteral labetolol can be given at the time of a hypertensive crisis and is well tolerated by fetal and maternal hemodynamics. Labetalol appears to be an effective agent in the management of mild to moderate pregnancy-induced hypertension. The data from this study suggest possible advantages and no apparent disadvantages for the fetus during its use[30]. It is concluded that atenolol and labetolol are safe and they are usually effective in the control of the hypertension complicating pregnancy. Labetolol has not been associated with fetal growth restriction to the same extent as atenolol, possibly because of its less specific and less potent effects[31].

Calcium channel blockers

Maternal indication

Calcium channel blockers are used for the management of systemic hypertension, vessel spasm associated with subarachnoid hemorrhage, arrhythmias and anti-angina (see more details under anti-arrhythmics). Calcium channel blockers, such as nifedipine and amlodipine, inhibit entry of calcium into cells leading to vasodilatation and hypotension. They also have a negatively inotropic effect on the myocardium and hence reduce its oxygen consumption. As an anti-arrhythmic, they work by shortening the refractory period. Diltiazem and verapamil are used for this latter indication.

Maternal and fetal outcome

Nifedipine slow release (SR) (40–120 mg per day) is the most commonly used calcium channel blocker for treatment of hypertension. It is effective in treatment of chronic hypertension and in acute severe cases. Capsules of nifedipine that are broken in the mouth for a rapid effect absorbed through the buccal mucosa are dangerous as they can cause a precipitous fall in BP, especially when given to someone taking magnesium sulfate[32]. Calcium channel blockers tend to be initiated in late pregnancy, but have been safely used throughout pregnancy without associated tetratogenic risks[33]. Nicardipine was shown to be as effective as labetolol in reducing BP in severe hypertension, and well tolerated, although moderate maternal tachycardia was noted with nicardipine[34].

Hydralazine

Maternal indication

Hydralazine is a centrally acting vasodilator that has been effectively used in the management of severe hypertension for many years. However, available data do not support its use as a first-line treatment in severe hypertension in pregnancy. When compared to labetolol or nifedipine SR, hydralazine appears to be inferior in outcome, not only in effecting a sustained reduction in BP, but also in its association with greater numbers of cesarean sections and placental abruptions[35].

Diuretics

Maternal indications

Diuretics are widely used in the management of systemic hypertension, but have not been widely used in pregnancy because they attenuate the healthy increase in maternal plasma volume, especially during pre-eclampsia. Loop diuretics are used for management of pulmonary edema.

Maternal and fetal outcome

Women with pre-eclampsia are already volume depleted, despite interstitial edema. Reducing the intravascular volume would further compromise placental insufficiency as well as aggravating hypertension by stimulating the renin–angiotension system. Although a reduction in plasma volume due to diuretics has not been associated with increased perinatal morbidity[36], some adverse effects in mother and fetus have made clinicians less inclined to use this class of medication[37]. Diuretic use has been associated with a difference in neonatal birth weight and preterm deliveries but this risk depends upon the indication for use. For example, pregnant women with hypertension had reduced birth weight[38]. Pregnancy does not preclude the use of diuretics to reduce or control blood pressure in women whose hypertension predated conception or manifested before mid-pregnancy. Diuretics are therefore safe and efficacious agents that can markedly potentiate the response to other antihypertensive agents and are not contraindicated in pregnancy except in settings where utero-placental perfusion is already reduced, e.g. pre-eclampsia and intrauterine growth restriction.

Other antihypertensives

Angiotensin-converting enzyme inhibitors and angiotensin II receptor antagonists (sartans)

Angiotensin-converting enzyme inhibitors (ACE inhibitors) and angiotensin II receptor antagonists (sartans) are effective antihypertensive drugs widely used outside of pregnancy, especially in association with renal disease of almost any etiology, apart from renal artery stenosis. However, they are not recommended during pregnancy as they are teratogenic[39]. Women taking ACE inhibitors and who are planning pregnancy should therefore switch to another antihypertensive if it is considered equally efficacious. Others, who may miss the protective effect of ACE inhibitors unless they are able to conceive quickly, can be advised to stop the ACE inhibitor as soon as they know they are pregnant, in the first trimester[39].

ACE inhibitors prescribed to the mother are associated with fetal cardiac and neurological abnormalities when given in the first trimester and reduced renal blood flow, oligohydramnios and renal failure, if prescribed in the second and third trimesters[40].

Alpha blockers, e.g. prazosin[41], have a good safety profile in pregnancy. Vasodilators such as *minoxidil*[42,43] are associated with fetal abnormalities and are to be avoided.

Adjuvant to antihypertensive or prophylactic treatment

Calcium supplementation

A Cochrane meta-analysis on calcium supplementation during pregnancy has shown a reduction in the risk of pre-eclampsia compared to placebo. The effects are greatest for women at high risk of hypertension and in women with low baseline calcium dietary intake. Calcium supplementation reduced the risk of having lighter than 2500 g babies and showed a modest reduction in systolic and diastolic BP. The recommendation from this review is to consider calcium supplementation, although a positive impact on maternal and fetal morbidity has not been confirmed[44].

Low-dose aspirin in pre-eclampsia

(See next section).

A summary of antihypertensive medication and their commonly prescribed dosage is given in Table 13.3.

Vitamin supplementation

Antioxidant vitamins, vitamin C (1000 mg) and vitamin E (400 IU), given from mid-pregnancy, had been shown to reduce the risk of later pre-eclampsia in a small study[106]. However, subsequent larger studies have failed to show benefit[107]. Indeed, not only was there no difference in the rate of pre-eclampsia, there were more low-birth-weight babies in the mothers who received antioxidant vitamins. This observation has been confirmed in a systematic review that has shown that there is no risk reduction of pre-eclampsia, neonatal loss, small-for-gestation infants, but alarmingly a suggestion of greater risk for preterm birth in the women who received these vitamins[108]. Vitamin supplementation should not be used in pregnancy unless new evidence comes to support its use, possibly at lower doses from randomized trials.

Table 13.3 **Summary of antihypertensive medication and their commonly prescribed dosage**

Drug	*Dose*	*Comments*
Methyldopa	500–1000 mg twice/three times daily	A safe drug in pregnancy, but with a poor side-effect profile
Labetolol	100–400 mg twice/three times daily	Similar in efficacy and safety to methyldopa and better tolerated
Beta-blockers	Various	Fetal bradycardia, low birth weight, when excessively used throughout pregnancy
Calcium channel blockers	Various	Nifedipine SR, a safe and effective treatment
Alpha-blockers	Various	Small, but reassuring safety data in pregnancy
Alpha 2 agonist (clonidine)	0.1–0.8 mg bd/qds	Limited data
Thiazide diuretics	Various	Reduced volume expansion, suggestion of fetal growth restriction
Angiotensin Converting Enzyme Inhibitor (ACEI)	Contraindicated	Fetal abnormalities in all trimesters. Can stop immediately *after* pregnancy diagnosis
All blockers	Contraindicated	Anuria and renal failure in fetus and fetal abnormalities

ANTICOAGULATION AND ANTIPLATELET AGENTS

Aspirin low dose (60–150 mg daily)

Aspirin inhibits thromboxane A2 in the cyclo-oxygenase pathway of arachidonic acid and, hence, prevents platelet aggregation. In addition, thromboxane A2 is a mediator of endothelium dysfunction and promotes vasoconstriction. Therefore, inhibition of this mediator has been positively associated with improved endothelial function and blood flow.

Pre-eclampsia

There is evidence that, at least in part, endothelial dysfunction is responsible for pre-eclampsia. By inhibiting thromboxane A (TAX2), not only does aspirin prevent platelet aggregation, but it also prevents the vasocontrictive effect of TAX2 and therefore can improve endothelial function. On this hypothesis, several trials have been conducted. Although some earlier studies were cautious about use of aspirin in prevention of pre-eclampsia[45–47,] more recent data based on larger studies and systematic reviews favor the use of low-dose aspirin in women at high risk of pre-eclmpsia.[48,49] Treatment with low-dose aspirin, initiated at 12–14 weeks of gestation, reduces the frequency of pregnancy-induced hypertension and pre-eclampsia and hypertension[50]. The most recent data from a meta-analysis of individual patient data have shown a significant 10% reduction in the relative risk of both pre-eclampsia and preterm birth before 34 weeks' gestation in patients on antiplatetelet agents compared with control. The data indicated a 10% reduction in the relative risk of the baby being small for gestational age and a 9% reduction in the relative risk of stillbirth or baby death before discharge. One of the early concerns about the use of antiplatelet agents during pregnancy was the possibility of an increase in bleeding problems for mother and fetus. This concern has been allayed by results from trials, including two that reported follow-up of the children at around 2 years of age and the results of a case-control study that indicate that aspirin use in early pregnancy does not result in an increased risk of congenital abnormalities in infants[50,51]. No change in the risk of postpartum or antepartum hemorrhage between women on antiplatelet agents and controls was found, nor was there an effect on infant bleeding[52]. Encouragingly, no adverse outcome in respect of gestation and birth weight is reported[53].

A follow-up study of the neonates of the CLASP study for 18 months, where low-dose aspirin was started after the first trimester, showed no adverse effects in respect of congenital malformations, neuromotor or developmental delay[54]. Available evidence suggests that low-dose aspirin (<150 mg/day) during the second and third trimesters is safe for both mother and fetus. Postpartum use of low-dose aspirin by breast-feeding mother is also safe for the neonate.

Concerns of aspirin and fetal development and complications

Aspirin crosses the placenta[55,56]. Early studies on ingestion of anti-inflammatory dose of aspirin by pregnant women has been associated with an increased risk of fetal and neonatal hemorrhage[57,58]. It has also been demonstrated that low-dose aspirin has antiplatelet effects on the fetus and newborn[59], although no major hemorrhages were observed in a large number of infants born to mothers who used low-dose aspirin as prophylaxis for pre-eclampsia[60,61].

Low-dose aspirin in pregnancy can be considered a safe drug without any adverse effect on the newborn. Several studies in mothers exposed to low-dose aspirin have shown a significantly lower thromboxane concentration on the first day of life, however, on the fourth day the level of serum thromboxane in the cases exposed reached the values of the unexposed ones[62].

No increased risk of congenital malformation was found from a large case-control data set from Hungary. A systematic review and a retrospective study reported on an increase in cases of gastroschisis with use of aspirin in the first trimester, although the dose is unclear in these reports[63,64].

Daily administration of low-dose aspirin during the second and third trimesters of pregnancy does not alter uteroplacental or fetoplacental hemodynamics and does not appear to cause significant constriction of the ductus arteriosus[65,66].

Daily maternal ingestion of 60 mg of aspirin does not decrease fetal urine output or amniotic fluid volume[67].

Heparin, warfarin and thrombolytics

These drugs are used as prophylaxis against thrombosis, for treatment of thromboembolic disease and as rescue therapy following coronary artery disease or pulmonary embolus. Low molecular weight heparin, unfractionated heparin and thrombolytic drugs do not cross the placenta and appear safe to use in pregnancy, but warfarin does cross the placenta and can cause teratogenic harm and later fetal bleeding.

Heparin

Neither unfractionated heparin (UFH) nor low molecular weight heparin (LMWH) cross the placenta[68,69] or are secreted in breast milk, and there is no evidence of teratogenesis or risk of fetal bleeding with these drugs. Prolonged use of UFH in pregnancy is associated with bone demineralization, symptomatic osteoporosis and heparin-induced thrombocytopenia (HIT) in the mother. LMWH has substantially less effect on bone mineral density and carries a substantially lower risk of HIT than UFH. LMWH is now the anticoagulant of choice in pregnancy; its safety and efficacy have been demonstrated in observational studies[70–72] and systematic reviews[73]. The lack of evidence of HIT in these studies and reviews supports the recent recommendation that platelet count need not be monitored in pregnant women treated exclusively with LMWH and not previously exposed to UFH. However, these data relate predominantly to dalteparin, enoxaparin and nadroparin; less data are available on other LMWHs, such as tinzaparin.

Warfarin

Risks of warfarin to the fetus are well established. It causes a fetopathy as well as major bleeds in mother and fetus. Coumarins, such as warfarin, are teratogenic in the first trimester and are associated with a risk of fetal bleeding in the second and third trimesters[74,75]. Coumarin embryopathy is associated with coumarin exposure between 6 and 9 weeks' gestation and occurs in about 5% of embryos exposed during that period[74]. The risk appears to be dose dependent[10]. Mid-facial hypoplasia and other skeletal abnormalities are associated with ectopic calcification. Prenatal exposure to coumarins is also associated with an increased risk of minor neurological dysfunction and low intelligence[76]. Coumarins are not secreted in breast milk in clinically significant concentrations and are safe to use during lactation.

Thrombolysis

Healthy pregnancy is a procoagulant state. Deep vein thrombosis and pulmonary embolus are 4–6 times more common in pregnancy[75]. The rate of ischemic stroke during pregnancy is not increased compared to the age-matched controls, although this risk is increased immediately postpartum (RR 2.5). Thrombosed mechanical cardiac valves are rare, but mitral valve thrombosis is more common during pregnancy. Anticoagulation with warfarin is more effective than with heparin but, of course, warfarin is worse for the fetus and a difficult decision needs to be made by clinician and patient[77]. Twice-daily high-dose LMW heparin, aiming for a high anti-Xa assay, may be the solution.

Thrombolytic therapy with tissue plasminogen activator (rt-PA) is an approved therapy for ischemic stroke, myocardial infarction, pulmonary embolism and thrombosis of cardiac valve prosthesis. Prospective randomized controlled trials of thrombolytic agents in pregnant women are scarce. The best available data are case reports and case series. Due to its large molecular weight rtPA does not cross placenta.

For pregnant women who have a stroke, thrombolytic therapy is the only approved therapy to establish reperfusion. In the case of myocardial infarction, percutaneous angioplasty is the preferred treatment despite X-ray exposure. Thrombolytic therapy of pulmonary embolism is applied in severe cases and is as effective as surgical thrombectomy. In cases of thrombosed cardiac valvular prosthesis, surgery is the alternative to thrombolysis. According to expert opinion cardiac surgery using the cardiopulmonary bypass circuit exposes mother and child to a greater risk than thrombolytic therapy[78].

In conclusion, currently available data are not sufficient to derive guidelines for rt-PA thrombolysis in pregnancy. The moderate rate of maternal and fetal complications and the absence of teratogenicity and fetotoxicity make thrombolysis a valuable therapeutic option in some pregnant patients with stroke, thrombosed cardiac valvular prosthesis, acute myocardial infarction and pulmonary embolism.

ANTI-ARRHYTHMICS IN PREGNANCY

During pregnancy, a number of rhythm disturbances can occur in the mother and the fetus. They may range from benign ectopic beats to life-threatening arrhythmias. An increased incidence of cardiac arrhythmias during pregnancy can be in part explained by the hormonal, metabolic and hemodynamic changes. The increased number of women with congenital cardiac defect who now reach reproductive age due to advances in cardiac surgery are also a group who are prone to cardiac arrhythmias and hence contribute to the rise in number of rhythm disturbances seen in pregnancy[79]. The most common arrhythmias in the pregnant mother are simple ventricular and atrial ectopics[80] and, in the fetus, they tend to be the supraventricular tachycardias[81].

General approach to treatment of cardiac arrhythmias

In the setting of a structurally normal heart and minimally symptomatic arrhythmias (premature ventricular or atrial beats), no treatment is required. When symptoms are more marked, conservative treatment such as vagal stimulation either by carotid sinus message or Valsalva maneuver may help terminate supraventricular tachycardias. Patients should be advised to avoid stimulants such as caffeine and alcohol. At the other extreme is a hemodynamically compromised patient who will need to be electrically DC cardioverted (mostly at 50–100 J)[82–85]. Of course, there are those cases in which drug therapy is required, pacemakers for bradycardias or implantable cardioverters. Radiofrequency ablation in patients with frequent supraventricular and ventricular arrhythmias should be considered prior to pregnancy.

Narrow complex tachycardias (QRS complex less than 0.12 seconds and heart rate of greater then 100 bpm)

Narrow complex tachycardias include atrial flutter or fibrillation, both of which are uncommon in pregnancy, and atrial premature beats.

Rate control can be achieved by beta-blockers (see section on hypertension) or calcium channel blockers. Atrial premature beats (APBs) are benign in pregnant women. Patient reassurance and avoidance of exacerbating conditions or drugs should be advised. In troublesome symptomatic cases, beta-blockers are used. Adenosine bolus intravenously has been used with a rapid onset and short half-life and no tetratogenicity has been reported[86]. During labor, this treatment has caused increased uterine contractility, maternal hypotension and fetal bradycardia, and monitoring the fetal heart rate when attempting to terminate maternal tachycardia is recommended.

Calcium antagonists

These cross the placenta and are excreted in breast milk with concentrations varying from 23 to 94% of that of the mother. Verapamil can be used in the acute and chronic treatment of supraventricular tachycardias, both in mother and fetus and no evidence of teratogenicity has been reported. However, maternal and/or fetal hypotension, bradycardia and A-V block have been described[85].

Broad complex tachycardia (QRS complexes greater than 0.12 seconds)

Diagnosis is most important as the drugs used in the treatment of supraventricular tachycardia may be deleterious to patients with ventricular tachycardias (VT).

Sustained VT (greater than 30 seconds) is rare in pregnant women. Nevertheless, in a hemodynamically compromised patient, DC cardioversion (50–100J) should be carried out. If this is unsuccessful, higher energy shock is mandatory (100–360)[87]. If the patient is stable, VT should be treated with pharmacological agents such as intravenous procainamide or lidocaine. Neither of these two agents is known to be teratogenic to the fetus. There are a few reports on increased myometrial tone and decreases in utero-placental flow with fetal bradycardia, but lidocaine use in early pregnancy is not associated with fetal defects[88]. Magnesium sulfate is effective in life-threatening ventricular arrhythmias[89] and is given intravenously over a few minutes. Adverse effects associated with magnesium sulfate include as maternal hypothermia and fetal bradycardia[90].

Ventricular fibrillation and flutter

Prompt DC cardioversion (100–360J) is the required life-saving treatment. It has been used many times during pregnancy for many different reasons, without apparent harm to the fetus.

Ventricular premature beats (VPB)

VPB in pregnant women with a structurally normal heart are benign and no therapy apart from reassurance is required. If symptomatic, beta-blockers are the treatment of choice. There is no indication to treat with amiodarone or other class III drugs as the risks outweigh the benefits.

Amiodarone is contraindicated during pregnancy, due to fetal hypothyroidism, growth restriction and premature delivery[91–93].

Table 13.4 **Reported adverse effect on the fetus from anti-arrhythmic drugs**

Anti-arrhythmic drugs	*Adverse effect on the fetus*
Adenosine	None reported except one case of bradycardia
Amiodarone	Hypothyroidism, fetal growth restriction, prematurity
Beta-blocker e.g. sotolol	Fetal growth restriction in high doses, bradycardia, hyperbilirubinemia, hypoglycemia, uterine contractions
Digoxin	None reported
Diltiazem	None reported
Disopyramide	Uterine contractions
Lidocaine	Central nervous system depression
Mexiletine	Bradycardia, low birth weight, low Apgar score
Phenytoin	Neuro-developmental delay and 'hydantoin syndrome'
Procainamide	None reported
Quinidine	Thrombocytopenia, eighth cranial nerve damage (at toxic doses)
Verapamil	Heart block, hypotension

Bradyarrhythmias

Bradycardias are rare in pregnancy. If they occur, it may be secondary to supine hypotensive syndrome of pregnancy with uterine compression of inferior vena caval return of blood with paradoxical sinus slowing.

Other bradyarrhythmias, if persistent and symptomatic, would require treatment. If necessary, a pacemaker is recommended.

A summary of reported adverse effect on the fetus from anti-arrhythmic drugs is given in Table 13.4.

ASTHMA

Inhaled corticosteroids and selective beta$_2$-agonists are the preferred drugs for the prevention and management of all levels of persistent asthma during pregnancy[94]. Airway inflammation is present in nearly all cases and therefore inhaled corticosteroids have been advocated as first-line therapy for patients with mild asthma[95].

There is no evidence linking inhaled corticosteroid use and increases in congenital malformations or adverse perinatal outcomes[96]. Because there are more data on budesonide during pregnancy than on other inhaled corticosteroids, the NAEPP (National Asthma Education Prevention Program) considered it to be the preferred medication. However, if a woman is well controlled by a different inhaled corticosteroid before pregnancy, it seems reasonable to continue that medication during pregnancy.

Inhaled beta$_2$-agonists

Inhaled beta$_2$-agonists are currently recommended for treatment of asthma in pregnancy. Excessive use of beta$_2$- agonists is associated with tremor, tachycardia and palpitations. Increased usage of bronchodilators could be an indicator of the need for additional anti-inflammatory therapy; chronic use of short acting beta$_2$-agonists has been associated with an increased risk of death[97]. Beta$_2$-agonists appear to be safe in pregnancy[94] and no significant relationship has been found between the use of inhaled beta$_2$-agonists and adverse pregnancy outcomes.

Cromolyn

Cromolyn sodium is virtually devoid of significant side effects; it blocks both the early and late phase pulmonary response to allergen challenge as well as preventing the development of airway hyperresponsiveness. Cromolyn does not have any intrinsic bronchodilator or antihistaminic activity. Compared with inhaled corticosteroids, the time to maximal clinical benefit is longer for cromolyn. Cromolyn seems to be less effective than inhaled corticosteroids in reducing objective and subjective manifestations of asthma. Cromolyn appears to be safe during pregnancy[98].

Theophylline

Theophylline is an alternative treatment for mild persistent asthma and an adjunct treatment for the management of moderate and severe persistent asthma during pregnancy[94]. High doses have been observed to cause jitteriness, tachycardia and vomiting in mothers and neonates[99]. Theophylline is only indicated for chronic therapy and is not effective for the treatment of acute exacerbations during pregnancy. Theophylline has anti-inflammatory actions that may be mediated through inhibition of leukotriene production and its capacity to stimulate PGE2 production. It may potentiate the efficacy of inhaled corticosteroids. Safety of theophylline at a serum concentration of 5–12 g/ml during pregnancy has been confirmed[94], as no differences were seen in asthma exacerbations or perinatal outcome in a cohort receiving theophylline compared with a cohort receiving inhaled beclomethasone[100].

Leukotriene receptor antagonists

Leukotrienes are arachidonic acid metabolites that have been implicated in transducing bronchospasm, mucous secretion and increased vascular permeability. The leukotriene receptor antagonists zafirlukast and montelukast are both pregnancy category B (see Table 13.2). It should be noted that there are minimal data regarding the efficacy or safety of these agents during human pregnancy, but so far what exists is reassuring.[101]

Oral corticosteroid

Oral corticosteroid use during pregnancy in patients who have asthma has been associated with an increased incidence of pre-eclampsia, preterm delivery and low birth weight[98,102–104]. A recent prospective study found that systemic corticosteroids resulted in a deficit of about 200 g in birth weight compared with controls and those exclusively treated with beta$_2$-agonists[105]. However, it is difficult to separate the effects of the oral corticosteroids on these outcomes from the effects of severe or uncontrolled asthma. When indicated for the long-term management of severe asthma or exacerbations during pregnancy, it is recommended that oral corticosteroids should be used[94].

For acute exacerbations, prednisolone may be given up to 40 mg per day. Once the peak expiratory flow volume reaches 70% of personal best, the daily dosage of parenteral or oral corticosteroid can be reduced[94].

IMMUNOSUPRESSANTS

Many diseases that require immnuosuppression may also themselves negatively influence pregnancy outcome and neonatal health. In diseases with involvement of major organ systems or systemic disease activity, intrauterine growth restriction, preterm delivery and low-birth-weight babies increase perinatal mortality.

Indications for treatment during pregnancy are: ongoing need for immunosuppression in cases of transplantation, control of disease activity and prevention of a flare of an autoimmune disorder in mother, in order to assure a good outcome.

Unfortunately, the lack of evidence due to a small number of poorly powered controlled studies of drug performance and neonatal outcome remains the constant theme to this chapter.

Systemic corticosteroids

Corticosteroids are used in the acute flare of chronic conditions, such as rheumatic disease, autoimmune disease, inflammatory bowel disease and vasculitis. They are also used acutely in asthma and anaphylactic shock. The most widely prescribed corticosteroids are prednisolone, oral or IV dexamethasone, betamethasone or methylprednisolone. The mother is given betamethasone or dexamethasone to accelerate fetal lung maturation if preterm delivery is expected.

Mode of action

Corticosteroids are anti-inflammatory and immunosuppressant drugs. Their formulations differ in that some are fluorinated and readily cross the placenta. Most preparations have both glucocorticoid and mineralocorticoid potency, but there is variation in the ratio of these two substances. Betamethasone and dexamethasone cross the placenta readily. Up to ninety percent of prednisolone and methylprednisolone is inactivated by the placenta.

Maternal and fetal outcome

There is an association with cleft palate in animal studies[109], although cohort studies have not reproduced these findings in humans[110]. A meta-analysis of epidemiological studies found an increase in the incidence of oral clefts after first trimester exposure[111]. Long-term follow-up studies of children who were exposed to corticosteriods during pregnancy have not shown significant neurodevelopmental delay, contrary to animal studies[112]. In one small study, specifically looking at very low-birth-weight neonates, there was an association with delayed neurodevelopment when followed up to a corrected age of 18–22 months[113].

Late pregnancy exposure to high-dose steroids may cause preterm labor. Other seldom reported side effects are growth restriction, neonatal cataracts, adrenal suppression in the neonate and increased risk of infection[114–116].

Breast feeding

Breast feeding is safe for neonates whose mother takes prednisolone with only clinically insignificant amounts of the drug being concentrated in breast milk[117,118]. Several reports of children who were breast fed while their mothers were on long-term treatment with steroids (prednisolone, methylprednisolone) have not shown any adverse effects[119].

Recommendations

First trimester prednisolone 15 mg/day (5–10% of prednisolone in maternal plasma). After placental development, all corticosteroids are partly inactivated by 11-beta-hydroxylase of the placenta with relative protection for the fetus.

If a pregnant mother has been on more than 7.5 mg prednisolone daily during her pregnancy, supplemental hydrocortisone should be given during labor or any other physically stressful procedure.

Azathioprine

Azathioprine is a purine antimetabolite, used as an immunosuppressant agent for prevention of transplant rejection and suppressing inflammatory bowel disease, rheumatoid disorders, autoimmune hepatitis. Azathioprine prevents cell proliferation and inhibits many lymphocyte functions.

Placental transfer

Azathioprine (AZA) crosses the placenta, but the fetal liver lacks the enzyme to metabolize it to the active metabolite. Toxicity induced by AZA is ascribed to the metabolites 6-methylmercaptopurine (6-MMP) (hepatotoxicity), 6-thioinosine-triphosphate (6-TITP) (e.g. pancreatitis) and 6-TGN (myelotoxicity), respectively. Therefore, monitoring of 6-MMP and 6-TGN levels in red blood cells (RBC) during AZA treatment has been proposed as a strategy to optimize efficacy and minimize toxicity of therapy[120]. When measured in the RBC of mother and infant directly after delivery, the 6-TGN concentration was slightly lower in the RBC of the infant than the mother. No 6-MMP could be detected in the infant. This may suggest that the placenta may act as a barrier to AZA and its metabolite[121] (two case studies).

Maternal and fetal outcome

The use of AZA during pregnancy is relatively safe[122]. No recurring birth defects in the offspring of women with renal transplants on AZA and corticosteroids have been noted[123,124]. Pregnant women with SLE who took AZA to control their disease had reduced rates of pregnancy losses and did not cause congenital abnormalities[125], although a cohort study of women with inflammatory bowel disease treated with AZA has shown an increased risk of preterm birth and congenital abnormality compared to controls[126].

Breast feeding

Although a controversial issue until recently, breast feeding in mothers on azathioprine appears to be safe. Active metabolites of azathioprine have not been detected in breast milk, or neonatal blood[127]. No adverse effects of azathioprine, such as fetal growth restriction, psychomotor development, blood counts or frequency of infections, were detected in children from allograft recipient mothers who breast fed their babies for 6–24 months[119,127–129].

Recommendation

AZA is safe in pregnancy and during breast feeding, but should be used at the minimum effective dose.

Aminosalicylates (ASA)

Aminosalicylates interfere with folate metabolism (inhibit dihydrofolate reductase). The most commonly used ASA is sulfasalazine. Sulfasalazine is the combination of ASA and sulfapyridine, the latter molecule is the carrier for the active molecule which is cleaved off by the colonic bacteria in the gut and helps with its local action. The main indication for its use in pregnancy is in mothers with inflammatory bowel disease.

Placental transfer

Both sulfasalazine and sulfapyridine cross the placenta as determined by cord blood concentrations and evaluation against the maternal serum concentrations[130].

Fetal outcome

ASA have been associated with a risk of congenital cardiovascular defects and oral cleft palate during first trimester exposure[131]. However, the largest amount of data on inflammatory bowel disease comprising over 2000 pregnancies suggests no increase in birth defects, pathological jaundice or small-for-gestational-age babies[132,133]. There is one case report on neonatal neutropenia exposed antenatally to sulfasalzine[134].

Breast feeding

Forty to 50% of the maternal serum concentrations of ASA are detected in breast milk[135]. High doses of drug have been detectable in the serum of the infant[136]. Although sulfasalazine is safe in breast feeding, caution must be practiced in preterm neonates.

Recommendation

Females of reproductive age who are on sulfasalzine should be also prescribed folate supplementation and continue throughout their pregnancy, according to clinical need.

Methotrexate

Methotrexate (MTX) is an antimetabolite inhibitor of dihydrofolate reductase and therefore folic acid synthesis. It also directly inhibits folic-acid-dependent enzymes and cell-mediated immune reactions and therefore acts like an immunosuppressant. It is used to treat rheumatic disorders, vasculitis and inflammatory bowel disorders.

Placental transfer

Methotrexate does cross the placenta and is contraindicated in pregnancy[137].

Fetal outcome

Lack of folic acid early in pregnancy can lead to neural tube defects in the offspring. Although the published literature reports normal birthweights of infants whose mothers had been on MTX during the first trimester of pregnancy, there is an association with increased miscarriages and congenital malformations[138,139].

Breast feeding

Methotrexate is secreted in the breast milk, although 10-fold less concentrations than found in the serum, there are no published data on its effects in the neonate[140].

Recommendations

MTX is contraindicated during pregnancy and, when prescribed to women of reproductive age, it should be combined with a safe contraception method. Folate therapy should be taken prenatally and continued throughout pregnancy.

Mycophenolate mofetil

Mycophenolate mofetil (MM) is an inhibitor of purine synthesis and is used in severe RA, lupus nephritis and transplantation.

Fetal outcome

MM is associated with miscarriages and congenital malformations such as cleft palate, micrognathia, hypoplastic nails[141,142].

Breast feeding

MM is transferred into breast milk, therefore lactation should be avoided while taking this medication[143].

Recommendations

Due to very limited experience, it is advised that MM should not be taken during pregnancy and ideally be discontinued before conception is attempted[144].

Cyclophosphamide

Cyclophosphamide is an alkylating agent which is used to treat a variety of malignancies as well as the vasculitic diseases.

It is teratogenic in all animal species. The risk of congenital malformations based on cancer studies is estimated at approximately 20%. Birth defects after the first trimester of pregnancy have been reported with facial, skin and musculoskeletal and visceral organ anomalies, growth retardation and developmental delay during childhood[145]. Given in the first trimester (lupus nephritis), it is reported to be associated with an increased rate of miscarriage, congenital anomalies in the second trimester and with pancytopenia in the newborn[146].

Breast feeding

It is excreted in the breast milk and therefore it should be avoided during lactation[147].

Recommendations

Cyclophosphamide is a human teratogen. Attempts at conception should be delayed until 3 months after cessation of therapy.

Cyclosporin A

Cyclosporin prevents graft rejection in organ transplant recipients. It has profoundly advanced survival[148] in transplant recipients and until the advent of tacrolimus was a standard component of most immunosuppressant regimens used to prevent graft rejection in transplant recipients[149]. It is also used to treat numerous autoimmune diseases such as SLE, polymyositis and rheumatoid arthritis (RA).

Cyclosporin is a calcineurin inhibitor that attenuates T-cell-mediated responses by preventing formation of interleukin-2 (IL-2)[150].

Placental transfer and fetal outcome

Cyclosporin crosses the placenta and is found in fetal blood[151].

The rate of congenital abnormalities among women who used cyclosporin either during part of their pregnancies or throughout pregnancy is no different to that of the general population[152,153]. Renal and liver function were also normal in neonates exposed in utero[154].

The major problems with cyclosporin are prematurity and low birth weight[153]. Reassuringly, it has generally shown follow-up of children born to recipients of cyclosporin did not show any abnormality of their immune system, contrary to what had been observed in rodents[155].

Breast feeding

Breast feeding while on cyclosporin A is not recommended, although there have been no reports of adverse outcomes in infants who have been breast fed[142,155]. Almost one sixth of cyclosporin in the breast milk is found in the neonates. Cyclosporin is not associated with any nephrotoxic side effects in infants[156].

Recommendations

Cyclosporin has been the treatment of choice in transplant patients and patients with autoimmune disorders. Monitoring of cyclosporin plasma concentrations to keep levels at the lower limit of normal recommended.

Antimalarial drugs

Antimalarial drugs, such as hydroxychloroquine, interfere with lysosome presentation and processing of antigens. Hydroxychloroquine (HCQ) is stored in the liver and has a long half-life of 8 weeks, so discontinuation even early in pregnancy does not prevent fetal exposure. It is the most commonly prescribed antimalarial agent in the treatment of rheumatoid arthritis (RA), Systemic Lupus Erythematosus (SLE) and other connective tissue disorders.

Placental transfer and fetal outcome

Hydroxychloroquine does cross the placenta. There are concerns of accumulation in the melanin-containing structures in the fetal uveal tract and inner ear[157]. However, follow-up studies of those children exposed to antimalarials in utero have not disclosed impairment in growth or visual or hearing abnormalities[158]. There has been no report of congenital malformation in over 500 pregnancies exposed to chloroquine or hydroxychloroquine during the first trimester[158,159].

Breast feeding

Hydroxychloroquine is found in human breast milk and the infant may be exposed to 2% of maternal dose/kg/day[160]. No ocular complications of any of the children who were exposed to hydroxychloquine through breast milk in their infancy has been reported[161].

Recommendations

Withdrawal of antimalarial treatment in non-pregnant and pregnant patients with SLE increases the risk of a lupus flare[162,163]. Since HCQ has not been associated with any fetal malformation or side effects in infancy, it should be continued during pregnancy and breast feeding.

Tacrolimus

Tacrolimus is a calcineurin inhibitor used as an immunosuppressive agent in transplantation.

Placental transfer and fetal outcome

Tacrolimus crosses the placenta and the drug level should be frequently monitored during pregnancy. The experience with tacrolimus is more limited than cyclosporin. There are, however, now many successful pregnancies in patients with kidney, liver and pancreas transplantation[142,164,165]. There is evidence for preterm delivery but, in most cases, the birth weight was appropriate for the gestational age. No more congenital abnormalities are observed in pregnancies on tacrolimus than in the general population[165].

Breast feeding

Tacrolimus is excreted in the breast milk[166].

Recommendations

Tacrolimus now has a good safety record in pregnancy and has surpassed cyclosporin as the immunosuppresant of choice for solid organ transplant patients. Drug levels should be kept at the lower level of normal as the plasma volume expansion of pregnancy naturally lowers the drug concentration.

Tumour necrosis factor antagonists

Tumour necrosis factor antagonists (anti-TNF) are inhibitors of a cytokine that mobilizes neutrophil proliferations. Examples are infliximab and etanercept. They are used in treatment of RA, inflammatory bowel disease, juvenile idiopathic arthritis, psoriatic arthritis and ankylosing spondylitis.

Fetal outcome

The reported outcomes in a population of women on infliximab prior to conception and in their first trimester has shown similar outcomes to a general pregnant population with 15% miscarriages, 15% therapeutic termination and 70% live births; for those continue beyond the first trimester, no congenital abnormalities were reported[167]. In a prospective study of 244 RA patients on anti-TNF, there were three unexpected pregnancies on treatment but none showed embryo toxicity, teratogenicity or increased loss. However, caution should be used when anti-TNF agents are used during pregnancy, as human experience is still extremely limited. The potential risk should be balanced against the known risks associated with disease modifying antirheumatic drugs (DMARDs) and steroid therapy. Large registries will be necessary before firm conclusions can be drawn[168].

Breast feeding

On the limited data, infliximab could not be detected in the breast milk with the standard assays[169], but a separate study showed etanercept to be detectable[170].

Interferon-beta 1

Interferon-beta is an immunomodulating drug. It is used to prevent relapses in multiple sclerosis.

Placental transfer and fetal outcome

Data available on the transfer of interferon-beta across the placenta are limited, however one ex vivo study has shown no transfer of interferon-alpha[171].

From animal studies, no teratogenicity with high doses are reported[172]. There are no data on breast feeding. It is recommended to stop interferon-beta before conception, although its use is not a reason for terminating an otherwise normal pregnancy.

Intravenous immunoglobulin

Intravenous immunoglobulin is used with great efficacy in autoimmune diseases, especially some of the neurological disorders such as multiple sclerosis, Guilian-Barré syndrome and myasthenia gravis[173]. In addition, it has been widely used to treat idiopathic thrombocytopenic purpura in pregnancy with a low rate of side effects.

A summary of immunosuppressant drugs and their effects is given in Table 13.5.

ENDOCRINE DISORDERS

Diabetes mellitus

Type-1 and type-2 diabetes mellitus can precede pregnancy and are associated with an increased risk of congenital abnormalities[175]. Interestingly, women with gestational diabetes mellitus (GD) are also at increased risk of having offspring affected by congenital abnormalities, including neural tube defects[175]. This likely reflects subclinical impaired glucose tolerance in the first trimester, which is only identified as clinical GD in the second half of pregnancy when maternal glucose tolerance is tested. Women with pre-pregnancy diabetes mellitus are advised to take a higher dose of folic acid, 5 mg daily instead of the standard folic acid 400 μg daily.

Insulin is the therapy which has been most widely used for the treatment of all forms of diabetes in pregnancy[176]. There are now reassuring safety data on newer insulin analogues, especially insulin lispro, to show it is safe and does not to cross the placenta[177]. Due to the safety of insulin in pregnancy, most women who were on oral hypoglycemic agents, such as sulfonylureas and metformin, pre-pregnancy were switched to insulin. However, since the 1970s, countries with low resources have been successfully using oral hypoglycemic agents to manage GD and type-2 diabetes in pregnancy[178]. More recently, glyburide and glipizide have been shown to be as effective as insulin on pregnancy outcome in the management of GD[179–183]. It appears that glyburide is actively transported from the fetal circulation back to the mother by placental enzymes[184,185]. A switch back to insulin from glyburide is, however, more likely in those women who have early onset GD, the highest fasting glucose levels, older age and multiparity[181,186].

Table 13.5 **Summary of immunosuppressant drugs and their effects**

Drug	*Placental transfer*	*Adverse effects on the fetus*	*Compatibility with breast feeding*
Prednisolone	Yes (1:10)*	Considered safe	Yes
Fluorinated steroids e.g. betamethasone, dexamethasone	Yes	Prolonged use associated with fetal growth restriction and oligohydramnios	Yes
Cyclosporin A	Yes	Possible abnormal immune system development	Yes
Azathioprine	Yes	Intrauterine growth restriction (IUGR), neonatal lymphopenia, hypogammaglobulinemia	Yes
Hydroxychloroquine	Yes	None reported	Yes
Methotrexate	Yes	Cranial and CNS abnormalities; limb defects	No
Cyclophosphamide	Yes	Embryopathy, craniofacial defects, distal limb defects, growth restriction	No
Sulfasalazine	Yes	None apparent	Yes
Tacrolimus	Yes	None apparent	Unknown
Mycophenolate mofetil	Yes	Embryopathy, cranofacial and distal limb defects	No
Beta-inteferon	Unknown	Insufficient data	Unknown
Intravenous immunoglobulin	Yes	None apparent	Unknown
Anti-TNA	Yes	Insufficient data	Insufficient data

*The placenta inactivates 90% of prednisolone and fetal blood levels are 10% of maternal

Metformin is often used to treat type-2 diabetes and polycystic ovary syndrome. Women find themselves conceiving on metformin and, until recently, were advised to switch to insulin during pregnancy. There is accumulating evidence that metformin is safe to take throughout pregnancy for women with type-2 diabetes and that it is as effective as insulin for the management of GD[187]. The results and follow-up of a trial comparing the use of metformin with insulin in pregnancy are soon to be published[188].

Maternal thyroid disease

Thyroid disease is a common problem in young women and therefore common during pregnancy. Approximately 2.5% of females will have clinical or subclinical hypothyroidism and 0.2% will have an overactive thyroid. Treatment of hypothyroidism in pregnancy is important to prevent a poor perinatal outcome. Whether subclinical hypothyroidism causes neurodevelopmental delay in the offspring is still unclear[189]. The management of hyperthyroidism in pregnancy is important for the fetus because of the effects of antithyroid drugs (thionamides; propylthiouracil, carbimazole and methimazole) on the developing fetal thyroid.

Maternal hypothyroidism

Maternal hypothyroidism, defined by an elevated serum thyroid stimulating hormone (TSH) and low free thyroxine (T4), is associated with a poor perinatal outcome and neurodevelopmental delay in the infant[190]. Replacement of thyroid hormone to keep the TSH in the normal range (just under 2.0 mU/l) prevents adverse perinatal outcome[190].

An increase in thyroid replacement therapy is necessary in 25–50% of hypothyroid women and therefore a check of maternal thyroid function is necessary in the first trimester. An automatic increase in thyroxine dose in early pregnancy is likely to overtreat many women, whereas an appropriate adjustment according to a TSH level would accurately guide maternal requirements with little delay. Excessive maternal thyroxine crosses the placenta and can be toxic to the fetus[191]. Occasionally, women have an isolated low free thyroxine (T4) level associated with a normal serum TSH. These women have the same perinatal outcome as those who have normal thyroid biochemistry[192]. However, mothers with low T4 at 12 weeks' gestation have been shown to have 3-week-old neonates with reduced neonatal behavioral scores and this may translate into delayed neurodevelopment at 2 years of age, unless thyroid function is corrected later in pregnancy[193,194]. Studies that attempted to address this issue included women with overt biochemical hypothyroidism TSH >10 mU/l and low serum T4[195] and may have exaggerated the need for routine first trimester screening of hypothyroidism. The European Endocrine Society recommends screening women at high risk of hypothyroidism (women with a family or personal history of thyroid disease and history of other autoimmune disease) in the first trimester[190]. As 30% of women who have subclinical hypothyroidism are at low risk of the condition, this will miss a significant minority of women[196]. Clinical suspicion of hypothyroidism in early pregnancy should give a low threshold for doing a simple test of thyroid function.

Hyperthyroidism

During the first trimester, transient hyperthyroxemia (raised T4) is evident in two-thirds of women with hyperemesis gravidarum, which affects about 1% of all pregnancies. The pathogenesis of hyperemesis is not clear, but in part relates to increased TSH receptor sensitivity to HCG. These women are not clinically hyperthyroid, but need to be treated with anti-emetics (see later), *not* antithyroid drugs.

Most women will be known to have autoimmune hyperthyroidism before they conceive. They will be on antithyroid treatment, either propylthiouracil (PTU) or carbimazole/methimazole (CBZ). All these drugs cross the placenta and can induce hypothyroidism in the developing fetus. This can lead to fetal goiter and fetal hypothyroidism. Balancing this risk are thyroid stimulating hormone (TSH)-receptor antibodies which also cross the placenta and stimulate the fetal thyroid to cause fetal and transient neonatal hyperthyroidism in 1–10% of cases[197]. Euthyroid mothers, who have been treated for Graves' disease, still have thyroid simulating antibodies that can potentially cross the placenta to cause neonatal hyperthyroidism.

Similar doses of PTU and CBZ have the same effect on fetal thyroid function[198]. There are sporadic reports of fetal anomalies such as aplasia cutis, choanal atresia and esophageal atresia with CBZ and, therefore, for this reason, rather than any functional affect on the fetal thyroid, PTU should be chosen over CBZ, but the latter need not be avoided if PTU cannot be tolerated[199]. After explaining these possible associations, it is the author's practice to recommend women who conceive on CBZ to remain on this drug rather than switch to PTU[200].

A pragmatic approach to management is to use the lowest effective dose of antithyroid drug to keep maternal thyroid function tests at the upper end of normal. Regimens that use a high-dose antithyroid drug to block completely maternal thyroid activity and additional thyroxine, a block and replace regimen, expose the fetus to unnecessary high doses of antithyroid drug and should be avoided. Symptomatic women with palpitations and tachycardia can safely use propranolol, usually 20–40 mg three times daily to normalize maternal hyperdynamic cardiovascular state.

ANTI-EPILEPSY DRUGS IN PREGNANCY

Epilepsy affects up to 2% of the population at some time during the first 25 years of life and has a population prevalence of approximately 0.6%, including women of reproductive years[201]. Good control of epilepsy is essential for maternal and fetal well-being. Poorly controlled epilepsy is associated with increased maternal and fetal morbidity and mortality[202]. Most women with epilepsy are diagnosed before conception and some no longer require treatment, while others will take a single or multiple anti-epilepsy drugs (AEDs). Fetal toxicity due to older-generation AEDs, phenytoin, carbamazepine, sodium valproate, has been known about for many years, and causes much anxiety for the pregnant mother[203]. The majority of women who take AEDs do however have a normal pregnancy and a healthy baby. Useful information about specific AEDs and doses of drug that are feto-toxic has come from several registries of women with epilepsy from around the world[9,204,205].

In a review of 128049 pregnant women who had their infants screened at delivery, women who have epilepsy, but who do not require treatment, do not have an increased risk of having a child with a congenital malformation[206]. However, those who took a single anti-epilepsy drug (AED) throughout pregnancy had an increased risk (OR 2.8; 95% CI 1.1–9.7) of having an infant with a major congenital malformation compared with women who did not take an AED[206]. Women who took two or more AEDs had an OR 4.2 (95% CI, 1.1–5.1). In order to try to combat this increased risk of major congenital malformation, women who take AEDs in pregnancy are encouraged to take high-dose folic acid 5 mg daily from before conception and until delivery. However, animal studies have shown that folic acid has no effect on preventing AED-induced neural tube defect, suggesting that this malformation occurs through a different mechanism. Specifically, folic acid 5 mg taken at the time of conception and throughout pregnancy has also failed to prevent neural tube defects in women taking sodium valproate[207]. It is possible that vitamin B6, which is low in women taking sodium valproate, may need to be supplemented in order to prevent a neural tube defect[207]. There may also be a genetic vulnerability to neural tube defects that eventuates in those fetuses exposed to adverse environmental conditions, e.g. exposure to AED[208].

Carbamazepine, phenytoin, phenobarbitone, primidone and oxcarbazepine induce hepatic enzymes. It has been suggested that maternal and fetal clotting may be compromised as a consequence and, therefore, women taking these AEDs after 34 weeks' gestation should be given 10 mg vitamin K(1) daily until delivery. Although this measure is widely practiced, there is evidence that it is unnecessary[209]. Neonatal hemorrhage is more common in women with alcohol abuse and maybe maternal vitamin K supplementation should be reserved for women with additional causes for hepatic enzyme induction.

Maternal serum AED levels were previously routinely used to guide drug dose during pregnancy. However, this led to an inevitable increase in treatment as drug concentration fell due to gestational plasma volume expansion. The fetus then sometimes became exposed to an unnecessarily increased concentration of teratogen. Lamotrogine and oxcarbazepine are induced during pregnancy and it has been suggested that levels of these drugs should be measured to keep in clinical control of the epilepsy[210]. With these exceptions, AED dose can usually be adjusted according to clinical response after discussion with the mother. Poor compliance is, however, common in pregnancy and when suspected, or if there is treatment failure, then drug levels or hair sampling may be useful[211].

Large registries of AED use in pregnancy have, to date, captured useful information on the most widely used drugs for epilepsy in pregnancy[205]. This includes sodium valproate, carbamazepine and lamotrogine. The UK register prospectively followed up 3607 pregnancies and found the greatest malformation prevalence of 6.2% (95% CI 4.6–8.2%) with sodium valproate monotherapy while carbamazepine monotherapy caused 2.2% (1.4–3.4%) and lamotrogine 3.2% (2.1–4.9%) compared with 3.5% (1.8–6.8%) in infants born to mothers with epilepsy, but who did not take AEDs[212]. Newer AEDs were not sufficiently well represented in the registry for meaningful interpretation. It is important therefore to remember that the absence of evidence of harm does not translate into the absence of harm; a property that is often pushed in newly released drugs before sufficient data can be accumulated.

Sodium valproate

Sodium valproate is an effective AED for the control of all forms of seizures and is therefore widely used. A prospective study of over 400 women has shown that the risk of congenital malformation with sodium valproate was dose dependent[9]. Women who took sodium valproate, <1100 mg daily, had a similar incidence of fetal malformation (3.6%) as women who took no AEDs during pregnancy (3.1%)[9]. Women who took a higher dose of sodium valproate (>1100 mg/day) had a 35.5% risk of fetal malformation. Women taking the higher dose of sodium valproate were, however, also more likely to be taking other AEDs at the same time. Again, the use of folic acid peri-conception, appeared to have no impact on reducing the incidence of fetal malformation in women who took sodium valproate[9].

Sodium valproate also has a negative effect on the neurodevelopment of children born to mothers who took the drug during pregnancy[213]. These later observations have taken years to be recognized by pediatricians and neurologists. The extent of this association appears to be strongest with sodium valproate compared with other AEDs[214], but many complex confounding issues need to be considered before we can be sure of this retrospective observation.

Recommendations

Advice at this time is to optimize a woman's anti-epilepsy drugs before conception, aiming for the lowest effective dose of a single AED. Peri-conceptual high-dose folic acid appears to be ineffective at preventing neural tube defects caused by AEDs. Until this is a definitive observation, folic acid 5 mg daily is probably worth taking. Supplemental vitamin B6 may be a more effective prophylactic against neural tube defects caused by AEDs, but awaits further study. Supplemental vitamin K appears to be unnecessary in women taking enzyme-inducing AEDs.

Fetal anticonvulsant syndromes

Children born to mothers who take anti-epilepsy drugs (AEDs) have been recognized as having a collection of features that, taken together, have been labeled as a fetal anticonvulsant syndrome (FACS). This is said to be particularly evident for phenytoin, carbamazepine and valproate[215].

Children born to mothers taking phenytoin during pregnancy are at risk of fetal hydantoin syndrome. This syndrome is characterized by growth restriction, microcephaly, mental deficiency, nail and digit hypoplasia, typical facial appearance (see later), rib anomalies and abnormal palmar creases[216]. Not all fetuses exposed to phenytoin are at risk of the syndrome as they have an enzyme, epoxide hydrolase, that can eliminate pathological oxidative metabolites. Fetuses that are homozygous for the recessive allele of epoxide hydrolase have low enzyme activity and are at risk of fetal hydantoin syndrome[217]. This vulnerability to fetal hydantoin syndrome is well illustrated by a case report of a mother with epilepsy taking phenytoin and who was pregnant with heteropaternal dizygotic twins. Each twin had different levels of epoxide hydrolase enzyme activity, which led to only one twin developing the fetal hydantoin syndrome[218]. This case report is an example of how genetic variability in drug metabolism can have a catastrophic outcome. Pharmacogenetics may evolve so that knowledge of an individual's genetic ability to metabolize a drug could be used to tailor the dose or selection of drug.

Carbamazepine is associated with a similar FACS to fetal hydantoin syndrome[219]. This similarity may result from both drugs being metabolized to an epoxide intermediate, which is itself teratogenic rather than the drug.

Dysmorphic facial features are also associated with valproate exposure and include medial deficiency of eyebrows, infraorbital grooves, broad nasal bridge, anteverted nose, abnormal philtrum and a thin upper lip[215]. It has been claimed that dysmorphic facial features correlate with verbal intelligence in valproate-exposed children[215]. However, an expert panel of dysmorphologists identified only 47% of children exposed to AEDs in utero as having fetal FACS and 45% of unexposed children as having these facial features[215]. The specificity and sensitivity of assessing children with fetal anticonvulsant syndrome according to facial features cannot therefore be very high[220]. Furthermore, most children grow out of them by the time they are 16 years old[215].

TREATMENT OF DEPRESSION

Depression is a common problem during and after pregnancy, affecting approximately 10% of women[221]. The decision to continue or initiate antidepressant treatment needs to balance the potential risk to the fetus from the drugs with the risk of leaving the mother untreated, a potentially life-threatening condition[202]. Treatment for depression includes three main classes of drug: tricyclic antidepressants, selective serotonin reuptake inhibitors (SSRIs) and monoamine oxidase inhibitors (MAOIs).

Selective serotonin reuptake inhibitors (SSRIs)

Since their introduction in the 1980s, SSRIs have become the most widely prescribed long-term antidepressants[222]. SSRI use in pregnancy has increased accordingly. A study from the Netherlands used prescribing databases to record 310/14902 (2.1%) pregnancies in which the mother took SSRIs[223]. Almost 90% of SSRIs were being taken long term. Paroxetine was the most widely prescribed (58%), followed by fluoxetine (22%), fluvoxamine (13%), citalopram (8%) and sertraline (4%)[223].

Initial small cohort studies concluded that there was no association between SSRIs taken during pregnancy and congenital malformations[224]. Subsequently, exposure to SSRIs in the first trimester has been linked to an increased risk of a non-specific pattern of congenital malformations; RR 1.34 (95% CI 1.00–1.79) for first-month exposure and 1.84 (1.25–2.71) for second- and third-month exposure[225]. This potentially weak teratogenic affect appears to be dose related. A Canadian 'medicines and pregnancy' registry has shown that women who take paroxetine >25 mg daily, but not lower doses, during the first trimester have a RR 3.1 (CI; 1.0–9.4) of fetal cardiac malformation[11].

Persistent pulmonary hypertension of the newborn has been found to be more common in the infants of mothers who took SSRIs during the second half of pregnancy, but not in the first half[226]. It is estimated that 1:100 infants born to mothers who take SSRIs after 20 weeks' gestation will have a neonate affected by PPHN[226]. Further studies are needed to clarify this risk with dose and type of SSRI.

Tricyclic antidepressants

Tricyclic antidepressants, especially amitriptyline and nortriptyline, have been safely used in pregnancy and during breast feeding for many years. There is no increased risk of congenital malformation with their use in the first trimester[227]. Tricyclic antidepressant use at the time of delivery can lead to a neonatal withdrawal syndrome of irritability, tachycardia and tachypnoea[228]. Often, however, this is a time when these drugs need to be continued by the mother to prevent life-threatening depression.

Lithium

Lithium is an effective treatment for bipolar disorders (manic depression). Its use in pregnancy suggests it is a weak teratogen, especially at high doses. Cardiac malformations, specifically Ebstein's anomaly, have been recognized in the fetuses of mothers taking lithium[229]. Its efficacy as a mood stabilizer and the rarity of associated congenital malformations usually dictate its continued use through pregnancy.

VACCINATION AND PREGNANCY

The administration of vaccines during pregnancy poses a number of concerns to physicians and patients about the risk of transmitting a virus to a developing fetus. This risk is primarily theoretical. Live virus vaccines are generally contraindicated in pregnant women.

No evidence shows an increased risk from vaccinating pregnant women with inactivated virus or bacterial vaccines or toxoids[230]. Therefore, if a patient is at high risk of being exposed to a particular disease, if infection would pose a risk to the mother or fetus, and if the vaccine is unlikely to cause harm, the benefits of vaccinating a pregnant woman usually outweigh the potential risks.

A summary of recommendations of immunizations during pregnancy is given in Table 13.6.

Table 13.6 **Summary of recommendations of immunizations during pregnancy**

Considered safe	*Special recommendations dependent on circumstances*	*Contraindicated during pregnancy or safety not established*
Tetanus and diphtheria	Anthrax	BCG
Toxoids (Td)	Hepatitis A	Measles*
Hepatitis B	Japanese encephalitis	Mumps*
Influenza	Pneumococcal	Rubella*
Meningococcal	Polio (IPV)	Varicella*
Rabies	Typhoid (parenteral and Ty21a*)	
	Vaccinia*	
	Yellow fever*	

* = Live, attenuated vaccine; BCG = bacille de Calmette-Guérin; IPV = inactivated polio virus. Adapted from Guidelines for vaccinating pregnant women. Recommendations of the Advisory Committee on Immunization Practices (ACIP). Atlanta, Ga.: Centers for Disease Control and Prevention, 2002

Breast feeding

No vaccination is contraindicated in breast feeding[230].

CONCLUSION

Prescribing in pregnancy for maternal health is done with limited evidence and often on the assumption of apparent lack of harm to the developing offspring. Studies of therapeutic management of maternal conditions are, with few exceptions, small and have short periods of follow up. To provide optimal care of the sick pregnant mother, we need better information about safe prescribing during pregnancy. Women who may have life-threatening conditions should neither be denied effective treatment nor given a drug that will harm their offspring. Sometimes compromise is as harmful as no treatment, for example in limited or tapered treatment of depression.

The challenge to obtain information on safe prescribing in pregnancy is to develop prospective, multicenter (international) observational studies that can document the timing and dosage of drugs used in pregnancy. Neonatal and childhood follow-up is necessary to document long-term adverse outcomes that are not evident at birth and may take years to evolve. To attribute teratogenicity wrongly to a drug and deny its use in pregnancy is as detrimental to maternal health as is prescribing a known teratogen to a mother and harming her offspring.

REFERENCES

1. Oakley GP, Jr. Frequency of human congenital malformations 3. *Clin Perinatol* **13**(3):545–554, 1986.
2. Williams DJ. Physiological changes of normal pregnancy. In *Oxford textbook of medicine*, 4th edn, DA Warrell (ed.), pp. 383–385. Oxford: Oxford University Press, 2003.
3. Myllynen P, Pasanen M, Vahakangas K. The fate and effects of xenobiotics in human placenta. *Expert Opin Drug Metab Toxicol* **3**(3):331–346, 2007.
4. Gedeon C, Koren G. Designing pregnancy centered medications: drugs which do not cross the human placenta. *Placenta* **27**(8):861–868, 2006.
5. Huang SA, Dorfman DM, Genest DR, Salvatore D, Larsen PR. Type 3 iodothyronine deiodinase is highly expressed in the human uteroplacental unit and in fetal epithelium. *J Clin Endocrinol Metab* **88**(3):1384–1388, 2003.
6. Wilson JG. Current status of teratology: general principles and mechanisms

derived from animal studies. In *Handbook of teratology, general principles and etiology*, JG Wilson, FC Fraser (eds), pp. 47–74. New York: NY Plenium Press, 1977.
7. Moore KL, Persaud TV. *The developing human: clinically orientated embryology*, 6th edn. Philadelphia: WB Saunders, 1998.
8. Iqbal MM, Sobhan T, Ryals T. Effects of commonly used benzodiazepines on the fetus, the neonate, and the nursing infant. *Psychiatr Serv* **53**(1):39–49, 2002.
9. Vajda FJ, O'Brien TJ, Hitchcock A et al. Critical relationship between sodium valproate dose and human teratogenicity: results of the Australian register of anti-epileptic drugs in pregnancy. *J Clin Neurosci* **11**(8):854–858, 2004.
10. Vitale N, De Feo M, De Santo LS, Pollice A, Tedesco N, Cotrufo M. Dose-dependent fetal complications of warfarin in pregnant women with mechanical heart valves. *J Am Coll Cardiol* **33**(6):1637–1641, 1999.
11. Berard A, Ramos E, Rey E, Blais L, St Andre M, Oraichi D. First trimester exposure to paroxetine and risk of cardiac malformations in infants: the importance of dosage. *Birth Defects Res B Dev Reprod Toxicol* **80**(1):18–27, 2007.
12. Bajoria R, Sooranna SR, Contractor SF. Differential binding of warfarin to maternal, foetal and non-pregnant sera and its clinical implications. *J Pharm Pharmacol* **48**(5):486–489, 1996.
13. Report of the National High Blood Pressure Education Program Working Group on High Blood Pressure in Pregnancy. *Am J Obstet Gynecol* **183**(1):S1–S22, 2000.
14. Geographic variation in the incidence of hypertension in pregnancy. World Health Organization International Collaborative Study of Hypertensive Disorders of Pregnancy. *Am J Obstet Gynecol* **158**(1): 80–83, 1988.
15. Brown MA, Lindheimer MD, de Swiet M, Van Assche A, Moutquin JM. The classification and diagnosis of the hypertensive disorders of pregnancy: statement from the International Society for the Study of Hypertension in Pregnancy (ISSHP). *Hypertens Pregnancy* **20**(1):IX–XIV, 2001.
16. Abalos E, Duley L, Steyn DW, Henderson-Smart DJ. Antihypertensive drug therapy for mild to moderate hypertension during pregnancy. *Cochrane Database Syst Rev* (1): CD002252, 2007.
17. Sibai BM. Diagnosis and management of gestational hypertension and preeclampsia. *Obstet Gynecol* **102**(1): 181–192, 2003.
18. von Dadelszen P, Ornstein MP, Bull SB, Logan AG, Koren G, Magee LA. Fall in mean arterial pressure and fetal growth restriction in pregnancy hypertension: a meta-analysis. *Lancet* **355**(9198):87–92, 2000.
19. Sibai BM. Treatment of hypertension in pregnant women. *N Engl J Med* **335**(4):257–265, 1996.
20. Waterman EJ, Magee LA, Lim KI, Skoll A, Rurak D, von Dadelszen P. Do commonly used oral antihypertensives alter fetal or neonatal heart rate characteristics? A systematic review. *Hypertens Pregnancy* **23**(2):155–169, 2004.
21. Sibai BM, Gonzalez AR, Mabie WC, Moretti M. A comparison of labetalol plus hospitalization versus hospitalization alone in the management of preeclampsia remote from term. *Obstet Gynecol* **3**(Pt 1): 323–327, 1987.
22. Montan S, Anandakumar C, Arulkumaran S, Ingemarsson I, Ratnam SS. Effects of methyldopa on uteroplacental and fetal hemodynamics in pregnancy-induced hypertension. *Am J Obstet Gynecol* **168**(1 Pt 1):152–156, 1993.
23. Sibai BM, Mabie WC, Shamsa F, Villar MA, Anderson GD. A comparison of no medication versus methyldopa or labetalol in chronic hypertension during pregnancy. *Am J Obstet Gynecol* **162**(4): 960–966, 1990.
24. Cockburn J, Moar VA, Ounsted M, Redman CW. Final report of study on hypertension during pregnancy: the effects of specific treatment on the growth and development of the children. *Lancet* **1**(8273):647–649, 1982.
25. Butters L, Kennedy S, Rubin PC. Atenolol in essential hypertension during pregnancy. *Br Med J* **301**(6752):587–589, 1990.
26. Magee LA, Duley L. Oral beta-blockers for mild to moderate hypertension during pregnancy. *Cochrane Database Syst Rev* (3): CD002863, 2003.
27. Easterling TR, Carr DB, Brateng D, Diederichs C, Schmucker B. Treatment of hypertension in pregnancy: effect of atenolol on maternal disease, preterm delivery, and fetal growth. *Obstet Gynecol* **98**(3):427–433, 2001.
28. Bayliss H, Churchill D, Beevers M, Beevers DG. Anti-hypertensive drugs in pregnancy and fetal growth: evidence for 'pharmacological programming' in the first trimester? *Hypertens Pregnancy* **21**(2):161–174, 2002.
29. Lip GY, Beevers M, Churchill D, Shaffer LM, Beevers DG. Effect of atenolol on birth weight. *Am J Cardiol* **79**(10): 1436–1438, 1997.
30. Pickles CJ, Symonds EM, Broughton PF. The fetal outcome in a randomized double-blind controlled trial of labetalol versus placebo in pregnancy-induced hypertension. *Br J Obstet Gynaecol* **96**(1):38–43, 1989.
31. Lardoux H, Gerard J, Blazquez G, Chouty F, Flouvat B. Hypertension in pregnancy: evaluation of two beta blockers atenolol and labetalol. *Eur Heart J* (Suppl G):35–40, 1983.
32. Magee LA, Miremadi S, Li J et al. Therapy with both magnesium sulfate and nifedipine does not increase the risk of serious magnesium-related maternal side effects in women with preeclampsia. *Am J Obstet Gynecol* **193**(1):153–163, 2005.
33. Magee LA, Schick B, Donnenfeld AE et al. The safety of calcium channel blockers in human pregnancy: a prospective, multicenter cohort study. *Am J Obstet Gynecol* **174**(3):823–828, 1996.
34. Elatrous S, Nouira S, Ouanes BL et al. Short-term treatment of severe hypertension of pregnancy: prospective comparison of nicardipine and labetalol. *Intensive Care Med* **28**(9):1281–1286, 2002.
35. Magee LA, Cham C, Waterman EJ, Ohlsson A, von Dadelszen P. Hydralazine for treatment of severe hypertension in pregnancy: meta-analysis. *Br Med J* **327**(7421):955–960, 2003.
36. Sibai BM, Grossman RA, Grossman HG. Effects of diuretics on plasma volume in pregnancies with long-term hypertension. *Am J Obstet Gynecol* **150**(7):831–835, 1984.
37. Barron WMLM. Management of hypertension during pregnancy. In *Hypertension: pathophysiology, diagnosis and management*, 2nd edn, JHBB Laragh (ed.), pp. 2427–2450. New York: Raven Press Ltd, 1995.
38. Olesen C, de Vries CS, Thrane N, MacDonald TM, Larsen H, Sorensen HT. Effect of diuretics on fetal growth: a drug effect or confounding by indication? Pooled Danish and Scottish cohort data. *Br J Clin Pharmacol* **51**(2):153–157, 2001.
39. Cooper WO, Hernandez-Diaz S, Arbogast PG et al. Major congenital malformations after first-trimester exposure to ACE inhibitors. *N Engl J Med* **354**(23):2443–2451, 2006.
40. Vendemmia M, Garcia-Meric P, Rizzotti A et al. Fetal and neonatal consequences of antenatal exposure to type 1 angiotensin II receptor-antagonists. *J Matern Fetal Neonatal Med* **18**(2):137–140, 2005.
41. Bourget P, Fernandez H, Edouard D et al. Disposition of a new rate-controlled formulation of prazosin in the treatment of hypertension during pregnancy: transplacental passage of prazosin. *Eur J Drug Metab Pharmacokinet* **20**(3):233–241, 1995.
42. Carson RG, Feenstra ES. Toxicologic studies with the hypotensive agent minoxidil. *Toxicol Appl Pharmacol* **39**(1): 1–11, 1977.
43. Kaler SG, Patrinos ME, Lambert GH, Myers TF, Karlman R, Anderson CL. Hypertrichosis and congenital anomalies associated with maternal use of minoxidil. *Pediatrics* **79**(3):434–436, 1987.
44. Atallah AN, Hofmeyr GJ, Duley L. Calcium supplementation during pregnancy for preventing hypertensive disorders and related problems. *Cochrane Database Syst Rev* **1**: CD001059, 2002.

45. CLASP: a randomised trial of low-dose aspirin for the prevention and treatment of pre-eclampsia among 9364 pregnant women, CLASP (Collaborative Low-dose Aspirin Study in Pregnancy) Collaborative Group, *Lancet* **343**(8898): 619–629, 1994
46. ECPPA: randomised trial of low dose aspirin for the prevention of maternal and fetal complications in high risk pregnant women, ECPPA (Estudo Colaborativo para Prevencao da Pre-eclampsia com Aspirina) Collaborative Group. *Br J Obstet Gynaecol* **103**(1):39–47, 1996.
47. Dekker GA, Sibai BM. Low-dose aspirin in the prevention of preeclampsia and fetal growth retardation: rationale, mechanisms, and clinical trials. *Am J Obstet Gynecol* **168**(1 Pt 1):214–227, 1993.
48. Coomarasamy A, Honest H, Papaioannou S, Gee H, Khan KS. Aspirin for prevention of preeclampsia in women with historical risk factors: a systematic review. *Obstet Gynecol* **101**(6):1319–1332, 2003.
49. Duley L, Henderson-Smart DJ, Knight M, King JF. Antiplatelet agents for preventing pre-eclampsia and its complications. *Cochrane Database Syst Rev* **1:** CD004659, 2004.
50. Vainio M, Kujansuu E, Iso-Mustajarvi M, Maenpaa J. Low dose acetylsalicylic acid in prevention of pregnancy-induced hypertension and intrauterine growth retardation in women with bilateral uterine artery notches. *Br J Obset Gynaecol* **109**(2):161–167, 2002.
51. Norgard B, Puho E, Czeizel AE, Skriver MV, Sorensen HT. Aspirin use during early pregnancy and the risk of congenital abnormalities: a population-based case-control study. *Am J Obstet Gynecol* **192**(3):922–9233, 2005.
52. Askie LM, Duley L, Henderson-Smart DJ, Stewart LA. Antiplatelet agents for prevention of pre-eclampsia: a meta-analysis of individual patient data. *Lancet* **369**(9575):1791–1798, 2007.
53. Tarim E, Bal N, Kilicdag E, Kayaselcuk F, Bagis T, Kuscu E. Effects of aspirin on placenta and perinatal outcomes in patients with poor obstetric history. *Arch Gynecol Obstet* **274**(4):209–214, 2006.
54. Low dose aspirin in pregnancy and early childhood development: follow up of the collaborative low dose aspirin study in pregnancy, CLASP collaborative group. Br *J Obstet Gynaecol* **102**(11):861–868, 1995
55. Jacobson RL, Brewer A, Eis A, Siddiqi TA, Myatt L. Transfer of aspirin across the perfused human placental cotyledon. *Am J Obstet Gynecol* **165**(4 Pt 1):939–944, 1991.
56. Shen J, Wanwimolruk S, Wilson PD, Seddon RJ, Roberts MS. A clinical trial of a slow-release formulation of acetylsalicylic acid in patients at risk for preeclampsia. *Br J Clin Pharmacol* **35**(6):664–667, 1993.
57. Rumack CM, Guggenheim MA, Rumack BH, Peterson RG, Johnson ML, Braithwaite WR. Neonatal intracranial hemorrhage and maternal use of aspirin. *Obstet Gynecol* **58**(5 Suppl):52S–56S, 1981.
58. Stuart MJ, Gross SJ, Elrad H, Graeber JE. Effects of acetylsalicylic-acid ingestion on maternal and neonatal hemostasis. *N Engl J Med* **307**(15):909–912, 1982.
59. Leonhardt A, Bernert S, Watzer B, Schmitz-Ziegler G, Seyberth HW. Low-dose aspirin in pregnancy: maternal and neonatal aspirin concentrations and neonatal prostanoid formation. *Pediatrics* **111**(1):e77–e81, 2003.
60. Low-dose aspirin in prevention and treatment of intrauterine growth retardation and pregnancy-induced hypertension. Italian study of aspirin in pregnancy. *Lancet* **341**(8842):396–400, 1993.
61. Sibai BM, Caritis SN, Thom E et al. Prevention of preeclampsia with low-dose aspirin in healthy, nulliparous pregnant women. The National Institute of Child Health and Human Development Network of Maternal-Fetal Medicine Units. *N Engl J Med* **329**(17):1213–1218, 1993.
62. Valcamonico A, Foschini M, Soregaroli M, Tarantini M, Frusca T. Low dose aspirin in pregnancy: a clinical and biochemical study of effects on the newborn. *J Perinat Med* **21**(3):235–240, 1993.
63. Kozer E, Nikfar S, Costei A, Boskovic R, Nulman I, Koren G. Aspirin consumption during the first trimester of pregnancy and congenital anomalies: a meta-analysis. *Am J Obstet Gynecol* **187**(6): 1623–1630, 2002.
64. Werler MM, Sheehan JE, Mitchell AA. Maternal medication use and risks of gastroschisis and small intestinal atresia. *Am J Epidemiol* **155**(1):26–31, 2002.
65. Grab D, Paulus WE, Erdmann M et al. Effects of low-dose aspirin on uterine and fetal blood flow during pregnancy: results of a randomized, placebo-controlled, double-blind trial. *Ultrasound Obstet Gynecol* **15**:19–27, 2000.
66. Di Sessa TG, Moretti ML, Khoury A, Pulliam DA, Arheart KL, Sibai BM. Cardiac function in fetuses and newborns exposed to low-dose aspirin during pregnancy. *Am J Obstet Gynecol* **171**(4): 892–900, 1994.
67. Maher JE, Owen J, Hauth J, Goldenberg R, Parker CR Jr, Copper RL. The effect of low-dose aspirin on fetal urine output and amniotic fluid volume. *Am J Obstet Gynecol* **169**(4):885–888, 1993.
68. Forestier F, Daffos F, Capella-Pavlovsky M. Low molecular weight heparin (PK 10169) does not cross the placenta during the second trimester of pregnancy study by direct fetal blood sampling under ultrasound. *Thromb Res* **34**(6): 557–560, 1984.
69. Forestier F, Daffos F, Rainaut M, Toulemonde F. Low molecular weight heparin (CY 216) does not cross the placenta during the third trimester of pregnancy. *Thromb Haemost* **57**(2):234, 1987.
70. Ellison J, Walker ID, Greer IA. Antenatal use of enoxaparin for prevention and treatment of thromboembolism in pregnancy. *Br J Obstet Gynaecol* **107**(9):1116–1121, 2000.
71. Hunt BJ, Doughty HA, Majumdar G et al. Thromboprophylaxis with low molecular weight heparin (Fragmin) in high risk pregnancies. *Thromb Haemost* **77**(1):39–43, 1997.
72. Nelson-Piercy C, Letsky EA, de Swiet M. Low-molecular-weight heparin for obstetric thromboprophylaxis: experience of sixty-nine pregnancies in sixty-one women at high risk. *Am J Obstet Gynecol* **176**(5):1062–1068, 1997.
73. Greer IA, Nelson-Piercy C. Low-molecular-weight heparins for thromboprophylaxis and treatment of venous thromboembolism in pregnancy: a systematic review of safety and efficacy. *Blood* **106**(2):401–407, 2005.
74. Bates SM, Greer IA, Hirsh J, Ginsberg JS. Use of antithrombotic agents during pregnancy: the Seventh ACCP Conference on Antithrombotic and Thrombolytic Therapy. *Chest* **126**(3 Suppl):627S–644S, 2004.
75. Greer IA. Thrombosis in pregnancy: maternal and fetal issues. *Lancet* **353**(9160):1258–1265, 1999.
76. Wesseling J, Van Driel D, Heymans HS et al. Coumarins during pregnancy: long-term effects on growth and development of school-age children. *Thromb Haemost* **85**(4):609–613, 2001.
77. Chan WS, Anand S, Ginsberg JS. Anticoagulation of pregnant women with mechanical heart valves: a systematic review of the literature. *Arch Intern Med* **160**(2):191–196, 2000.
78. Alpert JS. The thrombosed prosthetic valve: current recommendations based on evidence from the literature. *J Am Coll Cardiol* **41**(4):659–660, 2003.
79. Perloff JK. Pregnancy and congenital heart disease. *J Am Coll Cardiol* **18**(2):340–342, 1991.
80. Shotan A, Ostrzega E, Mehra A, Johnson JV, Elkayam U. Incidence of arrhythmias in normal pregnancy and relation to palpitations, dizziness, and syncope. *Am J Cardiol* **79**(8):1061–1064, 1997.
81. Krapp M, Kohl T, Simpson JM, Sharland GK, Katalinic A, Gembruch U. Review of diagnosis, treatment, and outcome of fetal atrial flutter compared with supraventricular tachycardia. *Heart* **89**(8):913–917, 2003.
82. Walsh KA, Ezri MD, Denes P. Emergency treatment of tachyarrhythmias. *Med Clin North Am* **70**(4):791–811, 1986.

83. Cox JL, Gardner MJ. Treatment of cardiac arrhythmias during pregnancy. *Prog Cardiovasc Dis* **36**(2):137–178, 1993.
84. Lee RV, Rodgers BD, White LM, Harvey RC. Cardiopulmonary resuscitation of pregnant women. *Am J Med* **81**(2): 311–318, 1986.
85. Page RL. Treatment of arrhythmias during pregnancy. *Am Heart J* **130**(4): 871–876, 1995.
86. Elkayam U, Goodwin TM. Adenosine therapy for supraventricular tachycardia during pregnancy. *Am J Cardiol* **75**(7): 521–523, 1995.
87. Finlay AY, Edmunds VDC. cardioversion in pregnancy. *Br J Clin Pract* **33**(3):88–94, 1979.
88. Elkayam U, Gleicher N. *Cardiac problems in pregnancy*, 3rd edn. New York: Wiley-Liss, 1998.
89. Varon ME, Sherer DM, Abramowicz JS, Akiyama T. Maternal ventricular tachycardia associated with hypomagnesemia. *Am J Obstet Gynecol* **167**(5):1352–1355, 1992.
90. Cardosi RJ, Chez RA. Magnesium sulfate, maternal hypothermia, and fetal bradycardia with loss of heart rate variability. *Obstet Gynecol* **92**(4 Pt 2): 691–693, 1998.
91. De Wolf D, De Schepper J, Verhaaren H, Deneyer M, Smitz J, Sacre-Smits L. Congenital hypothyroid goiter and amiodarone. *Acta Paediatr Scand* **77**(4): 616–618, 1988.
92. Magee LA, Downar E, Sermer M, Boulton BC, Allen LC, Koren G. Pregnancy outcome after gestational exposure to amiodarone in Canada. *Am J Obstet Gynecol* **172**(4 Pt 1):1307–1311, 1995.
93. Widerhorn J, Bhandari AK, Bughi S, Rahimtoola SH, Elkayam U. Fetal and neonatal adverse effects profile of amiodarone treatment during pregnancy. *Am Heart J* **122**(4 Pt 1):1162–1166, 1991.
94. National Institutes of Health, National Heart, Lung, and Blood Institute, National Asthma Education and Prevention Program. Working group report on managing asthma during pregnancy: recommendations for pharmacologic treatment, update 2004. Available at: http://www.nhlbi.nih.gov/health/prof/lung/asthma/astpreg.htm.
95. Haahtela T, Jarvinen M, Kava T et al. Comparison of a beta 2-agonist, terbutaline, with an inhaled corticosteroid, budesonide, in newly detected asthma. *N Engl J Med* **325**(6):388–392, 1991.
96. Kallen B, Rydhstroem H, Aberg A. Congenital malformations after the use of inhaled budesonide in early pregnancy. *Obstet Gynecol* **93**(3):392–395, 1999.
97. Spitzer WO, Suissa S, Ernst P et al. The use of beta-agonists and the risk of death and near death from asthma. *N Engl J Med* **326**(8):501–506, 1992.
98. Schatz M, Dombrowski MP, Wise R et al. The relationship of asthma medication use to perinatal outcomes. *J Allergy Clin Immunol* **113**(6):1040–1045, 2004.
99. Arwood LL, Dasta JF, Friedman C. Placental transfer of theophylline: two case reports. *Pediatrics* **63**(6):844–846, 1979.
100. Dombrowski MP, Schatz M, Wise R et al. Randomized trial of inhaled beclomethasone dipropionate versus theophylline for moderate asthma during pregnancy. *Am J Obstet Gynecol* **190**(3): 737–744, 2004.
101. Bakhireva LN, Jones KL, Schatz M et al. Safety of leukotriene receptor antagonists in pregnancy. *J Allergy Clin Immunol* **119**(3):618–625, 2007.
102. Bracken MB, Triche EW, Belanger K, Saftlas A, Beckett WS, Leaderer BP. Asthma symptoms, severity, and drug therapy: a prospective study of effects on 2205 pregnancies. *Obstet Gynecol* **102**(4):739–752, 2003.
103. Perlow JH, Montgomery D, Morgan MA, Towers CV, Porto M. Severity of asthma and perinatal outcome. *Am J Obstet Gynecol* **167**(4 Pt 1):963–971, 1992.
104. Schatz M, Zeiger RS, Hoffman CP et al. Perinatal outcomes in the pregnancies of asthmatic women: a prospective controlled analysis. *Am J Respir Crit Care Med* **151**(4):1170–1174, 1995.
105. Bakhireva LN, Jones KL, Schatz M, Johnson D, Chambers CD. Asthma medication use in pregnancy and fetal growth. *J Allergy Clin Immunol* **116**(3): 503–509, 2005.
106. Chappell LC, Seed PT, Briley AL et al. Effect of antioxidants on the occurrence of pre-eclampsia in women at increased risk: a randomised trial. *Lancet* **354**(9181):810–816, 1999.
107. Poston L, Briley AL, Seed PT, Kelly FJ, Shennan AH. Vitamin C and vitamin E in pregnant women at risk for pre-eclampsia (VIP trial): randomised placebo-controlled trial. *Lancet* **367**(9517):1145–1154, 2006.
108. Polyzos NP, Mauri D, Tsappi M et al. Combined vitamin C and E supplementation during pregnancy for preeclampsia prevention: a systematic review. *Obstet Gynecol Surv* **62**(3): 202–206, 2007.
109. Pinsky L, Digeorge AM. Cleft palate in the mouse: a teratogenic index of glucocorticoid potency. *Science* **147**: 402–403, 1965.
110. Fraser FC, Sajoo A. Teratogenic potential of corticosteroids in humans. *Teratology* **51**(1):45–46, 1995.
111. Park-Wyllie L, Mazzotta P, Pastuszak A et al. Birth defects after maternal exposure to corticosteroids: prospective cohort study and meta-analysis of epidemiological studies. *Teratology* **62**(6):385–392, 2000.
112. Adams DF, Ment LR, Vohr B. Antenatal therapies and the developing brain. *Semin Neonatol* **6**(2):173–183, 2001.
113. Vohr BR, Wright LL, Dusick AM et al. Neurodevelopmental and functional outcomes of extremely low birth weight infants in the National Institute of Child Health and Human Development Neonatal Research Network, 1993–1994. *Pediatrics* **105**(6):1216–1226, 2000.
114. Kozlowska-Boszko B, Soluch L, Rybus J, Lao M, Durlik M, Gaciong Z. Does chronic glucocorticosteroid therapy in pregnant renal allograft recipients affect cortisol levels in neonates?. *Transplant Proc* **28**(6):3490–3491, 1996
115. Kraus AM. Developmental cataracts. *NY State J Med* **75**(10):1757–1758, 1975.
116. Reinisch JM, Simon NG, Karow WG, Gandelman R. Prenatal exposure to prednisone in humans and animals retards intrauterine growth. *Science* **202**(4366):436–438, 1978.
117. Rayburn WF. Glucocorticoid therapy for rheumatic diseases: maternal, fetal, and breast-feeding considerations. *Am J Reprod Immunol* **28**(3–4):138–140, 1992.
118. Greenberger PA, Odeh YK, Frederiksen MC, Atkinson AJ Jr. Pharmacokinetics of prednisolone transfer to breast milk. *Clin Pharmacol Ther* **53**(3):324–328, 1993.
119. Grekas DM, Vasiliou SS, Lazarides AN. Immunosuppressive therapy and breastfeeding after renal transplantation. *Nephron* **37**(1):68, 1984.
120. Dubinsky MC, Lamothe S, Yang HY et al. Pharmacogenomics and metabolite measurement for 6-mercaptopurine therapy in inflammatory bowel disease. *Gastroenterology* **118**(4):705–713, 2000.
121. de Boer NK, Jarbandhan SV, de Graaf P, Mulder CJ, van Elburg RM, van Bodegraven AA. Azathioprine use during pregnancy: unexpected intrauterine exposure to metabolites. *Am J Gastroenterol* **101**(6):1390–1392, 2006.
122. Francella A, Dyan A, Bodian C, Rubin P, Chapman M, Present DH. The safety of 6-mercaptopurine for childbearing patients with inflammatory bowel disease: a retrospective cohort study. *Gastroenterology* **124**(1):9–17, 2003.
123. Williamson RA, Karp LE. Azathioprine teratogenicity: review of the literature and case report. *Obstet Gynecol* **58**(2): 247–250, 1981.
124. Successful pregnancies in women treated by dialysis and kidney transplantation. Report from the Registration Committee of the European Dialysis and Transplant Association. *Br J Obstet Gynaecol* **87**(10):839–845, 1980.
125. Ramsey-Goldman R, Mientus JM, Kutzer JE, Mulvihill JJ, Medsger TA Jr.

Pregnancy outcome in women with systemic lupus erythematosus treated with immunosuppressive drugs. *J Rheumatol* **20**(7):1152–1157, 1993.

126. Norgard B, Pedersen L, Christensen LA, Sorensen HT. Therapeutic drug use in women with Crohn's disease and birth outcomes: a Danish nationwide cohort study. *Am J Gastroenterol* **102**(7): 1406–1413, 2007.
127. Moretti ME, Verjee Z, Ito S, Koren G. Breast-feeding during maternal use of azathioprine. *Ann Pharmacother* **40**(12):2269–2272, 2006.
128. Coulam CB, Moyer TP, Jiang NS, Zincke H. Breast-feeding after renal transplantation. *Transplant Proc* **14**(3): 605–609, 1982.
129. Gardiner SJ, Gearry RB, Roberts RL, Zhang M, Barclay ML, Begg EJ. Exposure to thiopurine drugs through breast milk is low based on metabolite concentrations in mother-infant pairs. *Br J Clin Pharmacol* **62**(4):453–456, 2006.
130. Jarnerot G, Into-Malmberg MB, Esbjorner E. Placental transfer of sulphasalazine and sulphapyridine and some of its metabolites. *Scand J Gastroenterol* **16**(5):693–697, 1981.
131. Hernandez-Diaz S, Werler MM, Walker AM, Mitchell AA. Folic acid antagonists during pregnancy and the risk of birth defects. *N Engl J Med* **343**(22):1608–1614, 2000.
132. Mogadam M, Dobbins III, WO, Korelitz BI, Ahmed SW. Pregnancy in inflammatory bowel disease: effect of sulfasalazine and corticosteroids on fetal outcome. *Gastroenterology* **80**(1):72–76, 1981.
133. Norgard B, Czeizel AE, Rockenbauer M, Olsen J, Sorensen HT. Population-based case control study of the safety of sulfasalazine use during pregnancy. *Aliment Pharmacol Ther* **15**(4):483–486, 2001.
134. Levi S, Liberman M, Levi AJ, Bjarnason I. Reversible congenital neutropenia associated with maternal sulphasalazine therapy. *Eur J Pediatr* **148**(2):174–175, 1988.
135. Jarnerot G, Into-Malmberg MB. Sulphasalazine treatment during breast feeding. *Scand J Gastroenterol* **14**(7): 869–871, 1979.
136. Ambrosius CL, Rasmussen SN, Hansen SH, Bondesen S, Hvidberg EF. Salazosulfapyridine and metabolites in fetal and maternal body fluids with special reference to 5-aminosalicylic acid. *Acta Obstet Gynecol Scand* **66**(5):433–435, 1987.
137. Sweiry JH, Yudilevich DL. Transport of folates at maternal and fetal sides of the placenta: lack of inhibition by methotrexate. *Biochim Biophys Acta* **821**(3):497–501, 1985.
138. Ostensen M, Hartmann H, Salvesen K. Low dose weekly methotrexate in early pregnancy. A case series and review of the literature. *J Rheumatol* **27**(8): 1872–1875, 2000.
139. Chakravarty EF, Sanchez-Yamamoto D, Bush TM. The use of disease modifying antirheumatic drugs in women with rheumatoid arthritis of childbearing age: a survey of practice patterns and pregnancy outcomes. *J Rheumatol* **30**(2):241–246, 2003.
140. Johns DG, Rutherford LD, Leighton PC, Vogel CL. Secretion of methotrexate into human milk. *Am J Obstet Gynecol* **112**(7):978–980, 1972.
141. Le Ray C, Coulomb A, Elefant E, Frydman R, Audibert F. Mycophenolate mofetil in pregnancy after renal transplantation: a case of major fetal malformations. *Obstet Gynecol* **103**(5 Pt 2):1091–1094, 2004.
142. Armenti VT, Radomski JS, Moritz MJ et al. Report from the National Transplantation Pregnancy Registry (NTPR): outcomes of pregnancy after transplantation. *Clin Transp* :121–130, 2002.
143. Petri M. Immunosuppressive drug use in pregnancy. *Autoimmunity* **36**(1):51–56, 2003.
144. European best practice guidelines for renal transplantation. Section IV: Long-term management of the transplant recipient. IV.10. Pregnancy in renal transplant recipients. *Nephrol Dial Transplant* **17**(Suppl 4):50–55, 2002.
145. Enns GM, Roeder E, Chan RT, Ali-Khan CZ, Cox VA, Golabi M. Apparent cyclophosphamide (cytoxan) embryopathy: a distinct phenotype?. *Am J Med Genet* **86**(3):237–241, 1999.
146. Mirkes PE. Cyclophosphamide teratogenesis: a review. *Teratog Carcinog Mutagen* **5**(2):75–88, 1985.
147. Wiernik PH, Duncan JH. Cyclophosphamide in human milk. *Lancet* **1**(7705):912, 1971.
148. Weber M, Deng S, Olthoff K et al. Organ transplantation in the twenty-first century. *Urol Clin North Am* **25**(1):51–61, 1998.
149. Sims CJ. Organ transplantation and immunosuppressive drugs in pregnancy. *Clin Obstet Gynecol* **34**(1):100–101, 1991.
150. Burckart GJ, Venkataramanan R, Ptachcinski RJ et al. Cyclosporine pharmacokinetic profiles in liver, heart, and kidney transplant patients as determined by high-performance liquid chromatography. *Transplant Proc* **18**(6 Suppl 5):129–136, 1986.
151. Di Paolo S, Monno R, Stallone G et al. Placental imbalance of vasoactive factors does not affect pregnancy outcome in patients treated with cyclosporine A after transplantation. *Am J Kidney Dis* **39**(4):776–783, 2002.
152. Bar OB, Hackman R, Einarson T, Koren G. Pregnancy outcome after cyclosporine therapy during pregnancy: a meta-analysis. *Transplantation* **71**(8):1051–1055, 2001.
153. Lamarque V, Leleu MF, Monka C, Krupp P. Analysis of 629 pregnancy outcomes in transplant recipients treated with Sandimmun. *Transplant Proc* **29**(5):2480, 1997.
154. Shaheen FA, al Sulaiman MH, al Khader AA. Long-term nephrotoxicity after exposure to cyclosporine in utero. *Transplantation* **56**(1):224–225, 1993.
155. Di Paolo S, Schena A, Morrone LF et al. Immunologic evaluation during the first year of life of infants born to cyclosporine-treated female kidney transplant recipients: analysis of lymphocyte subpopulations and immunoglobulin serum levels. *Transplantation* **69**(10):2049–2054, 2000.
156. Nyberg G, Haljamae U, Frisenette-Fich C, Wennergren M, Kjellmer I. Breastfeeding during treatment with cyclosporine. *Transplantation* **65**(2): 253–255, 1998.
157. Phillips-Howard PA, Wood D. The safety of antimalarial drugs in pregnancy. *Drug Saf* **14**(3):131–145, 1996.
158. Costedoat-Chalumeau N, Amoura Z, Duhaut P et al. Safety of hydroxychloroquine in pregnant patients with connective tissue diseases: a study of one hundred thirty-three cases compared with a control group. *Arthritis Rheum* **48**(11):3207–3211, 2003.
159. Borden MB, Parke AL. Antimalarial drugs in systemic lupus erythematosus: use in pregnancy. *Drug Saf* **24**(14): 1055–1063, 2001.
160. Canadian Consensus Conference on hydroxychloroquine, *J Rheumatol* **27**(12): 2919–2921, 2000.
161. Motta M, Tincani A, Faden D, Zinzini E, Chirico G. Antimalarial agents in pregnancy. *Lancet* **359**(9305):524–525, 2002.
162. A randomized study of the effect of withdrawing hydroxychloroquine sulfate in systemic lupus erythematosus. The Canadian Hydroxychloroquine Study Group. *N Engl J Med* **324**(3):150–154, 1991.
163. Cortes-Hernandez J, Ordi-Ros J, Paredes F, Casellas M, Castillo F, Vilardell-Tarres M. Clinical predictors of fetal and maternal outcome in systemic lupus erythematosus: a prospective study of 103 pregnancies. *Rheumatology (Oxford)* **41**(6):643–650, 2002.
164. Kainz A, Harabacz I, Cowlrick IS, Gadgil SD, Hagiwara D. Review of the course and outcome of 100 pregnancies in 84 women treated with tacrolimus. *Transplantation* **70**(12):1718–1721, 2000.
165. Kainz A, Harabacz I, Cowlrick IS, Gadgil S, Hagiwara D. Analysis of 100

pregnancy outcomes in women treated systemically with tacrolimus. *Transpl Int* **13**(Suppl 1):S299–S300, 2000.
166. Jain A, Venkataramanan R, Fung JJ et al. Pregnancy after liver transplantation under tacrolimus. *Transplantation* **64**(4):559–565, 1997.
167. Burt MJ, Frizelle FA, Barbezat GO. Pregnancy and exposure to infliximab (anti-tumor necrosis factor-alpha monoclonal antibody). *J Gastroenterol Hepatol* **18**(4):465–466, 2003.
168. Roux CH, Brocq O, Breuil V, Albert C, Euller-Ziegler L. Pregnancy in rheumatology patients exposed to anti-tumour necrosis factor (TNF)-alpha therapy. *Rheumatology (Oxford)* **46**(4): 695–698, 2007.
169. Stengel JZ, Arnold HL. Is Infliximab safe to use while breastfeeding? *World J Gastroenterology* **14**:3085–3087, 2008.
170. Ostensen M, Eigenmann GO. Etanercept in breast milk. *J Rheumatol* **31**(5): 1017–1018, 2004.
171. Waysbort A, Giroux M, Mansat V, Teixeira M, Dumas JC, Puel J. Experimental study of transplacental passage of alpha interferon by two assay techniques. *Antimicrob Agents Chemother* **37**(6):1232–1237, 1993.
172. Walther EU, Hohlfeld R. Multiple sclerosis: side effects of interferon beta therapy and their management. *Neurology* **53**(8):1622–1627, 1999.
173. Haas J. High dose IVIG in the post partum period for prevention of exacerbations in MS. *Mult Scler* **6**(Suppl 2):S18–S20, 2000.
174. Cines DB, Blanchette VS. Immune Thrombocytopenic Purpura. *N Engl J Med* **346**:995–1008, 2002.
175. Allen VM, Armson BA, Wilson RD et al. Teratogenicity associated with preexisting and gestational diabetes. *J Obstet Gynaecol Can* **29**(11):927–934, 2007.
176. Chen R, Ben Haroush A, Weissman-Brenner A, Melamed N, Hod M, Yogev Y. Level of glycemic control and pregnancy outcome in type 1 diabetes: a comparison between multiple daily insulin injections and continuous subcutaneous insulin infusions. *Am J Obstet Gynecol* **197**(4): 404–405, 2007.
177. Gonzalez C, Santoro S, Salzberg S, Di Girolamo G, Alvarinas J. Insulin analogue therapy in pregnancies complicated by diabetes mellitus. *Expert Opin Pharmacother* **6**(5):735–742, 2005.
178. Coetzee EJ, Jackson WP. The management of non-insulin-dependent diabetes during pregnancy. *Diabetes Res Clin Pract* **1**(5):281–287, 1985.
179. Feig DS, Briggs GG, Koren G. Oral antidiabetic agents in pregnancy and lactation: a paradigm shift? *Ann. Pharmacother* **41**(7):1174–1180, 2007.
180. Jacobson GF, Ramos GA, Ching JY, Kirby RS, Ferrara A, Field DR. Comparison of glyburide and insulin for the management of gestational diabetes in a large managed care organization. *Am J Obstet Gynecol* **193**(1):118–124, 2005.
181. Kahn BF, Davies JK, Lynch AM, Reynolds RM, Barbour LA. Predictors of glyburide failure in the treatment of gestational diabetes. *Obstet Gynecol* **107**(6):1303–1309, 2006.
182. Langer O, Conway DL, Berkus MD, Xenakis EM, Gonzales O. A comparison of glyburide and insulin in women with gestational diabetes mellitus. *N Engl J Med* **343**(16):1134–1138, 2000.
183. Langer O, Yogev Y, Xenakis EM, Rosenn B. Insulin and glyburide therapy: dosage, severity level of gestational diabetes, and pregnancy outcome. *Am J Obstet Gynecol* **192**(1):134–139, 2005.
184. Gedeon C, Behravan J, Koren G, Piquette-Miller M. Transport of glyburide by placental ABC transporters: implications in fetal drug exposure. *Placenta* **27**(11–12):1096–1102, 2006.
185. Kraemer J, Klein J, Lubetsky A, Koren G. Perfusion studies of glyburide transfer across the human placenta: implications for fetal safety. *Am J Obstet Gynecol* **195**(1):270–274, 2006.
186. Ramos GA, Jacobson GF, Kirby RS, Ching JY, Field DR. Comparison of glyburide and insulin for the management of gestational diabetics with markedly elevated oral glucose challenge test and fasting hyperglycemia. *J Perinatol* **27**(5):262–267, 2007.
187. Ekpebegh CO, Coetzee EJ, van der ML, Levitt NS. A 10-year retrospective analysis of pregnancy outcome in pregestational type 2 diabetes: comparison of insulin and oral glucose-lowering agents. *Diabet Med* **24**(3): 253–258, 2007.
188. Rowan JA, Hague WM, Gao W, Battin MR, Moore MP and the MiG Trial Investigators. Metformin versus insulin for the treatment of gestational diabetes. *N Engl J Med* **358**:2003–2015, 2008.
189. Casey BM. Subclinical hypothyroidism and pregnancy. *Obstet Gynecol Surv* **61**(6):415–420, 2006.
190. Abalovich M, Amino N, Barbour LA et al. Management of thyroid dysfunction during pregnancy and postpartum: an Endocrine Society Clinical Practice Guideline. *J Clin Endocrinol Metab* **92**(8 Suppl):S1–S47, 2007.
191. Anselmo J, Cao D, Karrison T, Weiss RE, Refetoff S. Fetal loss associated with excess thyroid hormone exposure. *J Am Med Assoc* **292**(6):691–695, 2004.
192. Casey BM, Dashe JS, Spong CY, McIntire DD, Leveno KJ, Cunningham GF. Perinatal significance of isolated maternal hypothyroxinemia identified in the first half of pregnancy. *Obstet Gynecol* **109**(5):1129–1135, 2007.
193. Kooistra L, Crawford S, van Baar AL, Brouwers EP, Pop VJ. Neonatal effects of maternal hypothyroxinemia during early pregnancy. *Pediatrics* **117**(1):161–167, 2006.
194. Pop VJ, Brouwers EP, Vader HL, Vulsma T, van Baar AL, de Vijlder JJ. Maternal hypothyroxinaemia during early pregnancy and subsequent child development: a 3-year follow-up study. *Clin Endocrinol (Oxf)* **59**(3):282–288, 2003.
195. Haddow JE, Palomaki GE, Allan WC et al. Maternal thyroid deficiency during pregnancy and subsequent neuropsychological development of the child. *N Engl J Med* **341**(8):549–555, 1999.
196. Vaidya B, Anthony S, Bilous M et al. Detection of thyroid dysfunction in early pregnancy: universal screening or targeted high-risk case finding?. *J Clin Endocrinol Metab* **92**(1):203–207, 2007.
197. Kamijo K. TSH-receptor antibodies determined by the first, second and third generation assays and thyroid-stimulating antibody in pregnant patients with Graves' disease. *Endocr J* **54**(4):619–624, 2007.
198. Momotani N, Noh JY, Ishikawa N, Ito K. Effects of propylthiouracil and methimazole on fetal thyroid status in mothers with Graves' hyperthyroidism. *J Clin Endocrinol Metab* **82**(11):3633–3636, 1997.
199. Chattaway JM, Klepser TB. Propylthiouracil versus methimazole in treatment of Graves' disease during pregnancy. *Ann Pharmacother* **41**(6): 1018–1022, 2007.
200. Clark SM, Saade GR, Snodgrass WR, Hankins GD. Pharmacokinetics and pharmacotherapy of thionamides in pregnancy. *Ther Drug Monit* **28**(4): 477–483, 2006.
201. Christensen J, Vestergaard M, Pedersen MG, Pedersen CB, Olsen J, Sidenius P. Incidence and prevalence of epilepsy in Denmark. *Epilepsy Res* **76**(1):60–65, 2007.
202. Lewis G. Saving Mothers' Lives. The 7th report of the confidential enquiries into maternal deaths United Kingdom. CEMACH, 2007.
203. Tomson T, Battino D. Teratogenicity of antiepileptic drugs: state of the art. *Curr Opin Neurol* **18**(2):135–140, 2005.
204. Meador KJ, Baker GA, Finnell RH et al. In utero antiepileptic drug exposure: fetal death and malformations. *Neurology* **67**(3):407–412, 2006.
205. Tomson T, Battino D, French J et al. Antiepileptic drug exposure and major congenital malformations: the role of pregnancy registries. *Epilepsy Behav* **11**(3):277–282, 2007.
206. Holmes LB, Harvey EA, Coull BA et al. The teratogenicity of anticonvulsant drugs. *N Engl J Med* **344**(15):1132–1138, 2001.

207. Candito M, Naimi M, Boisson C et al. Plasma vitamin values and antiepileptic therapy: case reports of pregnancy outcomes affected by a neural tube defect. *Birth Defects Res A Clin Mol Teratol* **79**(1):62–64, 2007.
208. Finnell RH, Gould A, Spiegelstein O. Pathobiology and genetics of neural tube defects. *Epilepsia* **44**(Suppl 3):14–23, 2003.
209. Kaaja E, Kaaja R, Matila R, Hiilesmaa V. Enzyme-inducing antiepileptic drugs in pregnancy and the risk of bleeding in the neonate. *Neurology* **58**(4):549–553, 2002.
210. Harden CL. Pregnancy and epilepsy. *Semin Neurol* **27**(5):453–459, 2007.
211. Williams J, Myson V, Steward S et al. Self-discontinuation of antiepileptic medication in pregnancy: detection by hair analysis. *Epilepsia* **43**(8):824–831, 2002.
212. Morrow J, Russell A, Guthrie E et al. Malformation risks of antiepileptic drugs in pregnancy: a prospective study from the UK Epilepsy and Pregnancy Register. *J Neurol Neurosurg Psychiatr* **77**(2): 193–198, 2006.
213. Vinten J, Adab N, Kini U, Gorry J, Gregg J, Baker GA. Neuropsychological effects of exposure to anticonvulsant medication in utero. *Neurology* **64**(6):949–954, 2005.
214. Adab N, Kini U, Vinten J, Ayres J et al. The longer term outcome of children born to mothers with epilepsy. *J Neurol Neurosurg Psychiatr* **75**(11):1575–1583, 2004.
215. Kini U, Adab N, Vinten J, Fryer A. Clayton-Smith J on behalf of the Liverpool and Manchester Neurodevelopment Study Group. Dysmorphic features: an important clue to the diagnosis and severity of fetal anticonvulsant syndromes. *Arch Dis Fetal Neonatal Ed* **91**:F90–F95, 2006.
216. Adam J, Vorhee CV, Middaugh LD. Developmental toxicity of anticonvulsants: human and animal evidence on phenytoin. *Neurotoxicol Teratol* **12**:203–214, 1990.
217. Buehler BA, Delimont D, van Waes M, Finnell RH. Prenatal prediction of risk of the fetal hydantoin syndrome. *N Engl J Med* **329**:1660–1661, 1993.
218. Phelan MC, Pellock JM, Nance WE. Discordant expression of fetal hydantoin syndrome in heteropaternal dizygotic twins. *N Engl J Med* **307**:99–101, 1982.
219. Jones KL, Lacro RV, Johnson KA, Adams J. Pattern of malformation in the children of women treated with carbamazepine during pregnancy. *N Engl J Med* **320**:1661–1666, 1989.
220. Perucca E, Tomson T. Prenatal exposure to antiepileptic drugs. *Lancet* **367**: 1467–1469, 2006.
221. Bennett HA, Einarson A, Taddio A, Koren G, Einarson TR. Prevalence of depression during pregnancy: systematic review. *Obstet Gynecol* **103**(4):698–709, 2004.
222. Meijer WE, Heerdink ER, Leufkens HG, Herings RM, Egberts AC, Nolen WA. Incidence and determinants of long-term use of antidepressants. *Eur J Clin Pharmacol* **60**(1):57–61, 2004.
223. Bakker MK et al. *Br J Clin Pharm epub ahead of print* , 2007.
224. Kulin NA, Pastuszak A, Sage SR et al. Pregnancy outcome following maternal use of the new selective serotonin reuptake inhibitors: a prospective controlled multicenter study. *J Am Med Assoc* **279**(8):609–610, 1998.
225. Wogelius P, Norgaard M, Gislum M et al. Maternal use of selective serotonin reuptake inhibitors and risk of congenital malformations. *Epidemiology* **17**(6): 701–704, 2006.
226. Chambers CD, Hernandez-Diaz S, Van Marter LJ et al. Selective serotonin-reuptake inhibitors and risk of persistent pulmonary hypertension of the newborn. *N Engl J Med* **354**(6):579–587, 2006.
227. Altshuler LL, Cohen L, Szuba MP, Burt VK, Gitlin M, Mintz J. Pharmacologic management of psychiatric illness during pregnancy: dilemmas and guidelines. *Am J Psychiatr* **153**(5):592–606, 1996.
228. Webster PA. Withdrawal symptoms in neonates associated with maternal antidepressant therapy. *Lancet* **2**(7824):318–319, 1973.
229. Giles JJ, Bannigan JG. Teratogenic and developmental effects of lithium. *Curr Pharm Des* **12**(12):1531–1541, 2006.
230. Guidelines for vaccinating pregnant women. Recommendations of advisory committee on immunization practice. Centers for disease control and prevention, Atlanta, 2002.

CHAPTER 14

The perinatal postmortem

Phil Cox

KEY POINTS

- The perinatal postmortem is still a key part of the investigation of fetal loss
- The role of the postmortem is wider than just identifying the cause of death
- Most postmortems are performed with written consent of the parents. In the UK, the consent process is governed by the Human Tissue Act (2004) and its Codes of Practice
- The postmortem examination always requires histological examination of tissues and often includes other tests
- In cases of fetal hydrops, fetal akinesia and any other situation where metabolic disease is a possibility, the postmortem should be performed within 48 hours of death to give the best chance of reaching a definitive diagnosis
- Injection studies of monochorionic twin placentas may provide additional information relating to the cause of discordant growth
- Many intrapartum stillbirths and neonatal deaths show signs of compromise prior to the onset of labor

INTRODUCTION

In contrast to other areas of medicine, clinically driven (rather than medicolegal) postmortem examination remains a key element in the investigation of disorders of fetal and perinatal life. Although autopsy rates have fallen in many countries in recent years, the rates of consented postmortem are still much higher for fetal and neonatal deaths than in pediatric or adult deaths[1].

The aim of this chapter is not to be a comprehensive description of the pathology of the fetal and neonatal period. Instead the intention is to cover a number of areas relevant to the practicing obstetrician or specialist in fetal medicine.

Perinatal pathology is a distinct subspecialty of histopathology, dealing with a very different spectrum of disease to either adult or pediatric practice, which is mostly focused on the examination of biopsies or surgical specimens from live patients. The perinatal pathologist needs a sound knowledge of obstetrics, fetal medicine, neonatal pediatrics and genetics. Perinatal pathology also requires a different mindset from other branches of pathology. The 'patient' is not the baby being examined, but the mother and other members of the baby's family, whose future reproductive choices and obstetric care may be influenced by the findings of the autopsy. In addition, in contrast to biopsy or surgical pathology, there is generally only one chance to perform the examination with no opportunity to take additional samples. A repeat biopsy or re-examination of the sample (or in this case the baby) is generally not possible, therefore, the initial examination must gather all the information and samples necessary to reach or exclude all possible diagnoses for a given clinical situation. Most, if not all, perinatal pathologists will have been in the situation of wishing they had taken that extra sample that would have clinched the diagnosis. This tends to lead to very detailed examination and extensive sampling of tissues in even apparently straightforward cases. Protocols, such as that produced in the UK by the Royal College of Pathologists[2], may be helpful in ensuring that important findings are not missed.

In the UK and many other English-speaking economically developed countries, the majority of perinatal autopsies are performed by full-time, specialist perinatal pathologists who often provide a tertiary referral service to a number of obstetric/neonatal units. In contrast, in much of the European mainland, these cases are typically examined by general histopathologists with a degree of specialist expertise in this area, although specialist pathologists are becoming more common here as well.

REASONS FOR PERFORMING A PERINATAL POSTMORTEM

One typically thinks of a postmortem examination as being performed to identify the cause of death of the individual. However, in the perinatal arena, this is not always the case and is rarely the sole motivation.

The functions of the perinatal autopsy are:

- to identify cause of death
- to identify fetal genetic disease
- to identify potentially recurrent maternal disease
- audit of clinical care
- research
- teaching.

In a case of antepartum stillbirth, one might imagine that finding the cause of death was the only aim of the examination. While the examination may highlight features, such as mild growth restriction, which indicate a suboptimal intrauterine environment, often the precise cause of the death cannot be determined. However, the examination also serves to exclude (or occasionally suggest) an underlying chromosomal or genetic disorder, may indicate a possible maternal condition requiring treatment in a future pregnancy, and can provide an audit of the obstetric care received by the mother. The findings may help to defend or support a claim of medical negligence and can help to educate clinicians, leading to changes in management protocols.

Where pregnancy has been terminated following a prenatal diagnosis of fetal abnormality, the cause of death is not the issue. The postmortem serves to confirm the antenatal findings and identify additional abnormalities, which may allow a definitive diagnosis to be reached. Increasingly, this can lead to confirmation of a specific mutation at the DNA level, allowing early prenatal testing in subsequent pregnancies.

In many areas of fetal and perinatal pathology there is huge scope for research. The information collected at a full postmortem and the tissues taken for diagnosis are a valuable resource for research, often requiring relatively unsophisticated methods.

THE VALUE OF THE PERINATAL POSTMORTEM

With the ever-increasing resolution of ultrasound scanning machines and the availability of other imaging modalities, such as magnetic resonance imaging (MRI), to fetal medicine specialists it is tempting to believe that postmortem examination is unlikely to provide any relevant additional information. However, studies comparing postmortem findings to clinical diagnosis and/or antenatal ultrasound assessment universally show a clear and substantial benefit from the postmortem with regards to providing additional, clinically important information. Studies of stillbirths and neonatal deaths show significant additional information arising from the postmortem in 14–46% of cases, with the postmortem leading to a major change in the cause of death in around 10%[3–9]. Earlier studies comparing ultrasound to postmortem showed substantial numbers of false positive diagnoses by ultrasound. More recently, it appears that the false positive rate has fallen to a low level in expert hands, however, we have shown that postmortem continues to identify diagnostically significant additional findings in around 27% of cases scanned at a tertiary fetal medicine unit[10].

The postmortem should not, however, be regarded as the ultimate and only arbiter of fact. Some abnormalities that may be clearly demonstrated by ultrasound scan can be difficult to confirm at postmortem. This is particularly true of abnormalities of the brain, such as mild ventricular dilatation, which may be impossible to confirm in the presence of maceration following fetocide[11]. Thus, findings at antenatal scan and postmortem should be viewed as complementary investigations rather than one necessarily overriding the other. Regular review meetings between fetal medicine specialists and their perinatal pathology colleagues can facilitate this.

It is also worthy of note that the studies cited above are based on centers with specialist expertise in perinatal pathology. It has also been shown that perinatal postmortems performed by pathologists with no expertise or experience in this field are of substantially less, and sometimes no value[12,13].

AUTHORIZATION FOR POSTMORTEM

In most economically developed countries, postmortem examination can only be performed with appropriate authorization. In the UK, as in many other countries, this can come from one of two sources. The authorization may be given by the state legal authorities (the coroner, fiscal or other similar individual) under certain specified circumstances, or it can be given by the family of the deceased, in the form of (usually) written consent.

In the UK, the coroner's jurisdiction does not extend prior to the completion of birth and only applies to babies who have shown signs of life after birth. Therefore, terminations of pregnancy, antepartum and intrapartum fetal deaths are not the concern of the coroner (although occasionally the police may be involved). Babies born spontaneously prior to viability may show signs of life at birth but, generally, it is acceptable to give the cause of death as extreme prematurity. However, any baby who is born with signs of life, for whom a cause of death cannot be determined clinically, must be referred to the coroner. Similarly, any baby dying suddenly and unexpectedly falls under the coroner's jurisdiction. In the UK, the coroner or fiscal can authorize a postmortem examination without the need for parental consent and there is no right of objection. The scope of this examination is limited to determining the cause of death. It is illegal to remove any samples or tissue for other purposes, such as research or teaching, without consent from the family.

The legislation varies in different countries and even between England and Scotland, and it is important to be conversant with the law in the jurisdiction in which you are practicing, as there may be serious sanctions, or at the very least severe censure, for breaching the regulations.

The large majority of perinatal autopsies are performed with parental consent, a so-called 'hospital autopsy'. The rules governing consent for autopsy vary from country to country, but recent years have seen major changes to the laws governing the use of human tissue, including postmortem examination, in many countries.

In England and Wales, consented postmortem examination is governed by the Human Tissue Act (2004)[14]. This established a Human Tissue Authority (HTA)[15] to regulate the use of human tissue. A similar, although not identical, law and authority is in place in Scotland[16].

The Human Tissue Authority licenses organizations that undertake postmortem examinations and other activities involving human tissue. They have also produced a number of statutory Codes of Practice relating to these activities[17].

The Code of Practice relating to postmortem consent lays down the standards for obtaining postmortem consent, including who can give consent, who can obtain consent and what the discussion with the family prior to consent being given should include. This and the other HTA Codes of Practice have the force of statute and thus anyone wishing to seek consent for postmortem must adhere to them. It should be noted that the Human Tissue Act applies to all postmortem examinations, regardless of the gestation and includes previable fetuses. While the Human Tissue Act does not apply outside England and Wales, the principles laid down by the HTA in the Codes of Practice regarding obtaining parental consent are generally sound and are worthy of scrutiny by anyone who may have to obtain consent for postmortem, if similar documents are not available in the jurisdiction in which you practice. Many readers will be aware of the upheaval caused in the UK and elsewhere as a result of past failure to ensure that consent for postmortem was given in the light of a proper understanding by the relatives of what they were consenting to and why. Avoidance of such problems is to be strongly recommended.

THE POSTMORTEM EXAMINATION

The postmortem examination will usually be performed by a medically trained pathologist, often assisted by a trained mortuary technician. In some countries, non-medical personnel have been trained to be able to perform the examination and report the findings to the pathologist. The examination should be performed in an appropriately equipped facility, with excellent lighting and access to some form of magnifier and equipment of appropriate size for the examination to be performed. It is generally difficult to perform an adequate examination in a facility designed and equipped for adult autopsies.

Postmortem delay

The examination should be performed as soon as is practical. Ideally, this would be within 48 hours of the delivery, however, the delay is often longer, as a result of the time required to obtain consent, organize transfer of the body to the regional center, etc. On the whole, this is not a major problem. There will be some deterioration in the quality of the tissues on histological examination, but this is rarely sufficient to interfere with reaching a diagnosis. There is a fall in the success rate of tissue culture for karyotyping with increasing delay[18]. If the delay is likely to be greater than 3 or 4 days, it is advisable to take samples shortly after birth/death at the hospital of origin, to increase the chance of successful culture. There is also likely to be a fall in the yield of cultures of pathogenic bacteria, as well as a small increase in the chance of cultures yielding bacterial contaminants[18]. Providing that the body is adequately refrigerated, and samples for cytogenetics are taken within 3 days, the postmortem can reasonably be carried out within 7 days of the delivery/death, and even examinations performed later than this may still yield useful information.

Clinical information

It is essential that the person requesting the postmortem supply the pathologist with as much relevant clinical information as possible. Sending the hospital notes can be helpful, but it may difficult to glean the necessary information if the notes are voluminous or poorly written. Thus, many centers provide a detailed request form outlining the information required (Fig. 14.1). Properly completed, this can be of great assistance to the pathologist. There is sadly a tendency to leave parts of the form blank when the information is not to hand or assumed to be unimportant. This can lead to deficiencies in the examination or errors in interpretation of the findings. It is important to inform the pathologist of any particular areas of interest as these may require special techniques to be employed and may be omitted if a specific problem is not highlighted in the request.

External examination

Once the consent has been checked and baby's identity confirmed, the examination commences with the recording of the body weight and standard measurements such as crown–heel and crown–rump length, occipitofrontal circumference and foot length. Other measurements such as inner and outer canthal distances, chest and abdominal circumference may also be helpful in some situations. These can be compared to standard charts to help assess gestation, growth and normality.

External examination is performed next. The baby is examined to determine whether there are any congenital malformations. It is important to examine the orifices for patency, the mouth for palatal clefts and the hands and feet for missing or extra digits and syndactyly. Any of these anomalies are easily overlooked in small fetuses, unless a careful examination is performed, if necessary under a magnifying lens or dissecting microscope. The external phenotypic sex of the fetus is frequently misdiagnosed by the inexperienced before 18 weeks' gestation. It is important to inform clinical staff if a discrepancy is recognized, as parents frequently give a first name to even very small fetuses. Informing the parents that their little boy was, in fact, a little girl several weeks after a funeral has been held, can be a cause of great upset.

Assessment of the degree of maceration may give a guide to the time of fetal demise in stillborn infants[19–21]. This may be important, particularly when the quality of antenatal care is being called into question. While it is not possible to give a precise timing of death, it is usually possible to provide some approximate assessment of when the baby died. The stages of maceration and related duration of retention following fetal demise are shown in Table 14.1. Assessment of the degree of

Table 14.1 **Timing of fetal death related to macroscopic appearance of the fetus[19–21]**

Time since fetal demise	*Features*
<8 hours	Reddened skin
8–48 hours	Skin slippage, blistering and peeling
2–7 days	Extensive skin peeling, red serosanguinous effusions in body cavities
8–14 days	Yellow brown liver, turbid effusions in body cavities
>2 weeks	May be mummified

Birmingham Women's Health Care **NHS**
NHS Trust
DEPARTMENT OF HISTOPATHOLOGY

CLINICAL INFORMATION FOR FETAL / PERINATAL POST MORTEM

Please attach **Mother's** sticker here Family Name:..................... First Name:........................ D.o.B.: / / Reg No............................ Consultant:........................	Please attach **Baby's** sticker here Family Name:..................... First Name:........................ D.o.B.: / / Reg No............................ Consultant:........................

Ethnic origin: ___________ father's ethnic origin (if known) ______ Baby's Sex: M/F/?

REFERRING HOSPITAL:_______________ Ward: ___________

HOSPITAL OF BIRTH (if different) ___________

RELEVANT HISTORY:

Mother's Height: cm

Booking weight kg

PREVIOUS PREGNANCIES: G: ___ P: ____

date gestation labour sex outcome

1.___________________________________

2.___________________________________

3.___________________________________

4.___________________________________

5.___________________________________

THIS PREGNANCY: booked/unbooked LMP _________ EDD __________ BMI ____________

Gestation: by dates:_______/40 by scan:_______/40 weeks Blood group: ___, RhD pos/neg

HBsAg pos/neg Antibodies ________________________

Serum screening results: ________________________________ Medications _______________________

Abnormal USS findings(or send report) ____

____

Antenatal diagnostic procedures/results: ____

____

____ Karyotype: ____________________

threatened abortion: no/yes when _______________	severe anaemia no / yes
antepartum haemorrhage: no / yes when __________	infection risk: low/high(reason) ___________
hypertension: no / yes max b.p.________________	maternal pyrexia: no / yes when _________
pre-eclampsia: no / yes when ________________	other problem: ______________________

LABOUR: onset: spont / medical/none. IOL for: IUD/TOP/other___________ Fetocide: y/n date: ___________

Presentation: vertex/breech/other:__________ Liquor volume: normal / reduced / increased; colour:_________

Rupture of membranes: date ______ time_____ Augmentation (Syntocinon): yes/no

1st stage __h __min 2nd : __h __min Fetal heart last heard (S/B): date ______ time______

Fetal distress: yes/no specify: ____

Fig. 14.1 Clinical information form for perinatal postmortem.

DELIVERY: spontaneous / assisted (forceps / ventouse) / CS (elective/emergency) date ________ time______
DEATH: date _______________ time_____________

Baby: birth weight _______g Apgars: 1st min ____ 5th min ____ 10th min ____

ABNORMALITIES NOTED: nil / ____

____

____

RESUSCITATION: nil / mucus extraction / oxygen / mask / intubation / other ____________________

____ Surfactant: yes / no

For liveborn infants:

NEONATAL PROBLEMS:

1. ______________________________
2. ______________________________
3. ______________________________
4. ______________________________
5. ______________________________

PROCEDURES:

1. ______________________________
2. ______________________________
3. ______________________________
4. ______________________________
5. ______________________________

BRIEF SUMMARY OF LATER SYMPTOMS / TREATMENTS AND MAJOR INVESTIGATIONS (including CPAP/ventilation, IV therapy, fits, episodes of collapse, pneumonia, pneumothorax, bleeding problems, type of feeding etc.; **If complex course, please send photocopy of relevant pages of notes):**

SUSPECTED CAUSE(S) OF DEATH:

DEATH REGISTERED AS: livebirth / stillbirth / not registered (miscarriage)

ANY OTHER RELEVANT INFORMATION / SPECIAL POINTS TO BE NOTED AT POST MORTEM:

Referring Doctor / Midwife: ____________________________ Contact number / bleep No____________

ALL BABIES AND PLACENTAS SHOULD BE SENT FRESH IN LEAKPROOF, OPAQUE CONTAINERS UNLESS THERE IS AN INFECTIOUS HAZARD (in this case phone to discuss whether the specimen should be fixed in 10% formalin before transportation)

IT IS ESSENTIAL TO SEND THE PLACENTA WITH A FETUS / INFANT.

ALL SPECIMENS MUST BE CLEARLY LABELLED AND ACCOMPANIED WITH A COMPLETED REQUEST AND CONSENT FORM

Fig. 14.1 (Continued)

histological autolysis of the tissues can also help to determine the timing of death (Table 14.2)[22]. However, it should be noted that autolysis and some features of maceration may progress after delivery, and thus may be affected by the postmortem delay, especially if the baby is not stored in a refrigerator for significant periods after birth. The appearance of maceration can also be accelerated in hydropic fetuses and in the presence of infection[23].

Imaging

It is advisable to record any major anomalies with a camera (digital or otherwise). It is our practice to take one general image of every baby we examine, with additional images of anomalies. These images can be very useful when discussing findings with colleagues in obstetrics and, in particular, our clinical geneticists. Similarly, it should be standard practice to obtain a full skeletal X-ray, at least an anteroposterior view, in every baby. Spinal abnormalities are particularly likely to go unrecognized without routine radiographs, but other skeletal abnormalities may also be missed. In cases of skeletal dysplasia and other skeletal malformations, good quality radiographs are mandatory.

Magnetic resonance imaging may occasionally be useful. The images in well-preserved fetuses can be excellent. This is particularly true for cases of cerebral ventriculomegaly, where it may be difficult to identify the cause of ventricular dilatation at postmortem[24]. Unfortunately, but not unexpectedly, the images obtained from macerated fetuses are of lesser quality and, in such cases, carefully conducted postmortem examination can provide useful information, where MRI is uninformative.

Internal examination

Internal examination of the fetus should be performed through incisions that will be hidden under normal baby clothes, to minimize the distress caused to parents who may wish to view the body after the examination has been completed. It should be stressed to parents that neither the face nor the extremities are disturbed by the examination.

As with any procedure, it is important that a standard technique is followed, with variations as appropriate to deal with the precise situation. It is essential that a systematic examination of all of the major organs be performed, to identify structural abnormalities and relationships to other components of the organ system. In this way, subtle abnormalities will not be missed. As with the external examination, photography should be employed liberally to record abnormalities, in order to facilitate future diagnostic discussions. Organ weights should be routinely recorded and compared to normal standards for body weight and/or gestation. This can give important information regarding fetal growth and gestation and clues to underlying pathology.

Histology

Histological examination of all of the major organs must be performed as a routine. Even in severely macerated fetuses, vital information can frequently be obtained, which otherwise would go unrecognized. Tissue samples are fixed in formalin and processed to impregnate the tissue with paraffin wax and then sections, around 4 μm in thickness, are cut from the resulting tissue blocks, mounted on glass slides and stained to visualize the cellular structure (Fig. 14.2). In most cases, routine staining of slides with hematoxylin and eosin is sufficient but, on occasions, special stains and immunohistochemistry can be useful. It should be standard practice to store all histological tissue blocks and slides for at least 25 years, to allow review in case the diagnosis is queried, new information comes to light or new tests become available. These blocks and slides are also a valuable tool for audit, quality control, teaching and diagnostic research. In the UK, use for these additional purposes requires specific consent from the family.

Table 14.2 **Timing of fetal demise related to histological appearance of tissues[22]**

Time since fetal demise	*Histological appearance*
4 hours	Loss of nuclear basophilia in isolated renal cortical tubular cells
24 hours	Loss of nuclear basophilia in isolated cells in liver and inner half of myocardium
48 hours	Loss of nuclear basophilia in isolated cells in outer half of myocardium
96 hours	Loss of nuclear basophilia in isolated bronchial epithelial cells and in all cells of liver
1 week	Loss of nuclear basophilia in isolated tracheal cartilage cells and in all cells of GI tract and adrenals
4 weeks	Loss of nuclear basophilia in all cells in kidney

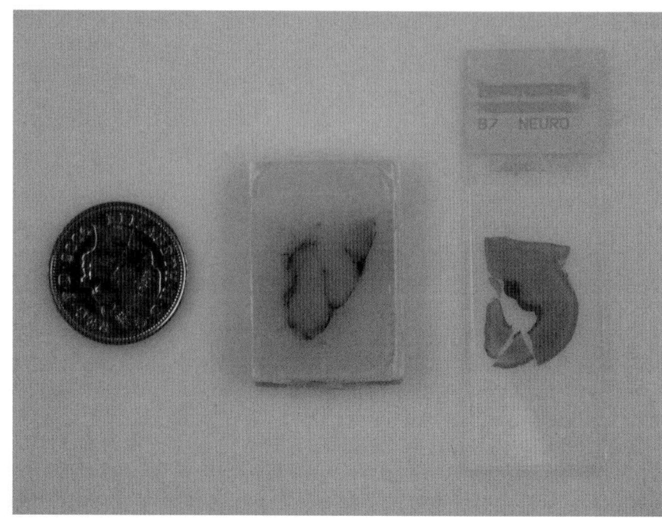

Fig. 14.2 Paraffin tissue block and histological slide.

Other investigations

In addition to the external and internal examination and histology, the perinatal postmortem frequently includes a variety of further tests. Where infection is suspected, bacterial, or occasionally viral cultures may be sent. Samples for karyotyping should be sent from any baby with congenital malformations, unless normal chromosomes have been shown antenatally. Many laboratories request confirmatory samples from babies shown to have an abnormal karyotype on amniocentesis or chorion villus sampling. Routine karyotyping of normally formed stillborn babies and spontaneous or missed miscarriages is of questionable value, and will not be undertaken by many laboratories, due to a very low rate of detection of an abnormal karyotype.

It is preferable to sample both fetal skin and placental tissue (taken through the fetal placental surface, close to the center of the placenta). The skin sample will unequivocally give the fetal karyotype, but is less likely to grow successfully in culture, especially following intrauterine death (naturally occurring or iatrogenic). Placental samples are more likely to grow than skin, as maternal placental perfusion continues after fetal death. However, there is a greater chance of cultural artefacts and also, if the fetus is female, it is impossible to be certain whether the cultured cells are of fetal or maternal origin.

Advances in technology have increased the possibility of some level of chromosome analysis from quite severely macerated fetuses. Techniques such as quantitative fluorescent polymerase chain reaction (QF-PCR) and fluorescent in situ hybridization (FISH) allow a limited analysis of the karyotype to identify the major common trisomies and sex chromosome aneuplodies in tissues that will not grow in culture. In the future, comparative genomic hydridization (CGH) and microarray studies may remove the need for cell culture and microscope-based cytogenetics completely.

It is good practice to save frozen tissue, typically liver, from fetuses with congenital malformations, unless they have already been shown to have an abnormal karyotype. This can be used as a source of DNA for genetic tests and may also be used for other tests such as biochemical assays for abnormalities of the sterol pathway (e.g. Smith–Lemli–Opitz syndrome) and PCR for viruses. DNA may also be routinely extracted from samples sent for karyotyping, but then other, non-genetic tests are not possible.

Biochemical tests of enzyme activity in fetal tissues, such as liver and muscle, in suspected metabolic disorders, are not possible unless the postmortem is performed within a few hours of death. Assays of enzyme activity for some, but far from all, metabolic disorders may be performed on cultured placental or skin fibroblasts. However, some enzymes or specific isoforms are not expressed in fibroblasts, therefore, if a metabolic disorder is a suspected prior to delivery, efforts should be made to obtain the necessary samples as soon as possible after birth.

The placenta

The placenta is a vital part of any fetal or perinatal autopsy. The placenta should always be submitted to the laboratory for examination with the baby. In cases of stillbirth and spontaneous miscarriage, the placenta alone may be sufficient to provide the cause of death/pregnancy loss and failure to submit it to the laboratory is seriously poor practice. In these cases, the postmortem without the placenta is only a partial examination. If at all possible, the placenta should also be sent for examination in cases of neonatal death, although if the baby appears well at birth, it is often disposed of. Babies born in poor condition and those born very prematurely should also have their placenta examined to try to identify the cause of their condition and, in the case of prematurity, to alert the neonatal unit to the possibility of congenital infection. Even following termination of pregnancy for congenital malformations, examination of the placenta has a role. In addition to providing tissue for karyotyping and fibroblast culture, the placenta occasionally can help make a diagnosis. Examples include cytomegalovirus infection, amniotic bands and placental mesenchymal dysplasia indicating Beckwith–Wiedemann syndrome (Fig. 14.3).

Laboratories differ as to whether they prefer to receive the placenta in the fresh state, or following formalin fixation. The preference of our unit is for submission fresh, as we find examination easier, and this allows sampling for cytogenetics as indicated. If fixed placentas are preferred, then the submitting obstetric unit must take the cytogenetics sample, into suitable transport medium, before fixation and either send it to the pathologist with the fixed placenta or directly to the cytogenetics department.

Examination of the placenta should follow a standard protocol[25]. As a minimum, the weight of the placental disk should be recorded, after removal of the cord and membranes, along with its dimensions in three planes. The length and diameter of the umbilical cord, the site of insertion into the placental disk, number of vessels and presence of knots or other lesions should be detailed. The appearance of the membranes and fetal surface should be documented, particularly looking for signs of infection. The maternal surface should be examined and any defects, suggesting retention of placental tissue in utero, should be noted. There is often some degree of superficial calcification, but this is of little significance. Following slicing of the disk at approximately 1 cm intervals, the overall appearance and any localized lesions should be recorded. Samples should be taken for histology. As a minimum, these should include a transverse section of umbilical cord, a roll of membranes and two full thickness sections of the placental disk. Additional samples

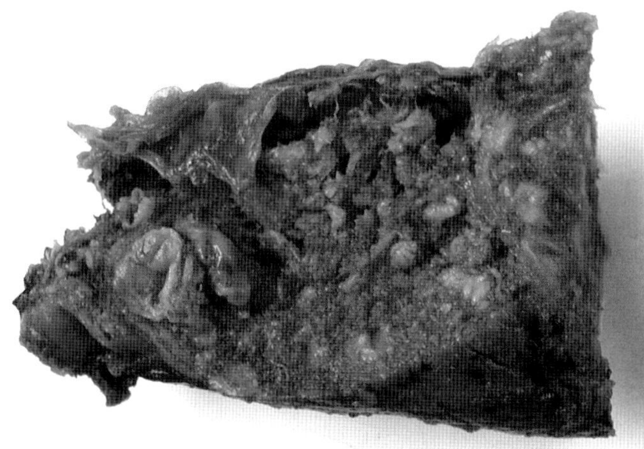

Fig. 14.3 Coarse, hydropic villi, suggestive of molar pregnancy in a case of placental mesenchymal dysplasia.

should be taken as indicated by the clinical situation and findings. Readers are referred to textbooks of placental pathology for a more detailed discussion of the pathological examination of the placenta[25,26].

Umbilical cord coiling has been the focus of considerable interest in recent years. Studies appear to show that the normal cord coiling index (CCI – complete twists per cm) is 0.17 (±0.009)[27]. Abnormal cord coiling below 10th centile (0.07) or above 90th centile (0.30) has been shown to be associated with adverse perinatal outcome[28]. Increased CCI has been found to be more common in birth asphyxia, intrauterine growth restriction and thrombosis along with a range of other complications, while low CCI is more common in association with chromosome abnormalities, fetal death, amniotic infection and premature delivery. It is currently unclear whether there is a causal relationship between these variations in cord coiling and any or all of the different complications.

THE POSTMORTEM IN SPECIAL SITUATIONS

In this final section, I will highlight the role of postmortem in a few relatively common special situations.

Intrauterine growth restriction

Intrauterine growth restriction (IUGR) is a common problem. The antenatal detection of IUGR is notoriously difficult, although serial growth measurements may indicate a tailing off in fetal growth[29]. However, undetected IUGR may be present in 40–50% of stillborn infants[30,31]. At postmortem, there are two key issues to address. The first is to determine whether the fetus truly shows growth restriction and the second is to identify the cause.

The body weight is used as the main clinical indicator of IUGR. Weight centiles by gestation are available for a number of different populations and ethnic groups. However, crude birth weight cannot distinguish whether a baby whose weight is on the 5th centile is well nourished but genetically small or growth restricted and genetically larger. Similarly, a baby whose weight is on the 50th centile may be well grown and of average size or undergrown and genetically large. The use of customized birth-weight centiles attempts to overcome this problem by correcting for factors such as ethnic origin, maternal height, weight and parity[32,33]. Customized centile calculators are freely available on the Internet[34]. However, even a low customized birth-weight centile is not conclusive proof of IUGR, as there will be a range of normal birth weight for any given set of maternal parameters. A variety of cut-offs have been used in the literature to separate normally grown from IUGR babies. The 10th centile is likely to identify most IUGR babies, but may also include a significant number of small, normally grown ones. Using the 3rd centile will reduce the number of false positives, but increase the number of true IUGR babies who are missed (false negatives).

The pathologist has the luxury at postmortem of invoking other evidence to support or refute the diagnosis of IUGR in a small baby and also to identify growth failure in babies with a 'normal' birth weight.

Pathological diagnosis of IUGR

Postmortem examination may demonstrate a number of pieces of evidence of impaired fetal nutrition and intrauterine stress that can help to put together a case for the presence of IUGR.

A baby showing severe IUGR will not only have a low birth-weight centile, but may also show a reduction in other growth parameters such as body length and femur length. Thus, a baby of 28 weeks' gestation, based on a dating scan, may only be the size of a 24 weeker. Typically, this is accompanied by a relatively large head circumference compared to the body length.

This pathologist's preferred indicator of IUGR is the ratio of brain weight to liver weight (brain-to-liver ratio, BLR). This is a reflection of the redirection of blood flow to the brain at the expense of the liver and other organs in babies suffering nutritional impairment, the brain-sparing effect.

The BLR is approximately 3:1 in a normally grown well-nourished fetus. Impaired fetal nutrition leads to a loss in weight of the liver, with a relatively maintained brain weight. Thus, the ratio increases with IUGR[35]. Precisely what level of BLR should be regarded as evidence of IUGR is not clearly defined. Most pathologists would regard a BLR of less than 4:1 as probably normal and one of over 6:1 as indubitably abnormal. A ratio of >5 correlates well with low birth-weight centile[36]. Of course, as with almost anything in medicine there are complicating factors. There is some evidence that maceration may differentially affect the weights of certain organs.[37] Thus the liver may lose a greater proportion of its weight than the brain and this may cause a significant increase in the BLR. Conversely, the brain of a severely macerated fetus may be impossible to remove intact and thus the recorded weight may be artificially low, leading to a normal BLR in a clearly IUGR fetus. Furthermore, vascular engorgement of the internal organs, for example, in a baby dying after placental abruption, can artificially increase the liver weight and mask an elevated BLR. Thus, an elevated BLR cannot be used as the sole criterion for diagnosis of IUGR and it always advisable to look for other evidence of fetal compromise.

Fetuses truly showing IUGR typically show one or more other markers indicating a period of intrauterine stress prior to death. The thymus is particularly sensitive to intrauterine stress. Such stress may be caused by any persistent abnormality of the intrauterine environment, for example chronic anemia, infection, fetal hydrops. However, chronic stress changes are almost universally present in IUGR babies. The thymus undergoes atrophy and is thus lighter than would be expected for the body weight, based on standard charts. Histologically, the thymic cortex shows patchy to generalized atrophy with blurring of the cortico-medullary junction, while the Hassall's corpuscles in the medulla become more prominent and may undergo cystic degeneration or calcification[38] (Fig. 14.4).

The adrenals may also show a response to chronic stress. This is less common than for the thymus, but also comprises a degree of atrophy with reduced weight and there is microscopic fatty change in the fetal cortical zone[39]. In severe cases, this may be extensive. As with thymic stress changes, the adrenal response is not specific for IUGR and milder cases may show normal adrenals.

Overall, it is probably wise to base a diagnosis of IUGR on the combined evidence of birth weight (ideally customized), BLR and signs of chronic intrauterine stress in the thymus and adrenals.

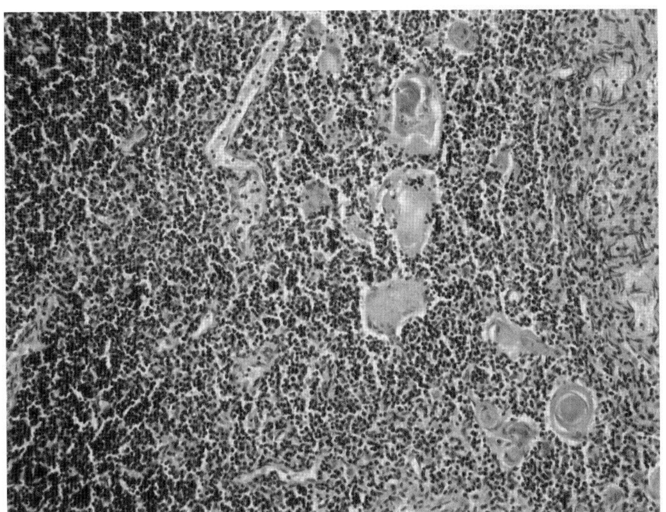

Fig. 14.4 Thymus showing atrophy of the cortex and prominent Hassall's corpuscles in a term infant with IUGR.

The second question to answer, once it has been decided that the baby's growth is restricted, is what is the cause?

By far the majority of IUGR is due to problems in the utero-placental unit. Therefore, examination of the placenta is absolutely essential in cases of intrauterine death. Most cases will be a consequence of inadequate maternal blood flow in the intervillous space, uteroplacental ischemia, with deficient transfer of oxygen and nutrients to the fetus. This may be a consequence of poor trophoblastic invasion and physiological conversion of the maternal spiral arteries. There is a resulting failure to increase the maternal blood supply to the intervillous space sufficiently to support the growth of the developing fetus. This may be associated with clinical signs of pre-eclampsia, but also often is not. In a still poorly defined group of mothers with uteroplacental ischemia, with or without pre-eclampsia, there may be an underlying thrombotic tendency, either as a result of anti-phopsholipid antibodies, or due to an inherited prothrombotic disorder, such as Factor V Leiden or anti-thrombin III deficiency[40]. This is more likely to be the case in IUGR starting before 24 weeks' gestation than later in pregnancy[41].

In cases of uteroplacental ischemia, the placenta is often lighter than expected for the gestation and weight of the baby. This can be assessed by comparison to standard charts, or by calculating the ratio of fetal weight to placental weight (feto-placental ratio, FPR). The normal FPR changes with gestation from 3.1 at 24 weeks to 7.2 at term[42], and thus it is important to compare to the normal for the gestation. However, the standard charts of normal placental weight for gestation are relatively crude, while the author has not found FPR to be especially helpful. Besides a typically small, lightweight placenta, utero-placental ischemia also leads to macroscopic and microscopic pathology in the placental parenchyma. Histologically, the chorionic villi usually show changes in response to uteroplacental ischemia. They give an appearance of advanced villous maturation, with small terminal villi often showing increased numbers of syncytiotrophoblastic knots, stromal fibrosis and reduced vascularity (Tenney Parker change). The terminal villi often appear relatively sparse. Areas of placental infarction are common and may involve a substantial proportion of the placenta. The significance of a given percentage of placental infarction is dependent on the size of the placenta and health of the remaining villi. For example, infarction of 30% of an otherwise healthy 500 g placenta would still leave 350 g of healthy villous parenchyma to support fetal growth, whereas 10% infarction in an already ischemic placenta of 250 g might be sufficient to lead to severe IUGR or fetal death. It is therefore vital to record the trimmed weight of the placenta, the percentage of infarction and the histological condition of the viable parenchyma. It may be possible to demonstrate the underlying pathology in the maternal decidual vessels. If maternal spiral arteries are present in the sections of the placental base, they may show evidence of failure to undergo the normal physiological conversion, with persistence of small muscular arteries. There may also be fibrinoid necrosis of converted or unconverted arteries and the characteristic lesion of acute atherosis with infiltration of the vessel wall by fat-laden foamy macrophages.

A number of other, less common, pathological disorders of the placenta may also underlie IUGR. Diffuse lesions of the placental parenchyma, such as villitis of unknown etiology[42] (idiopathic chronic villitis), massive perivillous fibrin deposition/maternal floor infarction[43,44] and massive histiocytic intervillositis[44] may all be associated with IUGR and antepartum (and occasionally intrapartum) fetal death. Minor degrees of chronic villitis, perivillous fibrin and histiocytic intervillositis are often seen in placentas from healthy infants. It is therefore the extent of the change and volume of uninvolved parenchyma that determines whether the fetus suffers ill effects, rather than the mere presence of the lesion and, on occasions, the significance of the changes may be difficult to judge. Nonetheless, when any of these changes is sufficiently severe to result in fetal compromise or death, the mother carries a significantly increased risk, up to 20% with chronic villitis[45], of suffering recurrent disease in subsequent pregnancies. There may also be an association between some cases of massive perivillous fibrin deposition/maternal floor infarction and maternal autoimmune disease/antiphospholipid syndrome[46].

In IUGR due to cytomegalovirus infection, the placenta shows a characteristic lymphoplasmacytic chronic villitis, in which viral inclusions may, or may not, be identified. Toxoplasmosis may show a chronic villitis, which may be lymphocytic or predominantly histiocytic and, occasionally, the typical cysts may be identified in the villi, subchorionic connective tissue or amniotic epithelium.

In recent years, there has been much interest in the entity of fetal thrombotic vasculopathy (FTV)[47]. This disorder is characterized by thrombotic lesions in the fetal circulation and fibrosis of the associated villi. Very similar vascular changes may be seen consequent upon fetal death and differentiating between antemortem thrombosis and postmortem vascular changes may be difficult. Some authors believe that FTV may account for a large proportion of stillbirths and may also be responsible for many cases of cerebral palsy and fetal distress[48]. The author remains to be convinced of this, however, there are undoubtedly cases of IUGR and fetal death that are clearly the result of progressive thrombotic occlusion of the fetal circulation during fetal life. In such cases, the placenta shows groups of fibrotic, avascular villi, often involving whole lobules of the placenta, widely distributed through the placenta, with intervening areas of normal parenchyma (Fig. 14.5). The vessels in stem villi and often the chorionic plate contain thrombotic lesions of differing ages. The cause of such cases is often not readily apparent. Some may be due to localized disturbance to the blood flow in

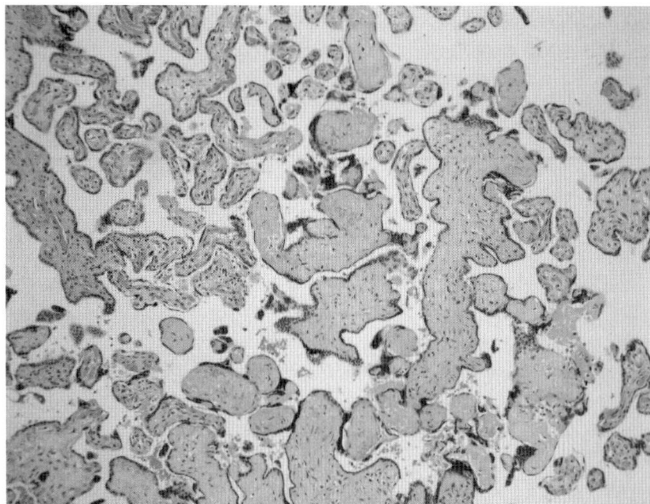

Fig. 14.5 Groups of avascular villi in a placenta with fetal thrombotic vasculopathy.

the umbilical cord or chorionic plate vessels, for example cord knots[49]. However, unless this is clearly the case, it is probably wise to seek a family history of thromboses and, if the child is alive, there may be a case for testing for prothrombotic disorders for, although the frequency of a positive diagnosis is relatively low, the implications for future pregnancies are serious.

Symmetrical versus asymmetrical IUGR

Traditionally, fetal growth restriction is regarded as either symmetrical or asymmetrical. Symmetrical growth restriction is characterized by equal delay of growth of all organs, whereas in asymmetrical IUGR, there is relative preservation of brain growth compared to other organs such as the liver. Symmetrical IUGR is said to reflect very early growth failure or reduced growth potential, for example due to early congenital infection or chromosome abnormality, so-called hypoplastic growth restriction, whereas asymmetrical IUGR is classically the result of problems of fetal nutrition in the third trimester (malnutrition type IUGR). In its classical form, a symmetrically IUGR fetus has a body weight below the 3rd centile for the gestation. However, the brain:liver weight ratio is normal and the weights of other organs are in proportion to the body weight. Apart from the discrepancy between gestation and body weight, the only pointer to symmetrical IUGR may be the maturity of the organs, which will be appropriate for the gestation. Thus the brain, while small, shows a pattern of gyral development in keeping with gestation and, at the histological level, the maturity of organs such as the kidneys and lungs is appropriate for the gestation and more advanced than the body and organ weights would suggest.

In practice, pure symmetrical IUGR is rare among stillbirths. Even fetuses with chromosome abnormalities frequently show an asymmetrical pattern of IUGR with an elevated BLR. This may be a reflection of impaired placental function as part of the generalized abnormality of development. The most striking example of this is seen in digynic triploidy, where the placenta is tiny and the fetus shows extreme asymmetrical IUGR, often with a BLR of close to 20. Equally, babies whose nutrition is impaired from the late second trimester onwards will show some hypoplastic features, with a reduction in other growth parameters as well as body weight. However, the BLR is always markedly elevated.

Table 14.3 **Mechanisms of fetal hydrops and examples of causes for the various mechanisms**

Mechanism of hydrops	*Examples*
Fetal anemia	Blood group isoimmunization (Rh/ABO/Le) Parvovirus B19 infection Alpha thalassemia Hemorrhage (external/internal) Dyserythropoietic disorders
Pump malfunction	Some congenital heart malformations Cardiomyopathy (endocardial fibroelastosis/other) Cardiac arrhythmia
High output failure	Congenital tumor (e.g. teratoma) Arteriovenous malformation Hemangioma/chorangioma Twin–twin transfusion syndrome
Obstruction to venous return	Thoracic/abdominal mass (e.g. congenital cystic adenomatoid malformation) Atresia/stenosis of ductus venosus
Hypoproteinemia/liver failure	Congenital hemochromatosis Storage disease Other congenital liver disease
Lymphatic abnormalities	Congenital lymphangiectasia
Chromosome abnormality	Monosomy X (Turner's syndrome) Trisomy 21 (Down's syndrome)

Fetal hydrops

Fetal hydrops, the combination of generalized skin edema with effusions in one or more body cavities, is the endpoint of a number of pathological processes which interfere with the normal regulation of tissue fluid via Starling's forces. Textbooks of perinatal pathology give very long lists of potential causes of fetal hydrops, however, these can readily be grouped under a small number of headings (Table 14.3). While examples have been listed against particular mechanisms, the list is not exhaustive and, in many situations, more than one mechanism operates.

Investigation of fetal hydrops should be regarded as a multidisciplinary effort. It is likely that the presence of fetal hydrops will have been identified, if it was present, at either the dating scan or midtrimester anomaly scan. Later onset hydrops may only be recognized at birth or when a scan is performed to assess fetal growth or to confirm intrauterine death (IUD). When hydrops is identified while the fetus is alive, a range of tests should have been performed in utero. The fetal karyotype should have been checked. If Doppler studies have indicated the possibility of fetal anemia, isoimmunization due to blood group incompatibility should have been excluded, maternal serology or fetal samples should have been sent to look for Parvovirus B19 infection and a Kleihauer test performed to identify fetomaternal hemorrhage. A fetal echocardiogram may also have been performed to look for a structural abnormality of the heart and cardiac arrhythmia.

The postmortem needs to cover as many of the possibilities not already investigated as feasible. It is therefore essential that the pathologist be supplied with a full history and list of the investigations already undertaken. The examination must be systematic in order not to miss rare causes. For example, atresia of the ductus venosus will be missed unless specifically looked for[50]. Since metabolic disease is among the differential diagnosis of hydrops, it is important that the postmortem is not delayed, as this may lead to failure of fibroblast culture and thus prevent a definitive diagnosis being reached. The examination should ideally be undertaken within 24 hours of birth, and definitely within 72 hours, as after that time the success of fibroblast culture falls dramatically. The placenta is absolutely vital to the examination and must be sent fresh to the laboratory. Failure to send it verges on negligent, and will certainly lead to a very unhappy pathologist. A team approach to the investigation of fetal hydrops should lead to a diagnosis in the majority of cases, but it should be recognized that in a small proportion the cause will remain idiopathic.

Table 14.4 **Origins of fetal akinesia and examples of causes of each mechanism**

Origin of akinesia	*Example*
Brain/spinal cord	Acquired disease (e.g. hypoxia, infection, toxic) Developmental abnormality (e.g. variant spinal muscular atrophy, olivopontocerebellar hypoplasia)
Peripheral nerve	Deficient myelination
Motor end plate	Maternal myasthenia gravis Fetal acetylcholine receptor subunit mutations
Muscle	Nemaline myopathy Centronuclear/myotubular myopathy Glygogen storage disease (type IV, type VII)
Skin	Restrictive dermopathy
External restriction	Prolonged oligohydramnios Large uterine fibroids
Chromosome abnormality	Trisomy 18, trisomy 15 mosaic

Fetal akinesia

Fetal movements are necessary for normal development. Lack of normal fetal movement (fetal akinesia) results in abnormal posture, joint contractures and frequently pulmonary hypoplasia. The phenotypes resulting from fetal akinesia go by a confusing array of names. These include:

- fetal akinesia deformation sequence (FADS)[51]
- fetal akinesia/hypokinesia sequence (FAHS)
- arthrogryposis multiplex congenita
- pena-Shokeir syndrome type 1
- lethal multiple pterygium syndrome (LMPS)[52].

The last three denote different phenotypes, resulting from progressively earlier onset of akinesia and with somewhat different genetic implications. The investigation of fetal akinesia has many aspects in common with fetal hydrops. There are many recognized causes, but these can be grouped together under a much smaller number of headings based on the site of the problem (Table 14.4). The list of causes below is far from exhaustive and only highlights the extensive nature of the investigation required.

As with fetal hydrops, the postmortem in fetal akinesia should not be delayed. It is essential to obtain fibroblasts on which to perform a full karyotype and also for storage in case a metabolic disorder is suspected. Ideally, samples of liver and muscle should also be snap frozen in liquid nitrogen for enzyme assay, and frozen muscle may be submitted for specialized histological examination as for a postnatal muscle disorder. This becomes less useful with increasing postmortem delay. Electron microscopy may also be helpful, particularly for the diagnosis of congenital nemaline myopathy, as the tiny nemaline rods in fetal muscle may not be readily demonstrated in histological sections. Detailed examination of the brain and spinal cord is essential, but becomes increasingly difficult, the longer the interval between death and postmortem.

The large majority of cases are due to disorders of the central nervous system or of skeletal muscle[53]. A timely and full postmortem examination may pinpoint the precise cause of fetal akinesia and allow a diagnosis to be made at the genetic level. However, in a significant proportion of cases, in particular when suboptimal tissue preservation limits the array of tests possible, it may not be possible to be more precise than 'probably neurogenic', i.e. brain/spinal cord/nerve, or 'probably myopathic'. This in itself is useful, however, since experience indicates that the risk of recurrence is significantly greater in the myopathic group than in the probable neurogenic cases, as a result of more autosomal recessive disorders in the myopathic group[54].

Monochorionic twins

Twin pregnancy and the complications of monochorionic twinning are dealt with elsewhere in this volume.

The perinatal pathologist may particularly contribute to investigation of the cause of growth discordance in monochorionic twins and also to assessment following intrauterine demise of one or both twins. In cases of single twin demise, this may help to understand the actual or potential consequences for the surviving twin.

Central to these investigations is examination of the placenta, although postmortem examination following death of one or both twins may also be highly informative.

In the vast majority of monochorionic twin placentas, there are vascular connections (anastomoses) between the respective circulations of the twins[55]. There may be direct connections between arteries or veins in the chorionic plate (arterio-arterial (AA) and veno-venous (VV) anastomoses), or there may be connections at the capillary level such that a group of placental villi receives its arterial blood supply from one twin but drains to the other (AV anastomoses) (Fig. 14.6). The pattern of anastomoses is laid down at an early stage of placental development, but the factors determining how many anastomoses form and of which types, is not understood.

Documentation of the number and types of anastomoses can help to inform the discussions regarding the complications of a particular twin pregnancy. Our practice is to perform injection studies of the fetal placental circulation in cases of complicated monochorionic twin prengnancy. Both arterial and venous circulations are injected with molten 1% agar solution colored with one of four tissue-marking dyes via a cannula. AA and VV anastomoses can be directly visualized, while AV anastomoses can be inferred from the presence of an area supplied by an artery from one twin, but drained by a vein to the other. Such preparations can be photographed to help to inform discussion in fora such as perinatal mortality meetings and can be used for research studies.

The anastomotic pattern can have serious consequences for the twins as the pregnancy proceeds. Chronic twin–twin transfusion syndrome (TTTS) is probably initiated, and to a large extent maintained, by an imbalance in blood flow across the anastomoses. Studies have shown that placentas from cases of TTTS typically lack AA and VV anastomoses and AV anastomoses are scarce and flow is predominantly from the smaller (donor) twin to the larger (recipient) one[56,57]. However, in many cases with well-documented growth discordance, this typical anastomotic pattern is not present. In part this is probably a reflection of our incomplete understanding of the pathogenesis of TTTS, which is likely to be more complex than a simple net transfusion of blood from one twin to the other. Nonetheless, major deviation from this classical pattern should bring the cause of growth discordance into question, since not all discordant twin growth is the consequence of TTTS[57]. There may be growth restriction of one twin as a consequence of poor implantation of part of the placenta, e.g. over a uterine scar or fibroid or in the lower segment, there may be a velamentous cord insertion, the small twin may be served by a very small placental territory, or may have congenital abnormalities. Alternatively, the larger twin may be discordant for a genetic disorder associated with growth restriction or overgrowth such as Russell–Silver syndrome or Beckwith–Wiedemann syndrome respectively[58]. In some cases of growth discordance, in which the placental territory of the smaller twin is particularly diminutive, the anastomotic pattern may suggest that there was likely to have been net flow towards the small twin, which may have been keeping it alive (so-called co-twin rescue)[57]. Such twins are especially likely to die following laser ablation of anastomotic connections.

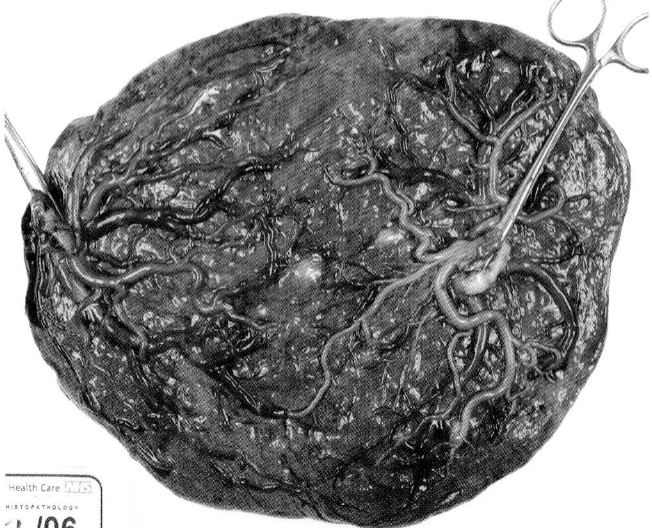

Fig. 14.6 Monochorionic diamniotic twin placenta following injection to show feto–fetal anastomoses.

In cases of single IUD in a pair of monochorionic twins, assessment of the placenta can be very helpful in advising of the likely risk of neurological sequelae in the survivor. Damage to the surviving twin is the result of a sudden drop in blood pressure in the circulation of the sick twin as it dies, leading to a major transfusion of blood into the dead twin's circulation, so called acute twin–twin transfusion[59]. Often this is sufficient to cause death of the other twin but, if it survives, there is a serious risk of neurological sequelae. Clearly, if there are no anastomoses, the survivor is likely to be protected from damage. Large studies have shown a high rate of co-twin death and neurological problems if AA and especially VV anastomoses are present, presumably because these direct connections allow rapid shift of blood into the stagnant circulation of the dead twin, resulting in acute hypotension in the survivor[57]. AV anastomoses appear to be less of a problem in this regard, which is probably due to the connection being at the capillary level, thus allowing less flow. However, the author is aware of perfectly healthy surviving monochorionic twins following single co-twin death whose placentas contained large AA or VV anastomoses, demonstrating the difference between statistical risk and individual cases.

The use of laser ablation of anastomoses as treatment for TTTS is becoming more widely used. Pathological examination of the placenta following delivery is often requested to document laser sites and to assess the completeness of destruction of anastomotic vessels. Injection studies can be very helpful in highlighting ablated areas and interrupted vessels and demonstrating connections which had escaped the laser. This is a useful form of audit of this relatively new procedure.

Intrapartum/early neonatal death

It is helpful to consider intrapartum and early neonatal deaths together as many of the same considerations apply. Such cases often, although not exclusively, follow a prolonged or unduly rapid labor in which signs of fetal compromise may have been apparent. Instrumental delivery with forceps or Ventouse may have been attempted and, if this failed, cesarean section may have proved difficult. Such cases frequently show signs of acute asphyxia and, depending on the difficulty of the delivery, there may be signs of birth trauma. Asphyxial signs include intense congestion of the internal organs with small hemorrhages on the pleural and epicardial surfaces and within the thymus gland. Hemorrhage may also be present in the portal tracts of the liver, the kidneys and adrenal glands. Meconium may be present in the major airways and stomach. The brain is typically mildly swollen and intensely congested and may show scattered tiny hemorrhages in the white matter. Traumatic lesions are particularly associated with instrumental deliveries, but may occur in spontaneous vaginal deliveries, particularly with breech presentation and in large babies, where there may be fractures due to shoulder dystocia. Many traumatic lesions are not sufficient to account for death, but are a marker of a difficult delivery. Exceptions to this include massive subaponeurotic hemorrhage, massive intracranial hemorrhage, for example due to tearing of a major venous sinus, major skull fractures and brain injury from misapplied forceps, occipital osteodiastasis with brain stem trauma and spinal cord transection from rotational forceps delivery or breech presentation. Where major trauma is not identified, death is often likely to have been due to a combination of asphyxia and trauma and it may be difficult to separate the contribution of these two factors[60].

It has been well demonstrated, in a number of studies, that many intrapartum and early neonatal deaths show evidence of pre-existing compromise, prior to the onset of labor[61]. In around one-third of such infants there is histological evidence of hypoxic–ischemic brain injury, which pre-dates the onset of labor. It is likely therefore, that many of these babies are ill prepared to cope with the stresses of labor.

Among the most problematic cases to resolve are the small numbers of infants who present as fresh stillbirths or in a severely compromised state following an apparently normal labor. While a review of the labor record and cardiotocographs may show that the signs of compromise were present during labor but missed in some of these, in others there truly are no premonitory signs. Postmortem should be encouraged in such cases, despite the undoubted highly charged emotions of family and staff surrounding such a devastating event. While it must be acknowledged that in some cases no cause can be identified, the pathologist may identify unsuspected infection, evidence of a previous serious hypoxic–ischemic brain injury or rarely metabolic disease or congenital malformations. Placental examination is absolutely vital but, all too often, in the furore surrounding the delivery it is discarded and vital information can be lost. Even if consent for postmortem is not granted, examination of the placenta may reveal the cause of death, for example tearing of vasa praevia leading to exsanguination, placental abruption or unsuspected severe amniotic infection.

CONCLUSION

Despite adverse publicity in the early 21st century, resulting in a fall in rates of postmortem in many countries of the economically developed world, the perinatal postmortem remains an important part of modern obstetric care. Many parents value the detailed information such an examination provides on the cause of death or congenital abnormalities of their baby. This information can be essential for accurate genetic counseling and may help guide the management of future pregnancies.

Changes to the law in the UK and elsewhere have made the rules governing obtaining consent for postmortem more robust, which it is hoped will provide families with sufficient information to come to an informed decision and ensure they have confidence in the procedure. Pathologists too can operate with greater confidence that they are acting in accordance with the family's wishes.

In order that perinatal postmortems provide useful information, it is essential that they are performed by pathologists with special expertise in this area, with access to special investigations such as cytogenetics and molecular genetics. Postmortems undertaken by general pathologists who examine the occasional baby are no longer acceptable and parents have the right to expect better. In particular, there are a variety of situations, such as fetal hydrops, fetal akinesia and intrapartum/early neonatal death, where the specialist knowledge of the perinatal pathologist may be critical to reaching the correct diagnosis. Sadly, an inadequately performed postmortem cannot be repeated in the same way as a blood test or biopsy on a live patient, unless the problem recurs in one of the mother's subsequent pregnancies. While it is acknowledged that a regional center for perinatal pathology may not be a possibility everywhere, large obstetric units should work with their pathology colleagues to ensure that a specialist perinatal pathology service is available and adequately funded either locally or on a regional basis.

REFERENCES

1. Adappa R et al. Perinatal and infant autopsy. *Arch Dis Child Fetal Neonatal Ed* **92**(1):F49–F50, 2007.
2. Guidelines on autopsy practice. Report of a working group of The Royal College of Pathologists Appendix 6. Guidelines for autopsy investigation of fetal and perinatal death. The Royal College of Pathologists, 2002.
3. Amini H et al. Comparison of ultrasound and autopsy findings in pregnancies terminated due to fetal anomalies. *Acta Obstet Gynecol Scand* **85**(10):1208–1216, 2006.
4. Faye-Petersen OM, Guinn DA, Wenstrom KD. Value of perinatal autopsy. *Obstet Gynecol* **94**(6):915–920, 1999.
5. Gordijn SJ, Erwich JJ, Khong TY. Value of the perinatal autopsy: critique. *Pediatr Dev Pathol* **5**(5):480–488, 2002.
6. Killeen OG et al. The value of the perinatal and neonatal autopsy. *Ir Med J* **97**(8):241–244, 2004.
7. Meier P et al. Perinatal autopsy: its clinical value. *Obstet Gynecol* **67**(3):349–351, 1986.
8. Shen-Schwarz S, Neish C, Hill LM. Antenatal ultrasound for fetal anomalies: importance of perinatal autopsy. *Pediatr Pathol* **9**(1):1–9, 1989.
9. Boyd PA et al. Autopsy after termination of pregnancy for fetal anomaly: retrospective cohort study. *Br Med J* **328**(7432):137, 2004.
10. Johns N et al. A comparative study of prenatal ultrasound findings and postmortem examination in a tertiary referral centre. *Prenat Diagn* **24**(5):339–346, 2004.
11. Piercecchi-Marti MD et al. Value of fetal autopsy after medical termination of pregnancy. *Forensic Sci Int* **144**(1):7–10, 2004.
12. Thornton CM, O'Hara MD. A regional audit of perinatal and infant autopsies in Northern Ireland. *Br J Obstet Gynaecol* **105**(1):18–23, 1998.
13. Vujanic GM et al. Perinatal and infant postmortem examinations: how well are we doing? *J Clin Pathol* **48**(11):998–1001, 1995.

14. Human Tissue Act, in 2004 Chapter 30. 2004: England & Wales.
15. Human Tissue Authority. cited; Available from: http://www.hta.gov.uk/.
16. Human Tissue Act (Scotland) 2006, in 2006 asp4. 2006: Scotland.
17. Codes of Practice. cited; Available from: http://www.hta.gov.uk/guidance/codes_of_practice.cfm.
18. Kyle PM et al. High failure rate of postmortem karyotyping after termination for fetal abnormality. *Obstet Gynecol* **88**(5):859–862, 1996.
19. Bain AD. *The perinatal autopsy, in neonatal medicine*, F Cockburn, CM Drillen (eds), pp. 820–834. Oxford: Blackwell Scientific Publications, 1974.
20. Langley FA. The perinatal postmortem examination. *J Clin Pathol* **24**(2):159–169, 1971.
21. Genest DR, Singer DB. Estimating the time of death in stillborn fetuses: III. External fetal examination: a study of 86 stillborns. *Obstet Gynecol* **80**(4):593–600, 1992.
22. Genest DR, Williams MA, Greene MF. Estimating the time of death in stillborn fetuses: I. Histologic evaluation of fetal organs: an autopsy study of 150 stillborns. *Obstet Gynecol* **80**(4):575–584, 1992.
23. Wigglesworth JS. The macerated stillborn fetus. In *Perinatal pathology*, pp. 78-86. Philadelphia: WB Saunders Co, 1984.
24. Cohen M et al. Less invasive autopsy: benefits and limitations of the use of magnetic resonance imaging in the perinatal post-mortem. *Pediatr Dev Pathol* **1**, 2007.
25. Baergen R. Macroscopic evaluation of the second and third trimester placenta. In *Manual of Benirschke and Kaufmann's Pathology of the human placenta*, pp. 23-44. New York: Springer, 2004.
26. Faye-Petersen OM, Heller DS, Joshi VV. *Handbook of placental pathology*, 2nd edn. London: Informa Healthcare, p. 254 2005.
27. van Diik CC et al. The umbilical coiling index in normal pregnancy. *J Matern Fetal Neonatal Med* **11**(4):280–283, 2002.
28. de Laat MW et al. The umbilical coiling index, a review of the literature. *J Matern Fetal Neonatal Med* **17**(2):93–100, 2005.
29. Gardosi J, Francis A. Controlled trial of fundal height measurement plotted on customised antenatal growth charts. *Br J Obstet Gynaecol* **106**(4):309–317, 1999.
30. Gardosi J et al. Classification of stillbirth by relevant condition at death (ReCoDe): population based cohort study. *Br Med J* **331**(7525):1113–1117, 2005.
31. Froen JF et al. Restricted fetal growth in sudden intrauterine unexplained death. *Acta Obstet Gynecol Scand* **83**(9):801–807, 2004.
32. Gardosi J et al. An adjustable fetal weight standard. *Ultrasound Obstet Gynecol* **6**(3):168–174, 1995.
33. Gardosi J et al. Customised antenatal growth charts. *Lancet* **339**(8788):283–287, 1992.
34. Gestation Network: Centile Calculator. cited; Available from: http://www.gestation.net/birthweight_centiles/birthweight_centiles.htm.
35. Gruenwald P. Growth and maturation of the foetus and its relationship to perinatal mortality. In *Perinatal problems*, NR Butler, ED Albermann (eds), pp. 141–161. Edinburgh: Livingstone, 1969.
36. Lyon V et al. Unadjusted and customised weight centiles in the identification of growth restriction among stillborn infants. *Br J Obstet Gynaecol* **111**(12):1460–1463, 2004.
37. Maroun LL, Graem N. Autopsy standards of body parameters and fresh organ weights in nonmacerated and macerated human fetuses. *Pediatr Dev Pathol* **8**(2): 204–217, 2005.
38. Wigglesworth JS. Hemopoietic and lymphoreticular systems. In *Perinatal pathology*, pp. 366-380. Philadelphia: WB Saunders Co, 1984.
39. Becker MJ, Becker AE. Fat distribution in the adrenal cortex as an indication of the mode of intrauterine death. *Hum Pathol* **7**(5):495–504, 1976.
40. Verspyck E et al. Thrombophilia and fetal growth restriction. *Eur J Obstet Gynecol Reprod Biol* **113**(1):36–40, 2004.
41. Kupferminc MJ et al. Mid-trimester severe intrauterine growth restriction is associated with a high prevalence of thrombophilia. *Br J Obstet Gynaecol* **109**(12):1373–1376, 2002.
42. Gruenwald P, Minh HN. Evaluation of body and organ weights in perinatal pathology. II Weight of body and placenta of surviving and of autopsied infants. *Am J Obstet Gynecol* **82**:312–319, 1961.
43. Bane AL, Gillan JE. Massive perivillous fibrinoid causing recurrent placental failure. *Br J Obstet Gynaecol* **110**(3):292–295, 2003.
44. Boyd TK, Redline RW. Chronic histiocytic intervillositis: a placental lesion associated with recurrent reproductive loss. *Hum Pathol* **31**(11):1389–1396, 2000.
45. Redline RW, Abramowsky CR. Clinical and pathologic aspects of recurrent placental villitis. *Hum Pathol* **16**(7): 727–731, 1985.
46. Bendon RW, Hommel AB. Maternal floor infarction in autoimmune disease: two cases. *Pediatr Pathol Lab Med* **16**(2):293–297, 1996.
47. Baergen R. Fetal thrombotic vasculopathy. In *Manual of Benirschke and Kaufmann's pathology of the human placenta*, pp. 392-402. New York: Springer, 2004.
48. Redline RW, Pappin A. Fetal thrombotic vasculopathy: the clinical significance of extensive avascular villi. *Hum Pathol* **26**(1):80–85, 1995.
49. Redline RW. Clinical and pathological umbilical cord abnormalities in fetal thrombotic vasculopathy. *Hum Pathol* **35**(12):1494–1498, 2004.
50. Siven M et al. Agenesis of the ductus venosus and its correlation to hydrops fetalis and the fetal hepatic circulation: case reports and review of the literature. *Pediatr Pathol Lab Med* **15**(1):39–50, 1995.
51. Moessinger AC. Fetal akinesia deformation sequence: an animal model. *Pediatrics* **72**(6):857–863, 1983.
52. Vestermark B. Arthrogryposis multiplex congenital: a case of neurogenic origin. *Acta Paediatr Scand* **55**(1):117–120, 1966.
53. Porter HJ. Lethal arthrogryposis multiplex congenital (fetal akinesia deformation sequence, FADS). *Pediatr Pathol Lab Med* **15**(4):617–637, 1995.
54. Quinn CM, Wigglesworth JS, Heckmatt J. Lethal arthrogryposis multiplex congenita: a pathological study of 21 cases. *Histopathology* **19**(2):155–162, 1991.
55. Robertson EG, Neer KJ. Placental injection studies in twin gestation. *Am J Obstet Gynecol* **147**(2):170–174, 1983.
56. Bajoria R, Wigglesworth J, Fisk NM. Angioarchitecture of monochorionic placentas in relation to the twin-twin transfusion syndrome. *Am J Obstet Gynecol* **172**(3):856–863, 1995.
57. Denbow ML et al. Placental angioarchitecture in monochorionic twin pregnancies: relationship to fetal growth, fetofetal transfusion syndrome, and pregnancy outcome. *Am J Obstet Gynecol* **182**(2):417–426, 2000.
58. Sagot P et al. Russell-Silver syndrome: an explanation for discordant growth in monozygotic twins. *Fetal Diagn Ther* **11**(1):72–78, 1996.
59. Fusi L et al. Acute twin-twin transfusion: a possible mechanism for brain-damaged survivors after intrauterine death of a monochorionic twin. *Obstet Gynecol* **78**(3 Pt 2):517–520, 1991.
60. Wigglesworth JS. Intrapartum and early neonatal death: the interaction of asphyxia and trauma. In *Perinatal pathology*, pp. 87-103. Philadelphia: WB Saunders Co, 1984.
61. Becher JC et al. The Scottish perinatal neuropathology study: clinicopathological correlation in early neonatal deaths. *Arch Dis Child Fetal Neonatal Ed* **89**(5): F399–F407, 2004.

SECTION 4

Epidemiology

15 Epidemiological techniques in fetal medicine 197
James P Neilson and Zarko Alfirevic

CHAPTER 15

Epidemiological techniques in fetal medicine

James P Neilson and Zarko Alfirevic

KEY POINTS

- Routinely collected perinatal datasets can generate useful information and important hypotheses, e.g. the 'Barker hypothesis', as long as the quality of data is sound
- The *likelihood ratio* describes the usefulness of a screening or diagnostic test
- The *randomized controlled trial* is the least biased method of assessing the effectiveness of clinical interventions. It has been little used in fetal medicine but reports are increasing
- The details of good clinical trial methodology are now well established. It is critically important to avoid *selection bias* by ensuring *allocation concealment*
- *Research synthesis* allows the reader to review the totality of relevant evidence on a particular topic. Systematic reviews can be performed of randomized controlled trials ('reviews of effectiveness'), screening and diagnostic tests, or other types of scientific literature. Meta-analysis may, or may not, be a component of a systematic review
- The *Cochrane Database of Systematic Reviews* is the largest source of high quality systematic reviews of healthcare interventions

INTRODUCTION

The science of epidemiology (the study of the distribution and causes of diseases in populations) has produced tools that are increasingly applied in the clinical arena and there is an emerging specialism of 'clinical epidemiology'. This chapter will explore those tools and the concepts that underpin them and will illustrate their application with reference to diagnostic and screening tests and therapeutic interventions in fetal and perinatal medicine. Fetal medicine is itself a young specialism and its short history and rapid progress have inevitably resulted in some errors and blind alleys. It is incumbent on 'fetal physicians' of the future to try to ensure that lessons are learned from past mistakes and that future progress is based on sound scientific foundations to ensure that the application of fetal medicine contributes more good than harm. In the words of Murray Enkin[1]:

> In most fields of medical care, persons come to a doctor because they are ill and seek a cure or relief. In obstetrics, pregnant women come to us healthy but with an iatrogenic belief that obstetrical care will further improve the excellent outcomes that nature has already provided for them. The professionally engendered nature of our care increases our responsibility. The presence of the baby, who has no choice in the matter, doubles it.

Care during pregnancy and childbirth has been among the vanguard areas of clinical activity in moving towards 'evidence-based' clinical practice. The basis of this process, the production of systematic reviews of scientifically rigorous studies, has been likened in scale and importance to the Human Genome Project[2].

ROUTINE DATASETS

Previous generations of perinatal epidemiologists mostly concentrated on large datasets either collected routinely or derived for a specific research project. It is undeniable that important insights have been derived from such studies, although misleading evidence has also emerged from the 'data dredging' of such resources. In contrast, the modern perinatal epidemiologist is much more likely to try to address a specific hypothesis (or hypotheses), either through generating clinical experiments, notably randomized controlled trials or by studying the results of a number of different clinical experiments, to reach the most informative and least biased conclusion (through 'systematic reviews' and meta-analysis).

Previous studies of routinely collected data about maternal deaths and, more recently, perinatal deaths, have been informative and may have contributed to lessening incidences of these disasters. Routine datasets continue to prove useful in a number of ways, e.g. generating hypotheses (some of which are best tackled definitively by a randomized controlled trial), identifying patterns of disease distribution in populations, and by identifying rare problems. Thus, the 'Barker hypothesis' linking undernutrition at critical stages of fetal life with adult diseases including coronary artery disease[3] has been generated by the study of routinely collected data on birthweights and placental weights and neonatal measurements, and linking these findings with health and disease in later adult life. Routinely collected maternity records in Iceland have proven valuable for population studies of inheritance of genetic predisposition to pre-eclampsia[4]. Records in Scotland have provided important insights into twin births[5], recurrent pregnancy complications[6] and subsequent fertility[7].

PERINATAL MORTALITY SURVEYS

The classification of perinatal mortality should have value in identifying both research and clinical service priorities in perinatal medicine. Different systems of classification have been used. It is bizarre that the current system in England, Wales and Northern Ireland still uses an anachronistic classification that fails to differentiate between growth-retarded and normally grown stillbirths[8]. Sixteen percent of stillbirths and 22% of neonatal deaths are due to congenital abnormalities[8].

The concept of 'avoidability' has been applied for many years in Britain to the scrutiny of maternal deaths in the triennial Confidential Enquiry reports[9]. This has, more recently, been applied to national studies of subsets of perinatal deaths as well, thus highlighting, in a study of intrapartum deaths, the problems of a lack of senior clinical involvement and of failure to anticipate certain complications (including exaggerated response to oxytocic drugs, cord prolapse, shoulder dystocia and difficulties with delivery of the second twin).

However, as these studies lack adequate controls, one has to be careful not to over-interpret the associations between adverse outcomes and elements of clinical care.

DIAGNOSTIC TESTS

It is important to draw a clear distinction between screening tests, which are often relatively crude tests applicable to large populations to help identify clinically unsuspected disease, and diagnostic tests, which are usually much more precise and which are applied for specific clinical reasons.

The performance of tests can be assessed by calculating sensitivity, specificity and predictive values (Table 15.1). The *sensitivity* denotes the proportion of women with the condition who have a positive test result; the *specificity* denotes the proportion of women without the condition who have a negative test result. The optimal balance of sensitivity and specificity will depend on individual aims and circumstances. The ultrasound diagnosis of structural fetal defects, for example, should be highly specific to avert unwanted termination of pregnancies in which the fetuses are, in fact, normal; a screening test for fetal neural tube defects or chromosomal abnormalities can accommodate a lower level of specificity because final decisions about intervention are based on diagnostic tests (e.g. ultrasound or amniocentesis) that are triggered by the abnormal screening test result. The relationship between sensitivity and specificity can be displayed figuratively in *receiver operator curves* (ROCs), the term being derived from radar technology during the Second World War. ROCs are useful in identifying the optimal trade-off between sensitivity and specificity for a given test so as to pinpoint the best cut-off value to differentiate 'normal' from 'abnormal' test results in a screening program.

Table 15.1 **Relationship between tests and disease (or other adverse outcome)**

Test	*Disease*	
	Present	*Absent*
Positive	True postive (a)	False positive (b)
Negative	False negative (c)	True negative (d)

Sensitivity = a/a + c. Specificity = d/b + d. Positive predictive value = a/a + b. Negative predictive value = d/c + d

The *predictive value* of a test is influenced by the prevalence of the condition in question in the population being studied; thus, the positive predictive value of a raised maternal serum alpha-fetoprotein result will be greater in a Celtic population with a higher incidence of neural tube defects. The more sensitive a test is, the better is the negative predictive value; the more specific a test is, the better is the positive predictive value.

The *likelihood ratio* (LR) is another measure of the value of a diagnostic test that is increasingly gaining popularity, as it seems to be more intuitive for clinicians. It combines the sensitivity and specificity of a test and expresses it as a ratio rather than percentage. The higher the likelihood ratio the more likely is that the patient with positive test will have the condition (disease) of interest and vice versa. If the likelihood ratio is 1, the pre-test probability of the disease has not changed despite the diagnostic test being performed – clearly a useless test. There is no magic LR cut-off above which the test should be considered clinically useful. Sometimes a simple test (e.g. a question) with relatively low LR may be clinically useful. On the other hand, an invasive and expensive diagnostic test with LR above 6 may not be cost-effective, especially if the treatment triggered by this test has high morbidity.

CASE STUDIES

Case series or even single case reports can be useful in generating hypotheses that can be tested in experimental studies. Thus, a case report, describing an association between fetal nuchal translucency during the first trimester and chromosomal abnormality[10], spawned a large and important program of work[11]. A potential problem with case studies is that these are sometimes seen as providing in themselves the basis for changing clinical practice. An example was the uncontrolled case series of the use of fetoscopically directed ablation of anastomostic vessels in twin–twin transfusion syndrome[12]. However, a subsequent randomized controlled trial comparing laser ablation with amnioreduction was performed much later[13]. Although not perfect from the standpoint of clinical trial methodology, this was a landmark study in fetal medicine.

A recent innovation has been the construction of case series of rare problems through the regular mailing of maternity units – an approach used in pediatrics for some years. Included in the current portfolio of the UKOSS Project based in the National Perinatal Epidemiology Unit, Oxford, UK, are fetomaternal alloimmune thrombocytopenia and fetal gastroschisis[14].

Historical control studies

When a case series is collected outside the confines of a planned experimental study, a temptation exists to compare outcome with a control group identified with hindsight; one such model is the historical control group, i.e. a similar group of patients or pregnancies treated or observed before the intervention in question was introduced; another model would be a comparison group treated at a different hospital, or by a different doctor. Both models carry a major risk of bias and of misleading conclusions. In the case of historical controls, many changes may have occurred over the timescale of the observed period as to alter prognosis. Thus, one study that encouraged inappropriately optimistic expectations of the widespread use of electronic fetal heart rate monitoring during labor was a small, historical control study[15].

EXPERIMENTAL STUDIES

Case-control studies

A major section of this chapter will be devoted to the methodology of the randomized controlled trial (RCT) because this is the gold standard method of assessing the effectiveness of clinical interventions[16]. However, it must be recognized that not all important questions in fetal medicine can be addressed by the randomized controlled trial. Thus, the question of whether high-dose vitamin A is a teratogen cannot, for ethical reasons, be resolved by randomly allocating half of a group of women in early pregnancy to exposure to vitamin A. Here, the case-control study that has been widely used with benefit in human cancer studies may be helpful.

Randomized controlled trials

Not all interventions can be evaluated by randomized trials – one cannot foresee, for example, randomized trials of fetal transfusion for severe fetal anemia in early pregnancy or of immediate delivery for prolonged fetal bradycardia in labor. However, different methods of fetal transfusion, of techniques of caesarean section would be obvious candidates for further evaluation.

Randomization

The randomized controlled trial is a simple but powerful method of avoiding *systematic errors*, or *bias*, by ensuring that experimental (study) groups and control groups are comparable in all important respects other than in their exposure to the intervention being tested. By random allocation, the experimenter accounts not only for known confounding variables, but also for factors that are unknown but are also potentially important determinants of final outcome.

Random allocation depends on allocation solely on the basis of chance – metaphorically on the basis of the flip of a coin, but not on the actuality of the flip of the coin which can, of course, be flipped again if the doctor did not get the side he or she favored. A potentially important trial of electronic fetal heart rate monitoring in a setting with significant risk of intrapartum death was weakened by the use of such a method[17]. The trial report described markedly unbalanced overall numbers in the two groups (electronic monitoring: 746; intermittent auscultation: 682) as well as dramatic differences in the number of women having had labor induced (16% versus 7%) or augmented (52% versus 38%), suggesting the operation of *selection bias*.

The essence of secure randomization requires that those involved in the study cannot know in advance to which group a particular woman will be allocated on entering a trial. Thus, the use of hospital case numbers or date of birth will not adequately conceal the direction of allocation and if a clinician has preconceptions about the effectiveness of the two treatment options, he or she may be influenced in whether or not that woman is actually asked to participate thus distorting the nature of two comparison groups. These methods of participant allocation to the study groups are sometimes called 'quasi-random' and with current concepts of good trial methodology should not be used[18].

Even apparently robust methods of random allocation, such as the commonly employed sealed opaque envelope to be opened only after the woman has consented to entering the trial, have been known to be abused on occasion. The gold standard method, used now in most large trials, is telephone randomization in which someone based at a remote site gives randomization instructions only after basic descriptive data about the woman and confirmation of eligibility criteria have been recorded on computer. Electronic communication may be particularly difficult in parts of the developing world and randomized trials may be particularly important in such settings because rates of both maternal and fetal mortality may be high. The Collaborative Eclampsia Trial[19], which for the first time demonstrated the indisputable pre-eminence of magnesium sulfate as the anticonvulsant of choice for eclampsia, took place mainly in developing countries and used identical boxes containing either magnesium sulfate or diazepam or phenytoin with appropriate administration equipment to be opened when a woman had an eclamptic fit, and had a system to monitor the use of these numbered boxes. Increasingly, web based randomizsation procedures have been used to good effect.

Explanatory versus pragmatic trials

There are two types of randomized trial; both are valid and the appropriate trial design will depend on the question to be answered, but the differences between the two represent a common source of confusion. The *explanatory trial* assesses *efficacy* – the performance of the intervention under ideal circumstances; the *pragmatic trial* assesses *effectiveness* – performance under what may be less than optimal, but real life, circumstances.

The Term Breech Trial[20] was a pragmatic trial that compared the outcome after planned cesarean section or planned vaginal delivery for fetuses presenting by the breech at term. Ninety percent of women in the planned cesarean section group were delivered by cesarean section; 57% in the planned vaginal delivery group delivered vaginally. Clinicians were required to consider themselves 'skilled' at vaginal breech delivery, with confirmation by their head of department. Randomization was controlled in Toronto, Canada, with a computerized system accessed by touch tone telephone. The trial showed a considerable short/medium term advantage to babies in the planned cesarean section group (perinatal mortality or neonatal mortality or serious neonatal morbidity: 1.6% versus 5%, relative risk 0.33, 95% confidence intervals 0.19–0.56). There were no significant differences in maternal mortality or serious maternal morbidity. Nor were there significant differences in neurodevelopmental delay among babies followed until 2 years of age[21].

The Term Breech Trial has had a major impact on clinical practice in many countries but has also generated considerable controversy[22,23], mainly around the issue of *generalizability*. Can the results of a large trial performed in diverse settings with differing levels of facility and expertise be applied to the correspondents' institution and practice? That is a necessary consideration with any trial. The Term Breech Trial team was well aware of this[24].

Sample size calculations

Type I errors occur when the results of a trial suggest a difference when, in fact, none exists; *a type II* error occurs when the results do not suggest a difference although one does, in fact, exist. The principal protection against both types of error lies in planning, in advance, an adequate sample size for the trial based on knowledge of baseline incidence of the primary outcome and a realistic judgment on what would prove to be a clinically useful change in the incidence by the new treatment. Another way to describe the importance of pre-specified sample size calculations is to compare a study that has confirmed predicted reduction in perinatal mortality following an intervention with a study that has merely observed a difference between the two groups looking at the data in retrospect. Clearly, the former should carry much weight with a clinician trying to decide whether to use the intervention or not.

Underpowered trials may still be useful, as long as they are of sound methodology, as the results can be included in meta-analysis[25].

Data monitoring

It is also a principle of good clinical trial design and execution to ensure that an independent panel of experts will have access to interim results to advise whether or not a trial should continue. A charter now exists to guide the workings of data monitoring committees[26]. Advice may be given to abort a trial early if there is overwhelming evidence that either the treatment group or the control group are at significant advantage or disadvantage on the basis of treatment. Thus, in both the Term Breech Trial[20] and the Magpie Trial[27](magnesium sulfate versus placebo for pre-eclampsia), recruitment was stopped earlier than planned on the recommendation of the Data Monitoring Committees because of large, clinically and statistically significant differences in the primary outcomes between the randomized groups.

Data monitoring committees may also have to decide if further recruitment to a trial can be ethically justified in a pursuit of prespecified sample size, where the tested intervention is clearly ineffective. Such a trial may be abandoned on grounds of futility.

What is bad practice is for the researchers themselves continually to monitor the results because of the possibility of stopping a trial once a 'statistically significant' result is obtained as this is likely to produce a type I error.

Factorial design

It may be possible to answer two questions rather than one through factorial design. Thus, a trial of women with pre-eclampsia might comprise four groups with different patterns of administration of Drug A (an anticonvulsant) and Drug B (an antihypertensive) and placebo: 1 (A + B), 2 (A/no B), 3 (no A/B), 4 (no A/no B). Comparison of the outcomes from groups 1 + 2 versus groups 3 + 4 addresses the value of Drug A; comparison of the outcomes from groups 1 + 3 versus groups 2 + 4 addresses the value of Drug B. The ORACLE trial[28], testing antibiotics in preterm, pre-labor rupture of membranes and preterm labor, used a factorial design.

'Intention to treat'

It is a feature of pragmatic trials (but not explanatory trials) that a woman may not receive the treatment or test to which she had been allocated. There are several reasons why this may happen – she might have delivered before the intervention could be implemented, she might have had second thoughts about involvement in the trial, or there may have been a mistake. Lack of appropriate treatment may, however, reflect the nature of the treatment. A course of drug treatment, for example, may have such unpleasant side effects that women stop taking medication. Since the fundamental aim of the pragmatic trial is to test the *policy* of allocating women to the treatment schedule in question, whether or not they actually receive the treatment in full, it is vital that analyses are based on 'intention to treat' to include *all* women allocated to the two groups.

The potential dangers of not including all randomized women in analyses can be illustrated by considering early trials of thyrotropin-releasing hormone (TRH) as a possible method of enhancing the effects of antenatal corticosteroids on fetal lung maturation before possible preterm delivery[29]. A meta-analysis (see below) included seven trials of TRH and demonstrated a statistically significant reduction in the incidence of respiratory distress among 'optimally treated babies' (i.e. a full course of TRH treatment with delivery occurring >24 hours and <10 days post-treatment)[30]. However, only three of the trials[31–33] reported all babies included in an 'intention to treat' analysis and the pooled results from these showed no beneficial impact on the incidence of respiratory distress syndrome. Similar trends were also seen in perinatal deaths – these could only be explained if there were disadvantages from TRH treatment to babies who remained *in utero* for more than 10 days. One could, for example, envisage pregnancies in which there is uteroplacental insufficiency with associated fetal physiological compensation by circulatory readjustment and metabolic thrift, in which a sudden boost of TRH-stimulated increased metabolic rate may not best serve the long-term interests of the baby.

Publication bias

Publication bias is 'the systematic, preferential publication of studies with statistically significant positive results over intermediate studies (frequently, researchers inappropriately term these 'negative studies'), or studies that show a statistically significant negative outcome[34]. Trial registration at inception in a central database is at least a partial solution and many journals now require such registration. Standardized methods of reporting trials (CONSORT guidelines)[35] further aid transparency.

SYSTEMATIC REVIEWS

The importance of reviews to inform busy clinicians is obvious as we are now swamped by a huge primary medical literature and all of us struggle to keep up to date even with our special areas of clinical or scientific interest. Unfortunately, we are all too often ill served by conventional *narrative* reviews whether published in books or in journals: they are frequently out of date at the time of publication if the topic is progressing rapidly; different 'experts' can reach entirely different conclusions after reviewing the same topic; as readers, we are usually not informed how the reviewer chose to select certain references and ignore others. As a consequence, we cannot be sure if the review can be trusted or not. The answer is the scientific or systematic review that, in contrast, is based on an explicit and rigorous process that includes:

- a clear description of the objectives
- explicit criteria for including studies
- an attempt to identify all relevant studies, whether published or not
- explicit description of why apparently relevant studies have not been considered
- extraction of data
- pooling of data from similar studies (meta-analysis)
- description of results
- drawing appropriate conclusions and discussing implications for clinical practice and future research.

Meta-analysis

In the perinatal field, large numbers of women or babies are usually needed to address important research questions about outcomes that may be rare, though important (e.g. fetal death). Such questions may be tackled by mounting very large studies or by pooling data from a number of different trials of similar structure and purpose – *meta-analysis*. Meta-analysis is a component of systematic reviews and there are now several examples of such analyses providing clear guidance about the value of interventions during pregnancy to try to optimize fetal outcome, e.g. corticosteroid treatment before likely preterm delivery[36], or the use of Doppler ultrasound to investigate umbilical artery waveforms in high-risk pregnancies[37].

There are debates about whether large single trials are preferable to the meta-analysis of results from several smaller trials. Whatever may be better, clinically important differences, without explanation, are rare in the obstetric arena[38].

The Cochrane Collaboration

The Cochrane Collaboration is an international network of individuals and institutions committed to producing up-to-date systematic reviews of the effectiveness of healthcare measures[39]. Cochrane reviews tend to be of better quality than other systematic reviews[40]. The Collaboration is based on the principles of genuine collaboration, equity and inclusiveness, and it consists of four dimensions – review groups, centers, fields, and methodology and software development groups. The centers are scattered around the world and provide support for review groups based within their geographical area of responsibility; each center also has responsibility for some strategic activity for the collaboration, e.g. trial registration, training of reviewers, software production. The 'fields' deal with large generic issues that transcend the interests of any one review group, e.g. children, the elderly, people living in developing countries. The review groups produce the systematic reviews and have expanded greatly in number since their genesis in the perinatal field; there are now, for example, productive review groups in the fields of stroke, infectious diseases, schizophrenia and menstrual disorders and subfertility. The pregnancy and childbirth group, based in Liverpool but with a large international panel of review authors, is the most productive group worldwide with >300 published systematic reviews. The review group administrative staff coordinate electronic and hand searching of the relevant literature for randomized controlled trials (including identification of unpublished material and non-English language literature).[41]

Until recently, the building blocks for Cochrane systematic reviews have been exclusively randomized controlled trials both because of the scientific strength of this method of assessing clinical interventions and because of the methodological difficulties of dealing with other types of scientific data (e.g. qualitative research data). However, the Cochrane Collaboration will soon start to publish systematic reviews of screening and diagnostic tests; one of the pilot projects is a review of screening tests for fetal Down's syndrome. Systematic reviews of non-RCTs of relevance to fetal medicine specialists have already been published by others. Topics have included prognosis for twins following intrauterine death of a co-twin[42], and value of fetal urine analysis in urinary tract obstruction[43].

The main product of the Cochrane Collaboration is the Cochrane Database of Systematic Reviews which is published in electronic form at 3-monthly intervals within the 'Cochrane Library', together with databases of clinical trials, methodological papers, and abstracts of other systematic reviews. Published pregnancy and childbirth reviews have, to date, been all *aggregate reviews* – based on published reports. *Individual patient data (IPD) meta-analyses* are much more resource-intensive but allow much more sophisticated exploration of subgroups. The first perinatal IPD review – of low-dose aspirin – has been published recently.[44]

Perinatal medicine provided prototype models for development of other Cochrane review groups. The first, pilot database produced was the Oxford Database of Perinatal Trials which followed the publication of the milestone book, *Effective Care in Pregnancy and Childbirth*[45]. The Oxford Database was developed by Sir Iain Chalmers and colleagues at the National Perinatal Epidemiology Unit, Oxford, UK, and was successful in demonstrating that such a project was feasible and that it would attract, as reviewers, committed people from many different countries and several different professional backgrounds.

Iain Chalmers continues to be active in retirement, documenting the history of controlled clinical trials (the James Lind Library) and promoting partnerships between patients and professionals to identify important uncertainties about treatment effects (the James Lind Alliance) in part to inform the research agenda.[46]

EVIDENCE-BASED MEDICINE

Given the limited resources of all healthcare systems, there is increasing pressure to deliver care according to clinical

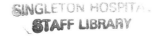

effectiveness. This should also, of course, be an imperative to all clinicians attempting to provide a high-quality service. As more and more interventions are scrutinized in robust clinical trials, and as more and more topics are reviewed systematically, it is now possible to identify treatments that are effective and which should be used widely; those that are ineffective or frankly harmful and which should be discarded; and those about which we are uncertain of effectiveness and which should be considered for future research agendas. Through the incorporation of sound evidence into clinical guidelines, clinical epidemiology is making a tangible impact on the way that care is structured and delivered in fetal and perinatal medicine.

REFERENCES

1. Enkin MW. The need for evidence-based obstetrics. *Evidence-Based Med* **1**:132–133, 1996.
2. Naylor CD. Grey zones of clinical practice: some limits to evidence-based medicine. *Lancet* **345**:840–842, 1995.
3. Barker DJP. The origins of the developmental origins theory. *J Intern Med* **261**:412–417, 2007.
4. Arngrimsson R, Sigurardottir S, Frigge ML et al. A genome-wide scan reveals a maternal susceptibility locus for pre-eclampsia on chromosome 2p13. *Hum Mol Genet* **8**:1799–1805, 1999.
5. Smith GC, Shah I, White IR, Pell JP, Dobbie R. Mode of delivery and the risk of delivery-related perinatal death among twins at term: a retrospective cohort study of 8073 births. *Br J Obstet Gynaecol* **112**:1139–1144, 2005.
6. Smith GC, Shah I, White IR, Pell JP, Dobbie R. Previous preeclampsia, preterm delivery, and delivery of a small for gestational age infant and the risk of unexplained stillbirth in the second pregnancy: a retrospective cohort study, Scotland, 1992–20001. *Am J Epidemiol* **165**:194–202, 2007.
7. Smith GC, Wood AM, Pell JP, Dobbie R. First cesarean birth and subsequent fertility. *Fertil Steril* **85**:90–95, 2006.
8. Confidential Enquiry into Maternal and Child Health. Perinatal Mortality 2005: England, Wales and Northern Ireland. London: CEMACH, 9, 2007.
9. Lewis G et al. Saving mothers' lives 2003–2005. *The Seven Report of the Confidential Enquiries into Maternal Deaths in the United Kingdom*. London: CEMACH, 2007.
10. Szabo J, Gellen J. Nuchal fluid accumulation in trisomy 21 detected by vaginosonography in first trimester. *Lancet* **336**:1133, 1990.
11. Kagan KO, Avgidou K, Molina FS, Gajewska K, Nicolaides KH. Relation between increased fetal nuchal translucency thickness and chromosomal defects. *Obstet Gynecol* **107**:6–10, 2006.
12. De Lia JE, Kuhlmann RS, Harstad TW, Cruikshank DP. Fetoscopic laser ablation of placental vessels in severe previable twin–twin transfusion syndrome. *Am J Obstet Gynecol* **172**:1202–1211, 1995.
13. Senat MV, Deprest J, Boulvain M, Paupe A, Winer N, Ville Y. Endoscopic laser surgery versus serial amnioreduction for severe twin-to-twin transfusion syndrome. *N Eng J Med* **351**:182–184, 2004.
14. UK Obstetric Surveillance System (UKOSS). www.npeu.ox.ac.uk/ukoss
15. Edington PT, Sibanda J, Beard RW. Influence on clinical practice of routine intra-partum fetal monitoring. *Br Med J* **3**:341–343, 1975.
16. Chalmers I. Evaluating the effects of care during pregnancy and childbirth. In *Effective care in pregnancy and childbirth*, I Chalmers, M Enkin, MJNC Keirse (eds), pp. 3–38. Oxford: Oxford University Press, 1989.
17. Vintzileos AM, Antsaklis A, Varvarigos I, Papas C, Sofatzis I, Montgomery JT. A randomized trial of intrapartum electronic fetal heart rate monitoring versus intermittent auscultation. *Obstet Gynecol* **81**:899–907, 1993.
18. Schulz KF, Grimes DA. Allocation concealment in randomized trials: defending against deciphering. *Lancet* **359**:614–618, 2002.
19. The Eclampsia Trial Collaborative Group. Which anticonvulsant for women with eclampsia? *Lancet* **345**:1455–1463, 1995.
20. Hannah ME, Hannah WJ, Hewson SA, Hodnett ED, Saigal SWillan AR for the Term Breech Trial Collaborative Group. Planned caesarean section versus planned vaginal birth for breech presentation at term: a randomized controlled trial. *Lancet* **356**:1375–1383, 2000.
21. White H, Hannah ME, Saigal S et al. for the 2-year infant follow-up Term Breech Trial Collaborative Group. Outcomes of children at 2 years after planned cesarean birth versus planned vaginal birth for breech presentation at term: The International Randomized Term Breech Trial. *Am J Obstet Gynecol* **191**:864–871, 2004.
22. Glezerman M. Five years to the term breech trial: the rise and fall of a randomized controlled trial. *Am J Obstet Gynecol* **194**:20–25, 2006.
23. Kotaska A. Inappropriate use of randomized trials to evaluate complex phenomena: case study of vaginal breech delivery. *Br Med J* **329**:1039–1042, 2004.
24. Hofmeyr J, Hannah M. Five years to the term breech trial: the rise and fall of a randomized controlled trial. *Am J Obstet Gynecol* **195**:22, 2006.
25. Schulz KF, Grimes DA. Sample size calculations in randomized trials: mandatory and mystical. *Lancet* **365**:1348–1353, 2005.
26. DAMOCLES Study Group. A proposed charter for clinical trial data monitoring committees: helping them to do their job well. *Lancet* **365**:711–722, 2005.
27. Altman D, Carroli G, Duley L, Farrell B, Moodley J, Neilson JP for the Magpie Trial Collaborative Group. Do women, and their babies, benefit from magnesium sulphate? The Magpie Trial: a randomized placebo-controlled trial. *Lancet* **359**:1877–1890, 2002.
28. Kenyon S, Taylor DJ, Tarnow-Mordi W for the ORACLE Collaborative Group. Broad spectrum antibiotics for preterm, prelabour rupture of fetal membranes: the ORACLE randomized trial. *Lancet* **357**:979–988, 2001.
29. Liggins GC, Schellenberg JC, Manzai M, Kitterman JA, Lee CC. Synergisms of cortisol and thyrotropin-releasing hormone in lung maturation in fetal sheep. *J Appl Physiol* **65**:1880–1884, 1988.
30. Crowther CA, Alfirevic Z, Haslam RR. Thyrotropin-releasing hormone added to corticosteroids for women at risk of preterm birth for preventing neonatal respiratory disease. *Cochrane Database of Systematic Reviews* (2), CD 000019, 2004.
31. Jikihara H, Sawada Y, Imai S et al. Maternal administration of thyrotropin-releasing hormone for prevention of neonatal respiratory distress syndrome. In *Proceedings of 6th Congress of the Federation of the Asia-Oceania Perinatal Societies, Perth, Western Australia* p. 87, 1990.
32. Knight DB, Liggins GC, Wealthall SE. A randomized controlled trial of antepartum thyrotropin-releasing hormone and betamethasone in the prevention of respiratory distress in preterm infants. *Am J Obstet Gynecol* **171**:11–16, 1994.
33. The Actobat Study Group. Australian Collaborative Trial of Betamethasone and Thyrotropin Releasing Hormone (ACTOBAT) for the prevention of neonatal respiratory disease. *Lancet* **345**:877–882, 1995.
34. Abaid LN, Grimes DA, Schulz KF. Reducing publication bias through trial registration. *Obstet Gynecol* **109**:1434–1437, 2007.
35. Moher D, Schulz KF, Altman D. CONSORT Group. The CONSORT statement: revised recommendations for improving the

quality of reports of parallel-group randomized trials 2001. *Explore (NY)* **1**:40–45, 2005.

36. Roberts D, Dalziel S. Antenatal corticosteroids for accelerating fetal lung maturation for women at risk of preterm birth. *Cochrane Database of Systematic Reviews* (3), CD 004454, 2006.
37. Alfirevic Z, Neilson JP. Doppler ultrasonography in high-risk pregnancies: systematic review with meta-analysis. *Am J Obstet Gynecol* **172**:1379–1387, 1995.
38. Cappelleri JC, Ioannidis JPA, Schmid CH et al. Large trials vs meta-analysis of smaller trials. How do their results compare? *J Am Med Assoc* **276**:1332–1338, 1996.
39. Chalmers I, Dickersin K, Chalmers T. Getting to grips with Archie Cochrane's agenda. *Br Med J* **305**:786–787, 1992.
40. Sheikh L, Johnston S, Thangaratinam S, Kilby MD, Khan KS. A review of the methodological features of systematic reviews in maternal medicine. *BMC Med* **5**:10, 2007.
41. Moher D, Fortin P, Jadad AR et al. Completeness of reporting of trials in languages other than English: implications for conduct and reporting of systematic reviews. *Lancet* **347**:363–366, 1996.
42. Ong SS, Zamora J, Khan KS, Kilby MD. Prognosis for the co-twin following single-twin death: a systematic review. *Br J Obstet Gynaecol* **113**:992–998, 2006.
43. Morris RK, Quinlan-Jones E, Kilby MD, Khan KS. Systematic review of accuracy of fetal urine analysis to predict poor postnatal renal function in cases of congenital urinary tract obstruction. *Prenat Diagn* Jul 4; epub ahead of print, 2007.
44. Askie LM, Duley L, Henderson-Smart DJ, Stewart LA on behalf of the PARIS Collaborative group. Antiplatelet agents for prevention of pre-eclampsia: a meta-analysis of individual patient data. *Lancet* **369**:1791–1798, 2007.
45. Chalmers I, Enkin M, Keirse MJNC (eds). *Effective Care in Pregnancy and Childbirth.* Oxford: Oxford University Press, 1979.
46. The James Lind Library. www.jameslindlibrary.org/

SECTION 5

Ethics

16 Ethical issues in maternal–fetal medicine 207
Susan Bewley

Ethical issues in maternal–fetal medicine

CHAPTER 16

Susan Bewley

KEY POINTS

- This chapter deals with the moral actors, objects and acts in maternal–fetal medicine and analyses the moral frameworks used by different ethical camps
- It explains the difference between descriptive and prescriptive ethics, intuition and rationality, and theory and practice
- The scientific and analytical tools of philosophy and ethical questions are explained
- The difference and tensions between duties, rights and goals are examined
- The moral status of fetal life cannot be tackled in isolation from the moral value of maternal life and maternal autonomy
- The 'fetus is a patient' is a proud medical description but the powerful language also contains a hidden and flawed moral claim
- Ethics (as the highest standard) and law (as the lowest standard) govern everyday medical practice
- Practical tips are given on how to stay out of ethical trouble and keep reflective and up-to-date, with an extensive bibliography and useful websites

INTRODUCTION

Discussions about ethics often seem irrelevant to practicing doctors: some are full of jargon and concepts that are alienating or cliquey; others appear to be an attack on an aspect of medical practice; often they fail to provide answers to real and pressing clinical problems. Why would one wish to submit oneself to the painful accusation or realization of being unethical? Maternal–fetal medicine specialists know that ethics are relevant as we deal with precious and vulnerable lives, complex family decision making and future children and adults. We are questioned publicly about our ethics. In difficult cases, we may also experience a visceral sinking or queasy feeling of 'am I doing something wrong here?'

It is not possible in a small space to do justice to the depth and breadth of ethical issues in maternal–fetal medicine. A reading list at the end of the chapter points the interested reader to more detailed texts, books and journals. There are both great theoretical and elaborate individual problems. To illustrate this, Table 16.1 provides a list of contentious issues in this relatively new and rapidly developing medical field. Technological developments are bound to increase the list. Another approach starts with case-based scenarios which are rich with complexity. A case study below shows an example of an everyday case that poses ethical, as well as medical, problems for the participants. This chapter will attempt to draw a structure for discussions of all types of ethical issues in maternal–fetal medicine.

Case study

Jane, an illiterate 15-year-old single primigravida living in a mobile caravan with her mother on welfare, is found to have a male fetus with megacystis and anhydramnios at 24 weeks' gestation. Apparently, the 18-week anomaly scan was normal. The provisional diagnosis is posterior urethral valves and possible 'prune-belly'. There is severe hydronephrosis and the kidney parenchyma is echogenic with a few cysts. Serial urine sampling shows relatively poor, but some, renal function. The previous week, the trainee talked optimistically about shunting without mentioning the poor long-term outlook and Jane is very keen to do everything possible to help the baby. However, even though the poor outlook has now been spelled out, she appears unrealistic about the possibility of neonatal death due to pulmonary hypoplasia or how she would manage long-term renal dialysis and childhood problems. She says, 'I love my baby and want everything possible to be done. I'm sure it'll be alright – the baby's moving OK'. Jane's mother understands the low likelihood of survival and is pressing Jane to terminate

Table 16.1 **Examples of current ethical issues in maternal–fetal medicine**

Occurring at any time
Genetic knowledge – whose is it?
Property rights in genes, cells, etc.
Rights to know paternity
Requests for futile treatments
Iatrogenic creation of medical problems
Experimental treatments
Risk/benefit calculations for long-term or second-generation harm
Informed consent
Research
Occurring pre-pregnancy
Contraception (coil, morning-after pill)
Egg and sperm donation or selling
In vitro fertilization
Embryo research
Preimplantation genetic diagnosis
Creation of sibling savior
Surrogacy
Xenotransplantation
Artificial placenta
Cloning
Hybrids
Occurring first and second trimester
Abortion – rights and wrongs
Embryo reduction
Screening ('search and destroy'?)
Invasive testing risks
Selective reduction in multiple and discordant pregnancies
Experimental fetal therapy
(Maternal)–fetal surgery
Occurring third trimester
Decisions re salvage or abandoning babies at edge of viability
Late karyotyping
Third-trimester termination and feticide
Monitoring during delivery
Enforced cesareans
Requested non-medically indicated interventions
Umbilical cord blood banking
Fetal and placental tissue donation
Occurring in neonatal life
Prematurity and sequelae
Withdrawal of intensive neonatal treatment
Value of the handicapped
Concept of the 'worthless life'
Infanticide

the pregnancy; 'You have always been slow, which is why you had special schooling. It'll be me bringing this child up with my angina and diabetes, and what if I die? If the baby lives and is ill, we won't be able to manage. This child isn't meant for the world and it'll be cruel to prolong its agony. You should end the pregnancy now, or at least just leave it be and let Nature decide'.

The case illustrates a number of problems. There is an *uncertain prognosis* and procedures would be *invasive* with *risks of harm* to mother and baby. Who is the *patient* and to whom are *obligations* owed? Is Jane *competent* to give *informed consent*? If the doctor takes all or some of the *responsibility for decision making*, is this medical *paternalism* or appropriate? Will the child have a *worthwhile life*? How does one handle the *family dynamics*? Would *late abortion* or early induction be wrong? Will *prematurity* add or *create harm*? What will *prolong life*? How does one *alleviate suffering*? Should *resource implications* be considered? What are the *legal limits* to medical behavior? What should a *good doctor* do?

WHY SHOULD WE CONSIDER ETHICS?

We all need to consider ethics for several reasons:

- to decide whether an action is right or wrong
- to guide us in the future when a dilemma occurs
- to know the extent of our professional obligations
- for society to set boundaries of unacceptable behavior through guidelines or laws.

An understanding of ethics may help doctors in a variety of ways. We may become aware of the underlying concepts guiding our everyday behavior. There is then a basis for formulating questions about future actions and working out consistent and credible answers when asked to justify what we do or will do.

Ethics and law, although they have many parallels and connections, are not the same. An action may be legal but unethical: for example, walking past and ignoring an injured child in the street. An action may be ethical but not legal: for example, breaking into a neighbor's house that is on fire. The 'mercy-killing' claim is that the ending of a life of a terminally ill patient with intractable pain at their request would be an ethical act to relieve suffering, athough still illegal. At the simplest level, medical ethics is about the *highest* achievable standard of behavior ('How can I be a good doctor?'), whereas law concerns itself with the *lowest* acceptable practice ('What is the lowest standard before redressing grievances or removing registration?'). Law is invoked to limit personal and professional judgments and freedoms when personal or professional ethics are not enough. Law and ethics are intertwined. For example, some legal precepts, such as basic human rights, *habeas corpus* or the principle that personhood is conferred at birth, reflect sound moral positions and go well beyond the grievance-resolution aspect of the law.

DESCRIPTIVE AND PRESCRIPTIVE ANALYSIS

An ethical analysis may have two parts:

1. *Descriptive. What is* the basis or foundation of the rules of behavior? How does this or that group of doctors behave? Classically, we find different ethical cultures and laws in

different countries, for example with regard to truth telling and abortion.

2. *Prescriptive. What should be* the basis of the rules? For example, is abortion the taking of innocent life and absolutely wrong or is it a justifiable killing to prevent maternal harm? In an increasingly egalitarian world, should fathers have more rights to make decisions about their offspring when in utero, and if not, why not?

These are similar to an individual's questions 'What *do* I do?' and 'What *should* I do?' A discrepancy between what I do and what I should do creates a pressure to change (either my belief or my behavior). This is what makes the study of ethics so profoundly disturbing. Inconsistencies in your belief systems may be revealed or a behavior may be wrong. We may realize that we have previously been acting unethically or harming patients in our care. Patients can be harmed in a variety of ways: physically (for example, through disease, side effects of treatment or negligent treatment); mentally (for example, through unsympathetic communication); and ethically. Patients are harmed ethically if they are treated without respect, against consent or merely as a 'means' to an end rather than as 'ends' in themselves (this last comes from Kant's categorical imperative[1]). Examples of patients being ethically harmed would include being put into a research trial without their knowledge or being examined under anesthetic without consent. They might not know what had occurred, nor suffer any physical or mental harm, but they would still have been wronged. Thus, being a good doctor is more than being good technically; it also includes respectful communication and an ethical approach. If I have not been acting ethically, it must be better to address that problem now rather than carry on regardless.

Within the question 'what should I do?' are two further distinctions:

1. between an *intuition* and a *rational* argument
2. between *theory* and *practice*.

Intuition and rational argument

For rationality: we have to overcome many gut reactions or instincts as doctors as they obstruct good medical practice. There is a social taboo about performing intimate examinations (for example a digital rectal examination, especially on a semi-stranger), but both the doctor and patient overcome the taboo by rational thought. We develop rituals to help both us and the patients overcome the instinctive upset and revulsion. We learn to hide our intense dislike of certain individuals or groups as it is unprofessional and inappropriate. An immediate instinct or intuition about the right course of action in a new and difficult ethical situation may equally be based on prejudice or ignorance. The 'yuk factor' may give way on deeper thought and reflection. Philosophers are practitioners trained in the art and science of argument and can be extremely helpful in untangling and clarifying complex problems. However, they are theoreticians and may well belong to a particular school of thought or analysis. The facts of a case may not fit tidily into a rule or algorithm, so doctors should not unthinkingly follow their prescriptions.

For intuition: intuitions are worth some attention as they have evolved over many years and are often quicker than conscious thought processes, but they are fallible. Intuition may be related to 'pattern recognition' or caring about people. Rationality can lead to cold, calculated and maybe ultimately amoral behavior. For example, if two men both require life-saving treatment and one is employed and childless but the other unemployed with several children, is it rational to treat only the first (as the cost to society is more likely to be recouped) or the second (as a worker is more easily replaced than a father)? Would a lottery or toss of a coin be fair? Or would we like a system with cheaper, but less effective treatments where both are given a chance? And what if it's the waiting list for a one-off transplant? We may want more than mere calculations to guide our morality. If an intuition and rational argument do not match, one will have to give way, or both will have to be examined further to find the flaw.

Theory and practice

It is important to keep up a two-way dialogue between theory and practice. It is possible for health professionals to become bogged down or overwhelmed with the morass of real-life complexity. Highbrow ethical analysis might be dismissed as out of touch, ivory tower, academic nonsense. Sometimes professionals can become so involved with the feelings of the participants that they lose objectivity or the need for principles. They might not 'see the wood for the trees' and yet talking through the problem can clarify the issues. It is also possible for philosophers or medical ethicists to be insensitive to human life and concerns. They might then miss out on examples or observations that refine, enrich or enlighten their theories. The most productive dialogue combines a mixture of both types of expertise. Doctors should not be afraid to open their practice to scrutiny, as they may well have detailed information that empowers others to follow or defend their practice. Sometimes it must be tempting to ask someone else, maybe the ethics committee or board, to take away the awful responsibility for hurting patients, saying no to their demands for treatment or drawing boundaries for discussions or decisions. There are days when it would be comforting for someone else to be the expert or do the ethics. The problem is that ethics is embedded in medical practice, it is not an 'add-on'. Ethical responsibility is bound within many everyday medical decisions which turn on the medical facts, and doctors have the expertise of doctoring. They should not be so arrogant as to act alone, but nor should they be intimidated by ethical experts.

HOW CAN PHILOSOPHERS OR ETHICISTS HELP?

Doctors look to science and scientific methods (e.g. genetics, pharmacology, epidemiology) to support their understanding of diseases and medicines. In a similar way, we can look to moral philosophy and its methodology to help understand ethical problems. Medical ethics is a branch of moral philosophy. Philosophers are experts in argument and have available certain tools to help.

First, philosophers *analyze words* and issues. They may draw our attention to the sloppiness of talking about 'euthanasia' for example. There may be many different topics under discussion: terminal care, relief of pain, the doctrine of double effect (acceptability of a good action, such as increasing pain relief, with the unintended but known side effect of shortening life), withdrawal of life support, active killing on request, or involuntary killing without consent. All the concepts (killing, intention, consent, etc.) are themselves divisible into parts and require much closer analysis.

Philosophers are used to *drawing distinctions*, or seeing morally relevant differences between situations. Consistency is a necessity in good arguments. If there is an appropriate ethical action (or maybe a range of actions) for situation A, and situation B is essentially the same, then the ethical action(s) should be the same. If, however, there is some discernible difference between A and B, then it might be justified to act differently. For example, one might consider that it is acceptable to induce labor early and without fetal monitoring for a lethal fetal anomaly. There are a number of different lethal anomalies. Are there distinctions between types of lethal anomaly and, if so, are these morally relevant distinctions? If there were three anomalies that were lethal at birth, one month or one year respectively, would it be right to deliver all three at 30 weeks' gestation for severe maternal distress? Extra suffering might be caused to the babies surviving for a month and a year if labor was induced (by adding prematurity to the problems of the newborns' short life). On the other hand, both maternal and neonatal suffering might be relieved by induction and death during or shortly after labor. The short life of suffering before inevitable death is lessened. Thus, the type of anomaly, the accuracy of prognosis and the likely treatment effects might be a relevant distinction. A 'distinction without a difference' would be when two babies had different anomalies, say, but with exactly the same prognosis, when it is the prognosis that is weighed in the judgment about the right course of action.

Philosophers are also expert in the *use of logic*. They might point out that an argument does not flow logically when going from A to B to F and thus to conclusion G. Unlike mathematics where if A = B, and B = C, then A = C, in language the following argument is wrong. 'Grass is green. Green is a colour. Therefore grass is a colour.' They pin down the elements of an argument and find the jumps, leaps of faith or rhetoric that may be emotionally persuasive or even comforting for doctors, but not necessarily logical.

Lastly, philosophers conduct *thought experiments*. These can sometimes seem ridiculous or trite, but are actually devices to separate the strands of an argument and examine them individually. Thought experiments are similar to controlled experiments in the laboratory where one variable is changed at a time to see its effect on the whole. It is to unpack our thoughts that they ask such unreal questions as 'Would you perform an invasive prenatal test for eye color?' A thought experiment that tests the lengths to which we really sign up to 'informed consent' or 'beneficence' might be: 'When would you refuse to do an amniocentesis?' Would it be at a 1 in 100 risk of aneuploidy, 1 in 1000, 1 in 10000 or never (if it is the mother's informed choice)? 'What if a mother asked for a second (or third) amniocentesis when she already has a negative result?' Would you continue and do an unnecessary invasive procedure with a risk of fetal loss on maternal request because that is the mother's informed choice? Would you refuse, saying you know what's best and must not cause harm? In which case, are you being paternalist? Or, can you get out of the dilemma by suggesting the woman's choice does not have to be respected as it is not rational? In which case, are you really a believer in informed choices, or only those choices that agree with yours?

You can see from the above that what makes a good philosopher or medical ethicist is not necessarily someone who has *answers*, but someone who has *tools* to help ask the right questions. Someone who does not merely assert but justifies or explains. Good scientists are those who use sound and transparent methodology to test hypotheses, and whose results are consistent and reproducible. Philosophy can be seen as a scientific discipline in this way also. Good philosophers would not claim to be right or ethically superior, but would be rigorous, scientific and consistent. Like scientists, they should be prepared to abandon a hypothesis if it proves to be flawed. This can be alarming for doctors if someone apparently persuasively makes an argument and then says 'maybe I am totally wrong' and takes the opposite line in the next moment. As clinicians, we must take decisions and actions that affect people's lives and feel confident when we act, advise, prescribe or operate. It is difficult to live with the uncertainty of medicine, let alone the worries of being unethical. We need some psychological certainty that we are acting ethically (unless we are uncaring psychopaths!). This can create a conflict or tension when doctors deal with academic ethicists if they dissect our actions and ideology from what seems a safe and theoretical environment. If an action is questioned we may well feel defensive, uncomfortable, or even terrible and guilty.

It could be said that good philosophers pay more attention to the process than outcome. They would not just accuse doctors of being unethical or tell them how to behave. They would point out that, on the facts and arguments presented, a certain conclusion cannot be sustained and why it cannot. This may be discomforting, but allows for growth and learning. Doctors are responsible for their actions and may have to take a longer and harder route to gain understanding and wisdom, rather than 'I was only doing what everyone else does' or 'I was only following orders'.

WHAT IS AN ETHICAL QUESTION?

What makes something an *ethical* issue? Ethics is the science of morals, the branch of philosophy that is concerned with human character and conduct. Thus any, and every, action within a doctor–patient relationship will have an ethical dimension. It is an inescapable fact of our everyday working life. Indeed, we take this so much for granted that we stop noticing it. For example, there are systems of morals or rules of behavior that are ingrained. We have a duty of confidentiality and so should not talk in public lifts, nor tell our patients' stories to journalists. The obligation to obtain consent means we would not hold protesting patients down to do vaginal examinations or amniocenteses. We only appear to notice ethics when a conflict or problem arises, but it is always there.

What makes a conversation between a midwife and a pregnant woman about Down's screening an ethical issue, whereas determining the decor in the labor ward is not? We need to look at the three essential ingredients: an actor, an object and an act.

1. The actor and object both have moral value
2. There has to be a relationship between them and
3. Something happens (including doing nothing if one could have done something).

Table 16.2 **Examples of ethical issues and components**

Actor	*Object*	*Act*	*Duty*	*Right*	*Goal*
Mother	Fetus	Smoking	Mother's duty not to harm fetus	Either right to be born unharmed or no real 'right' as non-autonomous	Minimize number of damaged babies born
Doctor	Patient	Telling a secret	Doctor's duty of confidentiality	Patient's right to confidentiality	Confidentiality maintains trust in, and efficacy of, the medical profession
Surgeon	Patient	Operation	Touching is an assault unless prior consent	Right to bodily integrity. Consent can override	Must maximize health outcomes. Consent a device

There are three main philosophical frameworks which all consider parts of this basic equation. They place major emphasis on one or other central tenet; the duties (crucially of the actor), the rights (crucially of the object) or the consequences (of the action). There are variations in views within each system, but they argue in different ways – that the ultimate 'good' occurs via adherence to a moral code derived from religious or secular authority (duty-based), protecting the right-bearer (rights-based) or the maximizing of good consequences (goal-based). We will consider who might be *actors* and *objects* of moral concern, then *special relationships* and, lastly, the *frameworks* of moral philosophy. The components of an issue of moral concern are shown in the following figure.

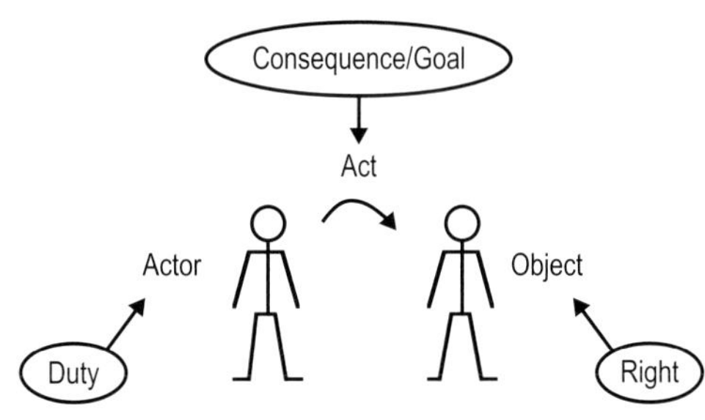

Table 16.2 gives examples of ethical issues and different views on the reasons that mothers should not smoke or doctors should maintain confidentiality or obtain consent.

THE 'PLAYERS' IN MATERNAL–FETAL MEDICINE

Table 16.3 contains examples of who or what might be an actor or object of moral concern. The 'objects' are divided into two lists: those that are autonomous and those that are non-autonomous. The meaning of autonomy is the power or right of self-government: the doctrine that the human will carries its guiding principle within itself[2]. The word 'autonomy' derives from the Greek for 'self-rule' and thus refers to beings that have self-awareness, can think and formulate actions.

Table 16.3 **Possible actors and objects of moral concern**

Actors (autonomous)	*Objects (autonomous)*	*Objects (non-autonomous)*
Doctor	Patient	Genes
Patient	Pregnant women	Gametes
Mother	Older child	Embryo
Father	Relative	Fetus
Donor	Mother	Neonate
Surrogate	Father	Young child
Relative	Doctor	Unconscious patient
Researcher	Researcher	Mentally incompetent
Government	Taxpayer	Animals
State	Donor	Future generations
Legal system	Surrogate	Precious commodities
Manager	Oppressed groups	
Taxpayer		
Pregnant women		
Pressure groups		
Interest groups		
Pharmaceutical companies		

We can see from the list that there will be many possible variations in the actor–object–act group, but that most actors and objects of moral concern are humans or groups of humans. Many appear on both lists. The only distinction between the lists is that it is a necessary, but not sufficient, condition to have a will or self-awareness or ability to formulate an action to appear on the 'actor' list. There are objects of moral concern without this that appear only on the objects list. Interestingly, some may appear temporarily on the object list, for example small children or unconscious patients, for whom others have to make decisions. However, at a later time, when they grow up or regain consciousness, they may also appear as actors. Others, such as the severely mentally disabled, may have to have some important decisions made on their behalf, although this should always be tested and not assumed. Some would dispute whether any moral value at all should be given to certain players on the object list (see later, 'What is the value or moral status of fetal life?'). What are the qualities that make something an agent or object of moral concern? Let us start with adult humans who have full moral worth.

WHAT GIVES ADULT HUMANS MORAL VALUE?

Let us agree that adult human life is of value and adults should not be wantonly or unjustly killed. What are the qualities that make us worthy of such moral consideration? There are a variety of reasons why adult human life may be of value:

1. *'We are part of God's creation and therefore sacred.'* This is also referred to as the 'sanctity of life' argument. The major problem with this argument is the absence of the quality of 'universalizability'. Any conclusions drawn from a religious view will not be generalizable or appeal to people of different, or no, religions. There is also still a debate about when God's creation started, or when the sanctity of life takes effect, although many religions hold that it starts at conception.
2. *'Humans are of value because we are human.'* Unfortunately, this is not enough as it is a circular argument. What really matters is what distinguishes us from other animals, and does that hold for all human forms? Why would the possession of human DNA be particularly valuable? What happens if and when we get mixtures?
3. *'Our ability to feel pleasure, happiness, or form relationships is enough to justify protection.'* What then happens about humans who cannot have these feelings or animals who can?
4. *'We have the ability to suffer and feel pain.'* Conversely, it can be argued that it is the ability to suffer which creates a duty in others not to cause needless or unjustified suffering. This might be a reason to protect humans and higher-order animals from suffering, but would not necessarily create a duty to preserve life.
5. *'We are self-conscious and self-aware.'* These qualities appear to distinguish us from animals and make human life full and worth living. They are required to formulate intentions and motives, take responsibility and feel conscience. These may be the prerequisites for morality to avoid killing adult humans, either (a) because these are very special qualities or (b) because adults then themselves value their lives. The qualities of self-conciousness and awareness may be used to justify moral status for the whole species, even if some members do not have them. The argument would be that because humans have self-consciousness the *whole human race* is of higher moral value. By contrast, if self-awareness were used as a determinant of *individual moral worth* then some humans, for example infants, or those with severe dementia or brain damage, would not have moral worth. In addition, if a person did not value his or her own life, then the worth might diminish, or the duties to that individual would be lowered (e.g. voluntary euthanasia).
6. Another higher function of adult humans is the *ability to form plans or express preferences* or aspirations. 'Utilitarians' say that the fulfilment of preferences, desires or aspirations is the greatest moral goal (maybe not individual preference satisfaction, but perhaps societal).

Then there may be a question of whether all humans are equal. Does one person have more moral value than another because of a greater degree of intelligence, capability, sensitivity or strength of desire to be fulfilled? Generally, most philosophers sign up to equality of adults' moral value, although some consider that some humans lose it through incapacity (e.g. the embryo or mentally handicapped) or heinous behavior (e.g. the criminal). It may be that the judgment about moral value is multilayered. Adult humans are important because they have all the qualities from (1) to (6). There may be some moral responsibility, but lesser or different, towards small animals because of (4) (the ability to suffer or feel pain).

What does 'moral value' confer? Most societies and religions agree that, at a minimum, (a) life should not be taken unjustly and (b) there is a general right not to be interfered with. There are many other protections and rights and they may follow a hierarchy. For example, although it is both wrong to kill and wrong to lie, it would be right to lie about someone hiding in your house to protect them from being killed by a murderous intruder. However, there are still very vigorous debates between people holding the same basic starting assumptions about the value of life, let alone different ones. These debates range from the rights and wrongs of capital punishment, to the ethics of a 'just war' to voluntary euthanasia.

If we could understand or analyze what gives adult human life value, we might be in a position to look at the smallest and earliest of human lives and their value. Do we value embryos or fetuses:

- for the same qualities as adults?
- for having those qualities in small amounts – and therefore counting, but not as much as adults?
- for the potential to have adult qualities – and does that mean they count now or not? or,
- for completely different reasons?

WHAT IS THE VALUE OR MORAL STATUS OF FETAL LIFE?

With respect to comparison with adults there are only three possible answers to this question – full, some or none – although many reasons can be put forward as to why it should be any of these answers.

Moral status	*Example*
Full	Adult human
Some	Animal
None	Inanimate object (e.g. chair)

Although some maternal–fetal medicine specialists, parents or ethicists may talk about the fetus as if it were of a certain value, it is important to be clear into which category they fall. For example, some argue for full moral status on the 'sanctity of life' argument, which would entail doctors doing everything possible to increase, prolong or preserve fetal life. The moral status is intrinsic to the fetus and nothing makes killing or abortion right. Others would argue that the fetus has full moral status because the mother cares for it. The moral status thus derived extrinsically obliges doctors to do good ('beneficence'). The problem with this argument is that if a mother did not care then there would be no status and the doctor would be released from medical obligations. In this argument, the group 'fetus' actually has *no* intrinsic moral worth.

A doctor and mother may care for and value fetuses but still accept abortion for fetal abnormality. They might believe either (a) that abnormality diminishes moral status (from full status to some or none) or (b) that no fetus has full moral status and protection against being killed. Most Western democracies with abortion law appear to accord the fetus 'some' moral status, in that life cannot be taken during pregnancy wantonly but nor is it absolutely protected.

HOW DOES FETAL MORAL WORTH CHANGE WITH TIME?

There is a time, most would agree, when there is no object of moral concern. The change from nothing to becoming an object of moral concern can only occur in one of three ways; suddenly, stepwise or gradually.

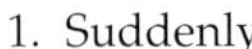

1. Suddenly

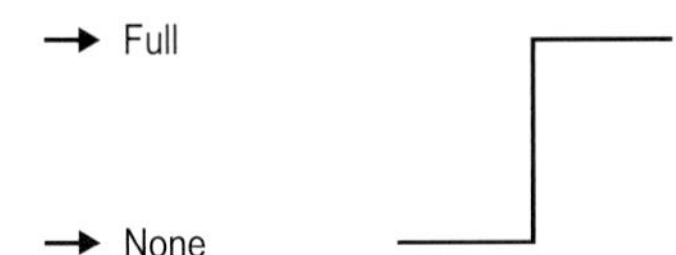

This sudden change might occur at conception (strict Catholic view), implantation, development of the neural tube (British Human Fertilisation and Embryology Act view for protection of human embryos against experimentation), viability ('fetus as a patient' view) or birth (woman's right to control her body view). Used strictly, sudden change allows a relatively simple analysis and resolution of problems in any dispute.

2. Stepwise

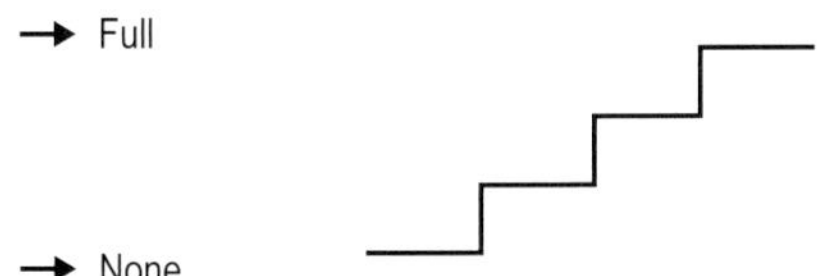

This view might correspond to the relationship of the mother to the developing fetus (e.g. status increasing in step with the pregnancy test and knowledge of pregnancy, quickening, first scan, birth and developmental milestones), or to a series of important physiological events (e.g. implantation, formation of the neural tube, development of sensory cortical connections, viability, birth). Each step brings the fetus closer to adult status and ethical protection may increase stepwise also.

3. Gradually

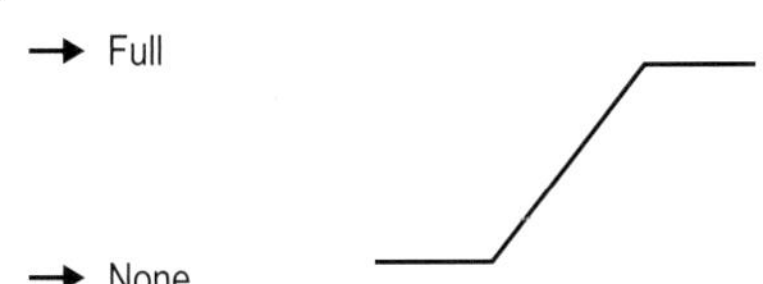

This might correspond to a developmental biological viewpoint, where status increases gradually with gestation, until a maximum is reached. The maximum could be being recognizably human, having the ability to sense pain or lay down memory, birth or self-awareness. Depending on the quality, full moral status might be reached before or after birth.

The stepwise and gradual views mean that each decision has to be individually weighed and balanced, and are similar in that they require more complex judgments to be made. What is acceptable ethically at 10 weeks might not be at 20 or 30 weeks. For example, with increasing gestation there will have to be a correspondingly greater justification for termination.

DOES BIRTH MAKE A DIFFERENCE?

Does birth make a difference to moral value? Intuitively it does, but is there a rational explanation? It is obvious that birth makes a difference to the mother as the fetus is now outside her body. For example, if one is weighing countering claims in situations where maternal behavior is damaging or the mother is refusing beneficial intervention, removal of the child once born does not involve forcible incarceration or invasion of the mother. Thus, after birth, any inhibition against violating the pregnant woman's autonomy and rights is removed. But does birth itself change the moral status of the fetus/child? We know that the mother undergoes labor and delivery and puts work and effort into this. The baby undergoes a rapid and major adaptation to extrauterine life, becomes physically separate and breathes on his or her own, although is still extremely dependent. The baby enters the family and society and is given a name. Many powerful and important social events occur, but are any of these morally relevant? This is of particular interest to pediatricians who find it inexplicable, if not abhorrent, that they are involved in life-saving exercises for babies who are at such a low gestation that obstetricians may consider them previable. Thus, at gestations around 24 weeks, obstetricians may, in different cases, pass a baby to a neonatologist or offer late termination, accept maternal refusal of cesarean section, decide not to monitor in labor, or deny classical cesarean section for fetal reasons.

WHAT ARE THE OBLIGATIONS OF OTHERS AND SPECIAL RELATIONSHIPS?

To whom do we owe a duty of care or responsibility? And what is its extent? The concept of 'special relationships' that bring extra and specific moral considerations into play is important. The most basic relationship is that of two strangers. What rights and responsibilities flow from a relationship of two strangers? How and why would the relationship of a mother to her child or two strangers be different? A stranger might be expected to keep a promise made to another, but not to buy all their clothes or wake repeatedly to feed every night, which would be expected of a mother for her child.

A doctor's duty to a patient is more than that of the stranger's. It may be characterized as doing one's best to increase life and decrease suffering. It may be characterized as respecting autonomy by fulfilling informed choices with regard to health outcomes, depending on the framework in which morality is being structured. However, being a doctor does not necessarily mean that one's duties to strangers or one's own children change or increase. Doctors may be concerned about the public health or be altruistic about global charity, but do they actually have a moral duty to improve the health of others at some distance from themselves? This has implications when it comes to balancing conflicts of interests between patients. Doctors must have regard for all the patients in their clinic and have to ration their time. They have an equal duty of care to all the patients in a clinic. They may spend more or less than the allocated appointment time with each according to their medical problems, but cannot spend two hours with the first one and always keep the rest waiting or shorten their appointments. Do doctors also have to ration their use of resources or costs, potentially depriving their patients of the best care, because other patients (not theirs) also have a claim to the limited resources? What does the implicit promise 'As your doctor, I will do my best for you' mean? There may be equal claims by patients on society, insurers or the state, or on doctors who manage budgets and priorities. Do doctors on the frontline fight for the needs of all 'their' individual patients or make decisions about competing needs? The same doctor may sit in the morning on a committee allocating resources and sit in a clinic in the afternoon with a patient denied that resource. Where does the responsibility lie? Or do we shift responsibility by using comfortable psychological devices so that we do not have to face unpalatable facts about limited resources?

Even if we agree that there is an ethical duty to care for a patient, the extent of this duty will be different for different individuals such as the doctor, nurse, relative, ward cleaner and passer-by. The standard, of doing one's best, might be the same, but that would entail different amounts or actions from a generalist versus a specialist, or a junior versus a senior doctor.

FRAMEWORKS FOR ANALYSIS

Normally, before communicating, discussing, arguing or negotiating with another person, we make sure we speak the same language and work out whether we are starting from the same or different places. The reader must realize that, in the fields of ethics and moral philosophy, it is very easy to be mistaken that two people are speaking the same language or have the same concepts or assumptions. There are fundamental differences in approaches between individuals, philosophers and proponents of certain intellectual thoughts. They may use the same words differently or with different shades of meaning. For example, some may not include embryos on the 'moral worth' list at all. If embryos are included, one person might do so because they are intrinsically worthwhile themselves, but another might argue that embryos are worthwhile as someone else cares for them. One view is that embryos have intrinsic worth, which could be absolute, and the other is that they have extrinsic value, but maybe not as much as a living child. These differences will lead to very different views about the disposal of spare artificially created embryos even between two people agreeing they are of moral worth.

Not only are there differences about who or what appears on the moral agent and object lists and why, but then there are differences about how to analyze why some action is right or wrong. Most people agree that altruism and truth telling are good and that murder and breaking promises are wrong, but they might give different reasons why. The answer to 'why?' may then lead to a difference of opinion, for example, regarding the next issue of payment for, or research on, human embryos.

The three main theoretical moral frameworks primarily examine the motives and intentions of the actor (duty-based), the object (rights-based) or the effects of the act (consequence- or goal-based). There are variations within each philosophical system, but their underlying bases are fundamentally different. The ultimate aim or value is: being good by adherence to moral rules (duty-based), protection of the right-bearer (rights-based) or the maximizing of good consequences (goal-based). Careful listening or analysis can identify these different appeals.

In duty-based (or deontological) systems, conscience and motive are paramount. Originating from religion, and God judging the actor, there are also secular, humanist versions. The category of the moral good overrides all other benefits (or losses). We have a duty not to undertake certain actions, even if they would produce states of affairs that would benefit us. These duties actually come before our rights, as well: the rights of others flow from our duties not to harm them, not the reverse. This is actually very close to the duty of first do no harm in medical ethics, which most doctors find understandable. By contrast, a consequentialist judges by whether things turn out well or badly, and the consequences (especially in medicine) are often beyond our control. In deontology, we have duties and obligations to others and any purported 'rights' they possess flow secondarily from the duty. That is, the 'right to life' exists as there is a duty not to kill. Typically, fetuses may have a 'right to life' even though they have no self-expression. Doctors are not allowed to kill even if that is what the patient requests. The exception is when a doctor uses the Doctrine of Double Effect. This is invoked when a doctor uses a drug such as morphine with a good intended effect (pain relief), but a known but non-intended side effect (life-shortening). 'Rights' do not really have much force in duty-based systems, although they are powerful rhetorically and politically. In a duty-based system, abortion can only be acceptable if fetuses do not have full moral worth. While deontology often appears harsh or abstract, in fact it is neither, in part because it does allow good intentions to matter. As Kant said, if there were only the good will, it would shine like a jewel in its own right.

In rights-based systems, by contrast, 'rights' are inherently held by people and duties flow secondarily from the right. They have largely been described in the 20th century within political philosophy[3]. For example, if one has a right to vote, this makes a very powerful political claim on others to provide that right. These kinds of strong rights have the quality of being able to be waived. For example, you might have a 'right to vote' or a 'right of association' but can choose not to use either of them. True rights can only be held by those capable of making autonomous choices. In rights-based systems, fetuses can have no rights as they cannot make choices or waive their rights. Thus they do not count at all. In obstetrics, women may claim certain rights (for example, to prenatal diagnosis or to choose the method of delivery). If one operates in a strong rights-based system, when rights exist doctors are obliged to provide the services. One might ask on what basis is there a right? For example, is there a right to reproduce, or a right to have a healthy child? Is there a fundamental right not to be interfered with, in which case clearly we should not stop women choosing to get pregnant or perform forcible abortion or sterilization, but this is not the same as a right to get help.

In goal-based systems, an action is not inherently right or wrong as it depends on the outcome or consequence. This consequentialist or utilitarian approach was developed in the 19th century from the work of Mill and Bentham[1,4]. The ultimate purpose of morality is to increase the sum of happiness, or maximization of pleasure or preferences. Modern utilitarians might not say that preference satisfaction is the greatest moral goal, at least not individual preference satisfaction, but perhaps societal. We should be acting for the maximization of good outcomes. When it is impossible to work out all the possible consequences of an action, a rule might be invoked that generally has that effect. If there were a rule, such as 'do not kill', it does not exist because we should not kill as killing is inherently wrong, but because having such a rule means the world is a better place in which to live. Some killings will actually be judged as right (for example, of people who do not wish to live or dictators who cause harm). It is in utilitarianism that no-one has inherent value. Value is related to qualities possessed by the subject, such as sentience, preferences or ability to feel pain. A major criticism of utilitarianism is that of sacrificing one for the many, or overall benefit. Concepts of speciesism and replacement children belong here. Utilitarianism can be very attractive to doctors, as we spend our lives making harm/benefit calculations on the individual level and responding to parents' views of the worth of their fertility or offspring.

Spotting where an argument comes from means it can be weighed in its context. It is somewhat similar to giving one's vote to a politician: it helps to know which party they belong to and thus how their presentation of the concepts of freedom, choice or equality of opportunity might be colored.

'THE FETUS AS A PATIENT'

An example of identifying the philosophical framework being used occurs in the debate about 'the fetus as a patient'. A popular view in maternal–fetal medicine holds that 'the fetus is a patient'. Does this have any *ethical* meaning? Chervenak and McCullough[5,6], in particular, have written a number of papers in the obstetric literature putting forward one particular model of maternal–fetal ethics. It is important to realize that, although this model dominates the American obstetric literature and claims to be 'ethically justified', it is not definitive and is far from being generally accepted in philosophical circles[7].

The particular argument about fetuses (and counterargument) runs thus:

- *Argument*: no-one can agree on the independent moral status of the fetus. There are diametrically opposed views. At one extreme, there is a belief in the 'sanctity of life', usually from conception, which is utterly opposed to abortion. At the other extreme, notions of 'personhood' are used to define moral status, which does not come until the child has interests, self-realization or sentience, etc. This latter view is not the same argument used by the ultra-feminists to defend abortion or the 'right to choose'. But those whose moral outlook depends on 'personhood' accept abortion, as the fetus does not have it while in utero. Despite philosophers' best efforts there is no resolution nor any likelihood of resolution of this issue.
- *Counterargument*: yes, there is disagreement about fundamental values. However, the existence of an impasse is not a justification for taking one side or the other. Does the concept of 'the fetus as a patient' end up being another version of one or other side of this impasse or is it a new view entirely that breaks the deadlock?
- *Argument*: we need to break the deadlock. So what do we agree upon? We all agree that the child is a patient to whom we have obligations. Therefore let us work backwards in time to identify our patients (to whom doctors have obligations).
- *Counterargument*: we might well agree that we have obligations to treat children but, as explained above, we might have different underlying reasons for our agreement. If we go further back in time, the reasons and agreement may become uncoupled. If we work back far enough, through child, baby, neonate, fetus, embryo and egg we may find that the thing we are dealing with has changed its nature and thus its moral status.
- *Argument*: patients are those we can benefit, i.e. this starts at about 24 weeks when the fetus becomes viable.
- *Counterargument*: first, it is not at all clear that 'patients are those we can benefit'. This is clearly too broad in that we can benefit pet cats and dogs by being kind to them, but that does not make them patients. A more traditional definition is that 'patients are those under the care of a doctor' (whether we can benefit them or not). Otherwise, we might find that we have obligations to unwilling and unwitting patients; those people who are unwell and can be benefited but who have not gone to see a doctor. Secondly, it is also paternalistic; even if patients do not want doctors to benefit them, doctors are obliged to, thus making a nonsense of informed consent. Thirdly, is it a plausible claim that moral worth is determined by whether a doctor can benefit you? Would that mean that the size of a doctor's obligation relates to the amount he or she can do for you? And why should it? Another interesting possibility would be that the very sick and dying would not be patients, or would count less than the remediably unwell, as doctors cannot benefit them. Are there obligations only to patients with treatable problems but not untreatable ones? Some would consider it reprehensible to walk past the beds of dying patients as they still require care even when cure is impossible. Or could it be that we only have a symbolic need to care for the vulnerable? And lastly, fetuses can be helped well before 24 weeks so viability is not relevant to the concept of 'the fetus as a patient' (excepting for the ability to separate the fetus from mother by delivery, or enforced cesarean, which can be only be attempted after viability). The ability to survive when separate from the mother is not the starting time for fetal benefit. For example, cervical cerclage and in-utero blood transfusions for isoimmunization can be administered much earlier. Particularly in the first trimester, when fetal vulnerability is greatest, teratogenic drugs can cause harms well before 24 weeks. If a mother requested thalidomide for hyperemesis, this view suggests that a doctor might prescribe it under autonomy-based obligations to the mother at a time when she has not conferred status and the doctor has no beneficence-based obligations to the fetus. Doctors must have obligations not to cause harm at a time before the 'fetus as a patient' view starts.
- *Argument*: if the mother confers status and protection to her fetus beforehand, we will then also have beneficence-based obligations to fetus before 24 weeks.
- *Counterargument*: the mother can confer or grant status to the fetus as and when she sees fit. This suggests that the status is optional, which means the fetus must actually be worth nothing intrinsically. There are only three views on

independent moral status of the fetus (as described earlier): none, some or full. The 'sanctity of life' view gives fetuses full moral value. The 'personhood' view gives them none. There are views in between that take neither side of the impasse. But what is the 'fetus as a patient' view in this scheme? A view where value is *extrinsic* or *dependent* is actually one with a starting point of none (the default option) unless some property is identified. In this case, the property that the fetus has that determines medical obligation is either (a) the ability to be helped, or (b) the mother conferring status (possibly as she has religious views or a sentimental attachment). Thus, the concept of the 'fetus as a patient' does not break the deadlock of fundamental values. Any particular fetus may or may not have value depending on external facts. There is no intrinsic worth. The view merely shifts the starting point to 24 weeks (if and when a fetus can be helped) where the deadlocked views are at conception and personhood. As an aside, it is not clear that the wider 'fetus as patient' camp think the fetus only becomes a patient at viability (rather that using this as a political device while actually believing that moral status starts at conception – from when the conceptus can be helped, and thus be a patient). Moral responsibilities cannot be determined by technological changes in the age of viability; this is symptomatic of what philosophers call the naturalistic fallacy, the assumption that what can be done ought to be done.

- *Argument*: various algorithms can then be devised to answer specific queries about the ethical permissibility of various treatments depending on gestation, and whether we have obligations to patients.
- *Counterargument*: if women do not do what obstetricians consider as the best for their fetus, the 'fetus as a patient' argument can be used to enforce treatments in late pregnancy, on the basis of the mother's purported 'beneficence-based obligations' (i.e. the obligations she has to help her fetus). The argument can be used to justify cesareans against consent. Thus, in reality, the 'fetus as a patient' (as already described and understood) is not a compromise view at all. It is a view that gives fetuses no intrinsic status and ends up conceptually being, in some senses, both anti-fetus and anti-mother. This happens as a consequence of overstating the role of the doctor on whose judgment of benefit moral status turns. Superficially, the view could be very appealing to doctors, who are shown a path between extreme views that appears to provide easy and comfortable solutions to difficult questions. But the doctor is given an intimation of omnipotence and the view should be rejected, even if, in part, it is our own fault for devising the medical slogan or concept of fetuses as patients. If the preceding steps are not accepted, no algorithm has to be followed.

Whatever the view on fetal moral status during pregnancy, and the rights or wrongs of abortion, one can argue that there is a separate and different obligation not to harm the child-to-be or adult who will eventually be born. There is an interesting difference in the obligations not to kill and not to harm when applied to adults and fetuses. In adult life, it is generally worse to kill than to harm because, even though damaged, the adult is still alive. However, during pregnancy it might be permissible to kill a fetus that has some moral worth if the argument is made that the abortion is of a lesser moral being and justified by some risk to the mother. However, at the same gestation that abortion might be allowable, it might not be permissible to harm the fetus for the sake of the mother (for example, giving thalidomide for hyperemesis). This explains why we cannot tolerate the induction of labour at 30 weeks for mere maternal discomfort as the fetus will later become a damaged moral being of full moral worth.

Conclusion

Although superficially logical, the 'fetus as a patient' is a simplistic argument with many flaws[7] and ultimately not a compromise at all. It relies on the powerful medical language and rhetoric of 'the fetus as a patient', used by medical practitioners and by fetal medicine pioneers themselves. This image may have helped promote and consolidate the emergent field of fetal medicine to point out to others that there are specific diseases and syndromes of fetuses. What is more, there are investigations and treatments that specialists can apply. Fetal life and the importance of helping fetuses, which we can do increasingly, have been drawn to public attention. However, to move from mere descriptions of medical advances to a redefinition of the relative moral worth of mothers and fetuses is a leap too far. It is interesting to consider that the ethical argument promoted here developed in the context of a particular fundamentalist religious viewpoint which gained ground at a similar time during the 1980s and 1990s in the USA and now threatens to overthrow abortion rights there altogether. The language of the 'fetus as a patient' chimes with a hardline political view, associated with the rise of extreme right-wing politics and a reaction against women's civic gains. Obstetricians elsewhere in the world may not know the political background and the strategic aims of 'the fetus as patient' movement nor be aware that the logical upshot is the outlawing of abortion altogether.

In the real world, law guides us through the competing arguments and claims when there is no compromise moral position. Because of the uniqueness of pregnancy, with one being within the body of another, there are no other parallels to draw upon and few choices between accepting that the mother counts more or the fetus counts more. It has been argued that a 'hands-off' approach to pregnancy actually increases maternal altruistic behavior and good pregnancy outcomes. Although there remain countries where women are not treated as equal citizens with men, we can see that in most jurisdictions, the fetus is usually afforded some legal protection but does not become a person in law, at least, until birth, whereas the mother is always a person. The law takes a symbolic stand and makes good and practical sense, because pregnancy and birth themselves are risky for the mother[8]. Although there are a lot of arguments around the question of what viability means for clinicians, especially in fetal medicine and perinatology, the law also usually distinguishes between abortion of a fetus and euthanasia of a neonate. This has been explored in great detail and settled more firmly again recently in the UK in a comprehensive and excellent expert review[8,9].

The most important conclusion for maternal–fetal medicine specialists is that the moral status of fetal life cannot really be tackled in isolation from the moral value of maternal life and maternal autonomy. We cannot make the fetus our sole and primary focus and dismiss the mother, nor vice versa.

'HOW SHOULD I ACT?'

Having explained some of the concepts behind language, and some of the philosophical approaches, practitioners on the frontline still have to find an answer to 'what do I do *now*?' They have both ethical and legal obligations and the following section explains how these are described and then makes some simple practical recommendations.

ETHICS – THE HIGHEST IDEAL OF BEHAVIOR?

How might one work towards a high ideal of behavior?

PROFESSIONAL ETHICS OR ETIQUETTE

The original description of a doctor's duty came from Hippocrates and, over the centuries, this has become the *Hippocratic tradition*. In the 18th and 19th centuries, codes of etiquette were drawn up that may have had more to do with professional demarcation than patient care. Many critics of medicine are particularly angry about the paternalism and authoritarianism that they feel is implicit in this tradition. One can try to act according to sets of rules devised by the profession. This might include professional codes of conduct (e.g. the GMC's *Duties of a doctor*[10]), international declarations (e.g. the Nuremberg Code[11] or the Declaration of Helsinki[12]) or specialty guidelines (e.g. RCOG guidelines on enforced treatment of pregnant women[13]). These might work most of the time but, inevitably, are general rather than specific and do not encourage independent thinking. The original Hippocratic Oath is now old-fashioned and inconsistent, although there are attempts to update it. The value of professional rules is that they are drawn up by experts and can guide professionals who are too busy, tired or lazy to think. They also encourage consistency between practitioners and public accountability and transparency.

VIRTUE ETHICS

Virtue theorists[14] consider that *virtues* should be inculcated and nourished in doctors and that this, rather than rules or intellect, will produce ethical doctors[15]. Virtues might include motivation, judgment and rapport, or self-effacement, self-sacrifice, compassion and integrity. Other virtues might be knowledge, compassion, decisiveness, consistency, punctuality and responsibility. Vices might include being ideological, incompetent, prejudiced, irrational, inconsistent, irresponsible or weak. Unfortunately, merely being 'virtuous' is not enough as a guide. Are there better virtues to cultivate? How does one achieve them? How much self-sacrifice is the minimum, reasonable or supererogatory (more than is required, for the sake of greater perfection)? Are doctors who work tirelessly for their patients, never take holidays and neglect their own families commendable or not?

PRINCIPLES AND ALGORITHMS

In the late 20th century, four principles, it is claimed, should guide and cover all ethical medical decision making[16]. These are *beneficence* (doing good), *non-maleficence* (avoiding harm), *respect for autonomy* and *justice*. Unfortunately, no guidance is given on which should give way when they clash, nor why doctors should follow them. If respect for autonomy overrides all other considerations, this is significantly different from doctors' traditional duties to look after best interests, especially for the vulnerable, non-autonomous or autonomy threatened (for example, the sick, ill, delirious, frightened and anxious). Should doctors be more concerned about justice because they are doctors, or should they be equally concerned just like other citizens? This matters when it comes to the distribution of scarce medical resources or rationing. Doctors have to ration their time in a clinic or on a ward round even when they have an equal obligation to all the patients; they cannot be leisurely with the first few and rush the rest, and they may need to give an unexpectedly complex patient some more time and take it off another less sick patient's consultation. Should a doctor fight for his or her individual patient (over the interests of the next doctor's patient) or should a doctor accept rationing (as a just and fair way of delivering services) and accept that the patient might get a second-best or 'good-enough' treatment or no treatment at all? It is not clear how far each of the principles goes in the individual special relationship. Algorithms have been devised[17,18], but either they merely describe all ethical dimensions to a problem or they are drawn up with a ranking of priorities already in mind. For example, most algorithms will finally make beneficence give way to autonomy or vice versa.

DUTY-, GOAL- AND RIGHTS-BASED PHILOSOPHIES

The frameworks as described are fundamentally mutually incompatible. This is not necessarily a counsel of despair as there may always be some fundamental underlying conflicts in human society that cannot be glossed over. The work of philosophers now is in assessing what is a good untangling, or an acceptable reason to veer in one direction or another. Whereas an algorithm may claim to give an answer to a problem, analytic philosophers can at least clarify what issues are at stake and who or what is being excluded or overridden in a decision.

LAW – THE LOWEST STANDARD OF BEHAVIOR?

Enough of the theorizing, agonizing, introverted detailed analysis, the seeing all points of view and 'on the one hand this, … and on the other hand that, …'. What about real life and decision making? A marvellous thing about medicine is that it is real and active. We have to make decisions and ignore certain information or interpretations, or order tests and treatments with good and harmful side effects. But inevitably people get hurt and conflicts arise. Law is concerned with sorting out grievances and damage within a society. What does the law do?

- It sets limits by defining unacceptable behavior
- It criminalizes the extremes
- It is used to settle grievances or provide recompense for negligence
- It may have a symbolic function in setting standards.

In maternal–fetal medicine, the most relevant criminal law usually relates to abortion and assault, though manslaughter may be relevant in maternal death. Negligence is usually a civil offence with financial recompense available. Law does not have to have the quality of 'generalizability' that is demanded of ethics. It varies greatly around the world. The main requirement of doctors is not to break local law. Law does not necessarily encourage ethical behavior, nor lead to good medical practice, but sets a lowest common denominator below which the worst doctor should not fall. There is a view that excess concern about negligence claims leads to an overinvasive, non-holistic and expensive type of 'defensive' medical practice, that is not actually in the individual patient's interest (and therefore not ethical!). It is self-evident that, when things go wrong (as they inevitably will due to the poor outcomes of diseases and treatments, let alone bad or unlucky judgment calls or negligent practice), that patients might ask themselves 'could this have been avoided?'. There is no evidence that a doctor who practices defensively, or even well, will keep law suits down. There is some evidence that doctors who appear rushed, dismissive or are poor communicators get more complaints, and thus more legal problems when outcomes are bad. If a claim is made, the doctor-defendant's lawyers are greatly helped by good documentation and standard practice. Thus, even only from the self-interested point of view, a doctor practicing ethically and to a high medical standard is unlikely to fall foul of the lawyers. There are lawyers working on both sides, for the plaintiff and the defendant, and it is best not to get too worked up about them. All of us, as citizens, have to have the security of legal mechanisms to address grievances, although it can be extremely personally upsetting to receive complaints.

When doctors are expected by the State to do something that is unethical, such as be involved in punishment of criminals, torture or labeling dissidents as mentally ill, they may find themselves in terrible personal conflict or danger. They have to heed a higher ethical calling and look for help and support from colleagues around the world. National medical organizations have been expelled from worldwide medical bodies for their toleration of persecution or abuse of doctors. Organizations such as Physicians for Human Rights or the World Medical Assembly may be helpful[19,20].

REAL-LIFE ETHICAL TROUBLE

When looking through notes of obstetric disasters, we often find a string of events, a series of small failures and many different people involved. It is rare to find that care was otherwise ideal and well documented but for one single mistake. Ethical crises are very similar. Many occur after miscommunication, muddled advice, poor medicine and in a muddied cultural context. If one starts at the beginning of the story and untangles it, the ethical component or dilemma is often smaller and more circumscribed than at first it appeared. Good medical practice will keep practitioners out of most ethical trouble. Table 16.4 contains examples of behavior that gets doctors into trouble. Avoid such behavior!

HOW TO GET OUT OF ETHICAL TROUBLE

First, avoid getting into trouble (see above). Document your concerns closely and contemporaneously. If stuck, get second opinions (medical, legal, or refer to your clinical ethics

Table 16.4 **How to get into ethical trouble in maternal–fetal medicine**

Dealing with the patient
Do not read the referral letter
Assume you are a good communicator
Be rushed and too busy to pay full attention
Do not listen to the patient
Instead of the patient, find out what her husband or family want
Assume you and the patient share ethical and cultural values
Assume the patient is too stupid to understand concepts
Use medical jargon to ensure non-comprehension
Personality factors
Determine the patient's wishes by her clothes, educational level, income or demeanor
Assume everyone is monogamous, married or part of a happy family
Have fixed views about the world
Have strong and unyielding views about abortion, handicap, motherhood
Divide women into 'good' and 'bad'
Denigrate other doctors and health professionals
Be ignorant of the law (but certain you know it)
Have no idea about the effect of own personality on others
Respond excessively to gratitude
Be blissfully ignorant and complacent
Love media attention
Practical issues
Work on partial information
Stick to traditions and practices you learnt ten years ago
Do tests before working out the consequences of results you might obtain
Do large numbers of tests 'just in case'
Do not speak to colleagues (general practitioner, midwife, etc.)
Discuss cases loudly, especially in the hospital lift
Pay no attention to others' concerns
Assume you are the best (and only) doctor around
Get second opinions only from people who agree with you
Be pressurized to get answers *now*
When you do not know, guess!
Do new procedures 'for the sake of it' or because you need practice to help other patients
Confuse experimentation, research and audit
Special responsibilities of the Head of Department
Set a bad example and consider it leadership
Delegate the work to inexperienced juniors, and push people beyond their competence
Spend much time away and out of department
Pay no attention to facilities, equipment, servicing
Have no interest in protocols or procedures
Be ignorant of your department's numbers, workload, referral times, delays and complaints
Delegate complaints and policy to others
Blame everyone else when things go wrong

committee if you have one). It is important to recognize the morally 'queasy' feeling. You do not feel quite right, or are being pressurized to do something unusual or out of your depth. Although stopping is difficult, proceeding may get you and the patient into deeper water nevertheless. It is quite acceptable to say: 'This is a difficult and complex problem and I would like to take advice about the best way to proceed. We will meet again on …' If feeling cornered, or emotionally blackmailed, one can always say: 'It would be unprofessional for me to carry on without reviewing the situation'. Often just taking stock or talking through a problem makes it vanish or at least manageable. Many problems continue to evolve, and take twists and turns, over time and with deepening relationships with the patient. Sometimes trying to solve a number of small issues one at a time achieves more progress than grander plans. Table 16.5 contains a variety of actions to improve your ethical expertise.

It is vitally important to *know your medicine* as many legal and ethical problems revolve around the medical facts. If there is a problem when offering a risky treatment, or rationing it, the problem may well become moot and go away if the complication rate proves to be 5% rather than 95% or vice versa. No-one can make an individual ethical decision or judgment without medical knowledge. It is this body of knowledge that is the justification for health professionals making ethical decisions in the first place. There is nobody else who can make medical ethical decisions *instead* of doctors, although there are several players who may make them *with* doctors (principally the patient). Indeed, it can be considered an abdication of one's responsibility to the patient to leave such decision making to committees at one remove.

When there is a conflict, identify:

- What are the issues?
- Who are the relevant parties?
- What are the vested interests or pressures?

Table 16.5 **Improving your own ethical expertise**

Outside experts
Professional codes of conduct and guidelines
Specialty organizations (associations, colleges, unions)
Medical defense organizations
Ethics committees
University departments of philosophy, law, theology
Hospital religious advisers
Ethical education
Read ethics articles, books and journals
Attend ethics courses
Obtain an ethics, law or philosophy degree
Make friends: religious advisers, educationalists, philosophers, 'wise' men and women
Identify ethics within usual case discussions
Be proactive – set up regular multidisciplinary ethics meetings and seminars
Read and take part in informed public debate and outside opinion

Try to divide a problem into its medical, legal, social, psychological, communication and ethical components. You may need advice from several sources, each appropriate to their part. Get expert advice from relevant experts, not reflex opinions from your friends. Do not get specialist medical advice from a generalist. Do not ask for ethical advice from a lawyer nor infer religious beliefs from a distant relative.

Do not be pressured into acting beyond your level of competence. This means being self-reflective about skills and their maintenance, continuing your medical education and referring on to other specialists when it is in the patient's interests. Examine your own personal difficulties and beliefs and where they may interact differently from your colleagues. Just because you feel strongly that you are right does not mean you will be the best doctor for the patient. Be open, transparent and ready for criticism. If you want to reflect about your practice, invite nurses, midwives, colleagues, juniors and visitors in to watch you and ask 'how could that have been improved?' If they do not make suggestions, challenge you or make you uncomfortable then you may not be creating the right or safe conditions for open discussion. Beware if you have a powerful or fragile personality that does not look as if it is genuinely ready to receive advice or criticism. On the other hand, do not be disabled by self-reproach or guilt as these too can lead to decision paralysis.

When things go wrong, find the source and put the systems right for next time. Are risk assessment, counseling and support services available in your unit? Particularly when things go wrong, keep communicating with the patients, demonstrate your continuing concerns by visiting the baby on the baby unit or offering a follow-up appointment, and make sure you have unhurried and uninterrupted time to listen and discuss.

Constantly ask 'what could I do better?'

CONCLUSIONS

- Every day is full of ethical decisions and practices.
- Doctors should not view ethics as an optional 'add-on' or something highly specialist.
- There are ethical skills that can be developed, honed and applied usefully to patient care.
- There are many sources of help for ethical difficulties including wise counsels, philosophers, lawyers, defense organizations, books, journals and patient organizations.
- An understanding of basic principles will enable doctors to examine their own practice critically and safely, defend such practice publicly and diminish their reliance on self-styled 'ethical experts'.
- Do not believe that there are easy solutions!

ACKNOWLEDGMENT

I would like to thank my teachers, particularly Ms Sophie Botros and Professor Sir Ian Kennedy, and colleagues, particularly Professor Donna Dickenson and Revd Peter Haughton, for helpful insights and guidance in the development of this chapter. The errors are all mine.

REFERENCES

1. Kant NR. Respect for persons. In *The moral philosophers: an introduction to ethics*, 2nd edn. Oxford University Press: Oxford, 1998.
2. Davidson GW, Seaton MA, Simpson J (eds). *The Wordsworth Concise English Dictionary*, p. 64. Edinburgh: Chamber, 1994.
3. Griffin J. *Well-being: its meaning, measurement and moral importance*. Oxford: Oxford University Press, pp. 224–253, 1986.
4. Raphael DD. *Moral philosophy*. Oxford: Oxford University Press, 1990.
5. Chervenak FA, McCullough LB. The fetus as a patient: an essential ethical concept for maternal–fetal medicine. *J Mat Fet Med* **5**:115–119, 1996.
6. McCullough LB, Chervenak FA. *Ethics in obstetrics and gynecology*. Oxford: Oxford University Press, 1994.
7. Callahan JC. First steps in preventative ethics. *Hastings Centre Report* **26**(2):45–46, 1996.
8. Warren MA. The moral significance of birth. *Hypatia* **4**:48–65, 1989.
9. Nuffield Council on Bioethics. *Critical care decisions in fetal and neonatal medicine: ethical issues*. London: Latimer Trend & Co Ltd, 2006.
10. General Medical Council. *Good Medical Practice*, 2006.
11. Katz J. *Experimentation with Human Beings*. Russell Sage Foundation, pp. 292–306, 1972.
12. World Medical Association. *Declaration of Helsinki* 1964 (amended 1975, 1983, 1989, 1996, 2000). http://www.wma.net/e/policy/b3.htm.
13. Royal College of Obstetricians and Gynaecologists. *RCOG Ethics Guidelines. Court authorized obstetric intervention: a consideration of the law and ethics* , 2006.
14. Hursthouse R. *On virtue ethics*. Oxford: Oxford University Press, 1999.
15. Brewin T. How much ethics is needed to make a good doctor? *Lancet* **341**:161–163, 1993.
16. Beachamp TL, Childress JF. *Principles of biomedical ethics*, 5th edn. Oxford: Oxford University Press, 2001.
17. Seedhouse D, Lovett L. *Practical medical ethics*. Chichester: John Wiley, 1992.
18. Johnson AG. *Pathways in medical ethics*. London: Edward Arnold, 1990.
19. Anon. Health and human rights. *Lancet* **350**:586–587, 1997.
20. Williams JR. *Medical ethics manual*. World Medical Association France:Ferney Voltaire. 2005 (downloadable free from http://www.wma.net/)

Further reading: Books & journal articles

- Ashcroft RE, Dawson A, Draper H, McMillan J (eds). *Principles of health care ethics*, 2nd edn. Chichester: John Wiley, 2007.
- Bewley S, Ward RH. *Ethics in obstetrics & gynaecology*. London: RCOG Press, 1994.
- Berkowitz JM. How I was almost aborted: reflections on a prenatal brush with death. *J Med Eth* **17**:136–137, 1991.
- Berkowitz RL. From twin to singleton. *Br Med J* **313**:373, 1996.
- Boss JA. First trimester prenatal diagnosis: earlier is not necessarily better. *J Med Eth* **20**:146–151, 1994.
- Boyd K, Callaghan B, Shotter E. *Life before birth. consensus in medical ethics*. London: SPCK, 1986.
- Boyd K, Higgs R, Pinching A. *The new dictionary of medical ethics*. London: BMJ Publishing, 1997.
- Chervenak FA, McCullough LB. An ethically justified, clinically comprehensive management strategy for third-trimester pregnancies complicated by fetal anomalies. *Obstet Gynecol* **75**:311–316, 1990.
- Chervenak FA, McCullough LB. An ethically justified algorithm for offering, recommending, and performing cesarean delivery and its application in managed care practice. *Obstet Gynecol* **87**:302–305, 1996.
- Cohen CB. 'Give me children or I shall die!' New reproductive technologies and harm to children. *Hastings Centre Report* **26**(2): 19–27, 1996.
- Dickenson D (ed.). *Ethical issues in maternal-fetal medicine*. Cambridge UP, 2002.
- Dickenson D. *Property in the body: Feminist perspectives*. Cambridge University Press, 2007.
- Draper H. Women, forced caesareans and antenatal responsibilities. *J Med Eth* **22**:327–333, 1996.
- Finnis J, Cohen M, Nagel T, Scanlon T (eds). *The rights and wrongs of abortion. A philosophy & public affairs reader*. Princeton, NJ: Princeton University Press, 1974.
- Fisk NM, Fordham K, Abramsky L. Elective late fetal karyotyping. *Br J Obstet Gynaecol* **103**:468–470, 1996.
- Garwood-Gowers A, Tingle J. *Healthcare law: the impact of the human rights act 1998*. Cavendish Publishing Ltd, 2001.
- Grundstein-Amado R. Teaching medical ethics. Values education: a new direction for medical education. *J Med Eth* **21**: 174–178, 1995.
- Evans D, Evans M. *A decent proposal. Ethical review of clinical research*. Chichester: John Wiley, 1996.
- Gillon R. *Philosophical medical ethics*. Chichester: John Wiley & Sons, 2003.
- Glover J. *Causing death and saving lives*. Penguin Books, 1990.
- Harris J. *The value of life. Introduction to medical ethics*. London: Routledge, 2001.
- Heyd D. *Genethics: moral issues in the creation of people*. Berkeley: University of California Press, 1992.
- Heyd D. Prenatal diagnosis: whose right?. *J Med Eth* **21**:292–297, 1995.
- Kallenberg K, Forslin L, Westerborn O. The disposal of the aborted fetus – new guidelines: ethical considerations in the debate in Sweden. *J Med Eth* **19**:32–36, 1993.
- Kennedy I. The law and ethics of informed consent and randomised controlled trials. *Treat me right*, pp. 213–224. Oxford: Clarendon Press, 1988.
- Kuhse H, Singer P. *Should the baby live? The problem of handicapped infants*. Oxford: Oxford University Press, 1987.
- Lee R, Morgan D. *Human fertilisation and embryology: regulating the reproductive revolution*. Blackstone Press, 2001.
- Mason K, Laurie G (eds). *Mason & McCall Smith's law and medical ethics*, 7th edn. Oxford University Press: Oxford, 2006.
- Mathieu D. *Preventing prenatal harm: should the state intervene*, 2nd edn. Georgetown University Press, 1996.
- Nuffield Council on Bioethics. *Genetic screening: ethical issues*. London: NCB, 1993.
- O'Hear A. *An introduction to the philosophy of science*. Oxford: Clarendon Press, 1991.
- Parker M, Dickenson DL. *The Cambridge medical ethics workbook: case studies, commentaries and activities*, 2001.
- Pinkerton JV, Finnerty JJ. Resolving the clinical and ethical dilemma involved in fetal–maternal conflicts. *Am J Obstet Gynecol* **175**:289–295, 1996.
- Rodeck CH, Bewley S. Late abortion for fetal abnormality. In *Ethics in obstetrics and gynaecology*, S Bewley, RH Ward (eds), pp. 262–267. London: RCOG Press, 1994.
- Spar D. *The baby business how money, science, and politics drive the commerce of conception*. Harvard Business School Press, 2006.
- Sutton A. *Prenatal diagnosis: confronting the ethical issues*. London: The Linacre Centre, 1990.
- Swartz M. Pregnant woman vs. fetus: a dilemma for hospital ethics committees. *Cambridge Quart. Healthcare Ethics* **1**:51–62, 1992.
- Thomasma DC, Muraskas J, Marshall PA, Myers T, Tomich P, O'Neill JA. The ethics of caring for conjoined twins: the Lakeberg twins. *Hastings Centre Report* **26**(4):4–12, 1996.
- Thornton JG. Measuring patients' values in reproductive medicine. *Contemp Rev Obstet Gynaecol* **1**:5–12, 1988.
- Wells C. On the outside looking in: perspectives on enforced Caesareans. In *Feminist perspectives on health care law*, S Sheldon, M Thomson (eds). Cavendish, 1998.

Journals relevant to medical law and ethics

- *Bioethics*
- *Bulletin of Medical Ethics*
- *Cambridge Quarterly of Healthcare Ethics*
- *Hastings Center Reports*
- *Journal of Law and Medicine*
- *Journal of Medical Ethics*
- *Medical Law Review*
- *Medico-legal Journal*
- *Oxford Journal of Legal Studies*
- *Law Quarterly Review*
- *Philosophy & Public Affairs*

Useful websites

- Bioethics.Net (Centre for bioethics, University of Pennsylvannia) http://www.bioethics.net/
- Bulletin of Medical Ethics http://www.bullmedeth.info/index.html
- Canadian Bioethics Society http://www.bioethics.ca/
- Council of Europe's Treaties: Bioethics http://conventions.coe.int/
- ENGLEMED (independent daily news reports of health & medicine) http://www.englemed.demon.co.uk/
- The English Server – Philosophy http://www.eserver.org/philosophy/
- The Ethics Connection (Markkula Center for Applied Ethics, Santa Clara University) http://www.scu.edu/Ethics/
- Ethics Updates http://ethics.sandiego.edu/
- European Court of Human Rights http://www.echr.coe.int/
- The Hastings Center (for Bioethics), Garrison, New York http://www.thehastingscenter.org/
- Human Rights Internet http://www.hri.ca/welcome.asp
- International Association of Bioethics (IAB) http://bioethics-international.org
- The Internet encyclopedia of philosophy www.utm.edu/research/iep
- Journal of Applied Philosophy Online Index http://www.pdcnet.org/ijap.html
- Journal of Medical Ethics (JME) http://jme.bmj.com/
- Kennedy Institute of Ethics, Georgetown University, Washington. D.C. http://www.georgetown.edu/research/kie/
- National Reference Centre for Bioethics Literature www.georgetown.edu/research/nrcbl
- The Nuffield Trust Bioethics Reports http://www.nuffieldbioethics.org
- The Philosopher's Magazine Online http://philosophers.co.uk/index.htm
- Philosophy resources on the internet http://www.epistemelinks.com/index.asp
- Philosophy around The Web http://users.ox.ac.uk/~worc0337/phil_index.html
- UK Central Office for Research Ethics Committees www.corec.org.uk
- UK Clinical Ethics Network www.ethics-net.org.uk
- United Nations High Commissioner for Human Rights http://www.ohchr.org/english/
- WHO Publications (inc ethics) http://www.who.int/pub/en/
- World Wide Legal Information Association (WWLIA) http://www.wwlia.org/

SECTION 6

Prenatal screening and diagnosis

17 Conveying information about screening 225
Louise Bryant, Shenaz Ahmed and Jenny Hewison

18 Parental reaction to prenatal diagnosis and subsequent bereavement 234
Jane Fisher and Helen Statham

19 Prenatal screening for open neural tube defects and Down's syndrome 243
James E Haddow, Glenn E Palomaki, Jacob A Canick and George J Knight

20 Ultrasound screening for fetal abnormalities and aneuploidies in the first and second trimesters 265
Fionnuala M Breathnach and Fergal D Malone

21 Non-invasive screening and diagnosis from maternal blood 282
Olav Lapaire, Sinuhe Hahn and Wolfgang Holzgreve

22 Invasive diagnostic procedures 292
Boaz Weisz and Charles Rodeck

23 Cytogenetics 305
Caroline M Ogilvie

24 Mendelian genetics – the old and the new 318
J Michael Connor

25 Preimplantation genetic diagnosis 323
Joyce C Harper and Joy D A Delhanty

26 Hemoglobinopathies 331
John M Old

27 Prenatal screening for thalassemias 344
Mary Tang and Kwok-Yin Leung

28 Cystic fibrosis 349
Mary Porteous and Jon Warner

29 Inborn errors of metabolism 357
Wim J Kleijer and Frans W Verheijen

CHAPTER 17

Conveying information about screening

Louise Bryant, Shenaz Ahmed and Jenny Hewison

KEY POINTS

- Provision of good quality information is essential, but not sufficient, to support informed screening choices
- Not all women and their partners wish to be autonomous decision makers. Many may value decision making with guidance from clinicians
- Information is valued in its own right and not always as an input to decision making
- Diversity of attitudes toward termination of pregnancy within different faith groups indicates that clinicians need to consider the beliefs and preferences of individuals
- Current information aids have been largely based on clinical perceptions of necessary information rather than on the actual needs of women and their partners
- Many women would value the provision of balanced information about the quality of life of an affected child and their family
- A number of good quality information resources have recently been made available to clinicians and the public
- Good quality information may help inform screening choices but may not alleviate anxiety following a positive result
- Many people find risk information difficult to integrate with their personal situation. Presentation of risk information in multiple formats can facilitate understanding
- If more than one test is available for the same condition, then information needs to be given about their relative advantages and disadvantages
- The role of ultrasound in screening needs to be made very clear, as non-reassuring findings from this source can be particularly distressing
- People who wish to have screening for one condition may not wish to have it for another condition; procedures need to ensure that individual choices are enabled and respected

INTRODUCTION

This chapter aims to provide clinicians with the key points relevant to patient information provision in relation to prenatal screening. It will consider why good practice in information giving is so important, what women and their partners need to know, and important technology specific considerations that are relevant to supporting informed patient decisions.

WHY IS INFORMATION GIVING SO IMPORTANT?

For most of its history, the explicit goal of prenatal screening has been to reduce the incidence of disability in the population[1,2]. Disabilities such as Down's syndrome have been viewed as a public health problem in much the same way as heart disease or tuberculosis[3]. It is only relatively recently that there have been efforts at a policy level to promote reproductive choice rather than test uptake as the preferred measure of a screening programme's success[4,5]. The UK National Screening Committee recognize 'there is a responsibility to ensure that people who accept an invitation [for screening] do so on the basis of informed choice' (p. 1)[6]. The published objectives of the UK National Down's syndrome screening program go even further stating that 'the primary aim [of the program] is to allow parents to make informed choices concerning their pregnancy outcome'[7]. This change in emphasis reflects, among other things, the general rise in consumerism in society and concerns around litigation[8]; in the context of prenatal testing emphasizing informed choice also distances the process from unwanted eugenic associations[9,10].

The term 'informed choice' is used in this chapter in preference to informed consent. Choosing to have prenatal screening for thalassemia or Down's syndrome is not directly equivalent to consenting to surgical procedures or even cancer screening, although many of the issues are related. Informed consent starts from the assumption that, based on his or her expertise, a clinician recommends a course of action to which the individual is asked to consent. An informed choice, on the other hand, starts from the assumption that the decision about the best course of action is still to be made and that the patient rather than the clinician should make it. In most cases, the only therapeutic intervention on offer following a diagnosis of abnormality is termination of pregnancy. For this reason, there is a growing acceptance that prenatal testing decisions should reflect the values of the individual woman and her partner, and that screening information materials should aim to be balanced and non-directive[11,12].

ASSUMPTIONS ABOUT 'INFORMED CHOICE'

There are a number of assumptions behind the concept of informed choice that need to be considered before we move on. One assumption is that pre-test information is all that is required to enable an informed choice. In addition to provision of information, an informed choice cannot be said to have been made unless the information is understood, the individual has competence in the relevant area and has control over the decision[13]. Another assumption is that people use, or want, pre-test information to make an informed decision. Not everyone wants to make healthcare choices and some people would prefer doctors to maintain this role[14–18].

Literature on 'desire for information' and 'desire to make decisions' indicates that, while people want more information on whatever medical procedure is facing them, many people prefer the health professional to make the final decision[19,20]. It has been suggested that decision making in a medical context lies on a continuum, from 'doctors know best' to the independent decision maker who uses the clinician only as a source of information (Figure 17.1)[21]. In between lie those people who are more likely to value shared decision making, or who value support from clinicians in exploring their views before making a decision.

Here lies a paradox; if some individuals are looking towards the health professional to make a choice for them, then why provide them with information aimed at informed decision making? Providing information on the choices available could result in women being faced with complex and difficult decisions and

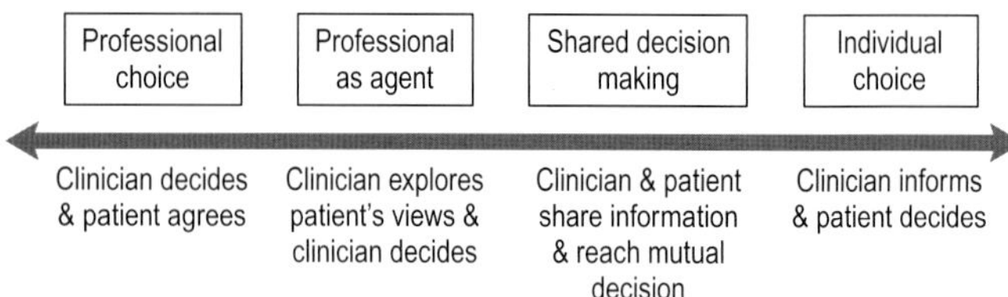

Fig. 17.1 The continuum of decision making in medical settings. (From Emery J 2001 Is informed choice in genetic testing a different breed of informed decision making? A discussion paper. *Health Expectations*. **4**: 81–86, with permission.)

it could be considered unethical to force people to make decisions they may not want to make[22]. However, there is some evidence that people view 'information' and 'consent' as two separate issues; valuing information because they want to be informed about the prenatal tests, not necessarily because they want to use the information to make decisions about the tests[23]. Therefore, it is important to provide pre-test information to women and their partners, irrespective of the way in which they choose to make their decisions.

A third assumption lies in the perceived high value of autonomy. Patient autonomy is generally accepted in Western societies as an important element of healthcare, but evidence demonstrates that patients from many other cultures place less value and emphasis on this construct[24,25]. In some cultures, the family plays a more pivotal role in healthcare decisions[23,26–30]. Overall, there is no evidence that people from different ethnic origins share the value of 'autonomous informed choice' in the prenatal testing context.

INFORMATION GIVING AND ETHNIC MINORITY POPULATIONS

A number of authors have commented on how provision of prenatal screening services in the UK may be affected by health professionals' beliefs that certain ethnic groups would not terminate an affected pregnancy[31–33]. This is understandable given much of the literature, which suggests that Muslim and African-Caribbean populations are most likely to decline prenatal diagnosis and termination of pregnancy because of their religious convictions[34–39]. However, while religion is an important factor in decision making about termination of pregnancy, it is not always the overriding factor[40]. People make prenatal testing decisions based on their own moral values and beliefs which, in turn, are influenced by personal experiences, perceptions and information about quality of life for, and with, a child with a condition[41–43]. It is therefore important to move away from stereotypical views of ethnicity or religion, recognize diversity within different faith groups and consider the beliefs and preferences of individuals[40].

THE INFORMATION NEEDS OF WOMEN AND THEIR PARTNERS

Research shows that women welcome up-to-date, accurate information delivered in a format that is understandable and timely. Information interventions delivered before prenatal screening decisions are made have not been found to significantly increase anxiety[44]. A slight rise of anxiety is a natural response to an increased awareness of the risk of disability and there is some evidence that in the pre-screening phase this may result in improved decision making and satisfaction with decision outcome[45].

For an informed screening decision to take place, there are a number of information components that have been considered to be essential[46–48]. Therefore, as a minimum, information should make clear:

- the purpose of the test
- what the procedure for testing involves
- any risks associated with the test
- the implications of the possible test results
- information about the target condition(s).

A recent collaboration of members of the public, people with personal experience of genetic conditions, clinicians and information providers has attempted to extend this list. Using the DISCERN methodology, the collaboration defined a set of criteria by which the quality of genetic screening information can be judged[49]. The DISCERN methodology has been widely used as a way to appraise the quality of lay health information on treatment choices in a wide range of conditions[50,51]. The criteria developed are also useful as a guideline for information provision in the prenatal testing context (Table 17.1).

Information that meets the DISCERN criteria is important to support an informed screening choice, to understand screening test results and (potentially) support future reproductive decisions around diagnostic testing and termination. However, the range of criteria also supports the argument that many people value information about genetic testing (and therefore screening) in its own right and not just as input to decision making. While the criteria have been developed with some consumer involvement, there is no guarantee that this list, although seemingly comprehensive, will meet everyone's information needs

Table 17.1 **DISCERN criteria for assessing the quality of information on genetic testing**

Information should provide:
■ An explanation of the background and effects of the condition
■ Any treatment and management options for the condition
■ Explanation of risk in simple terminology
■ The nature of the test (screening, diagnostic)
■ The testing procedure
■ The accuracy of test results
■ What happens after the test and potential follow-up tests
■ Who will have access to test results (especially in relation to genetic information)
■ Indication that decision making can be shared (with clinicians, family)
■ Psychosocial consequences of testing (anxiety, the range of reactions experienced)
■ Potential consequences of (genetic) information for family and partner
■ Additional sources of support and information

Adapted from Shepperd et al. 2006[49]

or that providing this information will ensure an informed choice will be made. Individual women will have different requirements and preferences in this regard and, as noted above, the role of formal information giving in influencing screening choices has yet to be established.

Information provided as part of a screening program has usually been based on clinicians' perceptions of what is important to know. A strong evidence base is lacking as to what might be specifically useful during prenatal screening decision making, although some research has tried to address this. A study investigating information recall in genetic counseling found that those being counseled more frequently judged information about family implications of the condition to be more important than did health professionals, while health professionals more frequently judged information about test, diagnosis and prognosis to be more important than their counselees[52]. An important factor in women's decisions about termination of pregnancy is a perception of the quality of the life of a child with the condition[53]. A particular concern is whether or not a child would experience 'suffering' as a result of the condition or its medical treatment:

> If I thought I was going to be having a child who's [going to have] a condition where they had to endure hellish treatment time after time after time, you know, really, really painful treatment... that would make me really think carefully about whether I would terminate because that is quality of life...[53]

The need for balanced information on potential quality of life for a child with the tested-for condition has been found to be important elsewhere and parents want to know what parenting a child with the tested-for conditions may be like[40]. Information about the tested-for condition has often had less priority than information about the testing process and any information provided has tended to have a medical or clinical focus. For example, a study of patient information leaflets about Down's syndrome screening showed that information about the chromosomal origins of the condition was almost always included, whereas information about emotional and social impacts on family was almost always missing[54]. The recently developed National Screening Committee leaflet has rectified this situation (see Information Resources section below). Knowledge of even relatively common conditions such as Down's syndrome has been shown to be low as many people have little personal experience of meeting or interacting with people with disabilities and their families[44]. For this reason, it is essential that balanced information based on the lived experience of families and individuals with a tested-for condition is made available at the screening stage[55].

INFORMATION RESOURCES

Time restrictions within the clinical setting make it unrealistic for clinicians to provide, in person, all the information that a woman and her partner may need. Those individuals delivering prenatal screening may also not be best placed to provide the condition related information that women and their partners may need. Language barriers may also reduce the ability of clinicians to convey adequate information to support an informed decision. This section provides some current sources of good quality information that may be of benefit to health professionals responsible for supporting prenatal testing decisions:

- The National Screening Committee's prenatal screening leaflet for Down's syndrome has been translated into seventeen languages (Arabic, Bengali, Chinese, Farsi, French, Greek, Gujarati, Hindi, Polish, Portuguese, Punjabi, Somali, Sorani, Spanish, Turkish, Urdu, Vietnamese) and is available at www.screening.nhs.uk/downs/women.htm. The content of this leaflet has been developed with a member of the UK Down's Syndrome Association.
- The UK-based charity DIPEx provides web-based information that includes personal experiences of health and illness. It is supported by the UK National Screening Committee and is aimed at patients, their carers, family and friends. One DIPEx module looks at experiences of prenatal screening generally (www.dipex.org/antenatalscreening) and another module focuses specifically on screening for sickle cell and thalassemia (www.dipex.org/sicklecellandthalassaemia). The DIPEx modules contain interviews with women and couples who have undergone prenatal screening. Website users can watch, listen to or read these interviews, some of which are in other languages (French, Mirpuri, Portuguese, Sylheti, Urdu).
- AnSWeR (Antenatal Screening Web Resource) funded by the Wellcome Trust, aims to provide information about the lives of people with a disability and their families. The resource focuses on five conditions: cystic fibrosis, Down's syndrome, neural tube defects, Klinefelter's syndrome and Turner's syndrome and contains interviews with affected individuals and family members. Website users can listen to or read these interviews, which are currently all in English. AnSWeR is available at http://www.antenataltesting.info

UNDERSTANDING AND CONVEYING INFORMATION ABOUT RISK

A major concern of screening practitioners has been how to convey information about screening-related risks and the comparison of different risks. Understanding of risk has been seen as important not only for making informed screening choices but also for understanding screening results and (potentially) for making decisions about further testing. However, the mathematical concepts of population screening and risk that underlie screening tests are not ones that most people deal with during their everyday lives. For this reason, research that shows many people struggle to understand risk and probability in relation to screening tests is unsurprising[44,56,57]. Current practice restricts the offer of diagnostic testing to women whose screening risk exceeds a predetermined cut-off value, the latter reflecting policy decisions about the optimum trade-off between detection and safety for the screened population as a whole. The rationale behind the choosing of a specific risk cut-off for offering invasive tests is probably understood by only a tiny percentage of those involved.

Researchers and practitioners have attempted to improve the way in which risk information is presented in screening information. Pictorial representations may help promote concrete visualization of conceptual mathematical constructs. For example, the Paling Pallette was designed to help health professionals explain comparative risks in a way that is appropriate in the prenatal screening context (Figure 17.2)[58]. There is some evidence that understanding of residual risk in 'screen negatives' can be enhanced by presenting screening test results in numbers (such as 1 in 800) rather than in non-specific word terms (such as a 'low risk' result)[59]. Some have also recommended providing multiple formats of the same information, for example, a 1 per 100 chance of an affected pregnancy should also be presented as a 1% chance of the baby being affected and a 99% chance that the baby will not be affected[60,61].

Providing alternative framings of the same risk information may also help to reduce certain decision-making biases associated with 'negative' and 'positive' presentations of risk values[62].

Severely anxious reactions to screen positive results have often been attributed to women misunderstanding the 'correct' meaning of a screening test result[57]. This has partly driven the search to find the optimal way to deliver risk information so that women can understand risk appropriately. The assumption is that correct understanding of risk will reduce anxiety in the majority of screen positives, as well as ensuring women realize the residual risk inherent in a screen negative result. 'Misunderstandings' may also reflect a need for people to simplify risk-related information in order to make difficult decisions more manageable. For example, people often find the 'one in something' test result hard to relate to their personal situation and a common strategy is to dichotomize any risk; the baby is either affected or it is not. It is also important to note that, while conveying information on risk is important, the information needed to support informed choice is not necessarily that which can alleviate anxiety associated with screening results. An acutely anxious result is probably a natural and appropriate, if unpleasant, response to a potential 'risk' to the health of the fetus[44]. One study reported on a health professional familiar with serum screening who received a positive screening result.

> Although because of her education she knew that few positive results indicated real abnormality, her first thought on learning of her positive result was 'disaster'. That evening she was unable to sleep and felt like crying desperately. The next day she described herself as being 'out of control'. Simply having technical knowledge did not prevent a negative emotional reaction (p. 104)[63].

Women offered an invasive test following a screen positive result can of course decline it and a significant minority does. The lower the individual's screening risk, the more likely she is to decline further testing[64]. This suggests that even if women do not fully understand the mathematics of screening, they do use risk information in a more basic sense when making decisions about invasive testing. Some have interpreted this as showing that women consider safety to be more important than detection, but such a simple conclusion would not be justified.

The views of women not currently offered invasive testing because their screening risk is considered too low to justify the associated miscarriage risk must also be examined if a full picture is to be obtained. A number of hypothetical studies have shown 'unmet demand' for diagnostic testing among such women and this has been supported more recently by studies of actual uptake rates of women[64–68]. Clearly, for some women in some circumstances, detection is more important than miscarriage risk, given that the latter risk is known not to be substantial. The logical conclusion of this body of work is that all

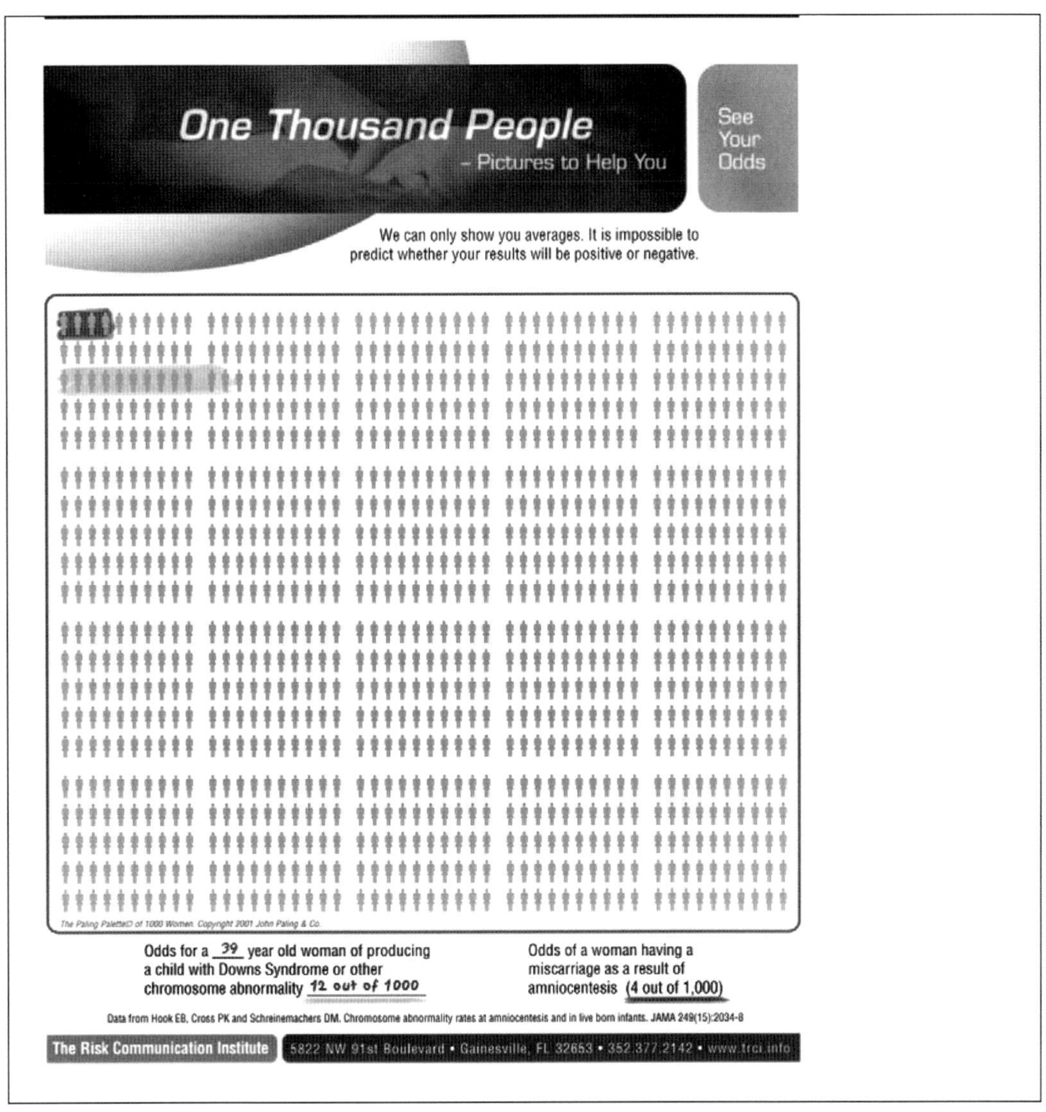

Fig. 17.2 The Paling palette. ©John Paling 2001.

women, not just those deemed to be at high risk, should be given information about their individual risk and supported in deciding whether or not to have an invasive test. Currently, such a policy would require significant attitude change among staff, many of whom would feel strongly that miscarriage risk can only be justified in restricted circumstances. In a patient centered NHS, this may be a necessary development for the future.

TECHNOLOGY-SPECIFIC CONSIDERATIONS

Although many of the information needs associated with screening tests apply across all protocols, there are also some technology-specific issues that must be considered. Increasingly, for many women and their partners, the choice is not only whether or not to have a screening test but also 'which test to have'? Practitioners are familiar with the idea that women must be helped to find their own balance between safety and certainty, but that simple tension is being superseded by a much more complicated set of costs and benefits arising from the proliferation of different testing protocols. The need to meet National Screening Committee standards does help to keep the number of variants down, but there is still a range of possibilities available that may be confusing to women and their partners, most of whom will be in unfamiliar decision-making territory.

There is currently no requirement by the National Screening Committee that women be given information about all the screening variants currently in use in the NHS or in the private sector. Indeed, some have argued that, in a national screening program, women should only be informed about, and offered, the safest and/or most cost-effective test. In a program predicated on choice, that approach is difficult to justify in principle, even if – in the information era – it could be sustained in practice. In reality, women learn about the various alternatives in an ad hoc way, depending on what is offered locally and on their own initiative.

Some of the ways in which screening protocols differ are likely to be meaningful to women and their partners and have the potential to make important contributions to decision making. This adds to the debate about how much information should be provided about screening tests and what aspects of information are most important to convey. The most salient dimensions on which screening protocols currently differ, and what relevance these may have for information provision, are now discussed.

First-versus second-trimester screening

The increase in chorionic villus sampling rates following first-trimester screening confirms the findings of attitude studies, namely that many women prefer an earlier, slightly more risky diagnostic test to a later, very slightly safer one[69]. This is largely due to the fact that termination is generally more acceptable to women if carried out in the first rather than the second trimester[70]. It may be that only basic information about relative safety is sufficient for most women to make a choice between a first-trimester test and a second (or integrated) one. Potentially, 'lay' concepts of risk and probability may be most influential on testing choices, although the information needs of women in this position have not been systematically studied.

Muslim women also have particular information needs regarding the timing of screening tests. Termination of pregnancy for a condition such as Down's syndrome is regarded by religious authorities as permissible under Islam, but only before 'breathing the soul' takes place at 120 days' gestation[71]. Like all women, Muslim women hold their own individual opinions about testing and termination for congenital conditions, but many do (or would) choose termination if circumstances permit[72,73]. First-trimester testing offers Muslim women distinctively different reproductive choices and the information provided about their screening options needs to reflect that.

Combined integrated and contingent screening

Soon after first-trimester serum and ultrasound markers were identified, it was established that for a given detection rate, the false positive rate could be reduced by using combinations of both first- and second-trimester markers. 'Integrated' testing of this kind offers a clear benefit to women who would otherwise have only had access to a second-trimester test, but if first-trimester testing is available, then women must trade-off a small gain in safety against a non-trivial delay in obtaining the test result. This highlights once more the general problem of how much information women need to have to enable them to make an informed choice, but it also raises the difficult question of how far women's individual preferences for different testing regimens can be incorporated into testing programs. Take for example, the issue of 'combined' versus 'contingent' screening.

Properly conducted, combined screening (using first-trimester serum and ultrasound markers) already achieves very satisfactory levels of test performance. The number of invasive procedures indicated by combined screening can be reduced further by incorporating information from second-trimester markers into the risk calculation for women with intermediate results; a form of 'contingent' screening[74]. Women whose overriding consideration is minimizing the chance of miscarriage will understand the logic soon enough, but others will wish to compare the marginal costs and benefits of waiting, and many will need help in doing that.

In the NHS, the use of combined screening has been constrained by the limited availability of appropriate ultrasonography resources. A different form of 'contingent' screening has been proposed to circumvent this problem in which a nuchal translucency scan is only offered to women who cannot be given a 'reassuring' result on the basis of first-trimester serum results alone; second-trimester serum measurement is offered to those whose combined risk remains at an intermediate level[75]. All forms of contingent screening share the disadvantage of incorporating one or more intermediate stages into the giving of results, making the process more drawn out over time (see Chapter 19). Inevitable questions arise about the information that should be included in intermediate results and about how best to support women and their partners through a protracted and uncertain process. Best information giving and support practice in this unfamiliar protocol will take time to establish. The development of a decision aid designed to take people beyond the present and into the potential consequences of each test option may be appropriate in this situation. Decision aids in healthcare have been shown to improve knowledge of treatment options, create realistic expectations of the pros and cons of each, and increase involvement in the decision-making process[76].

Ultrasound screening

The increasing use of ultrasound technology in screening brings with it particular challenges in relation to information provision. Scanning is very popular with women and their partners because of the opportunity it affords of 'seeing the baby' and, in the event, most scans are reassuring experiences that parents remember with pleasure. The first information challenge is to convey that the true purpose of scanning is to look for problems and that problems identified can be serious or minor, common or rare. The second challenge is how to convey that, unlike screening for a specific condition, scanning is a very open-ended investigation, with many different possible outcomes. It needs to be explained that while a scan can sometimes function as a diagnostic test and identify some problems with certainty, in many other instances the scan only functions as a screening test and further invasive diagnostic testing may be indicated.

Because of their variable and often uncertain prognostic significance, the identification of 'soft markers' using ultrasound scanning can lead to particular difficulties in relation to information giving. An approach where women are informed about each and every soft marker seen on a scan has been criticized for causing unnecessary anxiety, and leading to an inappropriate use of invasive testing[77].

Evidence also suggests that a non-reassuring result from an ultrasound scan may cause more enduring psychological distress than an equivalent result from serum screening. This problem was first identified in a qualitative study of 'false positives' arising from soft marker screening in the second trimester but has since been confirmed in a randomized comparison of serum and ultrasound screening in the first trimester[78,79]. The reasons are unknown why women find false positive screening results harder to put behind them when the data come from a scan, but the contrast with the anticipated pleasurable scan experience may be partly responsible. It is known that the adverse psychological effects of being a 'false positive' can linger even after the birth of an unaffected child, so women undergoing ultrasound screening do need to be prepared for that, even though the information may be unwelcome, and itself a possible cause of some disquiet.

The NSC's Fetal Anomaly Screening program has produced a detailed booklet for women about the purpose of scanning and the kinds of problems it can identify which is available on the Antenatal Screening and Newborns Programs website (http://www.screening.nhs.uk/anpublications). Detailed information about most conditions that can be screened for using ultrasound is not included in the National Screening Committee booklet, because there are just too many of them for this to be practicable. In this case, the previously raised issues about how clinicians convey information about screened-for conditions comes into play. At the time of writing, the National Screening Committee is also developing explicit guidance for clinicians on the ways in which information about soft markers should and should not be used in the justification of diagnostic testing and how explanations about the use of soft markers should be given to women and their partners.

Screening for multiple conditions

The difficulties of explaining that ultrasound can identify many different kinds of problems were mentioned in the section above, but the issue of how to ensure informed choice when screening is being offered for multiple conditions is a more general one. In the UK, the National Screening Committee currently has a screening program for hemoglobinopathies as well as for Down's syndrome, and screening programs for other conditions such as cystic fibrosis and fragile X are also under consideration. It cannot be assumed that an individual woman's views about testing and termination will be the same for all conditions, so the information provided must support separate decision making for each condition[72].

Few people are likely to confuse the condition of Down's syndrome with, say thalassemia, but they might easily forget why fathers might need testing for one condition but not the other, which condition was likely to recur in future pregnancies, what being a carrier meant, why gestation was more important in some screening circumstances than others, and so on. The fact that the first step in many screening pathways is a maternal blood test simplifies the task of information giving in some ways, but highlights too the difficulty of characterizing informed choice. Any assessment of informed choice that is weighted towards procedural aspects of testing is unlikely to be able to detect differences between conditions. Reliance on self-assessment of understanding becomes even more problematical than usual given the multiple possibilities for misunderstanding alluded to above. Obtaining a generic consent to testing for groups of conditions with similar characteristics (for example 'moderate learning difficulties') has been suggested, as a means of avoiding 'information overload'[80]. This is unlikely to be acceptable to women as perception of severity is relative not absolute and closely linked to personal experiences and values[72].

MEASURING INFORMED CHOICE

Research evaluating screening programs and associated information interventions would clearly benefit from a reliable and valid measure of informed choice. In response to this need, the 'Multi-dimensional Measure of Informed Choice' (MMIC) was developed, its aim being to measure values in relation to screening choices as well as knowledge[12]. Based on a widely used model of health behavior, the MMIC measures three aspects of a screening decision:

1. knowledge about the condition and the test characteristics (characterized as good or poor)
2. attitude towards having the screening test (characterized as positive or negative)
3. the screening 'behavior' (screening uptake: yes or no).

An informed choice is considered to be one where knowledge is good and the screening behavior (acceptance or decline) is consistent with the expressed attitude (positive or negative). Studies using the MMIC have so far demonstrated rates of informed choice (as defined by the measure) of between 20% and 60% depending on the population assessed: rates of informed choice being lowest in some ethnic groups and in 'socially disadvantaged' women[81–83].

In its current format, however, the measure cannot yet be considered a satisfactory instrument for measuring a complex construct like informed choice[83]. The ten knowledge items focus mainly on characteristics of the screening test with five out of eight items being concerned with understanding risk. The MMIC only assesses knowledge in relation to a single condition, thereby over-simplifying the link between the procedure and the range of conditions than can potentially be screened for using a single blood sample. The attitude items in the MMIC consider only attitudes towards undergoing the test (pleasant/unpleasant, for example) and do not capture values that many would consider important in a screening decision, such as views on termination of pregnancy. Furthermore, the emphasis on attitude–behavior consistency does not reflect the range of potential influences on actual screening uptake, for example the role of partner and family, language barriers and the organizational factors which affect access to services[84]. Further development in this area is needed as it is important to be able to validate the impact of information interventions on informed screening choices.

CONCLUSIONS

This chapter has aimed to demonstrate that while the provision of good quality information is essential in the prenatal screening situation, facilitating an informed choice goes beyond the delivery of a simple information intervention. The information needs of individuals and couples are diverse and new technologies bring fresh challenges to the information provider. Not all women wish to make 'autonomous' choices but instead value the clinician's input to the decision-making process. A range of resources to support the clinician facilitate informed choice currently exists, and more are in the process of being developed. Ultimately, however, flexibility of approach is required to meet the information needs of women and their partners in relation to screening, and this in itself is a significant challenge.

REFERENCES

1. Stein Z, Susser M, Guterman AV. Screening programme for prevention of Down's syndrome. *Lancet* **1**(7798):305–310, 1973.
2. Mikkelsen M. The incidence of Down's syndrome and progress towards its reduction. *Philos Trans Roy Soc Lond* **319**:315–324, 1988.
3. Wilson JMG, Jungner G. *Principles and practice of screening for disease* (Public health papers, 34). Geneva: WHO, 1968.
4. Raffle AE. Information about screening: is it to achieve high uptake or to ensure informed choice? *Hlth Expect* **4**:92–98, 2001.
5. Council of Europe. Recommendation No. R(90)13 of the Committee of Ministers to member states on prenatal genetic screening, prenatal genetic diagnosis and associated genetic counselling. *Int Dig Hlth Legislat* **41**:615–624, 1990.
6. UK National Screening Committee. *Second Report of the UK National Screening Committee.* London, available at http://www.nsc.nhs.uk/pdfs/secondreport.pdf: Department of Health, 2000.
7. NHS Antenatal and Newborn Screening Programmes. *Down's Syndrome Screening Programme Objectives*. London: NHS, 2006.
8. Charles C, Whelan T, Gafni A. What do we mean by partnership in making decisions about treatment? *Br Med J* **319**:780–782, 1999.
9. Williams C, Alderson P, Farsides B. What constitutes 'balanced information' in the practitioners' portrayals of Down's syndrome? *Midwifery* **18**:230–237, 2002.
10. Human Genetics Commission. *Making babies: reproductive decisions and genetic technologies*. London: Human Genetics Commission, 2006.
11. Bekker HL. Genetic testing: facilitating informed choices. In *Encyclopaedia of the human genome*, DN Cooper, N Thomas (eds), pp. 926–930. New York: Nature Publishing Group-Macmillan Publishers Ltd, 2003.
12. Marteau TM, Dormandy E, Michie S. A measure of informed choice. *Hlth Expect* **4**:99–108, 2001.
13. Kent GG. The role of psychology in the teaching of medical ethics: the example of informed consent. *Med Educ* **28**:126–131, 1994.
14. Deber RB, Kraetschmer N, Irvine J. What role do patients wish to play in treatment decision making? *Arch Int Med* **156**:1414–1420, 1996.
15. Mazur DJ, Hickam DH. Patients' preferences for risk disclosure and role in decision making for invasive medical procedures. *J Gen Int Med* **12**:114–117, 1997.
16. McKinstry B. Do patients wish to be involved in decision making in the consultation? A cross sectional survey with video vignettes. *BrMed J* **321**:867–871, 2000.
17. Robinson A, Thomson R. Variability in patient preferences for participating in medical decision making: implication for the use of decision support tools. *Qual Hlth Care* **10**(Suppl 1):i34–i38, 2001.
18. Schneider CE. *The practice of autonomy: patient, doctors, and medical decisions*. New York: Oxford University Press, 1998.
19. Ende J, Kazis L, Ash A, Moskowitz MA. Measuring patients' desire for autonomy: decision making and information-seeking preferences among medical patients. *J Gen IntMed* **4**:23–30, 1989.
20. Fallowfield L. Offering choice of surgical treatment to women with breast cancer. *Patient Educ Counsell* **30**:209–214, 1997.
21. Emery J. Is informed choice in genetic testing a different breed of informed decision-making? A discussion paper. *Hlth Expect* **4**:81–86, 2001.
22. Jepson RG, Forbes CA, Sowden AJ, Lewis RA. Increasing informed uptake and non-uptake of screening: evidence from a systematic review. *Hlth Expect* **4**:116–130, 2001.
23. Ahmed S, Green JM, Hewison J. Antenatal thalassaemia carrier testing: women's perceptions of 'information' and 'consent'. *J Med Screen* **12**:69–77, 2005.
24. Bowman KW, Hui E. Bioethics for clinicians: 20. Chinese bioethics. *Can Med Assoc J* **163**:481–1485, 2000.
25. Jafarey AM, Farooqui A. Informed consent in the Pakistani milieu: the physician's perspective. *J Med Ethics* **31**:93–96, 2005.
26. Berg JW, Applebaum PS, Lidz CW, Meisel A. *Informed consent: legal theory and clinical practice*. Oxford: Oxford University Press, 2001.
27. Berger JT. Culture and ethnicity in clinical care. *Arch Int Med* **158**:2085–2090, 1998.
28. Blackhall LJ, Murphy ST, Frank G, Michel V, Azen S. Ethnicity and attitudes toward patient autonomy. *J Am Med Assoc* **274**:820–825, 1995.
29. Elliot AC. Health care ethics: cultural relativity of autonomy. *J Transcult Nurs* **12**:326–330, 2001.
30. Lambris A. Informed consent for all? Not quite! A comparison of informed consent in the United States and Japan. *Temple Internat Comp Law J* **17**:237–259, 2003.
31. Atkin K, Ahmad WIU. Genetic screening and haemoglobinopathies: ethics, politics and practice. *Soc Sci Med* **46**:445–458, 1998.
32. Modell B, Harris R, Lane B et al. Informed choice in genetic screening for thalassaemia during pregnancy: audit from a national confidential inquiry. *Br Med J* **320**:337–341, 2000.
33. Anionwu EN, Atkin K. *The politics of sickle cell and thalassaemia*. Buckingham: Open University Press, 2001.
34. Durosinmi MA, Odebiyi AI, Adediran IA, Akinola NO, Adegorioye DE, Okunade MA. Acceptability of prenatal diagnosis of sickle cell anaemia (SCA) by female patients and parents of SCA patients in Nigeria. *Soc Sci Med* **41**:433–436, 1995.
35. de Montalembert M, Guilloud-Bataille MM, Ducros A et al. Implications of prenatal diagnosis of sickle cell disease. *Genet Counsel* **7**:9–15, 1996.
36. Zahed L, Bou-Dames J. Acceptance of first-trimester prenatal diagnosis for the haemoglobinopathies in Lebanon. *Prenat Diagn* **17**:423–428, 1997.
37. Ahmed S, Saleem M, Sultana N, Raashid Y, Waqar A, Anwar M. Prenatal diagnosis of beta-thalassaemia in Pakistan: experience in a Muslim country. *Prenat Diagn* **20**:378–383, 2000.
38. Alkuraya FS, Kilani RA. Attitude of Saudi families affected with hemoglobinopathies towards prenatal screening and abortion and the influence of religious ruling (Fatwa). *Prenat Diagn* **21**:448–451, 2001.
39. Kagu MB, Abjah UA, Ahmed SG. Awareness and acceptability of prenatal diagnosis of sickle cell anaemia among health professionals and students in North Eastern Nigeria. *Niger J Med* **13**:48–51, 2004.
40. Ahmed S, Atkin K, Hewison J, Green JM. The influence of faith and religion and the role of religious and community leaders in prenatal decisions for sickle cell disorders and thalassaemia major. *Prenat Diagn* **26**:801–809, 2006.
41. Wertz DC, Rosenfield JM, Janes SW, Erbe RW. Attitudes towards abortion among parents of children with cystic fibrosis. *Am J Pub Hlth* **81**:992–996, 1991.
42. Snowdon C, Green JM. *New reproductive technologies: attitudes and experiences of carriers of recessive disorders*. Cambridge: Centre for Family Research, University of Cambridge, 1994.
43. Henneman L, Bramsen I, Van Os TAM et al. Attitudes towards reproductive issues and carrier testing among adult patients and parents of children with cystic fibrosis (CF). *Prenat Diagn* **21**:1–9, 2001.
44. Green JM, Hewison J, Bekker HL, Bryant LD, Cuckle HS. Psychosocial aspects of genetic screening of pregnant women and newborns: a systematic review. *Hlth Technol Assess* **8**:33, 2004.
45. Bekker HL, Hewison J, Thornton JG. Understanding why decision aids work: linking process with outcome. *Patient Educ Counsel* **50**:323–329, 2003.
46. Reid M. Consumer-oriented studies in relation to prenatal screening tests. *Eur J Obstet Gynecol Reprod Biol* **28**(Suppl):79–92, 1988.
47. Royal College of Physicians. *Prenatal diagnosis and genetic screening: community*

and service implications. London: Royal College of Physicians, 1989.
48. Royal College of Obstetricians and Gynaecologists. *Termination of pregnancy for fetal abnormality in England, Wales and Scotland*. London: Royal College of Obstetricians and Gynaecologists, 1996.
49. Shepperd S, Farndon P, Grainge V et al. DISCERN-Genetics: quality criteria for information on genetic testing. *Eur J Hum Genet* **14**:1179–1188, 2006.
50. Charnock D, Shepperd S, Needham G, Gann B. DISCERN – an instrument for judging the quality of consumer health information on treatment choices. *J Epidemiol Commun Hlth* **53**:105–111, 1999.
51. Shepperd S, Charnock D, Cook A. A 5-star system for rating the quality of information based on DISCERN. *Hlth Informat Lib J* **19**(4):201–205, 2002.
52. Michie S, French D, Allanson A, Bobrow M, Marteau TM. Information recall in genetic counselling: a pilot study of its assessment. *Patient Educ Counsel* **32**:93–100, 1997.
53. Hewison J, Green J, Cuckle H, Mueller R, Thornton J. *Social and ethnic difference in attitudes and consent to prenatal testing: Report to the ESRC*. University of Leeds, 2005.
54. Bryant LD, Murray J, Green JM, Hewison J, Sehmi I, Ellis A. Descriptive information about Down syndrome: a content analysis of serum screening leaflets. *Prenat Diagn* **21**:1057–1063, 2001.
55. Parens E, Asch A. The disability rights critique of prenatal genetic testing. *The Hastings Center Report* **29**, 1999.
56. Bramwell R, West H, Salmon P. Health professionals' and service users' interpretation of screening test results: experimental study. *Br Med J* **333**:284–286, 2006.
57. Heyman B, Hundt G, Sandall J et al. On being at higher risk: a qualitative study of prenatal screening for chromosomal anomalies. *Soc Sci Med* **62**:2360–2372, 2006.
58. Paling J. Strategies to help patients understand risks. *Br Med J* **327**:745–748, 2003.
59. Marteau TM, Saidi G, Goodburn S, Lawton J, Michie S, Bobrow M. Numbers or words? A randomized controlled trial of presenting screen negative results to pregnant women. *Prenat Diagn* **20**(9):714–718, 2000.
60. Sullivan A. Involving parents: information and informed decisions. In *Midwife's guide to antenatal investigations*, A Sullivan, L Kean, A Cryer (eds), pp. 17–29. Edinburgh: Elsevier, 2006.
61. Gigerenzer G, Edwards A. Simple tools for understanding risks: from innumeracy to insight. *Br Med J* **327**:741–744, 2003.
62. Marteau TM. Framing of information: its influence upon decisions of doctors and patients. *Br J Soc Psychol* **28**:89–94, 1989.
63. Santalahti P, Latikka AM, Ryynanen M, Hemminki E. Women's experiences of prenatal serum screening. *Birth* **23**(2):101–107, 1996.
64. Nicolaides KM, Chervenak FA, McCullough LB, Avgidou K, Papageorghiou A. Evidence-based obstetric ethics and informed decision-making by pregnant women about invasive diagnosis after first-trimester assessment of risk for trisomy 21. *Am J Obstet Gynecol* **193**(2):322–326, 2005.
65. Mulvey S, Zachariah R, McIlwaine K, Wallace EM. Do women prefer to have screening tests for Down syndrome that have the lowest screen-positive rate rate or the highest detection rate? *Prenat Diagn* **23**:828–832, 2003.
66. Caughey AB, Washington AE, Gildengorin V, Kuppermann M. Assessment of demand for prenatal diagnostic testing using willingness to pay. *Obstet Gynecol* **103**(3):539–545, 2004.
67. Marini T, Sullivan J, Naeem R. Decisions about amniocentesis by advanced maternal age patients following maternal serum screening may not always correlate clinically with screening results: need for improvement in informed consent process. *Am J Med Genet* **109**:171–175, 2002.
68. Mueller VM, Huang T, Summers AM, Winsor SHM. The influence of risk estimates obtained from maternal serum screening on amniocentesis rates. *Prenat Diagn* **25**:1253–1257, 2005.
69. Spencer K, Aitken D. Factors affecting women's preferences for type of prenatal screening test for chromosomal anomalies. *Ultrasound Obstet Gynecol* **24**:735–739, 2004.
70. Learman LA, Drey EA, Gates EA, Kang M-S, Washington AE, Kupperman M. Abortion attitudes of pregnant women in prenatal care. *Am J Obstet Gynecol* **192**:1939–1947, 2005.
71. Abdel Haleem MAS. Medical ethics in Islam. In *Choices and decisions in healthcare*, A Grubb (ed.), pp. 1–20. Chichester, West Sussex: Wiley, 1993.
72. Hewison J, Green JM, Ahmed S et al. Attitudes to prenatal testing and termination of pregnancy for fetal abnormality: a comparison of white and Pakistani women in the UK *Prenat Diagn* **27**:419–430, 2007.
73. Zlotogora J. Parental decisions to abort or continue a pregnancy with an abnormal finding after an invasive prenatal test. *Prenat Diagn* **22**:1102–1106, 2002.
74. Benn P, Wright D, Cuckle H. Practical strategies in contingent sequential screening for Down syndrome. *Prenat Diagn* **25**:645–652, 2005.
75. Wright D, Bradbury I, Cuckle H et al. Three-stage contingent screening for Down syndrome. *Prenat Diagn* **26**:528–534, 2006.
76. O'Connor AM, Stacey D, Entwistle V et al. Decision aids for people facing health treatment or screening decisions. *Cochrane Database System Rev* Art. No. CD001431. DOI: 10.1002/14651858.CD001431, 2003.
77. Getz L, Kirkengan AL. Ultrasound screening in pregnancy: advancing technology, soft markers for fetal chromosomal aberrations, and unacknowledged ethical dilemmas. *Soc Sci Med* **56**:2045–2057, 2003.
78. Baillie C, Smith J, Hewison J, Mason G. Ultrasound screening for chromosomal abnormality: women's reactions to false positive results. *Br J Hlth Psychol* **5**:377–394, 2000.
79. Weinans MJN, Kooij L, Muller M, Bilardo KM, Van Lith JM, Tymstra T. A comparison of the impact of screen-positive results obtained from ultrasound and biochemical screening for Down syndrome in the first trimester: a pilot study. *Prenat Diagn* **24**:347–351, 2003.
80. Elias S, Annas G. Generic consent for genetic screening. *N Engl J Med* **330**:1611–1613, 1994.
81. Dormandy E, Michie S, Hooper R, Marteau TM. Low uptake of prenatal screening for Down syndrome in minority ethnic groups and socially deprived groups: a reflection of women's attitudes or a failure to facilitate informed choices? *Int J Epidemiol* **34**:346–352, 2005.
82. Rowe HJ, Fisher JRW, Quinlivan JA. Are pregnant Australian women well informed about prenatal genetic screening? A systematic investigation using the Multidimensional Measure of Informed Choice. *Aus NZ J Obstet Gynaecol* **46**:433–439, 2006.
83. Gourounti K, Sandall J. Do pregnant women in Greece make informed choices about antenatal screening for Down's syndrome? A questionnaire survey. *Midwifery* **24**:153–162, 2008.
84. Jepson RG, Hewison J, Thompson A, Weller D. Patient perspectives of information and choice in cancer screening: a qualitative study in the UK. *Soc Sci Med* **65**:890–899, 2007.

CHAPTER 18

Parental reaction to prenatal diagnosis and subsequent bereavement

Jane Fisher and Helen Statham

KEY POINTS

- This chapter deals with diagnosis of fetal abnormality and subsequent pregnancy loss from the parent perspective. It explores the impact on parents and how clinicians can provide the best possible care in these difficult circumstances
- It is crucial not to underestimate the distress caused by the diagnosis of a problem in an unborn baby. It is important that information is communicated clearly and sensitively with acknowledgment of the shock and sadness it will evoke in parents
- Parents need time both to assimilate the diagnosis and to decide on the next steps. There will be added difficulty if the prognosis is uncertain
- Parents may need help in creating a framework for their decision making when struggling with whether to continue or end the pregnancy. In the absence of a firm evidence base on how parents make decisions, a supportive individualized approach to care will best enable parents to make the decision they can best live with
- Those continuing a pregnancy after a diagnosis will have concerns as parents-to-be and these should not be overlooked due to focus on the affected baby
- Those undergoing a termination for abnormality appreciate being prepared for the practical and emotional issues they may face and being presented with choices they may have during the process. Good follow-up care can lead to recognition of complicated grief and the provision of intervention when necessary
- It is important to involve partners fully and to address the support needs they may have
- A subsequent pregnancy after a loss requires careful management and coordinated support so that parents can cope with the inevitable anxieties and conflicting emotions
- In order to provide high quality care in the context of loss due to fetal abnormality, clinicians need access to specialized training and appropriate support

INTRODUCTION

For the majority of women who undergo prenatal testing, the results confirm the absence of certain abnormalities. Thus many of those who had entered pregnancy at increased risk because of a specific indication (e.g. family history, age or use of prescribed medication), or who were more generally anxious can gain welcome reassurance for the remainder of the pregnancy, although no tests can guarantee a healthy baby. For other women and their partners, the tests reveal a fetal abnormality. Immediately and irreversibly, parents lose the healthy baby of their dreams and expectations. Then, in a state of shock and distress, they may have to make difficult decisions about the future of the pregnancy – whether to continue or to terminate.

Our understanding of the impact of a diagnosis, decision making and the consequences derives from two distinct but related types of data. Experiential accounts in both newspapers[1], academic literature[2,3] and from support groups such as ARC in the UK (Antenatal Results and Choices www.arc-uk.org) have been central to informing professional perceptions of parents' responses. As well as describing parents' emotions and reactions, the earlier accounts were largely responsible for informing major changes in care that have occurred over the last 20 years.[4] Psychological studies, on the other hand, have sought to theorize over decision making and quantify morbidity, particularly in response to termination, with the aim of identifying factors associated with adverse outcomes (reviewed in Statham et al.[5] and Statham[6]). This chapter will summarize what is known from both data sources and argue that, in the absence of conclusive, research-based evidence, health professionals are best advised to care for parents in a very individualized way during the management of such a complex process.

Throughout the chapter, we have chosen to use the word 'baby' to describe the fetus. Though we are aware that some parents and many clinicians prefer to talk about a fetus, in our experience, the majority of women and couples in a wanted pregnancy conceptualize their fetus as a baby from early gestation, with the wide range of associated meanings prospective parents ascribe to it.

BREAKING BAD NEWS

However 'prepared' parents might be for the possibility of fetal abnormality, perhaps after a worrying screening result, when the problem is confirmed, we cannot underestimate the impact this has on them. There is no evidence to suggest that the behavior of clinicians can ameliorate the pain women and their partners experience when told of an abnormality. We do know that sensitive individualized care, from the point of diagnosis, which is carefully coordinated and coupled with good communication, can help parents take some positive memories from a difficult experience and will avoid adding to existing distress[7].

Effective communication from clinicians involves more than choosing the right words. When shock makes assimilation of information hard for parents, a clear, carefully paced explanation of the anomaly and the prognosis is crucial. Perhaps the most overlooked skill that is required at this sensitive time is listening. Only by actively listening and responding to parents and involving them in discussions are clinicians truly able to assess the meaning the diagnosis has for them and come to an agreement on the most appropriate care pathway.

Parents have reported to ARC that they appreciate a clinician who is open and honest with them. This includes honesty about the possible outcomes of any finding and honesty about the limits of his/her professional knowledge regarding the diagnosis; with the proviso that every attempt will be made to locate and give parents as much information as possible and as quickly as possible[7]. It may also be necessary to acknowledge the distress for parents of having to wait for more information or further tests.

Shock manifests itself in a variety of ways, but for most it will mean that their ability to absorb complex information will be severely impaired. As a result, explanations need to be as jargon-free as possible, logically sequenced with pausing to check that parents are able to take in the essential information. It can be useful for them to have written information to take away to consolidate what has been said, as well as details of someone they can contact between appointments with any concerns. It is helpful if parents experience good continuity of care and consistent information. This is best achieved by ensuring there are clear channels of communication between all staff involved in both local and referral units.

IMPACT OF PRENATAL DIAGNOSIS

Bereavement following prenatal diagnosis arises first from the loss of a 'normal' expected baby after diagnosis of abnormality. The physical death of the baby occurs either as a result of termination or as a consequence of the abnormalities, though many abnormalities are discovered which, when the pregnancy continues, do not lead to death but to some degree of physical and/or intellectual impairment.

> Right now I am grieving for the healthy baby that I never had, a little brother for my son who would have been so excited to have a little baby in the house, and for the healthy little bundle that my husband and I wanted so desperately. (ARC Email Support Group Posting.)

Parents may need time to face the reality of the diagnosis and its implications. It may be difficult for them to grasp fully the implications in the space of a single consultation. Some will feel the need to have the abnormality confirmed by a second opinion. This should not be seen as undermining the initial clinical judgment. For some parents, it is an important part of the process of accepting the reality of the situation. Some parents report that knowing that they sought a range of opinion was key in helping them come to terms with their loss.

Another challenge for parents and their clinicians is dealing with uncertainty. Definite prognoses can only usually be given in cases of lethal malformations. Even in these circumstances, parents often have to deal with the uncertainty of when exactly their baby will die. As the advance of antenatal testing technology outstrips our ability to provide clear diagnoses, findings with uncertain outcomes are likely to increase. We need to bear in mind that many parents are making a decision about the future of a pregnancy based on probabilities rather than hard facts, which adds to the difficulty.

DECISION MAKING AFTER A PRENATAL DIAGNOSIS

Gathering formal research evidence about the process of decision making as the decision is being made is challenging. In all but a minority of specialist centers, positive diagnoses are infrequent, making recruitment to research before a diagnosis is made difficult and presenting many ethical challenges. What we know about decision making is therefore derived from descriptive studies that report how obstetric and sociodemographic factors correlate with decisions, and retrospective accounts of how decisions were made. When decision making is difficult, parents often choose to talk to supportive groups such as ARC, especially given the known difficulties that health professionals have in this area with pressures of both time and the fear of being 'directive'[8].

The options available to parents depend on the nature of the abnormality and the law relating to abortion. If termination is not legal at all in a particular jurisdiction, or is not legal in a specific case, either because of the 'severity' of the abnormality or the gestation at diagnosis, parents can only continue with the pregnancy; this will be discussed below (Continuing the pregnancy after a diagnosis).

The factors that have been investigated in the context of relationship with the decision to terminate or continue with a pregnancy include gestational age, severity of the abnormality, the appearance of structural abnormalities, maternal age, who counsels the parents and cultural factors (reviewed in Statham[6]). This review highlighted the variation in results between studies and cautioned that the nature of the different study populations did not allow for the assumption to be made that any particular factor was predictive of a decision[9]. As observed by Mansfield and colleagues[9], observed rates of termination may reflect how and to whom testing was offered, test uptake, prior attitudes of those undergoing tests and attitudes of those undertaking pre- and post-test counselling. For example, women may be more likely to terminate after an earlier diagnosis because women who are more inclined towards termination do more to ensure they get earlier diagnosis. These women may well be older because they know they are at increased risk of a baby with Down's syndrome[10].

All studies show that increasing severity of malformation is associated with an increased likelihood of termination[9,11–16]. Many authors have concentrated on termination rates for different karyotype abnormalities. In 20 studies reviewed by Mansfield[9], overall termination rates were 92% for Down's syndrome, 72% for Turner's syndrome and 58% for Klinefelter's syndrome. For the latter condition, rates in 8 studies varied between 36 and 92% while, in a later German study[17], only 4 of 23 cases (17%) were terminated, whereas in Israel termination rates for sex chromosome anomalies are 80%[18] and a recent American report showed 70% termination rate[16].

While data about the conditions for which parents are more likely to choose termination are interesting, they tell us little about the process of decision making nor how difficult it is for the parents to make their decision. The role of health professionals in decision making has been discussed since the early suggestion, not supported by significant results[19], that termination rates after the diagnosis of sex-chromosome anomalies were higher when parents were counseled by an obstetrician rather than a geneticist. Obstetricians have reported themselves to be more directive than genetic counselors[20] and may have less accurate information about relatively rare conditions[21]. Health professionals will be part of the source of information about the nature of the condition and its likely prognosis, but there is little research evidence about how parents perceive the way they are given this information. Furthermore, the increased availability of information from a range of sources, such as the Internet, may make the role of health professionals less significant.

The important issue of how parents make decisions is little understood. Marteau and Dormandy[22] observed in 2001 that: 'in contrast to the great volume of research on women's decisions about prenatal testing, there is a dearth of research on women's decisions following the diagnosis of a fetal abnormality' and little has changed since that time. Again we would argue that there are practical and ethical constraints to obtaining this information concurrently with the decision making but such narrative accounts as are available[2,3,23–25] attest to the immense difficulty in making the decision even for parents who know what they want to do. What emerges from these accounts is the way parents consider and balance the impact of the abnormality on the child, on themselves and on other immediate family members (including those not yet born) in the context of any prior attitudes and beliefs they may hold about abortion. Such data as are available that consider parents' subsequent feelings about their decision suggest that few parents regret their decisions, although this work is mostly in the context of a decision to terminate[26–30].

In the absence of a firm evidence base, the question arises as to how clinicians might best support parents so they are enabled to make a decision that they can best live with[31]. Some parents who are reeling from the shock of the diagnosis and struggling with what to do may look for direction from their obstetric team. They know they have to make the final decision, but this can feel particularly onerous, accompanied as it often is by an overwhelming desire to make the right decision; one that they will be best able to live with in the future[32]. We need to keep in mind that, when faced with the choice between continuing with the pregnancy in the knowledge that their baby will die or be disabled and ending their baby's life, it comes down to deciding between options that can feel equally bleak. Parents have to weigh up painful scenarios and judge which might be the least worst path; this as well as dealing with the intense emotional impact of the diagnosis. Behind the question *what should I do?* or *what would you do?* there is often a quest for acknowledgment of the magnitude of their dilemma and sometimes a search for acceptance of the decision they have tentatively made. There has been recent debate about whether a clinician's disclosure is valid as parents will use it among many other contributory factors in their decision making and not be unduly influenced[8]. Clinicians may be on safer ground empathizing with the difficulty the parents face and helping them to weigh up the competing benefits and harms in a way that means they can make the decision that is appropriate in their individual circumstances.

We would urge caution around assuming that the diagnosis of a lethal condition somehow makes the decision easier. Parents have to contend with the devastating news that their baby will not survive, coupled with the fact that they can choose the timing of their baby's death.

> I will never forget the desolation we felt. We were faced not only with the fact that our baby was going to die, but also that we had to play a part in deciding the timing of his death. (Mother describing diagnosis of anencephaly ARC News October 2002.)

Another assumption that can be unhelpful is that an earlier diagnosis makes it easier; this is pertinent in the current quest to bring many screening tests into the first trimester. Parents still have to come to terms with the loss of, what is in most cases, a much-wanted baby. Also they may have less recourse to external support, as many couples will have delayed announcement of the pregnancy until the first trimester is over.

It may be helpful to explore some of the factors parents bring to their decision making. We know that severity of the abnormality and the related quality of life for the baby are most often mentioned by parents as being high on the list of contributory factors. Apart from lethal conditions, parents are rarely offered certainty in either case. After a diagnosis of Down's syndrome, parents may be able to access good information on possible related health conditions and general prospects, but no one can tell them the level of learning disability their child will have. Some parents feel able to cope with the possibility of a child at the higher end of the spectrum but feel differently about the prospect of raising a child with severe difficulties. 'Quality of life' is difficult to measure and inevitably subjective. How parents view their potential child's quality of life will be colored by their own experience and lifestyle. In terms of the medical information clinicians give to parents, given the impossibility of being entirely value-free when providing a long-term prognosis, it helps if the description is as clear, jargon-free and unbiased as possible. Parents appreciate being signposted to other sources of information which could include condition-specific support groups and reputable websites. Parents who have access to the Internet will almost always take up their own search, so it is worth pointing them to reliable sites.

During the decision-making process, as well as thinking about their baby, parents will be thinking about themselves, as individuals and as a couple, and about their personal circumstances. They will be considering the impact of having a baby with special needs on their family life, including on existing and prospective siblings and wider family and social networks. Their chosen lifestyle, work and financial status may also have a bearing. They may have particular religious, moral or cultural values that play a part in their decision making, in which case an appointment with a faith leader may be helpful. It will always be useful to have a member of their care team who they can easily access for support through the process.

Depending on the gestation and legal parameters, there may be an added pressure of limited time. It is essential that, when possible, parents are afforded the time they need to make a decision with any unavoidable restrictions explained and the difficulty that this adds acknowledged.

> But how, as ... a human being you make those sorts of decisions, you know, Do I stick a needle in my baby's heart and kill him now? Do I give birth to him and then sort of hope that he doesn't die, have a heart attack and drop dead at the age of 5, you know? Or, if he survives it all, which is the best you hope for, how will he live with the burden of this knowledge of this terrible incurable thing? ...And I remember sort of going round in circles in my head between these things ...and thinking, what am I going to choose, you know? Which of these three just awful, very different scenarios is the one that I feel I could live with, or that I could choose him to have to live with?' (Mother of baby diagnosed with congenital heart disease http://www.dipex.org/antenatalscreening interview AN04.)

> Throughout we never felt pressurized into doing anything; we always felt that we had choices and that we were totally in control. There was no pressure or emotional blackmail at any stage from the initial phone call, to have the amniocentesis, or the termination, it was our decision. I cannot express how impressed with the sincerity, support, compassion and professionalism of all the staff involved in our baby's journey. (Mother of baby diagnosed with Down's syndrome ARC News August 2005.)

CONTINUING THE PREGNANCY AFTER A DIAGNOSIS

Research into the impact of continuing a pregnancy after a confirmed prenatal diagnosis was, until recently, relatively rare compared with that on the experiences of termination[5]. Much research focused on babies where a lethal abnormality had been discovered and there was some suggestion that, in this situation, the decision not to terminate may be better for a woman's emotional well-being because women who continue a pregnancy could avoid the guilt they might have felt had they terminated. For many women, however, the thought of continuing a pregnancy with a baby that they know will die is as unthinkable as termination is for others[33], and the important issue is that parents are enabled to make the right decision for them, as discussed above. Care for parents continuing a pregnancy has been reported as poor during the remainder of the pregnancy[34]. The development of planned palliative care programs for women, with intense pregnancy support[35] and clear planning around the birth of the baby and for the neonatal period is clearly to be welcomed for the small number of women who will choose this option, but as we have seen above, most women terminate after the diagnosis of serious malformations.

There are, however, very many parents who continue pregnancies after the diagnosis of one of the many anomalies that are not lethal and where termination might not even be offered, e.g. cleft lip or renal pelvic dilatation. Sometimes, babies will have conditions that need ongoing monitoring, sometimes there will be treatment available and other times there will be no treatment but, in all situations, the parents have lost the normal baby they had expected, will be adjusting to the uncertainty of the remainder of the pregnancy and after the baby is born, and will be experiencing many complex emotions[36]. In a growing base of qualitative data, researchers have now begun to explore the nature and experience of an ongoing pregnancy after a prenatal diagnosis, as well as how to care for the mother who remains a pregnant woman but who can appear to be forgotten when antenatal care focuses on the health of the baby[33,37]. Both Finnemore[38] and Edwins[39] discussed the implications for health professionals caring for parents and reinforced earlier recommendations[34] around communication, sensitivity and organization. Finnemore[38] identified uncertainty as the main characteristic of the experience of continuing: the remainder of the pregnancy is the time to try to resolve uncertainties with psychological coping strategies such as grieving, denial[39] and seeking information. Issues of shock at diagnosis[38], grief for the loss of the expected healthy baby[39] and isolation from family and health professionals after the decision to continue[40], have been highlighted. Even in the Republic of Ireland, a country where prenatal diagnosis is undertaken but termination of pregnancy is not legal, recent data suggest that systems of care for parents continuing pregnancies are not ideal to meet women's needs[7]. The DIPEX website (http://www.dipex.org/antenatalscreening) has many accounts of parents experiences, one of which has been recently published:

> ... It's quite vicious because you've got two stages of grieving. We had, we grieved for our baby when he was born and died so quickly, but also in September when we were diagnosed we had to grieve for the baby that we thought we were going to have. We had three months of having to get used to the idea that he wasn't going to see his first day at school, you know, I wasn't going to take him to see football matches or motor races or whatever. And that's, you have to allow yourself to grieve for that as well. It's, and it is very, very difficult. (Father describing continuing a pregnancy after a diagnosis of trisomy13[41].)

TERMINATION AFTER A DIAGNOSIS

At a time when parents are in a state of emotional turmoil, it can be sometimes be tempting to those caring for them to try to protect them from further distress by not going into detail about what the termination process entails. This is counterproductive in two main ways. Denying parents information at a time when they feel circumstances are out of their control can exacerbate this feeling of helplessness and vulnerability. Furthermore, they could be denied certain choices that may be open to them regarding how the process is managed. Many women report that gentle preparation for what was to come helped to allay some of their fears and many parents have commented that the ARC parents' handbook both provides them with information and enables them to formulate questions[4]. Their questions may include when and where the procedure will take place. This will often be dictated by gestation. If the termination is to be performed under general anesthetic on a gynecological or general ward, the mother may need to be prepared for the fact that she is likely to be surrounded by patients undergoing a range of procedures, including those who may be ending unwanted pregnancies. She may wish to talk about the exact nature of the procedure, and the fact that there will not be a recognizable body to see. In this instance, it might be appropriate to discuss possible ways of remembering the baby, perhaps by keeping a scan picture.

In the UK, most women after 13 weeks of gestation have a medical induction. The thought of laboring to deliver a dead baby is understandably painful for women to contemplate. However, this procedure does allow those women and couples who want to the opportunity to see and hold their baby. It can be especially hard to cope with being on a maternity ward and the sound of live babies or being near to women giving birth in happier circumstances. Parents speak positively of the provision of a private room with facilities for a partner to stay.

In the immediate aftermath of a termination for abnormality, women need to be prepared for possible lactation and bleeding. As well as being alerted to the probable physical consequences, some will want to know how they might expect to feel afterwards. It is hard to generalize as women and their partners describe a range of emotions, see below (Psychological effects of termination). For some, the intensity of their emotions is frightening and it can help if they are enabled to access support from those who have experience of this kind of bereavement or those who have had undergone a similar experience in order to 'normalize' their emotional responses.

From the moment the decision to end the pregnancy has been made, some parents are concerned about the implications for future pregnancies, this often includes worry about risks associated with the proposed method of termination. They may have questions as to when they can plan to try to conceive again. Conventional medical wisdom suggests that women wait at least two to three cycles before trying again and many advocate a longer wait to allow for grieving and some degree of emotional recovery. Despite the soundness of such advice, for some women, the desire to be pregnant again is all-consuming and the only way they foresee of moving forward from their loss. This will need particularly careful handling if information from postmortem results is expected to have implications for future pregnancies.

In certain cases, a feticide will be performed. This is a profoundly symbolic act for parents and professionals alike[42]. It demands a high degree of competence, confidence and sensitivity on the part of the clinician to help the parents through this part of the process. Some fathers have reported significant distress if they witness the fatal injection on screen and it is advisable to check that he is prepared for what he may see and that his support needs are not overlooked[43,44]. While some parents remain haunted by this experience, many describe it as a difficult part of a difficult process and some experience relief that it represents an end to their baby's suffering or clear point of death.

> And it is done. I am in shock. I have killed my beloved child. I have lain there and allowed them to do this. And I am relieved. (Mother describing feticide ARC News August 2005.)

PSYCHOLOGICAL EFFECTS OF TERMINATION FOR WOMEN

Early reports of women's experiences of termination for abnormality described emotions of sadness, anger and guilt[45–49]. These reports helped raise awareness among health professionals that, although parents actively chose to terminate, the pregnancy was wanted and, as with other perinatal losses, parents were bereaved[48]. A number of features of termination after prenatal diagnosis might have compounded grief, e.g. the isolation of women[27], their ignorance about how terminations would take place[24,27,50], poor care in hospital and no care or support after the event[28,51]. Around this time, attitudes towards the full range of perinatal deaths were changing with an increasing emphasis on all aspects of care and encouraging parental involvement with the process – making decisions, seeing and holding the baby, grieving. Grief, however, became something that could be measured and a plethora of studies have used a variety of psychological measures to describe women's emotional state after termination. The main aim of the majority of these studies has been to identify factors predictive of 'adverse' psychological reactions in order to target supportive interventions.

In a review of data, Statham[6] identified two clear findings. First, psychological distress is high in the short term after termination and secondly, this distress declines over time for most women. Signs of grieving, however, remain for many women for a long time, even when they do not show clinical signs of distress (see below, Follow-up). Beyond these very broad, and perhaps self-evident conclusions, research in this area (and in perinatal grief research more widely) is characterized by inconsistencies in methodologies, study populations and findings[52–54].

It has been widely presumed that obstetric aspects of the pregnancy and termination, in particular, the method of termination, the gestational age and the lethality of the condition that has been diagnosed, will influence the response to the termination with later terminations through induced labor for non-lethal conditions being associated with the worst outcomes. However, where these factors have been investigated, the findings have varied across studies: gestational age was found to correlate with psychological reaction in some studies[55,56] and not in others[57,58]. More recent studies have also varied in their findings. In an interesting series of studies, Korenromp and colleagues[59,60] have shown different results with different subsets of their study population of 254 women. With all women, there is a small effect of gestational age on grief[59], whereas with the population whose partner also took part, there is no effect[60]. These authors also report an increased likelihood of intrusive thoughts after later terminations measured 2–7 years post termination, whereas Davies and colleagues[61] found significantly increased post-traumatic stress symptoms with later terminations at 6 weeks post termination but not at 6 months or one year. Our own recent research found no effect when looking at scores on measures of grief and depression over 14 months, but many women expressed a preference for early termination and many of those who had an early termination believed that they were lucky to have been able to have an early diagnosis[43]. Similar variability of findings across studies is found for method of termination[62] and severity of the malformation[6]. For example, Korenromp's recent studies both do[59] and do not[60] find an effect of having or not having a lethal malformation.

This degree of variation between studies is seen for most of the putative predictor variables and most outcomes[6]. With regard to characteristics of care during a termination, there is little research evidence on which to base conclusions as to their impact on maternal well-being. Certainly care has changed and it is widely believed to be much improved, but it has not been possible to conduct research in this area once new practices were introduced based on what parents reported they wanted[63].

Making sense of the many disparate findings in this area must lead us to think about the issues in a different way. Thus, a typical comment by Geerinck-Vercammen[64] that: 'seeing the child and saying farewell and the medical and psychosocial support received from professional caregivers were of great value for the interviewees', appears in conflict with the findings of other studies that suggest that women experiencing a variety of perinatal losses who choose to avoid rituals around death and make less use of mementoes have lower grief scores[53,65–67]. Perhaps the issue is in measurement and in trying to apply the evidence-based medicine paradigm to something that is not merely complicated, but complex[68]. Enkin[68] goes on to describe problems that have 'multiple, interrelated, interconnected, interwoven, hopelessly tangled causes' which, because they are not 'tidy', demand a new way of looking at them. An alternative approach may be to focus not just on the idea that it is perception of the pregnancy loss that predicts psychological adjustment but that characteristics of the parents, including internal resources and coping strategies and their perceptions of relationship and other social support, are important[69]. Most of the available data do show a consistent positive effect of perceived social support, especially from a partner[6,43,59] and negative consequences for women with previous mental health problems, i.e. women with supportive partners are less likely in the short term after a termination to report higher scores on measures of grief and depression, women with previous mental health difficulties are more likely[6].

But, as yet, research has not found, and may never provide us with conclusive evidence on the choices that will best aid emotional recovery. We would recommend that parents are offered options around ways of remembering their baby and helped to decide what they, as individuals, feel best able to cope with.

> We had decided not to see Jonathan; my heart was already broken and I knew I couldn't cope with seeing him – it wasn't that I didn't love him, I did with all my heart, I just didn't want to remember him like that. I wish somebody had explained the emotional side of this terrible situation, the overwhelming feelings I had when I felt him being born. I knew I was a mother – no one could take that away from me. (Mother after termination after a diagnosis of renal abnormalities ARC News December 2005.)

PARTNERS

It is not unusual for care in the context of pregnancy loss to be concentrated on the mother. Similarly, there has been little research undertaken with fathers[43,60]. The limited findings show high levels of grief immediately after a termination but mostly this is not as high as found for mothers and levels fall more quickly for most men. Fathers will admit to neglecting or denying their own needs as they try to take on a supportive or practical role. It must be remembered that they too have suffered a significant loss, evoking feelings that are often in danger of being subsumed in the needs of the mother. An added burden for many is the agony of watching their partner suffer physically and emotionally and being powerless to assuage the pain. For men raised in a culture where males are not encouraged to express emotions, it can be especially difficult to articulate their feelings and needs. It is therefore incumbent upon those health professionals caring for the couple to make every effort to include the father at all times and to encourage him to seek support if appropriate.

> My feelings were of frustration, powerlessness and anger mixed with a lot of compassion for Julia and, of course, more guilt. Through the intense emotion of this meeting I remember the gratitude I felt to the specialist for not judging us for our decision one way or the other… (From 'Giddeon's story'[70].)

> When our world fell apart, I subconsciously assumed the strong role – dealing with the outside world, showing a brave face but, in retrospect, not realizing that by hiding my own grief I was giving the impression of being uncaring. This may not ring true for all men, but I bet it does for quite a few. (Father after a termination for Down's syndrome and heart defect ARC News July 2003.)

FOLLOW-UP AND THE SUBSEQUENT PREGNANCY

We have discussed previously that, for most women, grief and depression decrease over time post termination without any intervention. How best to facilitate this is yet another area that we cannot discuss from a firm evidence base, but similar arguments may apply as to those discussed above that bereavement is complex[68]. There are a number of examples in the literature describing supportive interventions for women which appear to have face-validity[71–73], with many of the recommendations emphasizing choices. Experiences over many years with parents who have contacted ARC suggest that it is the offering of choices that may be important. Rather than imposing 'the right way' to grieve[63], professionals caring for parents should enable and encourage them to consider what they wish to do and what care they would like, after informing them of what their options might be. However, ways of caring for parents have not been evaluated, and probably cannot be evaluated and it must be remembered that so-called 'supportive interventions' in other fields have not necessarily shown the expected improved outcomes[74]. A recent review entitled 'Grief work, disclosure and counselling: Do they help the bereaved?[75] concludes that there is no evidence that social support, emotional disclosure, experimentally induced emotional disclosure and grief interventions change the *course* of adjustment to bereavement (of a spouse) for the majority of the bereaved. Where the bereavement is perceived as traumatic, interventions may be more useful and the review concluded that grief counseling should be focused rather than given to all. In general terms, those experiencing 'complicated grief' that persists are more likely to have high distress in the immediate aftermath of the bereavement. These may be individuals who eventually seek out grief counseling but to whom it could perhaps be offered earlier if health professionals know parents well enough to recognize their symptoms.

There is an opportunity to pick up first indications of complicated grief at follow-up appointments to assess physical recovery or to discuss postmortem results. These appointments can be a daunting prospect for women. It will usually be the first time they have returned to the hospital since their termination. They may have to sit in a waiting area with expectant mothers or revisit the room where their baby's abnormality was first explained. For these reasons, it can be helpful if the consultation is arranged for a time when there will be an empty waiting room or, if practicable, an alternative venue offered.

When a couple do successfully conceive again, the initial joy is often tempered by conflicting and difficult feelings. These may include feelings of guilt at trying to 'replace' or fear of forgetting the baby that died. There are often worries about the recurrence of the abnormality, either based on fact if it is an inheritable condition, or based not on fact but on very real anxiety. In light of this, they will have concerns about the management of this pregnancy and the testing options open to them. Many will be keen to have their care overseen by the same clinical team, in the knowledge that they found the problem last time and sometimes because they are among the few for whom the lost pregnancy was 'real'. Others will want to treat this pregnancy completely differently and avoid contact with those who were involved in what are painful memories. Whoever is involved in the management of a pregnancy after a loss, it is crucial that they are aware of the woman/couple's previous experience. In the UK, it is common to put a teardrop-shaped sticker clearly visible on the maternity notes to indicate a previous loss, but this should be done with the woman's knowledge and consent.

Anxieties in a subsequent pregnancy do not necessarily subside completely when the moment of the previous diagnosis has passed or when all possible testing has revealed no major problems. Some women find the gestational weeks after the time the previous loss took place difficult because it is 'uncharted water' or evokes guilt as the previous baby did not make it this far. Others, having had a bad experience in pregnancy, find it almost impossible to believe they will have a happy outcome. For many, even the birth of a healthy child is tinged with sadness as it serves as a reminder of 'what should have been' in the previous pregnancy. In short, the majority of parents in the pregnancy after a loss will need extra support and carefully coordinated care from their obstetric team.

STAFF ISSUES

Working with distressed parents takes its personal toll on clinicians, however skilled or experienced they are. Indeed, whatever strategies clinicians employ to mitigate against this, if they find themselves able to cut off completely from the sadness of the situation, it will be important to reflect on the quality of care they are able to offer. The majority of women who see obstetricians ultimately have positive outcomes, which can make the rarer occasions when losses due to fetal abnormality do occur, harder to manage. Just as women and partners may express feelings of failure as they have been unable to produce a healthy baby, in some circumstances, there may be a sense of professional 'failure' surrounding the pregnancy loss.

We would argue for the provision of specialized training for clinicians to help them develop the requisite skills to provide the very best individualized care; along with appropriate support to ensure they are able to manage the emotional dimension without becoming inured to the impact of prenatal diagnoses on parents.

REFERENCES

1. Statham H. Cold comfort. *The Guardian* 24 March, 1987.
2. Brown J. The choice. *J Am Med Assoc* **262**:2735, 1989.
3. Green R. Letter to a genetic counselor. *J Genet Counsel* **1**(1):55–69, 1992.
4. ARC. *A handbook to be given to parents when an abnormality is diagnosed in their unborn baby*, 5th edn. London: Antenatal Results & Choices, 2007.
5. Statham H, Solomou W, Chitty L. Prenatal diagnosis of fetal abnormality: psychological effects on women in low-risk pregnancies. *Bailliere's Clin Obstet Gynaecol* **14**(4):731–747, 2000.
6. Statham H. Prenatal diagnosis of fetal abnormality: the decision to terminate the pregnancy and the psychological consequences. *Fetal Maternal Med Rev* **13**:213–247, 2002.
7. Lalor JG, Devane D, Begley CM. Unexpected diagnosis of fetal abnormality: women's encounters with caregivers. *Birth* **34**(1):80–88, 2007.
8. Baylis F, Downie J. Professional recommendations: disclosing facts and values. *J Med Ethics* **27**(1):20–24, 2001.
9. Mansfield C, Hopfer S, Marteau TM. Termination rates after prenatal diagnosis of Down syndrome, spina bifida, anencephaly, and Turner and Klinefelter syndromes: a systematic literature review. *Prenat Diagn* **19**:808–812, 1999.
10. Kramer RL, Jarve RK, Yaron Y et al. Determinants of parental decisions after the prenatal diagnosis of Down syndrome. *Am J Med Genet* **79**:172–174, 1998.
11. Verp MS, Bombard AT, Simpson JL, Elias S. Parental decision following prenatal diagnosis of fetal chromosome anomalies. *Am J Med Genet* **29**:613–622, 1988.
12. Drugan A, Greb A, Johnson MP et al. Determinants of parental decisions to abort for chromosome abnormalities. *Prenat Diagn* **10**:483–490, 1990.
13. Pryde PG, Isada NB, Hallak M, Johnson MP, Ogders AE, Evans MI. Determinants of parental decision to abort or continue after non-aneuploid ultrasound-detected fetal abnormalities. *Obstet Gynecol* **80**:52–56, 1992.
14. Evans MI, Pryde PG, Evans WJ, Johnson MP. The choices women make about prenatal diagnosis. *Fetal Diagn Ther* **8**:70–80, 1993.
15. Schechtman KB, Gray DL, Baty JD, Rothman SM. Decision-making for termination of pregnancies with fetal anomalies: analysis of 53,000 pregnancies. *Obstet Gynecol* **99**(2):216–222, 2002.
16. Brian L, Shaffer ABC, Norton ME. Variation in the decision to terminate pregnancy in the setting of fetal aneuploidy. *Prenat Diagn* **26**(8):667–671, 2006.

17. Meschede D, Louwen F, Nippert I, Holzgreve W, Miny P, Horst J. Low rates of pregnancy termination for prenatally diagnosed Klinefelter syndrome and other sex chromosome polysomies. *Am J Med Genet* **80**(4):330–334, 1998.
18. Sagi M, Meinger V, Reshef N, Dagan J, Zlotogora J. Prenatal diagnosis of sex chromosome aneuploidy: possible reasons for high rates of pregnancy termination. *Prenat Diagn* **21**(6):461–465, 2001.
19. Holmes-Seidel M, Ryynanen M, Lindenbaum RH. Parental decisions regarding termination of pregnancy following prenatal detection of sex chromosome anomalies. *Prenat Diagn* **7**:239–244, 1987.
20. Marteau TM, Drake H, Bobrow M. Counselling following diagnosis of a fetal abnormality: the differing approaches of obstetricians, clinical geneticists, and genetic nurses. *J Med Genet* **31**:864–867, 1994.
21. Abramsky L, Hall S, Levitan J, Marteau TM. What parents are told after prenatal diagnosis of a sex chromosome abnormality: interview and questionnaire study. *Br Med J* **322**:463–466, 2001.
22. Marteau TM, Dormandy E. Facilitating informed choice in prenatal testing: how well are we doing? *Am J Med Genet* **106**:185–190, 2001.
23. Rapp R. XYLO: a true story. In *Test-tube women: what future for motherhood?* R Arditt, R Duelli-Klein, S Minden (eds), pp. 313–328. London: Pandora Press, 1984.
24. Statham H. Professional understanding and parents' experience of termination. In *Prenatal diagnosis and screening*, DJH Brock, CH Rodeck, MA Ferguson-Smith (eds), pp. 697–702. London: Churchill Livingstone, 1992.
25. Statham H. Parents' reactions to termination of pregnancy for fetal abnormality: from a mother's point of view. In *Prenatal diagnosis: the human side*, L Abramsky, J Chapple (eds), pp. 157–172. London: Chapman & Hall, 1994.
26. Beeson D, Golbus MS. Decision making: whether or not to have prenatal diagnosis and abortion for X-linked conditions. *Am J Med Genet* **20**:107–114, 1985.
27. White-van Mourik MCA, Connor JM, Ferguson-Smith MA. Patient care before and after termination of pregnancy for neural tube defects. *Prenat Diagn* **10**:497–505, 1990.
28. Elder SH, Laurence KM. The impact of supportive intervention after second trimester termination of pregnancy for fetal abnormality. *Prenat Diagn* **11**:47–54, 1991.
29. Korenromp MJ, Tedema-Kuiper HR, van Spijker HG, Christiaens GCML, Bergsma J. Termination of pregnancy on genetic grounds: coping with grieving. *J Psychosomat Obstet Gynaecol* **13**:92–105, 1992.
30. White-van Mourik MCA, Connor JM, Ferguson-Smith MA. The psychosocial sequelae of a second-trimester termination of pregnancy for fetal abnormality. *Prenat Diagn* **12**:189–204, 1992.
31. ARC. *Supporting parents' decisions: a handbook for professionals*. London: Antenatal Results & Choices, 2005.
32. van Berkel D, van der Weele C. Norms and prenorms on prenatal diagnosis: new ways to deal with morality in counseling. *Patient Educ Counsel* **37**(2):153–163, 1999.
33. Statham H, Solomou W, Green JM. Continuing a pregnancy after the diagnosis of an anomaly: parents' experiences. In *Prenatal diagnosis: the human side*, 2nd edn, L Abramsky, J Chapple (eds), pp. 182–196. Cheltenham: Nelson Thornes, 2003.
34. Chitty LS, Barnes CA, Berry C. Continuing with pregnancy after a diagnosis of lethal abnormality: experience of five couples and recommendations for management. *Br Med J* **313**:478–480, 1996.
35. Breeze AC, Lees CC, Kumar A, Missfelder-Lobos HH, Murdoch EM. Palliative care for prenatally diagnosed lethal fetal abnormality. *Arch Dis Child Fetal Neonatal Ed* 092122, 2006.
36. Jones S, Statham H, Solomou W. When expectant mothers know their baby has a fetal abnormality: exploring a crisis of motherhood through qualitative data mining. *J Soc Work Res Evaluat* **6**(2):195–206, 2005.
37. ARC. *Supporting you throughout your pregnancy: a handbook for parents after prenatal diagnosis*. London: Antenatal Results and Choices, 2003.
38. Finnemore P. Future imperfect: coping and communication in continuing pregnancy after diagnosis of fetal abnormality: Middlesex University, 2000.
39. Edwins J. From a different planet: women who choose to continue their pregnancy after a diagnosis of Down's syndrome. *Pract Midwife* **3**(4):21–24, 2000.
40. Redlinger-Grosse K, Bernhardt BA, Berg K, Muenke M, Biesecker BB. The decision to continue: the experiences and needs of parents who receive a prenatal diagnosis of holoprosencephaly. *Am J Med Genet* **11**:369–378, 2002.
41. Locock L. The parents' journey: continuing a pregnancy after a diagnosis of Patau's syndrome. *Br Med J* **331**(7526):1186–1189, 2005.
42. Statham H, Solomou W, Green J. Late termination of pregnancy: law, policy and decision making in four English fetal medicine units. *Br J Obstet Gynaecol* **113**(12):1402–1411, 2006.
43. Statham H, Solomou W, Green JM. *When a baby has an abnormality: a study of parents' experiences*. Cambridge: Centre for Family Research, University of Cambridge, 2001.
44. Robson F. 'Yes! – a chance to tell my side of the story': a case study of a male partner of a woman undergoing termination of pregnancy for foetal abnormality. *J Health Psychol* **7**(2):183–193, 2002.
45. Blumberg BD, Golbus MS, Hanson KH. The psychological sequelae of abortion performed for a genetic indication. *Am J Obstet Gynecol* **122**:799–808, 1975.
46. Donnai P, Charles N, Harris R. Attitudes of patients after 'genetic' termination of pregnancy. *Br Med J* **282**:621–622, 1981.
47. Leschot NJ, Verjaal M, Treffers PE. Therapeutic abortion on genetic grounds. *J Psychosomat Obstet Gynaecol* **1-2**:47–56, 1982.
48. Lloyd J, Laurence KM. Sequelae and support after termination of pregnancy for fetal malformation. *Br Med J* **290**:907–909, 1985.
49. Jorgensen C, Uddenberg N, Ursing Z. Ultrasound diagnosis of fetal malformation in the second trimester: the psychological reactions of the women. *J Psychosomat Obstet Gynaecol* **4**:31–40, 1985.
50. Laurence KM. *Sequelae and support for termination carried out for fetal malformation*. Amsterdam: The Free Woman, 1989.
51. Kenyon S. Support after termination for fetal abnormality. *Midwives Chron Nurs Notes* **101**:190–191, 1988.
52. Zeanah CH. Adaptation following perinatal loss: a critical review. *J Am Acad Child Adoles Psychiatr* **28**(3):467–480, 1989.
53. Hunfeld J. The grief of late pregnancy loss: a four year follow up. PhD Thesis: Erasmus University, 1995.
54. Toedter LJ, Lasker JN, Janssen HJ. International comparison of studies using the perinatal grief scale: a decade of research on pregnancy loss. *Death Stud* **25**(3):205–228, 2001.
55. Black RB. A 1 and 6 month follow-up of prenatal diagnosis patients who lost pregnancies. *Prenat Diagn* **9**:795–804, 1989.
56. Iles S. The loss of early pregnancy. *Bailliere's Clin Obstet Gynaecol* **3**(4):769–790, 1989.
57. Zeanah CH, Dailey JV, Rosenblatt MJ, Saller DN, Jr. Do women grieve after terminating pregnancies because of fetal anomalies? A controlled investigation. *Obstet Gynecol* **82**(2):270–275, 1993.
58. Salvesen KA, Oyen L, Schmidt N, Malt UF, Eik-Nes SH. Comparison of long-term psychological responses of women after pregnancy termination due to fetal anomalies and after perinatal loss. *Ultrasound Obstet Gynecol* **9**:80–85, 1997.
59. Korenromp MJ, Christiaens GCML, van den Bout J et al. Long-term psychological consequences of pregnancy termination for fetal abnormality: a cross-sectional study. *Prenat Diagn* **25**:253–260, 2005.
60. Korenromp MJ, Page-Christiaens GCML, van den Bout J et al. Psychological consequences of termination of pregnancy

for fetal anomaly: similarities and differences between partners. *Prenat Diagn* **25**:1226–1233, 2005.

61. Davies V, Gledhill J, McFadyen A, Whitlow B, Economides D. Psychological outcome in women undergoing termination of pregnancy for ultrasound-detected fetal anomaly in the first and second trimesters: a pilot study. *Ultrasound Obstet Gynecol* **25**(4):389–392, 2005.
62. Burgoine GA, Van Kirk SD, Romm J, Edelman AB, Jacobson SL, Jensen JT. Comparison of perinatal grief after dilation and evacuation or labor induction in second trimester terminations for fetal anomalies. *Am J Obstet Gynecol* **192**(6):1928–1932, 2005.
63. Leon IG. Perinatal loss. A critique of current hospital practices. *Clin Pediatr (Phila)* **31**(6):366–374, 1992.
64. Geerinck-Vercammen CR, Kanhai HHH. Coping with termination of pregnancy for fetal abnormality in a supportive environment. *Prenat Diagn* **23**(7):543–548, 2003.
65. Hughes PM, Turton P, Evans CDH. Stillbirth as risk factor for depression and anxiety in the subsequent pregnancy: cohort study. *Br Med J* **318**:1721–1724, 1999.
66. Lasker JN, Toedter LJ. Predicting outcomes after pregnancy loss: results from studies using the Perinatal Grief Scale. *Illness, Crisis Loss* **8**(4):350–372, 2000.
67. Hughes P, Turton P, Hopper E, McGauley GA, Fonagy P. Disorganised attachment behaviour among infants born subsequent to stillbirth. *J Child Psychol Psychiatry* **42**(6):791–801, 2001.
68. Enkin MW, Glouberman S, Groff P, Jadad AR, Stern A. Beyond evidence: the complexity of maternity care. *Birth* **33**(4):265–269, 2006.
69. Lang A, Goulet C, Amsel R. Explanatory model of health in bereaved parents post-fetal/infant death. *Int J Nurs Stud* **41**(8):869–880, 2004.
70. Don A. *Fathers feel too*. London: Bosun Publishing on behalf of Sands, 2005.
71. Magyari PA, Wedehase BA, Ifft RD, Callanan NP. A supportive intervention protocol for couples terminating a pregnancy for genetic reasons. *Birth Defects Orig Art Ser* **23**(6):75–83, 1987.
72. Landenburger G, Delp KJ. An approach for supportive care before, during, and after selective abortion. *Birth Defects Orig Art Ser* **23**(6):84–88, 1987.
73. Fox R, Pillai M, Porter H, Gill G. The management of late fetal death: a guide to comprehensive care. *Br J Obstet Gynaecol* **107**(1):4–10, 1997.
74. Morrell CJ, Spiby H, Stewart P, Walters S, Morgan A. Costs and benefits of community postnatal support workers: a randomised controlled trial. *Hlth Technol Assess* **4**:6, 2000.
75. Stroebe W, Schut H, Stroebe MS. Grief work, disclosure and counseling: do they help the bereaved? *Clin Psychol Rev* **25**(4):395–414, 2005.

Prenatal screening for open neural tube defects and Down's syndrome

CHAPTER 19

James E Haddow, Glenn E Palomaki, Jacob A Canick and George J Knight

KEY POINTS

- This chapter deals with the prenatal detection of open neural tube defects (ONTD) and Down's syndrome, through use of maternal serum biochemical markers, either alone or combined with selected sonographic markers during the first and/or second trimesters
- The field of prenatal screening is traced from it origins in the 1970s, when ONTD identification was the primary focus, through the present, when greatest emphasis and recent progress have involved detection of Down's syndrome
- About 80% of open spina bifida cases (the ONTD being sought primarily) can be detected via elevated alpha-fetoprotein (AFP) measurements in maternal serum during the second trimester. This level of detection requires that about 4% of all pregnancies be classified as screen positive and offered diagnostic testing
- Maternal serum screening for Down's syndrome began as a supplement to ONTD screening, about 10 years later, after discovery that second-trimester AFP levels were lower in the presence of Down's syndrome. Initially, only 25% of affected pregnancies were detectable, but screening efficiency improved steadily over the succeeding years, with identification of additional serum markers, raising detection to 80%
- In the first trimester, biochemical markers (pregnancy-associated plasma protein A (PAPP-A) and the free-beta subunit of human chorionic gonadotrophin (free-beta hCG)) and ultrasound measurement of nuchal translucency thickness were found useful for detecting Down's syndrome. This offered the option for Down's syndrome (but not ONTD) screening to be performed earlier
- Currently, 'integrated screening' is the most effective strategy. This calls for biochemical and ultrasound measurements from both trimesters to be merged into a single interpretive risk statement. With this approach, about 90% of Down's syndrome cases can be detected at a 2% screen positive rate

HISTORY AND OVERVIEW: HOW PRENATAL SCREENING BEGAN AND EVOLVED

The era of prenatal screening began in 1972, when Brock and Sutcliffe reported that alpha-fetoprotein (AFP) measurement was useful as a marker for detecting open neural tube defects (open spina bifida and anencephaly) in the fetus[1]. This initial discovery was limited to AFP levels in amniotic fluid, but it set the stage for the subsequent discovery of an association between fetal open neural tube defects and elevated AFP levels in maternal serum[2,3]. Considerable overlap was found between maternal serum AFP levels in affected and unaffected pregnancies, however. For that reason, maternal serum AFP measurement, while useful as a screening test, could not be used for diagnostic purposes. Pregnancies identified as being at high risk for open neural tube defects by virtue of elevated maternal serum AFP levels require diagnostic studies, such as AFP and acetylcholinesterase measurements in amniotic fluid and/or fetal scanning by an expert sonographer. A large-scale collaborative study was promptly organized in the UK to determine how to apply second-trimester maternal serum AFP measurements most appropriately in population settings. The report of that study, in 1977, contained the scientific principles that continue to serve as guidelines for screening programs[4].

Initially, ultrasound played only a limited role in the screening process, with its greatest contribution being reliable gestational dating[5]. While anencephaly was readily visualized with available technology, the spinal defect associated with spina bifida was difficult to visualize directly and could not be relied upon[6]. In 1986, however, sonography revealed an abnormal fetal head shape in the presence of spina bifida, called the 'lemon sign', along with a second abnormality in the cerebellum – the 'banana sign'[7]. These two 'fruit signs' are readily visualized, and the false positive rate is sufficiently low that they can be considered diagnostic. These signs are now used in some antenatal diagnostic centers as a primary screening test and, in others, for diagnostic purposes, in conjunction with AFP serum screening.

In 1984, second-trimester serum AFP values were reported to be lower among women with Down's syndrome fetuses[8]. This discovery was made possible by the availability of prospectively obtained AFP measurements from large numbers of women being screened for open spina bifida, in combination with documentation of pregnancy outcome. The initial observation was rapidly confirmed and a model developed for adding an interpretation about Down's syndrome to the existing AFP screening report[9]. Information from the AFP measurement could be converted into a likelihood ratio and used to modify a woman's age-related risk. This allowed screening for Down's syndrome to be extended to women of all ages, for the first time. AFP alone, however, detected only 25% of the Down's syndrome cases at a 5% false positive rate (roughly comparable to using maternal age alone and offering diagnostic testing only to the 5% of oldest pregnant women). For that reason, a search began for more effective markers.

Two new Down's syndrome-associated second-trimester serum markers, human chorionic gonadotropin (hCG) and unconjugated estriol (uE3), were discovered in 1987[10] and 1988[11]. Subsequently, it was shown that information from these measurements could be combined with AFP and maternal age to improve substantially screening performance[12]. Now, 60–70% of the Down's syndrome cases could be identified, at the same 5% false positive rate. Free-beta hCG, a metabolic product of hCG, was also found effective as a screening marker and could be used in place of hCG[13]. These new markers were rapidly incorporated into the routine of prenatal screening, but the search continued for even more effective second-trimester screening markers, and also for markers that might be useful in the first trimester. A fourth second-trimester serum marker, dimeric inhibin A (DIA), was reported in 1996 and added to the screening panel by many centers[14].

Another major advance came with the discovery of first-trimester ultrasound and serum markers. Nuchal translucency thickness, an ultrasound measurement, identifies 60% of the Down's syndrome cases at a 5% false positive rate, when performed at 11 through 13 weeks' gestation[15,16]. Pregnancy-associated plasma protein-A (PAPP-A) identifies 36%, and free-beta hCG 37%[16]. When used together, they detect about 80% of the Down's syndrome cases, again at a 5% false positive rate. This is comparable to, or slightly better than, the combined performance of the four above-mentioned second-trimester serum markers. With detection rates having reached this level in both first and second trimesters, emphasis began to shift toward reducing the false positive rate, so that diagnostic procedure-related losses could be minimized.

In 1999, it was demonstrated that information from first- and second-trimester screening tests performed in the same woman could be combined into a single interpretation. The integrated test is more discriminatory than stand-alone testing in either trimester, alone[17]. In this configuration, the serum and ultrasound measurements were capable of detecting 85% of the Down's syndrome cases, at only a 1% false positive rate. This remains the most effective screening policy at the present time but, viewed in the historical context, more improvements might still be anticipated.

This chapter discusses all aspects of screening for open spina bifida and Down's syndrome that are briefly summarized in this introduction, with emphasis placed on current and anticipated future practice. The same analytic principles underlie calculations for both spina bifida and Down's syndrome screening and, for that reason, AFP is used as an example for many of the mathematical calculations and also for demonstrating modeling.

SCREENING FOR OPEN NEURAL TUBE DEFECTS

Why alpha-fetoprotein is useful as a marker for open neural tube defects

AFP was discovered in 1956 by Bergstrand and Czar. They observed an extra electrophoretic band in the α-1 region in fetal serum[18]. This extra α-1 band represented a protein not normally found in adults and was labeled alpha-1 fetoprotein. AFP is thought to be related evolutionarily to albumin. Genes for the two proteins are located on chromosome 4 and AFP has a similar molecular weight (69000 daltons) and structure to albumin[19,20]. In spite of this structural similarity, antisera raised to AFP in a variety of animal species do not cross-react with albumin. AFP antisera can, therefore, be used to develop immunoassays for analyzing AFP in body fluids that also contain albumin. The circulating half-life of AFP is approximately 4 days in the human adult.

AFP is synthesized in the fetal liver and yolk sac and is the dominant serum protein early in fetal life. It reaches a peak fetal serum concentration of approximately 300 mg/dl late in the first trimester. Thereafter, its concentration decreases steadily, but the fetal liver continues to produce AFP at a constant rate until approximately 30 weeks' gestation, after which production falls precipitously (Fig. 19.1)[21]. No functional role has been defined for AFP during fetal development. In three documented pregnancies, the fetuses produced minimal or no AFP, most

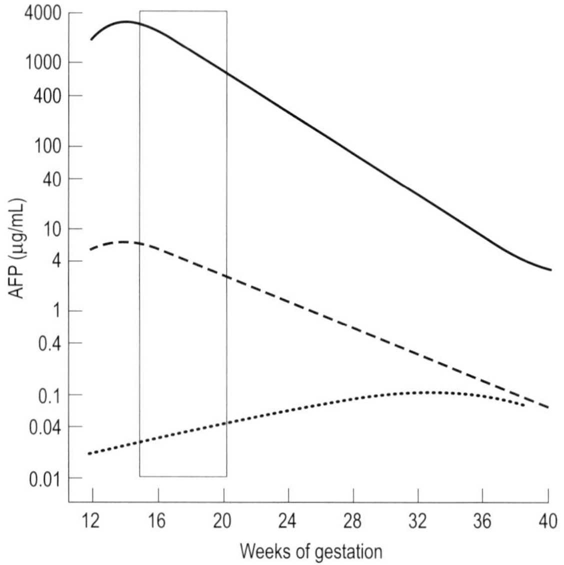

Fig. 19.1 Changes in AFP levels in fetal serum, amniotic fluid and maternal serum during gestation. The AFP values (μg/ml) are plotted on the logarithmic y-axis versus completed week of gestation. The levels of AFP in fetal serum, amniotic fluid and maternal serum are shown by the solid, dashed and dotted curves, respectively. The region enclosed in the rectangle indicates the gestational age range of 15 to 20 weeks. (Figure adapted from Seppala M, *Ann NY Acad Sci*, 1974:259:59.)

probably as a result of a gene deletion similar to that seen with analbuminemia[22]. All three pregnancies went to term and were associated with healthy newborns of normal weight.

How AFP reaches amniotic fluid

The fetal kidney normally allows measurable concentrations of AFP to escape into fetal urine, which then is excreted into amniotic fluid. Peak amniotic fluid AFP concentration is found at around 12 weeks' gestation, after which levels steadily decrease, averaging 10% per gestational week during the second trimester[23]. This normally occurring background AFP makes it necessary to establish gestational age-specific reference ranges, prior to measuring and interpreting amniotic fluid AFP levels for diagnostic purposes (see Fig. 19.1, boxed region, dashed line). Falsely elevated AFP levels can be present when amniotic fluid is contaminated by fetal blood[23]. This can make interpretation difficult, even when fetal blood contamination is identified. However, most false positive AFP results can be resolved by measuring acetylcholinesterase[24]. Although rarely used today because of the ability of high resolution ultrasound to identify open spina bifida, repeat atraumatic amniocentesis, carried out a minimum of 10 days later, will, as a rule, yield normal AFP levels in unaffected pregnancies[25].

The exposed membrane and blood vessel surfaces found with open neural tube defects allow AFP to transudate into amniotic fluid, roughly in proportion to the size of the exposed areas[23,25]. The same is true for open ventral wall defects (omphalocele and gastroschisis). Gastroschisis always lacks a covering membrane, and nearly all cases are associated with AFP elevations[26]. Omphalocele is covered with a membrane and sometimes skin, as well; the amount of AFP that transudates into amniotic fluid is, therefore, more variable among cases. Congenital nephrosis, a rare autosomal recessive condition, is characterized by high concentrations of amniotic fluid AFP[27]. About 20% of the cases of fetal spina bifida are classified as being closed, meaning that they are covered with skin or a thick membrane[28]. Such cases cannot be detected by AFP measurement but may be detected by ultrasound.

Diagnostic studies

The same mathematical principles that were developed for maternal serum AFP screening were subsequently applied to amniotic fluid AFP measurements in the Second UK Collaborative Study[23] and to amniotic fluid acetylcholinesterase measurements[24]. Performance characteristics of these diagnostic studies could then be described both separately and in combination, as defined by detection rates, false positive rates, and the odds of being affected, given a positive result. When acetylcholinesterase (AChE) measurements became available for diagnostic purposes, nearly all of the false positive amniotic fluid AFP measurements could be identified, with only minimal loss of detection.

Diagnostic ultrasound studies in the 1970s initially were directed at visualizing the fetal spine defects, themselves[6]. This often proved difficult and was much less reliable than the amniotic fluid AFP and AChE measurements. The 1986 discovery of alterations in fetal head shape (the 'lemon' sign) and in cerebellum (the 'banana' sign) in the presence of open spina bifida markedly improved the ability of ultrasound to provide reliable diagnostic information[7]. Methods for combining information from ultrasound and biochemical diagnostic studies have been proposed for interpretive purposes[29]. Some centers now use ultrasound measurement almost exclusively to diagnose open spina bifida.

How AFP reaches the maternal circulation

AFP normally reaches the maternal circulation by two routes, about two-thirds by transplacental diffusion and the remainder by transamnionic diffusion. When excess AFP resulting from fetal disorders is present in amniotic fluid, it reaches the maternal circulation by transamnionic diffusion. The restrictive amnionic membrane, in combination with a relatively high transplacental diffusion of normal background AFP, however, makes measurement of AFP in maternal serum both a less sensitive and a less specific test for the presence of open fetal malformations[4].

Gestational dating and maternal serum AFP levels

Once assay conditions have been optimized, gestational dating is the most important potential source of variability that can be taken into account for improving the screening performance of AFP measurement. If all pregnancy dates were to be verified by ultrasound prior to screening, the false positive rate would be approximately 40% lower than if only menstrual dates were available. The detection rate for open neural tube defects would also be slightly improved. A further improvement in detection would be gained if all of the ultrasound-derived dates were based only on biparietal diameter (BPD) measurements. This improvement is due to the BPD measurements of fetuses with open spina bifida being smaller, on average, than unaffected pregnancies[5]. This artefact makes the gestational age-adjusted maternal serum AFP measurements of these affected pregnancies appear higher and raises detection by approximately 10%, at a given false positive rate.

Maternal serum AFP screening for open spina bifida

Screening methodology along with expected detection rates and false positive rates are discussed in an upcoming section on mathematical principles. In summary, once maternal serum AFP levels are converted to multiples of the median (MoM), it is possible to detect 70% of open spina bifida pregnancies by classifying about 2% of all screened pregnancies as having an elevated result (2.5 MoM or higher). Alternatively, an AFP MoM cut-off level of 2.0 MoM can identify 80% of open spina bifida cases with a correspondingly higher false positive rate of about 4.0%.

Unexplained maternal serum AFP elevations and pregnancy outcome

Even when screening conditions have been optimized, there still remain falsely elevated maternal serum AFP measurements that cannot be explained. In such cases, the amniotic fluid AFP measurement is not elevated and/or no fetal defect is observed via ultrasound (i.e. the pregnancy is unaffected by a fetal malformation). This excess AFP in the maternal circulation is most probably transplacental in origin. One source is fetomaternal hemorrhage, sometimes associated with placental hematoma and/or infarcts. In one study, increased numbers of fetal red blood cells were demonstrated in the maternal circulation in a high proportion of women with maternal serum AFP elevations[30]. The integrity of the placental membrane interface might also be compromised by conditions such as fetal hydrops; this disorder has been found occasionally in association with maternal serum AFP elevation[31]. Placental lacunae have been described sonographically, as well, suggesting the possibility that excess AFP may somehow diffuse from these 'lakes' into the maternal circulation[32]. Most commonly, there is no explanation for falsely elevated maternal serum AFP measurements, but the high rate of low birth-weight deliveries (three times as high as with normal maternal serum AFP measurements) and late fetal death (12 times as high as with normal maternal serum AFP measurements) indicates fetal or placental compromise[33]. Rarely, a malignant tumor in the pregnant woman (most notably, hepatoma) may give rise to a maternal serum AFP elevation, sometimes reaching levels of several thousand nanograms per milliliter[34]. Maternal serum AFP elevation can also be found during the recovery phase from acute hepatitis[35]. Although some elevated AFP levels will be explained by the conditions discussed above, the most common finding is a normal pregnancy outcome.

The impact of screening on the birth prevalence of open neural tube defects

In the 30 years since AFP screening was first introduced, the birth prevalence of both anencephaly and open spina bifida has fallen sharply. This fall can be attributed in part to a lower incidence of these disorders during early pregnancy in the UK and USA, but prenatal screening is the major reason for this reduction. Figure 19.2 shows the pattern of live birth prevalence of anencephaly and spina bifida in the UK over a 40-year period[36]. The number of live births recorded with either defect between 1965 through 1969 is 15710. This has been reduced to 751 live births between 2000 and 2004, a more than 20-fold reduction.

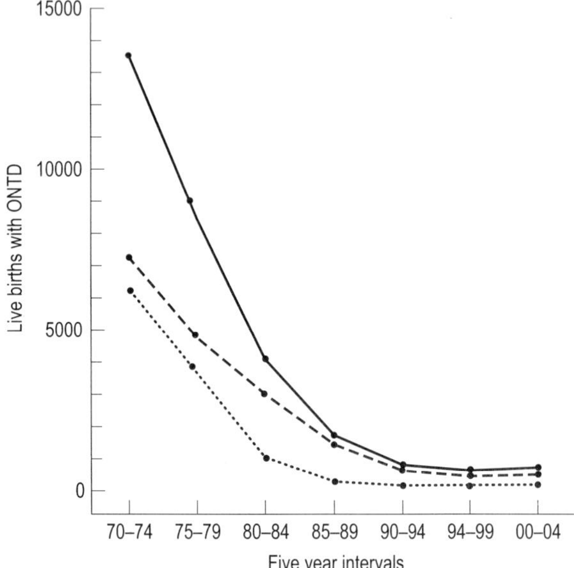

Fig. 19.2 A graphic display of the reduction in the live birth prevalence of open neural tube defects (ONTD). The horizontal axis shows time in 5-year intervals. The solid line connects the estimated number of live births of open spina bifida and anencephaly combined for England and Wales in each of the 5-year intervals. The dashed line connects the estimates for open spina bifida alone. The dotted line connects the estimates for anencephaly alone.

The impact of folic acid supplementation/fortification on the incidence of open neural tube defects

Folic acid supplementation is now known to provide protection against the development of most open neural tube defects, when taken by women during the months immediately before becoming pregnant and continuing through early pregnancy[37]. A daily supplement of 4 mg is recommended for women known to be at high risk because of a previous affected pregnancy. The greatest overall reduction in the rate of occurrence of those disorders would be achieved by fortifying the diets of all women in the childbearing years with at least 0.4 mg of folic acid, daily[38]. Introduction of folic acid fortification into the food supply has taken variable amounts of time in different countries. For example, in the USA and Canada, partial fortification of grain products began in 1997[39,40], while in the UK, a mandatory fortification policy was recommended in May of 2007. In the absence of general folate fortification of the food supply, the intake of folic acid supplements must rely on individual women's initiatives and on ongoing dissemination about the need for folic acid supplements by the health community.

MATHEMATICAL PRINCIPLES

An innovative system for normalizing and analyzing data, originally applied to AFP measurements, was developed as part of the First UK Collaborative Study[4]. That system is now used worldwide by prenatal screening laboratories to interpret all serum and amniotic fluid measurements, and by many laboratories to interpret nuchal translucency measurements.

Converting analyte values to multiples of the median – the first component

Concentrations of prenatal screening analytes change constantly throughout pregnancy. For example, AFP concentrations in maternal serum increase by about 15% per week during the most favorable time for detecting open neural tube defects (15–20 weeks' gestation). Converting these values to multiples of a gestational age-specific median value (MoM) normalizes for this gestational age effect. A laboratory first obtains measurements on sera received routinely from 300 to 500 women. Measurements are initially expressed in mass units (e.g. ng/ml) or international units (e.g. IU/ml). Weighted log-linear regression analysis is used to calculate an equation to determine median levels for the analyte in question for each gestational week. Each woman's measurement is then divided by the median value for the appropriate gestational age resulting in a multiple of the median (MoM). The overall median value in a population of women is, by definition, 1.00 MoM. For example, if the median value for AFP at 16 weeks' gestation is 30 ng/ml, a value of 15 ng/ml is assigned an MoM of 0.5; half the central value. A value of 45 ng/ml translates into

1.50 MoM; one and one-half times the central value. Figure 19.3 summarizes these computations graphically.

Using MoM as a normalizing function serves several practical purposes:

- MoM values are a common currency. Different laboratories can, therefore, compare data, even when assays do not yield identical mass unit results
- The population distribution of analyte measurements is described in unified terms
- Analyte values from the laboratory's own population, expressed as MoM, can be reliably compared with published distributions (this avoids the need for each laboratory to obtain its own measurements from affected pregnancies, before beginning to screen)
- A single cut-off can be used for neural tube defect screening, rather than separate cut-offs for each gestational week
- Other variables, such as maternal weight or race, can be taken into account without disturbing the format used for test interpretation
- Conversion to a MoM value is the starting point for calculating patient-specific risk for neural tube defects, Down's syndrome and other chromosomal abnormalities.

Population parameters – the second component

This second component of the analytic system uses Gaussian distributions of MoM values from unaffected pregnancies and from pregnancies with the condition being screened for. Each of these distributions can be summarized by two parameters; the logarithmic mean MoM (equivalent to the geometric mean, or the median) and the logarithmic standard deviation. The population parameters describe the relationship between the affected

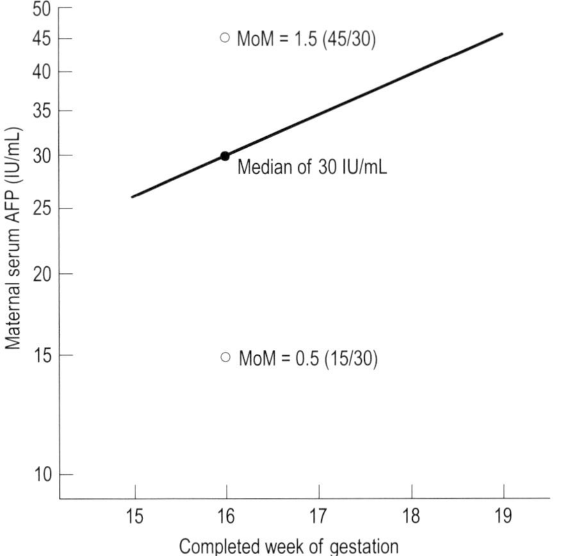

Fig. 19.3 Converting analyte results to multiples of the median (MoM). The completed week of gestation is shown on the horizontal axis while the maternal serum AFP levels are shown on the vertical logarithmic axis. The solid line indicates the results of a log-linear regression analysis generating the smoothed median levels for each week of gestation. The median for 16 weeks is shown as a filled circle. The two open circles represent AFP measurements in two women, with the results in mass units (45 and 15) being converted to MoM units (1.5 and 0.5, respectively).

and unaffected populations and allow direct determination of screening test performance. Most screening programs do not attempt to determine their own parameters but, instead, rely on published parameters derived from carefully conducted studies that have sufficient study subjects to be reliable. This is because establishing reliable parameters for any given analyte requires ascertainment of all affected pregnancies, including those not detected by screening. In addition, the number of affected pregnancies missed by screening (but ascertained at birth) must be adjusted upward to account for spontaneous fetal losses between the time of screening and term (to avoid overestimation of the detection rate). Parameters used by any screening program should be made available for review, upon request.

Determining detection rates, false positive rates and individual risks – the third component

The third component of the analytic system uses the population parameters to determine detection and false positive rates for a single marker at any specified MoM cut-off. For example, if a screening program uses a maternal serum AFP cut-off of 2.5 MoM, the approximate detection rate for open spina bifida is 70% and the false positive rate is 2%. Using a cut-off of 2.0 MoM, that same program would detect 80% of the spina bifida cases, at a 4% false positive rate. AFP standard deviations for both affected and unaffected populations have become smaller since the 1980s, primarily as a result of improved assays and more reliable gestational dating. The net effect has been to reduce the false positive rate at any given AFP MoM cut-off, with little or no adverse effect on the detection rate.

A further analysis involves calculating the odds of being affected given a positive result (OAPR). Using open spina bifida as the example, this calculation combines data derived from the overlapping Gaussian distributions of AFP measurements with knowledge of how frequently open spina bifida occurs in the pregnancy population. In this example, the screening program's AFP cut-off is 2.5 MoM and the frequency of open spina bifida in the population is 1:1000. Overall, 10 women per 10 000 will have an affected pregnancy and the remaining women (9990, or about 10 000) will have unaffected pregnancies. Seven of the 10 women with affected pregnancies will be screen positive (70% detection rate), along with about 200 women with unaffected pregnancies (2% false positive rate). The OAPR in this group of 207 women is 7:200, or about 1:30. The PPV of 7 in 207, or 1 in 31, is almost identical. The detection and false positive rates for the screened population as a whole can be shown visually by drawing a vertical line from the 2.5 MoM cut-off to intersect the overlapping distributions of affected and unaffected populations (Fig. 19.4). The proportions of affected and unaffected populations to the right of that line (the areas under the curves) represent the collective detection and false positive rates for all women with serum AFP values above that cut-off. The OAPR will vary, depending upon factors such as the prevalence of open spina bifida in different geographic locations.

The cumulative OAPR provides useful information for programmatic decision making (e.g. how many diagnostic procedures are needed to detect one case of open spina bifida). For counseling purposes, however, it is important to calculate individualized OAPR (risk), based on a woman's specific MoM value, because her risk will be greater at a higher AFP MoM.

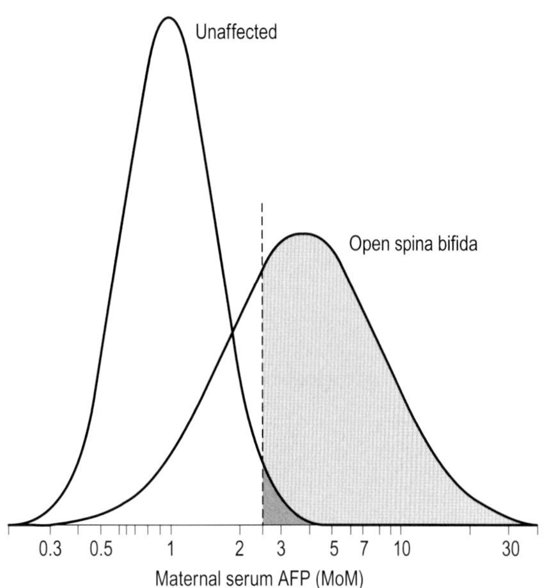

Fig. 19.4 Overlapping distributions of maternal serum AFP (MSAFP) levels in unaffected pregnancies and pregnancies affected with open spina bifida, showing the collective detection and false positive rates. The collective detection and false positive rates for open spina bifida screening can be visualized by using a vertical (dashed) line drawn at the screening cut-off level on the relative distributions of the two populations (i.e. the areas under each curve are equivalent). The large shaded area indicates the proportion of open spina bifida pregnancies detected (detection rate of 70%). The small darker area indicates the proportion of unaffected pregnancies with levels above the cut-off (false positive rate of 2%).

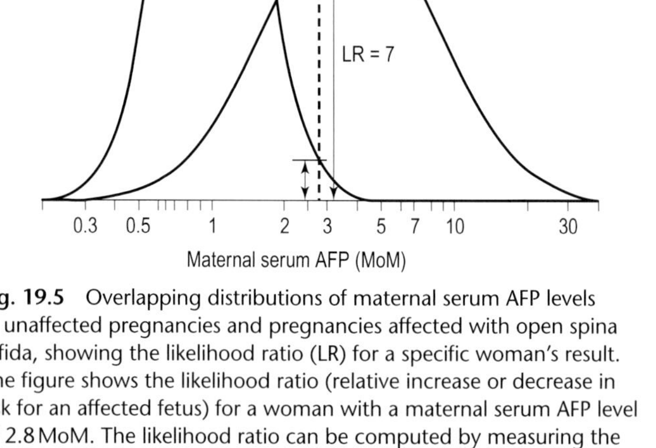

Fig. 19.5 Overlapping distributions of maternal serum AFP levels in unaffected pregnancies and pregnancies affected with open spina bifida, showing the likelihood ratio (LR) for a specific woman's result. The figure shows the likelihood ratio (relative increase or decrease in risk for an affected fetus) for a woman with a maternal serum AFP level of 2.8 MoM. The likelihood ratio can be computed by measuring the height of each curve (open spina bifida and unaffected). In this example, the height of the affected curve is seven times higher than that of the unaffected curve.

An AFP MoM value of 4.5, for example, carries a considerably higher risk than a value of 2.6 MoM.

Individualized risks are calculated by multiplying the population risk for open spina bifida by a likelihood ratio. The likelihood ratio is calculated from measurements of the distances from the baseline at the specified AFP MoM to the points of intersection with the respective Gaussian curves. Figure 19.5 graphically displays these distances for a woman with an AFP of 2.8 MoM. The distance to the intersection with the curve of affected pregnancies is seven times greater than the distance to the curve of unaffected pregnancies, yielding a likelihood ratio (LR) of seven. This means that the woman is seven times more likely to have an affected pregnancy than women in the general population. If the population background prevalence is one per 1000, the woman's individual risk is 7:1000 or about 1:140 (positive predictive value (PPV) of 1 in 141). Individualized risk for Down's syndrome using multiple markers, discussed later, is also calculated by multiplying risk (based on maternal age) by a likelihood ratio, which is calculated by combining measurements (expressed as MoM) for each marker used in the screening protocol.

In addition to developing the mathematical principles of screening and presenting a rational system upon which to base screening policy decisions, the First UK Collaborative Study also defined the optimal time in gestation for open spina bifida screening (16–18 weeks) and the boundaries beyond which screening was either ineffective (<15 weeks) or not feasible due to constraints on follow-up diagnostic testing and decision making (>21 or 22 weeks).

SCREENING FOR DOWN'S SYNDROME

The relationship between maternal age and Down's syndrome

The relationship between a pregnant woman's age and her risk for a Down's syndrome birth was first reported in the early 1950s by LS Penrose. Since then, observational studies have aimed to estimate more accurately this risk by year of maternal age[41,42]. Among the three more recent studies that performed summary analyses of published age-specific data[43–46], there is good agreement on risk estimates for pregnant women between the ages of 20 and 45. The curve fit for the largest, and most up-to-date, study is shown in Figure 19.6. Birth prevalence (solid curve in Fig. 19.6) increases from about 1:1500 in 20-year-old women to about 1:900 in 30-year-old women. Thereafter, birth prevalence increases more rapidly, reaching about 1:350 by age 35 (indicated by the thin vertical and lower horizontal line), 1:85 by age 40 and 1:35 by age 45. The most recent data suggest that birth prevalence does not increase appreciably after age 45 (not shown on Fig. 19.6).

Gestational age also influences the risk for a woman to have a pregnancy affected by Down's syndrome, because a greater proportion of Down's syndrome pregnancies is spontaneously lost than normal pregnancies. Historically, the best estimates of this preferential fetal loss have been derived by comparing the birth prevalence with the prevalence found at the time when diagnostic testing is performed (i.e. amniocentesis at 16 weeks',

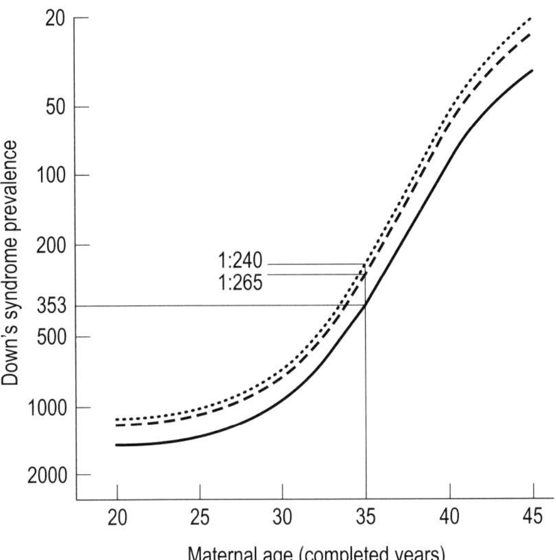

Fig. 19.6 Maternal age-associated Down's syndrome risk at three times in gestation. The solid line in the figure shows the relationship between maternal age (x-axis) and Down's syndrome birth prevalence (as an odds) on the logarithmic y-axis. The vertical thin line at 35 completed years of age shows the associated birth prevalence of 1:353. The dashed line shows the corresponding prevalence at the time of amniocentesis (about 16 weeks' gestation). For a 35-year-old woman, this risk is about 1:265. The dotted line shows the corresponding prevalence at the time of CVS (about 10 weeks' gestation). For a 35-year-old woman, this risk is about 1:240. The text contains sufficient information to derive corresponding numbers for any maternal age.

or chorionic villus sampling (CVS) at 10 weeks' gestation) – most often in women age 35 and older. An estimated 23% of Down's syndrome pregnancies are lost spontaneously between 16 weeks and term, while 43% are lost between 10 weeks and term[47]. Thus, risks will be higher for any given maternal age, the earlier in pregnancy that testing is performed. Furthermore, the most recent information suggests that older women with an affected pregnancy will experience a spontaneous loss more often than younger women[48]. At age 25, for example, the estimated loss rates from 10 and 16 weeks' gestation onwards are 23% and 19%, respectively. At age 35, these rates increase to 32% and 25%, while at age 45, the rates are 44% and 33%. Figure 19.6 shows two additional maternal age-related curves appropriate for women at about 10 weeks' gestation (dotted curve) and at 16 weeks' gestation (dashed curve). The corresponding risks (shown by the thin horizontal lines) are 1:265 and 1:240, respectively. Table 19.1 contains these three sets of risks by maternal age in completed years that could be used for counseling.

Over the past two decades, both the average maternal age at delivery and the proportion of deliveries to women age 35 and older have been increasing[49]. In 1980, for example, the mean age at delivery in the USA was 25.0 years, with about 5% of women age 35 and older. These values increased to 26.4 years and 9% in 1990, and 27.2 years and 13% in 2000. The mean age at delivery, however, differs by country, ranging, in 2000, from a low of 24 years in the Slovak Republic to 29 years in Switzerland. Maternal age distributions also differ by maternal race in the USA. Among African Americans, non-Hispanic Caucasians and Asian Americans, the average maternal ages at delivery were approximately, 25, 27 and 30 years, respectively. Although no definitive study has been reported, there do not appear to be substantial differences in the age-associated risk of Down's syndrome by maternal race. For now, the a priori Down's syndrome risk is determined by the woman's age at the estimated time of delivery and her gestational age at the time of risk calculation, and this is the basis for all further risk calculations that will be described in the following sections.

Table 19.1 **Maternal age-specific Down's syndrome risks at three times in pregnancy**

Maternal age (completed years)	*Down's syndrome risk (1:n) at*		
	Term[1]	*16 weeks*[2]	*10 weeks*[3]
20	1477	1211	1152
21	1461	1184	1125
22	1441	1168	1110
23	1415	1147	1090
24	1382	1120	1064
25	1340	1085	1032
26	1287	1029	978
27	1221	977	928
28	1141	901	856
29	1047	827	775
30	939	733	686
31	821	632	591
32	696	536	494
33	572	435	401
34	456	346	315
35	353	265	240
36	267	197	179
37	199	147	131
38	148	108	96
39	111	80	71
40	85	60	53
41	67	47	41
42	54	38	32
43	45	31	27
44	39	26	22
45	35	23	19

[1]Using Morris JK et al.,[45] where $P = 1/((1 + \exp^{(7.330-4.211)})/(1 + \exp^{(-0.282*(\text{age}-37.23))}))$; [2]adjusted using fetal loss rates from Table 1[48]

Until recently, it was recommended that a woman's age be used as a screening test for Down's syndrome and that the age of 35 years at delivery be used as a cut-off level for offering amniocentesis or CVS. However, an important upward shift in maternal age at delivery has occurred between 1980 and 2000, and this has substantially influenced both the detection and false positive rates at that age cut-off. In 1980, women age 35 and older accounted for about 5% of all pregnancies, and all of these women were candidates for diagnostic testing. The false positive rate for using age as a screening test was thus about 5%, at that time (after the cases of Down's syndrome were subtracted). The associated detection rate was about 25%, meaning that 25% of all Down's syndrome pregnancies occurred among women age 35 and older. In 1990, the false positive rate increased to 9% and the detection rate to 42%. In 2000, these rates were 13% and 54%, respectively. The emergence of other, more efficient screening strategies in recent years now makes it possible to achieve a higher detection of Down's syndrome, in combination with a considerably lower false positive rate, as described elsewhere in this chapter. As a consequence, a fixed maternal age cut-off level (e.g. age 35 or older at term) is no longer recommended as a Down's syndrome screening test[50].

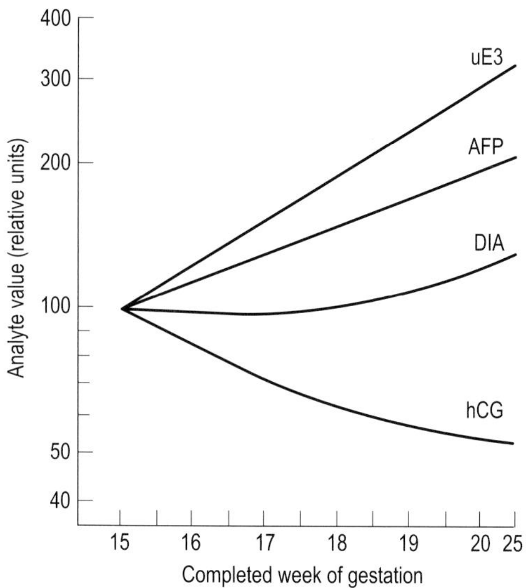

Fig. 19.7 Median levels of maternal serum markers used in second-trimester screening for unaffected pregnancies. The four second-trimester markers (uE3 = unconjugated estriol, AFP = alpha-fetoprotein, DIA = dimeric inhibin-A and hCG = human chorionic gonadotropin). Each marker change over the 15–20-week gestational age range is shown relative to the value observed at 15 weeks' gestation (100 units). For example, the AFP measurements increase 15% per week. Levels of DIA are less influenced by gestational age at collection than the other three markers.

Second-trimester serum screening for Down's syndrome

Markers in the second trimester

The possibility that analytes measured in maternal serum might be useful in risk assessment of Down's syndrome was first demonstrated in 1984, when serum AFP levels were found to be lower in the presence of this chromosome disorder[8]. The index case in this discovery was a woman who delivered an infant with trisomy 18. Serum AFP had been measured in the second trimester to screen for open defects, and the AFP value was very low. Based on this clue, Merkatz and colleagues examined AFP levels in pregnancies with fetal chromosomal abnormalities. They found maternal serum AFP levels to be lower in both Down's syndrome and trisomy 18 pregnancies than in unaffected pregnancies. A second retrospective observational study not only confirmed this observation, but also determined that AFP and maternal age were independent indicators of risk, thereby allowing an algorithm to be developed that assigned Down's syndrome risks to younger women for screening purposes, for the first time[9].

In the late 1980s, human chorionic gonadotropin (hCG), a placental product, was found to be elevated, and unconjugated estriol (uE3), a product of the fetoplacental unit, was found to be low in maternal serum from Down's syndrome pregnancies in the second trimester[10–12,51]. As a consequence, a more effective algorithm that used AFP, uE3, and hCG in combination with maternal age (the so-called triple test) was developed and introduced for routine screening purposes[12]. In 1994, the placental product, dimeric inhibin A (DIA), was found to be elevated in maternal sera during the second trimester, in the presence of Down's syndrome[52], leading to the development of a quadruple marker algorithm[14].

Marker distributions and univariate performance

Patterns of change in maternal serum marker levels are well characterized during the second trimester (15–20 weeks' gestation) (Fig. 19.7). AFP and uE3 increase in concentration in a log-linear fashion, AFP at a rate of about 15% per week and uE3 at a rate of about 25% per week. Levels of hCG decrease non-linearly, reaching a low plateau by about 19 weeks. In contrast, DIA levels have a shallow U-shaped pattern, with a nadir at 17 gestational weeks.

As with AFP in screening for neural tube defects, the effect of gestational age is normalized by establishing day-specific medians for each of the markers and by dividing each woman's value by the appropriate median to calculate the MoM. In Down's syndrome pregnancies, approximate median MoM values for AFP, uE3, hCG and DIA are 0.7, 0.7, 2.0 and 2.0, respectively.

The distribution of MoM values can then be compared in unaffected and Down's syndrome pregnancies, as shown in Figure 19.8. For a given marker, the shape of a distribution (unaffected or Down's syndrome) is defined by the mean of the log MoM values (comparable to the median MoM) and the corresponding standard deviation of the log MoM values. The overlapping distributions allow us to judge the degree of separation between unaffected and Down's syndrome populations for each marker. Univariately, hCG and DIA are the most effective second-trimester markers (approximately 45% DR at a 5% FPR), uE3 is next best (approximately 35% DR at a 5% FPR), and AFP is least effective (approximately 25% DR at a 5% FPR).

Variants of hCG as second trimester markers

In 1987, the free-alpha subunit of hCG was found to be elevated in Down's syndrome pregnancies[10], followed by free-beta hCG in 1990, and hyperglycosylated hCG (found predominantly in choriocarcinoma) in 1999. The latter two variants were proposed to be superior to hCG as maternal serum markers for Down's syndrome[53,54]. In Down's syndrome pregnancies, the median free-alpha hCG value is approximately 1.3 MoM, and its univariate performance is similar to that of AFP[55]. Median values for free-beta hCG (2.3 MoM) and hyperglycosylated

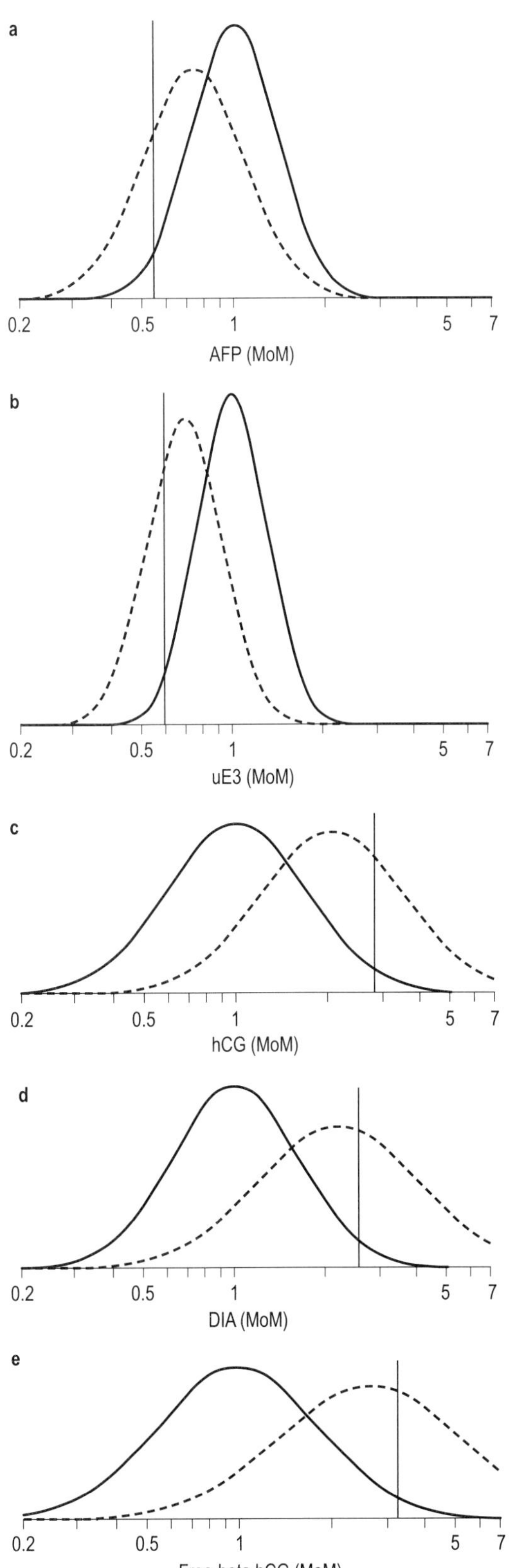

Fig. 19.8 The distributions of second-trimester maternal serum levels of AFP, uE3, hCG, dimeric inhibin A and free-beta hCG in unaffected and Down's syndrome pregnancies. The distributions of these measurements in unaffected pregnancies are shown with solid lines; Down's syndrome pregnancies with dashed lines. The vertical lines drawn from each baseline indicate a false positive rate of 5%, resulting in detection rates for (a) AFP, (b) uE3, (c) hCG, (d) DIA and (e) free-beta hCG of 25%, 35%, 45%, 45% and 45%, respectively.

hCG (3.5 MoM) in Down's syndrome pregnancies are higher than for hCG (2.0 MoM), but their distributions are broader, with the result that univariate performance among the three markers is similar. Reference ranges and overlapping distributions for free-beta hCG are also contained in Figure 19.8; this marker will perform similarly to hCG and DIA (approximately 45% DR at a 5% FPR).

Multiple markers, likelihood ratios and risk calculation

As described for AFP in screening for open spina bifida, the overlapping distributions allow a likelihood ratio for Down's syndrome to be calculated for a given marker level. With the knowledge that the serum marker values are largely (but not totally) independent of each other, the likelihood ratios for each marker in an individual can be combined by multiplying them together and accounting for the correlations between each marker pair in affected and unaffected pregnancies. The composite likelihood ratio is multiplied by the maternal age-related risk to give a final patient-specific risk. This statistical algorithm is known as multivariate Gaussian distribution analysis. Usually, but not always, correlations between marker pairs attenuate the final, group likelihood ratio, so that simply multiplying the likelihood ratios together is not sufficient.

Figure 19.9 shows the likelihood ratios and risks that will be calculated for three different combinations of quadruple marker values in a 30-year-old woman. In the first example, the MoM value for each marker is in the direction of higher risk (each likelihood ratio is greater than 1). This woman's risk of 1 in 733 (based on age) increases to 1 in 55, as a result of testing. In the second, the MoM value for each marker is located at the point of intersection between the unaffected and Down's syndrome curves. In this case, each likelihood ratio is 1, and the combination of measurements yields a risk for Down's syndrome equal to the age-related risk of 1 in 733. In the third example, the MoM value for each marker is 1.00, the most common result in unaffected pregnancies (each likelihood ratio less than 1). This combination of measurements lowers the risk to 1 in 9500.

Second-trimester screening performance

An easy to remember estimate of screening performance (detection rate at a 5% false positive rate) using combinations of second trimester markers with maternal age is: double markers (AFP + hCG) – 60%; triple markers (AFP + hCG + uE3) – 70%; quadruple markers (AFP + hCG + uE3 + inhibin A) – 80%. These estimates are based on results from several carefully constructed case-control studies and two recent clinical trials[14,56–58]. They assume that gestational age is estimated by ultrasound, rather than last menstrual period, and that marker values are adjusted for maternal weight. A more detailed discussion of recent clinical trial results is presented later in this chapter.

First-trimester serum and ultrasound screening for Down's syndrome

The desire for earlier screening

Screening in the first trimester is desirable for reasons of patient privacy and the greater availability and safety of pregnancy

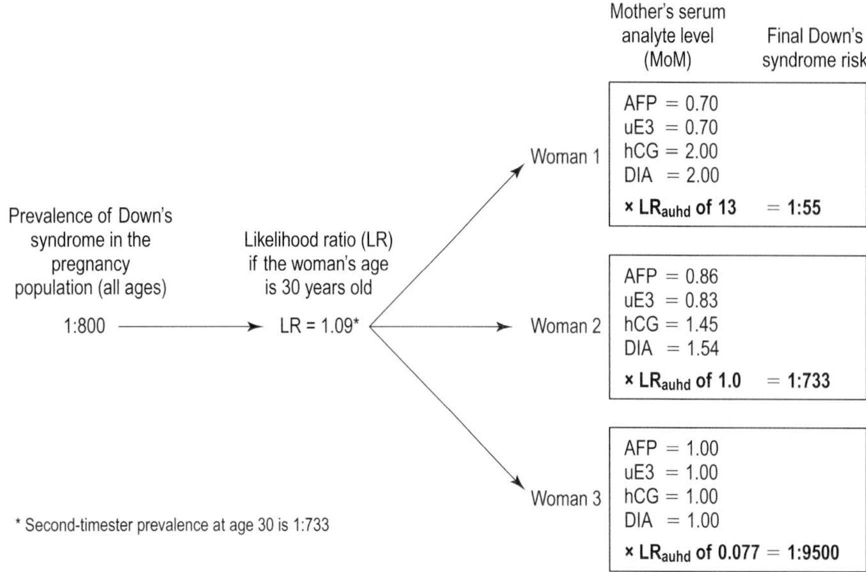

Fig. 19.9 The process of computing Down's syndrome risk for three 30-year-old women with different levels of AFP, uE3, hCG, and DIA. The three examples provide some insight into how extensively the biochemical measurements can alter a pregnant woman's age-related risk for Down's syndrome.

termination procedures. However, certain issues must be satisfied to justify a move to earlier screening:

1. the first-trimester screening test is at least as good as available second-trimester tests
2. the earlier screening test is readily accessible
3. diagnostic testing for women with a first-trimester *screen positive* result is acceptable and readily available.

Serum markers in the first trimester

Second-trimester serum screening markers have been evaluated to determine how they perform in the first trimester[59,60]. Univariately, free-beta hCG is the most effective of these markers in the first trimester. It is useful as early as 9 gestational weeks and improves in performance as gestation increases[16,57,61]. hCG and inhibin A begin to be informative at 11 weeks, and performance improves steadily during the succeeding 2 weeks[16,57,62]. In contrast, neither AFP nor uE3 is informative in the first trimester.

The most informative first-trimester serum marker is pregnancy-associated plasma protein-A (PAPP-A), a large glycoprotein tetramer secreted by the placenta[63]. On average, PAPP-A is about 2 to 2.5 times lower in Down's syndrome than in unaffected pregnancies (0.4–0.6 MoM). It is most effective at 8 and 9 weeks. Thereafter, median PAPP-A values in affected pregnancies move progressively toward 1.0 MoM and this marker is no longer useful by 14–15 weeks[16,57,61,64]. Figure 19.10 shows gestational age-related changes in median levels for each of the first trimester markers among pregnancies with Down's syndrome.

Ultrasound measurement of fetal nuchal translucency (NT)

The measurement of fetal NT in the first trimester is discussed in detail by Breathnach and Malone in Chapter 20 of this text. In screening for Down's syndrome, NT is usually measured between the 11th and 13th gestational week (measurement as early as the 10th week may be acceptable). NT normally increases with gestation in a log-linear fashion (as calibrated by increasing crown–rump length). This gestational age effect is taken into account by dividing an individual's NT millimeter value by the median NT established for the corresponding crown–rump length, thereby converting it to MoM.

NT performance as a Down's syndrome marker declines slowly between 10 and 13 weeks' gestation, although, on average, the NT level in Down's syndrome cases is approximately 2.0 MoM. This level is proportionally similar to the increased and decreased levels seen, on average, for second trimester hCG, free-beta hCG, inhibin A and first trimester PAPP-A (two times lower). In spite of this, however, NT is more effective than these serum markers, because the distribution of NT values in unaffected pregnancies (as measured by the standard deviation) is considerably narrower. In Figure 19.11, the overlapping distributions in unaffected and affected pregnancies are shown for each of the first-trimester markers at 12 weeks' gestation. The much narrower NT distribution among unaffected pregnancies yields a considerably lower false positive rate for a comparable detection rate. For example, at a 50% detection rate, the false positive rate for hCG or inhibin A is in the range of 5% to 8%, but the false positive rate for NT is under 2%.

The issue of what reference data are best used to normalize NT measurement is currently under review. The Fetal Medicine Foundation has long proposed that a single set of NT medians, based on tens of thousands of data points, be used by all sonographers[65]. In that system, the assumption is that all sonographers measure NT in exactly the same way, and that all will obtain the same result. An alternative method, in which individual sonographers or sonography centers establish their own sets of NT medians, was first proposed in a UK study[57] and then used in a USA clinical trial[64]. Both studies showed that, on average, the performance of NT-based screening was improved by using operator- or center-specific medians, rather than a single median equation.

Each method of NT normalization requires ongoing quality review. Quality assurance programs have been, and continue to be, developed to deal with the subjective nature of NT measurement and the need for objective quality maintenance. Quality

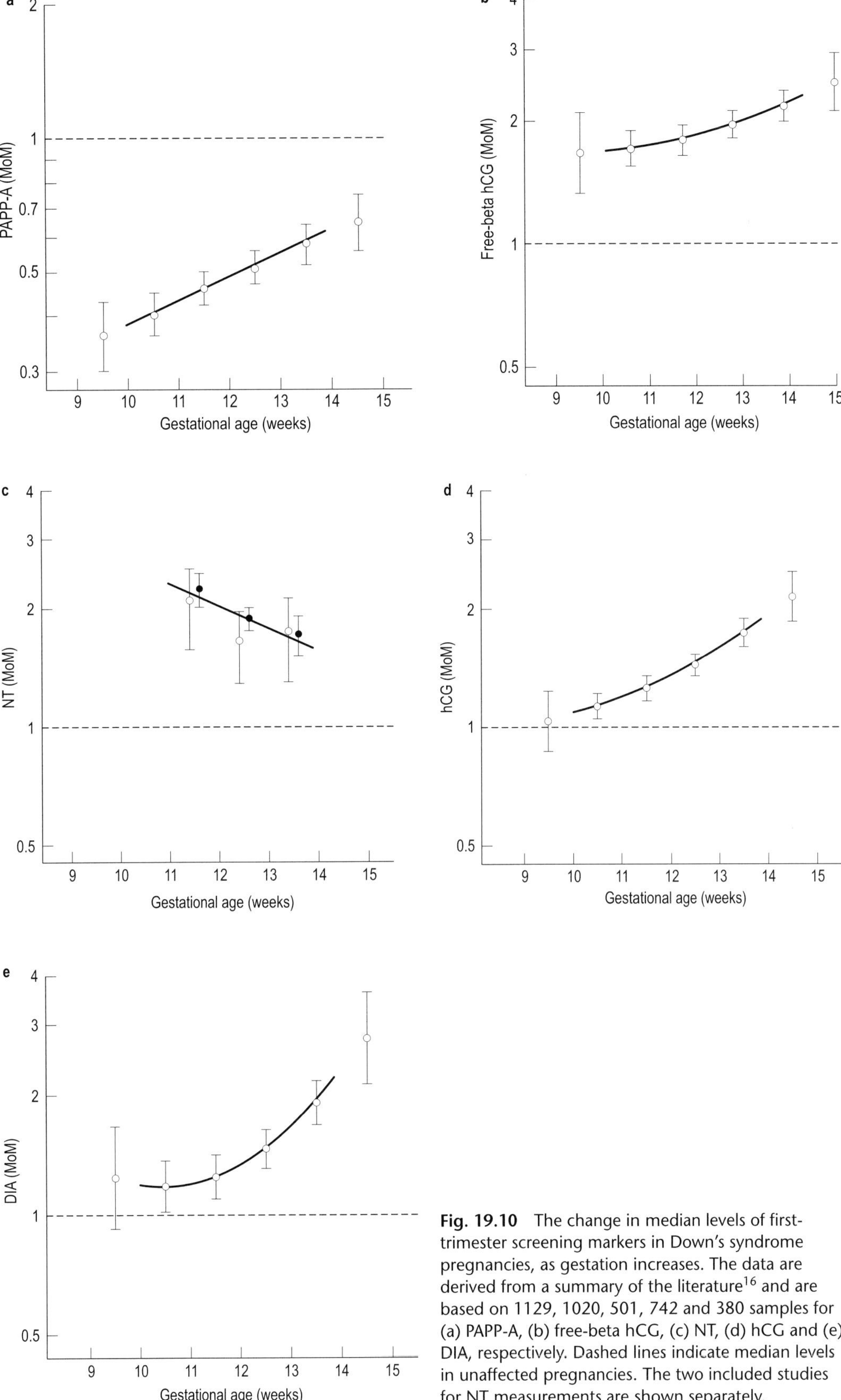

Fig. 19.10 The change in median levels of first-trimester screening markers in Down's syndrome pregnancies, as gestation increases. The data are derived from a summary of the literature[16] and are based on 1129, 1020, 501, 742 and 380 samples for (a) PAPP-A, (b) free-beta hCG, (c) NT, (d) hCG and (e) DIA, respectively. Dashed lines indicate median levels in unaffected pregnancies. The two included studies for NT measurements are shown separately.

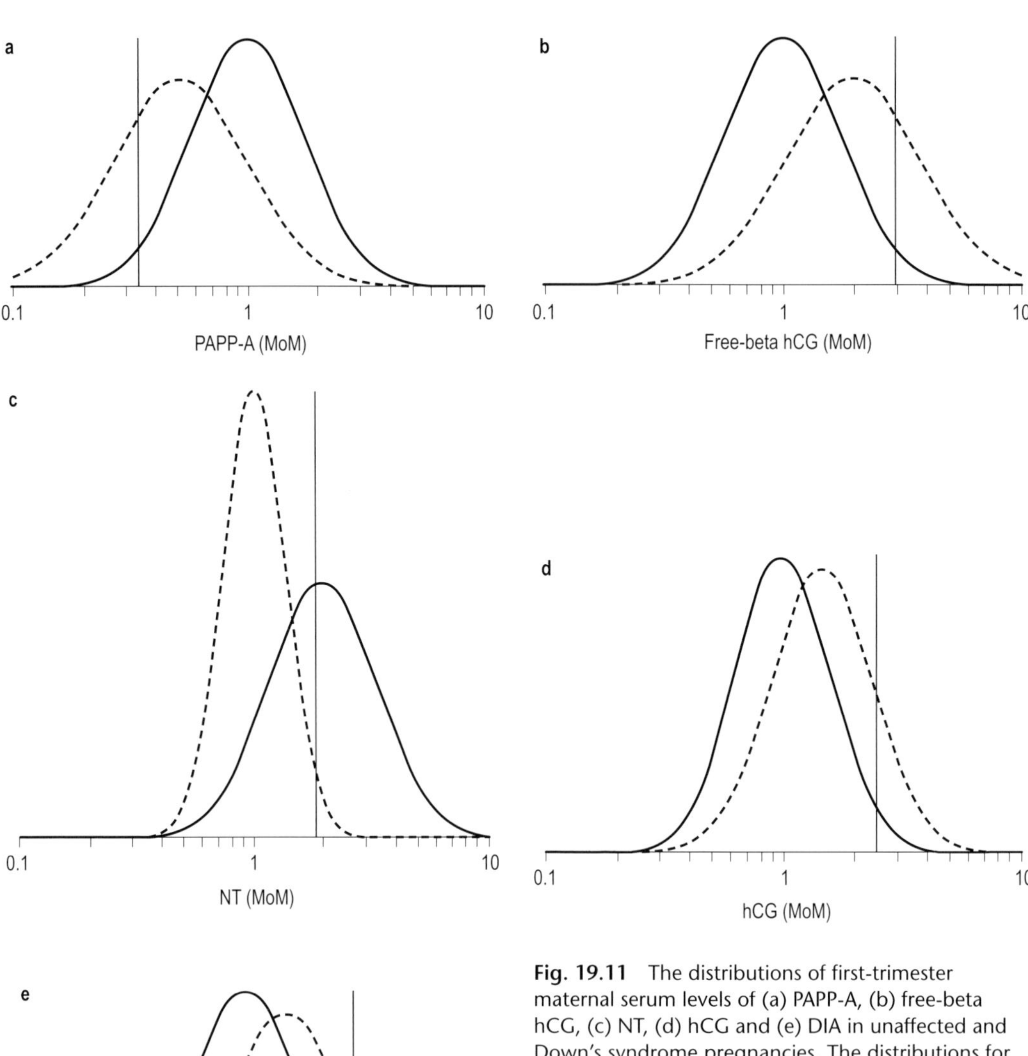

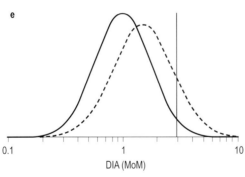

Fig. 19.11 The distributions of first-trimester maternal serum levels of (a) PAPP-A, (b) free-beta hCG, (c) NT, (d) hCG and (e) DIA in unaffected and Down's syndrome pregnancies. The distributions for each marker in unaffected and Down's syndrome pregnancies are shown as solid and dashed curves, respectively. These plots correspond to the parameters reported for 12 completed weeks' gestation.[16] The solid vertical lines drawn from each baseline indicate a false positive rate of 5%. At that false positive rate, the detection rates for PAPP-A, free-beta hCG, hCG, inhibin A and NT are 36%, 37%, 21%, 20% and 61%, respectively.

assurance issues for NT measurement today are reminiscent of those faced more than 20 years ago for serum markers, including the use of medians and calculation of patient-specific risk. For serum screening markers, quality assurance and monitoring, as well as external proficiency testing, have become routine. Similar programs are now being implemented for fetal ultrasound measurements.

First-trimester screening performance

The most widely accepted first-trimester screening method (the 'combined test') calls for offering ultrasound and serum markers together, at 11–13 completed weeks, including NT, serum PAPP-A and free-beta hCG (or hCG itself), in combination with maternal age. The consensus screening performance estimate for this approach is an 83–86% detection rate, at a 5% false positive rate[50,57,64]. Serum markers, or NT alone, do not achieve the performance level of second-trimester serum markers. At a fixed 5% false positive rate, the detection rate for NT with maternal age is approximately 68%, and for the serum markers with maternal age, approximately 63%. Some studies report detection rates of 92–94% for the combined test at a 5% false positive rate[66,67]. It is unclear why these studies show higher performance than expected, but ascertainment and enrolment bias should be considered.

Integrated screening for Down's syndrome

Concept of the integrated test

In 1999, Wald and colleagues proposed that information from first- and second-trimester screening markers be combined into a single risk estimate that utilized information from all of the markers[17]. The 'integrated' screening result is reported only after all the markers have been measured, allowing the collective information to be most effectively used. This single, final estimate of risk keeps the false positive rate at a minimum and avoids confusion that might be caused by releasing potentially conflicting interim results based on partial results (from first-trimester markers). In addition, screening for neural tube defects with AFP in the second trimester is preserved, and assessment of trisomy 18 risk is optimal, with both first- and second-trimester markers contributing to the risk calculation. The risk algorithm for the integrated test is based on known parameters of each marker at its optimal performance time in gestation, and also takes into account correlations among both first- and second-trimester markers. The full form of the integrated test includes NT and PAPP-A measurement in the first trimester and quadruple marker measurement in the second, along with maternal age. When NT measurement is not available, the serum-only form of the integrated test can be offered to estimate patient-specific risk. Free-beta hCG (or hCG) is measured only in the second trimester in the integrated test, because it is a more effective marker at that time. Criticisms of the integrated test center on the policy that interim results, based on first trimester marker values, not be reported and that:

- women would prefer an earlier test
- the requirement to wait until the second trimester for a result is not an advance in screening
- options for termination of pregnancy are safer and less stressful in the late first trimester than in the early second trimester.

These criticisms are moot, if screen-positive women prefer to wait for amniocentesis rather than undergo CVS for diagnostic purposes, and there are indications that this may be the case[68].

Integrated screening performance

At a fixed 5% false positive rate, the detection rate for Down's syndrome is approximately 94% for the full integrated test and 85% for the serum-only integrated test. Thus, the serum integrated test provides women lacking access to NT measurement with a test that is equivalent to the most effective first-trimester test (that includes NT). In practical terms, all screen positive women will be offered an invasive diagnostic procedure, no matter what combination of tests is used. If the screening result is reported early, CVS should be available but, by the end of the first trimester or beginning of the second trimester, amniocentesis is the procedure of choice. Whichever diagnostic test is chosen, the risk of losing the pregnancy due to the procedure is on the order of 0.5–1.0%[69], although most clinicians believe that amniocentesis is safer than CVS[70].

Safety in screening

Now that a screening test can provide a detection rate above 90% at the established 5% false positive rate, it is reasonable to consider reducing the false positive rate so that fewer women will need to consider an invasive diagnostic procedure, whether CVS or amniocentesis. If a new target false positive rate of 2% were to be chosen, 90% of the Down's syndrome cases could be detected, and 60% fewer women would need to consider invasive testing. If a 1% false positive rate were to be set for the full integrated test, an 85% detection rate could still be achieved, and 80% fewer women would need to consider invasive diagnostic testing. That compares favorably with the 5% false positive rate needed to achieve 85% detection, using either the first-trimester combined test or the serum-only integrated test. Any other current screening test would require a 10% or higher false positive rate to achieve that level of detection. Figures 19.12 and 19.13 summarize relative screening performance for various first-trimester, second-trimester and integrated Down's syndrome screening protocols. Figure 19.12 shows detection rates at a fixed false positive rate of 5%, while Figure 19.13 shows false positive rates at a fixed detection rate of 85%. In both figures, the estimates from two large clinical trials are shown for comparison[57,64].

Variants of the integrated test

Since the introduction of the integrated test, various modifications that include aspects of first-trimester screening have been suggested and implemented. The goal has been to maintain the

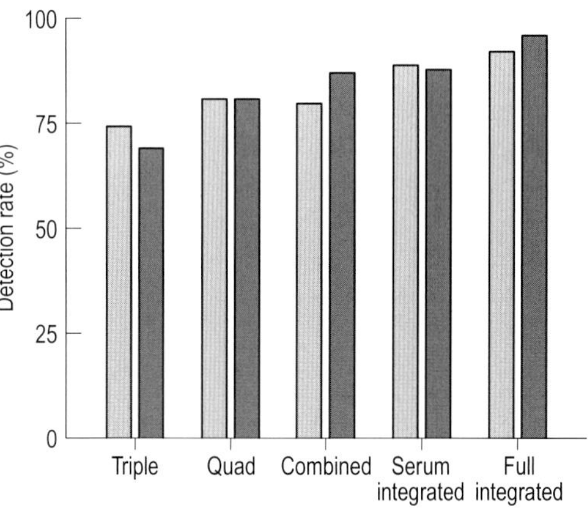

Fig. 19.12 Performance results of various screening tests in the SURUSS and FASTER studies, as shown by detection rates for a fixed 5% false positive rate. The detection rates provided by the SURUSS trial[57] are light gray, while those for the FASTER trial[64] are dark gray.

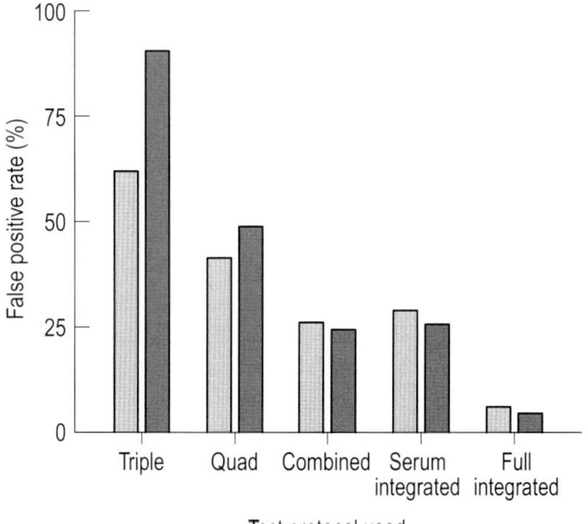

Fig. 19.13 Performance results of various screening tests in the SURUSS and FASTER studies, as shown by false positive rates needed to attain an 85% detection rate. The false positive rates provided by the SURUSS trial[57] are light gray, while those for the FASTER trial[64] are dark gray.

benefits of improved screening performance provided by the integrated test, while allowing for some women to get screening results in the first trimester.

The sequential approach

The most readily achievable variant of the full integrated test is a sequential test, in which the markers measured in the first trimester (either NT and PAPP-A, or NT, PAPP-A and free-beta hCG) are used to assess an interim risk[71–73]. If that interim risk is sufficiently high, such women are informed of their *screen positive* result and offered early diagnostic intervention. All women below the high initial risk cut-off continue on to the second stage of the integrated test and receive a full integrated risk report, with either a screen positive or screen negative result. There are three keys to keeping a sequential test simple and efficient:

1. Set the first-trimester risk cut-off high, so that no more than 1% of screened women will initially be identified as screen positive. A risk cut-off of 1 in 25 yields a *screen positive* rate of 0.5%, while a risk cut-off of 1 in 50 places about 1.0% of screened women in that category.
2. Release only the risks of the *screen positive* women after the first stage, so that the remaining women will not worry about their risk status and will continue to the second stage of the integrated test unencumbered by doubt.
3. Measure only NT and PAPP-A in the first trimester, rather than all three first-trimester combined markers. This will reduce the number of assays needed and will make the test more transparent to the individual being tested, although the first part of the test will be slightly less efficient.

Performance estimates are encouraging for the sequential approach. If the first-stage risk cut-off achieves a 0.5% false positive rate, and the second-stage risk cut-off (typically 1 in 100) achieves a 1.0% false positive rate, approximately 55% of the Down's syndrome cases will be identified at the first stage along with an additional 30% at the second stage, generating an overall detection rate of 85% for a 1.5% false positive rate. This approach appears to provide only slightly lower performance than the full integrated test and allows for a majority of cases to be identified earlier in gestation. Intervention trials will determine if this approach works as well as predicted.

The contingent approach

Another variant of the integrated test that appears to provide efficient screening performance, allow more women to be given an early result, and generate cost savings, is called contingent screening[72–76]. In this test, two risk cut-offs are assigned at the first stage, a very high risk cut-off, as in the sequential approach, and a low risk cut-off. After patient-specific risks are calculated using the first-trimester markers (NT and PAPP-A or NT, PAPP-A and free-beta hCG), three categories of screening results are released:

1. a very high risk, *screen positive* result, as in the sequential test
2. an intermediate risk result (falling between the high and the low risk cut-off) requiring second-trimester screening, with an integrated interpretation
3. a low risk, *screen negative* result, in which no further screening is indicated.

Only those with an intermediate risk are asked to return in the early second trimester to complete the integrated test.

The choice of a risk cut-off to identify the *screen positive* group in the first trimester will again be very high (1 in 25 or 1 in 50). The choice of risk cut-off to identify the *screen negative* group will generally be in the range of 1 in 1000 to 1 in 3000. Using the contingent method, as many as 70–80% of all women screened will be assigned risks below the low cut-off and will thus be provided early reassurance about their risk of Down's syndrome in their pregnancies. The intermediate risk group will be offered the opportunity to complete the integrated test, and a small subset of them will be identified as *screen positive* after the test is completed.

Category 2, the intermediate risk group, comprising between 20 and 30% of all women screened, should also be considered *screen positive*, since these women are alerted to consider further testing (the second stage of the integrated test) and are thereby faced with all the concerns and anxieties that any *screen positive* group might have. In addition, the contingent test protocol calls for all women who complete the first stage of the test to be issued an individualized risk report. With this report in hand, women with a high intermediate risk (e.g. 1 in 55) may opt for diagnostic testing, rather than waiting for the completion of the integrated test, while women with a high negative risk (e.g. 1 in 2100 if the cut-off is 1 in 2000) may request the full integrated test (to get a better risk estimate). This could create considerable confusion and complexity, obviating any cost savings that contingent screening might theoretically offer. As with the sequential approach, intervention trials will determine how well this approach works in a screening environment.

Results of validation trials

The results of a number of independent validation trials have been published within the past 5 years. Two trials have been designed to compare first, second and integrated screening protocols in the same women, while others have focused primarily on first-trimester screening protocols. Only the comparison studies are able to control for biases such as early pregnancy intervention, incomplete ascertainment and the association of abnormal marker values with compromised pregnancies, by comparing pregnancy outcome at the same point after all screening tests have been completed.

The two trials that compared different screening methods were SURUSS (serum, urine, ultrasound study) in the UK[57] and FASTER (first- and second-trimester evaluation of risk) in the USA[64]. SURUSS was an observational study in which more than 48000 women were enrolled and more than 100 Down's syndrome cases ascertained. Serum markers were assayed in a nested case/control set of stored first- and second-trimester samples, and NT ultrasound methods and results were reviewed. In contrast, FASTER was a composite observational and intervention trial, involving more than 36000 women. Once again, more than 100 Down's syndrome cases were ascertained. All women were offered first-trimester screening with NT, PAPP-A and free-beta hCG and were asked to return for second-trimester serum quadruple marker testing. Results were reported only after both the first-trimester combined test and the second-trimester quadruple test were completed. If a woman was *screen positive* by either of the tests, she was offered diagnostic intervention by amniocentesis.

Table 19.2 **Detection rates (DR) of various screening tests in SURUSS and FASTER at fixed false positive rates of 1% and 5%**

	DR (%) in SURUSS		*DR (%) in FASTER*	
Screening test	*@ 1% FPR*	*@ 5% FPR*	*@ 1% FPR*	*@ 5% FPR*
2nd trim triple	56	77	45	70
2nd trim quad	64	83	60	81
1st trim combined	72	86	73	87
Serum integrated	73	87	73	88
Full integrated	86	94	88	96

SURUSS[57,82], FASTER[64]

Table 19.3 **False positive rates of various screening tests in SURUSS and FASTER, needed to attain an 85% detection rate (DR)**

	FPR (%) to attain 85% DR	
Screening test	*in SURUSS*	*in FASTER*
2nd trim triple (15–18 weeks)	9.3	13.6
2nd trim quad (15–18 weeks)	6.2	7.3
1st trim combined		
11 weeks	4.3	3.8
12 weeks	6.0	4.8
13 weeks	7.7	6.8
Serum integrated		
11 weeks	3.9	3.6
12 weeks	4.9	4.4
13 weeks	5.6	5.2
Full integrated		
11 weeks	0.9	0.6
12 weeks	1.3	0.8
13 weeks	2.1	1.2

For tests that include 1st trimester markers, screening performance is shown for each week of gestation[57,64,82]

Tables 19.2 and 19.3 show results from the two studies. In Table 19.2, the detection rates of various screening tests are given at fixed 1% and 5% false positive rate. In Table 19.3, the false positive rates needed to attain a detection rate of 85% are given. The major findings are the striking similarity of results between the two studies and the close approximation of performance estimates of the various tests to those reported in previous studies.

Other clinically useful refinements to screening protocols

Prenatal screening for Down's syndrome is widespread, with more than 2 million women tested each year in the USA alone. Given the amount of data generated, laboratories have identified several important covariates that influence levels of serum analytes used for Down's syndrome (or ONTD) screening. These include, but are not limited to, the method of dating, maternal weight, multiple gestation, family history, maternal race and maternal smoking status. Other covariates reported include maternal diabetic status, fetal sex and assisted reproduction. This section will briefly review five of these.

Method of gestational dating

The most common methods of dating a pregnancy include using the first day of the last menstrual period (LMP) and various ultrasound measurements (US). In the first trimester, dating is usually based on the crown–rump length (CRL) while, in the second, dating can be based on biparietal diameter (BPD) or long bone measurements (e.g. humeral or femur length). It is generally acknowledged that CRL measurements in the first trimester are the most accurate for predicting the date of delivery, usually to within 7 days. As fetuses grow, the variability of ultrasound measurements increases and the reliability decreases, so that the use of multiple ultrasound measurements in the early second trimester is generally considered to be accurate to within about 10 days. On average, US dating of pregnancies results in more accurate assignment of MoM levels (as all Down's syndrome markers vary by gestational age) and this results in more accurate Down's syndrome risk assignments and improved screening performance.

Dating pregnancies solely by BPD aids in the detection of ONTD, due to the artefact described above. In addition, BPD and CRL measurements both reliably reflect gestational age in Down's syndrome pregnancies and these are the ultrasound measurements that should be used for dating, to optimize screening performance. In contrast, the shorter long bone measurements found in Down's syndrome fetuses at any given gestational age may, if used for dating, actually reduce Down's syndrome detection[77], due to the systematically lower risk assigned to affected fetuses.

Maternal weight

As screening became widespread, it soon became apparent that women whose weight was very low were more likely to be screen positive for ONTD, while very heavy women were almost never screen positive. Table 19.4 shows a clear relationship between the AFP median MoM in various weight categories and maternal weight. This is a dilution effect

Table 19.4 **The relationship between maternal weight and maternal serum AFP MoM levels**

Maternal weight		*Number of observations*	*AFP Median (MoM)*
Group	*Average*		
80–99	95	364	1.41
100–119	112	5080	1.23
120–139	130	13450	1.10
140–159	149	12657	1.00
160–179	168	7265	0.93
180–199	188	3919	0.85
200–219	208	2322	0.80
220–239	228	1249	0.75
240–259	248	662	0.70
260–279	268	371	0.67
280–299	288	148	0.64
300–350	316	98	0.61
All	154	47585	1.00

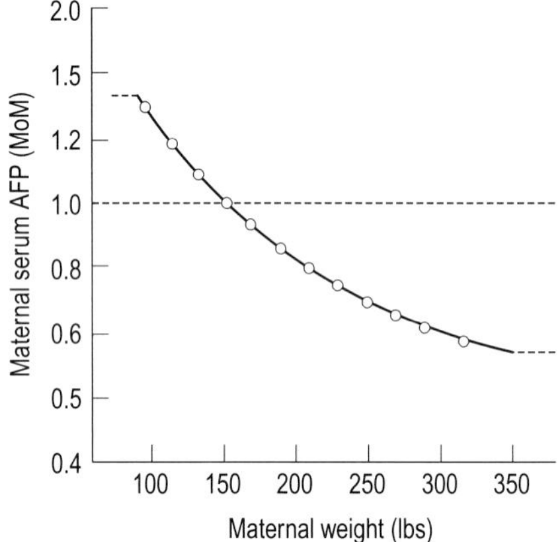

Fig. 19.14 The relationship between maternal weight and maternal serum AFP measurements. The maternal weights (in categories) are plotted on the horizontal axis with the corresponding median AFP values on the logarithmic vertical axis. The curved line shows the fitted regression line. The dashed line at 1.0 MoM indicates the overall average AFP level in the population studied. The horizontal dotted lines show truncation limits used for computing the expected AFP MoM at extreme maternal weights (<90 pounds and >350 pounds).

(a constant amount of AFP produced by the fetus diluted into a varying maternal blood volume). Figure 19.14 is a graphic display of the relationship, with a fitted curve based on a reciprocal model (expected MoM = 106.68*(1/weight-in-pounds) +0.282). Maternal weight adjustment of serum analytes is done by dividing the unadjusted MoM level by the expected median MoM level for that woman's weight. One woman in Figure 19.3 has an observed AFP value of 0.5 MoM. If she weighed 200 pounds, the median MoM value for that weight category

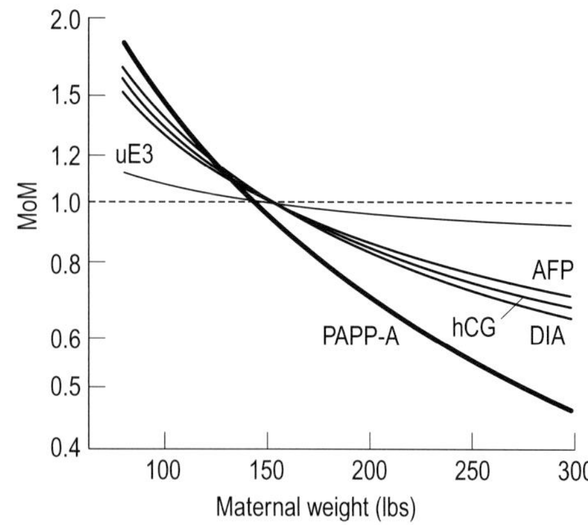

Fig. 19.15 The relationship between selected serum markers and maternal weight. The figure shows three distinctly different maternal weight effects. The strongest relationship is with PAPP-A; the weakest with uE3. Most other markers, including AFP, hCG and DIA are intermediate.

would be 0.82 (106.68 * 1/200 + 0.282). Her weight adjusted MoM, therefore, would be 0.61 (0.5/0.82).

The effect of maternal weight has also been studied for the other serum markers. Figure 19.15 shows the maternal weight effect for several maternal serum screening markers. Performing weight adjustment routinely will result in more accurate risk assignments and improved Down's syndrome detection, as well as improved ONTD and trisomy 18 detection (see below). Preliminary data (not shown) indicate the maternal weight effect for a given marker is similar between trimesters (e.g. the maternal weight relationship for hCG is the same in the first and second trimesters).

Multiple gestation

Serum marker levels in multiple gestations represent contributions from all of the fetuses. This is borne out in studies of average analyte levels in twin pregnancies, where median levels are about 2.0 MoM, compared to 1.0 MoM in singleton pregnancies. uE3 is an exception; the observed level in unaffected twin pregnancies is about 1.7 MoM. Twin pregnancies are most often discordant for Down's syndrome. Algorithms to assign 'pseudo risks' for twin pregnancies have been implemented successfully, but serum markers are considerably less good in predicting Down's syndrome risk in twin pregnancies.

Unlike serum markers, NT measurements are fetal-specific, allowing separate risks to be assigned for each fetus. Using chorionicity as a surrogate for zygosity, the two NT measurements in a monochorionic pregnancy can be considered a repeated measure, with the average NT (or geometric mean) being used as the estimate for the pregnancy. In a dichorionic pregnancy, each fetus is assigned a separate risk and the pregnancy's risk is the sum of the two.

Family history

Women with a personal (or family) history of Down's syndrome (or other chromosomal abnormality) have a higher recurrence risk[78]. About 95% of Down's syndrome pregnancies have a trisomy 21 karyotype and the additive risk in such circumstances is approximately 0.54% (about 1:200). If the previous Down's syndrome pregnancy was caused by an unbalanced translocation, the recurrence risk will depend on the origin of the translocation (i.e. de novo, maternal or paternal).

Maternal race/ethnicity

Virtually all data regarding maternal race are based on self-reporting. When comparing marker levels between racial groups, it is important to account for other systematic differences, such as maternal weight. As a group, Asian Americans are lightest (about 135 pounds), followed by Hispanic and non-Hispanic Caucasians (about 150 pounds) and African Americans (about 165 pounds). These differences in weight (along with any differences in other important covariates, such as method of dating) need to be accounted for in any analysis of race/ethnicity. Important differences in analyte levels by race (without adjustment for maternal weight) have been reported for African Americans (10–20% higher AFP and hCG levels and 10% lower DIA levels)[79]. Among Asian Americans, hCG levels are about 12% higher. Effects for other analytes/racial groups are either smaller or have not been studied extensively. Some screening programs routinely adjust analyte levels for maternal race (e.g. divide AFP MoM levels by 1.15 if the woman reports being African American), or derive separate reference data (medians) by race/ethnicity.

Maternal smoking status

First- and second-trimester hCG and free-beta hCG levels are about 25% lower in smokers and DIA measurements are 50–60% higher[80]. This effect is independent of cigarettes smoked and is consistent across the gestational weeks. Although the effect on the analyte levels is large, the effect on the Down's syndrome risk is less extreme because of a 'canceling' effect; lower hCG measurements are associated with decreased risks, while higher DIA measurements are associated with increased risk. While early reports suggested a lower age-associated risk of Down's syndrome among smokers, more recent studies do not support this observation[81].

Risk cut-off levels in Down's syndrome screening

Selecting risk cut-off levels and examining the trade off

Screening programs throughout the world have adopted a variety of Down's syndrome risk cut-off levels, such as a term risk of 1:250 (Britain)[82], a term risk of 1:300 (Germany)[83], a second-trimester risk of 1:295 (Japan)[84] and, in the USA, a second-trimester risk of 1:270[85]. The rationale for choosing the risk cut-off of 1:270 in the USA was its equivalence to the 35-year-old age cut-off used for Down's syndrome screening based on maternal age[85]. This, in turn, was chosen in the 1970s because it best approximated the risk of miscarriage resulting from amniocentesis. Prior practice not only drove the choice of a cut-off level for serum screening, but also represented for many the 'correct' risk for screening, including newer protocols that incorporate nuchal translucency measurements. Other programs make choices based on keeping the number of invasive diagnostic procedures within reasonable limits, typically 5–10%, taking into account limits in resources available for both the screening and diagnostic steps.

Selecting a risk cut-off level makes explicit the choice that must be made between increasing the detection rate versus reducing false positives, as improved Down's syndrome screening protocols are developed. Some have argued that current cut-offs should be retained to maintain consistency and avoid confusion. This approach fails to take advantage of the relatively large reduction in the false positive rate with only a marginal loss in the detection rate that can be achieved by raising the risk cut-off level.

Risk cut-off levels for specific screening combinations

These trade-offs can be appreciated by examining tests that can achieve at least an 80% detection rate at a 5% false positive rate (quadruple, combined, serum integrated and full integrated testing) at selected risk cut-off levels (Table 19.5). The data in Table 19.5 are based on the findings reported in SURUSS. Most screening programs in the USA have continued to use the risk of a 35-year-old woman as a cut-off for the combined test (approximately 1:215 in the first trimester, 1:300 in the second), which yields a detection of 84% for a 5.5% false positive rate. If the risk cut-off level were reset to 1:179, the detection rate would remain essentially unchanged (83%), but the false positive rate would be reduced to 4.7%. Lowering the cut-off level further to 1:143 would slightly reduce detection to 81%, but would significantly reduce false positives to 3.8%. The impact of adjusting the risk cut-off level for integrated testing is even more dramatic. If the 1:300 second-trimester risk is used, detection is 91% at a 3.4% false positive rate. A cut-off level of 1:200

Table 19.5 **Down's syndrome detection rates (DR) and false positive rates (FPR) for four screening strategies at three risk cut-off levels[1]**

	Second trimester Down's syndrome risk cut-off level (first trimester)					
	1:200 (1:143)		*1:250 (1:179)*		*1:300 (1:215)*	
	DR	*FPR*	*DR*	*FPR*	*DR*	*FPR*
Quadruple	82	4.7	84	5.7	86	6.6
Combined	81	3.8	83	4.7	84	5.5
Serum integrated	83	4.1	85	5.0	86	5.8
Integrated	89	2.4	90	3.0	91	3.4

[1]An expanded version of this table is available in the SURUSS report[57]

lowers detection slightly to 89%, but the corresponding false positive rate is lowered to 2.4% (a reduction of 29%).

Internal quality control and external quality assessment

Selecting kits

Maternal serum screening markers are measured by immunoassays. The protein analytes AFP, hCG and its free-beta subunit, PAPP-A and dimeric inhibin A are almost always measured by two-site immunometric assays using monoclonal antibodies. This method allows for a wide concentration range, high analytic sensitivity and high specificity. The commercial assays are highly correlated with each other (with occasional exceptions), but there are systematic differences in mass unit values of 10–50% between manufacturers. These differences are unimportant, provided kit-specific median values are used to calculate patient-specific multiples of the median, as described earlier. In general, all of the immunoassays perform well, but it is the laboratory's responsibility to monitor their performance to identify systematic shifts attributable to new reagent lots, instrument maintenance or updates, or standard recalibration by the manufacturer, and take appropriate action, as needed[86]. Methods for performing internal quality control have been promulgated by professional organizations, such as the College of American Pathologists, Clinical and Laboratory Standards Institute (formerly NCCLS) and the American College of Medical Genetics[86–88].

Epidemiologic monitoring

A powerful adjunct to these traditional methods is epidemiologic monitoring[89]. This process uses data gathered from the screened population as a quality control measure, e.g. the screen positive rate. This is variously called the false positive rate, the initial positive rate, or the positive rate and is readily determined by screening programs. Screen positive rates should fall within specified limits for any given marker protocol. In screening for open spina bifida, the screen positive rate is the percentage of women with an AFP MoM value equal to or above a MoM cut-off. For example, at a cut-off of 2.0 MoM, the screen positive rate should be between 3 and 5%, and rates outside of this range need to be investigated. A positive rate of 7% indicates that the AFP median values are too low, thereby causing inappropriately high MoM values to be assigned to individual women. Determination of the detection rate is beyond the capabilities of most programs.

In Down's syndrome screening, the screen positive rate is the percentage of women with a risk equal to, or greater than, a specified cut-off level. The positive rate is influenced by all of the analytes used in the risk calculation and therefore does not provide information on which analyte(s) are responsible, if this rate is too high or too low. Consequently, it is necessary to monitor each assay separately. This is accomplished by determining the median of all of the MoM values from the screened population. If median values are correct, the median MoM (the grand MoM) will by definition be 1.0, within statistical limits. In addition to demonstrating that a new set of medians is correct, the grand MoM is used on an ongoing basis to identify assay shifts due to new kit lots or instrument recalibration. Figure 19.16 shows an example of this monitoring for AFP over

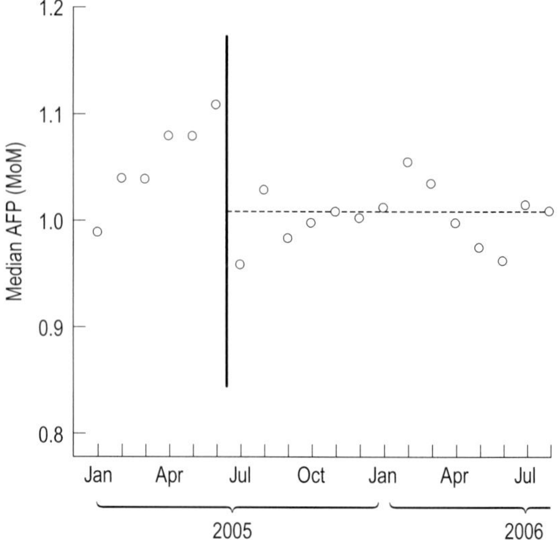

Fig. 19.16 Epidemiologic monitoring of the maternal serum AFP MoM level. Each monthly median AFP MoM level is indicated by an open circle. In the first half of 2005, a trend toward higher values is evident. In June (solid vertical line), new medians were computed. Over the next 14 months, the median AFP MoM was acceptable, with random fluctuations around an average of 1.02.

an 18-month time period. The monthly grand MoM is steadily rising, because the assay is yielding lower and lower AFP values, as the reagents age. In June 2005, the medians were adjusted and the median MoM fell back to more acceptable limits. In practice, each analyte, including nuchal translucency measurement, is monitored in the same way. Deviations from the expected 1.0 MoM, typically outside the limits of 0.90 and 1.10, require that corrective action be taken.

Although monitoring the grand MoM is essential for individual analytes for Down's syndrome screening, the screen positive rate should nonetheless be monitored, just as for open spina bifida screening. The screen positive rate can vary considerably, depending on the selection of markers, the percentage of pregnancies dated by ultrasound measurements, the maternal age distribution of the screened population and the risk cut-off selected[89]. In general, rates range from 3% to 9%. These rates are considerably higher if screening is offered primarily to older women[89]. Professional organizations require that screen positive rates and the grand MoM be monitored for both open spina bifida and Down's syndrome.

External proficiency testing

Mandatory proficiency testing programs that monitor laboratory performance are offered by organizations such as the US College of American Pathologists (www.cap.org) and the UK National External Quality Assessment Scheme (NEQAS). Regulatory bodies review the proficiency testing performance of individual laboratories during periodic inspections. Recently, programs have been developed that offer proficiency testing for first-trimester serum markers, including incorporation of nuchal translucency measurements into the risk calculation (information available at www.ipmms.org), the ability of laboratories to calculate and judge the acceptability of center- and sonographer-specific nuchal translucency measurements, and also to combine both first- and second-trimester markers for integrated testing.

Professional standards and guidelines

Various professional organizations have promulgated standards and guidelines that contain detailed requirements for screening laboratories[87,88]. Obtaining reliable NT measurements requires specialized training and certification. Several programs have been established to educate and qualify sonographers to make this measurement accurately, such as the NTQR program administered in the USA (www.ntqr.org) and the Fetal Medicine Foundation Program in the UK (www.fetalmedicine.com) and in the USA (www.fetalmedicine.com/usa).

Absolute agreement between sonographers is unrealistic, meaning that either sonographer-specific or center-specific medians are likely to be required to achieve optimal performance[64]. Epidemiologic monitoring of these parameters, both within a prenatal center and externally by professional organizations can be applied in the same manner as for serum markers. The laboratory is a logical choice to monitor and analyze these parameters and provide feedback to sonographers, because it is the recipient of all NT measurements used in the risk calculations. However, laboratories may be reluctant to take on this role, given the investment of time and expertise. Furthermore, laboratories lack authority to effect change when sonographers with poor performance are identified. For monitoring to be effective, the laboratory and sonographers need to work together and a sonographer (or center) who submits NT measurements that fail to meet established criteria would need to be prepared to take remedial action.

PRENATAL TESTING FOR TRISOMY 18

Introduction

Trisomy 18 is a relatively uncommon chromosome abnormality, with a birth prevalence of about 1 in 8000. Its prevalence increases with maternal age; the approximate age-specific birth prevalence is often expressed as being 1/10 that of Down's syndrome. For example, term risk for Down's syndrome for women at an average age of 35 years is 1:353. The corresponding risk for trisomy 18 is approximately 1:3530. Fetuses affected with trisomy 18 are often spontaneously miscarried during pregnancy (one study estimates the loss rate to be 70% from the mid-second trimester to term)[90]. Undiagnosed trisomy 18 pregnancies that remain viable are often delivered by emergency cesarean section, due to fetal distress[91]. More than half of all liveborn infants with trisomy 18 die by 10 days; more than 90% by 100 days. On average, females survive longer than males. Given this short span of survival, it would be difficult to justify the medical, social and financial costs of a screening program focused exclusively on trisomy 18, but routine trisomy 18 identification can be justified as an add-on to Down's syndrome screening[92]. In this chapter, detection of trisomy 18 is considered 'prenatal testing', rather than 'prenatal screening'.

Second-trimester prenatal testing for trisomy 18

At the time when maternal serum AFP measurement was recognized as a prenatal screening test for Down's syndrome, several small studies documented that AFP levels were even lower in trisomy 18 pregnancies. As long as AFP was the only marker used with maternal age, women identified as screen positive for Down's syndrome were also at increased risk for trisomy 18. In the early 1990s, uE3 and hCG measurements were added as screening markers (the triple test) and serum uE3 levels were shown to be lower in both Down's syndrome and trisomy 18 pregnancies. In contrast, however, hCG levels were higher in Down's syndrome pregnancies, but lower in trisomy 18 pregnancies[93]. A separate algorithm for detecting trisomy 18 was therefore implemented in screening laboratories throughout North America, based on fixed MoM cut-off levels[93]. MoM cut-off levels of 0.75, 0.60 and 0.55 for AFP, uE3 and hCG identified 60% of trisomy 18 pregnancies, with a false positive rate of 0.4%. The positive predictive value was 6% (1 in 17 screen positive pregnancies was affected with trisomy 18). Many programs in Europe did not use uE3 measurements as part of Down's syndrome screening and the lack of this marker seriously hampers trisomy 18 detection. Although the algorithm performed as expected[85], it did not account for the maternal age effect and did not properly account for borderline results (e.g. AFP and uE3 low, but hCG levels just above the fixed MoM cut-off level). Figure 19.17 shows the distribution of AFP, uE3 and hCG levels in 98 second-trimester trisomy 18 pregnancies collected as part of a nine center collaborative study[94]. The resulting multivariate algorithm is still widely used today in second-trimester screening programs. Several prospective trials demonstrated its effectiveness[85,95]. Maternal serum dimeric inhibin-A measurements are not useful for this purpose[96].

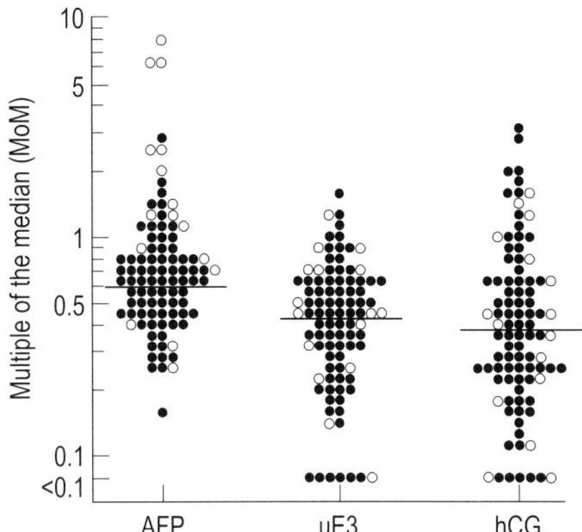

Fig. 19.17 Levels of three second-trimester maternal serum markers in 94 pregnancies affected with trisomy 18. The levels of AFP, uE3 and hCG in MoM are displayed on the vertical logarithmic scale. Open circles indicate that the pregnancy was also affected with either omphalocele or an open neural tube defect. The thin horizontal lines indicate the median MoM levels of 0.62, 0.42 and 0.36 for AFP, uE3 and hCG, respectively.

First-trimester prenatal testing for trisomy 18

In the late first trimester, nuchal translucency measurements average larger in the presence of trisomy 18. One large study[97] recorded all trisomy 18 cases (50 affected pregnancies) detected in the first trimester due to elevated NT measurements, but did not account for the fact that two-thirds or more of the missed cases with lower NT measurements would have spontaneously

Table 19.6 **Estimated detection rates (DR) and false positive rates (FPR) for trisomy 18 testing using either a second-trimester or an integrated serum algorithm**

Second-trimester serum algorithm[1]			*Integrated serum algorithm*[2]		
DR	*FPR*	*OAPR*[3]	*DR*	*FPR*	*OAPR*
60	<0.1	>1:6	60	<0.1	>1:4
70	0.13	1:8	70	<0.1	>1:4
80	0.54	1:20	80	<0.1	>1:4
90	2.63	1:100	90	0.10	1:6
67	0.1	1:5	90	0.1	1:4
73	0.2	1:10	92	0.2	1:8
76	0.3	1:14	93	0.3	1:12
78	0.4	1:8	94	0.4	1:15

[1]Maternal age in combination with measurements of AFP, uE3 and hCG.
[2]Maternal age in combination with first trimester PAPP-A, and the three second trimester markers.
[3]Odds of being affected given a positive test result (OAPR) computed using a second trimester trisomy 18 prevalence of 1:3500.

miscarried prior to term (an important bias relating to the trimester of ascertainment). This means that trisomy 18 cases with lower NT measurements are under-represented by a factor of three or more. Until this bias can be adequately accounted for, any trisomy 18 algorithm that included the NT information contained in this study would result in a substantial overestimation of test performance. As a result, the assigned risks and estimates of first-trimester screening performance may not be reliable. This study, and others, also presented information about maternal serum markers and trisomy 18, including PAPP-A and free-beta hCG; both are very low in the presence of trisomy 18. The same biases of ascertainment discussed above for NT measurements are also present in the studies of biochemical markers, but to a lesser extent.

Integrated prenatal serum testing for trisomy 18

Acceptable data are available on a limited basis for first-trimester serum markers in relation to trisomy 18 and this information can be combined with the second-trimester triple test to create a serum integrated screening protocol for trisomy 18[98]. Table 19.6 shows expected detection and false positive rates using serum integrated testing (the triple markers and a first-trimester PAPP-A measurement) and compares those rates with triple marker test performance at selected second-trimester risk cut-off levels. If the false positive rate were to be held relatively low (e.g. 0.2%), the triple marker algorithm would detect about 70% of trisomy 18 pregnancies, as opposed to about 90% for the serum integrated test.

REFERENCES

1. Brock DJ, Sutcliffe RG. Alpha-fetoprotein in the antenatal diagnosis of anencephaly and spina bifida. *Lancet* **2**:197–199, 1972.
2. Wald NJ, Brock DJ, Bonnar J. Prenatal diagnosis of spina bifida and anencephaly by maternal serum-alpha-fetoprotein measurement. A controlled study. *Lancet* **1**:765–767, 1974.
3. Brock DJ, Bolton AE, Scrimgeour JB. Prenatal diagnosis of spina bifida and anencephaly through maternal plasma-alpha-fetoprotein measurement. *Lancet* **1**:767–769, 1974.
4. Wald NJ, Cuckle H, Brock DJH, Peto R, Polani PE, Woodford FP. Maternal serum-alpha-fetoprotein measurement in antenatal screening for anencephaly and spina bifida in early pregnancy. Report of UK collaborative study on alpha-fetoprotein in relation to neural-tube defects. *Lancet* **1**:1323–1332, 1977.
5. Wald N, Cuckle H, Boreham J, Stirrat G. Small biparietal diameter of fetuses with spina bifida: implications for antenatal screening. *Br J Obstet Gynaecol* **87**:219–221, 1980.
6. Campbell S, Pryse-Davies J, Coltart TM, Seller MJ, Singer JD. Ultrasound in the diagnosis of spina bifida. *Lancet* **1**:1065–1068, 1975.
7. Nicolaides KH, Campbell S, Gabbe SG, Guidetti R. Ultrasound screening for spina bifida: cranial and cerebellar signs. *Lancet* **2**:72–74, 1986.
8. Merkatz IR, Nitowsky HM, Macri JN, Johnson WE. An association between low maternal serum alpha-fetoprotein and fetal chromosomal abnormalities. *Am J Obstet Gynecol* **148**:886–894, 1984.
9. Cuckle HS, Wald NJ, Lindenbaum RH. Maternal serum alpha-fetoprotein measurement: a screening test for Down's syndrome. *Lancet* **1**:926–929, 1984.
10. Bogart MH, Pandian MR, Jones OW. Abnormal maternal serum chorionic gonadotropin levels in pregnancies with fetal chromosome abnormalities. *Prenat Diagn* **7**:623–630, 1987.
11. Canick JA, Knight GJ, Palomaki GE, Haddow JE, Cuckle HS, Wald NJ. Low second trimester maternal serum unconjugated oestriol in pregnancies with Down's syndrome. *Br J Obstet Gynaecol* **95**: 330–333, 1988.
12. Wald NJ, Cuckle HS, Densem JW et al. Maternal serum screening for Down's syndrome in early pregnancy. *Br Med J* **297**:883–887, 1988.
13. Hallahan T, Krantz D, Orlandi F et al. First trimester biochemical screening for Down's syndrome: free beta hCG

versus intact hCG. *Prenat Diagn* **20**:785–789; discussion. 2000. 790–781
14. Wald NJ, Densem JW, George L, Muttukrishna S, Knight PG. Prenatal screening for Down's syndrome using inhibin-A as a serum marker. *Prenat Diagn* **16**:143–153, 1996.
15. Nicolaides KH, Azar G, Byrne D, Mansur C, Marks K. Fetal nuchal translucency: ultrasound screening for chromosomal defects in first trimester of pregnancy. *Br Med J* **304**:867–869, 1992.
16. Palomaki GE, Lambert-Messerlian GM, Canick JA. A summary analysis of Down's syndrome markers in the late first trimester. *Adv Clin Chem* **43**:177–210, 2007.
17. Wald NJ, Watt HC, Hackshaw AK. Integrated screening for Down's syndrome on the basis of tests performed during the first and second trimesters. *N Engl J Med* **341**:461–467, 1999.
18. Bergstrand CG, Czar B. Demonstration of a new protein fraction in serum from the human fetus. *Scand J Clin Lab Invest* **8**:174, 1956.
19. Harper ME, Dugaiczyk A. Linkage of the evolutionarily-related serum albumin and alpha-fetoprotein genes within q11-22 of human chromosome 4. *Am J Hum Genet* **35**:565–572, 1983.
20. Ruoslahti E. Isolation and biochemical properties of alpha-fetoprotein. In *Prevention of neural tube defects: the role of alpha-fetoprotein*, BF Crandall, M Brazier (eds), pp. 9–16. New York: Academic Press, 1978.
21. Tomasi TB, Jr. Structure and function of alpha-fetoprotein. *Annu Rev Med* **28**:453–465, 1977.
22. Greenberg F, Faucett A, Rose E et al. Congenital deficiency of alpha-fetoprotein. *Am J Obstet Gynecol* **167**:509–511, 1992.
23. Amniotic-fluid alpha-fetoprotein measurement in antenatal diagnosis of anencephaly and open spina bifida in early pregnancy. Second report of the UK Collaborative Study on alpha-fetoprotein in relation to neural-tube defects. *Lancet*, **2**, 651–662, 1979.
24. Wald N, Cuckle H, Nanchahal K. Amniotic fluid acetylcholinesterase measurement in the prenatal diagnosis of open neural tube defects. Second report of the Collaborative acetylcholinesterase study. *Prenat Diagn* **9**:813–829, 1989.
25. Haddow JE, Miller WA. Prenatal diagnosis of open neural tube defects. In *Methods in cell biology. Prenatal diagnosis: cell biological approaches*, S Latt, G Darlington (eds), pp. 68–93. New York: Academic Press, 1982.
26. Goldfine C, Haddow JE, Knight GJ, Palomaki GE. Amniotic fluid alpha-fetoprotein and acetylcholinesterase measurements in pregnancies associated with gastroschisis. *Prenat Diagn* **9**:697–700, 1989.
27. Ryynanen M, Seppala M, Kuusela P et al. Antenatal screening for congenital nephrosis in Finland by maternal serum alpha-fetoprotein. *Br J Obstet Gynaecol* **90**:437–442, 1983.
28. Althouse R, Wald N. Survival and handicap of infants with spina bifida. *Arch Dis Child* **55**:845–850, 1980.
29. Sensitivity of ultrasound in detecting spina bifida, *N Engl J Med*, **324**, 769–772, 1991.
30. Los FJ, de Wolf BT, Huisjes HJ. Raised maternal serum-alpha-fetoprotein levels and spontaneous fetomaternal transfusion. *Lancet* **2**:1210–1212, 1979.
31. Carrington D, Gilmore DH, Whittle MJ et al. Maternal serum alpha-fetoprotein – a marker of fetal aplastic crisis during intrauterine human parvovirus infection. *Lancet* **1**:433–435, 1987.
32. Perkes EA, Baim RS, Goodman KJ, Macri JN. Second-trimester placental changes associated with elevated maternal serum alpha-fetoprotein. *Am J Obstet Gynecol* **144**:935–938, 1982.
33. Haddow JE, Knight GJ, Kloza EM, Palomaki GE. Alpha-fetoprotein, vaginal bleeding and pregnancy risk. *Br J Obstet Gynaecol* **93**:589–593, 1986.
34. Haddow JE, Thompson DK, Kloza EM. Maternal hepatoma detected during serum AFP screening. *Lancet* **2**:806–807, 1980.
35. Kew MC, Purves LR, Bersohn I. Serum alpha-fetoprotein levels in acute viral hepatitis. *Gut* **14**:939–942, 1973.
36. Morris JK, Wald NJ. Prevalence of neural tube defect pregnancies in England and Wales from 1964 to 2004. *J Med Screen* **14**:55–59, 2007.
37. Prevention of neural tube defects: results of the Medical Research Council Vitamin Study. MRC Vitamin Study Research Group. *Lancet* **338**:131–137, 1991.
38. Recommendations for the use of folic acid to reduce the number of cases of spina bifida and other neural tube defects, *MMWR Recomm Rep*, **41**, 1–7, 1992.
39. Food and Drug Administration. Final Rule. Food Standards: Amendment of standards of identity for enriched grain products to require addition of folic acid. *Fed Regist* **61**:8781–8797, 1996.
40. Palomaki GE, Williams J, Haddow JE. Comparing the observed and predicted effectiveness of folic acid fortification in preventing neural tube defects. *J Med Screen* **10**:52–53, 2003.
41. Hook EB. Estimates of maternal age-specific risks of Down-syndrome birth in women aged 34–41. *Lancet* **2**:33–34, 1976.
42. Hook EB, Lindsjo A. Down's syndrome in live births by single year maternal age interval in a Swedish study: comparison with results from a New York State study. *Am J Hum Genet* **30**:19–27, 1978.
43. Cuckle HS, Wald NJ, Thompson SG. Estimating a woman's risk of having a pregnancy associated with Down's syndrome using her age and serum alpha-fetoprotein level. *Br J Obstet Gynaecol* **94**:387–402, 1987.
44. Hecht CA, Hook EB. Rates of Down's syndrome at livebirth by one-year maternal age intervals in studies with apparent close to complete ascertainment in populations of European origin: a proposed revised rate schedule for use in genetic and prenatal screening. *Am J Med Genet* **62**:376–385, 1996.
45. Morris JK, Mutton DE, Alberman E. Revised estimates of the maternal age specific live birth prevalence of Down's syndrome. *J Med Screen* **9**:2–6, 2002.
46. Morris JK, Wald NJ, Mutton DE, Alberman E. Comparison of models of maternal age-specific risk for Down's syndrome live births. *Prenat Diagn* **23**: 252–258, 2003.
47. Morris JK, Wald NJ, Watt HC. Fetal loss in Down's syndrome pregnancies. *Prenat Diagn* **19**:142–145, 1999.
48. Savva GM, Morris JK, Mutton DE, Alberman E. Maternal age-specific fetal loss rates in Down's syndrome pregnancies. *Prenat Diagn* **26**:499–504, 2006.
49. Matthews TJ, Hamilton BE. Mean age of mother, 1970–2000. National Vital Statistics Reports; Vol. 51, No. 1. Hyattsville, Maryland: National Center for Health Statistics, 2002.
50. ACOG Practice Bulletin No. 77. screening for fetal chromosomal abnormalities. *Obstet Gynecol* **109**:217–227, 2007.
51. Wald NJ, Cuckle HS, Densem JW et al. Maternal serum unconjugated oestriol as an antenatal screening test for Down's syndrome. *Br J Obstet Gynaecol* **95**:334–341, 1988.
52. Canick JA, Lambert-Messerlian GM, Palomaki GE et al. Maternal serum dimeric inhibin is elevated in Down's syndrome pregnancy. *Am J Hum Genet* **55**:A9, 1994.
53. Macri JN, Kasturi RV, Krantz DA et al. Maternal serum Down's syndrome screening: free beta-protein is a more effective marker than human chorionic gonadotropin. *Am J Obstet Gynecol* **163**:1248–1253, 1990.
54. Shahabi S, Oz UA, Bahado-Singh RO et al. Serum hyperglycosylated hCG: a potential screening test for fetal Down's syndrome. *Prenat Diagn* **19**:488–489, 1999.
55. Wald NJ, Densem JW, Smith D, Klee GG. Four-marker serum screening for Down's syndrome. *Prenat Diagn* **14**:707–716, 1994.
56. Wald NJ, Hackshaw AK, George LM. Assay precision of serum alpha fetoprotein in antenatal screening for neural tube defects and Down's syndrome. *J Med Screen* **7**:74–77, 2000.
57. Wald NJ, Rodeck C, Hackshaw AK, Walters J, Chitty L, Mackinson AM. First and second trimester antenatal screening for Down's syndrome: the results of the serum, urine and ultrasound screening study (SURUSS). *J Med Screen* **10**:56–104, 2003.

58. Haddow JE, Palomaki GE, Knight GJ, Foster DL, Neveux LM. Second trimester screening for Down's syndrome using maternal serum dimeric inhibin A. *J Med Screen* **5**:115–119, 1998.
59. Cuckle HS, Wald NJ, Barkai G et al. First-trimester biochemical screening for Down's syndrome. *Lancet* **2**:851–852, 1988.
60. Spencer K. Evaluation of an assay of the free beta-subunit of choriogonadotropin and its potential value in screening for Down's syndrome. *Clin Chem* **37**:809–814, 1991.
61. Spencer K, Crossley JA, Aitken DA, Nix AB, Dunstan FD, Williams K. Temporal changes in maternal serum biochemical markers of trisomy 21 across the first and second trimester of pregnancy. *Ann Clin Biochem* **39**:567–576, 2002.
62. Canick JA, Lambert-Messerlian GM, Palomaki GE et al. Comparison of serum markers in first-trimester Down's syndrome screening. *Obstet Gynecol* **108**:1192–1199, 2006.
63. Brambati B, Lanzani A, Tului L. Ultrasound and biochemical assessment of first trimester pregnancy. In *The embryo*, M Chapman, GJ Grudzinskas, T Chard (eds), pp. 181–194. Berlin: Springer, 1991.
64. Malone FD, Canick JA, Ball RH et al. First-trimester or second-trimester screening, or both, for Down's syndrome. *N Engl J Med* **353**:2001–2011, 2005.
65. Snijders RJ, Thom EA, Zachary JM et al. First-trimester trisomy screening: nuchal translucency measurement training and quality assurance to correct and unify technique. *Ultrasound Obstet Gynecol* **19**:353–359, 2002.
66. Spencer K, Spencer CE, Power M, Dawson C, Nicolaides KH. Screening for chromosomal abnormalities in the first trimester using ultrasound and maternal serum biochemistry in a one-stop clinic: a review of three years prospective experience. *Br J Obstet Gynaecol* **110**:281–286, 2003.
67. Nicolaides KH, Spencer K, Avgidou K, Faiola S, Falcon O. Multicenter study of first-trimester screening for trisomy 21 in 75 821 pregnancies: results and estimation of the potential impact of individual risk-orientated two-stage first-trimester screening. *Ultrasound Obstet Gynecol* **25**:221–226, 2005.
68. Wapner R, Thom E, Simpson JL et al. First-trimester screening for trisomies 21 and 18. *N Engl J Med* **349**:1405–1413, 2003.
69. Seeds JW. Diagnostic mid trimester amniocentesis: how safe? *Am J Obstet Gynecol* **191**:607–615, 2004.
70. Eddleman KA, Malone FD, Sullivan L et al. Pregnancy loss rates after midtrimester amniocentesis. *Obstet Gynecol* **108**:1067–1072, 2006.
71. Maymon R, Betser M, Dreazen E, Padoa A, Herman A. A model for disclosing the first trimester part of an integrated Down's syndrome screening test. *Clin Genet* **65**:113–119, 2004.
72. Palomaki GE, Steinort K, Knight GJ, Haddow JE. Comparing three screening strategies for combining first- and second-trimester Down's syndrome markers. *Obstet Gynecol* **107**:367–375, 2006.
73. Wald NJ, Rudnicka AR, Bestwick JP. Sequential and contingent prenatal screening for Down's syndrome. *Prenat Diagn* **26**:769–777, 2006.
74. Cuckle H. Integrating antenatal Down's syndrome screening. *Curr Opin Obstet Gynecol* **13**:175–181, 2001.
75. Wright D, Bradbury I, Benn P, Cuckle H, Ritchie K. Contingent screening for Down's syndrome is an efficient alternative to non-disclosure sequential screening. *Prenat Diagn* **24**:762–766, 2004.
76. Benn P, Wright D, Cuckle H. Practical strategies in contingent sequential screening for Down's syndrome. *Prenat Diagn* **25**:645–652, 2005.
77. Wald NJ, Smith D, Kennard A et al. Biparietal diameter and crown-rump length in fetuses with Down's syndrome: implications for antenatal serum screening for Down's syndrome. *Br J Obstet Gynaecol* **100**:430–435, 1993.
78. Foundation for Blood Research, Adjusting risk for a family history of Down's syndrome. Available at: http://www.fbr.org/edu/cap/cap_ds_famhx_fp-b_2002.pdf.Accessed: July 23, 2007.
79. Wald NJ, Kennard A, Hackshaw A, McGuire A. Antenatal screening for Down's syndrome. *J Med Screen* **4**:181–246, 1997.
80. Crossley JA, Aitken DA, Waugh SM, Kelly T, Connor JM. Maternal smoking: age distribution, levels of alpha-fetoprotein and human chorionic gonadotrophin, and effect on detection of Down's syndrome pregnancies in second-trimester screening. *Prenat Diagn* **22**:247–255, 2002.
81. Rudnicka AR, Wald NJ, Huttly W, Hackshaw AK. Influence of maternal smoking on the birth prevalence of Down's syndrome and on second trimester screening performance. *Prenat Diagn* **22**:893–897, 2002.
82. Wald NJ, Rodeck C, Hackshaw AK, Rudnicka A. SURUSS in perspective. *Br J Obstet Gynaecol* **111**:521–531, 2004.
83. Gasiorek-Wiens A, Tercanli S, Kozlowski P et al. Screening for trisomy 21 by fetal nuchal translucency and maternal age: a multicenter project in Germany, Austria and Switzerland. *Ultrasound Obstet Gynecol* **18**:645–648, 2001.
84. Onda T, Tanaka T, Yoshida K et al. Triple marker screening for trisomy 21, trisomy 18 and open neural tube defects in singleton pregnancies of native Japanese pregnant women. *J Obstet Gynaecol Res* **26**:441–447, 2000.
85. Palomaki GE, Knight GJ, Haddow JE, Canick JA, Saller DN, Jr, Panizza DS. Prospective intervention trial of a screening protocol to identify fetal trisomy 18 using maternal serum alpha-fetoprotein, unconjugated oestriol, and human chorionic gonadotropin. *Prenat Diagn* **12**:925–930, 1992.
86. NCCLS SC1-L Evaluation Protocols. NCCLS Specialty Collection, 2003, Wayne, PA.
87. College of American Pathologists. Available at: http://www.cap.org/apps/docs/laboratory_accreditation/checklists/chemistry_and_toxicology_october 2006.doc.Accessed: July 9.
88. Palomaki GE, Bradley LA, McDowell GA. Technical standards and guidelines: prenatal screening for Down's syndrome. *Genet Med* **7**:344–354, 2005.
89. Knight GJ, Palomaki GE. Epidemiologic monitoring of prenatal screening for neural tube defects and Down's syndrome. *Clin Lab Med*, 2003; **23**: 531-551, xi.
90. Hook EB. Chromosome abnormalities and spontaneous fetal death following amniocentesis: further data and associations with maternal age. *Am J Hum Genet* **35**:110–116, 1983.
91. Schneider AS, Mennuti MT, Zackai EH. High cesarean section rate in trisomy 18 births: a potential indication for late prenatal diagnosis. *Am J Obstet Gynecol* **140**:367–370, 1981.
92. Hackshaw AK, Kennard A, Wald NJ. Detection of pregnancies with trisomy 18 in screening programmes for Down's syndrome. *J Med Screen* **2**:228–229, 1995.
93. Canick JA, Palomaki GE, Osathanondh R. Prenatal screening for trisomy 18 in the second trimester. *Prenat Diagn* **10**:546–548, 1990.
94. Palomaki GE, Haddow JE, Knight GJ et al. Risk-based prenatal screening for trisomy 18 using alpha-fetoprotein, unconjugated oestriol and human chorionic gonadotropin. *Prenat Diagn* **15**: 713–723, 1995.
95. Benn PA, Leo MV, Rodis JF, Beazoglou T, Collins R, Horne D. Maternal serum screening for fetal trisomy 18: a comparison of fixed cutoff and patient-specific risk protocols. *Obstet Gynecol* **93**:707–711, 1999.
96. Lambert-Messerlian GM, Saller DN, Jr, Tumber MB, French CA, Peterson CJ, Canick JA. Second-trimester maternal serum inhibin A levels in fetal trisomy 18 and Turner syndrome with and without hydrops. *Prenat Diagn* **18**:1061–1067, 1998.
97. Tul N, Spencer K, Noble P, Chan C, Nicolaides K. Screening for trisomy 18 by fetal nuchal translucency and maternal serum free beta-hCG and PAPP-A at 10–14 weeks of gestation. *Prenat Diagn* **19**:1035–1042, 1999.
98. Palomaki GE, Neveux LM, Knight GJ, Haddow JE. Maternal serum-integrated screening for trisomy 18 using both first- and second-trimester markers. *Prenat Diagn* **23**:243–247, 2003.

Ultrasound screening for fetal abnormalities and aneuploidies in first and second trimesters

CHAPTER 20

Fionnuala M Breathnach and Fergal D Malone

KEY POINTS

- The focus for this chapter is the contribution that obstetric ultrasound makes to the field of fetal medicine
- The relative merits of a variety of screening programmes are discussed. The RCOG recommends a two-scan program; the first primarily for dating and the second between 18 and 20 weeks for detection of congenital anomalies
- The role of the genetic sonogram in adjusting risk assignment for aneuploidy, through identification of either major structural malformations or 'soft markers', is explored
- The identification of multiple soft markers is far more predictive of aneuploidy than demonstration of any marker in isolation
- First-trimester sonography is now meeting a demand for earlier detection of chromosomal abnormalities and, increasingly, the potential for identifying major structural defects in the first trimester is being realized

INTRODUCTION

Medical ultrasound has its origins in the method that was used first to detect icebergs following the sinking of the Titanic in 1912 and subsequently to detect submarines during the First World War[1]. Its application to medicine was pioneered by Wild[2], who studied the potential of ultrasound in the evaluation of breast masses. The field of obstetric ultrasound owes its origins to the vision and foresight of obstetrician Ian Donald and engineer Tom Brown in the Queen Mother's hospital in Glasgow[3], where the first sonographic studies of the fetus were carried out in 1957. These investigators recognized that:

> The pregnant uterus offers considerable scope for this kind of work because it is a cystic cavity containing a solid foetus.

Until it became apparent that ultrasound waves could be transmitted through water-soluble jelly, the scan was performed with the transducer being lowered into a bucket of water with a latex rubber base. Against this background, the ensuing 50 years have witnessed how the development of obstetric ultrasound has revolutionized prenatal care and given rise to fetal medicine as a subspecialty that offers immense diagnostic and therapeutic capabilities.

'ROUTINE' PRENATAL ULTRASOUND

As the potential of ultrasound in diagnosing fetal abnormalities became apparent in the 1970s, many countries explored the merit of offering ultrasound screening on a universal basis such that prenatal ultrasound has become an integral component of obstetric care today. There is, however, a lack of consensus on the most appropriate schedule for prenatal ultrasound. In 1980, the Federal Republic of Germany introduced a two-stage ultrasound screening program[4]. The Royal College of Obstetricians and Gynaecologists (RCOG) subsequently recommended a single routine scan[5].

In 1984, the National Institutes of Health (NIH) convened a conference to reach a consensus on the question of whether ultrasound examination should be performed on all pregnant women[6]. Recognizing that routine ultrasonography has not been shown to reduce perinatal morbidity or mortality, the panel recommended that ultrasound should be employed only where clinically indicated. Furthermore, a proposal was put forward that large-scale randomized controlled trials of routine ultrasound screening during pregnancy should be conducted in the USA. Such a study was presented by the Routine Antenatal Diagnostic Imaging with Ultrasound (RADIUS) group in 1993[7]. This study randomized 15000 low-risk women to timed routine prenatal ultrasound at 15–22 weeks' gestation and again at 31–35 weeks' gestation, or ultrasonography reserved for specific clinical indications alone. In spite of enhanced detection of congenital anomalies in the screened group, there were no appreciable differences in the rate of adverse perinatal outcome (death or serious perinatal morbidity) between the two groups. The findings of this study are in contrast to those of the Helsinki ultrasound trial[8], which found that perinatal mortality was significantly lower in babies born to women who had routine ultrasonography and that almost half of this reduction was attributed to the detection of major malformations. A further five major European studies[9–13] addressed this same issue and offered evidence of the potential benefits of routine scanning. Nonetheless, a meta-analysis of published studies of routine scanning indicates that, although routine scanning does result in enhanced detection rates for structural anomalies, it does not translate into an increase in the live birth rate, nor a decrease in perinatal morbidity[14]. An inherent bias in the studies that report a reduction in perinatal mortality as a result of routine prenatal ultrasound is that the reduction in perinatal mortality results from termination of pregnancies affected by severe congenital malformations rather than improved survival of affected fetuses.

Against the background of controversy that surrounds whether ultrasound screening should be offered on a routine basis, and what benefits may be realized by such screening, the RCOG has revised its previous guideline to include recommendations that screening should be undertaken only after the objectives have been identified clearly for the woman prior to the scan and that a two-scan program is considered to be the ideal, the first primarily for dating in the first trimester and the second between 18 and 20 weeks, for detection of congenital anomalies[15].

It is likely that perinatal morbidity and mortality outcomes are not at the forefront of patients' minds when undergoing mid-trimester fetal anatomy sonography. Increasingly, women request prenatal ultrasound even in the absence of specific clinical indications and do so motivated by factors other than concern about mortality or morbidity. Non-medical reasons cited by patients for requesting prenatal ultrasound include wanting to identify the baby's gender, wanting to 'see the baby', to experience the pregnancy as 'more real' and to involve the father[16,17]. The relative importance of these factors in influencing a patient to request prenatal ultrasound is not necessarily in line with factors that influence any decision making. These factors should be acknowledged in any evaluation of the value of prenatal ultrasound to the patient.

MID-TRIMESTER FETAL ANATOMY SCAN

Routine sonographic survey of fetal anatomy has gained widespread acceptance as a screening tool both for structural fetal malformations and for aneuploidy. While screening for aneuploidy is increasingly taking the form of combined serum and sonographic screening at earlier gestations, the 18–20-week scan retains its role as a key tool for identification of major structural malformations. The prenatal diagnosis of organ-specific anomalies is dealt with in Section 7 (Chapters 30–38). A comprehensive 'check-list' for the routine anomaly scan is outlined in Table 20.1.

Table 20.1 **Checklist for mid-trimester anatomy scan**

Fetal number	
Fetal cardiac activity	
Gestational age & fetal biometry	Biparietal diameter, head circumference, abdominal circumference, femur length
Intracranial structures	Falx cerebri, cavum septum pellucidum, skull bones, lateral ventricles (anterior & posterior horns), choroid plexi, cerebellum/vermis, nuchal fold, cisterna magna
Face	Orbits, nose, jaw, lips, palate, profile
Diaphragm	Right & left
Heart	Fetal heart rate, position, axis, four-chamber view, interventricular septum, foramen ovale, mitral valve, tricuspid valve
Great vessels	Left ventricular outflow tract, right ventricular outflow tract, aortic arch, ductal arch
Abdomen	Stomach, kidney (right & left), bladder, abdominal wall
Spine	Ossification centers & covering skin, (coronal, sagittal & axial views)
Extremities	Long bones, hands, ankle alignment, sole of foot
Umbilical cord	Insertion & vessel number
Amniotic fluid volume	
Placenta	Site & distance from internal os
Maternal anatomy	Uterus & adnexae

Factors affecting the sensitivity of ultrasound

The sensitivity of routine mid-trimester ultrasound for the detection of structural malformations shows wide variation. Interobserver variability in the interpretation of sonographic findings was the subject of a study conducted by Smith-Bindman et al.,[18] who used a test series of clinical cases to compare physicians' interpretations. Reassuringly, this group identified 'moderate to substantial' agreement between physicians in their reporting of the presence of anomalies for all organ systems. Importantly, however, the participating physicians were all described as being highly experienced, a fact that may render the findings of this study less applicable to some practices.

The sensitivity of ultrasound for the detection of structural anomalies also varies according to the organ system studied. Reported sensitivities are highest (exceeding 90%) for CNS abnormalities[18,19] and lower for diaphragmatic hernia and renal tract anomalies (62–66%)[18,19]. With increasing experience and improved ultrasound resolution, detection rates have improved in recent years. A 16-year prospective study of prenatal diagnosis of fetal abnormalities including over half a million registrable births in units that have offered anomaly scanning since the beginning of the study period (mid-1980s) has demonstrated improved diagnostic accuracy over time, with prenatal detection rates for spina bifida seen to have increased from 56% to 84% during the study period, bilateral renal agenesis from 52% to 93% and hypoplastic left heart from 12% to 88%[19].

In spite of these varying sensitivities, management decisions regarding whether to continue or to terminate a pregnancy are reliant upon the accuracy of ultrasound diagnoses. To this end, postmortem examination retains a pivotal role in validating sonographic performance. Indeed, additional information may come to light on the basis of a post-termination postmortem and such information may have implications in the arena of genetic counseling.

Ultrasound screening performance may be hindered by factors such as maternal obesity[20–22]. Furthermore, maternal obesity, even in the absence of diabetes, has been associated with an increased risk for fetal structural anomalies[23–26]. A study that focused on suboptimal ultrasonographic visualization of the fetal heart during routine anatomy scanning at 18–20 weeks' gestation found that suboptimal cardiac visualization was directly related to maternal body mass index, with reports of suboptimal visualization increasing from 12.4% in non-obese women to 46.6% in those with morbid obesity[27]. Various tactics have been used to surmount this problem, including the use of 3-dimensional ultrasonography[28], the use of harmonic imaging[29] and, indeed, transumbilical placement of the vaginal probe[21]. More simply, repeat targeted cardiac evaluation at 24 weeks in circumstances in which suboptimal views have been obtained at 18–20 weeks has been shown to be worthwhile as a strategy for obtaining satisfactory cardiac views and reducing the rate of inadequate cardiac visualization by 80–90%[30].

The duration of the ultrasound assessment will also impact on the acquisition of a satisfactory anatomic survey. This is not typically recorded in clinical practice. An increase in organ system visualization with increasing duration of examination has been demonstrated in one study[31], which documented that a complete anatomic survey was achieved within 10 minutes in just 8% of study subjects, increasing to 81% within 30 minutes. This same study identified gestational age as a further factor influencing sonographic visualization, with rates of complete anatomic surveys increasing from 67% at 16–18 weeks to 96% at 20–22 weeks. These findings are replicated in a trial that randomized patients to undergo an anomaly scan at 18, 20 or 22 weeks and found that there was a significantly lower percentage of completed examinations at 18 weeks' gestation (76%) than at 20 or 22 weeks (90% and 88% respectively), with no significant difference in scan performance between the latter two gestations. A reduction in the requirement for repeat examinations and greater efficiency in the time taken for each scan may therefore favor selecting 20–22 weeks' gestation as the optimal time for the anatomy scan rather than 18 weeks. Such a strategy, however, does present a trade-off for those who favor the provision of earlier diagnosis.

THE 'GENETIC SONOGRAM' AT 15–20 WEEKS

Anatomic survey of the fetus serves to identify structural abnormalities as outlined above, but also plays a critical role in the detection of chromosomal abnormalities, through identification of either major anomalies associated with certain aneuploid conditions, or so-called 'soft markers' for aneuploidy.

Until recent times, protocols directed at prenatal detection of chromosomal aneuploidy relied upon offering amniocentesis to women over the arbitrary age of 35 years. Owing to the recognition that selection of candidates for amniocentesis on the basis of maternal age alone is ineffective as a screening method for aneuploidy, a policy change has been observed in recent years. This change has further been fuelled by the view that the well-established iatrogenic fetal loss rate associated with amniocentesis, although low (perhaps as low as 1 in 1600)[32], is becoming less acceptable to patients, particularly as the majority of these iatrogenic losses are normal euploid pregnancies. The recognition of maternal serum marker patterns associated with aneuploidy and the evolution of the 'genetic sonogram' have addressed this demand. Hence patients can be offered amniocentesis if deemed 'high risk' on the basis of a combination of preliminary screening tests, to include maternal age, maternal serum markers and sonographic findings.

The 'genetic sonogram', was developed in the mid-1990s[33–36] and describes the application of second-trimester sonography to adjust risk assignment for chromosomal aneuploidy through identification of either major structural malformations or 'soft-markers' associated with aneuploidy. The term 'soft markers' refers to sonographic findings that are widely regarded as variants of normal, that do not confer any clinical ill-effects in their own right and are commonly seen to resolve as pregnancy advances[37,38]. Nonetheless, these traits are known to have an association with aneuploidy. That association is most marked where multiple soft markers are observed[39–41]. The collective term 'sonographic markers of fetal aneuploidy' (SMFAs)[42] has been applied to these markers and characteristic patterns of association have been observed for trisomies 21, 18 and 13 with considerable overlap in these patterns (Table 20.2).

While recognition of a major structural malformation with a known link to an autosomal trisomy, or identification of a multiplicity of soft markers, is likely to prompt a diagnostic test, interpretation of isolated soft marker significance requires some correlation with other risk factors, such as maternal age, obstetric or family history and maternal serum testing results. The genetic sonogram has developed for the purpose of providing patients with a refined, individualized risk-estimate in order to facilitate decision making on invasive testing and thereby minimize iatrogenic fetal loss. While some patients deemed high-risk on the basis of age or maternal serum screening will be given an even higher risk-estimate if sonographic markers are identified, many more will have their risk estimate reduced by 60–80%[40,41,43] if their second-trimester genetic sonogram identifies no markers of aneuploidy. The benefit of this strategy lies not only in the capacity to offer reassurance, but also in the consequent reduction in requests for amniocentesis. However, this is a controversial area and, in the UK, the current policy is not to adjust a Down's risk derived from a nationally recognized screening program on the basis of soft markers.

MAJOR STRUCTURAL ANOMALIES ASSOCIATED WITH ANEUPLOIDY

An infant with trisomy 21 displays a range of well-described phenotypic features including excess skin at the back of the neck, muscle hypotonia, a flattened facial profile (Fig. 20.1), short stature, dysplasia of the middle phalanx of the fifth digit, prominent epicanthic folds and a simian crease of the palm[44]. Those features most readily amenable to prenatal diagnosis are the commonly observed associated major structural

Table 20.2 **Sonographic markers for fetal aneuploidy**

	Trisomy 21	*Trisomy 18*	*Trisomy 13*
Structural abnormalities	Cardiac abnormalities Duodenal atresia Brachycephaly Hydrocephalus Clinodactyly Cystic hygroma & hydrops	Cardiac abnormalities Esophageal atresia Strawberry-shaped head Diaphragmatic hernia Omphalocele Meningomyelocele Agenesis corpus callosum Facial clefting Talipes Rocker-bottom foot Radial aplasia Overlapping digits Umbilical cord cyst Cystic hygroma & hydrops	Cardiac abnormalities Diaphragmatic hernia Omphalocele Holoprosencephaly Facial clefting Cyclopia Agenesis corpus callosum Rocker-bottom foot Polydactyly Talipes Cystic hygroma & hydrops
Soft markers	Nuchal fold thickening Ventriculomegaly Short femur or humerus Hypoplastic nose Echogenic bowel Pyelectasis Sandal gap toes	Choroid plexus cysts Enlarged cisterna magna Ventriculomegaly Short femur or humerus Hypoplastic nose Echogenic bowel Pyelectasis Single umbilical artery	Echogenic intracardiac foci Enlarged cisterna magna Ventriculomegaly Pyelectasis Single umbilical artery

Adapted from Breathnach et al., *Am J Med Genet* **145**(1):62–72, 2007

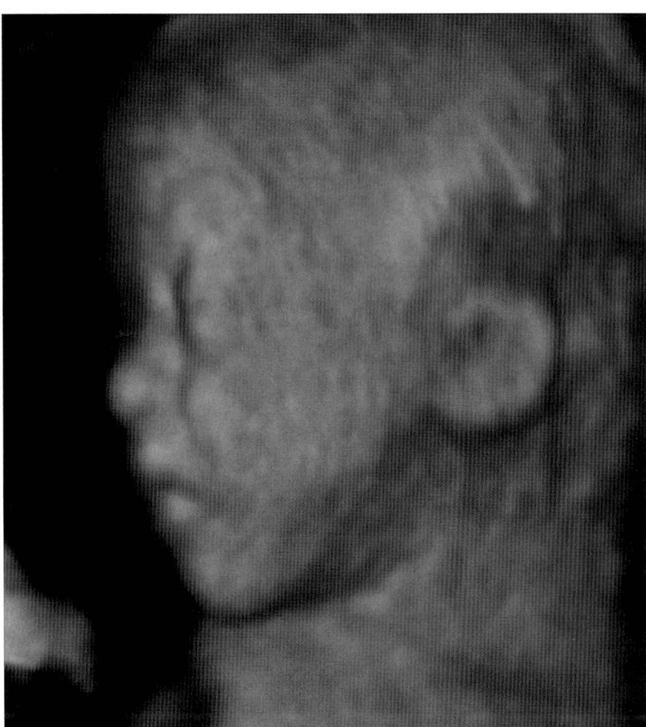

Fig. 20.1 Flattened facial profile in trisomy 21.

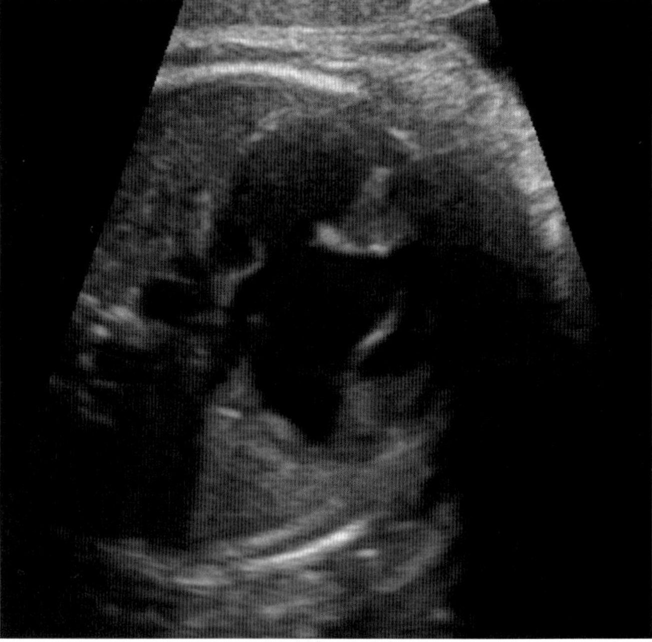

Fig. 20.2 Atrioventricular septal defect.

malformations such as cardiac anomalies (atrioventricular septal defect (Fig. 20.2), ventricular septal defect and tetralogy of Fallot), duodenal atresia (Fig. 20.3), cystic hygroma (Fig. 20.4), hydrops and hydrocephalus. Likelihood ratios are used to compute the risk of trisomy 21 in a pregnancy in which one of these structural malformations is present, as illustrated by the studies included in Table 20.3. The reported incidence of congenital heart defects in trisomy 21 is 46–65%, rendering this the most common class of major structural anomaly associated with this condition[46–48]. Incorporation of a thorough evaluation of the heart optimizes the performance of the genetic sonogram as a screening tool for aneuploidy. DeVore and co-workers[49] incorporated the following set of cardiac structural changes into their genetic

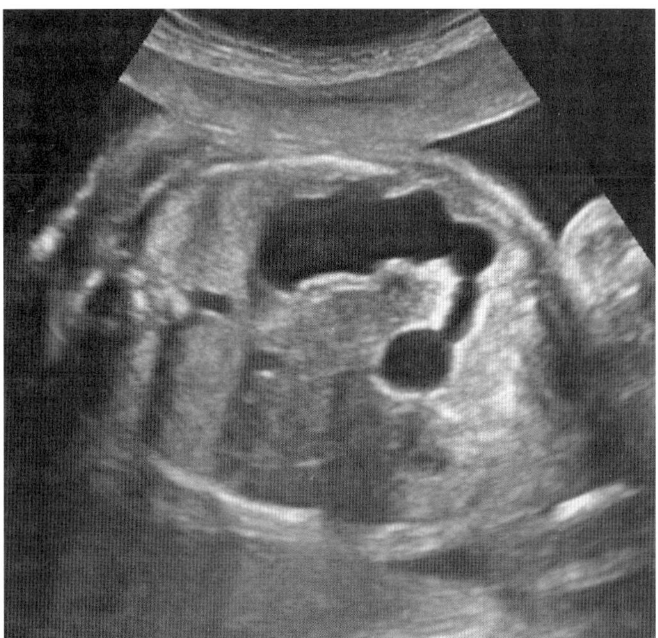

Fig. 20.3 'Double bubble' sign of duodenal atresia.

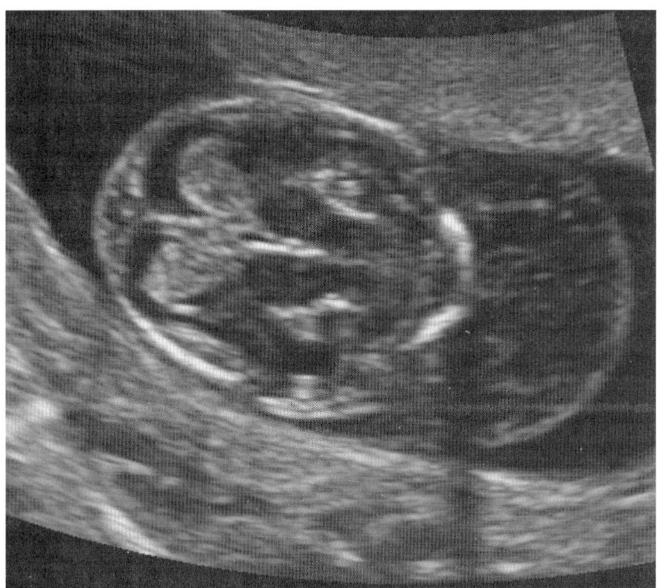

Fig. 20.4 Cystic hygroma.

Table 20.3 **Likelihood ratios for trisomy 21 associated with major structural malformations**

Study	*T21 Cases*	*Likelihood ratio*	*95% CI*
Vergani et al. 1999[45]	22	30	15–65
Nyberg et al. 2001[42]	186	28	15–54
Bromley et al. 2002[40]	164	22	11–46

Adapted from Breathnach et al., *Am J Med Genet* **145**(1):62–72, 2007

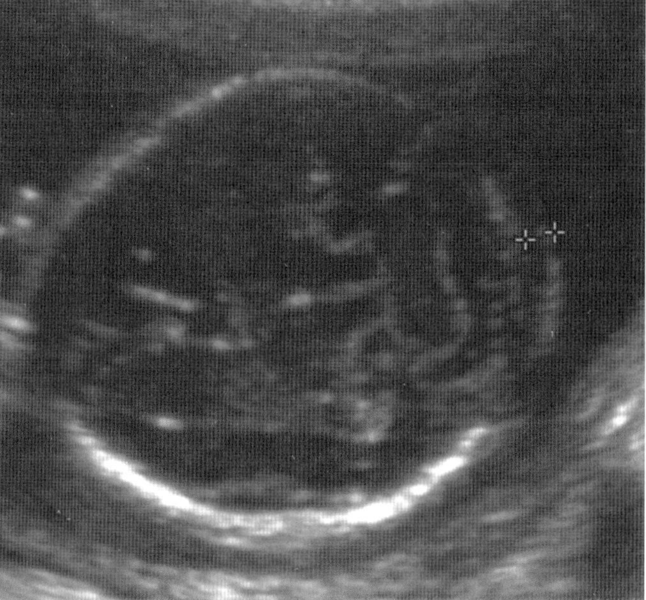

Fig. 20.5 Nuchal fold.

sonogram: right-to-left ventricular disproportion, ventricular septal defect, tricuspid regurgitation and pericardial effusion. These authors reported a resultant increase in the detection rate for trisomy 21 from 65% to 91%. In this analysis, fetal echocardiography also contributed to the identification of trisomy 13 and 18 cases (increased detection from 57% to 95%). For these aneuploidies, DeVore reported an overall false-positive rate of 13%. Identification of an atrioventricular septal defect (AVSD) is particularly suggestive of an abnormal karyotype (trisomy 21 in particular) and should prompt consideration for amniocentesis even when identified in isolation. Trisomy 21 has been reportedly identified in up to 50% of fetuses with isolated AVSD but without other sonographic abnormalities[50].

'SOFT' SONOGRAPHIC MARKERS FOR ANEUPLOIDY

Many major structural anomalies associated with aneuploidy, including cardiac defects, go undetected on prenatal ultrasound screening. Improved detection rates can be achieved by incorporating the aforementioned 'soft markers' into the sonographic screen for aneuploidy. The soft markers associated with the three most common autosomal trisomies are outlined in Table 20.2.

The first soft marker identified for trisomy 21 was thickening of the nuchal fold[51], a marker that retains its superior predictive value for trisomy 21 over all other soft markers. The sonographic view described for nuchal fold measurement requires an axial plane through the posterior fossa (Fig. 20.5). Calipers are placed from the outer aspect of occipital bone to the outer skin limit. Where a cut-off of 6mm is used, a meta-analysis has demonstrated a 17-fold increase (CI 8–35) in the risk of trisomy 21[52]. The definition of nuchal fold thickening has varied slightly since its original description. Most investigators now consider a cut-off of 5mm to be significant before 18 weeks' gestation, and 6mm thereafter[53–55].

Aside from nuchal fold thickening, the most commonly utilized panel of 'soft markers' for aneuploidy includes

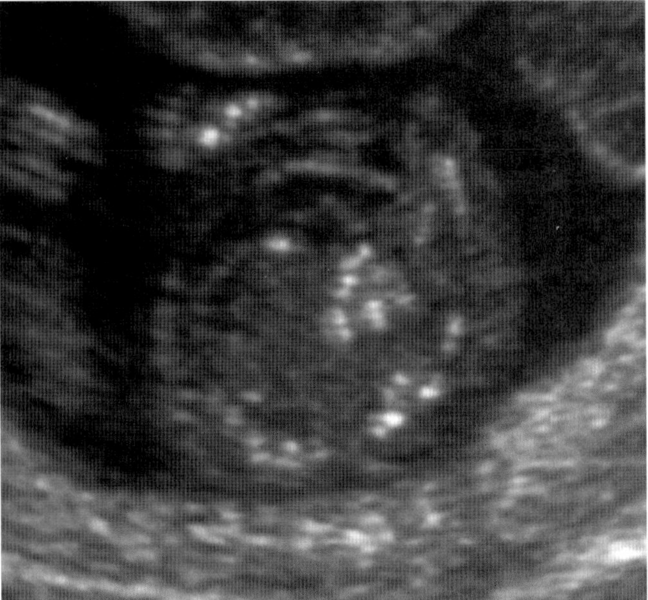

Fig. 20.6 Echogenic bowel.

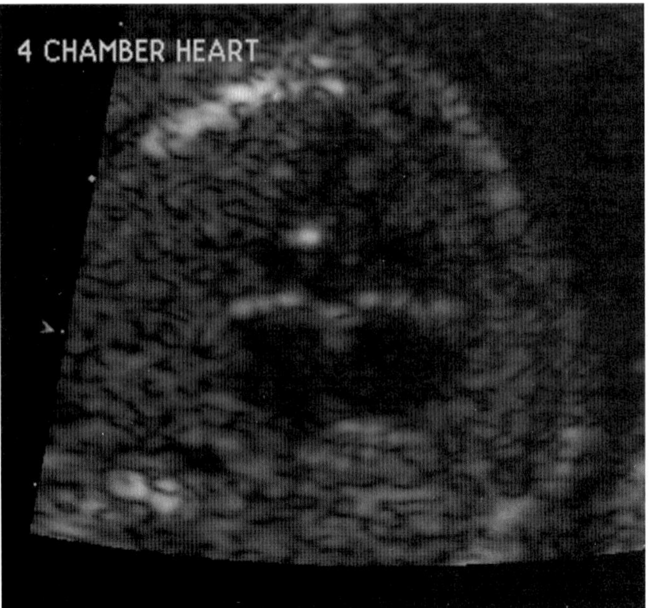

Fig. 20.7 Echogenic intracardiac focus.

echogenic bowel, echogenic intracardiac foci and renal pyelectasis (Figs. 20.6–20.8). Bowel that is as bright as adjacent bone is termed 'echogenic'. Although an association between echogenic bowel and aneuploidy is established, other causes for bowel echogenicity, such as infection, cystic fibrosis and bleeding should be considered[56,57]. An echogenic intracardiac focus comprises an area of calcified papillary muscle leading to a discrete dot in the left or, less commonly, the right ventricle. Again, the echogenicity is described as being as bright as bone. The prevalence of this marker in Asian populations approaches 30%[58]. Renal pyelectasis is identified when the anteroposterior diameter of either renal pelvis exceeds 3 mm between 15 and 20 weeks' gestation. With the exception of nuchal fold, soft markers in isolation have little significance in terms of aneuploidy risk.

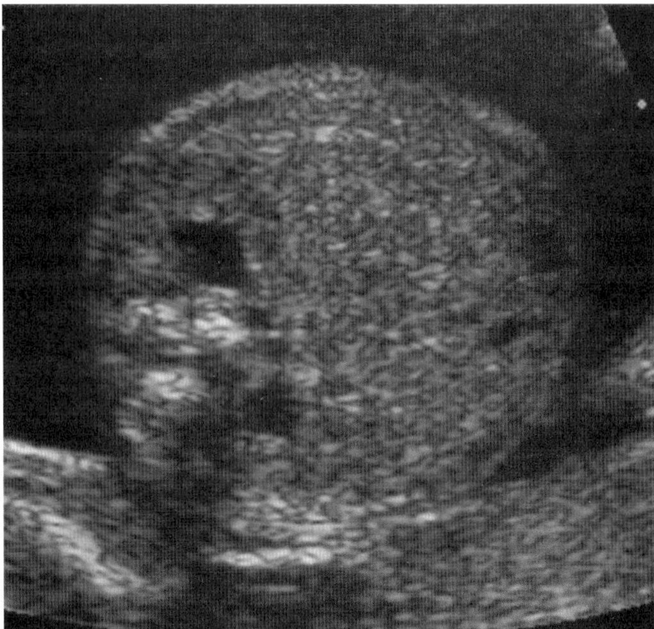

Fig. 20.8 Renal pyelectasis.

BIOMETRIC MARKERS FOR ANEUPLOIDY

The growth restriction observed in aneuploid pregnancies is most marked with trisomy 18 and trisomy 13. Although generally less striking, this feature is shared with trisomy 21 and translates into short stature as a phenotypic feature of this condition. Consequently, the prenatal identification of a short femur and humerus, as defined by an observed-to-expected length of <0.9[59,60], have been incorporated into the panel of markers for trisomy 21. The utility of such limb shortening as a marker for trisomy 21 is only helpful when observed in combination with other sonographic markers[61]. The shortened humerus length, although less prevalent, has been shown to be more predictive of trisomy 21 than a shortened femur[62]. Ethnic variation in long bone biometry impacts on the utility of these markers in populations that are not homogeneous and creates some limitation to the applicability of these markers in varied clinical settings.

OTHER SOFT SONOGRAPHIC MARKERS

A range of less commonly sought soft markers for aneuploidy has been described. Skeletal markers include wide lateral flare of the iliac bones, clinodactyly, 'sandal gap' toe, nasal bone hypoplasia and brachycephaly.

Wide lateral flare of the iliac bones is seen as a prenatally detectable characteristic of the trisomy 21 fetus[63,64] and can be demonstrated in a transverse image of the fetal pelvis, in which the angle formed between the iliac crests ('the iliac angle') is measured. However, this marker is subject to high rates of inter-observer variation and changes significantly according to the level at which the angle is measured, such that this marker has not been incorporated into the routine panel of markers studied for the genetic sonogram.

Close inspection of the fetal hand can yield signs of aneuploidy. Hypoplasia of the middle phalanx of the fifth digit (clinodactyly) (Fig. 20.9) is a recognized phenotypic feature

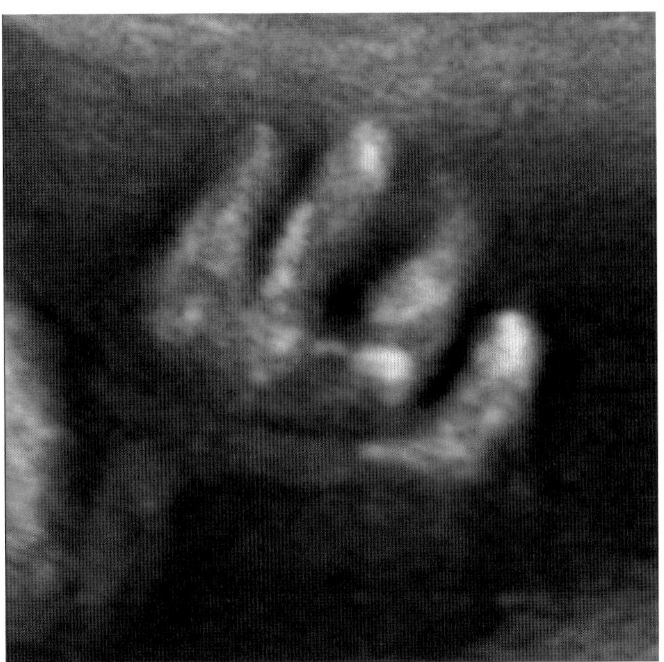

Fig. 20.9 Clinodactyly.

of trisomy 21 and its prenatal detection was first described by Benacerraf and colleagues[65]. In recent times, clinodactyly has displayed improved performance as a marker for trisomy 21, with a sensitivity of 17.1% and false positive rate of 3% reported by Deren and colleagues[66], in contrast to the high false-positive rate of 18% identified by the original authors.

A wide space between the first and second toes, such that the first toe is angled outward ('sandal gap toe') in infants with trisomy 21 is an additional phenotypic feature potentially amenable to prenatal identification[67,68]. However, its reported sensitivity in the second trimester, at just 3%[68], renders this marker unsuitable for widespread clinical application.

The identification of nasal bone hypoplasia in the second trimester has been cited by Cicero and colleagues[69] as a highly sensitive and specific marker for trisomy 21. This assertion is not, however, universally supported, perhaps owing to variations in the definition of this marker. Cicero and colleagues describe nasal bone hypoplasia as a feature of 62% of trisomy 21 fetuses and approximately 1% of chromosomally normal fetuses where the nasal bone was considered to be hypoplastic if it was either absent or 'strikingly small' (less than 2.5 mm). Published normative data[70] describe the nasal bone length increasing with gestation from a mean of 4.7 mm at 15 weeks to 8.2 mm at 22 weeks. Table 20.4 illustrates the varied reported sensitivities and false-positive rates according to differing definitions of hypoplasia. By comparing various nasal bone criteria, Obido and colleagues[71] found that the optimal nasal bone threshold associated with trisomy 21 was a biparietal diameter/nasal bone length ratio of 11 or greater. Irrespective of the definition used, however, an important prerequisite to consider is the angle of insonation of the fetal nose, which should be between 45° and 135° to avoid false shortening or lack of visualization of the nasal bone[72].

The term 'brachycephaly' refers to an abnormal skull shape and is assumed to reflect frontal lobe hypoplasia in individuals with trisomy 21. When identifiable on prenatal ultrasound,

Table 20.4 **Nasal bone hypoplasia as a second-trimester marker for trisomy 21**

Study	Definition	Sensitivity	False-positive rate	Positive LR
Bromley et al. 2002[40]	Absence of nasal bones	37%	0.5%	83
Bromley et al. 2002[40]	BPD/NBL ratio <10	81%	11%	8
Cicero et al. 2003[69]	Absence or hypoplasia (<2.5 mm)	62%	1.2%	51
Odibo et al. 2004[71]	BPD/ NBL ratio <11	50%	7%	7.1
Vintzileos et al. 2003[72]	Absence of nasal bones	41%	0%	–

it may prove useful as a screening tool. Although this feature has demonstrated some screening potential in retrospective studies using the 'cephalic index' (the biparietal diameter over the occipital frontal diameter)[40,73,74], it has yet to be evaluated prospectively. A comparable marker for trisomy 18 is the 'strawberry-shaped' cranium[75].

Evidence also supports an association between delayed fusion of the amnion and chorion (persisted separation after 17 weeks' gestation) and chromosomal abnormality, typically trisomy 21[76,77]. This sonographic finding is, however, too rare to represent a clinically useful marker.

In routine practice in unselected populations, the above 'other' sonographic markers have not undergone sufficient evaluation for inclusion in the routine panel of markers sought at the genetic sonogram.

VARIABILITY IN SONOGRAPHIC MARKER DETECTION

The applicability of the genetic sonogram to risk adjustment for fetal aneuploidy in women identified as 'high risk' on the basis of age or serum screening results is dependent on reliability and reproducibility of identified sonographic markers.

Wide variation in the detection rates of sonographic markers for trisomy 21 has been identified in a systematic review[78]. Reported rates of echogenic bowel ranged from 12 to 22% and thickened nuchal fold from 40 to 75% (false-positive rate <2%) among second-trimester fetuses with trisomy 21. This lack of uniformity in reported detection rates may result from the inherent subjectivity of soft marker evaluation, which may be improved by strict standardization of definitions used. By contrast, a study conducted by Smith Bindman and colleagues identified less marked inter-observer variation[18]. Among experienced practitioners, these investigators found moderate agreement in the reporting of sonographic markers for aneuploidy. In comparing their findings with inter-observer variability for other imaging modalities such as mammography and emergency medicine radiology, prenatal screening performed similarly.

Maternal and fetal variables that influence detection rates include gestational age, fetal gender and maternal body mass index. Advancing gestational age has a positive correlation with the detection of sonographic markers in trisomic fetuses, as illustrated by Taslimi and colleagues[79], who observed improved detection of sonographic markers with advancing gestation, rising from 12% at 15 weeks' gestation to greater than 60% after 18 weeks.

The influence of fetal gender on sonographic marker detection is less clear. Male fetuses have been shown to exhibit a significantly increased frequency of renal pelvis dilatation when compared with females[80]. A comparable inter-gender difference has not been demonstrated for other markers.

The influence of maternal body habitus on the sonographic detection of abnormalities, as discussed above, applies equally to the detection of soft markers, with increased maternal body-mass index posing technical challenges for some examinations.

SIGNIFICANCE OF INDIVIDUAL SOFT MARKERS

Computing a risk estimate for aneuploidy based on the identification of sonographic soft markers requires a validated knowledge of the risk conferred by each individual marker. The accuracy of the genetic sonogram in detecting cases of trisomy 21 has been the subject of many published studies (Table 20.5). An analysis representing 13 such studies[68], concluded that identification of at least one soft marker conferred an overall sensitivity of 77% for the detection of trisomy 21 with a false-positive rate of 13%. Similar overall sensitivity (72%) was reported by a collaborative 8-center group that studied a cohort of 176 cases of trisomy 21 and further identified nuchal fold thickening (greater than 5 mm) as the superior sonographic soft marker for aneuploidy, being identified in almost half of trisomy 21 fetuses.

The identification of multiple soft markers is far more predictive of aneuploidy than demonstration of any marker in isolation[83–86]. The comparative prevalence of isolated and multiple markers in aneuploid and euploid populations has been evaluated by Nyberg[43], as illustrated in Table 20.6. Given the high prevalence of isolated soft markers in the euploid population (which translates into a false positive rate for aneuploidy of 11–17%), the management of isolated soft markers has become a contentious issue. Where more than one soft marker is identified, the link with aneuploidy is sufficiently robust to justify invasive testing. In an analysis of 186 fetuses with trisomy 21, Nyberg and colleagues identified an isolated soft marker (panel outlined in Table 20.7) in 22.6% of trisomy 21 cases and 11.3% of euploid controls, while 2 or more markers were observed in 15.1% of cases and just 1.6% of normal controls. By contrast, although the identification of choroid plexus cysts is reported to have an association with trisomy 18, the published absolute risk of trisomy 18 where this marker is identified in isolation ranges from 0 to 3.6%[86–88], at the lower end of the scale in unselected populations.

Three large analyses that have explored the association between individual soft markers and aneuploidy report comparable likelihood ratios for various markers[40,43,52]. The association

Table 20.5 **Performance of genetic sonogram for detection of trisomy 21**

Study	*Reference*	*Sensitivity* (%)*	*FPR (%)*	*Positive LR*
Benacerraf (1994)	82	73	4.0	18
DeVore (1995)	33	87	7.4	12
Nadel (1995)	34	80	4.0	20
Bahado-Singh (1996)	83	71	14	5
Bahado-Singh (1998)	84	60	4.5	13
Deren (1998)	66	63	13	5
Verdin (1998)	147	82	10	8
Vintzileos (1995)	36	82	13	6
Sohl (1999)	74	67	19	4
Vergani (1999)	45	59	5.3	11
DeVore (2000)	41	91	14	N/A
Smith-Bindman (2001)	52	69	8.0	9
Nyberg (2001)	42	69	14	5
Bromley (2002)	40	81	12	7
Hobbins (2003)	67	72	N/A	N/A

*Refers to presence of major structural abnormality or soft marker or both.
Table adapted from Breathnach et al., *Am J Med Genet* **145**(1):62–72, 2007

Table 20.6 **Isolated versus multiple sonographic markers for trisomy 21**

	Trisomy 21	*Normal*	*LR*
No markers	31%	87%	0.4
One marker	23%	11%	2
Two markers	15%	2%	10
≥3 markers	15%	0.1%	115

Nyberg et al. 2001[43]

between pyelectasis or shortened femur as isolated soft markers for trisomy 21 did not reach statistical significance in 2 of the 3 studies; however, when identified in conjunction with other soft sonographic markers, both were found to carry a significant association with trisomy 21. Similarly, several authors have suggested that an echogenic intracardiac focus found in isolation should not warrant any amendment to the patient's individual risk assignment for aneuploidy[89,90]. The assertion of the authors of the largest meta-analysis to date[52], summarizing 59 studies pertaining to sonographic markers for trisomy 21, is that overall sensitivity of isolated soft markers, including

Table 20.7 **Sonographic markers for trisomy 21:Likelihood ratios and 95% CI when marker isolated**

	Smith-Bindman[52]	Nyberg[43]	Bromley[40]	DeVore[41]
Number T21 cases	1930	186	164	80
Nuchal fold	17 (8–38)	11 (6–22)	–	53.4 (27–107)
Short humerus	7.5 (5–12)	5.1 (2–17)	5.8 (1–34)	
Short femur	2.7 (1–6)	1.5 (0.8–3)	1.2 (0.5–3)	
Echogenic bowel	6.1 (3–13)	6.7 (3–17)	–	7.4 (4–15)
EICF	2.8 (2–6)	1.8 (1–3)	1.4 (0.6–4)	
Pyelectasis	1.9 (0.7–5)	1.5 (0.6–4)	1.5 (1–11)	7.6 (4–16)

EICF: echogenic intracardiac focus

a thickened nuchal fold, is too low to justify use as a practical screening test for trisomy 21. Furthermore, the authors state that if soft markers are incorporated into screening paradigms for trisomy 21 and thereby contribute to invasive fetal tests, the resultant procedure-related fetal loss rate would exceed the number of cases of trisomy 21 detected and indeed, that detection rates would fall. This assertion has been challenged by others[91], who argue that while this meta-analysis may support the widely held belief that soft markers contribute poorly to aneuploidy detection when identified in isolation, the screening performance of combined markers is a different matter and has been well validated in screening paradigms. More important is the acknowledgement that the absence of soft markers can dramatically reduce a patient's risk assignment for aneuploidy and provide reassurance without recourse to invasive testing for many patients.

APPLICATION OF SOFT MARKER IDENTIFICATION IN PRACTICE

The interpretation of the significance of individual soft markers should always take a patient's a priori risk into account. Several models have been described; all with the objective of correlating soft marker identification with other risk factors (namely, maternal age and/or serum analyte results). This strategy should minimize the number of invasive tests pursued on the basis of identification of isolated soft markers incidentally noted in low-risk women.

Benacerraf and colleagues[80,92] proposed a simple sonographic scoring index for this purpose. A score of 2 was assigned where a major structural abnormality or a thickened nuchal fold was identified, illustrating the weight assigned to these markers which, even when detected in isolation, would prompt consideration of an invasive diagnostic test. Soft markers other than nuchal fold thickening were each allocated a score of 1. The panel of soft markers included short femur, short humerus, pyelectasis, echogenic intracardiac focus, echogenic bowel and choroid plexus cysts. The authors demonstrated that, where amniocentesis was reserved for fetuses scoring ≥2, 73% of fetuses with trisomy 21 and 85% of fetuses with trisomy 18 could be identified with a false-positive rate of 4%.

An alternative scoring model, termed the Age-Adjusted Ultrasound Risk Assessment (AAURA), was devised by Nyberg and colleagues[85]. This model uses likelihood ratios to compute an individual patient-specific risk, by combining the presence or absence of sonographic markers with the a priori risk based on maternal age. Using one or more markers, these authors identified 68.3% of fetuses with trisomy 21, with a 12.5% false-positive rate.

The AAURA and a modified form of the Index Scoring System (incorporating maternal age, with a score of 1 assigned to women over 36 and 2 to women aged 40 or more) have demonstrated equivalent screening performance in a comparative study[93] with the AAURA detecting approximately half of all trisomy 21 fetuses at a 5% false-positive rate. The study identified that the addition of maternal age to the standard index scoring system further improved sensitivity (74% versus 68%) but at the expense of higher false-positive rates (42% versus 24%). Although the more complex AAURA model computes a more individualized risk than the Index Scoring System, this comparative study demonstrates no real difference in screening performance between the two models.

Using likelihood ratios (LR), two different approaches have been proposed by Nyberg and Nicolaides to calculate a revised risk. The Nyberg method requires multiplication of the a priori risk by the likelihood ratio associated with any identified marker or markers. The latter calculation, proposed by Nicolaides, further takes into account the significance of absent markers. The practical application of these two approaches in fact yields similar results, as illustrated by this example: A 39-year-old woman has an a priori age-related trisomy 21 risk of 1 in 100. The genetic sonogram identifies an isolated thickened nuchal fold. Applying the Nyberg method, the LR associated with this marker[11] is multiplied by her a priori risk (0.01) to give a revised risk of $0.01 \times 11 = 0.11$, or 'one in nine'. Applying the Nicolaides method in the same scenario requires multiplication of her a priori risk by a positive LR of 53.1 associated with nuchal fold thickening and also by the negative LRs associated with absent markers (i.e. combined negative LRs $0.7 \times 0.9 \times 0.6 \times 0.9 \times 0.8 = 0.272$) associated with the absence of short humerus, echogenic bowel, short femur, pyelectasis and echogenic intracardiac focus respectively. The same woman's revised risk is computed by multiplying these risks ($0.01 \times 53.1 \times 0.272$) to arrive at a risk of 0.14 or 'one in seven'. The likelihood ratios applicable to each method are outlined in Tables 20.7 and Table 20.8. It is worth noting the consistently wide confidence intervals surrounding the point estimates of these likelihood ratios, inferring that, while the identification of one or more markers may be an effective screening tool, the actual computed risk is only an approximation.

Replacing maternal age-determined a priori risk with a risk derived from biochemical screening (serum analytes plus maternal age) has formed the basis of a scoring system adopted more recently by several authors[35,54,81,82].

Table 20.8 Clinical example to compare Nicolaides and Nyberg methods of incorporating genetic sonogram markers into fetal aneuploidy risk assessment

A priori risk 1 in 100	
Genetic sonogram: isolated nuchal fold	
Nicolaides method	*Nyberg method*
Positive likelihood ratio (LR) = 53.1	Positive likelihood ratio (LR) = 11
But no short humerus, echogenic bowel (EB), short femur, pyelectasis, echogenic intracardiac focus (EIF)	No short humerus, echogenic bowel (EB), short femur, pyelectasis, echogenic intracardiac focus (EIF)
Negative LRs = 0.7 × 0.9 × 0.6 × 0.9 × 0.8 = 0.272	Negative LRs not calculated
Revised risk = 0.01 × 53.1 × 0.272 = 0.14	Revised risk = 0.01 × 11 = 0.11
= 1 in 7	**= 1 in 9**

If sonographic markers are to be combined with serum analyte markers for the purpose of providing a single risk-estimate, it is important that these markers are proven to be predictors of aneuploidy independent of the serum markers and that if correlations do exist between sonographic and biochemical markers, as suggested by Souter and colleagues[94], that correlation coefficients can be computed to overcome this concern. Such correlations include lower estriol levels in the presence of fetal cystic hygroma, higher estriol and lower alphafeto-protein (AFP) levels with EICF and a positive correlation between NF and maternal serum hCG. The complexity of these proposals only goes to emphasize the rationality of the program proposed in the UK by the National Screening Committee which has set targets for sensitivity (75%) and false-positive rate (3%) for Down's syndrome screening tests. As these tests now approach a 90% detection rate and only small numbers of Down's syndrome fetuses survive up to 20 weeks' gestation, the need for soft marker scanning will greatly diminish, if not disappear.

ANEUPLOID CONDITIONS OTHER THAN TRISOMY 21

The multiplicity of structural malformations, coupled with the marked intrauterine growth restriction, observed in trisomy 18, render this condition readily amenable to prenatal sonographic detection in 80–100% of cases,[95–98] as illustrated in Table 20.9. The incidence of major cardiac abnormalities among trisomy 18 fetuses exceeds 90%. Abnormalities of virtually all other organ systems have been described, as outlined in Table 20.2.

Choroid plexus cysts (CPCs) have been identified in approximately one-third of T18 fetuses in the second trimester in contrast to 1–2% of the euploid population. An association with trisomy 21 has not been demonstrated, such that the identification of choroid plexus cysts in cases of trisomy 21 has been attributed to coincidence[99]. A meta-analysis[100,101] has identified a likelihood of trisomy 18 of 13.8 times the a priori risk in fetuses with isolated choroid plexus cysts diagnosed in the second trimester. These investigators support offering genetic amniocentesis to women with this isolated sonographic finding only if maternal age at delivery was 36 years or older, or when the risk for trisomy 18 detected by serum multiple marker screen exceeded one in 3000. A further meta-analysis[102] has estimated that CPC confers a likelihood ratio of 8.6 for trisomy 18.

Table 20.9 The genetic sonogram and rarer trisomies

Study	*Trisomy*	*Detection rate*
Lehman 1995[103]	13	91% (30/33)
Nyberg 1993[95]	18	83% (39/47)
DeVore 2000[97]	18	97% (29/30)
Yeo 2003[98]	18	100% (38/38)

Adapted from Breathnach et al., *Am J Med Genet* **145**(1):62–72, 2007

The myriad of structural anomalies observed in trisomy 13 and triploidy again render these conditions amenable to prenatal identification as evidenced by detection rates that approach 90–100%[103,104]. Severe, early onset asymmetrical intrauterine growth restriction is the hallmark of triploidy[105], with oligohydramnios and a small placenta being characteristic of the condition where the surplus set of chromosomes is maternally derived, while a partial molar or hydropic placental appearance is more typical of a paternally derived extra set of chromosomes. Other sonographic abnormalities observed in triploidy include ventriculomegaly, Dandy-Walker malformation, agenesis of the corpus callosum, cardiac anomalies, micrognathia, echogenic bowel, renal malformations, thickened nuchal fold, neural tube defects, talipes and syndactyly of the 3rd and 4th digits[105,106].

FIRST-TRIMESTER SCREENING FOR ANEUPLOIDY

While mid-trimester sonography has witnessed immense improvements in identification of structural abnormalities as well as subtle signs of aneuploidy, there has, in recent times, been a demand for earlier detection of abnormalities. This drive toward first-trimester diagnosis has been fueled by the recognition of first-trimester serum markers (pregnancy-associated plasma protein-A (PAPP-A) and the free β-subunit of human chorionic gonadotrophin (fβhCG)) for aneuploidy, and the evolution of nuchal translucency as a first-trimester screening tool. Several reports of small series of high-risk pregnancies in the early 1990s demonstrated an association between nuchal translucency thickening and fetal aneuploidy[107–110]. Screening based on nuchal translucency alone, however, was soon superseded by a combined approach: utilizing NT in combination with maternal age and serum markers PAPP-A and fβhCG. Today, while a wide range of screening paradigms exists, comprising algorithms that include an expanding panel of sonographic and serum markers at varying gestations, the combined test that incorporates NT, PAPP-A and fβHCG represents one of the most widely adopted screening strategies for aneuploidy. Screening strategies incorporating serum markers are discussed in detail in Chapter 19.

It is worth noting that the first-trimester NT scan offers several benefits in addition to the refinement of aneuploidy risk. A range of abnormalities other than aneuploidy has been associated with increased nuchal translucency. These include cardiac anomalies, diaphragmatic hernia, skeletal dysplasia, fetal anaemia and abnormal lymphatic drainage associated with neuromuscular disorders[111]. Therefore, identification of an increased NT measurement should prompt not only the offer of a diagnostic test for aneuploidy, but also, in the case of a normal karyotype, a thorough anatomic survey for structural anomalies and a detailed fetal echocardiogram.

ACCURATE NUCHAL TRANSLUCENCY MEASUREMENT

Given the subtlety of first-trimester nuchal translucency, precision in the standard technique described for acquiring this measurement and adherence to strict criteria used to attain reproducible results are paramount. A proper sagittal view of the spine is required. This is generally achievable with transabdominal ultrasound but may require a transvaginal approach. The scan machine should be equipped with a video-loop function. The fetal crown–rump length should lie between 45 mm and 84 mm, in accordance with a gestational age of 11–13 weeks. The magnification should be such that the fetus occupies at least three-quarters of the image. Accepting that at this gestation fetal skin and amnion may be indistinguishable, care must be taken to observe the fetus 'lifting off' the amnion. The nuchal translucency should be measured with the fetus in a neutral position, avoiding hyperextension or indeed hyperflexion of the fetal neck (Fig. 20.10). Nuchal translucency measurement is thus achieved by placing the callipers on the lines corresponding to skin and soft tissue overlying the fetal cervical spine to attain the maximum thickness at this level.

With strict adherence to these principles, both inter- and intra-observer variability in NT measurements can be minimized to less than 0.5 mm[112,113].

PERFORMANCE OF FIRST-TRIMESTER COMBINED SCREENING

A series of pooled studies[114], comprising a study population of 209 603, has reported a collective 86% detection rate for trisomy 21 using first-trimester combined screening, for a false-positive rate of 5%. Two notable large prospective studies have demonstrated improved detection rates and lower false-positive rates achievable with first-trimester combined screening when compared with its second-trimester equivalent. The serum, urine and ultrasound screening study (SURUSS)[115] and first- and second-trimester evaluation of risk for fetal aneuploidy (FASTER)[116] trials allowed comparative analyses of first and second-trimester screening strategies in large unselected populations.

The performance of first-trimester combined screening is reportedly not consistent across the 11th–14th week. The FASTER investigators[116] reported a maximum performance of the screen for trisomy 21 at 11 weeks' gestational age, with detection rates dropping from 87% at 11 weeks to 82% at 13 weeks at a set false-positive rate of 5%.

The principal advantage of first-trimester screening for the majority of women lies in its potential to provide earlier reassurance, or indeed earlier diagnosis of aneuploidy, affording couples who choose to terminate an affected pregnancy the enhanced safety and privacy of doing so at an earlier gestation. However, recognizing the 30% spontaneous fetal loss rate after 12 weeks for trisomy 21 pregnancies[117], a potential disadvantage of earlier screening is the detection of aneuploid fetuses that would otherwise have been destined to miscarry, thereby overstating the real detection rate for liveborn aneuploid infants. Nonetheless, according to de Graaf and co-authors[118], the vast majority (97.8%) of women who opt for prenatal screening declare a preference for screening to be carried out in the first rather than second trimester. This demand is now being met in many countries by one-stop clinics that offer rapid risk assessment techniques.

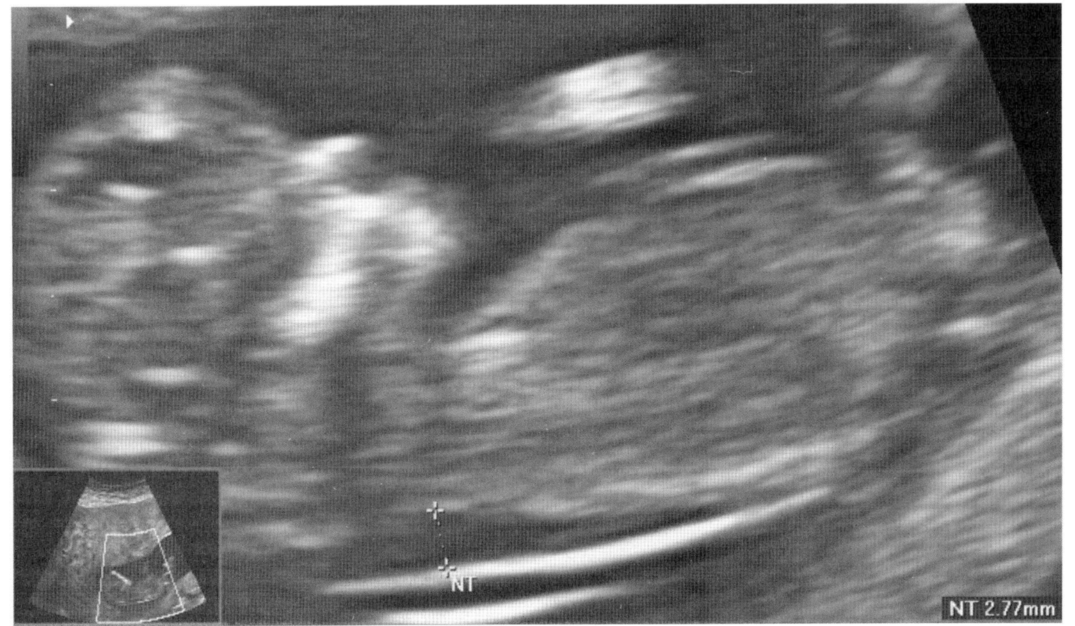

Fig. 20.10 Nuchal translucency.

SEPTATED CYSTIC HYGROMA

Recently, investigators have identified cystic hygromas as entities distinct from simple nuchal translucency thickening. In the FASTER study, cystic hygroma was strictly defined as an enlarged hypoechoic space at the back of the fetal neck, extending along the length of the fetal back, with clearly visible septations[119]. The incidence of cystic hygroma in this unselected population (median age 30.1 years) was 1 in 285. Aneuploidy was confirmed in approximately 50% of cases, of whom 40% had trisomy 21. Of the remaining euploid fetuses, half had major structural malformations and the majority of the remaining pregnancies had normal outcomes at a median follow-up of 25 months. These studies support the belief that septated cystic hygromas are indicative in their own right of a sufficiently high risk for aneuploidy to warrant the immediate offer of an invasive diagnostic test. If chromosomal analysis is normal, a detailed mid-trimester anatomic survey and fetal echocardiograph should be performed.

FETAL NASAL BONE IN THE FIRST TRIMESTER

The assertion that absence of the nasal bone during the first trimester served as a marker for trisomy 21 began with a large prospective trial in a high-risk population undergoing chorionic villus sampling[120]. The nasal bone was absent in 73% of trisomy 21 fetuses and in only 0.5% of euploid pregnancies. Given the high prevalence of this marker in affected pregnancies and rarity of this marker in euploid fetuses, these authors deduced that nasal bone assessment would significantly improve the performance of first-trimester ultrasound for trisomy 21. They estimated that 85% and 93% of trisomy 21 cases would be detected at false-positive rates of 1% and 4% respectively. The same group of investigators conducted a retrospective analysis that suggested a 97% detection rate for trisomy 21 could be achieved for a false-positive rate of 5% by incorporating nasal bone measurements into existing combined (NT and serum biochemistry) screening protocols[121].

When applied to general population screening in the FASTER study, the performance of this marker was, however, disappointing[122], as 9 of 11 fetuses with trisomy 21 had nasal bones present. Significant variability has been observed in nasal bone assessment, thereby limiting its applicability as a screening tool. For example, Cicero et al.[123] included not only cases in which the nasal bone was completely absent, but also those in which they observed the nasal bone as hypoplastic. Other authors[124] have strictly considered the nasal bone absent if there is no evidence whatsoever of its presence. For these reasons, nasal bone evaluation has not been incorporated into routine screening protocols in unselected populations.

FIRST-TRIMESTER DOPPLER ASSESSMENT OF THE DUCTUS VENOSUS

Reversed flow in the ductus venosus, a fetal vessel with a pulsatile waveform carrying oxygenated blood from the umbilical vein to inferior vena cava, has been associated both with aneuploidy and with congenital heart disease[125,126]. The utility of this marker was investigated by Nicolaides and colleagues[127] in a multicenter review which pooled the results of six studies assessing the relationship between ductus venosus flow and aneuploidy. Abnormal ductus venosus flow was identified in 82% of aneuploid fetuses with a false positive rate of 5%. Although these results are promising, the sometimes technically challenging nature of this marker may preclude its applicability to general population screening. The role of first-trimester Doppler assessment of the ductus venosus may, like that of nasal bone assessment, be restricted to high-risk pregnancies in specialist centres.

FIRST-TRIMESTER TRICUSPID REGURGITATION

Regurgitation across the tricuspid valve in the first trimester was demonstrated as having a link with fetal aneuploidy by Huggon and colleagues[128]. The majority of the 262 high-risk patients in this study had an increased nuchal translucency. Tricuspid regurgitation (TR) was identified by pulsed Doppler in 70 cases. The prevalence of aneuploidy in those who screened positive for tricuspid regurgitation was 83%, while 35% of those without TR were aneuploid, thus underpinning the high-risk nature of this cohort. This observation was further studied by Faiola and co-investigators[129], whose cohort of 742 high-risk pregnancies was scanned by pediatric cardiologists at 11–13 + 6 weeks' gestation. These investigators applied a strict definition for tricuspid regurgitation, in that it had to occupy at least half of systole and reach a velocity of over 80 cm/s. Tricuspid regurgitation was thus identified in 65% of fetuses with trisomy 21 and in 8.5% of chromosomally normal cases, with a likelihood ratio of TR for cardiac defects of 8.4. Again this screening tool has been validated in high-risk groups only.

ANATOMIC SURVEY IN THE FIRST TRIMESTER

The anatomic survey for structural abnormalities has traditionally been carried out at 18–20 weeks' gestation, as described above. However, with improved ultrasound resolution, and with recourse to the transvaginal probe, the potential of the 11–14 week sonographic examination to serve as a tool for identifying major structural fetal defects is increasingly being tested.

Transabdominal sonographic evaluation of fetal limb biometry between 10 and 14 weeks has been studied by De Biasio and colleagues[130], who report 98% success in measuring the humerus, ulna, femur and tibia and 93% success in obtaining foot measurements at this gestation. Intracranial structures can also be visualized and have an appearance that differs in some respects from mid-trimester scans. The lateral ventricles appear relatively large, while their cavities are filled with the choroid plexus. The cerebellum has been demonstrated by the 11th week in an entire cohort of patients in one study, and in 80% of patients by the 10th week[131]. Spinal views can also be studied during this examination, as evidenced by a study by Braithwaite and colleagues[132], who successfully obtained images of the vertebrae and overlying skin in both transverse and coronal sections in all of their cohort at 12 and 13 weeks' gestation.

The fetal bladder can be imaged from 11 weeks' gestation[133], but demonstration of the kidneys prior to 12 weeks is unreliable[134]. As expected, the reported success of early fetal echocardiography improves as gestation advances from 11 to 14 weeks. Haak and co-investigators[135] achieved a complete cardiac evaluation (including four-chamber view, pulmonary trunk, three-vessel view, aortic root, long axis aorta and crossing arteries) in 20% of cases at 11 weeks, rising to 97.6% of cases at 13 weeks.

Thus a range of major structural abnormalities are amenable to detection at 10–14 weeks, including anencephaly, some skeletal dysplasias, cardiac anomalies, omphalocele, megacystis and diaphragmatic hernia[136]. A recent prospective study of 1148 singleton unselected pregnancies[137] reported detection rates of 50% (7/14) for major structural defects in a structured examination of the fetal anatomy at this gestation. One concern that has been raised is that transient ultrasound findings in the first trimester that had resolved by the second-trimester scan (such as abdominal cysts and pericardial effusion) resulted in a false-positive rate of 18% in this study. Reservations surrounding the feasibility of conducting a complete anatomic survey at the time of NT screening have been raised in another study[138], that reported successful completion of an anatomic survey in just 33% of first-trimester fetuses, where this examination was conducted by sonographers at the same time as the NT scan.

Given that many anatomic structures, particularly intracranial structures, have not developed fully until later in gestation, it is unlikely that screening for structural anomalies at 11–14 weeks will replace the 18–20-week scan. However, where satisfactory images of selected structures can be obtained, the potential to provide early diagnosis or early reassurance will continue to attract researchers to expand the capabilities of the 11–14-week scan.

THREE-DIMENSIONAL ULTRASOUND

The advent of three-dimensional ultrasound, with capabilities to generate and store volumetric data, offers additional possibilities in the arena of prenatal diagnosis. This most recent obstetric imaging modality has proven useful as an adjunctive tool in the evaluation of facial abnormalities[139–141], talipes[142], skeletal dysplasias[143] and spinal anomalies.[144] In a comparative study of 2D and 3D modalities[145], the latter offered diagnostic advantages in 51% of fetal anomalies and had an impact on prenatal management in 5% of cases.

A key advantage of three-dimensional ultrasound is the ability to store volumetric data, thereby facilitating review and manipulation of the images by many specialists who may be remote from the patient. Nonetheless, this modality is time consuming and has yet to establish its role as a screening tool for anomalies in routine clinical practice.

CONCLUSION

Upon reporting his first series of obstetric images in 1958, Ian Donald declared that: 'The fact that recordable echoes can be obtained at all has both surprised and encouraged us...', a sentiment not uncommon to those embarking on obstetric ultrasound to this day. Undoubtedly, this pioneer of obstetric ultrasound would be astounded at the immense advances achieved in this field since his early experiments, and at the pace with which state-of-the-art technology has become integrated into routine obstetric practice today. In spite of recent advances in our understanding of maternal serum biochemical patterns associated with aneuploid conditions and the evolution of non-invasive diagnostic techniques for analyzing fetal cells in maternal blood, ultrasound remains at the forefront of prenatal diagnosis with its capacity to offer a global view of fetal health and timely diagnosis of a wide range of anomalies.

REFERENCES

1. McNay MB, Fleming JE. Forty years of obstetric ultrasound 1957–1997: from A-scope to three dimensions. *Ultrasound Med Biol* **25**(1):3–56, 1999.
2. Wild JJ. The use of ultrasonic pulses for the measurement of biologic tissues and the detection of tissue density changes. *Surgery* **27**(2):183–188, 1950.
3. Donald I MJ, Brown TG. Investigation of abdominal masses by pulsed ultrasound. *Lancet* **1**(7032):1188–1195, 1958.
4. Mutterschaftsrichtlinien. Beilage Nr 4-80 zumo Bundesanzeiger Nr 22. Feb(Suppl). 1980.
5. RCOG. Report of the RCOG Working Party on the Routine Ultrasound Examination in Pregnancy. 13–16, 1984.
6. Office of Medical Applications of Research, National Institutes of Health. The use of diagnostic ultrasound imaging during pregnancy. *J Am Med Assoc* **252**: 669–672, 1984.
7. Ewigman BG, Crane JP, Frigoletto FD, LeFevre ML, Bain RP, McNellis D. Effect of prenatal ultrasound screening on perinatal outcome. RADIUS Study Group. *N Engl J Med* **329**(12):821–827, 1993.
8. Saari-Kemppainen A, Karjalainen O, Ylostalo P, Heinonen OP. Ultrasound screening and perinatal mortality: controlled trial of systematic one-stage screening in pregnancy. *Lancet* **336**: 387–391, 1990.
9. Chitty LS, Hunt GH, Moore J, Lobb MO. Effectiveness of routine ultrasonography in detecting fetal structural abnormalities in a low risk population. *Br Med J* **303**:1165–1169, 1991.
10. Levi S, Hyjazi Y, Schapps JP et al. Sensitivity and specificity of routine antenatal screening for congenital anomalies by ultrasound: the Belgian multicentric study. *Ultrasound Obstet Gynecol* **1**:102–110, 1991.
11. Luck CA. Value of routine ultrasound scanning at 19 weeks: a 4-year study of 8849 deliveries. *Br Med J* **304**:1474–1478, 1992.
12. Rosendahl H, Kivinen S. Antenatal detection of congenital malformations by routine ultrasonography. *Obstet Gynecol* **73**:947–951, 1989.
13. Shirley IM, Bottomley F, Robinson VP. Routine radiographer screening for fetal abnormalities by ultrasound in an unselected low-risk population. *Br J Radiol* **65**:564–569, 1992.
14. Bucher HC, Schmidt JG. Does routine ultrasound scanning improve outcome in pregnancy? Meta-analysis of various outcome measures. *Br Med J* **307**: 13–17, 1993.
15. RCOG. Ultrasound screening for fetal abnormalities. Report of the RCOG working party, 1997.
16. Santalahti P, Aro AR, Hemminki E, Helenius H, Ryynanen M. On what grounds do women participate in prenatal screening? *Prenat Diagn* **18**: 153–165, 1998.

17. Stephens MB, Montefalcon R, Lane DA. The maternal perspective on prenatal ultrasound. *J Fam Pract* **49**:601–604, 2000.
18. Smith-Bindman R, Hosmer WD, Caponigro M, Cunningham G. The variability in the interpretation of prenatal diagnostic ultrasound. *Ultrasound Obstet Gynecol* **17**:326–332, 2001.
19. Richmond S, Atkins J. A population-based study of the prenatal diagnosis of congenital malformation over 16 years. *Br J Obstet Gynaecol* **112**:1349–1357, 2005.
20. Wolfe H, Sokol R, Martier SM, Zador I. Maternal obesity: a potential source of error in sonographic prenatal diagnosis. *Obstet Gynecol* **76**:339–342, 1990.
21. Rosenberg JC, Guzman ER, Vintzileos AM, Knupel RA. Transumbilical placement of the vaginal probe in obese pregnant women. *Obstet Gynecol* **85**:132–134, 1995.
22. DeVore GR, Medearis AL, Bear MB, Horenstein J, Platt LD. Fetal echocardiography: factors that influence imaging of the fetal heart during the second trimester of pregnancy. *J Ultrasound Med* **12**:659–663, 1993.
23. Waller DK, Mills JL, Simpson JL et al. Are obese women at higher risk for producing malformed offspring? *Am J Obstet Gynecol* **170**:541–548, 1994.
24. Queisser-Luft A, Kieninger-Baum D, Menger H, Stolz G, Schlaefer K, Merz E. Does maternal obesity increase the risk of fetal abnormalities? Analysis of 20,248 newborn infants of the Mainz Birth Register for detecting congenital abnormalities. *Ultraschall Med* **19**:40–44, 1998.
25. Watkins ML, Botto LD. Maternal prepregnancy weight and congenital heart defects in offspring. *Epidemiology* **12**: 439–446, 2001.
26. Watkins ML, Rassmussen SA, Honein MA, Botto LD, Moore CA. Maternal obesity and risk for birth defects. *Pediatrics* **111**:1152–1158, 2003.
27. Hendler I, Blackwell SC, Bujold E et al. The impact of maternal obesity on midtrimester sonographic visualization of fetal cardiac and craniospinal structures. *Int J Obes Relat Metab Disord* **28**:1607–1611, 2004.
28. Wang PH, Chen GD, Lin LY. Imaging comparison of basic cardiac views between two- and three-dimensional ultrasound in normal fetuses in anterior spine positions. *Int J Cardiovasc Imaging* **18**:17–23, 2002.
29. Treadwell MC, Seubert DE, Zador I, Goyert GL, Wolfe HM. Benefits associated with harmonic tissue imaging in the obstetric patient. *Am J Obstet Gynecol* **182**:1620–1623, 2000.
30. Hendler I, Blackwell SC, Bujold E et al. Suboptimal second-trimester ultrasonographic visualization of the fetal heart in obese women. *J Ultrasound Med* **24**:1205–1209, 2005.
31. Catanzarite V, Delaney K, Wolfe S et al. Targeted mid-trimester ultrasound examination: how does fetal anatomic visualization depend upon the duration of the scan? *Ultrasound Obstet Gynecol* **26**:521–526, 2005.
32. Eddelman KA, Malone FD, Sullivan L et al. Pregnancy loss rates after mid-trimester amniocentesis. *Obstet Gynecol* **108**:1067–1072, 2006.
33. DeVore GR, Alfi O. The use of colour Doppler ultrasound to identify fetuses at increased risk for trisomy 21: an alternative for high-risk patients who decline genetic amniocentesis. *Obstet Gynecol* **85**:378–386, 1995.
34. Nadel AS, Bromley B, Frigoletto FD, Jr, Benacerraf BR. Can the presumed risk of autosomal trisomy be decreased in fetuses of older women following a normal sonogram?*J Ultrasound Med* **14**:297–302, 1995.
35. Nyberg DA, Luthy DA, Cheng EY, Sheley RC, Resta RG, Williams MA. Role of prenatal ultrasonography in women with positive screen for Down syndrome on the basis of maternal serum markers. *Am J Obstet Gynecol* **173**:1030–1035, 1995.
36. Vintzileos AM, Egan JF. Adjusting the risk for trisomy 21 on the basis of second-trimester ultrasonography. *Am J Obstet Gynecol* **172**:837–844, 1995.
37. Achiron R, Lipitz S, Gabbay U, Yagel S. Prenatal ultrasonographic diagnosis of fetal heart echogenic foci: no correlation with Down syndrome. *Obstet Gynecol* **89**(6):945–948, 1997.
38. Bromley B, Benacerraf BR. The resolving nuchal fold in second trimester fetuses: not necessarily reassuring. *J Ultrasound Med* **14**:253–255, 1995.
39. Nicolaides KH, Snijders RJ, Gosden CM, Berry C. Ultrasonographically detectable markers for fetal aneuploidy. *Lancet* **340**:704–707, 1992.
40. Bromley B, Lieberman E, Shipp TD, Benacerraf BR. The genetic sonogram: a method of risk assessment for Down syndrome in the second trimester. *J Ultrasound Med* **21**(10):1087–1096, 2002.
41. Devore GR. Trisomy 21: 91% detection rate using second-trimester ultrasound markers. *Ultrasound Obstet Gynecol* **16**:133–141, 2000.
42. Nyberg DA, Souter VL. Sonographic markers for fetal trisomies: second trimester. *J Ultrasound Med* **20**(6):655–674, 2001.
43. Nyberg DA, Souter VL, El-Bastawissi A, Young S, Luthhardt F, Luthy DA. Isolated sonographic markers for detection of fetal Down syndrome in the second trimester of pregnancy. *J Ultrasound Med* **20**: 1053–1063, 2001.
44. Hall B. Mongolism in newborn infants. *Clin Pediatr* **5**:4–12, 1966.
45. Vergani P, Locatelli A, Piccoli MG et al. Best second trimester sonographic markers for detection of trisomy 21. *J Ultrasound Med* **18**(7):469–473, 1999.
46. Stoll C, Alembik Y, Dott B, Roth MP. Study of Down syndrome in 238 942 consecutive births. *Ann Genet* **41**:44–51, 1998.
47. Khoury MJ, Erickson JD. Improved ascertainment of cardiovascular malformations in infants with Down syndrome, Atlanta 1968 through 1989. Implications for the interpretation of increasing rates of cardiovascular malformations in surveillance systems. *Am J Epidemiol* **136**:1457–1464, 1992.
48. Paladini D, Lamberti A, Tartaglione A, Liguoir M, Teodoro A. The association between congenital heart disease (CHD) and Down syndrome (DS) in the fetus. *Ultrasound Obstet Gynecol* **12**(105): Suppl.I, 1998.
49. DeVore GR. The genetic sonogram: its use in the detection of chromosomal abnormalities in fetuses of women of advanced maternal age. *Prenat Diagn* **21**:40–45, 2001.
50. Langford K, Sharl G, Simpson JL. Relative risk of abnormal karyotype in fetuses found to have an atrioventricular septal defect (AVSD) on fetal echocardiography. *Prenat Diagn* **25**:137–139, 2005.
51. Benacerraf BR, Jr, Laboda LA. Sonographic diagnosis of Down syndrome in the second trimester. *Am J Obstet Gynecol* **153**:49–52, 1985.
52. Smith-Bindman R, Hosmer W, Feldstein VA, Deeks JJ, Goldberg JD. Second-trimester ultrasound to detect fetuses with Down syndrome: a meta-analysis. *J Am Med Assoc* **285**:1044–1055, 2001.
53. Locatelli A, Piccoli MG, Vergani P, Mariani E, Ghidini A, Mariana S. Critical appraisal of the use of nuchal fold thickness measurements for the prediction of Down syndrome. *Am J Obstet Gynecol* **82**(1):192–198, 2000.
54. Bahado-Singh RO, Oz A, Kovanci E et al. A high-sensitivity alternative to 'routine' genetic amniocentesis: multiple urinary analytes, nuchal thickness and age. *Am J Obstet Gynecol* **180**(1 Part 1):169–173, 1999.
55. Gray DL, Crane JP. Optimal nuchal skin-fold thresholds based on gestational age for prenatal detection of Down syndrome. *Am J Obstet Gynecol* **171**:1282–1286, 1994.
56. Hill LM, Fries J, Hecker J, Grzybek P. Second-trimester echogenic small bowel: an increased risk for adverse perinatal outcome. *Prenat Diagn* **14**(9):845–850, 1994.
57. MacGregor SN, Tamura R, Sabbagha R, Brenhofer JK, Kambich MP, Pergament E. Isolated hyperechoic fetal bowel: significance and implications for management. *Am J Obstet Gynecol* **173**(4):1254–1258, 1995.
58. Shipp TD, Bromley B, Lieberman E, Benacerraf BR. The frequency of fetal echogenic intracardiac foci with respect to maternal race. *Ultrasound Obstet Gynecol* **15**:460–462, 2000.
59. Benacerraf BR, Gezman R, Frigoletto FJ. Sonographic identification of second-trimester fetuses with Down Syndrome. *N Engl J Med* **317**:1371–1376, 1987.

60. Lockwood C, Krinsky A, Blakemore K et al. A sonographic screening method for Down Syndrome. *Am J Obstet Gynecol* **157**:803–808, 1987.
61. Grandjean H, Sarramon MF. Femur/foot length ratio for detection of Down syndrome: results of a multicenter prospective study. *Am J Obstet Gynecol* **173**(1):16–19, 1995.
62. Fitzsimmons J, Droste S, Shepard TH, Pascoe-Mason J, Chinn A, Mack LA. Long-bone growth in fetuses with Down syndrome. *Am J Obstet Gynecol* **161**(5):1174–1177, 1989.
63. Bork MD, Egan JF, Cusick W, Borgida AF, Campbell WA, Rodis JF. Iliac wing angle as a marker for trisomy 21 in the second trimester. *Obstet Gynecol* **89**(5 Part 1): 734–737, 1997.
64. Shipp TD, Bromley B, Lieberman E, Benacerraf BR. The second-trimester fetal iliac angle as a sign of Down's syndrome. *Ultrasound Obstet Gynecol* **12**(1):15–18, 1998.
65. Benacerraf BR, Osathanondh R, Frigoletto FD. Sonographic demonstration of hypoplasia of the middle phalanx of the fifth digit: a finding associated with Down syndrome. *Am J Obstet Gynecol* **159**: 181–183, 1988.
66. Deren O, Mahoney MJ, Copel JA, Bahado-Singh RO. Suble ultrasonographic anomalies: do they improve the Down syndrome detection rate? *Am J Obstet Gynecol* **178**(3):441–445, 1998.
67. Hobbins JC LD, Persutte WH et al. An eight-center study to evaluate the utility of mid-term genetic ultrasounds among high-risk pregnancies. *J Ultrasound Med* **22**:33–38, 2003.
68. Yeo L, Vintzileos AM. The use of genetic sonography to reduce the need for amniocentesis in women at high risk for Down syndrome. *Semin Perinat* **27**(2): 152–159, 2003.
69. Cicero S, Sonek JD, McKenna DS, Croom CS, Johnson L, Nicolaides KH. Nasal bone hypoplasia in trisomy 21 at 15-22 weeks' gestation. *Ultrasound Obstet Gynecol* **21**: 15–18, 2003.
70. Guis F, Ville Y, Vincent Y, Doumerc S, Pons JC, Frydman R. Ultrasound evaluation of the length of the nasal bones throughout gestation. *Ultrasound Obstet Gynecol* **5**:304–307, 1995.
71. Odibo AO, Sehdev HM, Dunn L, McDonald R, Macones GA. The association between fetal nasal bone hypoplasia and aneuploidy. *Obstet Gynecol* **104**:1229–1233, 2004.
72. Vintzileos AM, Walters C, Yeo L. Absent nasal bone in the prenatal detection of fetuses with trisomy 21 in a high-risk population. *Obstet Gynecol* **101**(5):903–908, 2003.
73. Sohl B, Scioscia A, Budorick NE, Moore TR. Utility of minor ultrasonographic markers in the prediction of abnormal fetal karyotype at a prenatal diagnostic center. *Am J Obstet Gynecol* **181**:898–903, 1999.
74. Winter TC, Reichman JA, Luna JA et al. Frontal lobe shortening in second-trimester fetuses with trisomy 21: usefulness as an ultrasound marker. *Radiology* **207**(1):215–222, 1998.
75. Nicolaides KH, Salvesen DR, Snijders RJ, Gosden CM. Strawberry-shaped skull in fetal trisomy 18. *Fetal Diagn Ther* **7**(2): 132–137, 1992.
76. Appelman Z, Zalel Y, Fried S, Caspi B. Delayed fusion of amnion and chorion: a possible association with trisomy 21. (Letter). *Ultrasound Obstet Gynecol* **11**(4):303–304, 1998.
77. Bromley B, Shipp TD, Benacerraf BR. Amnion-chorion separation after 17 weeks' gestation. *Obstet Gynecol* **94**: 1024–1026, 1999.
78. Shipp TD, Bromley B. Second trimester ultrasound screening for chromosomal abnormalities. *Prenat Diagn* **22**:296–307, 2002.
79. Taslimi MM, Acosta R, Cheuh J et al. Detection of sonographic markers of fetal aneuploidy depends on maternal and fetal characteristics. *J Ultrasound Med* **24**:811–815, 2005.
80. Wax JR, Cartin A, Pinette MG, Blackstone J. Does the frequency of soft sonographic aneuploidy markers vary by fetal sex? *J Ultrasound Med* **24**:1059–1063, 2005.
81. Benacerraf BR, Nadel A, Bromley B. Identification of second-trimester fetuses with autosomal trisomy by use of a sonographic scoring index. *Radiology* **193**:135–140, 1994.
82. Bahado-Singh RO, Deren O, Hunter D, Copel J, Mahoney MJ. Risk of Down syndrome and any clinically significant defect in pregnancies with abnormal triple-screen and normal targeted ultrasonographic results. *Am J Obstet Gynecol* **175**(4 Part 1):824–829, 1996.
83. Bahado-Singh RO, Oz A, Kovanci E et al. New Down syndrome screening algorithm: ultrasonographic biometry and multiple serum markers combined with maternal age. *Am J Obstet Gynecol* **179** (6 Part 1):1627–1631, 1998.
84. Vintzileos AM, Campbell WA, Guzman ER, Smulian JC, McLean DA, Ananth CV. Second-trimester ultrasound markers for detection of trisomy 21: which markers are best? *Obstet Gynecol* **89**:941–944, 1997.
85. Nyberg DA, Luthy DA, Resta RG, Nyberg BC, Williams MA. Age-adjusted ultrasound risk assessment for fetal Down syndrome during the second trimester: description of the method and analysis of 142 cases. *Ultrasound Obstet Gynecol* **12**:8–14, 1998.
86. Gupta JK, Cave M, Lilford RJ et al. Clinical significance of fetal choroid plexus cysts. *Lancet* **346**:724–729, 1995.
87. Chitty LS, Chudleigh P, Wright E, Campbell S, Pembrey ME. The significance of isolated choroid plexus cysts in an unselected population: the results of a multicenter study. *Ultrasound Obstet Gynecol* **12**:391–397, 1998.
88. Snijders RJM. Isolated choroid plexus cysts: should we offer karyotyping? *Ultrasound Obstet Gynecol* **8**:223–224, 1996.
89. Anderson N, Jyoti R. Relationship of isolated fetal intracardiac echogenic focus to trisomy 21 at the mid-trimester sonogram in women younger than 35 years. *Ultrasound Obstet Gynecol* **21**: 354–358, 2003.
90. Prefumo F, Presti F, Mavrides E et al. Isolated echogenic foci in the fetal heart: do they increase the risk of trisomy 21 in a population previously screened by nuchal transluency? *Ultrasound Obstet Gynecol* **18**(2):126–130, 2001.
91. Hobbins JC, Bahado-Singh RO, Lezotte DC. The genetic sonogram in screening for Down syndrome. *J Ultrasound Med* **20**:569–572, 2001.
92. Benacerraf BR, Frigoletto FD, Jr. Sonographic scoring index for prenatal detection of chromosomal abnormalities. *J Ultrasound Med* **11**(9):449–458, 1992.
93. Winter TC, Uhrich SB, Souter VL, Nyberg DA. The 'genetic sonogram': comparison of the index scoring system with the age-adjusted US risk assessment. *Radiology* **215**:775–782, 2000.
94. Souter VL, Nyberg DA, El-Bastawissi A, Zebelman A, Luthhardt F. Correlation of ultrasound findings and biochemical markers in the second trimester of pregnancy in fetuses with trisomy 21. *Prenat Diagn* **22**:175–182, 2002.
95. Nyberg DA, Kramer D, Resta RG et al. Prenatal sonographic findings of trisomy 18: review of 47 cases. *J Ultrasound Med* **2**(2):103–113, 1993.
96. Shields LE, Carpenter LA, Smith KM, Nghiem HV. Ultrasonographic diagnosis of trisomy 18: is it practical in the early second trimester? *J Ultrasound Med* **17**(5):327–331, 1998.
97. DeVore GR. Second trimester ultrasonography may identify 77 to 97% of fetuses with trisomy 18. *J Ultrasound Med* **19**(8):565–576, 2000.
98. Yeo L, Guzman ER, Day-Salvatore D, Walters C, Chavez D, Vintzileos AM. Prenatal detection of fetal trisomy 18 through abnormal sonographic features. *J Ultrasound Med* **22**(6):581–590, 2003.
99. Bromley B, Lieberman R, Benacerraf BR. Choroid plexus cysts: not associated with Down syndrome. *Ultrasound Obstet Gynecol* **8**(4):223–224, 1996.
100. Gross SJ, Shulman LP, Tolley EA et al. Isolated fetal choroid plexus cysts and trisomy 18: a review and meta-analysis. *Am J Obstet Gynecol* **172**(1 Part 1): 83–87, 1995.
101. Yoder PR, Sabbagha RE, Gross SJ, Zelop CM. The second-trimester fetus with isolated choroid plexus cysts: a

meta-analysis of risk of trisomies 18 and 21. *Obstet Gynecol* **93**:869–872, 1999.

102. Walkinshaw S. Fetal choroid plexus cysts: are we there yet? *Prenat Diagn* **20**:657–662, 2000.
103. Lehman CD, Nyberg DA, Winter TCI, Kapur RP, Resta RG, Luthy DA. Trisomy 13 syndrome: prenatal US findings in a review of 33 cases. *Radiology* **194**(1): 217–222, 1995.
104. Benacerraf BR, Miller WA, Frigoletto FDJ. Sonographic detection of fetuses with trisomies 13 and 18: accuracy and limitations. *Am J Obstet Gynecol* **158**(2):404–409, 1988.
105. Jauniaux E, Brown R, Rodeck C, Nicolaides KH. Prenatal diagnosis of triploidy during the second trimester of pregnancy. *Obstet Gynecol* **88**(6): 983–989, 1996.
106. Mittall TK, Vujanic GM, Morrissey BM, Jones A. Triploidy: antenatal sonographic features with post-mortem correlation. *Prenat Diagn* **18**(12):1253–1262, 1998.
107. Johnson MP, Johnson A, Holzgreve W et al. First-trimester simple hygroma: cause and outcome. *Am J Obstet Gynecol* **168**:156–161, 1993.
108. Hewitt B. Nuchal translucency in the first trimester. *Aust NZ J Obstet Gynaecol* **33**:389–391, 1993.
109. Shulman LP, Emerson D, Felker R, Phillips O, Simpson J, Elias S. High frequency of cytogenetic abnormalities with cystic hygroma diagnosed in the first trimester. *Obstet Gynecol* **80**:80–82, 1992.
110. Nicolaides KH, Azar G, Byrne D, Mansur C, Marks K. Fetal nuchal translucency: ultrasound screening for chromosomal defects in first trimester of pregnancy. *Br Med J* **304**:867–869, 1992.
111. Souka AP, Von Kaisenberg CS, Hyett JA et al. Increased nuchal translucency with normal karyotype. *Am J Obstet Gynecol* **192**:1021–1055, 2005.
112. Schuchter K, Wald NJ, Hackshaw AK, Hafner E, Liebhart E. The distribution of nuchal translucency at 10–13 weeks of pregnancy. *Prenat Diagn* **18**:281–286, 1998.
113. Pajkrt E, de Graaf IM, Mol BW, van Lith JM, Bleker OP, Bilardo CM. Weekly nuchal translucency measurements in normal fetuses. *Obstet Gynecol* **91**:208–211, 1998.
114. Rosen T, D'Alton ME. Down syndrome screening in the first and second trimesters: What do the data show? *Semin Perinat* **29**:367–375, 2005.
115. Wald NJ, Rodeck C, Hackshaw AK, Walters J, Chitty L, Mackinson AM. First and second trimester antenatal screening for Down's syndrome: the results of the Serum, Urine and Ultrasound Screening Study (SURUSS). *Health Technol Assess* **7**:1–77, 2003.
116. Malone FD, Canick JA, Ball RH et al. First-trimester or second-trimester screening, or both, for Down's syndrome. *N Engl J Med* **353**(19):2001–2011, 2005.
117. Snijders RJM, Sundberg K, Holzgreve W, Henry G, Nicolaides KH. Maternal age and gestation-specific risk for trisomy 21. *Ultrasound Obstet Gynecol* **13**: 167–170, 1999.
118. de Graaf IM, Tijmstra T, Bleker OP, van Lith JM. Women's preference in Down syndrome screening. *Prenat Diagn* **22**:624–629, 2002.
119. Malone FD, Nyberg DA et al. First-trimester septated cystic hygroma; prevalence, natural history and pediatric outcome. *Obstet Gynecol* **106**(2):288–294, 2005.
120. Cicero S, Curcio P, Papageorghiou A et al. Absence of nasal bone in fetuses with trisomy 21 at 11–14 weeks of gestation: an observational study. *Lancet* **358**: 1665–1667, 2001.
121. Cicero S, Bindra R, Rembouskas G et al. Integrated ultrasound and biochemnical screening for trisomy 21 using fetal nuchal translucency, absent fetal nasal bone, free beta-hCG and PAPP-A at 11–14 weeks. *Prenat Diagn* **23**:306–310, 2003.
122. Malone FD, Ball RH, Nyberg DA et al. First trimester nasal bone evaluation for aneuploidy in the general population. *Obstet Gynecol* **104**:1222–1228, 2004.
123. Cicero S, Rembouskas G, Vandecruys H et al. Likelihood ratio for trisomy 21 in fetuses with absent nasal bone at the 11–14 week scan. *Ultrasound Obstet Gynecol* **23**:218–223, 2004.
124. Orlandi F, Rossi C, Orlandi E et al. First-trimester screening for trisomy-21 using a simplified method to assess the presence or absence of the fetal nasal bone. *Am J Obstet Gynecol* **192**:1107–1111, 2005.
125. Matias A, Gomes C, Flack N, Montenegro N, Nicolaides KH. Screening for chromosomal abnormalities at 10–14 weeks: the role of ductus venosus blood flow. *Ultrasound Obstet Gynecol* **12**:380–384, 1998.
126. Matias A, Montenegro N, Areias JC et al. Anomalous fetal venous return associated with major chromosomopathies in the late first trimester of pregnancy. *Ultrasound Obstet Gynecol* **11**:209–213, 1998.
127. Nicolaides KH, Spencer K, Avgidou K et al. Multicenter study of first trimester screening for trisomy 21 in 75,821 pregnancies: results and estimation of the potential impact of individual risk-oriented two-stage first trimester screening. *Ultrasound Obstet Gynecol* **25**:221–226, 2005.
128. Huggon IC, DeFigueiredo DB, Allan LD. Tricuspid regurgitation in the diagnosis of chromosomal anomalies in the fetus at 11-14 weeks of gestation. *Heart* **89**:1071–1073, 2003.
129. Faiola S, Tsoi E, Huggon IC, Allan LD, Nicolaides KH. Likelihood ratio for trisomy 21 in fetuses with tricuspid regurgitation at the 11 to 13 + 6-week scan. *Ultrasound Obstet Gynecol* **26**: 22–27, 2005.
130. De Biasio P, Prefumo F, Lantieri PB, Venturini PL. Reference values for fetal limb biometry at 10–14 weeks of gestation. *Ultrasound Obstet Gynecol* **19**:588–591, 2002.
131. Blass HG, Eik-Nes SH, Kiserud T, Hellevik LR. Early development of the hindbrain: a longitudinal ultrasound study from 7 to 12 weeks of gestation. *Ultrasound Obstet Gynecol* **5**: 151–160, 1995.
132. Braithwaite JM, Armstrong MA, Economides DL. Assessment of fetal anatomy at 12 to 13 weeks of gestation by transabdominal and transvaginal sonography. *Br J Obstet Gynaecol* **103**: 82–85, 1996.
133. Rosati P, Guariglia L. Transvaginal sonographic assessment of the fetal urinary tract in early pregnancy. *Ultrasound Obstet Gynecol* **7**:95–100, 1996.
134. Bronshtein M, Yoffe N, Brandes JM, Blumenfeld Z. First and early second-trimester diagnosis of fetal urinary tract anomalies using transvaginal sonography. *Prenat Diagn* **10**:653–666, 1990.
135. Haak MC, Twisk JW, Van Vugt JM. How successful is fetal echocardiographic examination in the first trimester of pregnancy? *Ultrasound Obstet Gynecol* **20**:9–13, 2002.
136. Souka AP. Diagnosis of fetal abnormalities at the 10–14 weeks scan. *Ultrasound Obstet Gynecol* **10**:429–442, 1997.
137. Souka AP, Pilalis A, Kavalakis I et al. Screening for major structural abnormalities at the 11- to 14-week ultrasound scan. *Am J Obstet Gynecol* **194**:393–396, 2006.
138. McAuliffe FM, Fong KW, Toi A, Chitayat D, Keating S, Johnson J. Ultrasound detection of fetal anomalies in conjunction with first-trimester nuchal translucency screening: a feasibility study. *Am J Obstet Gynecol* **193**:1260–1265, 2005.
139. Pretorius DH, Nelson TR. Fetal face visualization using three-dimensional ultrasound. *J Ultrasound Med* **13**: 349–356, 1995.
140. Shih JC, Shyu MK, Lee CN, Wu CH, Lin GJ, Hsieh FJ. Antenatal depiction of the fetal ear with three-dimensional ultrasonography. *Obstet Gynecol* **91**: 500–505, 1998.
141. Merz E, Weber G, Bahlmann F, Mric-Tesanic D. Application of transvaginal and abdominal three-dimensional ultrasound for the detection or exclusion of malformations of the fetal face. *Ultrasound Obstet Gynecol* **9**:237–243, 1997.
142. Budorick NE, Pretorius DH, Johnson DD, Tartar MK, Nelson TR.

Three-dimensional ultrasound of the fetal distal lower extremity: normal and abnormal. *J Ultrasound Med* **17**: 649–660, 1998.

143. Pretorius DH, Garjian KV, Budorick NE, Cantrell CJ, Johnson DD, Nelson TR. Three-dimensional ultrasound of fetal skeletal dysplasias. *Radiology* **209**(Suppl):188, 1998.

144. Johnson DD, Pretorius DH, Riccabona M, Budorick NE, Nelson TR. Three-dimensional ultrasound of the fetal spine. *Obstet Gynecol* **89**:434–438, 1997.

145. Dyson RL, Pretorius DH, Budorick NE et al. Three-dimensional ultrasound in the evaluation of fetal anomalies. *Ultrasound Obstet Gynecol* **16**: 321–328, 2000.

146. Verdin SM, Economides DL. The role of ultrasonographic markers for trisomy 21 in women with positive serum biochemistry. *Br J Obstet Gynaecol* **105**(1):63–67, 1998.

CHAPTER

21 Non-invasive screening and diagnosis from maternal blood

Olav Lapaire, Sinuhe Hahn and Wolfgang Holzgreve

KEY POINTS

- The appearance of fetal cells in maternal circulation was first reported in 1893 by Georg Schmorl in Germany
- During the first phase of the research on non-invasive prenatal diagnosis, the major focus was on the enrichment of fetal cells from maternal blood and the search for the 'ideal' fetal target cell
- The final results of a multicenter study (the so-called NIFTY trial), revealed that the sensitivity and specificity of the cell-based methods were not satisfactory for aneuploidy detection, mainly because of the difficulty to detect reliably a third copy of a chromosome on the background of abundant disomic maternal cells
- In 1997, the first publication on cell-free fetal DNA extracted from maternal blood had opened a new perspective in prenatal diagnosis
- Circulating cell-free fetal DNA in the maternal circulation provides indirect clues to the underlying physiology and pathology during all trimesters
- In the case of the non-invasive prenatal diagnosis of the fetal Rhesus D status, the overall diagnostic accuracy of 97% based on cell-free fetal DNA analysis was excellent from the beginning with a slight limitation when the test was done before 12 weeks of gestation
- Cell-free fetal DNA has also been used to detect the Y chromosome, paternally inherited autosomal dominant conditions and autosomal recessive conditions when the parents carry different mutations
- Pre-eclampsia, one of the most important pregnancy-related diseases associated with major sequelae, is associated with a significantly increased amount of fetal material shed into the maternal circulation
- A new approach, using placentally derived cell-free fetal mRNA from maternal plasma, may serve as an additional promising pathway for the detection of fetal aneuploidies in a non-invasive manner

INTRODUCTION

Prenatal diagnosis for the detection of fetal aneuploidies by invasive procedures and malformations by ultrasound has been implemented since the 1970s. Due to the elevated risk of abortion, however, which at present is 0.5–1%, many pregnant women do not wish to have an invasive procedure. It has been calculated that out of 10 000 women in a standardized screening program, 45 fetuses will be lost through invasive testing. This is one of the major reasons why research groups world-wide are searching for new, effective, risk-free and reliable methods as well as additional markers for prenatal diagnosis. The basis for this is the retrieval of fetal material from maternal blood, either through enrichment of fetal cells, cell-free deoxyribonucleic acid (DNA) or cell-free ribonucleic acid (RNA).

Therefore, the passage of fetal material, with a spectrum from intact cells to cell-free DNA (cfDNA), across the so-called 'placental' barrier has become a focus of intense research over the past 15 years[1–4]. This started originally with the strong motivation to develop non-invasive prenatal diagnosis when appropriate molecular technologies became available. In the meantime, however, it has become clear that the presence of fetal material in the circulation of pregnant women is not only of interest for the field of prenatal diagnosis, but may have an immediate (e.g. pre-eclampsia) as well as long-term (e.g. scleroderma) impact on maternal health[5,6].

The appearance of fetal cells in maternal circulation was first reported in 1893. The German pathologist Georg Schmorl found cells in the lung capillaries of women who had died from pre-eclampsia, which resembled syncytiotrophoblast cells from fetal placenta[7].

He first documented the presence of fetal cells in the maternal body and emphasized the importance of the placenta in eclampsia. Although his classic paper, written in 1893, is widely cited today, few investigators have actually read the paper, as it was published in German[8]. Georg Schmorl was remarkably astute in his assessment of the pathologic changes that were seen in the 17 women on whom he performed complete autopsies. He found similar severe changes in all of the women, implying a common pathogenesis. This was in direct contrast to the then dominant doctrine. He was the first to observe the presence of emboli containing multinucleated syncytial giant cells in the lungs of the women and speculated that they were of placental origin. To support his hypothesis he performed animal experiments. He also recognized that fetomaternal trafficking occurred in normal gestations but was increased in pregnancies affected by eclampsia. Using sophisticated molecular techniques, we can now precisely confirm what Schmorl so elegantly described and speculated about.

A few decades later in the 1950s, the group of Gordon Douglas in New York[9] already suggested that a 'low-grade' cell traffic from the fetal to the maternal side might be a physiologic phenomenon which is somehow exaggerated in pre-eclampsia/eclampsia. However, these authors were unable to prove their theory based on cytological methods alone and only the advent of chromosome-specific probes, especially for the Y chromosome, made it possible to objectify the changes quantitatively. Based on these new investigations at the beginning of the 1990s, particularly using fluorescence in situ hybridization (FISH) (Fig. 21.1) and the polymerase chain reaction (PCR), it is now established that, on average, roughly one in a million cells in the maternal circulation is of fetal origin.

Later, by incorporating the work of the plant and cancer geneticists Philippe Anker and Maurice Stroun[10,11] from Geneva, the group of Dennis Lo[12], at that time in Oxford, now in Hong Kong, showed that cell-free DNA from the fetus can also be found in the maternal circulation, and that this phenomenon can be used clinically for the non-invasive diagnosis of some genetic conditions of the fetus. The methodology to detect very small amounts of 'foreign' DNA sequences in plasma and serum has been further improved[13–15]. Circulating cell-free nucleic acids in plasma and serum are now novel biomarkers with promising clinical applications in different medical fields, including prenatal diagnosis[16] or oncology[17]. Furthermore, the levels of cfDNA are elevated in acute medical emergencies, including trauma and stroke[18], and are indicators of disease severity. The presence of cell-free fetal DNA (cffDNA) in maternal blood has opened a new perspective in prenatal diagnosis. Circulating cell-free fetal DNA in the maternal circulation provides indirect clues to the underlying physiology and pathology during all trimesters.

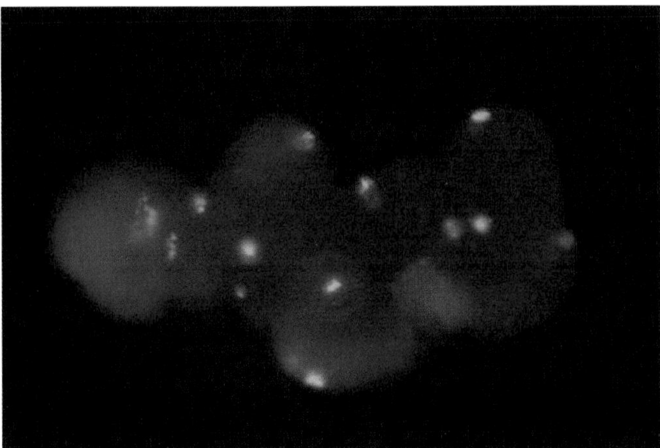

Fig. 21.1 FISH analysis of fetal male cells using probes against the centromeric regions of chromosome X and chromosome Y. Therefore female (maternal) cells are represented by two green (spectrum green) FISH signals whereas male (fetal) cells show one green (spectrum green) and one red (spectrum orange) signal.

The improvements of the techniques have allowed detection of minute amounts of genetic microchimerism and even in urine the ready detection of donor-specific single nucleotide polymorphisms of renal transplant recipients by matrix-assisted laser desorption/ionization time-of-flight mass spectrometry[19,20] as an early marker for organ rejection. The sensitivity and clinical power of the current techniques are further illustrated by the recent observation that cfDNA and corticotropin-releasing-hormone mRNA are increased in women with preterm delivery but not in those who respond to tocolysis[21,22]. There was also a report of postpartum monitoring of plasma cell-free DNA in a case of placenta increta where the decrease of fetal DNA in a patient's peripheral blood correlated well with her clinical improvement after delivery[23].

FETOMATERNAL TRAFFIC AS THE BASIC ELEMENT FOR NON-INVASIVE PRENATAL DIAGNOSIS

In the first phase of the research on non-invasive prenatal diagnosis, many years and efforts were spent on enrichment and depletion techniques and on the search for the 'ideal' fetal target cell[24,25]. Syncytiotrophoblast cells were found to have technical disadvantages of often being multinucleated with no specific antibody available for their enrichment. Recently, however, there was a preliminary report of the correct diagnosis of sex in fetal trophoblast cells isolated from cervical mucus during early pregnancy[26], so this cell type remains of interest. Lymphocytes, which are used postnatally for genetic investigations, turned out to be present only in smaller numbers early in gestation, and there were concerns about diagnostic errors from previous pregnancies due to their potential longevity. Bianchi[27] pointed out the advantages of using fetal nucleated erythrocytes: they can be enriched by a suitable antibody (anti-transferrin, CD71), they are abundantly present in fetal blood during early gestation and they have a short half-life, thus excluding interference from previous pregnancies. World-wide, considerable effort was then devoted to develop efficient enrichment and/or depletion techniques, but it finally had to be realized that during every such step to increase specificity, some of the precious fetal cells are lost. On the other hand, the cell-based approach led to the first report of a successful non-invasive diagnosis of a fetal trisomy[28]. Based on the rarity of the fetal cells in the maternal blood, it was clear from the beginning, however, that this revolutionary form of prenatal diagnosis needed to be rigorously tested, before a widespread clinical application could be considered.

The National Institutes of Health (NIH) initiated a large-scale study with four US-American and our Swiss center to evaluate different cell-based techniques for non-invasive prenatal diagnosis and to develop them further at the same time[29]. The results of this NICHD study (the so-called NIFTY trial), however, revealed that the sensitivity and specificity of the cell-based methods were not satisfactory for aneuploidy detection, mainly because of the difficulty to detect reliably a third copy of a chromosome against the background of abundant disomic maternal cells[30]. Up to now, erythroblasts cannot be reproducibly expanded[31]. Furthermore, we found recently that the nucleus of a fetal erythrocyte disintegrates some time before it disappears from the cell, thus making FISH from fetal cells in maternal circulation rather unreliable[32]. The NIFTY framework proved to be very useful and also allowed the international collaborative group to make interlaboratory comparisons of different techniques[33] and to scrutinize quickly newly proposed methods, such as the use of intact fetal cells from maternal plasma[34].

NON-INVASIVE PRENATAL DIAGNOSIS FROM 'BENCH TO BEDSIDE'

As opposed to this ultimately disappointing experience with the prenatal diagnosis of aneuploidies from intact fetal cells, the analysis of fetal DNA sequences in the maternal plasma is a success story which has finally resulted in the transition of non-invasive prenatal diagnosis from 'the bench to the bedside'. An ideal clinically relevant constellation are the Rhesus negative pregnant women with a Rhesus positive partner where, in the case of heterozygosity of the male partner, 50% of the offspring will be Rhesus negative. Whereas the cell-based approach for the detection of the Rhesus gene already showed high specificity but again, based on the rarity of the fetal cells in maternal blood, a lower sensitivity[35], the overall diagnostic accuracy based on cfDNA analysis was excellent from the beginning with a slight limitation when the test was done before 12 weeks of gestation. In the meantime, more than 8000 cases of non-invasive prenatal RHD genotypings have been reported with an amazing diagnostic accuracy of around 97%[36–42]. A recently published meta-analysis pooled the data from 37 publications reporting non-invasive Rhesus genotyping using fetal DNA obtained from maternal plasma or serum. This meta-analysis confirmed the high accuracy of 94.8%, including 16 most recent studies that reported 100% diagnostic accuracy in their fetal Rhesus D genotyping[43]. There is even consideration in some European countries to offer the new non-invasive test in a cost-effective way to all Rhesus negative women in order to save the prepartum anti-D prophylaxis in those cases where the child has been found prenatally to be Rhesus negative. In most places, the non-invasive Rhesus-test has already been handed over from the research to the service laboratories primarily within the blood banks, e.g. in Bristol, UK or Amsterdam, the Netherlands[40,44].

Using multiplex PCR, we have also shown that the Rhesus factor can be reliably examined together with SRY sequences[35], and the diagnostic accuracy for fetal gender based on cfDNA real time PCR (Fig. 21.2) is already more accurate than ultrasound prediction[45]. Fetal non-invasive sexing from cfDNA has been used clinically already in hundreds of cases at risk for X-linked conditions, including Duchenne muscular dystrophy, hemophilia and a host of others[46,47]. Not surprisingly, however, there is already some concern that this risk-free reliable approach for fetal gender detection could be used for sex selection outside the context of X-linked diseases[48,49]. This could be a major issue in regions of the world with obvious gender preference, but also a major topic of the EU-funded SAFE network.

Following the positive example with the non-invasive diagnosis of the Rhesus factor, autosomal dominant diseases transmitted by the father are also excellent candidates for a prenatal diagnosis from maternal plasma because, like in the Rhesus constellation, the mutation of interest is not present in the mother. The first successful non-invasive diagnoses of achondroplasia[50,51] and myotonic dystrophy[52] have been reported, and these individual case reports with a new method of prenatal diagnosis remind us of the introductory phases of amniocentesis in the late 1960s and chorionic villus sampling (CVS) in the middle 1980s, before large-scale individual center or multicenter collaborative series were published.

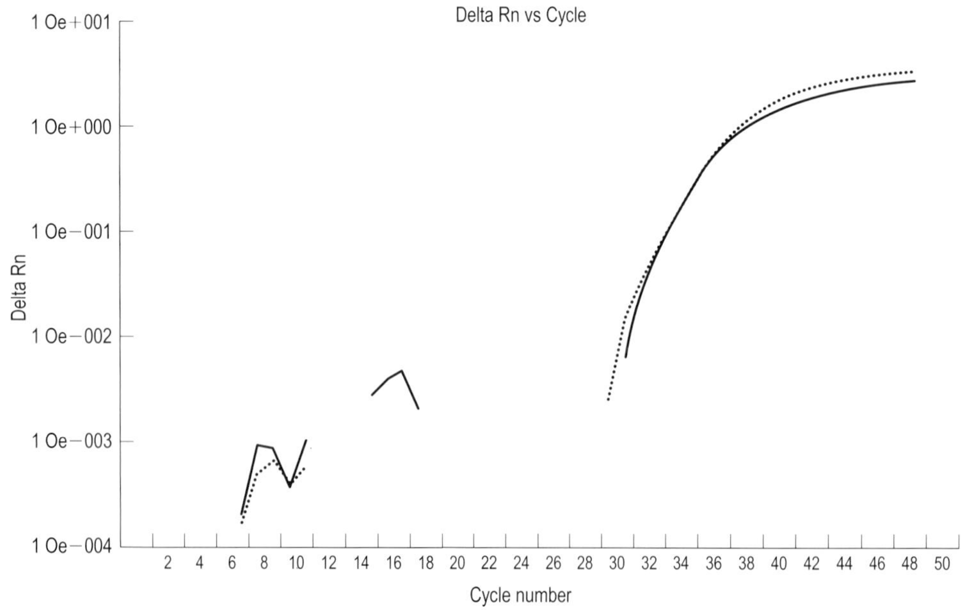

Fig. 21.2 Results of a real-time PCR, using a SRY-specific probe to detect male fetal DNA extracted from maternal plasma. Sample was run in duplicate. On the vertical axis, the fluorescence intensity (Delta Rn) is the normalized reporter signal (Rn).

A challenge is posed by autosomal recessive conditions because, here, both parents most often carry the same mutation. Fetal compound heterozygosity due to different parental mutations, however, are frequent in some populations, for instance in cystic fibrosis or beta-thalassemia, and have been approached successfully by excluding the paternal mutation[53,54]. Also, the non-invasive prenatal diagnosis of alpha-thalassemia was reported recently[55]. Our group has shown that various molecular biological tricks, such as size separation of the fetal and maternal DNA as well as PNA clamping to amplify specifically the mutant rather than the wild type allele, have contributed significantly to the now very high diagnostic accuracy[53].

It is interesting to know that the total amount of fetal DNA in the maternal circulation is not affected by maternal age, fetal sex or previous blood donations[56], but some elevation of cfDNA is found in pregnancies with aneuploid fetuses[57]. This latter observation could potentially lead to a new screening algorithm for the detection of aneuploidy. A further step towards a molecular identification of chromosomal abnormalities could be the use of short tandem repeats (STR)[58].

In summary, the field of prenatal diagnosis from maternal blood has not met the original goal of a non-invasive diagnostic approach to chromosomal anomalies but, at the same time, an ever increasing list of high-risk single gene diseases can now be detected by using cfDNA as the source.

IMMEDIATE CONSEQUENCES OF THE INFLUX OF FETAL MATERIAL INTO THE MATERNAL CIRCULATION

One of the first examples reported regarding an immediate (defined as during an ongoing pregnancy) effect of the passage of fetal cells into the maternal periphery came from an observation in dermatology. Based on the fact that, on the one side, in transplant recipients sometimes the skin can show signs of microchimerism, defined by the presence of fetal cells in maternal organs and blood, without any detectable graft-versus-host reaction or graft rejection. On the other side, there are characteristic skin disorders which develop specifically during pregnancy, e.g. polymorphic eruptions of pregnancy (PEP), for which a group in Paris[59] used Y-chromosome-specific sequences from the SRY gene to prove fetal–maternal cell traffic in a disease with disseminated pruritic skin papules, plaques and vesicles that heal spontaneously after delivery and associated with a significant increase of pregnancy complications, especially pre-eclampsia[60]. Interestingly, our own group had previously reported evidence of immune reactions in skin biopsies of PEP-patients[61], but the group of Aractingi in Paris was the first to identify the association of PEP with the haploidentical cells from a previously born child in some affected women[59].

CELL-FREE FETAL DNA: A PROMISING MARKER FOR PRE-ECLAMPSIA

Another pregnancy-related disease associated with major sequelae on the maternal as well as the fetal side is pre-eclampsia, whose etiology is not fully understood even today[62]. This condition, characterized by the development of hypertension usually by mid or late gestation (BP $\geq$ 140 mmHg systolic and/or $\geq$90 mmHg diastolic)[64] as well as a de novo proteinuria, is among the three most frequent etiologies of maternal mortality in the world and, in developed countries, it is responsible for up to a quarter of all the antenatal admissions to neonatology wards with a share of 25% among all very low birth weight (VLBW) babies[63]. Furthermore, there is increasing evidence that pregnancy-related growth restriction of the unborn child can be a major risk factor in adult life and other sequelae such as hypertension and atherosclerosis[64]. Our hypothesis, that this condition may also be related to abnormal fetomaternal cell traffic, originated by chance, because in a series of aneuploidies which we studied to develop non-invasive prenatal diagnosis, within the control group of euploid pregnancies we had a good number of pre-eclampsia patients, due to the fact that we are a tertiary center for high-risk pregnancies. These patients with pre-eclampsia within the control group had, to our surprise, a significantly increased amount of nucleated erythrocytes after triple density gradient and MACS enrichments in their peripheral blood[65]. Following this observation, in a blinded study in the same year, we confirmed that there is a significant difference in the number of fetal cells in the blood of women without and with manifest pre-eclampsia[66]. Lo et al.[67] reported a similar quantitative increase when looking at cfDNA in the serum of women with pre-eclampsia, and all other groups who subsequently studied fetal cells or cfDNA in women with pre-eclampsia confirmed these findings of a significantly increased amount of fetal material in the maternal circulation[68,69]. In our laboratory, we then extended this concept by not only analyzing the levels of cell-free fetal DNA in the plasma of about 300 women by a real-time PCR assay for the SRY gene but, at the same time, quantifying the total circulatory maternal DNA by a real-time PCR assay for the ubiquitous glyceraldehyde-3-phosphate dehydrogenase (GAPDH) gene, which is present in all genomes[70]. Looking at the results of this study, we could verify our second hypothesis, that an increase in maternal DNA reflecting her own endothelial cell damage follows the rise of the fetal DNA in the maternal plasma, because we could indeed find a significant increase of maternal total DNA and even a 'dose relationship' in the sense that the most severe cases (including those with associated HELLP syndromes) had the highest rise of fetal and subsequently maternal DNA in the maternal circulation. Maternal circulatory cell-free DNA levels increased only after the onset of pre-eclampsia symptoms, whereas the increase in the fetal DNA was found consistently to precede the onset of pre-eclampsia[71].

There have been many efforts to develop a reliable predictive test for pre-eclampsia so that better surveillance and earlier referral of at risk cases to perinatal centers would be possible and that interventional studies with new preventive approaches could be better targeted. So far, however, systematic reviews of screening tests for pre-eclampsia have shown no convincing progress[72,73]. Currently, the combination of uterine artery Doppler ultrasound and consideration of maternal factors (birth order, weight etc.) can provide the best estimate of risk[74]. After it was shown clearly by others and us that nucleated erythrocytes[75], as well as circulatory fetal DNA in maternal plasma[76], are elevated before pre-eclampsia develops (around 20 weeks), Levine et al.[77], using the same type of technology, studied stored samples which had been longitudinally obtained in a calcium pre-eclampsia trial. They also found an increase of fetal cfDNA after 17 weeks in patients who later developed pre-eclampsia. The observed second peak in their study can be related to the impaired clearance of fetal DNA from maternal plasma[78]. These findings correlate well with the recently reported increase of the circulating soluble endoglin, which is an anti-angiogenic protein, acting together with the circulating soluble fms-like tyrosine kinase 1, because this rise also begins 2–3 months before the onset of pre-eclampsia[79,80]. A multicenter trial under the coordination of the Maternal and Perinatal Health Programme of the WHO has just started to work out the predictive values of these early pre-eclampsia markers in 12 400 women in our and 5 other medical centers. It remains to be seen whether fetal DNA alone or, more likely, the combination with other early markers (e.g. uterine artery Doppler, Activin A, soluble fms-like tyrosine kinase 1 (sFlt1) and soluble endoglin, both antiangiogenic proteins, or placental growth factor (PlGF), a proangiogenic protein) could have a better performance in prediction than single marker testing, similar to first-trimester aneuploidy screening[81–83]. From our view, one of the most promising candidates for use in a combined algorithm to calculate prospectively the risk for pre-eclampsia together with cfDNA is Activin A which belongs to the TGF-beta family and may have a role in the appropriate proliferation, generation, differentiation and invasion of trophoblast cells. High levels of circulatory activin A in pre-eclampsia have been observed in several studies[84] and in those women at risk who later developed pre-eclampsia[85].

Although pre-eclampsia is not a monocausal condition and the manifestation depends upon many intervening variables, it is widely accepted that it originates from a placentation deficiency early in gestation, especially a so-called 'trophoblast invasion impairment'[86]. In pregnancies which later develop pre-eclampsia, the invasion of the placental bed by the cytotrophoblast is too shallow for the spiral arteries to be modified properly, and it is limited by increased apoptosis[87]. This also leads to the increased impedance to blood flow in the spiral arteries which can be detected by ultrasound Doppler investigations of the uterine arteries preceeding the development of pre-eclampsia[88]. Usually, the process of trophoblast invasion is completed by 20 weeks of gestation and, in the case of failure, which is typical for pre-eclampsia, a hypoxic dysfunctional placenta releases material into the circulation which causes the clinical symptoms similar to a systemic inflammatory response[89–92].

The group of Redman and Sargent[93] showed that even normal third-trimester pregnancies are characterized by a remarkable activation of peripheral blood leukocytes and this is further increased in pre-eclampsia which, therefore, can be considered to be 'an excessive maternal inflammatory response to pregnancy'[94]. An interesting observation in support of an inflammatory type sequence in pre-eclampsia is the fact that patients who receive dexamethasone in the presence of a HELLP syndrome may have an improvement of their symptoms, although this is not a sufficient treatment[95]. Interestingly, in studies on septicemia during pregnancy in mini-pigs, we had previously shown that pregnancy was characterized by an increased response to the endotoxin applied[96]. In the meantime, the sequence of events from the placental shedding of intact cells all the way to free DNA has become more and more clear. A model showed the normal turnover of villous trophoblast comprises differentiation of cytotrophoblast and fusion with the syncytiotrophoblast, subsequent aging and packaging of apoptotic material into syncytial knots, which are then deported in the maternal circulation and, ultimately, are removed by her own granulocytes, especially in the lung. If there is trophoblast invasion impairment, this normally highly controlled cascade may fail, leading to the release of aponecrotic material, which may induce an inflammation-like reaction in the mother. Markers for oxidative stress can be found in the placental tissues in association with the increased placental debris[89–97]. We have evidence that the increased amount of cfDNA in the maternal circulation stems from the placenta itself and not the increased traffic. The major effect is not due the increased numbers of fetal nucleated erythrocytes but to the placental impairment[98]. Redman and Sargent[99], as well as our group[100], have shown that the so-called syncytiotrophoblast microvilli (STBM) prepared from normal placenta could disrupt the growth and proliferation of endothelial cells in vitro and in vivo. Similar to STBMs, fetal cells and cfDNA were found to be present in significantly increased amounts in pre-eclamptic women[101]. We also found in vivo support for this theory in ethnic Tibetans and recently migrated Han Chinese in Lhasa, Tibet (altitude 3650 m) in comparison to Han Chinese living in Guangshou (altitude 7 m) in that the circulatory fetal DNA levels were significantly higher in normal pregnancies of Tibetans and Han women living in Tibet in comparison to Han women at sea level. In both groups there was an increase in the presence of pre-eclampsia and the highest increase could be observed in the Han women living in Tibet probably indicating their limited degree of adaptation to the low oxygen content[102].

Regarding the 'disease' of pre-eclampsia in the pregnant woman following her placental 'disease', endothelial dysfunction or pathological endothelial cell activation can be considered as the hallmark of the peripheral problems with enhanced platelet aggregation, endothelial cell permeability, increased T-cell and granulocyte microparticles[103,104]. Whereas the systemic vascular endothelial cell dysfunction cannot be detected easily clinically, in the kidney, the glomerular endothelial involvement results in the characteristic symptoms of pre-eclampsia[105]. We have suggested placentally derived interleukin-1 as one of the potential mediators of the maternal inflammatory response in pre-eclampsia[106]. If this sequence of the placental disease leading through the release of debris to the maternal response is accepted, it is not difficult to understand that intervening variables such as diabetes or hypertension causing pre-existing maternal endothelial cell damage can lower the peripheral threshold for developing symptoms.

Because the elevated plasma cfDNA most likely is derived from cell turnover and should be associated with histones, we examined the circulatory nucleosomes by ELISA[107]. The levels in the study groups with early and late onset pre-eclampsia were significantly higher than in a matched normotensive control group, and the concentrations correlated with the cfDNA as well as the total maternal DNA.

The latest hint towards a similarity between an inflammatory type of an overreaction to the influx of 'hostile' material in pre-eclampsia came from investigations in our laboratory regarding the so-called 'neutrophil extracellular DNA lattices' in pre-eclampsia[108]. Brinkmann et al. had reported in *Science* (2004) that peripheral neutrophils treated with bacterial endotoxin, inflammatory cytokine IL8 or phorbol ester rapidly formed intricate extracellular networks termed 'neutrophil extracellular traps' (NET)[109]. These fibrous extracellular lattices contain DNA. We found that placentally derived interleukin 8 and STBMs also efficiently activated neutrophils and triggered NET formation. Interestingly, large numbers of NETs were present directly in the intervillous space of the pre-eclamptic placentas which we examined. In a study on retrospective samples, we likewise found that plasma elastase concentrations were significantly elevated in the pre-eclampsia study group as compared to controls[108]. It can therefore be speculated that the generation of NET in pre-eclampsia may not only contribute to the increased levels of maternal circulatory cfDNA, but could also be involved with the clotting of the intervillous space and the increased placental impedance characteristic of Doppler examination of the uterine artery in patients with toxemia of pregnancy.

With any statement on the etiology and pathophysiology of pre-eclampsia, however, we have to be careful. Pre-eclampsia has been called the 'disease of theories', and every (new) theory has to go along at least with the epidemiologic facts known about this peculiar condition. We think that the following key observations in pre-eclampsia are in good agreement with the pathophysiologic model of increased influx of placental debris having a direct toxic effect and, at the same time, an immunological tolerance inducing effect in the mother.

Key observations in pre-eclampsia

- It is the disease of primiparity and primipaternity (the pregnant women has not been exposed to the genome of her partner)[110]
- Increased risk when condoms were used prior to pregnancy[111]
- Increased risk after ovum donation (the whole genome is foreign to the pregnant woman)[112]
- Increased risk with surgically obtained sperm[113]
- Decreased risk after prior blood transfusion[114]
- Decreased risk after an extended exposure to the partner's semen, even orally[115]
- Decreased risk in association with HIV-related immunodeficiency[116]

Since pregnancy in general can be considered as an 'immunological miracle' in that the mother does not reject her usually only haploidentical fetus[117], based on a number of mechanisms causing immune tolerance[118], an uncontrolled increased influx of fetal material into her circulation automatically causes her problems. From all the epidemiological findings in pre-eclampsia mentioned above it has even been speculated that, from an evolutionary point of view, a pregnancy advantage may have been placed on long-term rather than short-term relationships. Regarding the genetic influence on the pathophysiology of pre-eclampsia and the fetoplacental cell traffic, it is clear that the trophoblast invasion should be governed by many genes and safeguarded by some redundant mechanisms.

Although there is a familial component to pre-eclampsia[119,120] and candidate regions for genes possibly involved were identified[121], pre-eclampsia is clearly not a single gene but a multifactorial disorder. The new possibility, however, to study placental and fetal gene expression by analyzing fetal mRNA has already shown interesting results. In a parallel assessment of circulatory fetal DNA and corticotropin-releasing-hormone mRNA, we found both to be increased in pre-eclampsia especially in the early onset group[122,123]. It will be exciting to study further candidate genes and their epigenetic regulation on the DNA-, RNA- and protein-levels non-invasively by examining the maternal peripheral blood.

CURRENT ADVANCES IN NON-INVASIVE PRENATAL DIAGNOSIS FOR DOWN'S SYNDROME

The accurate and efficacious detection of fetal aneuploidies with non-invasive techniques, particularly trisomy 21, represents a long-aspired goal in prenatal diagnosis. Various routes and approaches have been explored in the past three decades but, to date, none has had any significant clinical impact as it was not possible to overcome inherent technical hindrances.

The first main route pursued was the detection of the rare fetal cells circulating in maternal blood[124].

Some few years later, the discovery of cell-free fetal DNA (cff-DNA) in maternal plasma and serum opened a new promising route for the non-invasive determination of fetal genetic traits. The advantage of this material was that it is far more substantial than the limited number of trafficking fetal cells (up to 1000-fold), and that it can be readily examined by conventional or real-time PCR for various fetal loci which are completely absent from the maternal genome, e.g. the Y chromosome or the fetal RhD gene in Rhesus negative pregnant women. This approach has been shown to be so successful for such fetal loci that it is already being successfully used clinically[125].

The major drawback of cff-DNA in maternal blood is that it only represents 3–5% of the total circulatory DNA, which renders the characterization of fetal loci less disparate from maternal ones, such as point mutations or those which could be used to determine fetal aneuploidies.

Although these technical challenges may be overcome in part by the enrichment of cff-DNA due to their smaller size (<300 base pairs) than fragments of maternal origin[126], or by selecting epigenetically modified cff-DNA sequences[127], these approaches have not yet been useful for the detection of fetal Down's syndrome.

By a very innovative further exploration of their discovery of placentally derived cell-free fetal mRNA (cff-RNA) in maternal plasma, Lo and colleagues recently published a new approach for the detection of fetal aneuploidies in a non-invasive manner[128].

Two main advantages of cff-RNA over cff-DNA are that it is possible to select for placenta-specific species not expressed by any maternal tissues, and that cff-RNA species are present in higher abundance than the corresponding cff-DNA locus. Hence, the analysis of cff-RNA can be viewed in the same way as the analysis of fetal genes completely absent from the maternal genome, e.g. RhD and SRY, in that there is no maternal background 'noise' to be concerned with.

With this approach, the authors were able to identify genes expressed in the placenta, but which were not detectable in maternal blood cells[129]. Due to the importance of prenatal detection of Down's syndrome, they focused on genes located on chromosome 21 and determined that placentally derived transcripts of the *PLAC4* (placenta specific 4) gene were readily detectable in maternal plasma in all three trimesters of pregnancy. As no expression was detected in the plasma of non-pregnant individuals, it was hypothesized that the *PLAC4* gene may serve as an ideal target for the evaluation of chromosome 21 levels.

A caveat with this approach is that simple bulk quantitative analysis of *PLAC4* mRNA levels would not yield sufficient information for the accurate determination of fetal chromosome 21 ploidy. Hence, an alternative strategy or technology had to be sought. This technological breakthrough was provided by the advent of mass spectrometry systems such as the Mass Array™ system developed by Sequenom Inc., USA (www.sequenom.com), which permits the detection and quantitation of nucleotide sequences differing by as little as one base[130].

With the availability of such tools, Lo and colleagues then reasoned that it would be possible to enumerate chromosome

21 copy numbers by quantifying the allelic ratio of *PLAC4* mRNA transcripts using a SNP locus in this gene.

In this manner, if the fetus had a normal complement of chromosome 21, then the allelic ratio of the *PLAC4* transcripts would be 1:1. However, in case of a trisomy there would either be 2 copies of SNP allele A and one copy of SNP allele G or vice-versa. Hence, the allelic ratio of the transcripts would theoretically be 2:1 or 1:2, indicative of the karyotypic imbalance.

In their analysis, in which 10 cases with trisomy 21 were examined, Lo and colleagues observed that this approach may indeed be feasible, in that they observed a remarkably clear discrimination between case (n = 10) and control samples (n = 56), yielding a sensitivity of 90%. Furthermore, Down's syndrome could be excluded in 96% of the unaffected cases.

The road leading to the development of an efficacious non-invasive detection of fetal aneuploidies has been long and hard, involving a number of dead-ends and detours. The most surprising part of this exploration is that, in the end, a rank outsider may turn out to be the winning strategy, in the form of cff-RNA rather than the two previously more promising candidates, fetal cells or cff-DNA. The reasons are that few scientists could have foretold that mRNA exists in a stable cell-free form in plasma, nor that it could be used to determine chromosomal copy numbers. The first issue which needs to be resolved is whether this technique can be transferred to other laboratories and whether it can be verified in independent studies. Once this has been established, the accuracy and reliability will need to be ascertained in large multicenter studies.

In this context, it is worth noting that a number of previous high-profile reports, all of which appeared to be very promising, could not be verified in independent studies or failed to achieve clinically sound results when examined on a large scale. This became most evident during the NIFTY study.

However, should the method developed by Lo and colleagues pass all these hurdles and be ascertained to be sound by a number of independent studies, wherein it is repeatedly demonstrated that fetal aneuploidies can be detected with high degrees of accuracy, then the *Holy Grail* of prenatal diagnosis will finally have been attained.

REFERENCES

1. Holzgreve W, Garritsen HS, Ganshirt-Ahlert D. Fetal cells in the maternal circulation. *J Reprod Med* **37**:410–418, 1992.
2. Ganshirt-Ahlert D, Burschyk M, Garritsen HS et al. Magnetic cell sorting and the transferrin receptor as potential means of prenatal diagnosis from maternal blood. *Am J Obstet Gynecol* **166**:1350–1355, 1992.
3. Simpson JL, Elias S. Isolating fetal cells from maternal blood. Advances in prenatal diagnosis through molecular technology. *J Am Med Assoc* **270**: 2357–2361, 1993.
4. Lo YM, Lo ES, Watson N et al. Two-way cell traffic between mother and fetus: biologic and clinical implications. *Blood* **88**:4390–4395, 1996.
5. Barinaga M. Cells exchanged during pregnancy live on. *Science* **296**:2169–2172, 2002.
6. Hahn S, Huppertz B, Holzgreve W. Fetal cells and cell free fetal nucleic acids in maternal blood: new tools to study abnormal placentation? *Placenta* **26**:515–526, 2005.
7. Schmorl G. *Pathologisch-anatomische Untersuchungen über Puerperal-Eklampsie.* Leipzig: FCW Vogel, 1893.
8. Lapaire O, Holzgreve W, Oosterwijk Jc, Brinkhaus R, Bianchi DW. Georg Schmorl on trophoblasts in the maternal circulation. *Placenta* **28**(1):1–5, 2007.
9. Douglas GW, Thomas L, Carr M, Cullen NM, Morris R. Trophoblast in the circulating blood during pregnancy. *Am J Obstet Gynecol* **78**:960–973, 1959.
10. Anker P, Mulcahy H, Chen XQ, Stroun M. Detection of circulating tumour DNA in the blood (plasma/serum) of cancer patients. *Cancer Metastasis Rev* **18**:65–73, 1999.
11. Stroun M, Maurice P, Vasioukhin V et al. The origin and mechanism of circulating DNA. *Ann NY Acad Sci* **906**:161–168, 2000.
12. Lo YM, Corbetta N, Chamberlain PF, Rai V, Sargent IL, Redman CW, Wainscoat JS. Presence of fetal DNA in maternal plasma and serum. *Lancet* **350**:485–487, 1997.
13. Garvin Am, Holzgreve W, Hahn S. Highly accurate analysis of heterozygous loci by single cell PCR. *Nucleic Acids Res* **26**:3468–3472, 1998.
14. Li Y, Wenzel F, Holzgreve W, Hahn S. Genotyping fetal paternally inherited SNPs by MALDI-TOF MS using cell-free fetal DNA in maternal plasma: influence of size fractionation. *Electrophoresis* **27**:3889–3896, 2006.
15. Li Y, Holzgreve W, Din E, Vitucci A, Hahn S. Cell-free DNA in maternal plasma: is it all a question of size? *Ann NY Acad Sci* **1075**:81–87, 2006.
16. Bianchi DW. Circulating fetal DNA: its origin and diagnostic potential – a review. *Placenta* **25**:S93–101, 2004.
17. Deligezer U, Erten N, Akisik EE, Dalay N. Circulating fragmented nucleosomal DNA and caspase-3 mRNA in patients with lymphoma and myeloma. *Exp Mol Pathol* **80**:72–76, 2006.
18. Lam NY, Rainer TH, Chan LY, Joynt GM, Lo YM. Time course of early and late changes in plasma DNA in trauma patients. *Clin Chem* **49**:1286–1291, 2003.
19. Li Y, Hahn D, Holzgreve W, Hahn S. Ready detection of donor-specific single-nucleotide polymorphisms in the urine of renal transplant recipients by matrix-assisted laser desorption/ionization time-of-flight mass spectrometry. *Clin Chem* **51**:1903–1904, 2005.
20. Li Y, Hahn D, Wenzel F, Holzgreve W, Hahn S. Detection of SNPs in the plasma of pregnant women and in the urine of kidney transplant recipients by mass spectrometry. *Ann NY Acad Sci* **1075**:144–147, 2006.
21. Zhong XY, Holzgreve W, Hoesli I, Hahn S. Circulatory corticotropin-releasing hormone mRNA concentrations are increased in women with preterm delivery but not in those who respond to tocolytic treatment. *Clin Chem* **51**:635–636, 2005.
22. Farina A, LeShane ES, Romero R et al. High levels of fetal cell-free DNA in maternal serum: a risk factor for spontaneous preterm delivery. *Am J Obstet Gynecol* **193**:421–425, 2005.
23. Jimbo M, Sekizawa A, Sugito Y et al. Placenta increta: postpartum monitoring of plasma cell-free fetal DNA. *Clin Chem* **49**(9):1540–1541, 2003.
24. Ganshirt-Ahlert D, Borjesson-Stoll R, Burschyk M et al. Detection of fetal trisomies 21 and 18 from maternal blood using triple gradient and magnetic cell sorting. *Am J Reprod Immunol* **30**:194–201, 1993.
25. Troeger C, Holzgreve W, Hahn S. A comparison of different density gradients and antibodies for enrichment of fetal erythroblasts by MACS. *Prenat Diagn* **19**:521–526, 1999.
26. Mantzaris D, Cram D, Healy C, Howlett D, Kovacs G. Preliminary report: Correct diagnosis of sex in fetal cells isolated from cervical mucus during early pregnancy. *Aust NZ J Obstet Gynaecol* **45**:529–532, 2005.
27. Bianchi DW, Flint AF, Pizzimenti MF, Knoll JH, Latt SA. Isolation of fetal DNA from nucleated erythrocytes in maternal

blood. *Proc Natl Acad Sci USA* **87**:3279–3283, 1990.

28. Elias S, Price J, Dockter M et al. First trimester prenatal diagnosis of trisomy 21 in fetal cells from maternal blood. *Lancet* **340**:1033, 1992.
29. Holzgreve W, Garritsen HS, Tercanli S, Miny P, Nippert I, Ganshirt D. Noninvasive prenatal diagnosis. Strategy for a clinical trial. *Ann NY Acad Sci* **731**:253–256, 1994.
30. Bianchi DW, Simpson JL, Jackson LG et al. Fetal gender and aneuploidy detection using fetal cells in maternal blood: analysis of NIFTY I data. National Institute of Child Health and Development Fetal Cell Isolation Study. *Prenat Diagn* **22**:609–615, 2002.
31. Zimmermann B, Holzgreve W, Zhong XY, Hahn S. Inability to clonally expand fetal progenitors from maternal blood. *Fetal Diagn Ther* **17**:97–100, 2002.
32. Babochkina T, Mergenthaler S, De Napoli G et al. Numerous erythroblasts in maternal blood are impervious to fluorescent in situ hybridization analysis, a feature related to a dense compact nucleus with apoptotic character. *Haematologica* **90**: 740–745, 2005.
33. Johnson KL, Dukes KA, Vidaver J et al. Interlaboratory comparison of fetal male DNA detection from common maternal plasma samples by real-time PCR. *Clin Chem* **50**:516–521, 2004.
34. Bischoff FZ, Hahn S, Johnson KL et al. Intact fetal cells in maternal plasma: are they really there? *Lancet* **361**:139–140, 2003.
35. Troeger C, Zhong XY, Burgemeister R et al. Approximately half of the erythroblasts in maternal blood are of fetal origin. *Mol Hum Reprod* **5**:1162–1165, 1999.
36. Faas BH, Beuling EA, Christiaens GC, von dem Borne AE, van der Schoot CE. Detection of fetal RHD-specific sequences in maternal plasma. *Lancet* **352**:1196, 1998.
37. Lo YM, Hjelm NM, Fidler C et al. Prenatal diagnosis of fetal RhD status by molecular analysis of maternal plasma. *N Engl J Med* **339**:1734–1738, 1998.
38. Zhong XY, Holzgreve W, Hahn S. Detection of fetal Rhesus D and sex using fetal DNA from maternal plasma by multiplex polymerase chain reaction. *Br J Obstet Gynaecol* **107**:766–769, 2000.
39. Gautier E, Benachi A, Giovangrandi Y et al. Fetal RhD genotyping by maternal serum analysis: a two-year experience. *Am J Obstet Gynecol* **192**:666–669, 2005.
40. Van der Schoot CE, Soussan AA, Koelewijn J, Bonsel G, Paget-Christiaens LG, de Haas M. Non-invasive antenatal RHD typing. *Transfus Clin Biol* **13**(1-2):53–57, 2006.
41. Rijnders RJ, Christiaens GC, Bossers B, Van Der Smagt JJ, Van Der Schoot CE, De Haas M. Clinical applications of cell-free fetal DNA from maternal plasma. *Obstet Gynecol* **103**:157–164, 2004.
42. Moise KJ. Fetal RhD typing with free DNA in maternal plasma. *Am J Obstet Gynecol* **192**:663–665, 2005.
43. Geifman-Holtzman O, Grotegut CA, Gaughan JP. Diagnostic accuracy of noninvasive fetal Rh genotyping from maternal blood – a meta-analysis. *Am J Obstet Gynecol* **195**:1163–1173, 2006.
44. Illanes S, Avent N, Soothill Pw. Cell-free fetal DNA in maternal plasma: an important advance to link fetal genetics to obstetric ultrasound. *Ultrasound Obstet Gynecol* **25**:317–322, 2005.
45. Martinhago CD, De Oliveira RM, Tomitao Canas M de C et al. Accuracy of fetal gender determination in maternal plasma at 5 and 6 weeks of pregnancy. *Prenat Diagn* **26**:1219–1223, 2006.
46. Costa JM, Benachi A, Gautier E, Jouannic JM, Ernault P, Dumez Y. First-trimester fetal sex determination in maternal serum using real-time PCR. *Prenat Diagn* **21**:1070–1074, 2001.
47. Santacroce R, Vecchione G, Tomaiyolo M et al. Identification of fetal gender in maternal blood is a helpful tool in the prenatal diagnosis of haemophilia. *Haemophilia* **12**:417–422, 2006.
48. Smith RP, Lombaard H, Soothill PW. The obstetrician's view: ethical and societal implications of non-invasive prenatal diagnosis. *Prenat Diagn* **26**:631–634, 2006.
49. Kaiser J. Prenatal diagnosis: an earlier look at baby's genes. *Science* **309**:1476–1478, 2005.
50. Saito H, Sekizawa A, Morimoto T, Suzuki M, Yanaihara T. Prenatal DNA diagnosis of a single-gene disorder from maternal plasma. *Lancet* **356**:1170, 2000.
51. Li Y, Holzgreve W, Page-Christiaens GC, Gille JJ, Hahn S. Improved prenatal detection of a fetal point mutation for achondroplasia by the use of size-fractionated circulatory DNA in maternal plasma--case report. *Prenat Diagn* **24**:896–898, 2004.
52. Amicucci P, Gennarelli M, Novelli G, Dallapiccola B. Prenatal diagnosis of myotonic dystrophy using fetal DNA obtained from maternal plasma. *Clin Chem* **46**:301–302, 2000.
53. Li Y, Di Naro E, Vitucci A, Zimmermann B, Holzgreve W, Hahn S. Detection of paternally inherited fetal point mutations for beta-thalassemia using size-fractionated cell-free DNA in maternal plasma. *J Am Med Assoc* **293**:843–849, 2005.
54. Saker A, Benachi A, Bonnefont JP et al. Genetic characterisation of circulating fetal cells allows non-invasive prenatal diagnosis of cystic fibrosis. *Prenat Diagn* 2006.
55. Tungwiwat W, Fucharoen S, Fucharoen G, Ratanasiri T, Sanchaisuriya K. Development and application of a real-time quantitative PCR for prenatal detection of fetal alpha(0)-thalassemia from maternal plasma. *Ann NY Acad Sci* **1075**:103–107, 2006.
56. Zhong XY, Hahn S, Kiefer V, Holzgreve W. Is the quantity of circulatory cell-free DNA in human plasma and serum samples associated with gender, age and frequency of blood donations? *Ann Hematol* **86**:139–143, 2007.
57. Zhong XY, Burk MR, Troeger C, Jackson LR, Holzgreve W, Hahn S. Fetal DNA in maternal plasma is elevated in pregnancies with aneuploid fetuses. *Prenat Diagn* **20**:795–798, 2000.
58. Samura O, Sohda S, Johnson KL et al. Diagnosis of trisomy 21 in fetal nucleated erythrocytes from maternal blood by use of short tandem repeat sequences. *Clin Chem* **47**:1622–1626, 2001.
59. Aractingi S, Berkane N, Bertheau P et al. Fetal DNA in skin of polymorphic eruptions of pregnancy. *Lancet* **352**:1898–1901, 1998.
60. Holmes RC, Black MM. The specific dermatoses of pregnancy: a reappraisal with special emphasis on a proposed simplified clinical classification. *Clin Exp Dermatol* **7**:65–73, 1982.
61. Holzgreve W, Vakilzadeh F. Herpes gestationis: clinical and optic immunofluorescence findings. *Zentralbl Gynakol* **104**:1462–1467, 1982.
62. Sibai B, Dekker G, Kupferminc M. Pre-eclampsia. *Lancet* **365**:785–799, 2005.
63. Roberts JM, Pearson GD, Cutler JA, Lindheimer MD. Summary of the NHLBI Working Group on Research on Hypertension During Pregnancy. *Hypertens Pregnancy* **22**:109–127, 2003.
64. Sattar N, Greer IA. Pregnancy complications and maternal cardiovascular risk: opportunities for intervention and screening? *Br Med J* **325**:157–160, 2002.
65. Ganshirt D, Smeets FW, Dohr A et al. Enrichment of fetal nucleated red blood cells from the maternal circulation for prenatal diagnosis: experiences with triple density gradient and MACS based on more than 600 cases. *Fetal Diagn Ther* **13**:276–286, 1998.
66. Holzgreve W, Ghezzi F, Di Naro E, Ganshirt D, Maymon E, Hahn S. Disturbed feto-maternal cell traffic in preeclampsia. *Obstet Gynecol* **91**:669–672, 1998.
67. Lo YM, Leung TN, Tein MS et al. Quantitative abnormalities of fetal DNA in maternal serum in preeclampsia. *Clin Chem* **45**:184–188, 1999.
68. Jansen MW, Korver-Hakkennes K, van Leenen D et al. Significantly higher number of fetal cells in the maternal circulation of women with pre-eclampsia. *Prenat Diagn* **21**:1022–1026, 2001.

69. Farina A, Sekizawa A, Iwasaki M, Matsuoka R, Ichizuka K, Okai T. Total cell-free DNA (beta-globin gene) distribution in maternal plasma at the second trimester: a new prospective for pre-eclampsia screening. *Prenat Diagn* **24**:722–726, 2004.
70. Zhong XY, Laivuori H, Livingston JC et al. Elevation of both maternal and fetal extracellular circulating deoxyribonucleic acid concentrations in the plasma of pregnant women with preeclampsia. *Am J Obstet Gynecol* **184**:414–419, 2001.
71. Zhong XY, Holzgreve W, Hahn S. Circulatory fetal and maternal DNA in pregnancies at risk and those affected by preeclampsia. *Ann NY Acad Sci* **945**:138–140, 2001.
72. Stamilio DM, Sehdev HM, Morgan MA, Propert K, Macones GA. Can antenatal clinical and biochemical markers predict the development of severe preeclampsia? *Am J Obstet Gynecol* **182**:589–594, 2000.
73. Conde-Agudelo A, Villar J, Lindheimer M. World Health Organization systematic review of screening tests for preeclampsia. *Obstet Gynecol* **104**:1367–1391, 2004.
74. Yu CK, Smith GC, Papageorghiou AT, Cacho AM, Nicolaides KH. An integrated model for the prediction of pre-eclampsia using maternal factors and uterine artery Doppler velocimetry in unselected low-risk women. *Am J Obstet Gynecol* **195**:330, 2006.
75. Holzgreve W, Li JJ, Steinborn A, Kulz T, Sohn C, Hodel M, Hahn S. Elevation in erythroblast count in maternal blood before the onset of preeclampsia. *Am J Obstet Gynecol* **184**:165–168, 2001.
76. Zhong XY, Holzgreve W, Hahn S. The levels of circulatory cell free fetal DNA in maternal plasma are elevated prior to the onset of preeclampsia. *Hypertens Pregnancy* **21**:77–83, 2002.
77. Levine RJ, Qian C, Leshane ES et al. Two-stage elevation of cell-free fetal DNA in maternal sera before onset of preeclampsia. *Am J Obstet Gynecol* **190**:707–713, 2004.
78. Lau TW, Leung TN, Chan LY et al. Fetal DNA clearance from maternal plasma is impaired in preeclampsia. *Clin Chem* **48**:2141–2146, 2002.
79. Venkatesha S, Toporsian M, Lam C et al. Soluble endoglin contributes to the pathogenesis of preeclampsia. *Nat Med* **12**:642–649, 2006.
80. Levine RJ, Lam C, Qian C et al. Soluble endoglin and other circulating antiangiogenic factors in preeclampsia. *N Engl J Med* **355**:992–1005, 2006.
81. Venkatesha S, Toporsian M, Lam C et al. Soluble endoglin contributes to the pathogenesis of preeclampsia. *Nat Med* **12**:642–649, 2006.
82. Levine RJ, Lam C, Qian C et al. Soluble endoglin and other circulating antiangiogenic factors in preeclampsia. *N Engl J Med* **355**:992–1005, 2006.
83. Farina A, Sekizawa A, Sugito Y et al. Fetal DNA in maternal plasma as a screening variable for preeclampsia: a preliminary nonparametric analysis of detection rate in low-risk nonsymptomatic patients. *Prenat Diagn* **24**:83–86, 2004.
84. Holzgreve W, Hahn S. Novel molecular biological approaches for the diagnosis of preeclampsia. *Clin Chem* **45**:451–452, 1999.
85. Troeger C, Holzgreve W, Ladewig A, Zhong XY, Hahn S. Examination of maternal plasma erythropoietin and activin A concentrations with regard to circulatory erythroblast levels in normal and preeclamptic pregnancies. *Fetal Diagn Ther* **21**(1):156–160, 2006.
86. Pijnenborg R, Ball E, Bulmer JN, Hanssens M, Robson SC, Vercruysse L. In vivo analysis of trophoblast cell invasion in the human. *Methods Mol Med* **122**:11–44, 2006.
87. Kadyrov M, Kingdom JC, Huppertz B. Divergent trophoblast invasion and apoptosis in placental bed spiral arteries from pregnancies complicated by maternal anemia and early-onset preeclampsia/intrauterine growth restriction. *Am J Obstet Gynecol* **194**:557–563, 2006.
88. Matijevic R, Johnston T. In vivo assessment of failed trophoblastic invasion of the spiral arteries in pre-eclampsia. *Br J Obstet Gynaecol* **106**: 78–82, 1999.
89. Redman CW, Sargent IL. Placental debris, oxidative stress and pre-eclampsia. *Placenta* **21**:597–602, 2000.
90. Roberts JM, Hubel CA. Is oxidative stress the link in the two-stage model of pre-eclampsia? *Lancet* **354**:788–789, 1999.
91. Tjoa ML, Cindrova-Davies T, Spasic-Boskovic O, Bianchi DW, Burton GJ. Trophoblastic oxidative stress and the release of cell-free feto-placental DNA. *Am J Pathol* **169**:400–404, 2006.
92. Orozco AF, Bischoff FZ, Horne C, Popek E, Simpson JL, Lewis DE. Hypoxia-induced membrane-bound apoptotic DNA particles: potential mechanism of fetal DNA in maternal plasma. *Ann NY Acad Sci* **1075**:57–62, 2006.
93. Redman CW, Sacks GP, Sargent IL. Preeclampsia: an excessive maternal inflammatory response to pregnancy. *Am J Obstet Gynecol* **180**:499–506, 1999.
94. Sacks GP, Studena K, Sargent K, Redman CW. Normal pregnancy and pre-eclampsia both produce inflammatory changes in peripheral blood leukocytes akin to those of sepsis. *Am J Obstet Gynecol* **179**:80–86, 1998.
95. Martin JN Jr, Thigpen BD, Rose CH, Cushman J, Moore A, May WL. Maternal benefit of high-dose intravenous corticosteroid therapy for HELLP syndrome. *Am J Obstet Gynecol* **189**(3):830–834, 2003.
96. Beller FK, Schmidt EH, Holzgreve W, Hauss J. Septicemia during pregnancy: a study in different species of experimental animals. *Am J Obstet Gynecol* **151**:967–975, 1985.
97. Many A, Hubel CA, Fisher SJ, Roberts JM, Zhou Y. Invasive cytotrophoblasts manifest evidence of oxidative stress in preeclampsia. *Am J Pathol* **156**:321–331, 2000.
98. Zhong XY, Holzgreve W, Hahn S. Cell-free fetal DNA in the maternal circulation does not stem from the transplacental passage of fetal erythroblasts. *Mol Hum Reprod* **8**:864–870, 2002.
99. Redman CW, Sargent IL. Latest advances in understanding preeclampsia. *Science* **308**:1592–1594, 2005.
100. Gupta AK, Holzgreve W, Hahn S. Microparticle-free placentally derived soluble factors downmodulate the response of activated T cells. *Hum Immunol* **66**:977–984, 2005.
101. Knight M, Redman CW, Linton EA, Sargent IL. Shedding of syncytiotrophoblast microvilli into the maternal circulation in pre-eclamptic pregnancies. *Br J Obstet Gynaecol* **105**:632–640, 1998.
102. Zhong Xy, Wang Y, Chen S et al. Can circulatory fetal DNA be used to study placentation at high altitude? *Ann NY Acad Sci* **1022**:124–128, 2004.
103. Taylor RN, de Groot CJ, Cho YK, Lim KH. Circulating factors as markers and mediators of endothelial cell dysfunction in preeclampsia. *Semin Reprod Endocrinol* **16**:17–31, 1998.
104. VanWijk MJ, Nieuwland R, Boer K, van der Post JA, VanBavel E, Sturk A. Microparticle subpopulations are increased in preeclampsia: possible involvement in vascular dysfunction? *Am J Obstet Gynecol* **187**:450–456, 2002.
105. Moran P, Lindheimer MD, Davison JM. The renal response to preeclampsia. *Semin Nephrol* **24**:588–595, 2004.
106. Rusterholz C, Gupta AK, Huppertz B, Holzgreve W, Hahn S. Soluble factors released by placental villous tissue: interleukin-1 is a potential mediator of endothelial dysfunction. *Am J Obstet Gynecol* **192**:618–624, 2005.
107. Zhong XY, Gebhardt S, Hillermann R, Tofa KC, Holzgreve W, Hahn S. Circulatory nucleosome levels are significantly increased in early and late-onset preeclampsia. *Prenat Diagn* **25**:700–703, 2005.
108. Gupta AK, Hasler P, Holzgreve W, Gebhardt S, Hahn S. Induction of neutrophil extracellular DNA lattices by placental microparticles and IL-8 and their presence in preeclampsia. *Hum Immunol* **66**:1146–1154, 2005.

109. Brinkmann V, Reichard U, Goosmann C et al. Neutrophil extracellular traps kill bacteria. *Science* **303**(5663):1532–1535, 2004.
110. Hahn S, Gupta AK, Troeger C, Rusterholz C, Holzgreve W. Disturbances in placental immunology: ready for therapeutic interventions? *Springer Semin Immunopathol* **27**:477–493, 2006.
111. Klonoff Cohen HS, Savitz DA, Cefalo RC, McCann MF. An epidemiologic study of contraception and preeclampsia. *J Am Med Assoc* **262**:3143–3147, 1989.
112. Soderstrom-Anttila V, Hovatta O. An oocyte donation program with goserelin down-regulation of voluntary donors. *Acta Obstet Gynecol Scand* **74**(4):288–292, 1995.
113. Wang JX, Knottnerus AM, Schuit G, Norman RJ, Chan A, Dekker GA. Surgically obtained sperm, and risk of gestational hypertension and pre-eclampsia. *Lancet* **359**:673–674, 2002.
114. Feeney JG, Tovey LA, Scott JS. Influence of previous blood-transfusion on incidence of pre-eclampsia. *Lancet* **1**(8017):874–875, 1997.
115. Robillard PY, Hulsey TC, Perianin J, Janky E, Miri EH, Papiernik E. Association of pregnancy-induced hypertension with duration of sexual cohabitation before conception. *Lancet* **344**(8928):973–975, 1994.
116. Hahn S, Gupta AK, Troeger C, Rusterholz C, Holzgreve W. Disturbances in placental immunology: ready for therapeutic interventions? *Springer Semin Immunopathol* **27**:477–493, 2006.
117. Medawar PB. Immunological tolerance. *Science* **133**:303–306, 1961.
118. Uckan D, Steele A, Cherry B et al. Trophoblasts express Fas ligand: a proposed mechanism for immune privilege in placenta and maternal invasion. *Mol Hum Reprod* **3**(8):655–662, 1997.
119. O'Shaughnessy KM, Ferraro F, Fu B, Downing S, Morris NH. Identification of monozygotic twins that are concordant for preeclampsia. *Am J Obstet Gynecol* **182**:1156–1157, 2000.
120. Lie RT, Rasmussen S, Brunborg H, Gjessing HK, Lie-Nielsen E, Irgens LM. Fetal and maternal contributions to risk of pre-eclampsia: population based study. *Br Med J* **316**:1343–1347, 1998.
121. Laivuori H, Lahermo P, Ollikainen V et al. Susceptibility loci for pre-eclampsia on chromosomes 2p25 and 9p13 in Finnish families. *Am J Hum Genet* **72**: 168–177, 2003.
122. Zhong XY, Gebhardt S, Hillermann R, Tofa KC, Holzgreve W, Hahn S. Parallel assessment of circulatory fetal DNA and corticotropin-releasing hormone mRNA in early- and late-onset preeclampsia. *Clin Chem* **51**:1730–1733, 2005.
123. Zhong XY, Holzgreve W, Gebhardt S et al. Minimal alteration in the ratio of circulatory fetal DNA to fetal corticotropin-releasing hormone mRNA level in preeclampsia. *Fetal Diagn Ther* **21**:246–249, 2006.
124. Hahn S, Holzgreve W. Prenatal diagnosis using fetal cells and cell-free fetal DNA in maternal blood: what is currently feasible? *Clin Obstet Gynecol* **45**:649–656, 2002.
125. Chiu RW, Lo YM. Noninvasive prenatal diagnosis by analysis of fetal DNA in maternal plasma. *Methods Mol Biol* **336**:101–109, 2006.
126. Li Y, Zimmermann B, Rusterholz C, Kang A, Holzgreve W, Hahn S. Size separation of circulatory DNA in maternal plasma permits ready detection of fetal DNA polymorphisms. *Clin Chem* **50**:1002–1011, 2004.
127. Chan KC, Ding C, Gerovassili A et al. Hypermethylated RASSF1A in maternal plasma: a universal fetal DNA marker that improves the reliability of noninvasive prenatal diagnosis. *Clin Chem* **52**:2211-1218, 2006.
128. Lo YM, Tsui NB, Chiu RW et al. Plasma placental RNA allelic ratio permits noninvasive prenatal chromosomal aneuploidy detection. *Nat Med* **13**:218–223, 2007.
129. Ng EK, Tsui NB, Lau TK et al. mRNA of placental origin is readily detectable in maternal plasma. *Proc Natl Acad Sci USA* **100**:4748–4753, 2003.
130. Ding C, Chiu RW, Lau TK et al. MS analysis of single-nucleotide differences in circulating nucleic acids: Application to noninvasive prenatal diagnosis. *Proc Natl Acad Sci USA* **101**:10762–10767, 2004.

CHAPTER

22 Invasive diagnostic procedures

Boaz Weisz and Charles Rodeck

KEY POINTS

- Amniocentesis is used from 15 weeks onwards for prenatal diagnosis of chromosomal abnormalities, single gene disorders, fetal lung maturity, fetal infections and inflammation
- Early amniocentesis (11–13 weeks) is not used in clinical practice due to increased risk of fetal loss rate and abnormalities
- The fetal loss rate associated with midtrimester amniocentesis is still not established and is probably between 0.5–1.0%. Newer studies show an even lower loss rate
- CVS is used from 10 weeks onwards for prenatal diagnosis of single gene defects and chromosomal abnormalities. It is especially relevant for families with mendelian disorders that wish to have an early prenatal diagnosis
- CVS can be done transabdominally or transcervically. Villi can be obtained by each route by aspiration or biopsy
- CVS is associated with a slightly increased risk of fetal loss compared with amniocentesis. However, the exact increase in risk is difficult to assess because of the natural miscarriage rate between 10 and 16 weeks (which is high in aneuploidy fetuses)
- In equally experienced hands both the transcervical and the transabdominal routes have a similar fetal loss rate (about 1–2%)
- The indications for fetal blood samplings and other invasive procedures are now limited due to the availability of less invasive or non-invasive methods

INTRODUCTION

Prenatal diagnosis of chromosomal abnormalities and genetic disorders by invasive procedures has become a major part of the practice of fetal medicine. Ultrasound guided chorionic villus sampling (CVS), amniocentesis and, to a lesser extent, placental biopsy (late CVS) and fetal blood sampling (FBS) are used routinely in fetal medicine units for prenatal diagnosis. Other fetal tissue biopsies such as skin, liver and muscle biopsy are used only rarely. In this chapter, we discuss the indications, the specific technical aspects and the procedure-related risks of each technique.

AMNIOCENTESIS

During the last four decades, amniocentesis in the second trimester of pregnancy has become the routine method to exclude chromosomal abnormalities of the fetus. The first reports about amniocentesis date back to 1881–82 when this technique was used for amniotic fluid drainage in cases of polyhydramnios in singleton and especially multiple pregnancies. In the 1930s, amniocentesis was used in France for abortion induction by introducing hypertonic saline. The introduction of conventional amniocentesis is usually associated with a publication by Bevis in 1952[1] who used it to evaluate the severity of Rhesus incompatibility. Fuchs and Riis (1956)[2] performed amniocentesis for determination of fetal sex by Barr body staining and Steele and Breg (1966)[3] cultured amniocytes and performed chromosome analysis. Valenti et al (1968)[4] reported the first prenatal diagnosis of Down's syndrome. The development of cytogenetics, the demand for prenatal diagnosis and the continuous improvement of ultrasound technology were factors in bringing amniocentesis into routine clinical practice. The first report of a fairly large series of some 150 amniocenteses in the second trimester appeared in 1970[5]. These early procedures were performed without sonographic localization of the amniotic sac and needle. With improvements in real-time ultrasound, pre-amniocentesis scanning evolved into the present-day standard practice of concurrent ultrasound guided amniocentesis.

Indications for amniocentesis

The historical indication for amniocentesis was to monitor fetuses with red cell alloimmunization by measuring the levels of bilirubin in the amniotic fluid[6]. Nowadays, this method has been replaced by non-invasive Doppler evaluation of the peak-systolic velocity in the middle cerebral artery (MCA) which was proven to be more sensitive and more accurate for the diagnosis of severe fetal anemia[7].

The most common indication for amniocentesis nowadays is cytogenetic analysis of the fetal chromosomes. Amniocentesis is widely available and the population selected for this invasive procedure is determined by maternal age,[8] screening tests[9,10] or purely maternal request. Many screening tests rely on second-trimester serum markers and the timing of obtaining the results of these tests corresponds with the timing of midtrimester amniocentesis. Most laboratories can report reliable karyotyping within 3 weeks from the procedure. Newer techniques such as polymerase-chain reaction (PCR) (see Chapter 23) or fluorescent in-situ hybridization (FISH)[11] can facilitate partial results within 2 days. These techniques can be used also for the detection of microdeletions in cases with known anomalies (such as the 22q11 which is associated with velocardiofacial syndromes). Recent advances in the technology of comparative genomic hybridization (CGH) and microarrays are being made. Array-CGH studies have revealed extensive inter-individual copy number variation of genomic segments, unanticipated complexity of apparently balanced translocations, and new phenotypes associated with DNA deletions and duplications. These observations will affect future counseling for prenatal diagnosis[12].

Single gene disorders with known mutations can also be diagnosed by amniocentesis, but it is used much less often than CVS for this indication because of the later gestational age and the lower yield of DNA obtained from amniocytes than from chorionic villi. These tests are performed in known parental carriers or in cases where sonographic findings are indicative, i.e. hyperechogenic bowel (cystic fibrosis), skeletal dysplasias (FGF R_3 mutations).

Another common indication for amniocentesis is diagnosis of fetal infections such as cytomegalovirus (CMV), toxoplasmosis and varicella. The presence of these microorganisms is detected in the amniotic fluid by PCR, antigen assays or specific cultures. In cases of suspected maternal infection, amniocentesis is done in order to diagnose fetal infection. The timing of amniocentesis in such cases is crucial since some pathogens (such as CMV) are secreted into the amniotic fluid by fetal urination after 22 weeks of gestation. It is recommended to postpone amniocentesis for at least 6 weeks from maternal infection[13]. Amniocentesis is also used in certain units in order to diagnose the presence of amniotic infection (with intact membranes) in cases of preterm labor. Although in dispute, some advocate sampling of amniotic fluid for the presence of mycoplasma and ureoplasma, as well as the presence of various cytokines, in specific cases of preterm labor[14].

Another indication for amniocentesis in late gestation, which is more common in the USA than in other countries, is evaluation of fetal lung maturity. This is usually performed when the reasons for induced delivery are not absolute and in order to avoid iatrogenic respiratory distress syndrome or transient tachypnea of the newborn. Amniotic fluid is analyzed by various methods (lecithin/sphingomylein (L/S) ratio, percent phosphatidylglycerol (%PG), lamellar body count (LBC) and surfactant-to-albumin ratio (TDx-FLM(II)) in amniotic fluid) which are strongly correlated with fetal lung maturity[15].

Technique of amniocentesis

Early amniocentesis refers to a procedure performed at 11–14 weeks of gestation. The Canadian Early and Mid-trimester Amniocentesis Trial (CEMAT) randomly allocated pregnant women to either early amniocentesis (between 11(+0) and 12(+6) gestational weeks(days)) or midtrimester (between 15(+0) and 16(+6) gestational weeks(days)) amniocentesis. This study showed a significant difference in total fetal losses for early amniocentesis compared with midtrimester amniocentesis (7.6% versus 5.9%; difference 1.7%, one-sided CI 2.98%, P = 0.012). There was also a significant increase in talipes equinovarus in the early amniocentesis group compared with the midtrimester amniocentesis group (1.3% versus 0.1%, P = 0.0001). Since this study (as well as others) showed that early amniocentesis is associated with an increased risk of fetal loss and talipes equinovarus, the usage of early amniocentesis for prenatal diagnosis has been restricted only to special circumstances[16].

Midtrimester amniocentesis, which is performed after 15 weeks of gestation, is the 'conventional' amniocentesis nowadays. Between weeks 15 and 17 of pregnancy, the total amount of amniotic fluid is about 200 ml and the uterus can be reached transabdominally without major risk of tranversing the bladder or bowel. In the beginning, it was performed without ultrasound guidance, but later it was used to select the site for needle insertion: after removal of the transducer, the needle was inserted immediately. Nowadays, the sonographically monitored technique consisting of the continuous visualization of the needle during the entire procedure is the only acceptable method (Fig. 22.1). A comparison between both techniques has shown that the sonographically monitored amniocentesis was associated with significantly fewer bloody taps and repeated needle insertions[17]. Most centers use the 'free-hand' technique but needle guides can be attached to the transducer.

When looking at the loss rates after transplacental, compared to non-transplacental amniocentesis, no difference between the two groups was found[18,19]. Although Golbus et al.[20] did not detect an increased rate of rhesus sensitization in 300 Rh-negative women not given anti-D after amniocentesis compared to 650 controls, most investigators have accepted an increased risk[21,22], so that, usually, the administration of 100–300 μg of anti-D is standard in most countries after amniocentesis.

Amniocentesis for twin pregnancies has been established for about 30 years[23], but the exact methodology varies between centers. Several techniques have been described for amniocentesis in twins. The most common technique is the use of two different needles inserted separately and sequentially into each amniotic cavity, under ultrasound guidance. Misdiagnosis using such a technique has been reported and might involve up to 3.5% of samples[24]. In order to reduce the risk of re-sampling the first sac from a different angle, some have advocated the use of Indigo carmine in order to dye the amniotic fluid of the first sac[24]. However, the injection of a foreign substance into the amniotic cavity is of concern and has been associated with fetal

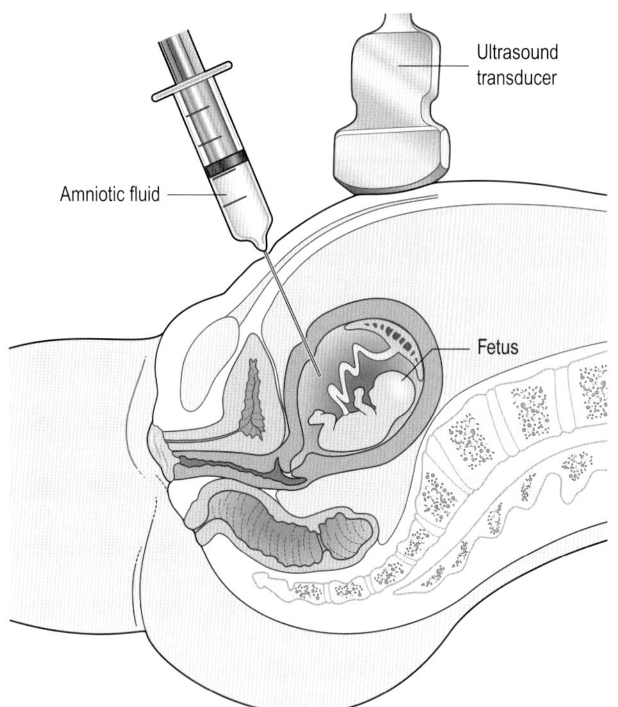

Fig. 22.1 Schematic picture of amniocentesis by free-hand technique.

intestinal atresias[25,26]. Many favor an instillation-free sampling technique. In our opinion, and that of others[27,28], the high-resolution ultrasound equipment available today makes instillation of dye unnecessary. It could be reserved for cases in which it is difficult to demonstrate the septum clearly (such as in amniotic fluid volume discordance), and for higher order multiple pregnancies[29] (in which every sac that has been aspirated has dye instilled). Another technique which may avoid the possibility of sampling twice from the same amniotic cavity in twin pregnancies is the single needle technique[30–34]. The septum dividing the two amniotic cavities is identified, and the needle is inserted into the first sac close to the septum. After aspiration of fluid and careful labeling of the container, the needle is then inserted *through the septum* into the second sac. This technique is less widely used, as it may be difficult to enter the second sac due to 'tenting' of the septum. There are two other potential problems: contamination of the second fluid with cells from the first sac and the possible risk of creating a pseudomonoamniotic twin pregnancy with its associated complication of cord entanglement[34].

Complications of amniocentesis

Amniocentesis is associated with increased pregnancy loss rate, which deters physicians and healthcare givers from recommending it to all pregnant women. However, the exact percentage of increased loss rate is still in dispute. Most of the figures of pregnancy loss rate after amniocentesis are drawn from case-control studies. There is only one randomized study that assessed the risk of second-trimester amniocenteses. In this Danish randomized study[35], 4606 women between 25 and 34 years were evaluated and all procedures were performed with a 20-gauge needle by very experienced investigators. A spontaneous abortion rate of 1.7% after the procedure was significantly higher than that of the control group (0.7%, $P < 0.01$). Therefore, the procedure-related loss rate was 1.0%. This figure of 1% is used in many fetal medicine units for counseling before amniocentesis. However, this methodology was not repeated in other studies assessing the procedure-related fetal loss and recent studies are all case-controlled. Some studies have shown a small, non-significant increase in fetal loss rate (0.3–0.6%) in patients undergoing amniocentesis[36–38]. Many centers (as well as the Centers for Disease Control and Prevention-USA[39,40]) nowadays, use the figure of 0.5% for counseling the procedure related fetal loss rate. A meta-analysis published by Seeds[41] evaluating 29 reports (68 119 procedures) concluded that contemporary amniocentesis with concurrent ultrasound guidance is associated with a procedure-related loss rate of 0.33% (95% CI, 0.09, 0.56) in a comparison of all studies to all available control subjects and 0.6% (95% CI, 0.31, 0.90) when restricting the analysis to studies that were case controlled.

A recent study which assessed the outcome of patients in the FASTER study[42] has shown a negligible, non-significant 0.06% increased risk of fetal loss rate after amniocentesis. Such a negligible procedure-related risk has been the basis for debates and new insights regarding this procedure. In our opinion, it is logical and well supported by the literature that both improvement in the technique and better ultrasound imaging should decrease the procedure-related fetal loss rate; however, it is still very premature to use such a low loss rate (of less than 0.1%) for routine counseling and more studies are needed in order to establish these figures.

Fetal injury that is attributed to midtrimester amniocentesis is rare and the association to the procedure is rarely proven. The risk of direct fetal needle injury often is presumed to be reduced with the use of simultaneous ultrasound guidance, but several case reports document or attribute cases of fetal injury to the amniocentesis needle, despite the use of simultaneous guidance for the procedure[43,44]. Isolated case reports of corneal perforation, ileocutaneous fistula, ileal atresia, gangrene of a limb, porencephalic cyst, patellar tendon disruption, and even peripheral nerve injury have been attributed to amniocentesis needle injury at midtrimester genetic amniocentesis, but the attribution has been generally by association only and not on the basis of direct evidence.

Maternal death due to amniocentesis is extremely rare. The cause of death is usually *Escherichia coli* sepsis and disseminated intravascular coagulation[45]. Fever, pain and uterine tenderness after an amniocentesis should be promptly evaluated and confirmation of intra-amniotic infection by amniocentesis may be considered if the diagnosis is in question.

Counseling before amniocentesis

1. The various indications for amniocentesis are detailed above. When the amniocentesis is being done to rule out Down's syndrome, it is essential that the patient is counseled regarding her background risks and about the best screening tests available, i.e. integrated, combined or sequential tests.
2. The risks of amniocentesis should be discussed, especially the risk of *fetal loss*. Since the exact risk is not well established, in our opinion, patients should be counseled that the estimated risk of fetal loss is

1/100–1/200, although new encouraging studies suggest that the risk may be smaller.
3. Patients should be warned of signs of amnionitis and encouraged to seek medical care in cases of post-procedure fever, rupture of membranes, painful contractions or vaginal bleeding.

CHORIONIC VILLUS SAMPLING (CVS)

Chorionic villi were first obtained in termination of pregnancy patients by Mohr[46] and Hahnemann[47]. The first clinical cases, done 'blindly' for fetal sexing, were reported from China[48]. Ultrasound-guided chorionic villus sampling (CVS) was developed during the early to mid-1980s[49–54] and involves the aspiration or biopsy of placental tissue. Although midtrimester amniocentesis is still the most common method for prenatal diagnosis, CVS is becoming more accepted, mostly due to the potential to identify patients with higher risks of having chromosomal abnormalities in early stages of pregnancy. CVS can be performed at any stage during pregnancy (e.g. CVS in the first trimester and placental biopsy in late pregnancy)[55].

The benefits of diagnosis of chromosomal abnormalities and genetic disorders in the first trimester are obvious and include reassurance and reduced stress throughout pregnancy in high-risk populations (with normal CVS results) on the one hand, and the potential of having an early termination of pregnancy before fetal movements have been felt with lesser clinical and social sequelae[56] on the other hand. This is especially relevant to high-risk situations, such as patients with parental balanced translocations and monogenic disorders who have mostly had an affected pregnancy before and usually prefer to have early prenatal diagnosis.

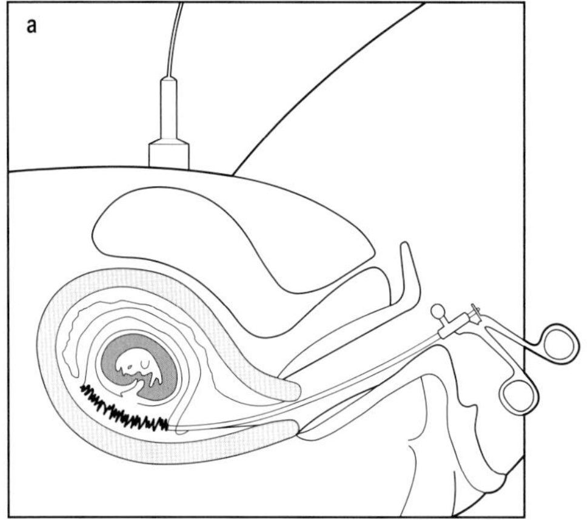

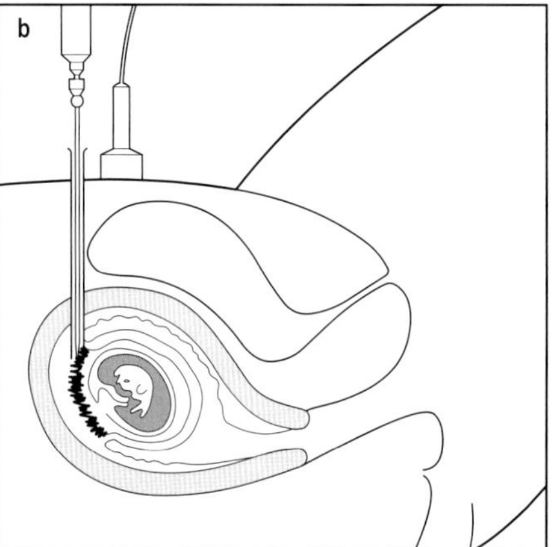

Fig. 22.2 Schematic depiction of frequently used CVS techniques. (a) Transcervical catheter aspiration; (b) transabdominal puncture.

Indications for CVS

The two main indications for CVS are:

1. DNA analysis for single gene defects
2. fetal karyotyping.

Previously, the latter was done for high-risk cases based on maternal age or past history of aneuploidy. In recent years, with the introduction of early anomaly scans, nuchal translucency (NT) measurements and the early combined screening tests, women with increased risk for aneuploidy are identified during the first trimester. The ability to screen for aneuploidies in such an early stage of pregnancy has caused a general decrease in the rate of invasive procedures since many women that were considered as 'high risk' based on their age alone, were now considered to have a low risk due to normal NT, fetal anatomy and biochemical markers[57]. On the other hand, the introduction of early screening tests has caused, in some centers, an increase in the rate of early (CVS) versus later (amniocentesis) invasive assessments[58]. In most clinical settings nowadays, women can be screened by ultrasound (NT and fetal anatomy survey) between 11 and 14 weeks of gestation and blood can be taken simultaneously for biochemical screening (see chapter 19) for the integrated test. At this point, an anatomic evaluation of the fetus is also performed and sonographic markers for Down's syndrome (omphalocele, absence of nasal bone, short femur etc.) can be detected. The result of the screening test is usually available within days. Whenever the risk is considered to be high (either due to screening test or due to an anatomical abnormality), the couple is counseled about the possibilities of having a diagnostic test. Such an invasive test can be performed without delay by CVS.

The chorionic villi are an excellent source of DNA and can be utilized for most of the molecular studies without prior culturing. Therefore, CVS is the method of choice for prenatal diagnosis of monogenic disorders with a significant morbidity and high recurrence risk (25% for carriers of autosomal recessive disorders, 50% for male fetuses carrying an X-linked disorder). Many genetic disorders are routinely diagnosed by CVS, such as hemoglobinopathies[59], hemophilia A and B[60], storage disorders, Duchenne muscular dystrophy[61], chronic granulomatous syndrome and many other abnormalities[62].

Techniques of CVS

It is possible to obtain chorionic villi as early as 8 weeks of gestation. However, several clusters of limb reduction defects were reported in association with very early CVS[63]. The consensus now is to only perform CVS after 10 weeks' gestation. Prior to performing the CVS, an ultrasound evaluation to assess gestational age (to ensure that the gestational age is satisfactory, e.g. crown–rump length (CRL) >30 mm), fetal number and viability

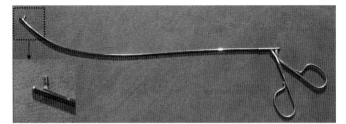

Fig. 22.3 Curved biopsy forceps, which are ideally suited for single-operator technique.

and placental position, should be performed. When the CRL is 45–84 mm, an NT measurement should be obtained if not previously taken.

There are two routes of performing CVS: transabdominal (TA) and transcervical (TC) (see Fig. 22.2). The choice of the route is usually decided on a case-by-case basis depending on placental site. Anterior and fundal placentas are usually easily accessed transabdominally while lower, posterior located placentas are more accessible transcervically. Patient and operator preference may also be factors. Both TA- and TC-CVS can be done by either aspiration of villi or obtaining a biopsy.

The transcervical route was the first to be developed, initially endoscopically. Aspiration of villi was described in the mid-1970s by a group in China[48]. In that report, the procedure which was done for fetal sexing, was performed without endoscopic or ultrasound guidance. Ultrasound guided transcervical CVS was first described in the early 1980s[49,51–53]. For the transcervical approach, a polyethylene catheter with obturator or malleable metal catheter is introduced through the cervix and guided to the placental chorion frondosum under continuous ultrasound surveillance[52,53]. Negative pressure is applied with a syringe or pump and a sample is aspirated. This procedure is usually done by two operators; while the first scans transabdominally and guides the procedure, the second inserts the transcervical catheter and retrieves the transcervical sample. Another instrument for transcervical CVS is the curved biopsy forceps (Fig. 22.3)[64], which has been used by one of the authors (CHR) since 1986 and which is ideally suited for a single-operator technique and for a posterior palcenta (Fig. 22.4a). The transcervical approach has the advantage of minimal patient discomfort[65]. Contraindications for the transcervical route are active vaginal bleeding and cervical infections. Forceps and cannula have been evaluated in several transcervical CVS trials[66–68]. When a cannula was used, operators obtained an inadequate sample (less than 5 mg) more often. Compared with forceps, cannulae had to be re-inserted more often and inserting a cannula was more painful. Multiple insertions also increase the risk of miscarriage. When different types of cannulae were compared, the Portex cannula was more likely to result in an inadequate sample and a difficult or painful procedure when compared with either the silver or aluminum cannula respectively[67,68]. The Cochrane review[69] concludes that, although there is some evidence to support the use of small forceps for transcervical chorionic villus sampling, the evidence is not strong enough to support change in practice for clinicians who have become familiar with aspiration cannulae. A recent review that compared instruments for transcervical CVS concluded that the use of biopsy forceps was better tolerated by women, provided

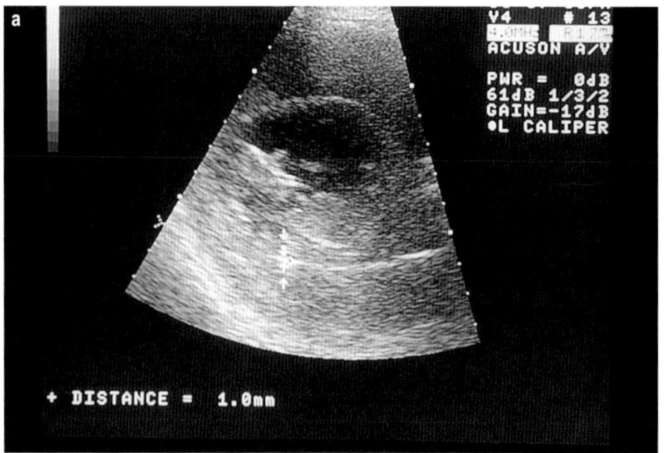

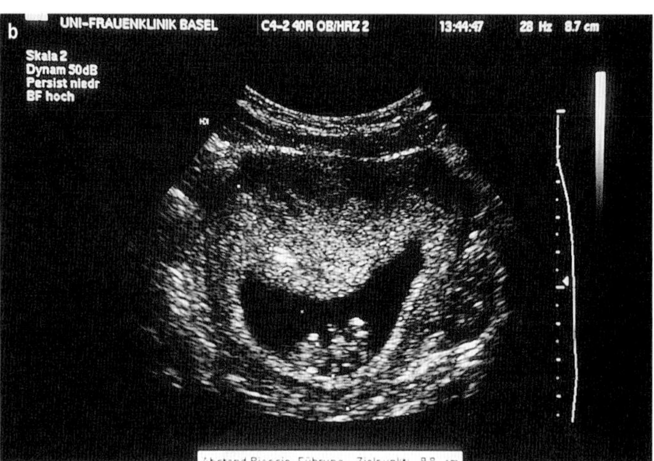

Fig. 22.4 Sonograms taken at the time of chorionic villus samplings. (a) Transcervical technique; (b) transabdominal technique.

culturable tissue after fewer instrument passes and with a more efficient learning curve[70].

Transabdominal CVS (Fig. 22.4b) was first described by Smidt-Jensen and Hahnemann[54]. Most centers perform the transabdominal aspiration by a free-hand technique while some use a needle guide on the ultrasound probe. It is usually performed by two operators (although it can be performed by a single operator). The first operator scans the pregnant mother, identifies the placenta and the fetus and introduces a needle into the placenta. The other operator aspirates the sample. Unlike amniocentesis (where the needle is inserted perpendicular to the amnion), the introduction of the needle should be done in a plane through the long axis of the placenta parallel, if possible, to the chorionic plate. The needle is introduced into the area of the chorion frondosum, which contains the most mitotically active cells. Transabdominal CVS is usually performed under local anesthesia. The needle used for aspiration is a 19–20 g needle[71]. In the single needle technique, the needle is inserted to the target area, the stylet is withdrawn from the needle, a syringe containing tissue culture medium is attached to the needle and suction is applied (usually by the second operator) as the needle is moved up and down through the placenta until it is thought that an adequate amount of tissue is obtained. The needle must be removed from the patient in order to inspect the sample and to ensure that an adequate

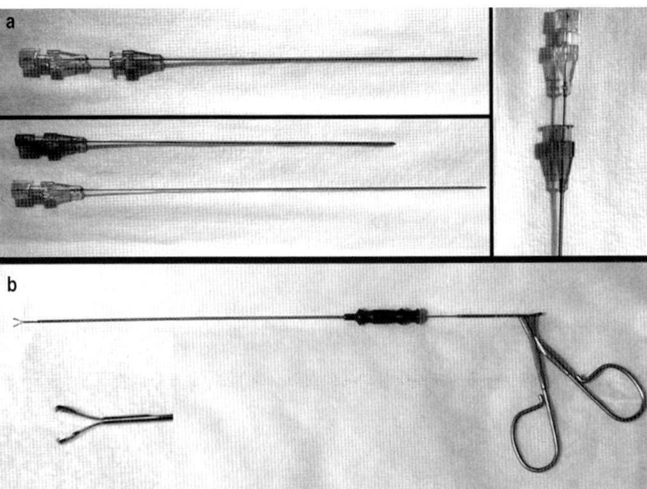

Fig. 22.5 (a) Double-needle technique – a larger 18 g needle is inserted into the sampling area of the placenta. The stylet is withdrawn, followed by passage of a 20 g needle down the 18 g needle and aspiration by the inner needle. (b) Transabdominal forceps which can be passed through an 18 g guide needle.

quantity of chorionic villi has been obtained. The disadvantage of this method is that when the sample is inadequate (about 1 in 10 cases), the procedure has to be repeated from the start (i.e. additional uterine entry). Alternatively, with the double-needle technique (Fig. 22.5a), a larger 18 g needle is inserted into the sampling area of the placenta. The stylet is withdrawn, followed by passage of a 20 g needle down the 18 g needle and aspiration by the inner needle. By this method, several sequential samples can be taken (usually two) without re-introducing a needle into the uterus. A few groups prefer the use of transabdominal forceps which can be passed through an 18 g guide needle and a small, but clean biopsy can be taken (Fig. 22.5b)[72]. There are no published studies comparing the various instruments used for transabdominal CVS.

Complications of CVS

Vaginal bleeding

Vaginal spotting (1–4%) or bleeding (<1%) before 20 weeks' gestation[73], is the most common immediate complication and it is mainly observed after transcervical sampling (up to 20% of cases) probably due to use of a tenaculum[74–76]. This complication is not noted after 20 weeks and CVS is not associated with increased mid- and late-trimester bleeding[77]. Other sequelae due to injury to the placental circulation include retro-placental hematomas and subchorionic hemorrhage. Significant amniotic fluid leakage after CVS is about 2–4 times less frequent when compared to early amniocentesis[78]. In a study surveying maternal complications in 1984 women after CVS (and 47 584 controls), CVS was not associated with severe pregnancy complications such as placental abruption or placenta previa[79].

Infections

Intrauterine infection (bacterial, viral and fungal) after CVS is extremely rare (<0.2%)[80–82] but it may lead to severe maternal illness and requires immediate uterine evacuation.[83,84] In a study where blood cultures were taken after CVS, 2/49 versus 0/65 patients having TC- and TA-CVS, respectively, had positive cultures. This may suggest that TC-CVS should be done after proper prophylaxis in patients with increased risk of endocarditis[85].

Fetal loss

The benefits of earlier diagnosis of fetal genetic abnormalities by chorionic villus sampling (CVS) or early amniocentesis must be set against higher risks of pregnancy loss and possibly diagnostic inaccuracies of these tests when compared with second-trimester amniocentesis. Fetal loss rate attributed to CVS is generally considered to be small (1–3%). The data used for determining the associated risks of fetal loss due to CVS are presented in the literature as case series with detailed outcome and comparative studies of CVS group versus amniocentesis (Table 22.1) and transabdominal versus transcervical CVS (Table 22.2). Unfortunately, no study has randomly evaluated CVS versus non-sampled (with same risk) patients. The fetal loss rates surveyed in this review are based on the report of the Cochrane database[86] and on several studies which were not included in that review.

Based on the presented data, CVS is associated with a slightly increased risk of fetal loss when compared to amniocentesis. Noteworthy, that excluding the results of the MRC study[77], CVS is associated with no more then 1% extra risk of fetal loss when compared to midtrimester amniocentesis. The risks of fetal loss rate in the tables should not be compared between the studies since each study had its own criteria for total fetal loss (although most have described fetal loss <28 weeks' gestation). Moreover, while some have included only cytogenetically normal fetuses, others have evaluated a mixed population. The risk of fetal loss after CVS can also be obtained from the studies comparing CVS with early (10–14 weeks) amniocentesis. Most of theses studies point to a relatively small risk of fetal loss (2–3%) associated with CVS on the one hand and a significantly increased risk of fetal loss in the early amniocentesis group on the other hand. Single-operator experience presents an estimated fetal loss rate after CVS of about 2–3%[54] Although, single operator experience shows that the results (fetal loss rate) of early procedures are better in the hands of skilled operators, this remains controversial. It is possible that very skilled operators could abolish the observed difference in pregnancy loss between early and later procedures. However, it is difficult to see how such 'experts' can produce local data that would prove to their patients that, in their hands, early procedures are equally safe as second-trimester amniocentesis. Such data would have to include thousands of women with complete information on the outcome of pregnancy (not just for several weeks after the procedure) with an adequate 'control' group. Transabdominal CVS is considered by many to be safer than the transcervical route. However, this observation is heavily influenced by the data from the Danish study[87]. Increase in pregnancy loss following transcervical procedure has not been replicated in other trials comparing transcervical and transabdominal procedures[65,76,88,89]. Based on these studies, as well as many single center reports and private communication, we believe that the poor results from the Danish study (where the Portex cannula was used) would not be repeated if the operators were equally good at the techniques being compared.

Table 22.1 **Fetal loss rate (FLR): CVS versus conventional amniocentesis**

#	Ref.	Group 1 Description	Group 2 Description	Group 1 FLR	Group 2 FLR		Remarks
1	[105,136] Canadian study	CVS-TC (1191)	Amnio (1200)	5.4%	4.3%	NS	Randomized. Total fetal loss
2	[77] MRC study	CVS (1609) TC-72%, TA-28%	Amnio (1592)	9.0%	6.0%	0.02	Randomized. SFL <28 weeks
3	[87]	CVS-TA (1027)	Amnio (1042)	3.1%	1.7%	NS	Randomized. Total fetal loss rate
4	[137]	CVS-TC (399)	Amnio (382)	3.1%	4.1%	NS	Randomized. SFL <22 weeks
5	[138]	CVS-TC By biopsy forceps (314)	Amnio (358)	2.2%	2.8%	NS	Randomized – disconnected when screening was introduced
6	[139]	CVS-TA (819)	Amnio (771)	2.9%	1.0%	NS	Single center report. Total fetal loss rate
7	[140]	CVS-TC (356)	Amnio (356)	2.9%	0.9%	NS	Single center report. Total fetal loss rate

SFL = Spontaneous fetal loss rate

Table 22.2 **Fetal loss rate after CVS**

#	Ref.	Group 1 Description	Group 2 Description	Group 1 FLR	Group 2 FLR		Remarks
1	[65]	CVS-TC (60)	CVS-TA (60)	3.3%	3.3%	NS	Randomized FLR <28 weeks
2	[88]	CVS-TC (489)	CVS-TA (595)	4.8%	4.0%	NS	Partly randomized SFL <28 weeks for cytogenetically normal fetuses
3	[76] NICHD	CVS-TC (1846)	CVS-TA (1816)	2.7%	2.6%	NS	Randomized trial SFL <28 weeks for cytogenetically normal fetuses
4	[87]	CVS-TC (1010)	CVS-TA (1027)	7.7%	3.1%	P < 0.001	Randomized trial
5	[141]	CVS-TC (1442)	CVS-TA (138)	4.3%	4.2%	NS	TC and TA CVS by biopsy forceps. Single center experience
6	[107]	CVS-TA	None	1.64%	–	–	Single center experience
7	[73]	CVS TA and TC	None	2.7%	–	–	Single center experience

FLR = Fetal loss rate, SFL= Spontaneous fetal loss rate

Fetal abnormalities

In general, the rate of fetal abnormalities after CVS is not different than in the general population[86]. Several case reports and cohort studies in the early 1990s have suggested a possible association between early CVS and a cluster of limb defects and oromandibular hypogenesis[63,90]. However, these findings were not repeated in other studies[91]. The background risk of limb reduction defects (LRD) in the general population is low and varies between 1.6 and 4/10 000[92]. In an evaluation of CVS safety presented by the WHO[93], LRD cases were observed in 115 cases (5.3/10 000). Another meta-analysis found an overall rate of 7.4/10 000 cases of LRD post CVS[94] and concluded that the risk is increased by up to 6-fold compared to the general population. It has been suggested that an early procedure might significantly increase the risk of LRD. However, only some of the published studies contain sufficiently detailed information regarding gestational age at sampling to enable gestation specific risk. Evaluation of 106 383 patients with known gestational age has found 42 cases of LRD (3.9/10 000). The risk of LRD following CVS performed at 8 weeks' gestation was 3–4-fold increased compared to 11 weeks'gestation. Other studies have found that the risk of LRD for procedures performed before 9 weeks' gestation was increased by 11- to 21-fold. The variation between studies is dependent on methodology and on the criteria applied for the diagnosis of transverse limb deficiencies[94–96]. The existence of a specific gestational age limit for LRD post CVS is debated. While the WHO has concluded that the risk is evident only prior to 8 weeks of gestation, the view of Firth et al.[97] is that there is a continuum of risk which diminishes with gestational age. This risk approaches the levels of background risk only at 11 weeks' gestation. Nonetheless, since the association of LRD is still debated, and these abnormalities are still rare even after CVS at 7 weeks' gestation, some advocate that the use of very early CVS should not be completely abolished[98]. This is especially relevant to patients with high risk of genetic abnormalities on the one hand and tolerable view on termination of pregnancy at very early stages on the other hand. In this case, very early CVS, such as performed for Orthodox Jewish patients[99] is an option for prenatal diagnosis (although preimplantation diagnosis is more suitable when available).

The possible mechanisms of LRD following CVS are unknown. However, there are three principal theories:

1. Vascular disruption caused by hemodynamic disturbances,[63] vasoactive peptides or embolism[100,101]
2. Amnion puncture with subsequent compression and entanglement of the fetus[102]
3. Immunological mechanisms causing increased apoptotic cell death.[103]

It is speculated that technical aspects of the procedure may have a bearing on the amount of placental trauma associated with the sampling procedure and the risk of limb deficiency. However, the rarity of limb deficiency following CVS means that none of the existing trials have the power to clarify the effect of technical factors on the risk. It remains unresolved whether the risk of limb deficiency differs for transabdominal versus transcervical sampling. Given the weight of current evidence supporting an association between early sampling and limb deficiency, it would be unethical to conduct a trial to investigate this prospectively. It would seem prudent, however, to take all reasonable steps to limit placental trauma and sample size to the minimum consistent with the sampling enabling successful prenatal diagnosis[104].

Laboratory aspects of CVS

In the early development of CVS, its reliability was questioned due to a high rate of incorrect results, maternal contamination and misinterpretation due to mosaicism. Nowadays, CVS is considered to be a reliable method of prenatal diagnosis with a high rate of success and accuracy. The laboratory failure rate of 2.3% in the early 1990s was significantly higher compared to amniocentesis[105]. It has declined to an estimate rate of less then 0.5%[106,107]. Maternal contamination occurs in less then 1% of cases and usually does not limit the possibilities of accurate diagnosis[107]. One of the most interesting observations that CVS has revealed is confined placental mosaicism (CPM). This is the occurrence of mosaicism limited only to placental tissue. The rate of CPM is about 1–2% in CVS done in the first trimester. While CPM was initially considered a drawback in the usage of CVS for prenatal evaluation, it is considered today as an important marker for pregnancies at increased risk for growth retardation or genetic abnormalities. Two main mechanisms leading to CPM are: trisomic rescue (trisomic conceptus with loss of chromosome in the embryonic cell line), and mitotic error originally confined to the placenta. The most significant at the clinical level is the correction of aneuploidy, the trisomic zygote rescue[108]. The most significant complication of CPM involves the pattern of uniparental disomy (UPD), e.g. when both chromosomes originate from the same parental origin. This is theoretically the case in about a third of CPM cases (each one of the triple chromosomal sets can be lost at 'rescue'). UPD has clinical consequences if the chromosome involved carries an imprinted gene in which expression is dependent on the parent of origin. This is best exemplified by the gene encoded on chromosome 15 that, when deleted, may cause Prader Willi syndrome with uniparental paternal disomy and Angelman syndrome with maternal disomy. Consequently, all cases that involve CPM of chromosome 15 should be evaluated for UPD. Other chromosomes that may have imprinted genes and should raise the possibility of UPD are 7,11,14 and 22[109,110]. There is also evidence that CPM (unrelated to UPD) might alter placental function leading to fetal growth restriction. This is especially relevant to chromosome 16 where placental trisomy affects growth of both uniparental and biparental disomy fetuses is a similar manner[111].

If mosaicism is found on either culture or direct preparation, follow-up amniocentesis should be offered. Only about 10–40% of the mosaic results will be confirmed as true mosaicism involving the fetus. A decision of termination of pregnancy should not be done on the basis of mosaicism found on CVS. However, when mosaicism is found in chorionic tissue culture, a normal amniocentesis result is associated with a false negative rate of about 6% and mosaic fetuses were reported to be born after normal amniotic fluid analysis[112]. In such cases, follow-up with serial scanning and possibly fetal biopsy should be considered.

Counseling before CVS

Counseling patients before CVS is extremely important and should emphasize the following issues:

1. The *indication*, i.e. the need for an invasive diagnosis in general and CVS in particular. CVS is especially valuable for patients with very high risk of abnormality such as a single gene disorder (with 25–50% risk of transmission) or chromosomal translocations. Although CVS should be available to lower-risk and high-risk patients who wish to

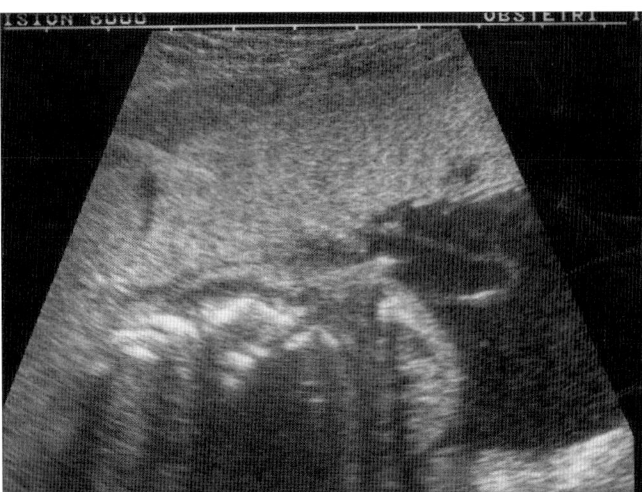

Fig. 22.6 Fetal blood sampling from the umbilical vein at the cord insertion of an anterior placenta.

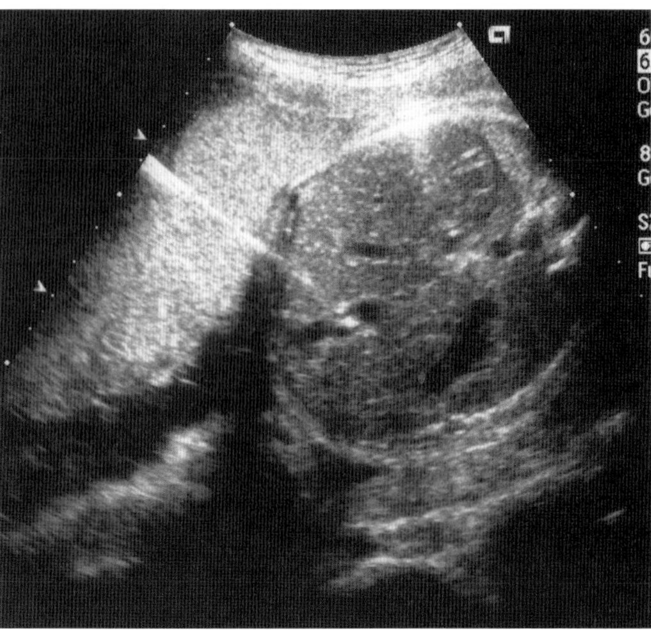

Fig. 22.7 Fetal blood sampling from the intrahepatic umbilical vein.

have chromosomal analysis, the alternative of amniocentesis should be fully explained in these cases.

2. The risks of CVS should be discussed, especially the risk of *fetal loss*. The risk of maternal infection and fetal abnormality is extremely low and the sequelae of such complications need not be routinely addressed during counseling, unless the patient asks.
3. *Failure of laboratory results* – specific data should be given. When PCR is used for rapid diagnosis, patients can be reassured that the chances of laboratory failure with both techniques (PCR and full karyotype) are extremely small.
4. *Confined placental mosaicism* and the need of another intervention (amniocentesis) in order to reach a final diagnosis in approximately 1–2%.

FETAL BLOOD SAMPLING (FBS)

FBS was originally performed by fetoscopy and this technique was used for prenatal diagnosis of fetal hemoglobinopathies and hemophilias. Rodeck and Campbell originally described a technique for pure fetal blood sampling in the second trimester of pregnancy combining fetoscopy with real-time ultrasound[113]. This technique was replaced by an ultrasound-guided approach as described by Daffos and others[114]. FBS, like amniocentesis, can be performed either by the free-hand technique or with the help of a needle guide. While, in most cases, the umbilical vein is punctured close to its placental insertion, in some cases fetal blood is obtained by puncture of the intrahepatic umbilical vein[115] (Figs. 22.6 and 22.7). The procedure-related fetal loss rate is about 0.8–2.5%[116–119].

The most common indications for FBS include the detection of inherited genetic diseases, hemoglobinopathies, congenital infections, rapid karyotyping in cases of structural fetal abnormality, evaluation of the acid–base balance in growth-restricted fetuses and the evaluation of the hematologic status in alloimmunized fetuses.

In recent years, fetal blood sampling has declined in frequency for several reasons. Amniocentesis is nowadays the gold standard for diagnosis of fetal infections (especially CMV[13]) by polymerase-chain-reaction (PCR) assays. Rapid karyotyping from fetal blood is being replaced by amniocentesis combined with rapid diagnostic techniques such as fluorescent in situ hybridization (FISH) and PCR (as discussed in this chapter). FBS for karyotyping is reserved for cases with severe oligohydramnios or anhydramnios, although late CVS may be an alternative. The use of FBS for fetal anemia is also unnecessary since non-invasive assessment has become well established[7]. FBS is now performed only when fetal blood transfusion is most likely. FBS is still needed for the evaluation of fetuses at risk of alloimmune thrombocytopenia. However, new studies are limiting its role only to severe cases or before vaginal birth is attempted[120].

FBS in twin pregnancies is performed for the same indications as singletons. A recent study has described FBS (mainly for hemoglobinopathies) in 84 twin pregnancies[121]. The overall procedure-related fetal loss (up to 2 weeks post procedure) was 8.2%, about 4-fold higher then the associated risk of FBS in singletons. The fetal loss rate was higher in fetuses diagnosed with fetal anomalies, although this group was too small for statistical evaluation.

FETAL TISSUE BIOPSY

Fetal liver biopsy

Fetal liver biopsy was the only means of diagnosing fetuses with inborn errors of the urea cycle, e.g. ornithine transcarbamylase deficiency[122,123], carbamoylphosphate synthetase deficiency[124] and other disorders expressed only in the liver such as von Gierke glycogen-storage disease type IA[125] and primary hyperoxaluria type I[126]. However, most of these conditions are now diagnosable by DNA analysis[127] (without the need for histology and enzymatic assays) of cells extracted from either chorionic villi or amniocytes. Direct genetic analysis of chorionic villi is feasible, fast and specific and can be regarded as the method of choice for first-trimester diagnosis in urea cycle disorders[128] and glycogen-storage disease Ia[129]. Yet, some rare liver enzymatic abnormalities are still not detectable by DNA analysis and fetal liver biopsy is still needed for those cases.

The procedure was originally performed with a fetoscopic approach[122] which was later replaced by an ultrasound-guided procedure. The optimal gestational age is between 17 and 22 weeks. With local anesthesia, a 17-gauge thin-walled needle is introduced into the right lobe of the fetal liver under continuous ultrasonographic guidance. An inner biopsy needle is then passed into the liver parenchyma, a syringe is attached and fetal liver is aspirated. In a personal series of about 20 cases, there were no diagnostic errors or fetal losses (CH Rodeck, unpublished results).

Fetal skin biopsy

Skin biopsy used to be the only way to diagnose serious dermatological diseases such as epidermolysis bullosa (EB), oculocutaneous albinism or harlequin ichthyosis[130]. This procedure was also initially done under direct vision fetoscopically[131], but is now performed with ultrasound guidance. With small biopsies the wound healing is remarkably good so that scars often can hardly be recognized after birth[132]. Fetal skin samples are examined by light and transmission electron microscopy. The development of monoclonal and polyclonal antibodies to various basement membrane components has enabled immunohistochemical tests to complement ultrastructural analysis in establishing an accurate diagnosis, especially in cases of EB. Fetal skin biopsy is now rarely required because, increasingly, the genodermatoses are becoming diagnosable by DNA methods applied to chorionic villi[133]. However, fetal skin biopsy remains an important tool that can be used with reasonably high levels of safety and confidence in skin lesions and genodermatoses with as yet undiscovered genetic mutations.

Fetal muscle biopsy

Duchenne muscular dystrophy (DMD) is a relentless progressive disorder, leading to severe disability during childhood and death in adolescence or early adulthood. In most families, prenatal diagnosis is readily achieved by molecular detection of DNA deletions using chorionic villi or amniocytes, or by linkage analysis. In some cases, however, molecular methods fail to provide a definitive diagnosis and, in such cases, in utero fetal muscle biopsy may serve as a diagnostic option[134,135].

Fetal muscle is obtained at 20–22 weeks' gestation by directing a 14-gauge (Tru-Cut) biopsy needle through the maternal abdomen and obliquely into the fetal gluteal region. Local anesthesia and maternal sedation are usually used. Real-time ultrasonography is essential for continuous visualization as with all invasive procedures. After sampling, the specimens are verified for the presence of muscle fibers and immunoblotting or immunofluorescence is used to determine the presence or absence of dystrophin.

CONCLUSION

The 40-year history of invasive procedures has seen a rise and then a fall in the degree of invasiveness of the procedures. Amniocentesis still remains the gold standard for karyotyping, especially now that rapid diagnostic methods are available. Invasive procedures may become obsolete when reliable noninvasive prenatal diagnosis becomes available.

REFERENCES

1. Bevis DCA. The antenatal prediction of haemolytic disease of the newborn. *Lancet* **i**:395–398, 1952.
2. Fuchs F, Riis P. Antenatal sex determination. *Nature* 177:330, 1956.
3. Steel MW, Breg WR. Chromosome analysis of human amniotic fluid cells. *Lancet* **i**:383–385, 1966.
4. Valenti C, Schutta EJ, Kehaty T. Prenatal diagnosis of Down's syndrome. *Lancet* **ii**: 220, 1968.
5. Nadler HL, Gerbie AB. Role of amniocentesis in the intrauterine detection of genetic disorders. *N Engl J Med* **282**(11):596–599, 1970.
6. Liley AW. The technique and complications of amniocentesis. *Northwest Med* **59**:581–586, 1960.
7. Oepkes D, Seward PG, Vandenbussche FP et al. Doppler ultrasonongraphy versus amniocentesis to predict fetal anemia. *N Engl J Med* **355**(2):156–164, 2006.
8. Hook EB, Cross PK, Jackson L, Pergament E, Brambati B. Maternal age-specific rates of 47, +21 and other cytogenetic abnormalities diagnosed in the first trimester of pregnancy in chorionic villus biopsy specimens: comparison with rates expected from observations at amniocentesis. *Am J Hum Genet* **42**(6):797–807, 1988.
9. Wald NJ, Rodeck C, Hackshaw AK, Walters J, Chitty L, Mackinnon AM. First and second trimester antenatal screening for Down's syndrome: the results of the serum, urine and ultrasound screening study (SURUSS). *J Med Screen* **10**(2):56–104, 2003.
10. Malone FD, Canick JA, Ball RH et al. First-trimester or second-trimester screening, or both, for Down's syndrome. *N Engl J Med* **353**(19):2001–2011, 2005.
11. D'Alton ME, Malone FD, Chelmow D, Ward BE, Bianchi DW. Defining the role of fluorescence in situ hybridization on uncultured amniocytes for prenatal diagnosis of aneuploides. *Am J Obstet Gynecol* **176**(4):769–774, 1997.
12. Van den Veyver I, Beaudet AL. Comparative genomic hybridization and prenatal diagnosis. *Curr Opin Obstet Gynecol* **18**(2):185–191, 2006.
13. Leisnard C, Donner C, Brancart F, Gosselin F, Delforge ML, Rodesch F. Prenatal diagnosis of congenital cytomegalovirus infection: prospective study of 237 pregnancies at risk. *Obstet Gynecol* **95**(6 pt 1):881–888, 2000.
14. Yoon BH, Romero R, Lim JH et al. The clinical significance of detecting Ureaplasma urealyticum by the polymerase chain reaction in the amniotic fluid of patients with preterm labor. *Am J Obstet Gynecol* **189**(4):919–924, 2003.
15. Karcher R, Sykes E, Batton D et al. Gestational age-specific predicted risk of neonatal respiratory distress syndrome using lamellar body count and surfactant-to-albumin ratio in amniotic fluid. *Am J Obstet Gynecol* **193**(5):1680–1684, 2005.
16. Randomised trial to assess safety and fetal outcome of early and midtrimester amniocentesis. The Canadian Early and Mid-trimester Amniocentesis Trial (CEMAT) Group. *Lancet* **351**: 242–247, 1998.
17. Romero R, Jeanty P, Reece EA et al. Sonographically monitored amniocentesis

to decrease intraoperative complications. *Obstet Gynecol* **65**(3):426–430, 1985.
18. Bombard AT, Powers JF, Carter S, Schwartz A, Nitowsky HM. Procedure-related fetal losses in transplacental versus nontransplacental genetic amniocentesis. *Am J Obstet Gynecol* **172**(3):868–872, 1995.
19. King CW, Leung TN, Leung TY et al. Risk factors for procedure-related fetal losses after mid-trimester genetic amniocentesis. *Prenat Diagn* **26**(10):925–930, 2006.
20. Golbus MS, Stephens JD, Cann HM, Mann J, Hensleigh PA. Rh isoimmunisation following genetic amniocentesis. *Prenat Diagn* **2**(3):149–156, 1982.
21. Murray JC, Karp LE, Williamson RA, Cheng EY, Luthy DA. Rh isoimmunisation related to amniocentesis. *Am J Med Genet* **16**(4):527–534, 1983.
22. Miles JH, Kaback MM. Prenatal diagnosis of hereditary disorders. *Pediatr Clin North Am* **25**(3):593–618, 1978.
23. Bang J, Nielsen H, Philip J. Prenatal karyotyping of twins by ultrasonically guided amniocentesis. *Am J Obstet Gynecol* **123**(7):695–696, 1975.
24. Jenkins TM, Wapner RJ. The challenge of prenatal diagnosis in twin pregnancies. *Curr Opin Obstet Gynecol* **12**(2):87–92, 2000.
25. Nicolini U, Monni G. Intestinal obstruction in babies exposed in utero to methylene blue. *Lancet* **336**:1258–1259, 1990.
26. van der Pol JG, Wolf H, Boer K et al. Jejunal atresia related to the use of methylene blue in genetic amniocentesis in twins. *Br J Obstet Gynaecol* **99**(2): 141–143, 1992.
27. Pruggmayer MR, Jahoda MG, van der Pol JG et al. Genetic amniocentesis in twin pregnancies: results of a multicenter study of 529 cases. *Ultrasound Obstet Gynecol* **2**(1):6–10, 1992.
28. Cragan JD, Martin ML, Khoury MJ, Fernhoff PM. Dye use during amniocentesis and birth defects. *Lancet* **341**(8856):1352, 1993.
29. Hausknecht RU, Yeh HC, Godmilow L. Prenatal genetic diagnosis in a triplet gestation. *Obstet Gynecol* **58**(3):382–385, 1981.
30. Antsaklis A, Souka AP, Daskalakis G, Kavalakis Y, Michalas S. Second-trimester amniocentesis vs. chorionic villus sampling for prenatal diagnosis in multiple gestations. *Ultrasound Obstet Gynecol* **20**(5):476–481, 2002.
31. Taylor MJ, Fisk NM. Prenatal diagnosis in multiple pregnancy. *Baillieres Best Pract Res Clin Obstet Gynaecol* **14**(4):663–675, 2000.
32. Jeanty P, Shah D, Roussis P. Single-needle insertion in twin amniocentesis. *J Ultrasound Med* **9**(9):511–517, 1990.
33. Buscaglia M, Ghisoni L, Bellotti M et al. Genetic amniocentesis in biamniotic twin pregnancies by a single transabdominal insertion of the needle. *Prenat Diagn* **15**(1):17–19, 1995.
34. van Vugt JM, Nieuwint A, van Geijn HP. Single-needle insertion: an alternative technique for early second-trimester genetic twin amniocentesis. *Fetal Diagn Ther* **10**(3):178–181, 1995.
35. Tabor A, Philip J, Madsen M, Bang J, Obel EB, Norgaard-Pedersen B. Randomised controlled trial of genetic amniocentesis in 4606 low-risk women. *Lancet* **1**(8493):1287–1293, 1986.
36. Antsaklis A, Papantoniou N, Xygakis A, Mesogitis S, Tzortzis E, Michalas S. Genetic amniocentesis in women 20–34 years old: associated risks. *Prenat Diagn* **20**(3):247–250, 2000.
37. Tongsong T, Wanapirak C, Sirivatanapa P, Piyamongkol W, Sirichotiyakul S, Yampochai A. Amniocentesis-related fetal loss: a cohort study. *Obstet Gynecol* **92**(1):64–67, 1998.
38. Mungen E, Tutuncu L, Muhcu M, Yergok YZ. Pregnancy outcome following second-trimester amniocentesis: a case-control study. *Am J Perinatol* **23**(1):25–30, 2006.
39. CDC publishes report on chorionic villus sampling and amniocentesis. *Am Fam Physician* **52**(4):1210, 1995.
40. Chorionic villus sampling and amniocentesis: recommendations for prenatal counseling. Centers for Disease Control and Prevention. *MMWR Recomm Rep* **44**(RR-9):1–12, 1995.
41. Seeds JW. Diagnostic mid trimester amniocentesis: how safe? *Am J Obstet Gynecol* **191**(2):607–615, 2004.
42. Eddleman KA, Malone FD, Sullivan L et al. Pregnancy loss rates after midtrimester amniocentesis. *Obstet Gynecol* **108**(5):1067–1072, 2006.
43. Fines B, Ben Ami TE, Yousefzadeh DK. Traumatic prenatal sigmoid perforation due to amniocentesis. *Pediatr Radiol* **31**(6):440–443, 2001.
44. Ahluwalia J, Lowenstein E. Skin dimpling as a delayed manifestation of traumatic amniocentesis. *Skinmed* **4**(5):323–324, 2005.
45. Thorp JA, Helfgott AW, King EA, King AA, Minyard AN. Maternal death after second-trimester genetic amniocentesis. *Obstet Gynecol* **105**(5 Pt 2):1213–1215, 2005.
46. Mohr J. Foetal genetic diagnosis: development of techniques for early sampling of foetal cells. *Acta Pathol Microbiol Scand* **73**:73–77, 1968.
47. Hahnemann N. Early prenatal diagnosis: a study of biopsy techniques and cell culturing from intra-embryonic membranes. *Clin Genet* **6**:294–306, 1974.
48. Department of Obstetrics & Gynaecology, Tietung Hospital of Anshan Iron and Steel Company, Anshan, China. Fetal sex prediction by sex chromation of chorionic villi cells during early pregnancy. *China Med J* **1**(2):117–126, 1975.
49. Kazy Z, Sztigar AM, Bacharev VA. [Chronionic biopsy under immediate real-time (ultrasonic) control]. *Orv Hetil* **121**(45):2765–2766, 1980.
50. Niazi M, Coleman DV, Loeffler FE. Trophoblast sampling in early pregnancy. Culture of rapidly dividing cells from immature placental villi. *Br J Obstet Gynaecol* **88**(11):1081–1085, 1981.
51. Kazy Z, Rozovsky IS, Bacharev VA. Chorionic biopsy in early pregnancy: a method of early prenatal diagnosis for inherited disorder. *Prenat Diagn* **2**:39–45, 1982.
52. Ward RH, Modell B, Petrou M, Karagozlu F, Douratsos E. Method of sampling chorionic villi in first trimester of pregnancy under guidance of real time ultrasound. *Br Med J* **286**:1542–1544, 1983.
53. Rodeck CH, Morsman JM, Nicolaides KH, McKenzie C, Gosden CM, Gosden JR. A single-operator technique for first-trimester chorion biopsy. *Lancet* **2**(8363):1340–1341, 1983.
54. Smidt-Jensen S, Hahnemann N. Transabdominal fine needle biopsy from chorionic villi in the first trimester. *Prenat Diagn* **4**(3):163–169, 1984.
55. Nicolaides KH, Rodeck CH, Soothill PW, Warren RC, Gosden CM. Why confine chorionic villus (placental) biopsy to the first trimester? *Lancet* **i**:543–544, 1986.
56. White-van Mourik MC, Connor JM, Ferguson-Smith MA. The psychosocial sequelae of a second-trimester termination of pregnancy for fetal abnormality. *Prenat Diagn* **12**(3):189–204, 1992.
57. Chasen ST, McCullough LB, Chervenak FA. Is nuchal translucency screening associated with different rates of invasive testing in an older obstetric population? *Am J Obstet Gynecol* **190**(3):769–774, 2004.
58. Zoppi MA, Ibba RM, Putzolu M, Floris M, Monni G. Nuchal translucency and the acceptance of invasive prenatal chromosomal diagnosis in women aged 35 and older. *Obstet Gynecol* **97**(6):916–920, 2001.
59. Petrou M, Modell B. Prenatal screening for haemoglobin disorders. *Prenat Diagn* **15**(13):1275–1295, 1995.
60. Ljung RC. Prenatal diagnosis of haemophilia. *Baillieres Clin Haematol* **9**(2):243–257, 1996.
61. Prigojin H, Brusel M, Fuchs O et al. Detection of Duchenne muscular dystrophy gene products in amniotic fluid and chorionic villus sampling cells. *FEBS Lett* **335**(2):223–230, 1993.
62. Chan V, TK CJ. Prenatal diagnosis of common single gene disorders by DNA technology. *Hong Kong Med J* **3**(2):173–178, 1997.
63. Firth HV, Boyd PA, Chamberlain P, MacKenzie IZ, Lindenbaum RH, Huson SM. Severe limb abnormalities

after chorion villus sampling at 56–66 days' gestation. *Lancet* **337**(8744):762–763, 1991.

64. Vaughan JI, Rodeck C. Interventional procedures. In *Ultrasound in obstetrics and gynaecology*, KC Dewbury, HB Meire, DO Cosgrove (eds), pp. 557–606. London: Churchill Livingstone, 2001.
65. Bovicelli L, Rizzo N, Montacuti V, Morandi R. Transabdominal versus transcervical routes for chorionic villus sampling. *Lancet* **2**(8501):290, 1986.
66. Pons JC, Fernandez H, Eydoux P et al. Chorionic villus sampling (CVS). Randomized study of efficacy of two transcervical biopsy methods: aspiration canulas and small forceps. *Eur J Obstet Gynecol Reprod Biol* **32**(3):187–194, 1989.
67. Mackenzie WE, Holmes DS, Webb T, Whitehouse C, Newton JR. A randomized study of three cannulas for transcervical chorionic villus sampling. *Am J Obstet Gynecol* **154**(1):34–39, 1986.
68. Barkai G, Rabinovici J, Chaki R et al. Transcervical chorionic villi sampling: a comparison between the silver cannula and the Portex catheter. *Gynecol Obstet Invest* **27**(2):70–73, 1989.
69. Alfirevic Z, von Dadelszen P. Instruments for chorionic villus sampling for prenatal diagnosis. *Cochrane Database Syst Rev* **1**:CD000114, 2003.
70. von Dadelszen P, Sermer M, Hillier J et al. A randomised controlled trial of biopsy forceps and cannula aspiration for transcervical chorionic villus sampling. *Br J Obset Gynaecol* **112**(5):559–566, 2005.
71. Brambati B, Oldrini A, Lanzani A. Transabdominal chorionic villus sampling: a freehand ultrasound-guided technique. *Am J Obstet Gynecol* **157**(1): 134–137, 1987.
72. Fortuny A, Borrell A, Soler A et al. Chorionic villus sampling by biopsy forceps. Results of 1580 procedures from a single centre. *Prenat Diagn* **15**(6):541–550, 1995.
73. Brambati B, Tului L, Alberti E. Prenatal diagnosis by chorionic villus sampling. *Eur J Obstet Gynecol Reprod Biol* **65**(1): 11–16, 1996.
74. Rhoads GG, Jackson LG, Schlesselman SE et al. The safety and efficacy of chorionic villus sampling for early prenatal diagnosis of cytogenetic abnormalities. *N Engl J Med* **320**(10):609–617, 1989.
75. Brambati B, Tului L, Cislaghi C, Alberti E. First 10,000 chorionic villus samplings performed on singleton pregnancies by a single operator. *Prenat Diagn* **18**(3): 255–266, 1998.
76. Jackson LG, Zachary JM, Fowler SE et al. A randomized comparison of transcervical and transabdominal chorionic-villus sampling. The U.S. National Institute of Child Health and Human Development Chorionic-Villus Sampling and Amniocentesis Study Group. *N Engl J Med* **327**(9):594–598, 1992.
77. Medical Research Council European trial of chorion villus sampling. MRC working party on the evaluation pf chorion villus sampling. *Lancet* **337**(8756):1491–1499, 1991.
78. Philip J, Silver RK, Wilson RD et al. Late first-trimester invasive prenatal diagnosis: results of an international randomized trial. *Obstet Gynecol* **103**(6):1164–1173, 2004.
79. Cederholm M, Haglund B, Axelsson O. Maternal complications following amniocentesis and chorionic villus sampling for prenatal karyotyping. *Br J Obset Gynaecol* **110**(4):392–399, 2003.
80. Paz A, Gonen R, Potasman I. Candida sepsis following transcervical chorionic villi sampling. *Infect Dis Obstet Gynecol* **9**(3):147–148, 2001.
81. Dong ZW, Li Y, Zhang LY, Liu RM. Detection of Chlamydia trachomatis intrauterine infection using polymerase chain reaction on chorionic villi. *Int J Gynaecol Obstet* **61**(1):29–32, 1998.
82. Brambati B, Matarrelli M, Varotto F. Septic complications after chorionic villus sampling. *Lancet* **1**(8543):1212–1213, 1987.
83. Fisk NM, Anderson JC. Avoidance of maternal morbidity in acute intrauterine infection following chorionic villus sampling. *Obstet Gynecol* **69**(3 Pt 2): 501–503, 1987.
84. Barela AI, Kleinman GE, Golditch IM, Menke DJ, Hogge WA, Golbus MS. Septic shock with renal failure after chorionic villus sampling. *Am J Obstet Gynecol* **154**(5):1100–1102, 1986.
85. Silverman NS, Sullivan MW, Jungkind DL, Weinblatt V, Beavis K, Wapner RJ. Incidence of bacteremia associated with chorionic villus sampling. *Obstet Gynecol* **84**(6):1021–1024, 1994.
86. Alfirevic Z, Sundberg K, Brigham S. Amniocentesis and chorionic villus sampling for prenatal diagnosis. *Cochrane Database Syst Rev* **3**:CD003252, 2003.
87. Smidt-Jensen S, Permin M, Philip J et al. Randomised comparison of amniocentesis and transabdominal and transcervical chorionic villus sampling. *Lancet* **340**(8830):1237–1244, 1992.
88. Brambati B, Terzian E, Tognoni G. Randomized clinical trial of transabdominal versus transcervical chorionic villus sampling methods. *Prenat Diagn* **11**(5):285–293, 1991.
89. Borrell A, Costa D, Delgado RD et al. Transcervical chorionic villus sampling beyond 12 weeks of gestation. *Ultrasound Obstet Gynecol* **7**(6):416–420, 1996.
90. Burton BK, Schulz CJ, Burd LI. Limb anomalies associated with chorionic villus sampling. *Obstet Gynecol* **79**(5 (Pt 1)): 726–730, 1992.
91. Monni G, Ibba RM, Lai R et al. Early transabdominal chorionic villus sampling in couples at high genetic risk. *Am J Obstet Gynecol* **168**(1 Pt 1):170–171, 1993.
92. Halliday J, Lumley J, Sheffield LJ, Lancaster PA. Limb deficiencies, chorion villus sampling, and advanced maternal age. *Am J Med Genet* **47**(7):1096–1098, 1993.
93. Evaluation of chorionic villus sampling safety: World Health Organization/ Pan American Health Organisation consultation on CVS. *Prenat Diagn* **19**(2):97–99 1999.
94. Olney RS, Khoury MJ, Alo CJ et al. Increased risk for transverse digital deficiency after chorionic villus sampling: results of the United States Multistate Case-Control Study, 1988–1992. *Teratology* **51**(1):20–29, 1995.
95. Botto LD, Olney RS, Mastroiacovo P et al. Chorionic villus sampling and transverse digital deficiencies: evidence for anatomic and gestational-age specificity of the digital deficiencies in two studies. *Am J Med Genet* **62**(2):173–178, 1996.
96. Mastroiacovo P, Botto LD. Chorionic villus sampling and transverse limb deficiencies: maternal age is not a confounder. *Am J Med Genet* **53**(2):182–186, 1994.
97. Firth H, Boyd PA, Chamberlain P, MacKenzie IZ, Huson SM. Limb defects and chorionic villus sampling. *Lancet* **347**(9012):1406–1408, 1996.
98. Papp C, Papp Z. Chorionic villus sampling and amniocentesis: what are the risks in current practice? *Curr Opin Obstet Gynecol* **15**(2):159–165, 2003.
99. Wapner RJ, Evans MI, Davis G et al. Procedural risks versus theology: chorionic villus sampling for Orthodox Jews at less than 8 weeks' gestation. *Am J Obstet Gynecol* **186**(6):1133–1136, 2002.
100. Rodeck CH, Sheldrake A, Beattie B, Whittle MJ. Maternal serum alphafetoprotein after placental damage in chorionic villus sampling 1. *Lancet* **341**(8843):500, 1993.
101. Rodeck CH. Fetal development after chorionic villus sampling. *Lancet* **341**(8843):468–469, 1993.
102. Kaufman MH. Hypothesis: the pathogenesis of the birth defects reported in CVS-exposed infants. *Teratology* **50**(6):377–378, 1994.
103. van dZ, de Heer E, Mentink MM, Vermeij-Keers C. Immunological factors responsible for pathogenetic cell degeneration in pregnancy. *Teratology* **42**(4):421–435, 1990.
104. Firth H. Chorion villus sampling and limb deficiency--cause or coincidence? *Prenat Diagn* **17**(13):1313–1330, 1997.
105. Lippman A, Tomkins DJ, Shime J, Hamerton JL. Canadian multicentre

randomized clinical trial of chorion villus sampling and amniocentesis. Final report. *Prenat Diagn* **12**(5):385–408, 1992.

106. Los FJ, van den BC, Wildschut HI et al. The diagnostic performance of cytogenetic investigation in amniotic fluid cells and chorionic villi. *Prenat Diagn* **21**(13):1150–1158, 2001.
107. Brun JL, Mangione R, Gangbo F et al. Feasibility, accuracy and safety of chorionic villus sampling: a report of 10741 cases. *Prenat Diagn* **23**(4):295–301, 2003.
108. Kalousek DK, Vekemans M. Confined placental mosaicism and genomic imprinting. *Baillieres Best Pract Res Clin Obstet Gynaecol* **14**(4):723–730, 2000.
109. Kotzot D. Complex and segmental uniparental disomy (UPD): review and lessons from rare chromosomal complements. *J Med Genet* **38**(8):497–507, 2001.
110. Ledbetter DH, Engel E. Uniparental disomy in humans: development of an imprinting map and its implications for prenatal diagnosis. *Hum Mol Genet* **4**(Spec No):1757–1764, 1995.
111. Kalousek DK. Pathogenesis of chromosomal mosaicism and its effect on early human development. *Am J Med Genet* **91**(1):39–45, 2000.
112. Phillips OP, Tharapel AT, Lerner JL, Park VM, Wachtel SS, Shulman LP. Risk of fetal mosaicism when placental mosaicism is diagnosed by chorionic villus sampling. *Am J Obstet Gynecol* **174**(3):850–855, 1996.
113. Rodeck CH, Campbell S. Sampling pure fetal blood by fetoscopy in second trimester of pregnancy. *Br Med J* **2**(6139):728–730, 1978.
114. Daffos F, Capella-Pavlovsky M, Forestier F. Fetal blood sampling via the umbilical cord using a needle guided by ultrasound. Report of 66 cases. *Prenat Diagn* **3**(4):271–277, 1983.
115. Nicolini U, Nicolaidis P, Fisk NM, Tannirandorn Y, Rodeck CH. Fetal blood sampling from the intrahepatic vein: analysis of safety and clinical experience with 214 procedures. *Obstet Gynecol* **76**(1):47–53, 1990.
116. Daffos F, Capella-Pavlovsky M, Forestier F. Fetal blood sampling during pregnancy with use of a needle guided by ultrasound: a study of 606 consecutive cases. *Am J Obstet Gynecol* **153**(6): 655–660, 1985.
117. Nicolaides P, Nicolini U, Fisk NM, Tannirandorn Y, Nasrat H, Rodeck CH. Fetal blood sampling from the intrahepatic vein for rapid karyotyping in the second and third trimesters. *Br J Radiol* **64**(762):505–509, 1991.
118. Weiner CP, Okamura K. Diagnostic fetal blood sampling-technique related losses. *Fetal Diagn Ther* **11**(3):169–175, 1996.
119. Antsaklis A, Daskalakis G, Papantoniou N, Michalas S. Fetal blood sampling: indication-related losses. *Prenat Diagn* **18**(9):934–940, 1998.
120. Yinon Y, Spira M, Solomon OE et al. Antenatal noninvasive treatment of patients at risk for alloimmune thrombocytopenia without a history of intracranial hemorrhage. *Am J Obstet Gynecol* **195**(4):1153–1157, 2006.
121. Antsaklis A, Daskalakis G, Souka AP, Kavalakis Y, Michalas S. Fetal blood sampling in twin pregnancies. *Ultrasound Obstet Gynecol* **22**(4):377–379, 2003.
122. Rodeck CH, Patrick AD, Pembrey ME, Tzannatos C, Whitfield AE. Fetal liver biopsy for prenatal diagnosis of ornithine carbamyl transferase deficiency. *Lancet* **2**(8293):297–300, 1982.
123. Holzgreve W, Golbus MS. Prenatal diagnosis of ornithine transcarbamylase deficiency utilizing fetal liver biopsy. *Am J Hum Genet* **36**(2):320–328, 1984.
124. Piceni SL, Bachmann C, Pfister U, Buscaglia M, Nicolini U. Prenatal diagnosis of carbamoyl-phosphate synthetase deficiency by fetal liver biopsy. *Prenat Diagn* **8**(4):307–309, 1988.
125. Golbus MS, Simpson TJ, Koresawa M, Appelman Z, Alpers CE. The prenatal determination of glucose-6-phosphatase activity by fetal liver biopsy. *Prenat Diagn* **8**(6):401–404, 1988.
126. Danpure CJ, Jennings PR, Penketh RJ, Wise PJ, Cooper PJ, Rodeck CH. Fetal liver alanine: glyoxylate amniotransferase and the prenatal diagnosis of primary hyperoxaluria Type 1. *Prenat Diagn* **9**:271–280, 1989.
127. Rozen R, Fox J, Fenton WA, Horwich AL, Rosenberg LE. Gene deletion and restriction fragment length polymorphisms at the human ornithine transcarbamylase locus. *Nature* **313**(6005):815–817, 1985.
128. Haberle J, Koch HG. Genetic approach to prenatal diagnosis in urea cycle defects. *Prenat Diagn* **24**(5):378–383, 2004.
129. Qu Y, Abdenur JE, Eng CM, Desnick RJ. Molecular prenatal diagnosis of glycogen storage disease type Ia. *Prenat Diagn* **16**(4):333–336, 1996.
130. Nicolini U, Rodeck CH. Fetal Blood and Tissue Sampling. In: Parental Diagnosis and Screening, eds: DJH Brock, CH Rodeck, M Ferguson-Smith, pp. 39–51. Churchill Livingstone, 1992.
131. Rodeck CH, Eady RA, Gosden CM. Prenatal diagnosis of epidermolysis bullosa letalis. *Lancet* **1**(8175):949–952, 1980.
132. Lorenz HP, Longaker MT, Perkocha LA, Jennings RW, Harrison MR, Adzick NS. Scarless wound repair: a human fetal skin model. *Development* **114**(1):253–259, 1992.
133. McGrath JA, Dunnil MG, Christiano AM, Lake BD, Atherton DJ, Rodeck CH et al. First trimester DNA-based exclusion of recessive dystrophic eqidermolysis bullosa from chorionic villus sampling. *Br J Dermatol* **134**(4):734–739, 1996.
134. Nevo Y, Shomrat R, Yaron Y, Orr-Urtreger A, Harel S, Legum C. Fetal muscle biopsy as a diagnostic tool in Duchenne muscular dystrophy. *Prenat Diagn* **19**(10):921–926, 1999.
135. Evans MI, Hoffman EP, Cadrin C, Johnson MP, Quintero RA, Golbus MS. Fetal muscle biopsy: collaborative experience with varied indications. *Obstet Gynecol* **84**(6):913–917, 1994.
136. Multicentre randomised clinical trial of chorion villus sampling and amniocentesis. First report. Canadian Collaborative CVS-Amniocentesis Clinical Trial Group. *Lancet* **1**(8628):1–6, 1989.
137. Ammala P, Hiilesmaa VK, Liukkonen S, Saisto T, Teramo K, von Koskull H. Randomized trial comparing first-trimester transcervical chorionic villus sampling and second-trimester amniocentesis. *Prenat Diagn* **13**(10): 919–927, 1993.
138. Borrell A, Fortuny A, Lazaro L, Costa D, Seres A, Pappa S et al. First-trimester transcervical chorionic villus sampling by biopsy forceps versus mid-trimester amniocentesis: a randomized controlled trial project. *Prenat Diagn* **19**(12): 1138–1142, 1999.
139. Palo P, Piiroinen O, Honkonen E, Lakkala T, Aula P. Transabdominal chorionic villus sampling and amniocentesis for prenatal diagnosis: 5 years' experience at a university centre. *Prenat Diagn* **14**(3):157–162, 1994.
140. Shalev E, Weiner E, Yanai N, Shneur Y, Cohen H. Comparison of first-trimester transvaginal amniocentesis with chorionic villus sampling and mid-trimester amniocentesis. *Prenat Diagn* **14**(4):279–283, 1994.
141. Fortuny A, Borrell A, Soler A, Casals E, Costa D, Carrio A et al. Chorionic villus sampling by biopsy forceps. Results of 1580 procedures from a single centre. Prenat Diagn, **15**(6):541–550, 1995.

CHAPTER 23

Cytogenetics

Caroline M Ogilvie

KEY POINTS

- Amniotic fluid, fetal blood and chorionic villus biopsy are all samples that can be cultured and tested for chromosome abnormality. Amniotic fluid is the preferred sample type in most cytogenetic laboratories
- Types of chromosome abnormality include autosomal trisomies, sex chromosome aneuploidy, triploidy, mosaicism for a cell line with aneuploidy or triploidy, diandry leading to molar pregnancies, balanced or unbalanced structural rearrangements of the autosomes or sex chromosomes, extra structurally abnormal chromosomes, uniparental disomy and copy number variants
- Chromosome abnormalities may arise de novo or may be inherited in the same or different form from one parent. Prognosis for the fetus can be difficult to assess in some cases
- Chromosome abnormalities in prenatal samples have traditionally been detected by G-banded chromosome analysis, but new molecular techniques are opening up alternative strategies for diagnosis. These techniques include FISH, QF-PCR, MLPA and microarrays
- Targeted prenatal testing for the common trisomies and, where indicated, for sex chromosome imbalance, is being introduced in some areas
- Future prospects include the possibility of non-invasive diagnosis, already feasible for unique paternal genetic sequences

INTRODUCTION

Chromosomes were first identified and named in the 19th century, but the correct human chromosome complement (46, comprising 22 pairs of autosomes and one pair of sex chromosomes) was not established until 1956[1,2], heralding the beginning of the modern cytogenetic era. This breakthrough was followed closely by the discovery that Down's syndrome was associated with the presence of an extra chromosome[3]. Other syndromes caused by abnormalities of whole chromosome copy number were identified shortly afterwards[4–7], and the development in 1969 of techniques for banding chromosomes[8] allowed the detection of more subtle structural chromosome abnormalities. The application of these discoveries to prenatal diagnosis was obvious, and the culture and karyotyping of cells from amniotic fluid (or, more recently, chorionic villi) to identify fetuses with chromosome abnormalities has been carried out since the late 1960s or early 1970s.

Chromosomes for karyotype analysis are arrested at the metaphase stage of the cell cycle, following DNA replication; at this point, the DNA is highly condensed, and the chromosomes consist of two identical chromatids, held together at the centromere. The centromere is a specialized structure for the attachment of the spindle apparatus which separates the chromatids at mitosis, and is visualized as a constriction in the chromosome. Some chromosomes have the centromere in the middle (metacentric), some nearer one end (submetacentric) and, in some, the centromere is almost at the end of the chromosome (acrocentric). The short and long arms of each chromosome (either side of the centromere) are designated 'p' and 'q' respectively. The short arms of the acrocentric chromosomes mostly comprise genetically inactive material, and vary considerably in size in the normal population. Conventionally, the chromosomes are numbered in approximate size order, with chromosome 1 being the largest; a karyotype is a pictorial representation with the chromosomes arranged in pairs in number order (Fig. 23.1). Most cytogenetics laboratories use trypsin digestion and Giemsa staining to visualize the chromosome bands; this results in so-called 'G-banded' chromosomes (GTG banding) with dark-staining bands representing gene poor regions, and pale bands which represent gene-rich regions. Other types of staining are occasionally carried out to characterize, for instance, specifically heterochromatic regions (heterochromatin comprises highly condensed DNA which

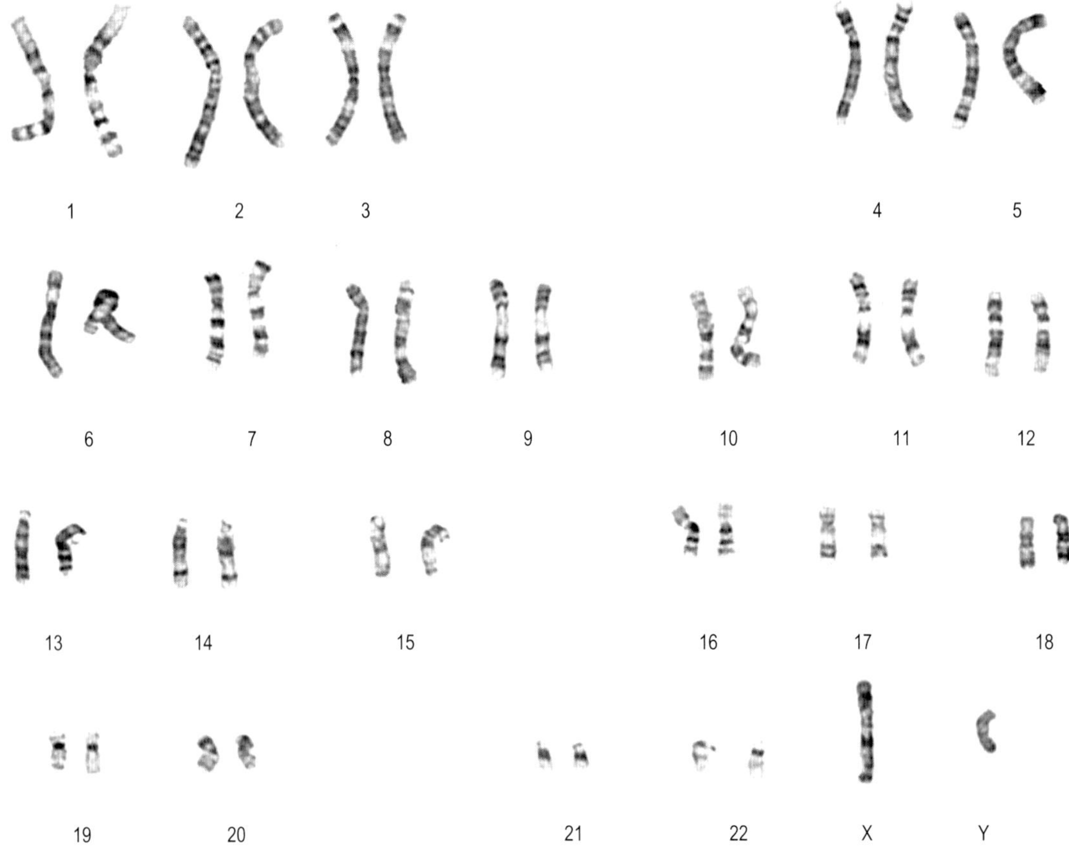

Fig. 23.1 Normal male karyotype, showing GTG-banded chromosomes.

is not transcriptionally active, and contains long stretches of repetitive sequences, also known as satellite DNA). Originally, these karyotypes were generated by photographing the chromosome spreads, then cutting out the individual chromosomes and pasting them into the karyotype. This procedure is now nearly always done using digital photography and a computer. 'Karyotype' also refers to the string of letters and numbers which describes the chromosome constitution: 46,XX or 46,XY for chromosomally normal females and males respectively. Abnormal karyotypes are described according to an international convention[9] which can sometimes be difficult to interpret; however, chromosome abnormalities should always be fully described in the text of the cytogenetics report.

REFERRAL INDICATIONS FOR CYTOGENETIC ANALYSIS

Because of the known association between maternal age and Down's syndrome[10], early prenatal samples were generally from women with raised maternal age. Since then, the advent of more specific Down's syndrome screening tests[11], detailed ultrasound anomaly scanning, and specific mutation tests for monogenic disease, prenatal samples are now referred for a number of different reasons (see other chapters in this book); however, in general, around 65–70% of samples are still tested because of a raised risk of Down's syndrome.

PRENATAL SAMPLES

Amniotic fluid, fetal blood and chorionic villus biopsy are all samples that can be cultured and tested for chromosome abnormality. In general, fetal blood sampling is only carried out for confirmation of fetal karyotype following equivocal findings from other sample types. Amniotic fluid is the preferred sample type in most cytogenetic laboratories, as the vast majority of cells are derived directly from fetal tissue, whereas the cell lineages contributing to the chorionic villi diverge from those making up the fetus itself at an early stage in embryogenesis, and can sometimes be cytogenetically different. The chorionic villi comprise an outer, cytotrophoblast layer, and an inner, mesenchymal core. The mesenchyme is closer in embryological origin to the cell lineages comprising the fetal tissues, and culture of material from chorionic villi samples preferentially selects mesenchyme-derived cells for karyotype analysis. The occurrence of confined placental mosaicism (CPM), where abnormal or normal cell lines may be present only in the placenta, compromises interpretation of cytogenetic results from chorionic villi biopsies (see section on mosaicism). In addition, these samples are technically demanding to prepare, as they require careful cleaning in order to remove contaminating maternal decidua. However, the benefits of early diagnosis of abnormality and hence earlier termination of pregnancy are considered by some professionals to outweigh the disadvantages of diagnosis from chorionic villi.

Table 23.1 Incidence of specific chromosome aneuploidies

Chromosome abnormality	*Incidence per live births*	*Incidence per amniocentesis*	*Incidence per spontaneous losses*
Trisomy 21 (Down's syndrome)	1/800 (0.12%)	1/86	1/60 (1.7%)
Trisomy 18 (Edwards' syndrome)	1/3000 (0.03%)	1/400	1/140 (0.7%)
Trisomy 13 (Patau's syndrome)	1/5000 (0.02%)	1/1350	1/60 (1.7%)
45,X (Turner's syndrome)	1/5000 (0.02%)	1/2200	1/16 (6.3%)
47,XXY (Klinefelter's syndrome)	1/1000 (0.01%)	1/600	1/400

Data from Miller & Therman[12]

TYPES OF CHROMOSOME ABNORMALITY

Autosomal aneuploidy

Whole chromosome aneuploidy (abnormal copy number) is detectable by standard cytogenetic analysis of banded chromosomes using light microscopy; the cell culture protocols necessary mean that the results of such analysis may not be available for 2–3 weeks. Whole chromosome aneuploidy results in extensive genomic imbalance and is in general incompatible with live birth, with the well-known exceptions of trisomy 21 (Down's syndrome), trisomy 13 (Patau's syndrome) and trisomy 18 (Edwards' syndrome). These trisomies usually arise following meiotic errors in gametogenesis, although post-zygotic mitotic error can also generate an apparently non-mosaic trisomy. Table 23.1 shows the incidence of these aneuploidies at live birth, prenatal diagnosis and in products of conception following miscarriage. Rapid methods of detecting these aneuploidies are now available (see below), leading to their identification within 24–48 hours.

Sex chromosome aneuploidy

Sex chromosome aneuploidy is found at prenatal diagnosis in approximately 1 in 300 samples[13]. Most sex chromosome imbalance is compatible with survival of the fetus to term, despite the large genomic imbalance that might be predicted. This is due to the phenomenon of X inactivation, whereby in normal females, one X chromosome undergoes a process of inactivation called lyonization which 'switches off' most of the genes[14]. However, some X chromosome genes escape inactivation and are therefore present as two active copies in normal females. These genes include those in the 'pseudoautosomal regions' (PAR1 and PAR2, at the end of the short and long arms respectively of the sex chromosomes). Outside PAR1 and PAR2, about 15% of genes escape inactivation[15] and it is the abnormal copy number of these genes that is very likely the cause of the abnormal phenotype found in individuals with sex chromosome aneuploidy.

These aneuploidies can be detected by karyotype analysis and also by some of the rapid testing methods described below.

Karyotype 45,X

This karyotype is associated with Turner's syndrome in liveborn individuals. However, it is also the most common karyotype abnormality found in products of conception (see Table 23.1). A pregnancy found to have 45,X at prenatal diagnosis may therefore be considered likely to abort spontaneously; those fetuses that survive to term may have a normal cell line in some tissues and some may be very mildly affected.

Karyotype 47,XXY

This karyotype gives rise to Klinefelter's syndrome. One of the two X chromosomes is always inactivated and therefore the genetic imbalance is trisomy for X chromosome genes that escape inactivation and are also found on the Y chromosome. As the phenotype in Klinefelter's syndrome is vary variable, a finding of 47,XXY at prenatal diagnosis gives rise to significant problems for professionals and parents in counseling and decision making as to whether or not to terminate the pregnancy.

Karyotype 47,XYY

Originally thought to result in behavior problems and impaired mental development, it is now recognized that, although approximately 50% of individuals known to have XYY have some form of mild learning difficulty, most have an IQ within the normal range[13]. As in the case of fetuses with a Klinefelter karyotype, a diagnosis at prenatal testing of 47,XYY is problematic for professionals and parents.

Very rarely, polysomy of the sex chromosomes (for instance, 48,XXXX or 48,XXXY) is found. Interestingly, even when there are more than two X chromosomes, the X inactivation mechanism always leaves only a single X chromosome in the fully active state; the mechanism for this process is not completely understood. Such sex chromosome polysomies are usually associated with significant developmental delay.

Triploidy and hydatidiform moles

Triploidy is unerringly detected by either karyotype analysis or quantitative fluorescence polymerase chain reaction (QF-PCR), but not by multiplex ligation-dependent probe amplification (MLPA) or microarrays.

Full triploidy

The normal human chromosome complement is diploid, as there are two sets of chromosomes – one inherited from the mother and the other from the father. Triploidy, where the fetus has a complete extra set of chromosomes, is found in approximately 1 in every 1500 pregnancies[16]. The extra set of chromosomes may originate from either the mother (digyny) or the father (diandry); recent data indicate that the phenotype of the fetus cannot be correlated with the parent of origin of the extra set of chromosomes[17]. Digynic triploidy arises from the failure of the oocyte to expel the second polar body at fertilization, while diandric triploidy is thought to be due to dispermic fertilization, although may occasionally arise from fertilization with a diploid sperm. The diandric triploid state may result in a partial molar pregnancy but, if this is avoided, the diandric or digynic triploid fetus may survive well into pregnancy[18], although few survive till term and no non-mosaic liveborn is known to have survived the neonatal period.

Mosaic triploidy

Triploidy may occur in mosaic form; mechanisms for mosaic triploidy include: fusion of two zygotes, one normal and one triploid, to give a chimeric fetus; delayed fertilization of a zygote with a second sperm; and re-incorporation of the second polar body into the fertilized egg[19]. Mosaic triploidy may be viable to term, depending on the proportion and distribution of the two cell lines. A case has been reported of mosaic triploidy detected at chorionic villus testing, where the triploid cell line was only present in extraembryonic tissues; the pregnancy resulted in a normal infant[19].

Complete hydatidiform moles

These pregnancies are diploid, but both sets of chromosomes are derived from the father. Most are due to fertilization of an anucleate egg by a single sperm, followed by doubling of the paternal chromosomes; very rarely, molar pregnancies arise following fertilization of an anucleate egg by two different sperm. Molar pregnancies are generally sporadic in their etiology; however, recurrence in families has been documented[20] and, in some cases, biparental inheritance has been demonstrated. This is thought to be due to mutation of a gene involved in the pathway leading to the 'reprogramming' of imprinted genes in the maternal germline, resulting in gametes with paternally imprinted chromosomes. Complete molar pregnancies have an associated risk of choriocarcinoma.

Partial hydatidiform moles

Some diandric triploid conceptuses result in partial molar pregnancies. These are not thought to be associated with any risk of choriocarcinoma. A partial molar pregnancy has been described with triploidy mosaicism, where the triploid cell line was confined to the placenta, while the diploid fetus survived to term[21].

Chromosomal mosaicism

Chromosomal mosaicism is the presence within one sample of two or more cell lines with different karyotypes. This mosaicism may arise when a trisomy conception is followed by 'trisomy rescue', generating a normal cell line by the loss of one chromosome, or when post-zygotic error generates an abnormal cell line following a normal conception. Mosaicism for trisomy 21, 13 and 18 is found in around 0.2% of all prenatal samples[22], but occurs at a much higher prevalence in chorionic villi; a number of studies has been published detailing audits of mosaicism in these prenatal samples, all reporting levels of mosaicism of between 1 and 2%[23–26]. The finding of mosaic aneuploidy in a chorionic villus sample may represent CPM (see above), leading to difficulties in counseling, as the abnormal cell line may not be present in the fetus. The risk of an abnormal fetus (either full trisomy or mosaic trisomy) will depend on the distribution of the abnormal cell line in the placental cell lineages. So-called 'direct' preparations sample cells from the cytotrophoblast, and are therefore considered to be inadequate as a stand-alone test. QF-PCR (see below) tests DNA extracted from whole villi, and is therefore more likely to detect all major cell lines present in the sample. Although analysis of cultured cells from the mesoderm is generally a good indicator of fetal karyotype, there have been published reports of discrepancies, leading to misdiagnosis of the fetal status[27–29]. Where mosaicism in chorionic villus samples is found, follow-up testing by amniotic fluid or fetal blood sampling is recommended[27].

Mosaic trisomy for any chromosome has the potential to result in a newborn with congenital abnormality; mosaic trisomies and monosomies are well documented for a number of chromosomes other than 21, 13 and 18[30]. Such mosaicism found at chorionic villus testing is very often followed by a normal follow-up amniotic fluid or fetal blood result. Although in these cases the presence of the abnormal cell line in the fetus can never be completely excluded, most practitioners would consider the most likely explanation of the original finding to be an example of CPM. However, if the mosaicism is confirmed on follow-up, the pregnancy outcome will depend on the level and distribution of the abnormal cell lines in the fetal tissues.

Autosomal structural rearrangements

In general, structural rearrangements are identified by traditional karyotype analysis and may be 'balanced' (i.e. no loss or gain of material can be visualized by light microscopy) or 'unbalanced'.

Balanced reciprocal translocations

These rearrangements typically involve heterologous exchange of the terminal portions of chromosome arms (Fig. 23.2) and are usually carried in an apparently balanced form in phenotypically normal individuals. It is estimated that approximately 1 in 500 people is a reciprocal translocation carrier[32]. A fetus that has inherited an apparently balanced reciprocal translocation from one parent is unlikely to have phenotypic abnormality associated with this finding. However, de novo apparently balanced rearrangements have a risk of associated phenotypic abnormality, due to the possibility of submicroscopic loss of material or gene disruption at the breakpoints. This risk has been estimated to be between 3 and 5% above the population background risk of congenital abnormality[30]. A prospective study by Warburton et al.[33] established that approximately 1 in 2000 pregnancies has a de novo reciprocal translocation,

Any carrier of a reciprocal translocation has a reproductive risk, due to the possibility of the formation of chromosomally abnormal gametes at meiosis, when the translocated chromosomes may not segregate together to the daughter cells,

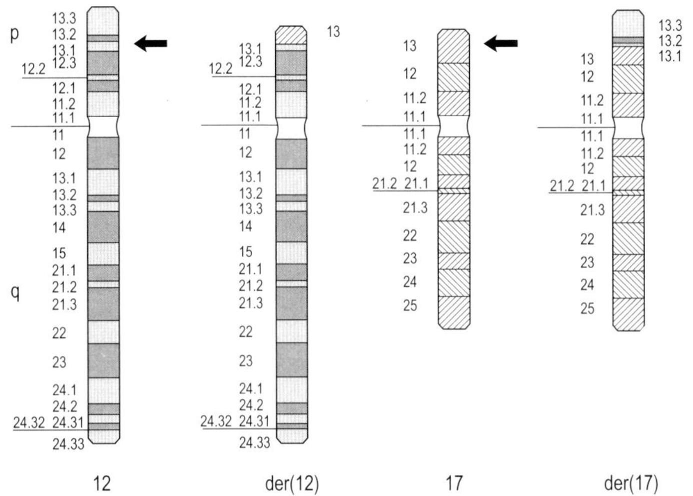

Fig. 23.2 Ideogram representation of a balanced reciprocal translocation[31] between the short arms of chromosomes 12 and 17. Arrows show the breakpoints on the normal homologues. Chromosome 12 material is dotted, chromosome 17 material is cross-hatched. Chromosome band numbers are shown. Derivative (rearranged) homologues are denoted der(12) and der(17).

resulting in genetic imbalance (Fig. 23.3). Familial reciprocal translocations are generally unique to the kindred in which each occurs, making reproductive risk assessment problematic; such assessment is usually based on a combination of the obstetric history in the family, the likely imbalance associated with abnormal meiotic segregation, plus any instances in the literature of liveborn individuals with similar imbalance. All rearrangements are likely to have some reproductive consequences for carriers; genetic counseling is recommended at an appropriate age.

Robertsonian translocations

A Robertsonian translocation is the fusion in the centric region of two acrocentric chromosomes, with no loss of euchromatic material (Fig. 23.4). These translocations occur with a prevalence of approximately 1 in 1000 in the general population[30]. By far the most common are the heterologous forms, i.e. those involving two different chromosomes; at meiosis, these rearrangements form trivalents, segregation of which may result in gametes nullisomic or disomic for one of the chromosomes involved in the rearrangement. The risks of miscarrriage or viable abnormality are dependent on the chromosomes making up the translocation. The most common Robertsonian translocation is between chromosomes 13 and 14. This form makes up approximately 75% of all Robertsonians and may be associated with infertility or recurrent spontaneous abortions; interestingly, at prenatal diagnosis for female carriers, fetuses with the balanced form are more commonly found than those with normal chromosomes[34], although theoretically the incidence should be the same. The other important Robertsonian is that between chromosomes 14 and 21 which, although far less common than the 13;14, has significance because of the risk of trisomy 21 (Down's syndrome). Female carriers have a 15% risk of trisomy 21 at prenatal diagnosis and a 10% risk of liveborn trisomy 21[35]. For male carriers, the risk of trisomy 21 conception is less than 0.5%. Trisomy arising as a result of a parental balanced rearrangement is known as 'translocation trisomy'.

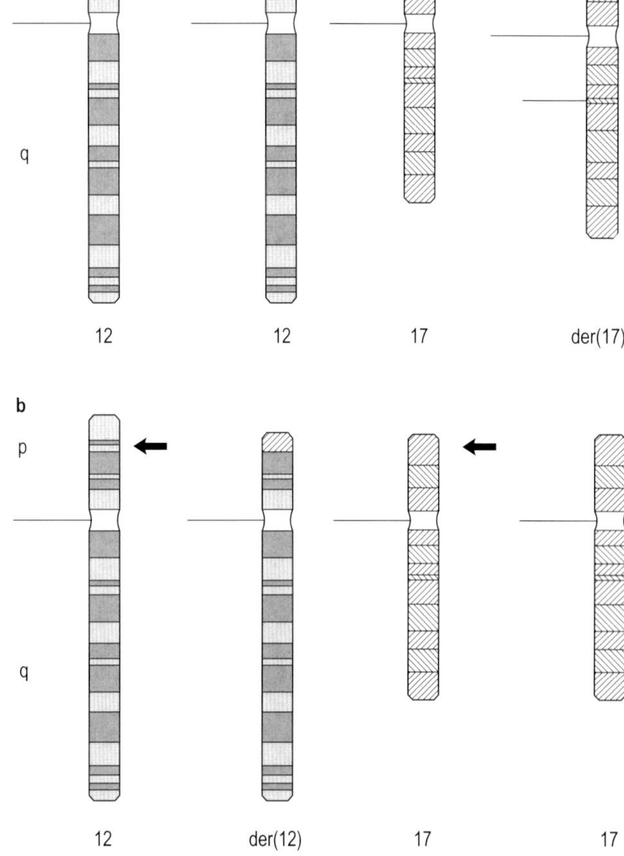

Fig. 23.3 Ideogram representation of expected imbalance from the balanced translocation shown in Figure 23.2. (a) Adjacent 1 segregation resulting in trisomy for the translocated segment of chromosome 12 and monosomy for the translocated segment of chromosome 17. (b) Adjacent 1 segregation resulting in trisomy for the translocated segment of chromosome 17 and monosomy for the translocated segment of chromosome 12.

De novo Robertsonian translocations, found in around 1/9000 pregnancies[33], are very unlikely to be of phenotypic significance, as the breakpoints lie within heterochromatic regions. Homologous Robertsonian translocations nearly always arise de novo and carriers have a near 100% risk of trisomy in their offspring.

Other autosomal structural rearrangements

Peri- and paracentric inversions and intrachromosomal insertions are other chromosome rearrangements that may be found at prenatal diagnosis. If inherited in the apparently balanced form from a normal parent, these anomalies are considered to be of little or no phenotypic significance. However, de novo rearrangements, found in approximately 1 in 10000 pregnancies, carry the same empiric risk of abnormal outcome as above (3–5%)[33]. There are reproductive risks associated with these rearrangements.

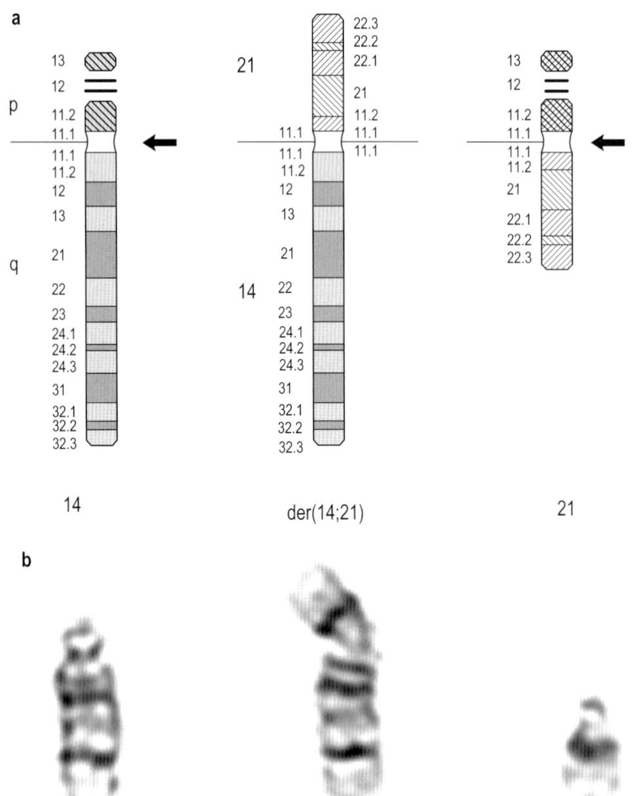

Fig. 23.4 (a) Ideogram representation of a balanced Robertsonian translocation between chromosomes 14 and 21. Chromosome 14 is shown dotted, chromosome 21 cross-hatched. Arrows indicate the breakpoints on the normal homologues. Chromosome band numbers are shown. (b) Partial karyotype of the Robertsonian translocation shown in (a); chromosomes are GTG banded.

Unbalanced autosomal rearrangements

Abnormal segregation of a parental balanced translocation at meiosis, or meiotic recombination within an inversion loop in the case of familial pericentric inversions, gives rise to genetic imbalance in gametes and hence in the resulting embryo and fetus. Such imbalance is likely to be detected by traditional karyotype analysis, although for some very rare cases of submicroscopic or cryptic rearrangements, other techniques such as fluorescence in situ hybridization (FISH; see below) may be necessary to detect associated prenatal imbalance. For most translocation and inversion carriers, specific FISH tests can be designed allowing the detection or exclusion within 24–48 h of imbalance arising from the rearrangement[36] (see FISH section). Whether de novo or arising from a familial balanced rearrangement, unbalanced rearrangements detected by traditional karyotype analysis are almost invariably associated with poor pregnancy outcomes (except in the case of CNVs – see below) – either miscarriage or livebirth with congenital abnormality.

Structural rearrangements involving the sex chromosomes

Females may carry a structurally rearranged X chromosome, either balanced or unbalanced, and yet have a normal phenotype, due to preferential inactivation of the abnormal X chromosome. A female fetus inheriting an abnormal X chromosome cannot, however, be assumed to be without congenital abnormalities, although preferential inactivation of the abnormal X is likely. In these pregnancies, careful ultrasound monitoring is usually recommended. Where the rearrangement gives rise to imbalance of the PAR1 region, disturbances in growth patterns are likely, due to the presence of the *SHOX* gene in this region; similarly, reduced fertility or infertility may result from monosomy for regions (Xq13-q22 and Xq22-q27) containing genes essential for normal ovarian function[37], as some of these genes escape inactivation. Imbalance for part of the X chromosome is nearly always lethal in a male fetus.

A special case of X chromosome rearrangement is that of the ring X chromosome, where the ring may be very small, and either replace a normal X chromosome, or be supernumerary. These rings are often lost during cell division, leading to mosaic karyotypes; in addition, monosomy for many of the genes escaping inactivation will give rise to a Turner-like phenotype in those cases where the ring replaces a normal X chromosome. However, if the ring chromosome is not inactivated, either because it lacks the X inactivation locus, or for other reasons, the phenotype may be very severe. This is thought to be due to functional disomy for genes that are normally inactivated.

Structural rearrangements of the Y chromosome do not usually result in abnormal phenotype, providing that function of the *SRY* gene remains unimpaired, although fertility may be compromised. If the rearrangement has been inherited from a normal father, this provides reassurance. However, structurally abnormal Y chromosomes may be present in mosaic form, along with a 45,X cell line; in these cases, abnormalities of sexual development may be found[38].

Rearrangements involving autosomes and sex chromosomes are more complex, due to the potential for the heterochromatization involved in X inactivation to spread into the autosomal regions of the derivative X chromosome. For this reason, in most X;autosome translocation carriers, the normal X chromosome is inactivated, allowing functionally normal copy number for genes on both the X chromosome and the translocated autosome.[39] Most de novo X;autosome translocations are thought to originate at paternal meiosis[40]; only the PAR1 regions of the X and Y chromosomes pair, leaving the rest of the X chromosome free to undergo illegitimate rearrangement with other chromosomes. Y;autosome translocations, provided they are balanced, do not usually result in abnormal phenotype[38], although infertility is to be expected; this is because the translocation is likely to interfere with the pairing of the PAR1 regions at male meiosis, leading to spermatogenic arrest.

Sex chromosome/phenotype discordance

Interruption to the normal development of phenotypic sex can be due to mutations or imbalance for genes along the sexual differentiation pathways. In particular, mutation in, or loss of, the *SRY* gene can give rise to XY females and, conversely, phenotypic males may have a 46,XX karyotype. This is sometimes due to a cryptic rearrangement between the terminal regions of the short arms of the X and Y chromosomes, whereby the *SRY* gene is translocated onto the tip of the X chromosome short arm during male meiosis. A FISH probe for the *SRY* gene is available and can be used to visualize the position of the gene on the chromosomes. Individuals with this rearrangement generally have normal development of male secondary sexual characteristics, but are invariably infertile.

Extra structurally abnormal chromosomes (ESACs)

In the early days of cytogenetics, these supernumerary chromosomes were designated 'marker chromosomes' if they were too small to be identified by traditional chromosome banding techniques. With the advent of more sophisticated techniques such as FISH, identification of the origin and approximate genetic content of these chromosomes is now expected, whether detected prenatally or postnatally[41]. The phenotypic consequences of these ESACs will depend on their genetic content, and thus the extent of genetic imbalance present in the carrier. As in the case of chromosome rearrangements, the presence of the same anomaly in a parent is reassuring. However, unlike chromosome rearrangements, ESACs are frequently present in mosaic form; differences in the frequency and distribution of the ESAC may lead to abnormal phenotype in the fetus, where none exists in the carrier parent. In addition, very recent studies[42] indicate that, in some cases, the carrier parent may in fact be genetically balanced, by carrying a chromosome deleted for the sequences present in the ESAC. If the fetus has not inherited the same deleted chromosome along with the ESAC, then there may be significant risk of phenotypic abnormality.

The most common ESACs found in the population are those derived from chromosome 15; these ESACs and their associated phenotypic consequences have been extremely well studied[43] and, with full characterization and appropriate inheritance studies, it is now possible to predict the phenotypic outcome in most prenatal cases of chromosome 15-derived ESACs. Other ESACs which have a known outcome are bisatellited dicentric ESACs derived from chromosome 22. The formation of these chromosomes is mediated by low-copy repeat regions in the proximal region of the chromosome 22 long arm and the genetic content is therefore generally predictable; the imbalance associated with these ESACs gives rise to cat-eye syndrome (OMIM #115470). However, for many ESACs, especially those that have arisen de novo (de novo ESACs are found in around 1 in 2500 pregnancies[33]), it is difficult to predict phenotype, even with fairly detailed knowledge of the genetic content, due to the relative rarity of these findings and the likely lack of reported cases with similar imbalance.

The frequency of ESACs at birth is approximately 0.07% and the overall risk of congenital abnormalities associated with ESACs is 13%[33].

Uniparental disomy (UPD)

Individuals or fetuses with UPD have both homologues of a chromosome originating from one parent, with no contribution from the other parent for that chromosome[44]. This can arise due to errors at meiosis, or very rarely can be the result of early mitotic error, generating a trisomy cell line, followed by correction due to loss of one of the chromosomes[26,45]. Clinical phenotype arises when the chromosome in question contains imprinted genes, i.e. where the parent of origin of the chromosome determines whether the genes are active or silenced. For instance, a gene that is in the active state on a maternally inherited chromosome but inactive on the paternal chromosome will be functionally monosomic in a normal person. UPDmat will result in functional disomy for the gene, and UPDpat will result in functional nullisomy. UPDmat and UPDpat for the same chromosome will therefore in most cases give rise to different clinical features. The finding of mosaic or full trisomy in a chorionic villus sample, followed by a normal result on amniocentesis should be followed by testing for UPD, if the trisomic chromosome is known to be associated with a UPD phenotype (for instance, UPD for chromosomes 6, 7, 11, 14, 15 and 16 is associated with specific phenotypic abnormalities). In addition, the presence of an ESAC may indicate rescue of a trisomy conception, and hence a risk of UPD. The Association of Clinical Cytogeneticists (ACC) (http://www.cytogenetics.org.uk/) guidelines recommend UPD testing where trisomy mosaicism for chromosomes 7, 11, 14, or 15 has been found in chorionic villi and in cases of homologous and non-homologous Robertsonian translocations involving chromosomes 14 and 15. Cases with ESACs originating from chromosomes 7, 11, 14 or 15 should also be tested for UPD. However, empiric evidence suggests that mosaic trisomy 16 pregnancies may have an adverse outcome even if UPD 16 in the fetus is excluded; this is thought to be due to placental insufficiency caused by the abnormal cell line, or to cryptic mosaicism for trisomy 16 in fetal tissue[46]. UPD testing requires blood samples from both parents; DNA from these samples, along with DNA from the prenatal sample, is tested by PCR amplification of polymorphic microsatellite markers along the chromosome of interest. The lengths of the microsatellites are then compared to establish bi- or uni-parental inheritance. This testing may be carried out in a molecular genetics laboratory, but is increasingly a test offered from within cytogenetics laboratories, especially those which offer the PCR-based QF-PCR rapid test, which uses the same technology (see QF-PCR section).

Copy number variants (CNVs)

Variation in the length of heterochromatic (inactive) chromosome regions has long been understood to be of little or no significance. However, more recently, it has become clear that some euchromatic chromosome regions contain genes that are not copy number sensitive. Multiple copies of some chromosome regions, leading to chromosome imbalance detectable by karyotype analysis, have been found in individuals with normal phenotype[47]. While these regions have been characterized and described in the literature, it remains possible that that there are more as yet undescribed, especially as the quality of chromosome preparations improves and the skill of cytogenetic analysts increases. It is therefore important that the detection at prenatal testing of any apparent imbalance should be followed by parental karyotyping to establish whether the imbalance has arisen de novo or has been inherited from a phenotypically normal parent.

CYTOGENETIC TECHNIQUES AND THEIR APPLICATIONS

Full karyotype analysis

In the first days of prenatal diagnosis, karyotype analysis (see Fig. 23.1) was the only method available for the detection of

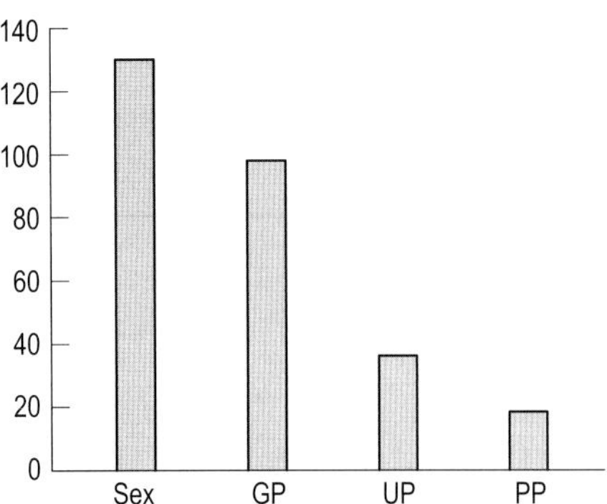

Fig. 23.5 Karyotype abnormalities found in a total of 24 891 pregnancies referred for raised risk of Down's syndrome, excluding those that would be detected by rapid testing for trisomy 13, 18 and 21. Sex = sex chromosome abnormalities; GP = good prognosis (such as inherited rearrangements); UP = uncertain prognosis (such as ESACs); PP = poor prognosis. Data from Mackie Ogilvie et al.[48].

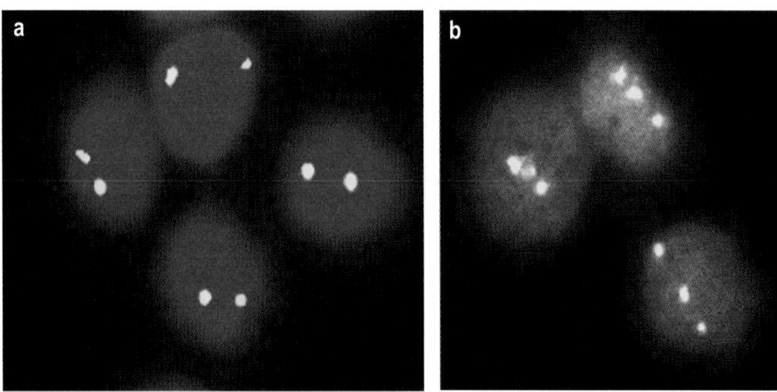

Fig. 23.6 Uncultured amniotic fluid cells tested by FISH with a probe for the centromere of chromosome 18. (a) Normal signal pattern, (b) trisomy 18.

chromosome abnormality. Modern culture and banding and staining techniques currently lead to average reporting times of around 10–14 days, although sometimes results may be available after 7–10 days. Most preparations are of sufficient quality to detect imbalance greater than around 4–5 megabases (Mb); it is important that professionals and patients understand that small regions of imbalance, with potentially profound significance for the fetus, will not be detected by this test. It has been the case that karyotyping of newborns with congenital anomalies has revealed chromosome abnormalities not detected prenatally. This is likely to be due to the more extended chromosomes produced by postnatal blood samples, and hence to the better resolution achieved. Karyotype analysis of prenatal samples will occasionally identify unexpected findings such as chromosome rearrangements, ESACs, or areas of CNV, some of which will be benign, some will have an unknown prognosis, and some will be predictive of a poor pregnancy outcome (Fig. 23.5).

Karyotype analysis is generally carried out on every prenatal sample, regardless of referral indication. However, concerns have been raised about the cost of the test, which is very labor intensive and requires highly skilled analysts. In addition, the equivocal nature of some of the findings leads to parental anxiety and, on occasion, to potentially unnecessary pregnancy terminations[48]. For these reasons, it has been suggested that more direct testing should be carried out, targeted to the specific referral indication. This issue is discussed further below.

Fluorescence in situ hybridization (FISH)

FISH utilizes DNA probes that are complementary to specific target regions within the genome. These regions may be highly repetitive sequences in heterochromatic regions, or may be 50–100 kilobases (Kb) of material, encompassing clinically important areas such as those associated with microdeletion syndromes. These DNA probes are labeled with fluorescent markers, then hybridized to chromosome spreads or interphase nuclei fixed to glass microscope slides. Examination of the slides under ultraviolet light shows the copy number of the targeted regions and, in the case of chromosome spreads, the location of the target sequence on the chromosomes.

In the prenatal arena, FISH is used to 'count' chromosomes in interphase nuclei, therefore bypassing the need for the lengthy culture protocols necessary for karyotype analysis[49,50]. For instance, a sample from a pregnancy at high risk of trisomy 18 can be tested with a FISH probe for chromosome 18 and trisomy confirmed or excluded within 24–48 hours (Fig. 23.6). Most centers using this approach would follow up the result with a full karyotype analysis.

Other applications of FISH include testing for microdeletion syndromes in pregnancies where the fetus shows specific abnormalities. For instance, conotruncal heart defects are associated with deletion in the proximal region of chromosome 22, giving rise to 22q11 deletion syndrome (also known as DiGeorge (OMIM #188400) or velocardiofacial syndrome (OMIM #192430)). It is now common practice to test all prenatal samples from pregnancies presenting with these cardiac defects using FISH with a probe for the critical region on chromosome 22[51]. Parents may choose to continue with the pregnancy even where the FISH test shows a deletion; however, knowledge of the genetic defect allows appropriate treatment to be initiated at delivery. FISH may similarly be used to confirm or exclude a microdeletion in pregnancies where previous offspring have carried a specific defect; even in cases where neither parent is a carrier, this test provides reassurance, and excludes the possibility of recurrence due to parental germ line mosaicism for the abnormality.

Carriers of balanced chromosome rearrangements have reproductive risks, which will be different for every rearrangement; in cases where there is significant risk of a fetus with associated imbalance compatible with survival to the end of the first trimester, rapid testing of a chorionic villus sample using FISH can be offered. Specific probes for the ends of every chromosome arm are available and a tailored test can be designed for the majority of chromosome rearrangements. These tests were originally designed and implemented for preimplantation testing of interphase nuclei from biopsied blastomeres[52–54]; preimplantation genetic diagnosis (PGD) is discussed in a separate chapter of this book. Since then, the same approach has been used to test uncultured prenatal material from carriers of chromosome rearrangements[36], confirming or excluding imbalance within 24–48 h.

Commercial FISH chromosome 'paints' are available. These comprise cosmid libraries of chromosome-specific sequences. Application of these paints allows the characterization of chromosomal material of unknown origin (Fig. 23.7), and can be effective in determining the prognosis for some cases of de novo chromosome abnormalities detected prenatally.

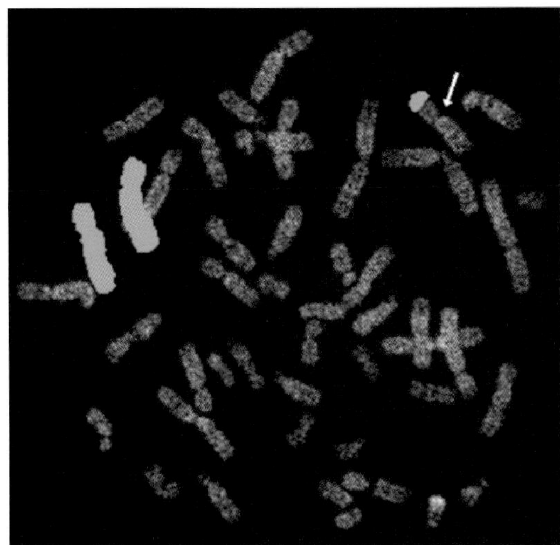

Fig. 23.7 Whole chromosome paint specific for chromosome 5, showing hybridization to both homologues of chromosome 5. Previously unidentified material on chromosome 8 (indicated by arrow) is shown to originate from chromosome 5.

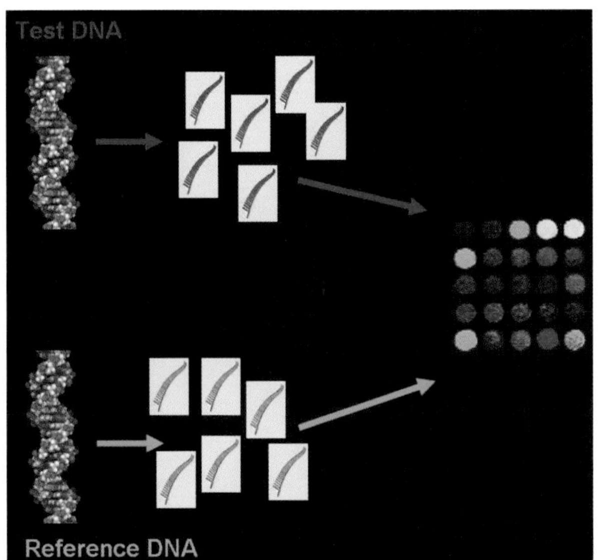

Fig. 23.8 Theory of microarray testing. Reference DNA is shown in green and test DNA in red. The box shows differential hybridization to the targets on the microarray, reflecting copy number differences between test and reference samples.

Microarray comparative genomic hybridization (CGH)

A sophisticated extension of the FISH approach is to fix small regions of the genome (usually either clones from bacterial artificial chromosomes (BACs), ≈100 Kb in length, or oligonucleotides (≈60 base pairs)) onto glass slides, to form microarrays, generally designed to include regions across the whole genome. Patient DNA is extracted, labeled with a fluorochrome, mixed with a reference DNA pool (labeled with a different fluorochrome), then hybridized to the microarray slide (Fig. 23.8). The two differentially labeled DNA pools compete for the targets on the microarray; if the patient has a deletion or duplication, this can be detected by a difference in the intensity ratio between the two different fluorochromes. This technology is still being

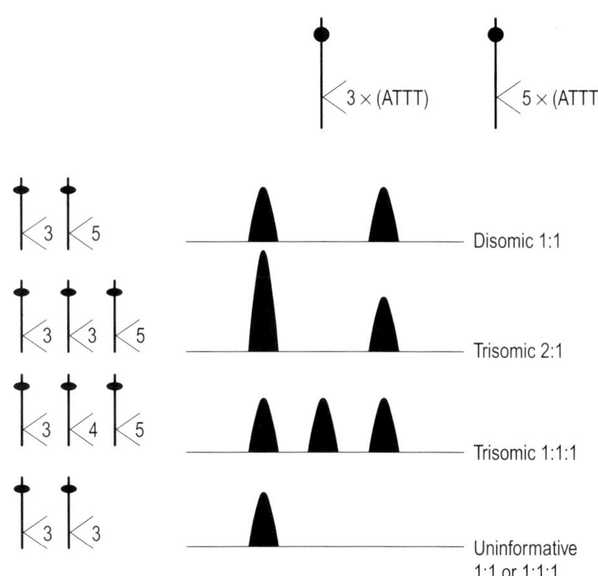

Fig. 23.9 Cartoon illustrating the theory of QF-PCR. ATTT is a representative tetranucleotide microsatellite; different combinations of repeat lengths are shown on the chromosomes at left, the electrophoretic peak patterns corresponding to these are shown in the middle, and the interpretation from the peak patterns is shown on the right.

developed and, although extensively used in genetic research, has yet to be generally implemented in diagnostic laboratories. Specific microarrays designed for prenatal diagnosis have been produced and marketed commercially, but their application has been hindered by concerns as to the accuracy of the test and the uncertainty as to the clinical significance of many areas of small segment imbalance, as well as by the current high cost of this test. CNVs detectable by karyotype analysis have been described (see above); a recent publication detailing sub-microscopic CNVs present in the normal population, detected by microarray analysis, underlines the prevalence of these variable areas[55], and much work needs to be done before a robust prenatal microarray, which detects only clinically significant imbalance, can be designed.

QF-PCR

Quantitative fluorescence polymerase chain reaction (QF-PCR) is a molecular diagnostic technique which has been introduced into many cytogenetic laboratories, usually for the purposes of rapid prenatal trisomy detection[56–58]. This elegant technology exploits the existence of 'microsatellite markers' throughout the genome. These microsatellites are stretches of DNA comprising repeat motifs of usually two, three or four nucleotides, and are polymorphic in the general population (for instance, for any individual, their two homologues of chromosome 21 are likely to have microsatellites of different lengths at any one locus); these microsatellite markers are used to provide genetic 'fingerprinting' for forensic testing.

QF-PCR utilizes primers specific to regions surrounding the microsatellites to amplify the DNA; PCR products of different sizes are then separated by capillary electrophoresis. The pattern of peaks produced can be used to infer the chromosome copy number in the sample (Figs 23.9 and 23.10). Prenatally,

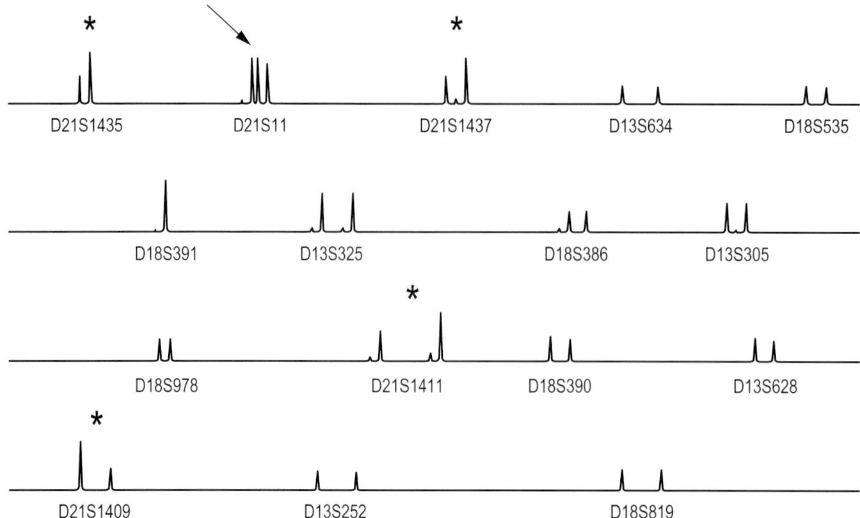

Fig. 23.10 Electrophoretogram showing the results of QF-PCR multiplex testing of markers on chromosome 13, 18 and 21. The marker names are shown. The sample tested showed trisomy 21, as indicated by the 2:1 or 1:2 peak ratios (starred) and the 3 allele peak pattern (arrowed). The markers for chromosomes 13 and 18 are either homozygous, or show normal 1:1 diallelic ratios.

this efficient and high-throughput technique is applied in the same way as FISH, i.e. for the rapid exclusion or confirmation of trisomy 13, 18 and 21, and for determining sex chromosome copy number abnormalities, where appropriate[59]. QF-PCR is very considerably cheaper and more efficient than FISH[60] and has economy of scale, meaning that a single center can offer this diagnostic service for a large catchment area. It has advantages over karyotyping in the detection of mosaicism (when the abnormal cell line is present at a level greater than or equal to 15%), as DNA is extracted from all cell types in the sample, rather than relying on the examination of clonal populations of only one cell type. In addition, it detects maternal cell contamination, which can be difficult to detect by other methods, especially where the fetus is female.

Commercial kits for QF-PCR have recently become available; some of these are CE-marked and therefore suitable for clinical diagnostics and the availability of such kits simplifies the introduction of rapid testing into cytogenetic laboratories, as development and validation of in-house protocols is no longer necessary.

Over 40000 cases of rapid diagnosis by QF-PCR have now been reported[57,61], with only a handful of cases where the diagnosis has been discordant with the karyotype result from cultured cells[62,63]. These discordant cases have all been the result of extreme mosaicism in chorionic villus biopsies and underline the problems associated with this sample type. Since the report of these discordant cases, the recommended protocols for laboratory preparation of chorionic villus samples have been revised to minimize these discrepancies[62,64].

a

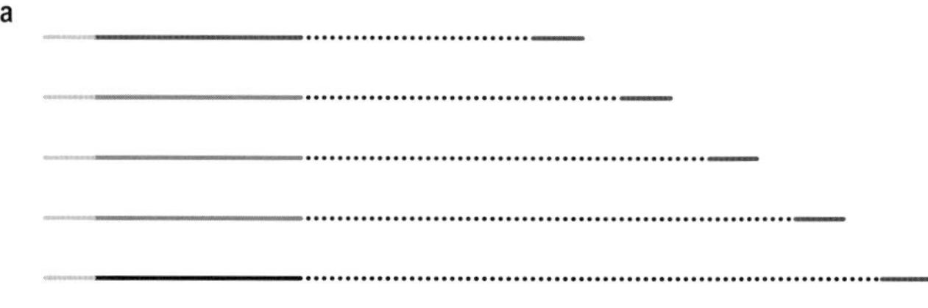

b

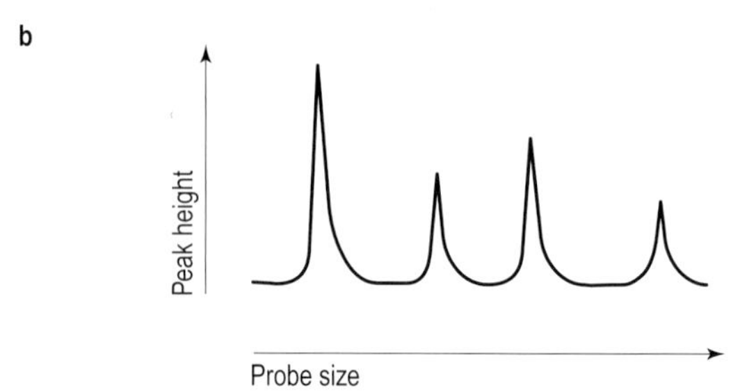

Fig. 23.11 Cartoon illustrating MLPA. (a) Region-specific probes, after ligation and dissociation from the target DNA, are shown in different shades, and have 'stuffer' fragments (shown by dotted line) to create different lengths of DNA. Each probe has the same PCR forward and reverse primer targets at each end, allowing amplification of all probes in a single PCR reaction. (b) Detail of an electrophoretic trace of PCR products. Peak heights for each probe are compared with the heights of the same probe in control samples to assess copy number in the test material.

MLPA

Multiplex ligation-dependent probe amplification (MLPA) is, like QF-PCR, a molecular method for counting copy number of stretches of DNA[65]. However, in this case, the technology relies on probes for specific genomic regions. The probes are formed of two parts which anneal end to end on the target sequence; a ligase enzyme joins the two parts of the probe together and, following disaggregation from the target DNA, PCR amplification is carried out, using specific primer targets spliced to each end of the probe. Each probe set provided in the commercial kits contains probes with a range of different sizes, but all with the same PCR primer sequences; this means that around 40 different targets can be tested simultaneously using only a single pair of PCR primers; the different products are then separated according to size by capillary electrophoresis (Fig. 23.11). As well as a number of applications for postnatal diagnosis, there is a commercial kit available specifically for prenatal detection of the common trisomies and this technique is in routine use in a number of centers, mostly in mainland Europe[66]. The disadvantage in comparison with QF-PCR is that maternal cell contamination is difficult to detect (and undetectable when the fetus is female) and, in addition, MLPA is unlikely to detect mosaicism[67].

Other molecular techniques

Other approaches for the detection of trisomies have been suggested, but none has so far been incorporated into clinical diagnostic service. These approaches include homologous gene quantitative PCR (HGQ-PCR)[68] and real-time PCR[69]. These techniques have some potential advantages over QF-PCR (for instance, they will be informative for all samples, as microsatellite markers are not required). However, these quantitative PCR approaches have limitations: while the QF-PCR approach exploits a 2:1 diallelic ratio and/or a qualitative triallelic result, the two other PCR approaches require a more subtle 3:2 dosage ratio to identify trisomy and, for this reason, may be less sensitive for the detection of trisomy mosaicism; in addition, triploidy and maternal cell contamination are not detectable if the fetus is female.

TARGETED TESTING

As technology has led to the introduction of new techniques for the detection of chromosome abnormalities, cytogeneticists and other professionals have been addressing the question as to the appropriate use of the different techniques for different referral indications. Karyotyping has long been regarded as the 'gold standard' of prenatal diagnosis, partly because it has always been used, and partly because it detects more abnormalities than more targeted tests such as FISH or QF-PCR. However, even more abnormalities could be discovered by testing for a range of microdeletion syndromes and subtelomere abnormalities using FISH or MLPA, or by testing for imbalance across the genome by using microarray technology, or by looking for single gene abnormalities such as ΔF508 mutations in the cystic fibrosis transmembrane regulator gene, or triplet repeat expansions in the Huntington gene. Most professionals consider it inappropriate to use these very detailed tests in the majority of cases, especially those where the referral indication is a raised risk of trisomy 21, and especially in the context of a state-funded health service. Financial implications are not the only consideration, however; there is also the uncertainty as to the significance to the fetus of some findings and the difficulty of ensuring fully informed consent from the patients.

This argument has now been extended to question the need for karyotype analysis on samples referred solely for raised risk of Down's syndrome. A number of publications have detailed audits of karyotype abnormalities found in prenatal samples in this referral group[48,70–74]. These audits suggest that rapid testing by FISH or QF-PCR without karyotype analysis for this group would mean that between one in 1000 and one in 1400 pregnancies would have a karyotype abnormality likely to lead to poor pregnancy outcome, which would not be detected by rapid testing. The advantage of this approach would be that parental concern over equivocal findings and, in some cases, potentially unnecessary pregnancy termination would be avoided and pre-test counseling would be greatly simplified. This proposal has been extensively discussed in the literature[48,50,70,72,73,75,76]; its adoption would underline a paradigm shift in prenatal diagnosis, from 'more knowledge is always better' to the benefits of targeted testing, where the outcome following an abnormal result can always be predicted and presented clearly to the patients. The UK National Screening Committee is shortly to be issuing guidelines on this subject.

FUTURE PROSPECTS

The most exciting way ahead for prenatal diagnosis of chromosome aneuploidy lies in the possibility of non-invasive investigations, i.e. the isolation of fetal cells[77] and/or DNA[78] from maternal blood, and the testing of this material. Developments in this area, especially for fetal sex and single gene defects, are progressing apace and are discussed in a separate chapter in this book. Determination of chromosome copy number, however, is more problematic; the use of FISH probes for chromosome 21 on fetal cells isolated from maternal blood can be used reliably only when a Y chromosome is also present in the cell, thus establishing fetal origin. QF-PCR technology has been shown in a research context[79] to be applicable to the ascertainment of chromosome copy number in fetal cells from maternal circulation, with around ten cells giving sufficient DNA for diagnosis. Fetal origin can be established by parallel testing of maternal cells from the same sample and comparison of allele sizes, regardless of the sex of the fetus.

Improvements in the isolation from maternal blood and identification of fetal cells and free fetal nucleic acids, extensive trials and streamlining of throughput will be necessary before this technology can be put in place for wide-scale screening of pregnant women for trisomy 21; even when in place, abnormal results may require confirmation by an invasive test before therapeutic pregnancy termination. However, this test could be applied to all pregnant women, allowing a much higher detection rate for Down's syndrome, with no concomitant risk to the pregnancy.

REFERENCES

1. Tijo H, Levan A. The chromosome numbers of man. *Hereditas* **42**:1–6, 1956.
2. Ford CE, Hamerton JL. The chromosomes of man. *Nature* **178**(4541):1020–1023, 956.
3. Lejeune J, Gautier M, Turpin R. Study of somatic chromosomes from 9 mongoloid children. *CR Hebd Seances Acad Sci* **248**(11):1721–1722, 1959.
4. Ford CE, Jones KW, Polani PE, De Almeida JC, Briggs JH. A sex-chromosome anomaly in a case of gonadal dysgenesis (Turner's syndrome). *Lancet* **1**(7075):711–713, 1959.
5. Jacobs PA, Strong JA. A case of human intersexuality having a possible XXY sex-determining mechanism. *Nature* **183**(4657):302–303, 959.
6. Patau K, Smith DW, Therman E, Inhorn SL, Wagner HP. Multiple congenital anomaly caused by an extra autosome. *Lancet* **1**:790–793, 1960.
7. Edwards JH, Harnden DG, Cameron AH, Crosse VM, Wolff OH. A new trisomic syndrome. *Lancet* **1**:787–790, 1960.
8. Caspersson T, Farber S, Foley GE et al. Chemical differentiation along metaphase

chromosomes. *Exp Cell Res* **49**(1):219–222, 1968.

9. ISCN. *An international system for human cytogenetic nomenclature*. Basle: S Karger, 2005.
10. Penrose LS. The relative aetiological importance of birth order and maternal age in mongolism. *Proc Roy Soc Lond* **115**:431–450, 1934.
11. Wald NJ, Bestwick JP, Morris JK. Cross trimester marker ratios: parameter estimates valid with no inconsistency. *Prenat Diagn* **26**(10):994, 2006.
12. Miller OJ, Therman E. *Human chromosomes*, 4th edn. New York: Springer-Verlag, 2001.
13. Linden MG, Bender BG. Fifty-one prenatally diagnosed children and adolescents with sex chromosome abnormalities. *Am J Med Genet* **110**(1): 11–18, 2002.
14. Lyon MF. The William Allan memorial award address: X-chromosome inactivation and the location and expression of X-linked genes. *Am J Hum Genet* **42**(1):8–16, 1988.
15. Carrel L, Cottle AA, Goglin KC, Willard HF. A first-generation X-inactivation profile of the human X chromosome. *Proc Natl Acad Sci USA* **96**(25):14440–14444, 1999.
16. Lindor NM, Ney JA, Gaffey TA, Jenkins RB, Thibodeau SN, Dewald GW. A genetic review of complete and partial hydatidiform moles and nonmolar triploidy. *Mayo Clin Proc* **67**(8):791–799, 1992.
17. McFadden DE, Robinson WP. Phenotype of triploid embryos. *J Med Genet* **43**(7): 609–612, 2006.
18. Daniel A, Wu Z, Bennetts B et al. Karyotype, phenotype and parental origin in 19 cases of triploidy. *Prenat Diagn* **21**(12):1034–1048, 2001.
19. Daniel A, Wu Z, Darmanian A, Collins F, Jackson J. Three different origins for apparent triploid/diploid mosaics. *Prenat Diagn* **23**(7):529–534, 2003.
20. Helwani MN, Seoud M, Zahed L, Zaatari G, Khalil A, Slim R. A familial case of recurrent hydatidiform molar pregnancies with biparental genomic contribution. *Hum Genet* **105**(1–2):112–115, 1999.
21. Sarno AP, Jr., Moorman AJ, Kalousek DK. Partial molar pregnancy with fetal survival: an unusual example of confined placental mosaicism. *Obstet Gynecol* **82** (4 Pt 2 Suppl):716–719, 1993.
22. Donaghue C, Mann K, Docherty Z, Ogilvie CM. Detection of mosaicism for primary trisomies in prenatal samples by QF-PCR and karyotype analysis. *Prenat Diagn* **25**(1):65–72, 2005.
23. Vejerslev LO, Mikkelsen M. The European collaborative study on mosaicism in chorionic villus sampling: data from 1986 to 1987. *Prenat Diagn* **9**(8):575–588, 1989.
24. Ledbetter DH, Zachary JM, Simpson JL et al. Cytogenetic results from the US Collaborative Study on CVS. *Prenat Diagn* **12**(5):317–345, 1992.
25. Wang BB, Rubin CH, Williams J, 3rd. Mosaicism in chorionic villus sampling: an analysis of incidence and chromosomes involved in 2612 consecutive cases. *Prenat Diagn* **13**(3):179–190, 1993.
26. Grati FR, Grimi B, Frascoli G et al. Confirmation of mosaicism and uniparental disomy in amniocytes, after detection of mosaic chromosome abnormalities in chorionic villi. *Eur J Hum Genet* **14**(3):282–288, 2006.
27. Smith K, Lowther G, Maher E, Hourihan T, Wilkinson T, Wolstenholme J. The predictive value of findings of the common aneuploidies, trisomies 13, 18 and 21, and numerical sex chromosome abnormalities at CVS: experience from the ACC UK Collaborative Study. Association of Clinical Cytogeneticists Prenatal Diagnosis Working Party. *Prenat Diagn* **19**(9):817–826, 1999.
28. Pindar L, Whitehouse M, Ocraft K. A rare case of a false-negative finding in both direct and culture of a chorionic villus sample. *Prenat Diagn* **12**(6):525–527, 1992.
29. Hahnemann JM, Vejerslev LO. Accuracy of cytogenetic findings on chorionic villus sampling (CVS) – diagnostic consequences of CVS mosaicism and non-mosaic discrepancy in centres contributing to EUCROMIC 1986–1992. *Prenat Diagn* **17**(9):801–820, 1997.
30. Gardner RJM, Sutherland GR. *Chromosome abnormalities and genetic counseling*, 3rd edn. New York: Oxford University Press, 2004.
31. Scriven PN. Communicating chromosome rearrangements and their outcomes using simple computer-generated color ideograms. *Genet Test* **2**(1):71–74, 1998.
32. Van Dyke DL, Weiss L, Roberson JR, Babu VR. The frequency and mutation rate of balanced autosomal rearrangements in man estimated from prenatal genetic studies for advanced maternal age. *Am J Hum Genet* **35**(2):301–308, 1983.
33. Warburton D. De novo balanced chromosome rearrangements and extra marker chromosomes identified at prenatal diagnosis: clinical significance and distribution of breakpoints. *Am J Hum Genet* **49**(5):995–1013, 1991.
34. Daniel A. Distortion of female meiotic segregation and reduced male fertility in human Robertsonian translocations: consistent with the centromere model of co-evolving centromere DNA/centromeric histone (CENP-A). *Am J Med Genet* **111**(4):450–452, 2002.
35. Stene J, Sten-gel-Rutowski S. Genetics risks of familial reciprocal and Robertsonian translocation carriers. In *The cytogenetics of mammalian autosomal rearrangements*, A Daniel (ed.), pp. 3–72. New York: Alan R. Liss, 1988.
36. Pettenati MJ, Von Kap-Herr C, Jackle B et al. Rapid interphase analysis for prenatal diagnosis of translocation carriers using subtelomeric probes. *Prenat Diagn* **22**(3):193–197, 2002.
37. Therman E, Laxova R, Susman B. The critical region on the human Xq. *Hum Genet* **85**(5):455–461, 1990.
38. Hsu LY. Phenotype/karyotype correlations of Y chromosome aneuploidy with emphasis on structural aberrations in postnatally diagnosed cases. *Am J Med Genet* **53**(2):108–140, 1994.
39. Waters JJ, Campbell PL, Crocker AJ, Campbell CM. Phenotypic effects of balanced X-autosome translocations in females: a retrospective survey of 104 cases reported from UK laboratories. *Hum Genet* **108**(4):318–327, 2001.
40. Powell CM, Taggart RT, Drumheller TC et al. Molecular and cytogenetic studies of an X-autosome translocation in a patient with premature ovarian failure and review of the literature. *Am J Med Genet* **52**(1): 19–26, 1994.
41. Liehr T, Mrasek K, Weise A et al. Small supernumerary marker chromosomes – progress towards a genotype-phenotype correlation. *Cytogenet Genome Res* **112** (1–2):23–34, 2006.
42. Baldwin EL, May LF, Justice AN, Martin CL, Ledbetter DH. Mechanisms and consequences of small supernumerary marker chromosomes: from Barbara McClintock to modern genetic counselling issues. *Am J Hum Genet* **82**:398–410, 2008.
43. Crolla JA, Harvey JF, Sitch FL, Dennis NR. Supernumerary marker 15 chromosomes: a clinical, molecular and FISH approach to diagnosis and prognosis. *Hum Genet* **95**(2):161–170, 1995.
44. Engel E, Antonarakis S. *Genomic imprinting and uniparental disomy in medicine. Clinical and molecular aspects*. New York: Wiley-Liss, 2002.
45. Robinson WP, Barrett IJ, Bernard L et al. Meiotic origin of trisomy in confined placental mosaicism is correlated with presence of fetal uniparental disomy, high levels of trisomy in trophoblast, and increased risk of fetal intrauterine growth restriction. *Am J Hum Genet* **60**(4):917–927, 1997.
46. Yong PJ, Marion SA, Barrett IJ, Kalousek DK, Robinson WP. Evidence for imprinting on chromosome 16: the effect of uniparental disomy on the outcome of mosaic trisomy 16 pregnancies. *Am J Med Genet* **112**(2):123–132, 2002.
47. Barber JC. Directly transmitted unbalanced chromosome abnormalities and euchromatic variants. *J Med Genet* **42**(8):609–629, 2005.
48. Mackie Ogilvie C, Lashwood A, Chitty L, Waters JJ, Scriven PN, Flinter F. The future of prenatal diagnosis: rapid testing or full karyotype? An audit of chromosome abnormalities and pregnancy outcomes for

women referred for Down's syndrome testing. Br J Obstetr Gynaecol In Press, 2005.

49. Klinger K, Landes G, Shook D et al. Rapid detection of chromosome aneuploidies in uncultured amniocytes by using fluorescence in situ hybridization (FISH). *Am J Hum Genet* **51**(1):55–65, 1992.
50. Lewin P, Kleinfinger P, Bazin A, Mossafa H, Szpiro-Tapia S. Defining the efficiency of fluorescence in situ hybridization on uncultured amniocytes on a retrospective cohort of 27407 prenatal diagnoses. *Prenat Diagn* **20**(1):1–6, 2000.
51. Raymond FL, Simpson JM, Mackie CM, Sharland GK. Prenatal diagnosis of 22q11 deletions: a series of five cases with congenital heart defects. *J Med Genet* **34**(8):679–682, 1997.
52. Scriven PN, Handyside AH, Ogilvie CM. Chromosome translocations: segregation modes and strategies for preimplantation genetic diagnosis. *Prenat Diagn* **18**(13):1437–1449, 1998.
53. Ogilvie CM, Braude P, Scriven PN. Successful pregnancy outcomes after preimplantation genetic diagnosis (PGD) for carriers of chromosome translocations. *Hum Fertil (Camb)* **4**(3):168–171, 2001.
54. Munne S, Sandalinas M, Escudero T, Fung J, Gianaroli L, Cohen J. Outcome of preimplantation genetic diagnosis of translocations. *Fertil Steril* **73**(6):1209–1218, 2000.
55. Redon R, Ishikawa S, Fitch KR, Feuk L, Perry GH, Andrews TD et al. Global variation in copy number in the human genome. *Nature* **444**(7118):444–454, 2006.
56. Mann K, Fox SP, Abbs SJ et al. Development and implementation of a new rapid aneuploidy diagnostic service within the UK National Health Service and implications for the future of prenatal diagnosis. *Lancet* **358**(9287):1057–1061, 2001.
57. Ogilvie CM, Donaghue C, Fox SP, Docherty Z, Mann K. Rapid prenatal diagnosis of aneuploidy using quantitative fluorescence-PCR (QF-PCR). *J Histochem Cytochem* **53**(3):285–288, 2005.
58. Cirigliano V, Ejarque M, Canadas MP et al. Clinical application of multiplex quantitative fluorescent polymerase chain reaction (QF-PCR) for the rapid prenatal detection of common chromosome aneuploidies. *Mol Hum Reprod* **7**(10): 1001–1006, 2001.
59. Donaghue C, Roberts A, Mann K, Ogilvie CM. Development and targeted application of a rapid QF-PCR test for sex chromosome imbalance. *Prenat Diagn* **23**(3):201–210, 2003.
60. Hulten MA, Dhanjal S, Pertl B. Rapid and simple prenatal diagnosis of common chromosome disorders: advantages and disadvantages of the molecular methods FISH and QF-PCR. *Reproduction* **126**(3):279–297, 2003.
61. Cirigliano V, Voglino G, Marongiu A et al. Rapid prenatal diagnosis by QF-PCR: evaluation of 30,000 consecutive clinical samples and future applications. *Ann NY Acad Sci* **1075**:288–298, 2006.
62. Waters JJ, Mann K, Grimsley, et al. Complete discrepancy between QF-PCR analysis of uncultured villi and karyotyping of cultured cells in the prenatal diagnosis of trisomy 21 in three CVS. *Prenat Diagn* In Press, 2007.
63. Waters JJ, Walsh S, Levett LJ, Liddle S, Akinfenwa Y. Complete discrepancy between abnormal fetal karyotypes predicted by QF-PCR rapid testing and karyotyped cultured cells in a first-trimester CVS. *Prenat Diagn* **26**(10):892–897, 2006.
64. Mann K, Kabba M, Donaghue C, Hills A, Mackie Ogilvie C. Analysis of a chromosomally mosaic placenta to assess the cell populations in dissociated chorionic villi: implications for QF-PCR aneuploidy testing. Prenat Diagn **27**:In Press, 2007.
65. Schouten JP, McElgunn CJ, Waaijer R, Zwijnenburg D, Diepvens F, Pals G. Relative quantification of 40 nucleic acid sequences by multiplex ligation-dependent probe amplification. *Nucl Acids Res* **30**(12):e57, 2002.
66. Gerdes T, Kirchhoff M, Lind AM, Larsen GV, Schwartz M, Lundsteen C. Computer-assisted prenatal aneuploidy screening for chromosome 13, 18, 21, X and Y based on multiplex ligation-dependent probe amplification (MLPA). *Eur J Hum Genet* **13**(2):171–175, 2005.
67. Mann K, Donaghue C, Fox SP, Docherty Z, Mackie Ogilvie C. Strategies for the rapid prenatal diagnosis of chromosome aneuploidy. *Eur J Hum Genet* **12**:907–915, 2004.
68. Deutsch S, Choudhury U, Sylvan A, Antonarakis SE. Detection of trisomy 21 and other aneuploidies by paralogous gene quantification. *Am J Hum Genet* **73**(5):318, 2003.
69. Zimmermann B, Holzgreve W, Wenzel F, Hahn S. Novel real-time quantitative PCR test for trisomy 21. *Clin Chem* **48**(2): 362–363, 2002.
70. Thein AT, Abdel-Fattah SA, Kyle PM, Soothill PW. An assessment of the use of interphase FISH with chromosome specific probes as an alternative to cytogenetics in prenatal diagnosis. *Prenat Diagn* **20**(4): 275–280, 2000.
71. Ryall RG, Callen D, Cocciolone R et al. Karyotypes found in the population declared at increased risk of Down's syndrome following maternal serum screening. *Prenat Diagn* **21**(7):553–557, 2001.
72. Leung WC, Lau ET, Lao TT, Tang MH. Can amnio-polymerase chain reaction alone replace conventional cytogenetic study for women with positive biochemical screening for fetal Down syndrome? *Obstet Gynecol* **101**(5 Pt 1):856–861, 2003.
73. Caine A, Maltby AE, Parkin CA, Waters JJ, Crolla JA. Prenatal detection of Down's syndrome by rapid aneuploidy testing for chromosomes 13, 18, and 21 by FISH or PCR without a full karyotype: a cytogenetic risk assessment. *Lancet* **366**(9480):123–128, 2005.
74. Chitty LS, Kagan KO, Molina FS, Waters JJ, Nicolaides KH. Fetal nuchal translucency scan and early prenatal diagnosis of chromosomal abnormalities by rapid aneuploidy screening: observational study. *Br Med J* **332**(7539):452–455, 2006.
75. Thilaganathan B, Sairam S, Ballard T, Peterson C, Meredith R. Effectiveness of prenatal chromosomal analysis using multicolor fluorescent in situ hybridisation. *Br J Obstet Gynaecol* **107**(2):262–266, 2000.
76. Ogilvie CM. Prenatal diagnosis for chromosome abnormalities: past, present and future. *Pathol Biol (Paris)* **51**(3):156–160, 2003.
77. Bianchi DW. Fetal cells in the maternal circulation: feasibility for prenatal diagnosis. *Br J Haematol* **105**(3):574–583, 1999.
78. Lo YM, Tein MS, Lau TK et al. Quantitative analysis of fetal DNA in maternal plasma and serum: implications for noninvasive prenatal diagnosis. *Am J Hum Genet* **62**(4):768–775, 1998.
79. Samura O, Pertl B, Sohda S et al. Female fetal cells in maternal blood: use of DNA polymorphisms to prove origin. *Hum Genet* **107**(1):28–32, 2000.

CHAPTER

24 Mendelian genetics – the old and the new

J Michael Connor

KEY POINTS

- Mendelian or single gene disorders are caused by mutations in one or both members of a gene pair
- These conditions have characteristic patterns of inheritance and often carry high recurrence risks for family members
- Completion of the human genome program and the resulting ability to analyze increasing numbers of single gene disorders at a molecular level has revealed many fallacies in our traditional teaching
- The true total number of human genes is 20–25 000 not 50–150 000 as originally predicted
- Gene mutations are not always stable and over 140 single gene disorders show this with consequent variation in disease severity within each family
- Most autosomal genes are expressed from both parental chromosomes as expected from classical Mendelian genetics but, in about 100, only the maternal or paternal gene is active
- Single gene disorders are not as distinct from other types of inherited disorder as was previously thought
- Few single gene disorders are truly only the product of one gene pair and influence from other genes is the norm although our knowledge about these is still limited
- The original belief that single gene disorders were the simplest type of inherited disorder is thus no longer the case and this contributed to the limited success of early attempts at gene therapy

INTRODUCTION

Inherited disorders may be caused by visible changes in the chromosomes (chromosomal disorders, e.g. Down's syndrome), by interactions of multiple genes often with environmental factors (multifactorial or part-genetic diseases, e.g. hypertension), by an accumulation of multiple genetic mutations often including visible changes to chromosomes (cumulative genetic diseases, e.g. cancer) or by mutations in single genes. This last category of genetic disease is the topic of this chapter. However, as will become apparent, the distinction from the other types of genetic disease is nowadays increasingly blurred.

Mendel, from plant breeding crosses, realized that some characteristics were genetically determined in a simple manner by a pair of genes (one on each of the partner chromosomes). Some characteristics were present if only one of the pair of genes was altered from the normal form, whereas others were only present if both members of the gene pair were altered. This type of simple inheritance applies to many human diseases and is either termed single gene inheritance or mendelian inheritance after its discoverer. Single gene disorders which show the disease when only one member of the gene pair is altered (mutated) are termed dominant and those which only show the disease when both members of the gene pair are mutated are termed recessive.

Aside from dominant and recessive single gene disorders, there is a further subdivision. Human single gene disorders include multiple conditions which are caused by mutations in genes on the X chromosome. These have very characteristic patterns of inheritance due to the fact that males have only one X chromosome (with an accompanying Y chromosome which has predominantly genes for male sex determination), whereas females have two X chromosomes. The remaining chromosomes in males and females can be paired and are termed the autosomes (numbered 1–22 in order of decreasing size). Thus, single gene disorders can be either due to mutations in autosomal genes and show dominant or recessive inheritance or be due to mutations in genes on the X chromosome (termed X-linked) and show dominant or recessive inheritance. Mutations in Y-linked genes can also occur but the resulting infertility precludes the expected characteristic pattern of inheritance from a father to all of his sons.

TRADITIONAL TEACHING ON SINGLE GENE DISORDERS

Numbers of single gene disorders

In older textbooks, the predicted number of human genes was generally estimated to be 50 000–150 000. At the same time, it was commonly believed that each gene would be matched to one protein and to one single gene disorder. It was also taught that once a gene had mutated, it was stable in the mutated form with a reverse mutation rate similar to the rare initial mutation rate.

Autosomal dominant inheritance

As indicated earlier, the affected person with an autosomal dominant disease has one mutant gene with a normal copy of the gene on the partner autosomal chromosome. He or she must hand on either the mutant or the normal gene and thus the recurrence risk for each child is 50% or 1 in 2. The gene is on an autosome rather than a sex chromosome and thus either sex can be affected with an equal degree of severity. In the family tree, these conditions are passed down from one generation to the next.

Although family members each have the same mutant gene, variable expression in the severity of the condition is commonly observed with autosomal dominant conditions. Further, some individuals with the mutant gene show no features of the disease and are said to be non-penetrant. This can be a particular problem when counseling apparently normal parents of an affected child. In this situation, the child may represent a new mutation in the gene (with a very low recurrence risk) or a parent may have the gene but be non-penetrant (and thus have a 50% recurrence risk). A further possibility is gonadal mosaicism. In this situation, an individual has two different cell lines. One cell line has a normal genetic constitution whereas the other has the mutant gene. If the cell line with the mutant gene is found in the gonad then the recurrence risk for each child is high. In contrast, if the cell line with the mutant gene is not found in the gonad (termed somatic mosaicism), then the recurrence risk is very low and equal to the new mutation rate. Depending on the condition, a mosaic person may show patchy or partial features of the disorder. The frequency of gonadal mosaicism differs between disorders. It is unclear why it is a frequent finding in some disorders such as fascioscapulohumeral muscular dystrophy and osteogenesis imperfecta whereas in others, such as achondroplasia, it is rare.

Autosomal recessive inheritance

In contrast to the autosomal dominant diseases, an autosomal recessive condition only occurs when both copies of the autosomal gene pair are mutant. The affected person inherits one copy of the mutant gene from each parent. The parents are outwardly normal despite carrying a single copy of the mutant gene as the effects are counterbalanced by the other normal copy of the gene. For these carrier parents the recurrence risk is high at 25% or 1 in 4. The condition can affect males or females with an equal degree of severity. In the family tree, these conditions usually occur in a single generation of a sibship (a group of brothers and sisters).

It is not unusual in some recessive disorders, such as sensorineural deafness, for two affected individuals to have children. For some, but not all of these couples, all of their children are deaf. This is to be expected if each parent has two copies of the same mutant gene. In other families where the parents are deaf but the offspring have normal hearing, the gene causing the deafness in the two parents is different and this is termed genetic or locus heterogeneity. These genetic look-a-likes cannot be distinguished clinically but can be identified by molecular genetic analysis.

The risk of an autosomal recessive condition is increased when there is parental consanguinity. Blood relatives are at an increased risk of sharing the same mutant genes for autosomal recessive conditions. Thus, parental consanguinity would be a clue that the disorder in the child was due to an autosomal recessive condition but it is not a prerequisite. Conversely, most children of parents who are consanguineous are healthy.

During human evolution there have been multiple factors (for example founder effects and selection pressures) which have influenced the carrier frequencies for autosomal recessive conditions in different populations. For example, the carrier frequency for sickle cell anemia is much higher in Africans than Caucasians and for cystic fibrosis is much lower in Africans than Caucasians.

X-linked recessive inheritance

X-linked recessive disorders have very characteristic patterns of inheritance. Males are affected with uniform severity and are linked in the family tree by outwardly normal females. These outwardly normal females who link the affected males are carriers of the mutant gene but its effects are counterbalanced by the normal copy of the gene on their partner X chromosome. For these carrier females, the recurrence risk is high with 50% or 1 in 2 of their sons being affected and 50% or 1 in 2 of their daughters being carriers.

While most female carriers are outwardly normal, some show mild features of the disease. This is caused by anomalous X-inactivation. Early in embryonic development, one of the X chromosomes in females is inactivated in each cell with the result that the female, like the male, has a single functional X chromosome in each cell. This process is normally random with on average half of the cells using the X chromosome inherited from the mother and half using the X chromosome from the father. If by chance the carrier mainly inactivates the normal X chromosome, mild features of the disease may be seen. This was useful for carrier detection in the days before modern molecular approaches became available.

X-linked dominant inheritance

In the family tree, an X-linked dominant disease can be easily mistaken for an autosomal dominant disorder but is identified by the facts that the affected males are more severely affected than the females and pass on the condition to all of their daughters but none of their sons. The recurrence risks are high for affected family members. An affected female will pass the condition on to, on average, 50% or 1 in 2 of her sons and daughters.

In some disorders due to mutant genes on the X chromosome, affected males are never or very rarely seen (e.g. incontinentia pigmenti and Goltz syndrome). This is thought to be due to the lethal effect in utero of the mutant gene in the male. An affected mother would hand the condition on to, on average, half of her daughters and would have an increased risk of early miscarriage.

NEW MENDELIAN GENETICS

Numbers of single gene disorders

With completion of the first human genome sequence in 2003, the true total of human genes is now known to be closer to 20–25 000[1,2] (as compared with the historical estimates of 50–150 000). The number is not yet exact as the boundaries of genes and the definition of functional sequences is still in progress. The total length of the DNA in each cell is 3164.7 million basepairs with 50–250 million basepairs per chromosome. Genes vary widely in size with an average of 3000 basepairs (3 kilobases, 3 kb) and the largest known gene is dystrophin (which when mutant causes Duchenne muscular dystrophy), which is 2.4 million basepairs in size (2.4 megabases, 2.4 Mb). Genes comprise only about 2% of the human genome; the remainder consists of non-coding regions, whose functions may include providing chromosomal structural integrity and regulating where, when, and in what quantity proteins are made. The total number of proteins produced by the genes is higher as there are many examples of the same gene producing more than one protein by alternative methods of transcription and translation[3]. At present, the function (s) are unknown for over 50% of the identified genes.

The availability of the normal sequence for each gene has allowed rapid progress in the delineation of the molecular pathology for each disorder[2,3]. Most conditions show molecular heterogeneity with multiple different mutations present in different patients (e.g. over 500 different mutations have been described in cystic fibrosis). Again, most conditions show genetic heterogeneity with more than one gene causing a similar or identical disease (e.g. multiple genes which when mutated can cause hereditary deafness).

Analysis of molecular pathology has also exposed the fallacy of the idea that mutations are always stable. This is exemplified by the common adult form of muscular dystrophy called myotonic dystrophy. This has long been known to be inherited as an autosomal dominant trait. In common with other autosomal dominant traits, it is expected to show variable expression of the features. For myotonic dystrophy, however, there was a tendency for the condition to show progressively more severe features as it passed down the generations (so-called anticipation). Thus, for a severely affected infant the mother might have mild muscle symptoms and her affected parent might only have adult onset cataracts (Fig. 24.1). Originally this apparent increase in severity was dismissed as a statistical fluke due to the way the families were identified. We now know that much of the clinical variation in myotonic dystrophy is due to instability of the genetic mutation in each individual. The mutation is a triplet repeat expansion in the gene for myotonic dystrophy and normally there are 5 to 37 repeats found in this gene. Once the number of repeats increases beyond 50, it becomes unstable with hundreds of repeats in adults with moderate disease and thousands of repeats in the congenitally affected children.

There are now 140 other examples of diseases caused by this type of unstable length mutation. In some of these, for example myotonic dystrophy, the expansion tends to increase in size when passed on by an affected mother, whereas in others, for example Huntington disease, the expansion tends to increase in size when passed on by an affected father[3].

Overlap of single gene disorders with chromosomal disorders

The smallest visible gain or loss from a chromosome when using a light microscope is 4 million base pairs of DNA (4 megabases). The average gene is about 3000 base pairs in length and thus a visible chromosomal change usually involves multiple genes. Smaller chromosomal changes are not visible with the light microscope, but can now be demonstrated by DNA analysis. These smaller changes are termed microdeletions and microduplications.

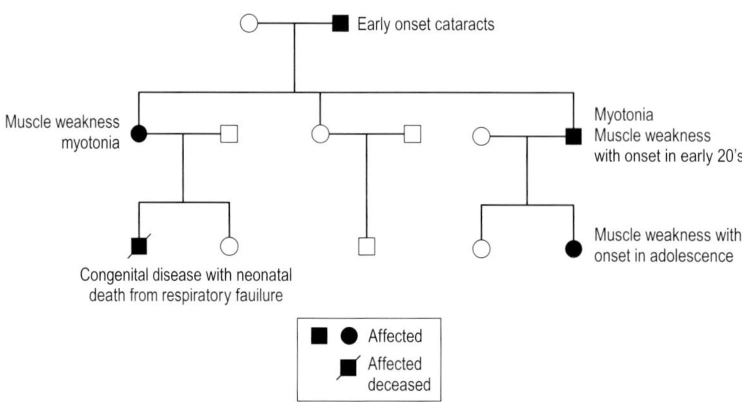

Fig. 24.1 Pedigree of a family with myotonic dystrophy demonstrating anticipation.

The smallest microdeletion would be the loss of a single base pair. If this lay within an important part of a gene this could cause a single gene disorder. A three base pair deletion is the commonest type of mutant gene seen in cystic fibrosis and, for some single gene disorders, such as Duchenne muscular dystrophy, larger deletions are the commonest type of molecular pathology. There is thus now a blurred boundary between single gene disorders and chromosomal disorders as a result of knowledge about the molecular basis of each.

Microdeletions can result in the loss of several neighboring genes and produce a contiguous gene disorder. For example, some patients with Duchenne muscular dystrophy also have X-linked adrenal hypoplasia when the deletion encompasses both of these genes. Coexistence of more than one single gene disorder in the same person is thus a clinical clue to the presence of a chromosomal microdeletion. Chromosomal deletions are commonly associated with learning difficulties. Unexpected coexistence of learning difficulties with a single gene disorder is a further clinical clue to the presence of a chromosomal deletion. For example, the presence of unexpected learning difficulties in a patient with polyposis coli and a chromosomal deletion of chromosome 5 was the clinical clue which led to the localization of the gene for polyposis coli[4].

Most autosomal genes are expressed from both parental chromosomes as expected from classical Mendelian genetics. However, a small number of genes (about 100) are expressed from only one parental gene, maternal or paternal depending on the gene. This phenomenon is termed genomic or genetic imprinting[5]. These imprinted genes are clustered into small regions on several chromosomes. One such region is on the long arm of chromosome 15. In part of this region, imprinted genes are paternally expressed/maternally silenced while neighboring genes are oppositely imprinted. A large DNA deletion in this region may cause Prader–Willi syndrome or the clinically very dissimilar Angelman syndrome, depending on whether the deletion is on the paternally or maternally transmitted chromosome. When it occurs on the paternal chromosome it causes Prader–Willi syndrome due to deletion of one or more paternally expressed imprinted genes. Conversely, when the deletion occurs on the maternal chromosome it causes Angelman syndrome due to functional loss of the maternally expressed genes.

Prader–Willi syndrome can also arise with apparently normal chromosomes. In this situation, the initial embryo is believed to have three copies of chromosome 15 (two from the mother and one from the father). Trisomy 15 is lethal but loss of one copy results in restitution of the normal chromosome number and this is termed trisomic rescue. If a paternal and maternal copy of chromosome 15 is retained, the child is normal but if both maternal copies of chromosome 15 are retained then Prader–Willi syndrome results due to lack of the paternally expressed genes from this region. This lack of a parental chromosome with both copies from the other parent is called uniparental disomy. Paternal uniparental disomy for chromosome 15 results in Angelman syndrome due to lack of maternally expressed genes from this region. Angelman syndrome can also be caused by point mutations in a key gene within this region, thus further blurring the boundary between single gene disorders and chromosomal disorders.

Hydatidiform moles and ovarian teratomas are extreme examples of diseases due to genomic imprinting. Benign ovarian teratomas are gynogenetic (i.e. no paternal contribution) in origin, arising from the parthogenetic development of unfertilized oocytes, whereas hydatidiform moles are androgenetic (i.e. no maternal contribution) and arise from fertilization of an 'empty' or defective oocyte by one or two sperm[5].

The nuclear chromosomes are not the only source of coding DNA in each cell. The typical human cell contains several hundred mitochondria which each possess their own DNA in the form of about 10 copies of a circular double helix of DNA in each mitochondrion. Each of these mitochondrial DNAs has 16569 base pairs and encodes for 37 mitochondrial proteins. Mutations in these genes can cause a variety of diseases which each show a characteristic pattern of inheritance[6]. Mitochondria are exclusively maternally inherited and so an affected mother passes the condition on to all of her children, whereas an affected father has normal children. The genes involved are concerned with mitochondrial energy production and their dysfunction typically affects tissues with high energy requirements (e.g. brain, skeletal muscle, heart, renal and endocrine systems). Usually, only a proportion of the cell's total mitochondria carry the mutant gene and thus the effect depends on the nature of the mutation, the tissue involved and the proportion of the mitochondria with the mutation in each cell. The clinical features thus tend to vary widely from one family member to the next and this often leads to initial misdiagnosis. The types of mutation in these mitochondrial chromosomal genes are no different from the types of mutation seen in other types of single gene disorders, which again blurs the boundary between single gene disorders and chromosomal disorders.

Overlap of single gene disorders with cumulative genetic disorders

In contrast to the other types of genetic disorder, for most cancers, the genetic mutations are not inherited and arise in somatic cells during adulthood as a result of exposure to environmental carcinogens. Multiple mutations are usually involved and this accumulation results in multiple steps which are reflected by the histopathological progression of a cancer. In 5–10% of some common cancers, including breast and colon cancer and in a higher percentage of certain rare cancer syndromes, the first mutation is inherited and, in these conditions, there is a high risk of cancer in relatives.

Formerly, these inherited forms of cancer could only be identified on the basis of pedigree analysis and large numbers of at-risk relatives had to be offered tumor surveillance even though many would turn out not to have the mutant gene. The management of these families has been greatly facilitated by mutation detection in the relevant genes using modern molecular genetic techniques. The types of mutation in these cancer-causing genes are no different from the types of mutation seen in other types of single gene disorders and so there is an overlap between mendelian disorders and cumulative genetic disorders.

Overlap of single gene disorders with part-genetic/multifactorial disorders

Unlike single gene disorders, part-genetic/multifactorial disorders do not show characteristic family trees. Often the affected individual is the only affected person in the family and the genetic contribution is demonstrated by showing an increased frequency in family members above the general population risk. There is probably a spectrum from true multifactorial disorders with many genes involved, each with a small but additive effect, to disorders with one or few genes involved with environmental triggers. Acute intermittent porphyria illustrates this point. This disorder is characterized by attacks of abdominal pain, constipation and psychiatric disturbances and is due to a mutation in a gene encoding an enzyme involved in hemoglobin biosynthesis. Attacks can be precipitated by certain drugs and, in the absence of such triggers, the patients are often asymptomatic. The family tree of a family with acute intermittent porphyria is usually not suggestive of an autosomal dominant trait and yet, with molecular testing, multiple family members will carry the same mutation with inheritance in this fashion. So is this a single gene disorder or actually the simplest type of multifactorial disorder with one gene and one environmental factor?

Single gene disorders commonly show genetic or locus heterogeneity. For example, inherited blindness due to retinitis pigmentosa can be caused by mutations in several different genes. In some families with retinitis pigmentosa, the condition can arise when a person is a carrier for two different recessive genes at different genetic locations[7]. This is termed digenic inheritance and the parents of the affected person will each be a carrier of one mutant gene and have normal vision. Digenic inheritance has also been demonstrated in inherited sensorineural deafness in which mutations in different deafness genes have been shown to interact in a synergistic manner[8].

Triallelic inheritance has been demonstrated in some families with Bardet–Biedel syndrome (BBS). This is a multisytem disorder characterized by obesity, retinal degeneration, polydactyly, malformations and developmental problems. Many families show autosomal recessive inheritance with genetic heterogeneity (nine gene loci so far identified). In some families with BBS, the condition only occurs when the patient has three mutant genes (two at one gene locus and one at another)[9].

The boundary between single gene disorders and multifactorial disorders is thus blurred. Information from studies of inbred animals have shown that the genetic background of an individual animal commonly influences the penetrance and expression of a mutant gene. Thus, it is likely that few conditions are truly single gene disorders and that influence from other genes is the norm. This is difficult to analyze but the contribution of a second gene to the risk of ovarian cancer in women carrying a mutation in the dominantly inherited breast/ovarian cancer gene (*BRCA1*) has been demonstrated[10].

Overlap of single gene disorders with inheritance of normal characteristics

The focus of this chapter has been on inherited diseases and it is easy to overlook the fact that the genes are responsible for normal inherited characteristics. Some of these characteristics, for example red–green colour blindness are inherited in a mendelian fashion, whereas for others, for example stature, part-genetic/multifactorial inheritance is apparent. Most of this variation is accepted as normal but there is a gray zone. For example, 1% of the population has a mutation in the gene for von Willebrand disease. A small proportion of these individuals are symptomatic with a hemorrhagic tendency, but the majority have few or no symptoms. This blurred boundary between normal genetic variation and genetic disease has hindered attempts to define the frequencies of genetic diseases.

CONCLUSION

It is always humbling to look at an older 'state of the art' textbook in the light of modern knowledge and, for genetics, the rapid pace of progress means that even quite recent teaching is erroneous. The traditional teaching about single gene disorders is clearly wrong in many respects and, increasingly, the distinction of single gene disorders from other types of inherited disease is blurred. The single gene disorders were originally viewed as the simplest types of inherited disease, but it is likely that few, if any, are caused by a single gene acting in isolation from other genes and the environment. This means that a full understanding of these conditions will take longer than originally anticipated once the human genome was sequenced. The bonus will hopefully be that this knowledge will speed up the understanding of the other types of genetic disorders which have been traditionally viewed as more complex.

REFERENCES

1. Human genome project information. Available http://www.ornl.gov/sci/techresources/Human_Genome/project/info.shtml
2. Online Mendelian Inheritance in Man (OMIM). Available http://www.ncbi.nlm.nih.gov/entrez/query.fcgi?db=OMIM
3. Antonarakis SE, Cooper DN. Mutations in human genetic disease. In *Emery and Rimoin's principles and practice of medical genetics*, 5th edn, DL Rimoin, JM Connor, RE Pyeritz, BR Korf (eds), pp. 101–128. Philadelphia: Churchill Livingstone Elsevier, 2007.
4. Bodmer WF, Bailey CJ, Bodmer J et al. Localisation of the gene for familial adenomatous polyposis on chromosome 5. *Nature* **328**:614–616, 1987.
5. Weksburg R, Sadowski P, Smith AC, Tycko B. Epigenetics. In *Emery and Rimoin's principles and practice of medical genetics*, 5th edn, DL Rimoin, JM Connor, RE Pyeritz, BR Korf (eds), pp. 81–100. Philadelphia: Churchill Livingstone Elsevier, 2007.
6. Wallace DC, Lott MT, Procaccio V. Mitochondrial genes in degenerative disease, cancer and aging. In *Emery and Rimoin's principles and practice of medical genetics*, 5th edn, DL Rimoin, JM Connor, RE Pyeritz, BR Korf (eds), pp. 194–298. Philadelphia: Churchill Livingstone Elsevier, 2007.
7. Kajiwara K, Berson E, Dryja T. Digenic retinitis pigmentosa due to mutations at the unlinked *peripherin/RDS* and *ROM1* loci. *Science* **264**:1604–1607, 1994.
8. Balciuiene J, Dahl N, Borg E et al. Evidence for digenic inheritance of nonsyndromic hererditary hearing loss in a Swedish family. *Am J Hum Genet* **63**:786–793, 1998.
9. Katsanis N, Ansley SJ, Badano JL et al. Triallelic inheritance in Bardet-Biedl syndrome, a Mendelian recessive disorder. *Science* **293**:2256–2259, 2001.
10. Phelan CM, Rebbeck TR, Weber BL et al. Ovarian cancer risk in BRCA1 carriers is modified by the HRAS1 variable number of tandem repeat (VNTR) locus. *Nat Genet* **12**:309–311, 1996.

CHAPTER 25

Preimplantation genetic diagnosis

Joyce C Harper and Joy DA Delhanty

KEY POINTS

- Biopsy is usually performed by removing 1–2 cells from the cleavage stage embryo, but the first/second polar body or trophectoderm cells can also be used
- The analysis of chromosomes is performed by FISH. This is the method of choice for sexing, for X-linked diseases, for the diagnosis of chromosomal abnormalities and for aneuploidy screening
- PCR is used for the diagnosis of monogenic disorders. Due to problems of contamination and allele drop out, methods usually include the mutation detection and informative markers
- Recent advances include the use of whole genome amplification for monogenic diagnosis and metaphase or array comparative genomic hybridization to analyze chromosomes
- There are several ethical issues surrounding PGD and, in some countries, PGD on cleavage stage embryos is prohibited. PGD is increasingly being used for disorders which are not routinely diagnosed at the prenatal stage

INTRODUCTION

The detection of genetic disease in the human embryo before implantation gives parents the chance of starting a pregnancy knowing that the baby will be free of the inherited disorder that is prevalent in their family. Pressure from several groups of patients for whom this approach held particular appeal led to the initiation of research towards this goal in the UK in the mid-1980s.

There are several groups of patients for whom preimplantation genetic diagnosis (PGD) is the preferred option. This includes patients who have already experienced prenatal diagnosis and the termination of an affected fetus, those who have moral or religious objections to termination of pregnancy, those who are carrying a translocation or other chromosomal abnormality and have experienced repeated miscarriages or infertility and those who are at risk of transmitting a genetic disease and are also infertile. More recently, some patients who themselves have a late onset disease, such as predisposition to inherited cancer where prenatal diagnosis is not normally indicated, have expressed a wish to have a healthy child by PGD. PGD has also been used for tissue typing so that the cord blood from the PGD baby can be used to treat an already existing ill child (savior siblings). World-wide, the use of PGD for sex selection for non-medical reasons is increasing.

THE APPROACH TO PREIMPLANTATION GENETIC DIAGNOSIS

The availability of in vitro fertilization (IVF) theoretically allows several approaches to genetic diagnosis at the preimplantation stage. These include polar body analysis or biopsy at the cleavage or blastocyst stage.

Polar body analysis

Initially, first polar body analysis to detect genetic disease appears attractive[1,2]. It allows preconception diagnosis and it is non-invasive of the embryo but, overall, the disadvantages outweigh the advantages. In the case of a mother who is a carrier for a monogenic disorder, the assumption would be that if the first polar body is positive for the mutant gene then the oocyte itself will carry the gene. However, the frequent crossing over between non-sister chromatids during first meiotic prophase in the human female leads to the situation where it is common to find the primary oocyte (and hence also the first polar body) carrying a chromosome that is heterozygous, with one chromatid bearing the mutation and the other normal. This situation is very difficult to detect technically, since there is a high probability that DNA from each chromatid will not amplify with equal efficiency during the polymerase chain reaction (PCR).

For many years, polar body analysis was only applied routinely by one center in the USA to avoid age-related aneuploidy in women aged 35 and above who were undergoing IVF treatment. The first, and/or in some cases, the second polar body was removed, spread on a slide and analyzed by fluorescent in situ hybridization (FISH) using DNA probes specific for chromosomes 18, 13/21 and X[3]. There were several difficulties with this approach. First, having carried out an enormous amount of work in dissecting and analyzing the first polar body, fewer than half of the analyzed oocytes were normally fertilized and available for transfer. Since a substantial proportion of aneuploidy involves chromatid anomalies, and some also arise at the second meiotic division, there was additional screening of the second polar body. Data from the ESHRE PGD Consortium has shown two trisomy 16 pregnancies resulting after first polar body biopsy for aneuploidy screening[4]. This is an unexpected finding since non-disjunction of chromosome 16 occurs during meiosis I and so should be detected by first polar body analysis. Data using probes for chromosomes 13,16,18,21 and 22 showed that the success rates overall in first and second polar body analysis amounted to 78%, meaning that almost one-quarter of the oocytes had to be discarded at the outset. The most frequent anomaly observed by far was the loss of a single chromatid from the first polar body; loss of a whole chromosome occurred with less than one-tenth of the frequency[5].

These data are completely at odds with that obtained from comprehensive research studies on human oocytes, which show chromatid and chromosome anomalies occurring with equal frequency[6]. The technique of comparative genomic hybridization (CGH), in which the whole genome is evaluated for chromosomal imbalance, has also been applied to testing of the first polar body in order to predict which mature oocytes are likely to have a normal karyotype; abnormal findings were confirmed by testing biopsied embryonic cells[7]. Due to legislation banning embryo biopsy in Germany and Italy, polar body biopsy for aneuploidy has recently been introduced to these two countries (in Italy only analysis of the first polar body is allowed).

Cleavage stage biopsy

The manipulation of embryos has been used in the bovine embryo transfer industry for many years. Adaptation of these techniques led to the successful biopsy of mouse[8] and human[9] embryos (Figure 25.1a).

In the human, the cryopresevation of embryos in IVF treatment cycles is routine, and from frozen embryo replacement cycles up to 50% of blastomeres can be destroyed and the embryo still is capable of producing a viable fetus. No increase in fetal abnormalities have been reported following transfer of cryopreserved embryos in which some cells have been destroyed by freezing/thawing. Studies examining the effect of embryo biopsy have shown that, at the eight-cell stage, removal of two cells was not detrimental to embryo metabolism or development[10] and is an efficient process with more than 90% of the embryos surviving. Biopsies performed at earlier stages (four cells) may alter the ratio of inner cell mass to trophectoderm cells which may be detrimental to embryo development[11]. Therefore, the main strategy used for embryo biopsy has been to biopsy embryos at the 6–10-cell stage, on day 3 post insemination. Removal of up to 25% of the embryo has been thought to be safe and not impair implantation or embryo development. To remove the blastomeres, acid Tyrodes solution, a laser or a mechanical method is used to drill a hole in the zona pellucida and the blastomeres are usually aspirated (Figure 25.1b)[4].

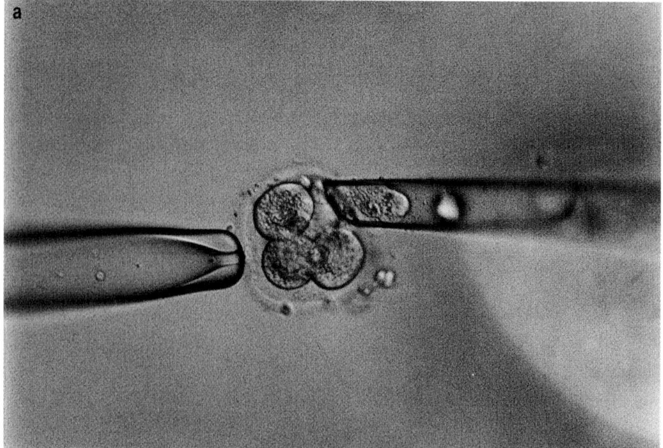

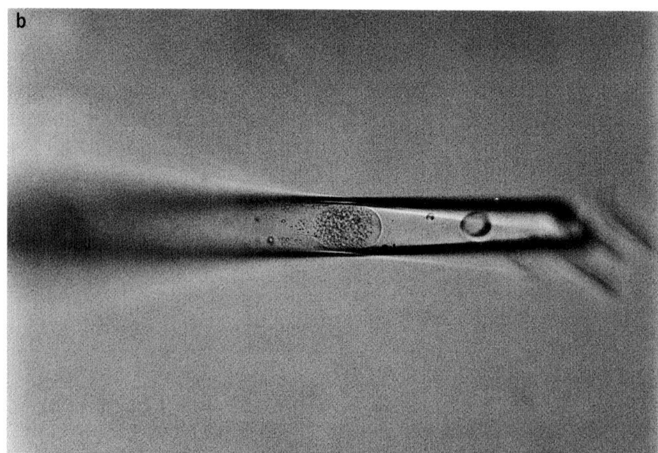

Fig. 25.1 (a) Cleavage stage embryo biopsy. (b) Blastomere aspiration. The blastomere can be seen in the capillary tube.

Two studies analyzed the pregnancies obtained from biopsied embryos after PGD[12,13]. Biochemical and ultrasound measurements showed that pregnancies did not show any significant developmental differences compared to controls, and deliveries, including birth weight and Apgar scores, were considered normal. Data from the ESHRE PGD Consortium have supported these findings[4,14–19].

Blastocyst biopsy

Blastocyst biopsy was first tried in murine blastocysts where a small slit was made in the zona pellucida and, as the blastomeres herniated through the slit, the cells were excised. Successful blastocyst biopsies have been performed in mice and primates with the delivery of healthy individuals[20,21]. In humans, blastocyst biopsy can be performed on day 5 or 6 post insemination[22,23]. Dokras et al.[22], using the herniation technique, examined human blastocyst viability by the production of human chorionic gonadotrophin (hCG) in vitro and found that the values for biopsied and non-biopsied controls were the same.

Development of this technique has been slow as more than 50% of cleavage stage human embryos arrest before the blastocyst stage[24]. For this reason, and since very little time would be available for the diagnosis, very few clinics use this approach[4], although one clinic has reported PGD cycles using blastocyst biopsy[25].

Blastocyst biopsy has the advantage that a larger number of cells can be removed from the outer trophectoderm (TE) layer without affecting the inner cell mass (ICM) from which the fetus later develops. However, TE may have diverged genetically from the ICM as in at least 1% of conceptions confined placental mosaicism (CPM) is observed, where the chromosome status of the embryo is different from the placenta. Also the TE is important in implantation. Removing a large percentage of this from the early blastocyst may adversely affect implantation.

CHROMOSOMAL ABNORMALITIES IN PREIMPLANTATION EMBRYOS

Since the successful generation of human preimplantation embryos in vitro, we have been able to examine chromosomes of early human embryos. As it is estimated that 60% of human conceptions are lost due to chromosome abnormalities, access to preimplantation embryos may eventually enable us to answer some of the questions as to why early human development is so error prone and have important consequences for PGD.

Karyotyping of human preimplantation embryos is problematic as it is difficult to arrest cells in metaphase but, using this technique, mosaicism, aneuploidy and ploidy abnormalities have been observed[26–29] and mosaicism with normal and aneuploid or polyploid cell lines appear to be the most common abnormality[28,30]. Early studies showed the existence of an embryo with trisomy 1[31], but this work highlights the problem with karyotyping, since from the eight-cell embryo, metaphase spreads were only obtained for two cells and so the possibility of mosaicism could not be explored.

With the application of fluorescent in situ hybridization (FISH) to interphase nuclei, we are able to examine the chromosome status of every cell within an embryo. The use of FISH with probes for chromosomes X and Y was developed to sex embryos for patients at risk of transmitting X-linked diseases[32,33]. Dual FISH gave the first indication of the frequency of chromosome mosaicism in diagnostic cleavage stage embryos[34].

FISH and comparative genomic hybridization (CGH) have been used for the analysis of chromosomes in human preimplantation embryos[35–39]. Studies on abnormally fertilized embryos (such as polyspermic embryos) have shown, as expected, that these embryos were highly abnormal[40], which is in agreement with the karyotype data obtained from such embryos[27].

Normally fertilized, normally developing embryos also show high levels of chromosomal abnormalities[37,41]. To try to categorize these abnormalities, the patterns have been divided into four groups[37,41]:

1. uniformly diploid for the chromosomes examined
2. uniformly abnormal, such as all cells with trisomy 21 (Down's syndrome)
3. mosaic, where usually both diploid cells and aneuploid, haploid or polyploid nuclei are present and can vary in proportion from mainly diploid to mainly abnormal
4. chaotic, where every nucleus shows a different chromosome complement.

From the FISH and CGH data a higher rate of chromosomally abnormal embryos has been observed than was previously reported from karyotyping data. However, since mosaic and chaotic embryos are common, if only one or two cells are analyzable from an embryo, then karyotyping would underestimate the level of chromosome abnormalities.

Chromosomal mosaicism has been observed in fetal development. Evidence from embryos has shown that the presence of two cell lines, as shown by mosaic embryos and in CPM, may arise due to abnormal chromosome segregation caused by a postzygotic event, or the chromosome loss from a trisomic embryo, which restores the diploid state (trisomic rescue)[42]. There are indications that these abnormal cells would most likely be found in the trophectoderm, and hence the placenta. First, only four cells from a blastocyst give rise to the embryo and so it would be unlikely that the abnormal cells would be found in the embryo; second, in most cases, a fetus with abnormal chromosomes will not be compatible with life. Interestingly, while mosaicism for trisomy of some of the non-sex chromosomes is compatible with postnatal life, the corresponding mosaic monosomies appear not to be although they are known in spontaneous abortion material[43].

With regard to chaotic embryos, these have been observed to reach the blastocyst stage of development, but are thought to fail to implant.

The accumulation of data on the chromosomal constitution of spare untransferred embryos from PGD cycles has revealed that, despite the fact that these are embryos from women of proven fertility, the incidence of postzygotic chromosomal anomalies is similar to that in embryos from routine IVF patients[27]. A second significant finding is that the incidence of the most bizarre type of anomaly, chaotically dividing embryos, is strongly related to the particular couple. In repeated cycles, certain couples regularly produced 'chaotic' embryos, while others did not, although the frequency of diploid mosaics was similar in both groups[37].

DIAGNOSIS OF MONOGENIC DISORDERS

PGD for monogenic disorders is now usually performed by fluorescent PCR with direct analysis of the mutation and linked or unlinked markers for contamination detection. However, the use of highly polymorphic linked markers alone presents an almost universal test for some disorders. The first clinical application was for couples at risk of transmitting cystic fibrosis (CF)[44,45]. Accurate detection of the common ΔF508 mutation was possible by using nested PCR to amplify the affected exon from single cells followed by heteroduplex formation[46,47]. The birth of the first unaffected child following embryo selection using this method was reported in 1992[44].

The list of disorders that can be diagnosed at the single-cell level is slowly increasing[4]. The ESHRE PGD Consortium showed that, up to 2004, the top ten diagnosed monogenic diseases were: autosomal recessive; cystic fibrosis, β-thalassemia, spinal muscular atrophy and sickle cell disease, autosomal dominant; myotonic dystrophy, Huntington's disease, Charcot Marie Tooth disease, and for the specific diagnosis of X-linked diseases; Duchenne muscular dystrophy (DMD), fragile X and hemophilia. PGD for the first autosomal dominant condition, Marfan's syndrome, was achieved in 1996[48]. Dominant disorders pose particular problems in diagnosis at the single-cell level and to minimize these, the authors incorporated primers for gender in a multiplex PCR reaction.

Potential sources of misdiagnosis in monogenic disorders are contamination by extraneous DNA (this could come from additional sperm that remain attached to the embryo) and analysis of sequences derived from a single chromosome only. This can be due to biopsy of a haploid cell, which may be found in about 15% of embryos or allele specific amplification failure so that DNA from the gene on one chromosome is not represented in the final reaction product. This is known as allele drop-out (ADO) and is a particular problem when amplifying the genome from single cells. If both parents are carrying the same gene mutation in a recessive disorder, ADO will not result in misdiagnosis of an affected embryo as unaffected, but problems can arise if the diagnosis relies on the detection of a common mutation, such as the three-base pair deletion causing CF, in one parent and a rare mutation in the other parent cannot be picked up. Here, the advantage of SSCP (single strand conformation polymorphism) is apparent since each DNA strand may be visualized and the absence of one allele is immediately obvious.

ADO is a major problem when diagnosing dominant disorders, as the failure of the mutant allele to amplify will lead to the diagnosis of a heterozygous (affected) embryo as homozygous normal. To overcome this problem, primers for a closely linked genetic polymorphism may be included in the reaction, providing an independent system for analysis. Multiplex PCR may be used to achieve this, but is not always feasible. A development that provides an alternative approach is that of whole genome amplification, first used in clinical PGD to diagnose the cancer predisposing disorder adenomatous polyposis coli (APC gene)[49]. A recent modification, multiple displacement amplification (MDA), amplifies the entire genome in a few hours by random hexamer priming of denatured DNA followed by strand displacement synthesis utilizing phi29 DNA polymerase[50]. The advantage for PGD is that it ensures amplification of the single genome so that methods of analysis are easier than performing a single cell diagnosis, however, levels of ADO can be very high. Renwick et al.[51] presented the first successful PGD cycles for CF and DMD using a method termed preimplantation genetic haplotyping (PGH). They used numerous polymorphic markers to haplotype the DNA, but this method requires DNA from affected relatives so that the phase can be established. This is not always possible, for example in the case of de novo mutations.

To eliminate the possibility of contamination by sperm released from the zona pellucida during the biopsy procedure, intracytoplasmic sperm injection (ICSI) should be used as the means of fertilization for the analysis of monogenic disorders[4]. A high percentage of cystic fibrosis carrier males have congenital absence of the vas deferens and sperm aspiration techniques are required to obtain the sperm, followed by ICSI for efficient fertilization.

EMBRYO SEXING TO AVOID X-LINKED DISEASE

Sexing for X-linked disease was intially one of the major indications for PGD[52]. X-linked recessive diseases account for 6–7% of monogenic defects and include conditions such as Duchenne muscular dystrophy (DMD), hemophilia and various mental retardation syndromes. The mother carries the mutation on one of her X chromosomes and so transmits the defective gene to half of her offspring. There are over 400 X-linked diseases. For some of these, the molecular nature of the mutation is known and a diagnosis of the disease is possible, either prenatally or postnatally. However, for many X-linked diseases, the exact mutation is unknown and so no direct genetic test is available. In these cases, it may be possible to establish which maternal X chromosome is carrying the mutation by DNA marker analysis (haplotyping) so that prenatal diagnosis may be offered. Therefore, for such X-linked diseases, PGD is used far less frequently than hitherto for embryo sexing.

The first cycles of PGD performed used PCR to amplify a Y-chromosome repeat sequence to sex embryos for patients carrying X-linked disease[53]. Using this method, embryos showing no signal were assumed to be female and such embryos were considered for transfer. A diagnostic error occurred in one of the first seven pregnancies that resulted and the pregnancy was terminated as no specific molecular test was available for this disease. This misdiagnosis may have been due to amplification failure, ADO, an anucleate cell (or failure to put the cell in the tube) or mosaicism where an XO cell was biopsied from an XY embryo. However, in addition, there are two drawbacks that apply when amplifying DNA from single blastomeres in order to sex the embryo. The first applies to any reaction involving PCR; that the risk of amplifying contaminating material is high. The second is that the presence of an amplified band only indicates that an X or Y chromosome is present and gives no information on copy number. For these reasons, the use of FISH is preferable. In the earliest report of this approach, five couples undergoing embryo sexing by FISH to avoid X-linked disease, no transfers took place for two of them despite the identification of X signals and no Y signals[34]. One embryo in this series was shown to be XO. Transfer of a potentially 45, X zygote could be disastrous when the aim is to avoid X-linked disease from the carrier mother, as the great majority of such embryos lack the paternal sex chromosome[54]. Since 45, X conceptuses are thought to occur with a frequency approaching 1%, such a finding will not be rare when carrying out preimplantation diagnosis. An extra advantage of FISH is that the risk of contamination is minimal as the nucleus can be observed all at stages of the process.

The FISH procedure can be efficiently performed in 2 h using directly labeled DNA probes[36,55]. Most laboratories use five-color FISH for embryo sexing with probes for chromosomes X, Y and three autosomes, and may include an additional round of FISH with more autosomal probes to provide information concerning aneuploidy and polyploidy. However, due to a number of misdiagnoses of sex by FISH (Table 25.1), it is always advisable to have the X and Y probes in the first round and to analyze two cells from each embryo to avoid problems due to mosaicism. Embryos that begin life with an XXY sex chromosome constitution, for example, may lose a chromosome in subsequent cell divisions to generate daughter cells with differing sexes[39].

DETECTION OF CHROMOSOME ABNORMALITIES

It is well known that 15% of all clinically recognized pregnancies spontaneously abort and, of these, 50% are chromosomally

Table 25.1 Misdiagnosis reported to the ESHRE PGD Consortium

Indication	*Method of diagnosis*	*Number of misdiagnosis reported to consortium*	*Total number of cycles to egg retrieval*
Sexing for X linked disease	FISH	2	858
Sexing for X linked disease	PCR	2	66
Translocations	FISH	3	2712
PGS	FISH	6	9153
Social sexing	FISH	1	497
Monogenic disorders	PCR	10	2599

Source: Harper et al., 2008[4]

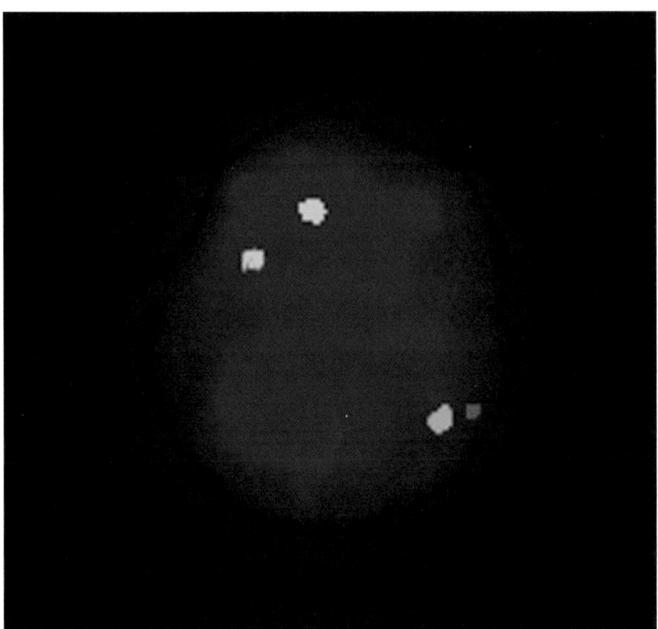

Fig. 25.2 Fluorescent in situ hybridization on a blastomere from a patient carrying an 18:21 translocation. Probes were used for the centromeric region of chromosome 18 (aqua), 18q telomeric probe (red) and 21q22.2 (green). The blastomere is monosomy 18 as there is only one aqua and one red signal.

abnormal, the most common abnormality being aneuploidy, which increases exponentially in the eggs of women over the age of 37. However, couples at the highest risk of a chromosomally abnormal conception are those where one partner carries a chromosomal rearrangement or is a gonadal mosaic for a trisomic chromosome. Such patients may have severe problems trying to achieve a normal pregnancy. Their history often shows either failure to obtain a pregnancy, repeated spontaneous miscarriages, or an affected pregnancy after prenatal diagnosis which may lead to repeated induced abortions. Therefore, for such couples, PGD may be an attractive option.

The most common strategy used to examine embryos from such patients uses cleavage stage embryo biopsy and interphase, multicolor FISH using appropriate combinations of alpha satellite and locus specific probes for the chromosomes in question[56–60] (Figure 25.2). To date, a few thousand couples have been treated in this way; the ESHRE PGD Consortium Data set VII lists over 500 cycles of treatment in 2004 alone[4]. The most striking observation relating to couples that resort to PGD because of problems conceiving due to rearranged chromosomes in a parent is the very high frequency of embryos that are abnormal on testing[4,56–62]. It is not uncommon for 70% of the embryos from these couples to be chromosomally abnormal. This observation perhaps provides some explanation for the unexpectedly poor reproductive history of these couples since rearrangements such as translocations are usually amenable to management by prenatal diagnosis. The anomalies seen relate not only to abnormal segregation of gametes in the carrier parent but also to random abnormalities arising postzygotically leading to extensive mosaicism. In this situation, there is a risk that the biopsied cell may not be representative of the whole embryo. Trisomic cells in diploid embryos have been observed and disomic cells have been seen in an otherwise trisomy 21 embryo. If a normal cell is biopsied, the embryo may be diagnosed as normal when it is affected. To reduce the chance of a misdiagnosis, for chromosome abnormalities, ideally only embryos where two nuclei are shown to be normal for the chromosomes analyzed should be replaced.

Aneuploidy screening

Aneuploidy screening (or preimplantation genetic screening – PGS) arose as a development of testing for chromosome anomalies. Since meiotic aneuploidy increases rapidly with rising maternal age, it seemed logical that screening embryos for the common trisomies would improve the pregnancy rate of older patients undergoing IVF – the advanced maternal age (AMA) group. Also, the prevalence of mosaicism suggested that such screening should improve the chances of success in couples with repetitive implantation failure (RIF). Screening is carried out using various combinations of probes, but usually including those for chromosomes 13,16,18,21 and 22; others such as 15 or X and Y may be added. PGS is now the most common indication for carrying out PGD; the ESHRE Data set VII lists over 2000 cycles for 2004[4].

However, the application of PGS remains controversial[63]. Its advocates claim improved implantation rates and reduced miscarriage rates[66], but randomized controlled trials have failed to prove that this is the case[64,65]. What is important is that it should only be applied to selected couples, those for whom the benefits are likely to exceed any reduction in implantation

Table 25.2 **The effect of monosomic or haploid chromosomal mosaicism on the single-cell diagnosis of dominant single-gene defects in the preimplantation embryo**

Dominant inheritance	*Embryo*	*Genotype*	*Minor cell line*	*Genotype*
Autosomal	Disomic (chromosomally normal)	wt/m (affected)	Haploid or monosomic for chromosome carrying the gene	**wt** or m
X-linked	Disomy	wt/m (female affected) m (male affected)	X-chromosome monosomic X- or Y-chromosome monosomic	**wt** or m no result or m

wt = wild type (normal allele); m = mutant allele; **wt** = misdiagnosis of an affected embryo as unaffected. Source: Delhanty and Handyside[68]

potential due to embryo biopsy, and that it should be carried out efficiently by experienced personnel, in much the same way as specific PGD is performed.

The potential for misdiagnosis and implication of mosaicism

The last published world data for PGD[4] showed pregnancy rates of 25% per cycle in which embryos are transferred, which are comparable to those for routine IVF and confirm the initial in vitro data that embryo biopsy on day 3 does not seriously affect preimplantation development[10]. Overall, the number of congenital abnormalities is similar to those reported for IVF.

Of more concern is that there have been at least 19 misdiagnoses among 1941 clinical pregnancies[4]. The first misdiagnosis of sex was almost certainly the result of amplification failure. The main problems with PCR are still caused by contamination and allele dropout. FISH misdiagnosis could be caused by contamination from a cumulus cell, mosaicism, or FISH error such as overlapping signals or failure of the probes to hybridize. Misdiagnosis can also be caused by human error (mislabeling of tubes, slides or transfer of the wrong embryo, but the possibility that the couple had unprotected intercourse and in vivo fertilization resulted, is always a possibility).

For PGD to be successful, the biopsied cell should be representative of the whole embryo. In the case of autosomal recessive disorders, where both parents are carriers for the same mutation, chromosomal mosaicism is unlikely to lead to misdiagnosis, since one or two extra or a missing copy of the relevant chromosome will not affect the detection of the mutation. Whereas for dominant conditions, autosomal or X linked, absence of one homologue in the biopsied cell could lead to failure to diagnose an affected embryo (Table 25.2). Mosaicism is also an important consideration when attempting to diagnose trisomies or monosomies at the preimplantation stage; the effect will depend upon whether the embryo was initially trisomic or normally disomic for the chromosome in question (Table 25.3). For both of these situations, it is advisable to analyze two independent blastomeres to obtain the most accurate result.

FUTURE DEVELOPMENTS

Research currently is focused on methods of detecting chromosome imbalance in the preimplantation embryo and on improving the reliability of monogenic diagnosis and extending the range of disorders amenable to specific diagnosis. In view of the frequency of chromosomal disorders in older women and in high-risk couples, methods for diagnosing abnormal copy numbers with reliability are urgently needed. Multicolor FISH with centromeric probes for up to 12 chromosomes has been used to screen IVF embryos prior to transfer in certain groups of patients[66] and polar body analysis is being applied for the same purpose. However, it has yet to be demonstrated that screening with a limited set of probes will enhance the ongoing pregnancy rate (see section on PGS).

Table 25.3 **The effect of chromosomal mosaicism on the single-cell diagnosis of chromosome copy number in the preimplantation embryo**

Embryo	*FISH signals per nucleus*	*Minor cell line*	*FISH signals per nucleus*
Disomic	• •	Monosomic or haploid	•
		Trisomic or triploid	• • •
Trisomic	• • •	Disomic or haploid	• • or •
		Tetrasomic or tetraploid	• • • • or • • • • • •

Inadvertent sampling of the minor cell line would always lead to misdiagnosis, but this would be serious only in the case of a trisomic embryo with a disomic (or haploid) cell line – • •. Source: Delhanty and Handyside[68]

The problem of gonadal trisomy mosaicism has been approached by developing locus-specific probes for use in conjunction with the relevant centromere probe. Problems due to translocations are less easily solved because of the many possible types of unbalanced gamete, including 3:1 disjunctions, that one needs to detect. The approach of using a combination of centromere and locus-specific probes that flank the breakpoint of one of the chromosomes has been applied[56,59]. It has become clear that, for diagnostic purposes, three is the maximum number of probes that can be reliably scored; probe combinations that include five probes are measurably less efficient.

It is clear that what is needed is a whole genome screen for aneuploidy, both for high-risk couples and older women having routine IVF treatment. Possible approaches that have been investigated include metaphase comparative genomic hybridization (m-CGH) by dual FISH of test and normal DNA onto normal metaphase chromosomes[57] following whole genome amplification from single blastomeres, and the use of fluorescent PCR primers for automated quantitative analysis of repeat sequences specific for the relevant chromosome region[58]. While m-CGH has given promising results[38,39], at the single-cell level, fluorescent PCR has proved to be an unreliable approach for the detection of chromosome imbalance[67]. Of the dominant monogenic disorders, some of the most frequent requests for preimplantation diagnosis are now for the inherited cancer predispositon syndromes, such as retinoblastoma, Li Fraumeni syndrome, neurofibromatosis I and II and familial adenomatous polyposis coli. Couples who are reluctant to terminate an otherwise normal pregnancy appear to be more willing to consider selection at the preimplantation stage.

REFERENCES

1. Verlinsky Y, Ginsburg N, Lifchez A, Valle J, Moise J, Strom C. Analysis of the first polar body: preconception genetic diagnosis. *Hum Reprod* **5**:826–829, 1990.
2. Munné S, Dailey T, Sultan KM, Grifo J, Cohen J. The use of first polar bodies for preimplantation diagnosis of aneuploidy. *Mol Hum Reprod* **1**:1014–1020, 1995.
3. Verlinsky Y, Strom C, Cieslak J, Kuliev A, Ivakhnenko V, Lifchez A. Birth of healthy children after preimplantation diagnosis of common aneuploidies by polar body fluorescent in situ hybridisation analysis. *Fertil Steril* **66**:126–129, 1996.
4. Harper JC, De Die C, Goosens V, et al. ESHRE PGD Consortium data collection VII: Cycles from January to December 2004 with pregnancy follow-up to October 2005. *Hum Reprod* **23**(3):478–480, 2008.
5. Kuliev A, Cieslak J, Verlinsky Y. Frequency and distribution of chromosome abnormalities in human oocytes. *Cytogenet Genome Res* **111**:193–198, 2005.
6. Fragouli E, Wells D, Thornhill A et al. Comparative genomic hybridisation analysis of human oocytes and polar bodies. *Hum Reprod* **21**:2319–2328, 2006.
7. Wells D, Escudero T, Levy B, Hirschhorn K, Delhanty JDA, Munné S. First clinical application of comparative genomic hybridization and polar body testing for preimplantation genetic diagnosis of aneuploidy. *Fertil Steril* **78**:543–549, 2002.
8. Wilton LJ, Shaw JM, Trounsen AO. Successful single-cell biopsy, and cryopreservation of preimplantation mouse embryos. *Fertil Steril* **51**:513–517, 1989.
9. Tarin JJ, Handyside AH. Embryo biopsy strategies for preimplantation diagnosis. *Fertil Steril* **59**:943–952, 1993.
10. Hardy K, Martin KL, Leese HJ, Winston RML, Handyside AH. Human preimplantation development *in-vitro* is not adversely affected by biopsy at the 8-cell stage. *Hum Reprod* **5**:708–714, 1990.
11. Tarin JJ, Conaghan J, Winston RML, Handyside AH. Human embryo biopsy on the 2nd day after insemination for preimplantation diagnosis: removal of a quarter of embryo retards cleavage. *Fertil Steril* **58**:970–976, 1992.
12. Soussis I, Harper JC, Handyside AH, Winston RML. Obstetric outcome of pregnancies resulting from embryos biopsied for preimplantation diagnosis of inherited disease. *Br J Obstet Gynaecol* **103**:784–788, 1996.
13. Soussis I, Harper JC, Kontogianni E et al. Pregnancies resulting from embryos biopsied for preimplantation diagnosis of genetic disease: biochemical and ultrasonic studies in the first trimester of pregnancy. *J Assist Reprod Genet* **13**:254–257, 1996.
14. ESHRE PGD Consortium steering committee. ESHRE Preimplantation Genetic Diagnosis (PGD) Consortium: preliminary assessment of data from January 1997 to September 1998. *Hum Reprod* **14**:3138–3148, 1999.
15. ESHRE PGD Consortium steering committee. ESHRE preimplantation genetic diagnosis (PGD) consortium: data collection II (May 2000). *Hum Reprod* **15**:2673–2683, 2000.
16. ESHRE PGD Consortium Steering Committee. ESHRE Preimplantation Genetic Diagnosis Consortium: data collection III (May 2001). *Hum Reprod* **17**:233–246, 2002.
17. Sermon K, Moutou C, Harper J et al. ESHRE PGD Consortium data collection IV: May-December 2001. *Hum Reprod* **20**:19, 2005.
18. Harper JC, Boelaert K, Geraedts J et al. ESHRE PGD Consortium data collection V: cycles from January to December 2002 with pregnancy follow-up to October 2003. *Hum Reprod* **21**:3–21, 2006.
19. Sermon KD, Michiels A, Harton G et al. ESHRE PGD Consortium data collection VI: Cycles from January to December 2003 with pregnancy follow-up to October 2004. *Hum Reprod* **22**(2):236–323, 2007.
20. Monk M, Muggleton Harris A, Rawlings E, Whittingham D. Preimplantation diagnosis of HPRT-deficient male and carrier female mouse embryos by trophectoderm biopsy. *Hum Reprod* **3**:377–381, 1988.
21. Summers PM, Campbell JM, Miller MW. Normal in vivo development of marmoset monkey embryos after trophectoderm biopsy. *Hum Reprod* **1**:89–94, 1988.
22. Dokras A, Sargent IL, Gardner RL, Barlow GH. Human trophectoderm biopsy and secretion of chorionic gonadotrophin. *Hum Reprod* **6**:1453, 1991.
23. Muggleton Harris AL, Glazier A, Wall M, Pickering SJ. Genetic diagnosis using polymerase chain reaction and fluorescent in situ hybridisation analysis of biopsied cells from both the cleavage and blastocyst stages of individual cultured human preimplantation embryos. *Hum Reprod* **10**:183–192, 1995.
24. Hardy K. Development of human blastocysts in vitro. In *Preimplantation embryo development*, B Bavister (ed.). Springer-Verlag, 1993.
25. McArthur SJ, Leigh D, Marshall JT, de Boer KA, Jansen RP. Pregnancies and live births after trophectoderm biopsy and preimplantation genetic testing of human blastocysts. *Fertil Steril* **84**:1628–1636, 2005.
26. Angell RR. Chromosome abnormalities in human preimplantation embryos. In *Development of preimplantation embryos and their environment*, pp. 181–187. New York: Alan R. Liss, 1989.
27. Plachot M, Mandelbaum J, Junca A-M, Grouchy J, de Salat-Baroux J, Cohen J. Cytogenetic analysis and developmental capacity of normal and abnormal embryos after IVF. *Hum Reprod* **4**(Suppl):99–103, 1989.
28. Zenzes MT, Casper RF. Cytogenetics of human oocytes, zygotes and embryos after in vitro fertilisation. *Hum Genet* **88**:367–375, 1992.
29. Jamieson ME, Coutts JRT, Connor JM. The chromosome constitution of human preimplantation embryos fertilised in vitro. *Hum Reprod* **9**:709–715, 1994.
30. Zenzes MT, Wang P, Casper RF. Chromosome status of untransferred (spare) embryos and probability of pregnancy after in vitro fertilisation. *Lancet* **340**:391–394, 1992.
31. Watt JL, Templeton AA, Messinis I, Bell L, Cunningham P, Duncan RO. Trisomy 1 in an eight cell human pre-embryo. *J Med Genet* **24**:60–64, 1987.
32. Griffin DK, Handyside AH, Harper JC et al. Clinical experience with preimplantation diagnosis of sex by dual fluorescent in-situ hybridisation. *J Assist Reprod Genet* **11**:132–143, 1994.
33. Munné S, Tang YX, Grifo J, Rosenwaks Z, Cohen J. Sex determination of human embryos using the polymerase chain reaction and confirmation by fluorescence in situ hybridization. *Fertil Steril* **61**:111–117, 1994.
34. Delhanty JDA, Griffin DK, Handyside AH et al. Detection of aneuploidy and chromosomal mosaicism in human embryos during preimplantation sex determination by fluorescent in-situ

hybridisation. *Hum Mol Genet* **2**:1183–1185, 1993.

35. Munné S, Lee A, Rosenwaks Z, Grifo J, Cohen J. Diagnosis of major chromosome aneuploidies in human preimplantation embryos. *Hum Reprod* **8**:2185–2191, 1993.
36. Harper JC, Coonen E, Ramaekers FCS et al. Identification of the sex of human preimplantation embryos in two hours using an improved spreading method and fluorescent in situ hybridisation using directly labelled probes. *Hum Reprod* **9**:721–724, 1994.
37. Delhanty JDA, Harper JC, Ao A, Handyside AH, Winston RML. Multicolour FISH detects frequent chromosomal mosaicism and chaotic division in normal preimplantation embryos from fertile patients. *Hum Genet* **99**:755–760, 1997.
38. Voullaire L, Slater H, Williamson R, Wilton L. Chromosome analysis of blastomeres from human embryos by using comparative genomic hybridization. *Hum Genet* **106**:210–217, 2000.
39. Wells D, Delhanty JDA. Comprehensive chromosomal analysis of human preimplantation embryos using whole genome amplification and single cell comparative genomic hybridization. *Mol Hum Reprod* **6**:1055–1062, 2000.
40. Coonen E, Harper JC, Ramaekers FCS et al. Presence of chromosomal mosaicism in abnormal preimplantation embryos detected by fluorescent in situ hybridisation. *Hum Genet* **54**:609–615, 1994.
41. Harper JC, Coonen E, Handyside AH, Winston RML, Hopman AHN, Delhanty JDA. Mosaicism of autosomes and sex chromosomes in morphologically normal, monospermic, preimplantation human embryos. *Prenat Diagn* **15**:1–49, 1995.
42. Daphnis D, Jerkovic S, Geye J, Craft I, Delhanty JDA, Harper JC. Detailed FISH analysis of day 5 human embryos reveals the mechanisms leading to mosaic aneuploidy. *Hum Reprod* **20**:129–137, 2005.
43. Lebedev IN, Ostroverkhova NV, Nikitina TV, Sukhanova NN, Nazarenko SA. Features of chromosomal abnormalities in spontaneous abortion cell culture failures detected by interphase FISH analysis. *Eur J Hum Genet* **12**:513–520, 2004.
44. Handyside AH, Lesko JG, Tarin JJ, Winston RML, Hughes MR. Birth of a normal girl after in vitro fertilisation and preimplantation diagnostic testing for cystic fibrosis. *N Engl J Med* **327**:905–909, 1992.
45. Ao A, Ray P, Harper JC, Lesko J et al. Clinical experience with preimplantation diagnosis of deltaF508 deletion in cystic fibrosis. *Prenat Diagn* **16**:137–142, 1996.
46. Lesko J, Snabes M, Handyside AH, Hughes M. Amplification of the cystic fibrosis DF508 mutation from single cells: applications toward genetic diagnosis of the preimplantation embryo. *Am J Hum Genet* **49**(4):223, 1991.
47. Liu J, Lissens W, Devroey P, Van Steirteghem A, Liebaers I. Efficiency and accuracy of polymerase-chain-reaction assay for cystic fibrosis allele delta F508 in single cell. *Lancet* **339**:1190–1192, 1992.
48. Harton GL, Tsipouras P, Sisson ME et al. Preimplantation genetic testing for Marfan syndrome. *Mol Hum Reprod* **2**:713–715, 1996.
49. Ao A, Wells D, Handyside AH, Winston RML, Delhanty JDA. Preimplantation genetic diagnosis of inherited cancer: familial adenomatous polyposis coli. *J Assist Reprod Genet* **15**:140–144, 1998.
50. Dean FB, Nelson JR, Giesler TL, Lasken RS. Rapid amplifcation of plasmid and phage DNA using Phi29 DNA polymerase and multiply-primed rolling circle amplification. *Genome Res* **11**:1095–1099, 2001.
51. Renwick PJ, Trussler J, Ostad-Saffari E et al. Proof of principle and first cases using preimplantation genetic haplotyping – a paradigm shift for embryo diagnosis. *Reprod Biomed Online* **13**:110–119, 2006.
52. Harper JC. Preimplantation diagnosis of inherited disease by embryo biopsy. An update of the world figures. *J Assist Reprod Genet* **13**(2):90–94, 1996.
53. Handyside AH, Kontogianni EH, Hardy K, Winston RML. Pregnancies from biopsied human preimplantation embryos sexed by Y-specific DNA amplification. *Nature* **244**:768–770, 1990.
54. Hassold T, Benham F, Leppert M. Cytogenetic and molecular analysis of sex chromosome monosomy. *Am J Hum Genet* **42**:534–541, 1988.
55. Harper JC, Delhanty JDA. FISH in preimplantation diagnosis. In *Methods in molecular biology, molecular diagnosis of genetic disease*, J Walker (ed.), pp. 259–268. New Jersey: Humana Press, 1996.
56. Conn CM, Harper JC, Winston RML, Delhanty JDA. Preimplantation diagnosis for trisomies 13, 14, 18 and 21 in translocation carriers using multicolour fluorescent in situ hybridisation. *Am J Hum Genet* **57**(Suppl. A):1611, 1995.
57. Conn C, Harper JC, Winston RML, Delhanty JDA. Preimplantation diagnosis of autosomal aneuploidy using multicolour fluorescent in situ hybridisation (FISH). *Eur J Hum Genet* **4**(Suppl. 1):125, 1996.
58. Conn C, Harper JC, Winston RML, Delhanty JDA. Infertile couples with Robertsonian translocations: preimplantation genetic analysis of embryos reveals chaotic cleavage divisions. *Hum Genet* **102**:117–123, 1998.
59. Munne S. Peimplantation genetic diagnosis of numerical and structural chromosome abnormalities. *Reprod Biomed Online* **3**:183–195, 2002.
60. Scriven PN, Handyside AH, Ogilvie CM. Chromosome translocations: segregation modes and strategies for preimplantation genetic diagnosis. *Prenat Diagn* **18**(13):1437–1449, 1998.
61. Simopoulou M, Harper JC, Fragouli E et al. Preimplantation genetic diagnosis of chromosome abnormalities: implications from the outcome for couples with chromosomal rearrangements. *Prenat Diagn* **23**:652–662, 2003.
62. Iwarsson E, Malgrem H, Inzunza J et al. Highly abnormal cleavage divisons in preimplantation embryos from translocation carriers. *Prenat Diagn* **20**:1047–1083, 2000.
63. Harper JC, Sermon K, Geraedts J, Vesela K et al. What next for Preimplantation Genetic Screening (PGS)? *Human Reproduction* **23**(3):478–480, 2008.
64. Staessen C, Platteau P, Van Assche E et al. Comparison of blastocyst transfer with or without preimplantation genetic diagnosis for aneuploidy screening in couples with advanced maternal age: a prospective randomized controlled trial. *Hum Reprod* **19**:2849–2858, 2004.
65. Mastenbroek S, Twisk M, Van Echten-arends J et al. Preimplantation genetic screening in women of advanced maternal age. *N Engl J Med* **357**(1):9–17, 2007, Epub Jul 4, 2007.
66. Munne S, Fischer J, Warner A, Chen S, Zouves C, Cohen J. Referring Centers PGD Group Preimplantation genetic diagnosis significantly reduces pregnancy loss in infertile couples: a multicenter study. *Fertil Steril* **85**(2):326–332, 2006.
67. Sherlock J, Cirigliano V, Pertl M, Tutschek B, Adinolfi M. Assessment of diagnostic quantitative fluorescent multiplex polymerase chain reaction assays performed on single cells. *Ann Hum Genet* **62**:9–23, 1998.
68. Delhanty JDA, Handyside AH. The origin of genetic defects in the human and their detection in the preimplantation embryo. *Hum Reprod Update* **1**(3):201–215, 1995.

CHAPTER 26

Hemoglobinopathies

John M Old

KEY POINTS

- This chapter deals with all aspects of prenatal diagnosis of the hemoglobinopathies: indications for prenatal diagnosis, the different types of globin gene mutations, the most commonly used molecular diagnostic techniques, the fetal samples to be used and guidelines for accurate fetal DNA diagnosis by PCR-based techniques
- The clinical states of the different types of α-thalassemia, β-thalassemia, δβ-thalassemia, Hb variants and their interactions are discussed
- All known thalassemia mutations and their phenotypes are summarized, together with the best analytical techniques for their detection
- Chorionic villus sampling is the procedure of choice for prenatal diagnosis of the hemoglobinopathies. Best practice guidelines and diagnostic pitfalls of CVS diagnosis are presented
- The current state of development of three new approaches to prenatal diagnosis is reviewed: preimplantation genetic diagnosis and the non-invasive methods using fetal cells in maternal blood and fetal DNA in maternal plasma
- The relative gene frequencies of β-thalassemia mutations in the UK population is compared to those of selected countries from the four major ethnic groups: Mediterranean, Asian Indian, Southeast Asian and African

INTRODUCTION

The hemoglobinopathies are a diverse group of autosomal recessive disorders characterized by either the synthesis of a structurally abnormal globin (the hemoglobin variants) or the reduced synthesis of one or more of the globin chains (the thalassemias)[1]. As a group they are the most common single-gene disorder in the world and are found at high frequencies in many populations as a result of positive selection pressure due to falciparum malaria. Individuals with the carrier state are easily identifiable, permitting the control of the serious hemoglobinopathies by a program of carrier screening, counseling and prenatal diagnosis. The most important disorders for which prenatal diagnosis is considered are α^0-thalassemia, β-thalassemia, sickle-cell anemia and various compound heterozygous states which result in a clinically significant disease (Table 26.1).

The hemoglobinopathies are regionally specific and each local population has its own characteristic spectrum of hemoglobin variants and thalassemia mutations. Therefore knowledge of the ethnic origin of a patient under study is often essential to enable the quick identification of the underlying molecular defects by the application of molecular biology techniques. This can be achieved in most cases as nearly all the globin gene mutations have now been identified and the particular mutations and their frequencies for most at-risk ethnic groups are known. The majority of the molecular defects can be diagnosed using a variety of techniques involving the analysis of DNA amplified by the polymerase chain reaction (PCR). PCR-based techniques provide a quick and sensitive approach to fetal DNA diagnosis and normally enable a result to be obtained in 2–3 days.

THE GLOBIN GENES

Hemoglobin is a tetrameric protein made up of two α-like (α or ζ) and two β-like (ε, γ, δ or β) globin chains. Each globin chain is synthesized from its own globin gene located in two gene clusters, the α-like globin genes on chromosome 16 and the β-like genes on chromosome 11. The α-like globin cluster includes an embryonic gene (ζ2), two fetal/adult genes (α1 and α2), several pseudogenes (ψζ1, ψα1 and ψα2) and a gene of undetermined function (θ1) arranged in the order ζ2-ψ 1-ψα2-πα1-α2-α1-θ. The β-globin cluster includes an embryonic gene (ε), two fetal genes ($^{G}\gamma$ and $^{A}\gamma$), two adult genes (β and δ) and a pseudogene (ψβ) in the order ε-$^{G}\gamma$-$^{A}\gamma$-ψβ-δ-β. Throughout development there are

Table 26.1 **Phenotypes of the thalassemias, sickle-cell disorders and various thalassemia/variant hemoglobin interactions**

Type	*Phenotype*	*DNA diagnosis*
Homozygous state		
α^0-thalassemia (--/--)	Hb Bart's hydrops fetalis	Gap-PCR, MLPA
α^+-thalassemia (-α/-α)	No clinical problems	Gap-PCR, MLPA
α^+-thalassemia ($\alpha^T\alpha/\alpha^T\alpha$)	Hb H disease or Hb H hydrops	DNA sequencing
β-thalassemia:		
β^0 or severe β^+ mutation	Thalassemia major	ASO, ARMS, Sequencing
Mild β^+ mutation	Thalassemia intermedia	ASO, ARMS, Sequencing
$\delta\beta^0$-thalassemia	Thalassemia intermedia	Gap-PCR, MLPA
HPFH	No clinical problems	Gap-PCR, MLPA
Hb Lepore	Variable: intermedia to major	Gap-PCR
Hb S	Sickle-cell disease	RE-PCR, ASO, ARMS
Hb C	No clinical problems	ASO, ARMS
Hb D-Punjab	No clinical problems	ASO, ARMS
Hb E	No clinical problems	ASO, ARMS
Compound heterozygous state		
α^0-thal/α^+-thal (--/-α)	Hb H disease	Gap-PCR, MLPA
α^0-thal/α^+-thal (--/$\alpha^T\alpha$)	Hb H disease or Hb H hydrops	Gap-PCR, MLPA
β^0-thal /severe β^+-thal	Thalassemia major	ASO, ARMS, Sequencing
Mild β^+-thal /β^0 or severe β^+-thal	Variable: intermedia to major	ASO, ARMS, Sequencing
$\delta\beta^0$-thal /β^0 or severe β^+-thal	Variable: intermedia to major	Gap-PCR, MLPA, PCR-β^T
$\delta\beta^0$-thal /mild β^+-thal	Mild thalassemia intermedia	Gap-PCR, MLPA, PCR-β^T
$\delta\beta^0$-thal /Hb Lepore	Thalassemia intermedia	Gap-PCR, MLPA, PCR-β^T
$\alpha\alpha\alpha$ /β^0 or severe β^+-thal	Mild thalassemia intermedia	Gap-PCR, PCR-β^T
Hb Lepore/β^0 or severe β^+-thal	Thalassemia major	Gap-PCR, MLPA, PCR-β^T
Hb C/β^0 or severe β^+	Variable: β-thal trait to intermedia	ASO, ARMS, Sequencing
Hb C/mild β^+-thal	No clinical problems	ASO, ARMS, Sequencing
Hb D/β^0 or severe β^+-thal	No clinical problems	ASO, ARMS, Sequencing
Hb E/β^0 or severe β^+-thal	Variable: intermedia to major	ASO, ARMS, Sequencing
Hb O-Arab/β^0-thal	Severe thalassemia intermedia	ASO, ARMS, Sequencing
Hb S/β^0 or severe β^+-thal	Sickle-cell disease	RE-PCR, ASO, ARMS
Hb S/mild β^+-thal	Usually mild sickle-cell disease	RE-PCR, ASO, ARMS
Hb S/Hb C	Sickle-cell disease, variable severity	RE-PCR, ASO, ARMS
Hb S/Hb D-Punjab	Sickle-cell disease	RE-PCR, ASO, ARMS
Hb S/Hb O-Arab	Sickle-cell disease	RE-PCR, ASO, ARMS
Hb S/HPFH	No clinical problems	RE-, Gap-PCR, MLPA
Hb E disorders		
Hb E + α^0-thal/α^+-thal (--/-α)	Similar to Hb H disease	Gap-PCR, ARMS
Hb EE + α^0-thal/α^+-thal (--/-α)	Severe thalassemia intermedia	Gap-PCR, ARMS
Hb EE + α^+-thal/α^+-thal ($\alpha^T\alpha/\alpha^T\alpha$)	Mild thalassemia intermedia	Gap-PCR, ASO

Hb = hemoglobin; thal = thalassemia; HPFH = hereditary persistence of fetal hemoglobin; PCR + polymerase chain reaction; MLPA = multiplex ligation-dependent probe amplification; RE = restriction enzyme; ASO = allele specific oligonucleotide; ARMS = amplification refraction mutation system a series of coordinated switches of production of one type of hemoglobin to another. During the first 8 weeks of intrauterine development, there is a switch from embryonic hemoglobin (Hb Gower 1 [$\zeta_2\varepsilon_2$], Hb Gower 2 [$\alpha_2\varepsilon_2$] and Hb Portland [$\zeta_2\gamma_2$]) to fetal haemoglobin (Hb F [$\alpha_2\gamma_2$]), which then switches at birth to adult hemoglobin (Hb A [$\alpha_2\beta_2$] and Hb A_2 [$\alpha_2\delta_2$]). By the end of the first year of life, the HbF level has dropped to less than 1% in normal individuals.

α-THALASSEMIA

Clinical states

α-Thalassaemia is characterized by a deficiency of α-globin chain synthesis. Defective gene expression may occur in either one globin gene (called α2- or α^+-thalassemia) or in both (α-1 or α^0-thalassemia) and thus there are four clinical states depending upon the number of functional α-globin genes (3, 2, 1 or 0).

Hb Bart's hydrops fetalis

The most severe form of α-thalassaemia is the homozygous state for α^0-thalassaemia, known as Hb Bart's hydrops fetalis syndrome. This condition results from a deletion of all four globin genes and an affected fetus cannot synthesize any α-globin to make Hb F or Hb A. Fetal blood contains only the abnormal hemoglobin Bart's (γ_4) and a small amount of Hb Portland. The resulting severe fetal anemia leads to asphyxia, hydrops fetalis and stillbirth or neonatal death, and prenatal diagnosis is always indicated in order to avoid the severe toxemic maternal complications that occur frequently in pregnancy with hydropic fetuses.

Hb H disease

Individuals with one functional α-gene have Hb H disease and are compound heterozygotes for α^+- and α^0-thalassemia. They have a moderately severe hypochromic microcytic anaemia and produce large amounts of Hb H (β_4) as a result of the excess β-chains in the reticulocyte. Patients with Hb H disease caused by deletion mutations (genotype --/-α) suffer from fatigue, general discomfort and splenomegaly, but they rarely require hospitalization and lead a relatively normal life.

However, patients with Hb H disease resulting from some of the non-deletion α^+-thalassemia mutations (genotypes --/$\alpha^T\alpha$ and $\alpha^T\alpha/\alpha^T\alpha$) may exhibit more severe symptoms with a possible requirement of recurrent blood transfusions and splenectomy. With some mutations in the α2-globin, cases of Hb H hydrops fetalis syndrome have been reported and couples at risk for this severe form of Hb H disease have opted for prenatal diagnosis and termination of an affected fetus[2]. In the UK, we have recently performed prenatal diagnosis for couples at risk for a fetus with Hb H hydrops fetalis resulting from the genotypes --^{SEA}/Hb Adana and PolyA (-AA)/PolyA (-AA)[3].

Asymptomatic states

Individuals with two functional α-globin genes (α^0-thalassemia trait or homozygous α^+-thalassemia) are characterized by a normal Hb A_2 level (<3.5%) and values for the mean cell hemoglobin (MCH) and mean cell volume (MCV) are clearly reduced below the normal range. The two genotypes have very similar phenotypes and can only be distinguished with certainty by DNA analysis. The detection of Hb Bart's in neonates[4] and the demonstration of occasional cells containing Hb H inclusion bodies in adults also signify the presence of α-thalassemia trait but, again, the tests do not clearly distinguish the various α-genotypes and do not detect all cases of α-thalassemia trait. Individuals with α^+-thalassaemia trait have three functional α-globin genes, with some having slightly reduced red cell indices, while others have red cell indices in the normal range.

In the UK, antenatal screening for α^0-thalassemia trait is performed using an algorithm which includes the ethnic origin of the mother[5]. This is designed to limit the number of investigations of suspected α-thalassemia in individuals of Indian, Pakistani and sub-Saharan African origin, in whom the clinically significant disorder of α^0-thalassemia is extremely rare and α^+-thalassemia is common.

Molecular defects

α^+-Thalassemia

Most individuals with α^+-thalassemia have a deletion of one of the two α-globin genes[6]. Although five different deletions have been identified, only two are commonly encountered in practice. These are the 3.7 kb deletion ($-\alpha^{3.7}$), which has reached high frequencies in the populations of Africa, the Mediterranean area, the Middle East, the Indian subcontinent and Melanesia, and the 4.2 kb deletion ($-\alpha^{4.2}$) which is commonly found in Southeast Asian and Pacific populations[7]. Various non-deletion defects have also been found to cause α^+-thalassemia and a total of 17 mutations have been described to date, mostly in populations from the Mediterranean area, Africa and Southeast Asia[8]. All of the mutations except one are located in the dominant α2-globin gene (denoted $\alpha^T\alpha$) and give rise to a more severe reduction in α-chain synthesis than in deletion α^+-thalassemia. The interaction of these non-deletional mutations with α^0-thalassemia results in severe Hb H disease or, in rare cases, Hb H hydrops fetalis syndrome[9].

α^0-Thalassemia

α^0-Thalassemia results from deletions which involve both α-globin genes and, to date, at least 14 different deletions have been described[8]. The deletions which have attained high gene frequencies are found in individuals from Southeast Asia and South China (--^{SEA}), the Philippine Islands (--^{FIL}), Thailand (--^{THAI}) and a few Mediterranean countries such as Greece, Cyprus and Turkey (--^{MED} and -(α)$^{20.5}$). Although an α^0-thalassemia mutation (--^{SA}) has been described in Asian Indians, it is extremely uncommon and no α^0-thalassemia deletions have been reported in individuals from sub-Saharan Africa, although α^0-thalassemia has been described, caused by a non-deletion α^+-thalassemia mutation linked to the 3.7 kb deletion gene. In Northern Europe, α-thalassemia occurs sporadically because of the lack of natural selection and several α^0-thalassemia deletions have been reported in single British families. However, one particular molecular defect (--^{BRIT}) appears to turn up fairly regularly in DNA samples referred to my laboratory for α-thalassemia investigations, especially from British individuals living in Cheshire and Lancashire.

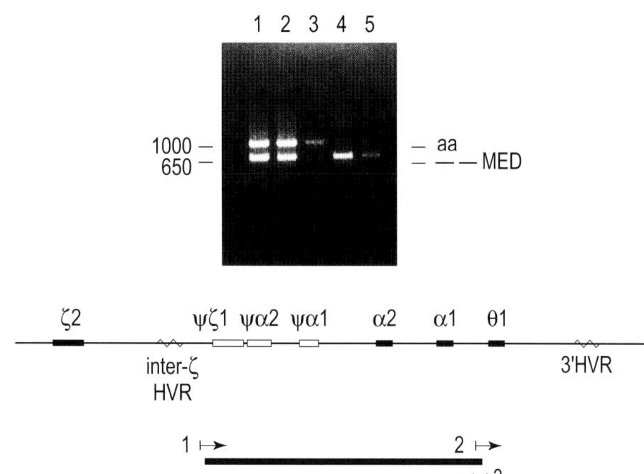

Fig. 26.1 Prenatal diagnosis for α⁰-thalassemia by GAP PCR. Lanes 1 and 2, maternal and paternal DNA heterozygous for the --^{MED} deletion gene; Lane 3, normal DNA; Lanes 4 and 5, fetal DNA showing homozygosity for α⁰-thalassemia. A diagram shows the location of the --^{MED} deletion within the α-globin gene cluster and the positions of primers 1 and 3 which amplify the mutant allele to give a 650 bp product and primers 2 and 3 which amplify only the normal allele to give a 1000 bp product.

Molecular diagnosis

Individuals with suspected α-thalassemia are normally screened first for the seven most common deletion alleles by the technique known as gap-PCR. Individuals with negative results are then screened for rare deletion α^0-thalassemia alleles by the technique called multiplex ligation-dependent probe amplification (MLPA), and/or by DNA sequence analysis for non-deletion α^+-thalassemia alleles.

Diagnosis of deletions by gap-PCR

The two most common α^+-thalassemia deletion genes, the -$\alpha^{3.7}$ and -$\alpha^{4.2}$ alleles, together with five α^o-thalassemia deletion genes, the --^{FILs}, --^{THAIs}, --^{MEDs}, -$(\alpha)^{20.5}$ and the --^{SEA} alleles, can be diagnosed by gap PCR[10–15] (Table 26.2). Gap PCR is the simplest of amplification techniques, using two primers complementary to the the DNA regions that flank the deletion to create a characteristic product that identifies the deletion gene. An example of the use of gap PCR for the prenatal diagnosis of the Mediterranean α^o-thalassemia mutation --^{MED} is illustrated in Figure 26.1.

Amplification of sequences in the α-globin gene cluster is technically more difficult than that of the β-globin gene cluster, requiring more stringent conditions for success due to the higher GC content. The addition of betaine and dimethyl sulfoxide to the PCR reaction in order to destabilize the GC-rich regions has improved the reliability of diagnosis. This has permitted the development of multiplex assays to detect heterozygosity and homozygosity of the seven deletion mutations[14,15], although great care is still needed in interpreting the results due to the possiblity of allele drop out. All prenatal diagnoses for α^o-thalassemia should be confirmed by a second technique such as MLPA.

Table 26.2 **Globin gene disorder deletions diagnosable by gap-PCR**

Disorder	*Deletion mutation*	*Distribution*
α^+-thalassemia	-$\alpha^{3.7}$	World-wide
	-$\alpha^{4.2}$	World-wide
α^0-thalassemia	-$(\alpha)^{20.5}$	Mediterranean
	--^{MED}	Mediterranean
β-thalassemia	--^{SEA}	Southeast Asian
	--^{THAI}	Thailand
	--^{FIL}	Philippines
	290 bp deletion	Turkey, Bulgaria
HPFH	532 bp deletion	Africa
	619 bp deletion	India, Pakistan
	1.4 kb deletion	Africa
	1.6 kb deletion	Croatia
	3.5 kb deletion	Thailand
	10.3 kb deletion	India
	45 kb deletion	Philippines
	Hb Lepore	Mediterranean
$\delta\beta^0$-thalassemia	Spanish	Spain
	Sicilian	Mediterranean
	Vietnamese	Vietnam
	Macedonian/Turkish	Mediterranean
$\gamma\delta\beta^0$-thalassemia	Indian	India, Bangladesh
	Chinese	Southern China
HPFH	HPFH 1	Africa
	HPFH 2	Ghana, Africa
	HPFH 3	India
	Hb Kenya	Kenya, Africa

Hb = hemoglobin; bp = base pairs; kb = kilobase pairs; HPFH = hereditary persistence of fetal hemoglobin

Diagnosis of deletions by MLPA

Other approaches have also been developed to provide quick simple, rapid, accurate and cost effective methods of screening for the deletion mutations. These include the use of real-time quantitative PCR[16], denaturing HPLC[17], real-time quantitative PCR[18] and the use of an oligonucleotide microarray[19,20]. However, the most useful recent development for the diagnosis of deletion mutations is the technique known as multiplex ligation-dependent probe amplification (MLPA)[21]. Two sets of 35 probes have been developed that can detect all known deletions located in the α-globin gene cluster on chromosome 16p13.3. This method detects rare and novel forms of deletional α-thalassemia that cannot be diagnosed by gap PCR and provides an excellent back-up diagnostic method for the common deletion mutations in prenatal diagnosis of homozygous α^o-thalassemia.

Diagnosis of point mutations

The non-deletion α^+-thalassemia mutations can be identified by PCR techniques following the selective amplification of the α-globin genes[22]. This technique allows the amplified product from each α-globin gene to be analyzed by a variety of techniques for known mutations, or by DNA sequence analysis for an unknown mutation[3]. Techniques for the direct detection of known point mutations include allele specific oligonucleotide hybridization or allele specific priming[23] or restriction enzyme analysis, useful for Hb Constant Spring[2].

β-THALASSEMIA

Clinical states

β-Thalassemia is characterized by a deficiency of β-globin chain synthesis. Individuals with β-thalassemia trait are essentially healthy, although they may have a slightly reduced Hb level and have typically low MCH and MCV values. In contrast to α-thalassemia, the Hb A_2 concentration in carriers is usually elevated above the normal range to a level of 3.5–7.0%. Exceptions are carriers with co-inherited δ-thalassemia trait[24] or the inheritance of a mild allele known as a silent β-thalassemia or normal Hb A_2 β-thalassemia[25]. Carriers with an unusually high level of Hb A_2 (7.0–9.0%) have a deletion mutation affecting the promoter region of the β-globin gene.

The majority of individuals homozygous for β-thalassemia have the transfusion-dependent condition called β-thalassemia major. This condition results from the homozygous state for a severe β-thalassemia mutation or, more commonly, the compound heterozygous state for two different severe mutations. At birth, β-thalassemia homozygotes are asymptomatic because of the high production of Hb F but, as this declines, affected infants present with severe anemia during the first or second year of life. Treatment is by frequent blood transfusion to maintain a hemoglobin level above 10 g/dl, coupled with iron chelation therapy to control iron overload, otherwise death results in the second or third decade from cardiac failure. This treatment does not cure β-thalassemia major, although some patients have now reached the age of 40 in good health and have married and produced children. With the prospects for gene therapy remaining as distant as ever, the only cure for β-thalassemia for the foreseeable future is bone marrow transplantation. Although this form of treatment has proved successful when carried out in young children, it is limited by the requirement of an HLA-matched sibling or relative.

Some individuals homozygous for β-thalassemia have a milder clinical condition called thalassemia intermedia. Such patients present later in life relative to those with thalassemia major and are capable of maintaining a hemoglobin level above 6 g without transfusion. Thalassemia intermedia is caused by a wide variety of genotypes and covers a broad clinical spectrum. Patients with a severe condition present between 2 and 6 years of age and, although they are capable of surviving with an Hb level of 5–7 g/dl they will not develop normally and are treated with minimal blood transfusion. At the other end of the spectrum are patients who do not become symptomatic until they reach adult life and remain transfusion independent with Hb levels of 8–10 g/dl. However, even these milder patients tend to accumulate iron with age and many thalassemia intermedia patients develop clinical problems relating to iron overload after the third decade.

Molecular defects

Unlike α-thalassemia, most β-thalassemia heterozygotes carry a non-deletion mutation. More than 200 point mutations or small insertions/deletions of DNA sequence in and around the β-globin gene have been described, in contrast to only 13 large deletions of 44 nucleotides or greater[24]. The mutations either reduce the expression of the β-globin gene (β^+-type) or result in the complete absence of β-globin (β^0-type). Many of the mutations have attained high frequencies through a positive selection mechanism due to malaria and these are listed in Table 26.3 for selected countries from the four main regions: the Mediterranean area, Asian India, Southeast Asia and Sub-Saharan Africa. For each region there are a small number of specific mutations which account for more than 90%, together with a larger number of mutations found with a very low gene frequency. With each country within a region having its own characteristic spectrum of mutations, knowledge of the ethnic origin of a patient simplifies the identification of the mutations, especially in countries like the UK with patients from all four regions (Table 26.3).

The majority of β^+- and β^0-type mutations have a severe phenotype, but a few β^+-type mutations result in a milder phenotype because of an increased amount of β-gene expression, and a couple of β^0-type mutations have a mild phenotype because they are linked to a genetic determinant which increases Hb F production. The β^+ mutations include the transcription mutations located in the promoter region upstream of the β-globin gene, such as the mutations at nucleotide −88, −87, −30, −29 and −28 listed in Table 26.3, the CAP + 1 site mutation, mutations between codon 24 and 27 such as the codon 24 mutation in Africans and the codon 26 mutation which creates Hb E, and the mutation at IVSI-6 mutation found in Mediterranean countries. The latter mutation, together with CAP + 1 found in Asian Indians, results in a borderline-raised Hb A_2 level of 3.5–4.0%, and carriers of these mutations may be mistaken for having α-thalassemia trait. However, these mutations do result in reduced MCV and MCH values, in contrast to three Mediterranean silent β-thalassemia mutations, −101 (C→T) and −92 (C→T) and IVSII-844 (G→C). Heterozygotes for these mutations exhibit normal MCV and MCH values in addition to a normal/borderline-raised Hb A_2 value and are often missed by hematological screening tests, thus having a truly silent type of β-thalassemia.

The mild β^+ mutations are characterized by having been identified in thalassemia intermedia patients in either the homozygous or compound heterozygous state. However, predicting the phenotype of thalassemia intermedia on the basis of a known genotype remains a problem. Homozygosity for a mild mutation nearly always results in intermedia, but the combination of a mild and severe mutation results in thalassemia major in some cases. In addition, the inheritance of ameliorating genetic factors such as α thalassemia, a high Hb F determinant, or other factors for which the molecular basis remains unclear[26] can result in a patient with a thalassemia major genotype developing thalassemia intermedia. Other causes of thalassemia intermedia include the compound heterozygosity for a β-thalassemia mutation and a triple or quadruple

Table 26.3 The relative gene frequencies of the common β-thalassemia mutations in selected countries in the four main thalassemia regions, compared with those found in the UK population[a]

Mutation	Mediterranean					South Asian				Southeast Asian				African	UK
	Spain	Italy	Greece	Turkey	Egypt	Pakistan	India	Sri Lanka	Bangladesh	China	Thailand	Malaysia	Indonesia	African-American	
−101 (C→T)		0.4	0.5	0.4											1.3
−88 (C→T)							0.3							24.3	4.8
−87 (C→G)		1.5	2.0	1.1	1.9										0.1
−30 (T→A)			0.1	3.1	1.5										
−29 (A→G)										2.3				68.4	2.3
−28 (A→G)										12.4	5.8	3.1			0.7
CAP + 1(A→ C)						1.2	1.0								4.8
CD5 (−CT)			0.3	2.3	1.9	2.1									3.2
CD6 (−A)	1.0	1.2	2.8	0.4	0.3										0.4
CD8 (−AA)	0.2		0.5	5.4	0.3										0.1
CD8/9 (+G)	14.1		0.1	1.6		24.1	12.0	2.0	10.0		0.2				9.8
CD15 (G→A)			0.1	0.2	0.1	3.3	0.7	1.0	10.0				6.8		3.7
CD16 (−C)						1.8	0.5	1.0							0.1
CD17 (A→T)										16.6	21.2	7.1	1.7		1.0
CD19 (A→G)											5.4	10.2			
CD24 (T→A)														2.4	0.2
CD30 (G→C)		0.1	0.1			2.3	1.0	1.0					1.7		2.4
IVSI-1 (G→A)	25.0	10.4	13.4	4.7	15.1			27.0					1.7		1.9
IVSI-1 (G→T)			0.1			10.4	23.0			1.3	3.8	9.4	10.2		1.6
IVSI-5 (G→C)		0.2		1.3		32.4	30.5	56.0	60.0	2.5		45.9	54.2	1.8	22.5
IVSI-6 (T→C)	9.4	10.1	8.4	11.3	19.7										2.2

Table 26.3 **(Continued)**

Mutation	*Mediterranean*					*South Asian*				*Southeast Asian*				*African*	*UK*
	Spain	*Italy*	*Greece*	*Turkey*	*Egypt*	*Pakistan*	*India*	*Sri Lanka*	*Bangladesh*	*China*	*Thailand*	*Malaysia*	*Indonesia*	*African-American*	
IVSI-110 (G→A)	10.2	23.5	42.5	39.7	28.5										5.5
CD39 (C→T)		41.0	19.6	4.4	2.1										3.4
CD41/42 (−TCTT)						6.3	7.0	2.0	20.0	42.3	40.2	7.1	1.7		9.0
CD71/72 (+A)										5.8	2.4	2.8			0.1
IVSII-1 (G→A)		3.9	2.0	6.3	2.2	0.6									2.3
IVSII-654 (C→T)					0.1					12.1	6.0	4.1	11.9		1.6
IVSII-745 (C→G)	1.5	5.2	4.8	3.2	3.7										1.7
619 bp deletion						13.1	20.0	0.2					8.7		1.7
Others	9.6	3.4	3.2	11.9	14.4	2.5	3.7	9.8	10.0	4.3	3.8	11.3	3.8	3.9	13.7

CD = codon; IVS = intervening sequence; bp = base pairs

[a]Data collected by J Old for the European Commission ITHANET Coordination Action project – Infrastructure for Thalassemia Research Network

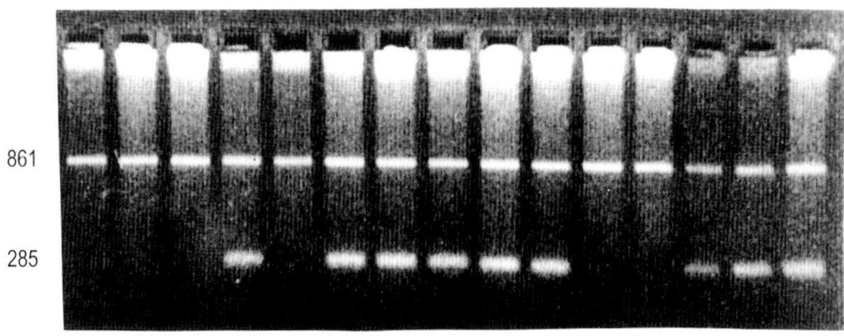

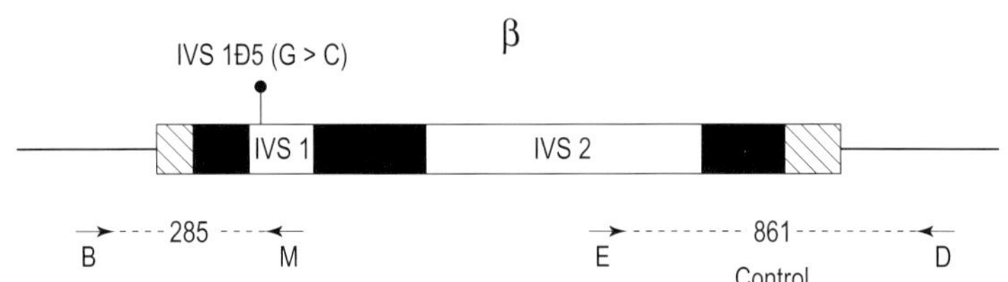

Fig. 26.2 Screening for the mutation IVS1-5 (G→C) by primer specific amplification. A diagram of the β-globin gene shows the location of the mutation and its specific ARMS primer (M) plus the positions of the common primer (B) and two control primers (E and D) which generate an 861 bp product. Above, an ethidium bromide stained gel shows the results of screening a number of heterozygous β-thalassemia individuals for IVS1-5 (G→C). The generation of the specific 285 bp product indicates an individual heterozygous for the mutation.

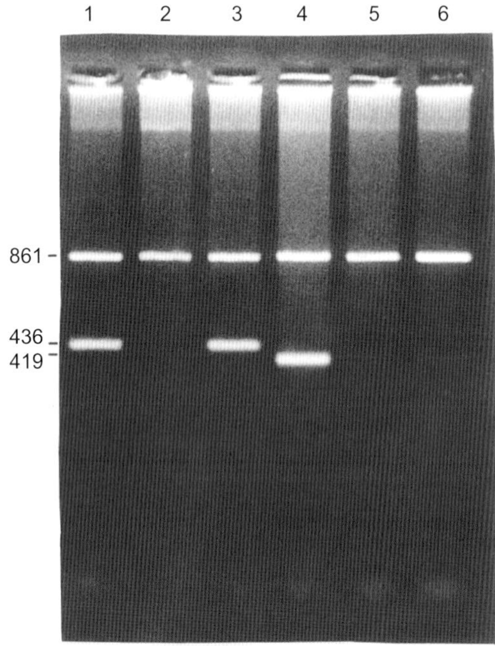

Fig. 26.3 Prenatal diagnosis for β-thalassemia using ARMS primers to detect the mutations IVS1-110 (G→A) and codon 39 (C→T). Lanes 1 and 6 show fetal DNA, lanes 2 and 4 maternal DNA and lanes 3 and 5 paternal DNA. The first three lanes show the results with an ARMS primer for codon 39 and lanes 4–6 show the results with an ARMS primer for IVS1-110. The upper band is the 861 bp control product. The results show the fetus was heterozygous for codon 39.

α-gene locus, and the heterozygous state for one of the rare β-thalassemia mutations in exon 3 which cause inclusion-body hemolytic anemia, sometimes called dominantly inherited β-thalassemia[27].

Molecular diagnosis

DNA sequences from the β-globin gene cluster are easily amplified under standard conditions and a wide variety of techniques have been developed and new ones are continually being published. However, most diagnostic laboratories use just one or two of the techniques described below, following a strategy which depends upon knowing the most prevalent mutations likely to be encountered in the ethnic group of the individual being screened. When the ethnic origin is not known, then direct sequencing may be the quickest method of identifying the mutation.

Allele-specific oligonucleotides

The hybridization of allele-specific oligonucleotide probes (ASOs) to amplified DNA bound to nylon membrane in the form of dots was the first PCR-based method to be developed[28]. The method gained widespread use, but is limited by the need for separate hybridizations to test for more than one mutation.

To overcome this problem the method of reverse dot blotting was developed, in which the roles of the oligonucleotide probe and target amplified DNA are reversed[29]. This procedure allows multiple mutations to be tested for in one hybridization reaction and has been applied to the detection of β-thalassemia mutations in Mediterraneans[30], African-Americans[31] and Thais[32], using a two-step procedure with one strip for the common mutations and the other for the less common ones.

The principle of reverse dot blotting has been brought up to date by the development of microarrays for the simultaneous detection of large numbers of β-thalassemia mutations[33,34]. Using the approach of tagged single-based extension and hybridization to glass, flow-through arrays have been developed by several groups for the detection of 17 and 23 β-globin mutations[35,36]. However, it is not yet clear whether these state-of-the-art methods will prove cheap enough to replace conventional techniques in the future and whether there will be a viable market for thalassemia mutation chips, because the diagnosis of the common mutations in most populations can be easily screened for by rapid low-tech methods and for which the additional screening capacity on the chip would be redundant.

Primer-specific amplification

A number of different methods have been developed based on the principle of primer-specific amplification, which is that a perfectly matched PCR primer is much more efficient in annealing and directing primer extension than one containing one or two mismatched bases. The method known as the amplification refractory mutation system (ARMS)[37] has been developed to a simple, cheap detection method for all the common β-thalassemia mutations in all four major ethnic groups[38]. The method provides a quick screening method which does not require any form of labeling as the amplified products are visualized simply by agarose gel electrophoresis and ethidium bromide staining (Figs 26.2 and 26.3), although fluorescent labels can be used[39]. The technique can be multiplexed to screen more than one mutation at the same time[40], and variations of the technique include competitive oligonucleotide priming (COP)[41] and the use of ARMS primers that differ in length, called the mutagenetically separated polymerase chain reaction (MS-PCR)[42].

Other techniques

Gap-PCR is useful for the diagnosis of some of the the β-thalassemia deletion mutations, as detailed in Table 26.1[43]. Restriction enzyme analysis (RE-PCR) is not so useful as only approximately 40 β-thalassemia mutations are known to create or abolish a restriction endonuclease site.

Unknown mutations

A number of techniques have been applied for the detection of β-thalassemia mutations without prior knowledge of the molecular defect, including denaturing gradient gel electrophoresis (DGGE)[44] and heteroduplex analysis by non-denaturing gel electrophoresis[45]. However, the most widely used method of identifying unknown mutations is direct DNA sequencing of the β-globin gene. This can now be done very efficiently in just three amplification reactions using an automated DNA sequencing machine utilizing fluorescence detection technology.

δβ-THALASSEMIA

Clinical states

δβ-Thalassemia and the deletion types of hereditary persistence of fetal hemoglobin (HPFH) are characterized by the complete absence of Hb A and Hb A_2 in homozygotes, and an elevated level of Hb F in heterozygotes. Both disorders are caused by large DNA deletions removing the β- and δ-globin genes but leaving either one or both γ-globin genes intact. More than 50 different deletion mutations have been identified[46] and they can be classified into the $(\delta\beta)^0$- and $(^A\gamma\delta\beta)^0$-thalassemias, HPFH conditions, fusion chain variants and $(\varepsilon\gamma\delta\beta)^0$-thalassemia.

The $(\delta\beta)^0$-thalassemias are characterized by the Hb F consisting of both $^G\gamma$- and $^A\gamma$-globin chains, with heterozygotes exhibiting an Hb F level of 5–15% and normal Hb A_2 levels. For the majority of mutations, the Hb F is heterogeneously distributed in the red cells. There is a reduction of the non-α-globin chains compared to α-globin and the red cells are hypochromic and microcytic. Homozygotes for this condition have thalassemia intermedia.

The $(^A\gamma\delta\beta)^0$-thalassemias are characterized by the Hb F containing only $^G\gamma$-globin chains as the $^A\gamma$-globin gene has been deleted in these conditions. Apart from this distinction, the phenotype of the heterozygous and homozygous states are identical to those for $(\delta\beta)^0$-thalassemia.

The deletional HPFH conditions can be regarded as a type of δβ-thalassemia in which the reduction in β-globin chain production is almost completely compensated for by the increased γ-globin chain production. Homozygous individuals have 100% F comprising of both $^A\gamma$- and $^G\gamma$-globin chains but, in contrast to $(\delta\beta)^0$-thalassemia homozygotes, they are clinically normal. Heterozygotes have an elevated Hb F level of 17–35%, usually higher than that found in δβ-thalassemia heterozygotes, and the Hb F is distributed uniformly (pancellular) in red cells that have near normal MCH and MCV values.

Two deletions in the β-globin gene cluster create a fusion Hb chain, as a result of unequal crossing over between different globin genes. Hb Lepore is a hybrid globin chain comprising δ and β globin sequences and is a β-thalassemia allele, while Hb Kenya comprises γ- and β-globin sequences and is an HPFH allele. Hb Lepore homozygotes have a severe disorder, similar to thalassemia major or severe thalassemia intermedia. Hb Kenya has only been observed in the heterozygous state and is similar to heterozygous HPFH, with individuals having 5–10% HbF, normal red cell morphology and balanced globin chain synthesis.

The $(\varepsilon\gamma\delta\beta)^0$ thalassemias are rare conditions that result from long deletions that start upstream of the β-globin gene cluster locus control region (LCR) and remove either all of the β-globin gene cluster or, in two cases, all but β-globin gene (which is inactivated as a result). In adult life, heterozygotes for this condition have a similar hematological picture to β-thalassemia trait with a normal Hb A_2 level. The homozygous condition is presumed to be incompatible with fetal survival.

Finally, there is a group of conditions called non-deletion HPFH in which heterozygous individuals have normal red cells and no clinical abnormalities and an elevated Hb F level as a result of a point mutation in the promoter region of the $^A\gamma$- or $^G\gamma$-globin gene in most cases. The %Hb F is variable, ranging from 1–3% in the Swiss type to 10–20% in the Greek type.

Molecular diagnosis

The δβ-thalassemia, Hb Lepore and HPFH deletion mutations were characterized originally by restriction enzyme mapping and Southern blotting, but Gap PCR is now used for the diagnosis of the common mutations (see Table 26.1)[43]. The technique is useful for the diagnosis of Hb Lepore (7), six δβ thalassemia alleles, three HPFH deletion mutations (82) and Hb Kenya. This technique provides a useful and simple screening method for distinguishing HPFH from δββ-thalassemia in Asian Indian, African and Mediterranean individuals. Individuals carrying a rare or novel δβ-thalassemia, εγδβ-thalassemia and HPFH deletion mutations can now be investigated by MLPA analysis[21].

ABNORMAL HEMOGLOBINS

The structural hemoglobin variants that cause clinical disorders can be divided into those that alter the oxygen-carrying properties of hemoglobin, unstable variants that produce a hemolytic anemia and a few that are ineffectively synthesized and thus result in the phenotype of thalassemia. Although most are not very common, three (Hb S, Hb C and Hb E) have reached gene frequencies high enough to cause major public health problems in many countries.

Hb S

Prenatal diagnosis is normally offered for the sickling disorders, which include the homozygous condition, called sickle-cell disease (SS) and the compound heterozygous states for the Hb S gene in association with β-thalassemia, Hb C, Hb D-Punjab and Hb O-Arab. Sickle-cell disease is characterized by a lifelong hemolytic anemia, the occurrence of acute exacerbations called crises, and a variety of complications resulting from an increased propensity to infection and the deleterious effects of repeated vaso-occlusive episodes. Hemoglobin SC disease can be mild, though it may be associated with ocular, CNS and bone complications and thrombotic problems in pregnancy. The interactions with Hb D-Punjab and Hb O-Arab are more severe, resulting in both cases in a disease indistinguishable from homozygous sickle-cell anemia. With active management, the proportion of patients expected to survive to 20 years of age is approximately 90%. The course of the illness is very variable, even within individual sibships, let alone different racial groups. The clinical course of sickle-cell β-thalassemia is also very variable, ranging from a disorder identical with sickle-cell anemia to a completely asymptomatic condition, depending on the severity of the β-thalassemia mutation.

The sickle mutation, codon 6 (A→T), is thought to have arisen independently at least four times in Africa and once in Asia because of its association with different β-globin gene haplotypes, named Benin, Bantu or CAR, Senegal, Cameroon and Saudi Arabian/Indian[47]. Epidemiological studies have shown that the CAR haplotype is associated with the most clinically severe condition[48]. The haplotype associated with the mildest course of the disease is the Saudi Arabian/Indian type. SS patients with this haplotype exhibit high levels of Hb F (10–25%) because this particular β^S mutation is linked to the −158 C→T mutation 5′ to the $^G\gamma$-globin gene which results in enhanced γ-chain production in response to anemic stress.

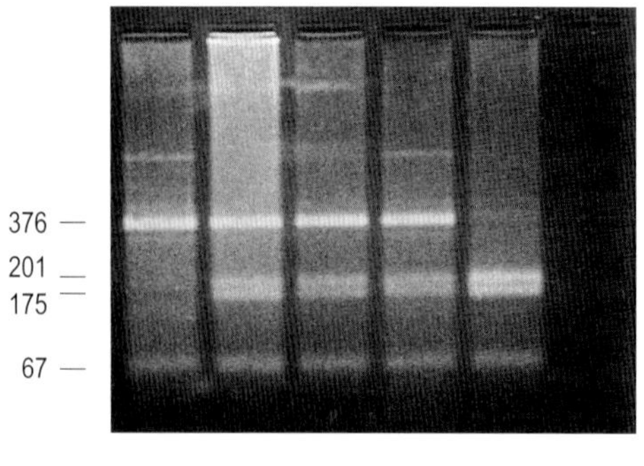

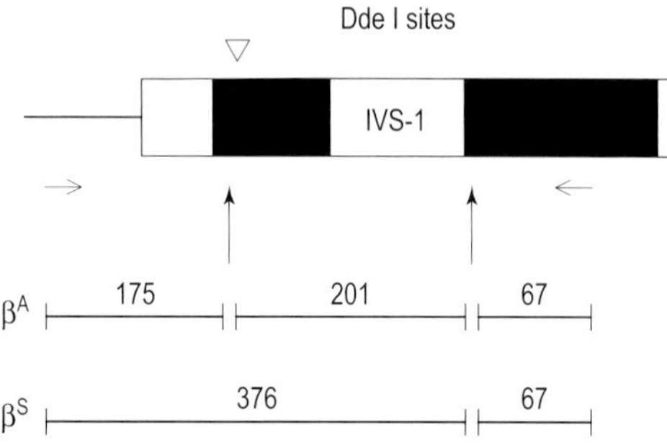

Fig. 26.4 Prenatal diagnosis of the sickle-cell mutation by amplification and digestion of the product with *Dde* I. An ethidium bromide stained agarose gel shows the digestion products observed from DNA from: Lane 1, a sickle-cell homozygote (S/S); Lanes 2 and 3, sickle-cell heterozygotes (parental samples); Lane 4, fetal DNA (A/S); Lane 5, a normal individual (A/A). The sickle mutation at codon 6 (shown by the triangle) is diagnosed by the presence of the 376 bp fragment.

Hb C

Hb C is found predominantly in West African countries and the frequency of heterozygous state has reached as high as 28% in some parts of Ghana. The heterozygous state is symptomless and the homozygous state is characterized by a variable hemolytic anemia due to the red cells being abnormally rigid and having a shortened lifespan, but is associated with no serious clinical disability. Hb C is clinically significant because of its interaction with Hb S.

Hb E

Hb E is extremely common in Southeast Asian countries. Hb E is associated with a mild β-thalassemia phenotype because the mutation activates a cryptic splice site producing an abnormal mRNA molecule. The homozygous state for Hb E is associated with no clinical disability and the importance of Hb E lies in its interaction with β-thalassemia. Compound heterozygotes have a variable clinical picture ranging from a disorder indistinguishable from β-thalassemia major to a mild form of β-thalassemia intermedia. As with Hb S, compound heterozygotes with a β^0-thalassemia allele exhibit the most severe disorder, while those with a β^+ allele may sometimes have a milder disorder[1].

Molecular diagnosis

The mutations giving rise to Hb S, Hb D-Punjab and Hb O-Arab may be diagnosed most easily and quickly by restriction endonuclease digestion of an amplified β-globin gene fragment (Fig. 26.4). The Hb S mutation abolishes a *Dde* I or *Mst* II site, Hb E abolishes an *Mnl* I site and Hb D-Punjab and Hb O-Arab both abolish an *Eco*R I site. The Hb C mutation does not affect a restriction site and must be diagnosed by dot blot analysis or ARMS.

PRENATAL DIAGNOSIS

An antenatal screening program for detection of at-risk couples should be able to identify by hematological and DNA testing the majority of carrier states for α^0-thalassemia, β-thalassemia, δβ-thalassemia, and the Hb variants S, C, D-Punjab, O-Arab and Lepore[49]. In the UK, there are two strategies for antenatal screening, one based on universal screening for high prevalence areas, and one based on ethnic origin of the woman and her partner for low prevalence areas. The screening algorithms and guidelines for referral of patients for DNA analysis can be found on the NHS Sickle Cell and Thalassemia Screening Program website (http://www.kcl-phs.org.uk/haemscreening).

Chorionic villus DNA

Chorionic villus sampling is the method of choice for providing fetal DNA as it is carried out in the first trimester of pregnancy and provides a good yield of DNA. The average sample taken between 10 and 12 weeks' gestation by transcervical or transabdominal aspiration yields 35 μg of fetal DNA. Villi collected by either method must be sorted by microscopic dissection to remove all traces of maternal tissue before DNA preparation. Sorted villi can then be transported to a DNA diagnosis laboratory in either tissue culture medium or, preferably, in a small volume of cell lysis buffer containing sodium dodecyl sulphate (SDS) and proteinase K, which lyses the villi in transit and provides a stable protective environment for the DNA for many days.

Amniotic fluid cell DNA

Amniocentesis is often used for couples who present themselves too late for prenatal diagnosis by chorionic villus sampling. Less fetal DNA is obtained from an amniotic fluid sample than from chorionic villi; a 10 ml sample will yield between 1.5 and 5 μg of DNA. Cultured cells should always be grown as a back up source of fetal DNA in case of diagnostic failure with the direct sample.

FETAL CELLS IN MATERNAL BLOOD

Fetal cells have long been known to be present in the maternal circulation and they provide an attractive non-invasive approach to prenatal diagnosis. However, attempts to isolate the fetal cells as a source of fetal DNA using immunological methods and cell sorting have had only moderate success in providing a population of cells pure enough for fetal DNA analysis. Until recently, analysis of fetal cells in maternal blood could only be applied for the prenatal diagnosis of β-thalassemia in women whose partners carried a different mutation, as reported for the diagnosis of Hb Lepore[50]. However, the development of the technique of isolation of single nucleated fetal erythrocytes by micromanipulation under microscopic observation[51] has permitted the analysis of both fetal genes in single cells from maternal blood. This approach has now been tried successfully for prenatal diagnosis in two pregnancies at risk for sickle-cell anemia and β-thalassemia[52]. However, the approach has proved subject to technical difficulties as well as being costly and time consuming, and is not widely applicable at the moment.

FETAL DNA IN MATERNAL PLASMA

The analysis of fetal DNA in maternal plasma is a simpler and more robust procedure than the analysis of DNA in fetal nucleated red cells in maternal blood as no enrichment process is involved[53]. Cells are removed from the plasma by simple centrifugation and then the DNA in the plasma may be purified by standard methods[54]. Fetal DNA has been detected in as little as 10 ml of maternal plasma at 11–17 weeks' gestation and is cleared very rapidly from the maternal plasma post partum[55]. The technique is being used for the prenatal diagnosis of sex-linked disease and fetal RhD blood group type. The approach can only be used to detect the paternally inherited mutation and thus for β-thalassemia it is limited in that it is only potentially applicable to couples in which the paternal mutation is different to the maternal mutation. It has been used for the prenatal exclusion of β-thalassemia major in eight fetuses at risk using allele specific primers for the detection of the CD 41/42 (-CTTT) mutation by real-time PCR[56], and the detection of homozygous α^0-thalassemia[57]. However, the further development of the method to detect both maternal and paternal linked polymorphisms may allow the technique to exclude maternal β-thalassemia mutations in the future[58].

PREIMPLANTATION DIAGNOSIS

Preimplantation genetic diagnosis (PGD) represents a 'state-of-the-art' procedure that allows at-risk couples to have disease-free children without the need to terminate affected pregnancies. PCR-based diagnostic methods can be potentially applied for preimplantation genetic diagnosis using three types of cells: polar bodies from the oocyte/zygote stage, blastomeres from cleavage stage embryos and trophoectoderm cells from blastocysts[59]. Although the technique requires a combined expertise in both reproductive medicine and molecular genetics, a small number of centers around the world are now set up to carry out this procedure for hemoglobin disorders, resulting in the birth of more than 50 healthy children. PGD has been used successfully for both α-thalassemia[60,61] and β-thalassemia[62,63]. The approach is especially useful for couples for whom religious or ethical beliefs will not permit the termination of pregnancy, and for couples who have already had one or more therapeutic abortions.

However, preimplantation genetic diagnosis is technically challenging, multistep and an expensive procedure. The PCR protocol must be able to diagnose the required genotype in single cells reliably and accurately and it also has to be optimized to minimize PCR failure and to avoid the problem of allele dropout which could lead to a misdiagnosis. Protocols designed to monitor the occurrence of allele dropout include multiplex PCR to detect both alleles that contribute to the genotype, such as denaturing gradient gel electrophoresis (DGGE), single strand conformation analysis (SSCA) and real-time PCR[64]. The birth of a healthy unaffected baby depends not only on an accurate diagnosis, but also on the success of each of the multiple stages of the assisted reproduction procedure. Overall, the success rate of the procedure is only 20–30% and thus this approach is not likely to be used routinely for the monitoring of pregnancies at risk for hemoglobin disorders. One specific use of this approach is to allow the birth of a normal child that is HLA identical to an affected sibling, thus permitting a possible cure by stem cell transplantation[63].

Diagnostic strategy

Since nearly all of the α- and β-thalassaemia mutations have been determined and most racial groups have only a few common mutations, it is now possible to offer prenatal diagnosis (PND) for almost every couple at risk for thalassemia. The best strategy is to determine the mutations in the parents before fetal sampling. However, provided the ethnic origin of each partner is known, it is possible to identify the parental mutations and perform a fetal diagnosis in 3–4 days in more than 95% of couples at risk for β-thalassemia without knowing the mutation. If one parent has a rare mutation that requires DNA sequencing to identify a mutation first, the prenatal diagnosis may take a little longer. Note that fresh parental samples blood are usually required for every PND, even when the mutations are known, in order to provide fresh control DNA samples.

DIAGNOSTIC PITFALLS

A problem with all PCR-based techniques used for fetal DNA diagnosis is the coamplification of maternal sequences. With chorionic villus samples this event can be avoided by the careful dissection of maternal decidua from the fetal trophoblast and by reducing the number of amplification cycles to 25, as shown by the experience of the Italian groups who have reported no misdiagnoses in 457 first-trimester fetal DNA analyses for β-thalassemia[65]. Uncultured amniotic fluid samples are more of a problem, with a recent study finding the presence of maternal cell contamination in 21% of samples compared with 0.2% in cultured fluid[66], and all such cases in which the fetal diagnosis is identical to the maternal genotype should be retested using a back-up culture[67] or checked by DNA polymorphism analysis to avoid the possibility of misdiagnosis. The presence of coamplified maternal DNA sequences may be revealed by the amplification of informative polymorphic markers[68], or by analyzing up to 12 short tandem repeat markers on a DNA sequencing machine[69]. Another potential source of error is the failure to amplify one of the target DNA alleles. This may be due to allele dropout, as with gap-PCR for α-thalassemia, or when the hybridization of a primer or probe is compromised by an unexpected change in the target DNA sequence[70].

ACKNOWLEDGMENTS

The β-thalassemia mutation frequency data presented in Table 26.3 was collected for the European Commission Coordination Action project 'Infrastructure for Thalassaemia Research Network' (ITHANET), and funding for this EC Coordination Action Contract no 026539 is gratefully acknowledged.

REFERENCES

1. Weatherall DJ, Clegg JB. *The thalassemia syndromes*, 4th edn. Oxford: Blackwell Scientific Publications, 2001.
2. Ko TM, Tseng LH, Hsieh FJ et al. Prenatal diagnosis of HbH disease due to compound heterozygosity for south-east Asian deletion and Hb Constant Spring by polymerase chain reaction. *Prenat Diagn* **13**:143–146, 1993.
3. Henderson S, Chapple M, Rugless M et al. Haemoglobin H hydrops fetalis syndrome associated with homozygosity for the alpha2-globin gene polyadenylation signal mutation AATAAA-->AATA- -. *Br J Haematol* **135**:743–745, 2006.
4. Rugless MJ, Fisher CA, Stephens AD et al. Hb Bart's in cord blood: an accurate indicator of alpha-thalassemia. *Hemoglobin* **30**:57–62, 2006.
5. Old JM. Screening and genetic diagnosis of haemoglobinopathies. *Scand J Clin Lab Invest* **66**:1–16, 2006.
6. Higgs DR, Vickers MA, Wilkie AOM et al. A review of the molecular genetics of the human α-globin gene cluster. *Blood* **73**:1081–1110, 1989.
7. Flint J, Harding RM, Boyce AJ, Clegg JB. The population genetics of the haemoglobinopathies. In *The haemoglobinopathies, Baillière's clinical haematology*, DR Higgs, DJ Weatherall (eds), pp. 215–262. London: Baillière Tindall and WB Saunders, 1993.
8. Higgs DR. α-Thalassaemia. In *The haemoglobinopathies, Baillière's clinical haematology*, DR Higgs, DJ Weatherall (eds), pp. 117–150. London: Baillière Tindall and WB Saunders, 1993.
9. Ko T, Hsieh FJ, Hsu PM et al. Molecular characterisation of severe α-thalassaemias causing hydrops fetalis in Taiwan. *Am J Med Genet* **39**:317–320, 1991.
10. Dode C, Krishnamoorthy R, Lamb J et al. Rapid analysis of -α$^{3.7}$ thalassaemia and ααα$^{anti\ 3.7}$ triplication by enzymatic amplification analysis. *Br J Haematol* **82**:105–111, 1992.
11. Baysal E, Huisman THJ. Detection of common deletional α-thalassaemia-2 determinants by PCR. *Am J Hematol* **46**:208–213, 1994.
12. Bowden DK, Vickers MA, Higgs DR. A PCR-based strategy to detect the common severe determinants of α-thalassaemia. *Br J Haematol* **81**:104–108, 1992.
13. Ko T-M, Li S-F. Molecular characterization of the --FIL determinant of alpha-thalassaemia (corrigendum for Ko, et al 1998). *Am J Hematol* **60**:173, 1999.
14. Liu YT, Old JM, Fisher CA et al. Rapid detection of α-thalassaemia deletions and α-globin gene triplication by multiplex PCRs. *Br J Haematol* **108**:295–299, 2000.
15. Chong SS, Boehm CD, Higgs DR et al. Single-tube multiplex-PCR screen for common deletional determinants of α-thalassemia. *Blood* **95**:360–362, 2000.
16. Sun CF, Lee CH, Cheng SW et al. Real-time quantitative PCR analysis for alpha-thalassemia-1 of Southeast Asian type deletion in Taiwan. *Clin Genet* **60**:305–309, 2001.
17. Ou-Yang H, Hua L, Mo HQ et al. Rapid, accurate genotyping of the common alpha (4.2) deletion based on the use of denaturing HPLC. *J Clin Pathol* **57**: 159–163, 2004.
18. Tungwiwat W, Fucharoen S, Fucharoen G et al. Development and application of a real-time quantitative PCR for prenatal detection of fetal alpha(0)-thalassemia from maternal plasma. *Ann NY Acad Sci* **1075**:103–107, 2006.
19. Zesong L, Ruijun G, Wen Z. Rapid detection of deletional alpha-thalassemia by an oligonucleotide microarray. *Am J Hematol* **80**:306–308, 2005.
20. Bang-Ce Y, Hongqiong L, Zhuanfong Z et al. Simultaneous detection of alpha-thalassemia and beta-thalassemia by oligonucleotide microarray. *Haematologica* **89**:1010–1012, 2004.
21. Harteveld Cl, Voskamp A, Phylipsen M et al. Nine unknown rearrangements in 16p13.3 and 11p15.4 causing alpha- and beta-thalassaemia characterised by high resolution multiplex ligation-dependent probe amplification. *J Med Genet* **42**: 922–931, 2005.
22. Molchanova TP, Pobedimskaya DD, Postnikov YV. A simplified procedure for sequencing amplified DNA containing the α-2 or α-1 globin gene. *Hemoglobin* **18**: 251–255, 1994.
23. Old J, Traeger-Synodinos J, Galanello R, et al. *Prevention of thalassaemias and other haemoglobin disorders*, volume 2. Nicosia, Cyprus: Thalassaemia International Federation, 2005.
24. Baysal E. The β-and δ-thalassemia repository. *Hemoglobin* **19**:213–236, 1995.
25. Rosatelli MC, Faa V, Meloni A et al. A promoter mutation, C→T at position −92, leading to silent β thalassaemia. *Br J Haematol* **90**:483–485, 1995.
26. Camaschella C, Mazza U, Roetto A et al. Genetic interactions in thalassemia intermedia: analysis of beta-mutations, alpha-genotype, gamma-promoters, and beta-LCR hypersensitive sites 2 and 4 in Italian patients. *Am J Hematol* **48**:82–87, 1995.

27. Kazazian HH, Jr, Dowling CE, Hurwitz RL et al. Dominant thalassemia-like phenotypes associated with mutations in exon 3 of the β-globin gene. *Blood* **79**:3014–3018, 1992.
28. Ristaldi MS, Pirastu M, Rosatelli C et al. Prenatal diagnosis of β-thalassaemia in Mediterranean populations by dot blot analysis with DNA amplification and allele specific oligonucleotide probes. *Prenat Diagn* **9**:629–638, 1989.
29. Saiki RK, Walsh PS, Levenson CH et al. Genetic analysis of amplified DNA with immobilized sequence-specific oligonucleotide probes. *Proc Nat Acad Sci USA* **86**:6230–6234, 1989.
30. Maggio A, Giambona A, Cai SP et al. Rapid and simultaneous typing of hemoglobin S, hemoglobin C and seven Mediterranean β-thalassaemia mutations by covalent reverse dot-blot analysis: application to prenatal diagnosis in Sicily. *Blood* **81**:239–242, 1993.
31. Sutcharitchan P, Saiki R, Huisman THJ et al. Reverse dot-blot detection of the African-American β-thalassaemia mutations. *Blood* **86**:1580–1585, 1995.
32. Sutcharitchan P, Saiki R, Fucharoen S et al. Reverse dot-blot detection of Thai β-thalassaemia mutations. *Br J Haematol* **90**:809–816, 1995.
33. Bang-Ce Y, Hongqiong L, Zhuanfong Z et al. Detection of alpha-thalassemia and beta-thalassemia by oligonucleotide microarray. *Haematologica* **89**:1010–1012, 2004.
34. Gemignani F, Perra C, Landi S et al. Reliable detection of beta-thalassemia and G6PD mutations by a DNA microarray. *Clin Chem* **48**:2051–2054, 2002.
35. Van Moorsel CH, van Wijngaraarden EE, Fokkema IF et al. Beta-globin mutation detection by tagged single-base extension and hybridization to universal glass and flow-through microarrays. *Eur J Hum Genet* **12**:567–573, 2004.
36. Lu Y, Kham SK, Tan PL et al. Arrayed primer extension: a robust and reliable genotyping platform for the diagnosis of single gene disorders: beta-thalassemia and thiopurine methyltransferase deficiency. *Genet Test* **9**:212–219, 2005.
37. Newton CR, Graham A, Heptinstall LE. Analysis of any point mutation in DNA. The amplification refractory mutation system (ARMS). *Nucleic Acids Res* **17**: 2503–2516, 1989.
38. Old JM. Haemoglobinopathies: community clues to mutation detection. In *Methods in molecular medicine. Molecular diagnosis of genetic diseases*, R Elles (ed.), pp. 69–184. Totowa: Humana Press, 1996.
39. Tan JA, Tay JS, Lin LI et al. The amplification refractory mutation system (ARMS): a rapid and direct prenatal diagnostic techniques for β-thalassaemia in Singapore. *Prenat Diagn* **14**:1077–1082, 1994.
40. Zschocke J, Graham CA. A fluorescent multiplex ARMS method for rapid mutation analysis. *Mol Cell Probes* **9**: 447–451, 1995.
41. Chehab FF, Kan YW. Detection of specific DNA sequence by fluorescence amplification: a colour complementation assay. *Proc Nat Acad Sci USA* **86**: 9178–9182, 1989.
42. Chang JG, Lu JM, Huang JM et al. Rapid diagnosis of β-thalassaemia by mutagenically separated polymerase chain reaction (MS-PCR) and its application to prenatal diagnosis. *Br J Haematol* **91**:602–607, 1995.
43. Craig JE, Barnetson RA, Prior J et al. Rapid detection of deletions causing δβ thalassemia and hereditary persistence of fetal hemoglobin by enzymatic amplification. *Blood* **83**:1673–1682, 1994.
44. Losekoot M, Fodde R, Harteveld CL et al. Denaturing gradient gel electrophoresis and direct sequencing of PCR amplified genomic DNA: a rapid and reliable diagnostic approach to beta thalassaemia. *Br J Haematol* **76**:269–274, 1991.
45. Savage DA, Wood NA, Bidwell JL et al. Detection of β-thalassaemia mutations using DNA heteroduplex generator molecules. *Br J Haematol* **90**:564–571, 1995.
46. Weatherall DJ, Clegg JB, Higgs DR et al. The haemoglobinopathies. In *The metabolic basis of inherited disease*, CR Scriver, AL Beaudet, WS Sly, D Valle (eds), pp. 2281–2339. New York: McGraw-Hill, 1989.
47. Kulozik AE, Wainscoat JS, Serjeant GR et al. Geographical survey of β^s-globin gene haplotypes: evidence for an independent Asian origin of the sickle-cell mutation. *Am J Hum Genet* **39**:239–244, 1986.
48. Powars DR. β^S-gene cluster haplotypes in sickle cell anemia. *Hematol/Oncol Clin N Am* **5**:475–493, 1991.
49. Old JM. Screening and genetic diagnosis of haemoglobinopathies. *Scand J Clin Lab Invest* **66**:1–16, 2006.
50. Camaschella C, Alfarano A, Gottardi E et al. Prenatal diagnosis of fetal hemoglobin Lepore-Boston disease on maternal peripheral blood. *Blood* **75**:2102–2106, 1990.
51. Sekizawa A, Watanabe A, Kimwa T et al. Prenatal diagnosis of the fetal RhD blood type using a single fetal nucleated erythrocyte from maternal blood. *Obstet Gynaecol* **87**:501–505, 1996.
52. Cheung M-C, Goldberg JD, Kan YW. Prenatal diagnosis of sickle cell anemia and thalassemia by analysis of fetal cells in maternal blood. *Nat Genet* **14**:264–268, 1996.
53. Lo YM. Fetal DNA in maternal plasma. *Ann NY Acad Sci* **906**:141–147, 2000.
54. Chiu RW, Lui WB, El-Sheikah A et al. Comparison of protocols for extracting circulating DNA and RNA from maternal plasma. *Clin Chem* **51**:2209–2210, 2005.
55. Lo YM, Zhang J, Leung TN et al. Rapid clearance of fetal DNA from maternal plasma. *Am J Hum Genet* **64**:18–24, 1999.
56. Chiu RW, Lau TK, Leung TN et al. Prenatal exclusion of β-thalassaemia major by examination of maternal plasma. *Lancet* **360**:998–1000, 2002.
57. Tungwiwat W, Fucharoen S, Fucharoen G et al. Development and application of a real-time quantitative PCR for prenatal detection of fetal alpha(0)-thalassemia from maternal plasma. *Ann NY Acad Sci* **1075**:103–107, 2006.
58. Lo YM. Recent developments in fetal nucleic acids in maternal plasma: implications to noninvasive prenatal fetal blood group genotyping. *Transfusion Clin Biol* **13**:50–52, 2006.
59. Kanavakis E, Traeger-Synodinos J. Preimplatation genetic diagnosis in clinical practice. *J Med Genet* **39**:6–11, 2002.
60. Chan V, Ng EH, Yam I, Yeung WS et al. Experience in preimplantation genetic diagnosis for exclusion of homozygous alpha degrees thalassemia. *Prenat Diagn* **26**:1029–1036, 2006.
61. Deng J, Peng WL, Li J et al. Successful preimplantation genetic diagnosis for alpha- and beta-thalassemia in China. *Prenat Diagn* **26**:1021–1028, 2006.
62. Monni G, Cau G, Usai V et al. Preimplantation genetic diagnosis for beta-thalassaemia: the Sardinian experience. *Prenat Diagn* **24**:949–954, 2004.
63. Kuliev A, Rechitsky S, Verlinsky O et al. Preimplantation diagnosis and HLA typing for haemoglobin disorders. *Reprod Biomed Online* **11**:362–370, 2005.
64. Vrettou C, Traegaer-Synodinos J, Tzetis M et al. Real-time PCR for single-cell genotyping in sickle cell and thalassemia syndromes as a rapid, accurate, reliable, and widely applicable protocol for preimplantation genetic diagnosis. *Hum Mutat* **23**:513–521, 2004.
65. Rosatelli MC, Tuveri T, Scalas MT et al. Molecular screening and fetal diagnosis of β-thalassaemia in the Italian population. *Hum Genet* **89**:585–589, 1992.
66. Winsor EJT, Silver MP, Theve R et al. Maternal cell contamination in uncultured amniotic fluid. *Prenat Diagn* **16**:49–54, 1996.
67. Wang X, Seaman C, Paik M et al. Experience with 500 prenatal diagnoses of sickle cell diseases: the effect of gestational age on affected pregnancy outcome. *Prenat Diagn* **14**:851–857, 1994.
68. Decorte R, Cuppens H, Marynen P et al. Rapid detection of hypervariable regions by the polymerase chain reaction technique. *DNA Cell Biol* **9**:461–469, 1990.
69. Stojilkovic-Mikic T, Mann K, Docherty Z et al. Maternal cell contamination of prenatal samples assessed by QF-PCR genotyping. *Prenat Diagn* **25**:79–83, 2005.
70. Chan V, Chan TPT, Lau K et al. False non-paternity in a family for prenatal diagnosis of β-thalassaemia. *Prenat Diagn* **13**:977–982, 1993.

CHAPTER

27 Prenatal screening for thalassemias

Mary Tang and Kwok-Yin Leung

KEY POINTS

- Non-invasive exclusion for homozygous α^0-thalassemia is possible by ultrasound examination for fetal cardiomegaly and placentomegaly from 12 weeks of pregnancy
- Ultrasound detection of suspected homozygous α^0-thalassemia needs confirmation by molecular diagnosis
- Screening for carriers of thalassemias and structural hemoglobin variants in regions with high prevalence of hemoglobinopathies helps at risk couples avoid morbidity and mortality related to these conditions
- Information on the significance of screening for hemoglobinopathies should be provided to pregnant women as an integral part of the antenatal screening
- Measurement of MCV and/or MCH is appropriate for antenatal thalassemia screening. An MCV cut-off of <80 fl or an MCH cut-off of <27 pg is appropriate for antenatal thalassemia screening
- Couples identified as α-α couples, β-β couples, α-αβ couples and carriers of structural hemoglobin variants should be counseled by experienced personnel and offered prenatal diagnostic tests to exclude major hemoglobinopathies affecting the fetus

α^0-THALASSEMIA MAJOR

A non-invasive approach consisting of serial two-dimensional ultrasound examinations can effectively reduce the need for invasive testing in the majority of unaffected pregnancies[1–4]. In an affected pregnancy, the ultrasonographic measurements of the fetal cardiothoracic ratio (CTR) and placental thickness (PT) are increased because of severe fetal anemia (Fig. 27.1, and see p. 522)[5–10]. Since α-globin-dependent hemoglobin F is the major hemoglobin of a fetus from 8 weeks' gestation onwards, anemia can occur in an affected fetus after this gestation.

Serial two-dimensional ultrasound examination

For all women at risk of carrying fetuses with homozygous α^0-thalassemia, the option of a non-invasive approach can be offered as an alternative to avoid invasive procedures in unaffected pregnancies. Serial ultrasound examinations are performed at 12–15, 18–20 and 30 weeks' gestation[4]. The fetal CTR is a ratio of the fetal transverse cardiac diameter taken at the level of the atrioventricular valves between the epicardial surfaces at diastole to the transverse fetal thoracic diameter[1]. PT is a measurement of the maximal placental thickness, with the transducer placed perpendicularly to the placenta and measurements taken in the longitudinal and transverse sections[5]. If there is fetal cardiomegaly (CTR ≥ 0.50, 0.52 and 0.59 at 12–15, 18 and 30 weeks' gestation respectively), and/or placentomegaly (>18 mm at 12 weeks' gestation), chorionic villus sampling or amniocentesis for fetal DNA analysis is performed for confirmation of α^0-thalassemia major[4]. Previously, early cordocentesis was performed for pregnancies with abnormal ultrasound findings that are highly specific of the disease[16]. Cordocentesis is technically feasible at 12–14 weeks' gestation with a free-hand technique using a 26- or 24-gauge spinal needle with a 20-gauge introducer[16], and hemoglobin study can be performed on the the fetal blood sample. This approach is of particular value in areas where resources for molecular studies are limited. The success rate of early cordocentesis was reported to be 97% in 59 fetuses studied[16]. However, 25% and 20% of the fetuses had bleeding from the cord and bradycardia, respectively[16]. The total fetal loss rate was 8% following early cordocentesis[16]. Because of the high complication rate, less invasive procedures (amniocentesis or chorionic villus sampling) have replaced early cordocentesis to exclude or confirm homozygous α^0-thalassemia. With the use of quantitative polymerase chain reaction, a rapid report can be available within 1–2 days after amniocentesis or chorionic villus sampling[17]. The reporting time is comparable to fetal hemoglobin pattern study following early cordocentesis.

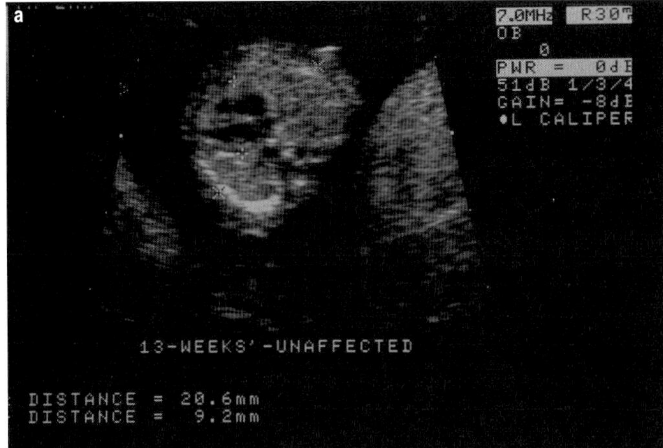

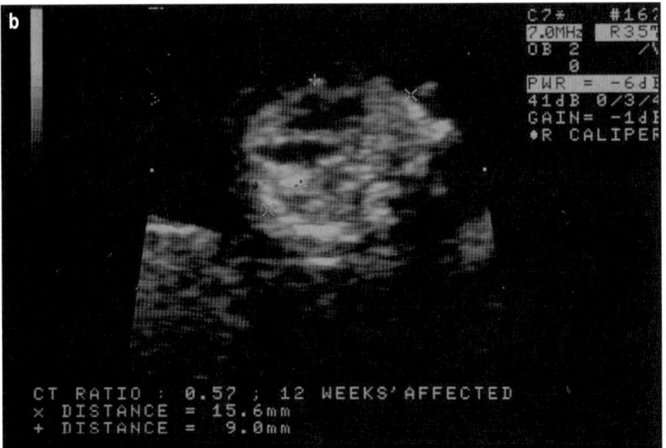

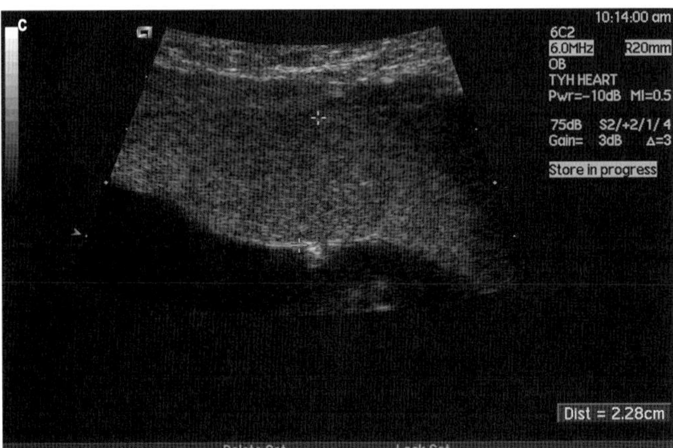

Fig. 27.1 Ultrasonography of (a) normal pregnancy and pregnancy affected by homozygous α^0-thalassemia at 12 weeks' gestation; (b) cardiomegaly with cardiothoracic ratio of 0.57; (c) placentomegaly with placental thickness of 22 mm.

The overall sensitivity and specificity of this non-invasive approach was 100% and 95.6%, respectively[4]. The major benefit in the use of this non-invasive approach was the avoidance of an invasive test in about 75%[4] of patients, while the cost saving was relatively small in comparison to the cost of the whole prenatal screening program for thalassemia[3]. This approach is applicable in singleton, as well as twin pregnancies[18], and can be used to confirm normality in pregnancies conceived after preimplantation genetic diagnosis[19].

There are several limitations of this non-invasive approach. First, the predictive values of the fetal CTR decrease with gestational age[4]. In advanced gestation, hydropic signs including ascites or pleural effusion are more apparent than cardiomegaly in affected pregnancies[4]. Measurement of the fetal middle cerebral artery peak systolic velocity (MCA-PSV) may be a more sensitive sonographic parameter in identifying affected fetuses[18, 20–21], although the usefulness of measurement of MCA-PSV at 12–13 weeks' gestation has not been proven because of extensive overlap of its values between affected and unaffected fetuses at such early gestation[22]. Second, the false positive rate of this non-invasive approach was about 3% because disorders like intrauterine growth restriction, congenital heart disease[4] and Hb H disease[23] can present with cardiomegaly and/or placentomegaly. Third, there is a risk of delaying the diagnosis of an affected pregnancy due to either lack of experience in the examination of the fetal heart or suboptimal image resolution obtained at early second trimester[4]. The use of this approach demands an accurate measurement of the fetal cardiothoracic ratio. Adequate training and subsequent quality control are essential. When the image quality of the fetal heart at 12 weeks' gestation is suboptimal, even with the use of transvaginal scan, rescan in 2–3 weeks will be a reasonable option if a woman still prefers ultrasound monitoring to an invasive testing[4]. The risk of delaying the diagnosis of an affected pregnancy till second trimester and the disadvantages of second-trimester pregnancy termination of an affected pregnancy should be balanced against the risk of an invasive testing.

If a woman opts for first-trimester combined Down's syndrome screening, normal maternal serum-free beta-human chorionic gonadotrophin (β-hCG) and pregnancy-associated placental protein A (PAPP-A) at 11–14 weeks' gestation is a reassuring sign of normality for fetuses at risk of homozygous α^0-thalassemia[11]. However, either two-dimensional ultrasonography or three-dimensional placental volumetry[12] is not predictive of affected pregnancies before 12 weeks' gestation. Immunofluorescence staining of fetal erythrocytes in maternal blood is a potentially useful but labor intensive non-invasive technique in the first trimester[13]. In affected pregnancies, positive staining with fluorescence-labeled monoclonal anti-zeta but not with anti-α-globin antibodies can identify fetal non-nucleated red blood cells in maternal blood. More recently, non-invasive testing for affected fetuses is feasible by examination of fetal DNA in maternal plasma using different techniques including a real-time quantitative semi-nested polymerase chain reaction (PCR) method[14] and a multiplex quantitative fluorescent PCR (QF-PCR) test[15]. The latter is a potentially rapid non-invasive test for simultaneous detection of homozygous α^0-thalassaemia by absence of both microsatellite markers located within breakpoints of the Southeast Asia deletion and exclusion of maternal contamination by absence of non-inherited maternal alleles[15].

β-THALASSEMIA MAJOR

Examination of the circulatory fetal DNA in maternal plasma as an alternative to invasive procedures has been investigated. In a situation where the male partner carrying the codon 41/42 (−CTTT) mutation, and the pregnant woman carrying another β-thalassemia mutation, Lo et al. suggested a non-invasive approach in which allele-specific primers and a fluorescent probe were used to detect or exclude paternal inherited codon

41/42 mutation in maternal plasma[24]. If the couples have the same β-thalassemia mutation, the analysis of single-nucleotide polymorphism linked to the β-globin locus may be useful[25].

However, a major technical challenge relates to the ability to discriminate fetal DNA from the coexisting background of maternal DNA in maternal plasma. The mean fractional fetal DNA concentration in maternal plasma is only 3.4% and 6.2% during early (late first to mid-second trimester) and late (late third trimester) pregnancies, respectively[26]. Absence of inheritance of paternal mutation in maternal plasma can be false negative due to fetal DNA degradation, DNA extraction failure, or PCR allele dropout[25]. Hence, the diagnostic reliability of fetal DNA analysis in maternal plasma depends on the sensitivity and specificity of the analytic system for the detection of fetal-specific markers. Lo et al. have developed a method based on single-allele base extension reaction (SABER) and mass array system (MS), which allowed reliable detection of fetal-specific alleles, including point mutations and single-nucleotide polymorphisms (SNP), in maternal plasma[25]. It has recently been shown that circulatory fetal DNA sequences are generally smaller (<300 base pairs) than comparable circulatory maternal DNA species (>500 base pairs)[27,28]. This phenomenon can be used selectively to enrich for fetal DNA molecules, which permits the detection of otherwise masked highly polymorphic fetal microsatellite markers[27]. Further studies are needed before this non-invasive approach can be used clinically.

SCREENING

With population migration, hemoglobinopathies are no longer regionally specific. The global prevalence of hemoglobinopathies prompts the need for pre-marital or antenatal screening of at-risk couples[29]. Obstetricians need to be aware of the ethnic origin of patients and offer pre-pregnant or prenatal screening tests for hemoglobinopathies for at-risk couples. Web-based population and genetic information on hemoglobin mutations and variants are available for easy reference[30]. The populations especially at risk include those from Africa, the Mediterranean area, the Middle East, the Indian subcontinent, Southeast Asia and the Pacific region[31].

Screening methods

Different methods have been implemented for screening hemoglobinopathies. Given the heterogeneity of hemoglobinopathies, a simple screening test for every variety of hemoglobinopathy has not been developed. A practical approach is to screen for the commonest and clinically important hemoglobinopathies in the region. The goal is to identify couples at risk and to detect early the severe forms of the disorder, i.e. homozygous α^0-thalassemia, transfusion dependent thalassemias and the sickling disorders, in order to avoid morbidity and mortality related to these conditions.

For populations with thalassemias as the major health problem, measurements of mean corpuscular volume (MCV) and mean corpuscular hemoglobin (MCH) have been adopted as screening parameters. For populations with predominant sickle-cell disease, hemoglobin electrophoresis is performed for carrier detection. Couples identified as carriers have 1 in 4 chance of having affected infants.

Thalassemia screening

An understanding in the hematological changes in thalassemia carriers provides the basis for screening based on MCV (or MCH). Hemoglobin (Hb) level is usually normal in α- and β-thalassemia carriers. In α^0-thalassemia carriers, the MCV is below 80 fl. Hb H granules may or may not be present on incubating the red cells with brilliant cresyl blue. Hb A_2 level and hemoglobin pattern are normal. α^0-Thalassemia carrier state can thus be diagnosed in the presence of low MCV and Hb H granules, and normal Hb A_2 level, but cannot be excluded in women with low MCV and normal hemoglobin pattern.

In α^+-thalassemia carriers (with single α-globin gene deletion or non-deletion α-globin gene mutation such as Hb Constant Spring), MCV between 80 and 85 fl has been found. The couple will have a chance of having a child with Hb H disease if the spouse carries α^0-thalassemia. Thus, antenatal thalassemia screening programs using an MCV cut-off of 80 fl would not be aiming at screening couples at risk of having children with Hb H disease.

β-Thalassemia carriers are diagnosed by the presence of low MCV (<80 fl) and raised Hb A_2. For β-thalassemia carriers with iron deficiency, Hb A_2 level may be normal. Thus, it is essential to exclude iron deficiency before excluding β-thalassemia carrier state based on the finding of low MCV and normal Hb A_2.

Both MCV and MCH are useful for screening α- and β-thalassemia. MCH has the theoretical advantage over MCV because it is more stable over time. Different MCV cut-offs, between 76 fl and 82 fl, have been used. With MCH, 27 pg seems to be the most acceptable cut-off. By genotyping archived samples from school children up to MCV of 85 fl, it has been shown that a MCV cut-off of 80 fl or MCH cut-off of 27 pg could detect all SEA deletion carriers and β-thalassemia carriers[32].

Timing of screening

Early screening allows time for workup and counseling of at-risk couples. In case termination of pregnancy needs to be considered, timely diagnosis of thalassemia major in the fetus is desirable. For populations with a high prevalence of α-thalassemia carriers, antenatal thalassemia screening should be offered to all pregnant women regardless of gestational age, in view of maternal risks associated with pregnancies with homozygous α^0-thalassemia.

Education and counseling as an integral part of screening

Education of health care professionals[33], information for couples, and informed consent are required before screening. Information for couples may be provided through various means, including pamphlets, video display, posting on website or explanation in person. The prognosis of affected infants, maternal risks associated with affected pregnancies, available support and therapy for affected infants, available invasive and non-invasive options for prenatal tests, test accuracy, limitation of prenatal tests in prenatal diagnosis, screening workflow, and need for confirmation testing at delivery, all need to be discussed with the at-risk couples.

Workup for screen-positive couples

Screen-positives are those whose MCV and/or MCH falls below the cut-off value. α^0-thalassemia trait, β-thalassemia trait or iron deficiency need to be excluded. Laboratory tests to look for the presence of Hb H inclusion bodies and elevation in Hb A2, and an iron study should be performed. The presence of Hb H inclusion bodies and elevation in Hb A2 (>3.5%) are diagnostic of α^0-thalassemia trait and β-thalassemia, respectively. Iron deficiency may account for the microcytosis and hypochromasia, but coexistence of β-thalassemia cannot be totally excluded.

Workup on the partner should begin with MCV and/or MCH. A positive screening result in the partner necessitates laboratory tests for the presence of Hb H inclusion bodies and elevation in Hb A2, and an iron study. The purpose is to identify whether the couple has the same type of thalassemia, i.e. whether they are α-α or β-β couples. In regions with high prevalence of both α- and β-thalassemia, up to 7% of β-thalassemia carriers are compound α- and β-thalassemia heterozygotes[34]. Couples discordant for α- and β-thalassemia (α-β couples) should therefore be offered a DNA study to exclude coexistent α-thalassemia in the partner with β-thalassemia.

When at-risk couples are identified, counseling and prenatal testing should be carried out by personnel and laboratories with experience in prenatal diagnosis[33].

REFERENCES

1. Lam YH, Ghosh A, Tang MHY, Lee CP, Sin SY. Early ultrasound prediction of pregnancies affected by homozygous α-thalassemia-1. *Prenat Diagn* **17**:327–332, 1997.
2. Lam YH, Tang MHY, Lee CP, Tse HY. Prenatal ultrasonographic prediction of homozygous type 1 alpha-thalassemia at 12–13 weeks of gestation. *Am J Obstet Gynecol* **180**:148–150, 1999.
3. Leung KY, Lee CP, Tang MHY et al. Cost-effectiveness of prenatal screening for thalassemia in Hong Kong. *Prenat Diagn* **24**:899–907, 2004.
4. Leung KY, Liao C, Li QM et al. A new strategy for prenatal diagnosis of homozygous alpha-thalassaemia. *Ultrasound Obstet Gynecol* **28**:173–177, 2006.
5. Ghosh A, Tang MHY, Lam YH, Fung E, Chan V. Ultrasound measurement of placental thickness to detect pregnancies affected by homozygous α-thalassemia-1. *Lancet* **344**:988–989, 1994.
6. Lam YH, Ghosh A, Tang MHY, Lee CP, Sin SY. Early ultrasound prediction of pregnancies affected by homozygous α-thalassemia-1. *Prenat Diagn* **17**:327–332, 1997.
7. Lam YH, Tang MHY, Lee CP, Tse HY. Prenatal ultrasonographic prediction of homozygous type 1 alpha-thalassemia at 12–13 weeks of gestation. *Am J Obstet Gynecol* **180**:148–150, 1999.
8. Tongsong T, Wanapirak C, Sirichotiyakul S. Placental thickness at midpregnancy as a predictor of Hb Bart's Disease. *Prenat Diagn* **19**:1027–1030, 1999.
9. Tongsong T, Wanapirak C, Sirchotiyakul S, Piyamongkol W, Chanprapaph P. Fetal sonographic cardiothoracic ratio at midpregnancy as a predictor of Hb Bart disease. *J Ultrasound Med* **18**:807–811, 1999.
10. Tongsong T, Wanapirak C, Sirchotiyakul S, Chanprapaph P. Sonographic markers of hemoglobin Bart disease at midpregnancy. *J Ultrasound Med* **23**:49–55, 2004.
11. Ong CY, Lee CP, Leung KY, Lau E, Tang MHY. Human chorionic gonadotropin and plasma protein-A in alpha0-thalassemia pregnancies. *Obstet Gynecol* **108** :651–655, 2006.
12. Chen M, Leung KY, Lee CP, Tang MHY, Ho PC. Use of placental volume measured by three-dimensional ultrasound for the prediction of fetal Hb-Bart's disease: a preliminary report. *Ultrasound Obstet Gynecol* **28**:166–172, 2006.
13. Lau ET, Kwok YK, Luo HY et al. Simple non-invasive prenatal detection of Hb Bart's disease by analysis of fetal erythrocytes in maternal blood. *Prenat Diagn* **25**:123–128, 2005.
14. Tungwiwat W, Fucharoen S, Fucharoen G, Ratanasiri T, Sanchaisuriya K. Development and application of a real-time quantitative PCR for prenatal detection of fetal alpha(0)-thalassemia from maternal plasma. *Ann NY Acad Sci* **1075**:103–107, 2006.
15. Ho SSY, Chong SS, Koay ESC et al. Microsatellite markers within $^{-SEA}$ breakpoints for prenatal diagnosis of Hb Bart's hydrops fetalis. *Clin Chem* **53**:173–179, 2007.
16. Lam YH, Tang MH. Prenatal diagnosis of haemoglobin Bart's disease by cordocentesis at 12–14 weeks – experience with the first 59 cases. *Prenat Diagn* **20**:900–904, 2000.
17. Chan V, Yip B, Lam YH, Tse HY, Wong HS, Chan TK. Quantitative polymerase chain reaction for the rapid prenatal diagnosis of homozygous alpha-thalassemia (Hb Bart's hydrops fetalis). *Br J Haematol* **115**:341–346, 2001.
18. Leung KY, Lee CP, Tang MHY, Chan HY, Chan V. Prenatal diagnosis of alpha-thalassaemia in a twin pregnancy. *Ultrasound Obstet Gynecol* **25**:201–202, 2005.
19. Chan V, Ng EH, Yam I, Yeung WS, Ho PC, Chan TK. Experience in preimplantation genetic diagnosis for exclusion of homozygous alpha degrees thalassemia. *Prenat Diagn* **26**:1029–1036, 2006.
20. Hernandez-Andrade E, Scheier M, Dezerega V, Carmo A, Nicolaides KH. Fetal middle cerebral artery peak systolic velocity in the investigation of non-immune hydrops. *Ultrasound Obstet Gynecol* **23**:442–445, 2004.
21. Leung WC, Oepkes D, Seaward G, Ryan G. Serial sonographic findings of four fetuses with homozygous alpha-thalassemia-1 from 21 weeks onwards. *Ultrasound Obstet Gynecol* **19**:56–59, 2002.
22. Lam YH, Tang MHY. Middle cerebral artery Doppler study in fetuses with homozygous α-thalassemia-1 at 12–13 weeks of gestation. *Prenat Diagn* **22**:56–58, 2002.
23. Leung KY, Lee CP, Tang MHY, Chan HY, Ma ESK, Chan V. Detection of increased middle cerebral artery peak systolic velocity in fetuses affected by hemoglobin H Quong Sze disease. *Ultrasound Obstet Gynecol* **23**:523–526, 2004.
24. Chiu RWK, Lau TK, Leung TN, Chow KCK, Chui DHK, Lo YMD. Prenatal exclusion of β thalassaemia major by examination of maternal plasma. *Lancet* **360**:998–1000, 2002.
25. Ding C, Chiu RWK, Lau TK et al. MS analysis of single-nucleotide differences in circulating nucleic acids: Application to noninvasive prenatal diagnosis. *Proc Natl Acad Sci USA* **101**:10762–10767, 2004.
26. Lo YMD, Tein MSC, Lau TK et al. Quantitative analysis of fetal DNA in maternal plasma and serum: implications for noninvasive prenatal diagnosis. *Am J Hum Genet* **62**:68–775, 1998.
27. Li Y, Zimmermann B, Rusterholz C, Kang A, Holzgreve W, Hahn S. Size separation of circulatory DNA in maternal plasma permits ready detection of fetal DNA polymorphisms. *Clin Chem* **50**:1002–1011, 2004.
28. Chan KC, Zhang J, Hui AB et al. Size distribution of maternal and fetal DNA in maternal plasma. *Clin Chem* **50**:88–92, 2004.

29. Vichinsky EP. Changing patterns of thalassemia worldwide. *Ann NY Acad. Sci* **1054**:18–24, 2005.
30. Giardine B, van Baal S, Kaimakis P et al. HbVar database of human hemoglobin variants and thalassemia mutations: 2007 update. *Hum Mutat* **28**:206, 2007.
31. Higgs DR, Thein SL, Wood WG. In *Distribution and population genetics of the thalassaemias in the thalassaemia syndromes*, DJ Weatherall, JB Clegg (eds), pp. 237–284. London: Blackwell Science, 2001.
32. Ma ESK, Chan AYY, Ha SY, Lau YL, Chan LC. Thalassaemia screening based on red cell indices in the Chinese. *Haematologica* **86**:1286–1287, 2001.
33. Antenatal screening programme from the NHS Thalassaemia and Sickle Cell Screening Programme at http://www.sickleandthal.org.uk/antenatal.htm
34. Lam YH, Ghosh A, Tang MH, Chan V. The risk of α-thalassaemia offspring of β-thalassaemia carriers in Hong Kong. *Prenat Diagn* **17**:733–736, 1997.

CHAPTER

28

Cystic fibrosis

Mary Porteous and Jon Warner

KEY POINTS

- Cystic fibrosis is a severe monogenic condition with a birth prevalence of 1 in 2500
- Routine, kit-based CFTR mutation testing will identify over 85% of cases and can form the basis for population antenatal and newborn screening programs
- Mutations in the CFTR gene give rise to a wide variety of phenotypes from classical CF to male infertility and caution must be exercised in interpretation of results
- Echogenic bowel, while associated with an increased risk of CF in the fetus, is a non-specific finding

CLINICAL OVERVIEW OF CYSTIC FIBROSIS

Cystic fibrosis (CF) is the most common life-shortening mendelian disorder found in children and in young adults of Caucasian descent. CF presents in a variety of ways and, although usually diagnosed within the first year of life, may occasionally escape detection until the second or later decades. In early infancy, a majority of patients present with a combination of respiratory symptoms, failure to thrive and steatorrhea. Some 10–15% of newborns with CF have meconium ileus and, when present, it is virtually diagnostic of CF.

Prophylactic antibiotic therapy to prevent bacterial colonization of the airways and regular physiotherapy in combination with the use of aerosolized mucolytic drugs, including recombinant human deoxyribonuclease, have helped delay the most serious complications experienced by CF patients. It is hard to make meaningful statements about life expectancy as therapies have dramatically improved over the lifetime of currently affected patients with ever more patients experiencing protracted survival to age 40 or 50 and sometimes beyond. Another problem in any predictions is the fact that the cystic fibrosis disease spectrum has widened with the advent of gene testing. Comparing a survey made by the British Paediatric Association covering 1977 to 1985, which suggested a median survival in the UK for boys of 21 years and for girls of 19 years[1], with the 2005 statistics from the Cystic Fibrosis Foundation (USA) patient registry, which suggests a predicted median sex independent life expectancy of 36.5 years, demonstrates dramatic improvements in therapy.

The diagnosis is made on a sweat test, a procedure in which sweating is stimulated by pilocarpine iontophoresis. The diagnosis is confirmed if the chloride ion concentration in the sweat is greater than 60 meq/l. CF shows an autosomal recessive mode of inheritance and, for Caucasian populations, epidemiological surveys show a birth prevalence ranging from about 1 in 1700 to about 1 in 6500. If the birth prevalence is assumed to be 1 in 2500, the gene frequency is 0.02 and the carrier frequency 0.04 or 1 in 25. Data from multiple prevalence and screening studies suggest a carrier frequency between 1 in 22 and 1 in 30 in populations of European ancestry[2–5].

THE CFTR GENE

The CF gene was identified in 1989 by a multicenter reverse mapping initiative[6–8] and is localized on the long arm of chromosome 7. It spans some 230 kb of genomic DNA and contains 27 exons. The gene product, the cystic fibrosis transmembrane conductance regulator (*CFTR*), has a calculated molecular mass of 170 000 Da and is an ATP-dependent membrane transport protein. *CFTR* comprises five domains of which two are membrane spanning, two nucleotide binding (which bind ATP) and one regulatory and is expressed in those tissues primarily involved in the disease process, such as pancreas, nasal polyps, lung, colon, sweat glands, placenta, liver and parotid gland. Variants resulting in an abnormal *CFTR* gene product compromise chloride ion transport in these key tissues.

The predominant mutant allele at the CF locus is a 3 base-pair deletion in exon 10, which removes a phenylalanine residue at position 508 of the 1480 amino acid sequence of CFTR. This allele, traditionally known as ΔF508 (F is the single letter code for phenylalanine), makes up 50–90% of mutations in Caucasian populations[9].

It is now known that CF is an extremely heterogeneous condition at the DNA level. Over 1500 different mutant alleles have been described (see http://www.genet.sickkids.on.ca/cftr/app).

Many pathogenic mutations are extremely rare. With the exception of ΔF508, only a few have been found at frequencies of more than 1% in the British population. Table 28.1[10] shows representative data for a well-studied UK population. A universal approach to describing the variation within human genetic sequences has recently been adopted. The Human Genetic Variation Society (HGVS) has produced a series of recommendations that apply to all human genetic variants (http://www.hgvs.org/rec.html). These descriptions are unambiguous as they relate to specific genomic DNA and transcript (cDNA) sequences defined by unique accession numbers. The mutation nomenclature in Table 28.1 is derived using accession number NM_000492.3 according to HGVS guidelines. We have provided the traditional nomenclature alongside the new names. Over time, the HGVS descriptions should supersede the older notation but, currently, both forms are encountered and archived notes are likely to be written in the older format.

For this and other populations of European ancestry, most commercial test kits will detect >85% of CF alleles. A typical test comprises 20–30 pathogenic mutations. For the Ashkenazi Jewish population, the inclusion of common founder mutation W1282X (p.Trp1282X) results in a higher detection rate (>90%). Non-European populations (African, Asiatic) achieve lower detection rates but also benefit from a significantly lower birth prevalence for cystic fibrosis of between 1/10 000 and 1/100 000.

It is possible to detect both normal and mutant CF alleles on any tissue which contains nucleated cells; in practice this means almost any fresh tissue with the exception of mature red blood cells. Typically, laboratories prepare DNA for analysis from whole blood specimens (EDTA) for the majority of referrals. Buccal scrapes and mouthwash specimens have proved useful where phlebotomy is problematic. DNA can be amplified from dried blood spots which are collected for use in newborn screening programs. For prenatal testing, DNA is routinely extracted from sorted fronds of chorionic villus biopsy. Laboratory detection of CF alleles is nearly always performed after prior amplification of the portion of the CF gene in which the relevant mutation lies. The standard technique used is the polymerase chain reaction (PCR), which employs a heat-stable DNA polymerase to produce between 10^7 and 10^9 copies of the target DNA sequence in a few hours. Many commercial PCR-based kits for detection of the more common CF alleles are now marketed. Not only is the PCR a quick and easy procedure, but it may also be applied to samples with an extremely low DNA content.

The ideal situation occurs when each parent carries a defined CF allele. In the UK, some 85–90% of CF heterozygotes carry an allele detectable by routine tests. Thus, for 70–80% of couples, both CF alleles are easily identified by the local genetics laboratory. Should one or both parental CF alleles mutations not be identified by routine tests, more extensive testing is generally offered. In the UK, complete gene sequencing and rearrangement analysis (MLPA) is offered by specialist laboratories and it is very rare when a parental allele remains unresolved for long. Linked markers can still have a key role to play in preimplantation genetic testing.

ECHOGENIC BOWEL AS A MARKER FOR CYSTIC FIBROSIS

Hyperechogenic bowel is seen in between 0.1 and 1.8% of pregnancies at second-trimester anomaly ultrasound scanning[10]. This is usually a transient observation, resulting from a temporary intestinal obstruction which resolves of its own accord later in pregnancy. If hyperechogenic bowel persists in successive ultrasound examinations, there is an increased risk of a serious underlying problem such as a karyotypic abnormality, congenital infection, intestinal obstruction or cystic fibrosis.

In the largest retrospective study investigating the link between hyperechogenic bowel and cystic fibrosis, in excess of 346 000 pregnancies where ultrasonography was performed were audited[11]. This French study took place over a 10-year period in an area with a high birth prevalence for cystic fibrosis (1/2987) and where >99% of CFTR mutations have been identified. A total of 142 diagnoses of hyperechogenic bowel were made. From this population, subsequent DNA testing identified 14 fetuses (10%) with two pathogenic CFTR variants with a prediction that they would develop cystic fibrosis. Where two pathogenic CF variants are involved, the resulting malfunction of the *CFTR* protein is thought to result in the dehydration of mucus secretions which, becoming viscous, block the bowel leading to meconium ileus. The carrier frequency in the study population was 1/27 but 11/142 (=1/13) fetuses with hyperechogenic bowel were shown to carry a single pathogenic mutation. This enrichment for CFTR carriers in cases of hyperechogenic bowel has been seen in other studies[12].

This study and others for Northern European populations give a 10–13% prior empirical risk of an eventual diagnosis of CF based on a severely echoic signal picked up in the second trimester. Estimating hyperechogenicity is highly subjective and operator dependent and outcome studies for other populations have given significantly lower detection rates of 3–5%. Noteworthy among many studies is one where a very much higher involvement of CF in hyperechogenic bowel was seen in patients of Asiatic origin (75%). The management of an isolated finding of hyperechogenic bowel during pregnancy remains problematic. DNA testing for pathogenic CF mutations may be helpful. We strongly recommend testing the parents of any fetus with a diagnosis of hyperechogenic bowel first. If both parents are shown to be carriers of pathogenic CF mutations, interpretation of any prenatal test result will be straightforward. If no pathogenic mutations are identified, then prenatal testing will not be helpful in refining the risk that the fetus will develop cystic fibrosis. The real dilemma is the identification of a single mutation positive parent. If prenatal testing shows the mutation is also present in the fetal DNA, then estimating the risk that the fetus will develop cystic fibrosis is problematic. Difficulties in determining precise values for echogenicity and an increased frequency of CF mutation carriers in fetuses diagnosed with hyperechogenic bowel make accurate risk estimates impossible. Empirical risk estimates in the literature range between 5% and 43% for this situation depending on multiple factors including ethnicity and its effect on test sensitivity[12,13].

PRESYMPTOMATIC TESTING IN CYSTIC FIBROSIS

Early diagnosis of cystic fibrosis, either through newborn screening or antenatal couple testing, offers couples the opportunity to make choices about future pregnancies. However, it also creates a major dilemma for some couples who are asked to make decisions before they have any personal experience of the clinical features of the disorder. It is hoped that early detection

Table 28.1 *CFTR* **mutation frequency for the 20 most common mutations among individuals clinically diagnosed with cystic fibrosis for the North of England**

	CFTR pathogenic variant		*Exon i = intron*	*Number*	*Frequency (%)*
Traditional name	*HGVS standard nomenclature*				
	Protein name	*Nucleotide name*			
DeltaF508	p.Phe508del	c.1521_1523delCTT	10	1420	81.0
G551D	p.Gly551Asp	c.1652G > A	11	62	3.5
G542X	p.Gly542X	c.1624G > T	11	20	1.1
621 + 1(G > T)	n/a	c.489 + 1G > T	i4	17	1.0
1898 + 1(G > A)	n/a	c.1766 + 1G > A	i12	16	0.9
R553X	p.Arg553X	c.1657C > T	11	13	0.7
R117H	p.Arg117His	c.350G > A	4	13	0.7
R560T	p.Arg560Thr	c.1679G > C	11	11	0.6
3272-26A > G	n/a	c.3140-26A > G	i17a	10	0.6
3659delC	p.Lys1177SerfsX15	c.3528delC	19	9	0.5
N1303K	p.Asn1303Lys	c.3909C > G	21	8	0.5
1717-1G > A	n/a	c.1585-1G > A	i10	7	0.4
2711delT	p.Phe861LeufsX3	c.2583delT	14a	7	0.4
G85E	p.Gly85Glu	c.254G > A	3	6	0.3
W1282X	p.Trp1282X	c.3846G > A	20	6	0.3
DeltaI507	p.Ile507del	c.1519_1521delATC	10	5	0.3
1154insTC	p.Phe342HisfsX28	c.1021_1022dupTC	7	5	0.3
V520F	p.Val520Phe	c.1558G > T	10	5	0.3
1078delT	p.Phe316LeufsX12	c.948delT	7	5	0.3
Q493X	p.Gln493X	c.877C > T	10	5	0.3
1461ins4	p.Ile444ArgfsX3	c.1326_1329dupAGAT	9	5	0.3
E60X	p.Glu60X	c.178G > T	3	3	0.2
1138insG	p.Ile336SerfsX28	c.1006dupG	7	3	0.2
4016insT	p.Ser1297PhefsX5	c.3889dupT	21	3	0.2
S549N	p.Ser540Asn	c.1646G > A	11	2	0.1
D579Y	p.Asp579Tyr	c.1735G > T	12	2	0.1
711 + 1G > T	n/a	c.579 + 1G > T	i5	2	0.1
300delA	p.Glu56AspfsX35	c.169delA	3	2	0.1
R1066H	p.Arg1066His	c.3197G > A	17b	2	0.1
D1152H	p.Asp1152His	c.3454G > C	18	2	0.1
2184delA	p.Lys684AsnfsX38	c.2052delA	13	2	0.1
Other known mutations				49	2.8
Unknown				27	1.6
			Total =	1754	100.0

Martin Schwarz, Personal communication May 2007

of cystic fibrosis will allow prompt treatment and therefore a better outcome for affected children. How do parents maintain optimism about the future for their affected child while deciding that the condition is so severe as to warrant prenatal diagnosis and termination of pregnancy? The increasing availability of preimplantation genetic diagnosis has increased reproductive choice, but may make conventional prenatal diagnosis harder for some CF couples to justify.

Family history of CF

Carrier testing has been available for many years for individuals with a family history of CF through direct mutation analysis when the mutation is known or using linked markers. Cascade testing – whereby a mutation is tracked through a family – has been a well-accepted method of genetic family investigation. However, the evidence suggests that it is effective only in motivated families. Current testing protocols discourage carrier testing of children and so young family members may not be tested at the same time as other relatives. Whether they seek testing at a later date will depend on whether they are re-contacted or actively seek out testing for themselves. In the past, there was an assumption that genetic registers might help in the efficient contacting of at risk individuals, but a combination of data protection and a change in role of the Regional Genetics Centers means that such help is likely to be scarce.

A typical carrier with an untested partner has a ≈1/92 risk of a pregnancy affected by cystic fibrosis. Testing of the partner with a commercial mutation detection kit able to detect ≈90% of common Northern European mutations will reduce the risk to 1/884. If a carrier's partner is shown also to be a carrier, then the risk of an affected pregnancy rises to one in four.

Antenatal population screening

Another approach to identifying couples at increased risk of an affected pregnancy is antenatal couple screening. This screening of individuals with no previous family history of cystic fibrosis depends on the availability of a test able to identify the majority of pathogenic CF mutations likely to be found in the target population. Ideally, such a test will make allowances for the patient's own ethnic background and any CFTR variants that are identified will be certain to have a strong predictive value. Antenatal screening programs have been running for several years in the USA and currently an estimated 30% of pregnant couples opt for cystic fibrosis testing when offered CF couple screening[14].

Such a program ran in Lothian from 1990 to 2004. At their booking appointment, women were offered the opportunity to participate through providing a mouthwash sample and taking a bottle for a mouthwash sample home to their partner. Initially, the woman's sample was tested for up to 9 CF mutations able to detect >80% alleles. If the woman's sample tested negative for these mutations, a negative report would be issued to her at her next midwife appointment. If a woman's sample failed to amplify or if she was shown to be a carrier, then her partner's sample would be tested. If the partner tested negative then a report would be issued at the next midwife appointment either advising the woman that she was a carrier while her partner was unlikely to be or that her sample failed to amplify and her husband was unlikely to be a carrier.

Couples identified as both being carriers would be contacted urgently by their midwife and offered the opportunity to come and discuss their results and options for prenatal diagnosis with the fetal medicine midwife and geneticist.

Initial publications about the Edinburgh antenatal screening program demonstrated an uptake rate of 70% of booking women. From 1990 to 1999, 67 of the 74 couples identified to be at 1 in 4 risk of an affected child opted for prenatal diagnosis. From these prenatal tests, 17 couples were identified as having an affected pregnancy and all of these opted to terminate the pregnancy. Over the last 3 years of the program the uptake rate dropped to around 60%. However, the percentage of couples opting for prenatal diagnosis was significantly lower at around 50%; and two couples told they had affected pregnancies elected not to terminate.

Wald and others[14] have argued that 'couple testing' for CF carrier status with calculation of a 'couple risk' is a cost effective way to deliver antenatal CF screening. Sequential testing with the woman's specimen tested first and only if a pathogenic mutation is identified testing the partner's specimen, may appear attractive but may lead to problems with inaccurate risk estimates. The false reassurance of a negative antenatal couple risk based on the testing of only one of the two parental specimens can be particularly challenging. Parents may be confused if a child with cystic fibrosis is identified shortly after birth by a newborn screening program when their antenatal screening test suggested a very low risk. With a robust process of obtaining informed consent for antenatal CF testing, parents can cope with the test's limitations and the unfortunate situation of an undiagnosed pathogenic variant. It is, however, harder to justify the low 'couple risk' calculated from a sequential testing scheme if the untested parent is subsequently shown to carry a common CF mutation.

In April 2001, American College of Medical Genetics (ACMG) recommended a panel of 25 pathogenic mutations for antenatal screening. To be selected, sequence variants had to be present in CF patients at a frequency >0.1%, were to be of strong predictive value and associated with classical CF rather than with less severe phenotypes from the CFTR associated disease spectrum. This panel proved very effective and, in many States, schemes have achieved the stated aim of detecting >80% of causative mutations involved in cystic fibrosis for the principal at risk populations. ACMG also recommended that the limitations of any mutation test (the fact that it cannot identify all pathogenic CF mutations) should be an integral part of the information provided to couples when obtaining informed consent for testing. A strong recommendation that both partners be tested simultaneously, with full disclosure to each of their test results, and the risk to the pregnancy was also made[15–17]. A flowchart demonstrating such a scheme is shown in Figure 28.1.

A minor revision of the initial ACMG 25 mutation panel recommendations in 2004 resulted in the removal of the variant p.Ile148Thr[16]. This sequence variant was shown to be greatly over represented in the carrier population and generally benign. The complex mutation R117H (p.Arg117His) remains in the ACMG mutation panel. The severity of this cystic fibrosis variant in exon 4 of *CFTR* is moderated by a second sequence involved in the splicing of exon 9 of *CFTR*. A polymorphic thymidine tract immediately upstream of the intron 8/exon 9 splice site influences exon 9 splicing efficiencies. Three lengths: 9T, 7T and 5T with decreasing splicing efficiencies are seen.

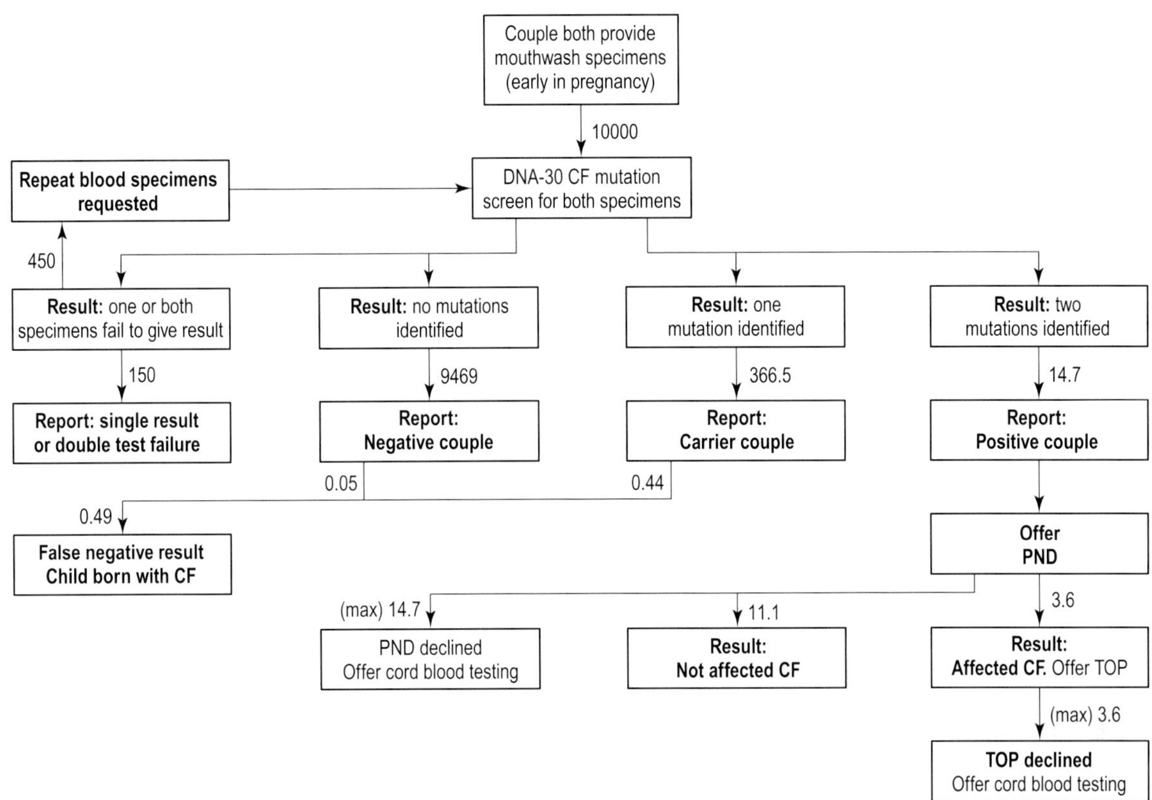

Fig. 28.1 Flow chart for a theoretical antenatal cystic fibrosis screening protocol. Estimated figures for 10 000 couples screened (0.89 mutation detection frequency).

Mis-splicing produces exon 9 deficient mRNA and a *CFTR* protein lacking cAMP dependent chloride channel function[17]. The CFTR mutation R117H (p.Arg117His) is seen in cis with (on the same chromosome as) both the 7T and 5T variants.

In Edinburgh, from a cohort of 38 infertile men with congenital bilateral absence of the vas deferens (CBAVD), all three patients with the genotype F508/R117H (p.Phe508del/p.Arg117His) have R117H in cis with the more efficient 7T variant. Apart from the infertility, which was under investigation and prompted the CF mutation screening test, these men were otherwise healthy. The R117H (p.Arg117His) variant is, however, frequently seen in clinically affected CF patients in Scotland with an allele frequency of ≈1.7%. Affected patients (n = 8) with the genotype R117H/F508 (p.Phe508del/p.Arg117His) all have R117H in cis with the 5T variant (R117H 5T).

Based on birth prevalence of CF in the Lothian region, the CF carrier frequency is 1 in 23. For 27 877 couples participating in the local antenatal screening program from 1993 to 1999, a total of 28 993 individuals were tested. A total of 1260 CF carriers would be predicted. The frequencies (observed/theoretical total) for the four most common mutations were 68.1% F508, 5.2% G551D, 4.0% G542X and 8.8% R117H. At 8.8% (n = 112), the R117H frequency is 5.2 times greater than in the CF affected population. As seen in Table 28.2, at least 86 /112 R117H are in cis with the 7T variant (or the more efficient 9T). A >3.3 fold excess of the more efficiently spliced R117H 7T over R117H 5T is seen in our R117H carrier population.

The use of a secondary test (reflex test) to determine the associated splicing efficiency for this variant was recommended by the ACMG. Primary testing is for a wide range of CF mutations with couples where R117H is identified in combination with a 'classical' CF mutation (e.g. F508) offered a secondary (reflex) test to clarify the T tract status. Reflex testing should be interpretable, offering couples accurate predictive information on the fetal phenotype.

Table 28.2 **Genotype frequencies in the normal population and for the 112 antenatal screening program carriers of R117H**

T tract genotype	*Frequency (%) in matched normal population (n = 200)*	*Frequency (%) in antenatal screening R117H carrier population (n = 112)*
5T/5T	0.5	–
5T/7T	9.0	21.4
5T/9T	0.5	1.8
7T/7T	68.5	61.6
7T/9T	20.0	15.2
9T/9T	1.5	–
5T allele	GTG**TTTTT**AAAC **AG**	
7T allele	GTG**TTTTTTT**AAAC **AG**	
9T allele	GTG**TTTTTTTTT**AAAC **AG**	

DNA sequence immediately upstream of exon 9 of *CFTR* splice site for 5T, 7T and 9T alleles.
T tract and **AG** splice acceptor in bold

Antenatal screening program couples where the mutation R117H is involved have proved difficult to counsel. For a couple with no family history of CF it is impossible to predict the CF status and fertility of any fetus that is a compound heterozygote involving R117H 7T and a severe CF mutation (>77% of outcomes involving R117H). Phenotypes range from male infertility (rare) to no discernable symptoms. Cystic fibrosis with a mild disease course, or male infertility can be predicted for the compound heterozygote involving R117H 5T. It is essential, however, to establish phase as some 25% of the 5T alleles might be low risk alleles not in cis with the R117H mutation. To establish phase, the parents of the R117H carrier or the fetus must be tested. The fetal phenotype cannot be predicted for >80% of test outcomes involving R117H. Testing of other family members is needed to clarify phase for R117H 5T including some unnecessary prenatal testing. On the basis of our analysis and our practical experience, we find it is impossible to obtain fully informed consent for testing during pregnancy. The mutation R117H was removed from the Edinburgh antenatal screening program in June 2000.

Test outcomes from antenatal screening require sensitive handling. Counseling by appropriately trained staff is essential to clarify residual risks, any implications to the immediate and extended family, as well as the significance of being a cystic fibrosis carrier. Another key element in a successful antenatal screening program is the production of clearly written accurate patient information.

Newborn screening

Newborn screening programs have been established across the UK based on immunoreactive trypsinogen (IRT) levels in dried blood spots (heel pricks) taken around the 6th day of life. In combination with sweat testing and mutation analysis, this means that most cystic fibrosis cases are identified within the first 2 months of life. As a consequence of this rapid detection, appropriate monitoring and therapy regimens can often be initiated early and the severity of some of the manifestations of the disease may be mitigated.

In Scotland, newborn screening for CF has been available since February 2003. The screening has been integrated within the existing screening program and is offered along with screening for phenylketonuria (PKU) and congenital hypothyroidism (CHT) as part of the routine heel prick test. A single laboratory in the Institute of Medical Genetics in Glasgow carries out testing of all bloodspot cards in Scotland and an uptake of over 99.8% has been achieved.

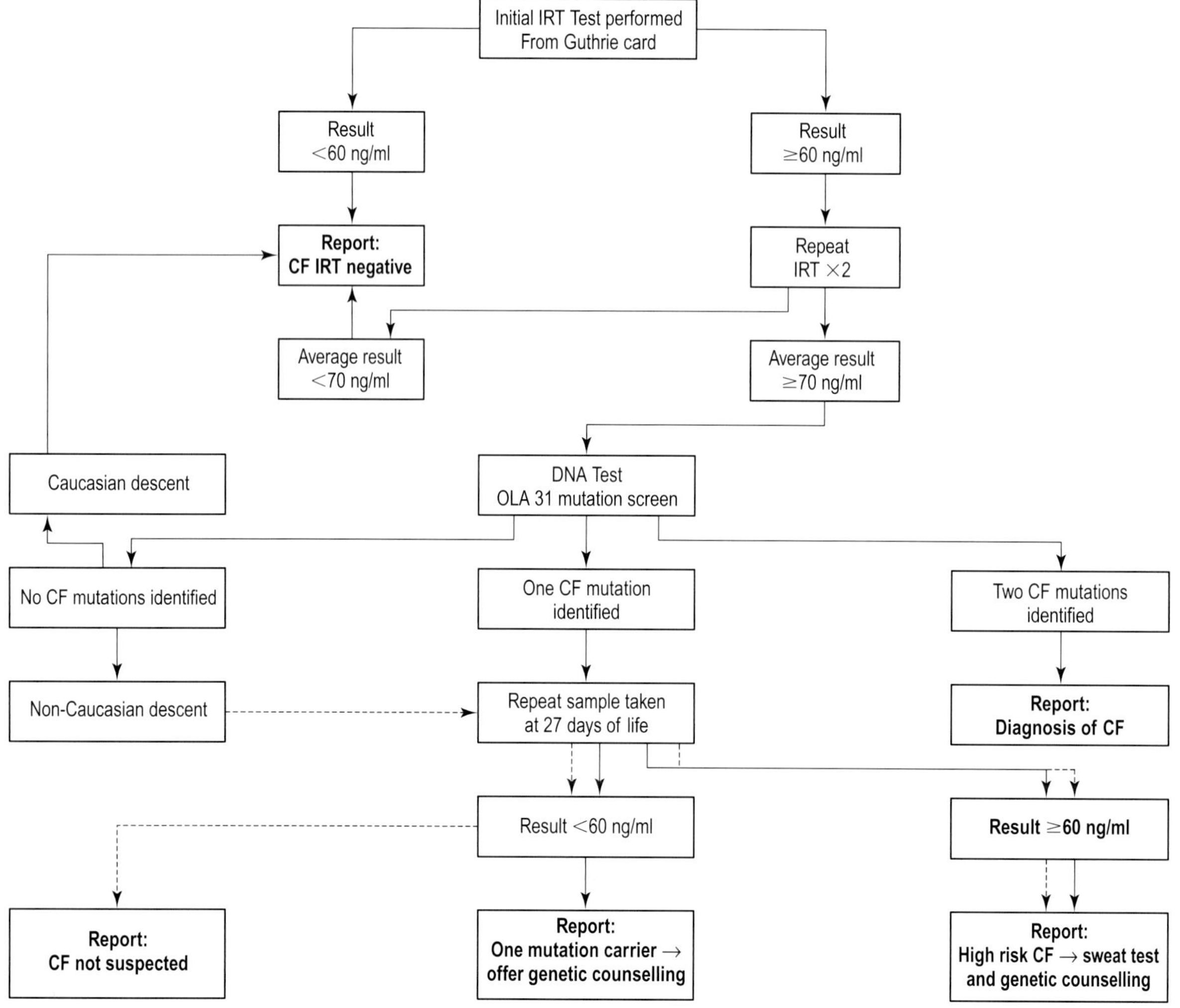

Fig. 28.2 Neonatal cystic fibrosis screening protocol (Glasgow).

For CF screening, immunoreactive trypsinogen (IRT) levels are measured on the heel prick dried blood spot taken around 6 days of life. DNA testing for 30 *CFTR* mutations is carried out when the IRT is raised above the 99.5 percentile, using the initial blood spot sample. If no mutations are identified, no further action is taken unless the child has non-European parents. CF is seen in ethnic minority populations but any cases may have pathogenic mutations not covered by the 30 mutation panel, so non-Caucasian babies with no mutation detected are offered a second IRT test at or near 27 days of life. Babies with 2 mutations are referred to the local CF pediatrician as confirmed cases of CF. A second blood spot sample is taken from babies with one mutation. If the IRT level for any second sample is in the normal range, a result will be issued 'CF not suspected' and, for babies with a single mutation present, notification of the carrier status of the child is made to the parents via the GP along with an offer of genetic counseling. If the IRT remains high, the baby will be referred to the CF pediatrician for a sweat test. The standard protocol followed in Scotland is summarized in Figure 28.2.

Between 2004 and 2007, only one confirmed case of cystic fibrosis has been 'missed' by the heel prick test. The DNA testing outcomes have been similar to those seen in other published programs. The majority of children who went on to be given a positive sweat test result had two pathogenic mutations that were identified by the 30 mutation panel. A small number of cases with a single mutation identified and a positive sweat test were sent to a specialist laboratory for CFTR gene sequencing and a second pathogenic variant was identified. The frequency of single mutation carrier newborns with a single raised IRT result was ≈1/14 which is almost twice the carrier estimation for the Scottish population derived from birth prevalence figures for cystic fibrosis. In particular, the variant R117H was frequently identified on a 7T splice background.

The 30 CFTR mutation panel includes several 'complex' mutations including R117H. Duplicate raised IRT results in specimens taken approximately 20 days apart and intermediate sweat test results (30–59 mEq/l) can be associated with the presence of a 'classical' severe mutation and a 'dominant mild' or 'complex' mutation such as R117H 7T. Care when reporting this variant as part of a pair of CF mutations is essential as phenotypic predictions are nigh impossible and range from no symptoms to male infertility. The predictive value of finding R117H 5T in combination with a classical CF mutation is more straightforward with a prognosis that the child will develop cystic fibrosis, albeit often with a milder disease course.

Preimplantation testing

For some couples faced with a high risk of having a child with cystic fibrosis, preimplantation genetic diagnosis (PGD) is the only acceptable reproductive option. Single blastomeres are biopsied from embryos produced by in vitro fertilization at around 3 days. Traditionally, PCR amplification was performed directly on single cell lysates using one or two amplimers near to or containing the regions of interest in the CFTR gene. More recently, whole genome amplification, in particular multiple displacement amplification (MDA), the generation of microgram quantities of DNA from single cells has become possible. This has revolutionized molecular testing in the PGD context allowing more complex analyses to be performed.

A multiplex PCR assay using 10 short tandem repeat markers (STRs) spanning the CFTR locus has been designed and adopted for PGD testing by Renwick et al.[19]. This simultaneous testing of multiple closely linked loci minimizes the possibility of false negative results as a consequence of allele dropout (ADO). Interpretable genotypes are achieved for most biopsies which leads to a greater choice of low-risk embryos for subsequent re-implantation and a correspondingly better chance of a achieving a viable pregnancy.

REFERENCES

1. British Paediatric Association Working Party on Cystic Fibrosis. Cystic fibrosis in the United Kingdom 1977–1985: an improving picture. *Br Med.J* **297**:1599–1602, 1988.
2. Schwarz MJ, Malone GM, Hayworth A et al. Cystic fibrosis mutation analysis: report from 22 UK regional genetics laboratories. *Hum Mutat* **6**:326–333, 1995.
3. Shrimpton AE, McIntosh I, Brock DJH. The incidence of different cystic fibrosis mutations in the Scottish population: effects on prenatal diagnosis and genetic counselling. *J Med Gene* **28**:317–321, 1991.
4. Comeau AM, Parad RB, Dorkin HL et al. Population-based newborn screening for genetic disorders when multiple mutation DNA testing is incorporated: a cystic fibrosis newborn screening model demonstrating increased sensitivity but more carrier detections. *Pediatrics* **113**:1573–1581, 2004.
5. National Newborn Screening and Genetics Resource Center. National newborn screening report 2000. San Antonio, TX: National Newborn Screening and Genetics Resource Center, 2003. Available at http://genes-r-us.uthscsa.edu/resources/newborn/00chapters.html.
6. Rommens JM, Iannuzzi MC, Kerem B et al. Identification of the cystic fibrosis gene: chromosome walking and jumping. *Science* **245**:1059–1065, 1989.
7. Riordan JR, Rommens JM, Kerem B et al. Identification of the cystic fibrosis gene: cloning and characterization of complementary DNA. *Science* **245**: 1066–1073, 1989.
8. Kerem B, Rommens JM, Buchanan JA et al. Identification of the cystic fibrosis gene: genetic analysis. *Science* **245**:1073–1080, 1989.
9. The Cystic Fibrosis Genetic Analysis Consortium. Worldwide survey of the ΔF508 mutation. *Am J Hum Genet* **47**:354–359, 1990.
10. Scotet V, Braekeleer M De, Audrézet M-P et al. Prenatal detection of cystic fibrosis by ultrasonography: a retrospective study of more than 346 000 pregnancies. *J Med Genet* **39**:443–448, 2002.
11. Schwarz M. Personal communication May 2007.
12. Bosco AF, Norton ME, Lieberman E. Predicting the risk of cystic fibrosis with echogenic fetal bowel and one cystic fibrosis mutation. *Obstet Gynecol* **94**:1020–1023, 1999.
13. Hodge SE, Lebo RV, Yesley AR, Cheney SM, Angle H, Milunsky J. Calculating posterior cystic fibrosis risk with echogenic bowel and one characterized cystic fibrosis mutation: avoiding pitfalls in the risk calculations *Am J Med Genet* **82**(4):329–335, 1999.
14. Wald NJ, George LM, Wald NM, Mackenzie I. Couple screening for cystic fibrosis. *Lancet* **338**(8778):1318–1391, 991.
15. Grody WW, Cutting GR, Klinger KW, Richards CS, Watson MS, Desnick RJ.

Laboratory standards and guidelines for population-based cystic fibrosis carrier screening. *Genet Med* **3**(2):149–154, 2001.

16. ACMG Cystic Fibrosis Carrier Screening Work Group, American College of Medical Genetics et al. Cystic fibrosis population carrier screening: 2004 revision of American College of Medical Genetics mutation panel. *Genet Med* **6**(5):387–391, 2004.
17. Amos J. *Technical standards and guidelines for CFTR mutation testing, 2006 edn.* American College of medical genetics available at http://www.acmg.net
18. Kiesewetter S, Macek M, Jr, Davis C et al. A mutation in CFTR produces different phenotypes depending on chromosomal background. *Nat Genet* **5**(3):274–278, 1993.
19. Renwick PJ, Lewis CM, Abbs S, Ogilvie CM. Determination of the genetic status of cleavage-stage human embryos by microsatellite marker analysis following multiple displacement amplification. *Prenat Diagn* **27**(3):206–215, 2007.

CHAPTER 29

Inborn errors of metabolism

Wim J Kleijer and Frans W Verheijen

KEY POINTS

- This chapter deals with the prenatal diagnosis of inborn errors of metabolism: indications, prerequisites, fetal samples to be used, analytical techniques, worldwide diagnostic experience and future developments
- 113 genetic metabolic diseases with known gene and primary protein defects are discussed
- Prenatal diagnosis has been reported for 104 metabolic disorders and is considered feasible for 9 others
- Biochemical analysis is practical and reliable for 81 diseases. DNA mutation analysis is preferred or needed for prenatal diagnosis of 32 other metabolic disorders, because enzyme or metabolite assay is cumbersome or less reliable
- Chorionic villus sampling appears to be the procedure of choice for 101 disorders, although cultured villus cells are needed for 5 assays
- Amniocentesis is recommended for biochemical analysis of 12 disorders

INTRODUCTION

Several thousands of human genetic disorders are caused by single gene mutations[1]; they comprise conditions varying from slight deviations from the normal phenotype to severe disabling conditions and disorders which are incompatible with life. In most of these disorders, metabolism is affected in at least some stage of development, but only in a minority of the disorders (some 500–1000) has the primary metabolic defect been established[1,2]. Mostly, the defective gene product concerns an enzyme, but coenzymes, activators, hormones, transporter or receptor proteins and structural proteins are also involved. The specific diagnosis of these disorders is often complicated by the fact that most are quite rare and, moreover, clinically heterogeneous. Patients with the same enzyme deficiency or even the same mutations may present with different manifestations; conversely, similar patterns of symptoms may be caused by deficiencies of different but often related enzymes. This requires, in addition to clinical investigations, specialized studies of metabolites in blood and urine and of enzymes in blood cells, cultured skin fibroblasts or tissues[2,3]. A precise diagnosis is needed as early as possible to allow adequate treatment, therapy and genetic counseling. Unfortunately, in spite of spectacular progress in recent years, options for effective therapy are still limited or absent for most severe metabolic diseases. The available options range from dietary treatment, as in phenylketonuria, to enzyme replacement therapy (ERT)[4], as for Gaucher disease, and, in the future, gene therapy, but all of these strategies exhibit severe limitations with respect to scope, effectiveness and the burden to patient and parents.

Parents faced with the high 25% recurrence risk in subsequent pregnancies may therefore refrain from having further children unless prenatal diagnosis is available with the option of termination of the affected pregnancy. More than 100 inborn errors of metabolism can be diagnosed prenatally from amniotic fluid or fetal tissue, mostly by testing the primary enzyme defect, sometimes by the demonstration of accumulating metabolites or storage material. Alternatively, DNA mutation analysis may be used, as the genes for nearly all inborn errors of metabolism have been characterized. However, this requires mutation analysis in the family, preferably prior to pregnancy, which may frequently not be possible or practical (see DNA analysis below).

INDICATIONS FOR PRENATAL DIAGNOSIS

The risk to a couple of having offspring with a metabolic disorder appears usually only after a first affected child has been born. The diagnosis of an autosomal recessive disorder establishes both parents as heterozygotes; in subsequent pregnancies their risk of recurrence is 25%. It is thus essential that the diagnosis is made as soon as possible to allow adequate counseling of the parents and prenatal diagnosis if wanted.

In general, there are few ways to prevent a first affected child. Although it is possible to detect heterozygosity by enzyme or mutation analysis, this is inefficient in the absence of an indication of an increased risk. For some disorders with high incidence in certain populations, screening for heterozygosity has been effective, e.g. for β-thalassemia in Sardinia and Cyprus by mutation analysis (see Chapter 27) and for Tay–Sachs disease in Ashkenazi Jewish populations in the USA and in Israel. Also, in families in which a metabolic disorder has been diagnosed in one or more patients, screening of their relatives together with their partners may be considered, especially in populations with a tradition of consanguineous marriage and in small closed communities.

For the much smaller, but important, group of X-linked recessive disease, the situation is quite different. The main indication for prenatal diagnosis of X-linked diseases is again the recurrence risk to mothers of patients. However, as soon as this mother is recognized as a carrier, all female relatives (e.g. sisters and daughters of the heterozygous mother) have a high risk of being heterozygote and thus that their sons will be affected. To some degree, carrier detection is possible for X-linked disorders by biochemical methods, but it is usually not possible to rule out heterozygosity with certainty. Prenatal diagnosis has, in the past, been indicated for all close female relatives of a patient with a severe X-linked disease. This policy has now changed as most genes are known, allowing reliable carrier detection by mutation or linkage analysis (see section on DNA analysis). The main advantage of this approach is the ability to exclude heterozygosity in females at risk, so that unnecessary prenatal analyses can be avoided.

PREREQUISITES FOR PRENATAL DIAGNOSIS

Before prenatal diagnosis can be offered, the diagnosis in the proband – usually the affected child in the family – must be precisely established. A clinical diagnosis alone is not sufficient as there are many groups of disorders with similar and overlapping clinical manifestations, but based on different primary enzyme defects. On the other hand, extensive clinical heterogeneity occurs among patients with the same enzyme deficiency, but sometimes with different levels of residual activity, which should be known before prenatal diagnosis is undertaken. For many disorders, demonstration of the primary enzyme defect is the preferred (or the only possible) approach for prenatal diagnosis. However, for some diseases, abnormal and specific metabolite patterns in amniotic fluid have proven to be indicative for the affected status of the fetus[5]. Characteristic patterns of metabolite concentrations in urine and/or blood are associated with several disorders of, for example, amino and organic acid metabolism. A clearly abnormal metabolite pattern in urine is, however, no guarantee for similar abnormalities in amniotic fluid of an affected fetus. This can only be established by the demonstration of these abnormalities in affected pregnancies. However, irrespective of the method used for prenatal diagnosis, enzyme or metabolite analysis, it is essential that a precise diagnosis of the disorder in the index patient has been established, not only by metabolite analysis, but if possible also by enzyme assay.

Although many enzyme deficiencies can be demonstrated primarily in blood cells, it is advantageous or necessary to have cultured fibroblasts available from the proband and often also from the parents for preparation for future prenatal analysis. If the disease has an early fatal outcome, it is essential to take a skin biopsy at the earliest occasion and store the cultured fibroblasts in a cell bank.

A further requirement for prenatal diagnosis by enzyme assay is that the enzyme is expressed in the available fetal material and that its deficiency is evident in an affected fetus. Both requirements are not always met. Several enzymes are only active in liver, muscle, blood or other tissues which are much less accessible than chorionic villi or amniotic fluid (cells). Even if the enzyme is active, its deficiency may theoretically be obscured by isoenzymes or other interfering enzymes which specifically act in the fetal cells. Therefore, at least one precedent, showing enzyme deficiency in an affected fetus, is needed before reliable prenatal diagnosis can be offered. Obviously, before undertaking prenatal diagnosis, the laboratory must establish the normal ranges of metabolites in the fluid or enzyme activities in villi and cultured fetal cells[5,6]. Reliable and sensitive (micro)methods must have been developed which are not vulnerable and allow accurate measurements even at low metabolite concentrations or, as far as enzyme assay is concerned, in the small amount of fetal material.

All these requirements can only be fulfilled efficiently if the few requests for prenatal diagnosis for each of the rare metabolic diseases are handled by relatively few specialized laboratories per country or even per continent. This will enable these few centers to gain and maintain experience and organize their service in such a way that they are ready any moment to accept and handle any request immediately. Expertise on the technical level, although essential, is not the only prerequisite. The whole logistics of the many steps involved should ideally be arranged according to an established scenario with optimal mutual communication and cooperation in a small team coordinated by the clinical geneticist. In many cases, it will, however, be necessary to send material over long distances to the laboratory, which is, if arranged carefully, perfectly possible.

CHORIONIC VILLI (CV)

The great advantages of chorionic villus sampling (CVS) are the early stage of sampling (10–12 weeks) and the immediate testing which provides definitive results within a day for many enzymes; for some metabolic tests and also for some DNA analyses, several days to a week are necessary. This means that an affected pregnancy can be terminated by aspiration as opposed to the prostaglandin induction of labor, which is necessary at 13 weeks or later.

Cells can be cultured efficiently from the villi, allowing the identification of those metabolic tests which can only be performed on cultured cells, or if necessary, to confirm previous results of the direct assay on the villi. A disadvantage of the use of long-term CV cultures, besides the much longer waiting time, is the occasional growth of maternal cells in these cultures. Although rare, this maternal cell contamination (MCC) may occur in 1–2% of the cultures[7,8]. A maternal blood sample is required to test for MCC in CV cultures and also in the directly used CV tissue. MCC may be excluded by the comparison of several genetic markers, so avoiding the risk of erroneous interpretation.

The suitability of CV for direct prenatal analyses has, in the past two decades, been demonstrated in large series, comprising a few thousand analyses for some 60 different metabolic disorders, with practically complete enzyme deficiencies in affected pregnancies[6,9–11]. This shows that the generally needed amount of 20 mg of pure fetal CV tissue can be reliably obtained without admixture of maternal tissue. CV can easily be sent in sterile culture medium at room temperature over long distances for

24–48 h. It is essential, however, that adequate selection, cleaning and primary examination of the quality and quantity of the villi is done immediately at the site of sampling.

AMNIOCENTESIS

Amniocentesis allows analysis of both the amniotic fluid and of cultured amniocytes. Approximately 100 metabolic diseases have been diagnosed prenatally in this way. Compared to CVS, the late stage of amniocentesis (16 weeks) and the 2–3 weeks needed to culture sufficient cells for biochemical analysis is a major disadvantage. For this reason, amniocentesis has largely been replaced by CVS for the diagnosis of metabolic disorders in high-risk pregnancies. However, amniocentesis remains indicated when the analysis of CV or cultured CV cells is not sufficiently reliable or when there is a need to confirm the initial results of the assay(s) on CV or CV cells. For some diseases, the analysis of metabolites in amniotic fluid either with or without combination with enzyme assay in the cells is a more attractive choice.

Direct measurement of metabolites in the fluid allows a rapid diagnosis within 1 or 2 days after amniocentesis in the 15th–16th week. The reliability of this approach has been demonstrated for a considerable number of diseases[5]. The possibility of earlier amniocentesis in the 12th–13th week has been investigated in a small number of centers[12] (see Chapter 22). This seems an advantage, especially for chemical analysis of the fluid, at least if this allows a definitive diagnosis without the need of further analysis of cultured amniocytes. In principle, early amniocentesis and CVS could be performed simultaneously, to allow direct enzyme assay and metabolite measurement as well[13].

FETAL BLOOD AND OTHER FLUIDS AND TISSUES

Fetal blood and tissues such as liver and skin offer the possibility to detect disorders which are not expressed in CV or amniotic fluid (cells) (see Chapter 22). Fetal blood sampling has been practiced for the diagnosis of hemoglobinopathies by globin chain analysis but the much earlier analysis of DNA from CV has replaced this approach. Fetal blood sampling may still be useful if the pregnancy is too advanced for amniocentesis and cell culture (e.g. late presentation, growth failure of amniocytes or ultrasound indication of abnormalities). However, in this situation placental biopsy may be a better choice.

Fetal liver biopsy has been carried out at 18–20 weeks of gestation for the assay of enzymes which are not expressed in CV or amniocytes. Thus diagnoses have been made for ornithine transcarbamylase deficiency, carbamoyl-phosphate synthetase, primary hyperoxaluria type I and glycogenosis I (see Tables 29.3, 29.4 and 29.6). As the genes involved in these disorders have been cloned, mutation or linkage analysis using DNA from CV is a better option if the mutations or informative markers in the family have been identified. Fetal skin biopsies have been used for the prenatal diagnosis of genodermatoses by light- or electronmicroscopy.

ENZYME ANALYSIS

Prerequisites for enzyme assays used in prenatal diagnosis are that they are accurate, sensitive, fast and relatively stable. Usually, the assays are performed directly in microliter volumes of cell or tissue homogenates using appropriate fluorogenic, chromogenic or radioactive substrates[6]. Some activities may, however, be assessed indirectly in intact cells or CV by tracing radiolabeled precursors through their metabolic pathways. Examples are the assay of decarboxylases by measuring the release of $[^{14}C]CO_2$ and of reactions which may be followed by the incorporation of the radioactive products into high-molecular macromolecules (i.e. proteins, nucleic acids, phospholipids)[6]. To allow reliable interpretation of the results, the enzyme activities in the fetal cells or villi from the pregnancy at risk are always compared with a set of appropriate controls from stored or simultaneously sampled fetal material and also with the activities in cultured fibroblasts of the proband, parents and controls. For direct enzyme assays in cell homogenates, samples can be used which have been stored at −80 °C. However, for metabolic tests using living cells or villi, also living controls are needed, which requires careful timing of sampling in the hospital and analysis in the laboratory. In all samples, a reference enzyme is tested simultaneously to check for possible loss of activity due to transport and further handling of the sample.

Most enzyme tests can be done equally well in CV and cultured amniotic fluid cells. Some enzymes have higher, others a lower activity in CV compared to amniocytes[6]. The latter is true for α-L-iduronidase, which is deficient in the Hurler syndrome; in this case, heterozygote levels of activity in CV may approach the patients' range, which may occasionally necessitate further analysis of cultured CV cells or occasionally even require amniocentesis.

METABOLITE ANALYSIS

For a few dozens of metabolic diseases, the (postnatal) diagnosis is indicated by elevated concentrations of specific metabolites in plasma and urine[3]. Similarly, prenatal diagnosis of several of these diseases is possible because of the demonstration of increased metabolite levels in amniotic fluid[5]. However, the postnatal diagnosis made from urine cannot be extrapolated to the prenatal situation as demonstrated by the normal levels of branched chain amino acids in amniotic fluid of fetuses affected with maple syrup urine disease. Also, fetal metabolite patterns may be influenced by maternal diet or condition. Therefore, the reliability of metabolite measurement for prenatal diagnosis must be established by determining the range of abnormal concentrations from other affected pregnancies. This has been accomplished for a considerable number of disorders which are listed below (see Tables 29.1–29.7).

As the concentration of the relevant metabolites in amniotic fluid is often low, their quantification may require special methods using reference compounds labeled with stable isotopes and gas chromatography/mass spectrometry[5]. For most purposes, rapid transport of the (sterile) centrifuged or unprocessed fluid at ambient temperature is adequate; for some, the centrifuged (cell-free) fluid must be sent while frozen on dry ice.

DNA ANALYSIS

The development of DNA technology has provided great diagnostic possibilities which are especially important for the numerous genetic disorders for which a primary protein defect or a secondary metabolic defect is not known or not easily detectable. Some of these disorders and the techniques used to demonstrate mutations or to show linkage of certain markers with the disease-causing gene are discussed in other chapters (23–28). In another category of disorder, specific metabolic defects are known but they are either not expressed in the available fetal material or the available assays are not fully specific or are technically vulnerable. Again DNA analysis, if reliable and practicable, will then be desirable, as indicated in the tables and in the text below. For the majority of the metabolic disorders listed and discussed in this chapter, rapid and reliable prenatal diagnosis is possible by enzyme or metabolic tests and the question may be raised, therefore, about role of DNA analysis. Nearly all genes involved have been cloned and sequenced and, for many of these disorders, numerous mutations have been identified. For many metabolic diseases only rare or unique mutations have been found, whereas for some other diseases one or more, relatively common, mutations have been identified besides rare mutations. Until recently, the search for mutations has mainly been undertaken in research institutes. For diagnostic use, the search for mutations in each newly diagnosed patient is still time-consuming and expensive, but the technology is rapidly developing to provide greater efficiency. A major potential use of mutation analysis is carrier detection, which is of great importance for females in families with X-linked diseases and for autosomal recessive disorders in affected families with consanguineous marriages or in populations with a high frequency of a specific mutation. In most other situations, carrier screening (in high-risk relatives and their low-risk partners) seems rather inefficient, even if a set of the most frequent mutations in the population is tested.

DIAGNOSTIC EXPERIENCE

The number of metabolic disorders which have been detected prenatally has expanded rapidly in the first two decades of prenatal diagnosis to more than a hundred. The discovery of primary enzyme (protein) defects has slowed down in the past 10 years; however, the number of other genetic disorders diagnosable by DNA analysis is now increasing rapidly. The number of pregnancies tested per disease correlates to its incidence, severity and probably the availability (and reliability) of pre- and postnatal diagnostic services. For most of the rare diseases, with the recurrence risk being the major indication for prenatal diagnosis, the number of analyses per year may vary worldwide from none to several dozens. For a few disorders with higher incidence in some populations and for which prenatal diagnosis is offered as a result of carrier screening, the numbers tested are higher (e.g. Tay–Sachs disease by enzyme assay and cystic fibrosis and sickle cell anemia by mutation analysis). The accuracy of prenatal diagnosis has been high for the majority of disorders. Pitfalls have been reported for some disorders, especially in the early stage of prenatal analysis and, for some, the prenatal analysis is still in an experimental stage.

In Tables 29.1–29.7 disorders are listed for which prenatal diagnoses have been made by biochemical analysis in affected pregnancies or for which prenatal diagnosis seems quite feasible. For some of the metabolic disorders listed the preferential use of DNA technology is indicated; genetic disorders without an identified metabolic defect but detectable by DNA analysis are not included. References for the diseases are given in the tables and in the text; to reduce their number, preference has been given to original first reports and more recent reports describing improved methods or larger series. Additional references may be found in previous reviews[14,15].

LYSOSOMAL STORAGE DISEASES

A considerable proportion of prenatal analyses made for metabolic disorders concern lysosomal storage diseases (50% in our center in Rotterdam). This group comprises approximately 45 diseases with a defect in the degradation of complex cellular constituents or in the transport of some small metabolites leading to the accumulation of these products in lysosomes. Although there is a wide clinical heterogeneity in each of these diseases, most of them include severe forms with progressive neurological and/or somatic anomalies which warrant prenatal diagnosis. Large numbers of prenatal diagnoses have been made for some disorders with a relatively high incidence such as Tay–Sachs disease (a few thousand[16]), Krabbe, Hurler, Hunter and Pompe disease (worldwide up to a thousand each); by contrast the numbers are very small for some extremely rare disorders such as Farber, Wolman.

Since the early 1990s, enzyme replacement therapy (ERT) for the non-neuronopathic (type 1) form of Gaucher disease has been introduced in many countries. Similar ERT programs have been approved for Fabry and mucopolysaccharidosis (MPS) types I (Hurler) and VI (Maroteaux-Lamy), whereas trials are ongoing for glycogenosis II (Pompe disease) and MPS II (Hunter). In spite of its successes, limitations of ERT clearly remain with respect to the prevention of long-term and especially neurologic effects and the life-long intravenous treatment means a burden to patient and family[4]. Therefore, the option of ERT does not eliminate the need for prental diagnosis.

Lipidoses (Table 29.1)

Sphingolipidoses

Using adequate and practicable fluorogenic artificial substrates for the enzyme assays, the prenatal diagnosis for GM1-gangliosidosis, Fabry, Gaucher, Sandhoff and Tay–Sachs disease is relatively uncomplicated: there is usually clear distinction between the enzyme deficiency which is characteristic for an affected fetus and the sometimes low levels of activity found in case of heterozygosity. For the X-linked Fabry disease, fetal sex determination is needed before a low α-galactosidase activity can be interpreted to indicate an affected male rather than a female carrier[17]. A potential complication in carrier detection and prenatal diagnosis of Tay–Sachs disease is the occurrence of a rare mutation in the hexosaminidase A gene, which causes low enzyme activity but no disease[32]. A similar phenomenon called 'pseudodeficiency' (PsD) is well known and much more frequent in metachromatic leukodystrophy (in 10–15% of normal alleles[32,33]). If PsD is suspected in one of the parents of a patient by the finding of very low arylsulfatase A activity, it is necessary to test for PsD mutations in this parent and in a subsequent prenatal analysis in this family. Special attention to the possible involvement of PsD is needed in enzyme-based testing for heterozygosity in individuals with a low population risk. The chance may then be high that a reduced enzyme activity is due to a PsD mutation rather than to a disease-causing

Table 29.1 Lysosomal storage diseases – disorders of (sphingo)lipid metabolism

Disease	*Defect*	*Sample[a]*	*Reference*
Fabry disease	α-Galactosidase	CV	Kleijer et al.[17]
Farber disease	Ceramidase	DNA (CV), AC	Fensom et al.[18]
Gaucher disease	β-Glucosidase	CV	Besley et al.[19]
GM1-gangliosidosis	β-Galactosidase	CV	Besley and Broadhead[20]
GM2-gangliosidosis (Sandhoff)	Hexosaminidase A + B	CV	Giles et al.[21]
GM2-gangliosidosis (Tay–Sachs)	Hexosaminidase A	CV	Grebner and Wenger[22]
Krabbe disease	Galactocerebrosidase	CV, VC, AC	Kleijer et al.[23]
Metachromatic leukodystrophy	Arylsulfatase A	CV, VC, AC	Fensom et al.[24]
Niemann–Pick type A (and B)	Sphingomyelinase	CV	Vanier et al.[25]
Niemann–Pick disease type C	Cholesterol transport	DNA, VC, AC	Vanier et al.[26]
Wolman disease/CESD	Acid lipase	CV	van Diggelen et al.[27]
Mucolipidosis:			
Type I (sialidosis)	Neuraminidase	AC	Sasagasako et al.[28]
Type II (I-cell disease)	Multiple lysosomal enzymes	AF, AC	Besley et al.[29]
Type IV	Accumulation of lipids	DNA, AC	Zeigler et al.[30]
Galactosialidosis	Protective protein/cathepsin A	(CV), AC	Kleijer et al.[31]

[a]CV = chorionic villi are indicated as the material of choice if suitable, additional samples are indicated only if they are occasionally needed or preferred; (CV) = possible on CV but positive cases not yet reported; VC = cultured chorionic villus cells; AF = amniotic fluid; AC = cultured amniocytes; DNA = analysis on DNA from chorionic villi

mutation: this is certainly true for metachromatic leukodystrophy but also for Tay–Sachs, Krabbe and Pompe disease and the Hurler and Sly syndromes[16,32–34]. Another complication in metachromatic leukodystrophy has been the low arylsulfatase A activity in CV and the interference of much higher activities of the interfering enzymes arylsulfatase B and C. This problem was solved by a simple modification of the assay: at 0 °C, the interfering enzymes were completely inactive, while considerable activity of arylsulfatase A remained[24].

Until recently, radiolabeled natural substrates have been preferred for the prenatal diagnosis of Krabbe[23], Niemann–Pick[25] and Wolman disease[27]. However, newly developed fluorogenic substrates and methods have now been shown to allow convenient and reliable prenatal diagnosis for Krabbe[35] and Niemann–Pick disease[36]. The relatively low galactosylceramidase activity in uncultured CV may occasionally create a problem in distinguishing between a true enzyme deficiency and a low heterozygote level. In rare cases, it may be necessary to exclude an affected fetus definitively by testing cultured villus cells or even amniocytes (in our center this has been necessary in five out of 133 pregnancies at risk tested for Krabbe disease on CV; Kleijer et al., unpublished). Alternatively, DNA analysis may be chosen if the mutations in the family are known. World-wide probably a thousand prenatal diagnoses have successfully been made for Krabbe disease on cultured amniocytes or fresh CV.

Niemann–Pick type C (NPC) is caused by mutations in the *NPC1* and *NPC2* genes, which affect intracellular trafficking of unesterified cholesterol. Definite postnatal diagnosis is achieved by the demonstration of accumulated cholesterol in lysosomes by staining with filipin to form a strongly fluorescent complex[37]. This filipin staining method is also adequate for prenatal diagnosis of the classical type of NPC using cultured CV or AF cells[26]. However, mutation analysis, using uncultured CV is the method of choice if possible for the classical type and probably the only reliable method for variant types[38]. Farber disease has been diagnosed on amniocytes[18] and excluded on CV[39] by direct acid ceramidase assay using radiolabeled ceramide. New indirect assays using cultured cells have been described to facilitate the (prenatal) diagnosis of this rare disease[40], but mutation analysis may be preferred for prenatal diagnosis[41].

Mucolipidoses

Prenatal diagnosis of sialidosis (or mucolipidosis I) by analysis of amniocytes has been reported[28]. Fresh CV are not suitable because of the very low activity and the instability of neuraminidase[31]. Galactosialidosis may be detectable by a secondary β-galactosidase deficiency in CV as previously shown on amniocytes[42]; however, it is also recommended to test the primary defective protein, cathepsin A, which is known to protect and activate β-galactosidase and neuraminidase by forming a complex with them. An affected fetus was recently diagnosed by cathepsin A deficiency in cultured CV cells[43], but this should also be feasible by using fresh CV[31]. I-cell disease (or mucolipidosis II) has been diagnosed in CV by measuring the responsible defect of phosphorylation of lysosomal enzymes[44], but a

Table 29.2 **Lysosomal storage diseases – disorders of glyco(lipo)protein and mucopolysaccharide metabolism**

Disease	*Defect*	*Sample*[a]	*Reference*
Glycoproteinoses:			
Aspartylglucosaminuria	Aspartylglucosaminidase	CV	Aula et al.[48]
Fucosidosis	α-Fucosidase	(CV), AC	Poenaru et al.[49]
α-Mannosidosis	α-Mannosidase	CV	Petushkova[50]
β-Mannosidosis	β-Mannosidase	(CV)	Kleijer et al.[51]
Salla/sialic acid storage disease	Sialic acid transport	CV	Lake et al.[52]
Schindler disease	α-*N*-acetylgalactosaminidase	(CV)	Van Diggelen et al.[53]
Ceroid lipofuscinosis	Accumulation of lipopigments		
Infantile (Santavuori)	Palmitoyl protein thioesterase	CV, DNA	De Vries et al.[54]
Late-Infantile (Jansky–Bielschowski)	Tripeptidyl peptidase I	CV, DNA	Kleijer et al.[55]
Juvenile (Batten)	CLN 3 protein	DNA	Munroe et al.[56]
Mucopolysaccharidoses (MPS) type:			
I Hurler	α-L-iduronidase	CV, VC, AF	Young et al.[57]
II Hunter	Iduronate 2-sulfatase	CV	Kleijer et al.[58]
IIIA Sanfilippo A	Heparansulfamidase	CV	Kleijer et al.[59]
IIIB Sanfilippo B	*N*-acetylglucosaminidase	CV	Minelli et al.[60]
IIIC Sanfilippo C	Acetyl-CoA: α-glucosaminide *N*-acetyltransferase	CV	Di Natale et al.[61]
IIID Sanfilippo D	*N*-acetylglucosamine 6-S'ase	(CV, AF)	Wang He et al.[62]
IVA Morquio A	*N*-acetylgalactosamine 6-S'ase	CV, AF, AC	Kleijer et al.[63]
IVB Morquio B	β-Galactosidase	(CV, AF, AC)	-
VI Maroteaux–Lamy	Arylsulfatase B	(CV)[b], AF, AC	Kleijer et al.[64]
VII Sly	β-glucuronidase	CV	Van Eyndhoven et al.[65]
Mucosulfatidosis	Multiple sulfatases	CV, (AF, AC)	Patrick et al.[66]
Other:			
Glycogenosis II (Pompe) (see Table 29.4)			
Cystinosis (see Table 29.6)			
Hydrops fetalis (see text)			

[a]CV = chorionic villi are indicated as the material of choice if suitable, additional samples are indicated only if they are occasionally needed or preferred; (CV) = possible on CV but positive cases not yet reported; VC = cultured chorionic villus cells; AF = amniotic fluid; AC = cultured amniocytes; DNA = analysis on DNA from chorionic villi

[b]Warning: interference by steroid sulfatase may cause false-negative diagnosis (Verheijen et al., 2008, in preparation)

more convenient and reliable approach is the demonstration of increased activities of several lysosomal enzymes in amniotic fluid (even at 10–12 weeks)[29,45] and of reduced activities of the same enzymes in cultured amniocytes[29,45] or CV cells.[45,46] Mucolipidosis type IV is caused by mutations in the MCOLN1 gene leading to defective lysosomal exocytosis[47] and accumulation of high-molecular products. Prenatal diagnosis has been made by electron microscopy and by phospholipid and ganglioside analysis of cultured amniocytes[30], but DNA analysis of CV would now be the method of choice.

Glycoproteinoses (Table 29.2)

The glycoproteinoses listed in Table 29.2 are rare diseases, although higher incidences occur for aspartylglucosaminuria[48] and Salla disease[67] in Finland. All disorders, except Salla disease, can be diagnosed by convenient and sensitive enzyme assays using fluorogenic substrates[68]. Prenatal diagnosis for these disorders is relatively uncomplicated. However, caution is needed with respect to residual enzyme activity in α-mannosidosis (K_M mutants)[50,69] and to greatly different levels of α-fucosidase activity in fibroblast-like and epithelial amniocytes (lower and higher activity respectively)[49] and CV (high activity)[5]. In fact, the experience is very limited, especially for fucosidosis (not diagnosed by CVS), β-mannosidosis (only one heterozygote diagnosed by CVS)[51] and Schindler disease[53] (not done).

Severe infantile sialic acid storage disease has been diagnosed by increased levels of free sialic acid in amniocytes and CV as detected by chemical assay and by electronmicroscopy[52,67]. In Salla disease, the lysosomal accumulation of free sialic acid is much less pronounced; the level in amniocytes seems too low for reliable diagnosis[67]. DNA analysis should be preferred for intermediate variants of this disorder[67].

Various types of neuronal ceroid lipofuscinosis (NCL) may be diagnosed prenatally by electronmicroscopic study of CV tissue[56], but special care and expertise is needed. The identification of genes and mutations in six types of NCL[70] has allowed prenatal diagnosis, e.g. for the infantile type (Santavuori, CLN1)[54], the late-infantile type (Jansky-Bielschowsky, CLN2)[55], the juvenile type (Batten, CLN3)[56] and the variant late-infantile type (vLINCL, CLN5)[71]. The infantile (CLN1) type as well as some juvenile and adult CLN1 variants are caused by a deficiency of palmitoyl protein thioesterase (PPT)[70]. The feasibility of prenatal diagnosis by using a newly developed, convenient enzyme assay was recently demonstrated[54]. In the authors' laboratory, four affected pregnancies showed complete deficiency of PPT activity in CV and in amniocyte, respectively[54].

Mucopolysaccharidoses (Table 29.2)

A general approach for the diagnosis of all MPS types is the two-dimensional electrophoresis of glycosaminoglycans in amniotic fluid. The reliability of this method was shown by the study of a large series of amniotic fluids from pregnancies at risk ($n = 72$) by Mossman and Patrick in 1982[72] and the successful use has been described in many of the literature references given in this section, e.g. in reports from the author's laboratory on MPS II[73], IIIA[59], IIIB[74], IIIC[75], IVA[76] and VII[77].

Artificial substrates are now available which allow convenient enzyme assays for the diagnosis of all MPS types[78]. Some of these substrates have only recently been developed and applied for pre- and postnatal diagnosis of MPS II[73], IIIA[59], IIIC[75], IIID[62] and IVA[76]. The first-trimester diagnosis of the Hurler syndrome in CV may occasionally be complicated as a result of the generally low activity of α-L-iduronidase in this tissue[57]. This hampers the distinction between affected fetuses and carriers with relatively low or even very low activity due to a 'pseudodeficiency allele'[79]. Further investigation of cultured CV cells or amniocentesis and GAG electrophoresis may then be necessary[80]. In our experience, this was necessary in 3 out of 75 pregnancies at risk for MPS I tested in the first trimester. As the Hunter syndrome is X linked, it is assumed that only male fetuses are at risk; the iduronate sulfatase activity in males will be normal or deficient but not intermediate. Therefore the diagnosis of an affected fetus is only justified after establishing the male fetal sex. Very low activity may occur in amniocytes[81] or in CV[82] from a female fetus due to non-random X-chromosome inactivation or selection of one cell type. The chance that the female fetus would be affected seems extremely small but is not impossible[83] and therefore ascertainment may be required by electrophoresis of glycosaminoglycans in amniotic fluid. Many unique mutations have been identified in the IDUS gene but, in 20% of the families, this concerns a large deletion or a gross rearrangement which allows rapid carrier detection in female relatives in these families[84].

The occurrence of four types of Sanfilippo disease, each caused by a different enzyme defect, emphasizes the general requirement to confirm a clinical diagnosis by enzyme investigation. This has become much easier since convenient artificial substrates for all four enzymes became available. Relatively few prenatal diagnoses have been reported, although the incidence of Sanfilippo disease may be as high as Hurler and Hunter disease. The reason is probably that, in the past, families were already completed before the diagnosis was made in the first affected child. The recent improvement of the enzyme assays should promote early postnatal diagnosis and prenatal diagnosis as well. First- and second-trimester diagnoses have been described for the types A[59], B[60,74,85] and C[61,75] but not yet for the extremely rare type D.

Few prenatal diagnoses have been made for the remaining MPS types and multiple sulfatase deficiency[66]. Diagnoses have been made in the first and the second trimester for Morquio A[63] and for Maroteaux–Lamy syndrome[64] as yet only in the second trimester, although enzyme analysis of CV is possible as well[78]. MPS VII (Sly) has been diagnosed in several pregnancies affected with fetal hydrops[65,77] and nuchal translucency[86]. α-Glucuronidase deficiency was also demonstrated in CV in the 12th week[65,86]. The occurrence of pseudodeficiency alleles should be considered and to anticipate complications in prenatal diagnosis, parental cells may be tested[87].

Hydrops fetalis (HF) and Nuchal translucency (NT)

Fetal hydrops is associated with a large number of genetic and non-genetic conditions (see Chapter 37). Blood group incompatibilities, cardiovascular diseases, chromosome abnormalities and hematologic disorders (e.g. α-thalassemia) are major causes but, in addition, lysosomal storage diseases and other metabolic disorders should be considered as a possible cause of HF in fetuses or newborns. Cases of HF have been described or briefly mentioned in a large number of reports which have been referred in reviews on HF in general[88,89] or in lysosomal diseases in particular[90,91]. The diseases are: Gaucher disease[88,89,92], GM_1-gangliosidosis[88,90,91], galactosialidosis[31,43,90,91], Niemann–Pick types A[93]and C[90], mucolipidosis I[28,88,90,93]and II[88,90,93], sialic acid storage disease[94–96], Farber disease[90]and the mucopolysaccharidoses I[90], IVA[88,90,97] and especially VII[65,77,88–91].

Other (non-lysosomal) metabolic causes of HF are disorders associated with hemolytic anemia such as α-thalassemia and deficiencies of glucose 6-phosphate dehydrogenase, glucose phosphate isomerase[89] and pyruvatekinase[98]. Further reports are on glycogenosis IV[99], long-chain 3-hydroxyacyl-coenzyme A dehydrogenase[100], Zellweger syndrome[101], Smith–Lemli–Opitz syndrome[102], congenital disorder of glycosylation type I[103], congenital erythropoietic porphyria[104] and hereditary hemochromatosis[105].

The incidence of HF due to lysosomal disorders (1%)[89] has probably been underestimated[91,93]. Until recently, metabolic disorders have not been screened when HF was indicated by ultrasound and after miscarriage or (still)birth. In such cases, it is essential that appropriate tissues, cells or fluids are sampled to allow routine screening for several (mainly lysosomal) disorders after the major causes of HF have been excluded[91,93,94].

Table 29.3 Peroxisomal disorders

Disease	*Defect*	*Sample[a]*	*Reference*
Peroxisomal biogenesis disorders			
Zellweger spectrum disorders (ZS, NALD and IRD)[b]	Generalized loss of peroxisomal functions due to mutations in PEX genes	CV, AC, DNA	Schutgens et al.[107]
RCDP[b] type 1	PEX7	DNA, VC, AC	
Single peroxisomal enzyme disorders			
RCDP[b] type 2 (DHAP-AT deficiency)	Dihydroxyacetonephosphate acyl transferase	CV, VC, AC	Schutgens et al.[107]
RCDP[b] type 3 (alkyl-DHAP synthase deficiency)	Alkyl-dihydroxyacetone phosphate synthase	CV, VC, AC	Brookhyser[108]
X-linked adrenoleukodystrophy	ALD-protein	DNA, VC, AC	Wanders et al.[109]
Acyl CoA oxidase deficiency	Acyl-CoA oxidase	DNA, VC, AC	Wanders et al.[110]
D-bifunctional protein deficiency	D-bifunctional protein	DNA, VC, AC	Paton et al. [111]
Primary hyperoxaluria type I	Alanine:glyoxylate aminotransferase	DNA, AF, FL	Danpure and Rumsby[112]

[a]CV = chorionic villi are indicated as the material of choice if suitable, additional samples are indicated only if they are occasionally needed or preferred; (CV) = possible on CV but positive cases not yet reported; VC = cultured chorionic villus cells; AF = amniotic fluid; AC = cultured amniocytes; FL = fetal liver; DNA = analysis on DNA from chorionic villi

[b]ZS, Zellweger syndrome; NALD, Neonatal adrenoleukodystrophy; IRD, Infantile Refsum disease; RCDP, Rhizomelic chondrodysplasia punctata

Several of the prenatal diagnoses reported in the references in this chapter became possible only after finding the metabolic cause of HF in a previous pregnancy.

Screening for metabolic disorders may similarly be considered after finding increased nuchal translucency (NT), which may be a herald of HF. Increased NT has been observed in several of the HF-associated disorders mentioned in this section[86,93,95,99,100].

However, in a report[106] of 13 pregnancies with fetuses affected with metabolic disorders which are occasionally associated with HF, the NT was normal.

PEROXISOMAL DISORDERS (TABLE 29.3)

Peroxisomal disorders are a group of diseases with often severe neurological involvement, caused by deficiences of one or more of the peroxisomal functions such as the β-oxidation of very long chain fatty acids (VLCFA), ether-phospholipid biosynthesis and glyoxylate detoxification etc. In some disorders (n = 4), there is a generalized loss of peroxisomal functions due to a complete or partial defect in peroxisomal biogenesis[113,114], whereas in others (n = 10), single peroxisomal enzymes are deficient[115]. Clinical and biochemical aspects of the 14 peroxisomal disorders have recently been reviewed[113–115]. Only the severe disorders which demand prenatal diagnosis are included in Table 29.3. Many prenatal diagnoses have been made for the generalized severe Zellweger syndrome[107] (many hundreds) and much smaller numbers for X-linked adrenoleukodystrophy (ALD) and some other disorders.[116] Several different methods may be used to demonstrate the metabolic abnormalities. For the peroxisome biogenesis disorders (ZS, NALD, IRD and RCDP, see Table 29.3) the methods of choice using fresh CV are dihydroxyacetonephosphate acyltransferase (DHAPAT) assay and immunoblot analysis of acyl-CoA oxidase and/or peroxisomal thiolase[113]. In families with relatively mildly affected patients with NALD and IRD, other methods may be needed such as the measurement of VLCFA levels, plasmalogen biosynthesis and immunofluorescence microscopy analysis of catalase, using cultured CV cells or amniocytes[115]. In cases of amniocentesis, the measurement of bile acid intermediates is a supplementary tool in the prenatal diagnosis of disorders in which bile acid biosynthesis is impaired[117]. In addition, RCDP may be detected by ultrasonography[118]. For X-linked ALD and other peroxisomal β-oxidation defects cultured CV or AF cells are needed to measure VLCFA levels (C26:0/C22:0 ratio) and β-oxidation of VLCFA[116,119]. However, this approach has not always been successful. Therefore, DNA mutation analysis is preferable both for prenatal diagnosis and for carrier detection in female family members, but this requires the search for a new mutation in practically each family[120]. The defective enzyme in hyperoxaluria type I (alanine: glyoxylate aminotransferase, AGT) is only expressed in liver. Prenatal diagnosis by fetal liver biopsy has been made but, clearly, the analysis of the AGT gene in DNA isolated from CV would be the method of choice whenever this is possible[112].

DISORDERS OF CARBOHYDRATE METABOLISM (TABLE 29.4)

Only limited use is made of prenatal investigation for galactosemia because this is a treatable disease. Unfortunately, the long-term results of treatment appear not completely satisfactory[135]. Sometimes prenatal diagnosis is requested to decide whether maternal galactose restriction during pregnancy should be continued or not; however, it seems questionable whether maternal restriction is effective at all[136]. Prenatal diagnosis of galactosemia is preferably done by enzyme assay in CV or by

Table 29.4 **Disorders of carbohydrate metabolism**

Disease	*Enzyme defect*	*Sample[a]*	*Reference*
Galactosemia	Galactose 1P-uridyltransferase	CV, AF, AC	Jakobs et al.[121]
Glycogenosis Ia	Glucose 6 P-ase	DNA, FL	Golbus et al.[122]
Glycogenosis Ib	Glucose 6 P-translocase	DNA	Lam et al.[123]
Glycogenosis II	Lysosomal α-glucosidase	CV, VC, AC	Kleijer et al.[124]
Glycogenosis III	Debranching enzyme	CV, VC, AC	Shin et al.[125]
Glycogenosis IV	Branching enzyme	DNA, VC, AC,	Brown and Brown[126]
Complex IV deficiency	Cytochrome C oxidase	CV, AC	Ruitenbeek et al.[127]
PC deficiency	Pyruvate carboxylase	CV, VC, AC	Van Coster et al.[128]
PDH deficiency	Pyruvate dehydrogenase (E1α)	DNA	Brown and Brown[129]
	PDH Protein X	DNA	Rouillac et al.[130]
GK deficiency	Glycerolkinase	AF, AC, (CV)	Borresen et al.[131]
PK deficiency	Pyruvate kinase	DNA, (FB)	Rouger et al.[132]
GPI deficiency	Glucose phosphate isomerase	CV, AC	Whitelaw et al.[133]
CDG[b] syndrome type Ia	Phosphomannomutase	DNA, CV, AC	Charlwood et al.[134]
CDG[b] syndrome type Ib	Phosphomannose isomerase	(CV)	-

[a]CV = chorionic villi are indicated as the material of choice if suitable, additional samples are indicated only if they are occasionally needed or preferred; (CV) = possible on CV but positive cases not yet reported; VC = cultured chorionic villus cells; AF = amniotic fluid; AC = cultured amniocytes; FB = fetal blood; FL = fetal liver; DNA = analysis on DNA from chorionic villi.

[b]CDG, congenital disorder of glycosylation

galactitol measurement in amniotic fluid[121]; both methods provide a reliable diagnosis within 1 or 2 days after sampling. The presence of a common mutation in the GALT gene will allow carrier detection in many families[137]. In several countries, galactosemia is now part of a neonatal screening program, which allows early treatment of the diagnosed patients.

The glycogen storage diseases (GSD) comprise more than 10 diseases, but prenatal diagnosis seems only relevant for the types I to IV[138]. Type II or Pompe's disease is a lysosomal storage disease caused by the deficiency of acid α-glucosidase (GAA). The incidence is relatively high and many hundreds of prenatal diagnoses have been made for the severe infantile form[124]. Direct enzyme analysis of CV is the method of choice not only because of the early result but also because of the high activity of GAA in CV compared to AF cells, which facilitates reliable diagnosis[124]. A few common mutations in the GAA gene are known, which is useful for carrier detection and for prenatal diagnosis in special cases[124].

As glucose 6-phosphatase is only expressed in liver, prenatal diagnosis by enzyme assay of GSD type Ia requires fetal liver biopsy[122]. Mutation analysis will thus be preferred if possible[139]. Similarly, mutation analysis is the method of choice for the prenatal diagnosis of GSD Ib[123]. Direct enzyme analysis in CV has successfully been used for the diagnosis of GSD III[125,140] but for type IV cultured amniocytes have mostly been used because the direct assay on CV may give inconsistent results[126,138]. Nevertheless, successful enzyme diagnosis using native villi has recently been reported[99]; DNA analysis may be preferred if possible[141]. In some cases, ultrasound examination showing increased nuchal translucency or fetal hydrops may also help[99].

Prenatal diagnosis for respiratory chain disorders, e.g. complex IV deficiency has been undertaken[127], but its general reliability remains to be established[142]. The potential for prenatal diagnosis of defective mitochondrial (mt) function which is encoded by mtDNA is limited. The occurrence of heteroplasmy (i.e. the presence of mtDNA molecules with and without a certain mutation in various proportions) makes the interpretation of both enzyme and mtDNA analysis difficult. Generally, an affected fetus is reliably indicated by enzyme deficiency at the level previously shown in fibroblasts of the index patient, but is not always excluded by normal results[142]. In the case of a respiratory chain defect caused by a mutation in a nuclear gene, reliable prenatal diagnosis can be effected by mutation analysis but, in practice, this concerns only a minority of families[143].

Two disorders of pyruvate metabolism are also mitochondrial but nuclear DNA encoded. Pyruvate carboxylase (PC) deficiency has been demonstrated in CV[128] and in AF cells[144]. Pyruvate dehydrogenase (PDH) deficiency is usually demonstrated in muscle tissue; the activity in fibroblasts, amniocytes and CV is probably not sufficiently specific to allow reliable diagnosis[129]. The major form of PDH deficiency (due to the defective E1α subunit) is X-linked; prenatal diagnosis will be possible in most families by DNA analysis[129,145] and reliable in the case of an affected or normal male and a non-carrier female, but the outcome is difficult to predict in case of a carrier female[145]. Prenatal diagnosis has also been reported for the autosomal recessive protein X deficiency form of PDH deficiency[130].

Another X-linked disorder, glycerolkinase (GK) deficiency, has been diagnosed by the demonstration of accumulated glycerol in AF and of the enzyme deficiency in AF cells[131] but direct or indirect enzyme testing of CV also seems feasible. The prenatal diagnosis of the red cell pyruvate kinase (PK) deficiency, which causes non-spherocytic hemolytic anemia, should preferably be attempted by DNA rather than by enzyme analysis of fetal erythrocytes. Polymorphisms and common mutations are known in different populations[146] and prenatal diagnosis has recently been reported[132]. Glucosephosphate isomerase (GPI) deficiency is another defect causing hemolytic anemia and occasionally fetal hydrops. Prenatal diagnosis by enzyme analysis in AF cells has been reported[133] and should be possible in CV as well[147].

Finally, Table 29.4 includes the congenital disorder of glycosylation (CDG) syndrome type Ia, which is caused by the primary deficiency of phosphomannomutase (PMM) and the much less frequent type Ib caused by phosphomannose isomerase deficiency. For type Ia, prenatal diagnosis on CV will be possible in most families[134], but not in families in which the index patient has high residual or even normal PMM activity[148]. For the milder and treatable type Ib, prenatal diagnosis will generally not be appropriate.

DISORDERS OF NUCLEOTIDE METABOLISM AND DNA REPAIR (TABLE 29.5)

The diagnosis of the X-linked Lesch–Nyhan syndrome by direct enzyme analysis in CV has been reported[149,159]and is rapid (1–2 days) and reliable[149,159]. Complications have been reported, which only emphasize the need for proper selection of the CV sample, establishment of the fetal sex and of sufficient experience with the hypoxanthine phosphoribosyltransferase (HPRT) assay in CV. In case of doubt (e.g. intermediate activity in a male fetus), cultured CV cells may be tested for confirmation. Mutation analysis is especially important for carrier detection in female relatives[160]. This is illustrated in our own results: only 11 affected fetuses were found in 92 pregnancies at risk. Probably more than half of these prenatal tests could have been prevented by timely exclusion of heterozygosity of the pregnant women.

Adenosine deaminase (ADA) and purine nucleoside phosphorylase (PNP) deficiencies have been demonstrated in CV[150,151] and in AF cells[161,162] from pregnancies at risk for these two rare immunodeficiencies. Dihydropyrimidine dehydrogenase (DHPDH) deficiency may not be detectable in CV, but prenatal diagnosis has been made by measurement of increased levels of thymine and uracil in AF[153]. Adenylosuccinase deficiency was recently diagnosed by mutation analysis[152]; and by analogy to patients' urine, accumulation of metabolites (S-Ado and SAICA-riboside) may be expected in amniotic fluid but has not yet been demonstrated[152]. Molybdenum cofactor deficiency, which results in the combined deficiency of xanthine and sulfite oxidase, can be diagnosed by testing the latter enzyme in CV[154,163]; in cases of amniocentesis enzyme assay in AF cells may be combined with S-sulfocysteine measurement in the fluid[164].

For the demonstration of the DNA repair defects in xeroderma pigmentosum (XP), trichothiodystrophy (TTD), Cockayne syndrome (CS) and also of ataxia telangiectasia (AT), several methods are available which all require cultured CV (or AF) cells rather than fresh CV. Repair of DNA damage may be studied by direct measurement of repair DNA synthesis (XP[155,165], TTD[156]) or by studying the recovery of RNA or DNA synthesis after UV exposure (CS[157,166], XP[165], TTD[156]). Mutation analysis of the DNA repair disorders is hampered by the involvement of multiple genes (8 for XP, 3 for TTD, 2 for CS) and the lack of diagnostic laboratories active in this field. AT is

Table 29.5 **Disorders of nucleotide metabolism and DNA repair**

Disease	*Defect*	*Sample*[a]	*Reference*
Lesch–Nyhan syndrome	Hypoxanthine phosphoribosyltransferase	CV, AC	Gibbs et al.[149]
ADA deficiency	Adenosine deaminase	CV, AC	Dooley et al.[150]
PNP deficiency	Purine nucleoside phosphorylase	CV, AC	Pérignon et al.[151]
Adenylosuccinase deficiency	Adenylosuccinase	DNA, (AF)	Marie et al. [152]
DHPDH deficiency	Dihydropyrimidine dehydrogenase	AF	Jakobs et al.[153]
Combined xanthine- and sulfite oxidase deficiency	Molybdenum cofactor/sulfite oxidase	CV, AF	Gray et al.[154]
Xeroderma pigmentosum	DNA repair	VC, AC	Halley et al.[155]
Trichothiodystrophy	DNA repair	VC, AC	Sarasin et al.[156]
Cockayne syndrome	DNA repair/transcription	VC, AC, DNA	Lehmann et al.[157]
Ataxia telangiectasia	Radioresistant DNA synthesis	VC, AC, DNA	Kleijer et al.[158]

[a]CV = chorionic villi are indicated as the material of choice if suitable, additional samples are indicated only if they are occasionally needed or preferred; (CV) = possible on CV but positive cases not yet reported; VC = cultured chorionic villus cells; AF = amniotic fluid; AC = cultured amniocytes; DNA = analysis on DNA from chorionic villi

demonstrated by increased, so-called radioresistant DNA synthesis (RDS) after X-irradiation of cultured CV or AF cells[158], but the test is undertaken in very few laboratories. Mutation analysis of the ATM gene may be preferred, but the large size of the gene and the lack of common mutations hamper the rapid detection of the mutations in patients[167]. The same RDS test can be used for the diagnosis of Nijmegen breakage syndrome, but for this disorder, mutation analysis would be more appropriate because of the smaller gene and the presence of a common mutation[168]. However, as for all metabolic disorders and especially in this group of DNA repair disorders, it is essential that the suspected biochemical defect is demonstrated in the proband in the family before prenatal diagnosis or even mutation analysis is considered.

DISORDERS OF AMINO ACID AND ORGANIC ACID METABOLISM (TABLE 29.6)

Many inborn errors of amino and organic acid metabolism appear in Table 29.6, but the list is not complete. Some disorders have already been listed in Table 29.3 and 29.4; other

Table 29.6 **Disorders of amino acid and organic acid metabolism**

Disease	*Enzyme defect*	*Sample*[a]	*Reference*
Phenylketonuria	Phenylalaninehydroxylase	DNA	Lidsky et al.[169]
Phenylketonuria II	Dihydropteridine reductase	AC	Blau et al.[170]
Phenylketonuria III	6-pyruvoyl tetrahydropterin synthase	AF, FB	Blau et al.[170]
Canavan disease	Aspartoacylase	DNA, AF	Bennett et al.[171]
Tyrosinemia I	Fumarylacetoacetase	DNA, CV, AF	Jakobs et al.[172]
Non-ketotic hyperglycinemia	Glycine cleavage system	DNA, CV	Hayasaka et al.[173]
Cystinosis	Lysosomal cystine transport	CV	Patrick et al.[174]
Maple syrup urine disease	BCKA decarboxylase	CV	Kleijer et al.[175]
Isovaleric acidemia	Isovaleryl CoA-dehydrogenase	CV, AF	Kleijer et al.[176]
3-MCC deficiency	3-methylcrotonyl CoA carboxylase	(CV, AF)	Jakobs et al.[5]
3-MGA deficiency	3-methylglutaconyl-CoA hydratase	(CV, AF)	Chitayat et al.[177]
3-HMG deficiency	3-hydroxy 3-methylglutaryl CoA lyase	CV, AF, AC	Chalmers et al.[178]
Multiple carboxylase deficiency	Holocarboxylase synthase	AF, AC	Packman et al.[179]
	Biotinidase	(CV)	Chalmers et al.[180]
Citrullinemia	Argininosuccinate synthetase	CV, AF	Kleijer et al.[181]
Argininosuccinic aciduria	Argininosuccinate lyase	CV, AF	Vimal et al.[182]
CPS deficiency	Carbamoyl phosphate synthetase	DNA, FL	Piceni Sereni et al.[183]
OTC deficiency	Ornithine carbamoyl transferase	DNA, FL	Rodeck et al.[184]
HHH syndrome	Ornithine transport	AC(CV)	Shih et al.[185]
Gyrate atrophy	Ornithine amino transferase	(CV, AC)	Shih et al.[185]
Propionic acidemia	Propionyl CoA carboxylase	CV, AF	Rolland et al.[186]
Methylmalonic aciduria	Methylmalonyl CoA mutase	AF, AC, CV	Fowler et al.[187]
Glutaric aciduria I	Glutaryl CoA dehydrogenase	CV, VC, AF	Christensen[188]
Glutaric aciduria II	ETF or ETF dehydrogenase	AF, AC	Yamaguchi et al.[189]
MCAD deficiency	Medium chain acyl CoA dehydrogenase	DNA, AC	Bennett et al.[190]
VLCAD deficiency	Very long chain acyl CoA dehydrogenase	CV, AC, DNA	Nada et al.[191]
LCHAD deficiency	Long chain 3-hydroxyacyl CoA dehydrogenase	CV, DNA	Von Döbeln et al.[192]

[a]CV = chorionic villi are indicated as the material of choice if suitable, additional samples are indicated only if they are occasionally needed or preferred; (CV) = possible on CV but positive cases not yet reported; VC = cultured chorionic villus cells; AF = amniotic fluid; AC = cultured amniocytes; FB = fetal blood; FL = fetal liver; DNA = analysis on DNA from chorionic villi

disorders have either been omitted or included but not discussed because prenatal diagnosis is seldom requested as they are rare or usually mild. Nowadays, several of these disorders are included in neonatal screening programs which allows early detection and treatment.

Phenylketonuria is a treatable disease for which prenatal diagnosis is, in most countries, rarely performed. However, as the limitations of treatment are becoming clear and since DNA analysis of CV has become available, this option may be considered more often[193]. Similarly, DNA analysis will be the method of choice for two of the urea cycle disorders (OTC and CPS deficiency) whenever this is possible[194]; the option of enzyme assay in fetal liver is clearly less favorable but its feasibility has been demonstrated[183,184,195]. DNA analysis will also be chosen for the prenatal diagnosis of Canavan disease if the mutations in the index patient can be found[196,197]; aspartoacylase activity in CV and AF cells is too low, but *N*-acetylaspartate measurement in AF at 16 weeks or later is probably reliable in most but not all cases[171,196,197]. Tyrosinemia type I can be diagnosed reliably in most but not in all pregnancies at risk by increased succinylacetone in AF[198], probably even by early amniocentesis[172], but also fumarylacetoacetase assay in CV[172] and mutation analysis have been used[199].

The diagnosis of non-ketotic hyperglycinemia has been made by the demonstration of a defective glycine cleavage system in CV[173]; however false-negative diagnoses have been reported[200], making mutation analysis preferable whenever possible[201].

For several disorders, tests have been designed to study the relevant metabolic pathways in native CV or in cultured cells; such tests are often more sensitive and more practicable than the direct enzyme assay in cell or tissue homogenates[6]. For example, the lysosomal transport defect in cystinosis can be demonstrated by studying the uptake and accumulation of free ^{35}S-cystine in intact cells or CV[174]; recently, however, direct quantitative measurement of cystine in CV and cultured cells was used[202]. Several disorders of leucine catabolism are amenable to prenatal diagnosis by direct or indirect enzyme assay or by measurement of specific metabolites. Increased metabolite levels have been demonstrated in amniotic fluid for isovaleric acidemia[176] and 3-hydroxymethylglutaric aciduria[203] but not for maple syrup urine disease[5]. The latter disorder can be reliably diagnosed by measuring the decarboxylation of radiolabeled leucine in intact CV, providing results within a day. Since the first reported first-trimester diagnosis[175], we have successfully investigated CV from 70 pregnancies at risk, finding 21 affected fetuses, mostly after long-distance transport of the samples. Several prenatal diagnoses of isovaleric acidemia have been made by showing strongly increased levels of isovalerylglycine in the amniotic fluid[176]; furthermore, we have diagnosed five affected fetuses in 15 pregnancies at risk by the demonstration of defective incorporation of radiolabeled isovaleric acid in proteins in CV[176]. Prenatal diagnosis of multiple carboxylase deficiency has been performed to allow prenatal treatment with biotin[204].

Incorporation tests using CV, as well as metabolite measurements in AF allow reliable prenatal diagnosis of two urea cycle disorders, citrullinemia and argininosuccinic aciduria. A collaborative European report[195] of prenatal diagnosis of urea cycle disorders has summarized the results in 183 pregnancies at risk, with 47 affected fetuses, for the two disorders together. Some pitfalls in this large series and in other reports[182,205] were mainly related to the use of cultured AF and CV cells or may have been caused by maternal tissue in the CV sample; they should be avoidable. Relatively large series for citrullinemia and argininosuccinic aciduria (n = 53; 13 affected) in the authors' laboratory revealed an unexpectedly high rate of recurrence for citrullinemia (39.5%). As these results were independent of the methods used (metabolites in AF, enzyme or DNA in CV, CVC and AFC) and the majority of diagnoses were confirmed by multiple tests, a hypothetical explanation was raised for the observed transmission ratio distortion[206].

Propionic acidemia can be diagnosed reliably both by direct assay of propionyl CoA carboxylase in CV[186] and by measurement of methylcitrate in AF at 14–16 weeks as usual[207] or earlier[186,13]. The direct assay of the defective mutase in CV for methylmalonic acidemia is possible[187] but not routinely available; fortunately, measurement of methylmalonic acid in AF allows a reliable diagnosis[207]. Both types of glutaric aciduria, I and II, can be diagnosed by increased concentrations of glutaric acid in amniotic fluid[189,207–209], whereas type I has also been diagnosed in the first trimester by glutaryl CoA dehydrogenase deficiency in CV[188]. By far the most prevalent disorder of mitochondrial fatty acid oxidation is the medium chain acyl-CoA dehydrogenase (MCAD) deficiency. Early diagnosis of this often mild or even asymptomatic disorder is indicated in families at risk to anticipate severe complications. Prenatal diagnosis is possible by direct or indirect enzyme assay in cultured AF cells[190]. However, as a single highly prevalent mutation (A985G) is responsible for MCAD deficiency, prenatal or immediate neonatal screening for this mutation will be applicable in most families[210]. MCAD is included in the neonatal screening programs in several countries including now, the UK. A common mutation is also present in LCHAD deficiency[211], but in contrast large mutational heterogeneity was reported for VLCAD deficiency[212]. Both disorders can however be diagnosed by direct enzyme assay[191,192,211,212] or by measurement of the production of the respective acylcarnitines[191].

OTHER DISORDERS (TABLE 29.7)

Most of the disorders listed in Table 29.7 can be diagnosed prenatally by metabolic and by DNA methods; for several, the DNA approach will be preferred if informative data are available. The first four disorders of the list are X linked. This makes the option of DNA-based carrier detection in females important for at least the two severe diseases, the Menkes[229] and Lowe[214] syndromes. Direct copper measurement in CV has provided many correct and early diagnoses for Menkes disease, but this method is susceptible to copper contamination[213]. Alternatively, cultured amniocytes may be used for uptake studies with ^{64}Cu or with the more practical radioisotope ^{110m}Ag[230]. Prenatal diagnosis for the Lowe syndrome has recently been reported, but the enzyme assay is available in very few laboratories[214]. To anticipate complications at birth (delay of labor and failure of cervix dilatation), fetal X-linked ichthyosis may easily be demonstrated in CV or placental biopsy material, but also the measurement of dihydroepiandrosterone sulfate in AF or specific steroid profiles in maternal urine and blood may be diagnostic[215]. For chronic granulomatous disease, DNA analysis will be preferred for prenatal diagnosis as the available tests of enzyme activity in neutrophils require fetal blood[231]. Prolidase

Table 29.7 Other disorders

Disease	*Defect*	*Sample*[a]	*Reference*
Menkes syndrome	Copper transport (ATPase)	DNA, AC, CV	Tønnesen et al.[213]
Lowe syndrome	Phosphatidyl inositol 4,5biP5Pase	DNA, AC, VC	Suchy et al.[214]
X-linked ichthyosis	Steroid sulfatase	CV, AF	Hähnel et al.[215]
Chronic granulomatous disease	NADPH-oxidase	DNA, FB	Huu et al.[216]
Congenital adrenal hyperplasia	21-hydroxylase	DNA, AF	Raux-Demay et al.[217]
Acute intermittent porphyria	Porphobilinogen deaminase	AC, DNA	Sassa et al.[218]
Congenital erythropoietic porphyria	Uroporphyrin I	AF, DNA	Ged et al.[219]
Familial hypercholesterolemia	LDL receptor	DNA, AC,	Brown et al.[220]
Leprechaunism	Insulin receptor	DNA, (CV), (AC)	Maassen et al.[221]
Hypophosphatasia	Alkaline phosphatase	DNA, CV	Brock and Barron[222]
Collagen disorders (E-D; OI)	Collagen	DNA, CV, VC	Raghunath et al.[223]
Prolidase deficiency	Prolidase	(CV), AFC	Mandel et al.[224]
Mevalonic aciduria	Mevalonate kinase	CV, AF, AC	Rolland et al.[225]
Smith–Lemli–Opitz syndrome	7-dehydrocholesterol reductase	CV, AF, AC	Mills et al.[226]
Sjogren–Larsson syndrome	Fatty aldehyde dehydrogenase	VC, AC	Rizzo et al.[227]
Cystic fibrosis	Cl transport (CFTR)	DNA, AF	Brock et al.[228]

[a]CV = chorionic villi are indicated as the material of choice if suitable, additional samples are indicated only if they are occasionally needed or preferred; (CV) = possible on CV but positive cases not yet reported; VC = cultured chorionic villus cells; AF = amniotic fluid; AC = cultured amniocytes; FB = fetal blood; DNA = analysis on DNA from chorionic villi; Cl = chloride

deficiency has been shown in amniocytes[224] but this should be possible in CV as well.

Mevalonic aciduria is caused by a defect in the first part of the cholesterol biosynthetic pathway and can be diagnosed prenatally by measurement of mevalonate kinase activity in CV or by mevalonate in amniotic fluid[232]. Smith–Lemli–Opitz syndrome can be diagnosed at the metabolite level (7-dehydrocholesterol)[226] using maternal urine[233], AF or CV or by enzyme assay (7-DHC-reductase) in CV[234] or by DNA analysis[233].

References are given in Table 29.7 for prenatal diagnoses made by biochemical analysis. However, for most of these disorders, the use of mutation or linkage analysis will be preferred, e.g. for congenital adrenal hyperplasia[235], the porphyrias[219], hypercholesterolemia[236], leprechaunism[237], hypophosphatasia[238] and the collagen disorders[223]. DNA analysis is also the method of choice for prenatal diagnosis of cystic fibrosis, but cases may remain where neither the mutations nor informative markers are available[239] (see Chapter 28). Microvillar enzyme testing in AF at 17–18 weeks then allows rapid prenatal diagnosis which may, in an experienced center, reduce the risk from 25% to 1–2%[240].

PAST, PRESENT AND FUTURE

The past decades have shown great progress in the prenatal diagnosis of inborn errors of metabolism in several respects. First, the number of disorders which can be diagnosed prenatally has increased rapidly to approximately 100 in the first two decades (1970–1990). In the past decade especially, DNA-based techniques have provided new ways to diagnose the thousands of disorders for which the primary protein defect is not known or difficult to assess. Also, for some of the disorders diagnosed currently through their defective metabolic functions, DNA analysis may provide more reliable or earlier results (examples have been given in the Tables). However, for the majority of the disorders discussed in this chapter, the metabolic tests are reliable, rapid and most importantly they are, in principle, applicable to all affected families. For these disorders, DNA analysis seems neither necessary nor advantageous and they would only be applicable in those families in whom disease-causing mutations have been demonstrated.

Secondly, the introduction of CVS has allowed a much earlier and often almost immediate diagnosis. For some diseases which are diagnosed by metabolite measurement, amniocentesis may be advanced by a few weeks[12,13].

Thirdly, the reliability of prenatal diagnosis has been increased by the expansion of available methods and of the experience acquired with them. The optimal combination can now be chosen from materials (CV, AF, cultured CV or AF cells) and methods (analysis at the DNA, protein or metabolite level) for each disorder and particular situation. More than one technique may occasionally be necessary to corroborate or clarify initial results.

Fourthly, DNA analysis has improved the prospects for heterozygote detection. In families with X-linked diseases, this is not only important to detect heterozygosity but also to avoid unnecessary prenatal diagnosis in female relatives of a patient, who appear not to be a carrier. For autosomal recessive disorders, the demonstration or exclusion of heterozygosity in relatives of a patient and their partners is possible and especially important in populations with one or more common mutations causing the disease concerned and in populations with a tradition of consanguineous marriage.

Non-invasive sampling methods have been a long-sought goal for prenatal diagnosis. One approach has been the isolation of intact fetal cells from maternal blood. However, successful biochemical study and probably also DNA analysis would require the isolation of much higher numbers of fetal cells than hitherto achieved[241]. Another approach, which needs further development to allow future applications, is the molecular analysis of cell-free fetal nucleic acids in maternal plasma[242].

On a small scale, preimplantation genetic diagnosis (PID) of genetic metabolic disorders has been performed in combination with in vitro fertilization (IVF) using DNA (micro)methods, but the approach will presumably remain limited to special situations (see Chapter 25). Biochemical (micro)methods are not suitable for PID.

REFERENCES

1. *Online Mendelian Inheritance in Man*, OMIM (TM). McKusick-Nathans Institute for Genetic Medicine, Johns Hopkins University (Baltimore, MD, USA.) and National Center for Biotechnology Information, National Library of Medicine (Bethesda).
2. Scriver CR, Beaudet AL, Sly WS, Valle D. *The metabolic and molecular bases of inherited disease*, 8th edn. New York: McGraw-Hill, 2001.
3. Blau N, Duran M, Blaskovics M, Gibson KM. *Physicians' guide to the laboratory diagnosis of inherited metabolic disease*, 2nd edn. Berlin: Springer, 2002.
4. Wraith JE. Limitations of enzyme replacement therapy: current and future. *J Inher Metab Dis* **29**:442–447, 2006.
5. Jakobs C, Ten Brink HJ, Stellaard F. Prenatal diagnosis of inherited metabolic disorders by quantitation of characteristic metabolites in amniotic fluid: facts and future. *Prenat Diagn* **10**:265–271, 1990.
6. Kleijer WJ. First-trimester diagnosis of genetic metabolic disorders. *Contr Gynecol Obstet* **15**:80–89, 1986.
7. Roberts E, Duckett DP, Lang GD. Maternal cell contamination in chorionic villus samples assessed by direct preparations and three different culture methods. *Prenat Diagn* **8**:635–640, 1988.
8. Ledbetter DH, Zachary JM, Simpson JL et al. Cytogenetic results from the US collaborative study on CVS. *Prenat Diagn* **12**:317–345, 1992.
9. Poenaru L. First trimester prenatal diagnosis of metabolic diseases: a survey in countries from the European community. *Prenat Diagn* **7**:333–341, 1987.
10. Besley GTN, Young EP, Fensom AH, Cooper A. First trimester diagnosis of inherited metabolic disease: experience in the UK. *J Inher Metab Dis* **14**:128–133, 1991.
11. Desnick RJ, Schuette JL, Golbus MS et al. First trimester biochemical and molecular diagnoses using chorionic villi: high accuracy in the US collaborative study. *Prenat Diagn* **12**:357–372, 1992.
12. Wilson RD. Early amniocentesis: a clinical review. *Prenat Diagn* **15**:1259–1273, 1995.
13. Chadefaux-Vekemans B, Rabier D, Cadoudal N et al. Prenatal diagnosis of some metabolic diseases using early amniotic fluid samples: report of a 15 years' experience. *Prenat Diagn* **26**: 814–818, 2006.
14. Kleijer WJ, Galjaard H. Praenatale Diagnostik genetisch bedingter stoffwechselleiden. In *Murken Praenatale Diagnostik und Therapie*, pp. 100–132. Stuttgart: Enke, 1987.
15. Besley GTN. Enzyme analysis. In *Prenatal diagnosis and screening*, DJH Brock, CH Rodeck, MA Ferguson-Smith (eds), pp. 127–145. Edinburgh: Churchill Livingstone, 1992.
16. Kaback M, Lim-Steele J, Dabholkar D, Brown D, Levy N, Zeiger K. Tay–Sachs disease – carrier screening, prenatal diagnosis, and the molecular era. An international perspective, 1970 to 1993. *J Am Med Assoc* **270**:2307–2315, 1993.
17. Kleijer WJ, Hussaarts-Odijk LM, Sachs ES, Jahoda MGJ, Niermeijer MF. Prenatal diagnosis of Fabry's disease by direct analysis of chorionic villi. *Prenat Diagn* **7**:283–287, 1987.
18. Fensom AH, Benson PF, Neville BRG, Moser HW, Moser AE, Dulaney JT. Prenatal diagnosis of Farber's disease. *Lancet* **ii**:990–992, 1979.
19. Besley GTN, Ferguson-Smith ME, Frew C, Morris A, Gilmore DH. First trimester diagnosis of Gaucher disease in a fetus with trisomy 21. *Prenat Diagn* **8**:471–474, 1988.
20. Besley GTN, Broadhead DM. Prenatal diagnosis of inherited metabolic disease by chorionic villus analysis: the Edinburgh experience. *J Inher Metab Dis* **12**(suppl 2):263–266, 1989.
21. Giles L, Cooper A, Fowler B, Sardharwalla IB, Donnai P. First trimester prenatal diagnosis of Sandhoff's disease. *Prenat Diagn* **8**:199–205, 1988.
22. Grebner EE, Wenger DA. Use of 4-methylumbelliferyl-6-sulpho-2-acetamido-2-deoxy-D-glucopyranoside for prenatal diagnosis of Tay–Sachs disease using chorionic villi. *Prenat Diagn* **7**:419–423, 1987.
23. Kleijer WJ, Mancini GMS, Jahoda MGJ et al. First-trimester diagnosis of Krabbe's disease by direct enzyme analysis of chorionic villi. *N Engl J Med* **311**:1257, 1984.
24. Fensom AH, Marsh J, Jackson M et al. First-trimester diagnosis of metachromatic leucodystrophy. *Clin Genet* **34**:122–125, 1988.
25. Vanier MT, Boué J, Dumez Y. Niemann–Pick disease type B: first-trimester prenatal diagnosis on chorionic villi and biochemical study of a foetus at 12 weeks of development. *Clin Genet* **28**:348–354, 1985.
26. Vanier MT, Rodriguez-Lafrasse C, Rousson R. Prenatal diagnosis of Niemann–Pick type C disease: current strategy from an experience of 37 pregnancies at risk. *Am J Hum Genet* **51**:111–122, 1992.
27. Van Diggelen OP, Von Koskull H, Ämmälä P, Vredeveldt GTM, Janse HC, Kleijer WJ. First trimester diagnosis of Wolman's disease. *Prenat Diagn* **8**:661–663, 1988.
28. Sasagasako N, Miyahara S, Saito N, Shinnoh N, Kobayashi T, Goto I. Prenatal diagnosis of congenital sialidosis. *Clin Genet* **44**:8–11, 1993.
29. Besley GTN, Broadhead DM, Nevin NC, Nevin J, Dornan JC. Prenatal diagnosis of mucolipidosis II by early amniocentesis. *Lancet* **335**:1164–1165, 1990.
30. Zeigler M, Bargal R, Suri V, Meidan B, Bach G. Mucolipidosis type IV: accumulation of phospholipids and gangliosides in cultured amniotic cells. A tool for prenatal diagnosis. *Prenat Diagn* **12**:1037–1042, 1992.
31. Kleijer WJ, Geilen GC, Janse HC et al. Cathepsin A deficiency in galactosialidosis: studies of patients and carriers in 16 families. *Pediatr Res* **39**:1067–1071, 1996.
32. Thomas GH. 'Pseudodeficiencies' of lysosomal hydrolases. *Am J Hum Genet* **54**:934–940, 1994.
33. Leistner S, Young E, Meaney C, Winchester B. Pseudodeficiency of arylsulphatase A: strategy for clarification of genotype in families of subjects with low ASA activity and neurological

symptoms. *J Inher Metab Dis* **18**:710–716, 1995.
34. Vervoort R, Gitzelmann R, Bosshard N, Maire I, Liebaers I, Lissens W. Low β-glucuronidase enzyme activity and mutations in the human β-glucuronidase gene in mild mucopolysaccharidosis type VII, pseudodeficiency and a heterozygote. *Hum Genet* **102**:69–78, 1998.
35. Grimm U, Zschiesche M, Widerschain G, Seidlitz G, Machill G. Use of a fluorogenic substrate, 6-hexadecanoylamino-4-methylumbelliferyl-β-D-galactopyranoside, in the diagnosis of Krabbe disease. *J Inher Metab Dis* **14**:940–941, 1991.
36. Van Diggelen OP, Voznyi YaV, Keulemans JLM et al. A new fluorimetric enzyme assay for the diagnosis of Niemann-Pick A/B, with specificity of natural sphingomyelinase substrate. *J Inher Metab Dis* **28**:33–741, 2005.
37. Vanier MT, Millat G. Niemann-Pick type C. *Clin Genet* **64**:269–281, 2003.
38. Vanier MT. Prenatal diagnosis of Niemann-Pick diseases types A, B and C. *Prenat Diagn* **22**:630–632, 2002.
39. Akhunov VS, Gargaun SS, Krasnopolskaya XD. First-trimester enzyme exclusion of Farber disease using a micromethod with [^{3}H] ceramide. *J Inher Metab Dis* **18**:616–619, 1995.
40. Chatelut M, Feuteun J, Harzer K et al. A simple method for screening for Farber disease on cultured skin fibroblasts. *Clin Chim Acta* **245**:61–71, 1996.
41. Bär J, Linke T, Ferlinz K, Neumann U, Schuchman EH, Sandhoff K. Molecular analysis of acid ceramidase deficiency in patients with Farber disease. *Hum Mut* **17**:199–209, 2001.
42. Kleijer WJ, Hoogeveen A, Verheijen FW et al. Prenatal diagnosis of sialidosis with combined neuraminidase and β-galactosidase deficiency. *Clin Genet* **16**:60–61, 1979.
43. Itoh K, Miharu N, Ohama K, Mizoguchi N, Sakura N, Sakuraba H. Fetal diagnosis of galactosialidosis (protective protein/cathepsin A deficiency). *Clin Chim Act* **266**:75–82, 1997.
44. Parvathy MR, Mitchell DA, Ben-Yoseph Y. Prenatal diagnosis of I-cell disease in the first and second trimesters. *Am J Med Sci* **297**:361–364, 1989.
45. Poenaru L, Mezard C, Akli S, Oury JF, Dumez Y, Boue J. Prenatal diagnosis of mucolipidosis type II on first-trimester amniotic fluid. *Prenat Diagn* **10**:231–235, 1990.
46. Falik-Zaccai TC, Zeigler M, Bargal R, Bach G, Borochowitz Z, Raas-Rothschild A. Mucolipidosis III type C: first-trimester biochemical and molecular prenatal diagnosis. *Prenat Diagn* **23**:211–214, 2003.
47. LaPlante JM, Sun M, Falardeau J et al. Lysosomal exocytosis is impaired in mucolipidosis type IV. *Mol Genet Metab* **89**:339–348, 2006.
48. Aula P, Mattila K, Piiroinen O, Ämmälä A, Von Koskull H. First-trimester prenatal diagnosis of aspartylglucosaminuria. *Prenat Diagn* **9**:617–620, 1989.
49. Poenaru L, Dreyfus J-C, Boué J, Nicolesco H, Ravise N, Bamberger J. Prenatal diagnosis of fucosidosis. *Clin Genet* **10**:60–264, 1976.
50. Petushkova NA. First-trimester diagnosis of an unusual case of α-mannosidosis. *Prenat Diagn* **11**:279–283, 1991.
51. Kleijer WJ, Geilen GC, Van Diggelen OP, Wevers RA, Los FJ. Prenatal analyses in a pregnancy at risk for β-mannosidosis. *Prenat Diagn* **12**:841–843, 1992.
52. Lake BD, Young EP, Nicolaides K. Prenatal diagnosis of infantile sialic acid storage disease in a twin pregnancy. *J Inher Metab Dis* **12**:152–156, 1989.
53. Van Diggelen OP, Schindler D, Kleijer WJ et al. Lysosomal α-N-acetyl-galactosaminidase deficiency: a new inherited metabolic disease. *Lancet* **ii**:804, 1987.
54. De Vries BBA, Kleijer WJ, Keulemans JLM et al. First-trimester diagnosis of infantile neuronal ceroid lipofuscinosis (INCL) using PPT enzyme assay and *CLN1* mutation analysis. *Prenat Diagn* **19**:559–562, 1999.
55. Kleijer WJ, Van Diggelen OP, Keulemans JLM et al. First-trimester diagnosis of late-infantile neuronal ceroid lipofuscinosis (LINCL) by tripeptidyl peptidase I assay and CLN2 mutation analysis. *Prenat Diagn* **21**:99–101, 2001.
56. Munroe PB, Rapola J, Mitchison HM et al. Prenatal diagnosis of Batten's disease. *Lancet* **347**:1014–1015, 1996.
57. Young EP. Prenatal diagnosis of Hurler disease by analysis of α-iduronidase in chorionic villi. *J Inher Metab Dis* **15**:224–230, 1992.
58. Kleijer WJ, Van Diggelen OP, Janse HC, Galjaard H, Dumez Y, Boue J. First trimester diagnosis of Hunter syndrome on chorionic villi. *Lancet* **ii**:472, 1984.
59. Kleijer WJ, Karpova EA, Geilen GC et al. Prenatal diagnosis of Sanfilippo A syndrome: experience in 35 pregnancies at risk and the use of a new fluorogenic substrate for the heparin sulphamidase assay. *Prenat Diagn* **16**:829–835, 1996.
60. Minelli A, Danesino C, Lo Curto F et al. First trimester prenatal diagnosis of Sanfilippo disease (MPSIII) type B. *Prenat Diagn* **8**:47–52, 1988.
61. Di Natale P, Pannone N, D'Argenio G, Gatti R, Ricci R, Lombardo C. First-trimester prenatal diagnosis of Sanfilippo C disease. *Prenat Diagn* **7**:603–605, 1987.
62. Wang He, Voznyi YaV, Boer AM, Kleijer WJ, Van Diggelen OP. A fluorimetric enzyme assay for the diagnosis of Sanfilippo disease type D (MPS IIID). *J Inher Metab Dis* **16**:935–941, 1993.
63. Kleijer WJ, Geilen GC, Garritsen V et al. First-trimester diagnosis of Morquio disease type A. *Prenat Diagn* **20**:183–185, 2000.
64. Kleijer WJ, Wolffers GM, Hoogeveen A, Niermeijer MF. Prenatal diagnosis of Maroteaux–Lamy syndrome. *Lancet* **ii**:50, 1976.
65. Van Eyndhoven HWF, Ter Brugge HG, Van Essen A, Kleijer WJ. β-Glucuronidase deficiency as cause of recurrent hydrops fetalis: the first early prenatal diagnosis by chorionic villus sampling. *Prenat Diagn* **18**:959–962, 1998.
66. Patrick AD, Young E, Ellis C, Rodeck CH. Multiple sulphatase deficiency: prenatal diagnosis using chorionic villi. *Prenat Diagn* **8**:303–306, 1988.
67. Aula N, Aula P. Prenatal diagnosis of free sialic acid storage disorders (SASD). *Prenat Diagn* **26**:655–658, 2006.
68. Voznyi YaV, Keulemans JLM, Kleijer WJ, Aula P, Gray GR, Van Diggelen OP. Applications of a new fluorimetric enzyme assay for the diagnosis of aspartylglucosaminuria. *J Inher Metab Dis* **16**:929–934, 1993.
69. Poenaru L, Girard S, Thepot F et al. Antenatal diagnosis in three pregnancies at risk for mannosidosis. *Clin Genet* **16**:428–432, 1979.
70. Mole SE, Williams RE, Goebel HH. Correlations between genotype, ultrastructural morphology and clinical phenotype in the neuronal ceroid lipofuscinosis. *Neurogenet* **6**:107–126, 2005.
71. Rapola J, Lähdetie J, Isosomppi J, Helminen P, Penttinen M, Järvelä. Prenatal diagnosis of variant late-infantile neuronal ceroid lipofuscinosis (vLINCL$_{FINNISH}$; CLN5). *Prenat Diagn* **19**:685–688.
72. Mossman J, Patrick AD. Prenatal diagnosis of mucopolysaccharidosis by two-dimensional electrophoresis of amniotic fluid glycosaminoglycans. *Prenat Diagn* **2**:169–176, 1982.
73. Keulemans JLM, Sinigerska I, Garritsen VH et al. Prenatal diagnosis of the Hunter syndrome and the introduction of a new fluorimetric enzyme assay. *Prenat Diagn* **22**:1016–1021, 2002.
74. Kleijer WJ, Huijmans JGM, Blom W et al. Prenatal diagnosis of Sanfilippo disease type B. *Hum Genet* **66**:287–288, 1984.
75. Wang He, Voznyi YaV, Huijmans JGM et al. Prenatal diagnosis of Sanfilippo disease type C using a simple fluorometric enzyme assay. *Prenat Diagn* **14**:17–22, 1994.
76. Zhao H, Van Diggelen OP, Thoomes R et al. Prenatal diagnosis of Morquio disease type A using a simple fluorometric enzyme assay. *Prenat Diagn* **10**:85–91, 1990.
77. Kagie MJ, Kleijer WJ, Huijmans JGM, Maaswinkel-Mooy P, Kanhai HHH. β-Glucuronidase deficiency as a cause of

fetal hydrops. *Am J Med Genet* **42**:693–695, 1992.

78. Fensom AH, Benson PF. Recent advances in the prenatal diagnosis of the mucopolysaccharidoses. *Prenat Diagn* **14**:1–12, 1994.
79. Aronovicz EL, Pan D, Whitley CB. Molecular genetic defect underlying α-L-iduronidase pseudodeficiency. *Am J Hum Genet* **58**:75–85, 1996.
80. Kleijer WJ, Thompson EJ, Niermeijer MF. Prenatal diagnosis of the Hurler syndrome: report on 40 pregnancies at risk. *Prenat Diagn* **3**:179–186, 1983.
81. Kleijer WJ, Mooy PD, Liebaers I, Van Der Kamp JJP, Niermeijer MF. Prenatal monitoring for the Hunter syndrome: the heterozygous female fetus. *Clin Genet* **15**:113–117, 1979.
82. Cooper A, Thornley M, Wraith JE. First-trimester diagnosis of Hunter syndrome: very low iduronate sulphatase activity in chorionic villi from a heterozygous female fetus. *Prenat Diagn* **11**:731–735, 1991.
83. Sukegawa K, Song X-Q, Masuno M et al. Hunter disease in a girl caused by R468Q mutation in the iduronate-2-sulfatase gene and skewed inactivation of the X-chromosome carrying the normal allele. *Hum Mutat* **10**:361–367, 1997.
84. Hopwood JJ, Bunge S, Morris CP et al. Molecular basis of mucopolysaccharidosis type II: mutations in the iduronate-2-sulphatase gene. *Hum Mutat* **2**:435–442, 1993.
85. Mossman J, Young EP, Patrick AD et al. Prenatal tests for Sanfilippo disease type B in four pregnancies. *Prenat Diagn* **3**:347–350, 1983.
86. Den Hollander NS, Kleijer WJ, Schoonderwaldt EM, Los FJ, Wladimiroff JW, Niermeijer MF. *In utero* diagnosis of mucopolysaccharidosis type VII in a fetus with an enlarged nuchal translucency. *Ultrasound Obstet Gynecol* **1:6**:87–90, 2000.
87. Vervoort R, Gitzelman R, Bosshard N, Maire I, Liebaers I, Lissens W. Low β-glucuronidase enzyme activity and mutations in the human β-glucuronidase gene in mild mucopolysaccharidosis type VII, pseudodeficiency and a heterozygote. *Hum Genet* **102**:69–78, 1998.
88. Machin AG. Hydrops revisited: literature review of 1,414 cases published in the 1980s. *Am J Med Genet* **34**:366–390, 1989.
89. Jauniaux E, Van Maldergem L, De Munter C, Moscoso G, Gillerot Y. Nonimmune hydrops fetalis associated with genetic abnormalities. *Obstet Gynecol* **75**:568–572, 1990.
90. Kattner E, Schäfer A, Harzer K. Hydrops fetalis: manifestation in lysosomal storage diseases including Farber disease. *Eur J Pediatr* **156**:292–295, 1997.
91. Kooper AJA, Janssens PMW, De Groot ANJA et al. Lysosomal storage disease in non-immune hydrops fetalis pregnancies. *Clin Chim Acta* **371**:179–182, 2006.
92. Tayebi N, Cushner SR, Kleijer WJ et al. Prenatal lethality of a homozygous null mutation in the human glucocerebrosidase gene. *Am J Med Genet* **73**:41–47, 1997.
93. Burin MG, Scholz AP, Gus R. Investigation of lysosomal storage diseases in nonimmune hydrops fetalis. *Prenat Diagn* **24**:653–657, 2004.
94. Piraud M, Froissart R, Mandon G, Bernard A, Maire I. Amniotic fluid for screening of lysosomal storage diseases presenting in utero (mainly as non-immune hydrops fetalis). *Clin Chim Acta* **248**:143–155, 1996.
95. Froissart R, Cheillan D, Bouvier R, Tourret S, Piraud M, Maire I. Clinical, morphological, and molecular aspects of sialic acid storage disease manifesting in utero. *J Med Genet* **42**:829–836, 2005.
96. Lemyre E, Russo P, Melancon SB, Gagné R, Potier M, Lambert M. Clinical spectrum of infantile free sialic acid storage disease. *Am J Med Genet* **82**:385–391, 1999.
97. Colmant C, Picone O, Froissart R, Labrune P, Senat M-V. Second-trimester diagnosis of mucopolysaccharidosis type IV A presenting as hydrops fetalis. *Prenat Diagn* **26**:750–752, 2006.
98. Ferreira P, Morais L, Costa R et al. Hydrops fetalis associated with erythrocyte pyruvate kinase deficiency. *Eur J Pediatr* **159**:481–482, 2000.
99. L'Herminé-Coulomb A, Beuzen F, Bouvier R et al. Fetal type IV glycogen storage disease: clinical, enzymatic, and genetic data of a pure muscular form with variable and early antenatal manifestations in the same family. *Am J Med Genet* **139A**:118–122, 2005.
100. Tercanli S, Uyanik G, Hösli I, Cagdas A, Holzgreve W. Increased nuchal translucency in a case of long-chain 3-hydroxyacyl-coenzyme A dehydrogenase deficiency. *Fetal Diagn Ther* **15**:322–325, 2000.
101. Christiaens GCML, De Pater JM, Stoutenbeek P, Dogtrop A, Wanders RJA, Beemer FA. First-trimester nuchal anomalies as a prenatal sign of Zellweger synsrome. *Prenat Diagn* **20**:520–521, 2000.
102. Maymon R, Ogle RF, Chitty LS. Smith-Lemli-Opitz syndrome presenting with persisting nuchal oedema and non-immune hydrops. *Prenat Diagn* **19**: 105–107, 1999.
103. De Koning TJ, Toet M, Dorland L et al. Recurrent nonimmune hydrops fetalis associated with carbohydrate-deficient glycoprotein syndrome. *J Inher Metab Dis* **21**:681–682, 1998.
104. Daikha-Dahmane F, Dommergues M, Narcy F et al. Congenital erythropoietic porphyria: prenatal diagnosis and autopsy findings in two sibling fetuses. *Pediatr Dev Pathol* **4**:180–184, 2001.
105. Kassem E, Dolfin T, Litmanowitz I, Regev R, Arnon S, Kidron D. Familial perinatal hemochromatosis: a disease that causes recurrent non-immune hydrops. *J Perinat Med* **27**:122–127, 1999.
106. De Biasio P, Prefumo F, Casagrande V, Stroppiano M, Venturini PL, Filocamo M. First-trimester fetal nuchal translucency and inherited metabolic disorders. *Prenat Diagn* **26**:77–80, 2006.
107. Schutgens RBH, Schrakamp G, Wanders RJA, Heymans HSA, Tager JM, Van Den Bosch H. Prenatal and perinatal diagnosis of peroxisomal disorders. *J Inher Metab Dis* **12**(suppl 1):118–134, 1989.
108. Brookhyser KM, Lipson MH, Moser AB, Moser HW, Lachman RS, Rimoin DL. Prenatal diagnosis of rhizomelic chondrodysplasia punctata due to isolated alkyldihydroacetonephosphate acyltransferase synthase deficiency. *Prenat Diagn* **19**:383–385, 1999.
109. Wanders RJA, Mooyer PW, Dekker C, Vreken P. X-linked adrenoleukodystrophy: improved prenatal diagnosis using both biochemical and immunological methods. *J Inher Metab Dis* **21**:285–287, 1998.
110. Wanders RJA, Schelen A, Feller N et al. First prenatal diagnosis of acyl-CoA oxidase deficiency. *J Inher Metab Dis* **13**:371–374, 1990.
111. Paton BC, Solly PB, Nelson PV, Pollard AN, Sharp PC, Fietz MJ. Molecular analysis of genomic DNA allows rapid, and accurate, prenatal diagnosis of peroxisomal D-bifunctional protein deficiency. *Prenat Diagn* **22**:38–41, 2002.
112. Danpure CJ, Rumsby G. Strategies for the prenatal diagnosis of primary hyperoxaluria type 1. *Prenat Diagn* **16**:587–598, 1996.
113. Wanders RJA, Waterham HR. Peroxisomal disorderes I: biochemistry and genetics of peroxisome biogenesis disorders. *Clin Genet* **67**:107–133, 2004.
114. Steinberg SJ, Dodt G, Raymond GV, Braverman NE, Moser AB, Moser HW. Peroxisome biogenesis disorders. *Biochim Biophys Acta* **1763**:1733–1748, 2006.
115. Wanders RJA, Waterham HR. Peroxisomal disorders: the single peroxisomal enzyme deficiencies. *Biochim Biophys Acta* **1763**:1707–1720, 2006.
116. Wanders RJA, Schutgens RBH, Van Den Bosch H, Tager JM, Kleijer WJ. Prenatal diagnosis of inborn errors in peroxisomal β-oxidation. *Prenat Diagn* **11**:253–261, 1991.
117. Stellaard F, Kleijer WJ, Wanders RJA, Schutgens RBH, Jakobs C. Bile acids in

amniotic fluid: promising metabolites for the prenatal diagnosis of peroxisomal disorders. *J Inher Metab Dis* **14**:353–356, 1991.

118. Sastrowijoto SH, Vandenberghe K, Moerman , Lauweryns JM, Fryns JP. Prenatal ultrasound diagnosis of rhizomelic chondrodysplasia punctata in a primigravida. *Prenat Diagn* **14**:770–776, 1994.
119. Moser AB, Moser HG. The prenatal diagnosis of X-linked adrenoleukodystrophy. *Prenat Diagn* **19**:46–48, 1999.
120. Imamura A, Suzuki Y, Song X-Q et al. Prenatal diagnosis of adrenoleukodystrophy by means of mutation analysis. *Prenat Diagn* **16**:259–261, 1996.
121. Jakobs C, Kleijer WJ, Allen J, Holton JB. Prenatal diagnosis of galactosemia. *Eur J Pediatr* **154**(suppl 2):S33–S36, 1995.
122. Golbus MS, Simpson TJ, Koresawa M, Appelman ZVI, Alpers CE. The prenatal determination of glucose-6-phosphatase activity by fetal liver biopsy. *Prenat Diagn* **8**:401–404, 1988.
123. Lam C-W, Sin S-Y, Lau ET, Lam Y-Y, Poon P, Tong S-F. Prenatal diagnosis of glycogen storage disease type Ib using denaturing high performance liquid chromatography. *Prenat Diagn* **20**:765–768, 2000.
124. Kleijer WJ, Van Der Kraan M, Kroos MA et al. Prenatal diagnosis of glycogen storage disease type II: enzyme assay or mutation analysis? *Pediatr Res* **38**:103–106, 1995.
125. Shin YS, Rieth M, Tausenfreund J, Endres W. First trimester diagnosis of glycogen storage disease type II and type III. *J Inher Metab Di* **12**(suppl 2):289–291, 1989.
126. Brown BI, Brown DH. Branching enzyme activity of cultured amniocytes and chorionic villi: prenatal testing for type IV glycogen storage disease. *Am J Hum Genet* **44**:378–381, 1989.
127. Ruitenbeek W, Sengers RCA, Trijbels JMF, Janssen AJM, Bakkeren JAJM. The use of chorionic villi in prenatal diagnosis of mitochondriopathies. *J Inher Metab Di* **15**:303–306, 1992.
128. Van Coster RN, Janssens S, Misson J-P, Verloes A, Leroy JG. Prenatal diagnosis of pyruvate carboxylase deficiency by direct measurement of catalytic activity on chorionic villi samples. *Prenat Diagn* **18**:1041–1044, 1998.
129. Brown RM, Brown GK. Prenatal diagnosis of pyruvate dehydrogenase E1*a* subunit deficiency. *Prenat Diagn* **14**:435–442, 1994.
130. Rouillac C, Aral B, Fouque F et al. First prenatal diagnosis of defects in the *HsPDX1* gene encoding Protein X, an additional lipoyl-containing subunit of the human pyruvate dehydrogenase complex. *Prenat Diagn* **19**:1160–1164, 1999.
131. Børresen AL, Hellerud C, Møller P, Søvik O, Berg K. Prenatal diagnosis of glycerol-kinase deficiency associated with a DNA deletion on the short arm of the X-chromosome. *Clin Genet* **32**:254–259, 1987.
132. Rouger H, Girodon E, Goossens M, Galacteros F, Cohen-Solal M, Mondor PK. Prenatal diagnosis of a frameshift mutation in the LR pyruvate kinase gene associated with severe hereditary non-spherocytic haemolytic anaemia. *Prenat Diagn* **16**:97–104, 1996.
133. Whitelaw AGL, Rogers PA, Hopkinson DA et al. Congenital haemolytic anaemia resulting from glucose phosphate isomerase deficiency: genetics, clinical picture, and prenatal diagnosis. *J Med Genet* **16**:189–196, 1979.
134. Charlwood J, Clayton P, Keir G, Mian N, Young E, Winchester B. Prenatal diagnosis of the carbohydrate-deficient glycoprotein syndrome type 1A (CDG 1A) by a combination of enzytmology and genetic linkage analysis after amniocentesis or chorionic villus sampling. *Prenat Diagn* **18**:693–699, 1998.
135. Waggoner DD, Buist NRM, Donnell GN. Long-term prognosis in galactosaemia: results of a survey of 350 cases. *J Inher Metab Dis* **13**:802–818, 1990.
136. Jakobs C, Kleijer WJ, Bakker HD, Gennip AH, Przyrembel H, Niermeijer MF. Dietary restriction of maternal lactose intake does not prevent accumulation of galactitol in the amniotic fluid of fetuses affected with galactosaemia. *Prenat Diagn* **8**:641–645, 1988.
137. Tyfield L, Reichardt J, Fridovich-Keil J et al. Classical galactosemia and mutations at the galactose-1-phosphate uridyl transferase (*GALT*) gene. *Hum Mutat* **13**:417–430, 1999.
138. Chen Y-T, Bali D, Sullivan J. Prenatal diagnosis in glycogen storage diseases. *Prenat Diagn* **22**:357–359.
139. Wong L-JC. Prenatal diagnosis of glycogen storage disease type 1a by direct mutation detection. *Prenat Diagn* **16**:105–108, 1996.
140. Maire I, Mandon G, Mathieu M. First trimester prenatal diagnosis of glycogen storage disease type III. *J Inher Metab Dis* **12**(suppl 2):292–294, 1989.
141. Akman HO, Karadimas C, Gyftodimou Y et al. Prenatal diagnosis of glycogen storage disease type IV. *Prenat Diagn* **26**:951–955.
142. Faivre L, Cormier-Daire V, Chrétien D et al. Determination of enzyme activities for prenatal diagnosis of respiratory chain deficiency. *Prenat Diagn* **20**: 732–737, 2000.
143. Thorburn DR, Dahl H-HM. Mitochondrial disorders: genetics, counseling, prenatal diagnosis and reproductive options. *Am J Med Genet* **106**:102–114, 2001.
144. Marsac C, Augereau CH, Feldman G, Wolf B, Hansen TL, Berger R. Prenatal diagnosis of pyruvate carboxylase deficiency. *Clin Chim Acta* **119**:121–127, 1982.
145. Lissens W, De Meirleir L, Seneca S et al. Mutations in the X-linked pyruvate dehydrogenase (E1) α subunit gene (*PDHA1*) in patients with a pyruvare dehydrogenase complex deficiency. *Hum Mutat* **15**:209–219, 2000.
146. Pissard S, Max-Audit I, Skopinski L et al. Pyruvate kinase deficiency in France: a 3-year study reveals 27 new mutations. *Br J Haematol* **133**:683–689, 2006.
147. Dallapiccola B, Novelli G, Ferranti G, Pachi A, Cristiani ML, Magnani M. First trimester monitoring of a pregnancy at risk for glucose phosphate isomerase deficiency. *Prenat Diag* **6**:101–107, 1986.
148. Matthijs G, Schollen E, Van Schaftingen E. The prenatal diagnosis of congenital disorders of glycosylation (CDG). *Prenat Diagn* **24**:114–116, 2004.
149. Gibbs DA, McFadyen IR, Crawford MD. First-trimester diagnosis of Lesch–Nyhan syndrome. *Lancet* **2**:1180–1183, 1984.
150. Dooley T, Fairbanks LD, Simmonds HA. First trimester diagnosis of adenosine deaminase deficiency. *Prenat Diagn* **7**:561–565, 1987.
151. Pérignon JL, Durandy A, Peter MO, Freycon F, Dumez Y, Griscelli C. Early prenatal diagnosis of inherited severe immunodeficiencies linked to enzyme deficiencies. *J Pediatr* **111**:595–598, 1987.
152. Marie S, Flipsen JWAM, Duran M et al. Prenatal diagnosis in adenylosuccinate lyase deficiency. *Prenat Diagn* **20**:33–36, 2000.
153. Jakobs C, Stellaard F, Smit LME et al. The first prenatal diagnosis of dihydropyrimidine dehydrogenase deficiency. *Eur J Pediatr* **150**:291, 1991.
154. Gray RG, Green A, Basu SN et al. Antenatal diagnosis of molybdenum cofactor deficiency. *Am J Obstet Gynecol* **163**:1203–1204, 1990.
155. Halley DJ, Keijzer W, Jaspers NG et al. Prenatal diagnosis of xeroderma pigmentosum (group C) using assays of unscheduled DNA synthesis and postreplication repair. *Clin Genet* **16**:137–146, 1979.
156. Sarasin A, Blanchet-Bardon C, Renault G, Lehmann A, Arlett C, Dumez Y. Prenatal diagnosis in a subset of trichothiodystrophy patients defective in DNA repair. *Br J Dermatol* **127**:485–491, 1992.
157. Lehmann AR, Francis AJ, Gianelli F. Prenatal diagnosis of Cockayne's syndrome. *Lancet* **i**:486–487, 1985.

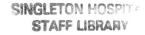

158. Kleijer WJ, Van Der Kraan M, Los FJ, Jaspers NGJ. Prenatal diagnosis of ataxia-telangiectasia and Nijmegen breakage syndrome by the assay of radioresistant DNA synthesis. *Int J Radiat Biol* **66**:S167–S174, 1994.
159. Kleijer WJ, Van den Berg P, Los FJ. Prenatal Diagnosis of Lesch-Nyhan syndrome. *Prenat Diagn* **24**:658–659, 2004.
160. Jinnah HA, De Gregorio L, Harris JC, Nyhan WL, O'Neill JP. The spectrum of inherited mutations causing HPRT deficiency: 75 new cases and a review of 196 previously reported cases. *Mutat Res* **463**:309–326, 2000.
161. Hirschhorn R, Beratis N, Rosen FS, Parkman R, Stern R, Polmar S. Adenosine deaminase deficiency in a child diagnosed prenatally. *Lancet* **1**:73, 1975.
162. Kleijer WJ, Hussaarts-Odijk LM, Los FJ, Pijpers L, de Bree PK, Duran M. Prenatal diagnosis of purine nucleoside phosphorylase deficiency in the first and second trimesters of pregnancy. *Prenat Diagn* **9**:401–407, 1989.
163. Johnson JL. Prenatal diagnosis of molybdenum cofactor deficiency and isolated sulfite oxidase deficiency. *Prenat Diagn* **23**:6–8, 2003.
164. Ogier H, Wadman SK, Johnson JL et al. Antenatal diagnosis of combined xanthine and sulphite-oxidase deficiency. *Lancet* **2**:1363–1364, 1983.
165. Cleaver JE, Volpe JPG, Charles WC, Thomas GH. Prenatal diagnosis of xeroderma pigmentosum and Cockayne syndrome. *Prenat Diagn* **14**:921–928, 1994.
166. Kleijer WJ, Van der Sterre MLT, Garritsen VH, Raams A, Jaspers NGJ. Prenatal diagnosis of the Cockayne syndrome: survey of 15 years experience. *Prenat Diagn* **26**:980–984.
167. Chessa L, Piane M, Prudente S et al. Molecular prenatal diagnosis of ataxia telangiectasia heterozygosity by direct mutational assays. *Prenat Diagn* **19**:542–545, 1999.
168. Muschke P, Gola H, Varon R et al. Retrospective diagnosis and subsequent prenatal diagnosis of Nijmegen breakage syndrome. *Prenat Diagn* **24**:111–113, 2004.
169. Lidsky AS, Guttler F, Woo SLC. Prenatal diagnosis of classical phenylketonuria by DNA analysis. *Lancet* **1**:549–551, 1985.
170. Blau N, Niederwieser A, Curtius HC. Prenatal diagnosis of atypical phenyketonuria. *J Inher Metab Dis* **12**(suppl 2):295–298, 1989.
171. Bennett MJ, Gibson KM, Sherwood WG et al. Reliable prenatal diagnosis of Canavan disease (aspartoacylase deficiency): comparison of enzymatic and metabolite analysis. *J Inher Metab Dis* **16**:831–836, 1993.
172. Jakobs C, Stellaard F, Kvittingen EA, Henderson M, Lilford R. First-trimester prenatal diagnosis of tyrosinemia type I by amniotic fluid succinylacetone determination. *Prenat Diagn* **10**:133–139, 1990.
173. Hayasaka K, Tada K, Fueki N, Aikawa J. Prenatal diagnosis of nonketotic hyperglycinemia: enzymatic analysis of the glycine cleavage system in chorionic villi. *J Pediatr* **116**:444–445, 1990.
174. Patrick AD, Young EP, Mossman J, Warren R, Kearney L, Rodeck CH. First trimester diagnosis of cystinosis using intact chorionic villi. *Prenat Diagn* **7**:71–74, 1987.
175. Kleijer WJ, Horsman D, Mancini GMS, Fois A, Boue J. First-trimester diagnosis of maple syrup urine disease on intact chorionic villi. *N Engl J Med* **313**:1608, 1985.
176. Kleijer WJ, van der Kraan M, Huijmans JGM, van den Heuvel CMM, Jakobs C. Prenatal diagnosis of isovaleric acidaemia by enzyme and metabolite assay in the first and second trimesters. *Prenat Diagn* **15**:527–533, 1995.
177. Chitayat D, Chemke J, Gibson KM et al. 3-Methylglutaconic aciduria: a marker for as yet unspecified disorders and the relevance of prenatal diagnosis in a 'new' type ('type 4'). *J Inher Metab Dis* **15**:204–212, 1992.
178. Chalmers RA, Tracey BM, Mistry J, Stacey TE, McFadyen IR. Prenatal diagnosis of 3-hydroxy-3-methylglutaric aciduria by GC-MS and enzymology on cultured amniocytes and chorionic villi. *J Inher Metab Dis* **12**:286–292, 1989.
179. Packman S, Cowan MJ, Golbus MS et al. Prenatal treatment of biotin-responsive multiple carboxylase deficiency. *Lancet* **i**:1435–1439, 1982.
180. Chalmers RA, Mistry J, Docherty PW, Stratton D. First trimester prenatal exclusion of biotinidase deficiency. *J Inher Metab Dis* **17**:751–752, 1994.
181. Kleijer WJ, Thoomes R, Galjaard H, Wendel U, Fowler B. First-trimester (chorion biopsy) diagnosis of citrullinaemia and methylmalonicaciduria. *Lancet* ii:1340, 1984.
182. Vimal CM, Fensom AH, Heaton D, Ward RHT, Garrod P, Penketh RJA. Prenatal diagnosis of argininosuccinicaciduria by analysis of cultured chorionic villi. *Lancet* ii:521–522, 1984.
183. Piceni Sereni L, Bachmann C, Pfister U, Buscaglia M, Nicolini U. Prenatal diagnosis of carbamoylphosphate synthetase deficiency by fetal liver biopsy. *Prenat Diagn* **8**:307–309, 1988.
184. Rodeck CH, Patrick AD, Pembrey ME, Tzannatos C, Whitfield AE. Fetal liver biopsy for prenatal diagnosis of ornithine carbamyl transferase deficiency. *Lancet* ii:297–300, 1982.
185. Shih VE, Laframboise R, Mandell R, Pichette J. Neonatal form of the hyperornithinaemia, hyperammonaemia, and homocitrullinuria (HHH) syndrome and prenatal diagnosis. *Prenat Diagn* **12**:717–723, 1992.
186. Rolland MO, Divry P, Mandon G et al. Early prenatal diagnosis of propionic acidaemia with simultaneous sampling of chorionic villus and amniotic fluid. *J Inher Metab Dis* **13**:345–348, 1990.
187. Fowler B, Giles L, Sardharwalla IB, Donnai P, Clayton JK. First trimester diagnosis of methylmalonic aciduria. *Prenat Diagn* **8**:207–213, 1988.
188. Christensen E. Prenatal diagnosis of glutaryl-CoA dehydrogenase deficiency: experience using first trimester chorionic villus sampling. *Prenat Diagn* **14**:333–336, 1994.
189. Yamaguchi S, Shimizu N, Orii et al. Prenatal diagnosis and neonatal monitoring of a fetus with glutaric aciduria type II due to electron transfer flavoprotein (β-subunit) deficiency. *Pediatr Res* **30**:439–443, 1991.
190. Bennett MJ, Allison F, Pollitt RJ et al. Prenatal diagnosis of medium-chain acyl-CoA dehydrogenase deficiency in family with sudden infant death. *Lancet* i:440–441, 1987.
191. Nada MA, Vianey-Saban C, Roe CR et al. Prenatal diagnosis of mitochondrial fatty acid oxidation defects. *Prenat Diagn* **16**:117–124, 1996.
192. Von Döbeln U, Venizelos N, Westgren M, Hagenfeldt L. Long-chain 3-hydroxyacyl-CoA dehydrogenase in chorionic villi, fetal liver and fibroblasts and prenatal diagnosis of 3-hydroxyacyl-CoA dehydrogenease deficiency. *J Inher Metab Dis* **17**:185–188, 1994.
193. Scriver CR, Clow CL. Avoiding phenylketonuria: why parents seek prenatal diagnosis. *J Pediatr* **113**:495–497, 1988.
194. Rapp B, Häberle J, Linnebank M et al. Genetic analysis of carbamoylphosphate synthetase I and ornithine transcarbamylase deficiency using fibroblasts. *Eur J Pediatr* **160**:283–287, 2001.
195. Kamoun P, Fensom AH, Shin YS et al. Prenatal diagnosis of the urea cycle diseases: a survey of the European cases. *Am J Med Genet* **55**:247–250, 1995.
196. Matalon R, Michals-Matalon K. Prenatal diagnosis of Canavan disease. *Prenat Diagn* **19**:669–670, 1999.
197. Gordon N. Canavan disease: a review of recent developments. *Eur J Paediatr Neurol* **5**:65–69, 2000.
198. Grenier A, Cederbaum S, Laberge C, Gagné R, Jakobs C, Tanguay RM. A case of tyrosinaemia type 1 with normal level of succinylacetone in the amniotic fluid. *Prenat Diagn* **16**:239–242, 1996.
199. Ploos van Amstel JK, Jansen RPM, Verjaal M, van den Berg IET, Berger R.

Prenatal diagnosis of type I hereditary tyrosinaemia. *Lancet* **344**:336, 1994.
200. Applegarth DA, Toone JR, Rolland MO, Black SH, Yim DKC, Bemis G. Non-concordance of CVS and liver glycine cleavage enzyme in three families with non-ketotic hyperglycinaemia (NKH) leading to false negative prenatal diagnoses. *Prenat Diagn* **20**:367–370, 2000.
201. Conter C, Rolland MO, Cheillan D, Bonnet V, Maire I, Froissart R. Genetic heterogeneity of the *GLDC* gene in 28 unrelated patients with glycine encephalopathy. *J Inherit Metab Dis* **29**:135–142, 2006.
202. Jackson M, Young E. Prenatal diagnosis of cystinosis by quantitative measurement of cystine in chorionic villi and cultured cells. *Prenat Diagn* **25**:1045–1047, 2005.
203. Mitchell GA, Jakobs C, Gibson KM et al. Molecular prenatal diagnosis of 3-hydroxy-3-methylglutaryl CoA lyase deficiency. *Prenat Diagn* **15**:725–729, 1995.
204. Suormala T, Fowler B, Jakobs C. Late-onset holocarboxylase synthetase-deficiency: pre- and post-natal diagnosis and evaluation of effectiveness of antenatal biotin therapy. *Eur J Pediatr* **157**:570–575, 1998.
205. Northrup H, Beaudet AL, O'Brien WE. Prenatal diagnosis of citrullinaemia: review of a 10-year experience including recent use of DNA analysis. *Prenat Diagn* **10**:771–779, 1990.
206. Kleijer WJ, Garritsen VH, Van der Sterre MLS, Berning C, Häberle J, Huijmans JGM. Prenatal diagnosis of citrullinemia and argininosuccinic aciduria: evidence for a transmission ratio distortion in citrullinemia. *Prenat Diagn* **26**:242–247, 2006.
207. Jakobs C. Prenatal diagnosis of inherited metabolic disorders by stable isotope dilution GC-MS analysis of metabolities in amniotic fluid: review of four years experience. *J Inher Metab Dis* **12**(suppl 2): 267–270, 1989.
208. Goodman SI, Gallegos DA, Pullin CJ et al. Antenatal diagnosis of glutaric acidemia. *Am J Hum Genet* **32**:695–699, 1980.
209. Shigematsu Y, Hata I, Nakai A et al. Prenatal diagnosis of organic acidemias based on amniotic fluid levels of acylcarnitines. *Pediatr Res* **39**:680–684, 1996.
210. Andresen BS, Bross P, Udvari S et al. The molecular basis of medium chain acyl-CoA dehydrogenase (MCAD) deficiency in compound heterozygous patients: is there a correlation between genotype and phenotype? *Hum Mol Genet* **6**:695–707, 1997.
211. Ijlst L, Ruiter JPN, Hoovers JMN, Jakobs ME, Wanders RJA. Common missense mutation G1528C in long-chain 3 hydroxyacyl-CoA dehydrogenase deficiency. *J Clin Invest* **4**:1028–1033, 1996.
212. Andresen BS, Olpin S, Kvittingen EA et al. DNA-based prenatal diagnosis for very-long-chain acyl-CoA dehydrogenase deficiency. *J Inher Metab Dis* **22**:281–285, 1999.
213. Tønnesen T, Gerdes AM, Damsgaard E et al. First-trimester diagnosis of Menkes disease: intermediate copper values in chorionic villi from three affected male fetuses. *Prenat Diagn* **9**:159–165, 1989.
214. Suchy SF, Lin T, Horwitz JA, O'Brien WE, Nussbaum RL. First report of prenatal biochemical diagnosis of Lowe syndrome. *Prenat Diagn* **18**:1117–1121, 1998.
215. Hähnel R, Hähnel E, Wysocki SJ, Wilkinson SP, Hockey A. Prenatal diagnosis of X-linked ichthyosis. *Clin Chim Acta* **120**:143–152, 1982.
216. Huu TP, Dumez Y, Marquetty C, Durandy A, Boue J, Hakim J. Prenatal diagnosis of chronic granulomatous disease (CGD) in four high risk male fetuses. *Prenat Diagn* **7**:253–260, 1987.
217. Raux-Demay M, Mornet E, Boue J et al. Early prenatal diagnosis of 21-hydroxylase deficiency using amniotic fluid 17-hydroxprogesterone determination and DNA probes. *Prenat Diagn* **9**:457–466, 1989.
218. Sassa S, Solish G, Levere RD, Kappas A. Studies in porphyria. IV. Expression of the gene defect of acute intermittent porphyria in cultured human skin fibroblasts and amniotic fluid cells: prenatal diagnosis of the porphyric trait. *J Exp Med* **142**:722–731, 1975.
219. Ged C, Moreau-Gaudry F, Taine L et al. Prenatal diagnosis in congenital erythropoietic porphyria by metabolic measurement and DNA mutation analysis. *Prenat Diagn* **16**:83–86, 1996.
220. Brown MS, Goldstein JL, Vandenberghe K et al. Prenatal diagnosis of homozygous familial hypercholesterolaemia. *Lancet* **i**:526–529, 1978.
221. Maassen JA, Lindhout D, Reuss A, Kleijer WJ. Prenatal analysis of insulin receptor autophosphorylation in a family with leprechaunism. *Prenat Diagn* **10**:13–16, 1990.
222. Brock DJH, Barron L. First-trimester prenatal diagnosis of hypophosphatasia: experience with 16 cases. *Prenat Diagn* **11**:387–391, 1991.
223. Raghunath M, Steinmann B, Delozier-Blanchet C, Extermann P, Superti-Furga A. Prenatal diagnosis of collagen disorders by direct biochemical analysis of chorionic villus biopsies. *Pediatr Res* **36**:441–448, 1994.
224. Mandel H, Abeling N, Gutman A et al. Prolidase deficiency among an Israeli population: prenatal diagnosis in a genetic disorder with uncertain prognosis. *Prenat Diagn* **20**:927–929, 2000.
225. Rolland MO, Cuisset L, Le Bozec J, Guffon N, Vianey-Saban C. First-trimester enzymatic and molecular prenatal diagnosis of mevalonic aciduria. *J Inherit Metab Dis* **28**:1141–1142.
226. Mills K, Mandel H, Montemagno R, Soothill P, Gershoni-Baruch R, Clayton PT. First trimester prenatal diagnosis of Smith–Lemli–Opitz syndrome (7-dehydrocholesterol reductase deficiency). *Pediatr Res* **39**:816–819, 1996.
227. Rizzo WB, Craft DA, Kelson TL. Prenatal diagnosis of Sjögren–Larsson syndrome using enzymatic methods. *Prenat Diagn* **14**:577–581, 1994.
228. Brock DJH, Clark HAK, Barron L. Prenatal diagnosis of cystic fibrosis by microvillar enzyme assay on a sequence of 258 pregnancies. *Hum Genet* **78**:271–275, 1988.
229. Tümer Z, Horn N. Menkes disease: underlying genetic defect and new diagnostic possibilities. *J Inher Meatb Dis* **21**:604–612, 1998.
230. Verheijen FW, Beerens CEMT, Havelaar AC, Kleijer WJ, Mancini GMS. Fibroblast silver loading for the diagnosis of Menkes disease. *J Med Genet* **35**:849–851, 1998.
231. Roos D, De Boer M, Kóker MY et al. Chronic granulomatous disease caused by mutations other than the common GT deletion in NCF1, the gene encoding the $p47^{phox}$ component of the phagocyte NADPH oxidase. *Hum Mutat* **27**:1218–1229, 2006.
232. Hoffmann GF, Sweetmann L, Bremer HJ et al. Facts and artefacts in mevalonic aciduria: development of a stable isotope dilution GCMS assay for mevalonic acid and its application to physiological fluids, tissue samples, prenatal diagnosis and carrier detection. *Clin Chim Acta* **198**:209–228, 1991.
233. Jezela-Stanek A, Malunowicz EM, Ciara E et al. Maternal urinary steroid profiles in prenatal diagnosis of Smith-Lemli-opitz syndrome: first patient series comparing biochemical and molecular studies. *Clin Genet* **69**:77–85, 2006.
234. Wanders RJA, Romeijn GJ, Wijburg F et al. Smith-Lemli-Opitz syndrome: Deficient Δ^7-reductase activity in cultured skin fibroblasts and chorionic villus fibroblasts and its application to pre- and postnatal detection. *J Inher Metab Dis* **20**:432–436, 1997.
235. Nimkarn S, New MI. Prenatal diagnosis and treatment of congenital adrenal hyperplasia. *Horm Res* **67**:53–60, 2007.
236. Vergotine J, Thiart R, Langenhoven E, Hillermann R, De Jong G, Kotze MJ. Prenatal diagnosis of familial hypercholesterolemia: importance of

DNA analysis in the high-risk South African population. *Genet Couns* **12**:121–127, 2001.
237. Desbois-Mouthon C, Girodon E, Ghanem N et al. Molecular analysis of the insulin receptor gene for prenatal diagnosis of leprechaunism in two families. *Prenat Diagn* **17**:657–663, 1997.
238. Mornet E. Hypophosphatasia: the mutations in the tissue-nonspecific alkaline phosphatase gene. *Hum Mutat* **15**:309–315, 2000.
239. Marcus-Soekarman D, Offermans J, Van den Ouweland AMW et al. Hyperechogenic fetal bowel: counseling difficulties. *Eur J Med Genet* **48**:421–425, 2005.
240. Claass AHW, Kleijer WJ, van Diggelen OP, van der Veer E, Sips HJ. Prenatal detection of cystic fibrosis: comparative study of maltase and alkaline phosphatase activities in amniotic fluid. *Prenat Diagn* **6**:419–427, 1986.
241. Bianchi DW, Simpson JL, Jackson LG et al. Fetal gender and aneuploidy detection using fetal cells in maternal blood: analysis of NIFTY I data. *Prenat Diagn* **22**:609–615, 2002.
242. Lo YMD. Recent advances in fetal nucleic acids in maternal plasma. *J Histochem Cytochem* **53**:293–296, 2005.

SECTION 7

Diagnosis and management of fetal malformations

30 Sonography of the fetal central nervous system 379
Gustavo Malinger and Gianluigi Pilu

31 The heart 412
Helena M Gardiner

32 Fetal lung lesions 429
N Scott Adzick

33 Congenital diaphragmatic hernia 437
Alan W Flake and Holly L Hedrick

34 Abdomen 447
Martin J Whittle

35 Kidney and urinary tract disorders 459
Marc Dommergues, Farida Daïkha-Dahmane, Françoise Muller, Marie Cécile Aubry, Stephen Lortat-Jacob, Claire Nihoul-Fékété, Yves Dumez – updated for the 2nd edition by Mark D Kilby

36 Fetal skeletal abnormalities 478
Lyn S Chitty, Louise Wilson and David R Griffin

37 Fetal hydrops 514
Jon Hyett

38 Fetal tumors 528
Mark P Johnson and Stephanie Mann

Sonography of the fetal central nervous system

CHAPTER 30

Gustavo Malinger and Gianluigi Pilu

KEY POINTS

- The basic examination of the fetal CNS by ultrasound using axial planes enables the visualization of the lateral ventricles and cerebellum and is used as a screening method for the detection of fetal malformations
- The detailed neurosonographic examination is indicated in fetuses with suspected brain anomalies or in patients at risk for the development of such anomalies
- Disorders of brain development occurring early in pregnancy are usually diagnosed during the late first or during the second trimester
- Disorders of neuronal proliferation, migration and organization are apparent only late in pregnancy or after delivery

INTRODUCTION

The introduction of ultrasound (US) in the field of prenatal diagnosis has enabled the diagnosis of an increasing number of CNS malformations and anomalies. As it may be expected, the pioneers in prenatal diagnosis described the most severe entities and those that developed early in pregnancy. The diagnosis of dorsal induction defects such as anencephaly and open neural defects[1–3] was followed by the diagnosis of patients with ventral induction defects[4] and proliferation disorders[5,6]. With the introduction of the transvaginal approach and the development of high-resolution transducers, a more detailed evaluation of the fetal brain facilitated the diagnosis of more subtle pathologies[7–10] and of pathologies that developed late in pregnancy such as migration disorders and brain insults[11]. Recently, fetal magnetic resonance imaging (MRI) of the brain has started to play an important role in cases when US is not conclusive or in order to confirm or refine the US diagnosis[12–14].

The prenatal diagnosis of CNS anomalies requires a thorough understanding of fetal brain anatomy[15] and the rapid developmental changes occurring during fetal life[16].

Major events in human brain development include: primary neurulation (3–4 weeks of gestation); prosencephalic development (2–3 months of gestation); neuronal proliferation (3–4 months of gestation); neuronal migration (3–5 months of gestation); organization (starting at around 5 months of gestation and continuing after birth) and myelination (starting around term and continuing after birth)[16]. Events or insults occurring before the 'termination period' may cause similar neurological deficits and those occurring after this period will not affect the developmental events that have ended by the time of the insult[17].

In the presentation and description of prenatal detectable CNS conditions, we will start with the description of the brain anatomy at different gestational ages, followed by a description of the brain malformations according with to their period of occurrence.

FETAL CNS ANATOMY – A DYNAMIC PATTERN

The rapid changes occurring in the fetal brain during pregnancy make the systematic evaluation of the brain anatomy a difficult task. We will present a description of the anatomical features seen at each of the three trimesters.

During the first trimester, the brain vesicles are the main landmarks visualized by ultrasound evaluation (Fig. 30.1). Around 10–11 weeks, the lateral ventricle choroid plexuses may be observed (Fig. 30.1)[18,19]. It is important to emphasize that only a very limited number of CNS malformations are expected to be diagnosed during this period.

The early second trimester offers an excellent window for a more complete study of the fetal brain and spine[20]. The examination may be performed using the transabdominal and/or transvaginal (TVS) approach; usually TVS provides better resolution. With a combination of these two approaches or by the use of 3D multiplanar US, orthogonal planes (axial, sagittal and coronal) are obtained (Figs. 30.2, 30.3). Axial planes are useful for assessment of cranial biometry and the measurement of the lateral ventricles, cerebellar transverse diameter and cisterna magna width. Coronal planes, at this early stage, may provide the first visualization of the anterior portion of the corpus callosum (Fig. 30.4) and help in ruling out cranial

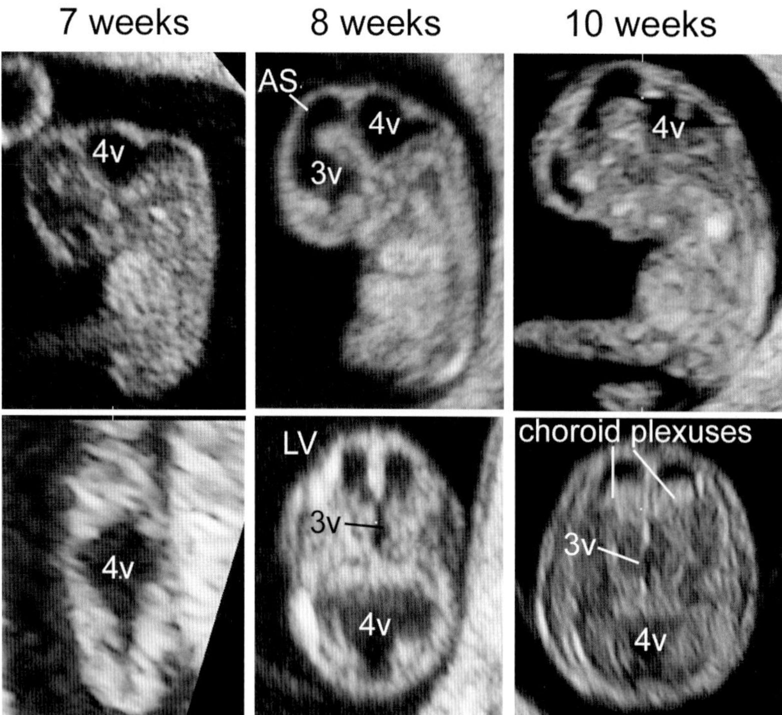

Fig. 30.1 Sonography of the embryonic and early fetal brain as demonstrated by sagittal sections (upper row) and axial sections (lower row). At *7 weeks' gestation* (transvaginal scan), the rhombencephalic vesicle, that will give rise to the fourth ventricle (4v) is usually the only demonstrable structure: at *8 weeks* (transvaginal scan) the remaing two primary vesicles of the brain can be demonstrated: the mesencephalic vesicle that will give rise to the acqueduct of Sylvius (AS), the prosencephalic vesicle that will develop into the third ventricle (3v); the tiny cavities of the lateral ventricles (LV) can also be seen; at *10 weeks*, the choroid plexuses of the lateral ventricles can be seen.

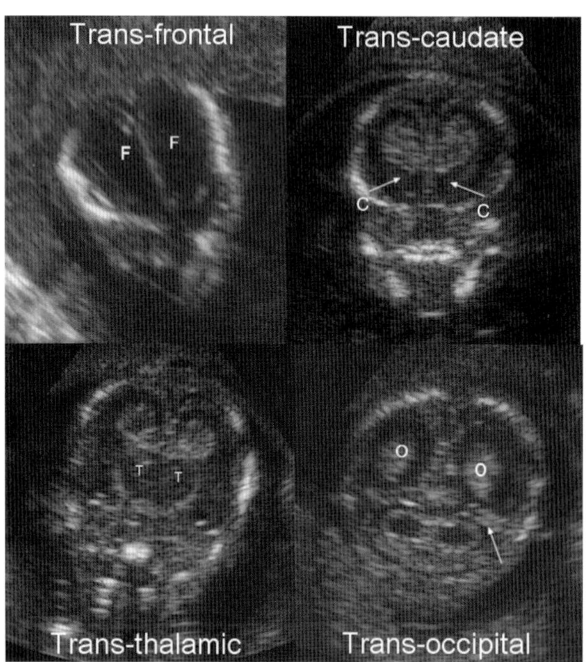

Fig. 30.2 Normal coronal planes at 16 weeks. A complete examination of the brain coronal planes should include at least these four views: transfrontal view shows the relatively large frontal horns of the lateral ventricle (F); transcaudate view shows the choroid plexuses filling completely the lateral ventricles and the caudate nucleus (C); transthalamic view shows the thalami (T); transoccipital view shows the cerebellar hemispheres, the tentorium (arrow) and the occipital horns of the lateral ventricles (O).

defects, such as encephalocele. Sagittal planes depict the lateral ventricles with the choroid plexus; the midline sagittal plane is usually not informative and the diagnosis of midline cerebellar anomalies should be avoided before the last weeks of the second trimester. Orthogonal planes of the spine during the early second-trimester examination enable good quality visualization of the vertebrae.

In the vast majority of countries, the study of the brain anatomy is done between 19 and 22 weeks of pregnancy. At this time, two different examinations may be performed: the basic brain scan or the detailed neurosonographic examination[15].

In the basic brain scan (Fig. 30.5), the visualization of three axial planes is required: the transventricular, transthalamic and transcerebellar planes. The transventricular plane is used for the assessment of the lateral ventricles and cavum septi pellucidi and includes a measurement of the lateral ventricle width at the level of the atrium. The transthalamic plane enables measurement of the biparietal diameter and head circumference, the third ventricle may be also depicted in this plane. The transcerebellar plane enables visualization of the cerebellar hemispheres and vermis, measurements of the cerebellar transverse diameter and the cisterna magna are performed. A normal basic brain examination is a very powerful tool in the diagnosis of fetal brain malformations; Filly et al.[21] showed that 97% of the fetuses with CNS malformations diagnosed during pregnancy have at least an abnormal finding in one of these three planes. On the other hand, we need to remember that a considerable number of brain anomalies may develop late in pregnancy and may be not evident at 19–22 weeks[11].

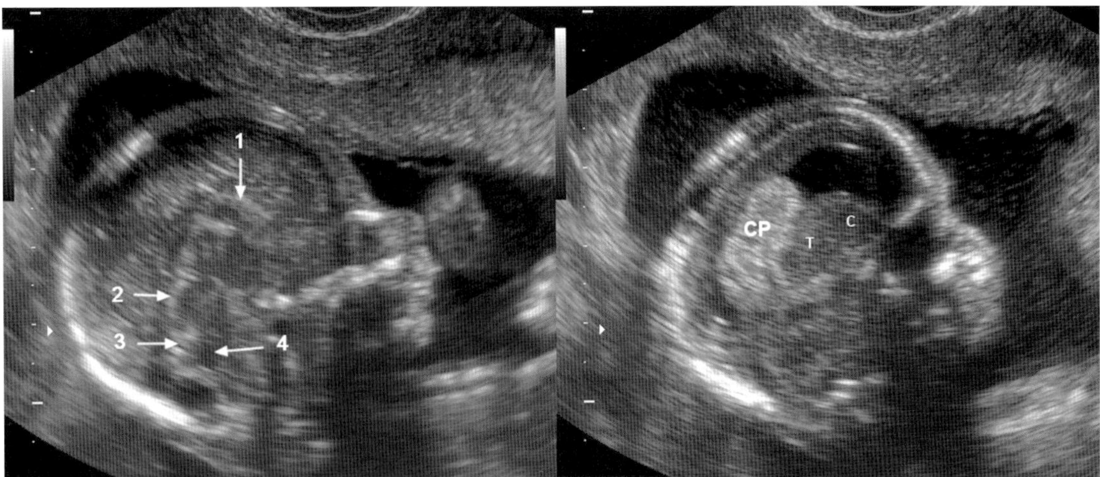

Fig. 30.3 Normal sagittal planes at 16 weeks. A complete examination of the brain sagittal planes should include the visualization of the mid-sagittal plane and at least two parasagittal views (one on each side of the brain). Using high-frequency TVS probes the midsagittal plane enables visualization of the primordium of the corpus callosum (1); the tectum (2); cerebellar vermis (3) and fourth ventricle (4). Parasagittal views enable visualization of the lateral ventricle with the echogenic choroid plexus (CP); thalamus (T) and caudate nucleus (C).

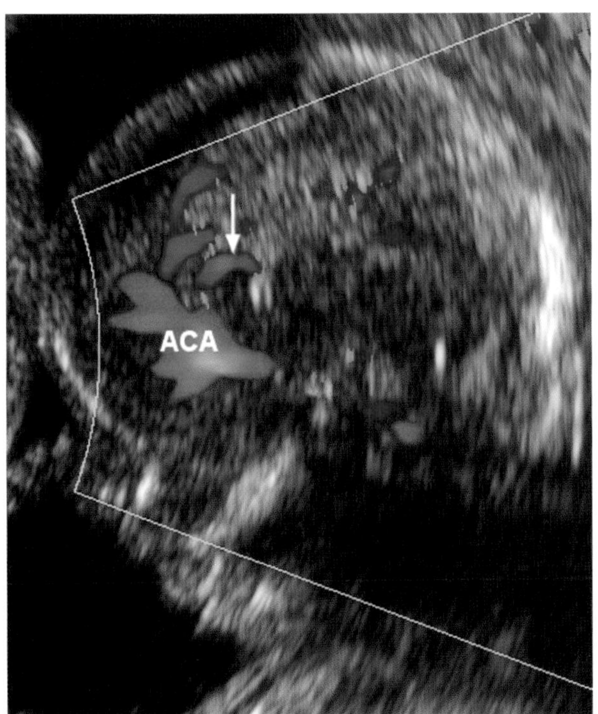

Fig. 30.4 Color Doppler mid-sagittal plane at 16 weeks showing the anterior cerebral artery (ACA) and the pericallosal artery (arrow).

A detailed neurosonographic examination may be indicated following the suspicion of the presence of a CNS anomaly; other indications include non-CNS malformations, suspected intra-uterine infection or a positive family history of CNS malformations. The examination is usually performed by combining the transabdominal and transvaginal approach during the second half of pregnancy and requires more technical expertise than the basic one. When the fetus is in a non-vertex presentation, an attempt at external version or the use of a transfundal approach is recommended. Using the transabdominal approach, we usually visualize axial and coronal planes and by the transvaginal approach, coronal and sagittal ones[15,22].

In addition to the information obtained from the axial planes during the basic examination, during the detailed examination, axial planes provide information on the development of the brain sulcation[23] and cerebellar folia and vermis. Coronal planes are obtained by sweeping the transducer through the anterior fontanelle, the sagittal suture and the posterior fontanelle; in this way parallel planes are obtained. The examination shows a large number of coronal views from the foremost anterior portion of the brain to the cisterna magna and, for didactic purposes, we describe four different coronal planes at the level of the caudate, thalamus, foramen of Monro and occipital lobes (Fig. 30.6).

We use three sagittal planes, one for the midline and one for each hemisphere at the level of the lateral ventricle (Fig. 30.7). Sweeping the transducer more laterally enables visualization of the Sylvian fissure and temporal lobe, but these images may be difficult to obtain late in pregnancy due to a decrease in the sagittal suture width and an increase of calcium in the skull bones. Difficult visualization of the posterior midline structures may be the first clue in the diagnosis of sagittal craniosynostosis.

DISORDERS OF PRIMARY NEURULATION

Neurulation occurs at the dorsal aspect of the embryo during the third and fourth gestational week. Primary neurulation refers to the formation of the brain and most of the spinal cord, while secondary neurulation comprises the development of the lower sacral and coccygeal portions of the spinal cord. The anterior end of the neural tube is definitively closed at 24 days post conception and the posterior end 2 days later. The caudal neural tube develops later and does not complete development until 7weeks of gestation.

Disorders of dorsal induction result in a wide range of congenital malformations with different degrees of severity. A considerable number of these disorders may be diagnosed during fetal life.

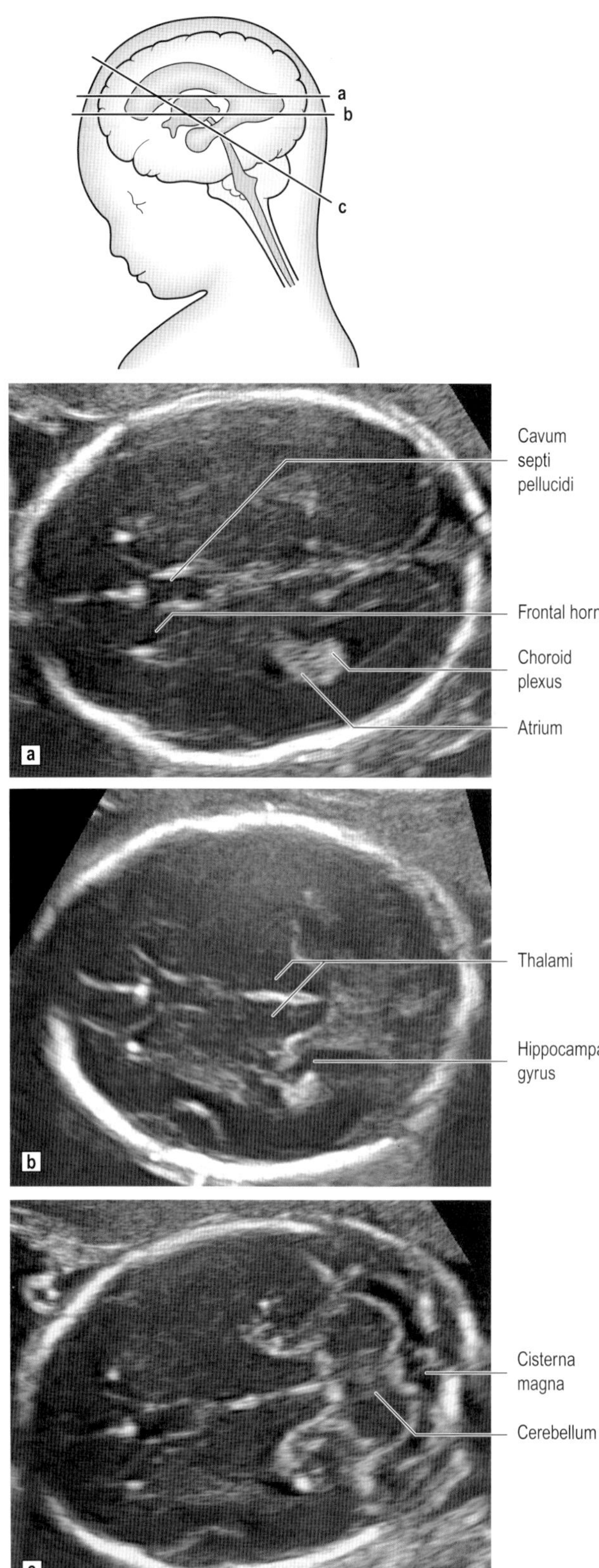

Fig. 30.5 Axial views of the fetal head: (a) transventricular plane; (b) transthalamic plane; (c) transcerebellar plane. Reproduced with permission from: International Society of Ultrasound in Obstetrics & Gynecology Education Committee: Sonographic examination of the fetal central nervous system: guidelines for performing the 'basic examination' and the 'fetal neurosonogram'. Ultrasound Obstet Gynecol. 2007 Jan;**29**(1):109–116.

Craniorachischisis

Craniorachischisis represents the most severe disorder of primary neurulation and is due to complete failure of neural tube formation without development of the skull, vertebrae and skin. Most cases are aborted early in pregnancy and present with associated malformations[24]. The incidence of this disease ranges from 10.7 per 10000 births in Northern China to 0.51 and 0.1 per 10000 births in Texas and Atlanta respectively[25].

Early prenatal diagnosis has been reported[26]. Myeloschisis shows a similar pattern involving only the posterior neural tube and in iniencephaly there is also involvement of the base of the cranium and cervical vertebrae but with normal closure of the anterior portion of the neural tube.

Anencephaly

Anencephaly is due to complete or incomplete failure of closure of the anterior end of the neural tube occurring before the 24th post conceptional day. Failure in the formation of the cranial bones with the presence brain tissue early in pregnancy and even the possible identification of apparently normal or malformed cerebral structures is called acrania or exencephaly. Controversy exists regarding the question of anencephaly and exencephaly being the same malformation or two different entities[27].

Anencephaly is considered a multifactorial disease influenced by a combination of genetic and environmental factors. Different factors have been reported to influence the prevalence of anencephaly, including geographical location, sex, race, maternal age, socioeconomic status, contact with possible teratogens and familial history[28–31]. Recently, three mutations in the VANGL1 gene in patients with familial and sporadic types of the disease have been reported[32].

Prenatal diagnosis relies on fetal ultrasound and, from a large population based study has an overall diagnostic accuracy close to 100%[33]. We need to emphasize that this may not be the case during the first trimester when some cases of anencephaly, particularly those representing exencephaly, may remain undiagnosed[34]. The diagnosis is made based on the absence of the cranium with the presence in some cases of almost normal brain tissue moving freely in the amniotic cavity; characteristically the eyes and ears are prominent (Fig. 30.8).

Since anencephaly is a lethal condition, termination of pregnancy should be offered; but continuation of pregnancy and delivery may be an acceptable alternative for patients who do not consider termination because of religious or ethical issues. In a study published recently, Jaquier et al.[35] showed that continuation of pregnancy and delivery did not increase maternal morbidity; in 20% of the cases there was intrauterine fetal death; 67% of the liveborn died within 24 hours and only 6 newborns survived more than 6 days (maximum 28 days).

Encephalocele

Encephalocele is considered a partial defect in closure of the anterior neuropore but this concept has not been definitively proved and some doubts remain regarding its pathogenesis[36].

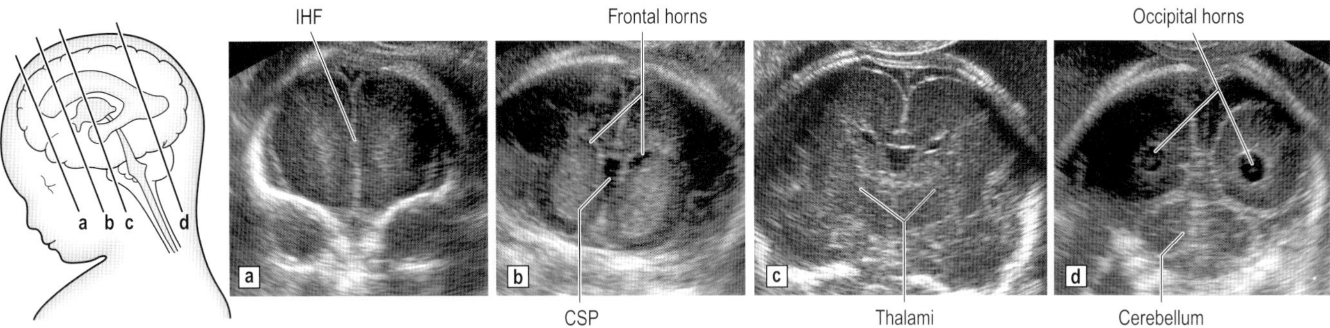

Fig. 30.6 Coronal views of the fetal head: (a) transfrontal plan; (b) transcaudate plane; (c) transthalamic plane; (d) transcerebellar plane (IHF, interhemispheric fissure). Reproduced with permission from: International Society of Ultrasound in Obstetrics & Gynecology Education Committee: Sonographic examination of the fetal central nervous system: guidelines for performing the 'basic examination' and the 'fetal neurosonogram'. Ultrasound Obstet Gynecol. 2007 Jan;**29**(1):109–16.

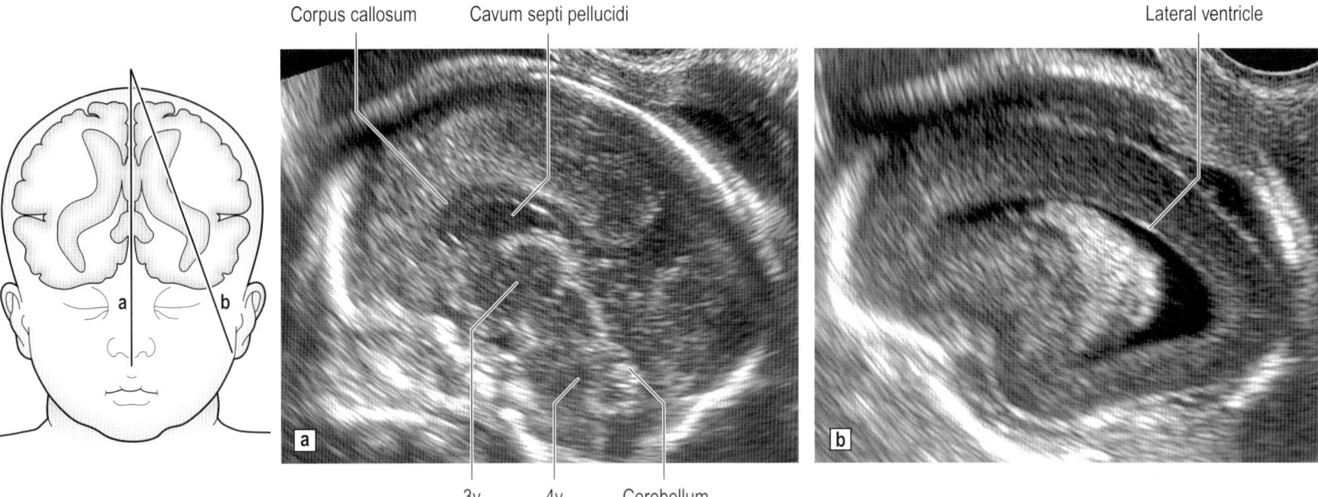

Fig. 30.7 Sagittal planes of the fetal head: (a) midsagittal plane; (b) parasagittal plane. (3v, 4v, third and fourth ventricle). Reproduced with permission from: International Society of Ultrasound in Obstetrics & Gynecology Education Committee: Sonographic examination of the fetal central nervous system: guidelines for performing the 'basic examination' and the 'fetal neurosonogram'. Ultrasound Obstet Gynecol. 2007 Jan;**29**(1):109–16.

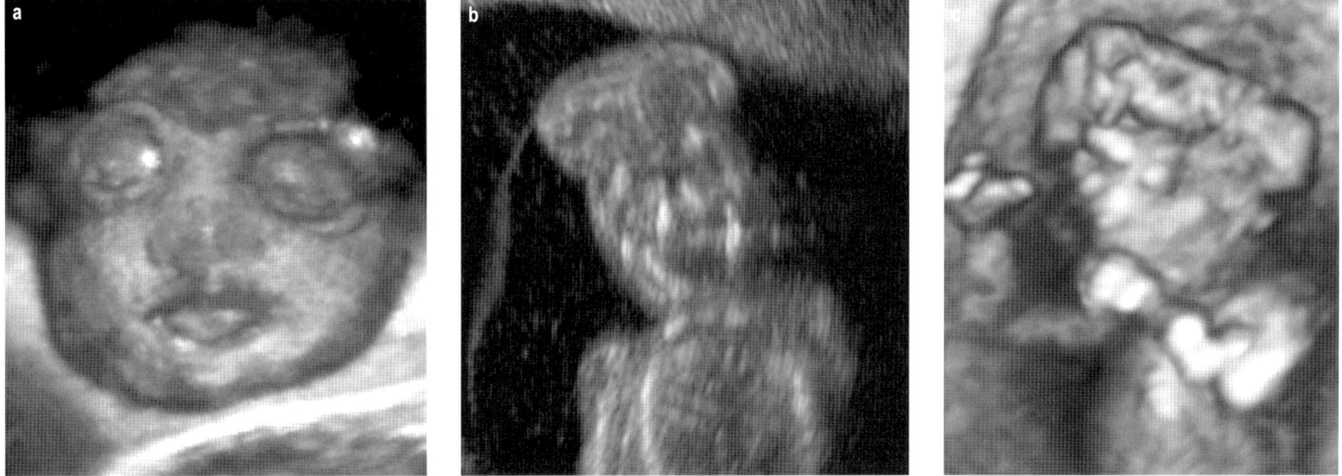

Fig. 30.8 Anencephaly in the third (a) and second trimester (b,c). (a, Courtesy of Renato Ximenes, Sao Paulo, Brasil.)

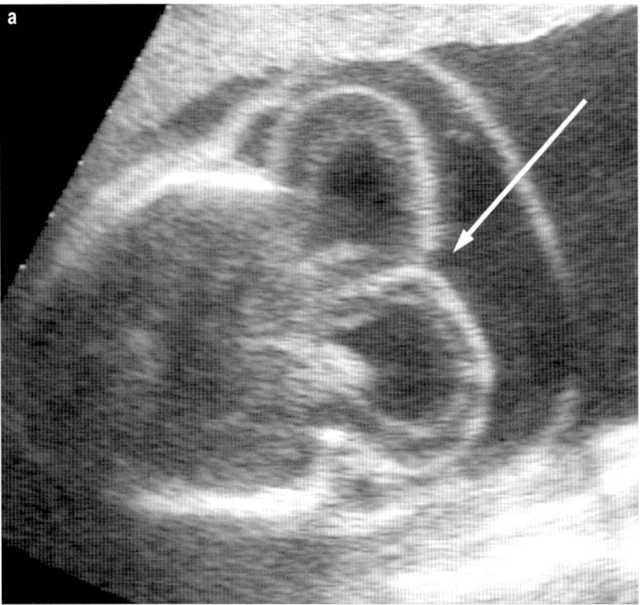

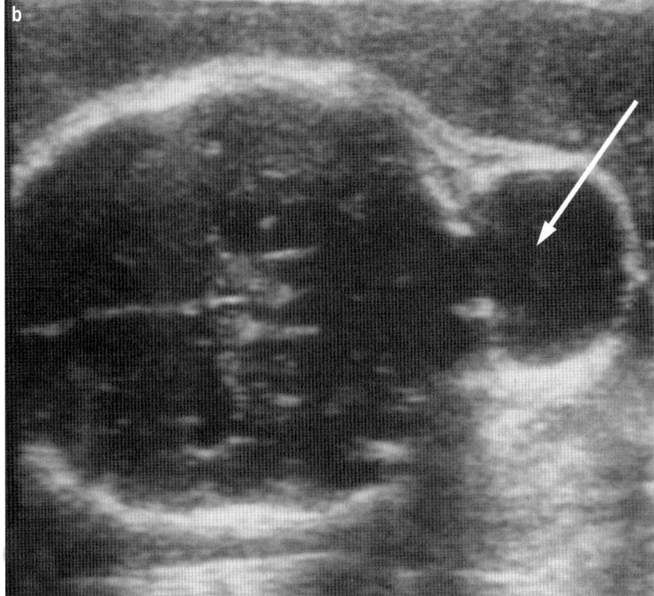

Fig. 30.9 Fetal cephaloceles: (a) encephalocele; (b) cranial meningocele.

When parts of the brain herniate through the defect, the terms encephalocele or cephalocele are used; when the sac is empty of brain contents the diagnosis is cranial meningocele.

In the vast majority of cases, the defect is in the midline and around 75% of them are occipital. Non-midline encephaloceles are usually caused by a disruption sequence. Encephaloceles and meningoceles are associated with an increased risk of CNS anomalies including ventriculomegaly, microcephaly and spina bifida and are also found in various genetic syndromes including Meckel–Gruber, Walker–Warburg and frontonasal dysplasia.

The prenatal diagnosis of these conditions is usually easy, particularly in cases with large defects, brain contents inside the sac or associated malformations (Fig. 30.9). Small defects and those positioned in atypical places may remain undiagnosed through pregnancy; elevated maternal serum alpha-fetoprotein (MSAFP) may be the only clue for the prenatal diagnosis in these occasions[37]. In most cases, MSAFP is normal because the defect is covered with skin. Differential diagnosis include skin and subcutaneous tumors and cysts[38], cervical cystic hygroma[39], cervical meningomyelocele[40] and Dandy–Walker malformation with a herniated cyst[41]; the diagnosis is usually based on the demonstration of a skull defect with or without brain contents inside the defect, in some cases color Doppler may show cerebral vessels inside the sac. An extremely rare type of cephalocele is the atretic cephalocele and, although it was never before diagnosed in the fetus, the sonographer must be aware of this condition since, although apparently innocuous, it is associated in some cases with other brain anomalies[42] that may remain undiagnosed during US and MRI fetal examinations.

The operative outcome of encephalocele depends on the presence of associated malformations, the coexistence of hydrocephalus and the presence of brain tissue in the sac[43]. Prenatally diagnosed cases have a very poor outcome[44,45]. In cases with isolated cranial meningocele the prognosis is much better[43].

Myelomeningocele

Myelomeningocele (MMC) is caused by a localized failure in the closure of the posterior neuropore, occurring usually in the lumbar region, the last portion of the neural tube to develop. The defect involves the spine, meninges, vertebrae and skin and may be open to the amniotic cavity or may comprise a cyst filled with CSF. As for anencephaly, MMC is considered a multifactorial disorder with an increased familial risk when the mother or one or more siblings are affected. Geographical location is another well know risk factor, with a great incidence in some parts of the UK[33] and China[46]. The incidence of MMC has declined during the last three decades, probably due to dietary and socioeconomic changes occurring in many regions of the world and to the gradual introduction of folic acid supplementation[30,47,48]. The prevalence of spina bifida reported on birth certificates in the USA declined from 24.88 (95% CI = 23.25–26.52) per 100 000 live births in 1991 to 20.09 (95% CI = 18.63–21.54) in 2001[49] (Table 30.1). A similar decrease occurred in Sweden between 1973 and 2003 from 55 per 100 000 newborns to 29 per 100 000 newborns; in the southern part of the country the prevalence of spina bifida starting from 1993 was half that of the rest of the country, the authors attribute this decline to the introduction of ultrasound screening[50].

Chromosomal anomalies appear to be more frequent in patients with open neural tube defects; in a multicenter study from Chile, Sepulveda et al. reported a 9% prevalence (6/66 fetuses) of karyotypic abnormalities among fetuses with spina bifida[51]. The true prevalence of chromosomal anomalies may be much higher as shown by Phillip et al.[52] in a study of embryos from triploid missed abortions; the authors found that 10 out of 18 embryos had spina bifida. The increased incidence of open neural tube defects (ONTD) after the use of certain medications, particularly valproic acid and carbamazepine in patients with seizure disorders, remains controversial[53,54].

Determination of the levels of alpha-fetoprotein (AFP) in the amniotic fluid and maternal serum has been the main tool

Table 30.1 Number of live births and prevalence* for spina bifida and anencephaly in United States, 1991–2001

	Spina bifida		*Anencephaly*		
Year	*No. cases*	*Prevalence (95% CI§)*	*No. cases*	*Prevalence (95% CI)*	*Total no. live births*
1991	887	24.88 (23.25–26.52)	655	18.38 (16.97–19.78)	3,564,453
1992	816	22.84 (21.27–24.41)	457	12.79 (11.62–13.96)	3,572,890
1993	896	25.15 (23.50–26.80)	481	13.50 (12.29–14.71)	3,562,723
1994	900	25.51 (23.85–27.18)	387	10.97 (9.88–12.06)	3,527,482
1995	975	27.98 (26.22–29.74)	408	11.71 (10.57–12.84)	3,484,539
1996	917	26.36 (24.65–28.07)	416	11.96 (10.81–13.11)	3,478,723
1997	857	24.70 (23.05–26.35)	434	12.51 (11.33–13.69)	3,469,667
1998	790	22.45 (20.88–24.01)	349	9.92 (8.88–10.96)	3,519,240
1999	732	20.72 (19.22–22.22)	382	10.81 (9.73–11.89)	3,533,565
2000	759	20.85 (19.37–22.33)	376	10.33 (9.28–11.37)	3,640,376
2001¶	733	20.09 (18.63–21.54)	343	9.40 (8.40–10.39)	3,649,061

*Per 100,000 live births. Excludes data for Maryland, New Mexico, and New York, which did not require reporting for spina bifida and anencephaly for certain years. §Confidence interval. ¶Data for 2001 are preliminary.
Source: National Vital Statistics System, National Center for Health Statistics, CDC

in the screening for open neural tube defects since its introduction more than 30 years ago[55,56]. The use of ultrasound for this purpose was described almost concomitantly[57], but now it replaces amniocentesis as the diagnostic method of choice in most circumstances[58–60]. The use of ultrasound as the primary method of screening has gained good acceptance, but results are still operator dependent[61,62]. The advantages of US over AFP screening reside in the possibility to reach the diagnosis early enough to have a surgical termination of pregnancy[63–65] and on the fact that US is not dependent on other tests or examinations for definitive diagnosis. In addition, ultrasound can estimate the level and severity of the lesion.

The ultrasonographic diagnosis of MMC is based on direct demonstration of the presence of a defect in the fetal back or neck and/or in the presence of indirect signs characteristic of MMC in the brain and skull.

Direct visualization of MMC depends on gestational age, fetal position, maternal habitus and US waves transmissibility, quality of the equipment, the approach used and, finally, on operator proficiency.

Case reports of early diagnosis of MMC have been reported using high-resolution transvaginal probes[66,67]. In a large study performed between 10 and 14 weeks, the authors failed to diagnose all the cases of spina bifida (29 MMC/61 972 patients) at this time but were able to diagnose 28 of them in follow-up examinations performed between 16 and 22 weeks; the remaining case was diagnosed at 32 weeks[68]. According to some studies, the presence of indirect signs early in pregnancy may precede direct demonstration of the MMC[65] but others have shown the opposite[67].

For direct demonstration of MMC, a careful examination of the spine should be performed using at least two sectional planes (Fig. 30.10). Axial planes enable stepwise visualization of single vertebrae and the presence of cystic protruding lesions, skin defects and/or abnormally wide distance between the transverse processes. Sagittal and coronal planes usually depict adjacent vertebrae and the presence of protruding cystic lesions or an interruption in skin and subcutaneous continuity; sagittal planes are also used in the evaluation of the extent of the defect by counting the number of vertebrae involved and their exact site.

Indirect signs for the presence of MMC are based on the association between this condition and Arnold–Chiari malformation type 2 (ACM2). ACM2 consists of elongation and descent of the cerebellum, pons and medulla through the foramen magnum with obliteration of the cisterna magna and is pathognomonic for MMC[69]. Other forms of classic ACM have been described. In type 1, only the cerebellar tonsils descend below the foramen magnum and it is usually not associated with ventriculomegaly; in type 3, the cerebellum is totally or partially positioned in an occipital or high cervical meningocele; finally, in type 4, the infratentorial structures are not displaced but the cerebellum is aplastic or hypoplastic with dilatation of the 4th ventricle and cisterna magna[70].

The US expression of ACM2 in the fetus was first described by Nicolaides et al.[1]. In their original paper they found that in 12 of 21 fetuses, in which an image of the cerebellum was available, the shape of the cerebellum was abnormal (the banana sign) and the cisterna magna was obliterated; in another 8 fetuses the cerebellum was not visualized in its normal location (Fig. 30.11). The authors also described the abnormal shape of the frontal bones due to scalloping (the lemon sign) (Fig. 30.11) and the associated presence of ventriculomegaly and small head circumference in a significant number of fetuses[1]. A review of papers published on this subject until 1991 showed that almost 100% (232 of 233 fetuses) with proven open MMC had at least one of the US signs described by Nicolaides and colleagues[72]. Another potentially helpful sign in

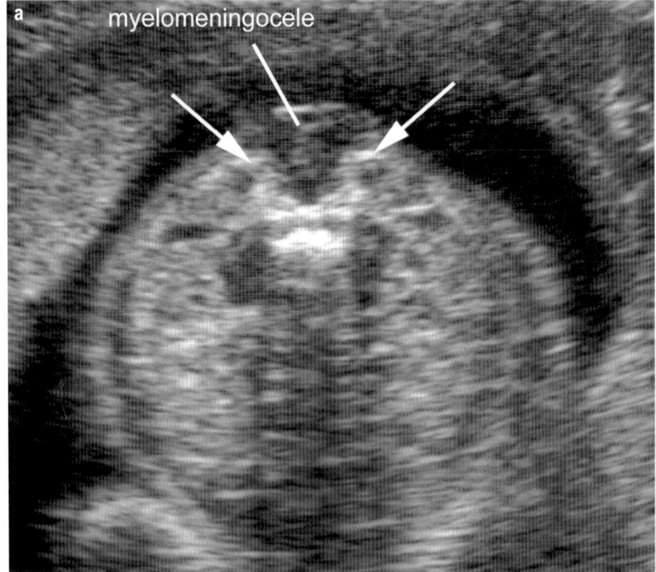

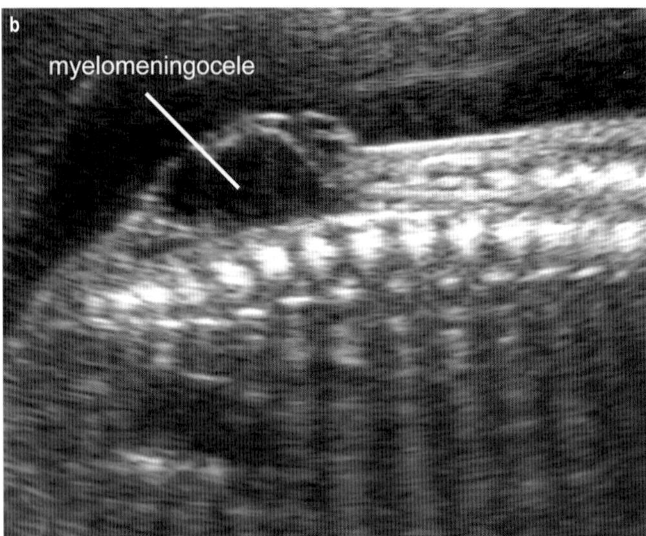

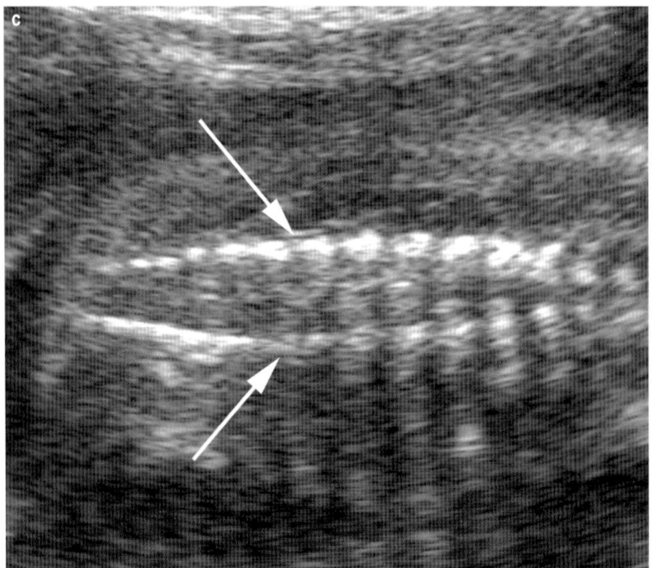

Fig. 30.10 Myelomeningocele in a midtrimester fetus.

the diagnosis of open MMC may be the absence of CSF around the brain.

False negative diagnosis may occur, as previously mentioned, when the examination is performed very early in pregnancy, but we have made the correct diagnosis based on the presence of the 'fruit' signs as early as 14 weeks. False negative diagnosis may be also the result of the presence of a closed NTD in which the covering skin is disrupted during delivery. A single false positive diagnosis has been reported in a fetus with tripoidy[73].

First- and second-trimester termination of pregnancy should be considered in keeping with the legal regulations of the country. In some countries, even third-trimester termination may be an option.

Alternatively, a non-interventional approach may be considered[74] with early, aggressive management in selected cases. By using this approach, McLaughlin and colleagues reported normal cognitive development in 79% of their patients and 72% were ambulatory[75]. Currently, in the USA, a large prospective study is being conducted to compare two approaches to the treatment of babies with spina bifida: surgery before birth and surgery after birth[76,77].

Evaluation of the extent and severity of MMC is important for an accurate prognosis and when considering intrauterine surgery, either by detailed ultrasound examination[78] or by fetal MRI[79]. Eventually, 3DUS will also become an important tool in the evaluation of spina bifida[40,80].

DISORDERS OF SECONDARY NEURULATION

Disorders of secondary neurulation represent an abnormal development of the lower sacral and coccygeal segments occurring after the 28th day post conception and are characterized by the presence of intact skin covering the defect[16]. The skin covering makes the diagnosis of these conditions particularly difficult and they are called closed or occult spinal dysraphisms.

Because of the caudal position of the lesion, the neural involvement is usually mild, affecting the conus medullaris or the filum terminalis. Malformations of the skeletal system, represented by laminar defects, widened spinal canal, sacral and limb anomalies, occur in as many as 85–90% of the patients[16]; and dermal lesions represented by subcutaneous lipomas, skin tags, vascular nevi, pori, hairy patches, hypertrichosis, meningoceles and 'cigarette burn' marks are present in 86% of the patients[81]. Different conditions have been described according to the time of occurrence and the presence or absence of a mass (Table 30.2).

Although prenatal diagnosis of some of these conditions has been sporadically reported, most cases are detected after delivery, during infancy or even in adulthood. Prenatal diagnosis is usually based on the visualization of a lumbosacral mass or some skeletal anomaly[82–84] (Fig. 30.12). The determination of the terminal part of the conus medullaris has been proposed as a possible screening method for the diagnosis of tethered cord, but it remains difficult to determine the exact position in relation to the lumbar vertebrae because of the difficulty in counting the sacral vertebrae[85]. Visualization of the conus terminalis ending at the level of the middle of the kidney may be considered with good certainty a sign of normality, but it should be used cautiously since it is probable that traction and downwards displacement occurs only after delivery.

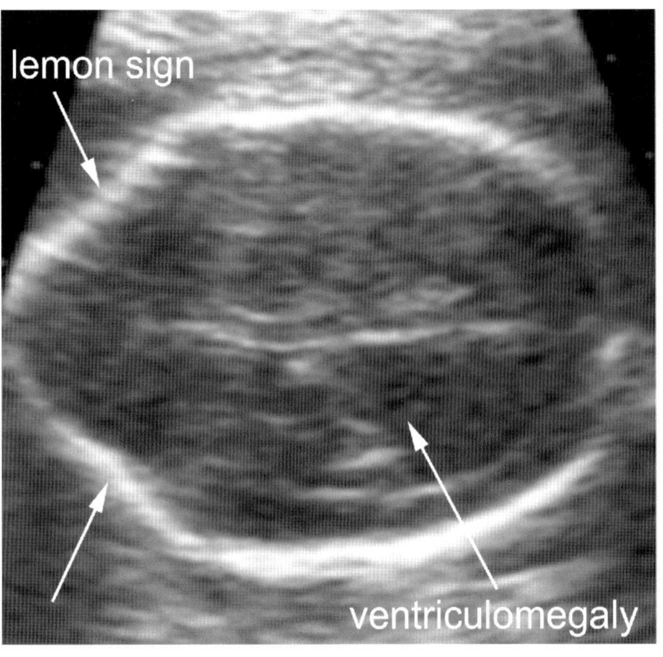

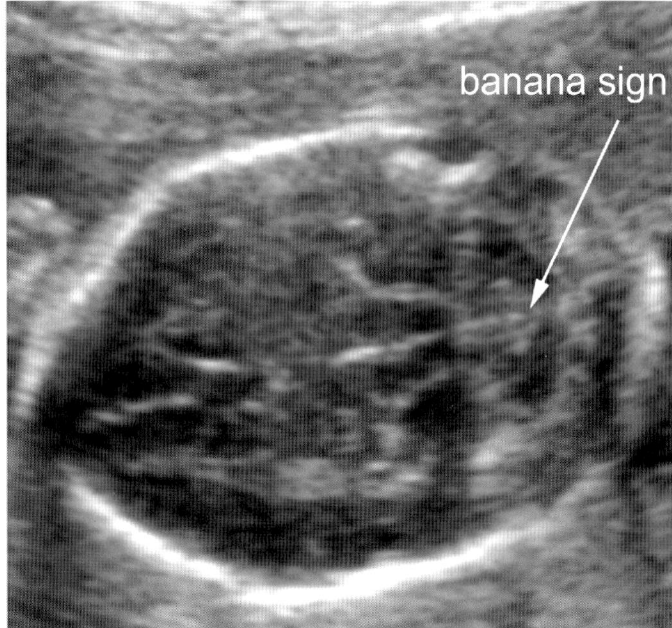

Fig. 30.11 The cranial signs associated with open spina bifida.

Table 30.2 **Clinical neuroradiological classification of spinal dysraphisms**

Open spinal dysraphisms
Myelomeningocele
Myelocele
Hemimyelomeningocele
Hemimyelocele
Closed spinal dysraphisms
With subcutaneous mass
Lipomas with dural defect
Lipomyelomeningocele
Lipomyelocele
Terminal myelocystocele
Meningocele
Without subcutaneous mass
Simple dysraphic states
Intradural lipoma
Filar lipoma
Tight filum terminale
Persistent terminal ventricle
Dermal sinus
Complex dysraphic states
Disorders of midline notochordal intergration
Dorsal enteric fistula
Neurenteric cysts
Diastematomyelia
Disorders of notochordal formation
Caudal agenesis
Segmental spinal dysgenesis

Rossi A, Biancheri R, Cama A, Piatelli G, Ravegnani M. Tortori-Donati P. Imaging in Spine and spinal cord malformations. Eur J Radiol. 2004 May;**50**(2):177–200.

Ventriculomegaly

Enlargement of the lateral cerebral ventricles (Fig. 30.13) can be regarded as a non-specific marker of abnormal brain development and is encountered with many different cerebral anomalies. Evaluation of the integrity of the cerebral lateral ventricles is therefore of particular importance while screening for fetal cerebral anomalies. Although many different approaches to the evaluation of the integrity of lateral ventricles have been proposed, measurement of the internal width of the atrium of the lateral ventricle at the level of the glomus of the choroid plexus is currently favored[86]. Under normal conditions, the measurement is less than 10 mm, while a value of more than 15 mm indicates *severe ventriculomegaly*, which is almost always associated with an intracranial malformation at birth. The outcome of these fetuses is variable and depends largely upon the underlying etiology of the ventricular dilatation. The available studies suggest that fetuses with isolated severe ventriculomegaly have an increased risk of perinatal death and a probability of severe neurologic sequelae in the range of 50% of survivors[87]. An intermediate value for the atrial width, 10–15 mm, is commonly referred to as *mild ventriculomegaly* and is associated with a much increased probability of cerebral and extracerebral malformations, aneuploidies and infections and therefore should be carefully evaluated in an expert center. Fetuses with isolated mild ventriculomegaly usually have a good outcome and, in most infants, the ventricles return to normal size during pregnancy. However, these infants also run an increased risk of neurologic compromise and, in some cases, develop severe cerebral anomalies in the last part of the gestation or after birth, including hydrocephalus, white matter injury and cortical plate abnormalities[88]. The risk is particularly increased when the atrial width is greater than 12 mm, when the dilatation affects both lateral ventricles and in females[88]. It has been suggested that the term mild ventriculomegaly should be limited only to cases with atrial measurements of 10–12 mm, while values of 12.1–15 mm should be

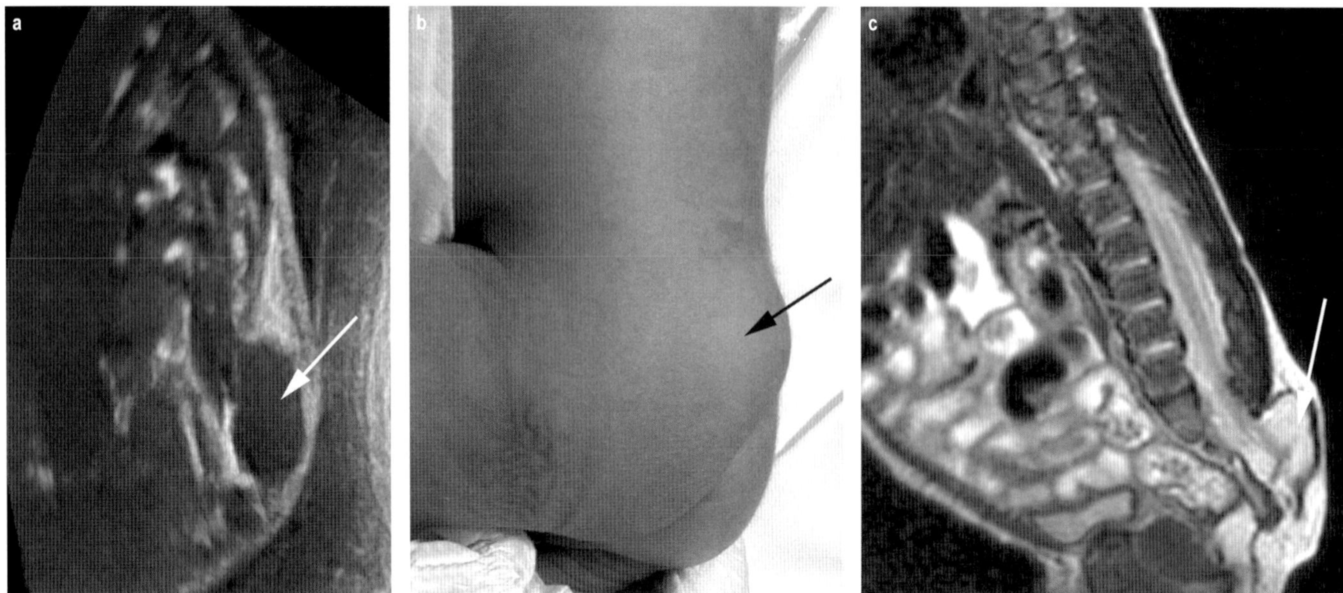

Fig. 30.12 Closed spina bifida with lipoma. (a, prenatal sonogram, b, postnatal appearance, c, magnetic resonance.)

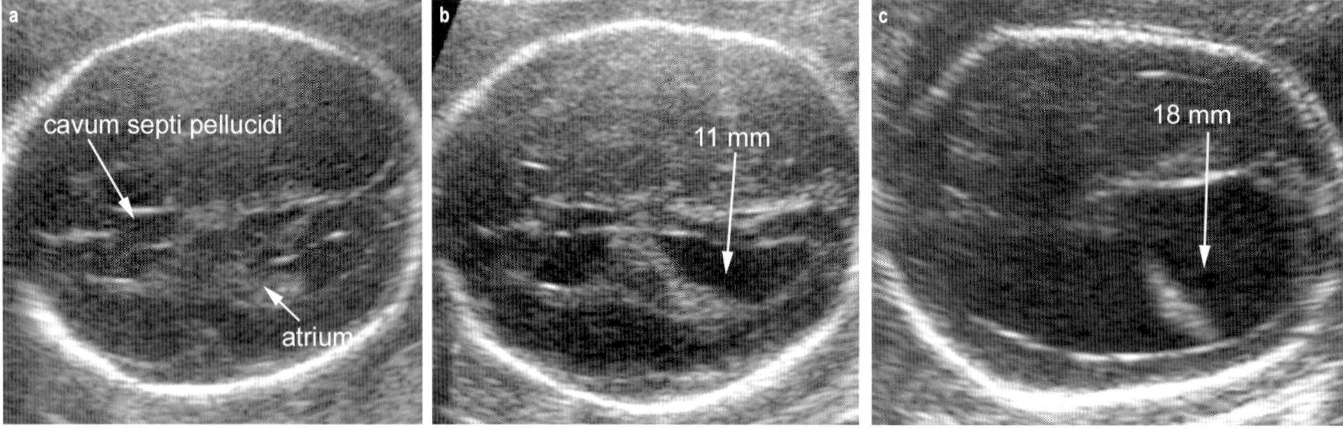

Fig. 30.13 (a) Normal transventricular scan demonstrating an atrium of lateral ventricle of normal size; (b) mild ventriculomegaly; (c) severe ventriculomegaly.

referred to as *moderate* ventriculomegaly, as they tend to have, in general, a worse outcome[89].

Congenital hydrocephalus has genetic implications. It should be stressed that the experience thus far indicates that antenatal ultrasound is unreliable for predicting the recurrence of isolated ventriculomegaly, and particularly of the X-linked variety, because, in many cases, enlargement of the lateral ventricles only develops late in gestation or after birth. DNA analysis for the X-linked variety is now available and should be considered, although the exact sensitivity remains uncertain[90–92].

When the diagnosis of severe ventriculomegaly is made prior to viability, many parents would probably request termination of pregnancy. In continuing pregnancies, no modifications of standard obstetric management are required. A cesarean section is recommended only in those cases with associated macrocrania. Cephalocentesis to reduce cranial size is associated with significant morbidity and is indicated only in cases with a presumption of a severe prognosis[93].

DISORDERS OF PROSENCEPHALIC DEVELOPMENT

The inductive processes leading to the development of the prosencephalon start by weeks 5–6 of pregnancy and consist of three sequential events, closely interconnected: formation, cleavage and midline development[16]. Anomalies occurring during this period lead to the development of a wide range of malformations, their severity closely related to the time of occurrence. Since ventral induction is closely related to facial development, many fetuses and children with prosencephalic disorders suffer from facial anomalies.

Disorders of prosencephalic formation

Disorders of prosencephalic formation, aprosencephaly and atelencephaly, are the most severe anomalies: aprosencephaly is the complete lack of development of the telencephalon and diencephalon and, in atelencephaly, the diencephalon is present but usually abnormal[94]. These are extremely rare anomalies and in all prenatally reported cases a different brain malformation was suspected in utero and the definitive diagnosis was reached only after pathological examination[95].

Disorders of prosencephalic cleavage

Disorders of prosencephalic cleavage, holoprosencephaly (HPE) and holotelencephaly, follow in the degree of severity; the different names refer to the involvement of both the diencephalon and telencephalon (holoprosencephaly) or only the telencephalon (holotelencephaly).

In two recent large population based studies, the reported prevalence of holoprosencephaly was between 1.09 and 1.7 per 10000 births and terminations[96,97]. In the study from the UK, chromosomal anomalies were found in 46% of the cases in which a karyotype was obtained, 96% of the fetuses were diagnosed or suspected before delivery and termination of pregnancy was performed in 80% of the cases[97]. The prevalence in aborted material has been found to be much higher, at 41 per 10000 induced abortions[98].

Odent et al.[99] (Table 30.3) found, by studying the records of 259 HPE cases, that one hundred (39%) had associated chromosomal abnormalities; 52 (20%) had non-chromosomal syndromes and 4 (1.5%) were related to maternal diabetes. In 79 (30.5%), a familial history of HPE with major or minor signs was obtained: based on these, of 79 non-syndromic non-chromosomal HPE sibships, the authors postulated transmission by an autosomal dominant mode of inheritance with a high but incomplete penetrance (82–88%) and a high proportion of sporadic cases (68%)[99]. Their model makes it possible to predict a recurrence risk of 13–14% following an isolated case.

Table 30.3 **Distribution of 258 holoprosencephalic records, from Ref[99], with permission**

Category	*No. of cases*	*Percentage (%)*
Chromosome abnormality	100	39
Syndromic nonchromosomal	52	20
Diabetic mothers	4	1.5
Incomplete information	23	9
Total	179	69.5
Nonchromosomal and nonsyndromic	79	30.5
Familial cases	23	
Minor signs in a parent	10	

The list of chromosomal aberrations found in patients with HPE includes more than 35 conditions, but only 7 are frequently described: trisomy 13, del(13q), del(18p), trisomy 18, tripoidy, dup(3p) and de1(7)(pter + q32)[100].

Several loci for holoprosencephaly have been mapped to specific chromosomal sites and the molecular defects in some cases of HPE have been identified[101]. Holoprosencephaly-1 (HPE1) maps to 21q22.3. HPE2, caused by mutation in the SIX3 gene maps to 2p21. HPE3, caused by mutation in the sonic hedgehog gene (SHH), maps to 7q36. HPE4, caused by mutation in the TGIF gene, maps to 18p11.3. HPE5, caused by mutation in the ZIC2 gene, maps to 13q32. HPE6 maps to 2q37.1. HPE7, caused by mutation in the PTCH1 gene, maps to 9q22.3. HPE8 maps to 14q13. HPE9, caused by mutation in the GLI2 gene, maps to 2q14.

Affected subjects may present with a very wide spectrum of brain disorders and associated facial anomalies. HPE has been classified into three different types: alobar, semilobar and lobar. Recently, a new variant, the middle interhemispheric variant, has also been described (Fig. 30.14)

Alobar HPE represents the most severe form and has the worst prognosis; a univentricular cavity is present and the hemispheres and the thalami are fused with midline structures being absent (Fig. 30.15). Semilobar HPE is also a severe malformation with a bad prognosis; the frontal ventricular horns form a single anterior ventricle but the occipital and temporal horns are separated; the frontal lobes and parts of the thalami are fused and there may be partial development of midline structures. Lobar HPE represents the mildest form; there is a common frontal ventricle with partial fusion of frontal gyri and almost normal midline structures (Fig. 30.16). The middle interhemispheric variant stands in between the lobar and alobar type (Fig. 30.17). All types of HPE are characterized by the absence of the septum pellucidum and fusion of the foremost anterior portion of the frontal horns[102].

The severity of facial anomalies is usually, but not always, related to the severity of brain findings[103]. Facial anomalies ranged from severe forms such as cyclopia and agnathia-astomia to very mild ones with minimal hypotelorism or the presence of a single central incisor (Table 30.4).

Prenatal diagnosis of HPE by US has been reported and criteria for diagnosis are well established[4]. The visualization of facial anomalies or severe ventricular dilatation are usually the first step in the diagnostic process, but a definitive diagnosis may still be difficult[102], particularly in cases of lobar HPE[104,105]. Early diagnosis of alobar HPE during the first and early second

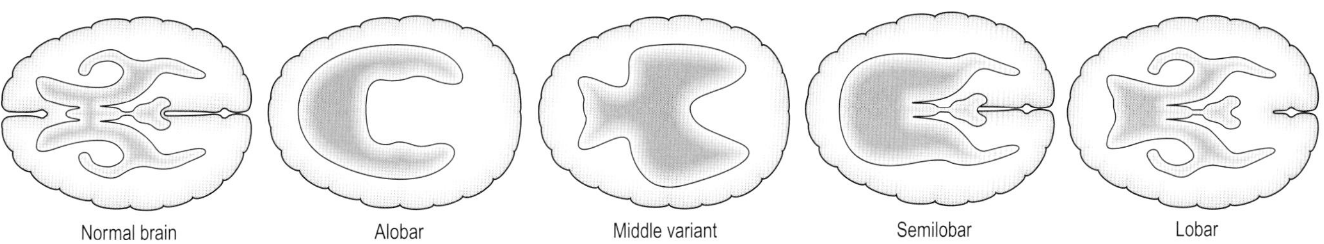

Fig. 30.14 Schematic representation of a normal brain compared with different varieties of holoprosencephaly.

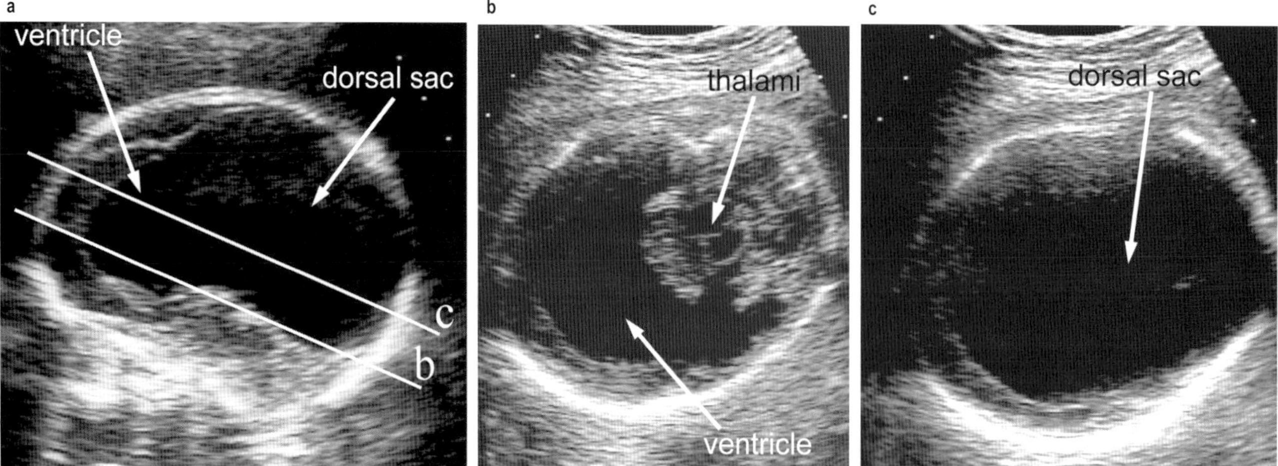

Fig. 30.15 Multiplanar sonography of alobar holoprosencephaly in the midtrimester. (a) median plane demonstrating the single ventricular cavity, that has a rim of cortex anteriorly and amply communicates posteriorly with a dorsal sac; (b) axial scan at the level of the thalamus, demonstrating the crescent-shaped single ventricle and the absence of the midline in the anterior cortex; (c) in a slightly craniad axial plane than the previous one, the communication between the ventricular cavity and the dorsal sac is demonstrated.

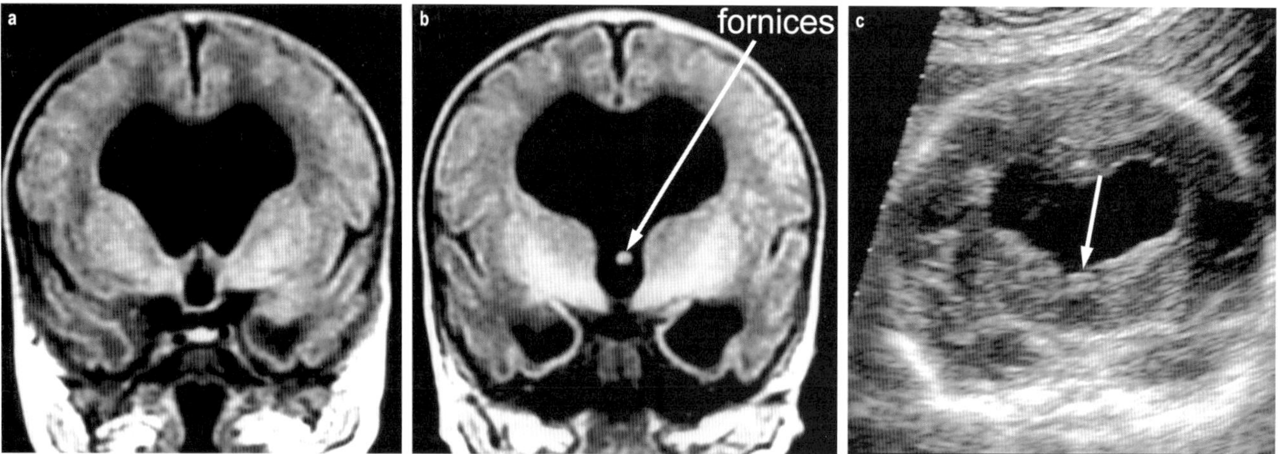

Fig. 30.16 Lobar holoprosencephaly. (a,b) Postnatal magnetic resonance; (c) prenatal ultrasound. The frontal horns are fused centrally, as well as the fornices (arrow) that form a thick fascicle running in the floor of the cavity.

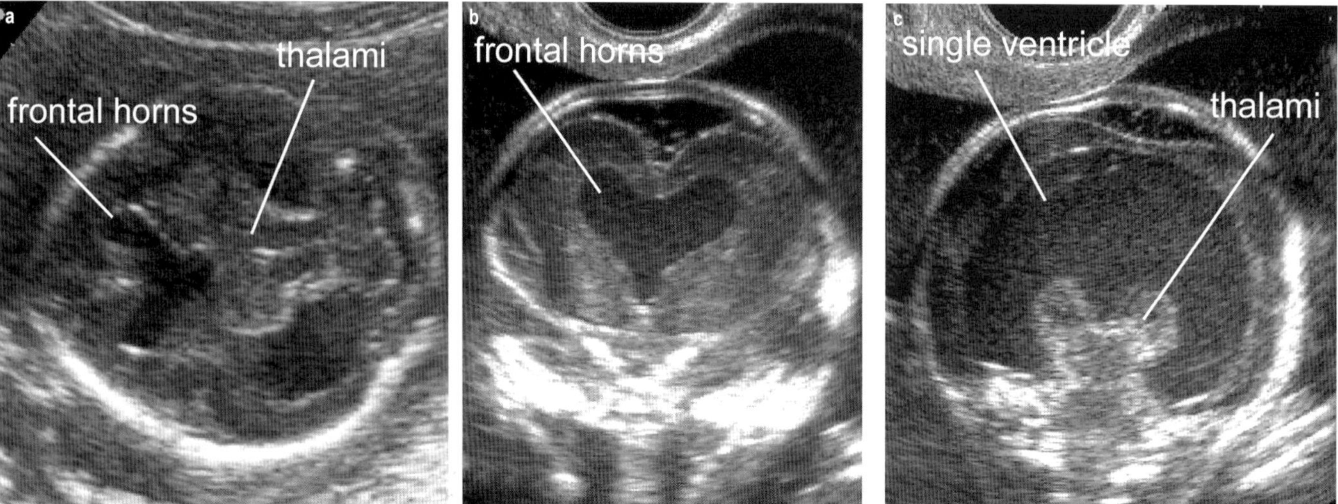

Fig. 30.17 Middle interhemispheric variant of holoprosencephaly in the axial (a), anterior coronal (b) and midcoronal plane (c). The frontal horns are well developed and there is a partial formation of the interhemispheric fissure. However, the midcoronal plane reveals a common ventricular cavity with hypoplastic undivided thalami.

Table 30.4 **Facial defects in holoprosencephaly**

Cyclopia	Single eye or single orbit Arrhinia with proboscis
Ethmocephaly	Extreme hypotelorism Arrhinia with proboscis
Cebocephaly	Orbital hypotelorism Proboscis-like nose, no cleft
Median cleft	Orbital hypotelorism Flat nose
Agnathia-astomia	Hypoplasia or absence of the mandible Small or absent mouth Abnormal position of the ears

trimester has been reported based on the visualization of a single ventricle[106,107] or cyclopia[108]. Blaas et al.[109] published a large series of prenatally diagnosed fetuses with HPE; the mean gestational age at detection was 21w + 3d weeks (range, 9w2d–37w2d); termination of the pregnancy was performed in 23 of the 30 cases (73%), one fetus died in utero and 4 died during or shortly after delivery, one child died at the age of 1 year 6 months and one child with frontonasal dysplasia was born in 1999, and was still alive at the age of 24 months.

Fetal MRI may have a role in the elucidation of particularly difficult cases of lobar HPE or some of the non-classical forms of HPE, i.e. middle interhemispheric variant of HPE[110].

DISORDERS OF PROSENCEPHALIC MIDLINE DEVELOPMENT

Disorders of prosencephalic midline development, agenesis of corpus callosum, agenesis of septum pellucidum and septo-optic dysplasia, usually have less severe presentations, but affected subjects may suffer from severe neurodevelopmental retardation, endocrinologic and visual disorders.

Agenesis of the corpus callosum

The corpus callosum (CC) is the biggest commissure connecting the hemispheres and is composed of axonal tracts connecting the right and left side of the brain. The CC starts its development relatively late in pregnancy at around 10 weeks and continues growing well after delivery. The anterior and hypothalamic commissures are the other two smaller commissures.

Anomalies of the commissures may include agenesis of all the structures or only individual structures.

Callosal fibers may be identified close to the lamina terminalis during the 10th gestational week, but the corpus callosum itself develops some weeks later. Histological studies have shown the presence of callosal fibers crossing the midline at 13 weeks, but recent studies, based on diffusion tensor magnetic resonance imaging (DTMRI), were able to demonstrate the presence of a clearly defined midline corpus callosum at around 15 weeks. At this time only the anterior portions – rostrum, genu and part of the body – are present[111]. In the same study, the CC was fully identified only 3–5 weeks later.

The exact prevalence of agenesis of the corpus callosum (ACC) is not known. In a rather old study based on the use of pneumoencephalograms, the prevalence was 0.7%[112]. The prevalence of ACC in children with mental retardation as demonstrated with computerized tomography was 2.3%[113].

A study based on the performance of cranial US in 2309 clinically normal term neonates found two cases of ACC[114]. These findings are in accordance with our findings in a large unpublished series of low-risk patients, assessed by US at 15–17 weeks and reassessed at 22–25 weeks with direct demonstration of the corpus callosum. In our patients, we found only one case of agenesis of the corpus callosum out of 2835 examinations.

Due to its relatively late formation, agenesis of the corpus callosum may be found in association with a vast number of brain anomalies, but it may also be an isolated finding[115]. It is important to remember that congenital callosal pathologies may also develop after prenatal insults such as infections[116] or ischemic processes[117].

The demonstration of the corpus callosum is possible with ultrasound, starting from around 18–20 weeks of gestation, but requires some degree of technical skill since it is not depicted using the standard axial planes but coronal and particularly sagittal ones (Fig. 30.18). In fetuses in vertex presentation the

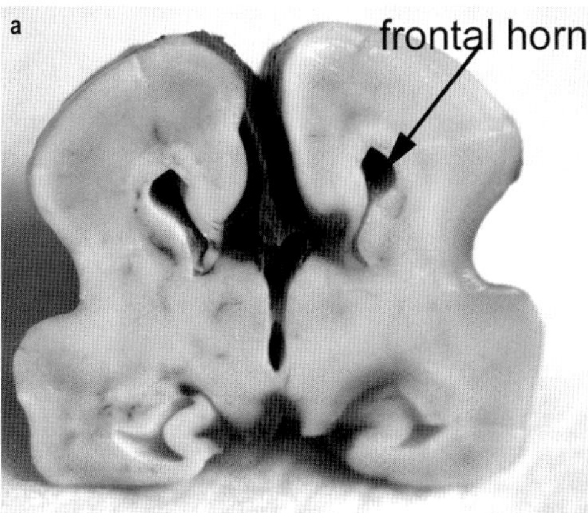

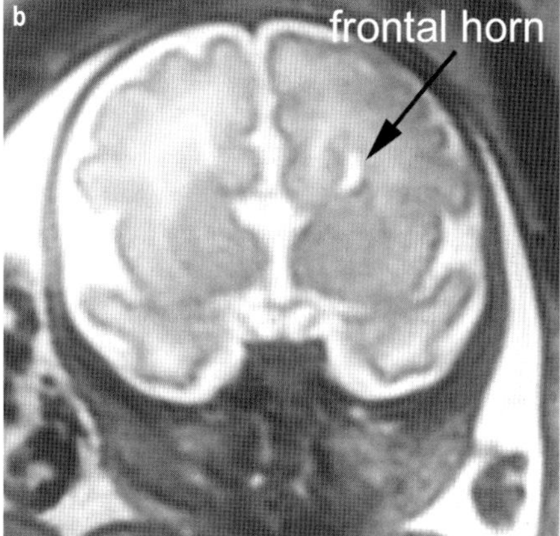

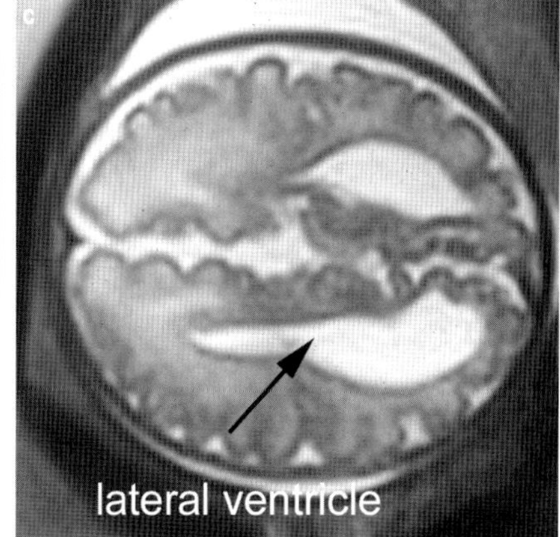

Fig. 30.18 Complete agenesis of the corpus callosum: (a) pathology in a midtrimester fetus; (b,c) magnetic resonance at 32 weeks. Apart from the absence of the corpus callosum, a number of abnormal findings can be appreciated including the increased separation of the hemispheres, the comma-shaped frontal horns and the teardrop shape of the lateral ventricles in the axial plane.

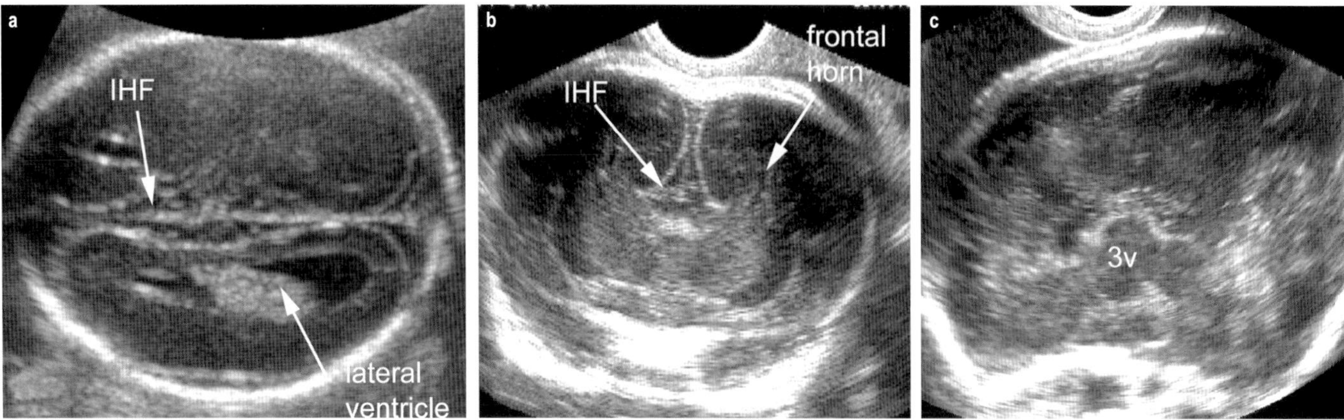

Fig. 30.19 Sonography of fetal agenesis of the corpus callosum. (a) In the axial plane the interhemispheric fissure (IHF) appears wider than usual without evidence of the cavum septi pellucidi; (b) in the coronal and sagittal plane, no corpus callosum and cavum septi pellucidi can be seen above the third ventricle (3v).

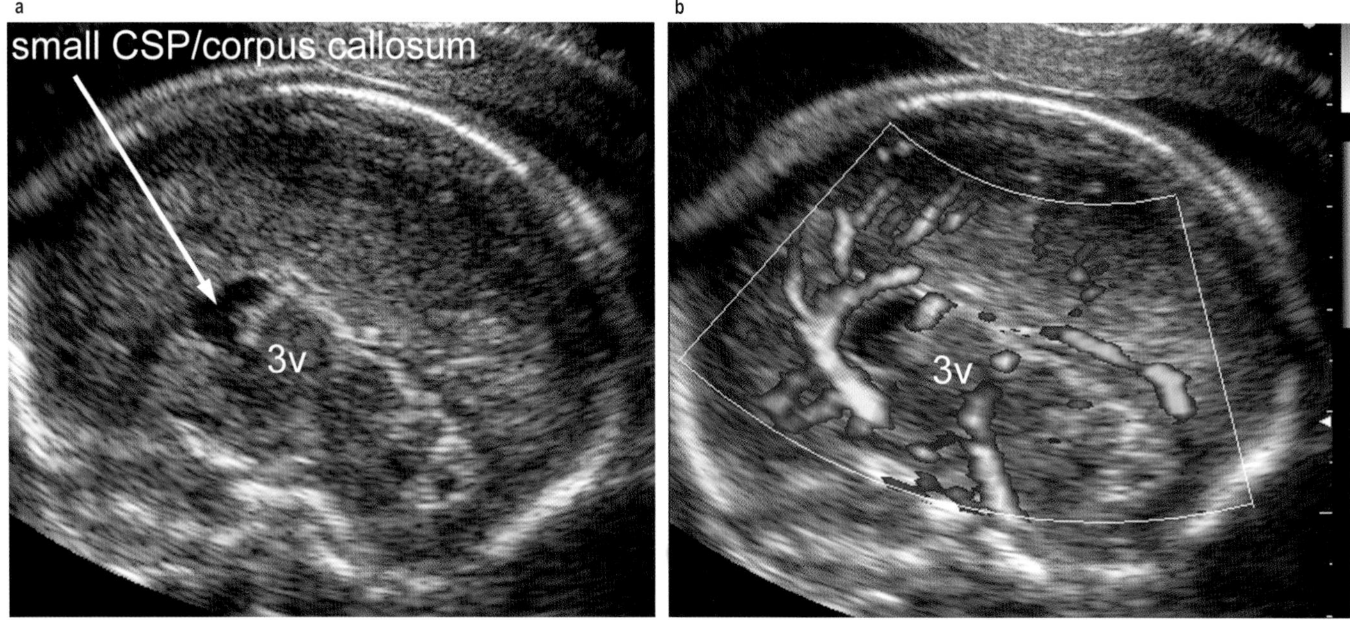

Fig. 30.20 Partial agenesis of the corpus callosum. (a) In this 21 weeks' fetus the corpus callosum/cavum septi pellucidi complex is much smaller than normal; in fact it does not extend entirely over the third ventricle, but only reaches about midway; (b) the corpus callosum appears thin and barely discernible with gray scale imaging and can be positively identified only when highlighted by the course of the pericallosal artery.

transvaginal approach is preferred[118]; in breech presentation we recommend a transfundal approach. Recently, the use of a 3D multiplanar technique has been also proposed[119].

Before 17–18 weeks it will not be possible to visualize the full length of the corpus callosum but, using coronal planes, we may be able to show the presence of at least the rostral portions through the presence of an interruption in the continuity of the inter-hemispheric fissure.

The anatomy of agenesis of the corpus callosum is variable. Figure 30.19 demonstrates the most typical type. The prenatal diagnosis of agenesis of the corpus callosum has been reported as case reports and in some series[11,119–121]. When using axial planes, the diagnosis is based on the presence of indirect signs: colpocephaly (tear-drop shape of the lateral ventricle with large and round occipital horn and sharp and pointed frontal horn); separated frontal horns and absence of the septum pellucidum (Fig. 30.20). Other indirect signs that are difficult or impossible to depict in axial planes are: elevation of the 3rd ventricle; radial sulci and gyri reaching the elevated 3rd ventricle and absence of normal developed pericallosal arteries[110]. In modern prenatal diagnosis, direct visualization of the midline and demonstration of the callosal pathology is needed for a definitive diagnosis (see Fig. 30.19). Particularly with partial agenesis, careful scanning in the sagittal view is necessary to make the diagnosis (see Fig. 30.20). In our hands, ultrasound provides a more detailed visualization of the corpus callosum than fetal MRI and also enables better measurements of callosal length and thickness. Some authors suggest that MRI may be more informative for the presence of associated anomalies and we believe that it may have a possible application in

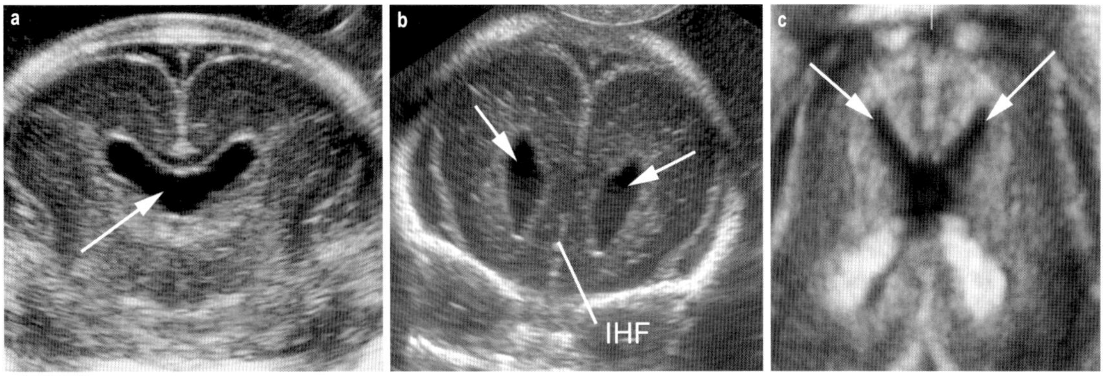

Fig. 30.21 Agenesis of the septum pellucidum: (a) coronal plane demonstrating the absence of the septum pellucidi with fusion of frontal horns; this condition can be differentiated from lobar holoprosencephaly because a more anteriorly oriented coronal plane (b) and an axial plane (c) demonstrate that the frontal horns are separated anteriorly and that there is a well-developed interhemipsheric fissure (IHF) in between the anterior hemispeheres.

cases of apparently isolated ACC as demonstrated by US when termination of pregnancy is an option.

Counseling regarding prognosis and risk of neurodevelopmental retardation after the prenatal diagnosis of ACC is based on the presence of associated anomalies. To rule out an associated malformation, the evaluation must include a detailed neurosonographic examination, a US search for non-CNS anomalies, fetal echocardiography, karyotype, TORCH tests and, finally, in cases with apparently isolated ACC, a fetal brain MRI. Knowledge of specific syndromes with ACC is also important[122]. When a syndrome or associated malformations is diagnosed, the prognosis is poor and termination of pregnancy should be considered.

Counseling in apparently isolated cases is more difficult since the available data, based on long-term follow-up of patients diagnosed prenatally, are scant. Moutard and collaborators have published the largest study on these patients based on long-term follow-up[120]. They performed neuropsychological evaluation of 17 children with ACC and found a progressive decrease in the IQ with age and an increase in slowness, attention difficulties and instability.

Septo-optic dysplasia and agenesis of the septum pellucidum

Agenesis of the septum pellucidum (ASP) is usually associated with brain anomalies, particularly cortical malformations and holoprosencephaly[102,123]. Among the cortical malformations, the association with schizencephaly is particularly frequent[124].

In these cases, the diagnosis of ASP and one of the associated malformations makes the counseling relatively easy because of the poor prognosis of these complex anomalies.

Apparently isolated cases of ASP may be due to septo-optic dysplasia (SOD) or represent an isolated anomaly. SOD is a rare condition characterized by optic nerve hypoplasia, pituitary hypoplasia and agenesis of the septum pellucidum. Known also as De Morsier syndrome, SOD can be caused by a mutation in the homeobox gene HESX1 or occur because of exposure to teratogens or viral infections. In the fetus, the differential diagnosis between SOD and isolated ASP may be attempted by evaluation of maternal urine and serum estriol levels, fetal blood assays for growth hormone, ACTH and prolactin, and visualization of the optic nerve size by MRI in a search for optic nerve hypoplasia[125].

The prenatal diagnosis of ASP (Fig. 30.21), either isolated[125,126] or with associated malformations[102,127,128], has been reported, thus enabling parental counseling.

DISORDERS OF NEURONAL PROLIFERATION

Neuronal proliferation occurs at the ventricular and subventricular zones starting during the second month of pregnancy. Neuroblast formation reaches its peak during the third to fourth month of gestation, followed by glial formation starting around the fifth month of gestation and continuing after delivery[16]. Neuroblast proliferation has been shown to occur in two different patterns. During the early stages, the stem cells migrate from the periphery of the ventricular zone to reach a position adjacent to the lateral ventricles and divide symmetrically to form new stem cells. The number of stem cells reaches its maximum during the second month of pregnancy; by this time, each 'proliferative unit' starts to produce successive asymmetric divisions resulting in the formation of a new stem cell and a post-mitotic neuronal cell[129]. Post-mitotic neuronal cells originating in a specific 'proliferative unit' are programmed to develop a specific task after reaching the cortex. The final size of the proliferative units is determined by the number of divisions of each stem cell during this crucial period of neurogenesis.

It is now clear that neuronal proliferation is temporally related to neuronal migration and organization and the three processes occur simultaneously[130]. This explains why insults occurring during the proliferation period affect not only proliferation but also neuronal migration and organization (Table 30.5).

Microcephaly

Microcephaly is defined postnatally as low brain weight; clinically this is associated with a small head circumference (HC) more than two standard deviations (SD) below the mean or below the third percentile. Such a broad definition obviously includes normal individuals. The smaller the head circumference, the higher the chances of associated mental retardation.

Table 30.5 **Classification of congenital microcephalies* and megalencephaly**

- I. Malformations due to abnormal neuronal and glial proliferation or apoptosis
  - A. Decreased proliferation/increased apoptosis or increased proliferation/decreased apoptosis
    - 1. Microcephaly with normal to thin cortex
      - a. Autosomal recessive microcephaly
        - i. Autosomal recessive microcephaly with normal or slightly short stature and high function
          - (a) MCPH1 mutations
          - (b) ASPM mutations
          - (c) CDKsRAP2 mutations
          - (d) CENPJ mutations
        - ii. Automal recessive microcephaly with normal or minor short stature and very poor function
          - (a) Profound microcephaly – Amish-type lethal microcephaly (SLC25A19 mutations)
          - (b) Less severe microcephaly with periventricular nodular heterotopia (ARFGEF2 mutations)
          - (c) Less severe microcephaly with abnormal frontal cortex and thin corpus callosum – Warburg micro syndrome (RABsGAP mutations)
      - b. Extreme microcephaly with simplified gyral pattern and normal stature
        - i. Extreme microcephaly with jejunal atresia
        - ii. Microcephaly with pontocerebellar hypopasia
      - c. Primary microcephaly (microcephaly vera), NOC
    - 2. Microlissencephaly (extreme microcephaly with thick cortex)
      - a. MLIS with thick cortex (Norman–Roberts syndrome)
      - b. MLIS with thick cortex, severe brainstem and cerebellar hypoplasia (Barth MLIS syndrome)
      - c. MLIS with severe, proportional short stature – Seckel ayndrome (ATR mutation)
      - d. MLIS with mildly to moderately thick (6- to 8-mm) cortex, callosal agenesis
    - 3. Microcephaly with polymicrogyria or other cortical dysplasias
      - a. Extreme microcephaly with diffuse or asymmetric polymicrogyria
      - b. Extreme microcephaly with ACC and cortical dysplasia
  - B. Increased proliferation
    - 1. Megalencephaly (anatomic)
    - 2. Megalencephaly-polymicrogyria-polydactyly-hydrocephalus syndrome

*Extreme microcephaly defined as −3 SD or smaller at birth. NOC = not otherwise classified; MLIS = microlissencephaly; ACC = agenesis of the corpus callosum. From Ref[124], with permission

The exact definition of microcephaly during the prenatal period is a matter of controversy since there is no consensus regarding the definition of abnormally small HC. Some authors propose the −2SD[130] cut-off while others propose the −3SD[6,131] cut-off. Using the −3SD definition, Chervenak et al. showed that the prenatal HC measurement was sensitive for diagnosis of microcephaly with no false negatives, −4SD was a specific test with no false positive cases[6]. Persutte recommends the use of the same definition based on the fact that it will include 0.1% of the population, an incidence that is more in accordance with the true incidence of the disease as found in epidemiological studies[131].

The incidence of microcephaly at birth is estimated to be in the range between 1:6250 and 1:8500 deliveries. The incidence is much higher, 1.6 per 1000 after the first year of life[6] due to progressive microcephaly following perinatal insults or due to a neurodegenerative metabolic or neurogenetic processes. Congenital microcephaly may present as an isolated finding, when it is known as primary microcephaly or microcephaly vera, or may be associated with a wide range of CNS and non-CNS pathologies[132].

The reported accuracy of ultrasound in the detection of microcephaly thus far has been limited, with high rates of both false positives and false negatives diagnoses[133–135].

The prenatal diagnosis of microcephaly, particularly in cases of primary microcephaly, is usually difficult before the 3rd trimester, furthermore, it is expected that, in many cases, prenatal US will fail to reach the diagnosis. Reece and Goldstein, in a study of 9600 low-risk pregnancies in which the brain was scanned for congenital anomalies, failed to diagnose all 5 cases of microcephaly[136].

Bromely and Benacerraf[133] found that 6 out of 7 fetuses with postnatally diagnosed microcephaly had normal head size measurements before 22 weeks of pregnancy and were diagnosed only after 27 weeks of gestation.

Two retrospective analyses of cases diagnosed prenatally have been published. Den Hollander et al. reported on 30 fetuses with prenatally diagnosed microcephaly[137]. The main referral indications were reduced head size or suspected IUGR (16 fetuses), intracranial anomalies (5 fetuses), and extracranial anomalies (3 fetuses). Mean gestational age at the time of referral was 27 weeks and, at the time of diagnosis, 28 weeks. Associated anomalies were present in 83.3% of the patients: holoprosencephaly (16.7%), chromosomal anomalies (23.3%), genetic syndromes (20%) and multiple anomalies (23.3%). Only 5 patients were considered to represent 'isolated microcephaly', but a careful analysis of these cases showed that three of them had other minor anomalies, one was probably associated with twin-to-twin transfusion syndrome with ventriculomegaly and one was diagnosed in a family with a previous history of microcephaly. The authors did not describe the number of fetuses with microcephaly diagnosed after delivery in their center.

Dahlgren and Wilson reviewed all cases of microcephaly diagnosed during a 10-year period at British Columbia Women's Hospital[138]. They found 45 patients; in 21, the diagnosis was made prenatally and confirmed postnatally. In 15 patients, the second-trimester ultrasound was available and 12 of these patients had a normal scan between 15 and 20 weeks of gestation. In 9 patients (43%), the etiologic cause of microcephaly remained unclear: possible viral infection based on placental signs of villitis or chorioamnionitis (4), multiple

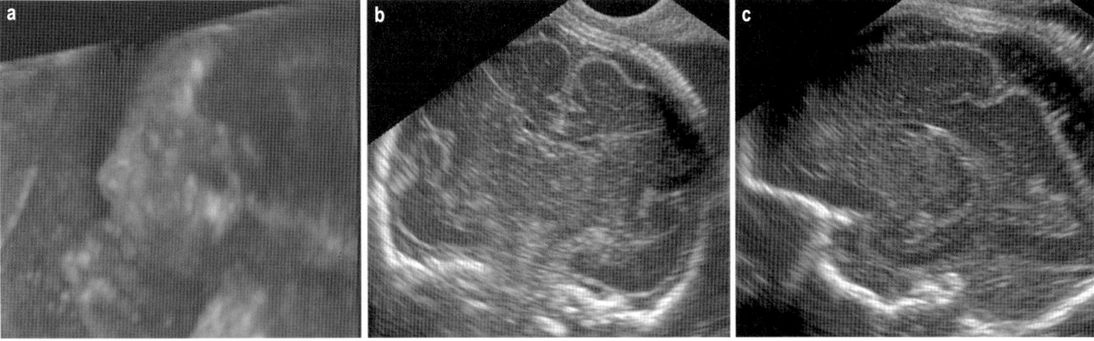

Fig. 30.22 Microcephaly: (a) sloping forehead in a fetus with a small head circumference increases the index of suspicion; (b,c) transvaginal neurosonogram in a 31 weeks' fetus with a small head circumference (247 mm = −3SD); (b) coronal view at the level of the Sylvian fissures, showing a simplified gyral pattern; (c) parasagittal view showing almost absolute lack of sulcation and an increase in the size of the subarachnoid space.

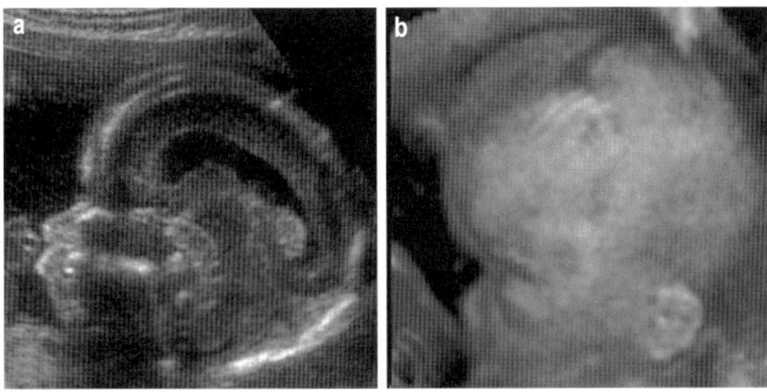

Fig. 30.23 Macrocephaly in a 20 weeks' fetus with chromosomal anomaly (46XX del [3q] 26.1–27.1). Head circumference: 203 mm (+2SD) (a) Sagittal transabdominal view showing frontal bossing, mild ventriculomegaly and micrognathia; (b) three-dimensional US of the fetal skull and face.

malformations (1), constitutional (1) and no specific etiology identified (3).

In some cases, the presence of microcephaly may be suspected based on additional sonographic findings like: small frontal lobe[139,140], enlarged subarachnoid space[140,141] and/or abnormal power Doppler demonstration of the anterior and middle cerebral arteries[140]. Our experience suggests that a sloping forehead (Fig. 30.22), although a rather subjective finding, may be of value in recognizing microcephaly[140]. The sensitivity and specificity of these findings in the diagnosis of microcephaly has never been evaluated, therefore its application for the diagnosis of microcephaly should be used with great caution if at all. In suspected cases, detailed neurosonographic examination and/or MRI may help in the diagnosis of abnormal gyration, heterotopia or subtle anomalies of the corpus callosum (Fig. 30.23).

The counseling dilemma for fetuses with a small HC remains difficult[142]. Mental retardation can safely be predicted in cases with associated US findings, abnormal karyotype or positive test for intrauterine infection. In fetuses with isolated small HC, an effort should be made to determine gyral normality in utero by US or MRI. Children with severe primary microcephaly may have a simplified gyral pattern that, in the most severe cases, may resemble lissencephaly. It is noteworthy that this pattern may develop late in pregnancy or even after delivery.

Primary microcephaly is genetically heterogeneous, with several loci currently mapped[143]. The advances in identifying genes associated with brain development will enable future prenatal molecular diagnosis in families at risk. The recurrence risk to parents of a child with primary microcephaly is 25%[143].

Macrocephaly

Macrocephaly is defined as a head circumference above the 98th percentile or more than 2 SD above the mean. In the absence of hydrocephaly or enlarged subarachnoid space, it is synonymous with megalencephaly. In a study of Swedish boys, it was found in 0.5% of the population and was associated with lower intelligence[144]. Other investigators found that the vast majority of children with megalencephaly have normal intelligence[145].

The most common form of megalencephaly is autosomal dominant and familial, and usually not associated with mental retardation. Yet, megalencephaly may be associated with many syndromes[146].

The prenatal diagnosis of macrocephaly has been occasionally reported[11,147–149]. The differential diagnosis in these cases is difficult. The demonstration of an enlarged subarachnoid space, particularly in the frontal region, in a fetus with macrocephaly is suggestive of benign enlargement of the subarachnoid spaces and is usually associated with a good prognosis (when the head circumference is normal or low, enlarged subarachnoid spaces may imply brain atrophy)[141]. The presence of ventriculomegaly, frontal bossing or associated malformations is an indication of a poor prognosis (see Fig. 30.23).

An essential part of the evaluation is measurement of the parents' head circumference. When one parent has a large head circumference, it is not immediately reassuring that the fetus has benign familial macrocephaly, since several syndromes that may combine macrocephaly and mental retardation can be inherited in an autosomal dominant fashion while the affected parent may only present with macrocephaly. These syndromes include neurofibromatosis type 1 (NF1), Sotos syndrome, Weaver syndrome, Cole-Hughes syndrome, and the inherited macrocephaly-hamartomas syndrome due to PTEN mutations. Therefore, a careful medical history of the affected parent should be obtained regarding neurological problems, developmental milestones, skin abnormalities, endocrine disorders and propensity for the development of tumors. The parent with macrocephaly should be examined with special attention to the skin (lipomas, macules, café au lait spots, neurofibromas) and

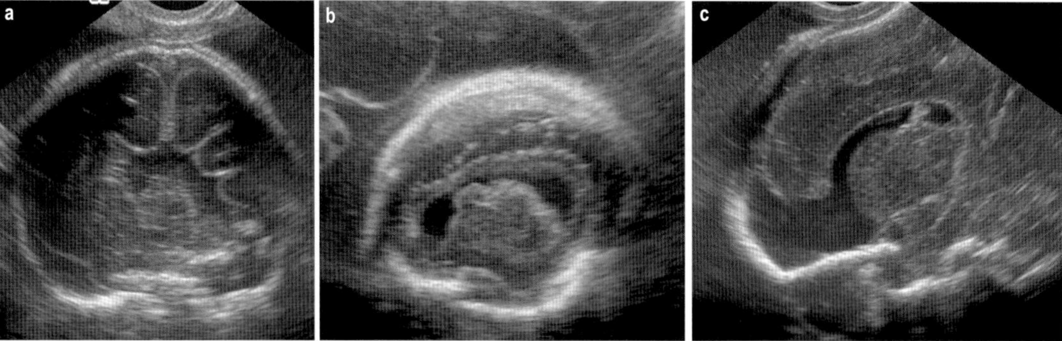

Fig. 30.24 (a) Thanatophoric dysplasia in a fetus at 23 weeks of gestation. TVS coronal plane shows bilateral abnormal overdeveloped sulci and gyri in the occipital lobes. (b) Lissencephaly in a 26 weeks' fetus in a twin pregnancy with hypoplastic left heart and microcephaly. Transabdominal parasagittal plane shows thin and irregular cortex surrounded by an increased amount cerebro-spinal fluid. (c) Frontal bilateral schizencephaly in a 25 weeks' fetus referred because of mild ventriculomegaly. Transvaginal parasagittal plane demonstrates the communication between the lateral ventricle and the subarachnoid space.

dysmorphic features. If there are specific findings in the parent, molecular diagnosis is now possible for NF1, Sotos syndrome and macrocephaly-hamartomas syndromes.

A large fetal head circumference is even more concerning when the parents have a normal head circumference. When it is associated with overgrowth, both Sotos and Weaver syndromes should be considered because most cases are sporadic. When it is observed in a fetus with short femur, skeletal dysplasias such as achondroplasia and hypochondroplasia are possible[11].

DISORDERS OF NEURONAL MIGRATION

Neuronal migration is an orderly process that starts at around 6 weeks' gestational age, but the exact time at which it ends remains controversial, but recent data suggest that it may occur between 24[150] and 30 weeks[151]. During this period, neurons multiply and move in successive waves from the periventricular germinal matrix through the cerebral cortex. As new waves of neurons reach the cortex, they position themselves close to the pia mater. By the end of this period, the fetal cortex is composed of six neuronal layers. Neuronal migration is closely associated with the development of the sulci and gyri since the number of neurons migrating in each successive wave rises exponentially and more space is needed at the surface of the cortex to accommodate them.

Our knowledge on migration disorders has been greatly increased since the advent of MRI and new genetic technologies. Classifications have been primarily based on data obtained from clinical, imaging or genetic aspects of these malformations in adult and pediatric populations[152,153]. Current classifications use all this information in a unified way[130,154].

Case reports[155–158] and small series of patients[159,160] diagnosed during pregnancy have been published. Recently, and following the description of normal fetal cortical development by MRI[161] and US[23,162,163], studies dealing with the prenatal diagnosis of malformations of cortical development (MCD) have described the different pathologic imaging patterns present during fetal life[110,164,165].

In the majority of prenatally diagnosed cases, the patient was referred for dedicated neurosonographic examination or for MRI because of the presence of abnormal cerebral or extracerebral findings, usually including multiple malformations with very reserved prognosis. However, the diagnosis of MCD in isolation remains an important factor in counseling and prenatal diagnosis in future pregnancies. Less severe cases, particularly those without ventriculomegaly usually remain undiagnosed. The fact that third-trimester evaluation of the brain is not routinely performed reduces the chance for diagnosis. Fong et al.[166], in a retrospective study of children born with Miller-Dieker syndrome, found that the disease was correctly diagnosed before delivery in only 3 out of 7 patients. The same group, in another study, proposed a method based on the demonstration of some of the major sulci as effective in the diagnosis of MCD[23].

Although MRI is considered the method of choice in the evaluation of both children and fetuses with suspected MCD, studies based on ultrasound examinations have proved to be effective at least in the more severe cases[165,167]. In the majority of the patients, a definitive etiologic diagnosis is possible only after delivery using the clinical, imaging, pathological and genetic data obtained.

Either by the use of ultrasound or MRI, the diagnosis of abnormal cortical development is based on the visualization of deviations from the normal sulcation patterns. Some of these abnormal patterns may be easy to identify (Fig. 30.24), but others require good knowledge of the normal sulcation patterns at different gestational ages (Fig. 30.25). The diagnosis will remain particularly difficult when the anomaly is isolated, focal or placed in a region of the brain of difficult access (temporal lobes, anterior portions of the frontal lobes).

DISORDERS OF CEREBELLAR DEVELOPMENT

The cerebellum starts its development by day 22 with the formation of the rhombencephalon and ends approximately 5 months after birth[168,169].

Different classifications of cerebellar malformations have been proposed based on the embryonic origin of the different structures affected[169,170], their imaging patterns[171] or genetics[172]. Although there is extensive research in this field, we have not yet reached a complete understanding of these diseases and very interesting breakthroughs should be expected in the near future.

We believe that presently the use of the embryologic classifications is easier to remember and helps in the understanding

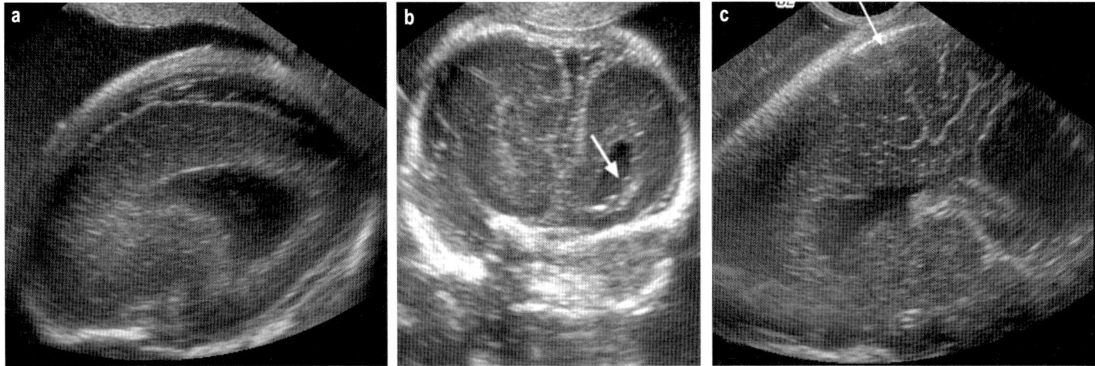

Fig. 30.25 (a) Lissencephaly in a fetus at 29 weeks referred because of mild bilateral ventriculomegaly. TVS parasagittal plane shows the enlarged ventricle, and lack of normal sulcation. (b) Periventricular heterotopia in a 22 weeks' fetus with agenesis of the corpus callosum. TVS coronal plane shows the irregular ventricular wall with the heterotopic nodule protruding into the lateral ventricle. (c) Pachygyria in a 40 weeks' fetus referred because of a large arachnoid cyst. Parasagittal plane shows normal sulcation in the posterior portion of the parietal lobe and abnormal sulcation in the anterior portion and frontal lobe. The arrow indicates the demarcation between the two zones.

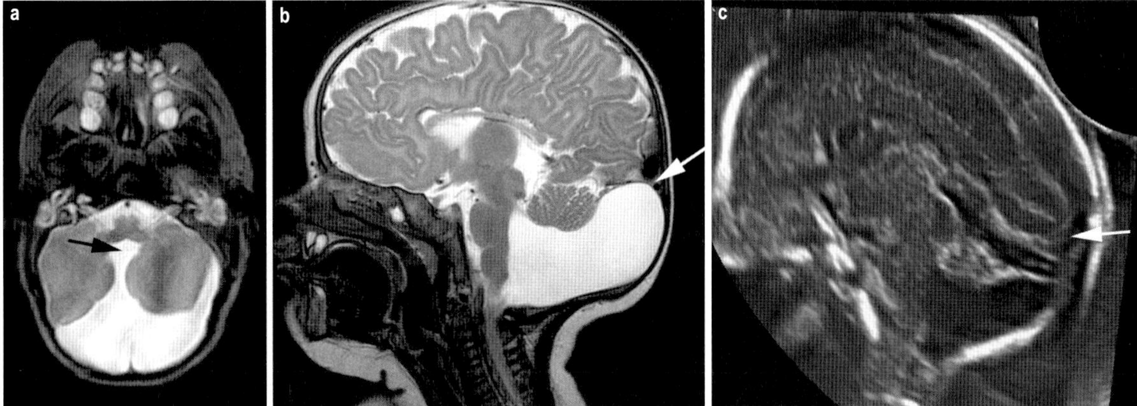

Fig. 30.26 Dandy–Walker malformation: (a,b) postnatal magnetic resonance demonstrating a large cisterna communicating with the area of the fourth ventricle (black arrow), rotation of the cerebellar vermis and superior displacement of the tentorium cerebelli and torcular herophilii (white arrow); (c) a similar case diagnosed antenatally; the arrow indicates the high position of tentorium and torcular.

of the different pathologies, the time of their occurrence and, more importantly, the limitations and possible pitfalls found in prenatal diagnosis of these conditions.

The different parts of the cerebellum develop from three different portions: the archicerebellum forms the flocculonodular lobe; the paleocerebellum the floculi of the hemispheres and the vermis; and the neocerebellum the cerebellar hemispheres excluding the flocculi[169]. Malformations of the paleocerebellum involve the vermis and malformations of the neocerebellum almost exclusively the cerebellar hemispheres. Involvement of the entire cerebellum is extremely rare producing cerebellar aplasia or may be found in conjunction with an involvement of the midbrain and the rest of the hindbrain or may be due to malformations associated with late prenatal degeneration[170].

Malformations of the paleocerebellum

Malformations of the paleocerebellum include Dandy–Walker malformation and isolated cerebellar vermis hypoplasia; 'molar tooth' sign associated malformations and rhomboencephalosynapsis may also be included in this category, but they are usually associated with other anomalies of the pons and midbrain.

Dandy–Walker malformation is exceedingly rare, with an estimated incidence of about 1:30 000 births, and is found in 4–12% of all cases of infantile hydrocephalus. However, minor variations of this condition are rather frequently encountered, as attested by the increasing number of reports, in both the prenatal and pediatric literature.

The term *Dandy-Walker syndrome or malformation* was originally introduced to indicate the association of:

1. ventriculomegaly of variable degree
2. a large cisterna magna
3. a defect in the cerebellar vermis through which the cyst communicates with the fourth ventricle.

In these cases, the axial planes demonstrate a large cisterna magna and a median V-shaped defect of the cerebellum that extends into the fourth ventricle. In the median plane, which is the most important one for the diagnosis, the cisterma magna extends superiorly, displacing the cerebellar vermis (which is frequently hypoplastic) and elevating above its normal position the *tentorium cerebelli* and the *torcular Herophili* (Fig. 30.26). The presence of ventriculomegaly is not essential to make the diagnosis because, in many cases, it has been found to develop only years after birth. Dandy–Walker malformation is frequently

Table 30.6 **Abnormalities associated with Dandy–Walker malformation**

Malformations	*Mendelian*	*Chromosomal*	*Environmental*
Holoprosencephaly	Warburg (AR)	45,X	Rubella
Agenesis of the corpus callosum	Aase-Smith (AD)	6p-	Coumadin
Neural tube defects	Ruvalcaba syndrome (AD/X-linked)	9q+	Alcohol
Cleft lip	Coffin-Siris (AR)	dup 5p	Cytomegalovirus
Congenital heart disease	Oro-facio-digital syndrome type II (AR)	dup 8p	Diabetes
Cornelia de Lange syndrome	Meckel Gruber syndrome (AR)	dup 8q	Isotretinoin
Goldenhar syndrome	Aicardi syndrome (X-linked dominant)	trisomy 9	
Kidney abnormalities	Ellis Van Creveld (AR)	triploidy	
Facial hemangiomas	Fraser cryptophthalmus (AR)	dup 17q	
Klippel-Feil syndrome			
Polysyndactyly			

AR/AD = autosomal recessive/autosomal dominant

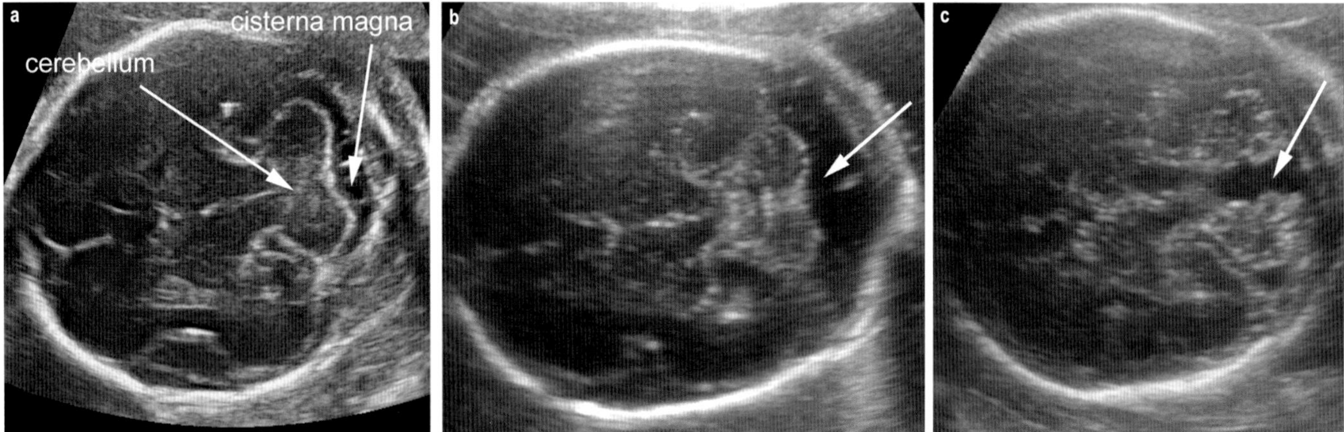

Fig. 30.27 The normal transcerebellar scan (a) compared with variations of the Dandy–Walker continuum; (b) an enlarged cisterna magna with a seemingly normal vermis; (c) a cerebellar 'cleft' suggesting a vermian defect.

associated with other neural defects, mostly with other midline anomalies, such as agenesis of the corpus callosum and holoprosencephaly. Other deformities include encephaloceles, polycystic kidneys, cardiovascular defects and facial clefting. Table 30.6 lists the most frequent associations. Cases with associated malformations have a poor prognosis. Recent experience with MRI in infants suggests that those cases in which the vermis appears hypoplastic have a subnormal intelligence in 85% of cases versus only 15% of those in which the vermis appears intact[173,174]. In the original study, the cerebellar vermis was considered normal if it was possible with MRI to document in the median plane three main anatomic landmarks: the fastigium point that corresponds to the posterior apex of the fourth ventricle and the two main fissures. A similar approach has also been suggested for antenatal studies. Both MRI and multiplanar, possibly transvaginal ultrasound can be used. It is expected, however, that the small size of the vermis and the difficulty in obtaining an exact median plane will represent major limiting factors, particularly in early gestation. We need to emphasize the importance of visualization of the pons and midbrain since involvement of these structures in the pathology carries a very poor prognosis.

The term *Dandy-Walker complex* (or *continuum*) has been used to indicate a spectrum of abnormal findings that share in common an enlargement of the cisterna magna and/or the impression of a V-shaped cleft in the cerebellar vermis in the axial plane (Figs. 30.27, 30.28)[173,175,176]. The current understanding of vermian malformations considers classical Dandy–Walker malformation (with a large cisterna magna and elevated tentorium) and vermian hypoplasia/dysgenesis (with a normal size cisterna magna) two separate and distinct entities with different etiologies and prognoses.

Distinction between an intact and a hypoplastic vermis is far from simple. Under normal conditions during mid-gestation, it is usually possible with either sonography or MRI sagittal planes to demonstrate the fastigium of the fourth ventricle and the two main fissures[173–175]. With hypoplasia of the vermis, these landmarks cannot be identified. Nomograms of

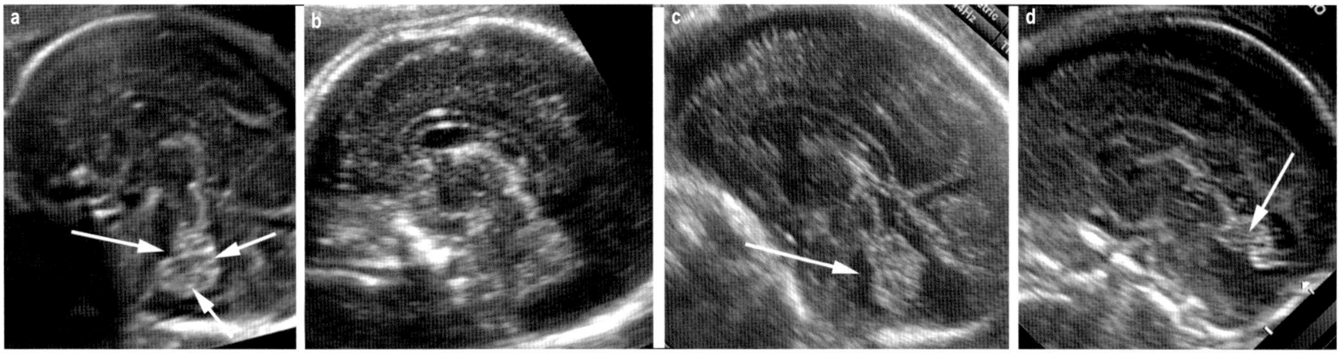

Fig. 30.28 The normal midsagittal view (a) demonstrating the main landmarks of the cerebellar vermis (fastigium of fourth ventricle and the two main fissures) (arrows) is compared with variations of the Dandy–Walker continuum: (b) enlargement of the cisterna magna with an intact vermis (megacisterna magna); (c) upward rotation (arrow) of a seemingly intact vermis (Blake's pouch cyst) and (d) upward rotation of an hypoplastic vermis (vermian hypoplasia).

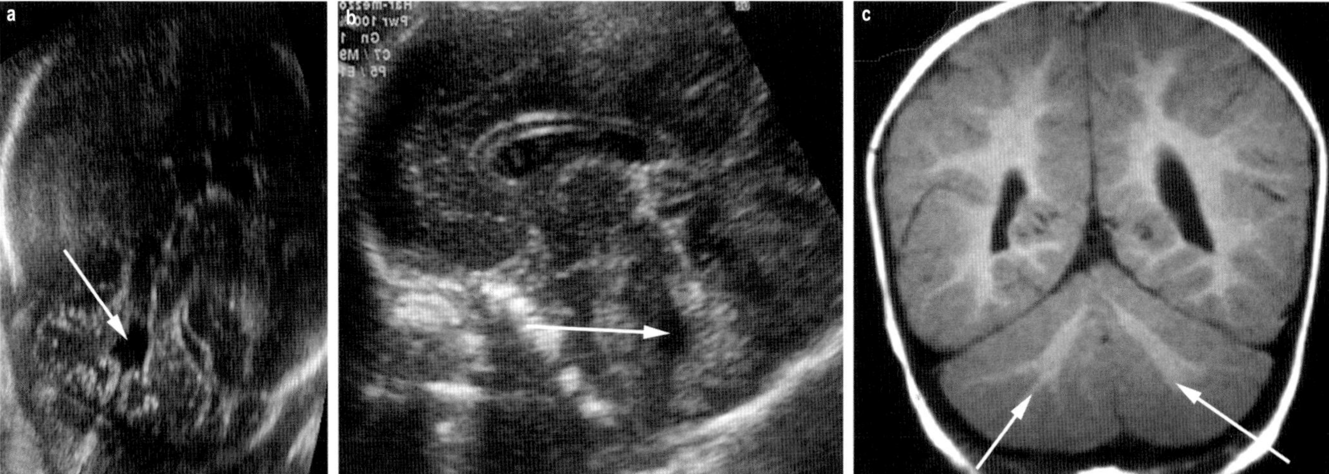

Fig. 30.29 Joubert syndrome. The sonographic findings are limited to the presence of a communication between the fourth ventricle and the cisterna magna (a) and an abnormal shape of the fourth ventricle (b). Postnatally, magnetic resonance demonstrates the absence of the cerebellar vermis. (Courtesy Philippe Jeanty, Nashville, Tennessee.)

the normal size of the vermis throughout gestation are also available[177].

The greatest diagnostic challenge is probably represented by molar tooth sign associated malformations and particularly by *Joubert syndrome*, a group of disorders with autosomal recessive transmission characterized by hypoplasia of the cerebellar vermis with the characteristic neuroradiologic molar tooth sign and neurologic symptoms, including dysregulation of breathing pattern, abnormal eye movements, developmental delay, retinal dystrophy and renal anomalies. Variable features include encephaloceles and polydactyly. In a pregnancy at specific risk, the condition can be suspected when a communication is seen between the fourth ventricle and a cisterna magna of normal size in the transverse plane (Fig. 30.29)[178]. In the absence of the vermis, the two hemispheres impinge on the midline and therefore the median plane is of little use, although at times it may demonstrate a fourth ventricle of slightly irregular shape[178]. In the absence of a positive familial history, this finding has a very low predictive value and most cases that we have seen were found to be normal at birth.

Caution is warranted while making the diagnosis of any vermian anomaly before 20–24 weeks' gestation since these 'suspected findings' frequently represent an artefact mimicking a vermian defect[179].

In general, meticulous scanning with a multiplanar approach is recommended in cases with a suspicion of a posterior fossa anomaly. The poor correlation that has been demonstrated in several studies between antenatal diagnosis and autopsy finding is probably related to the use of only axial planes that can be extremely misleading. In the axial plane, entities that are clinically different, such as Dandy–Walker malformation, vermian hypoplasia, Blake's pouch cyst cannot be distinguished.

As the diagnosis of posterior fossa anomalies depends upon section planes of the fetal head that are sometimes difficult to obtain, we have found that three-dimensional ultrasound is frequently of considerable help. Multiplanar slicing of a volume obtained from axial scans usually provide images of diagnostic quality[119].

Malformations of the neocerebellum

Neocerebellar dysgenesis is much rarer than paleocerebellar anomalies and is usually found in association with other CNS anomalies or with chromosomal anomalies. In some cases, particularly when unilateral, it may represent an acquired disorder[180].

Posterior fossa fluid collection

Mega-cisterna magna and posterior fossa arachnoid cyst are the main diagnoses to consider when a large posterior fossa with normal cerebellar structures is found.

Mega-cisterna magna is diagnosed when the cisterna magna depth is more than 10 mm, the cerebellar vermis appears intact, in normal position and without signs of pressure to surrounding structures (see Figs. 30.27, 30.28). Although this is a risk factor for associated malformations including aneuploidies (trisomy 18 in particular)[181,182], most isolated cases are of no consequence[119,175,183,184]. If there is the impression of a V-shaped cleft in the cerebellum in the axial plane and the median plane reveals a vermis that is intact, the diagnosis is most likely a *Blake's pouch cyst* and the prognosis is also usually good[184,185] (see Figs. 30.27, 30.28).

In our own experience, isolated mega-cisterna magna and Blake's pouch cyst represent the bulk of the posterior fossa anomalies that are diagnosed antenatally[119]. Although the data thus far are limited and the neurologic risk cannot be predicted precisely, it would seem that in the majority of these cases the prognosis is good.

Arachnoid cysts also carry an excellent prognosis, although they may occasionally produce complications related to increased pressure on surrounding structures that may cause ventriculomegaly and may need neurosurgical intervention in the neonatal period[22].

PRENATAL INSULTS

Destructive cerebral lesions

Many congenital anomalies of the brain are not the consequence of an embryogenetic malformative process but are due to a destructive process. The pathophysiology is frequently unclear and, in many cases, the etiology remains unknown. A link with a variety of obstetric complications is, however, frequently found.

Intracranial hemorrhage (ICH) is usually found at the level of the lateral ventricles, although it can occur in other anatomical locations. It is a frequent complication in the premature infant. Although rare, it may occur antenatally, as a consequence of coagulopathy, such as alloimmune thrombocytopenia, or trauma, or other unexplained factors. The sonographic appearance of an intracranial hemorrhage is extremely variable depending upon the severity and the timing of its occurrence (Fig. 30.30)[186]. Blood accumulated into the ventricles appears as an echogenic collection initially. With time, the blood clot retracts and demonstrates an anechoic core and there is frequently ventricular dilatation (grade 3 hemorrhage). Large hemorrhagic collections may be complicated by infarct and destruction of the surrounding white matter (grade 4 hemorrhage).

The prognosis is poor. In a review of the literature, perinatal death occurred in about 50% of cases and 50% of survivors had neurologic compromise at long-term follow-up. There was a correlation between the outcome and the grade of the hemorrhage. The prognosis was more favorable with grade 1 and 2 hemorrhages (hemorrhage limited to the germinal matrix or lateral ventricles without ventriculomegaly), with possible resolution in utero, but was usually severe with grade 3 and 4 lesions (intraventricular hemorrage associated with severe ventriculomegaly and white matter destruction, respectively)[186].

Congenital *porencephaly* is defined as the presence of cystic cavities within the brain matter. The cavities usually communicate with either the ventricular system, the subarachnoid space or both[187]. Loss of cerebral tissue may derive from a morphogenetic disorder (true porencephaly or *schizencephaly*). More frequently, it is the consequence of an intrauterine disruption (pseudoporencephaly or encephaloclastic porencephaly). The developmental form is typically bilateral and symmetrical and is frequently associated with microcephaly. In *pseudoporencephaly*, a unilateral lesion is usually found. In both cases, there is a wide variability in the size of the lesion[187]. Cerebrospinal fluid turnover is often impaired and hydrocephalus is present.

Hydranencephaly can be regarded as an extreme form of pseudoporencephaly. Most of the cerebral hemispheres are replaced by fluid. The brainstem and rhomboencephalic structures are usually spared. The head may be small, of normal size or extremely enlarged. The etiology is heterogeneous. Congenital infections, including toxoplasmosis and cytomegalovirus, and intrauterine strangulation or occlusion of the internal carotid arteries have been reported. Accurate antenatal

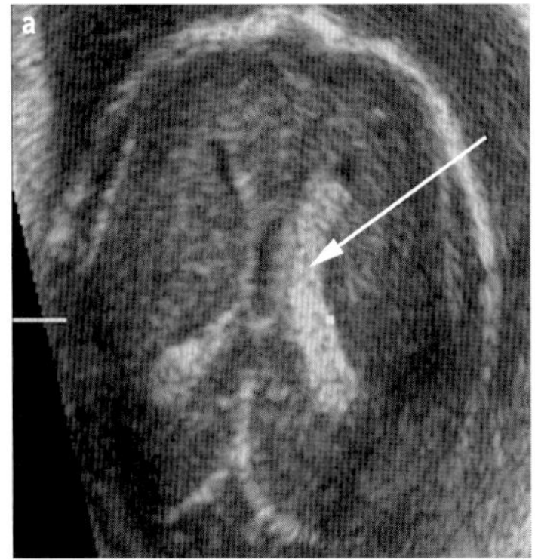

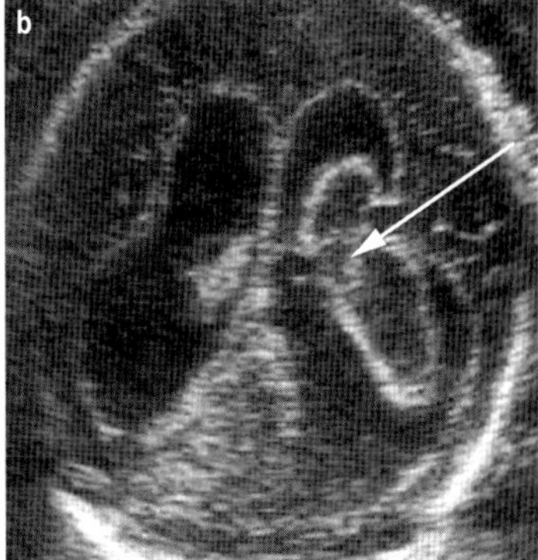

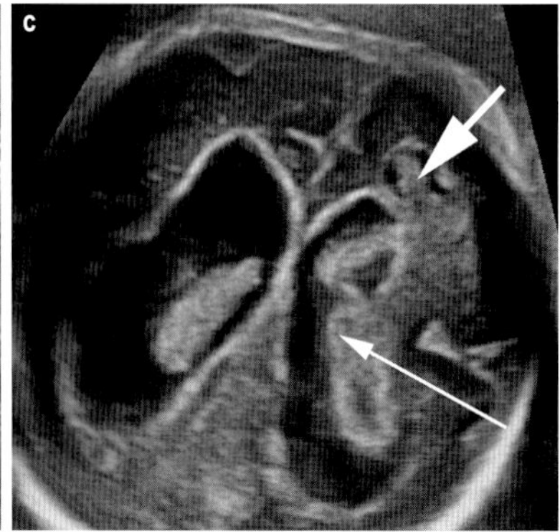

Fig. 30.30 Types of intracranial hemorrhage: (a) soon after the hemorrhage, the blood is intensely echogenic (arrow); this is grade II hemorrhage; (b) an old hemorrhage; the coronal scan demonstrates a typical blood clot and ventricular enlargement (grade 3 hemorrhage); (c) grade IV hemorrhage: the arrow indicates an intraventricular blood clot, the arrowhead a destructive lesion in the periventricular cortex.

diagnosis of both schizencephaly and porencephaly has been reported (Fig. 30.31). It should be stressed, however, that porencephaly is a disruption condition that usually occurs only in the third trimester.

The outcome of infants with a congenital destructive process of the brain is dictated by the size and location of the lesion. Extensive porencephaly, particularly if associated with hydrocephalus or microcephaly, and hydranencephaly have a uniformly poor outcome[187].

Periventricular leukomalacia is a degenerative disorder of the white matter that is most frequently encountered in premature infants and is frequently associated with a poor prognosis. The cystic variety of this condition has been described recently in the fetus. The diagnosis is made by demonstrating multiple small cysts close to the upper corner of the lateral ventricles (see Fig. 30.31)[188].

INTRAUTERINE INFECTIONS AFFECTING THE BRAIN

Although uncommon, intrauterine infections may severely affect the fetal brain. Infective agents that are potentially dangerous include not only the TORCH complex (toxoplasma, rubella, cytomegalovirus (CMV), herpes virus[189]), but other microorganisms may, in certain conditions, produce prenatal CNS damage including: bacteria (syphilis and probably also tuberculosis[190]), viral (varicella[191], congenital lymphocytic choriomeningitis virus[192] and echovirus[193]) and parasites (filariasis[194]).

Cytomegalovirus

Human cytomegalovirus is an endemic virus from the herpes virus group that produces cytoplasmatic inclusions after infecting human cells (see Chapter 44).

CMV infective fetopathy may produce different patterns of brain insults depending fundamentally on the time of infection and the virulence of the microorganism involved. Periventricular white matter involvement in the form of increased echodensity with or without cysts is consistently present and is usually accompanied by ventriculomegaly, intraventricular adhesions, calcifications, signs of vasculitis and/or microcephaly[116] (Fig. 30.32). Cortical, callosal and cerebellar involvement is also frequent.

In the newborn, the presence of positive ultrasound signs and/or microcephaly has been shown to carry a more than

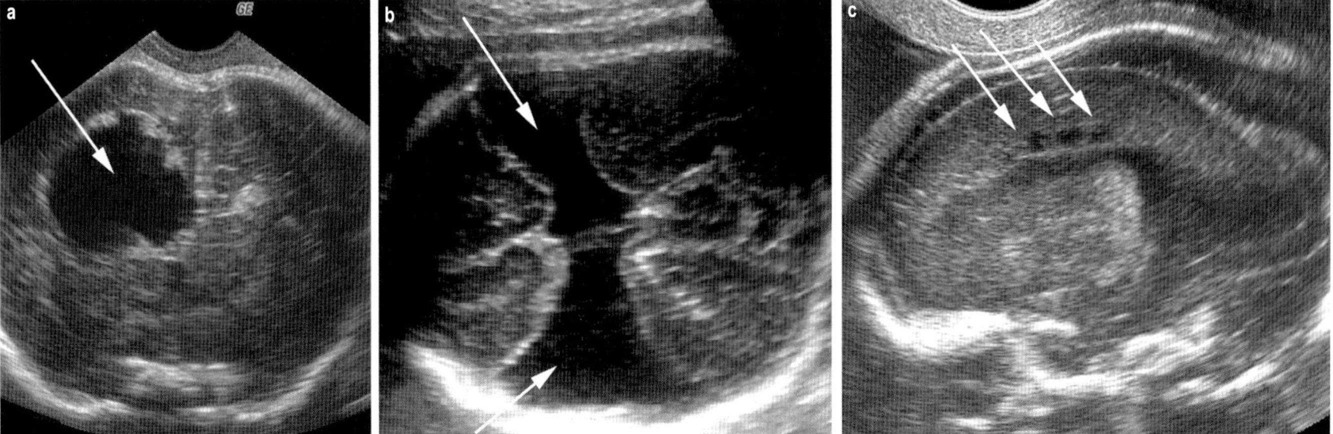

Fig. 30.31 Destructive lesions of the fetal brain: (a) porencephalic cyst; (b) schizencephaly; (c) periventricular leukomalacia.

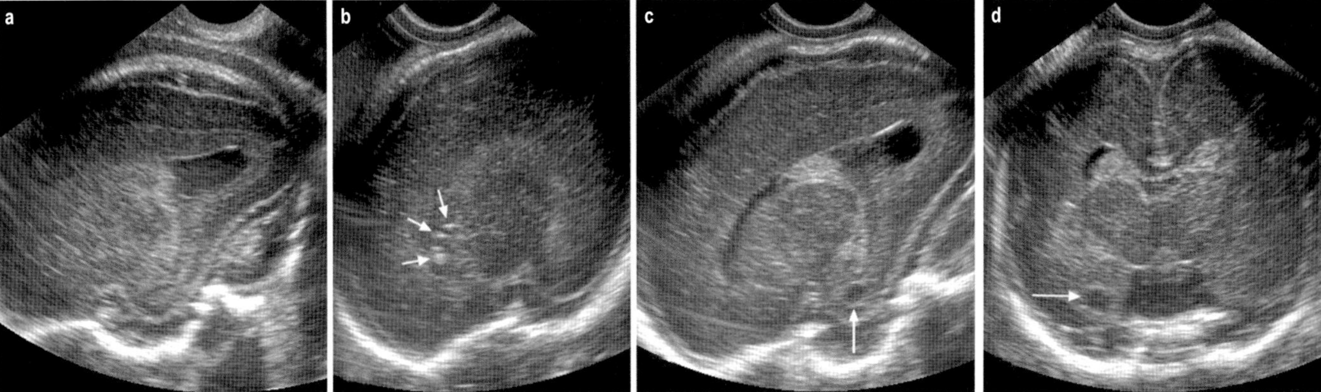

Fig. 30.32 First trimester CMV seroconversion in a 28 weeks' pregnancy showing: (a) periventricular hyperechogenic tissue, note the clear delineation between the affected periventricular zone and the rest of the brain; (b) periventricular punctuate hyperechogenicities, consistent with focal calcifications (arrows); (c) parasagittal view through the lateral ventricle showing the presence of a small temporal cyst (arrow). (d) Coronal view showing the temporal cyst (arrow).

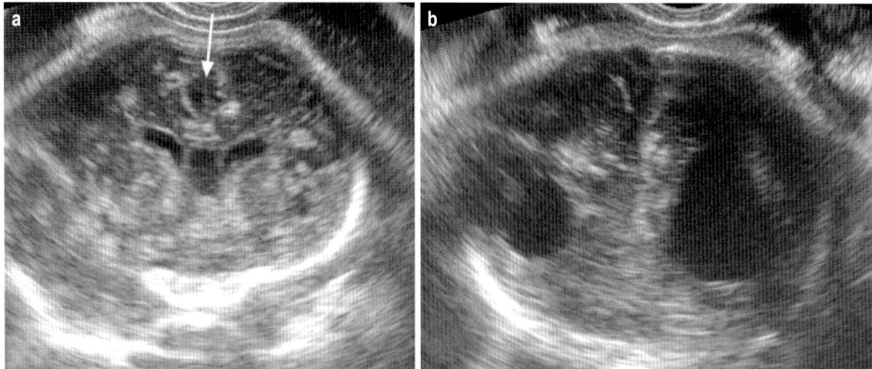

Fig. 30.33 Toxoplasmosis in a 34 weeks' fetus, postnatal serologic confirmation. (a) Coronal TVS plane at the level of the frontal horns of the lateral ventricles showing multiple nodular echodensities. The wide open intrahemispheric fissure (arrow) rises the suspicion of developing brain atrophy. (b) Coronal TVS plane at the level of the occipital horns showing asymmetric ventriculomegaly. (Courtesy of Dr Mauricio Herrera, Bogotà, Colombia.)

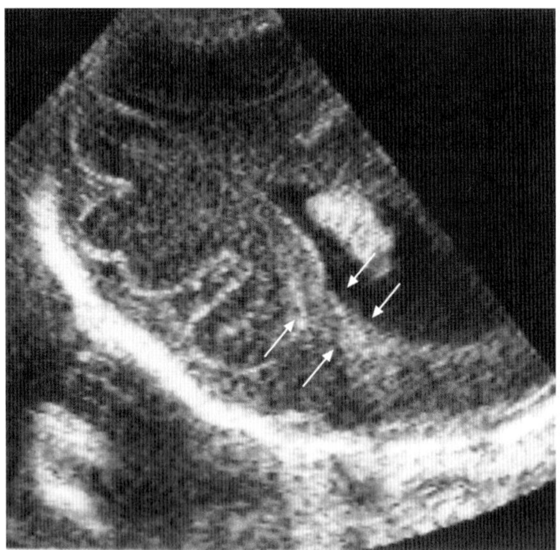

Fig. 30.34 Pachygyria in a 34 weeks' fetus with postnatal confirmation of congenital syphilis. Note the presence of ventriculomegaly and slightly echogenic and irregular periventricular white matter (arrows).

90% risk of neurodevelopmental delay and/or sensorineural hearing loss[195].

Toxoplasma gondii

Toxoplasma gondii is a parasite transmitted by consumption of infected raw meat or by exposure to oocysts (see Chapter 44). Only primary infection during pregnancy may produce fetal infection. The classical signs of congenital toxoplasma infection are chorioretinitis, calcifications and hydrocephalus, but the spectrum and severity of the disease is highly variable and may be difficult to differentiate from other intrauterine infections without amniocentesis (Fig. 30.33). Toxoplasma is the only infective fetopathy amenable to intrauterine treatment with spiramycin, sulfadiazine or a combination of sulfadiazine and pyrimethamine[196].

Syphilis

Although preconception or early first-trimester tests for syphilis are an integral part of routine pregnancy follow-up and early treatment of affected women has reduced almost to zero the incidence of congenital syphilis in industrialized countries, occasional cases may still occur (Fig. 30.34). As in other intrauterine infections affecting the brain, the insult depends on its time of occurrence (see Chapter 44).

VASCULAR ABNORMALITIES

Vascular anomalies of the fetal brain are rare and only a handful of cases has been described thus far. The majority of reports concentrate upon the vein of Galen vascular malformations. More recently, thrombosis of the dural sinuses has been described.

The term aneurysm of the vein of Galen indicates a spectrum of arteriovenous malformations, ranging from a single large aneurysmal dilatation of the vein of Galen to multiple communications between the vein and the carotid and vertebrobasilar systems[197]. Three types are described:

1. arteriovenous fistula
2. arteriovenous malformation with ectasia of the vein of Galen and
3. varix of the vein of Galen.

The arteriovenous fistula is frequently manifest in the fetal or neonatal period with high output heart failure due to cardiac overload. Both the ectasia and the varix tend to present later in life with bleeding episodes and are not associated with cardiac failure. Arteriovenous fistulae associated with a varix are not part of the definition when they are located elsewhere in the brain.

Prenatally, the typical finding is an elongated anechoic area at the level of the cistern of the vein of Galen, with color and pulsed Doppler evidence of turbulent venous and/or blood arterial flow[198]. The cerebral architecture may be intact, or it may be distorted because of the concomitance of ventriculomegaly, porencephaly and/or brain edema, that is inferred by increased echogenicity of the cortex. The dural sinuses and neck vessels are frequently enlarged, and signs of cardiac overload may be present, including cardiomegaly, hepatosplenomegaly, soft

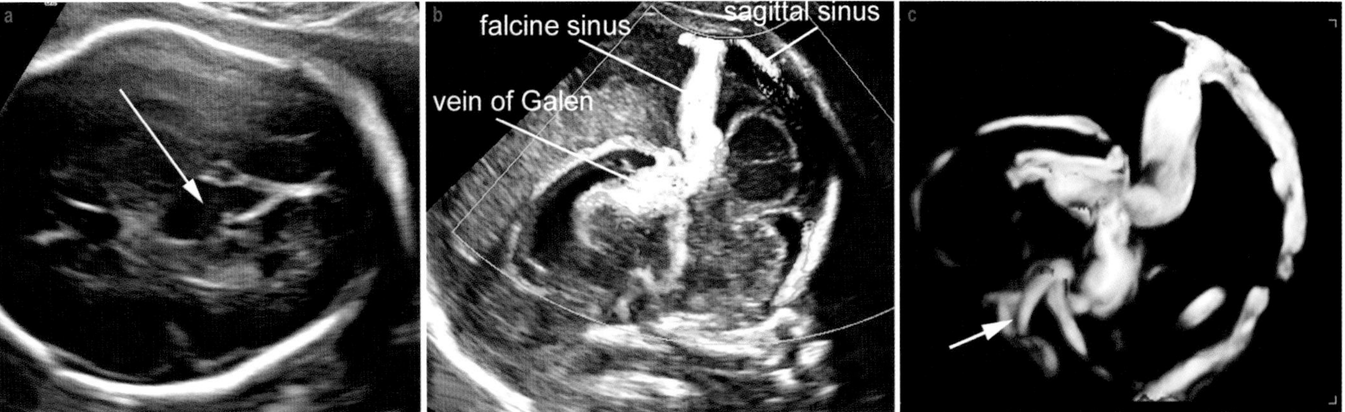

Fig. 30.35 Aneurysm of the vein of Galen: (a) 2-dimensional image obtained transabdominally with an axial approach demonstrating the aneurysm (arrow); (b) transvaginal color Doppler image demonstrating that the aneurysmatic vein of Galen does not enter the straight sinus but connects superiorly to the falcine sinus that drains into the superior sagittal sinus; (c) 3D color Doppler rendering of one ultrasound volume obtained from a transvaginal approach demonstrating in one single image the different elements of the vascular malformations, including the multiple anastosmoses between the arteries of the skull base (arrow) and the vein of Galen, which drains into the falcine sinus.

tissue edema, polyhydramnios and hydrops. Color Doppler may help in identifying the origin of the vessels feeding the lesion, an observation that may have practical implications for assessing the prognosis (Fig. 30.35). MRI has also been used in these cases.

Although vein of Galen aneurysms may become symptomatic in the elderly, they are more frequently seen in the neonatal period. The common clinical features in the neonate are cardiomegaly with congestive heart failure and increased intracranial pressure with hydrocephaly or cranial bruit. Focal neurological deficit, seizure and hemorrhages are less common findings. The available experience with prenatal diagnosis suggests a mortality rate in the range of 50% and a normal development in about 50% of survivors[187,198,199]. The outcome is strongly dependent upon the antenatal evidence of other intracranial abnomalities (hydrocephalus, brain edema, porencephaly) and/or hydrops. When any of these are found, the prognosis is always poor. In general, cases with normal postnatal development had isolated vascular lesions, without cerebral or cardiovascular compromise in utero, and were treated after birth with angiographic embolization[199].

Dural sinus thrombosis is a well-known entity in the neonatal period that has been documented in utero as well. The etiology includes trauma, systemic conditions such as sepsis, meningitis and dehydration and hypercoagulopathy caused by polycythemia or deficiency of physiological anticoagulants (antithrombin, protein C or protein S, factor V Leiden mutation). Prematurity and perinatal asphyxia are considered predisposing factors. A possible role of maternal pre-eclampsia has also been suggested. However, in up to 40% of cases the condition is idiopathic[200].

In the cases thus far diagnosed in utero, ultrasound revealed the dilated superior sagittal sinus containing a thrombus. Color Doppler demonstates the interruption of blood flow at the level of the dilated sinuses (Fig. 30.36)[200]. MRI and MRI angiography are the techniques of choice for the diagnosis after birth and have been used antenatally as well.

The clinical presentation of thrombosis of the dural sinuses in newborn infants is variable. Symptoms include seizures, unexplained irritability, macrocephaly or a bulging fontanelle. Postnatal studies reveal that, in general, thrombosis of the cerebral venous circulation is an important and under-recognized cause of seizures in term infants. The natural history is variable. In the absence of perinatal asphyxia, normal neurodevelopmental outcome is likely and the risk of seizure recurrence is low. A poor outcome should be expected especially in preterm neonates and in cases of secondary cerebral sinus thrombosis. Associated imaging signs such as infarction or ventricular hemorrhage are correlated with poor prognosis. Sequelae may also depend on the location of the thrombus. In a recent study, all patients with permanent neurologic disability had thrombosis of the deep veins with an associated deep cerebral infarction; in contrast, all patients with thrombosis without infarction or with superficial cortical venous infarction had uniformly a good outcome[201].

INTRACRANIAL CYSTS

Intracranial arachnoid cysts are an accumulation of clear cerebrospinal-like fluid between the dura and the brain substance. The histologic diagnosis is not always available and the term is frequently used to indicate any intracranial cyst located in the subarachnoid space.

Arachnoid cysts are found anywhere in the central nervous system including the spinal canal. The most frequent locations are the surface of the cerebral hemispheres in the sites of the major fissures (Sylvian, rolandic and interhemispheric), the region of sella turcica, the anterior fossa and the middle fossa. Less frequently, they are seen in the posterior fossa. Most of the cases diagnosed antenatally involve supratentorial cysts, in the midline, Sylvian fissure and ambient cistern. Arachnoid cysts may be primary (congenital) or secondary (acquired). Congenital types are believed to be formed by maldevelopment of the leptomeninges and do not freely communicate with the subarachnoid space. Acquired types are formed as the result of hemorrhage, trauma and infection and often communicate with the subarachnoid space. Arachnoid cysts have the potential to grow as the result of either some communication with the subarachnoid space from a ball valve mechanism or

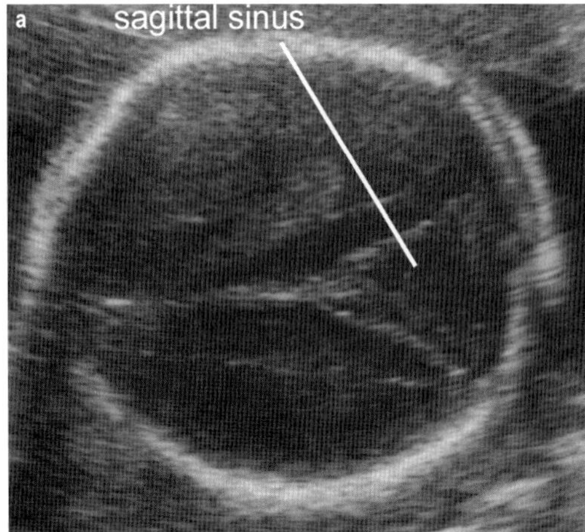

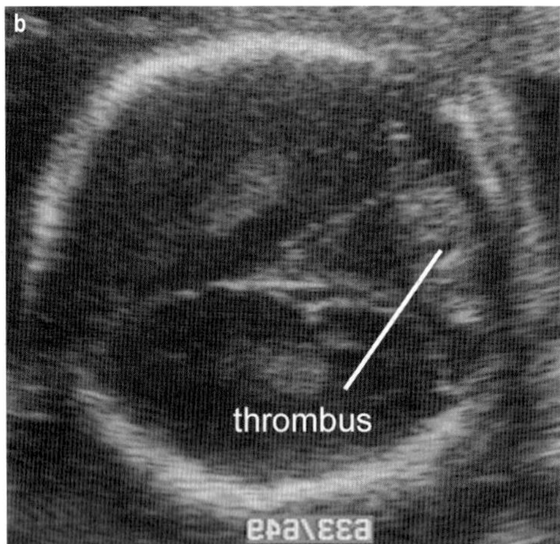

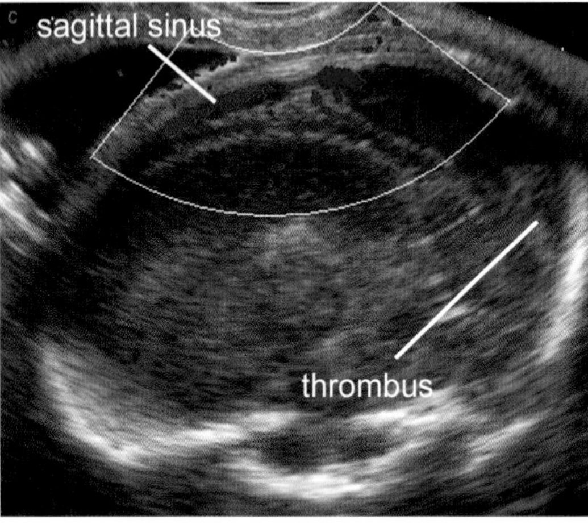

Fig. 30.36 Congenital thrombosis of the dural sinuses: (a) a large fluid collection is seen posteriorly to the brain (long arrow), corresponding to the dilated superior sagittal sinus, (b) within the greatly enlarged sinus a thrombus is seen as an echogenic mass; (c) color Doppler ultrasound demonstrates cessation of blood flow (arrow) within the enlarged portion of the superior sagittal sinus.

cerebrospinal fluid production by a choroid plexus-like tissue contained within the cyst wall. Large arachnoid cysts can cause obstructive ventriculomegaly by compressing the foramen of Monro, the aqueduct posteriorly, or blocking the basal cisterns. Hydrocephalus and macrocephaly are the most common presentations in the neonatal period. Arachnoid cysts have been reported very rarely in association with other anomalies. The list includes trisomy 18, tetralogy of Fallot, sacrococcygeal tumor and neurofibromatosis.

Ultrasound examination of arachnoid cysts demonstrates a well-defined anechoic lesion with adjacent mass effect, occasionally associated with hydrocephalus (Fig. 30.37). The majority of arachnoid cysts diagnosed in utero thus far have been recognized only in the third trimester. In a few cases, unremarkable sonograms had been obtained in the midtrimester. It is therefore likely that most of these lesions develop only in late gestation. Differentiating fetal arachnoid cysts from other intracranial fluid collections may be difficult at times. However, in the largest available series, multiplanar brain imaging and vaginal sonography of vertex fetuses were found to be extremely effective[187]. Porencephalic cysts are located inside the brain substance, whereas arachnoid cysts lie between the skull and brain surface. Furthermore, the majority of congenital porencephalic cysts communicate with the lateral ventricles. In schizencephaly, the fluid-filled collection connects the lateral ventricles to the subarachnoid space.

A posterior fossa arachnoid cyst is distinguished from the Dandy–Walker complex by demonstrating the integrity of the cerebellar vermis. Another useful clue is the demonstration that arachnoid cysts tend to be laterally positioned and result in an asymmetric posterior fossa.

In many cases, arachnoid cysts are asymptomatic, but they may cause epilepsy, mild motor or sensory abnormalities, or hydrocephalus. Hydrocephalus and macrocephaly are the most common presentations in the neonatal period.

The neurosurgical series suggest in general a good prognosis, with absence of symptoms in more than 70% of cases. The location of the cyst has influence on the final outcome. In one series, the temporal cysts were found to have the best outcome, with more than 90% of patients recovering completely or with only slight deficits, and there were no deaths. The other locations were associated with a significantly lower success rate. In particular, posterior fossa arachnoid cysts had the worst outcomes[202,203].

Glioependymal cysts are thought to derive from displaced neuroectodermal tissue and have the same ultrasound appearance as arachnoid cysts[204]. Differentiation between these two entities is usually possible only on the basis of histologic examination. The diagnosis of a gliopendymal cysts should, however, be considered when the cyst is in the midline and is associated with agenesis of the corpus callosum. The distinction may not be clinically relevant, as it is uncertain whether the prognostic implications are different.

Choroid plexus cysts appear as round sonolucent areas in the context of the choroid plexus of lateral ventricles (Fig. 30.38). They have been described with increasing frequency over the last years. Survey of low-risk pregnant patients indicates that the frequency of this finding in the midtrimester is in the range of 1%. However, the real incidence is probably dependent upon the resolution of the ultrasound equipment, the attention of the operator and the definition of choroid plexus cyst that is employed. On average, the incidence in most studies is in the range of 1%. However, figures as high as 3.6% have been reported[205,206].

Choroid plexus cysts may be unilateral or bilateral and, occasionally, are multiple. They are typically found at the level of the atrium of the lateral ventricles, less frequently within the bodies. When examined with high-resolution ultrasound

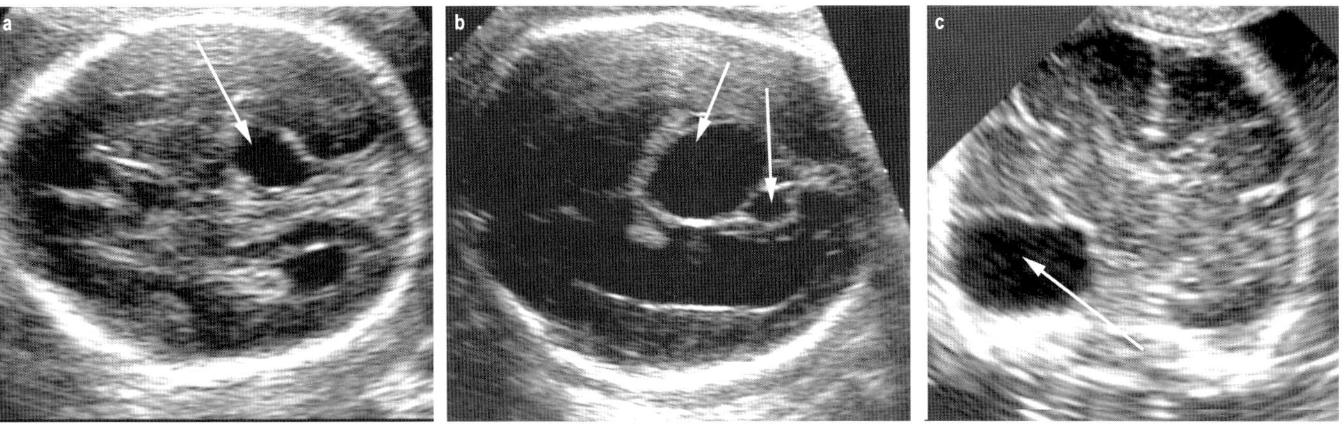

Fig. 30.37 Sonograms of fetuses with arachnoid cysts. (a) A small cyst in the ambient cistern; (b) a midline bilocular cyst; (c) a very large cyst arising from the Sylvian fissure.

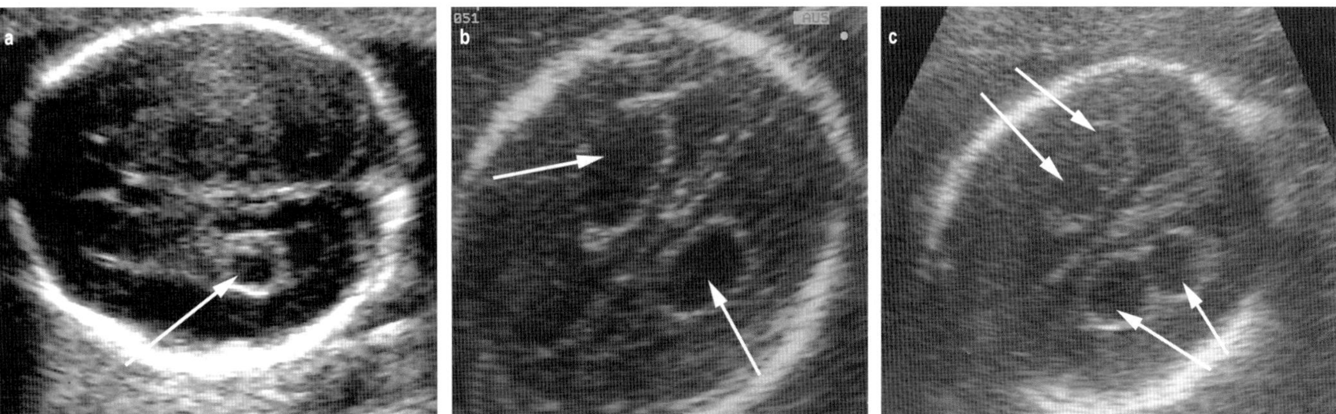

Fig. 30.38 Choroid plexus cyst: (a) single and small; (b) large bilateral; (c) multiple.

equipment, the choroid plexus often appears slightly heterogeneous. Choroid plexus cysts should measure at least 2 mm in diameter. Large cysts up to 14 mm may be seen, and usually contain internal septa.

The diagnosis of a choroid plexus cyst is readily made in the majority of cases by noting the typical location within the atria of lateral ventricles, with a normal appearance of the surrounding fetal brain. The only problem that can be encountered at times is differentiating a large choroid plexus cyst slightly distending the cavity of a ventricle from primary ventriculomegaly. In such cases, the most important clue is the demonstration that choroid plexus cysts have a thick echogenic wall and tend to have internal septations. In dubious cases, a follow-up scan may be useful as most choroid plexus cysts rapidly decrease in size and even disappear with advancing gestation. A localized intraventricular bleed may result in a blood clot resembling an abnormality of the choroid plexus. However, the clot is less regular than a choroid plexus cysts and the surrounding ventricle is usually enlarged.

Fetal choroid plexus cysts are benign findings that are, however, associated with an increased likelihood of trisomy 18. The available data do not indicate an association with other chromosomal aberrations, including trisomy 21[207,208]. In 80–90% of fetuses with trisomy 18, anatomic deformities will be detected by ultrasound[182]. On the basis of these data, a prudent approach is to perform a thorough sonographic examination of the fetus when a choroid plexus cyst is identified. This examination should include evaluation of the hands and feet and a thorough examination of the fetal heart. If an additional ultrasound abnormality is identified, chromosomal analysis should be offered. Otherwise, the woman may be counseled using the figures suggested by Snijders and co-workers[208], that is that the risk of trisomy 18 is increased 1.5 times over the baseline. Additional reassurance can be obtained by correlating ultrasound findings with serum biochemical markers.

From time to time, suggestions have been made that the risk of aneuploidy is related to the size of the cyst, whether it is unilateral or bilateral, whether it is persistent or disappears. From the available literature, no evidence supports any of these suggestions. Small cyst, unilateral cyst, transient cyst have all been documented in association with aneuploidies.

Isolated choroid plexus cysts do not modify standard obstetrical management. As no deleterious effect on the fetus has been thus far reported with this finding, there is no need in our opinion for follow-up scans. A handful of very large cysts of the choroid plexuses causing intracranial hypertension has been described in the neurosurgical literature, but these probably represent a separate clinical entity[209].

CONCLUSIONS

Modern ultrasound equipment yields a unique potential for the evaluation of the normal and abnormal fetal central nervous system. A large number of congenital anomalies can be consistently recognized. Transvaginal sonography is extending antenatal diagnosis to very early gestation. MRI can be used to improve the accuracy of the diagnosis in selected cases.

Nevertheless, there are many limits to the prenatal diagnosis of CNS anomalies. Some studies of low-risk patients undergoing basic examinations have reported sensitivities in excess of 80%[210,211]. However, these results probably overestimate the diagnostic potential of the technique. These surveys had invariably very short follow-up and almost only included open neural tube defects, whose recognition was probably facilitated by systematic screening with maternal serum alpha-fetoprotein. Pitfalls of prenatal ultrasound are well documented and occur for a number of reasons. One of the most important limitations is related to continuing brain development in the second half of gestation and into the neonatal period that limits the detection of anomalies such as microcephaly and cortical malformations. Furthermore, some cerebral lesions are not due to faulty embryological development but represent the consequence of acquired prenatal, perinatal and postnatal insults. Even in expert hands some types of anomalies may be difficult or impossible to diagnose in utero, in a proportion that is yet impossible to determine with precision[11].

On the other hand, when an anomaly is identified, counseling the parents and deciding a sensible obstetric management are frequently difficult. Some cerebral anomalies have outcomes that can be predicted with reasonable precision. This is certainly the case with catastrophic lesions such as anencephaly and severe holoprosencephaly, as well as with anomalies that are invariably detected at birth, such as spina bifida. There is, however, a large number of conditions that can be accurately identified in utero and yet have an unclear natural history. Agenesis of the corpus callosum, mild ventriculomegaly and minor variations of the Dandy–Walker continuum are examples that pose this dilemma.

REFERENCES

1. Nicolaides KH, Campbell S, Gabbe SG, Guidetti R. Ultrasound screening for spina bifida: cranial and cerebellar signs. *Lancet* **2**:72–74, 1986.
2. Kratochwil A, Schaller A. Obstetric diagnostics of anencephalus using ultrasound. *Geburtshilfe Frauenheilkd* **31**:564–567, 1971.
3. Michell R, Bradley-Watson P. The detection of fetal meningocele by ultrasound B scan. *J Obstet Gynaecol Br Commonw* **80**:1100–1101, 1973.
4. Pilu G, Romero R, Rizzo N, Jeanty P, Bovicelli L, Hobbins JC. Criteria for the prenatal diagnosis of holoprosencephaly. *Am J Perinatol* **4**:41–49, 1987.
5. Karp LE, Smith DW, Omenn GS, Johnson SL, Jones K. Use of ultrasound in the prenatal exclusion of primary microcephaly. *Gynecol Invest* **5**:311–316, 1974.
6. Chervenak FA, Jeanty P, Cantraine F et al. The diagnosis of fetal microcephaly. *Am J Obstet Gynecol* **149**:512–517, 1984.
7. Pilu G, Romero R, De Palma L et al. Antenatal diagnosis and obstetric management of Dandy-Walker syndrome. *J Reprod Med* **31**:1017–1022, 1986.
8. Pilu G, Reece EA, Romero R, Bovicelli L, Hobbins JC. Prenatal diagnosis of craniofacial malformations with ultrasonography. *Am J Obstet Gynecol* **155**:45–50, 1986.
9. Pilu G, De Palma L, Romero R, Bovicelli L, Hobbins JC. The fetal subarachnoid cisterns: an ultrasound study with report of a case of congenital communicating hydrocephalus. *J Ultrasound Med* **5**: 365–372, 1986.
10. Timor-Tritsch IE, Monteagudo A, Peisner DB. High-frequency transvaginal sonographic examination for the potential malformation assessment of the 9-week to 14-week fetus. *J Clin Ultrasound* **20**: 231–238, 1992.
11. Malinger G, Lerman-Sagie T, Watemberg N, Rotmensch S, Lev D, Glezerman M. A normal second-trimester ultrasound does not exclude intracranial structural pathology. *Ultrasound Obstet Gynecol* **20**:51–56, 2002.
12. Blaicher WPD, Bernaschek G. Magnetic resonance imaging and ultrasound in the assessment of the fetal central nervous system. *J Perinat Med* **31**:459–468, 2003.
13. Levine D, Barnes PD, Robertson RR, Wong G, Mehta TS. Fast MR imaging of fetal central nervous system abnormalities. *Radiology* **229**:51–61, 2003.
14. Malinger G, Ben-Sira L, Lev D, Ben-Aroya Z, Kidron D, Lerman-Sagie T. Fetal brain imaging: a comparison between magnetic resonance imaging and dedicated neurosonography. *Ultrasound Obstet Gynecol* **23**:333–340, 2004.
15. ISUOG guidelines. Sonographic examination of the fetal central nervous system: guidelines for performing the basic examination and the fetal neurosonogram. *Ultrasound Obstet Gynecol* **29**:109–116, 2007.
16. Volpe JJ. *Human brain development. Neurology of the newborn*. pp. 1–43. Philadelphia: WB Saunders Company, 1995.
17. Warkany J. *Congenital malformations*. Chicago: Year Book, 1971.
18. Blaas HG, Eik-Nes SH, Kiserud T, Berg S, Angelsen B, Olstad B. Three-dimensional imaging of the brain cavities in human embryos. *Ultrasound Obstet Gynecol* **5**: 228–232, 1995.
19. Blaas HG, Eik-Nes SH, Kiserud T, Hellevik LR. Early development of the hindbrain: a longitudinal ultrasound study from 7 to 12 weeks of gestation. *Ultrasound Obstet Gynecol* **5**:151–160, 1995.
20. Bronshtein M, Zimmer E. *Transvaginal sonography of the normal and abnormal fetus*. pp. 280. Casterton Hall: The Parthenon Publishing Group Limited, 2001.
21. Filly RA, Cardoza JD, Goldstein RB, Barkovich AJ. Detection of fetal central nervous system anomalies: a practical level of effort for a routine sonogram. *Radiology* **172**:403–408, 1989.
22. Malinger G, Lev D, Lerman-Sagie T. Normal and abnormal fetal brain development during the third trimester as demonstrated by neurosonography. *Eur J Radiol* **57**:226–232, 2006.
23. Toi A, Lister WS, Fong KW. How early are fetal cerebral sulci visible at prenatal ultrasound and what is the normal pattern of early fetal sulcal development? *Ultrasound Obstet Gynecol* **24**:706–715, 2004.
24. Polat I, Gul A, Aslan H et al. Prenatal diagnosis of pentalogy of Cantrell in three cases, two with craniorachischisis. *J Clin Ultrasound* **33**:308–311, 2005.
25. Johnson K, Suarez L, Felkner M, Hendricks K. Prevalence of craniorachischisis in a Texas-Mexico border population. *Birth Defects Res A Clin Mol Teratol* **70**:92–94, 2004.
26. Grange G, Favre R, Gasse B. Endovaginal sonographic diagnosis of craniorachischisis at 13 weeks of gestation. *Fetal Diagn Ther* **9**:391–394, 1994.
27. Achiron R, Malinger G, Tadmor O, Diamant Y, Zakut H. Exencephaly and anencephaly: a distinct anomaly or an embryologic precursor. In utero study by transvaginal sonography. *Isr J Obstet Gynecol* **1**:60–63, 1989.
28. Frey L, Hauser WA. Epidemiology of neural tube defects. *Epilepsia* **44**:4–13, 2003.

29. Lacasana M, Vazquez-Grameix H, Borja-Aburto V et al. Maternal and paternal occupational exposure to agricultural work and the risk of anencephaly. *Occup Environ Med* **63**:649–656, 2006.
30. Williams LJRS, Flores A, Kirby RS, Edmonds LD. Decline in the prevalence of spina bifida and anencephaly by race/ethnicity: 1995–2002. *Pediatrics* **116**:580–586, 2005.
31. Yen I, Khoury M, Erickson J, James L, Waters G, Berry R. The changing epidemiology of neural tube defects. United States, 1968–1989. *Am J Dis Child* **146**:857–861, 1992.
32. Kibar Z, Torban E, McDearmid JR et al. Mutations in VANGL1 associated with neural-tube defects. *N Engl J Med* **356**:1432–1437, 2007.
33. Richmond S, Atkins J. A population-based study of the prenatal diagnosis of congenital malformation over 16 years. *Br J Obstet Gynaecol* **112**:1349–1357, 2005.
34. Johnson SP, Sebire NJ, Snijders RJ, Tunkel S, Nicolaides KH. Ultrasound screening for anencephaly at 10-14 weeks of gestation. *Ultrasound Obstet Gynecol* **9**: 14–16, 1997.
35. Jaquier M, Klein A, Boltshauser E. Spontaneous pregnancy outcome after prenatal diagnosis of anencephaly. *Br J Obstet Gynaecol* **113**:951–953, 2006.
36. Rowland CA, Correa A, Cragan JD, Alverson CJ. Are encephaloceles neural tube defects? *Pediatrics* **118**:916–923, 2006.
37. Nadel AS, Green JK, Holmes LB, Frigoletto FDJ, Benacerraf BR. Absence of need for amniocentesis in patients with elevated levels of maternal serum alpha-fetoprotein and normal ultrasonographic examinations. *N Engl J Med* **323**:557–561, 1990.
38. Lau TK, Leung TN, Leung TY, Pang MW, Tam WH. Fetal scalp cysts: challenge in diagnosis and counseling. *J Ultrasound Med* **20**(2):175–177, 2001.
39. van Zalen-Sprock MM, van Vugt JM, van dHarten HJ, van Geijn HP. Cephalocele and cystic hygroma: diagnosis and differentiation in the first trimester of pregnancy with transvaginal sonography. Report of two cases. *Ultrasound Obstet Gynecol* **2**:289–292, 1992.
40. Malinger G, Lerman-Sagie T, Lev D, Tamarkin M, Kidron D. Case 49. TheFetus. net, 2001.
41. Lee W, Vettraino IM, Comstock CH et al. Prenatal diagnosis of herniated dandy-walker cysts. *J Ultrasound Med* **24**:841–848, 2005.
42. Martinez-Lage JF, Sola J, Casas C, Poza M, Almagro MJ, Girona DG. Atretic cephalocele: the tip of the iceberg. *J Neurosurg* **77**:230–235, 1992.
43. Martinez-Lage JF, Poza M, Sola J et al. The child with a cephalocele: etiology, neuroimaging, and outcome. *Childs Nerv Syst* **12**:540–550, 1996.
44. Budorick NE, Pretorius DH, McGahan JP, Grafe MR, James HE, Slivka J. Cephalocele detection in utero: sonographic and clinical features. *Ultrasound Obstet Gynecol* **5**:77–85, 1995.
45. Goldstein RB, LaPidus AS, Filly RA. Fetal cephaloceles: diagnosis with US. *Radiology* **180**:803–808, 1991.
46. Li Z, Ren A, Zhang L et al. Extremely high prevalence of neural tube defects in a 4-county area in Shanxi Province, China. *Birth Defects Res A Clin Mol Teratol* **76**:237–240, 2006.
47. Spina bifida and anencephaly before and after folic acid mandate – United States, 1995–1996 and 1999–2000. *Morb Mortal Wkly Rep* **53**:362-365, 2004.
48. Bower C, Raymond M, Lumley J, Bury G. Trends in neural tube defects 1980–1989. *Med J Aust* **158**:152–154, 1993.
49. Mathews TJ, Honein MA, Erickson JD. Spina bifida and anencephaly prevalence – United States, 1991–2001. *MMWR Recomm Rep* **51**:9–11, 2002.
50. Nikkila A, Rydhstrom H, Kallen B. The incidence of spina bifida in Sweden 1973–2003: the effect of prenatal diagnosis. *Eur J Public Health* **16**:660–662, 2006.
51. Sepulveda W, Corral E, Ayala C, Be C, Gutierrez J, Vasquez P. Chromosomal abnormalities in fetuses with open neural tube defects: prenatal identification with ultrasound. *Ultrasound Obstet Gynecol* **23**:352–356, 2004.
52. Philipp T, Grillenberger K, Separovic ER, Philipp K, Kalousek DK. Effects of triploidy on early human development. *Prenat Diagn* **24**:276–281, 2004.
53. Adab N, Tudur SC, Vinten J, Williamson P, Winterbottom J. Common antiepileptic drugs in pregnancy in women with epilepsy. *Cochrane Database Syst Rev* **3**, 2004.
54. Meador KJ, Baker GA, BakerFinnell RH et al. In utero antiepileptic drug exposure: fetal death and malformations. *Neurology* **67**:407–412, 2006.
55. Brock DJ, Sutcliffe RG. Alpha-fetoprotein in the antenatal diagnosis of anencephaly and spina bifida. *Lancet* **2**:197–199, 1972.
56. Wald NJ, Cuckle H, Brock JH, Peto R, Polani PE, Woodford FP. Maternal serum-alpha-fetoprotein measurement in antenatal screening for anencephaly and spina bifida in early pregnancy. Report of UK collaborative study on alpha-fetoprotein in relation to neural-tube defects. *Lancet* **1**:1323–1332, 1977.
57. Campbell S, Pryse-Davies J, Coltart TM, Seller MJ, Singer JD. Ultrasound in the diagnosis of spina bifida. *Lancet* **1**:1065–1068, 1975.
58. Kooper AJ, de Bruijn D, de van Ravenwaaij-Arts CM et al. Fetal anomaly scan potentially will replace routine AFAFP assays for the detection of neural tube defects. *Prenat Diagn* **27**:29–33, 2007.
59. Widlund K, Gottvall T. Routine assessment of amniotic fluid alpha-fetoprotein in early second-trimester amniocentesis is no longer justified. *Acta Obstet Gynecol Scand* **86**:167–171, 2007.
60. Vintzileos AM, Ananth CV, Fisher AJ et al. Cost-benefit analysis of targeted ultrasonography for prenatal detection of spina bifida in patients with an elevated concentration of second-trimester maternal serum alpha-fetoprotein. *Am J Obstet Gynecol* **180**:1277–1233, 1999.
61. Pilu G, Hobbins JC. Sonography of fetal cerebrospinal anomalies. *Prenat Diagn* **22**:321–330, 2002.
62. Boyd PA, Wellesley DG, De Walle HE et al. Evaluation of the prenatal diagnosis of neural tube defects by fetal ultrasonographic examination in different centres across Europe. *J Med Screen* **7**:169–174, 2000.
63. Blumenfeld Z, Siegler E, Bronshtein M. The early diagnosis of neural tube defects. *Prenat Diagn* **13**:863–871, 1993.
64. Blaas HG, Eik-Nes SH, Isaksen C. The detection of spina bifida before 10 gestational weeks using two- and three-dimensional ultrasound. *Ultrasound Obstet Gynecol* **16**:25–29, 2000.
65. Buisson O, De Keersmaecker B, Senat MV, Bernard JP, Moscoso G, Ville Y. Sonographic diagnosis of spina bifida at 12 weeks: heading towards indirect signs. *Ultrasound Obstet Gynecol* **19**:290–292, 2002.
66. Bernard JP, Suarez B, Rambaud C, Muller F, Ville Y. Prenatal diagnosis of neural tube defect before 12 weeks' gestation: direct and indirect ultrasonographic semeiology. *Ultrasound Obstet Gynecol* **10**:406–409, 1997.
67. Blaas HG, Eik-Nes SH, Isaksen CV. The detection of spina bifida before 10 gestational weeks using two- and three-dimensional ultrasound. *Ultrasound Obstet Gynecol* **16**:25–29, 2000.
68. Sebire NJ, Noble PL, Thorpe-Beeston JG, Snijders RJ, Nicolaides KH. Presence of the 'lemon' sign in fetuses with spina bifida at the 10-14-week scan. *Ultrasound Obstet Gynecol* **10**:403–405, 1997.
69. McKusick VA. Chiari malformation type II. *Online Mendelian Inheritance in Man.* OMIM; 2006.
70. McKusick VA. Chiari malformation type I: *Online Mendelian Inheritance in Man.* OMIM; 2007.
72. Watson WJ, Chescheir NC, Katz VL, Seeds JW. The role of ultrasound in evaluation of patients with elevated maternal serum alpha-fetoprotein: a review. *Obstet Gynecol* **78**:123–128, 1991.
73. Johnson DD, Nager CW, Budorick NE. False-positive diagnosis of spina bifida in a fetus with triploidy. *Obstet Gynecol* **89**:809–811, 1997.
74. Bruner JP, Tulipan N. Tell the truth about spina bifida. *Ultrasound Obstet Gynecol* **24**:595–596, 2004.

75. McLaughlin JFSD, Lamers JY, Stuntz JT, Hayden PW, Kropp RJ. Influence of prognosis on decisions regarding the care of newborns with myelodysplasia. *N Engl J Med* **312**:1589–1594, 1985.
76. Farmer DL, von Koch CS, Peacock WJ et al. In utero repair of myelomeningocele: experimental pathophysiology, initial clinical experience, and outcomes. *Arch Surg* **138**:872–878, 2003.
77. Bruner JP, Tulipan N, Reed G et al. Intrauterine repair of spina bifida: preoperative predictors of shunt-dependent hydrocephalus. *Am J Obstet Gynecol* **190**:1305–1312, 2004.
78. Bruner JP, Tulipan N, Dabrowiak ME et al. Upper level of the spina bifida defect: how good are we? *Ultrasound Obstet Gynecol* **24**:612–617, 2004.
79. Appasamy M, Roberts D, Pilling D, Buxton N. Antenatal ultrasound and magnetic resonance imaging in localizing the level of lesion in spina bifida and correlation with postnatal outcome. *Ultrasound Obstet Gynecol* **27**:530–536, 2006.
80. Quintero Mejia J. *Spina bifida, 3D*. TheFetus.net, 2003.
81. Schropp C, Sorensen N, Collmann H, Krauss J. Cutaneous lesions in occult spinal dysraphism – correlation with intraspinal findings. *Childs Nerv Syst* **22**:125–131, 2006.
82. Allen LM, Silverman RK. Prenatal ultrasound evaluation of fetal diastematomyelia: two cases of type I split cord malformation. *Ultrasound Obstet Gynecol* **15**:78–82, 2000.
83. Pierre-Kahn A, Sonigo P. Lumbosacral lipomas: in utero diagnosis and prognosis. *Childs Nerv Syst* **2003**:551–554, 2003.
84. Della Monica M, Nazzaro A, Lonardo F, Ferrara G, Di Blasi A, Scarano G. Prenatal ultrasound diagnosis of cloacal exstrophy associated with myelocystocele complex by the 'elephant trunk-like' image and review of the literature. *Prenat Diagn* **25**:394–397, 2005.
85. Zalel Y, Lehavi O, Aizenstein O, Achiron R. Development of the fetal spinal cord: time of ascendance of the normal conus medullaris as detected by sonography. *J Ultrasound Med* **25**:1397–1401, 2006.
86. Cardoza JD, Goldstein RB, Filly RA. Exclusion of fetal ventriculomegaly with a single measurement: the width of the lateral ventricular atrium. *Radiology* **169**:711–714, 1988.
87. Gupta JK, Bryce FC, Lilford RJ. Management of apparently isolated fetal ventriculomegaly. *Obstet Gynecol Surv* **49**:716–721, 1994.
88. Pilu G, Falco P, Gabrielli S, Perolo A, Sandri F, Bovicelli L. The clinical significance of fetal isolated cerebral borderline ventriculomegaly: report of 31 cases and review of the literature. *Ultrasound Obstet Gynecol* **14**:320–326, 1999.
89. Gaglioti P, Danelon D, Bontempo S, Mombro M, Cardaropoli S, Todros T. Fetal cerebral ventriculomegaly: outcome in 176 cases. *Ultrasound Obstet Gynecol* **25**:372–377, 2005.
90. Lyonnet S, Pelet A, Royer G et al. The gene for X-linked hydrocephalus maps to Xq28, distal to DXS52. *Genomics* **14**:508–510, 1992.
91. Serville F, Benit P, Saugier P et al. Prenatal exclusion of X-linked hydrocephalus-stenosis of the aqueduct of Sylvius sequence using closely linked DNA markers. *Prenat Diagn* **13**:435–439, 1993.
92. Rogers JG, Danks DM. Prenatal diagnosis of sex-linked hydrocephalus. *Prenat Diagn* **3**:269, 1983.
93. Chervenak FA, McCullough LB. Ethical analysis of the intrapartum management of pregnancy complicated by fetal hydrocephalus with macrocephaly. *Obstet Gynecol* **68**:720–725, 1986.
94. Harris CP, Townsend JJ, Norman MG et al. Atelencephalic aprosencephaly. *J Child Neurol* **9**:412–416, 1994.
95. Ippel PF, Breslau-Siderius EJ, Hack WW, van der Blij HF, Bouve S, Bijlsma JB. Atelencephalic microcephaly: a case report and review of the literature. *Eur J Pediatr* **157**:493–497, 1998.
96. Forrester MB, Merz RD. Epidemiology of holoprosencephaly in Hawaii, 1986–97. *Paediatr Perinat Epidemiol* **14**: 61–63, 2000.
97. Ong S, Tonks A, Woodward ER, Wyldes MP, Kilby MD. An epidemiological study of holoprosencephaly from a regional congenital anomaly register: 1995–2004. *Prenat Diagn* **27**:340–347, 2007.
98. Matsunaga E, Shiota K. Holoprosencephaly in human embryos: epidemiologic studies of 150 cases. *Teratology* **16**:261–272, 1977.
99. Odent S, Le Marec B, Munnich A, Le Merrer M, Bonaiti-Pellie C. Segregation analysis in nonsyndromic holoprosencephaly. *Am J Med Genet* **77**:139–143, 1998.
100. Cohen MM, Jr. Perspectives on holoprosencephaly: Part I. Epidemiology, genetics, and syndromology. *Teratology* **40**:211–235, 1989.
101. McKusick VA. Holoprosencephaly. *Online Mendelian Inheritance in Man*, OMIM, 2007.
102. Malinger G, Lev D, Kidron D, Heredia F, Hershkovitz R, Lerman-Sagie T. Differential diagnosis in fetuses with absent septum pellucidum. *Ultrasound Obstet Gynecol* **25**:42–49, 2005.
103. DeMeyer W, Zeman W, Palmer CG. The face predicts the brain: diagnostic significance of median facial anomalies for holoprosencephaly (archinencephaly). *Pediatrics* **34**:256–263, 1964.
104. Pilu G, Ambrosetto P, Sandri F et al. Intraventricular fused fornices: a specific sign of fetal lobar holoprosencephaly. *Ultrasound Obstet Gynecol* **4**:65–67, 1994.
105. Pilu G, Sandri F, Perolo A et al. Prenatal diagnosis of lobar holoprosencephaly. *Ultrasound Obstet Gynecol* **2**:88–94, 1992.
106. Bronshtein M, Wiener Z. Early transvaginal sonographic diagnosis of alobar holoprosencephaly. *Prenat Diagn* **11**:459–462, 1991.
107. Turner CD, Silva S, Jeanty P. Prenatal diagnosis of alobar holoprosencephaly at 10 weeks of gestation. *Ultrasound Obstet Gynecol* **13**:360–362, 1999.
108. Blaas HG, Eik-Nes SH, Vainio T, Isaksen CV. Alobar holoprosencephaly at 9 weeks gestational age visualized by two- and three-dimensional ultrasound. *Ultrasound Obstet Gynecol* **15**:62–65, 2000.
109. Blaas HG, Eriksson AG, Salvesen KA et al. Brains and faces in holoprosencephaly: pre- and postnatal description of 30 cases. *Ultrasound Obstet Gynecol* **19**:24–38, 2002.
110. Garel C. *MRI of the fetal brain. Normal development and cerebral pathologies*. Berlin: Springer, p. 267 2004.
111. Ren T, Anderson A, Shen WB et al. Imaging, anatomical, and molecular analysis of callosal formation in the developing human fetal brain. *Anat. Rec. A Discov. Mol. Cell. Evol. Biol* **288**:191–204, 2006.
112. Grogono JL. Children with agenesis of the corpus callosum. *Dev Med Child Neurol* **10**:613–616, 1968.
113. Jeret JS, Serur D, Wisniewski K, Fisch C. Frequency of agenesis of the corpus callosum in the developmentally disabled population as determined by computerized tomography. *Pediatr Neurosci* **12**:101–103, 1985–1986.
114. Wang LW, Huang CC, Yeh TF. Major brain lesions detected on sonographic screening of apparently normal term neonates. *Neuroradiology* **46**:368–373, 2004.
115. Davila-Gutierrez G. Agenesis and dysgenesis of the corpus callosum. *Semin Pediatr Neurol* **9**:292–301, 2002.
116. Malinger G, Lev D, Zahalka N et al. Fetal cytomegalovirus infection of the brain: the spectrum of sonographic findings. *Am J Neuroradiol* **24**:28–32, 2003.
117. Weinstein AS, Goldstein RB, Barkovich AJ. In utero disappearance of the corpus callosum secondary to extensive brain injury. *J Ultrasound Med* **22**:837–840, 2003.
118. Malinger G, Zakut H. The corpus callosum: normal fetal development as shown by transvaginal sonography. *Am J Roentgenol* **161**:1041–1043, 1993.
119. Pilu G, Segata M, Ghi T et al. Diagnosis of midline anomalies of the fetal brain with the three-dimensional median view. *Ultrasound Obstet Gynecol* **27**: 522–529, 2006.
120. Moutard ML, Kieffer V, Feingold J et al. Agenesis of corpus callosum: prenatal

diagnosis and prognosis. *Childs Nerv Syst* **19**:471–476, 2003.
121. Pilu G, Sandri F, Perolo A et al. Sonography of fetal agenesis of the corpus callosum: a survey of 35 cases. *Ultrasound Obstet Gynecol* **3**:318–329, 1993.
122. Paul LK, Brown WS, Adolphs R et al. Agenesis of the corpus callosum: genetic, developmental and functional aspects of connectivity. *Nat Rev Neurosci* **8**:287–299, 2007.
123. Belhocine O, Andre C, Kalifa G, Adamsbaum C. Does asymptomatic septal agenesis exist? A review of 34 cases. *Pediatr Radiol* **35**:410–418, 2005.
124. Raybaud C, Girard N, Levrier O, Peretti-Viton P, Manera L, Farnarie P. Schizencephaly: correlation between the lobar topography of the cleft(s) and absence of the septum pellucidum. *Childs Nerv Syst* **17**:217–222, 2001.
125. Lepinard C, Coutant R, Boussion F et al. Prenatal diagnosis of absence of the septum pellucidum associated with septo-optic dysplasia. *Ultrasound Obstet Gynecol* **25**:73–75, 2005.
126. Celentano C, Prefumo F, Liberati M et al. Prenatal diagnosis of septal agenesis with normal pituitary function. *Prenat Diagn* **26**:1075–1077, 2006.
127. Pilu G, Sandri F, Cerisoli M, Alvisi C, Salvioli GP, Bovicelli L. Sonographic findings in septo-optic dysplasia in the fetus and newborn infant. *Am J Perinatol* **7**:337–339, 1990.
128. Pilu G, Tani G, Carletti A, Malaigia S, Ghi T, Rizzo N. Difficult early sonographic diagnosis of absence of the fetal septum pellucidum. *Ultrasound Obstet Gynecol* **25**:70–72, 2005.
129. Rakic P. Specification of cerebral cortical areas. *Science* **241**:170–176, 1988.
130. Barkovich AJ, Kuzniecky RI, Jackson GD, Guerrin IR, Dobyns WB. A developmental and genetic classification for malformations of cortical development. *Neurology* **65**:1873–1887, 2005.
131. Persutte WH. Microcephaly. No small deal. *Ultrasound Obstet Gynecol* **11**: 317–318, 1998.
132. Jones KL. Microcephaly. In *Smith's recognizable patterns of human malformation,* KL Jones (ed.), pp. 776–777. Philadelphia: WB Saunders Company, 1997.
133. Bromley B, Benacerraf BR. Difficulties in the prenatal diagnosis of microcephaly. *J Ultrasound Med* **14**:303–306, 1995.
134. Chervenak FA, Rosenberg J, Brightman RC. A prospective study of the accuracy of ultrasound in predicting fetal microcephaly. *Obstet Gynecol* **69**:908–910, 1987.
135. Jaffe M, Tirosh E, Oren S. The dilemma in prenatal diagnosis of idiopathic microcephaly. *Dev Med Child Neurol* **29**:187–189, 1987.
136. Reece EB, Goldstein I. Three-level view of fetal brain imaging in the prenatal diagnosis of congenital anomalies. *J Matern Fetal Med* **8**:249–242, 1999.
137. den Hollander NS, Wessels MW, Los FJ, Ursem NT, Niermeijer MF, Wladimiroff JW. Congenital microcephaly detected by prenatal ultrasound: genetic aspects and clinical significance. *Ultrasound Obstet Gynecol* **15**:282–287, 2000.
138. Dahlgren L, Wilson RD. Prenatally diagnosed microcephaly: a review of etiologies. *Fetal Diagn Ther* **16**:323–326, 2001.
139. Goldstein I, Reece EA, Pilu G, O'Connor TZ, Lockwood CJ, Hobbins JC. Sonographic assessment of the fetal frontal lobe: a potential tool for prenatal diagnosis of microcephaly. *Am J Obstet Gynecol* **158**:1057–1062, 1988.
140. Pilu G, Falco P, Milano V, Perolo A, Bovicelli L. Prenatal diagnosis of microcephaly assisted by vaginal sonography and power Doppler. *Ultrasound Obstet Gynecol* **11**:357–360, 1998.
141. Malinger G, Lerman-Sagie T, Achiron R, Lipitz S. The subarachnoid space: normal fetal development as demonstrated by transvaginal ultrasound. *Prenatal Diagn* **20**:890–893, 2000.
142. Malinger G, Lev D, Lerman-Sagie T. Assessment of fetal intracranial pathologies first demonstrated late in pregnancy: cell proliferation disorders. *Reprod Biol Endocrinol* **1**:110, 2003.
143. Dobyns WB. Primary microcephaly: new approaches for an old disorder. *Am J Med Genet* **112**:315–317, 2002.
144. Petersson S, Pedersen NL, Schalling M, Lavebratt C. Primary megalencephaly at birth and low intelligence level. *Neurology* **53**:1254–1259, 1999.
145. Lorber J, Priestley BL. Children with large heads: a practical approach to diagnosis in 557 children, with special reference to 109 children with megalencephaly. *Dev Med Child Neurol* **23**:494–504, 1981.
146. Cohen MM. Mental deficiency, alterations in performance, and CNS abnormalities in overgrowth syndromes. *Am J Med Genet* **117C**:49–56, 2003.
147. Chen CP, Lin SP, Chang TY et al. Perinatal imaging findings of inherited Sotos syndrome. *Prenat Diagn* **22**: 887–892, 2003.
148. DeRosa R, Lenke RR, Kurczynski TW, Perssutte WH, Nemes J. In utero diagnosis of benign fetal macrocephaly. *Am J Obstet Gynecol* **161**:690–692, 1989.
149. Nyberg RH, Uotila J, Kirkinen P, Rosendahl H. Macrocephaly-cutis marmorata telangiectatica congenita syndrome--prenatal signs in ultrasonography. *Prenat Diagn* **52**:129–132, 2005.
150. de Graaf-Peters VB, Hadders-Algra M. Ontogeny of the human central nervous system: what is happening when? *Early Hum. Dev* **84**:257–266, 2006.
151. Gupta RK, Hasan KM, Trivedi R et al. Diffusion tensor imaging of the developing human cerebrum. *J Neurosci Res* **81**:172–178, 2005.
152. Leventer RJ, Phelan EM, Coleman LT, Kean MJ, Jackson GD, Harvey AS. Clinical and imaging features of cortical malformations in childhood. *Neurology* **53**:715–722, 1999.
153. Raymond AA, Fish DR, Sisodiya SM, Alsanjari N, Stevens JM, Shorvon SD. Abnormalities of gyration, heterotopias, tuberous sclerosis, focal cortical dysplasia, microdysgenesis, dysembryoplastic neuroepithelial tumour and dysgenesis of the archicortex in epilepsy. Clinical, EEG and neuroimaging features in 100 adult patients. *Brain* **118**:629–660, 1995.
154. Sarnat HB, Flores-Sarnat L. Molecular genetic and morphologic integration in malformations of the nervous system for etiologic classification. *Semin Pediatr Neurol* **9**:335–344, 2002.
155. Holzgreve W, Feil R, Louwen F, Miny P. Prenatal diagnosis and management of fetal hydrocephaly and lissencephaly. *Childs Nerv Syst* **9**:408–412, 1993.
156. McGahan JP, Grix A, Gerscovich EO. Prenatal diagnosis of lissencephaly: Miller-Dieker syndrome. *J Clin Ultrasound* **22**:560–563, 1994.
157. Mitchell LA, Simon EM, Filly RA. Antenatal diagnosis of subependymal heterotopia. *Am J Neuroradiol* **21**:296–300, 2000.
158. Righini A, Zirpoli S, Mrakic F, Parazzini C, Pogliani L, Triulzi F. Early prenatal MR imaging diagnosis of polymicrogyria. *Am J Neuroradiol* **25**:343–346, 2004.
159. Bornemann A, Pfeiffer R, Beinder E et al. Three siblings with Walker-Warburg syndrome. *Gen Diagn Pathol* **141**:371–375, 1996.
160. Saltzman DH, Krauss CM, Goldman JM, Benacerraf BR. Prenatal diagnosis of lissencephaly. *Prenat Diagn* **11**:139–143, 1991.
161. Garel C, Chantrel E, Brisse H et al. Fetal cerebral cortex: normal gestational landmarks identified using prenatal MR imaging. *Am J Neuroradiol* **22**:184–189, 2001.
162. Monteagudo A, Timor-Tritsch IE. Development of fetal gyri, sulci and fissures: a transvaginal sonographic study. *Ultrasound Obstet Gynecol* **9**:222–228, 1997.
163. Cohen-Sacher B, Lerman-Sagie T, Lev D, Malinger G. Developmental milestones of the fetal cerebral cortex. A longitudinal sonographic study.

Ultrasound Obstet Gynecol **27**:494–502, 2006.

164. Fogliarini C, Chaumoitre K, Chapon F et al. Assessment of cortical maturation with prenatal MRI: part II: abnormalities of cortical maturation. *Eur Radiol* **15**:1781–1789, 2005.
165. Malinger G, Kidron D, Schreiber L et al. Prenatal diagnosis of malformations of cortical development by dedicated neurosonography. *Ultrasound Obstet Gynecol* **29**:178–191, 2007.
166. Fong KW, Ghai S, Toi A, Blaser S, Winsor EJ, Chitayat D. Prenatal ultrasound findings of lissencephaly associated with Miller-Dieker syndrome and comparison with pre- and postnatal magnetic resonance imaging. *Ultrasound Obstet Gynecol* **24**:716–723, 2004.
167. Pellicer A, Cabanas F, Perez-Higueras A, Garcia-Alix A, Quero J. Neuronal migration disorders studied by cerebral ultrasound and colour Doppler flow imaging. *Arch Dis Child Fetal Neonatal Ed* **73**:F55–61, 1995.
168. Lemire R, Loeser J, Leech R, Alvord E. *Normal and abnormal development of the human nervous system*. Hagerstown: Harper and Row, 1975.
169. Altman NR, Naidich TP, Braffman BH. Posterior fossa malformations. *Am J Neuroradiol* **13**:691–724, 1992.
170. Parisi MA, Dobyns WB. Human malformations of the midbrain and hindbrain: review and proposed classification scheme. *Mol Genet Metabol* **80**:36–53, 2003.
171. Patel S, Barkovich AJ. Analysis and classification of cerebellar malformations. *Am J Neuroradiol* **23**:1074–1087, 2002.
172. Sarnat HB, Flores-Sarnat L. Integrative classification of morphology and molecular genetics in central nervous system malformations. *Am J Med Genet A* **126**:386–392, 2004.
173. Boddaert N, Klein O, Ferguson N et al. Intellectual prognosis of the Dandy-Walker malformation in children: the importance of vermian lobulation. *Neuroradiology* **45**:320–324, 2003.
174. Klein O, Pierre-Kahn A, Boddaert N, Parisot D, Brunelle F. Dandy-Walker malformation: prenatal diagnosis and prognosis. *Childs Nerv Syst* **19**:484–489, 2003.
175. Adamsbaum C, Moutard ML, Andre C et al. MRI of the fetal posterior fossa. *Pediatr Radiol* **35**:124–140, 2005.
176. Guibaud L, des Portes V. Plea for an anatomical approach to abnormalities of the posterior fossa in prenatal diagnosis. *Ultrasound Obstet Gynecol* **27**:477–481, 2006.
177. Malinger G, Ginath S, Lerman-Sagie T, Watemberg N, Lev D, Glezerman M. The fetal cerebellar vermis: normal development as shown by transvaginal ultrasound. *Prenat Diagn* **21**:687–692, 2001.
178. Doherty D, Glass IA, Siebert JR et al. Prenatal diagnosis in pregnancies at risk for Joubert syndrome by ultrasound and MRI. *Prenat Diagn* **25**:442–447, 2005.
179. Bromley B, Nadel AS, Pauker S, Estroff JA, Benacerraf BR. Closure of the cerebellar vermis: evaluation with second trimester US. *Radiology* **193**:761–763, 1994.
180. Malinger G, Zahalka N, Kidron D, Ben-Sira L, Lev D, Lerman-Sagie T. Fatal outcome following foetal cerebellar haemorrhage associated with placental thrombosis. *Eur J Paediatr Neurol* **10**:93–96, 2006.
181. Nyberg DA, Mahony BS, Hegge FN, Hickok D, Luthy DA, Kapur R. Enlarged cisterna magna and the Dandy-Walker malformation: factors associated with chromosome abnormalities. *Obstet Gynecol* **77**:436–442, 1991.
182. Nyberg DA, Kramer D, Resta RG et al. Prenatal sonographic findings of trisomy 18: review of 47 cases. *J Ultrasound Med* **12**:103–113, 1993.
183. Adam R, Greenberg JO. The mega cisterna magna. *J Neurosurg* **48**:190–192, 1978.
184. Tortori-Donati P, Fondelli MP, Rossi A, Carini S. Cystic malformations of the posterior cranial fossa originating from a defect of the posterior membranous area. Mega cisterna magna and persisting Blake's pouch: two separate entities. *Childs Nerv Syst* **12**:303–308, 1996.
185. Zalel Y, Gilboa Y, Gabis L et al. Rotation of the vermis as a cause of enlarged cisterna magna on prenatal imaging. *Ultrasound Obstet Gynecol* **27**:490–493, 2006.
186. Ghi T, Simonazzi G, Perolo A et al. Outcome of antenatally diagnosed intracranial hemorrhage: case series and review of the literature. *Ultrasound Obstet Gynecol* **22**:121–130, 2003.
187. Pilu G, Falco P, Perolo A et al. Differential diagnosis and outcome of fetal intracranial hypoechoic lesions: report of 21 cases. *Ultrasound Obstet Gynecol* **9**:229–236, 1997.
188. Ghi T, Brondelli L, Simonazzi G et al. Sonographic demonstration of brain injury in fetuses with severe red blood cell alloimmunization undergoing intrauterine transfusions. *Ultrasound Obstet Gynecol* **23**:428–431, 2004.
189. Hutto C, Arvin A, Jacobs R et al. Intrauterine herpes simplex virus infections. *J Pediatr* **110**:97–101, 1987.
190. Bailao LA, Osborne NG, Rizz iMC, Bonilla-Musoles F, Duarte G, Bailao TC. Ultrasound markers of fetal infection, Part 2: Bacterial, parasitic, and fungal infections. *Ultrasound Q* **22**:137–151, 2006.
191. Enders G, Miller E, Cradock-Watson J, Bolley I, Ridehalgh M. Consequences of varicella and herpes zoster in pregnancy: prospective study of 1739 cases. *Lancet* **343**:1548–1551, 1994.
192. Schulte D, Comer JA, Erickson BR et al. Congenital lymphocytic choriomeningitis virus: an underdiagnosed cause of neonatal hydrocephalus. *Pediatr Infect Dis J* **25**:560–562, 2006.
193. Haddad J, Messer J, Gut JP, Chaigne D, Christmann D, Willard D. Neonatal echovirus encephalitis with white matter necrosis. *Neuropediatrics* **21**:215–217, 1990.
194. Fonticella M, Lopez-Negrete L, Prieto A et al. Congenital intracranial filariasis: a case report. *Pediatr Radiol* **25**:171–172, 1995.
195. Ancora G, Lanari M, Lazzarotto T et al. Cranial ultrasound scanning and prediction of outcome in newborns with congenital cytomegalovirus infection. *J Pediatr* **150**:157–161, 2007.
196. Gras L, Wallon M, Pollak A et al. Association between prenatal treatment and clinical manifestations of congenital toxoplasmosis in infancy: a cohort study in 13 European centres. *Acta Paediatr* **94**:1721–1731, 2005.
197. Johnston IH, Whittle IR, Besser M, Morgan MK. Vein of Galen malformation: diagnosis and management. *Neurosurgery* **20**:747–758, 1987.
198. Sepulveda W, Platt CC, Fisk NM. Prenatal diagnosis of cerebral arteriovenous malformation using color Doppler ultrasonography: case report and review of the literature. *Ultrasound Obstet Gynecol* **6**:282–286, 1995.
199. Rodesch G, Hui F, Alvarez H, Tanaka A, Lasjaunias P. Prognosis of antenatally diagnosed vein of Galen aneurysmal malformations. *Childs Nerv Syst* **10**:79–83, 1994.
200. Visentin A, Falco P, Pilu G et al. Prenatal diagnosis of thrombosis of the dural sinuses with real-time and color Doppler ultrasound. *Ultrasound Obstet Gynecol* **17**:322–325, 2001.
201. Medlock MD, Olivero WC, Hanigan WC, Wright RM, Winek SJ. Children with cerebral venous thrombosis diagnosed with magnetic resonance imaging and magnetic resonance angiography. *Neurosurgery* **31**:870–876, discussion 876, 1992.
202. Marinov M, Undjian S, Wetzka P. An evaluation of the surgical treatment of intracranial arachnoid cysts in children. *Childs Nerv Syst* **5**:177–183, 1989.
203. Richard KE, Dahl K, Sanker P. Long-term follow-up of children and juveniles with arachnoid cysts. *Childs Nerv Syst* **5**:184–187, 1989.

204. Hassan J, Sepulveda W, Teixeira J, Cox PM. Glioependymal and arachnoid cysts: unusual causes of early ventriculomegaly in utero. *Prenat Diagn* **16**:729–733, 1996.
205. Chinn DH, Miller EI, Worthy LM, Towers CV. Sonographically detected fetal choroid plexus cysts. Frequency and association with aneuploidy. *J Ultrasound Med* **10**:255–258, 1991.
206. Gupta JK, Cave M, Lilford RJ et al. Clinical significance of fetal choroid plexus cysts. *Lancet* **346**:724–729, 1995.
207. Bromley B, Lieberman R, Benacerraf BR. Choroid plexus cysts: not associated with Down syndrome. *Ultrasound Obstet Gynecol* **8**:232–235, 1996.
208. Snijders RJ, Shawa L, Nicolaides KH. Fetal choroid plexus cysts and trisomy 18: assessment of risk based on ultrasound findings and maternal age. *Prenat Diagn* **14**:1119–1127, 1994.
209. Neblett CR, Robertson JW. Symptomatic cysts of the telencephalic choroid plexus. *J Neurol Neurosurg Psychiatr* **34**:324–331, 1971.
210. Ewigman BG, Crane JP, Frigoletto FD, LeFevre ML, Bain RP, McNellis D. Effect of prenatal ultrasound screening on perinatal outcome. RADIUS Study Group. *N Engl J Med* **329**:821–827, 1993.
211. Crane JP, LeFevre ML, Winborn RC et al. A randomized trial of prenatal ultrasonographic screening: impact on the detection, management, and outcome of anomalous fetuses. The RADIUS Study Group. *Am J Obstet Gynecol* **171**:392–399, 1994.

CHAPTER 31 The heart

Helena M Gardiner

KEY POINTS

- First-trimester diagnosis of structural cardiac malformation is now commonplace as a result of early screening initiatives. However, the majority of cardiac defects will continue to be detected after the second-trimester anomaly scan
- Antenatal detection of cardiac defects will improve if there is an emphasis on offering high quality cardiac screening for all pregnant women in their local setting, rather than the selection of a 'high-risk' group for specialized scanning
- Improved audit mechanisms are essential to monitor what is being achieved in screening and to plan and support the future needs of those caring for the fetus with congenital heart disease
- A multidisciplinary team is an essential component of a good service. Antenatal diagnosis creates an opportunity to counsel and plan for optimal management of complex cases which may include offering fetal therapy

INTRODUCTION

When fetal echocardiography initially became incorporated into clinical practice, early reports predicted that this subspecialty would reduce referrals for surgery for congenital heart disease (CHD) due to increased termination of pregnancy[1–3]. In contrast, improvements in surgical outcome have encouraged parents to continue with pregnancies that may have been terminated in the past[4–6].

Improved ultrasound technology and increased interest from fetal medicine specialists have resulted in first-trimester screening programs and increased detection rates of CHD, particularly in major centers, resulting in more detailed and earlier antenatal diagnoses and more comprehensive antenatal counseling[7,8]. There has been new enthusiasm for improved fetal therapy for arrhythmias, including pacing[9–12] and a refinement of interventional catheter techniques to open the stenosed or atretic aortic or pulmonary valve and the intact interatrial septum associated with hypoplastic left heart syndrome and simple transposition of the great arteries[13–16]. Fetal cardiac surgery on bypass has also been attempted for conditions thought hopeless because of progressive pulmonary hypoplasia. This chapter will explore current trends and progress in screening and detection of CHD with a guide to basic lesion-based counseling, a review of arrhythmias and advances in assessment and therapy.

SCREENING FOR CHD

Technical advances in obstetric ultrasound machines and improved training and education have resulted in new standards of screening for cardiac defects[17]. There is a new enthusiasm at ground level which has resulted in increased antenatal detection in several countries[18–21].

Nuchal translucency (NT) measurement forms part of early (11–13 week) screening programs: a combination of serum screening and NT gives an age-related risk for trisomy 21. Other chapters in this book deal with these screening strategies in more detail. An observation from the early nuchal translucency programs was that about one-third of fetuses with increased NT will also have CHD[22–24]. This has led to the introduction in some centers of cardiac scanning at the same time an increased NT is detected[8]. Perhaps more commonly, selected cases (usually those with an NT >3.5 mm that have a fourfold increased risk for CHD above baseline) are referred for a 14-week cardiac scan. The majority of hearts are still examined for the first time later in gestation, usually at the 20-week level 2 anomaly screening program offered almost universally in the UK.

The Royal College of Obstetricians and Gynaecologists in the UK have surveyed the protocols and practice of those screening the fetal heart (predominantly sonographers) and report that at least half are now routinely looking at the outflow tracts, even if they are not included in their departmental protocols[17]. This improvement in the basic examination has resulted in increased numbers of referrals for structural cardiac abnormalities, especially those affecting the great arteries, that are difficult or impossible to detect on the four-chamber view alone, such as transposition of the great arteries and tetralogy of Fallot[25].

Obstetric screening programs should detect 3.5 major CHD per 1000 screened women.

Major CHD has been defined as cases requiring surgery or intervention in the first year after delivery[3]. Detection rates from these screening programs range from about 25% to just over 80% in many teaching centers[18–21,26].

An increase in detection has an effect on the families and health professionals alike. The psychological impact of detection of abnormality is important, yet there is a disparity between improving diagnostic rates and the ability to manage its impact. Some sonographers admit to not wanting to detect cardiac abnormality because they find it difficult to cope with breaking this news to parents. Easy access to a second opinion is vital to support screening professionals and families alike. It is important to recognize that the antenatal screening program offers the best opportunity to detect CHD and the early postnatal examination often detects less than half of neonates with CHD[27].

Termination of pregnancy is offered to mothers when the fetus has aneuploidy. It is also discussed when the fetus has severe cardiac disease and a two-ventricle repair is unlikely. The outlook for a child who also has extracardiac malformations is often poor and accompanied by long hospital stays and significant morbidity. In the UK, it is possible to offer termination of pregnancy after the usual legal limit of 24 weeks of pregnancy to such cases under Clause E of the 1967 Termination of Pregnancy act. The proportion of women requesting termination of pregnancy is decreasing, in part as surgical results are improving and mortality approaches zero for many lesions[6] and also because the diagnosis is made rather late in pregnancy. Many women now have first-trimester integrated screening followed by their level 2 anomaly scan at 22 weeks. Any cardiac defect suspected at this time may not be confirmed until close to the 24-week limit of termination of pregnancy. For the more complicated cardiac cases, such as hypoplastic left heart syndrome, about two-thirds of mothers will choose a termination of pregnancy, but the overall rate in pregnancies with isolated cardiac defects likely to have a two-ventricle circulation is about 10%. However, it is possible that termination rates will increase in those where a first-trimester diagnosis is made.

WHO SHOULD BE REFERRED TO THE FETAL CARDIOLOGIST?

There is increasing recognition of the need to improve screening for congenital heart disease in the whole of the pregnant population and refine the current triage system that relies too heavily on so-called 'maternal risk factors' taken from the medical history to refer for a detailed fetal echocardiogram by a specialist[28]. Eighty-five percent of babies born with CHD have mothers with no 'maternal risk factors' and many publications confirm the finding that pregnancies at 'increased risk' have a relatively low yield of structural heart disease (usually about a 3%) compared to those showing sonographic abnormality. Triage can create a false sense of security suggesting that women whose babies have CHD will be removed from the general screening program by this process.

Diabetes, epilepsy and teratogenic drugs

Demographic trends towards increased obesity and type II diabetes make selection of these pregnant women for detailed fetal echocardiography unworkable because of limited specialist availability[17,29]. Similarly, women with epilepsy or depression may be treated with drugs that are potentially teratogenic for the heart. The risk of CHD (mostly ventricular septal defects and coarctation of the aorta) is thought to be dose dependent for sodium valproate and lamotrigine and a 2-fold increase in CHD has been described with paroxetine, a selective serotonin re-uptake inhibitor[30]. There is an approximate risk of 3% of CHD in the fetuses of these women, but as the skill base of sonographers has improved, it is preferable to examine these women within the current screening program and refer to a cardiologist if an abnormality is detected on ultrasound examination[31].

Family history of CHD

The triage depends very much on the quality of the history taken. For example, a family history of congenital heart disease is often documented, but poorly defined so individuals with minor or no congenital heart disease are misclassified as being at increased risk. However, more young adults with congenital heart disease are surviving to become parents and they have a risk between 3 and 10% of having a child with CHD[32,33]. It is important to inform young people about their heart disease throughout their care so they can provide this information to other health professionals later in life, especially when they consider becoming parents themselves. Because of their personal experience, it is best practice to offer them a first trimester specialist fetal cardiology scan, particularly if there is a history of left-sided obstructive disease.

TRAINING

There are many alternative practical ways in which screening standards can be established and monitored and these depend upon the setting. If there is a national screening program, there is the potential to introduce a basic screening protocol and for training to be regulated by a professional body[34].

Screening should now routinely include the more comprehensive ultrasound protocol of five transverse views of the fetal heart[31]. Details of how to perform a fetal cardiac scan are found in many textbooks and papers and obstetric screening programs will require access to educational support and training materials that can be obtained or downloaded from the web from sites such as http://www.tinytickers.org. Training needs to be underpinned by audit so that ascertainment rates can be compared at baseline and any improvement documented following training; however, support for audit is inadequate in clinical practice.

In some countries, practitioners are required to pass a series of ultrasound examinations or an 'exit' examination demonstrating competency. These examinations require an individual to demonstrate a gradation of skills in ultrasound which will qualify them to perform the more complex examinations such as Doppler of the fetal circulation and echocardiography.

FIRST-TRIMESTER SCREENING

First-trimester screening is discussed more extensively in Chapters 19–21. Its primary goal is to detect aneuploid fetuses. Universal early screening using any test which includes a nuchal translucency measurement will detect a subgroup of euploid individuals with CHD. It would be best practice to offer these women a fetal echocardiogram, either at the time of the nuchal test or at about 14 weeks, once the karyotype is known, to look for major CHD[7,8]. Early detailed echo increases the complexity of the examination and the time required to examine the fetal heart[35]. Moreover, this examination will need to be repeated by the fetal cardiologist at 20 weeks to ensure completeness of audit of these early scans.

Funding and technical expertise must be in place to support screening programs. This would include funding for trainers to run programs to improve existing skills in first- and second-trimester fetal echocardiography, to ensure that doctors and technicians are adequately trained to satisfy the demands of the screening program and accreditation requirements.

Universal early screening is planned for the UK and will generate a cohort of about 4700 euploid pregnancies with NT >98th centile a year. Most cases will be in addition to the current workload as 14-week cardiac scanning is still not commonplace. A conservative estimate is that a 10% expansion in the current number of pediatric cardiologists in the UK would be required just to cope with the new demand for the early and repeat fetal cardiac scans. Clearly, as this is not likely, there needs to be an adjustment in existing referral patterns to enable specialists to be able to support the new screening program.

What can realistically be detected at a cardiac scan?

The 12–14-weeks' gestation scan

The early fetal cardiac scan has been shown to be satisfactory for the detection of abnormalities of cardiac connections and detection of large septal defects[8,23,35]. Certain defects that are progressive, such as left heart hypoplasia or aortic and pulmonary stenosis, may not be obvious at this stage and will require a further detailed cardiac scan at 20 weeks' gestation. Furthermore, there may be difficulty in ascertaining some connections, such as those of the pulmonary veins, at 12–14 weeks and it is accepted as both desirable and best practice to repeat the scan at 20 weeks, and again in some cases later in gestation.

The 20-weeks' gestation scan

The 20-week scan should, if all five transverse views are obtained, be able to detect abnormalities of situs, cardiac connections, hearts showing chamber or great arterial disproportion and septal defects (Fig. 31.1). Commonly missed lesions

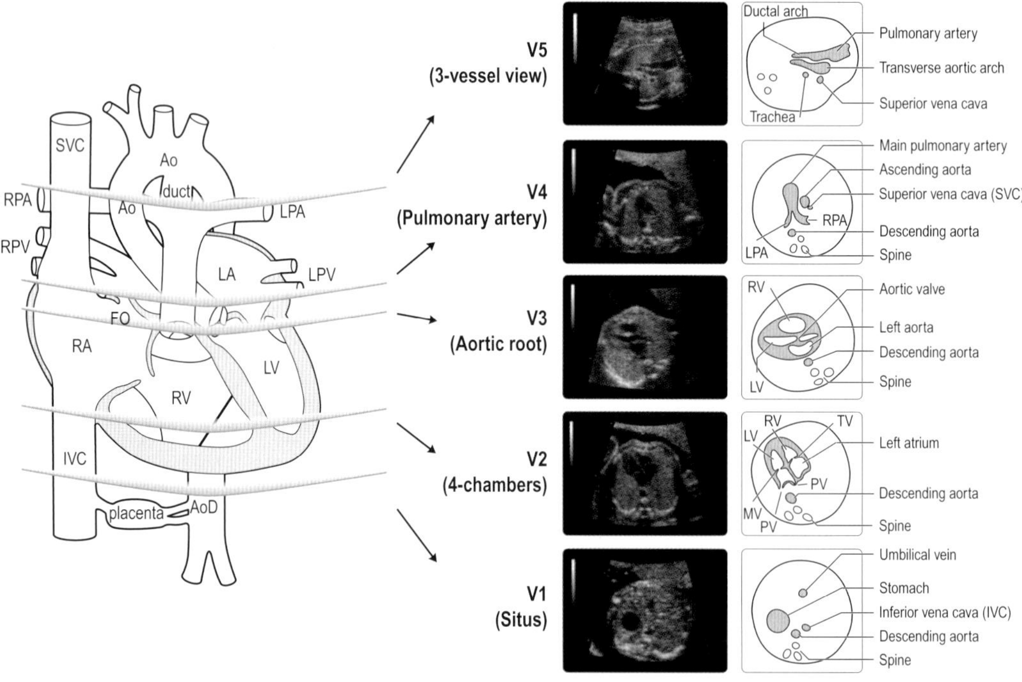

Fig. 31.1 Diagram illustrating the five transverse scanning planes through the fetal body. (V1) Abdominal situs: fetal lie must be determined so the left and right sidedness of structures can be assessed in order to diagnose complex cardiac malformations accurately. In normal situs, the aorta lies to the left and the inferior vena cava to the right of the spine. (V2) Four-chamber view: allows assessment of morphology and symmetry. The left atrium is characterized by the coronary sinus and the left atrial appendage and the right ventricle by the offsetting of the tricuspid valve with attachments to the septum and the moderator band. (V3 and V4) Great arterial crossover: the aorta arises first, sweeping to the fetal right and the pulmonary artery crosses over. The great arteries are usually easiest to differentiate by confirming early bifurcation, characteristic of the pulmonary artery. (V5) The three-vessel and trachea view enables a comparison of the transverse aortic arch and ductal arch. They should be of similar sizes. Additional vessels such as a persistent left superior caval vein or aberrant left subclavian artery may be identified at this level.

at screening include abnormalities of pulmonary venous connections (which are rare in isolation) and coarctation of the aorta which is not accompanied by marked ventricular or great arterial disproportion. It is probable that some cases of aortic and pulmonary stenosis may be mild at 20 weeks and will be missed by screening programs, but these cases may be duct dependent by term and may require early intervention. Small to moderate ventricular septal defects may not be readily appreciated but usually close spontaneously and do not usually cause any symptoms in the baby.

Because heart disease is often progressive, it is good practice to look at the fetal heart if women are referred for ultrasound scans later in pregnancy for other reasons such as fetal growth and placental position.

Counseling and further investigations

A positive screening result will usually be followed by a referral to a fetal medicine unit or pediatric cardiac center to confirm the diagnosis. It is important to exclude extracardiac malformations and aneuploidy (usually following an invasive test) and provide joint counseling from cardiologists, obstetricians and other specialists such as neonatal surgeons and geneticists. Improving surgical results for congenital heart disease[36] have altered the proportion of women choosing termination of pregnancy, but for all types of congenital heart disease the presence of extracardiac malformations or aneuploidy will worsen outcome[37].

Congenital cardiac malformations are complex but can be divided into broad categories as detailed below to assist initial counseling. These are, of course, just guidelines and the final counseling will depend on the fine morphological and physiological details of each case as well as the presence of associated aneuploidy or extracardiac malformations. Many questions are raised following the diagnosis of CHD by health professionals and families alike. They most often include the following: likelihood of associated aneuploidy and extracardiac malformation; progression of the lesion during pregnancy; likelihood of ductal dependency at birth; the timing and type of major cardiac surgery, specifically the need for and type of early surgery (occurring within days or weeks); surgical mortality and likelihood of repeat surgery in later childhood/adult life and, finally, the expected quality of life and life expectancy.

A summary of the problems associated with the broad categories of congenital heart disease are described in the next section and the major points are summarized in Table 31.1.

BROAD CLASSIFICATION OF CONGENITAL HEART DISEASE DETECTED ANTENATALLY

Shunts with balanced anatomy

Septal defects result in shunts which are usually right to left or bidirectional in the fetus but, usually, become left to right after birth as the pulmonary pressures fall. Babies with undiagnosed septal defects may present with symptoms of breathlessness and failure to thrive. In fetal life, morphological features such as the sizes of the inlet valves and flow patterns influence the relative growth of left and right ventricles to produce a balanced or unbalanced situation. CHD with balanced ventricles is likely to be suitable for a postnatal biventricular circulation but, if one ventricle is substantially smaller than the other, a univentricular or 'Fontan-type' route is usually the only surgical option[38]. Cardiac transplantation is a limited option in many countries, but there are some notable exceptions where it provides a realistic alternative to neonatal surgery for some lesions[39,40].

Atrial septal defect

Oval fossa atrial septal defects are rarely diagnosed in fetal life because patency of the oval foramen is essential for survival. The coexistence of extracardiac malformations such as in Holt-Oram may suggest an association. In conditions such as right atrial isomerism, there is often very little atrial septal tissue, but this is usually associated with complex CHD including atrioventricular septal defects[41].

If an isolated atrial septal defect is suspected, the easiest management plan is to arrange for a postnatal scan at about 3 months of age (provided the baby is well at delivery) as the diagnosis can be confirmed or refuted with confidence then. It is very common for a patent oval foramen to be present at birth and so an early scan is often not as definitive. If an atrial septal defect is present, surgery or interventional closure is usually planned before school age. Occasionally, a baby with an isolated atrial septal defect becomes symptomatic with breathlessness and failure to thrive earlier and requires surgical closure, which is carried out on bypass through a median sternotomy with extremely low morbidity and mortality. The interventional catheter approach is now more usual in many countries and is suitable if the defect is not too large and has a good rim of tissue surrounding it. The procedure can be performed with an overnight stay in most cardiology units and involves passing a catheter-mounted device through a sheath inserted into a femoral vein. There are size constraints because of the equipment used and usually babies <8 kg are thought unsuitable for this procedure[42].

Ventricular septal defect

Improved ultrasound technology has resulted in increased recognition of small ventricular septal defects (VSDs), some muscular and some perimembranous, which share the natural history of those detected postnatally in that most will close spontaneously[43]. The risk of aneuploidy is probably small in these cases (<1%) and karyotyping not usually thought worthwhile, although multiple extracardiac abnormalities may suggest a diagnosis of trisomy 13 or 18. A postnatal scan should be organized as antibiotic prophylaxis is advised until closure. A small number may never close but almost none require surgery. However, these young adults will require contact with an adult congenital heart disease unit so that they can be properly advised and supported in the future[32].

The natural method of closure is that tricuspid valve tissue becomes applied to the ventricular septum reducing the size and shunt of the defect. Sometimes the right coronary cusp of the aortic valve is involved in this attempt to close the defect which causes prolapse and aortic regurgitation in about 1% of persistent VSDs[43]. Aortic regurgitation may be progressive and lead to left ventricular dilatation and a reduction in function. For this reason, surgery on bypass is recommended to close the

Table 31.1 Association of aneuploidy and extracardiac malformations (ECM) and approximate outcomes of cardiac lesions

Lesion	*Aneuploid (%)*	*ECM (%)*	*Progression*	*Duct dependent*	*Neonatal surgery*	*Infant surgery*	*Childhood surgery*	*Repeat surgery*	*1-year survival (%)*	*5-year survival (%)*
Atrial septal defect	5	10	N	N	N	N	Y	N	>98	>98
Ventricular septal defect	46	30	N	N	N	Y	Y	N	>98	>98
Overriding aorta										
Tetralogy of Fallot	>10	30	Y	N*	N*	Y	N	N	>95	>95
Double outlet RV	21	<25	N*	N*	N*	Y	N*	N	>95	>95
Tetralogy/pulmonary atresia	>10	<25	Y	Y	Y	Y	Y	Y	83	71
Common arterial trunk	19	25	N	N	Y	N	Y	Y		
CAT/ interrupted arch	39	14	N	Y	Y	N	Y	Y	39	31
AVSD										
Balanced AVSD	46	>50	N	N	N	Y	N	N	>95	>90
Unbalanced AVSD	<25	<25	Y	Y	Y	Y	Y	Y	70–90	65–80
AVSD with isomerism	<1	>50	N	Y*	Y	Y	N*	Y	65–80	<50*
Absent connections										
Mitral atresia	18	<25	N	Y*	Y	Y	Y	Y	95	85
Tricuspid atresia	11	<10	N	Y*	Y	Y	Y	Y	95	85
Left-sided obstruction										
Hypoplastic left heart	7	10	N	Y	Y	Y	Y	Y	65–80	45–60
Coarctation of the aorta	<25	<25	N	Y	Y	N	Y	Y	>95	>95
Interrupted aortic arch	33	<25	N	Y	Y	N	Y	Y	66	61
Moderate aortic stenosis	10	10	Y	N	N	Y	N*	Y	90	>80
Critical aortic stenosis	10	10	Y	Y	Y	Y	Y	Y	65–85	45–60
Discordant ventriculoaterial connections										
Simple transposition	<1	1	N	Y	Y	N	N	N	98	98
Double discordancy	<1	1	N	N	N	Y	Y	Y	90	60–90
Right-sided obstruction										
Pulmonary stenosis	5	<10	Y	N	N	Y	N	N	>95	>95
Critical pulmonary stenosis	5	1	Y	Y	Y	Y	N*	Y	>95	68–90
Pulmonary atresia	5	1	Y	Y	Y	Y	N*	Y	73	68

*Usual outcome but if morphology is more complicated, the management and outcome are different. AVSD, atrioventricular septal defect; CAT, common arterial trunk; RV, right ventricle

defect and resuspend the aortic valve. This is a rare but well-recognized complication and it is wise to review children with perimembranous ventricular septal defects at about 10 years of age if the defect has not closed spontaneously.

Large ventricular septal defects

These will require postnatal evaluation to assess the significance of the shunt. This is probably best done as an outpatient at about 4–6 weeks of age once the pulmonary pressures have fallen, provided there is no suspicion of any coexisting lesion such as coarctation of the aorta. Large defects are reported to be associated with aneuploidy in 40% of cases in some series, but these figures are affected by referral bias and there is probably about at least a 10% risk. Infants tend to become symptomatic at about 4–6 weeks after delivery as pulmonary hypertension reduces permitting a left to right shunt. They can be managed medically by diuretics while surgery is planned. Surgery is performed on bypass through a median sternotomy. There is usually no need for any repeat procedure and outlook is good. Heart block is a rare complication of surgery as the conduction tissue runs around the defect but often this is transient and may be due to edema following surgery. If it occurs, it is managed by inserting a temporary pacing wire until sinus rhythm is re-established.

Multiple ventricular septal defects

Management and outcome is less certain for fetuses with multiple ventricular septal defects. Often, the shunt is substantial but closure of the defects may be very difficult because of their location. Expectant management includes pulmonary artery banding (performed off bypass) once the baby becomes symptomatic, usually between 4–6 weeks to allow the majority of the smaller defects to close spontaneously. The right ventricle hypertrophies in response to banding, which can sometimes make repair of multiple ventricular septal defects more difficult. Devices introduced by catheter may be used to close multiple defects in the lower trabecular septum and have become an attractive alternative to surgery[44]. Ventricular septal defects may be part of a complex of malformations, in particular, there is a well known association with coarctation of the aorta or interrupted aortic arch. These are duct-dependent lesions and will alter the management plan for the woman and her baby. Aneuploidy is reported in up to 46% and, if there are arch abnormalities, it is possible to examine the thymus and offer 22q11 testing if it is small or absent[37,45].

Overriding aorta

A series of malformations is characterized by an overriding aorta (Fig. 31.2). These include tetralogy of Fallot (with and without pulmonary atresia), double outlet right ventricles and common arterial trunk. These all have a moderate risk of aneuploidy (10–20%), particularly 22q11 deletion and extracardiac malformations (see Table 31.1). These cardiac lesions almost always require surgery on bypass in infancy. They are not usually duct dependent, except where there is associated pulmonary atresia or an interrupted aortic arch. Both tetralogy of Fallot with pulmonary atresia and common arterial trunk

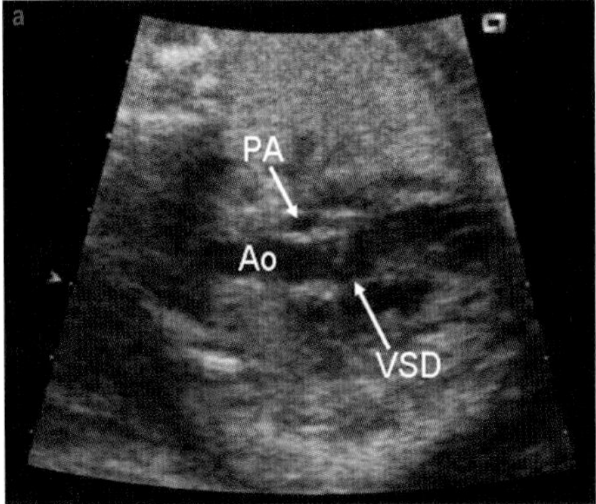

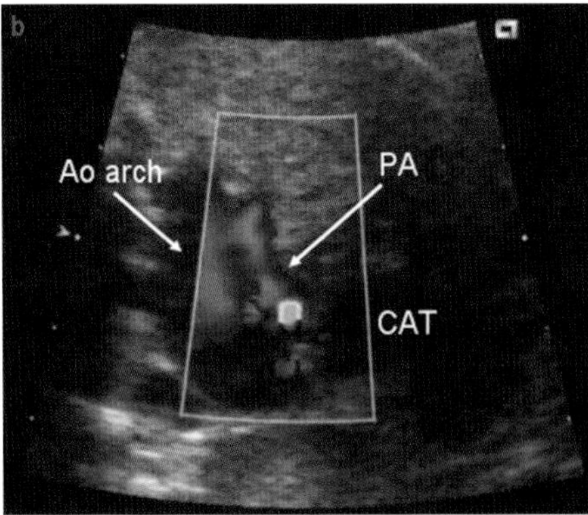

Fig. 31.2 Several conditions are characterized by an overriding aorta. (a) In tetralogy of Fallot, there is an aorta (Ao) overriding the interventricular septum with a large ventricular septal defect (VSD) and a smaller pulmonary artery (PA) which may be atretic. Pulmonary atresia with long segment muscular atresia may be difficult to differentiate from (b) a common arterial trunk (CAT) where there is a solitary outlet from the heart (Trunk) from which the aortic arch (Ao Arch) and branch pulmonary arteries arise (PA).

require early surgery. Tetralogy of Fallot will require immediate shunting if the pulmonary valve is atretic or within the first few weeks if the pulmonary arteries are very small. Common arterial trunk is usually repaired at about 6 weeks of age unless there is an associated interrupted aortic arch, as it behaves physiologically like a large ventricular septal defect. In tetralogy of Fallot, the pulmonary valve may become atretic during the pregnancy which will make the lesion duct dependent. However, this is usually identified on serial scans towards the end of pregnancy and appropriate planning can be instituted. Provided the ventricles are well balanced and the inlet valves not dysplastic (usually it is the tricuspid valve that shows redundant tissue), these conditions can be well managed at surgery with low risk of mortality.

Tetralogy of Fallot with pulmonary atresia is not easy to manage. This condition is characterized by abnormal pulmonary blood supply; the natural pulmonary arteries are small and often not connected to the right ventricle and the pulmonary blood supply may be supplemented by major aortopulmonary collaterals (MAPCAS). A child may require several operations on bypass to centralize the diffuse pulmonary blood supply and connect this back to the right ventricle using a conduit[46,47]. This lesion has one of the highest associations with 22q11 deletion in up to a third of cases[37]. Similarly, in the management of common arterial trunk, a prosthetic conduit or homograft is used to connect the centralized pulmonary arteries to the right ventricle. Any material that does not grow with the child will require replacement perhaps twice in childhood or adolescence[46]. Functional problems can occur later, particularly right ventricular failure and arrhythmias. These problems are seen in young adults whose surgery was many years ago and it is hoped that many of these later problems will not be seen in those operated on in the current era[48].

Atrioventricular septal defects

Atrioventricular septal defect is a defect characterized by a common atrioventricular junction and valve (Fig. 31.3). The septal defects are of variable size and may even be absent which makes detection of this condition more difficult[49,50,51]. It has a strong association with trisomy 21 and isomeric states (where there is bilateral right or left sidedness). It is wise to offer karyotyping for all lesions thought to have normal situs as cases of atrioventricular septal defects diagnosed in early fetal life have about a 100-fold increased risk of trisomy 21 above the age-related risk for an individual woman[52]. About 5% of cases of atrioventricular septal defect are associated with tetralogy of Fallot and this is suggestive of trisomy 21. There are several characteristics that may help to differentiate between the two conditions if an invasive test is declined. Fetuses with trisomy 21 may show soft ultrasound markers for aneuploidy and a double bubble if there is associated duodenal atresia. Those with right atrial isomerism may have the stomach and heart on opposite sides of the body. The atrioventricular septal defect is often associated with pulmonary stenosis or atresia and total anomalous pulmonary venous connections with bilateral superior caval veins.

Cardiac monitoring is important during pregnancy to ensure there continues to be good ventricular balance, mild or no atrioventricular valve regurgitation and no associated malformations, such as coarctation of the aorta, that make this a duct dependent lesion. If there is good balance, a biventricular circulation is anticipated, but the presence of abnormalities of the common valve, such as a dual orifice left atrioventricular valve, may preclude a biventricular circulation or cause troublesome stenosis. This may be difficult to diagnose until the time of surgery. Isolated atrioventricular septal defect or atrioventricular septal defect with tetralogy of Fallot are not duct dependent unless there is associated pulmonary atresia or coarctation of the aorta. These complications are usually diagnosed during pregnancy. Most cases will undergo surgery on bypass at about 3–6 months of age, earlier for those with trisomy 21 as they develop pulmonary vascular disease early. Operative mortality is low and outcome good unless there is significant atrioventricular valve regurgitation or a dual orifice left atrioventricular valve[49]. It is unusual to require repeat surgery later in life and, provided that ventricular function is good, outcome is determined by non-cardiac associations or right atrial isomerism as discussed below.

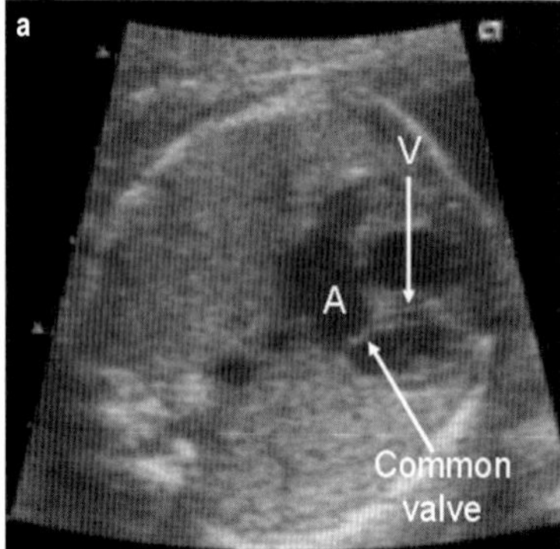

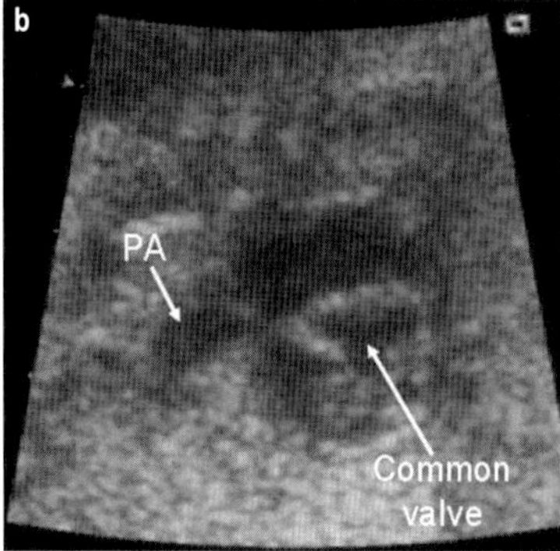

Fig. 31.3 The atrioventricular septal defect is characterized by a common atrioventricular junction and valve. The components of the septal defect may be variable in size with a moderate atrial (A) and ventricular component (V) as in this example. The short axis views show a common valve confirming the defect is an atrioventricular septal defect with a normally placed pulmonary artery (PA).

Shunts with unbalanced anatomy

Large septal defects may be associated with override or straddle of one of the inlet valves that favors flow into the left or right ventricle producing hypoplasia of structures associated with the opposite side such as aortic arch hypoplasia and coarctation. It is important to monitor cardiac growth serially as early scans may not detect straddle and initial counseling might be for a biventricular circulation but, later, it may become apparent that only a univentricular palliation is suitable. Unbalanced lesions are often duct dependent and, if in doubt, perinatal planning should include prostaglandin infusion and postnatal assessment (Fig. 31.4). If there is pulmonary atresia, the baby is usually managed by a systemic to pulmonary artery shunt first to secure a good pulmonary blood supply[46]. If coarctation of the aorta is present, the surgery may be staged with initial repair of the arch and pulmonary artery banding to reduce pulmonary blood flow allowing time to decide on circulatory outcome at a later date. Both these early procedures are usually performed off bypass through a thoracotomy. Any circulation that is unbalanced is likely to require later surgery to replace shunts, redirect systemic venous flow and replace conduits that do not grow with the body. The long-term objective is to separate the systemic and pulmonary circulations by a series of procedures known as the 'Fontan' route[38,53]. Later surgery depends on the specific lesion. If ventricular function is good and pulmonary vascular resistance is low, the outlook is reasonable. Later morbidity is caused by ventricular dysfunction, particularly if the systemic ventricle is a right ventricle, and arrhythmias[48].

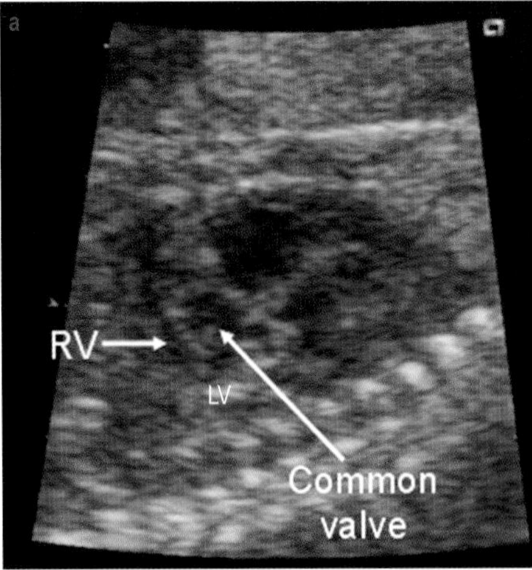

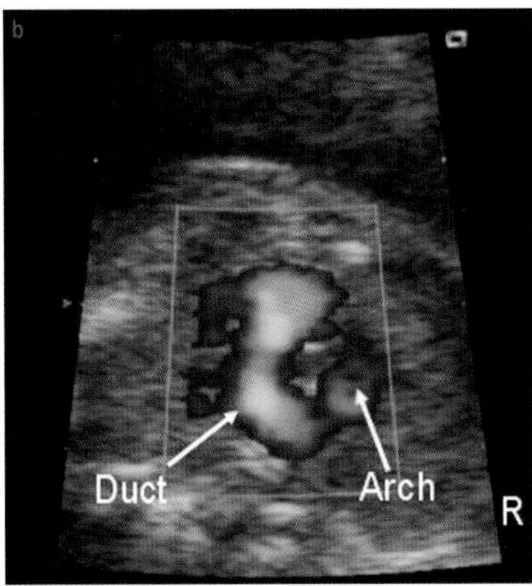

Fig. 31.4 This is an unbalanced atrioventricular septal defect with a small left ventricle (LV) which may be associated with a double inlet arrangement or a hypoplastic or atretic inlet mitral valve. Disproportion is an important characteristic of unbalanced conditions. In this example, the right ventricle (RV) forms the apex of the heart. The three-vessel view (b) demonstrated a normal arterial duct (Duct) and a smaller right aortic arch (Arch) with coarctation of the aorta.

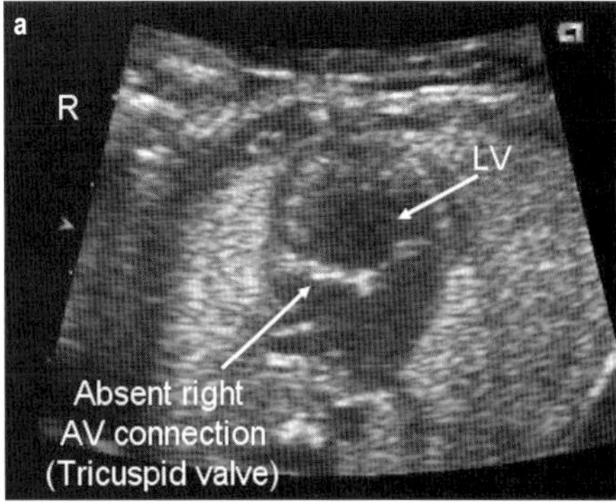

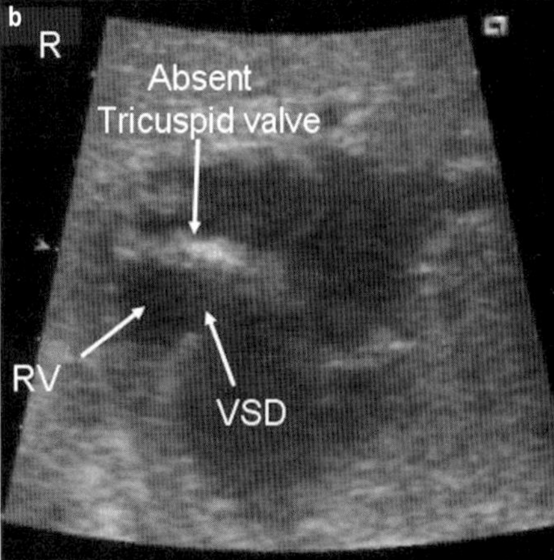

Fig. 31.5 This four-chamber view demonstrates tricuspid atresia (known as absent right atrioventricular connection). It is associated with severe ventricular disproportion with a large left ventricle (LV) and a rudimentary right ventricle (RV). This may be larger if there is a moderate or large ventricular septal defect (VSD) as in (b).

Absent or hypoplastic valves or chambers

Examples of absent or hypoplastic valves and chambers include hypoplastic left heart syndrome, pulmonary atresia with intact septum, tricuspid or mitral atresia with a variety of great arterial connections (Fig. 31.5). These lesions are usually identified at screening because there is one large and one rudimentary ventricle. These appearances are loosely termed 'single ventricle' hearts, although this morphological entity is a very unusual occurrence. Tricuspid atresia may be associated with pulmonary atresia and mitral atresia with aortic atresia (classical hypoplastic left heart syndrome). In mitral atresia, both great arteries may arise from the right ventricle via a double outlet right ventricle connection which may be associated with coarctation of the aorta if there is imbalance.

The appearances usually change little during pregnancy, but many are duct dependent and will require early systemic to pulmonary artery shunting to improve pulmonary blood flow or repair of arch obstruction (Fig. 31.4). The overall risk of aneuploidy is about 10% with a small incidence of 22q11 deletion[37].

Timing of the next stage of surgery depends on symptoms. The final pathway is to use the heart as a pump for the systemic oxygenated blood and divert the deoxygenated blood directly to the lungs. This is usually achieved in childhood and requires three staged procedures. There are many surgical variants but all these are variants of the Fontan circulation. Long-term outcome is uncertain for all but more so if the ventricle is a morphological right ventricle as later deterioration and possible failure of the systemic right ventricle occurs in many individuals with a systemic right ventricle[48] requiring long medical therapy or possibly cardiac transplantation[39,40].

Discordant ventriculoarterial connections

Simple transposition of the great arteries is more correctly described as discordant ventriculoarterial connections (Fig. 31.6). This lesion is usually associated with a very low risk of aneuploidy (<1%) or extracardiac malformation. It is a duct-dependent lesion and may be isolated, associated with a ventricular septal defect or arise as part of a more complex malformation. If there is an intact ventricular septum or only a small/moderate muscular ventricular septal defect, mixing of the pulmonary and systemic circulations depends on patency of the arterial duct and

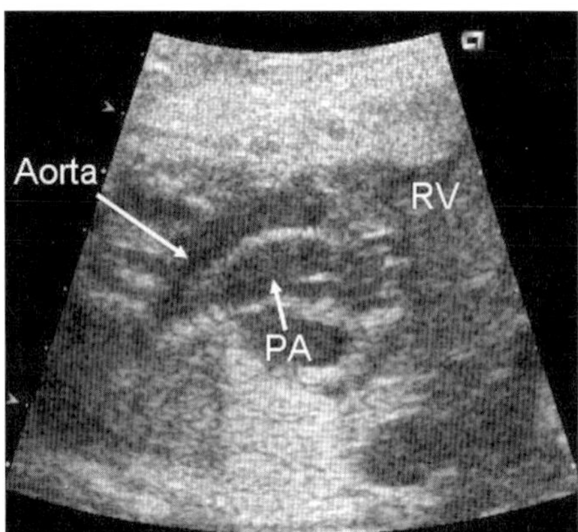

Fig. 31.6 Transposition of the great arteries shows a parallel relationship of the aorta and pulmonary arteries (PA) arising from the right (RV) and left ventricles respectively.

the interatrial communication (oval foramen). The interatrial septum may become thickened and close in utero, which may result in significant morbidity and possible intrauterine death[54]. If this is recognized early, balloon atrial septostomy should be attempted, as it is recognized that closure of the interatrial septum can result in pulmonary venous hypertension and hemorrhage. Some babies die in the perinatal period before they reach surgery. Paradoxically, administration of prostaglandin may worsen this situation by increasing the pulmonary circulation. For this reason, fetal therapy has been proposed to ameliorate the outcome for newborns with restrictive or closed interatrial septum[16].

The important morphological features to look for in cases of transposition of the great arteries during pregnancy are ventricular balance and equality of semilunar valve (pulmonary and aortic valves) size as pulmonary stenosis can occur that may preclude the arterial switch procedure after birth. The semilunar valves should be thin pliable leaflets as, following the arterial switch procedure, the pulmonary valve will become the new aortic valve. If there is significant stenosis or potential for stenosis, this surgery will not be attempted. The arterial switch is usually performed in the first week of life on bypass and the decision to perform a balloon atrial septostomy before this depends on symptoms, hypoxemia and surgical preference. Infants with a large ventricular septal defect and well-balanced ventricles and good semilunar valves are usually suitable for the switch procedure but it does not need to be performed early because there is usually good mixing of oxygenated and deoxygenated blood. There is a variety of coronary artery patterns associated with this lesion and these details can usually be verified using ultrasound after birth to aid surgical planning.

Surgical mortality approaches zero[6] and outcome after the arterial switch is excellent and usually no further surgery required but, sometimes, the branch pulmonary arteries are small or become kinked during the Lecompte maneuver, a surgical procedure to bring them anterior to the aorta. This complication may be treated by balloon dilatation, sometimes with stent implantation or, occasionally, surgery is required, particularly if the branches are relatively hypoplastic.

Double discordancy

In double discordancy (sometimes called congenitally corrected transposition of the great arteries), the circulation is

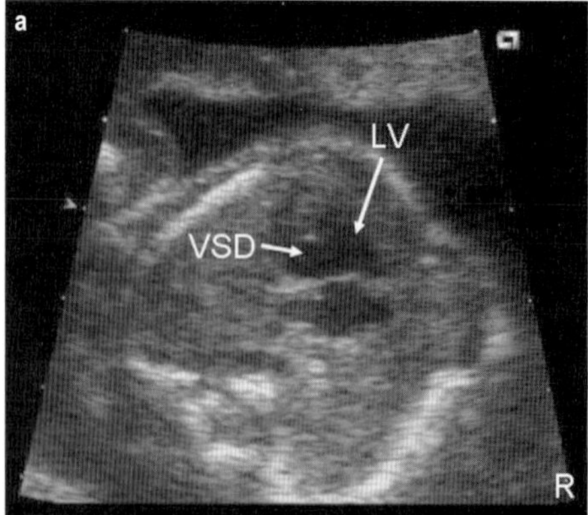

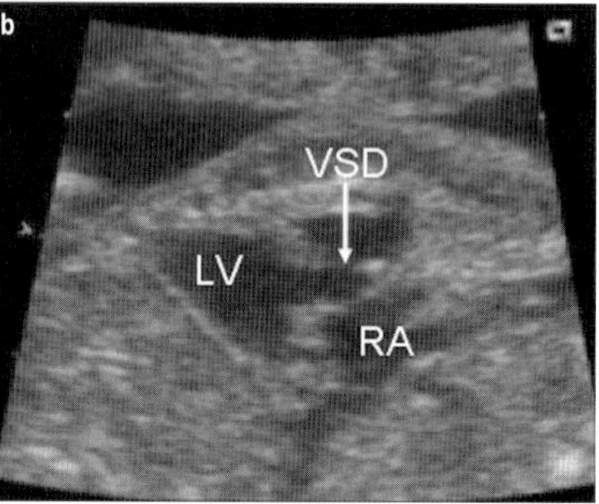

Fig. 31.7 (a) Double discordancy (or congenitally corrected transposition) is characterized by 'reverse off-setting' of the mitral and tricuspid valves as the morphological left ventricle (LV) lies on the fetal right (R) and is connected to the right atrium (RA) (b) and vice versa. Additional defects may include ventricular septal defects (VSD) and pulmonary stenosis.

physiologically normal because both atrioventricular and ventriculoarterial connections are discordant. That is the left atrium connects to the right ventricle and thence to the aorta and vice versa[55] (Fig. 31.7). This may be detected in fetal life because the heart is sometimes in the right chest or has an odd, rounded appearance as the right ventricle lies on the fetal left. The commonest associations are ventricular septal defect and pulmonary stenosis. Complete heart block is reported to develop in at least a third of individuals during childhood that were born with sinus rhythm[56]. If there is no ventricular septal defect or pulmonary stenosis, no surgery may be required, indeed, the diagnosis may not be made until adult life in such cases. Long-term outlook is dependent on right ventricular function and the presence of tricuspid valve dysplasia or Ebstein malformation. The right ventricle is in the systemic position and will not function long term as well as a left ventricle would. Any proposed surgery is complex, the ultimate correction being a double switch procedure[57]. This comprises a procedure to divert atrial flows to the opposite ventricle by means of interatrial baffles (the Mustard procedure) and an arterial switch procedure. The medium-term results of this procedure in carefully selected patients performed by very experienced surgeons are reasonable and it has been undertaken in infancy. Heart failure may best be treated by medical means or consideration for heart transplantation[40].

Isolated aortic or pulmonary valve stenosis

Aortic stenosis

The early signs of aortic stenosis may be subtle and can easily be missed at screening. Aortic stenosis is characterized by left ventricular dilatation in the early stages, with progressive outflow tract obstruction, the left ventricle suffers secondary damage resulting in endocardial fibroelastosis, poor function, reduced coronary perfusion and fibrosis and mitral regurgitation. Some cases will progress to hypoplastic left heart syndrome and these usually show reversal of flow in the transverse aortic arch progressing to aortic arch hypoplasia[13] (Fig. 31.8). The left ventricle may respond to this pressure load by continuing to grow relatively normally, dilate or become short, compared to the right side[59]. If there is mitral regurgitation, there may be left atrial enlargement and often the interatrial septum becomes thickened and closed producing abnormalities of pulmonary venous flow that lead to pulmonary venous arterialization and pulmonary hypertension[58]. This is a duct-dependent lesion termed 'critical aortic stenosis'. The treatment possibilities are twofold: if there is adequate left ventricular size and function, balloon aortic valvuloplasty is the treatment of choice and, if not, the three-stage 'Norwood' procedure is performed. There are now many variants to the surgery originally described by Norwood. However, they all result in a univentricular circulation. It may be possible in some cases to remove the fibrous lining of the left ventricle during this surgery and improve left ventricular filling which may permit continued growth of the ventricle in infancy. A reversal of the initial surgery may then be possible resulting in an eventual biventricular circulation. Aortic valve replacement is usually required later in life, so it is advantageous to use balloon catheter treatments in early life to reduce the risks associated with reoperation. If the stenosis is severe early in fetal life, it is more likely that the resultant left ventricular damage and reduction in growth velocity will determine that a univentricular outcome is the only possible route. If the aortic arch is also severely hypoplastic, the 'Norwood' procedure will be required to improve the blood supply to the cerebral circulation. Outcome for 'Norwood' results are variable and depend on case selection with those complicated by a restrictive or closed interatrial septum having worse results[58,60] as well as surgical skill, choice of procedure (Norwood, hybrid catheter procedure or transplantation) and institutional facilities. The 30-day survival is reported as >80% in several institutions, but 5-year survival following completion of surgery is often nearer to 45%[58,61–64].

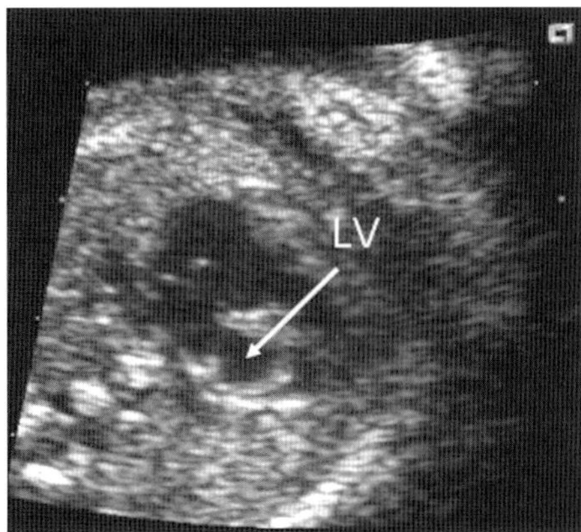

Fig. 31.8 In aortic atresia the aortic valve has no forward flow. If the mitral valve remains patent after the aortic valve has closed the ventricular response may result in a 'walnut-sized left ventricle' characterized by thick bright ventricular walls and a small cavity (LV). This form of hypoplastic left heart syndrome may have associated coronary artery abnormalities.

Pulmonary stenosis/atresia

Pulmonary stenosis presents with a range of severity and may progress to complete closure (atresia) in fetal life. It is associated with varying degrees of right ventricular hypoplasia (ranging from a ventricle consisting of one to three parts) and degrees of tricuspid valve dysplasia associated with tricuspid regurgitation[65]. The circulation and morphology can worsen significantly during pregnancy and result in fetal hydrops. A further complication is the association with right ventricular to coronary artery fistulae which may result in the coronary circulation being dependent on a high pressure right ventricle to perfuse the myocardium. Opening the pulmonary valve will decompress the right ventricle and may result in coronary artery steal and myocardial infarction.

Isolated pulmonary valve stenosis is successfully treated in postnatal life using balloon catheter techniques, but may not be successful if associated with Noonan syndrome where the valve is thickened or dysplastic[66]. This may be suspected either by a positive family history and/or the development of pleural effusions in the fetus. If the pulmonary valve closes during pregnancy, this becomes a duct-dependent lesion and requires careful planning for delivery with prostaglandin infusion prior to transfer for surgery. If right ventricular size is small or function is poor, a univentricular circulation may be the only option and, in most series of pulmonary atresia, only about one-third of children are able to go on to have a biventricular circulation. Five-year survival is about 68% overall in most large series[67]. Prediction of outcome using morphological measures such as tricuspid valve size has been proposed, but it is not uncommon for several years to elapse before the appropriate choice of final circulation (uni- or biventricular) is clear.

Ventricular or great arterial disproportion

Ventricular disproportion and/or great arterial disproportion may indicate a cardiac malformation, for example coarctation of the aorta, or it may be associated with normal variants such as persistence of the embryonic left superior caval vein draining to the coronary sinus (Fig. 31.9). It may also be an indicator of trisomy, intrauterine growth restriction or anemia. It is important to note that all cardiac malformations may be balanced or not and, therefore, a wide variety of malformations may show disproportion. About three-quarters of all cardiac lesions associated with disproportion are duct dependent and so they are important to recognize before birth so the team can plan for optimal perinatal care. The likelihood of aneuploidy and associated extracardiac malformations depends on the specific lesion and imbalance often worsens during pregnancy. As with all duct-dependent lesions, early surgery is common within days or weeks after delivery. The short- and long-term outcomes of surgery depend on specific circumstances.

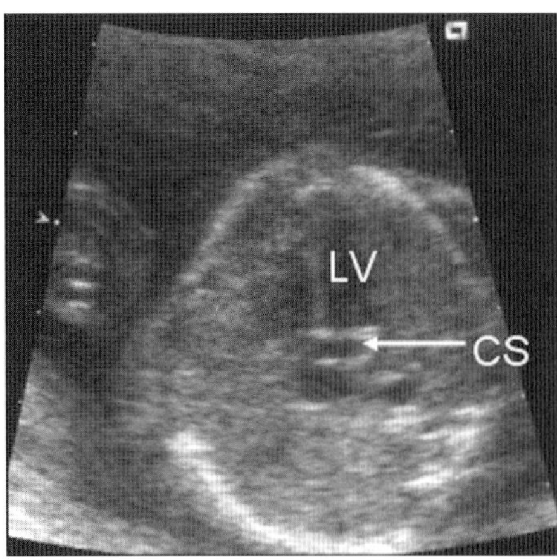

Fig. 31.9 A persistent left superior caval vein may be a normal variant. When it drains to the coronary sinus (CS), it may obstruct flow through the developing mitral valve and result in fetal cardiac disproportion with a smaller left (LV) than right ventricle in some cases, but not here. This is associated with an increased risk of cardiac malformations.

One of the most important conditions diagnosed on suspicion of disproportion, often with no other cardiac signs, is isolated coarctation of the aorta or interrupted aortic arch. If this is detected early it will be repaired within a few days of delivery, usually with good success. If it is not detected antenatally or before discharge to home, neonatal collapse may occur in the community and death is not uncommon[68]. Poor feeding and respiratory distress are common first signs of a cardiac problem. Surgery for coarctation is performed off bypass via a thoracotomy. Re-stenosis may occur and is often treated by balloon dilatation. Repeat surgery is sometimes required for re-coarctation or aneurysm formation at the site of operation. The medium- and long-term problems include later hypertension and need for replacement of the aortic valve that suffers from accelerated stenosis if it is bicuspid.

Heterotaxy syndromes

This complicated area is viewed differently by obstetricians and cardiologists, which may result in some confusion of terminology and definition. Cardiologists define the syndromes based on the morphology of the atrial appendages rather than presence or absence of the spleen, although they are associated characteristics of the syndromes. Arrangement of the atrial appendages can be inferred from the relative position of the aorta and inferior vena cava to the spine, but abnormality of arrangement is not essential to the diagnosis[69]. An individual with isomerism shows bilateral left or right sidedness of a variety of structures such as the lungs. Fetuses with right atrial isomerism have a poor outcome, while those with left atrial isomerism usually fare better. Isomerism is rarely associated with aneuploidy but, the commonly associated extracardiac malformations of biliary atresia and bowel malrotation, often seen in left atrial isomerism, have an important influence on outcome[41,69].

Left atrial isomerism

Cases of left atrial isomerism may have no cardiac malformation other than bilateral left atrial appendages. There is often an atrioventricular septal defect within normal great arteries. There may also be heart block or low atrial rhythm as the sinus node is a right atrial structure. The most usual finding is interruption of the IVC with azygous continuation to a persistent left superior caval vein which may drain into the coronary sinus which becomes enlarged, or to the right superior caval vein (see Fig. 31.9). The left side of the heart may be relatively small and associated with arch obstruction. Associated problems include heart block, biliary atresia and bowel malrotation. Antenatal diagnosis is useful in order to alert the pediatric team to these possible neonatal problems. If there is no heart block and no extracardiac problems, the outlook is good.

Right atrial isomerism

Right atrial isomerism has a poor prognosis as the cardiac lesions are more complex than in left atrial isomerism and there is usually functional asplenia. Less than half of affected children reach 2 years of age because of the combination of complex cardiac defects and infection[41]. The commonest cardiac lesion is atrioventricular septal defect, often with associated pulmonary stenosis or atresia. A further complication is that the pulmonary veins are draining anomalously as there are two morphological right atria. Postnatal treatment will involve early surgery on bypass to correct total anomalous pulmonary connections, especially if they are obstructed, and insert a systemic to pulmonary artery shunt if there is severe pulmonary stenosis or atresia. The ventricular balance can worsen during gestation and, if pulmonary atresia develops, it will become a duct-dependent lesion.

It is difficult to cover all variants that may occur in these conditions and these are dealt with well in the literature[41]. The important points are that antenatal assessment is difficult and often the situation is worse than appreciated. Counseling should be guarded and a multidisciplinary team is best placed to discuss the management of both cardiac and extracardiac problems.

Miscellaneous group

There is a group of unrelated conditions characterized by poor cardiac function or poor lung growth that may result in fetal hydrops and a high risk of intrauterine death. Overall, about 6% of fetuses with congenital heart disease suffer an intrauterine death. Examples include Ebstein malformation, absent pulmonary valve syndrome, complete heart block, dilated or hypertrophic cardiomyopathy, cardiac tumors (some of which may be associated with arrhythmia such as ventricular tachycardia), ventricular aneurysms and large pleural or pericardial effusions. The association with aneuploidy is moderate and there is a high likelihood of associated extracardiac malformation. These conditions usually worsen during gestation as heart function decreases. The conditions are not usually duct dependent, but delivery needs to be planned carefully as many of these babies are unstable and will need early surgery (within days or weeks). There is a well-recognized association of lung hypoplasia with Ebstein malformation and absent pulmonary valve syndrome which, if severe, has a very gloomy prognosis. It is important to counsel carefully in these conditions as the chances of intrauterine and neonatal death are high, and there may be no good surgical option for these babies. The specific timing and type of surgery will depend on the condition and, because of the relative rarity of these conditions, up-to-date information should be sought to inform decision making on individual cases.

Cardiac arrhythmias

Bradycardias

The differential diagnosis of fetal bradycardia presents a clinical dilemma, particularly if there are no personnel immediately available to distinguish between bradycardia due to fetal distress or a cardiac arrhythmia. Avoidance of the premature delivery of infants with complex heart disease and heart block is desirable as treatment is more difficult if complicated by small size and sickness due to respiratory disease. The differential diagnosis includes complete heart block that may be isolated or associated with congenital heart disease, long QT syndrome and conditions such as atrial bigeminy where the conduction of normal atrial beats is halved resulting in a fetal heart rate between 60 and 70 beats per minute[12,70,71]. This latter diagnosis is usually benign and self-limiting with the majority of babies having a normal heart rate by term (Fig. 31.10).

Fetuses presenting with atrial ectopic beats or tachyarrhythmias usually have structurally normal hearts. However, this is not the case for those with complete heart block, about half of whom have important heart malformations, often atrioventricular septal defects and/or left atrial isomerism[12]. The associated problems of those with isomerism have been dealt with above and their outlook is poor. In contrast, fetuses with isolated heart block do better. Their complete heart block is most often due to transference of anti-Ro/La antibodies across the placenta from a mother with connective tissue disease that may not have been previously diagnosed. Provided hydrops does not occur and cardiac function is good, many of these fetuses survive to term. The evidence of any effective antenatal therapy is limited: if the HR is below 55, maternal sympathomimetics such as salbutamol may be helpful but may be deleterious if the diagnosis is long QT syndrome[71]. Antenatal steroids may be useful to improve hydrops and reduce later fibrosis, but there is considerable debate on their effects on the degree of eventual heart block[72–75]. Immunoglobulin therapy may be more useful in altering the progression of block, but experience is limited.

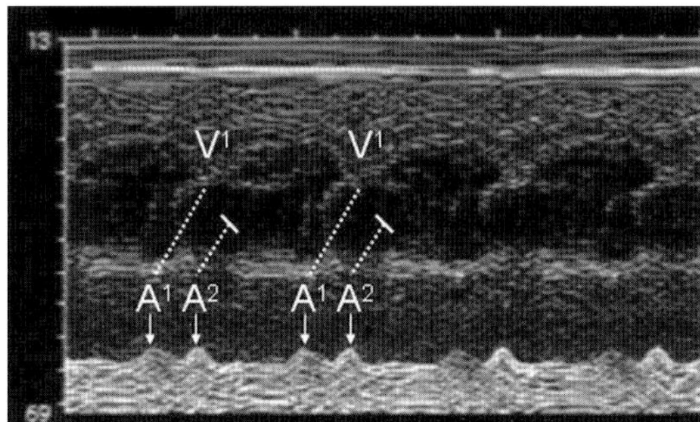

Fig. 31.10 This M-mode strip illustrates atrial bigeminy. This is characterized by coupled atrial beats only one of which, A1, is conducted to produce a ventricular beat, V1. The second atrial beat, A2, occurs during the refractory period and is blocked. This results in a ventricular rate of 60 to 70 beats per minute, but there is rarely hydrops and most cases resolve spontaneously without any need for pacing.

Many children function well initially but pacing is advised for those whose 24-hour tapes show the heart rate falls below 55 for sustained periods.

Tachycardias

Fetal tachycardia is usually amenable to medical therapy given to the mother[70,76]. Conventional antenatal assessment uses pulsed Doppler or M-mode to identify the relationship between the atrial and ventricular beats. Atrial tachycardias are common but ventricular tachycardias are more rare and may be associated with cardiomyopathy, ventricular tumors or long QT syndrome in the fetus[71]. Atrial tachycardias with one to one conduction are usually due to either an accessory pathway or atrial tachycardia and may be divided into those with long or short RP interval using Doppler methods to clarify the mechanism and allow the best medical therapy to be selected[76–78].

Most fetuses have short RP tachycardia which is usually responsive to oral digoxin given to the mother (in the absence of hydrops) or flecainide (in Europe), or verapamil in North America. Success of cardioversion is high in the absence of hydrops, but there is no consensus on drug choices. Atrial flutter is much more difficult to treat. It is diagnosed where there is an atrial rate of 400 bpm or more with variable degrees of block to the ventricles. All tachycardias may result in fetal hydrops and outcome is worsened with an average 25% mortality.

A meta-analysis of several published reports concluded that atrial flutter presents nearer to term than 'supraventricular tachycardia' and is less often associated with hydrops. While drug treatment is effective for supraventricular tachycardias, electrical cardioversion is really the only effective therapy for atrial flutter[79]. Mortality is similar for both conditions ranging from zero to 15%.

There are no controlled trials of therapy and the decision to treat is influenced by gestational age, the presence of sustained versus intermittent arrhythmia, evidence of fetal compromise and the type of arrhythmia. The management options include surveillance alone, drug therapy or delivery. It is important to remember that many of the drugs have a negative ionotropic action and are pro-arrhythmic and may cause harm. They exert their action on specific ion channels of the action potential or at the atrioventricular node.

Short RP tachycardia may be due to a re-entrant mechanism, such as an accessory pathway as seen in Wolf–Parkinson–White syndrome (WPW), and is usually effectively treated with digoxin or flecainide. Digoxin is favored by many because of long experience with it and its positive ionotropic action. It is a glycoside drug, used since 1978 in the treatment of fetal tachycardias. It works by blocking the A-V node and does not treat atrial tachycardia but increases atrioventricular block.

Flecainide is a class 1C drug used since 1988 and works to inhibit the fast sodium channels. It increases action potential duration and should be given slowly if used intravenously. It is important to monitor the maternal ECG response and this should be done pre-therapy and after the first dose. It is most useful if there is hydrops or digoxin fails to slow the ventricular rate.

Amiodarone is a useful class 3 drug working by prolonging the action potential. It is good for atrial and ventricular tachycardia but the main concern has been its possible effects on the fetal thyroid. It increases the levels of digoxin by about 50% and, if used in combination, digoxin dose should be reduced.

Sotolol causes non-selective beta blockade through class III action on the calcium channels. It is a mild negative ionotropic, but effective and is used as a first-line drug by some[80].

Verapamil is a class 4 drug acting on the calcium channels in the sinoatrial and atrioventricular nodes. It is favored in North America but is not used often in fetal or pediatric tachyarrhythmias in Europe because of its negative ionotropic effect. It increases digoxin levels by 50–70% and the dose of this should be reduced to avoid toxicity. It should be avoided in atrioventricular block.

Adenosine is short acting and can be given directly into the fetal circulation. It blocks adenosine receptors in the atrioventricular node so is useful for re-entrant tachycardias. It is a good diagnostic tool and may terminate a tachycardia but this is less likely if there is a high sympathetic drive associated with prolonged tachycardia and hydrops.

Long RP tachycardia may be more difficult to manage and may be due to atrial ectopic tachycardia or rarer conditions, such as persistent junctional reciprocating tachycardia (PJRT). These arrhythmias are more likely to respond to drugs like flecainide or sotolol but may not be easily controlled in the fetus, or even after birth in the neonate. It is good practice to liaise with a pediatric electrophysiologist when considering management options in a fetus with tachycardia, particularly choice of drug therapy.

Newer technologies such as fetal ECG, Doppler tissue imaging and magnetocardiography may help refine diagnosis and choice of and response to medical therapy[81–83]. Many fetuses without hydrops will respond well to oral therapy given to the mother. For those presenting with hydrops, therapy is more difficult and a proportion are refractory to treatment and die in utero[78]. Medium- and long-term outlook for survivors is good with the majority of them showing no further episodes. A postnatal ECG is helpful to determine whether there is an overt accessory pathway and the choice of postnatal drug therapy depends on the findings and the individual electrophysiologist's preference. Many prescribe therapy for 6 months or so and then stop it. Less than a third of children will have another episode of tachycardia and only a small proportion will require long-term therapy or later radiofrequency ablation for an additional pathway[78].

A large number of fetuses have atrial ectopic beats. These cause undue anxiety in mothers and health professional alike. They are commonplace and benign with only rare reports that they may trigger a tachycardia. In a series by Simpson et al., 195 fetuses with irregular rhythm were followed up, 157 had a normal ventricular rate and 37 subnormal ventricular rate due to multiple blocked beats. Eight of these babies developed sustained tachycardias either prenatally (n = 4) or postnatally (n = 4). Three babies had shown a normal ventricular rate and five a subnormal ventricular rate due to multiple blocked atrial ectopics.

A practical management strategy may include auscultation by the local obstetrician or midwife every 10–14 days with review in the cardiology center offered after 4 weeks depending on gestational age, frequency of ectopics with particularly close monitoring of multiple blocked atrial extrasystoles. The role of substances such as caffeine is not clear but often women find this unpalatable during pregnancy and decrease their intake spontaneously. There is usually no need for postnatal surveillance or therapy.

MANAGEMENT DURING PREGNANCY

Once a cardiac defect is detected, counseling with a multidisciplinary team is arranged. This will include the use of a cardiac liaison nursing team and genetic counseling where appropriate. Serial visits will be arranged, the frequency depending on the type of malformation detected and the ease of visiting the center for the family. At each visit it is wise to recheck the anatomy, the presence of extracardiac malformations and fetal growth and well-being in collaboration with the fetal medicine team. The perinatal management of the fetus may be altered by progression of disease[15]. For example, abnormalities of pulmonary venous flow may indicate increasing restriction of the interatrial septum with resultant pulmonary venous hypertension and the potential for pulmonary hemorrhage in the perinatal period that may result in morbidity and mortality in some[58]. Management of this complication may include offering the option for fetal intervention to open the interatrial septum[16] or urgent septostomy or surgical septectomy immediately after delivery. In conditions where a Fontan surgical route is anticipated, the development of tricuspid regurgitation is an adverse prognostic sign and may indicate that surgical options are reduced and outcome may be poorer than thought earlier. In common arterial trunk, the presence of truncal regurgitation may lead to worsening ventricular damage and impact negatively on surgery. Valvar stenosis may become atresia and lesions become duct dependent so that perinatal management is altered.

Timing of delivery and perinatal management

The majority of fetuses with congenital heart disease should be able to deliver normally at term. However, there is a substantial association with extracardiac malformations and growth restriction and early delivery may be precipitated by adverse Doppler findings. It is important to hold early discussions with the neonatal and surgical teams to plan perinatal management, for example exit strategies in cases of arch obstruction or thoracic tumors, management of twins discordant for abnormality and the use of prostaglandin or balloon atrial septostomy in preparation for transfer to the cardiac center. Where there is an associated malformation requiring early neonatal surgery, such as exomphalos, prioritization of procedures should be discussed and appropriate measures taken to arrange for the surgical procedures to be performed shortly after delivery.

Auditing outcomes

The general feedback to the primary screener and local obstetricians and geneticists is often poor. It is essential for local screeners to know what they detect and what they miss and lack of feedback significantly impedes audit of screening programs. A detailed postmortem by a perinatal pathologist is important in cases of fetal or neonatal demise. Local obstetricians will require detailed feedback so they can counsel mothers before the next pregnancy and in case of bereavement. It is common for bereavement counseling to be offered by the tertiary center that have performed the investigations and managed the pregnancy but, if this is the case, local obstetricians should not be left out of the loop. The genetics team is vital to provide post-pregnancy investigations and counseling and also to advise on the need for pre-pregnancy testing in a future pregnancy. Unfortunately, the fetal medicine team and neonatologists are not always informed of the outcome of specific cardiac cases which reduces their ability to provide a comprehensive service to families and to remain involved. A routine multidisciplinary debriefing session to consider the team approach to particular cases that may or may not have gone smoothly as planned, is not a routine part of practice, but one that may be extremely helpful and improve the clinical service.

NEW TECHNOLOGIES AND THERAPIES

Overall detection rates at screening are now improving and create an increased demand for consultation. One possible solution is to use telemedicine support to permit a more effective use of the specialist's time[84,85]. Telemedicine can provide diagnostic and educational support to referring centers. The tertiary center can triage cases remotely without the need for women to travel. This helps to restrict the cases that require a detailed examination and consultation by the fetal cardiologist to those with abnormalities rather than encourage the continuance of time-consuming, low-yield referrals of the traditional high-risk groups.

Imaging and functional assessment

Imaging improves year on year and enables an improved assessment of not only structural[86] but also functional developments. These allow better and more detailed diagnosis and perhaps guide prediction of outcome. Time intervals assessed by Doppler such as the Tei index allow an assessment of efficiency of fetal cardiac function[87]. Tissue Doppler measures velocities of the myocardium, thus permitting an assessment of myocardial shortening and lengthening. M-mode assessment of displacement of the atrioventricular ring reflects function of the long axis fibers of the heart that may be affected first in conditions of myocardial ischemia[88,89]. These methods may be useful in assessing function in fetuses with myocardial hypertrophy such as maternal diabetes[90].

Volume sets may allow better functional assessment than two-dimensional images as they are relatively free of geometric assumptions. Fetal gating remains difficult to achieve but automated image collection allows re-alignment of B-mode images according to their spatial and temporal domain and permits evaluation of a loop of 3-D fetal cardiac activity. The addition of color Doppler further enhances the diagnostic ability of the examination[86].

In countries where specialist consultations require long distance travel by pregnant women, the use of 3/4D volume sets sent over the Internet may allow the specialists to examine the data in more detail in their own center and provide a comprehensive report to the local center who can then counsel the woman appropriately and refer for a detailed assessment if necessary.

Electrophysiological assessment of the fetus

There have been several encouraging reports on the acquisition of fetal ECG using magnetocardiography[91] and non-invasive fetal ECG[92]. More recently, Doppler tissue imaging has described the mechanism of myocardial conduction in arrhythmias[83]. A better understanding of the normal development of electrical signaling in the fetus, developmental control mechanisms and response to therapy will improve our ability to make a detailed diagnosis of the mechanisms of tachycardia and bradycardia and to prescribe the best therapy before birth to terminate or manage arrhythmia that may save lives, particularly when there is fetal hydrops.

More sensitive monitoring in cases of emerging heart block may permit a better understanding of the mechanisms and permit objective evaluation of a therapeutic trial in cases secondary to anti-Ro/La antibody disease[93].

There is currently unsatisfactory management of the fetus with a low heart rate. They are at risk of developing hydrops and fetal death. Alternative management strategies include preterm delivery and postnatal pacing[12], maternal therapy with sympathomimetic drugs, or intrauterine pacing with variable success. Technical difficulties have impeded the progression of intrauterine pacing, but various groups are working on ways to pace the fetus with heart block and improved equipment and techniques may result in a minimally invasive deployment of a pacing system[94,95].

Valvuloplasty and balloon atrial septostomy in the fetus

Fetal cardiac therapy has been proposed for progressive cardiac disease with relatively poor prognosis such as critical aortic stenosis[96,97] and pulmonary atresia with intact ventricular septum[67,98].The procedures have been performed in fetal medicine units where the personnel are used to performing invasive procedures using a variety of techniques and approaches and where the pregnant woman can be appropriately managed[99]. The cardiac procedures have included cardiac valvuloplasty for aortic and pulmonary atresia or critical stenosis and balloon atrial septostomy for hypoplastic left heart syndrome or simple transposition of the great arteries with closed or restrictive interatrial communication[13–16]. The major reason for fetal intervention is to improve postnatal outcome and encourage a biventricular outcome, or the best possible univentricular circulation. To achieve this aim, prevention of secondary damage is desirable. Unfortunately, there are no animal models of progressive heart disease sufficiently similar to the human fetus to aid in developing comparable treatment strategies and so progress has been slow. Fetal therapy shows promise but selection criteria, timing of the procedure and comparative data on outcomes in treated and untreated control cases are required to ascertain its role.

CONCLUSIONS

The fetus with a structural cardiac malformation may now be detected in the first trimester. Earlier detection does not necessarily mean that there is an increased rate of termination of pregnancy, particularly in those with isolated cardiac problems. However, it results in an increased opportunity to counsel and plan for optimal management of complex cases. In order to achieve this goal, we require increased resources to develop and utilize experts from several disciplines working together in teams. These teams also need improved audit mechanisms to monitor what is being achieved and to plan and support the future needs of those caring for the fetus with congenital heart disease.

REFERENCES

1. Allan LD, Cook A, Sullivan I et al. Hypoplastic left heart syndrome: effects of fetal echocardiography on birth prevalence. *Lancet* **337**:959–961, 1991.
2. Cullen S, Sharland GK, Allan LD et al. Potential impact of population screening for prenatal diagnosis of congenital heart disease. *Arch Dis Child* **67**:775–778, 1992.
3. Bull C. Current and potential impact of fetal diagnosis on prevalence and spectrum of serious congenital heart disease at term in the UK. British Paediatric Cardiac Association. *Lancet* **354**(9186):1242–1247, 1999.
4. Schneider HE, Kreutzer J, Cohen MS et al. Intermediate-term outcome of neonates with critical aortic stenosis after valvotomy in the Ross era. *Circulation* **108**(Suppl IV):678, 2003.
5. Ashburn DA, McCrindle BW, Tchervebkov CI et al. Outcomes after the Norwood operation in neonates with critical aortic stenosis or aortic valve atresia. *J Thoracic Cardiovasc Surg* **5**: 1070–1076, 2003.
6. http://www.ccad.org.uk/paedanalysis.
7. Achiron R, Rotstein Z, Lipitz S et al. First-trimester diagnosis of fetal congenital heart disease by transvaginal ultrasonography. *Obstet Gynecol* **84**(1): 69–72, 1994.
8. Lombardi CM, Bellotti M, Fesslova V et al. Fetal echo at the time of the nuchal translucency scan. *Ultrasound Obstet Gynecol* **29**(3):249–257, 2007.
9. Carpenter RJ, Strasburger JF, Garson A et al. Fetal ventricular pacing for hydrops secondary to complete atrioventricular block. *J Am Coll Cardiol* **8**:1434–1436, 1986.
10. Walkinshaw SA, Welch CR, McCormack J et al. In utero pacing for fetal congenital heart block. *Fetal Diagn Ther* **9**(3):183–185, 1994.
11. Assad RS, Zielinsky P, Kalil R et al. New lead for in utero pacing for fetal congenital heart block. *J Thorac Cardiovasc Surg* **126**:300–302, 2003.
12. Donofrio MT, Gullquist SD, Mehta ID et al. Congenital complete heart block: fetal management protocol, review of the literature, and report of the smallest successful pacemaker implantation. *J Perinatol* **24**(2):112–117, 2004.
13. Tworetzky W, Wilkins-Haug L, Jennings RW et al. Balloon dilation of severe aortic stenosis in the fetus: potential for prevention of hypoplastic left heart syndrome: candidate selection, technique, and results of successful intervention. *Circulation* **110**(15):2125–2131, 2004.
14. Tulzer G, Arzt W, Franklin RC et al. Fetal pulmonary valvuloplasty for critical pulmonary stenosis or atresia with intact septum. *Lancet* **360**(9345):1567–1568, 2002.
15. Gardiner HM. Progression of fetal heart disease and rationale for fetal intracardiac interventions. *Semin Fetal Neonatal Med* **10**(6):578–585, Epub 2005 Oct 4, 2005.
16. Marshall AC, van der Velde ME, Tworetzky W et al. Creation of an atrial septal defect in utero for fetuses with hypoplastic left heart syndrome and intact or highly restrictive atrial septum. *Circulation* **110**(3):253–258, 2004.
17. UK National Screening Committee. *Antenatal ultrasound screening. Ultrasound survey of England: 2002*. Kettering: UK National Screening Committee, 2005. Available at: http://www.screening.nhs.uk/fetalanomaly/ultrasound_survey.pdf
18. Buskens E, Grobbee DE, Frohn-Mulder IME et al. Efficacy of routine fetal ultrasound screening for congenital heart disease in normal pregnancy. *Circulation* **94**:67–72, 1996.
19. Tegnander E, Eik-Nes SH, Johansen OJ et al. Prenatal detection of heart defects at the routine fetal examination at 18 weeks in a non-selected population. *Ultrasound Obstet Gynecol* **5**:372–380, 1995.
20. Hunter S, Heads A, Wyllie J et al. Prenatal diagnosis of congenital heart disease in the northern region of England: benefits of a training programme for obstetric ultrasonographers. *Heart* **84**(3):294–298, 2000.
21. Carvalho JS, Mavrides E, Shinebourne EA et al. Improving the effectiveness of routine prenatal screening for major congenital heart defects. *Heart* **88**:387–391, 2002.
22. Hyett J. Does nuchal translucency have a role in fetal cardiac screening? *Prenat Diagn* **24**:1130–1135, 2004.
23. Allan LD. The mystery of nuchal translucency. *Cardiol Young* **16**(1):11–17, 2006.
24. Makrydimas G, Sotiriadis A, Huggon IC et al. Nuchal translucency and fetal cardiac effects: a pooled analysis of major fetal echocardiography centres. *Am J Obstet Gynecol* **192**:89–95, 2005.
25. Chaoui R. The four-chamber view: four reasons why it seems to fail in screening for cardiac abnormalities and suggestions to improve detection rate. *Ultrasound Obstet Gynecol* **22**(1):3–10, 2003.
26. Stumpflen I, Stumpflen A, Wimmer M et al. Effect of detailed fetal echocardiography as part of routine prenatal ultrasonographic screening on detection of congenital heart disease. *Lancet* **348**:854–857, 1996.
27. Wren C, Richmond S, Donaldson L. Presentation of congenital heart disease in infancy: implications for routine examination. *Arch Dis Child Fetal Neonatal Ed* **80**:F49–53, 1999.
28. Small M, Copel JA. Indications for fetal echocardiography. *Pediatr Cardiol* **25**: 210–222, 2004.
29. Feig DS, Palda VA. Type 2 diabetes in pregnancy: a growing concern. *Lancet* **359**:1690–1692, 2002.
30. Källén BAJ, Olausson PO. Maternal use of selective serotonin re-uptake inhibitors in early pregnancy and infant congenital malformations. *Birth Defects Res Clin Mol Teratol* Jan 10, epub, 2007.
31. Yagel S, Cohen SM, Achiron R. Examination of the fetal heart by five short A -axis views: a proposed screening method for comprehensive cardiac evaluation. *Ultrasound Obstet Gynecol* **17**(5):367–369, 2001.
32. Gatzoulis MA. Adult congenital heart disease: education, education, education. *Nat Clin Pract Cardiovasc Med* **3**:2–3, 2006.
33. Burn J, Brennan P, Little J et al. Recurrence risks in offspring of adults with major heart defects: results from first cohort of British collaborative study. *Lancet* **351**: 311–316, 1998.
34. UKAS. Guidelines for professional working standards. *Ultrasound Practice*, 2001 (October) London.
35. Simpson JM, Jones A. Accuracy and limitations of transabdominal fetal echocardiography at 12–15 weeks of gestation in a population at high risk for congenital heart disease. *Brit J Obstet Gynaec* **107**(12):1492–1497, 2000.
36. Tworetzky W, McElhinney DB, Reddy VM et al. Improved surgical outcome after fetal diagnosis of hypoplastic left heart syndrome. *Circulation* **103**:1269–1273, 2001.
37. Wimalasundera RC, Gardiner HM. Congenital heart disease and aneuploidy. *Prenat Diagn* **24**:1116–1122, 2004.
38. Senzaki H, Masutani S, Kobayashi J et al. Ventricular after load and ventricular work in Fontan circulation: comparison with normal two-ventricle circulation and single-ventricle circulation with Blalock-Taussig shunts. *Circulation* **105**(24):2885–2892, 2002.
39. Chinnock RE, Cutler D, Baum M. Clinical outcome 10 years after infant heart transplantation. *Prog Pediatr Cardiol* **11**(2):165–169, 2000.
40. Webber SA, McCurry K, Zeevi A. Heart and lung transplantation in children. *Lancet* **368**:53–69, 2006.
41. Webber S. Atrial isomerism. In *Paediatric cardiology*, 2nd edn, RH Anderson, EJ Baker, FJ Macartney, ML Rigby, EA Shinebourne, M Tynan (eds). London: Churchill Livingstone, 2002.
42. Bjornstad PG, Holmstrom H, Smevik B et al. Transcatheter closure of atrial septal defects in the oval fossa: is the method applicable in small children? *Cardiol Young* **12**(4):352–356, 2002.

43. Turner SW, Hornung T, Hunter S. Closure of ventricular septal defects: a study of factors influencing spontaneous and surgical closure. *Cardiol Young* **12**(4): 357–363, 2002.
44. Knauth AL, Lock JE, Perry SB et al. Transcatheter device closure of congenital and postoperative residual ventricular septal defects. *Circulation* **110**(5):501–507, epub Jul 19, 2004.
45. Chaoui R, Korner H, Bommer C et al. Fetal thymus and the 22q11.2 deletion. *Prenat Diagn* **22**(9):839–840, 2002.
46. Amark KM, Karamlou T, O'Carroll A. et al. Independent factors associated with mortality, reintervention, and achievement of complete repair in children with pulmonary atresia with ventricular septal defect. *J Am Coll Cardiol* **47**(7):1448-1456, epub Mar 20, 2006.
47. Reinhartz O, Reddy VM, Petrossian E et al. Unifocalization of major aortopulmonary collaterals in single-ventricle patients. *Ann Thorac Surg* **82**(3):934–938, discussion 938–939 2006.
48. Davlouros PA, Niwa K, Webb G et al. The right ventricle in congenital heart disease. *Heart* **92**(Suppl 1):i27–38, 2006.
49. Craig B. Atrioventricular septal defect: from fetus to adult. *Heart* **92**:1879–1885, 2006.
50. Kaski JP, Wolfenden J, Josen M et al. Can atrioventricular septal defects exist with intact septal structures? *Heart* **92**:832–835, 2006.
51. ter Heide H, Thomson JDR, Wharton GA et al. Poor sensitivity of routine fetal anomaly ultrasound screening for antenatal detection of atrioventricular septal defect. *Heart* **90**:916–917, 2004.
52. Langford K, Sharland G, Simpson J. Relative risk of abnormal karyotype in fetuses found to have an atrioventricular septal defect (AVSD) on fetal echocardiography. *Prenat Diagn* **25**(2): 137–139, 2005.
53. Forbess JM, Cook N, Roth SJ et al. Ten-year institutional experience with palliative surgery for hypoplastic left heart syndrome: risk factors related to stage I mortality. *Circulation* **92**(suppl II):II-262–II-II-266, 1995.
54. Bonnet D, Coltri A, Butera G et al. Detection of transposition of the great arteries in fetuses reduces neonatal morbidity and mortality. *Circulation* **99**(7):916–918, 1999.
55. Sharland G, Tingay R, Jones A et al. Atrioventricular and ventriculoarterial discordance (congenitally corrected transposition of the great arteries): echocardiographic features, associations, and outcome in 34 fetuses. *Heart* **91**: 1453–1458, 2005.
56. Daliento L, Corrado D, Buja G et al. Rhythm and conduction disturbances in isolated, congenitally corrected transposition of the great arteries. *Am J Cardiol* **58**(3):314–318, 1986.
57. Devaney EJ, Charpie JR, Ohye RG et al. Combined arterial switch and Senning operation for congenitally corrected transposition of the great arteries: patient selection and intermediate results. *J Thorac Cardiovasc Surg* **125**(3):500–507, 2003.
58. Rychik J, Rome JJ, Collins MH et al. The hypoplastic left heart syndrome with intact atrial septum: atrial morphology, pulmonary vascular histopathology and outcome. *J Am Coll Cardiol* **34**:554–560, 1999.
59. Gardiner H. Response of the fetal heart to changes in load: from hyperplasia to heart failure. *Heart* **91**(7):871–873, 2005.
60. Vlahos AP, Lock JE, McElhinney DB et al. Hypoplastic left heart syndrome with intact or highly restrictive atrial septum outcome after neonatal transcatheter atrial septostomy. *Circulation* **109**:2326–2330, 2004.
61. Sano S, Ishino K, Kado H et al. Outcome of right ventricle-to-pulmonary artery shunt in first-stage palliation of hypoplastic left heart syndrome: a multi-institutional study. *Ann Thorac Surg* **78**:1951–1957, 2004.
62. Nilsson B, Mellander M, Sudow G et al. Results of staged palliation for hypoplastic left heart syndrome: a complete population-based series. *Acta Paediatr* **95**(12):1594–1600, 2006.
63. Artrip JH, Campbell DN, Ivy DD et al. Birth weight and complexity are significant factors for the management of hypoplastic left heart syndrome. *Ann Thorac Surg* **82**(4):1252–1257, discussion 1258–1259 2006.
64. Bacha EA, Daves S, Hardin J et al. Single-ventricle palliation for high-risk neonates. *J Thorac Cardiovasc Surg* **131**:163–171, 2006.
65. Daubeney PE, Delany DJ, Anderson RH et al. Pulmonary atresia with intact ventricular septum: range of morphology in a population-based study. *J Am Coll Cardiol* **39**(10):1670–1679, 2002.
66. Shaw AC, Kalidas K, Crosby AH et al. The natural history of Noonan syndrome: a long-term follow-up study. *Arch Dis Child* **92**(2):128–132, 2007.
67. Daubeney PE, Sharland GK, Cook AC et al. Pulmonary atresia with intact ventricular septum: impact of fetal echocardiography on incidence at birth and postnatal outcome. UK and Eire Collaborative Study of Pulmonary Atresia with Intact Ventricular Septum. *Circulation* **98**(6):562–566, 1998.
68. Franklin O, Burch M, Manning N et al. Prenatal diagnosis of coarctation of the aorta improves survival and reduces morbidity. *Heart* **87**:67–69, 2002.
69. Pasquini L, Tan T, Ho SY et al. The implications for fetal outcome of an abnormal arrangement of the abdominal vessels. *Cardiol Young* **15**:35–42, 2005.
70. Kleinman CS, Nehgme RA. Cardiac arrhythmias in the human fetus. *Pediatr Cardiol* **25**(3):234–251, 2004.
71. Duke C, Stuart G, Simpson JM. Ventricular tachycardia secondary to prolongation of the QT interval in a fetus with autoimmune mediated congenital complete heart block. *Cardiol Young* **15**(3):319–321, 2005.
72. Raboisson MJ, Fouron JC, Sonesson SE et al. Fetal Doppler echocardiographic diagnosis and successful steroid therapy of Luciani-Wenckebach phenomenon and endocardial fibroelastosis related to maternal anti-Ro and anti-La antibodies. *J Am Soc Echocardiogr* **18**(4):375–380, 2005.
73. Jaeggi ET, Fouron JC, Silverman ED et al. Transplacental fetal treatment improves the outcome of prenatally diagnosed complete atrioventricular heart block. *Circulation* **110**:1542–1548, 2004.
74. Copel JA, Buyon JP, Kleinman CS. Successful in utero therapy of fetal heart block. *Am J Obstet Gynecol* **173**:1384–1390, 1995.
75. Rosenthal E, Gordon PA, Simpson JM et al. Letter regarding article by Jaeggi et al, 'Transplacental fetal treatment improves the outcome of prenatally diagnosed complete atrioventricular block without structural heart disease'. *Circulation* **111**(18): e287-288, author reply e287–288, 2005.
76. Fouron J-C. Doppler and M-mode assessment of fetal tachyarrhythmia mechanisms. In *Conference proceedings advances in fetal and perinatal cardiology*, LK Hornberger, LD Allan (eds), pp. 47–50. Toronto: World congress in paediatric cardiology and surgery, 2001.
77. Andelfinger G, Fouron JC, Sonesson SE et al. Reference values for time intervals between atrial and ventricular contractions of the fetal heart measured by two Doppler techniques. *Am J Cardiol* **88**(12):1433–1436, 2001.
78. Simpson JM, Sharland GK. Fetal tachycardias: management and outcome of 127 consecutive cases. *Heart* **79**:576–581, 1998.
79. Krapp M, Kohl T, Simpson JM, Sharland GK, Katalinic A, Gembruch U. Review of diagnosis, treatment, and outcome of fetal atrial flutter compared with supraventricular tachycardia. *Heart* **89**(8):913–917, 2003.
80. Sonesson SE, Fouron JC, Wesslen-Eriksson E, Jaeggi E, Winberg P. Foetal supraventricular tachycardia treated with sotalol. *Acta Paediatr* **87**(5):584–587, 1998.
81. Zhao H, Strasburger JF, Cuneo BF et al. Fetal cardiac repolarization abnormalities. *Am J Cardiol* **98**(4):491–496, eEpub Jun 21 2006.
82. Taylor MJ, Smith MJ, Thomas M et al. Non-invasive fetal electrocardiography in singleton and multiple pregnancies. *Br J Obstet Gynaecol* **110**:668–678, 2003.
83. Rein AJ, O Donnell C, Geva T et al. Use of tissue velocity imaging in the diagnosis of fetal cardiac arrhythmias. *Circulation* **106**:1827–1833, 2002.

84. Dowie R, Mistry H, Young TA et al. Telemedicine in pediatric and perinatal cardiology: economic evaluation of a service in English hospitals. *IJTAHC* **23**(1):1–10, 2007.
85. Michailidis GD, Simpson JM, Karidas C et al. Detailed three-dimensional fetal echocardiography facilitated by an Internet link. *Ultrasound Obstet Gynecol* **18**(4):325–328, 2001.
86. Chaoui R, Hoffmann J, Heling KS. Three-dimensional (3D) and 4D color Doppler fetal echocardiography using spatio-temporal image correlation (STIC). *Ultrasound Obstet Gynecol* **23**(6):535–545, 2004.
87. Tei C. New non-invasive index for combined systolic and diastolic ventricular function. *J Cardiol* **26**:135–136, 1995.
88. Harada K, Tsuda A, Orino T et al. Tissue Doppler imaging in the normal fetus. *Int J Cardiol* **71**(3):227–234, 1999.
89. Gardiner HM, Pasquini L, Wolfenden J et al. Myocardial tissue Doppler and long axis function in the fetal heart. *Int J Cardiol* **113**(1):39–47, 2006.
90. Gardiner HM, Pasquini L, Wolfenden J et al. Increased periconceptual maternal glycosolated haemoglobin in diabetic mothers reduces fetal long axis cardiac function. *Heart* **92**(8):1125–1130, 2006.
91. Zhao H, Strasburger JF, Cuneo BF, Wakai RT. Fetal cardiac repolarization abnormalities. *Am J Cardiol* **98**(4):491–496, 2006.
92. Gardiner HM, Belmar C, Pasquini L et al. Fetal ECG: a novel predictor of atrioventricular block in anti-Ro positive pregnancies. *Heart* Nov 3, epub, 2006.
93. Zhao H, Cuneo BF, Strasburger JF, Huhta JC, Gotteiner NL, Wakai RT. Electrophysiologic characteristics of fetal AV block. *J Am Coll Cardiol*. **51**:77–84, 2008.
94. Kohl T, Szabo Z, Suda K et al. Fetoscopic and open transumbilical fetal cardiac catheterization in sheep. *Potential approaches for human fetal cardiac intervention. Circulation* **95**(4):1048–1053, 1997.
95. Kohl T, Muller A, Tchatcheva K et al. Fetal transesophageal echocardiography: clinical introduction as a monitoring tool during cardiac intervention in a human fetus. *Ultrasound Obstet Gynecol* **26**(7): 780–785, 2005.
96. Simpson JM, Sharland GK. Natural history and outcome of aortic stenosis diagnosed prenatally. *Heart* **77**:205–210, 1997.
97. Reich O, Tax P, Marek J et al. Long term results of percutaneous balloon valvuloplasty of congenital aortic stenosis: independent predictors of outcome. *Heart* **90**:70–76, 2004.
98. Dyamenahalli U, McCrindle BW, McDonald C et al. Pulmonary atresia with intact ventricular septum: management of, and outcomes for, a cohort of 210 consecutive patients. *Cardiol Young* **14**:299–308, 2004.
99. Kumar S, O' Brien A. Recent developments in fetal medicine. *Br Med J* **328**:1002–1006, 2004.

CHAPTER 32

Fetal lung lesions

N Scott Adzick

KEY POINTS

- This chapter reviews the prenatal diagnosis, natural history and modes of therapy for fetal lung lesions. There is a broad spectrum of clinical severity. The overall prognosis depends on the size of the thoracic mass and the secondary physiologic derangement
- Experimental studies in fetal animal models have elucidated the pathophysiological consequences of fetal intrathoracic masses and have demonstrated that fetal pulmonary resection is feasible. Experiments in non-human primates have led to the development of the necessary fetal surgical, anesthetic and tocolytic techniques prior to clinical use
- Thoracoamniotic catheter insertion and open fetal surgical resection are reserved for large fetal lung masses associated with fetal hydrops. The technical features of these procedures are reviewed
- In clinical scenarios where the fetal lung lesion is very large during the third trimester and it is anticipated that significant respiratory distress will be present at birth, the ex utero intrapartum therapy (EXIT) procedure can be performed using placental bypass during the fetal thoracotomy and lobectomy

INTRODUCTION

Prenatal diagnosis provides insight into the in utero evolution of fetal thoracic lesions such as congenital cystic adenomatoid malformation (CCAM), bronchopulmonary sequestration (BPS), congenital lobar emphysema and mediastinal teratoma. Serial sonographic study of fetuses with thoracic lesions has helped define the natural history of these lesions, determine the pathophysiologic features that affect clinical outcome and formulate management based on prognosis[1–6]. In 1998, we reported a series of more than 175 prenatally diagnosed cases from the Children's Hospital of Philadelphia and the University of California, San Francisco[7], and our clinical experience over the past 12 years at the Center for Fetal Diagnosis and Treatment at the Children's Hospital of Philadelphia now extends to more than 500 cases. We have found that the overall prognosis depends on the size of the thoracic mass and the secondary physiologic derangement: a large mass causes mediastinal shift, hypoplasia of normal lung tissue, polyhydramnios and cardiovascular compromise leading to fetal hydrops and death. Hydrops is a harbinger of fetal or neonatal demise and manifests itself as fetal ascites, pleural and pericardial effusions and skin and scalp edema.

Smaller thoracic lesions can cause respiratory distress in the newborn period and the smallest masses may be asymptomatic until later in childhood when infection, pneumothorax or malignant degeneration may occur. Large fetal lung tumors may regress in size on serial prenatal sonography illustrating that improvement can occasionally occur during fetal life[8–10]. In particular, many non-cystic BPSs dramatically decrease in size before birth and may not need treatment after birth.[7]

The finding that fetuses with hydrops are at very high risk for fetal or neonatal demise led us to perform either fetal surgical resection of the massively enlarged pulmonary lobe (fetal lobectomy) for cystic/solid lesions or thoracoamniotic shunting for lung lesions with a dominant cyst[7,11–13]. Lesions with associated hydrops diagnosed late in gestation may benefit from resection using an ex utero intrapartum therapy (EXIT) approach[14]. Recognition of cystic mediastinal masses may also first occur on fetal ultrasound. The fetus who develops progressive non-immune hydrops, cardiac failure or mediastinal shift with compression of developing lung tissue may benefit from in utero decompression or resection of a cystic mediastinal lesion[15]. The fetus with a lung mass but without hydrops has an excellent chance for survival with maternal transport, planned delivery and neonatal evaluation and surgery.

PRENATAL DIAGNOSIS AND NATURAL HISTORY

CCAM is characterized by an 'adenomatoid' increase of terminal respiratory bronchioles that form cysts of various sizes. Grossly, a CCAM is a discrete, intrapulmonary mass that contains cysts ranging in diameter from less than 1 mm to over 10 cm. Histologically, CCAM is distinguished from other lesions and normal lung by:

1. polypoid projections of the mucosa
2. an increase in smooth muscle and elastic tissue within cyst walls
3. an absence of cartilage (except that found in 'entrapped' normal bronchi)
4. the presence of mucous secreting cells, and
5. the absence of inflammation.

Although the tissue within these malformations does not function in normal gas exchange, there are connections with the tracheobronchial tree as evidenced by air trapping that can develop during postnatal resuscitative efforts. Cha has identified two histologic patterns of fetal CCAM, pseudoglandular and canalicular[16]. Stocker defined three types of CCAM (types I to III) based primarily on cyst size[17]. We have classified prenatally diagnosed CCAM into two categories based on gross anatomy and ultrasound findings[1]. Macrocystic lesions contain single or multiple cysts that are 5 mm in diameter or larger on prenatal ultrasound, whereas microcystic lesions appear as a solid echogenic mass on sonography. CCAM usually arises from one lobe of the lung and bilateral lung involvement is rare. We have learned that the overall prognosis depends primarily on the size of the CCAM rather than on the lesion type, and the underlying growth characteristics are likely to be important.[18]

Resected large fetal CCAM specimens demonstrate increased cell proliferation and markedly decreased apoptosis compared to gestational age-matched normal fetal lung tissue[19]. Examination of factors that enhance cell proliferation or downregulate apoptosis in CCAM may provide further insights into the pathogenesis of this tumor and may suggest new therapeutic approaches. With regard to cell proliferation, we examined the role of pneumocyte mitogens like keratinocyte growth factor (KGF) and platelet-derived growth factor (PDGF) in rapidly growing fetal CCAMs. CCAM-like lesions occur in transgenic mice that over-express KGF[20], but we found no differences in the expression of KGF protein or KGF mRNA in CCAM and normal lung. In contrast, fetal CCAMs that grew rapidly, progressed to hydrops and required in utero resection showed increased PDGF-B gene expression and PDGF-BB protein production compared to either normal fetal lung or term CCAM specimens[21].

Bronchopulmonary sequestrations are masses of non-functioning lung tissue that are supplied by an anomalous systemic artery and do not have a bronchial connection to the native tracheobronchial tree. On prenatal ultrasonography, a BPS appears as a well-defined echodense, homogeneous mass. Detection by color flow Doppler of a systemic artery from the aorta to the fetal lung lesion is a pathognomonic feature of fetal BPS[22]. However, if this Doppler finding is not detected, then an echodense microcystic CCAM and a BPS can have an identical prenatal sonographic appearance. Ultrafast fetal magnetic resonance imaging (MRI) may help differentiate CCAM from BPS[23]. Furthermore, we and others have also described prenatally diagnosed lung masses that display clinicopathologic features of both CCAM and sequestration – hybrid lesions – which suggests a shared embryologic basis for some of these lung masses[24,25]. The ability to differentiate intralobar and extralobar sequestration before birth is limited unless an extralobar sequestration is highlighted by a pleural effusion or is located in the abdomen. There are no diagnostic hallmarks for the specific prenatal diagnosis of an intralobar sequestration.

Congenital lobar emphysema can be distinguished prenatally from other cystic lung lesions on ultrasonography by increased echogenicity and reflectivity compared to a microcystic CCAM and the absence of systemic arterial blood supply compared to a BPS[26]. Progressive enlargement of these lesions prior to 28 weeks' gestation may be due to fetal lung fluid trapping in the lobe analogous to the air trapping seen postnatally. Late in gestation, lobar emphysema may regress in the size and the character of the mass rendering it indistinguishable from adjacent normal fetal lung[27]. Postnatal assessment is important because of the risk of postnatal air trapping in the emphysematous lobe. At the time of birth, the affected lobe may be radiopaque on chest radiography because of delayed clearance of fetal lung fluid. Prenatally diagnosed mainstem bronchial atresia results in massive lung enlargement, hydrops and fetal death; ultrafast fetal MRI demonstrates that the entire lung is involved and that there are dilated bronchi distal to the mainstem atresia[28].

Huge fetal lung lesions have reproducible pathophysiologic effects on the developing fetus. Esophageal compression by the thoracic mass causes interference with fetal swallowing of amniotic fluid and results in polyhydramnios. Polyhydramnios is a common obstetrical indication for ultrasonography, so a prenatal diagnostic marker exists for many large fetal lung tumors. Support for this concept comes from the absence of fluid in the fetal stomach in some of these cases and the alleviation of polyhydramnios after effective fetal treatment[2]. The hydrops is secondary to vena caval obstruction and cardiac compression from large tumors causing an extreme mediastinal shift. Like CCAMs, a fetal BPS can also cause fetal hydrops, either from the mass effect or from a tension hydrothorax that is the result of fluid or lymph secretion from the BPS[7]. Although there is some association of both polyhydramnios and hydrops with fetal lung lesions, our experience indicates that either can occur independently of the other.

Although sonographic prenatal diagnosis is becoming increasingly sophisticated, diagnostic errors are possible. Diaphragmatic hernia can be distinguished by careful sonographic assessment, an amniogram with or without a CT scan, or by ultrafast MRI[23]. We, and others, have experience with other fetal thoracic masses including bronchogenic and enteric cysts, mediastinal cystic teratoma, congenital lobar emphysema, hemangioma and bronchial atresia[29]. We have described two cases of intrathoracic gastric duplication cyst associated with hydrops that were treated with placement of a thoraco-amniotic shunt[30]. Several years ago, we had an unusual case of unilateral pulmonary agenesis in which the prenatal sonographic findings included a densely echogenic left lung mass with flattening of the left hemidiaphragm and a marked mediastinal shift to the right. A chest X-ray after birth revealed right-sided pulmonary agenesis and hyperinflation of the remaining left lung. A bronchoscopic evaluation demonstrated a long area of tracheobronchial stenosis to the solitary left lung. Retention of fetal lung fluid with overdistention of the left lung secondary to the high-grade airway obstruction during fetal life resulted in sonographic findings similar to those of a large microcystic CCAM.

Associated anomalies in our experience are very uncommon compared to some other reports[2]. This difference may reflect a referral bias of cases to our center for possible fetal or postnatal treatment, such that fetuses with associated anatomic anomalies may not be referred.

Although a large pulmonary lesion diagnosed in utero is an ominous finding, the natural history of prenatally diagnosed pulmonary lesions is variable. Approximately 15% of our CCAM lesions decreased in size during gestation and the majority (68%) of BPS lesions shrank dramatically before birth. Several other groups have also reported the involution of some pulmonary lesions[4,5,8–10], although the mass is invariably detectable by chest CT scan after birth[31]. Although regression of a lung lesion and associated hydrops has been reported, this is a very rare circumstance[6,32].

The exact mechanism by which these lesions shrink is unclear. The masses that shrank in our series and in other reported cases were usually echodense lesions. The echogenic appearance on ultrasonography is due to the large number of tissue/fluid interfaces. As the lung lesions decreased in size, they also became less echogenic implying that they were losing fluid/tissue interfaces. CCAMs and sequestrations usually do not communicate directly with the tracheobronchial tree, although abnormal channels to the airway and the gastrointestinal tract have been reported. Perhaps the lesions shrink due to decompression of fetal lung fluid through these abnormal channels. Another possible explanation is that the pulmonary lesions outgrow their vascular supply and involute. Initial impressions concerning the prognosis of large pulmonary lesions should be tempered with the understanding that they can shrink in size or even 'disappear'.

Recently, we have determined CCAM volume by sonographic measurement using the formula for a prolate ellipse (length × height × width × 0.52). A cystic adenomatoid malformation volume ratio (CVR) was obtained by dividing the CCAM volume by head circumference to correct for fetal size. We found that a CVR >1.6 is predictive of increased risk of hydrops with 80% of these CCAM fetuses developing hydrops. The CVR may be useful in selecting fetuses at risk for hydrops and thus need close ultrasound observation and possible fetal intervention[33]. By performing serial CVR measurements, we have learned that CCAM growth usually reaches a plateau by 28 weeks' gestation. For fetuses at less than 28 weeks, we recommend twice weekly ultrasound surveillance if the CVR >1.6, and initial weekly surveillance for fetuses with smaller CVR values.

THE EXPERIMENTAL BACKGROUND FOR CLINICAL FETAL SURGERY

Experimental studies have elucidated the pathophysiologic consequences of fetal intrathoracic masses and have demonstrated that fetal pulmonary resection is straightforward. Simulation of the thoracic mass effect with an intrathoracic balloon in the third-trimester fetal lamb resulted in pulmonary hypoplasia and death at term due to respiratory insufficiency, whereas lambs that underwent simulated resection of the mass by balloon deflation in the middle of the third trimester had sufficient lung growth to permit survival at birth.[34,35] In addition, we have shown that intrauterine pneumonectomy in fetal lambs is technically feasible at early and mid-gestation and can induce compensatory growth of the remaining lung by term[36].

Hydrops caused by large CCAM lesions has been attributed to direct mediastinal compression, obstruction of venous return, protein loss from the tumor, or unspecified humoral factors that increase capillary permeability. In order to study the etiology of hydrops associated with huge fetal lung masses, we created a fetal sheep model in which a surgically implanted intrathoracic tissue expander was gradually inflated over several days while monitoring fetal arterial, venous, intrathoracic and intra-amniotic pressures and while monitoring for sonographic indications of hydrops[37]. We found that balloon inflation resulted in hydrops as a result of cardiac venous obstruction and increasing central venous pressure. Simulation of prenatal resection of the fetal thoracic mass by deflating the expander resulted in complete resolution of the hydrops and return of pressures to normal.

Experiments in non-human primates led to the development of the necessary surgical, anesthetic and tocolytic techniques prior to clinical use and have shown that fetal intervention is safe for the mother and her future reproductive potential[38–40]. The salvage of human fetuses with a variety of serious birth defects by in utero intervention established a sound basis for open fetal surgery based on extensive animal studies[41].

THE FETAL SURGERY EXPERIENCE: TAPS, SHUNTS, RESECTIONS AND THE EXIT

Fetuses with life-threatening lung lesions were selected for prenatal treatment according to predetermined guidelines, including the gestational age of the fetus, the size of the intrathoracic lesion, maternal health and the development of fetal hydrops. The finding that fetuses with large tumors and hydrops are at high risk for fetal or neonatal demise led to several therapeutic maneuvers. Fetal thoracentesis alone was ineffective for treatment because of rapid reaccumulation of cyst fluid[42]. In rare cases, the aspirated cyst does not reaccumulate fluid. However, thoracentesis usually serves as a temporizing maneuver prior to shunt placement or resection.

Catheter shunt placement

Thoracoamniotic shunting was performed in cases that had a large predominant cyst as long as there was not a large solid component to the CCAM (Figs 32.1 and 32.2). Twenty years ago, Clark documented resolution of hydrops after 3 weeks of catheter drainage[43] and successful shunt placement has been reported in several other cases of unilocular CCAM lesions[2,5,44]. Eight years ago, our group reported the management of 9 hydropic CCAM pregnancies using thoracoamniotic shunting[45]. The mean pre- and post-shunting mass volumes were 46.3 and 18.1 ml, respectively, representing a 61% mean reduction in mass volume following shunt placement. Hydrops resolved following shunting in all cases. Average shunt to delivery time was 13 weeks 2 days and fetal or neonatal loss was 1/9. Our total experience is now 23 cases with 17 survivors[46]. We have also learned a gestational age of 20 weeks' gestation or less at thoracoamniotic shunt placement may increase the risk of postnatal chest wall abnormalities[47]. Multicystic or predominantly solid CCAM lesions do not lend themselves to catheter decompression and require resection.

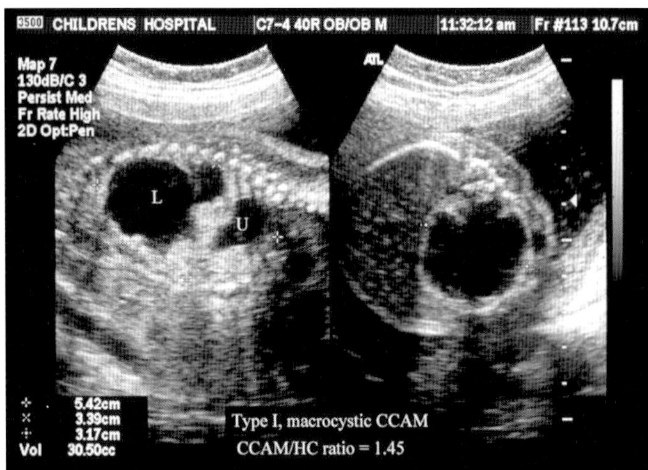

Fig. 32.1 Sonographic views of a 22-week gestation fetus with a congenital cystic adenomatoid malformation associated with ascites and polyhydramnios. Longitudinal view on the left shows two large cysts marked L (lower) and U (upper) that proved to communicate. Transverse view on the right shows the largest cyst. A thoracoamniotic shunt was placed.

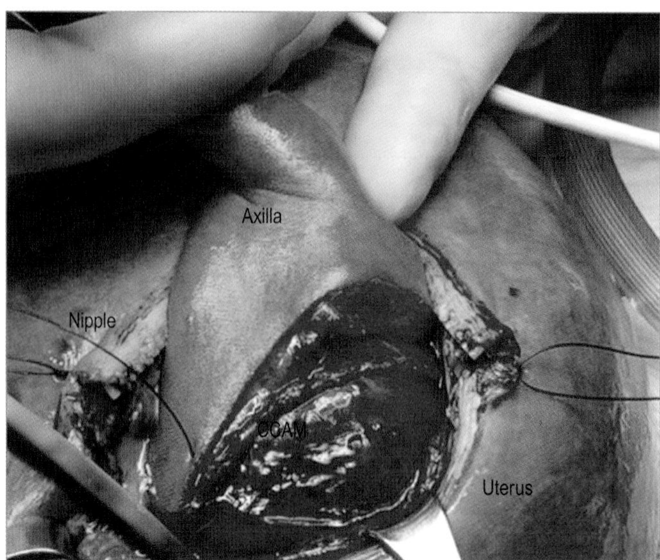

Fig. 32.3 Intraoperative photograph of a fetal surgical resection of congenital cystic adenomatoid malformation at 24 weeks' gestation.

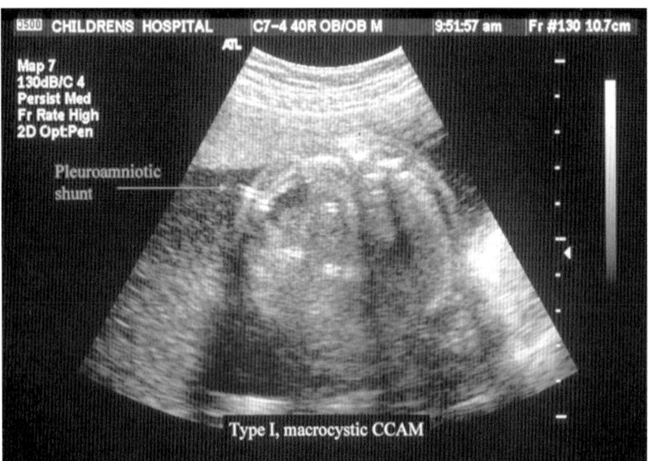

Fig. 32.2 Transverse view of the chest of the fetus shown in Fig. 32.1. A thoracoamniotic shunt (also known as a pleuroamniotic shunt) devised by Professor Charles Rodeck has been successfully placed percutaneously under sonographic guidance, resulting in complete decompression of the cysts in the fetal chest.

In 1998, we reported the treatment of 3 fetuses with a BPS and hydrops at 27, 29 and 30 weeks' gestation[7]. The hydrops appeared to be a consequence of a tension hydrothorax from fluid or lymph secretion by the mass. The hydrops resolved after weekly fetal thoracenteses in one case and thoracoamniotic shunt placement in the two other cases. All three survived after delivery at 33–35 weeks' gestation, required ventilatory support and subsequently underwent BPS resection. Another fetus with sequestration, hydrops and preterm labor diagnosed at 34 weeks' gestation was not treated prenatally and this baby died from pulmonary hypoplasia despite postnatal resection and the use of extracorporeal membrane oxygenation (ECMO) for 3 weeks.

Open fetal surgery for CCAM

For fetal surgery candidates, each family undergoes extensive discussion of the risks and benefits of fetal therapy for a lung tumor associated with hydrops. Fetal surgery candidates have a normal karyotype by amniocentesis or percutaneous umbilical blood sampling and no other anatomic abnormalities are present on detailed sonographic and echocardiographic survey[48]. Fetal surgical techniques have been previously described in detail[49] but, in brief, indomethacin and antibiotics are given preoperatively, isoflurane provides the necessary uterine relaxation and anesthesia for both mother and fetus, and a low transverse maternal laparotomy is performed. Sterile intraoperative sonography delineates both the fetal and placental position. The hysterotomy is facilitated by the placement of two large absorbable monofilament sutures parallel to the intended incision site and through the full-thickness of the uterine wall. A uterine stapler (US Surgical Corporation, Norwalk, CT) with absorbable Lactomer staples[50] is then directly introduced through this point of fixation and into the amniotic cavity using a piercing attachment on the lower limb of the stapler. The stapler is then fired thereby anchoring the amniotic membranes to the uterine wall and creating a hemostatic hysterotomy. The fetal chest is entered by a fifth intercostal space thoracotomy. Invariably, the lesion readily decompresses out through the thoracotomy wound consistent with increased intrathoracic pressure from the mass (Fig. 32.3). Using techniques developed in experimental animals, the appropriate pulmonary lobe(s) containing the lesion is resected[7]. The fetal thoracotomy is closed, the fetus is returned to the uterus, warmed Ringer's lactate containing antibiotics is instilled into the amniotic cavity and the uterine and abdominal incisions are closed in layers. Tocolysis with intravenous magnesium sulfate begins as the mother emerges from anesthesia. All fetal surgery mothers have a subsequent cesarean delivery.

The knowledge that hydrops is highly predictive of fetal or neonatal demise led to fetal surgical resection of a massive multicystic or predominantly solid CCAM (fetal lobectomy) in 24 cases at 21–31 weeks' gestation with 13 healthy survivors at

1–16 years follow-up. Resections involved a single lobectomy in 18 cases, right middle and lower lobectomies in 4 cases, extralobar BPS resection in one case, and one left pneumonectomy for CCAM. All cases had histologic confirmation of the diagnosis. In one multicystic case, a thoracoamniotic shunt failed to decompress adequately the mass effect prior to open fetal surgery. In the 13 fetuses that survived, fetal CCAM resection led to hydrops resolution in 1–2 weeks, return of the mediastinum to the midline within 3 weeks and impressive in utero lung growth. Follow-up developmental testing has been normal in all survivors.

There were 11 fetal deaths in the fetal surgery resection cases. In the first case, the mother had already developed the maternal 'mirror' syndrome[51,52]. The fetal operation was successful, the hydrops improved, but the placentomegaly and maternal hyperdynamic state remained and the fetus was delivered 1 week later. In cases 6 and 16, 21-week gestation fetuses became bradycardic and died 8 and 12 hours postoperatively; postmortem did not elucidate the cause of death in either case. In case 7, fetal death was due to uncontrolled intraoperative uterine contractions, which hallmarks this limitation of fetal surgery. In case 18, postoperative chorioamnionitis 10 days postoperatively led to early delivery and neonatal demise. Finally, in 6 other cases, massive hydrops was present at 21–24 weeks' gestation and all fetuses died intraoperatively, usually after developing profound bradycardia after delivery of the mass from the fetal chest. We believe that mass delivery and abrupt removal of cardiac compression resulted in pathophysiology similar to relief of pericardial tamponade with fetal hemodynamic collapse and reactive bradycardia. As such, we have modified our approach before beginning the fetal operation. Prior to the fetal thoracotomy, we now obtain fetal intravenous access, check a fetal blood gas and hematocrit, and pretreat with intravenous atropine and fluid volume (usually warm, fresh blood). We also use fetal echocardiography on a routine basis for all fetal surgery cases, regardless of lesion type, to monitor fetal myocardial performance, particularly since maternal–fetal general anesthesia is a fetal myocardial depressant[53].

With regard to maternal morbidity, there was one wound seroma and one wound infection that developed after cesarean delivery and each required drainage. There were two maternal blood transfusions of one unit of packed red blood cells. Two cases of mild postoperative interstitial pulmonary edema responded to furosemide diuresis. There was one case of chorioamnionitis that led to neonatal death. In one case, a uterine wound dehiscence was evident at the time of cesarean delivery in each of her two subsequent pregnancies. Thirteen mothers have delivered normal babies by planned cesarean delivery subsequent to the fetal surgery pregnancy.

These results demonstrate that fetal CCAM resection is technically feasible, reasonably safe, reverses hydrops over 1–2 weeks and allows sufficient lung growth to permit survival and normal postnatal development. The steep learning curve derived from our experience with more than 400 fetal surgery and fetoscopy cases for a variety of fetal anomalies has provided invaluable lessons regarding optimal maternal anesthesia and uterine relaxation, hysterotomy and fetal exposure techniques, intraoperative fetal monitoring and reliable methods for amniotic membrane and uterine closure.

In contrast, the unsuccessful fetal CCAM resection cases highlight remaining challenges. We learned in the first case that the maternal hyperdynamic state referred to as the 'mirror syndrome' cannot be reversed solely by treatment of the underlying fetal condition. This pre-eclamptic state is associated with molar pregnancies and fetal conditions that cause placentomegaly, and may be caused by a factor released by poorly perfused placental tissue that leads to endothelial cell injury[51,52]. Until the pathophysiology of the maternal mirror syndrome is understood, earlier intervention before the onset of placentomegaly and the related maternal pre-eclamptic state may be the only approach to salvage these doomed fetuses. A subsequent case illustrated that placentomegaly can regress after fetal surgical CCAM resection if clinical signs of the maternal 'mirror syndrome' are not present preoperatively.

Our clinical focus has shifted from the technical details of the fetal surgical procedure to the crucial need for better postoperative maternal–fetal monitoring, reliable intraoperative fetal intravascular access for fetal blood sampling and infusions, and intraoperative fetal echocardiographic hemodynamic assessment. The detection and treatment of preterm labor remains the 'Achilles heel' of fetal surgery. As a result of ongoing work in fetal animal models, the concept of a fetal intensive care unit with a specially trained cadre of physicians and nurses has become a clinical reality.

In the future, minimally invasive approaches to fetal lung lesions associated with hydrops may be possible. Laser therapy to fulgerate a fetal CCAM has been reported[54,55], but we believe that this approach is untenable given current technical limitations. For example, a mother carrying a 28-week gestation fetus with a large right-sided CCAM and hydrops was turned down for open fetal surgery by our group because of maternal psychosocial difficulties, and she decided to seek YAG laser therapy at another medical center. Using a percutanous technique under ultrasound guidance, a laser fiber was deployed in the fetal right chest and the procedure was repeated twice during the next 4 weeks. After birth, the baby died from pulmonary hypoplasia and had a severely caved-in right chest with multiple rib fractures as a result of the prenatally applied laser energy. It is possible that laser therapy or techniques such as radiofrequency thermal ablation will be clinically useful for fetal lung lesions associated with fetal hydrops if the result is a decrease in mass effect, but experimental studies in animal models to test these techniques rigorously should be mandatory prior to clinical trials[56]. Finally, it is possible that administration of a short course of maternal betamethasone may impair CCAM growth in some cases and lead to amelioration of hydrops[57].

The EXIT procedure for high-risk CCAM

In clinical scenarios where the CVR continues to be large during the third trimester and it is anticipated that significant respiratory distress may be present at birth, the EXIT procedure is considered using placental bypass during the fetal thoracotomy and lobectomy. At the time of EXIT delivery, only the head, neck and chest are delivered through the stapled hysterotomy (Fig. 32.4). The intrauterine volume is maintained with the lower fetal body and continuous amnioinfusion of warmed Ringers lactate to prevent cord compression and hypothermia. Uterine relaxation is maintained by high concentration of inhalational anesthetics to preserve the uteroplacental circulation and gas exchange between maternal, placental and fetal compartments. We reported 9 fetuses who underwent resection of fetal lung lesions during EXIT delivery[14]. The mean gestational age at EXIT delivery was 35.4 weeks. All lung masses remained

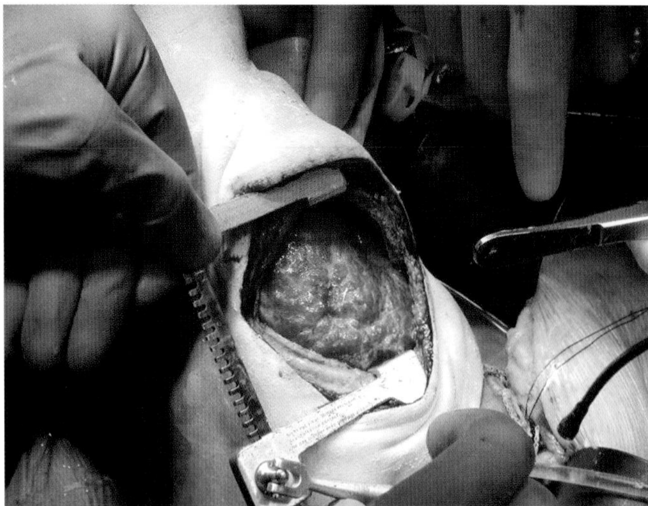

Fig. 32.4 Intraoperative photograph of a near-term resection of a large congenital cystic adenomatoid malformation during an ex utero intrapartum therapy (EXIT) procedure. The lower half of the fetus remains in the uterus and the fetus remains connected to the maternal–placental–fetal circulation.

large late in gestation with a mean CVR of 2.5 at initial presentation and 2.2 at EXIT. Some of the 9 fetuses demonstrated hydropic changes and/or polyhydramnios and had prenatal intervention including thoracentesis, thoracoamniotic shunt placement, amnioreduction and/or maternal betamethasone administration. Eight of the 9 neonates survived. The average time on placental bypass was 65 minutes. Postnatal complications included reoperation for air leak (n = 1) and death from bleeding and prematurity (n = 1). Extracorporeal membrane oxygenation (ECMO) was used successfully in 4 neonates for persistent pulmonary hypertension. Maternal complications included polyhydramnios (n = 5), preterm labor (n = 4) and chorioamnionitis (n = 1). One mother required a perioperative blood transfusion. We have learned that the EXIT procedure allows for controlled resection of large fetal lung masses at delivery, avoiding acute respiratory decompensation related to mediastinal shift, air trapping and compression of normal lung.

MANAGEMENT SUMMARY

We have learned from prenatal diagnosis that there is a wide spectrum of clinical severity for the fetus with a lung mass. Accurate prognostic information is necessary for providing appropriate management and parental counseling. If an associated life-threatening anomaly is present or if the mother is sick with the 'mirror' syndrome, then the family may choose to terminate the pregnancy. If fetus is not hydropic and an isolated fetal lung lesion is present, then the mother is followed by serial ultrasound and arrangements are made for the best possible care after birth. Some CCAMs and many BPSs will shrink in size, so it is important to try to differentiate these lesions using prenatal diagnostic criteria, although this is not always possible[7].

All fetuses with thoracic masses and without hydrops in our series survived in the setting of maternal transport, planned delivery and postnatal evaluation at a facility with ECMO capability. Many of the babies with large lesions at our center required ventilatory support and 10 babies needed treatment with ECMO. Interestingly, our impression is that these non-hydropic fetuses with lung masses have less lung hypoplasia and a much better prognosis than those with diaphragmatic hernia despite a similar degree of mediastinal shift as judged by prenatal sonography.

In asymptomatic neonates with a cystic lung lesion, we believe that elective resection is warranted because of the risks of infection and occult malignant transformation[58–62]. Malignancies consist mainly of pleuropulmonary blastoma in infants and young children and bronchioloalveolar carcinoma in older children and adults. After confirmation of CCAM location by postnatal chest CT scan with intravenous contrast, we recommend elective resection at one month of age or older. This age has been chosen because anesthetic risk in babies decreases after 4 weeks of age. An experienced pediatric surgeon can safely perform a lobectomy in infants with minimal morbidity. Early resection also maximizes compensatory lung growth. In contrast, we have usually followed patients with a tiny, asymptomatic, non-cystic BPS if we are confident of the diagnosis based on postnatal imaging studies. We do not favor the approach of catheterization and embolization for the treatment of larger BPS lesions.

If the fetus is hydropic at presentation or if hydrops develops during serial follow-up, then management depends upon the gestational age. For those hydropic fetuses greater than 32 weeks' gestation, early delivery should be considered so that the lesion can be resected using an EXIT strategy with resection of the mass during the EXIT procedure. For those hydropic fetuses less than 32 weeks' gestation, there is now an accepted therapeutic option which is to treat the lesion before birth.

REFERENCES

1. Adzick NS, Harrison MR, Glick PL et al. Fetal cystic adenomatoid malformation: prenatal diagnosis and natural history. *J Pediatr Surg* **20**:483–488, 1985.
2. Thorpe-Veeston JG, Nicolaides KH. Cystic adenomatoid malformation of the lung: prenatal diagnosis and outcome. *Prenat Diagn* **14**:677–688, 1994.
3. Sakala EP, Perrott WS, Grube GL. Sonographic characteristics of antenatally diagnosed extralobar pulmonary sequestration and congenital cystic adenomatoid malformation. *Obstet Gynecol Surv* **49**:647–655, 1994.
4. Miller JA, Corteville JE, Langer JC. Congenital cystic adenomatoid malformation in the fetus: natural history and predictors of outcome. *J Pediatr Surg* **31**:805–808, 1996.
5. Dommergues M, Louis-Sylvestre C, Mandelbrot L et al. Congenital adenomatoid malformation of the lung: when is active fetal therapy indicated? *Am J Obstet Gynecol* **177**:953–958, 1997.
6. Taguchi T, Suita S, Yamanouchi T. Antenatal diagnosis and surgical management of congenital cystic adenomatoid malformation of the lung. *Fetal Diagn Ther* **10**:400–407, 1995.
7. Adzick NS, Harrison MR, Crombleholme TM, Flake AW, Howell LJ. Fetal lung lesions: management and outcome. *Am J Obstet Gynecol* **179**:884–889, 1998.

8. Saltzman DH, Adzick NS, Benacerraf BR. Fetal cystic adenomatoid malformation of the lung: apparent improvement in utero. *Obstet Gynecol* **71**:1000–1003, 1988.
9. MacGillivray TE, Harrison MR, Goldstein RB, Adzick NS. Disappearing fetal lung lesions. *J Pediatr Surg* **28**:1321–1325, 1993.
10. Laberge JM, Flageole H, Pugash D. Outcome of the prenatally diagnosed congenital cystic adenomatoid lung malformation: a Canadian experience. *Fetal Diagn Ther* **16**:178–186, 2001.
11. Harrison MR, Adzick NS, Jennings RW et al. Antenatal intervention for congenital cystic adenomatoid malformation. *Lancet* **336**:965–967, 1990.
12. Kuller JA, Yankowitz J, Goldberg JD et al. Outcome of antenatally diagnosed cystic adenomatoid malformation. *Am J Obstet Gynecol* **167**:1038–1041, 1992.
13. Adzick NS, Harrison MR, Flake AW, Howell LJ, Golbus MS, Filly RA. Fetal surgery for cystic adenomatoid malformation of the lung. *J Pediatr Surg* **28**:806–812, 1993.
14. Hedrick HL, Flake AW, Crombleholme TM et al. The ex utero intrapartum therapy (EXIT) procedure for high risk fetal lung lesions. *J Pediatr Surg* **40**:1038–1043, 2005.
15. Merchant AM, Hedrick HL, Crombleholme TM et al. Management of fetal mediastinal teratoma: a report of two cases. *J Pediatr Surg* **40**:228–231, 2005.
16. Cha I, Adzick NS, Harrison MR, Finkbeiner WE. Fetal congenital cystic adenomatoid malformations of the lung: a clinicopathologic study of eleven cases. *Am J Surg Path* **21**:537–544, 1997.
17. Stocker TJ, Manewell JE, Drake RM. Congenital cystic adenomatoid malformation of the lung: classification and morphologic spectrum. *Hum Pathol* **8**:155–171, 1977.
18. Krieger PA, Ruchelli ED, Mahboubi S, Hedrick HL, Adzick NS, Russo PA. Fetal pulmonary malformations: defining histopathology. *Am J Surg Pathol* **30**: 643–649, 2005.
19. Cass DL, Yang EY, Liechty KW, Quinn TM, Crombleholme TM, Adzick NS. Increased cell proliferation and decreased apoptosis in congenital cystic adenomatoid malformation: insights into pathogenesis. *Surg Forum* **47**:659–661, 1997.
20. Simonet WS, DeRose ML, Bucay N. Pulmonary malformation in transgenic mice expressing keratinocyte growth factor in the lung. *Proc Natl Acad Sci* **92**:12461–12465, 1995.
21. Liechty KW, Quinn TM, Cass DL, Crombleholme TM, Flake AW, Adzick NS. Elevated PDGF-B in congenital cystic adenomatoid malformations requiring fetal resection. *J Pediatr Surg* **34**:805–810, 1999.
22. Hernanz-Schulman M, Stein SM, Neblett WW. Pulmonary sequestration: diagnosis with color Doppler sonography and a new theory of associated hydrothorax. *Radiology* **180**:817–821, 1991.
23. Quinn TM, Hubbard AM, Adzick NS. Prenatal magnetic resonance imaging enhances prenatal diagnosis. *J Pediatr Surg* **33**:312–316, 1998.
24. Cass DL, Crombleholme TM, Howell LJ, Stafford PW, Adzick NS. Cystic lung lesions with systemic arterial blood supply: a hybrid of congenital cystic adenomatoid malformation and bronchopulmonary sequestration. *J Pediatr Surg* **32**:986–990, 1997.
25. Mackenzie TC, Guttenberg ME, Nissenbaum HL, Johnson MP, Adzick NS. A fetal lung lesion consisting of bronchogenic cyst, bronchopulmonary sequestration, and congenital cystic adenomatoid malformation: the missing link? *Fetal Diagn Ther* **16**:193–195, 2001.
26. Ankermann T, Oppermann HC, Engler S et al. Congenital masses of the lung: cystic adenomatoid malformation versus congenital lobar emphysema. *J Ultrasound Med* **23**:1379–1384, 2004.
27. Olutoye O, Coleman B, Hubbard AM et al. Prenatal diagnosis and management of congenital lobar emphysema. *J Pediatr Surg* **35**:792–795, 2000.
28. Keswani SG, Crombleholme TM, Johnson MP et al. The prenatal diagnosis and management of mainstem bronchial atresia. *Fetal Diagn Ther* **20**:74–78, 2005.
29. Albright EB, Crane JP, Shackelford GD. Prenatal diagnosis of a bronchogenic cyst. *J Ultrasound Med* **7**:91–95, 1988.
30. Ferro MM, Milner R, Cannizzaro C, Rodriquez S, Bonifacino G, Adzick NS. Intrathoracic alimentary tract duplication cysts treated in utero by thoracoamniotic shunting. *Fetal Diagn Ther* **13**:343–347, 1998.
31. Winters WD, Effmann EL, Nghiem HV. Disappearing fetal lung masses: importance of postnatal imaging studies. *Pediatr Radiol* **27**:535–539, 1997.
32. daSilva OP, Ramanan R, Romano W. Nonimmune hydrops fetalis, pulmonary sequestration, and favorable neonatal outcome. *Obstet Gynecol* **88**:681–683, 1996.
33. Crombleholme TM, Coleman BG, Howell LJ et al. Elevated cystic adenomatoid malformation volume ratio (CVR) predicts outcome in prenatal diagnosis of cystic adenomatoid malformation of the lung. *J Pediatr Surg* **37**:331–338, 2002.
34. Harrison MR, Jester JA, Ross NA. Correction of congenital diaphragmatic hernia in utero I. The model: intrathoracic balloon produces fatal pulmonary hypoplasia. *Surgery* **88**:174–180, 1980.
35. Harrison MR, Bressack MA, Churg AM. Correction of congenital diaphragmatic hernia in utero II. Simulated correction permits fetal lung growth with survival at birth. *Surgery* **88**:260–268, 1980.
36. Adzick NS, Harrison MR, Hu LM, Davies P, Reid LM. Compensatory growth after pneumonectomy in fetal lambs: a morphologic study. *Surg Forum* **37**:309–311, 1986.
37. Rice HE, Estes JM, Hedrick MH, Bealer JF, Harrison MR, Adzick NS. Congenital cystic adenomatoid malformation: a sheep model. *J Pediatr Surg* **29**:692–696, 1994.
38. Harrison MR, Anderson J, Rosen MA. Fetal surgery in the primate I. Anesthetic, surgical, and tocolytic management to maximize fetal-neonatal survival. *J Pediatr Surg* **17**:115–122, 1982.
39. Nakayama DK, Harrison MR, Seron-Ferre M. Fetal surgery in the primate II. Uterine electromyographic response to operative procedure and pharmacologic agents. *J Pediatr Surg* **19**:333–339, 1984.
40. Adzick NS, Harrison MR, Anderson JV, Flake AW, Villa RL. Fetal surgery in the primate III. Maternal outcome after fetal surgery. *J Pediatr Surg* **21**:477–480, 1986.
41. Adzick NS, Nance ML. Medical progress: pediatric surgery. *N Engl J Med* **342**:1651-1657, 1726-1732, 2000.
42. Chao A, Monoson RF. Neonatal death despite fetal therapy for cystic adenomatoid malformation. *J Reprod Med* **35**:655–657, 1990.
43. Clark SL, Vitale DJ, Minton SD, Stoddard RA, Sabey P. Successful fetal therapy for cystic adenomatoid malformation associated with second trimester hydrops. *Am J Obstet Gynecol* **157**:294–297, 1987.
44. Bernaschek G, Deutinger J, Hansmann M, Bald R, Holzgreve W, Bollmann R. Feto-amniotic shunting: report of the experience of four European centres. *Prenatal Diagn* **14**:821–833, 1994.
45. Baxter JK, Johnson MP, Wilson RD et al. Thoracoamniotic shunts: pregnancy outcome for congenital cystic adenomatoid malformation and pleural effusion. *Am J Obstet Gynecol* **185**:S245, 1998.
46. Wilson RD, Baxter JK, Johnson MP et al. Thoracoamniotic shunts: fetal treatment of pleural effusions and congenital cystic adenomatoid malformations. *Fetal Diagn Ther* **19**:413–420, 2004.
47. Merchant AM, Peranteau WH, Wilson RD et al. Postnatal chest wall deformities after fetal thoracoamniotic shunting for congenital cystic adenomatoid malformation. *Fetal Diagn Ther* (in press).
48. Mahle WT, Rychik J, Tian ZY et al. Echocardiographic evaluation of the fetus with congenital cystic adenomatoid malformation. *Ultrasound Obstet Gynecol* **16**:620–624, 2000.
49. Adzick NS, Harrison MR. Fetal surgical techniques. *Sem Pediatr Surg* **2**:136–142, 1993.
50. Adzick NS, Harrison MR, Flake AW. Automatic uterine stapling devices in fetal

operation: experience in a primate model. *Surg Forum* **36**:479–480, 1985.

51. Creasy R. Mirror syndromes. In *Care of the fetus*, RC Goodlin (ed.), pp. 48–50. New York: Masson, 1979.
52. Langer JC, Harrison MR, Schmidt KG. Fetal hydrops and death from sacrococcygeal teratoma: rationale for fetal surgery. *Am J Obstet Gynecol* **160**:1145–1150, 1989.
53. Rychik J, Tian Z, Ewing S et al. Acute cardiovascular effects of fetal surgery in the human. *Circulation* **110**:1549–1556, 2004.
54. Fortunato S, Lombardo S, Dantrell J, Ismael S. Intrauterine laser ablation of a fetal cystic adenomatoid malformation with hydrops: the application of minimally invasive surgical techniques to fetal surgery. *Am J Obstet Gynecol* **177**:S84, 1997.
55. Bruner JP, Jarnagin BK, Reinisch L. Percutaneous laser ablation of fetal congenital cystic adenomatoid malformation: too little, too late? *Fetal Diagn Ther* **15**:359–363, 2000.
56. Milner R, Kitano Y, Olutoye O, Flake AW, Adzick NS. Radiofrequency thermal ablation (RTA): a potential treatment for hydropic fetuses with a large chest mass. *J Pediatr Surg* **35**:386–389, 2000.
57. Peranteau WH, Wilson W, Liechty KW, et al. The effect of maternal betamethasone on prenatal congenital cystic adenomatoid malformation growth and fetal survival. *Fetal Diagn Ther* (in press).
58. Benjamin DR, Cahill JL. Bronchoalveolar carcinoma of the lung and congenital cystic adenomatoid malformation. *Am J Clin Pathol* **95**:889–892, 1991.
59. Murphy JJ, Blair GK, Fraser GC. Rhabdomyosarcoma arising within congenital pulmonary cysts: report of three cases. *J Pediatr Surg* **27**:1364–1367, 1992.
60. d'Agnostino S, Bonoldi E, Dante S, Meli S, Cappellari F, Musi L. Embryonal rhabdomyosarcoma of the lung arising in cystic adenomatoid malformation. *J Pediatr Surg* **32**:1381–1383, 1997.
61. Ribet ME, Copin MC, Soots JG, Gosselin BH. Bronchioloalveolar carcinoma and congenital cystic adenomatoid malformation. *Ann Thorac Surg* **60**:1126–1128, 1995.
62. Granata C, Gambini C, Balducci T et al. Bronchioloalveolar carcinoma arising in a congenital cystic adenomatoid malformation in a child: case report and review of the literature. *Pediatr Pulmonol* **25**:62–66, 1996.

CHAPTER

33

Congenital diaphragmatic hernia

Alan W Flake and Holly L Hedrick

KEY POINTS

- CDH is a complex congenital anomaly that presents with a broad spectrum of severity that is dependent upon components of fixed pulmonary hypoplasia and reversible pulmonary hypertension
- While improvements in neonatal care have improved the overall survival of CDH in experienced centers, morbidity remains very high in a subset of CDH infants with severe CDH
- The most important prenatal negative prognostic predictor in left-sided CDH is the presence of herniated liver in the chest
- More accurate prenatal predictive parameters need to be developed to allow standardization of results between centers and appropriate design of clinical trials in CDH
- Thus far, all randomized trials comparing prenatal intervention to standard postnatal therapy have shown no benefit to prenatal intervention. While the recent non-randomized reports of success with balloon tracheal occlusion (and release) are provocative, prenatal therapy should not be widely adopted until a well-designed prospective randomized trial demonstrating efficacy is performed

INTRODUCTION

Congenital diaphragmatic hernia (CDH) is a developmental defect in the diaphragm that results in herniation of abdominal viscera into the chest. The frequency of CDH is approximately 1 in 2000–2500 live births. There is a spectrum of severity in CDH. The majority of affected neonates will present in the first few hours of life with respiratory distress that may be mild or so severe as to be incompatible with life. With the advent of antenatal diagnosis and improvement of neonatal care, survival has improved but there remains a significant risk of mortality and major morbidity in infants with severe CDH.

CDH was one of the first anomalies considered for prenatal intervention due to the compelling rationale for prevention of untreatable pulmonary hypoplasia at birth[1,2]. Despite years of effort by many investigators, the subject remains highly controversial. The controversies relate to three questions:

1. What is the 'natural history' of CDH?
2. Can we identify a subset of CDH fetuses that can be predicted to die or experience major morbidity despite optimal postnatal therapy?
3. Can prenatal intervention improve outcome in severe CDH?[3]

Despite nearly three decades of discussion and improved insight into this disorder, these questions remain unresolved. This chapter will discuss the pre-, peri- and postnatal considerations related to CDH in the context of standard postnatal therapy and experimental prenatal intervention.

ETIOLOGY

CDH is a simple anatomic defect, i.e. an opening in the diaphragm that leads to the devastating physiologic consequence of pulmonary hypoplasia. The pathophysiology of CDH is comprised of both fixed and reversible components. The fixed component is pulmonary hypoplasia which arises from interference with branching morphogenesis during lung development. Branching morphogenesis is the process by which airways and vascular structures in the lung arborize into a complete bronchopulmonary tree. A lung with severe hypoplasia has fewer branch points and therefore fewer airways, arteries, veins and alveolar structures than a normal lung. This results in fixed increased vascular resistance and decreased surface area for gas exchange[4,5]. In addition to the relatively fixed deficit from pulmonary hypoplasia, lungs in severe CDH also have markedly abnormal pulmonary vasculature. The peripheral pulmonary arteries are hypermuscular, with a thickened medial muscular layer that extends further distal on the arterioles than normal. The clinical correlate of this anatomic observation is increased pulmonary vasoreactivity accounting for the marked clinical lability of patients with severe CDH.

The resultant pulmonary hypertension results in persistence of the fetal circulation with shunting through the patent ductus arteriosus, or foramen ovale, with secondary hypoxemia and acidosis. As hypoxemia and acidosis stimulate further pulmonary vasospasm, a 'vicious cycle' is initiated with rapid clinical deterioration of the patient and inability to ventilate using conventional techniques[6]. Thus a combination of pulmonary hypoplasia and pulmonary vascular abnormality results in the still considerable mortality and morbidity of CDH.

EMBRYOLOGY OF CDH

In considering the embryology of CDH, both diaphragmatic and lung development must be considered. There are competing theories regarding the embryogenesis of CDH that have not been resolved. During embryogenesis, the diaphragm develops anteriorly as a septum between the heart and liver and then grows posteriorly. The final closure occurs at the left Bochdalek foramen between 8 and 10 weeks' gestation. At about 10 weeks, the bowel migrates from the yolk sac to the abdominal cavity. Theories regarding why the foramen of Bochdalek fails to close range from premature migration of the primitive gut from the yolk sac into the abdominal cavity, resulting in physical interference with closure of the foramen, to an undefined mesenchymal lesion resulting in the defect. Whatever the reason for failure of diaphragmatic closure, the prevailing theory is that visceral herniation results in 'compression' of the lung bud, resulting in the associated pulmonary hypoplasia. This theory is supported by observations in surgical models of CDH, where pulmonary hypoplasia can result purely as a consequence of visceral herniation and its severity is related to the timing of creation of the defect and the volume of visceral herniation[1,7,8]. An alternative theory has been proposed that CDH results from a primary defect in lung development. This theory arose from a study by Iritani[9] in the rat nitrofen model of CDH which demonstrated primary lung hypoplasia, prior to herniation of viscera into the chest and it was postulated that this led, by an unexplained mechanism, to failure of diaphragmatic development. This study was flawed however, by the administration of nitrofen from E5–E11 of gestation which likely resulted in an early direct effect of nitrofen on multiple tissues. Subsequent independent studies by Kluth[10] and Greer et al.[11] have demonstrated that the lung is structurally normal prior to compression by the viscera. Finally, there are human cases[12] and animal models[13] of severe lung hypoplasia or lung agenesis in which diaphragmatic development is normal. This discussion is far from complete and the interested reader is referred to a number of excellent review articles on this subject[14,15].

PULMONARY HYPOPLASIA

From the available evidence, it is reasonable to conclude that, in human CDH, pulmonary hypoplasia results, at least in part, from lung compression. The timing of herniation coincides with a critical period of lung development when bronchial and pulmonary artery branching occurs. A discussion of the potential molecular mediators of this process is beyond the scope of this chapter but has been recently reviewed by Rottier and Tibboel[16]. With increased severity of lung compression, there is a corresponding impact on lung branching morphogenesis resulting in a reduction of generations of bronchi and associated vascular structures. Morphometric analysis of non-surviving human infants and experimental lamb studies have confirmed the loss of pulmonary tissue and decreased bronchiolar branching[17]. In addition to a reduction of arterial branching, there is muscular hyperplasia of the pulmonary arterial tree[5] which results in a significant component of the postnatal pathophysiology of CDH. Pulmonary hypoplasia is most severe on the ipsilateral side but is also usually present on the contralateral side due to mediastinal shift and compression of the contralateral lung.

GENETICS OF CDH

Non-syndromic CDH is usually considered to be a sporadic condition and it has been estimated that less than 2% of such cases are familial[5]. The recurrence risk of non-syndromic CDH in the absence of a family history is low at 2%[18]. It is likely that CDH is genetically heterogeneous based on reports of syndromic cases of CDH caused by different genes and recurrent chromosome aberrations in CDH. Non-syndromic CDH has been considered to have multifactorial inheritance with gene mutations, environmental factors and their interactions contributing to the anomaly in susceptible individuals[19].

Associated anomalies are seen in from 25 to 58% percent of CDH cases[20] and include chromosomal abnormalities, congenital heart disease (CHD) and neural tube defects. In stillborn infants, associated anomalies are more common. These anomalies are often diagnosed prenatally and are associated with a very poor prognosis. In approximately 10% of cases of CDH with associated anomalies, there is an underlying syndrome diagnosis, so-called 'syndromic' CDH[19]. The majority of syndromic CDH patterns have not been ascribed to a specific gene mutation. However, there is a growing list of identified gene mutations responsible for specific patterns of syndromic CDH. In addition, chromosomal abnormalities are present in an estimated 33% of CDH patients with aneuploidies being the commonest reported cytogenetic abnormalities. CDH has been associated with cytogenetic aberrations in almost every chromosome.

There will undoubtedly be more genes identified that contribute to both syndromic and non-syndromic CDH. The currently recognized genetic associations of CDH have recently been thoroughly reviewed by Slavotinek[21] and by Holder et al.[22]. From a practical perspective, it is important to be aware of the high incidence of associated anomalies in CDH and to be as thorough as possible during the prenatal evaluation in seeking and recognizing patterns of syndromic CDH. All CDH pregnancies should have an amniocentesis performed for a high resolution G-banded karyotype and patients with multiple anomalies should have prenatal genetics consultation.

NATURAL HISTORY

For the purposes of this chapter, 'natural history' is defined as the outcome that can be expected for a population of newborns treated by whatever is considered optimal postnatal care in the environment in which they are born[3]. This, of course, is not the true natural history, which would be neonatal death for the majority of babies with CDH. Knowing the natural history, as defined, is useful to compare the efficacy of prenatal therapies to current standards of postnatal treatment. A requirement for any prenatal therapy should be that it improves upon the natural history of the disease. Although in theory, the natural history of CDH would include all conceptions that have CDH, when considering natural history in the context of potential prenatal therapy, it is much more meaningful to consider a limited population of patients, i.e. those fetuses with a prenatal diagnosis of isolated CDH that are referred for consideration of prenatal therapy. Even if one narrows down the population considered, defining a natural history for CDH is complicated by other variables contained within the definition. The concept of optimal postnatal care is dependent upon both the center where the fetus is delivered and by the time frame of the fetus' birth. There is wide variation in survival of neonates with isolated CDH that is due both to differences in the patient population and differences in the quality of postnatal care. Finally, the definition of optimal postnatal care is in constant evolution. The postnatal care of CDH today is not what it was even 5 years ago. Many centers in the USA and Europe are reporting improved survival of CDH[23–28] and this holds true even when stratified for severity by prenatal criteria. Thus, defining the natural history of CDH is a moving target that must be constantly updated and is both center and time dependent. The classic definition of natural history as a definable and concrete entity is naïve and misleading, particularly for an anomaly as complex as CDH.

The importance of this concept cannot be overemphasized, particularly in the current era where there is renewed enthusiasm by some investigators for prenatal intervention for CDH. Historical perspective on CDH and its treatment provides insight into the pitfalls of inadequately validated therapies. There have been numerous treatments proposed as successful for CDH without adequate comparison to the natural history of the disease. To prove efficacy, one needs a large series of patients that have clearly done better than a group of patients with similar stratification for severity, treated by optimal postnatal care, in the same centers where the therapy is being evaluated. In addition, what proves efficacious in a center with a CDH mortality of 60%, may not prove efficacious in a center with a baseline mortality of only 10%. In other words, one needs well-designed, randomized, controlled studies performed in multiple centers to assess any new treatment. To date, such a study has not proven that prenatal therapy can improve upon the natural history of CDH. Until such a study proves the benefit of prenatal therapy, it should be considered experimental and should not be adopted outside of well-designed studies by capable centers.

An all important aspect of natural history that is rarely emphasized is the morbidity of CDH. While many centers are touting improved survival of patients with severe CDH who would have been expected to die in previous years, it has become increasingly apparent that mortality is being replaced with morbidity in a subgroup of patients with very severe CDH[28–34]. Centers with the lowest mortality, may have the highest rates of neurologic and pulmonary morbidities. CDH is far from a solved clinical problem and improved survival should not necessarily be mistaken for success. There is increasing recognition by major centers in the USA and elsewhere that only comprehensive, multidisciplinary, long-term follow-up can assess the success or failure of treatment for CDH. Claims of minimal morbidity for populations of severe CDH patients should be viewed skeptically without long-term neurodevelopmental outcome data that can only be obtained with great effort, diligence and expense. It should be stated that the population of patients with the highest morbidity is precisely the population that might benefit most from prenatal treatment to prevent pulmonary hypoplasia. It is for this reason that, despite improvements in survival in CDH, prenatal therapy should still be investigated. The inclusion of morbidity outcomes and long-term follow-up should become the primary endpoints of trials of prenatal therapy for CDH, rather than focusing predominantly on mortality. This is particularly true for centers with very low mortality, as improvement in mortality would be difficult to achieve with prenatal treatment.

PRENATAL DIAGNOSIS

With the increase in the use of antenatal ultrasound, many cases of CDH are diagnosed prenatally. The definitive sonographic diagnosis of fetal CDH relies on the visualization of abdominal organs in the fetal chest and the sonographic hallmark of a left CDH is a fluid-filled stomach just behind the left atrium and ventricle in the lower thorax as seen on a transverse view. Other sonographic features that imply the presence of left CDH include the absence of the stomach below the diaphragm, mediastinal shift to the right and a small abdominal circumference. Right CDH is more frequently missed or misdiagnosed because the herniated viscera consists predominantly of the right lobe of the liver which may have similar echogenicity to the lung, or be confused with a solid mass in the chest such as a congenital cystic adenomatoid malformation (CCAM). With the advent of improved ultrasound technology, the liver can usually be directly visualized in the chest cavity (Fig. 33.1). However, if there is any doubt, the presence of liver in the chest on either side can be conclusively demonstrated by Doppler examination of the hepatic vasculature and umbilical vein. The appreciation of an elongated intra-abdominal portion of the umbilical vein, an abnormal position and bowing of the portal sinus, and visualization of portal venous and hepatic venous branches above the diaphragmatic ridge are all indicative of intrathoracic herniation of the liver[35]. In addition, on a cross-sectional view, a mid-thoracic or posterior thoracic position of the stomach with tissue visualized anteriorly between the stomach and heart strongly suggests liver in the chest (Fig. 33.2). Finally, magnetic resonance imaging (MRI) is being routinely used in many centers and can clearly visualize the extent of liver herniation (Fig. 33.3) removing any ambiguity.

Differential diagnosis

Thoracic lesions that should also be considered when the diagnosis of CDH is made prenatally by ultrasound include diaphragmatic eventration, congenital cystic adenomatoid malformation, bronchopulmonary sequestration, bronchogenic cysts, bronchial atresia, enteric cysts and teratomas. (See 'Congenital diaphragmatic hernia: prenatal diagnosis and management' section on differential diagnosis.)

Prenatal prediction of CDH severity

We feel that it is extremely important to obtain a complete and accurate assessment of the fetal patient with CDH by high resolution ultrasound, fetal MRI scan, echocardiography and amniocentesis for fetal karyotype assessment between 20 and 24 weeks' gestation. This allows for maximal information to be obtained from the imaging studies and allows comprehensive

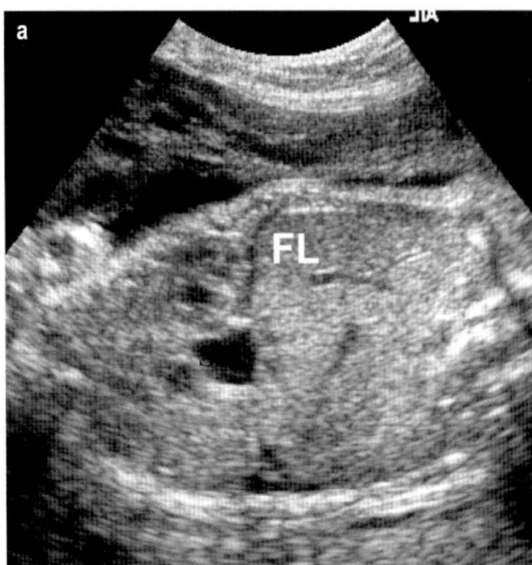

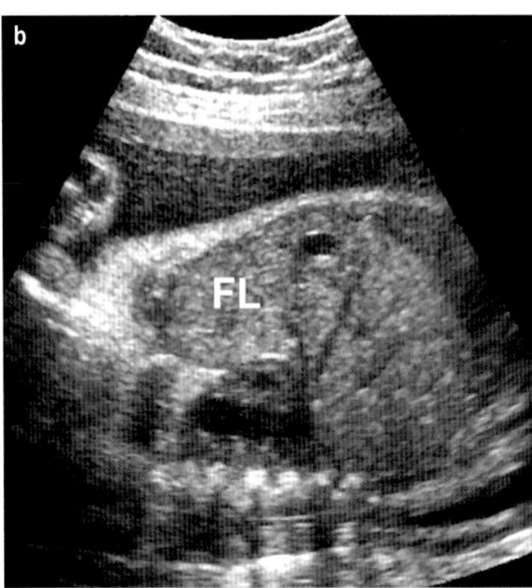

Fig. 33.1 Direct demonstration of fetal liver herniation into the chest by ultrasound. (a) Visualization of the diaphragm with stomach above and liver below the diaphragm consistent with a favorable prognosis CDH. (b) Once again the diaphragm can be seen well on the right side, but the left diaphragm is predominantly missing with herniation of a large amount of the left lobe of the liver into the chest, consistent with a poor prognosis CDH. FL: fetal liver.

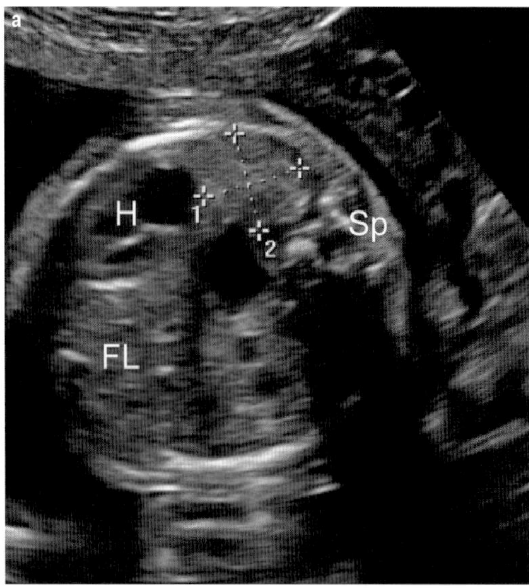

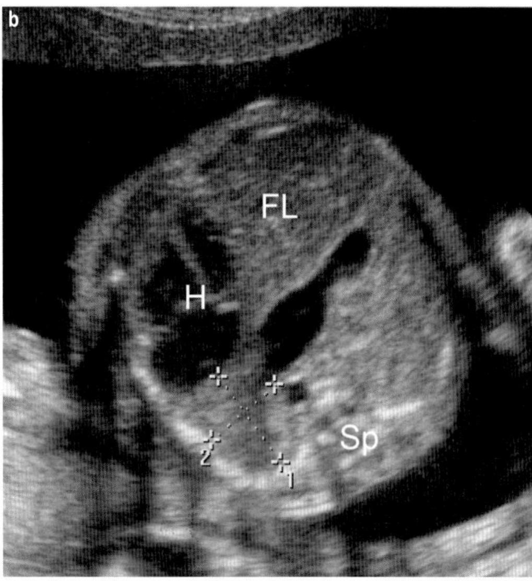

Fig. 33.2 Cross-sectional views of the fetal thorax in two fetuses with CDH at the level of a four-chamber view of the heart. The left lung is measured at its two longest perpendicular measurements, as depicted by the dotted lines, to calculate the LHR. On these cross-sectional views, the mid-thoracic or posterior thoracic position of the stomach with tissue visualized anteriorly between the stomach and heart demonstrated liver in the chest. FL: fetal liver; H: heart; Sp: spine.

non-directive counseling regarding CDH, including the option of elective termination. In order to provide optimal counseling, accurate prenatal prognostication is essential. Much effort has been directed toward identification of poor prognostic indicators in the fetus with CDH, often with conflicting results that are difficult to reconcile.

Associated anomalies

Obviously, the fetus with CDH in association with another major anomaly has a very poor prognosis. While there are recent reports of survivors of CDH associated with congenital heart disease, all of these reports are of patients with relatively mild CDH and biventricular cardiac anatomy[36,37]. The infant with severe CDH and univentricular CHD has a near 100% mortality and should be offered comfort care. Familial CDH (diaphragmatic agenesis), bilateral CDH, syndromic CDH and CDH associated with specific genetic abnormalities are all associated with very poor outcomes.

Liver herniation

In addition to patients with associated anomalies, the next clear poor prognostic factor is the presence of liver herniation. This is the single most reliable predictor of severity and mortality in CDH and has been validated by multiple centers[38–41]. With the advent of improved ultrasound technology and MRI, all fetuses that are prenatally diagnosed with CDH should have accurate assessment of the volume of liver in the chest. The presence of liver in the chest associated with a left-sided CDH is indicative of a large defect with early herniation of viscera resulting in severe pulmonary hypoplasia. In our most recent series, mortality of patients with 'liver up' was 65% compared to 7% when the liver is below the diaphragm. It was also highly predictive

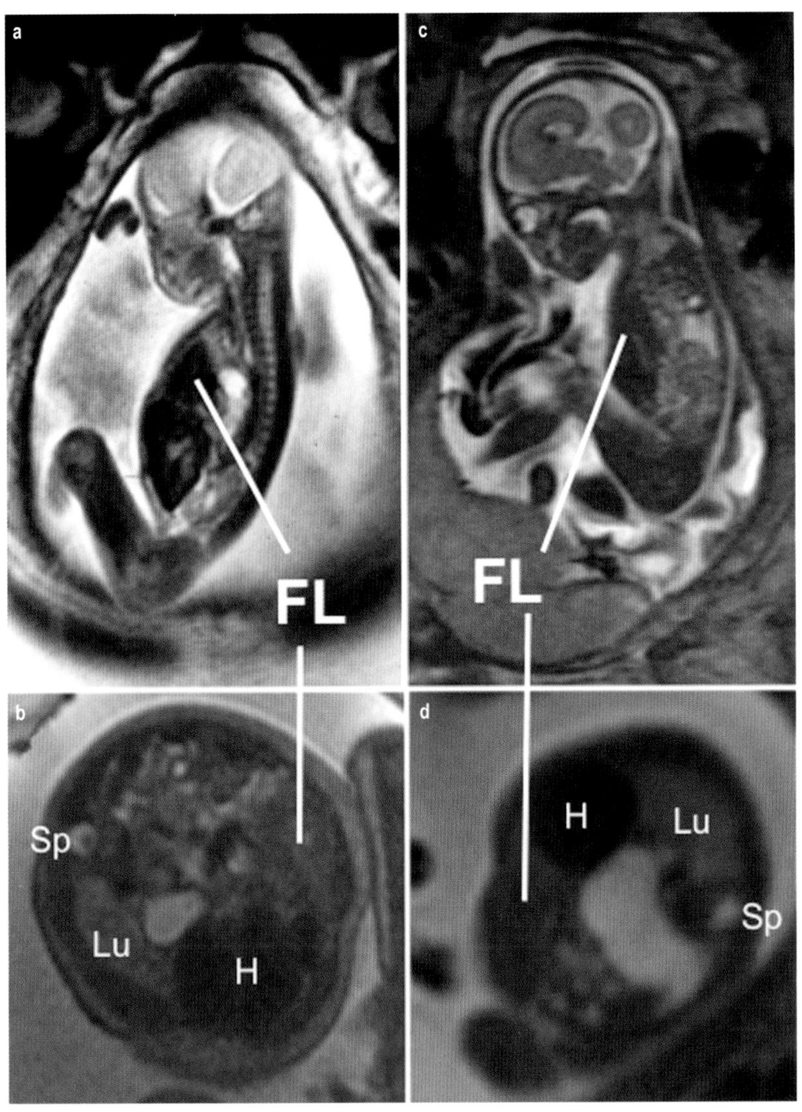

Fig. 33.3 Matched sagittal and cross-sectional views of two fetuses with liver in the chest. MRI clearly visualizes liver in the chest and allows accurate estimation of the extent of liver herniation. Lu: lung; FL: fetal liver; H: heart; Sp: spine.

of the need for extracorporeal membrane oxygenation (ECMO) with 80% of liver up patients requiring ECMO compared to 25% of those without liver herniation[42].

Measurements of lung volume

Extensive efforts continue to be made to correlate direct or indirect estimates of lung volume with outcome in CDH. This is complicated due to the relatively poor physiologic correlation between pulmonary vascular bed reactivity and lung volume. Thus, it is unlikely that lung volume alone, even if measured precisely, will ever provide exact correlation with outcome. In fact, this has been demonstrated in neonates, where accurate lung volumes derived from postnatal radiographs correlates poorly with clinical status[43–45]. Nevertheless, we feel that lung-volume-based prognostication plays a role in counseling patients with CDH, although this role needs to be validated at individual fetal treatment centers.

The most frequently cited measurement is the contralateral lung to head ratio or LHR. The controversy surrounding the utility of LHR measurements are representative of the issues related to all lung volume measurements. As originally described at UCSF (University of California, San Francisco), the LHR consists of a cross-sectional area of the right lung taken at the level of a four-chamber view of the heart calculated as the product of the two longest perpendicular linear measurements of the lung (see Fig. 33.2)[46]. Since its original description, the LHR has been claimed to be highly reliable as a prognostic indicator by several groups[40,47–50] and of minimal or no value by others[51,52]. Part of this may be explained by lack of standardization of the measurement (for instance, some groups have measured the greatest AP and lateral dimensions of the lung rather than the parameters above) and by clear operator variability, which is related to the volume of cases seen and experience of the sonographer. A more pervasive problem, however, is the practice of taking other centers' criteria and applying them out of context to one's own center[53,54]. The predictive value of the LHR is likely to depend upon the postnatal care provided and survival data for a given center. Given that the postnatal care and survival can vary dramatically between centers, it follows that the value of the LHR can only be validated within a center by the generation of data on a particular center's own patient population over time. This introduces the third major confounding factor in the application of the LHR. Over the past two decades, postnatal care has changed dramatically for the newborn with CDH. The introduction of delayed repair, permissive hypercapnia (or gentilation), ECMO and, more recently, a focus on treatment of pulmonary hypertension and cardiac decompensation, has had a dramatic impact on survival in many centers. Thus, LHR as a predictor of mortality becomes a moving target. As mortality improves, LHR becomes less predictive. This has been most evident in single center data from UCSF[46,49,55] and CHOP (Children's Hospital of Philadelphia)[42,50] over the years. As our survival has improved, the LHR number that predicts low survival has been moving downward. Currently at CHOP, we do not consider LHR to be independently predictive of survival or need for ECMO. The predictive value of the LHR independent of liver in the chest is nil and the additive predictive value when combined with liver in the chest is not statistically significant. Thus, the LHR value in our hands, is simply confirmatory of likely severity of a CDH but, in contrast to the past, no longer considered independently predictive of survival or major morbidities.

As LHR is a two-dimensional estimate of lung size, it is logical to think that perhaps a three-dimensional lung volume calculation would have higher predictive value. There have been a number of recent reports from several centers utilizing MRI-based volume rendering[56–62]. These techniques are highly technology dependent and modern MRI technology, allowing very rapid scanning and acquisition of closely spaced images, has resulted in the ability to render lung volumes accurately. Lung volumes (either right or combined) in CDH have been compared to normative lung volumes or fetal body volume to create a percentage of predicted lung volume as a parameter for prognostication. While recent reports have been promising, they require further validation in multiple centers with larger numbers of patients. The various methods will need to be compared for clinical value. In addition, the same caveats regarding specific predictive values apply for lung volumes. They will need to be validated internally for each center that utilizes this technology and what is predictive for one center may not be predictive for another. This is already seen in the variation in predictive values in the studies published thus far ranging from less than 15%[56] to less than 45%[60] predicted lung volume being predictive of death and/or increased morbidity. There have also been promising preliminary reports for volume rendering using 3D ultrasound in CDH[63].

As inferred above, many patients with adequate lung volumes for survival on the basis of gas exchange alone succumb or have significant morbidity related to the sequelae of unrelenting pulmonary hypertension. This raises doubts as to whether prenatal volume assessments will ever provide complete prognostic information for counseling families with a CDH fetus. What is needed to complete the prenatal assessment is information on the pulmonary vascular bed, allowing calculation of pulmonary vascular resistance and assessment of vascular reactivity. This can be approached by Doppler assessment of pulmonary blood flow and pulmonary vascular diameters in normal fetuses[64] but is extremely difficult technically in severe CDH infants at the gestational ages required for prenatal counseling, due to the marked anatomic perturbation and small size of the pulmonary arteries. Recently, the technique of 3D power Doppler has been applied to CDH with assessment of vascular indices by analysis of the Doppler histogram. The authors have claimed predictive value with this technique, but far more experience is needed[65].

PRE- AND PERINATAL MANAGEMENT

The prenatal management of CDH remains controversial. The first component of prenatal management involves the non-directive counseling process. This is best performed by a multidisciplinary team that has extensive experience with the pre-, peri- and postnatal issues related to CDH. The family must understand the severity of this anomaly and the expected pre- and postnatal events that may transpire. They should be clearly informed of the potential for poor outcome for a severe CDH infant, including death, and severe neurologic, pulmonary and gastrointestinal morbidity and the resulting impact on quality of life. Optimal prenatal counseling will result in anticipation and understanding of the events that follow and will allow the opportunity for informed decision making with respect to options of termination or, as an experimental option, prenatal therapy.

The standard of care remains expectant management with ultrasound surveillance for prenatal complications. Most pregnancies effected by isolated CDH will carry to term with the exception of a low incidence of stillbirth effecting from 3%[42] to 8%[66] of prenatally detected cases. In addition, a subset of fetuses with severe CDH will develop polyhydramnios related to herniation of the stomach into the chest with kinking of the gastroesophageal junction and will be at increased risk for preterm labor. This is particularly problematic in the CDH infant as the combination of prematurity with associated pulmonary immaturity and severe pulmonary hypoplasia is often lethal. We normally recommend ultrasound once per month prior to 32 weeks' gestation and more frequently as term approaches to observe for and manage polyhydramnios as required and for fetal biophysical profiles and non-stress tests to evaluate fetal well-being. We have not been able to prevent stillbirth with this approach but can avoid preterm labor with aggressive management of polyhydramnios.

Optimal perinatal management requires the efforts of a well-coordinated multidisciplinary team for optimal outcomes. We feel strongly that fetuses with known CDH should deliver at tertiary centers, preferably with ECMO capability (unless ECMO is not practiced in the region or country where the fetus is delivered) and immediate availability of neonatologists and pediatric surgeons. Transport of CDH infants is hazardous and can precipitate pulmonary vasospasm with resultant instability. We favor a planned vaginal delivery, unless there are obstetric indications for cesarean section, with induction of labor at around 38 weeks' gestation. This allows the care team to be prepared and avoids the potential for onset of labor without fetal monitoring. While we believe that vaginal delivery is beneficial for lung function, we have a very low threshold for cesarean delivery. Failure to progress, or evidence of fetal compromise should precipitate a prompt cesarean delivery as perinatal stress, hypoxia and acidosis can also induce pulmonary vasospasm.

In the delivery room, infants with CDH should be immediately intubated; blow-by oxygen and/or bag-masking lead to gastric/abdominal distension and compression of the lung and are therefore avoided. The infant should be ventilated with low peak pressure (goal, <25 cm H_2O) to minimize lung injury. Any delay in obtaining an airway can intensify the resultant acidosis and hypoxia, which can increase the risk of pulmonary hypertension. The downward spiral of hypoxia, hypercarbia and acidosis is difficult to reverse in this population.

A nasogastric tube connected to continuous suction is placed in the stomach for decompression of the abdominal contents. This can help expand available lung tissue.

The infant should have an umbilical artery line placed for frequent monitoring of blood gases and blood pressure and, if possible, an umbilical vein (UV) catheter for administration of fluids and medications. In patients with the liver in the chest, the UV catheter does not go through the ductus venosus and once the patient is stabilized, other venous access should be obtained.

Blood pressure support should be given to maintain arterial mean blood pressure levels ≥50 mmHg to minimize any right to left shunting. Support includes the use of isotonic fluids and inotropic agents such as dopamine and/or dobutamine.

The administration of surfactant therapy has been suggested in treating infants with CDH[67]. However, a report from the Congenital Diaphragmatic Hernia Registry did not find that surfactant improved outcomes[68]. Although this was not a prospective controlled trial and infants who received surfactant may have had more severe diseases, it does not appear that surfactant is beneficial in the treatment of CDH. We consider the use of surfactant in neonates ≤34 weeks' gestation with chest radiographic findings of alveolar atelectasis suggestive of respiratory distress syndrome.

While beyond the scope of this chapter the post-resuscitative management of CDH has changed significantly in the past several years with an emphasis on sparing of the lung parenchyma using strategies of permissive hypercapnia, high frequency ventilation and, if necessary, early institution of ECMO. Surgical repair is delayed to allow maximal resolution of pulmonary vascular reactivity.

Fetal intervention for CDH

The rationale for prenatal therapy is to prevent or reverse pulmonary hypoplasia and restore adequate lung growth for neonatal survival[1,8]. The initial prenatal approach consisted of patch closure of the diaphragmatic defect[69,70]. Fetuses with herniation of the left lobe of the liver could not be salvaged by this approach, because reduction of the herniated liver led to kinking of the umbilical vein. This approach was ultimately abandoned when a small clinical trial showed no survival advantage in fetuses with CDH without liver herniation, a relatively favorable prognostic group[66]. More recently, prenatal tracheal occlusion (TO) has been clinically applied as a treatment for CDH-induced lung hypoplasia. It has been recognized for many years that the dynamics of fetal lung fluid affect lung growth[71,72]. The lungs are net producers of amniotic fluid. Under normal circumstances, lung liquid volume and intratracheal pressure are maintained at fairly constant values by fetal laryngeal mechanisms[73]. Disruption of normal fetal lung fluid dynamics has a dramatic influence on lung growth. Increasing the egress of lung fluid by fetal tracheostomy, induced oligohydramnios, or cervical spinal cord transection results in pulmonary hypoplasia. Obstructing the egress of lung fluid by fetal TO results in large, fluid-filled lungs. The realization that this physiologic phenomenon might result in functional lungs and prevent CDH-induced pulmonary hypoplasia is relatively recent. Wilson and DiFiore demonstrated in the fetal lamb bilateral nephrectomy[74] and CDH[75] models, that TO could prevent pulmonary hypoplasia and, in fact, accelerate lung growth. These findings were confirmed by Hedrick and colleagues in a 75-day gestation fetal lamb CDH model, in which TO for only a 2-week period beginning at 120 days' gestation resulted in fetal lung growth and visceral reduction, with marked improvement of pulmonary function[76]. Dramatic lung growth has also been observed in both normal and the hypoplastic rat lungs seen in the nitrofen-induced model of CDH[77,78]. Lung growth appears proportional to level of transpulmonic pressure and can be further increased by lung pressurization[79]. In addition to parenchymal lung growth, TO reverses the high impedance to flow in the fetal pulmonary circulation and normalizes its physiological response to oxygen in the sheep model of CDH[64], supporting reversal of the vascular changes induced by CDH[80]. The obvious clinical implication of these studies is that TO might offer a relatively simple approach to accelerate lung growth in human fetuses with CDH. Further experimental work in the sheep model, however, demonstrated that TO had a detrimental effect on lung maturation causing disappearance of type II pneumocytes and secondary surfactant deficiency[81,82]. A number of studies demonstrated that TO with release at an interval prior to delivery could successfully induce significant lung growth and that release of TO restored type II pneumocytes and surfactant production[83–85], although there was evidence that lung function was not restored to normal and that the alveolar wall in TO lungs was abnormally thick resulting in a diffusion abnormality limiting gas exchange[86].

Based on the early experimental data on TO, clinical trials were initiated at UCSF[87]. The technique evolved from an open approach to a fetoscopic approach with uncontrolled case series suggesting an advantage for the fetoscopic approach and an improvement in survival of severe CDH[88]. This led to an NIH sponsored single center controlled, randomized, trial at UCSF comparing prenatal fetoscopic TO with postnatal care with selection criteria based on the LHR[55]. The trial demonstrated no benefit in the TO group in part due to the unexpected excellent survival of the control group. It was speculated that a lower LHR should been used for selection of a more severe group of CDH infants. During this trial, a non-randomized, prospective trial was performed at CHOP utilizing open technique to assure complete TO[50]. Selection of a severe group of CDH patients was based on liver up, and LHR predictive of 90% mortality in our contemporaneous institutional cohort. TO achieved a 33% survival (5/15 patients), but the survivors had significant neurologic and pulmonary morbidity leading us to abandon the approach. A particularly troubling observation of this trial was that even when dramatic lung growth occurred, lung function was impaired after delivery. These results were discouraging and, in general, have resulted in reduced enthusiasm in USA centers for prenatal TO as a treatment of CDH. However, during this USA saga, investigators in Europe[89–91] developed a truly minimally invasive approach to TO in the sheep model utilizing a deployable balloon technology through a single small trocar. This approach is now being applied by the Eurofetus study group in a multicenter clinical trial, that initially reported using only TO[92], and then TO and release[53,54]. The results have sparked renewed interest in TO as a treatment modality for CDH in the USA and Europe. However, close scrutiny and critical assessment of the Eurofetus trial will be necessary to determine whether TO changes the 'natural history' of CDH. Because of limitations inherent in the structure of this trial, it may be difficult to draw firm conclusions regarding efficacy of the approach. The group has thus far not published true, concurrent, same institutional controls to validate their selection criteria and survival comparisons. This is difficult because study subjects come from a wide range of institutions across Europe and return to their institutions for perinatal care. As there are vast differences in CDH survival at different institutions in Europe, this is a truly confounding factor for interpretation of results. The control data for LHR criteria that have been repeatedly used for comparison come from a retrospective analysis of a multicenter CDH registry consisting of 184 patients from 9 European centers and UCSF accrued between 1995 and 2004[40]. The patients were not equally distributed among centers, with the largest number of patients (77) derived from UCSF. Only 26 of the patients had LHRs of less than 1.0, and only 8 less than 0.9, with less than 1.0 being the entry criteria for the trial. For the many reasons discussed above, these control data are not applicable to the treatment population. No true, concurrent, same institutional control data that have been prospectively stratified for severity have been published. In addition, little information is available on long-term survival and associated morbidity with a single statement provided that the long-term survivors had 'no apparent developmental problems'. It is incumbent on the Eurofetus study group to publish detailed data on appropriate controls, to perform long-term developmental outcomes data, and to perform a randomized trial designed to address mortality and morbidity endpoints before publishing further preliminary uncontrolled data claiming benefit of this approach. Until then, judgment should be withheld regarding the efficacy of TO in improving the natural history of CDH.

Despite these reservations, the developments in minimally invasive TO as developed and applied by the Eurofetus group are exciting. It is unlikely that postnatal therapies can ever effectively treat the manifestations of severe lung hypoplasia and the compelling rationale for prevention of this devastating condition remains legitimate. While TO and release would appear to be the most promising prenatal strategy to date, the details of optimal application of this therapy still need development. Questions of timing of institution of TO and duration of TO for optimal effect have not been fully answered. Technologic improvements in occlusion devices are needed to allow complete TO without tracheal injury. Recent experimental findings of optimal lung growth with prenatal cyclical pressure induced strain[93] and the normalization of pulmonary morphometrics, including alveolar septal thickening by the addition of glucocorticoids to TO and release protocols[94], suggest promise for further improvement in the results of this intervention. The ultimate successful application of this technology will depend upon improvements in our ability to select fetuses who will benefit from prenatal intervention and the appropriate evaluation of each modification with well-designed clinical trials.

REFERENCES

1. Harrison M, Jester J, Ross N. Correction of congenital diaphragmatic hernia in utero. I . The model: intrathoracic balloon produces fatal pulmonary hypoplasia. *Surgery* **88**:174–182, 1980.
2. Harrison MR, Bjordal RI, Langmark F, Knutrud O. Congenital diaphragmatic hernia: the hidden mortality. *J Pediatr Surg* **13**:227–230, 1978.
3. Flake A. Fetal Surgery for congenital diaphragmatic hernia. *Semin Pediatr Surg* **5**:266–274, 1996.
4. Hislop A, Reid L. Persistent hypoplasia of the lung after repair of congenital diaphragmatic hernia. *Thorax* **31**:450–455, 1976.
5. Kitagawa M, Hislop A, Boyden EA, Reid L. Lung hypoplasia in congenital diaphragmatic hernia. A quantitative study of airway, artery, and alveolar development. *Br J Surg* **58**:342–346, 1971.
6. Mohseni-Bod H, Bohn D. Pulmonary hypertension in congenital diaphragmatic hernia. *Semin Pediatr Surg* **16**:126–133, 2007.
7. Adzick NS, Outwater KM, Harrison MR et al. Correction of congenital diaphragmatic hernia in utero. IV. An early gestational fetal lamb model for pulmonary vascular morphometric analysis. *J Pediatr Surg* **20**:673–680, 1985.
8. Harrison MR, Bressack MA, Churg AM, de Lorimier AA. Correction of congenital diaphragmatic hernia in utero. II. Simulated correction permits fetal lung growth with survival at birth. *Surgery* **88**:260–268, 1980.
9. Iritani I. Experimental study on embryogenesis of congenital diaphragmatic hernia. *Anat Embryol* **169**:133–139, 1984.
10. Kluth D, Tenbrinck R, von Ekesparre M et al. The natural history of congenital diaphragmatic hernia and pulmonary hypoplasia in the embryo. *J Pediatr Surg* **28**:456–462, discussion 462–453, 1993.
11. Allan DW, Greer JJ. Pathogenesis of nitrofen-induced congenital diaphragmatic hernia in fetal rats. *J Appl Physiol* **83**:338–347, 1997.
12. Greenough A, Ahmed T, Broughton S. Unilateral pulmonary agenesis. *J Perinat Med* **34**:80–81, 2006.
13. Whitsett JA. Disorders of lung morphogenesis. *Paediatr Resp Rev* **7** (Suppl 1):S248, 2006.
14. Clugston RD, Greer JJ. Diaphragm development and congenital diaphragmatic hernia. *Semin Pediatr Surg* **16**:94–100, 2007.
15. Greer JJ, Allan DW, Babiuk RP, Lemke RP. Recent advances in understanding the pathogenesis of nitrofen-induced congenital diaphragmatic hernia. *Pediatric Pulmonol* **29**:394–399, 2000.
16. Rottier R, Tibboel D. Fetal lung and diaphragm development in congenital diaphragmatic hernia. *Semin Perinatol* **29**:86–93, 2005.
17. DiFiore JW, Fauza DO, Slavin R, Wilson JM. Experimental fetal tracheal ligation and congenital diaphragmatic hernia: a pulmonary vascular morphometric analysis [see comments]. *J Pediatr Surg* **30**:917–923, discussion 923–914, 1995.
18. Norio R, Kaariainen H, Rapola J, Herva R, Kekomaki M. Familial congenital diaphragmatic defects: aspects of etiology, prenatal diagnosis, and treatment. *Am J Med Genet* **17**:471–483, 1984.
19. Enns GM, Cox VA, Goldstein RB, Gibbs DL, Harrison MR, Golabi M. Congenital diaphragmatic defects and associated syndromes, malformations, and chromosome anomalies: a retrospective study of 60 patients and literature review. *Am J Med Genet* **79**:215–225, 1998.
20. Skari H, Bjornland K, Haugen G, Egeland T, Emblem R. Congenital diaphragmatic hernia: a meta-analysis of mortality factors. *J Pediatr Surg* **35**: 1187–1197, 2000.
21. Slavotinek AM. The genetics of congenital diaphragmatic hernia. *Semin Perinatol* **29**:77–85, 2005.
22. Holder AM, Klaassens M, Tibboel D, de Klein A, Lee B, Scott DA. Genetic factors in congenital diaphragmatic hernia. *Am J Med Genet* **80**:825–845, 2007.
23. Langham MR, Jr., Kays DW, Beierle EA et al. Twenty years of progress in congenital diaphragmatic hernia at the University of Florida. *Am Surg* **69**:45–52, 2003.
24. Downard CD, Jaksic T, Garza JJ et al. Analysis of an improved survival rate for congenital diaphragmatic hernia. *J Pediatr Surg* **38**:729–732, 2003.
25. Boloker J, Bateman DA, Wung JT, Stolar CJ. Congenital diaphragmatic hernia in 120 infants treated consecutively with

permissive hypercapnea/spontaneous respiration/elective repair. *J Pediatr Surg* **37**:357–366, 2002.
26. Bysiek A, Zajac A, Budzynska J, Bogusz B. Evolution of diaphragmatic hernia management in the years 1991–2002. *Eur J Pediatr Surg* **15**:17–21, 2005.
27. Doyle NM, Lally KP. The CDH Study Group and advances in the clinical care of the patient with congenital diaphragmatic hernia. *Semin Perinatol* **28**:174–184, 2004.
28. Bagolan P, Casaccia G, Crescenzi F, Nahom A, Trucchi A, Giorlandino C. Impact of a current treatment protocol on outcome of high-risk congenital diaphragmatic hernia. *J Pediatr Surg* **39**:313–318, discussion 313–318, 2004.
29. Cortes RA, Keller RL, Townsend T et al. Survival of severe congenital diaphragmatic hernia has morbid consequences. *J Pediatr Surg* **40**:36–45, discussion 45–36, 2005.
30. Muratore CS, Kharasch V, Lund DP et al. Pulmonary morbidity in 100 survivors of congenital diaphragmatic hernia monitored in a multidisciplinary clinic. *J Pediatr Surg* **36**:133–140, 2001.
31. Hayward MJ, Kharasch V, Sheils C et al. Predicting inadequate long-term lung development in children with congenital diaphragmatic hernia: an analysis of longitudinal changes in ventilation and perfusion. *J Pediatr Surg* **42**:112–116, 2007.
32. Chen C, Jeruss S, Chapman JS et al. Long-term functional impact of congenital diaphragmatic hernia repair on children. *J Pediatr Surg* **42**:657–665, 2007.
33. Trachsel D, Selvadurai H, Bohn D, Langer JC, Coates AL. Long-term pulmonary morbidity in survivors of congenital diaphragmatic hernia. *Pediatr Pulmonol* **39**:433–439, 2005.
34. Chiu PP, Sauer C, Mihailovic A et al. The price of success in the management of congenital diaphragmatic hernia: is improved survival accompanied by an increase in long-term morbidity? *J Pediatr Surg* **41**:888–892, 2006.
35. Bootstaylor BS, Filly RA, Harrison MR, Adzick NS. Prenatal sonographic predictors of liver herniation in congenital diaphragmatic hernia. *J Ultrasound Med* **14**:515–520, 1995.
36. Cohen MS, Rychik J, Bush DM et al. Influence of congenital heart disease on survival in children with congenital diaphragmatic hernia. *J Pediatr* **141**:25–30, 2002.
37. Graziano JN. Cardiac anomalies in patients with congenital diaphragmatic hernia and their prognosis: a report from the Congenital Diaphragmatic Hernia Study Group. *J Pediatr Surg* **40**:1045–1049, 2005. discussion 1049–1050
38. Albanese CT, Lopoo J, Goldstein RB et al. Fetal liver position and perinatal outcome for congenital diaphragmatic hernia. *Prenat Diagn* **18**:1138–1142, 1998.
39. Fumino S, Shimotake T, Kume Y et al. A clinical analysis of prognostic parameters of survival in children with congenital diaphragmatic hernia. *Eur J Pediatr Surg* **15**:399–403, 2005.
40. Jani J, Keller RL, Benachi A et al. Prenatal prediction of survival in isolated left-sided diaphragmatic hernia. *Ultrasound Obstet Gynecol* **27**:18–22, 2006.
41. Kitano Y, Nakagawa S, Kuroda T et al. Liver position in fetal congenital diaphragmatic hernia retains a prognostic value in the era of lung-protective strategy. *J Pediatr Surg* **40**:1827–1832, 2005.
42. Hedrick HL, Danzer E, Merchant A et al. Liver position and lung-to-head ratio for prediction of extracorporeal membrane oxygenation and survival in isolated left congenital diaphragmatic hernia. *Am J Obstet Gynecol* In Press, 2007.
43. Cloutier R, Allard V, Fournier L, Major D, Pichette J, St-Onge O. Estimation of lungs' hypoplasia on postoperative chest X-rays in congenital diaphragmatic hernia. *J Pediatr Surg* **28**:1086–1089, 1993.
44. Holt PD, Arkovitz MS, Berdon WE, Stolar CJ. Newborns with diaphragmatic hernia: initial chest radiography does not have a role in predicting clinical outcome. *Pediatr Radiol* **34**:462–464, 2004.
45. Dimitriou G, Greenough A, Davenport M, Nicolaides K. Prediction of outcome by computer-assisted analysis of lung area on the chest radiograph of infants with congenital diaphragmatic hernia. *J Pediatr Surg* **35**:489–493, 2000.
46. Metkus AP, Filly RA, Stringer MD, Harrison MR, Adzick NS. Sonographic predictors of survival in fetal diaphragmatic hernia. *J Pediatr Surg* **31**:148–151, discussion 151–142, 1996.
47. Jani J, Peralta CF, Van Schoubroeck D, Deprest J, Nicolaides KH. Relationship between lung-to-head ratio and lung volume in normal fetuses and fetuses with diaphragmatic hernia. *Ultrasound Obstet Gynecol* **27**:545–550, 2006.
48. Laudy JA, Van Gucht M, Van Dooren MF, Wladimiroff JW, Tibboel D. Congenital diaphragmatic hernia: an evaluation of the prognostic value of the lung-to-head ratio and other prenatal parameters. *Prenat Diagn* **23**:634–639, 2003.
49. Keller RL, Glidden DV, Paek BW et al. The lung-to-head ratio and fetoscopic temporary tracheal occlusion: prediction of survival in severe left congenital diaphragmatic hernia. *Ultrasound Obstet Gynecol* **21**:244–249, 2003.
50. Flake AW, Crombleholme TM, Johnson MP, Howell LJ, Adzick NS. Treatment of severe congenital diaphragmatic hernia by fetal tracheal occlusion: clinical experience with fifteen cases. *Am J Obstet Gynecol* **183**:1059–1066, 2000.
51. Arkovitz MS, Russo M, Devine P, Budhorick N, Stolar CJ. Fetal lung-head ratio is not related to outcome for antenatal diagnosed congenital diaphragmatic hernia. *J Pediatr Surg* **42**:107–110, discussion 110–101, 2007.
52. Heling KS, Wauer RR, Hammer H, Bollmann R, Chaoui R. Reliability of the lung-to-head ratio in predicting outcome and neonatal ventilation parameters in fetuses with congenital diaphragmatic hernia. *Ultrasound Obstet Gynecol* **25**: 112–118, 2005.
53. Deprest J, Jani J, Cannie M et al. Prenatal intervention for isolated congenital diaphragmatic hernia. *Curr Opin Obstet Gynecol* **18**:355–367, 2006.
54. Deprest J, Jani J, Gratacos E et al. Fetal intervention for congenital diaphragmatic hernia: the European experience. *Semin Perinatol* **29**:94–103, 2005.
55. Harrison MR, Keller RL, Hawgood SB et al. A randomized trial of fetal endoscopic tracheal occlusion for severe fetal congenital diaphragmatic hernia. *N Engl J Med* **349**:916–1924, 2003.
56. Barnewolt CE, Kunisaki SM, Fauza DO, Nemes LP, Estroff JA, Jennings RW. Percent predicted lung volumes as measured on fetal magnetic resonance imaging: a useful biometric parameter for risk stratification in congenital diaphragmatic hernia. *J Pediatr Surg* **42**:193–197, 2007.
57. Bonfils M, Emeriaud G, Durand C et al. Fetal lung volume in congenital diaphragmatic hernia. *Arch Dis Child* **91**:F363–F364, 2006.
58. Cannie M, Jani JC, De Keyzer F et al. Fetal body volume: use at MR imaging to quantify relative lung volume in fetuses suspected of having pulmonary hypoplasia. *Radiology* **241**:847–853, 2006.
59. Gorincour G, Bouvenot J, Mourot MG et al. Prenatal prognosis of congenital diaphragmatic hernia using magnetic resonance imaging measurement of fetal lung volume. *Ultrasound Obstet Gynecol* **26**:738–744, 2005.
60. Hayakawa M, Seo T, Itakua A et al. The MRI findings of the right-sided fetal lung can be used to predict postnatal mortality and the requirement for extracorporeal membrane oxygenation in isolated left-sided congenital diaphragmatic hernia. *Pediatr Res* **62**:93–97, 2007.
61. Paek BW, Coakley FV, Lu Y et al. Congenital diaphragmatic hernia: prenatal evaluation with MR lung volumetry – preliminary experience. *Radiology* **220**:63–67, 2001.
62. Walsh DS, Hubbard AM, Olutoye OO et al. Assessment of fetal lung volumes and liver herniation with magnetic resonance imaging in congenital diaphragmatic hernia. *Am J Obstet Gynecol* **183**:1067–1069, 2000.

63. Ruano R, Martinovic J, Dommergues M, Aubry MC, Dumez Y, Benachi A. Accuracy of fetal lung volume assessed by three-dimensional sonography. *Ultrasound Obstet Gynecol* **26**:725–730, 2005.
64. Sylvester KG, Rasanen J, Kitano Y, Flake AW, Crombleholme TM, Adzick NS. Tracheal occlusion reverses the high impedance to flow in the fetal pulmonary circulation and normalizes its physiological response to oxygen at full term. *J Pediatr Surg* **33**:1071–1074, discussion 1074–1075, 1998.
65. Ruano R, Aubry MC, Barthe B, Mitanchez D, Dumez Y, Benachi A. Quantitative analysis of fetal pulmonary vasculature by 3-dimensional power Doppler ultrasonography in isolated congenital diaphragmatic hernia. *Am J Obstet Gynecol* **195**:1720–1728, 2006.
66. Harrison MR, Adzick NS, Estes JM, Howell LJ. A prospective study of the outcome for fetuses with diaphragmatic hernia [see comments]. *J Am Med Assoc* **271**:382–384, 1994.
67. Glick PL, Leach CL, Besner GE et al. Pathophysiology of congenital diaphragmatic hernia. III: Exogenous surfactant therapy for the high-risk neonate with CDH. *J Pediatr Surg* **27**: 866–869, 1992.
68. Van Meurs K. Is surfactant therapy beneficial in the treatment of the term newborn infant with congenital diaphragmatic hernia? *J Pediatr* **145**: 312–316, 2004.
69. Harrison MR, Adzick NS, Flake AW, Jennings RW. The CDH two-step: a dance of necessity. [Review]. *J Pediatr Surg* **28**:813–816, 1993.
70. Harrison MR, Adzick NS, Flake AW et al. Correction of congenital diaphragmatic hernia in utero: VI. Hard-earned lessons. *J Pediatr Surg* **28**:1411–1417, discussion 1417–1418, 1993.
71. Adzick N, Harrison M, Glick P, Villa R, Finkbeiner W. Experimental pulmonary hypoplasia and oligohydramnios: relative contributions of lung fluid and fetal breathing movements. *J Pediatr Surg* **19**:658–663, 1984.
72. Alcorn D, Adamson T, Lambert T et al. Morphologic effects of tracheal ligation and drainage in the fetal lamb lung. *J Anat* **123**:649–660, 1977.
73. Harding R, Bocking A, Sigger J. Influence of upper respiratory tract on liquid flow to and from fetal lungs. *J Appl Physiol* **61**:68–74, 1986.
74. Wilson JM, DiFiore JW, Peters CA. Experimental fetal tracheal ligation prevents the pulmonary hypoplasia associated with fetal nephrectomy: possible application for congenital diaphragmatic hernia. *J Pediatr Surg* **28**:1433–1439, discussion 1439–1440, 1993.
75. DiFiore JW, Fauza DO, Slavin R, Peters CA, Fackler JC, Wilson JM. Experimental fetal tracheal ligation reverses the structural and physiological effects of pulmonary hypoplasia in congenital diaphragmatic hernia. *J Pediatr Surg* **29**:248–256, discussion 256–247, 1994.
76. Hedrick MH, Estes JM, Sullivan KM et al. Plug the lung until it grows (PLUG): a new method to treat congenital diaphragmatic hernia in utero. *J Pediatr Surg* **29**:612–617, 1994.
77. Kitano Y, Davies P, von Allmen D, Adzick NS, Flake AW. Fetal tracheal occlusion in the rat model of nitrofen-induced congenital diaphragmatic hernia. *J Appl Physiol* **87**:769–775, 1999.
78. Kitano Y, Yang EY, von Allmen D, Quinn TM, Adzick NS, Flake AW. Tracheal occlusion in the fetal rat: a new experimental model for the study of accelerated lung growth. *J Pediatr Surg* **33**:741–1744, 1998.
79. Kitano Y, Flake A, Quinn T et al. Lung growth induced by tracheal occlusion in the sheep is augmented by airway pressurization. *J Pediatr Surg* **35**:216–222, 2000.
80. Kanai M, Kitano Y, von Allmen D, Davies P, Adzick NS, Flake AW. Fetal tracheal occlusion in the rat model of nitrofen-induced congenital diaphragmatic hernia: tracheal occlusion reverses the arterial structural abnormality. *J Pediatr Surg* **36**:839–845, 2001.
81. O'Toole SJ, Karamanoukian HL, Irish MS, Sharma A, Holm BA, Glick PL. Tracheal ligation: the dark side of in utero congenital diaphragmatic hernia treatment. *J Pediatr Surg* **32**:407–410, 1997.
82. O'Toole SJ, Sharma A, Karamanoukian HL, Holm B, Azizkhan RG, Glick PL. Tracheal ligation does not correct the surfactant deficiency associated with congenital diaphragmatic hernia. *J Pediatr Surg* **31**:546–550, 1996.
83. Bratu I, Flageole H, Laberge JM et al. Surfactant levels after reversible tracheal occlusion and prenatal steroids in experimental diaphragmatic hernia. *J Pediatr Surg* **36**:122–127, 2001.
84. Papadakis K, De Paepe ME, Tackett LD, Piasecki GJ, Luks FI. Temporary tracheal occlusion causes catch-up lung maturation in a fetal model of diaphragmatic hernia. *J Pediatr Surg* **33**:1030–1037, 1998.
85. Bin Saddiq W, Piedboeuf B, Laberge JM et al. The effects of tracheal occlusion and release on type II pneumocytes in fetal lambs. *J Pediatr Surg* **32**:834–838, 1997.
86. Davey MG, Hedrick HL, Bouchard S et al. Temporary tracheal occlusion in fetal sheep with lung hypoplasia does not improve postnatal lung function. *J Appl Physiol* **94**:1054–1062, 2003.
87. Harrison MR, Adzick NS, Flake AW et al. Correction of congenital diaphragmatic hernia in utero VIII: response of the hypoplastic lung to tracheal occlusion. *J Pediatr Surg* **31**:1339–1348, 1996.
88. Harrison MR, Mychaliska GB, Albanese CT et al. Correction of congenital diaphragmatic hernia in utero IX: fetuses with poor prognosis (liver herniation and low lung-to-head ratio) can be saved by fetoscopic temporary tracheal occlusion. *J Pediatr Surg* **33**: 1017–1022, discussion 1022–1013, 1998.
89. Benachi A, Dommergues M, Delezoide AL, Bourbon J, Dumez Y, Brunnelle F. Tracheal obstruction in experimental diaphragmatic hernia: an endoscopic approach in the fetal lamb. *Prenat Diagn* **17**:629–634, 1997.
90. Deprest JA, Evrard VA, Van Ballaer PP et al. Tracheoscopic endoluminal plugging using an inflatable device in the fetal lamb model. *Eur J Obstet Gynecol Reprod Biol* **81**:165–169, 1998.
91. Deprest J. Towards an endoscopic intra-uterine treatment for congenital diaphragmatic hernia. *Verhandelingen Koninklijke Acad Geneeskunde Belg* **64**: 55–70, 2002.
92. Deprest J, Gratacos E, Nicolaides KH. Fetoscopic tracheal occlusion (FETO) for severe congenital diaphragmatic hernia: evolution of a technique and preliminary results. *Ultrasound Obstet Gynecol* **24**: 121–126, 2004.
93. Nelson SM, Hajivassiliou CA, Haddock G et al. Rescue of the hypoplastic lung by prenatal cyclical strain. *Am J Respir Crit Care Med* **171**:1395–1402, 2005.
94. Davey MG, Danzer E, Schwarz U, Adzick NS, Flake AW, Hedrick HL. Prenatal glucocorticoids and exogenous surfactant therapy improve respiratory function in lambs with severe diaphragmatic hernia following fetal tracheal occlusion. *Pediatr Res* **60**:131–135, 2006.

CHAPTER 34

Abdomen

Martin J Whittle

KEY POINTS

- Normal fetal bowel has fairly unremarkable ultrasound appearances
- Diagnosis of many bowel conditions is often not possible at the routine screening scan at 18–22 weeks because the conditions often develop later in pregnancy
- In contrast, structural abnormalities such as anterior abdominal walls have a high rate of diagnosis at 18–22 weeks
- Bowel abnormalities are often not isolated and their presence should elicit a careful ultrasound review

INTRODUCTION

Abnormalities involving the gastrointestinal tract (GIT) account for about 15% of the congenital abnormalities identifiable by ultrasound. They have a wide range of incidence from about 1 in 2000 for gastroschisis to about 1 in 5000 for duodenal atresia together with some very rare conditions. Certainly not all abnormalities of the GIT will be detected by routine ultrasound examinations and detection rates are dependent on the type of lesion. Thus, only about a third of duodenal atresias are identified by an 18–to 20–week anomaly scan compared with virtually 100% of gastroschises. As with abnormalities in other organ systems, this failure of detection may arise for two main reasons. First, the lesion may not be apparent at the time of the scan because it develops later as the fetus matures and, secondly, there may be a technical failure. Some GIT abnormalities present clinically, for example, with the development of polyhydramnios and often not until the third trimester.

The relatively low incidence of abnormalities affecting the GIT is surprising given its fairly complex embryology. The primitive gut forms during the fourth post conceptual week. The epithelium is derived from the endoderm of the primitive gut and the muscular and fibrous elements of the digestive tract come from the splanchnic mesenchyme.

In this chapter, the description of each lesion will be preceded by a brief outline of the relevant embryology when this contributes to the understanding of the abnormality. In addition, the management issues surrounding the abnormality will be discussed.

NORMAL ULTRASOUND APPEARANCES

The gut is usually an unremarkable entity ultrasonically unless it is abnormal. At 20 weeks, the stomach should be seen and located in the left upper abdomen below the heart. The size of the stomach does not seem to have any particular significance, although a small stomach may be a feature of a tracheoesophageal atresia. The small bowel may be visible in about 40% of fetuses by 20 weeks and in all cases thereafter[1], but it should not appear echodense. Large bowel segments will be seen in all cases after about 25 weeks. As the fetus matures, the contents of the large bowel become sonolucent but the bowel itself is not dilated. Peristalsis can be seen from about 25 weeks in small bowel and about 30 weeks in large bowel. The normal small bowel diameter in the third trimester is less than 8 mm and in large bowel up to 18 mm^2.

Apart from the bowel, other structures in the abdomen include the liver and spleen, the former containing the gall bladder, a cystic structure usually visible from 20 weeks and located on the right side. The presence of a normal renal tract, including a bladder, should be confirmed in all examinations and the anterior abdominal wall confirmed as intact.

STRUCTURAL BOWEL ABNORMALITIES

Echogenic bowel

Sometimes the bowel may appear unusually echogenic and, although this is unlikely to be a structural problem, it may act as a marker for a more serious condition. This appearance of the bowel may arise either from echogenic contents or from edema or ischemia of the bowel wall. The echogenicity can be graded as follows:

- Grade 1 – less echogenic than iliac bone
- Grade 2 – as echogenic as iliac bone
- Grade 3 – more echogenic than iliac bone.

Grade 1 changes, in which the degree of echodensity was less than the fetal iliac crest, were not associated with problems, but greater degrees of density appeared to be[3].

In a review of echogenic bowel[4], the incidence was found to be about 1% of all pregnancies. Chromosome anomalies were found in about 9%, infection in about 3% and cystic fibrosis in 2%. Other cases were associated with a poor perinatal outcome (34%) and intrauterine growth restriction in 8%. However, in a population-based study[5], the incidence of chromosomal abnormality was less than 1% (1/108 cases) but cystic fibrosis was found in just under 2% (2/108).

Clearly, echogenic bowel has the potential to be associated with significant pathology. Its presence should lead to a careful search for other abnormalities and markers which, if present, would indicate the need to consider karyotyping. However, in isolation, the incidence of chromosomal abnormality probably does not justify karyotyping, particularly when the woman has already undergone a screening test for Down's syndrome. It is interesting to note that in one large population study in which the incidence of Grade 2 and 3 echogenic bowel was 0.1%, the incidence of Down's syndrome when echogenic bowel was an isolated feature was 1.7% (12/650). However, of this group about half had not undergone any prior screening[6].

Nevertheless, echogenic bowel should be considered a risk factor for cystic fibosis (see Chapter 28), fetal infection such as CMV (see Chapter 44) and intrauterine growth restriction and poor outcome requiring closer fetal surveillance.

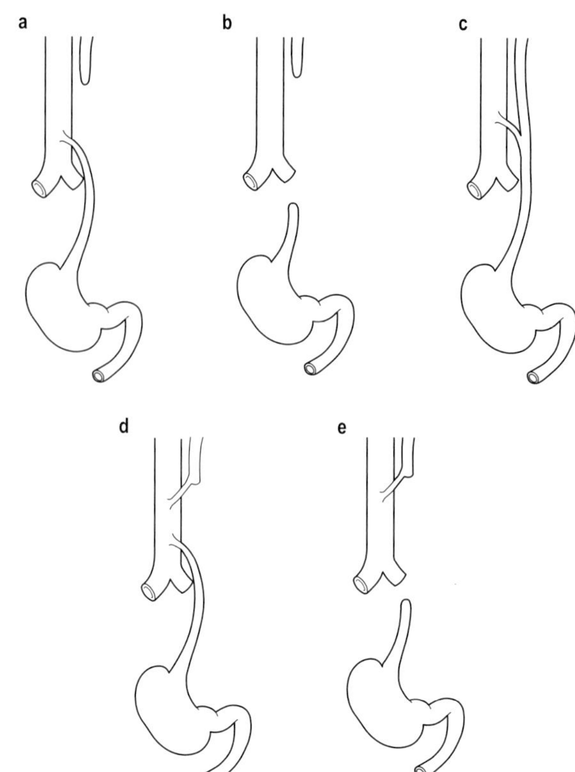

Fig. 34.1 The different types of tracheoesophageal fistulae.

Tracheoesophageal atresia

Embryology

The laryngeal-tracheal tube develops from the primitive esophagus through the formation of a laryngeal-tracheal groove in the ventral floor of the pharynx at about 26–27 days post conception. The complete separation of the esophagus from the respiratory tree occurs during the fourth and fifth weeks post conception (pc) and a failure of this process at this point leads to the development of a tracheoesophageal fistula. A further problem can arise from a failure of growth and elongation at the cranial end of the of the esophagus, which is initially a very short tube. This growth is completed by about 7 weeks pc and its velocity matches the rapid elongation of the embryo at this time. The epithelium of the esophagus proliferates and partially obliterates the lumen, recanalization of which is not complete until the end of the embryonic period.

Definition

Tracheoesophageal atresia is a rare condition occurring between 2 and 4 per 10000 births[7]. There are five main types, only two of which are identifiable on ultrasound because they are associated with an absent stomach, there being no communication between the upper gut and trachea[8]. In 80% of cases, the esophagus ends blindly and the stomach is connected to the lower end of the trachea. Figure 34.1 illustrates the common arrangements, with type (b) and type (e) being associated with an absent stomach on ultrasound. Type (a) occurs in about 90% of all cases. Because of the connections between the trachea and the lower end of the esophagus, the stomach becomes rapidly distended with air, once the baby is delivered.

Diagnosis

Polyhydramnios[9] is the most likely clinical alerting factor, but this may not become apparent until the third trimester. Ultrasound will confirm the polyhydramnios and, although the fetal stomach may be identified, its presence does not exclude tracheoesophageal fistula because of the high chance that the stomach will connect with the trachea. However, the stomach should always be visible at a 20-week screening scan so its absence must prompt a further evaluation at 24–26 weeks[10].

When tracheoesophageal fistula is suspected, the presence of associated abnormalities should always be sought and may be found in about 50–75% of fetuses[11]. These abnormalities will include cardiovascular defects in about 30%, defects of the anorectal and genitourinary systems each in about 20%. The combination of these abnormalities may amount to the VATER syndrome, which includes vertebral, anorectal, cardiac, esophageal anomalies, radial aplasia and the presence of a single umbilical artery. Karyotypic abnormalities may also exist and Down's syndrome has been reported in tracheoesophageal fistula with an incidence of between 6% and 9%[11].

The differential diagnosis of the ultrasound appearances is limited. If the absence of a fetal stomach is the only ultrasound feature apart from polyhydramnios, a careful search for the stomach elsewhere, namely in the chest, is important to exclude diaphragmatic hernia. The presence of the stomach on the wrong side is found in situs invertus.

Management

When the condition is suspected, a detailed ultrasound examination should exclude other abnormalities. It will usually be

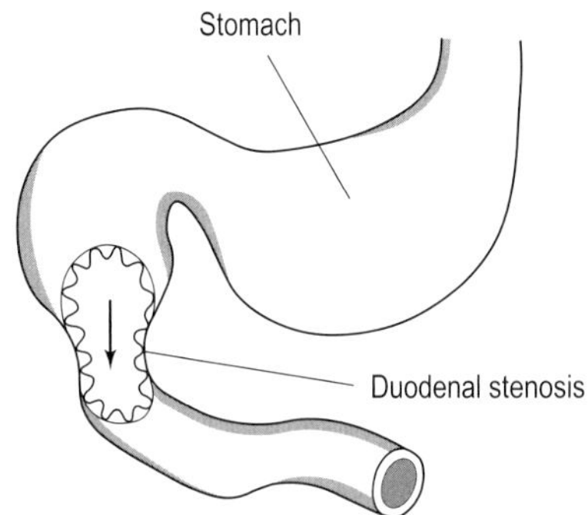

Fig. 34.2 The site of duodenal atresia.

appropriate to obtain a karyotype, especially if other anomalies exist. In the absence of other abnormalities, the prognosis can be favorable with about an 80% survival. The main surgical problem arises from the shortness of the esophagus and, if this is the case, a staged procedure may be required to achieve anastomosis.

The immediate neonatal management problem stems from the inhalation of milk and this can be prevented by checking that a balloon will pass into the stomach before oral feeding is commenced. It is essential that this simple test is performed whenever the risk of tracheoesophageal atresia exists, such as in the presence of clinical polyhydramnios.

Genetic counseling should indicate that isolated tracheoesophageal fistula is likely to be a sporadic event and that recurrence rates reflect those of the associated conditions. VATER itself is usually regarded as sporadic.

Duodenal obstruction

Embryology

During the development of the foregut, the proliferation of the endothelial lining during the fifth and sixth weeks leads initially to occlusion. Recanalization is usually complete by the end of the embryonic period, but a failure in this process will lead to the development of atresia. Another mechanism arises from the presence of an annular pancreas which may compress the duodenum externally and which is found in about 20% of duodenal atresias. Most atresias are found in the second and third part of the duodenum and comprise a web or membrane (Fig. 34.2).

Definition

Duodenal atresia arises in about 1 in 5000 pregnancies and may be associated with abnormalities of the bile duct[12,13]. Atresia is found in 40–60% of cases, the space between the two parts of the duodenum being filled by pancreas. Duodenal webs are found in about 40% of cases.

Diagnosis

The typical double bubble appearance arises from the enlarged stomach and the duodenal cap which becomes fluid filled[14,15] (Fig. 34.3). Usually, the diagnosis is not difficult but, interestingly, the double bubble is not always apparent at 20 weeks, presumably because the duodenal cap fills later in pregnancy and therefore only about 30% are suspected at this time. However,

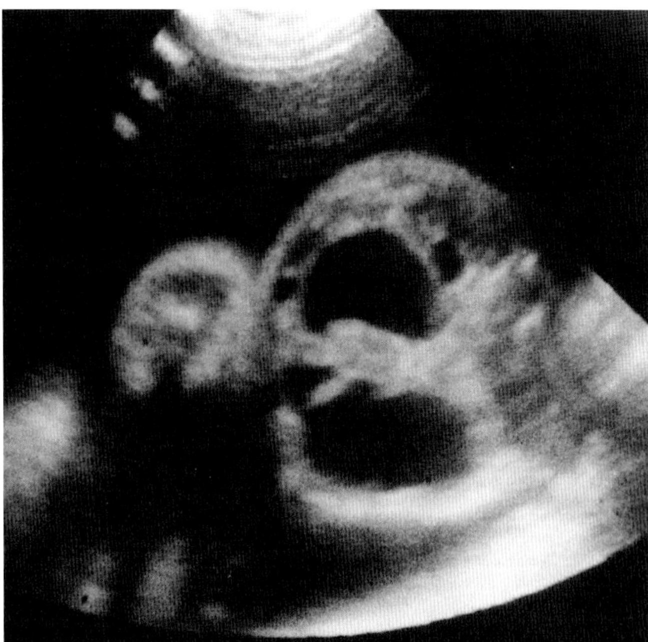

Fig. 34.3 Ultrasound appearance of duodenal atresia – 'double bubble'.

diagnosis in the first trimester has been reported[16]. The pyloric sphincter can usually be identified. Polyhydramnios is a constant finding and is often the initial indication for the scan.

A careful search for other anomalies must be made because duodenal atresia occurs as an isolated abnormality in only about 50% of cases. Cardiac abnormalities may be found in about 10–20%, skeletal changes in about a third and other intestinal abnormalities in about a quarter. Perhaps the best known association is with trisomy 21, although the literature gives a wide range of incidence but, when the duodenal atresia is isolated, the risk of Down's syndrome is reported from 15% to 30%[17]. However, the numbers of cases in these studies are very small and caution is required in interpreting these figures.

The diagnosis of duodenal atresia is not usually difficult, but other cystic structures may confuse the picture. Thus, structures such as a distended gallbladder or a choledochal cyst both lie more anterior than the duodenum but can be mistaken. Gut reduplication cysts or mesenteric cysts may be seen, but these are unlikely to cause diagnostic difficulties as they are not usually associated with polyhydramnios. An annular pancreas is one which surrounds the duodenum and may cause obstruction. The clue to its presence is from the presence of a further cyst in the head of the pancreas which is located behind the stomach. This cyst may arise from the abnormal drainage of an accessory pancreatic duct.

Management

In the absence of associated abnormalities, the outcome for duodenal atresia is excellent, with about 95% survival. Because the condition has a known association with Down's syndrome, there is a need to discuss karyotyping but, because the presentation is often late, the subsequent management, with a possible prospect of feticide, can be difficult and distressing for both parents and attendants. Surgical repair of the atresia is performed soon after birth and once the baby is stable[18].

Jejunal and ileal atresias

Embryology

Gut atresias which occur distal to the duodenum are more likely to have a vascular basis rather than a strictly embryological one.

Definition

These are rare conditions which occur with a frequency of about 1 in 10000 pregnancies. They are probably the consequence of a volvulus, a transparietal constriction or a parietal perforation and the resulting vascular occlusion causes a segment of bowel to become stenotic rather than atretic. Multiple forms may rarely be familial. The apple-peel type[19,20] is seen when the bowel is coiled around a vascular axis and it can be secondary to a volvulus which causes occlusion of the jejunal branches of the superior mesenteric arteries. Other structural fetal abnormalities are rare with jejunal atresia.

About a third of these atresias involve the ileum and, like the jejunum, the incidence of other abnormalities is rare, although the incidence of Down's syndrome may be increased and, in one study, had a relative risk close to that for duodenal atresia[21].

Diagnosis

The classical ultrasonic appearance of jejunal atresia is an intra-abdominal 'triple bubble' (Fig. 34.4). This is a bit of a misnomer since, in fact, there are more than three 'bubbles', and the phenomenon arises from the effect of the ultrasound 'cut' across the abdomen. The distended loops usually appear large and, as with other upper gut problems, there is usually polyhydramnios[22].

Ileal atresia may produce similar appearances and, although the small bowel distension may produce a typical honeycomb appearance, in fact, small and large bowel changes can be difficult if not impossible to distinguish. There is less likely to be polyhydramnios with ileal atresia.

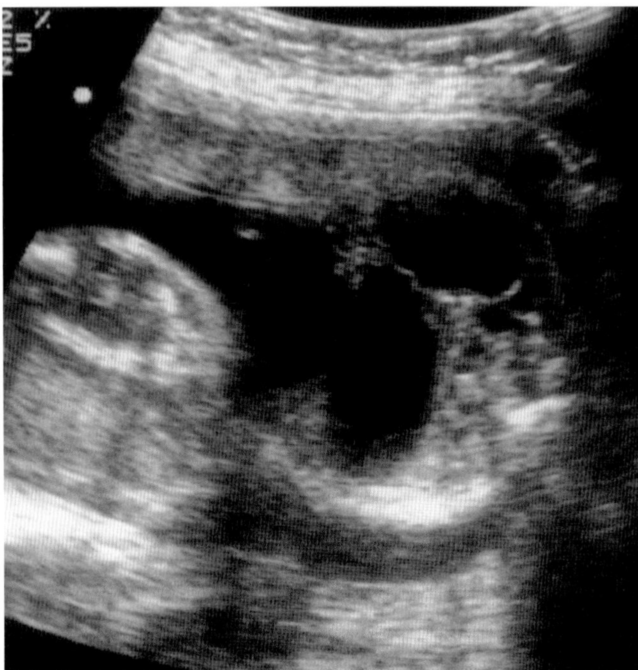

Fig. 34.4 Ultrasound appearance of jejunal atresia – 'triple bubble'.

Management

The prognosis for jejunal and ileal atresias is usually good, although dependent on the length of bowel which has to be resected. If very long sections have to be removed, the child may suffer from nutritional deficiencies as he or she gets older. Conversely, the rarity of associated problems considerably improves prognosis. Knowledge before birth that the lesions exist also allows a more timely surgical intervention after delivery and before the baby can become unwell from dehydration.

Imperforate anus

Embryology

The rectum and anus are developed from the division of the cloaca by the urorectal septum which develops caudally towards the cloacal membrane, fusion occurring by the end of the sixth week. The rectum and anus lie dorsal to the urogenital septum and the urogenital sinus ventrally. The proctodeum develops as a pit, external to the anal membrane which closes the primitive anal canal (Fig. 34.5).

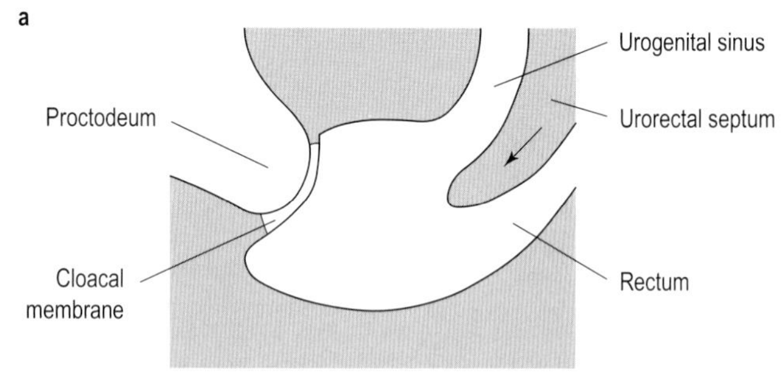

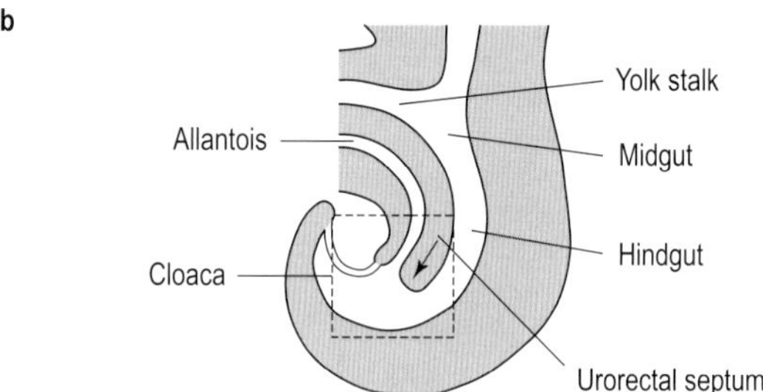

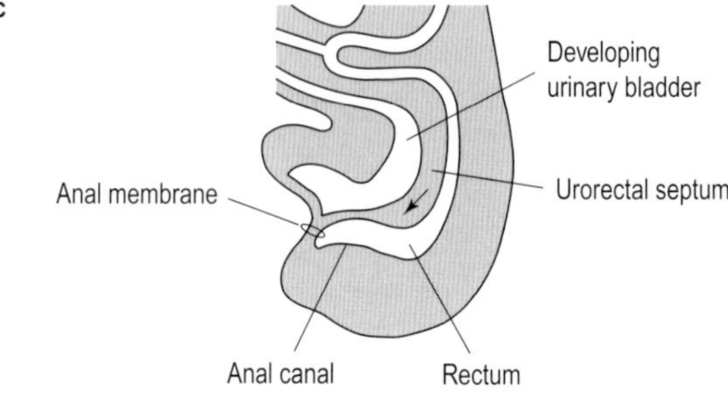

Fig. 34.5 A sequence showing the embryonic development of cloacal structures and showing the progressive downgrowth of the urorectal septum which divides the primitive cloaca.

Definition

The commonest abnormality is anal agenesis, which has an incidence of about 1 in 3000 and which is found in about 45% of all cases of imperforate anus. It is more common in males and usually arises as a failure of the urorectal septum to develop normally, this leading to incomplete separation of the cloaca into urogenital and anorectal portions. It is usually associated with a fistula which, in females, may open in the vulva and, in males, the urethra. A rare malformation is the 'covered anus', which is due to a failure of the anal membrane to perforate. These conditions are usually isolated but may be found in syndromes such as VATER.

Diagnosis

The ultrasound diagnosis of imperforate anus may not be possible although, in some cases, distended loops of bowel are observed in the fetal pelvis continuous with a fluid-filled, dilated rectum. There is no polyhydramnios unless abnormalities of the upper tract exist as well. Other bowel conditions may cause confusion and both Hirschsprung's disease and colonic atresia may provide similar ultrasound appearances[23,24].

Management

Prenatal diagnosis of imperforate anus is unusual. First, the ultrasound markers are unreliable and, secondly, clinical features, such as polyhydramnios do not usually occur. However, if other features compatible with VATER syndrome are apparent, then a careful examination of the fetal pelvis is advisable.

Once the baby is born, clinical examination should be undertaken to confirm the patency of the anus. If obstruction is confirmed, then a defunctioning colostomy procedure or immediate anatomical correction with primary anastomosis is required. Prognosis is good for low lesions but less certain with high ones, in which the risk of associated problems may be significant.

Bladder extrophy and cloacal extrophy

Embryology

The embryology has already been described for imperforate anus and it relates to the development of cloacal structures. In bladder extrophy, the problem is restricted to the bladder such that there is incomplete retraction of the cloacal membrane and a failure of mesodermal ridges to reinforce the lower abdominal wall. Once the cloacal membrane disintegrates the posterior wall of the primitive bladder becomes exposed and remains so.

The problems seem more profound in cloacal extrophy when disappearance of the cloacal membrane before the urogenital ridge divides the primitive cloaca, leads to exposure of both bladder and rectum.

Definition

Bladder extrophy exists when the anterior wall of the bladder is missing. It has an incidence of about 1 in 30 000 and occurs a little over twice as commonly in boys. It is associated with separation of the pubic bones, low set umbilicus and abnormalities of the external genitalia.

Cloacal extrophy comprises two hemibladders, each with its own ureter, separated by bowel which often ends blindly at the anus. Exomphalos occurs in about 85% of cases but, overall, the condition is exceedingly rare, with an incidence of 1 in 300 000.

Diagnosis

Neither of these conditions is readily diagnosed; however, the absence of a fetal bladder on ultrasound is likely to be the most reliable feature[25]. A bladder should always be visible at some time during an examination and its absence should raise suspicion that a serious problem exists. Both bladder and cloacal extrophy may be associated with other abnormalities, the latter particularly so, and it may well be these other features that eventually lead to the diagnosis.

Although ultrasound is the main method of diagnosis, fetoscopy directly to visualize the cloacal area has been attempted.

Management

The affected neonates need immediate treatment to close the defect. Whereas bladder extrophy can be repaired with reasonable success, although several operations may be required, cloacal extrophy is a major surgical challenge. Important peripheral issues may make it necessary to reassign gender in males. Long-term prognosis must be guarded, not only from the point of cloacal extrophy itself, but also the associated conditions.

Intestinal duplication

Definition

Duplications are rare and may have an incidence of about 1 in 4500[26]. They may be classified into those that are closed and cystic and those that are tubular and in communication with the intestinal lumen. The former are the most common and probably the ones most likely to be seen in the fetus. They are formed by failure of normal canalization, resulting in two lumina, and lie on the mesenteric side of the intestine.

Diagnosis

Their precise diagnosis in utero is not usually possible, although they can look like ovarian cysts, so the appearance of such cysts in the male fetus should increase suspicion. Alterations within the duplicated bowel may produce a variety of bizarre changes with calcification of the cyst wall (Fig. 34.6) and visible remnants of the cyst wall[27]. The cyst may become very large.

Management

Simple observation is all that is required in the antenatal period but, postnatally, careful assessment is advised since these reduplications can be the cause of intestinal obstruction.

FUNCTIONAL BOWEL ABNORMALITIES

These are generally very rare conditions which may occasionally be identified during routine ultrasound examinations.

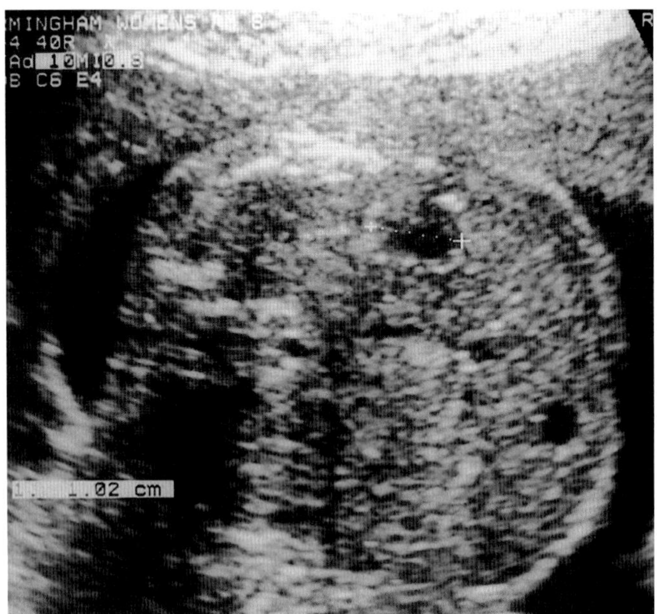

Fig. 34.6 Ultrasound appearances of a bowel duplication cyst in the left fetal hypochondrium.

Megacystis-microcolon-intestinal-hypoperistalsis syndrome (MMIHS)

Definition

This abnormality is associated with functional small bowel obstruction, intestinal malrotation, microcolon and an enlarged bladder with a non-obstructed renal tract. The condition is usually fatal in early life and affects predominantly females.

Diagnosis

Ultrasound diagnosis has been described[28]. The striking feature is the grossly distended bladder; dilated bowel is rare. The other odd feature is the amniotic fluid volume, with oligohydramnios being noted in early pregnancy but polyhydramnios in the latter weeks.

Management

Most of these children develop renal failure and the outlook is poor. Prune belly syndrome is a further complication.

Congenital chloridorrhea

This is an exceedingly rare condition in which there is impaired chloride transport in the bowel wall leading to gross dilatation of the terminal ileum and colon.

STRUCTURAL ABNORMALITIES OF THE LIVER

Embryology

The liver, gallbladder and biliary duct system arise from the foregut as a ventral bud at the fourth week. This hepatic diverticulum extends rapidly in between the layers of the ventral mesentery and divides into a large cranial component which becomes the liver and a smaller caudal one which gives rise to the gallbladder. The cranial portion divides many times to becomes the intrahepatic biliary system and this is surrounded by mesenchyme which differentiates into fibrous and hemopoietic tissue and the Kupffer cells.

The gallbladder arises from the caudal division of the hepatic diverticulum and is attached by the cystic duct to the duodenum. This duct is initially occluded but later canalizes to become the common bile duct. This lies initially on the ventral aspect of the duodenum, growth and rotation of which eventually place it dorsally. Although variations in liver lobulation are not uncommon, serious congenital malformations of the liver are rare. Abnormalities of the biliary tree, such as extrahepatic biliary atresia, are most serious and may occur in 1 in 20000 pregnancies arising from a failure of recanalization.

Hepatic cyst

Definition

The lining of the cyst usually comprises cuboidal or columnar epithelium and presumably arises from canalicular maldevelopment. These cysts seem to be very rare but can potentially be large enough to cause respiratory embarrassment following delivery. The cyst will appear in the right upper abdomen more frequently than the left and it should be possible to see that it is placed within the structure of the liver and separate from other surrounding organs[29]. Hepatic cysts need to be differentiated from other cystic structures, such as those associated with bowel reduplication, although these other cysts are much more likely to be mobile. Choledochal cysts will usually exist on the right side of the liver and pancreatic cysts will lie behind the stomach.

Management

Prior identification alerts the pediatrician to the possibility of respiratory embarrassment. The cysts themselves can be very large, but excision is usually possible and the prognosis is good.

Liver tumors are rare and arise mainly from the mesenchymal tissue which form the definitive liver.

Hepatic hamartoma

These tumors are primarily non-neoplastic malformations containing a variety of tissue types of mesenchymal origin. They are not locally destructive although may produce pressure effects. They are rare but will appear in the liver as cystic spaces which may be septated and very large[30,31].

Hepatic teratoma

Teratomas are rare fetal tumors, the commonest examples being sacrococcygeal tumors. Extragonadal sites, such as the liver, are particularly rare and, in these areas, the tumor may arise from both somatic cells or ectopic germ cells. The tumor comprises tissue from all three germ layers and may be cystic or solid. Histologically, teratomas can theoretically be differentiated from fetus in fetu by a lack of a notochord, but this has been disputed, and fetus in fetu may be part of the teratoma spectrum.

Hepatic hemangioma

Small hemangiomas are sometimes found incidentally at the time of necropsy and probably are of little significance. In the fetus, very large hepatic hemangiomas can be rarely seen[32,33]. These are benign tumors which will usually resolve following delivery. However, their size and their large vascular interconnections may provoke heart failure in the fetus with the development of hydrops. Under these circumstances, a fatal outcome becomes a possibility. Although these tumors will usually be detected incidentally, they may sometimes present with polyhydramnios as a secondary feature of hydrops. The appearance of the liver will suggest the diagnosis, and invasive investigations such as biopsy do not seem justifiable.

STRUCTURAL ABNORMALITIES OF THE BILIARY TREE

Gallstones

Gallstones are extremely rare in the fetus and, indeed, the neonate, although an incidence of about 1.5% is reported in pediatric populations. They may be associated with abnormalities of the biliary tree, hemolytic disease due to sickle cell hemoglobinopathy, thalassemia or spherocytosis. Apart from the associated causative factors, their presence probably have little significance.[34,35] The presence of echodense material within the gallbladder (sludge) can be sometimes clearly identified.

Gallbladder abnormalities

Abnormalities of the gallbladder are rare[36]. Agenesis and bilobing may occur in development and a left-sided gallbladder has been described. The gallbladder should be visible by 15–16 weeks and its absence may occur in the presence of other anomalies. External biliary atresia may present with an absent gall bladder and this has a poor prognosis. The simple congenital absence of the gallbladder usually carries a good prognosis. It may be enlarged in trisomy 13.

Choledochal cyst

Definition

Choledochal cysts arise probably as a weakness in the wall of the common bile duct, although other parts of the biliary tree, both intra- and extrahepatic, may be involved[37]. It is rare in the Western world, most cases being described from Japan. The cyst usually appears in the right half of the liver and the fetal gall bladder may be separately identified[38–40] (Fig. 34.7). The cyst must be distinguished from duodenal atresia and other cystic structures in the liver, mesentery and omentum.

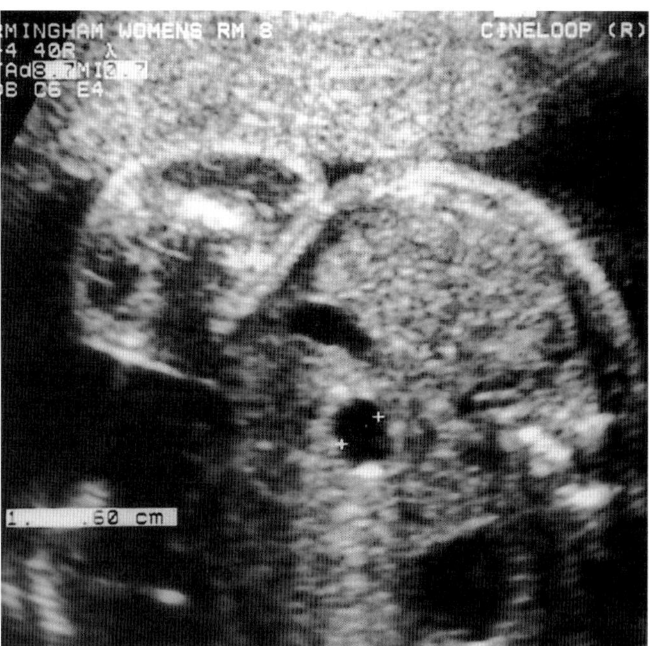

Fig. 34.7 Ultrasound appearances of a choledochal cyst shown between the two + marks.

Duodenal atresia will usually be associated with polyhydramnios, while intra-abdominal cysts will usually appear freely mobile within the abdominal cavity.

Management

There is little that needs to be done antenatally apart from confirmation of the diagnosis. Once the baby is born, further evaluation should establish the exact site of the cyst[41]. Usually, it is possible to excise the cyst but, failing this, it may be drained into a Roux jejunal loop. Long-term outcome is usually good, but ascending cholangitis, portal hypertension and malignancy in the cyst wall have been described.

INTESTINAL ACCIDENTS

Congenital volvulus

Embryology

Volvulus arises as a result of malrotation of the gut, and several types exist. One, the so-called left-sided colon, occurs as the result of total non-rotation of the gut, which leaves the gut prone to volvulus. A mixed rotation is one in which the cecum lies just inferior to the pylorus; volvulus in this circumstance leads to duodenal obstruction. In midgut volvulus, the intestine is attached to the posterior abdominal wall at only two points and the small intestines hang by a narrow mesentery containing the superior mesenteric arteries, an arrangement which is particularly likely to tort.

Definition

Volvulus may result in the necrosis of a large amount of bowel. The prognosis is poor, with about a 30% mortality[42].

The occurrence of fetal distress in the presence of the condition is recognized and may arise either as a feature of central shock or perhaps shock arising from loss of fluid; intra-abdominal hemorrhage is described.

Diagnosis

The appearance of a complex intra-abdominal mass is typical[43–45]. The bowel will become very distended and sonolucent as the bowel fills with fluid. Particulate matter may be observed within the bowel and peristalsis may cease. Ascites or hemoperitoneum may develop[46]. During the acute phase, fetal movements may cease but, if the baby survives, recovery is marked by the return of fetal activity; the affected bowel, however, remains dilated.

Management

The prospects for a successful outcome are poor. If the event occurs before 37 weeks, the immediate delivery of the baby is probably not indicated, but presentation after this time, may allow the baby to be rescued, although the prognosis is still grave.

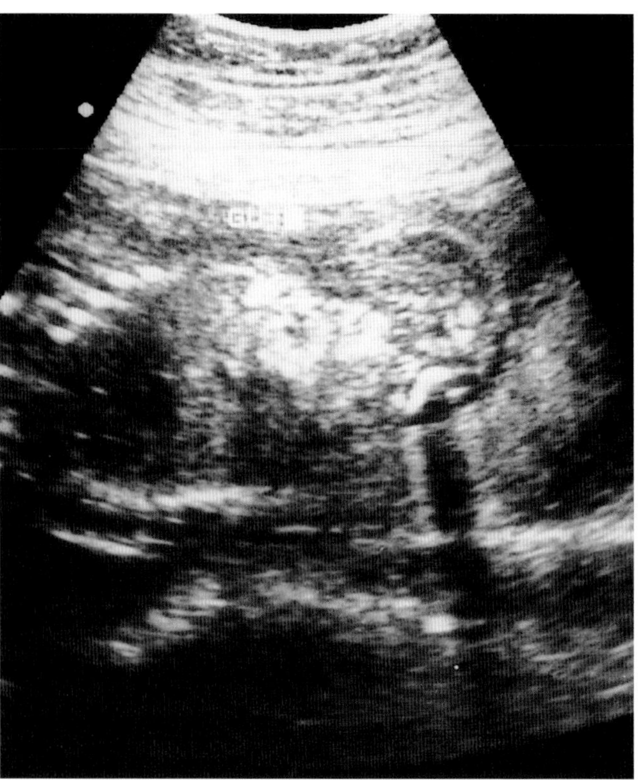

Fig. 34.8 Ultrasound appearances of 'bright gut' seen in some cases of cystic fibrosis.

Intestinal perforation

Definition

Perforation usually occurs as the result of bowel obstruction which may arise as the result of a vascular accident to the bowel such as volvulus, intussusception, or secondary to severe growth retardation. It is a rare event with a reported incidence of around 1 in 35 000 births[47]. Obstructive problems may also arise from meconium ileus as seen in cystic fibrosis or, later in pregnancy, Hirschsprung's disease, although intrauterine perforation in the latter condition is not reported.

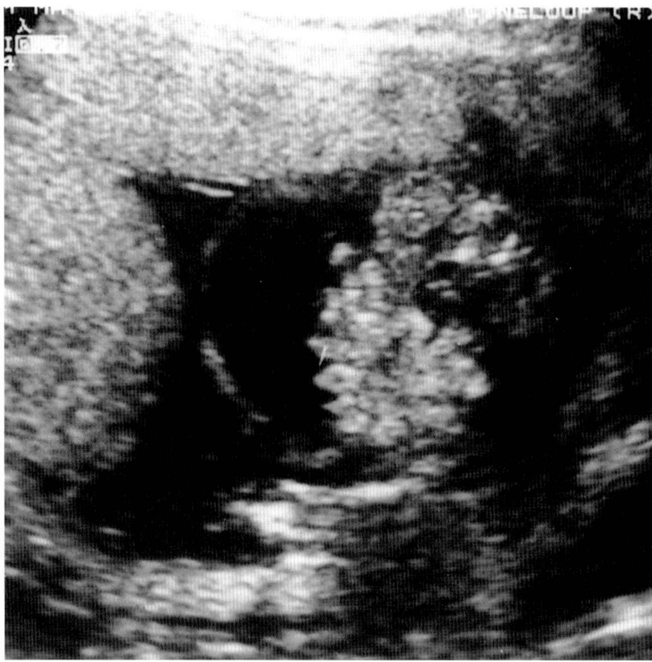

Fig. 34.9 Ultrasound appearances of ascites due to probable bowel perforation.

Diagnosis

The early diagnosis (15–17 weeks) of intestinal obstruction has been reported, although changes may be noted which are normal and only transient[48,49]. Evidence of possible meconium ileus may be seen from the presence of echogenic fetal bowel[3] (Fig. 34.8). Then ascites develops (Fig. 34.9) as a result of the peritoneal irritation arising from leaked meconium. There are probably two phases, the first being acute, in which generalized ascites forms, and the second, adhesive when the ascites begins to be walled-off, leading to the development of pseudoascites[50–52]. Under these circumstances, the gut often appears bound to the posterior abdominal wall rather than to be freely floating. Calcified deposits may appear on the peritoneal surfaces (Fig. 34.10)[53]. Further obstructive changes may appear, but spontaneous resolution is also observed.

The meconium peritonitis which arises from bowel perforation is probably secondary to meconium ileus. The commonest association is with cystic fibrosis (25–40%), an autosomal recessive condition due to a gene deletion on chromosome 7. Why this condition should be associated with spontaneous perforation is unclear, but it probably relates to transient obstruction[54]. The meconium which leaks from the bowel acts as an irritant, which produces peritonitis and ascites. Pseudoascites may develop because the ascites becomes walled-off by the inflammatory process. After time, the pseudoascites may disperse, in worst

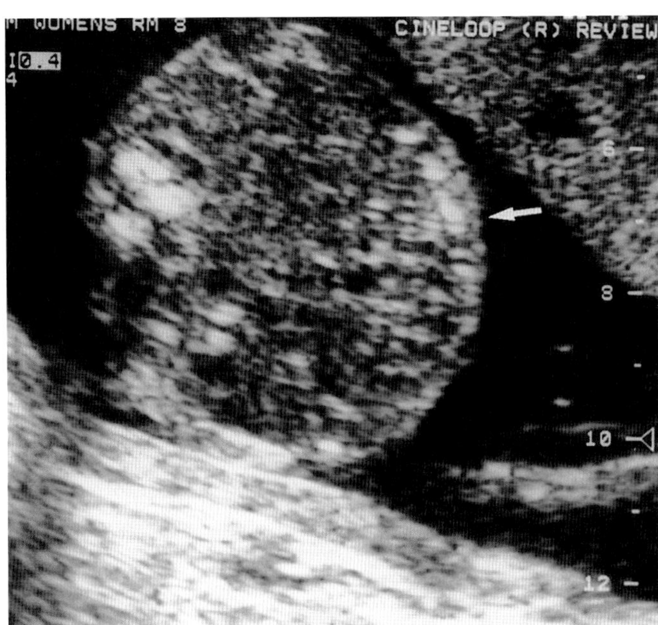

Fig. 34.10 Ultrasound appearance of intra-abdominal calcification.

cases leaving a scaphoid abdominal wall. Intra-abdominal calcification may remain. Meconium peritonitis is a serious condition with a mortality of about 60% in neonates who undergo surgery. In utero survival rates are hard to establish.

Management

Other causes of ascites need to be excluded and an assessment of fetal karyotype, a search for evidence of infection and screening the parents as carriers of cystic fibrosis may be indicated. There is no particular indication for elective delivery and, indeed, the prevention of prematurity should be the aim. Polyhydramnios is a common complication of bowel perforation and can be reduced often by the use of drugs such as indomethacin (15 mg orally tds) for 5 days.

Care should be taken at the time of delivery because the continuing presence of ascites may splint the baby's diaphragm and limit respiration to the extent that urgent paracentesis may be required. Following delivery, the baby will need careful evaluation and, if bowel obstruction persists, laparotomy.

MIDLINE HERNIATIONS

Exomphalos

Definition

Normally, the gut returns to the abdominal cavity by the 10th week pc, undergoing rotation at this time. Exomphalos has an incidence of about 1 in 5000 and results from defective embryological development. The severest conditions are associated with failure of the closure of the lateral fold by about 4 weeks pc. This results in a very large hernial sac containing liver and stomach and a defect in the abdominal wall which may include bladder and cloacal extrophy. In both large and small

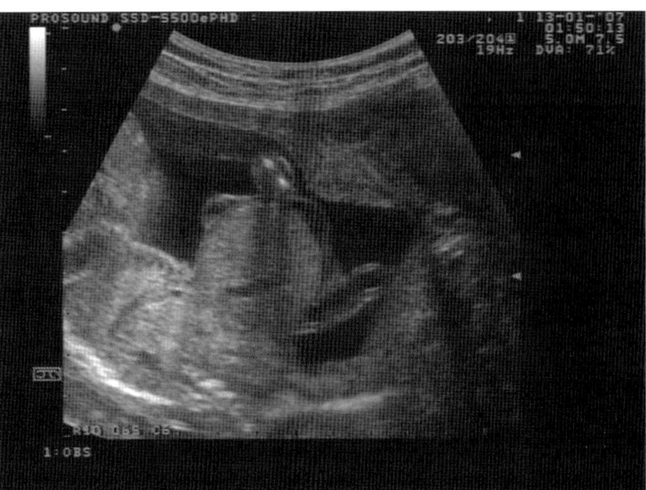

Fig. 34.11 Ultrasound appearance of exomphalos at 20 weeks. (Courtesy of Dr Pranav Pandya.)

exomphalos, the mass is covered by a layer of peritoneum and amnion. Because the mechanism by which the rectus muscles approach one another to close the circular defect left once the intestines have returned to the abdomen is defective, babies who have had their exomphalos repaired remain with a totally deficient anterior abdominal wall.

Diagnosis

Exomphalos should not usually be missed by an adequate screening scan[55] (Fig. 34.11); caution is necessary when the scan is performed prior to 11 weeks because the physiological sac may not have returned to the abdominal cavity by this time. However, minor defects which may amount to a small herniation of the sac into the base of the umbilical cord may be overlooked. This is important, since the small defects may be more likely associated with karyotypic anomalies. A major lesion is defined as one which exceeds 5 cm in diameter at term. The maternal serum alpha-fetoprotein levels may be elevated in about two-thirds of those cases with an exomphalos. Once an exomphalos has been diagnosed a detailed ultrasound examination of the rest of the baby is essential.

Management

Once identified, the presence of an exomphalos should elicit a detailed search for other abnormalities. The parents should be counseled that termination of pregnancy is an option for them but that, once it can be established as far as possible that the lesion is isolated, the prognosis might be as good as 90%, although not all studies support this figure[56]. It is important to exclude karyotypic and cardiac abnormalities, which are found in about 50% of cases of exomphalos[57,58]. Conditions such as Beckwith–Wiedemann syndrome, which is associated with macrosomia, macroglossia and enlarged, potentially malignant kidneys should be considered. The exclusion of cloacal abnormalities is also important, especially in the absence of a fetal bladder and, because ultrasound views of this area may be difficult, fetoscopy may have a limited role.

Delivery should be in a unit with appropriate neonatology support. Vaginal delivery is not generally contraindicated if the lesion is less than 5 cm, although concerns about major exomphalos and the need to time delivery may indicate a cesarean section.

Gastroschisis

Definition

Gastroschisis may arise from an embryological aberration of the right vitilline vessel. The gut is usually short and malrotated so the etiology is more complex than merely an abdominal defect. The incidence of the condition appears to be increasing and it is more common among women aged less than 20 years[59]. Smoking and drug abuse[60] are other possible factors. Importantly, other anomalies are rare and may only be found in about 5% of cases. Karyotypic abnormalities do not appear to be increased and occur at the background frequency for the mother's age. The pregnancy must be carefully monitored and evidence of bowel dilatation assessed. Intrauterine death is described, although the underlying etiology of this is uncertain. Babies with gastroschisis tend to be small for dates, about 30% weighing below the tenth centile.

Diagnosis

Gastroschisis is not usually missed so long as the anterior abdominal wall is carefully scrutinized[61] (Fig. 34.12). The important differential is with exomphalos but, in the case of gastroschisis, the bowel lies free in the amniotic cavity. The bowel can be some way from the fetus, often around the feet, so the whole amniotic cavity must be scanned. If serum screening is used, virtually 100% of gastroschisis will be detected from elevated maternal serum alpha-fetoprotein.

Management

Many centers plan early delivery at 37 weeks, although the evidence for this is not strong. Careful monitoring of the fetal status is required as intrauterine death can occur[62]. Reduced amounts of amniotic fluid seem to be a common feature, although the underlying cause of these changes is unclear. Should delivery be indicated, then an attempt at vaginal delivery should be made, there being no substantial evidence to suggest an advantage to cesarean section.

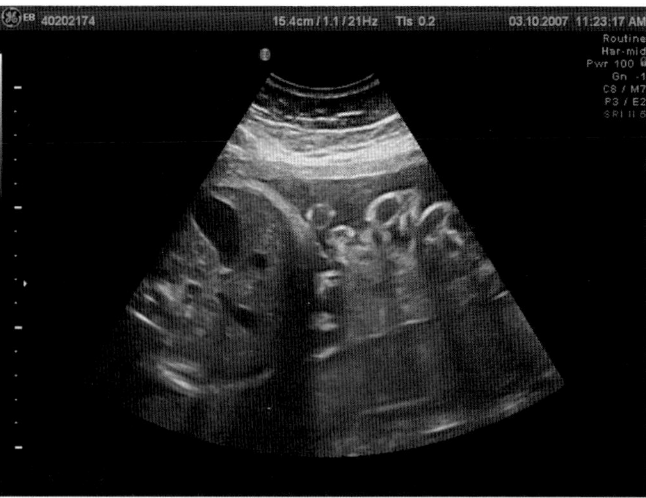

Fig. 34.12 Ultrasound appearances of gastroschisis at 20 weeks. (Courtesy of Dr Pranav Pandya.)

Pentalogy of Cantrell

Definition

The five features of this syndrome are defects of the pericardium, sternum, diaphragm and abdominal wall, together with displacement of the heart. The abnormality probably arises from an embryological defect which occurs between 14 and 18 days pc when there is a failure of ventromedial migration of paired mesodermal structures. Many variants of the syndrome have been described and other parts of the fetus such as the face and cranium can be affected.

Diagnosis

The bizarre collection of abnormalities should indicate the diagnosis[63–65]. The most striking abnormality is the displacement of the fetal heart outside the thorax. The anterior wall defect may be typical of either gastroschisis or exomphalos and may have features of both.

Management

This is an extremely severe abnormality which is likely to be fatal, although survivors are reported, probably in the lesser affected cases. It is likely that most couples may elect to terminate the pregnancy.

REFERENCES

1. Parulekar SG. Sonography of normal fetal bowel. *J Ultrasound Med* **10**:211–220, 1991.
2. Nyberg DA, Mack LA, Patton RM, Cyr DR. Fetal bowel: normal sonographic findings. *J Ultrasound Med* **6**:3–6, 1987.
3. Chitty LS, Griffin DR. The gastrointestinal tract. In *Ultrasound in obstetrics and gynaecology*, K Dewbury, H Meire, D Cosgrove (eds), pp. 352–354. London: Churchill Livingstone, 1993.
4. Sepulveda W, Sebire NJ. Fetal echogenic bowel: a complex scenario. *Ultrasound Obstet Gynaecol* **16**:510–514, 2000.
5. Patel Y, Boyd PA, Chamberlain P, Lakloo KF. Followup of children with isolated fetal echogenic bowel with particular reference to bowel related symptoms. *Prenat Diagn* **24**:35–37, 2004.
6. Simon-Bouy B, Muller F and the French Collaborative Group. Hyperechogenic fetal bowel and Down syndrome. Results of a French collaborative study based on 680 prospective cases. *Prenat Diagn* **22**:189–192, 2002.
7. Depaepe A, Dolk H, Lechat MF. EUROCAT Working Group The epidemiology of tracheo-oesophageal fistula and oesophageal atresia in Europe. *Arch Dis Child* **68**:743–748, 1993.
8. Harvard AC, MacDonald LM. Oesophageal atresia and other disorders

with a similar antenatal presentation. *Br J Radiol* **64**:557–558, 1991.
9. Pretorius DH, Drose JA, Dennis MA, Manchester DK, Manco-Johnson ML. Tracheoesophageal fistula in utero. Twenty two cases. *J Ultrasound Med* **6**:509–513, 1987.
10. Estroff JA, Parad RB, Share JC, Benacerraf BR. Second trimester prenatal findings in duodenal and esophageal atresia without tracheoesophageal fistula. *J Ultrasound Med* **13**:375–379, 1994.
11. van Heurn LWE, Cheng W, de Vries B et al. Anomalies associated with oesophageal atresia in Asians and Europeans. *Pediatr Surg Int* **18**:241–243, 2002.
12. Akhtar J, Guiney EJ. Congenital duodenal obstruction. *Br J Surg* **79**:133–135, 1992.
13. Athale AS, Vaishnav TV, Jhala PJ, Vohra P. Prenatal diagnosis of duodenal atresia by ultrasound. *Indian J Pediatr* **58**:145–147, 1991.
14. Collier D. Antenatal diagnosis of duodenal atresia by ultrasound: a case report. *Radiography* **48**:102–103, 1982.
15. Nelson LH, Clark CE, Fishburne JI, Urban RB, Penry MF. Value of serial sonography in the in utero detection of duodenal atresia. *Obstet Gynecol* **59**:657–660, 1982.
16. Petrikovsky BM. First trimester diagnosis of duodenal atresia. *Am J Obstet Gynecol* **171**:569–570, 1994.
17. Snijders RMJ, Nicolaides KH. Fetal abnormalities. In *Ultrasound markers for fetal chromosome defects*, RMJ Snijders, KH Nicolaides et al (eds), pp. 33–35. London: Parthenon Publishing Group, 1996.
18. Grosfeld JL, Rescorla FJ. Duodenal atresia and stenosis: reassessment of treatment and outcome based on antenatal diagnosis, pathological variance and longterm followup. *Wld J Surg* **17**:301–309, 1993.
19. Fletman D, McQuown D, Kanchana Poon V,Gyepes MI. 'Apple peel' atresia of the small bowel: prenatal diagnosis of the obstruction by ultrasound. *Pediar Radiol* **9**:118–119, 1980.
20. Lai PC, Jehng CH, Chiang LM et al. Jejunal atresia with 'apple peel' deformity: report of one case. *Acta Paediatr Sin* **32**:47–53, 1991.
21. Torfs CP, Christianson RE. Anomalies in Down syndrome individuals in a large population-based registry. *Am J Med Genetics* **77**:431–438, 1998.
22. Filkins K, Russo J, Flowers WK. Third trimester ultrasound diagnosis of intestinal atresia following clinical evidence of polyhydramnios. *Prenat Diagn* **5**:215–220, 1985.
23. Hallak M, Reiter AA, Smith LG, Dildy GA, Finegold MJ. Oligohydramnios and megacolon in the fetus with vesicorectal fistula and anal urethral atresia: a case report. *Am J Obstet Gynecol* **167**:79–81, 1992.
24. Miller SF, Angtuaco TL, Quirk JG, Hairston K. Anorectal atresia presenting as an abdominopelvic mass. *J Ultrasound Med* **9**:669–672, 1990.
25. Romero R, Pilu G, Jeanty P, Ghidini A, Hobbins J. Bladder extrophy and cloacal extrophy. In *Prenatal diagnosis of congenital anomalies*, R Romero (ed.), pp. 228–232. New York: Appleton and Large, 1988.
26. Michalsky M, Besner GE. Ailmentary duplication. *eMed J* **7**(8), 2006. http://www.author.emedicne.com/PED/topic2922.htm
27. Chitty LS, Griffin DR. The gastrointestinal tract. In *Ultrasound in obstetrics and gynaecology*, K Dewbury, H Meire, D Cosgrove (eds), p. 359. London: Churchill Livingstone, 1993.
28. Stamm E, King G, Thickman D. Megacystis-microcolon-intestinal hypoperistalsis syndrome: prenatal identification in siblings and review of the literature. *J Ultrasound Med* **10**:599–602, 1991.
29. Chung WM. Antenatal detection of hepatic cyst. *J Clin Ultrasound* **14**:217–219, 1986.
30. Foucar E, Williamson RA, Yiu-Chiu V, Varner MW, Kay BR. Mesenchymal hamartoma of the liver identified by fetal sonography. *Am J Radiol* **140**:970–972, 1983.
31. Hirata GI, Matsunaga ML, Medearis AL, Dixon P, Platt LD. Ultrasonographic diagnosis of a fetal abdominal mass: a case of a mesenchymal liver hamartoma and a review of the literature. *Prenat Diagn* **10**:507–512, 1990.
32. Nakamoto SK, Dreilinger A, Dattel B, Mattrey RF, Key TC. The sonographic appearance of hepatic haemangioma in utero. *J Ultrasound Med* **2**:239–241, 1983.
33. Sepulveda WH, Donetch G, Giuliano A. Prenatal diagnosis of fetal hepatic haemangioma. *Eur J Obstet Gynecol Reprod Biol* **48**:73–76, 1993.
34. Abbitt PL, McIlhenny J. Prenatal detection of gallstones. *J Clin Ultrasound* **18**:202–204, 1990.
35. Heijne L, Ednay D. The development of fetal gallstones demonstrated by ultrasound. *Radiography* **51**:155–156, 1985.
36. Bronshtein M, Weiner Z, Abramovici H, Filmar S, Erlik Y, Blumfeld Z. Prenatal diagnosis of gallbladder anomalies: report of 17 cases. *Prenat Diag* **13**:851–861, 1993.
37. Tsang TM, Tam PK, Chamberlain P. Obliteration of the distal bile duct in the development of congenital choledochal cyst. *J Pediatric Surg* **29**:1582–1583, 1994.
38. Ellia F, Dugue Mrechaud MD, Levrd G, Bonneau D, Magnin G. Choledochal cysts. *A rare parental diagnosis. J Gynecol Obstet Biol Reprod* **24**:400–404, (in French) 1995.
39. Gallivan EK, Crombleholme TM, D'Alton ME. Early prenatal diagnosis of choledochal cyst. *Prenat Diagn* **16**:934–937, 1996.
40. Bancroft JD, Bucuvalas JC, Ryckman FC, Dudgeon DL, Saunders RC, Schwarz KB. Antenatal diagnosis of choledochal cyst. *J Ped Gastero Nutr* **18**:142–145, 1994.
41. Baunin C, Mechinaud-Puget C, Fajadet P et al. Management of a biliary cyst disclosed prenatally. 2 cases. *Chir Pediatr (French)* **31**:160–163, 1990.
42. Crisera CA, Ginsburg HB, Gittes GK. Fetal midgut volvulus presenting at term. *J Pediatric Surg* **34**:1280–1281, 1999.
43. Cloutier MG, Fried AM, Selke AC. Antenatal observation of midgut volvulus by ultrasound. *J Clin Ultrasound* **11**:286–288, 1983.
44. Mercado MG, Bulas DI, Chandra R. Prenatal diagnosis and management of congenital volvulus. *Pediatr Radiol* **23**:601–602, 1993.
45. Samuel N, Dicker D, Feldberg D, Goldman JA. Ultrasound diagnosis and management of fetal intestinal obstruction and volvulus in utero. *J Perinat Med* **12**:333–337, 1984.
46. Witter FR, Molteni RA. Intrauterine intestinal volvulus with hemoperitoneum presenting as fetal distress at 34 weeks gestation. *Am J Obstet Gynecol* **155**:1080–1081, 1986.
47. Nyberg DA. Intraabdominal abnormalities. In *Diagnostic ultrasound of fetal abnormaities*, DA Nyberg, BS Mahoney, DH Pretorius (eds), pp. 342–394. St Louis: Mosby, 1990.
48. Bronshtein M, Zimmer EZ. Early sonographic detection of fetal obstruction and possible diagnostic pitfalls. *Prenat Diagn* **16**:203–206, 1996.
49. Slotnick RN, Abuhamad AZ. Prognostic implications of fetal echogenic bowel. *Lancet* **347**:85–87, 1996.
50. Shalev J, Frankel Y, Avigad I, Mashiach S. Spontaneous intestinal perforation in utero: ultrasonic diagnostic criteria. *Am J Obstet Gynecol* **144**:855–857, 1982.
51. Denholm TA, Crow HC, Edwards WH, Simmons GM, Marin-Padilla M, Bartrum RJ. Prenatal sonographic appearance of meconium ileus in twins. *Am J Roentgenol* **143**:371–372, 1984.
52. McGahan JP, Hanson F. Meconium peritonitis with accompanying pseudocyst: prenatal sonographic diagnosis. *Radiology* **148**:125–126, 1983.
53. Dunne M, Haney P, Sun CC. Sonographic features of bowel perforation and calcific meconium peritonitis in utero. *Pediatr Radiol* **13**:231–233, 1983.
54. Shalev J, Navon R, Urbach D, Mashiach S, Goldman B. Intestinal obstruction and cystic fibrosis: antenatal ultrasound appearance. *J Med Genet* **20**:229–230, 1983.
55. Lindfors KK, McGahan JP, Walter JP. Fetal exomphalos and gastroschisis: pitfalls in sonographic diagnosis. *Am J Roentgenol* **147**:797–800, 1986.
56. Morrow R, Whittle MJ, McNay MB, Raine PA, Gibson AA, Crossley J. Prenatal diagnosis and management of anterior abdominal wall defects in the west of Scotland. *Prenat Diagn* **13**:111–115, 1993.
57. Gilbert WM, Nicolaides KP. Fetal omphalocoele: associated malformations

and chromosomal defects. *Obstet Gynecol* **70**:633–635, 1987.
58. Snijders RJM, Sebire NJ, Souka A, Santiago C, Nicolaides KH. Fetal exomphalos and chromosomal defects: relationship to maternal age and gestation. *Ultrasound Obstet Gynecol* **6**:250–255, 1995.
59. Tan KH, Kilby MD, Whittle MJ, Beattie BR, Booth IW, Botting BJ. Congenital anterior abdominal wall defects in England and Wales, 1987–1993: retrospective analysis of OPCS data. *Br Med J* **313**:903–906, 1996.
60. Morrison JJ, Chitty LS, Peebles D, Rodeck CH. Recreational drugs and fetal gastroschisis: maternal hair analysis in the periconceptional period and during pregnancy. *Br J Obstet Gynaecol* **112**:1022–1025, 2005.
61. Langer JC, Khanna J, Caco C, Dykes EH, Nicolaides KH. Prenatal diagnosis of gastroschisis: development of objective sonographic criteria for prdicting outcome. *Obstet Gynecol* **81**:53–56, 1993.
62. Crawford RAF, Ryan G, Wright VM, Rodeck CH. The importance of serial biophysical assessment of fetal well being in gastroschisis. *Br J Obstet Gynaecol* **99**:899–902, 1992.
63. Abu-Yousef MM, Wray AB, Williamson RA, Bonsib SM. Antenatal diagnosis of variant of pentalogy of Cantrell. *J Ultrasound Med* **6**:535–538, 1987.
64. Ghidini A, Sirtori M, Romero R, Hobbins JC. Prenatal diagnosis of pentalogy of Cantrell. *J Ultrasound Med* **7**:567–572, 1988.
65. Zimmer EZ, Bronshtein M. Fetal midline disruption syndromes. *Prenat Diagn* **16**:65–69, 1996.

CHAPTER 35

Kidney and urinary tract disorders

Marc Dommergues, Farida Daïkha-Dahmane, Françoise Muller, Marie Cécile Aubry, Stephen Lortat-Jacob, Claire Nihoul-Fékété, Yves Dumez – updated for the 2nd edition by Mark D Kilby

KEY POINTS

- When a fetal renal anomaly is identified careful ultrasound examination is required to exclude other coexistent anomalies
- When other coexistent anomalies exist, then the risk of aneuploidy and single gene disorders as an underlying etiology should be considered and investigated
- Particularly in bilateral disease, regular sonographic follow-up should be arranged
- Quantitative measures of amniotic fluid volume give a surrogate marker of renal function (especially in bilateral disease) with oligohydramnios associated with increased perinatal morbidity and mortality
- Measures of renal function, such as analytes (i.e. Na^+, Ca^{2+}) may have use in individual cases, but systematic review of the literature indicates poor overall predictive value of chronic renal impairment when using such investigation
- In cases of severe bilateral renal disease and associated severe oligohydramnios, termination of pregnancy should be considered
- In ongoing pregnancies, multidisciplinary perinatal management should be planned with involvement of pediatric nephrologists and surgeons
- Post-delivery careful assessment of the baby should be performed. This may include radiological imaging of the urinary tract. In cases of perinatal death, post-mortem examination and fetal karyotyping/storage of DNA should be considered (if not performed prenatally)

EMBRYOLOGY

Kidneys, ureters and renal function

The urinary excretory system develops from the mesonephric duct, while the kidney itself differentiates from the metanephros[1–6]. Initially, the urogenital ridge is derived from the intermediate mesoderm on both sides of the primitive aorta. The intermediate mesoderm gives rise to a nephrogenic cord which forms the pronephros, mesonephros and metanephros. The pronephros and the mesonephros are transient embryonic structures, while the metanephros differentiates as a result of inductive interactions between the metanephric blastema and the ureteric bud, a caudal outgrowth of the Wolffian duct.

The Wolffian duct is initially connected to a transient structure, the mesonephros, and participates in the formation of the vas deferens, epididymis, efferent ductules and rete testis in the male. It degenerates in the female. The definitive kidney derives from the metanephros, formed caudal to the mesonephros in the fifth week of development. The ureter arises as a diverticulum from the lower mesonephric duct and grows in the direction of the metanephric blastema. The growing end of the ureter undergoes repeated dichotomous branching forming the collecting system of the kidneys: renal pelvis, major calyces, minor calyces, collecting ducts. The interaction of the distal end of the collecting duct (called the ampulla) with the metanephric mesenchyme is crucial to induce the differentiation of the nephrons. Nephrons appear first as cellular condensates around the ampulla that soon develop into comma-shaped and S-shaped bodies. One end of these S-bodies is connected with the collecting tubules. At the other end, their inferior cleft is invaded by capillaries to form the glomerulus. The rest of the S-bodies will form the proximal and distal convoluted tubules and the loops of Henle.

The branching process is completed by 20 weeks, but the induction of the mesenchyme by the epithelial ureteric structures is not completed before 32–36 weeks, accounting for the progressive maturation of fetal renal function. The maturation of renal function progresses further due to the enlargement of the existing nephrons.

Fetal urine production is thought to begin by 11–12 weeks, but the biochemistry of human fetal urine is not well documented until 16 menstrual weeks. Later in gestation, the analysis of the biochemistry of fetal urine suggests that the various functions of the kidney do not develop at the same time. At 20 weeks, the low protein content of fetal urine suggests that glomerular protein filtration is already mature. The virtual absence of fetal urinary glucose and phosphorus suggests that the tubular reabsorption of these substrates is also achieved by then[7–11]. The progressive maturation of tubular reabsorption of sodium and β2 microglobulin and of tubular secretion of calcium is more progressive during the second half of pregnancy.

Finally, from 30 weeks onward, a progressive increase in the fetal urinary elimination of the nitrogen compounds (urea, creatinine, and ammonia) probably results from an increase in fetal muscular mass[9].

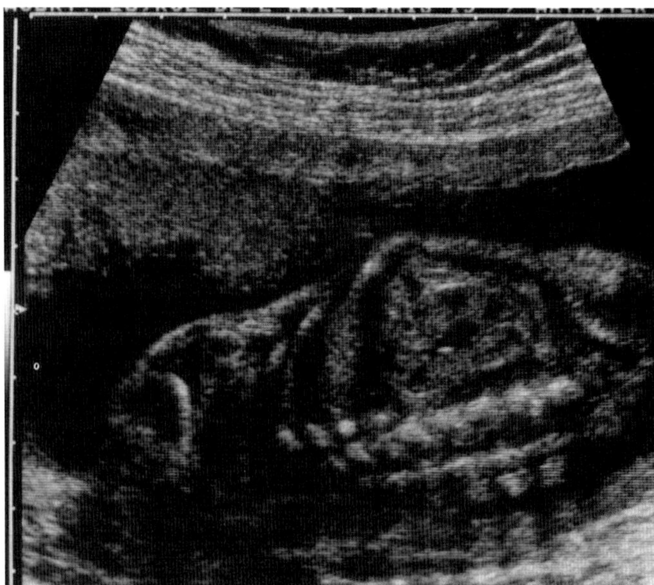

Fig. 35.1 Frontal cross-section of normal fetal kidney at 24 weeks demonstrating corticomedullary differentiation.

Bladder and external genitalia

The bladder is derived mainly from the cloacal endoderm. The anterior part of the bladder forming the urachus, however, derives from the allantois, accounting for anomalies such as the umbilical cysts resulting from persistently patent urachal structures.

The cloaca becomes separated into anterior and posterior portions by the rectovesical septum at 6 weeks of development. The anterior part of the cloaca becomes the urogenital sinus, which will form the major part of the bladder, while the posterior part will form the rectum. The most caudal part of the mesonephric duct, to which the ureters connect, becomes incorporated to the region of the trigone so that the ureters acquire an entrance into the bladder separate from the mesonephric duct. In males, the mesonephric duct empties via this ejaculatory duct which is the terminal part of the vas deferens into the prostatic urethra, while in females it degenerates[2].

The urethra is formed from the urogenital sinus in both sexes. In males, an additional contribution comes from the ectoderm of the genital tubercle, which becomes canalized as the distal urethra[2].

NORMAL SONOGRAPHIC DEVELOPMENT OF THE FETAL KIDNEYS AND URINARY TRACT

The fetal bladder can be identified from the late first trimester of pregnancy. Ultrasound examination between 11 and 14 weeks has identified the presence of a fetal bladder at this gestation in up to 93% of cases, with the bladder being identified in all 'normal fetuses' with a crown–rump length exceeding 67 mm. Therefore, the absence of bladder image using ultrasound can be considered as abnormal after this gestational age[12].

Fetal kidneys may be imaged by transvaginal ultrasound from 10 weeks[13] and from 11–12 weeks using transabdominal ultrasound. By this gestation, they appear homogeneously echogenic. Later, in gestational life, the medulla becomes hypoechogenic and can be distinguished from the renal cortex. This sonographic corticomedullary differentiation takes place by 24 weeks and, therefore, its absence can be considered as truly pathological only after that period (Fig. 35.1). The growth of fetal kidneys is grossly parallel to that of the fetus and can be evaluated on a quantitative manner based on sonographic charts[14,15]. Because sources of amniotic fluid other than fetal urine are predominant in early gestation, amniotic volume does not reflect fetal urinary output until the second trimester.

The images of the genital tubercle should be interpreted carefully in the first trimester[16] with the identification of a prominent genital tubercle not being specific to the male fetuses[17]. However, some centers have now performed fetal sexing in the first trimester by obtaining a mid-sagittal view of the fetuses and measuring the angle from the genital tubercle to a horizontal line through the lumbosacral skin surface. Male fetuses are detected when the angle exceeds 30°. Using this technique, the accuracy of fetal sexing increased from 70% at 11 weeks' gestation to 99% at 12 weeks'[18,19]. Later in gestation, the fetal gender is easy to establish. It is, however, essential to remember that females should be diagnosed by visualization of the labia not the absence of a phallus.

In boys, the urethral canal can be visualized by 26–27 weeks, and is even easier to see in the third trimester. In girls, although the vulval structure can be identified at 15 weeks and the vulva is clearly seen at 22 weeks, a detailed analysis of a vulval anomaly is often not feasible until 24 weeks.

Urinary tract anomalies

Prenatal detection of fetal urinary tract anomalies using real time, 2D high resolution ultrasound is relatively easy based on the identification of transonic images corresponding to the dilated urinary tract. However, frequently, it is not possible to ascertain the exact mechanism of the uropathy in utero, as an 'obstructive process' often cannot be imaged directly, and because urinary tract dilatations resulting from a vesicoureteral reflux do not differ from dilatations above a true urinary outflow obstruction.

In many cases of prenatal diagnosis of renal malformations, the exact pathological diagnosis may not be correctly delineated. Therefore, prenatal management of fetal uropathies mainly consists of the identification of these fetuses, monitoring progression during prenatal life and allowing immediate postnatal evaluation. The exclusion of associated structural anomalies (indicating the potential risk of associated aneuploidy or single gene defects) or ultrasound features that indicate a high probability of renal failure provide important prognostic information. This process is fundamental so that an organized rational perinatal management plan can be formulated in collaboration with pediatric surgeons and neonatologists.

CLASSIFICATION AND PATHOLOGY

Fetal urinary tract dilatation (of the pelvicalyceal, ureteric or urethrovesical systems) may result either from over distension of the filling system above an obstructive lesion or from increased urinary flow occurring as a consequence of reflux. It can on occasions be difficult to distinguish between these two broad pathologies and cohort studies have consistently indicated relatively small rates of false positive and negative diagnosis using real time ultrasound[20].

NEPHROLOGICAL CONSEQUENCES OF FETAL UROPATHIES

In cases of apparent fetal renal anomaly with no associated structural malformation, the prognosis depends on baseline diagnosis and progressive assessment of fetal renal function. This is important as a small but significant number of anomalies may be associated with renal dysplasia. It is not established whether renal dysplasia results from an early increase in the renal urinary pressure or whether it results from an abnormal embryological process simultaneous to the obstruction but not occurring as a true consequence of it. If the latter hypothesis is true, then attempts at intrauterine therapy based on vesicoamniotic shunting ought to be illogical. Our understanding of pathogenesis has thus been aided by a number of animal studies. Experimental data have suggested that, at least in the fetal lamb, renal lesions (similar to those encountered in the human) can be reproduced by ligating the fetal urinary tract during the first half of gestation and can be prevented by fetal urinary diversion[21–26]. In addition, a recent systematic review and meta-analysis of the literature on vesicoamniotic shunting in human pregnancies associated with severe lower urinary tract obstruction has demonstrated increased survival in the 'intervention group' with subgroup analysis indicating benefit predominantly in the group with predicted poor prognosis[27].

It is clear, however, that the problem of poor overall renal function may be associated predominantly with bilateral fetal renal pathology. This risk is less significant in the unilateral cases. In severe bilateral obstructions, a localized lesion such as posterior urethral valves or urethral atresia may be extremely deleterious. In the most severe forms, the uropathy is associated with microcystic parenchymal dysplasia and terminal renal failure early in the second trimester. Fetal anuria results in severe oligohydramnios, fetal urine being the main source of amniotic fluid production in the second and third trimester of pregnancy. Due to several mechanisms, the absence of amniotic fluid prevents the expansion of the fetal thorax, the establishment of amniotic fluid inhalation and may result in severe pulmonary hypoplasia. This complication is invariably lethal postnatally. Fetal demise may also occur in utero due to cord compression. Indeed, prospective follow up of babies with lower urinary tract obstruction (LUTO) to one year of age has demonstrated that normal amniotic fluid index (a surrogate marker of renal function) was a predictor of good renal function in infancy with poor amniotic fluid levels predicting poor renal function and often perinatal mortality[28].

In addition, the absence of amniotic fluid causes a combination of anomalies usually referred to as 'Potter's sequence'. The absence of fetal movements due to severe oligohydramnios results in a variety of limb deformations and specific dysmorphic features. There are prominent epicanthic folds that form characteristic semicircles arising on the forehead, a flattened nose, low set ears, bowing of the legs with inward rotation of the feet and large spade-shaped hands[29].

In some cases, fetal anuria may occur late in gestation, in the third trimester. Pulmonary hypoplasia at this time is unusual but neonatal demise, if it occurs, is often the result of the presence of progressive renal dysplasia and associated terminal neonatal renal failure. However, when the kidneys appear non-dysplastic and urinalysis may be reassuring, renal function may be good despite third-trimester oligohydramnios. Measurement of fetal urinary analytes has been utilized to aid prognostic information and to predict renal morbidity. There has been controversy over which (or if any) urinary analytes have good sensitivity and specificity for predicting postnatal renal function. There has been discussion in the literature as to whether such analytes should be used alone or in combination. In addition, as to whether first or serial fresh fetal urine samples give optimal information. A recent systematic review of data informing the use of fetal urinary analytes has shown that the literature is full of small, heterogeneous cohort studies. These utilize differing thresholds to indicate abnormality. The conclusion of this review indicated that there is insufficient evidence at the present time to advocate the use of fetal urinary analyte estimation in predicting long-term renal morbidity. However, the measurement of fetal urinary sodium and calcium appeared to show the most promise with concentrations of ≥95th centile for gestation being associated with poorer postnatal renal outcome[30].

In more moderate fetal renal dysfunction, the amniotic fluid volume remains normal during pregnancy. Prenatal ultrasonography may reveal moderately abnormal features in the structure of the renal parenchyma such as 'hyperechogenicity'. In such cases, when sonography is inconclusive, analysis of fetal urine may be useful in indicating associated abnormal renal function. Again, sensitivity and specificity is variable, dependent upon the type of fetal urinary analyte tested and the timing of the test[30]. In early postnatal evaluation, high serum creatinine values may be found but often decrease rapidly after any obstruction is relieved. In the neonatal period, serum and urinary measurements of renal function are of poor predictive value of renal function throughout childhood and adolescence. This underscores the need for future prospective studies to correlate prenatal findings with long-term postnatal follow up of these patients.

Nevertheless, it should be remembered that the great majority of fetuses with urinary tract dilatation will have normal renal function postnatally. This is of course most likely to be the case for unilateral lesions and, indeed, for many bilateral lesions of the upper urinary tract. These cases with a good postnatal outcome are characterized prenatally by normal amniotic fluid volume and the persistence of normal structure in the renal parenchyma. It should be emphasized that the size of the pelvic dilatation is not a bad prognostic marker and that huge dilatation may eventually be associated with normal urine output and low urinary pressure resulting from high compliance of the urinary tract walls.

OBSTRUCTIONS TO THE URINARY OUTFLOW

Obstructions at the ureteropelvic junction

Ureteric obstruction at the ureteropelvic junction[31] is the most common lesion of the fetal urinary tract. The obstruction may rarely be associated with compression by an ectopic vessel. It may also be seen in duplication or ectopy of the ureteric system.

Megaureter

True megaureter is the result of a dysfunction at the ureterovesical junction. Spontaneous relief of this dysfunction most commonly occurs in the first years of life[32].

Ureterocele

A ureterocele is a cystic dilatation of the distal intravesical ureter. Most ureteroceles arise from an abnormal location of the ureteral meatus in the bladder and are therefore termed ectopic. Ureteroceles are often associated with a double ureter (duplex system), the ureterocele at the lower ureteric orifice draining the upper pole of the duplex kidney. The lesion may be associated with obstruction accounting for the dilatation of the corresponding ureter and/or renal pelvis. A large ureterocele may obstruct the bladder neck, the disease then resembling an infravesical obstruction.

Obstruction of the bladder outlet (lower urinary tract obstruction; LUTO)

Obstruction of the bladder outlet usually occurs in the urethra and can lead to bladder dilatation with muscle hypertrophy and hydronephrosis. The kidneys may also be dysplastic, resulting in a variable association with chronic renal failure[33]. The severity of outflow obstruction is often reflected by the gestational age of presentation (early gestational diagnosis being associated with worse prognosis) and reflecting the ultimate outcome (both in terms of morbidity and mortality).

The most common cause of bladder obstruction (and perhaps the cause most amenable to treatment) is posterior urethral valves. The 'valves' consist of folds of mucosa along the posterior wall of the urethra, most often extending from the verumontanum and resulting in a very narrow urethral lumen. Urethral atresia is less common and results in lethal lesions with fetal anuria in the first and early second trimesters[34].

Reflux

Vesicoureteral reflux is a common disorder that is associated with dilatation of the ureters and calyceal filling systems in utero and is usually confirmed postnatally. Direct imaging of the reflux is sometimes possible during real time 2D ultrasonography. In the most severe cases, the bladder and ureters appear dilated due to a functional increase of the urinary outflow. The potential benefit of prenatal diagnosis of such cases is to avoid postnatal urinary infection and subsequent kidney damage. Postnatal assessment is essential and surgery may be required in the severe forms of reflux.

Complex cloacal anomalies

These anomalies result from the failure of the urogenital sinus to divide properly. Therefore fistulae form in vesicovaginal or urethrovaginal locations in females or urethrorectal locations in males. The association with anorectal atresia is frequent.

Urachal diverticulum

The urachus connects the bladder to the anterior wall in utero. The intrafunicular part of this canal can remain open in utero and result in a transonic cystic mass located in the cord, next to its fetal insertion. Although the cyst itself may disappear in utero, it may result in a vesicocutaneous fistula that should be managed appropriately in the neonatal period.

SONOGRAPHIC PRENATAL DIAGNOSIS OF FETAL UROPATHIES

The fetal uropathies may be classified according to the level of the dilatation[35–40]. In upper lesions, only the renal pelvises are dilated, while the ureters are also often involved in midlevel lesions. Upper and mid uropathies may be categorized as unilateral or bilateral. This is an important feature from a prognostic point of view as postnatal renal function will mostly likely be normal in unilateral cases. Dilatations of the upper urinary tract may correspond either to a ureteropelvic junction obstruction or to a ureteropelvic reflux. Similarly, a midlevel uropathy may be the morphological manifestation of a vesicoureteral reflux as well as a congenital megaureter.

The abnormalities of the fetal bladder on ultrasound examination may be present in low-level lesions, which comprise mainly posterior urethral valves or urethral obstruction. However, a dilated bladder may also be the hallmark for major vesicoureteral reflux, which increases the urine output through the bladder and therefore its volume. More complex urinary malformations, for example cloacal malformations, may be associated with bladder dilatation. This latter etiology is relatively more common in females and carries a high morbidity.

Pelvic dilatations and hydronephrosis

There is no universally accepted definition and grading of upper urinary tract dilatation in the fetus. One may define pyelectasis as a pelvic dilatation without calyceal involvement (Fig. 35.2), hydronephrosis being defined by the finding of dilated calyces. Grading systems have been proposed for this anomaly on ultrasound[41,42]. For instance[42], grade I corresponds to normal fetuses, grade II to pyelectasis (pelvis <15 mm) and grades III–V to hydronephrosis (pelvis >15 mm).

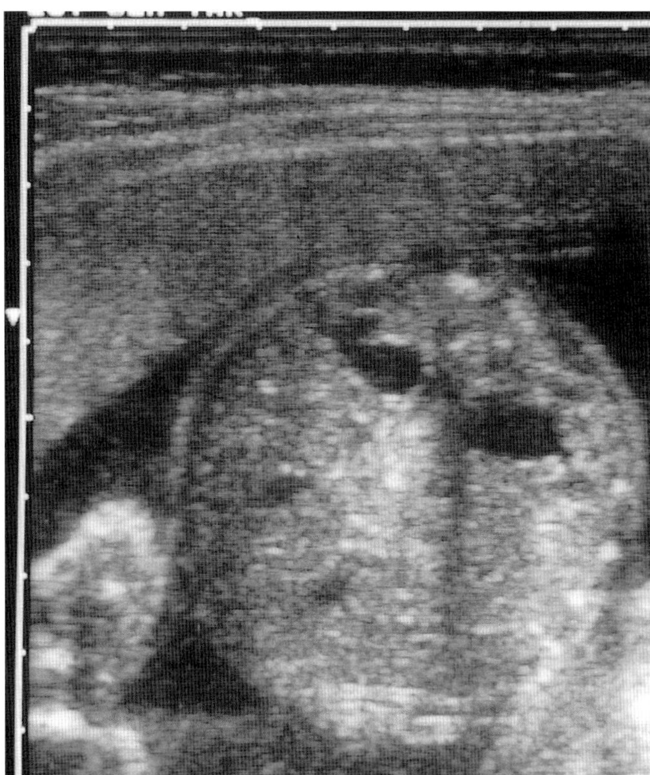

Fig. 35.2 Bilateral renal pelvis dilation at 23 weeks: transverse section.

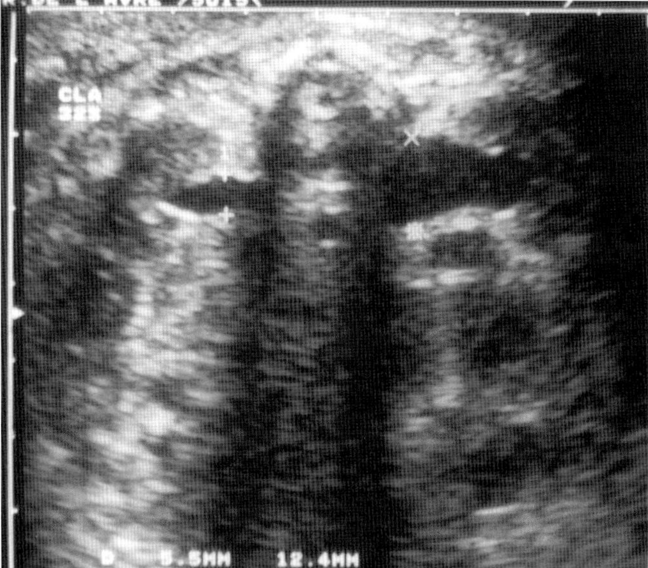

Fig. 35.3 Mild unilateral hydronephrosis in a 32-week fetus: transverse cross-section.

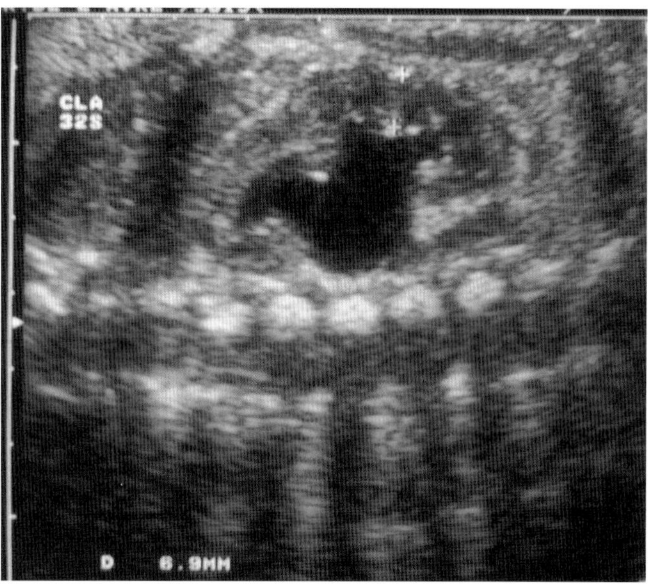

Fig. 35.4 Mild unilateral hydronephrosis in a 32-week fetus with ureteropelvic junction obstruction.

Pyelectasis

Moderate dilatation of the renal pelvic cavities is diagnosed by routine sonography in up to 2% of pregnancies (see Fig. 35.2). In the literature, pyelectasis is defined by an anteroposterior pelvic diameter exceeding 6 mm in the second trimester on a cross-sectional view and 8–10 mm in the third[43–49]. The quantitative definition of fetal pyelectasis should be stringent enough to avoid generating iatrogenic consequences due to an unacceptable rate of false positive diagnosis.

In most cases, isolated fetal pyelectasis is physiological. However, it may correspond to a mild reflux or to a ureteropelvic junction obstruction. Prenatal ultrasound follow-up should assess that the dilatation does not increase with gestation[50]. Postnatal evaluation is usually limited to renal sonography within the first 6 weeks of age. In case of unexplained symptoms such as fever occurring postnatally, the prenatal history should be kept in mind in order not to overlook a urinary tract infection[35,51,52]. However, the sensitivity of prenatal ultrasound remains low for the screening of reflux and most cases are picked up based only on postnatal symptoms.

Hydronephrosis

Fetal hydronephrosis may be defined by an anteroposterior pelvic size of more than 15 mm and/or calyceal involvement[41]. In mild hydronephrosis (grade III), the calyces are slightly dilated (Figs 35.3, 35.4). In larger dilatations of the upper urinary tract (grade IV), the calyces become round in shape (Fig. 35.5), but the ultrasonic calyceal images are distributed regularly and are connected with the renal pelvis. In contrast, ultrasound of the multicystic dysplastic kidney demonstrates an irregular pattern of cysts which are independent from the pelvis. In more severe cases (grade V), the calyceal images are no longer differentiated from the pelvis, because the calyces become involved in a large single transonic image (Fig. 35.6). The renal parenchyma may be considered as exceedingly thinned when it becomes less than 3 mm thick. However, this latter feature is not necessarily ominous, since large dilations with a thin parenchyma may be associated with a normal renal function.

At the parenchymal level, the presence or absence of a corticomedullary differentiation should be recorded, as well as the echogenicity of the parenchyma and the presence of cysts. Although subjective[53–56], the evaluation of the sonographic structure of the renal parenchyma may be a useful predictor of renal function.

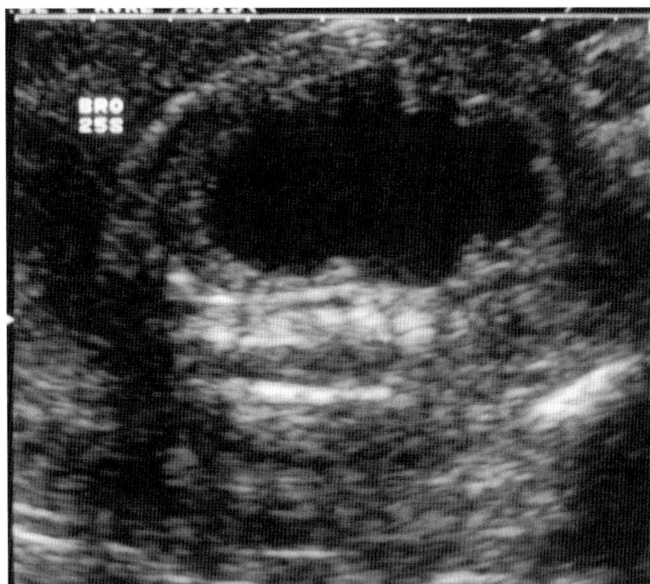

Fig. 35.5 Large unilateral hydronephrosis at 34 weeks (grade IV): cross-section.

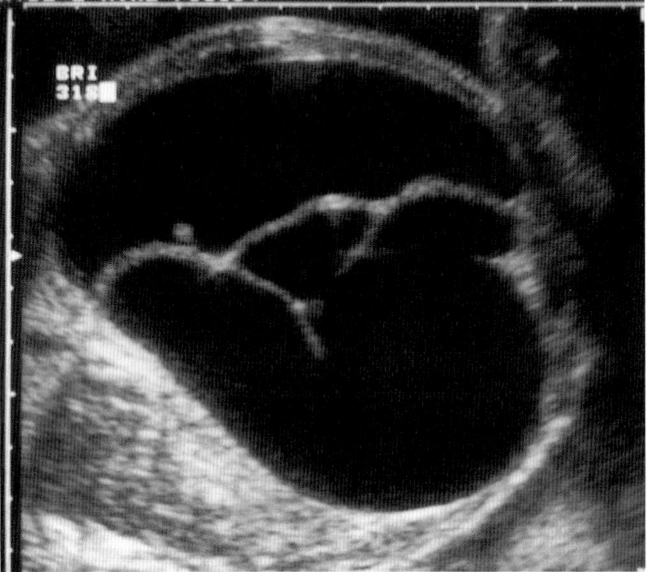

Fig. 35.6 Large hydronephrosis at 25 weeks (grade V).

Hydroureter

The ureter is normally not visualized on routine prenatal ultrasound examination of the fetus. A dilated ureter appears as a convoluted transonic image, located between the kidney and the bladder. Peristaltic activity is suggestive of a megaureter, but a dilated ureter may also be due to a vesicoureteral reflux[57].

Bladder dilatation

A dilated bladder which does not empty throughout sonographic examination is suggestive of an obstruction of its outlet. The ultrasound image of the fetal bladder can be easily confirmed by imaging the umbilical arteries on each side using color flow Doppler. The bladder dilatation is usually round in

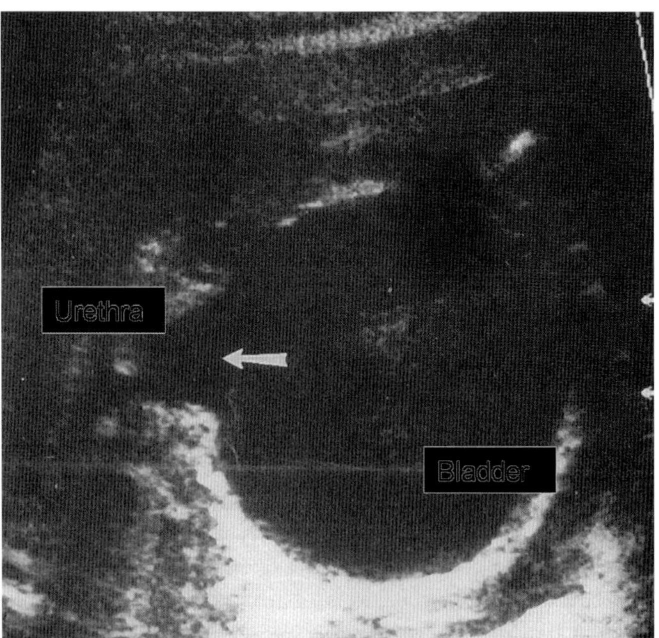

Fig. 35.7 A coronal section of a fetal bladder with a dilated proximal urethral in posterior urethral valves.

shape, but it may be larger above the umbilical arteries than below evoking the shape of the cork of a champagne bottle. The relatively smaller size of the dilated bladder below the umbilical arteries should not be mistaken for a dilated proximal urethra above posterior urethral valves. The image of a dilated urethra is specific to posterior urethral obstruction (Fig. 35.7).

At a later stage, bladder outlet obstruction can result in muscular hypertrophy that can be imaged as bladder wall thickness ($\geq$3 mm). Associated bladder diverticula may also be identified.

Although in males, posterior urethral valves are the most common cause of bladder dilatation, other etiologies are possible.

Urethral atresia cannot be directly imaged but is usually diagnosed by pathological post-mortem examination, this condition being associated with early ultrasound detection and anhydramnios[34] (Fig. 35.8). Its etiology is more frequently encountered in females than in males, in whom posterior urethral valves are the most common cause of low-level obstruction.

Urinary ascites and perirenal urinoma

Ascites may result from leakage of urine into the peritoneal cavity through a minor and usually unidentifiable disruption of the urinary tract wall. It is not specific to a given type of uropathy and is not necessarily an ominous finding. The urinary origin of the ascites is usually evident, the uropathy being identified by ultrasound. Similarly, disruption of the urinary tract in the retroperitoneal space may result in a urinoma, presenting as a transonic image surrounding renal tissue.

PRENATAL MANAGEMENT OF FETAL UROPATHIES

The prenatal diagnosis of a fetal uropathy is usually made at the mid-trimester detailed ultrasound scan with high sensitivity[58].

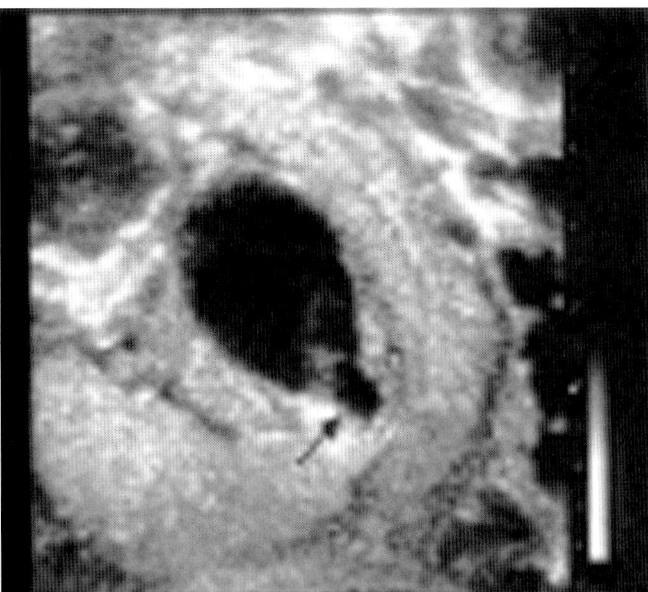

Fig. 35.8 Enlarged fetal bladder in a case of urethral atresia at 16 weeks[34].

When an abnormality is detected, a detailed assessment of the genitourinary tract should be performed, focusing on amniotic fluid volume, renal size, parenchyma, collecting system and bladder size[59]. However, over recent years there has been a trend to earlier diagnosis[34]. Once the prenatal diagnosis using ultrasound of a fetal uropathy is made, the single clinically relevant question is its prognosis. As discussed previously, to determine prognosis it is not necessary to determine exact pathology, which is more important for deciding postnatal management. Prenatally, the important factors relating to poor prognosis are gestational age at diagnosis at or before 24 weeks[60–62], severe oligohydramnios[63], evidence of renal dysplasia (cortical cysts, echogenic parenchyma)[64–66], association with other structural or chromosomal anomalies and female gender (indicating more complex cloacal plate anomalies)[67].

Screening for associated anomalies

Sonography

Extraurinary anomalies[68–70] should be excluded by ultrasound assessment of the fetus. Mild unilateral hydronephrosis is usually an isolated condition; bilateral hydronephrosis and lower urinary tract obstruction are, however, associated with other coexistent structural anomalies including cardiac, facial, abdominal wall defects, CNS anomalies and cloacal dysgenesis[58,64,67]. If there is severe oligohydramnios, amnioinfusion may be required to allow accurate evaluation of the fetus.

In some cases, the fetus obviously presents with major extraurinary anomalies, and a lethal outcome is relatively easy to predict. In such circumstances, the main task of the obstetrician is to provide adequate information to the parents and to emphasize the need for a post-mortem examination together with a fetal karyotype, in order to allow for appropriate genetic counseling for subsequent pregnancies.

Abdominal wall defects, such as bladder exstrophy, should be considered when no bladder is visualized on ultrasound while the amniotic fluid volume is normal[71,72]. The diagnosis of associated anomalies, however, may be more difficult. In cloacal malformations, for instance, prenatal diagnosis is based on the association of a variety of relatively minor signs that may appear only during the third trimester[73–76]. A uroenteric fistula may be diagnosed based on associated bowel dilatation containing hyperechogenic material. The direct image of an enlarged duplicated vagina is quite specific to a cloacal malformation[77], but this image sometimes appears only during the third trimester. It is possible to image the anal sphincter, but this does not rule out the diagnosis of anal atresia. The external genitalia should also be carefully imaged and may present as enlarged and fused labia 'floating' in the amniotic fluid. Overall, when a cloacal malformation is diagnosed in utero, the potential for surgical repair may be difficult to establish and should be discussed individually with the pediatric surgeon.

Microcolon-megacystis-intestinal hypoperistalsis syndrome[78–79] may be suspected on ultrasound evaluation of the fetus, based on the association of a large dilatation of the bladder with coexistent bowel dilatation. Unfortunately, the latter features may occur only in the late third trimester, which explains why this condition is easily overlooked prenatally, although it carries a severe postnatal prognosis due to poor intestinal function. This condition is more common in females and should thus be considered in a female with features of lower urinary tract obstruction but normal liquor volume. Recent literature reporting results of animal work has suggested a genetic basis to this condition being associated with an anomaly of the acetylcholinesterase receptor[80–83].

Karyotyping

Overall, the incidence of chromosomal anomalies is reported to be as high as 12% in fetal renal defects[69,70]. However, in many uropathies with chromosomal anomalies, additional extrarenal defects can be picked up by ultrasound. Therefore, the prevalence of chromosomal anomalies in truly isolated uropathies, such as posterior urethral valve, is probably relatively low. However, we believe that a karyotype should usually be performed when a fetal malformation is diagnosed. The aim of this strategy is to provide as accurate a prognostic evaluation as possible to these parents who will have to undergo the stress of planning the postnatal surgical program of a child yet unborn. Due to the relatively low prevalence of true fetal uropathies, this policy is not likely to raise the amniocentesis rate significantly in the general population. This is not the case when one considers pyelectasis as a potential indication for karyotyping. Indeed, this sonographic feature is often a variant of the normal and is found in up to 2% of normal pregnancies. This makes routine amniocentesis questionable in fetuses with isolated pyelectasis. When pyelectasis is associated with an other fetal anomaly, even minor, the risk of aneuploidy is increased by 10–20 times[45,84–86] and karyotyping is obviously indicated. In contrast, in cases with isolated pyelectasis, the risk of aneuploidy is increased by 1.2- to 6-fold only and the clinical relevance of this needs to be discussed[44,45–47,87–90].

Fetal renal function

In isolated bilateral uropathies, the prognosis and prenatal management are a function of a single parameter, renal function. Indeed, the best postnatal surgical repair will remain useless if the renal parenchyma is severely damaged during fetal life[91,92]. The evaluation of fetal renal function is based on sonography and then consideration may be given to invasive assessment with analysis of fetal urine, serum or amniotic fluid and renal biopsy. At present, fetal urinalysis is the most commonly used invasive investigation to inform prognosis.

Sonography evaluates the structure of renal parenchyma and the amniotic fluid volume[37]. Fetal urinalysis assesses the ability of the renal tubule to reabsorb a variety of compounds (sodium, β2 microglobulin, calcium, phosphorus, glucose)[7–9,93–98]. In the human fetus, urinalysis reflects renal function because, during fetal life, the mother supplies the fetus with balanced nutrients and fetal homeostasis is ensured without intervention of the kidneys. Therefore, the composition of fetal urine depends only on fetal renal function (filtration, excretion, reabsorption) and reflects renal potential. An estimate of normal values has been obtained by sampling urine in fetuses affected by a non-urinary disease or in normal fetuses prior to termination[95]. An alternative approach consisted of sampling fetuses with an obstructive uropathy who were subsequently found to have a normal renal function either at birth[11] or after a longer follow-up[7–9]. The next step was to characterize the fetal urine biochemical profiles that were associated with abnormal postnatal outcome. Studies have indicated that fetal urinary sodium or chloride values in excess of 100 mmol/l are predictive of fetal or perinatal death from terminal renal or pulmonary failure[65,95,99]. β2-Microglobulin levels >13 mg/l have been reported as being invariably associated with fatal outcome[97]. These studies are, however, looking at perinatal mortality as the main outcome which, as discussed, can be predicted by ultrasound alone.

Fetal urinalysis to predict postnatal renal function has generated much controversy[30]. A systematic review of diagnostic accuracy of fetal urinalysis found that the available studies differ in population, threshold for test, definition of outcome and are generally small case series or cohorts. Many studies do not report gestational age at testing, presence of poor predictive factors at diagnosis (e.g. oligohydramnios) or whether intervention occurred (e.g. vesicoamniotic shunting) thus, the studies are extremely heterogeneous[30]. From the results of the systematic review, the two most accurate tests were calcium >95th centile for gestation (positive likelihood ratio 6.65, 0.23–1.90.96; negative likelihood ratio 0.19, 0.05–0.74) and sodium >95th centile for gestation (likelihood ratio positive 4.46, 1.71–11.6; likelihood ratio negative 0.39, 0.17–0.88) (Fig. 35.9). Several authors have reported that sequential urinalysis may better reflect renal function secondary to decompression of the fetal bladder[98]. The conclusion of the systematic review was that the current evidence was insufficient to estimate the accuracy and usefulness of fetal urinalysis to predict postnatal renal function. Fetal urinalysis has also been used as an investigation to identify those patients that might benefit from vesicoamniotic shunting[100], with urinary sodium and calcium having the best accuracy[101–104], but further research is needed to determine the true value of this investigation. More recently, attention has focused on newer methods of analyzing fetal urine, such as proton nuclear magnetic resonance spectroscopy[102,103], to assess amino acid levels. These small case series showed amino acid measurement to be more accurate in predicting postnatal renal function than any of the other investigated analytes.

In contrast to the data from fetal urine, most compounds measurable in fetal blood do not reflect fetal renal function, since they cross the placenta and are cleared by the maternal kidney[105]. Serum microglobulins do not cross the placenta due to their molecular weight (MW < 40000 Da), but are still filtered by the glomerulus and can provide an estimation of glomerular rather than tubular function[106]. Several microglobulins have been investigated with the majority of work looking at β2 microglobulin and α1-microglobulin[107–110]. Advantages to measurement of β2-microglobulin and serum measurements are that levels do not seem to vary with gestational age, they reflect glomerular function and serial measurements can be performed even after shunting when there will be minimal fetal urine. Again the number of studies and subjects is still small and serum monitoring carries the distinct disadvantage of the requirement for fetal blood sampling. Fetal renal biopsy has been used to identify abnormal renal histology in utero but it is limited by its poor success rate in obtaining fetal renal tissue (50%). When this procedure was successful, renal histology added to the diagnosis in a third of cases[111].

Terminal renal failure in utero

The amniotic fluid volume reflects the fetal urinary output, at least in the second and third trimester. When severe oligohydramnios develops in a fetus with an obstructive uropathy, the diagnosis of fetal anuria and of terminal renal failure may be considered almost certain. This is sometimes evident relatively early in gestation, for instance in cases with urethral atresia. Severe oligohydramnios may also occur later in gestation, for instance in posterior urethral valves complicated by fetal renal failure. Severe oligohydramnios is usually associated with abnormal images of the renal parenchyma, such as loss of normal corticomedullary differentiation, hyperechogenicity, cortical cysts (Fig. 35.10). In such cases, fetal urinary biochemistry would confirm the diagnosis of renal failure, showing high fetal urinary levels of sodium and β2 microglobulin[95,101]. However, later in gestation, a relatively acute onset of oligohydramnios may occur in the fetus with non-dysplastic renal parenchyma and moderately altered urinalysis. The possibility of acute obstruction of the outflow should then be considered which might be managed by induction of labor or shunting.

Obviously normal renal function

The functional prognosis of unilateral uropathies is uniformly good, provided that the contralateral kidney is normal. In such cases, it is not necessary to invade the fetus to obtain biochemical data from the abnormal kidney regardless of its sonographic appearance.

Similarly, in upper obstruction with normal amniotic fluid volume and normal renal parenchyma, the functional prognosis is usually good and fetal urine sampling is unnecessary.

Uncertain renal function

In some cases, the functional status of the kidney cannot be established by sonography alone. This includes bilateral lesions with a moderately decreased amniotic fluid volume, or with mild alteration of the renal parenchyma. Moreover, in cases in which the prenatal diagnosis of posterior urethral valves is almost certain, the relatively high incidence of postnatal renal failure could argue in favor of fetal urine sampling, even in cases without any ominous sonographic finding.

As mentioned above, the prognostic value of fetal urinalysis can be understood only with reference to the criteria used to define the groups of postnatal outcome in prospective studies[7,96]. One of the pitfalls most often encountered in these studies is the lack of postnatal follow-up of children in whom a

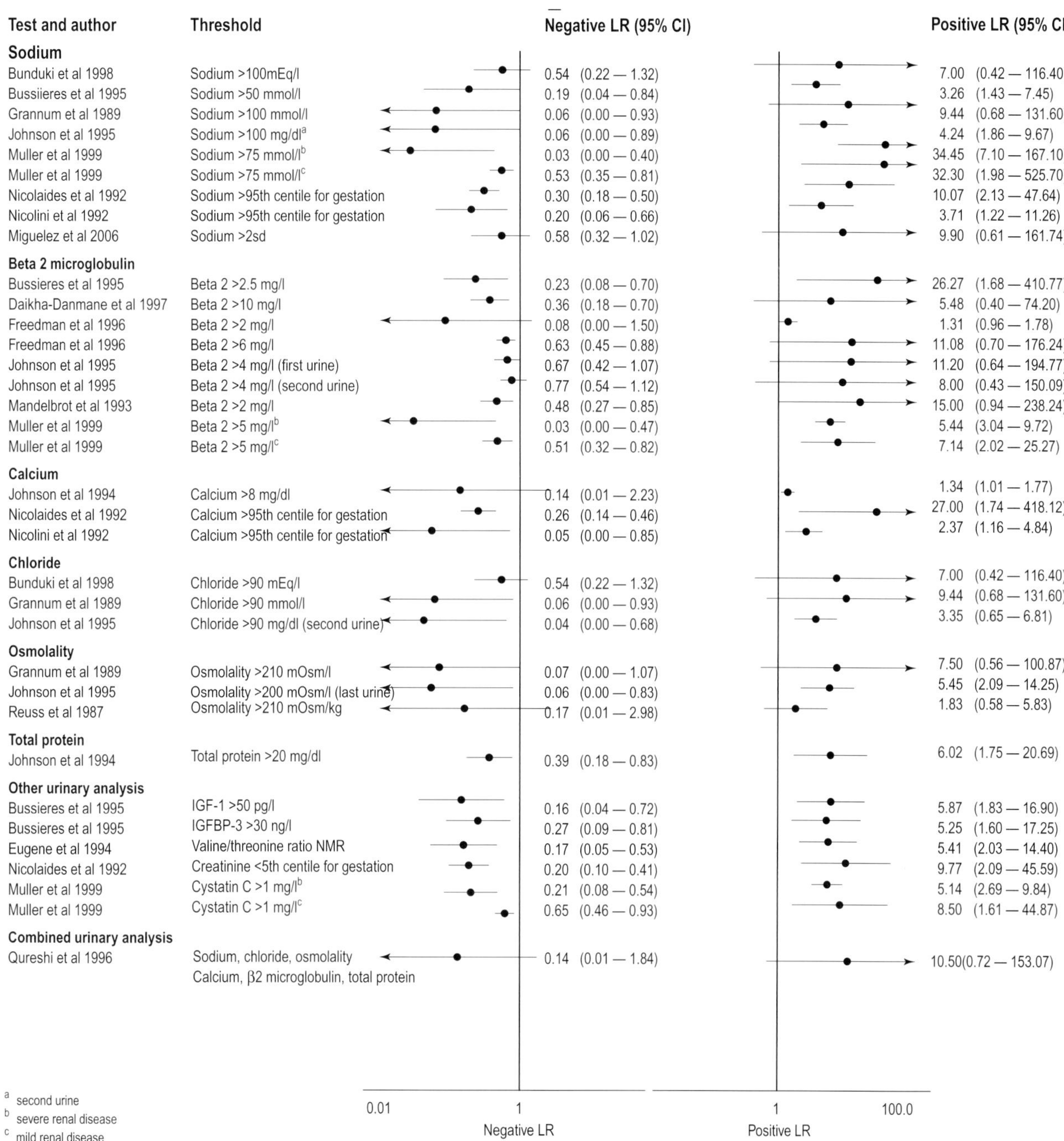

Test and author
Threshold
Negative LR (95% CI)
Positive LR (95% CI)
Sodium
Bunduki et al 1998 | Sodium >100mEq/l | 0.54 (0.22 — 1.32) | 7.00 (0.42 — 116.40)
Bussiieres et al 1995 | Sodium >50 mmol/l | 0.19 (0.04 — 0.84) | 3.26 (1.43 — 7.45)
Grannum et al 1989 | Sodium >100 mmol/l | 0.06 (0.00 — 0.93) | 9.44 (0.68 — 131.60)
Johnson et al 1995 | Sodium >100 mg/dl a | 0.06 (0.00 — 0.89) | 4.24 (1.86 — 9.67)
Muller et al 1999 | Sodium >75 mmol/l b | 0.03 (0.00 — 0.40) | 34.45 (7.10 — 167.10)
Muller et al 1999 | Sodium >75 mmol/l c | 0.53 (0.35 — 0.81) | 32.30 (1.98 — 525.70)
Nicolaides et al 1992 | Sodium >95th centile for gestation | 0.30 (0.18 — 0.50) | 10.07 (2.13 — 47.64)
Nicolini et al 1992 | Sodium >95th centile for gestation | 0.20 (0.06 — 0.66) | 3.71 (1.22 — 11.26)
Miguelez et al 2006 | Sodium >2sd | 0.58 (0.32 — 1.02) | 9.90 (0.61 — 161.74)
Beta 2 microglobulin
Bussieres et al 1995 | Beta 2 >2.5 mg/l | 0.23 (0.08 — 0.70) | 26.27 (1.68 — 410.77)
Daikha-Danmane et al 1997 | Beta 2 >10 mg/l | 0.36 (0.18 — 0.70) | 5.48 (0.40 — 74.20)
Freedman et al 1996 | Beta 2 >2 mg/l | 0.08 (0.00 — 1.50) | 1.31 (0.96 — 1.78)
Freedman et al 1996 | Beta 2 >6 mg/l | 0.63 (0.45 — 0.88) | 11.08 (0.70 — 176.24)
Johnson et al 1995 | Beta 2 >4 mg/l (first urine) | 0.67 (0.42 — 1.07) | 11.20 (0.64 — 194.77)
Johnson et al 1995 | Beta 2 >4 mg/l (second urine) | 0.77 (0.54 — 1.12) | 8.00 (0.43 — 150.09)
Mandelbrot et al 1993 | Beta 2 >2 mg/l | 0.48 (0.27 — 0.85) | 15.00 (0.94 — 238.24)
Muller et al 1999 | Beta 2 >5 mg/l b | 0.03 (0.00 — 0.47) | 5.44 (3.04 — 9.72)
Muller et al 1999 | Beta 2 >5 mg/l c | 0.51 (0.32 — 0.82) | 7.14 (2.02 — 25.27)
Calcium
Johnson et al 1994 | Calcium >8 mg/dl | 0.14 (0.01 — 2.23) | 1.34 (1.01 — 1.77)
Nicolaides et al 1992 | Calcium >95th centile for gestation | 0.26 (0.14 — 0.46) | 27.00 (1.74 — 418.12)
Nicolini et al 1992 | Calcium >95th centile for gestation | 0.05 (0.00 — 0.85) | 2.37 (1.16 — 4.84)
Chloride
Bunduki et al 1998 | Chloride >90 mEq/l | 0.54 (0.22 — 1.32) | 7.00 (0.42 — 116.40)
Grannum et al 1989 | Chloride >90 mmol/l | 0.06 (0.00 — 0.93) | 9.44 (0.68 — 131.60)
Johnson et al 1995 | Chloride >90 mg/dl (second urine) | 0.04 (0.00 — 0.68) | 3.35 (0.65 — 6.81)
Osmolality
Grannum et al 1989 | Osmolality >210 mOsm/l | 0.07 (0.00 — 1.07) | 7.50 (0.56 — 100.87)
Johnson et al 1995 | Osmolality >200 mOsm/l (last urine) | 0.06 (0.00 — 0.83) | 5.45 (2.09 — 14.25)
Reuss et al 1987 | Osmolality >210 mOsm/kg | 0.17 (0.01 — 2.98) | 1.83 (0.58 — 5.83)
Total protein
Johnson et al 1994 | Total protein >20 mg/dl | 0.39 (0.18 — 0.83) | 6.02 (1.75 — 20.69)
Other urinary analysis
Bussieres et al 1995 | IGF-1 >50 pg/l | 0.16 (0.04 — 0.72) | 5.87 (1.83 — 16.90)
Bussieres et al 1995 | IGFBP-3 >30 ng/l | 0.27 (0.09 — 0.81) | 5.25 (1.60 — 17.25)
Eugene et al 1994 | Valine/threonine ratio NMR | 0.17 (0.05 — 0.53) | 5.41 (2.03 — 14.40)
Nicolaides et al 1992 | Creatinine <5th centile for gestation | 0.20 (0.10 — 0.41) | 9.77 (2.09 — 45.59)
Muller et al 1999 | Cystatin C >1 mg/l b | 0.21 (0.08 — 0.54) | 5.14 (2.69 — 9.84)
Muller et al 1999 | Cystatin C >1 mg/l c | 0.65 (0.46 — 0.93) | 8.50 (1.61 — 44.87)
Combined urinary analysis
Qureshi et al 1996 | Sodium, chloride, osmolality Calcium, β2 microglobulin, total protein | 0.14 (0.01 — 1.84) | 10.50(0.72 — 153.07)
a second urine
b severe renal disease
c mild renal disease
0.01
1
Negative LR
1
100.0
Positive LR

Fig. 35.9 Forrest plots demonstrating individual results for index tests likely to be at least moderately useful in the prediction of postnatal chronic renal failure[30].

uropathy was diagnosed prenatally. The most severe cases, resulting in perinatal renal failure and often neonatal death by pulmonary hypoplasia secondary to prolonged intrauterine exposure to severe oligohydramnios, are easily recognized by sonography alone. In such cases, biochemistry only confirms the bad prognosis suggested by sonography. The most clinically relevant question is to identify among the children who will survive, i.e. grossly those with normal or slightly decreased amniotic fluid volume, who are at risk for developing postnatal renal failure and who will have normal renal function following surgical repair.

Establishing the prognostic value of any marker is made difficult by the fact that renal failure may occur relatively late, for instance during adolescence, which underscores the need for long-term follow-up of children in whom fetal urine analysis was performed in utero. Until such studies are completed, we must base our prenatal evaluation of renal function on cohorts with a shorter follow-up.

Management options

A plan of management should only be made after a full assessment of the fetus as described. This allows the prognosis to be established and appropriate management options to be discussed with the parents after they have been counseled by a multidisciplinary team, allowing them to make informed decisions. Options for management antenatally include interventions

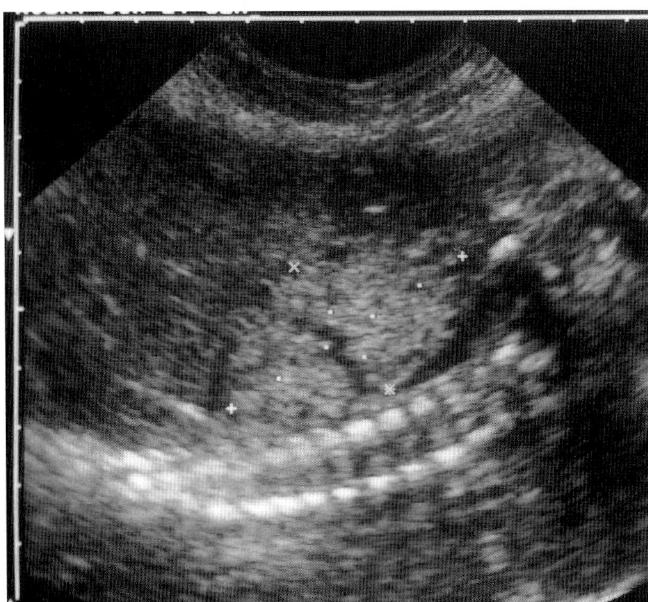

Fig. 35.10 Echogenic renal parenchyma with 'microcysts' and loss of normal corticomedullary differentiation.

such as termination of pregnancy, fetal therapy or merely observation. A management plan should include details of antenatal, intrapartum and postnatal care and follow-up.

Termination of pregnancy

In the most severe cases (i.e. babies with multiple malformations or terminal renal failure), the prognosis is unequivocally poor and most patients elect to have their pregnancy terminated. In this difficult situation, it is important to ensure that post-mortem examination can be implemented in order to provide genetic and postnatal counseling as it is recognized that parents terminating for fetal abnormality are more likely to suffer adverse psychological and social reactions[112].

Conservative management

The fetus with isolated antenatal hydronephrosis may be managed conservatively. A follow-up scan should be arranged in the third trimester to reassess renal pelvic dilatation and help determine postnatal care, due to the natural history of this condition.

Some parents, even when faced with a very poor prognosis for survival, will opt for conservative management. They should have follow-up scans antenatally to assess sonographic features and viability as there is a risk of intrauterine death. Parents should be counseled by a pediatrician as these babies, if they survive until birth, have a risk of pulmonary hypoplasia and renal failure. The mother should be booked for delivery in a unit with appropriate neonatal facilities. In the event of intrauterine death, post mortem should be discussed and postnatal follow up arranged.

Planning postnatal therapy

In contrast, when the uropathy is isolated and the renal parenchyma is not damaged, the parents should be encouraged to continue the pregnancy. During pregnancy, contact with the pediatrician who will be in charge of the baby postnatally is extremely useful to relieve the stress occasioned to the parents by the announcement of a fetal anomaly, even with a good prognosis. In more severe cases, we refer the couple prenatally to the pediatric urologist who will later treat the baby. This allows direct information concerning the timing of postnatal investigations, and also the anticipated surgical procedures. In this respect, the identification of posterior urethral valves is important prenatally, because this anomaly requires emergency endoscopic or surgical therapy. The option of delivery near to a neonatal surgical center should be offered to the mother, to avoid transferring the neonate elsewhere.

However, in many uropathies, no specific therapy is needed in the neonatal period, allowing the mother to deliver in the maternity hospital of her choice.

Fetal therapy

Experimental data in the fetal lamb demonstrated that complete urethral obstruction produced severe hydronephrosis, hydroureter, megacystis, urinary ascites and pulmonary hypoplasia but could not demonstrate renal dysplasia. Resolution of the findings occurred with decompression. Further experiments with ureteral compression showed renal dysplasia with decompression allowing recovery of renal function with an inverse relationship between length of obstruction and recovery of renal function on decompression[99,113,114]. Experiments in other models have shown restoration of amniotic volume allows improvement in respiratory function and that there may be specific mechanisms at play in congenital urinary tract obstruction (e.g. renin-angiotensin system)[114].

There is some controversy surrounding the applicability of animal models to human congenital disease, however, these experiments form the theoretical basis for intervention in the fetus.

From a technical point of view, restoring a normal urinary outflow in a fetus with posterior urethral valves can be achieved by different approaches. One could consider the direct destruction of the valves by electrocoagulation or laser ablation. This has been performed using a transvesical fetoscopic approach, but has many drawbacks[115,116]. First, once the endoscope is introduced into the fetal bladder, the valves are not easy to identify accurately. Second, it is difficult to be certain that surrounding tissue will not be damaged, especially when electrocoagulation is used in a small fetus. The other approach consists of bypassing the obstruction. Theoretically, performing a vesicostomy or a nephrostomy by direct fetal surgery would allow a better control of the quality of the bypass. For some conditions, the case for fetal surgery has been proven, e.g. congenital cystic adenomatoid malformation and sacrococcygeal teratoma. For obstructive uropathy, the case is less clear; open fetal surgery is extremely invasive with high complication rates for preterm labor, has adverse effects on future reproductive outcomes and a risk of neurological injury for the fetus. The last option consists of percutaneous ultrasound guided vesicoamniotic shunting. Briefly, one end of a double pigtailed catheter (Harrison or Rodeck design) is inserted into the bladder, the other end of the catheter being left in the amniotic cavity[10] (Fig. 35.11a and b). Although vesicocentesis is not usually a therapeutic procedure, early first-trimester bladder dilatation has regressed following bladder puncture[117]. These results should be interpreted cautiously since regression of urinary dilatation is also possible spontaneously, for instance in reflux.

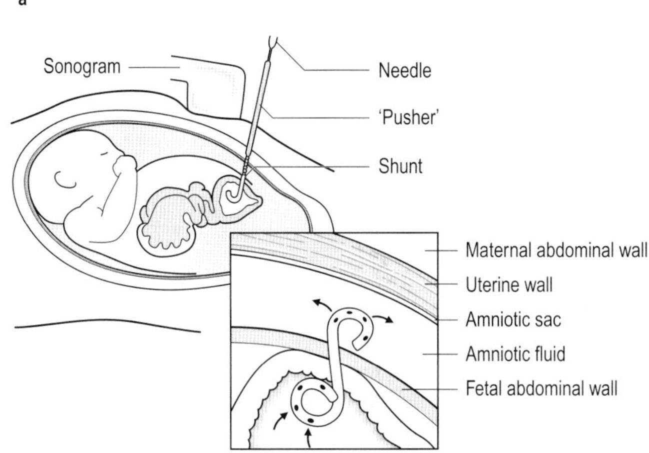

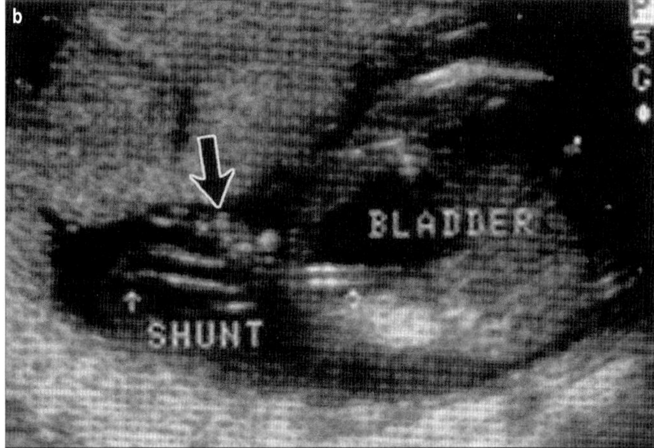

Fig. 35.11 A vesicoamniotic shunt in situ. (a) Schematic diagram; (b) ultrasound image.

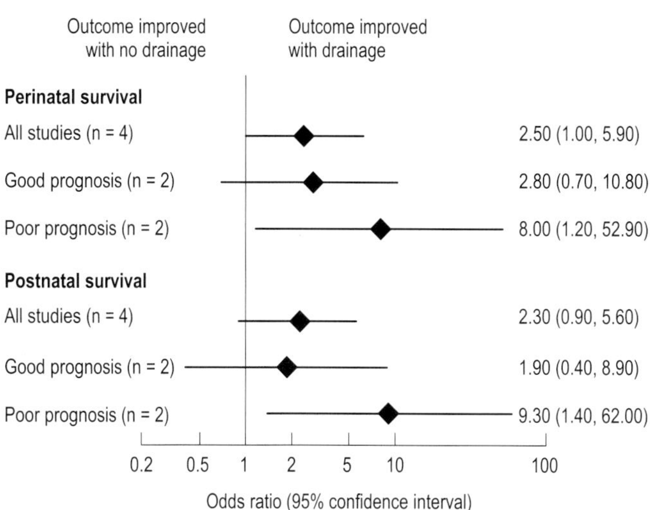

Fig. 35.12 Forrest plot demonstrating efficacy of vesicoamniotic shunting[27].

This approach is clearly less invasive than open surgery, but it is associated with complications (up to 40%) such as shunt blockage, shunt migration, preterm labor and miscarriage, amniorrhexis, intrauterine infection and fetal trauma (i.e. iatrogenic gastroschisis)[117,118]. The effectiveness of prenatal therapy for bladder outflow obstruction is also unproven. A systematic review and meta-analysis of the literature identified no randomized controlled trials but 16 observational studies. These were mainly small studies with different patient selection criteria, different surgical techniques and different outcome measures; their overall quality was poor. The heterogeneity within these studies leads to introduction of significant bias and inaccurate estimations of effectiveness. The meta-analysis demonstrated an improvement in overall perinatal survival with vesicoamniotic drainage in utero compared to no drainage (OR 2.5; 1.0–5.9; $P < 0.03$), with the subgroup of poor prognosis patients (ultrasound features and/or fetal urinalysis) showing the most improvement (OR 8.0; 1.2–52.9; $P < 0.03$) (Fig. 35.12). The conclusion of the authors, however, was that there was insufficient good quality evidence reliably to inform clinical practice[27]. This is a view which has recently been upheld by the National Institute for Health and Clinical Excellence (NICE) with the publication of interventional procedure guideline IP:202 (http://www.nice.org.uk/guidance/IPG202/?c=91520) which states that vesicoamniotic shunting should only be considered as part of a randomized controlled trial. PLUTO (percutaneous shunting in lower urinary tract obstruction) is a UK multicentered RCT coordinated by the University of Birmingham and is now recruiting. Further information can be found at www.pluto.bham.ac.uk.

KIDNEY ANOMALIES

Nosological classification and pathology

Fetal renal anomalies include anomalies of number, location, size and structure of the kidney. These malformations are primarily renal and may occur in the absence of a urinary tract defect. Some are rather common and easy to diagnose, for example renal agenesis or multicystic kidney disease. The diagnosis and prenatal management may be more difficult, as the prenatal structural anomalies of the kidney may be difficult to correlate to postnatal function.

As for uropathies, the prognosis is usually good in unilateral lesions, while bilateral anomalies associated with severe oligohydramnios are often associated with high perinatal mortality and morbidity. In bilateral cases with normal amniotic fluid, the long-term postnatal morbidity is often difficult to predict with certainty. Biochemical 'urinary analyte' markers, which have proved some degree of predictive accuracy of postnatal morbidity in uropathies, have not been as helpful in fetal nephropathies.

Anomalies of number

Renal agenesis

Renal agenesis can be uni- or bilateral. It may result from early degeneration of the ureteric bud, or from failed interaction between the ureteric bud and the blastema (Fig. 35.13). The corresponding adrenal gland takes a globoid shape and should not be misdiagnosed prenatally for a hypoplastic kidney[119]. It can sometimes be challenging not to mistake the adrenal gland for fetal kidney, especially in the presence of severe oligohydramnios.

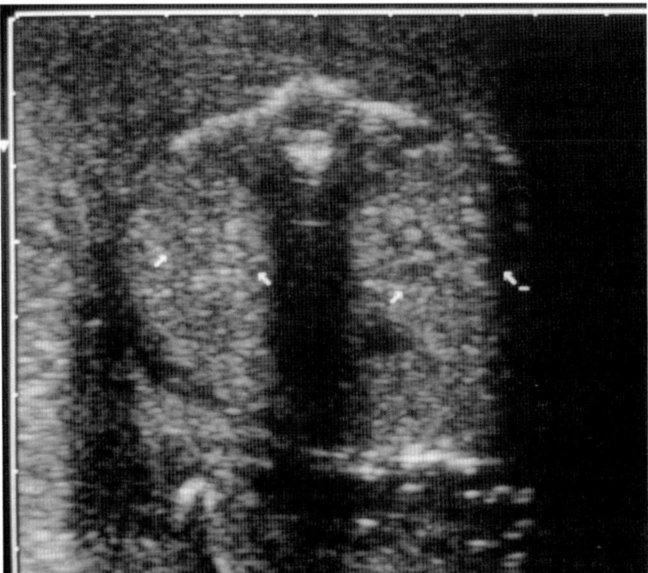

Fig. 35.13 Bilateral renal agenesis at 26 weeks. Severe oligohydramnios and adrenal glands filling the renal fossae.

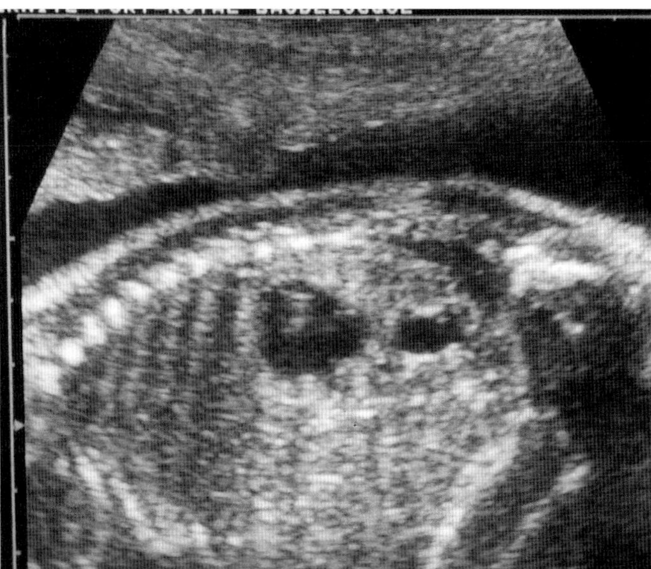

Fig. 35.14 Duplex renal filling system at 22 weeks.

Bilateral renal agenesis is a lethal condition resulting in the oligohydramnios sequence (pulmonary hypoplasia, dysmorphic face and limb deformities)[120]. It should be remembered that the amount of amniotic fluid often remains normal until the mid-second trimester, when fetal urine becomes the main source of amniotic fluid production[121].

Most cases of renal agenesis are sporadic, with a low risk of recurrence among subsequent sibs. However, familial cases have been reported with different types of inheritance[2].

In the absence of associated anomalies, unilateral renal agenesis occurs in approximately 1 in 3000 births and, as with other unilateral renal conditions, has a relatively good prognosis. The contralateral kidney is often enlarged. It may also be associated with minor genital anomalies such as Mullerian uterine malformations. More complex structural anomalies associated with renal agenesis include hypoplasia or absence of the fetal bladder, rectal atresia and lumbosacral vertebral anomalies. It may be associated with esophageal atresia and cardiac malformations, as part of the VACTERAL sequence.

Unilateral renal agenesis may occur with dysplasia of the contralateral kidney. This underscores the need for careful prenatal evaluation of the development of the contralateral kidney in fetuses with apparently isolated unilateral renal agenesis. The mode of inheritance is autosomal dominant with incomplete penetrance and a wide variability of expression, ranging from lethal cases with a single dysplastic kidney to unilateral renal agenesis with minor contralateral anomalies such as ureteropelvic junction obstruction. Increasingly, such cases are seen in conjunction with clinical geneticists so that detailed prospective evaluation of previous children may occur.

Duplex kidney

Duplex kidneys have two pelvicalyceal systems and are more common in female fetuses[122]. Duplication of the kidney results from premature division of the ureteric bud before it connects to the nephrogenic mesoderm (Fig. 35.14). This accounts for the association with a double or bifid ureter. The upper ureter usually enters the bladder more caudally and more medially than normal, and may also connect ectopically to the urethra, vagina, seminal vesicle or the rectum.

If this is detected prenatally, it is usually because there is associated obstruction or reflux which may be associated with parenchymal dysplasia. Therefore, a dilated pelvis or the abnormal structure of the dysplastic part of the kidney can be the hallmark for the prenatal diagnosis of this condition. It may be complicated by a distal ureter prolapsing into the bladder resulting in a ureterocele. In contrast, the ureter from the lower moiety may often reflux.

Supernumerary kidney

A third kidney may result from premature branching of the ureteric bud. Therefore it will have its own ureter and blood supply, and may be complicated by obstruction or dysplasia.

Abnormalities of position

Renal ectopy

Ectopic kidneys are usually displaced caudally towards the pelvis. One or both kidneys may be involved and it occurs in approximately 1 in 1200 births. Their shape can appear abnormal due to malrotation. This condition is asymptomatic, provided the renal parenchyma is well differentiated and free from dysplasia[123]. However, if the ectopic kidney is in the pelvis (its most common site) there is an increased risk of obstruction leading to hydronephrosis. In crossed renal ectopia, both kidneys are located on the same side and may be fused.

Horseshoe kidney

This anomaly results from the fusion of the kidneys, usually by their lower poles[124]. Fusion of both upper and lower poles results in ring kidney. When isolated, horseshoe kidneys are usually asymptomatic, but they may be associated with fetal aneuploidy (usually trisomy 18, Turner's syndrome or triploidy).

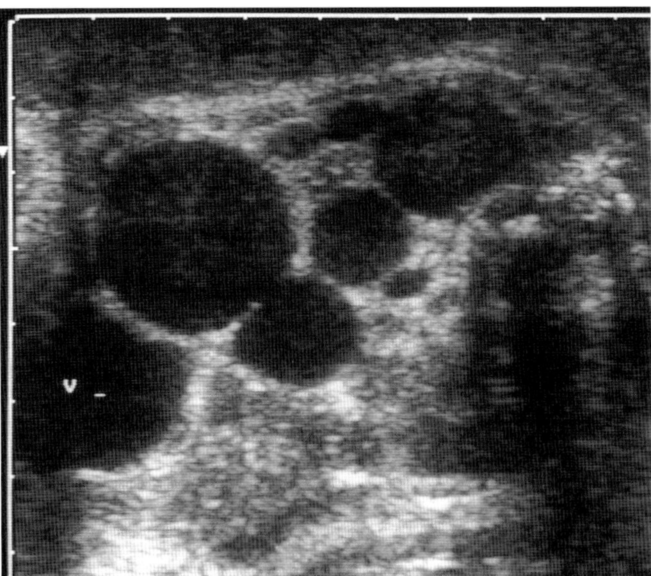

Fig. 35.15 Unilateral multicystic dysplastic kidney at 33 weeks (v marks the fetal bladder).

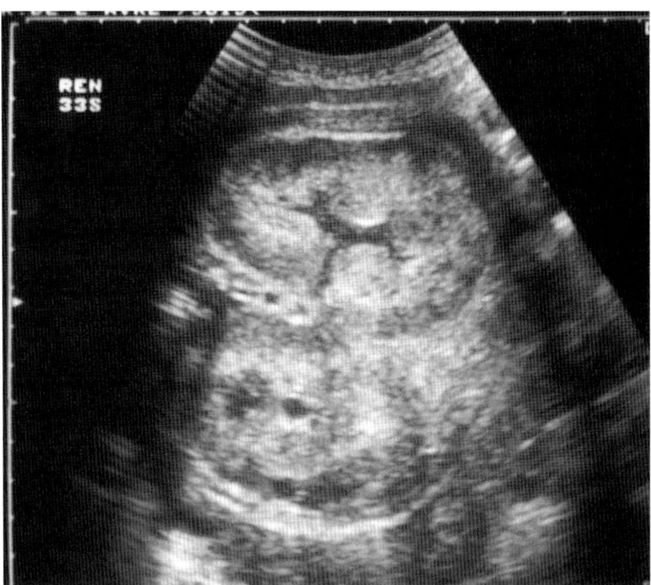

Fig. 35.16 Recessive polycystic renal disease at 33 weeks.

Isolated abnormalities of size and/or structure

Although growth charts are available[12,13], the assessment of renal size is usually made by subjective visual examination. However, growth charts may be useful to express the degree of kidney enlargement to aid diagnosis of a presumed renal anomaly or in cases where serial examinations are being performed for either a previous history of a renal anomaly or a presumed diagnosis.

Renal hypoplasia

Renal hypoplasia is defined as a kidney mass less than 2 SD below the mean. This condition is usually diagnosed postnatally, except in the most severe forms.

Multicystic dysplasia

Idiopathic multicystic dysplasia presents prenatally as a kidney which has lost its normal shape due to cysts of variable diameter (0.5–3 cm or more), which are not connected to each other or to the rest of the urinary tract. Some clusters of tubules, rudimentary glomeruli, primitive ducts and bars of metaplastic cartilage can be irregularly distributed within the loose mesenchyme. The ureter is usually atretic. While bilateral cases are lethal, unilateral ones have a good prognosis. However, associated renal anomalies, most commonly pelviureteric junction obstruction[125], have been reported in up to 40% of cases. More recently, a cohort study in women undergoing cystoscopy and/or colposcopy noted additional minor urogenital anomalies in up to 75% of cases[126]. Spontaneous involution of the multicystic kidney is usual in postnatal life and may exceptionally occur in utero. The size of the cysts is usually constant throughout fetal life, but very unusually, extremely large cysts may compress the fetal abdomen or cause dystocia and therefore require intrauterine decompression.

These macrocystic lesions (Fig. 35.15) are easy to differentiate from polycystic kidney diseases which present prenatally as enlarged hyperechogenic kidneys. The sonographic pattern of the latter conditions is due to the presence of microscopic cysts in the renal parenchyma.

Autosomal recessive polycystic kidney disease

This inherited disorder is also referred to as infantile polycystic kidney disease. It is characterized by enlarged kidneys which retain their normal shape, but the cut surface of which shows a spongy appearance due to the presence of elongated microcysts with a radial orientation extending from the medulla to the cortical surface. These cysts correspond to dilated collecting ducts[2]. The liver is always involved with portal fibrosis and proliferation of bile ducts.

In postnatal life, the diagnosis is easy to make based on typical anatomical features. The pathological diagnosis, however, may be far more difficult in second-trimester fetuses, underscoring the need for evaluation by an experienced pathologist familiar with fetal renal development in the event of a pregnancy termination.

In utero, the expression of the disease is variable[127–129]. Some fetuses remain sonographically normal and, in these, kidney enlargement will develop only in infancy and renal failure is anticipated to occur relatively late during the second decade of life. At the other end of the spectrum, recessive polycystic kidney disease may present in the second trimester as a premortem anuric fetus with absent amniotic fluid and dramatically enlarged hyperechogenic kidneys with no corticomedullary differentiation (Fig. 35.16). Intermediate forms are also possible, with a variable combination of kidney enlargement and late onset oligohydramnios[127]. The gene for this disorder has been mapped to chromosome 6p21–cen, with up to a hundred mutations of this gene being described[130].

Autosomal dominant polycystic kidney disease

This disease is often referred to as adult polycystic disease, because its clinical onset usually takes place in adulthood. This term, however, is misleading because the dominant polycystic disease may have an early and occasionally severe expression, even before birth. Due to the relatively high frequency of the mutation in the general population, dominant polycystic kidney is a common etiology of enlarged hyperechogenic kidneys in the fetus[131]. The diagnosis is easy when renal cysts are present in one of the parents. This useful clue may be lacking either because of the variability of expression of the disease itself (no cysts yet in young parents) or because the fetus may be affected by a new mutation.

Anatomically in the adult, the kidneys are enlarged and their surface is distorted by bulging macrocysts. During fetal life, however, the cysts are usually very small, resulting in a sonographic pattern of enlarged hyperechogenic kidneys very similar to that of the recessive disease. In the most severe cases, terminal renal failure occurs in utero, resulting in perinatal death. The diagnosis is made by postmortem examination showing both collecting tubules and nephronic cysts. The genes of the dominant polycystic kidney disease have been mapped to several loci on chromosome 16 (PKD1 locus) and to chromosome 4 (PKD2 locus)[132–135]. However, the most common form is mapped to the extreme distal portion of chromosome 16p.

Rare etiologies of fetal nephropathies

A number of rare conditions can present prenatally as enlarged kidneys. A precise diagnosis is seldom possible in utero and the identification of the disease will be based on postnatal follow-up or on post-mortem examination.

Renal tubular dysgenesis is a rare condition characterized by poorly developed or undeveloped proximal tubules leading to severe oligohydramnios[136]. It is thought to be due to a primary abnormality of the renin-angiotensin system. Its most common association is with the kidneys of babies complicated by severe twin-to-twin transfusion syndrome[137,138].

This lethal condition is probably inherited in an autosomal recessive fashion and should be recognized on fetal autopsy to provide adequate genetic counseling. Similar renal anomalies have been reported following prenatal exposure to angiotensin-converting enzyme (ACE) inhibitors. Prolonged exposure to indomethacin may also induce renal failure, probably by a different mechanism[139].

Nephroblastomatosis is characterized by the presence of nephrogenic rests of metanephric blastema in both kidneys[140]. It may be associated with overgrowth syndromes such as Beckwith–Wiedemann. Affected patients are at risk of developing Wilm's tumor.

Tumors, both benign and malignant, present exceptionally during fetal life as a rapidly growing solid heterogeneous mass[133]. These lesions may be associated with polyhydramnios and fetal magnetic resonance imaging may provide useful adjuvant information[141]. They are easy to distinguish from single transonic cysts similar to those observed in adults, which may also be recognized in utero but remain asymptomatic postnatally.

Fetal nephropathies associated with polyhydramnios

The Finnish type of congenital nephrotic syndrome may present prenatally as the association of polyhydramnios, enlarged placenta and moderate growth restriction. Moderate alterations of the renal parenchyma, such as hyperechogenicity, are inconstant, which makes prenatal diagnosis difficult in the absence of an index case[142–144]. In practice, one should consider performing a biochemical analysis of amniotic fluid in cases of unexplained polyhydramnios, which may occasionally lead to the diagnosis of fetal proteinuria (high concentration of alpha-fetoprotein and other proteins). Occasionally, anomalies in the electrolyte or aldosterone concentration of amniotic fluid may be suggestive of Bartter syndrome[145,146].

Cystic kidneys and multiple malformation syndromes

Cystic kidneys can be the hallmark of a number of multiple malformation anomalies of various origins. The Meckel–Gruber syndrome is one of the most common. In this recessive autosomal inherited lethal disorder, severe oligohydramnios occurs during the second trimester. The kidneys are markedly enlarged and their normal structure is replaced by multiple cysts[147]. Encephalocele and postaxial polydactyly are characteristic of the Meckel–Gruber syndrome, but may be difficult to pick up by ultrasound once severe oligohydramnios has occurred[148]. Severe oligohydramnios and enlarged dysplastic kidneys may be prominent sonographic features of trisomy 13 and trisomy 9.

Horseshoe kidney may be associated with trisomy 18, Turner's syndrome or triploidy.

The Laurence–Moon–Bardet–Biedl syndrome presents prenatally as the association of hyperechogenic kidneys with polydactyly. Growth is still normal prenatally in this syndrome. In contrast, in the Beckwith–Wiedemann syndrome, the enlarged kidneys are only one of the elements of a more generalized visceromegaly, suggestive when associated with an omphalocele.

Dysplastic kidneys may also be found in a variety of syndromes, but usually as a secondary symptom, for instance in short rib polydactyly associations.

PRENATAL DIAGNOSIS AND MANAGEMENT

As when any fetal structural anomaly is picked up by routine sonographic screening, the first step of prenatal management is to rule out associated anomalies, based on ultrasound and karyotyping. In isolated nephrological abnormalities, the prognosis then relies on the prediction of postnatal renal function. In cases with fetal renal failure indicated by severe oligohydramnios, the prognosis is obviously lethal. In unilateral isolated anomalies, the outcome is uniformly good. In those cases, however, in which bilateral nephrological anomalies are found together with a normal amniotic fluid volume, the long-term postnatal prognosis is virtually impossible to predict. Indeed, while biochemical fetal predictors of postnatal renal function have been evaluated in uropathies, these results cannot be transposed to fetal nephropathies. Our personal experience suggests that fetal urinary electrolytes are not accurate predictors of postnatal renal function in fetuses with bilaterally enlarged and hyperechogenic kidneys in whom the amount of amniotic fluid is normal. Conclusive data are lacking concerning the potential value of fetal serum β2- microglobulin.

Cases presenting with severe oligohydramnios

When severe oligohydramnios is diagnosed in the second or third trimester, the sonographic evidence that the kidneys are abnormal or absent is a key to the pathophysiological diagnosis. The renal anomalies are usually gross, such as undifferentiated hyperechogenic kidneys measuring more than 4 SDs above the mean. However, the evidence of a renal anomaly may be more difficult to obtain due to poor technical conditions. For instance, adrenals may mimic abnormal kidneys in renal agenesis, or an ectopic dysplastic kidney may be extremely difficult to identify by prenatal ultrasound. Nevertheless, because the outcome is obviously lethal, a precise etiology need not be known in order to provide adequate information for the parents and to decide to terminate the pregnancy if they find this option acceptable.

Before terminating the pregnancy, a karyotype should be obtained, either on fetal blood or on chorionic villi if the former tissue is not accessible. Amnioinfusion may be helpful to facilitate fetal blood sampling and to provide a more detailed review of associated anomalies. This can be of interest for prenatal management. For instance, if a small encephalocele and hexadactyly are diagnosed after amnioinfusion, the diagnosis of Meckel–Gruber syndrome is strongly suspected and fetal DNA should be stored for subsequent genetic diagnosis. Fetal DNA storage may also be immediately useful to the management of subsequent pregnancies. For instance, in isolated enlarged hyperechogenic kidneys, the diagnosis of recessive or dominant polycystic disease is strongly suspected. Stored fetal DNA would be used to perform linkage studies, which is a prerequisite before early genetic diagnosis by chorionic villus sampling in subsequent pregnancies. However, it must be stressed that this molecular genetic strategy would be in vain if the morphological diagnostic of the fetal index case was inaccurate, emphasizing the need to have fetal kidneys examined by a pathologist familiar with these diseases in fetuses.

The management of subsequent pregnancies based on early genetic diagnosis is technically satisfactory, but may raise difficult ethical problems, for instance in genetic disorders with extremely variable expression[149]. We have the experience of a couple in whom the first pregnancy was terminated because of a lethal form of dominant polycystic disease. One of the parents was found to have renal cysts following prenatal diagnosis of the fetal nephropathy. Fetal post-mortem examination confirmed the diagnosis of dominant polycystic disease and early genetic testing was requested by the parents for their subsequent pregnancy. Chorionic villi were sampled, demonstrating that the second child was carrying the mutation. However, this did not rule out the possibility that the child would remain symptom free for years. Eventually, the pregnancy was continued, amniotic fluid volume remained normal despite the presence of moderately enlarged hyperechogenic kidneys and an asymptomatic child was delivered.

Normal amniotic fluid

Unilateral lesion

The management of unilateral renal agenesis or multicystic disease should obviously be conservative, provided no extrarenal fetal anomaly is identified and the contralateral kidney remains normal. Postnatal follow-up should be explained to the parents, ideally by the pediatrician who will be in charge of the child. The development of the contralateral kidney is normal in the majority of cases, but should be monitored due to the possibility that a contralateral anomaly could be identified in the second trimester.

Exceptional situations, such as a renal tumor diagnosed in utero, should be discussed with the appropriate pediatric specialist in order to evaluate the potential for postnatal therapy.

Bilateral lesions

In the context of normal amniotic fluid volume, isolated enlarged hyperechogenic kidneys are the most common bilateral fetal nephrological anomaly[150]. In the absence of a family history, the etiological diagnosis is almost impossible to make in utero. When the amniotic fluid is and remains normal throughout gestation, postnatal survival can be anticipated, but it is not possible to obtain a precise prediction of morbidity and especially of the risks of renal failure in infancy. Relatively small size of the kidneys and the presence of a normal corticomedullary differentiation are reassuring and suggest the hypothesis of a transient nephromegaly. However, such findings may also be the hallmark of recessive polycystic kidney disease. Although chromosomal anomalies are not often encountered in these cases, a normal fetal karyotype is reassuring. Fetal renal biopsy has been proposed in such cases, but has not proved clinically useful so far. Indeed, even if the etiological diagnosis was made, for instance if one of the parents was found to have dominant polycystic disease, it would remain very difficult to predict when the affected child would develop clinical symptoms postnatally.

Because of the limitations of our prediction of postnatal outcome, the prenatal diagnosis of enlarged hyperechogenic kidneys may seem psychologically devastating to the parents. However, it may have a positive impact, because the early diagnosis of nephropathies may improve their prognosis, for instance by allowing early management of systemic hypertension in childhood.

ACKNOWLEDGMENTS

We thank Dr JP Aubury and Dr MC Aubry who provided some of the ultrasound images and Drs PJ Thompson and Katie Morris for their comments on the manuscript.

REFERENCES

1. Hamilton WJ, Boyd JD, Mossman HW. *Human embryology – prenatal development of form and function*. Baltimore: Williams & Wilkins Company, Macmillan Press, 1972.
2. Thorner P, Berstein J, Landing BH. Kidneys and lower urinary tract. In *Disease of the fetus and newborn*, GB Reed, AE Claireaux, F Cockburn (eds), pp. 609–630. London: Chapman and Hall, 1995.
3. Saxen L, Sariola H. Early organogenesis of the kidney. *Pediatr Nephrol* **1**:385–392, 1987.
4. Bard JBL, Woolf AS. Nephrogenesis and the development of renal disease. *Nephrol Dial Transplant* **7**:563–572, 1992.
5. Ekblom P. Renal development. In *The kidney: physiology and pathophysiology*, DW Seldin, G Giebisch (eds). New York: Raven Press, 1992.
6. Clapp WL, Abrahamson DR. Development and gross anatomy of the kidney. In *Renal pathology with clinical functional correlations*, CC Tisher, BM Brenner (eds). Philadelphia: JB Lippincott Company, 1994.
7. Muller F, Dommergues M, Mandelbrot L, Aubry MC, Nihoul-Fekete C, Dumez Y. Fetal urinary biochemistry predicts postnatal renal function in children with bilateral obstructive uropathies. *Obstet Gynecol* **82**(5):813–820, 1993.

8. Eugène M, Muller F, Dommergues M, LeMoyec L, Dumez Y. Evaluation of postnatal renal function in fetuses with bilateral uropathies by proton nuclear magnetic resonance spectroscopy. *Am J Obstet Gyneol* **170**:595–602, 1994.
9. Muller F, Dommergues M, Bussieres L et al. Development of human renal function: reference intervals for 10 biochemical markers in fetal urine. *Clin Chem* **42**(11):1855–1860, 1996.
10. Nicolini U, Rodeck C, Fisk N. Shunt treatment for fetal obstructive uropathy. *Lancet* **2**:1338–1339, 1987.
11. Nicolaides KH, Cheng HH, Snijders RJ, Moniz CF. Fetal urine biochemistry in the assessment of obstructive uropathy. *Am J Obstet Gynecol* **166**(3):932–937, 1992.
12. Sebire NJ, Von Kaisenberg C, Rubio C, Snijders RJ, Nicolaides KH. Fetal megacystis at 10–14 weeks of gestation. *Ultrasound Obstet Gynecol* **8**:387–390, 1996.
13. Bronshtein M, Yoffe N, Brandes JM, Blumenfeld Z. First and early second-trimester diagnosis of fetal urinary tract anomalies using transvaginal sonography. *Prenat Diagn* **10**:653–666, 1990.
14. Grannum P, Bracken M, Silverman R, Hobbins J. Assessment of fetal kidney size in normal gestation by comparison of ratio of kidney circumference to abdominal circumference. *Am J Obstet Gynecol* **136**:249–254, 1980.
15. Jeanty P, Dramaix-Wilmet M, Elkazen N, Hubinont C, Regemorter V. Measurement of fetal kidney growth on ultrasound. *Radiology* **144**:159–162, 1982.
16. Emerson DS, Felker RE, Brown DL. The sagittal sign – an early second trimester sonographic indicator of fetal gender. *J Ultrasound Med* **8**:293–297, 1989.
17. Reece EA, Winn HN, Wan M, Burdine C, Green J, Hobbins JC. Can ultrasonography replace amniocentesis in fetal gender determination during the early second trimester? *Am J Obstet Gynecol* **156**: 579–581, 1987.
18. Mazza V, Di Monte I, Pati M et al. Sonographic biometrical range of external genitalia differentiation in the first trimester of pregnancy: analysis of 2593 cases. *Prenat Diagn* **24**:677–684, 2004.
19. Efrat Z, Akinfenwa OO, Nicolaides KH. First-trimester determination of fetal gender by ultrasound. *Ultrasound Obstet Gynecol* **13**(5):305–307, 1999.
20. Broadley P, McHugo J, Morgan I, Whittle MJ, Kilby MD. The 4 year outcome following the demonstration of bilateral renal pelvidilation on prenatal renal ultrasound. *Br J Radiol* **72**(855): 265–270, 1999.
21. Beck AD. The effect of intra-uterine urinary obstruction upon the development of the fetal kidney. *J Urol* **105**:784–789, 1982.
22. Vallancien G, Beurton D, Szemat R et al. Etude expérimentale comparée des conséquences rénales du reflux vésico-urétéral et de l'obstruction urétérale chez le foetus de brebis. *J Urol Paris* **88**:27–30, 1982.
23. Glick PL, Harrison MR, Noall RA, Villa RL. Corrections of congenital hydronephrosis in utero III. Early mid-trimester ureteral obstruction produces renal dysplasia. *J Pediatr Surg* **18**(6): 681–687, 1983.
24. Pringle KC, Bonsib SM. Development of fetal lamb lung and kidney in obstructive uropathy: a preliminary report. *Fetal Ther* **3**:118–128, 1988.
25. Gonzalez R, Reinberg Y, Burke B, Wells T, Vernier RL. Early bladder outlet obstruction in fetal lambs induces renal dysplasia and the prune-belly syndrome. *J Pediatr Surg* **25**:342–345, 1990.
26. Peters CA, Carr MC, Lais A, Retik AB, Mandell J. The response of the fetal kidney to obstruction. *J Urol* **148**:503–509, 1992.
27. Clark TJ, Martin WL, Divakaran TG, Whittle MJ, Kilby MD, Khan KS. Prenatal bladder drainage in the management of fetal lower urinary tract obstruction: a systematic review and meta-analysis. *Obstet Gynecol* **102**:367–382, 2003.
28. Zaccara A, Giorlandino C, Mobili L et al. Amniotic fluid index and fetal bladder outflow obstruction. Do we really need more? *J Urol* **174**:1657–1660, 2005.
29. Potter EL. *Pathology of the fetus and infant*. Chicago: Year Book Medical Publishers, 1961.
30. Morris RK, Quinlan-Jones E, Kilby MD, Khan KS. Systematic review of accuracy of fetal urine analysis to predict poor postnatal renal function in cases of congenital urinary tract obstruction. *Prenat Diagn* **27(10)**:900–911, 2007.
31. Flake A, Harrison M, Sauer L, Adzick S, de Lorimier A. Ureteropelvic junction obstruction in the fetus. *J Ped Surg* **21**:1058–1063, 1986.
32. Liu HY, Dhillon HK, Yeung CK, Diamond DA, Duffy PG, Ransley PG. Clinical outcome and management of prenatally diagnosed primary megaureters. *J Urol* **152**(2 Pt 2):614–617, 1994.
33. Nakayama D, Harrison M, de Lorimier A. Prognosis of posterior urethral valves presenting at birth. *J Ped Surg* **21**:43–45, 1986.
34. Robyr R, Benachi A, Daikha-Dahmane F, Martinovich J, Dumez Y, Ville Y. Correlation between ultrasound and anatomical findings in fetuses with lower urinary tract obstruction in the first half of pregnancy. *Ultrasound Obstet Gynecol* **25**(5):478–482, 2005.
35. Persutte WH, Koyle M, Lenke RR, Klas J, Ryan C, Hobbins JC. Mild pyelectasis ascertained with prenatal ultrasonography is pediatrically significant. *Ultrasound Obstet Gynecol* **10**(1):12–18, 1997.
36. Hayden SA, Russ PD, Pretorius DH, Manco-Johnson ML, Clewell WH. Posterior urethral obstruction. Prenatal sonographic findings and clinical outcome in fourteen cases. *J Ultrasound Med* **7**(7):371–375, 1988.
37. Hobbins J, Romero R, Grannum P, Berkowitz R, Cullen M, Mahoney M. Antenatal diagnosis of renal anomalies with ultrasound. I. Obstructive uropathy. *Am J Obstet Gynecol* **148**:868–877, 1984.
38. Wladimiroff J, Scholtmeijer R, Stewart P, Sauer P, Niermeijer M. Prenatal evaluation and outcome of fetal obstructive uropathies. *Prenat Diagn* **8**:93–102, 1988.
39. Paduano L, Giglio L, Bembi B, Peratoner L, D'Ottavio G, Benussi G. Clinical outcome of fetal uropathy. I. Predictive value of prenatal echography positive for obstructive uropathy. *J Urol* **146**(4):1094–1096, 1991.
40. Paduano L, Giglio L, Bembi B, Peratoner L, Benussi G. Clinical outcome of fetal uropathy. II. Sensitivity of echography for prenatal detection of obstructive pathology. *J Urol* **146**(4): 1097–1098, 1991.
41. Fernbach SK, Maizels M, Conway JJ. Ultrasound grading of hydronephrosis: introduction to the system used by the Society for Fetal Urology. *Pediatr Radiol* **23**(6):478–480, 1993.
42. Grignon A, Filion R, Filatrault et al. Urinary tract dilatation in utero: classification and clinical applications. *Radiology* **160**:645–647, 1986.
43. Anderson N, Clautice-Engle T, Allan R, Abbott G, Wells JE. Detection of obstructive uropathy in the fetus: predictive value of sonographic measurements of renal pelvic diameter at various gestational ages. *Am J Roentgenol* **164**:719–723, 1995.
44. Dremsek PA, Gindl K, Voitl P et al. Renal pyelectasis in fetuses and neonates: diagnostic value of renal pelvis diameter in pre- and postnatal sonographic screening. *Am J Roentgenol* **168**(4): 1017–1019, 1997.
45. Corteville JE, Dicke JM, Crane JP. Fetal pyelectasis and Down syndrome: is genetic amniocentesis warranted? *Obstet Gynecol* **79**(5 Pt 1):770–772, 1992.
46. Bronshtein M, Bar-Hava I, Lightman A. The significance of early second-trimester sonographic detection of minor fetal renal anomalies. *Prenat Diagn* **15**(7):627–632, 1995.
47. Adra AM, Mejides AA, Dennaoui MS, Beydoun SN. Fetal pyelectasis: is it always 'physiologic'? *Am J Obstet Gynecol* **173**:1263–1266, 1985.
48. Morin L, Cendron M, Crombleholme TM, Garmel SH, Klauber GT, D'Alton ME. Minimal hydronephrosis in the fetus: clinical significance and implications for management. *J Urol* **155**:2047–2049, 1996.

49. Ouzounian JG, Castro MA, Fresquez M, al-Sulyman OM, Kovacs BW. Prognostic significance of antenatally detected fetal pyelectasis. *Ultrasound Obstet Gynecol* **7**(6):424–428, 1996.
50. Bobrowski RA, Levin RB, Lauria MR, Treadwell MC, Gonik B, Bottoms SF. In utero progression of isolated renal pelvis dilation. *Am J Perinatol* **14**(7):423–426, 1997.
51. Barker AP, Cave MM, Thomas DF et al. Fetal pelvi-ureteric junction obstruction: predictors of outcome. *Br J Urol* **76**: 649–652, 1995.
52. Thomas DF, Madden NP, Irving HC, Arthur RJ, Smith SE. Mild dilatation of the fetal kidney: a follow-up study. *Br J Urol* **74**(2):236–239, 1994.
53. Corteville JE, Gray DL, Crane JP. Congenital hydronephrosis: correlation of fetal ultrasonographic findings with infant outcome. *Am J Obstet Gynecol* **165**(2):384–388, 1991.
54. Gunn TR, Mora JD, Pease P. Antenatal diagnosis of urinary tract abnormalities by ultrasonography after 28 weeks' gestation: incidence and outcome. *Am J Obstet Gynecol* **172**(2 Pt 1):479–486, 1995.
55. Blachar A, Blachar Y, Livne PM, Zurkowski L, Pelet D, Mogilner B. Clinical outcome and follow-up of prenatal hydronephrosis. *Pediatr Nephrol* **8**(1): 30–35, 1994.
56. Hutton KA, Thomas DF, Davies BW. Prenatally detected posterior urethral valves: qualitative assessment of second trimester scans and prediction of outcome. *J Urol* **158**(3 Pt 2):1022–1025, 1997.
57. Caione P, Patricolo M, Lais A, Capitanucci ML, Capozza N, Ferro F. Role of prenatal diagnosis in the treatment of congenital obstructive megaureter in a solitary kidney. *Fetal Diagn Ther* **11**(3):205–209, 1996.
58. Wiesel A, Queisser-Luft A, Clementi M et al. Prenatal detection of congenital renal malformations by fetal ultrasonographic examination: an analysis of 709,030 births in 12 European countries. *Eur J Med Genet* **48**(2):131–144, 2005.
59. RCOG Working Party Report. *Ultrasound screening for fetal abnormalities*. London: RCOG, 2000. Ref Type: Electronic Citation.
60. Barker AP, Cave MM, Thomas DF et al. Fetal pelvi-ureteric junction obstruction: predictors of outcome. *Br J Urol* **76**(5): 649–652, 1995.
61. Hutton KA, Thomas DF, Davies BW. Prenatally detected posterior urethral valves: qualitative assessment of second trimester scans and prediction of outcome. *J Urol* **158**(3):1022–1025, 1997.
62. Mahoney BS, Callen PW, Filly RA. Fetal urethral obstruction: ultrasound evaluation. *Radiology* **157**:221–224, 1985.
63. Oliveira EA, Cabral AC, Pereira AK et al. Outcome of fetal urinary tract anomalies associated with multiple malformations and chromosomal abnormalities. *Prenat Diagn* **21**(2):129–134, 2001.
64. Anumba DO, Scott JE, Plant ND, Robson SC. Diagnosis and outcome of fetal lower urinary tract obstruction in the northern region of England. *Prenat Diagn* **25** (1): 7–13, 2005.
65. Crombleholme TM, Harrison MR, Golbus MS et al. Fetal intervention in obstructive uropathy: prognostic indicators and efficacy of intervention. *Am J Obstet Gynecol* **162**(5):1239–1244, 1990.
66. Estroff JA, Mandell J, Benacerraf BR. Increased renal parenchymal echogenicity in the fetus: importance and clinical outcome. *Radiology* **181**(1):135–139, 1991.
67. Oliveira EA, Rabelo EA, Pereira AK et al. Prognostic factors in prenatally-detected posterior urethral valves: a multivariate analysis. *Pediatr Surg Int* **18**(8):662–667, 2002.
68. Bois E, Feingold J, Benmaiz H, Briard ML. Congenital urinary tract malformations: epidemiologic and genetic aspects. *Clin Genet* **8**:37–47, 1975.
69. Cocchi G, Magnani C, Morini MS et al. Urinary tract abnormalities (UTA) and associated malformations: data of the Emilia–Romagna registry. *Eur J Epidemiol* **12**:493–497, 1996.
70. Nicolaides KH, Cheng HH, Abbas A, Snijders RJM, Gosden C. Fetal renal defects: associated malformations and chromosomal defects. *Fetal Diagn Ther* **7**:1–11, 1992.
71. Mirk P, Calisti A, Fileni A. Prenatal sonographic diagnosis of bladder exstrophy. *J Ultrasound Med* **5**:291–293, 1986.
72. Barth R, Filly R, Sondheimer F. Prenatal sonographic findings in bladder exstrophy. *J Ultrasound Med* **9**:359–361, 1990.
73. Nussbaum AR, Sanders RC, Gearhart JP. Obstructed uterovaginal anomalies: demonstration with sonography. Neonates and infants. *Radiology* **179**: 79–83, 1991.
74. Jaramillo D, Lebowitz RL, Hendren WH. The cloacal malformation: radiologic findings and imaging recommendations. *Radiology* **177**:441–448, 1990.
75. Mandell J, Lebowitz RL, Peters CA, Estroff JA, Retik AB, Benacerraf BR. Prenatal diagnosis of the megacystis-megaureter association. *J Urol* **148**(5):1487–1489, 1992.
76. Smith DP, Felker RE, Noe HN, Emerson DS, Mercer B. Prenatal diagnosis of genital anomalies. *Urology* **47**(1): 114–117, 1996.
77. Mirk P, Pintus C, Speca S. Ultrasound diagnosis of hydrocolpos: prenatal findings and postnatal follow-up. *J Clin Ultrasound* **22**(1):55–58, 1994.
78. Gillis DA, Grantmyre EB. Megacystis-microcolon-intestinal hypoperistalsis syndrome: survival of male infant. *J Ped Surg* **20**(3):279–281, 1985.
79. Mandell J, Blyth BR, Peters CA, Retik AB, Estroff JA, Benacerraf BR. Structural genitourinary defects detected in utero. *Radiology* **178**(1):193–196, 1991.
80. Lev-Lehman E, Bercovich D, Xu W, Stockton DW, Beaudet AL. Characterization of the human beta4 nAChR gene and polymorphisms in CHRNA3 and CHRNB4. *J Hum Genet* **46**(7):362–366, 2001.
81. Richardson C, Morgan J, Jasani B et al. Megacystis-microcolon-intestinal hypoperistalsis syndrome and the absence of the alpha3 nicotinic acetylcholine receptor subunit. *Gastroenterology* **121**(2):350–357, 2001.
82. Xu W, Gelber S, Orr-Urteger A et al. Megacystis, mydriasis and ion channel defect in mice lacking the alpha3 neuronal nicotinic acetylcholine receptor. *Proc Nat Acad Sci USA* **96**:5746–5751, 1999.
83. Xu W, Orr-Urteger A, Nigro F et al. Multiple autonomic dysfunction in mice lacking the beta2 and beta4 subunits of neuronal nicotinic acetylcholine receptors. *J Neurosci* **19**:9298–9905, 1999.
84. Benacerraf BR, Mandell J, Estroff JA, Harlow BL, Frigoletto FD, Jr. Fetal pyelectasis: a possible association with Down syndrome. *Obstet Gynecol* **76**(1): 58–60, 1990.
85. Benacerraf BR, Neuberg D, Bromley B, Frigoletto FD, Jr. Sonographic scoring index for prenatal detection of chromosomal abnormalities. *J Ultrasound Med* **11**(9):449–458, 1992.
86. Benacerraf BR, Nadel A, Bromley B. Identification of second-trimester fetuses with autosomal trisomy by use of a sonographic scoring index. *Radiology* **193**(1):135–140, 1994.
87. Snijders RJM, Sebire NJ, Faria M, Patel F, Nicolaides KH. Fetal mild hydronephrosis and chromosomal defects: relation to maternal age and gestation. *Fetal Diagn Ther* **10**:349–355, 1995.
88. Wickstrom E, Maizels M, Sabbagha RE, Tamura RK, Cohen LC, Pergament E. Isolated fetal pyelectasis: assessment of risk for postnatal uropathy and Down syndrome. *Ultrasound Obstet Gynecol* **8**(4):236–240, 1996.
89. Wickstrom EA, Thangavelu M, Parilla BV, Tamura RK, Sabbagha RE. A prospective study of the association between isolated fetal pyelectasis and chromosomal abnormality. *Obstet Gynecol* **88**(3):379–382, 1996.
90. Vintzileos AM, Campbell WA, Guzman ER et al. Second-trimester ultrasound markers for detection of trisomy 21: which markers are best? *Obstet Gynecol* **89**(6):941–944, 1997.
91. Reznik VM, Kaplan GW, Murphy JL et al. Follow-up of infants with bilateral renal disease detected in utero. Growth and renal function. *Am J Dis Child* **142**(4): 453–456, 1988.

92. Reznik VM, Murphy JL, Mendoza SA, Griswold WR, Packer MG, Kaplan GW. Follow-up of infants with obstructive uropathy detected in utero and treated surgically postnatally. *J Pediatr Surg* **24**(12):1289–1292, 1989.
93. Adzick NS, Harrison MR, Flake AW, Laberge JM. Development of a fetal renal function test using endogenous creatinine clearance. *J Pediatr Surg* **20**:602–607, 1985.
94. Glick PL, Harrison MR, Golbus MS et al. Management of the fetus with congenital hydronephrosis II: Prognostic criteria and selection for treatment. *J Pediatr Surg* **20**(4):376–387, 1985.
95. Nicolini U, Fisk NM, Rodeck CH, Beacham J. Fetal urine biochemistry: an index of renal maturation and dysfunction. *Br J Obstet Gynaecol* **99**: 46–50, 1992.
96. Wilkins IA, Chitkara U, Lynch L, Goldberg JD, Mehalek KE, Berkowitz RL. The nonpredictive value of fetal urinary electrolytes: preliminary report of outcomes and correlations with pathologic diagnosis. *Am J Obstet Gynecol* **157**(3):694–698, 1987.
97. Lipitz S, Ryan G, Samuell C et al. Fetal urine analysis for the assessment of renal function in obstructive uropathy. *Am J Obstet Gynecol* **168**:174–179, 1993.
98. Johnson MP, Corsi P, Bradfield W et al. Sequential urinalysis improves evaluation of fetal renal function in obstructive uropathy. *Am J Obstet Gynecol* **173**(1):59–65, 1995.
99. Glick PL, Harrison MR, Noall RA, Villa RL. Correction of congenital hydronephrosis in utero III. Early mid-trimester ureteral obstruction produces renal dysplasia. *J Pediatr Surg* **18**(6): 870–881, 1983.
100. Lissauer D, Morris RK, Kilby MD. Fetal lower urinary tract obstruction. *Semin Fetal Neonat Med* **12**(6):464–470, 2007.
101. Daïkha-Dahmane F, Dommergues M, Muller F et al. Development of human fetal kidney in obstructive uropathy: correlations with ultrasonography and urine biochemistry. *Kidney Int* **52**(1): 21–32, 1997.
102. Eugene M, Muller F, Dommergues M, Le ML, Dumez Y. Evaluation of postnatal renal function in fetuses with bilateral obstructive uropathies by proton nuclear magnetic resonance spectroscopy. *Am J Obstet Gynecol* **170**(2):595–602, 1994.
103. Foxall PJ, Bewley S, Neild GH, Rodeck CH, Nicholson JK. Analysis of fetal and neonatal urine using proton nuclear magnetic resonance spectroscopy. *Arch Dis Child Fetal Neonal Ed* **73**(3):F153–F157, 1995.
104. Johnson MP, Bukowski TP, Reitleman C, Isada NB, Pryde PG, Evans MI. In utero surgical treatment of fetal obstructive uropathy: a new comprehensive approach to identify appropriate candidates for vesicoamniotic shunt therapy. *Am J Obstet Gynecol* **170**(6): 1770–1776, 1994.
105. Nolte S, Mueller B, Pringsheim W. Serum alpha1-microglobulin and beta2-microglobulin for the estimation of fetal glomerular renal function. *Pediatr Nephrol* **5**(5):573–577, 1991.
106. Nicolini U, Spelzini F. Invasive assessment of fetal renal abnormalities: urinalysis, fetal blood sampling and biopsy. *Prenat Diagn* **21**(11):964–969, 2001.
107. Berry SM, Lecolier B, Smith RS et al. Predictive value of fetal serum beta2-microglobulin for neonatal renal function. *Lancet* **345**(8960), 1995.
108. Cagdas A, Aydinli K, Irez T, Temizyurek K, Apak MY. Evaluation of the fetal kidney maturation by assessment of amniotic fluid alpha-1 microglobulin levels. *Eur J Obstet Gynecol Reprod Biol* **90**(1):55–61, 2000.
109. Ciardelli V, Rizzo N, Farina A, Vitarelli M, Boni P, Bovicelli L. Prenatal evaluation of fetal renal function based on serum beta(2)-microglobulin assessment. *Prenat Diagn* **21**(7):586–588, 2001.
110. Cobet G, Gummelt T, Bollmann R, Tennstedt C, Brux B. Assessment of serum levels of alpha-1-microglobulin, beta-2-microglobulin, and retinol binding protein in the fetal blood. *A method for prenatal evaluation of renal function. Prenat Diagn* **16**(4):299–305, 1996.
111. Bunduki V, Saldanha LB, Sadek L, Miguelez J, Miyadahira S, Zugaib M. Fetal renal biopsies in obstructive uropathy: feasibility and clinical correlations–preliminary results. *Prenat Diagn* **18**(2):101–109, 1998.
112. Donnai P. Attitudes of patients after 'genetic' termination of pregnancy. *Br Med J* **282**:621–622, 1981.
113. Glick PL, Harrison MR, Adzick NS. Correction of congenital hydronephrosis in utero IV: in utero decompression prevents renal dysplasia. *J Pediatr Surg* **19**(6):649–657, 1984.
114. Harrison M, Ross N, Noall R, de Lorimier A. Correction of congenital hydronephrosis in utero I. The model: fetal urethral obstruction produces hydronephrosis and pulmonary hypoplasia in fetal lamb. *J Ped Surg* **18**:247–256, 1983.
115. Estes JM, MacGillivray TE, Hedrick MH, Adzick NS, Harrison MR. Fetoscopic surgery for the treatment of congenital anomalies. *J Pediatr Surg* **27**(8):950–954, 1992.
116. Quintero R, Hume R, Smith C et al. Percutaneous fetal cystoscopy and endoscopic fulguration of posterior urethral valves. *Am J Obstet Gynecol* **172**:206–209, 1995.
117. Rodeck CH, Nicolaides KH. Ultrasound guided invasive procedures in obstetrics. *Clin Obstet Gynaecol* **10**(3):515–539, 1983.
118. Manning FA, Harrison M, Rodeck CH. Catheter shunts for fetal hydronephrosis ad hydropcephalus. *N Engl J Med* **315**:336–340, 1986.
119. Sepulveda W, Stagiannis KD, Flack NJ, Fisk NM. Accuracy of prenatal diagnosis of renal agenesis with color flow imaging in severe second-trimester oligohydramnios. *Am J Obstet Gynecol* **173**(6):1788–1792, 1995.
120. Romero R, Cullen M, Grannum P et al. Antenatal diagnosis of renal anomalies with ultrasound III. Bilateral renal agenesis. *Am J Obstet Gynecol* **151**:38–43, 1985.
121. Bronshtein M, Amit A, Achiron R, Noy I, Blumenfeld Z. The early prenatal sonographic diagnosis of renal agenesis: techniques and possible pitfalls. *Prenat Diagn* **14**(4):291–297, 1994.
122. Winters WD, Lebowitz RL. Importance of prenatal detection of hydronephrosis of the upper pole. *Am J Roentgenol* **155**(1):125–129, 1990.
123. Meizner I, Yitzhak M, Levi A, Barki Y, Barnhard Y, Glezerman M. Fetal pelvic kidney: a challenge in prenatal diagnosis? *Ultrasound Obstet Gynecol* **5**(6):391–393, 1995.
124. Sherer D, Cullen J, Thompson H, Metlay L, Woods J. Prenatal sonographic findings associated with a fetal horseshoe kidney. *J Ultrasound Med* **9**:477–479, 1990.
125. Kleiner B, Filly RA, Mack L, Callen PW. Multicystic dysplastic kidney: observations of contralateral disease in the fetal population. *Radiology* **161**: 27–29, 1986.
126. Damen-Elias HA, Stoutenbeek PH, Visser GH, Nikkels PG, de Jong TP. Concomitant anomalies in 100 children with unilateral multicystic kidney. *Ultrasound Obstet Gynecol* **25**:384–388, 2005.
127. Wisser J, Hebisch G, Froster U et al. Prenatal sonographic diagnosis of autosomal recessive polycystic kidney disease (ARPKD) during the early second trimester. *Prenat Diagn* **15**(9): 868–871, 1995.
128. Reuss A, Wladimiroff JW, Stewart PA, Niermeijer MF. Prenatal diagnosis by ultrasound in pregnancies at risk for autosomal recessive polycystic kidney disease. *Ultrasound Med Biol* **16**(4): 355–359, 1990.
129. Barth RA, Guillot AP, Capeless EL, Clemmons JJ. Prenatal diagnosis of autosomal recessive polycystic kidney disease: variable outcome within one

family. *Am J Obstet Gynecol* **166**(2): 560–561, 1992.

130. Zerres K, Mücher G, Bachner L et al. Mapping of the gene for autosomal recessive polycystic kidney disease (ARPKD) to chromosome 6p21-cen. *Nat Genet* **7**:429–432, 1994.
131. Sinibaldi D, Malena S, Mingarelli R, Rizzoni G. Prenatal ultrasonographic findings of dominant polycystic kidney disease and postnatal renal evolution. *Am J Med Genet* **65**(4):337–341, 1996.
132. Germino GG, Weistat-Saslow D, Himmelbauer H et al. The gene for autosomal dominant polycystic kidney disease lies in the 750-Kb CpG-rich region. *Genomics* **13**:144–151, 1992.
133. The European Polycystic Kidney Disease Consortium. The polycystic kidney disease 1 gene encodes a 14 Kb transcript and lies within a duplicated region on chromosome 16. *Cell* **77**:881–894, 1994.
134. The American PKD1 Consortium. Analysis of the genomic sequence for the autosomal dominant polycystic kidney disease (PKD1) gene predicts the presence of a leucine-rich repeat. *Hum Mol Genet* **4**:575–582, 1995.
135. Kimberling WJ, Kumar S, Gabow PA, Kenyon JB, Connolly CJ, Somlo S. Autosomal dominant polycystic kidney disease: localization of the second gene to chromosome 4q13–q23. *Genomics* **18**:467–472, 1993.
136. Allanson JE, Pantzar JT, MacLeod PM. Possible new autosomal recessive syndrome with unusual renal histopathological changes. *Am J Med Genet* **16**:57–60, 1983.
137. Mahieu-Caputo D, Muller F, Joly D et al. Pathogenesis of twin-twin transfusion syndrome: the renin-angiotensin system hypothesis. *Fetal Diagn Ther* **16**(4): 241–244, 2001.
138. Kilby MD, Platt C, Whittle MJ, Oxley J, Lindop GB. Renin gene expression in fetal kidneys of pregnancies complicated by twin-twin transfusion syndrome. *Pediatr Dev Pathol* **4**(2):175–179, 2001.
139. Gloor JM, Muchant DG, Norling LL. Prenatal maternal indomethacin use resulting in prolonged neonatal renal insufficiency. *J Perinatol* **13**(6):425–427, 1993.
140. Ambrosino M, Hernanz Schulman M, Horii S, Raghavendra B, Genieser N. Prenatal diagnosis of nephro-blastomatosis in two siblings. *J Ultrasound Med* **9**:49–51, 1990.
141. Chen WY, Lin CN, Chao CS et al. Prenatal diagnosis of congenital mesoblastic nephroma in mid-second trimester by sonography and magnetic resonance imaging. *Prenat Diagn* **23**: 927–931, 2003.
142. Perale R, Talenti E, Lubrano G, Fassina A, Pavanello L, Rizzoni G. Late ultrasonographic pattern in congenital nephrotic syndrome of the Finnish type. *Ped Radiol* **18**:71, 1988.
143. Huttunen NP. Congenital nephrotic syndrome of the Finnish type. *Arch Dis Child* **51**:344–348, 1976.
144. Moore B, Pretorius D, Scioscia A, Reznik V. Sonographic findings in a fetus with congenital nephrotic syndrome of the Finnish Type. *J Ultrasound Med* **11**:113–116, 1992.
145. Sieck UV, Ohlsson A. Fetal polyuria and hydramnios associated with Bartter's syndrome. *Obstet Gynecol* **63**:22S, 1984.
146. Abramson O, Zmora E, Mazor M, Shinwell ES. Pseudohypoaldosteronism in a preterm infant: intrauterine presentation as hydramnios. *J Pediatr* **120**:129–132, 1992.
147. Rehder H, Labbé F. Prenatal morphology in Meckel's syndrome. *Prenat Diagn* **1**:161–172, 1981.
148. Dumez Y, Dommergues M, Gubler MC et al. Meckel–Gruber syndrome: prenatal diagnosis at 10 menstrual weeks using embryoscopy. *Prenat Diagn* **14**:141–144, 1994.
149. Zerres K, Hansmann M, Knopfle G, Stephan M. Prenatal diagnosis of genetically determined early manifestation of autosomal dominant polycystic kidney disease? *Hum Genet* **71**(4):368–369, 1985.
150. Carr MC, Benacerraf BR, Estroff JA, Mandell J. Prenatally diagnosed bilateral hyperechoic kidneys with normal amniotic fluid: postnatal outcome. *J Urol* **153**(2):442–444, 1995.
151. Bussieres L, Laborde K, Souberbielle JC, Muller F, Dommergues M, Sachs C. Fetal urinary insulin-like growth factor I and binding protein 3 in bilateral obstructive uropathies. *Prenat Diagn* **15**(11): 1047–1055, 1995.
152. Grannum PA, Ghidini A, Scioscia A, Copel JA, Romero R, Hobbins JC. Assessment of fetal renal reserve in low level obstructive uropathy. *Lancet* **1**(8632):281–282, 1989.
153. Muller F, Bernard MA, Benkirane A, Ngo S, Lortat-Jacob S, Oury JF, Dommergues M. Fetal urine cystatin C as a predictor of postnatal renal function in bilateral uropathies. *Clin Chem* **45**(12):2292–2293, 1999.
154. Miguelez J, Bunduki V, Yoshizaki CT, Sadek Ldos S, Koch V, Peralta CF, Zugaib M. Fetal obstructive uropathy: is urine sampling useful for prenatal counselling? *Prenat Diagn* **26**(1):81–84, 2006.
155. Freedman AL, Johnson MP, Gonzalez R. Fetal therapy for obstructive uropathy: past, present, future? *Pediatr Nephrol* **14**(2):167–176, 2000.
156. Mandelbrot L, Dumez Y, Muller F, Dommergues M. Prenatal prediction of renal function in fetal obstructive uropathies. *J Perinat Med* **19**(Suppl 1): 283–287, 1991.
157. Reuss A, Wladimiroff JW, Pijpers L, Provoost AP. Fetal urinary electrolytes in bladder outlet obstruction. *Fetal Ther* **2**(3):148–153, 1987.
158. Qureshi F, Jacques SM, Seifman B, Quintero R, Evans MI, Smith C, Johnson MP. In utero fetal urine analysis and renal histology correlate with the outcome in fetal obstructive uropathies. *Fetal Diagn Ther* **11**(5):306–312, 1996.

CHAPTER

36 Fetal skeletal abnormalities

Lyn S Chitty, Louise Wilson and David R Griffin

KEY POINTS

- Diagnosis of skeletal anomalies is challenging and requires time and a team approach, including clinical geneticists, pediatricians and pathologists. This chapter deals with the prenatal diagnosis of skeletal anomalies. It gives aids to diagnosis and categorizes conditions by sonographic findings in order to help the sonographer narrow the differential diagnoses
- The definitive diagnosis can sometimes be achieved prenatally following targeted molecular genetic or metabolic investigations, but it must usually await expert postnatal radiology
- Definitive diagnosis is essential in order to define recurrence risks (which can vary from <1% to 50%) and appropriate prenatal diagnosis in subsequent pregnancies. Parents and clinicians must be aware that diagnosis requires postnatal radiology and, where appropriate, pathology to achieve this
- In all cases, samples should be stored for DNA analysis, as increasingly, the genetic etiology for these conditions is being defined

INTRODUCTION

Congenital skeletal anomalies are not uncommon, occurring with an incidence of around 1:500. Many are amenable to prenatal detection using ultrasound. The underlying etiology is varied and includes:

- aneuploidy
- genetic syndromes
- skeletal dysplasias
- teratogens
- isolated anomalies secondary to disruption.

The sonographic detection of a fetus with a skeletal anomaly can present a challenging diagnostic dilemma, management options can be very varied and diagnosis may require biochemical, genetic or hematological investigation. Increasingly more sophisticated imaging such as magnetic resonance imaging (MRI) or computed tomography (CT) may elucidate features more easily interpreted by postnatal radiologists. Clinical genetic input is invariably useful, not only because the family history or parental examination may yield valuable clues to the diagnosis, but also this is a field which is evolving rapidly. This chapter will discuss the normal embryology and sonographic appearances of fetal limb development and go on to suggest a systematic approach to the diagnosis of fetal skeletal anomalies as well as describing some of the commoner conditions in more detail. Generalized skeletal dysplasias will be discussed as well as those groups of conditions associated with more localized limb anomalies which may or may not be part of a wider genetic syndrome. Accurate sonographic identification of skeletal abnormalities becomes increasingly important as more genes for skeletal conditions are identified, raising the potential for accurate prenatal diagnosis using molecular methods.

TERMINOLOGY

Fetal ultrasound diagnosis relies on the identification and accurate description of sonographic findings. Skeletal anomalies are associated with a range of genetic syndromes and dysplasias and discussion with other specialists (in particular clinical geneticists, radiologists and orthopedic surgeons) is necessary in order to try to define both the diagnosis and prognosis to inform accurate parental counseling. To be able to do this efficiently a good understanding of terminology is required. Normal bone nomenclature is illustrated in Figure 36.1. The terminology used in describing abnormalities of the limbs is given in Table 36.1.

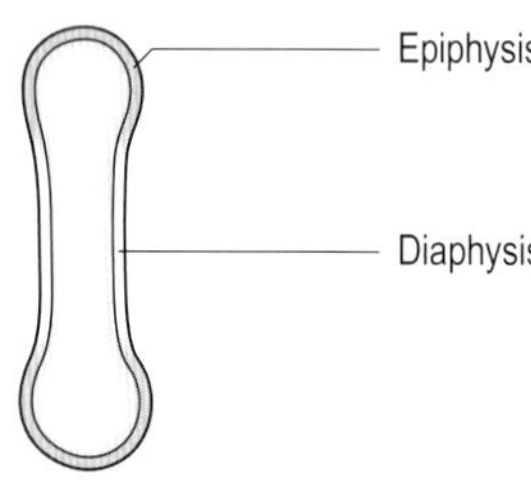

Fig. 36.1 Bone nomenclature.

Table 36.1 **Terminology used in describing skeletal abnormalities**

Achiria	Absent hand(s)		
Achiropodia	Absent hand(s) and feet		
Acromelia	Shortening of the distal segments of limbs, hands and feet		
Adactyly	Absent fingers and/or toes		
Amelia	Complete absence of one or more limbs from shoulder or pelvic girdle		
Apodia	Absent foot (feet)		
Arthrogryposis	Joint constractures developing before birth		
Brachydactyly	Short fingers		
Camptomelia	Bent limb or bent fingers		
Clinodactyly	Incurved 5th finger		
Ectrodactyly	Split hand(s) or feet (lobster claw deformity)		
Hemimelia	Absence of the distal arm or leg below the elbow or knee		
Kyphoscoliosis	Combination of lateral and anteroposterior curvature of the spine		
Kyphosis	Dorsal convex curvature of the spine		
Meromelia	Partial absence of a limb	Transverse Longitudinal Terminal Intercalary	Defect extending across the whole width of the limb Defects affecting one bone along an axis No bony part distal to the defect With recognizable parts distal to the defect
Mesomelia	Shortening of the middle segment of a limb (radius/ulna and tibia/fibula)		
Micromelia	Shortening of all long bones		
Oligodactyly	Absent or partially absent finger(s) and toe(s)		
Phocomelia	Hands and feet attached to shortened arm(s) and/or leg(s)		
Platyspondyly	Flattening of the vertebral bodies		
Polydactyly	Extra fingers or toes	Preaxial Postaxial	Extra digit on the radial or tibial side Extra digit on the ulna of fibular side
Rhizomelia	Shortening of the proximal long bones (femur and humerus)		
Scoliosis	Lateral curvature of the spine		
Syndactyly	Fused fingers +/− toes	Skin Osseous	Fu sed skin only Bony fusion
Talipes	Club-foot	Equinovalgus Equinovarus Equinus	Foot twisted outwards Foot twisted inwards Extended foot

Table 36.2 **Gestational age range for development of the human fetal skeleton**

Postmenstrual age (days)	*Upper limb development*	*Lower limb development*
40	Arm buds appear	
41–43		Lower limb bud appears
47–48	Elongated arm bud	
47–51	Hand paddle forms	
51–53	Fingers begin to separate	
54–56	Fingers distinct	
57–59		Toes appear
65–66	Fingers fully separated	
67–68		Toes fully separate

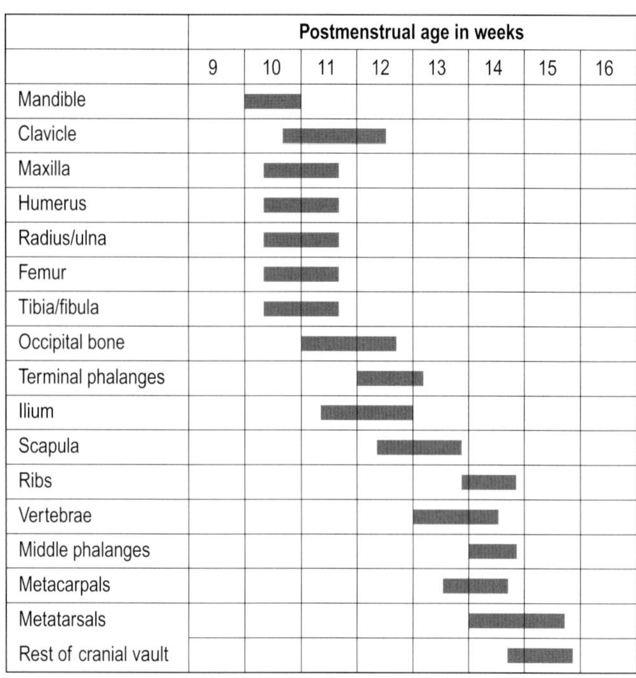

Fig. 36.2 Chart showing the appearance of skeletal structures using transabdominal ultrasound. Adapted from Brons et al.[2].

EMBRYOLOGY AND SONOGRAPHIC APPEARANCE OF THE NORMAL FETAL SKELETON

In the human, the upper limbs develop a few days in advance of the lower limbs, with the arm buds appearing at about five and a half postmenstrual weeks. Table 36.2 gives an outline of the early limb development in man[1].

The fetal skeleton forms in two ways: membranous ossification (clavicle and mandible) and intracartilanginous (endrochodral), when ossification occurs by calcium deposition in pre-existing cartilage matrix. Fetal ossification begins in the clavicle at around 8 weeks' gestation, followed by the mandible, vertebral bodies and neural arches around 9 weeks, the frontal bones at 10–11 weeks and the long bones around 11 weeks. Most skeletal structures can be identified sonographically by 14–15 weeks. The appearance of the ossification in the fetal skeleton has been studied both radiographically and sonographically, using transabdominal ultrasound and provides a useful indication of which structures should be identified when scanning in early pregnancy[2] (Fig. 36.2). Identification of anomalies of skeletal development requires not only detailed scanning but also aids such as charts of normal skeletal size, including length of long bones, clavicles, mandible, scapular, chest size, orbital diameters, renal size etc. Many of these can be found in the appendix[3–9]. Other workers have reported a range of charts for use in early pregnancy or when using transvaginal scanning[10].

CLASSIFICATION OF SKELETAL DYSPLASIAS

The genetic and pathological etiology of skeletal anomalies is wide and there have been several classifications used. These have evolved as the genetic and pathological understanding of these rare but complex disorders becomes clear. Classifications can be on clinical and/or radiological grounds[11], by molecular/genetic etiology or by structure and function of responsible genes and proteins (e.g. defects in structural proteins, metabolic pathways, transcription factors, etc.)[12] or a hybrid of both[13]. A classification based on sonographic findings is the most useful classification for the prenatal diagnostician (Table 36.3), but there can be considerable overlap in conditions and so a table listing the common diagnoses with gene location, where known, inheritance and main sonographic findings is also given (Table 36.4).

Clues to the diagnosis of skeletal anomalies

Risk factors for skeletal anomalies include:

- family history
- drugs in early pregnancy
- maternal disease
- abnormal findings on routine ultrasound.

Family history

Clearly, diagnosis in families where there has already been an affected child or when one parent is affected with a dominantly inherited condition can be more straightforward than interpretation of findings that arise de novo. Knowledge of the sonographic features and natural history of the condition can aid prenatal diagnosis, but parents do need to be aware that some conditions, e.g. achondroplasia, may present relatively late and not be amenable to diagnosis until well into the second trimester, with others being more variable, e.g. hypochondroplasia, and not obvious until after birth or in early childhood. For these reasons, molecular diagnosis using chorionic villus sampling may be preferable in families where the gene has been

Table 36.3 Classification of skeletal dysplasias according to major sonographic finding

Sonographic finding	*Condition*	*Other investigations to be considered*
Skull		
Hypomineralized	Osteogenesis imperfecta IIA and IIC Achondrogenesis type I Hypophospatasia (severe neonatal form)	(Phosphoethanolamine in parental urine)
Mild hypomineralization	Achondrogenesis type 2 Cleidocranial dysostosis Osteogenesis imperfecta IIB	
Cloverleaf	Thanatophoric dysplasia type II Occasionally in SRPSs (short ribbed polydactyly syndromes) Antley-Bixler Craniosynostosis syndromes (Pfeiffer/Crouzon/Saethre–Chotzen)	Screen for mutations in FGFR3 and 2 genes
Spine		
Hypomineralized	Achondrogenesis type I	
Disorganized	Jarcot Levine Syndrome Spondylocostal dysplasia Dyssegmental dysplasia Some chondrodysplasia punctatas Vertebral defects, Analatresia, Tracheo-Esophageal fistula and Radial dysplasia, or Vertebral anomalies, Analatresia, Cardiac malformations, Tracheo-Esophageal fistula, Renal anomalies and Limb anomalies (VATER/VACTERL)	
Face		
Frontal bossing	Thanatophoric dysplasia Achondroplasia Acromesomelic dysplasia	Screen for mutations in FGFR3 gene
Depressed nasal bridge	Chondrodysplasia punctatas Warfarin embryopathy	Drug history, mutations in ARSE gene, metabolic investigations – very long chain fatty acids and sterol profile, maternal history of autoimmune disease
Micrognathia	Spondylo-epiphyseal dysplasia congenita (SEDC) Stickler's syndrome Camptomelic dysplasia	
Cleft lip	Majewski syndrome Orofaciodigital Syndrome IV (OFD IV)	
Legs		
Isolated, straight short long bones	Intra-uterine growth restriction (IUGR) Constitutional short stature	Fetal and maternal Doppler
Femoral bowing	Camptomelic dysplasia Osteogenesis imperfecta Hypophospatasia	Karyotype – sex reversal in males
Talipes	Camptomelic dysplasia Diastrophic dysplasia	
Stippled epiphyses	Rhizomelic chondrodysplasia punctata Conradi Hunermann X-linked recessive chondrodysplasia punctata Warfarin embryopathy	Drug history, mutations in ARSE gene, metabolic investigations – very long chain fatty acids and sterol profile, maternal history of autoimmune disease

(Continued)

Table 36.3 Continued

Sonographic finding	*Condition*	*Other investigations to be considered*
Limb girdles		
Short clavicles	Camptomelic dysplasia Cleidocranial dysostosis	
Small scapula	Camptomelic dysplasia	
Hands		
Polydactyly	Jeunes asphyxiating thoracic dystrophy Ellis van Creveld syndrome Short ribbed polydactyly syndromes	
Short fingers/trident hand	Achondroplasia Acromesomelic dysplasia Thanatophoric dysplasia	
Thorax		
Narrow with short ribs	Short ribbed polydactyly syndromes Jeunes asphyxiating thoracic dystrophy Thanatophoric dysplasia Osteogenesis imperfecta types IIA, C and B Camptomelic dysplasia Achondrogenesis Hypochondrogenesis Paternal UPD14	
Beaded ribs	Osteogenesis imperfecta type IIA and C	
Polyhydramnios	Achondroplasia Thanatophoric dysplasia Paternal UPD14	

identified before pregnancy. With rapid advances in molecular genetics, the underlying genetic etiology for many of these conditions is known and it is imperative that tissue is available from affected pregnancies if parents are subsequently to be availed of early testing. In many conditions, multiple mutations in large genes can be responsible for the features and extensive genetic analysis prior to pregnancy is required before prenatal molecular testing can be offered. Many families may wish to avoid the risks associated with invasive prenatal testing. The advent of non-invasive testing using free fetal DNA in the maternal plasma will mean that parents will increasingly be able to get a diagnosis without risk as this technology progresses[14]. Nonetheless, genetic work-up prior to pregnancy will be required for this technology as well as for traditional invasive testing.

Drugs in early pregnancy

While drugs are now extensively tested before release onto the market, there are still those used regularly that may result in skeletal malformations if taken in early pregnancy (Table 36.5)[15]. Furthermore, there is good evidence that some recreational drugs, if used in early pregnancy, can cause skeletal anomalies, a postulated vascular effect being responsible for some drugs (e.g. cocaine).

Maternal disease

The most common maternal conditions that can result in fetal musculoskeletal anomalies (Table 36.6) include:

- diabetes
- myasthenia gravis
- myotonic dystrophy.

Other conditions, such as systemic lupus erythematous (SLE) and hypothyroidism, can also cause skeletal changes, but less commonly. Poorly controlled insulin-dependent diabetes is the most common maternal condition that can result in significant skeletal anomalies in the fetus, which include developmental field defects of the spine, caudal regression syndrome, deficiencies of the limbs (particularly femoral hypoplasia) and arthrogryposis, as well as anomalies of other viscera, in particular the urogenital tract[16]. In maternal myasthenia gravis, transmission of acetycholine receptor antibodies to the fetus can result in generalized arthrogryposis and neonatal or infant death[17]. In some instances, the antibodies are specific to the fetal subunit of the acetylcholine receptor and the mother may be asymptomatic. Myotonic dystrophy is an autosomal dominantly inherited condition which, when transmitted maternally to the fetus, can result in congenital myotonic dystrophy (CMD). Mothers who have clinically detectable neuromuscular manifestations

Table 36.4 Skeletal dysplasias: gene location, inheritance and sonographic findings

Diagnosis	*Gene/ location*	*Genetics*	*Gestation at presentation*	*Limbs*				*Thorax*		*Spine*	*Skull*	*Other features*
				Short	*Bowed*	*Fingers*	*Joints*		*Ribs*			
Achondrogenesis I	DTDST	AR	12	+++				Narrow	Short, ± beaded	Hypo	Hypo	Edema
Achondrogenesis II[22]	COL2A1	AD	12	++				Narrow	Short			
Achondroplasia[36,53,55,57]	FGFR3	AD	>24	+	± Mild	Short		± Small				Frontal bossing
Acromesomelic dysplasia	NPR2	AR	Around 22	+		Short		± Small				Frontal bossing
Beemer–Langer[66]	Unknown	AR	Around 20	+		Poly		Small	Short		Cloverleaf	
Camptomelic dysplasia[40,41,42]	SOX9	AD	16–20, var	Legs	Legs		Talipes	± Small				Micrognathia, cardiac defects, sex reversal in males
Conradi Hunermann Chondrodysplasia punctata (CDP)[52]	EBP	X-linked dominant	Var	+, Stippled						Stippled		
Diastrophic dysplasia[60,61]	DTDST	AR	>16	+		Hitch-hiker thumbs	Talipes					Micrognathia
Ellis van Creveld[33,39]	EVC	AR	From 16	+		Poly		Narrow	Short			Cardiac anomaly
Hypophosphatasia (severe neonatal form)[24–27,65,69]	TNSALP	AR	>12	++	++						Hypo	
Jeunes asphyxiating thoracic dystrophy		AR	From 16 variable	+		± Poly		Narrow	Short			CNS anomaly
Kneist	COL2A!	AD	Var	+	Mild			Short				Micrognathia, depressed nasal bridge

(Continued)

Table 36.4 Continued

Diagnosis	*Gene/ location*	*Genetics*	*Gestation at presentation*	*Limbs*				*Thorax*		*Spine*	*Skull*	*Other features*
				Short	*Bowed*	*Fingers*	*Joints*		*Ribs*			
Majewski[64,67]	Unknown	AR	>12	++	Ovoid tibia	Poly		Narrow	Short ++			Renal, cardiac, CNS, genital
Osteogenesis imperfecta IIA/C and IIC[30–33]	COL1A1 COL1A2	AD, gm	>12	+++	+++			Narrow	Short, beaded		Hypo	
Osteogenesis imperfecta IIB[30,32,33]	COL1A1 COL1A2	AD, gm	>16	++	+			(Narrow)	(Beaded)			
Osteogenesis imperfecta III[43,48]	COL1A1 COL1A2	AD, gm	20	+	Legs							
Osteogenesis imperfecta IV	COL1A1 COL1A2	AD, gm	>20		Mild, femora							
Rhizomelic CDP[50,51]	RCDP1,2,3	AR	20	Rhizomelic, stippled						Stippled		Nasal hypoplasia, cataracts
Saldino-Noonan[70]	Unknown	AR	>12	++		Poly		Narrow	Short ++			Renal, cardiac, genital
Spondylo-epiphyseal dysplasia congenita (SEDC)[35,36]	COL2A1	AD	>12	++				Short				Micrognathia
Thanatophoric dysplasia I[34,37]		AD	<16	Severe micomelia,	(Mild)	Short, trident		Small ++	Short ++		Normal	Frontal bossing
Thanatophoric dysplasia II		AD	<16	Severe micromelia	(Mild)	Short trident		Small ++	Short ++		Cloverleaf	Frontal bossing
X-linked recessive CDP[63]	ARSE	X-linked	Var	+, Stippled		Short				Stippled		Stippled larynx and trachea

Table 36.5 **Skeletal anomalies associated with drug use in early pregnancy**

Drug/substance	*Skeletal anomalies*	*Other sonographic findings*
Warfarin	Rhizomelic shortening of limbs, stippled epiphyses, kyphoscoliosis	Flat face, depressed nasal bridge, renal, cardiac and CNS anomalies
Sodium valproate	Reduction deformity of arms, polydactyly, oligodactyly, talipes	Cardiac and CNS anomalies
Methotrexate	Mesomelic shortening of long bones, hypomineralized skull, syndactyly, oligodactyly, talipes	CNS anomalies including neural tube defects, micrognathia
Vitamin A	Hypoplasia or aplasia of arm bones	CNS and cardiac anomalies, spina bifida, cleft lip and palate, diaphragmatic hernia, exomphalos
Phenytoin	Stippled epiphyses	Micrognathia, cleft lip, cardiac anomalies
Alcohol	Short long bones, reduction deformity of arm bones, preaxial polydactyly of hands, oligodactyly, stippled epiphyses	IUGR, cardiac anomalies
Cocaine	Reduction deformities of arms +/− legs, ectrodactyly, hemivertebrae, absent ribs	CNS, cardiac, renal anomalies, anterior abdominal wall defects, bowel atresias

Table 36.6 **Sonographic clues in the fetal skeleton to maternal disease**

Sonographic findings	*Maternal condition*	*Maternal diagnosis*
Caudal regression Femoral hypoplasia	Diabetes	Glucose tolerance test
Multiple joint contractures Arthrogryposis	Myasthenia gravis	Anticholinesterase antibodies
Talipes and polyhydramnios	Myotonic dystrophy	Examine for signs of myotonia, facial appearance, genetic referral
Short limbs, stippled epiphyses, depressed nasal bridge	Systemic lupus erythematous	Autoimmune screen, history

of myotonic dystrophy have between a 10–50% risk of having a baby with CMD[18,19]. In pregnancy, characteristic sonographic findings include talipes, decreased fetal movements/breathing and polyhydramnios. Affected neonates are very floppy and often have respiratory problems requiring ventilatory support. Mortality is high (20%). Most survivors have significant developmental delay and a reduced life expectancy. The finding of talipes and polyhydramnios in a euploid fetus should stimulate examination of the mother for signs of myotonic dystrophy. Maternal systemic lupus erythematosus (SLE) can cause a variety of problems in the fetus including limb shortening with stippled epiphyses, facial anomalies, in particular a depressed nasal bridge and an abnormal appearance of the spine secondary to extra calcification. Other findings can include bradycardias, growth retardation and hydrops[20].

Sonographic features of skeletal malformations

The first clue that there may be a skeletal anomaly present is often the identification of a short femur at the time of a scan for another reason, either a routine fetal anomaly scan at around 20 weeks' gestation or a scan later in pregnancy for other indications. Careful examination of the rest of the fetal anatomy can reveal further signs of a skeletal dysplasia (Table 36.7). If limb shortening appears to be isolated, then intrauterine growth retardation must be considered as a possible etiology. In these circumstances, review of maternal serum screening results for levels of pregnancy-associated placental protein A (PAPP-A), beta human chorionic gonadotrophin (beta-hCG) and maternal serum alpha-fetoprotein (MSAFP) and assessment of fetal and maternal Doppler can be useful diagnostic aids. In a 4-year period at University College London Hospital (UCLH), of 130 fetuses referred with 'abnormal' femora (short, bowed, hypoplastic), 42 fetuses were thought to have short straight femurs/limbs with no other sonographic abnormalities detected. Only two of these had a skeletal dysplasia. Many were normal and had either had an incorrect assignment of gestational age or familial short stature, but 31% had IUGR (Fig. 36.3).

Skull

The skull should normally be rugby-football in shape and cast a good acoustic shadow indicating normal mineralization. Decreased mineralization is indicated by an anechoic skull vault which casts little or no acoustic shadow (see Fig. 36.8a). Furthermore, the intracranial contents will be more clearly visualized than normal and, as the cerebral hemispheres appear

Table 36.7 **Sonographic examination required when suspecting a skeletal abnormality**

Anatomical part	*Features*
Long bones	Length Pattern of shortening Short trunk – short limbs predominantly Rhizomelic – mesomelic – acromelic Symmetrical – asymmetric Which bones Bowing/evidence of fractures Width Ossification Epiphyses for stippling
Spine	Length Mineralization Alignment (hemivertebrae) Organization (stippling)
Cranium	Shape Mineralization (acoustic shadow)
Face	Profile – frontal bossing Depressed nasal bridge Micrognathia Cleft lip Cleft palate Orbital diameters for hypo- or hypertelorism
Chest	Size Ribs – length shape beading (fractures)
Hands	Short fingers (trident hand) Camptodactyly Ectrodactyly Polydactyly Oligodactyly
Feet	Size Polydactyly
Joints	Contractures Pterygia Talipes Radial club hand
Associated abnormalities	Cardiac abnormalities Renal anomalies Intracranial abnormalities Genital anomalies
Fetal and maternal Doppler	Screen for IUGR

relatively anechoic, the appearances are not infrequently mistaken for cerebral ventriculomegaly. Careful examination will reveal the characteristic and hyperechoic normally located choroid plexus (see Fig. 36.8a). In conditions associated with

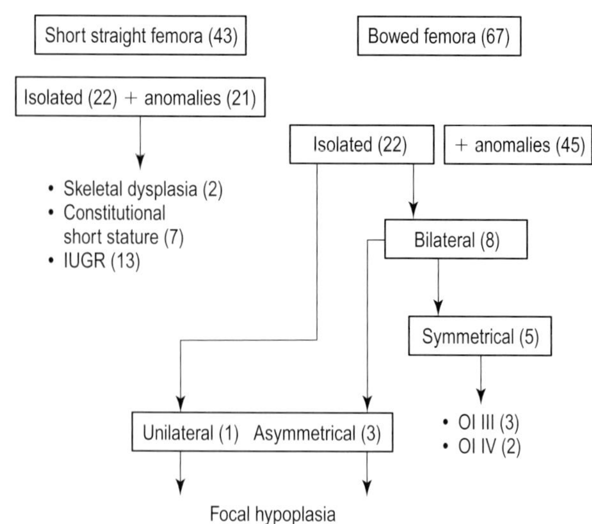

Fig. 36.3 Etiology of femoral abnormalities seen in a 4-year period at UCLH.

hypomineralization in later pregnancy, the skull shape can readily be deformed by pressure from the transducer. Variation in skull shape can be seen rarely in some craniosynostosis syndromes and the cloverleaf skull is seen in thanatophoric dysplasia type II (see Fig. 36.10i).

Spine

The spine should be examined carefully in all three orthogonal planes. There may be absent or decreased mineralization, but it must be remembered that ossification of the cervical and sacral vertebral bodies is a late event; the sacral vertebral bodies are not ossified until 27 weeks' gestation. Osseous maldevelopment as in hemivertebrae (Fig. 36.4a) can occur with or without associated rib anomalies. The appearance of general disorganization may indicate ectopic calcification seen in some chondrodysplasia punctatas (Fig. 36.4b,c) or bony abnormalities as in Jarcot Levin syndrome (Fig. 36.4d,e).

Face

Many skeletal dysplasias have associated facial anomalies. The face should be examined in the coronal view to exclude a cleft lip which, in some conditions such as oral facial digital syndrome type IV or Ellis van Creveld, can be very small and difficult to detect (Fig. 36.5a,b). An axial view of the palate should be visualized in order to detect significant degrees of cleft palate which can be associated with several dysplasias. A sagittal view will reveal micrognathia, flattening of the facial profile, frontal bossing or a depressed nasal bridge. Measurement of the mandible and orbital diameters can be useful, but may be more difficult to achieve in later pregnancy with increasing acoustic shadowing from surrounding bony structure (see appendix).

Long bones

Length of long bones should be checked against appropriate charts of long bone length (see appendix). The pattern of shortening is a useful diagnostic aid. There may be generalized shortening of all long bones (micromelia). It may be more marked in the proximal long bones (rhizomelia) or the forearms and

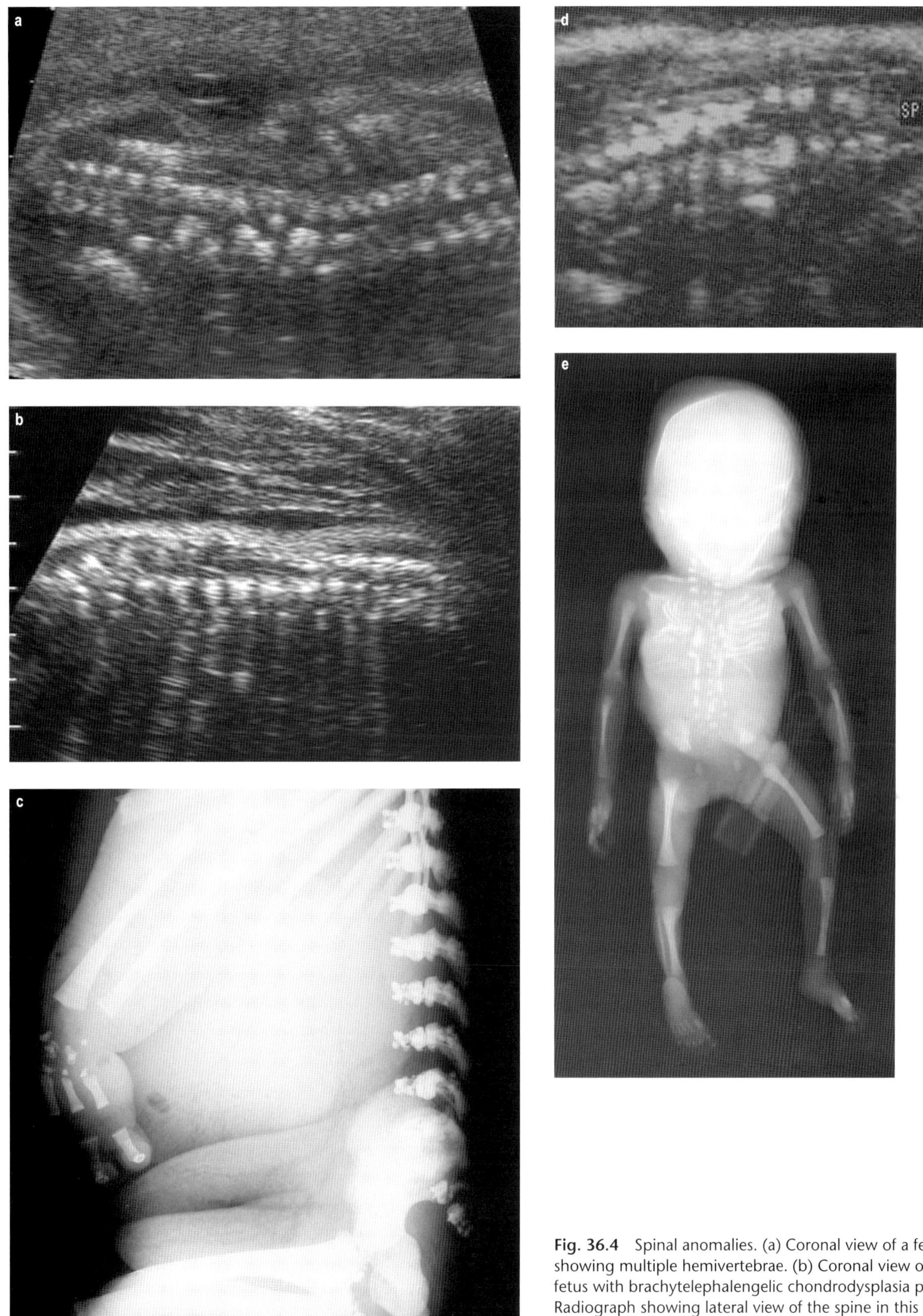

Fig. 36.4 Spinal anomalies. (a) Coronal view of a fetal spine showing multiple hemivertebrae. (b) Coronal view of a spine in a fetus with brachytelephalengelic chondrodysplasia punctata. (c) Radiograph showing lateral view of the spine in this neonate with brachytelephalengelic chondrodysplasia punctata. (d) Coronal view of a spine in a fetus with Jarcot Levin syndrome. (e) Radiograph of the fetus with Jarcot Levin syndrome.

lower legs (mesomelia). In some conditions, the changes may be confined to the legs (e.g. camptomelic dysplasia) or arms (e.g. Holt Oram). Deformation of the bones is a very useful diagnostic feature. The position and degree of bowing or fracturing should be noted, bones may appear short, thick and crumpled indicating severe degrees of fracturing and undermodeling (see Fig. 36.8d,e). Deformity, hypoplasia or absence of tibia, fibula, radius or ulna may be present. The ends of the bones should be carefully examined to exclude epiphyseal stippling that might indicate a chondrodysplasia punctata (see Figs 36.18, 36.19c,d). If stippling is identified, there are various metabolic and cytogenetic investigations that can be done in order to try to define the underlying etiology (see section on chondrodysplasia punctata below). Expanded metaphyses may be seen in Kniest syndrome.

Joints

The joints may be abnormal in a number of conditions and talipes, in particular, can be a feature of several dysplasias. There may be fixed flexion deformities, with or without webbing or pterygia.

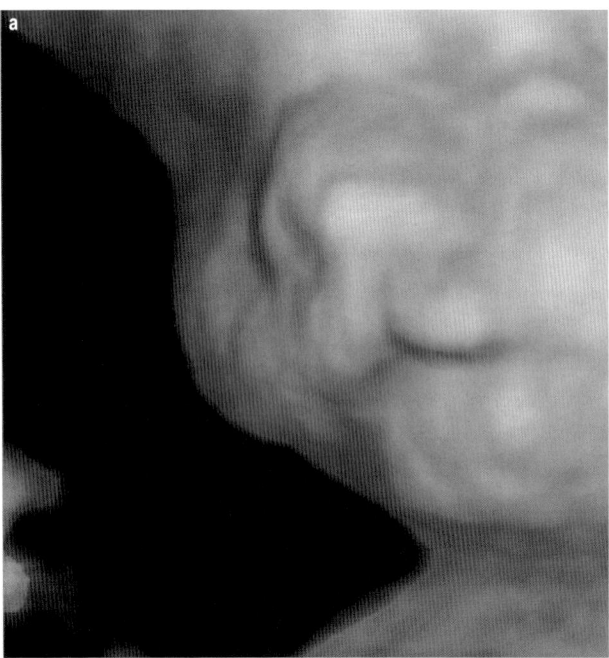

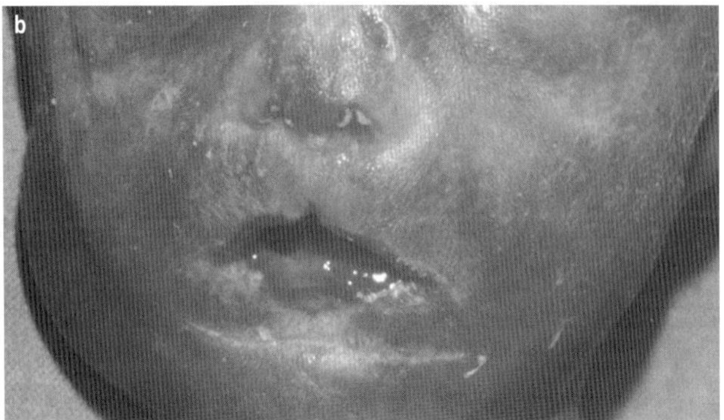

Fig. 36.5 Small midline cleft lip as may be found in Majewski, OFD IV or Ellis van Creveld. (a) 3D-ultrasound image showing the small cleft lip (arrow) in the axial plane. (b) Coronal view after birth.

Hands and feet

Polydactyly, either pre- or postaxial, can be a feature of a number of conditions (Fig. 36.6a,b). Oligodactyly, ectrodactyly and syndactyly are less common features (Fig. 36.6c,d,e) but are good clues to the diagnosis when present. Rocker bottom feet are seen in trisomy 18 and some of the contractural syndromes (Fig. 36.6f).

Limb girdles

The limb girdles, shoulder and pelvis, can be more difficult to examine. However, some skeletal dysplasias have hypoplastic clavicles (cleidocranial dysostosis) or scapulae (camptomelic dysplasia).

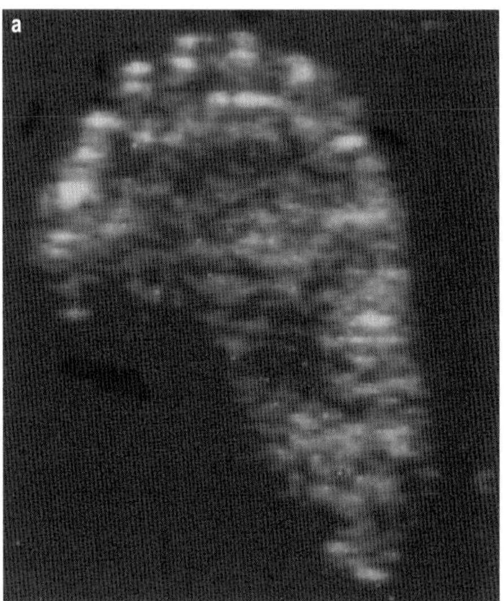

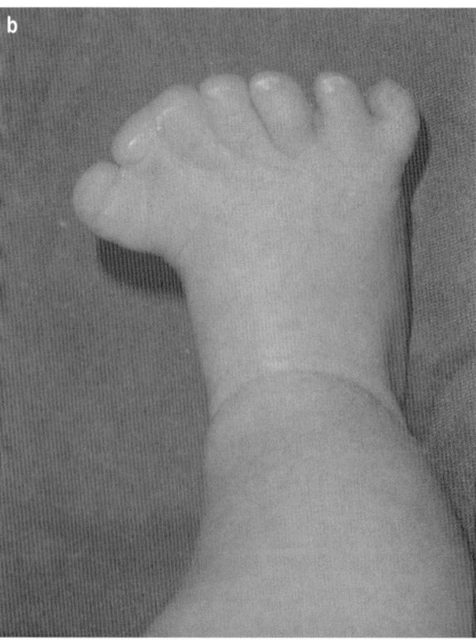

Fig. 36.6 Clues to the diagnosis that may be found in the hands and feet. (a) Ultrasound image of preaxial polydactyly of the feet in Greigs acrocephalopolysyndactyly. (b) The view of this foot after birth. (c) Oligodactyly in a case with Cornelia de Lange syndrome. (d) Ultrasound image showing the syndactyly resulting in the mitten hand seen in Apert syndrome. (e) The same hand as in (d) but visualized using 3D ultrasound. (f) Rocker bottom foot.

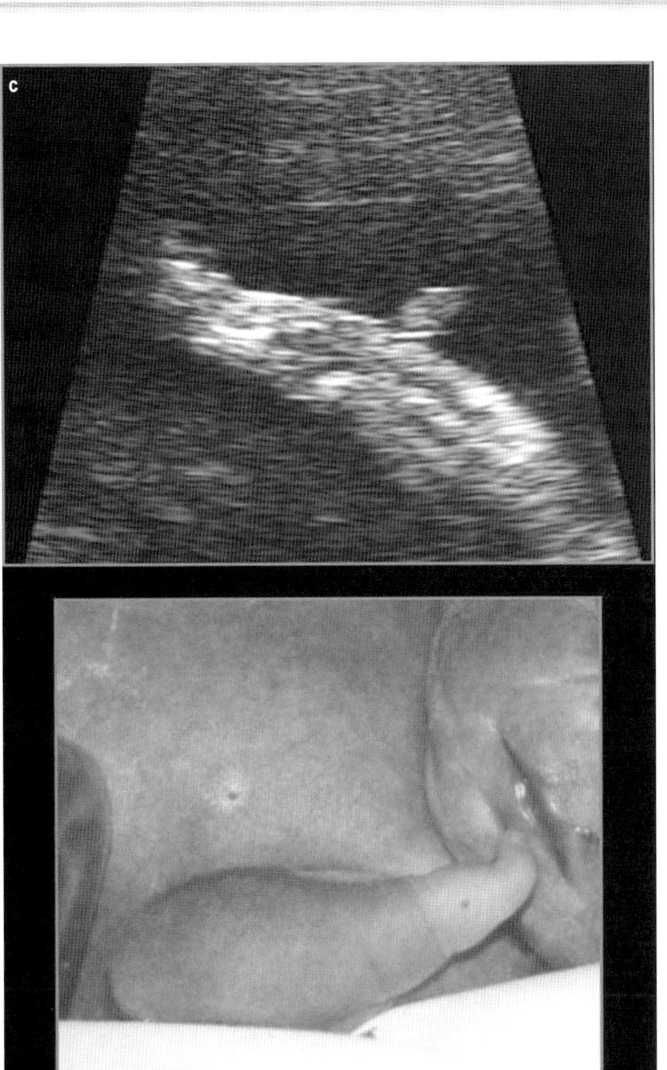

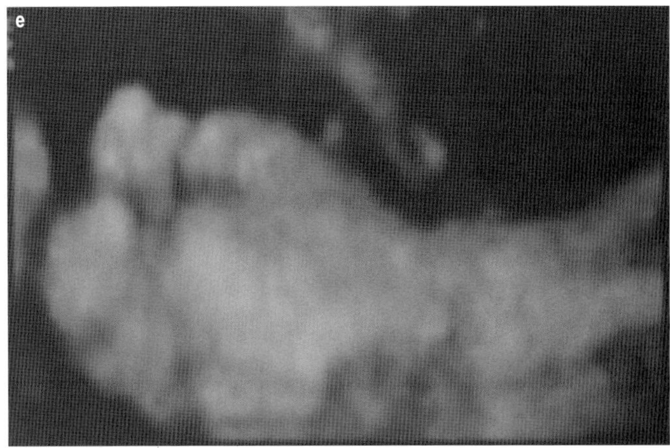

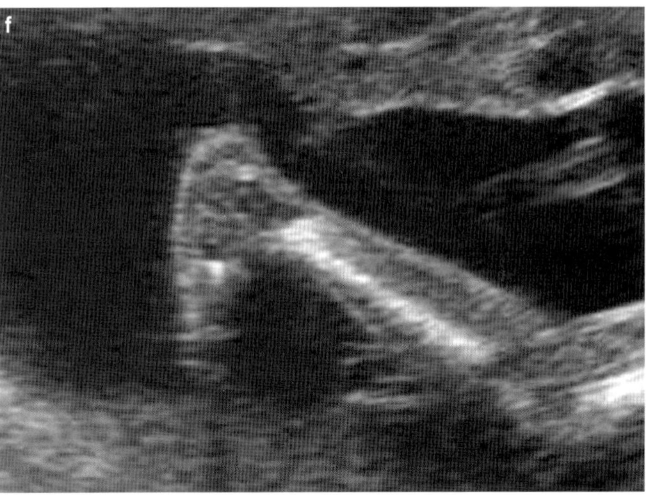

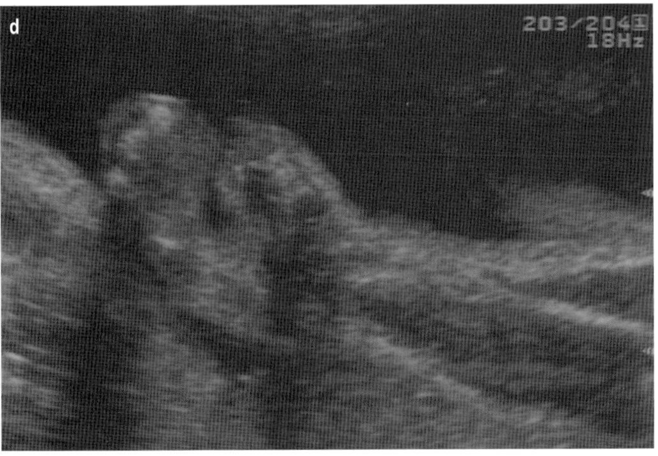

Fig. 36.6 Continued

Thorax

Many lethal dysplasias are associated with thoracic abnormalities. Nomograms of thoracic circumference are available (see appendix), but a small chest can often be inferred by observation alone. In normal circumstances, the thorax and abdomen should be approximately the same size viewed in the axial plane, and comparison can help indicate a small chest (see Figs 36.9d, 36.10c). The heart should normally occupy one third of the chest. If the ribs are short, the heart will appear to occupy a greater proportion of the chest when viewed in the axial plane and, when there is extreme shortening of the ribs, the heart may appear to lie outside the thoracic cavity (see Fig. 36.11b). In sagittal section, the thorax will be narrow and the abdomen protuberant, a configuration that has given rise to the expression 'champagne-cork

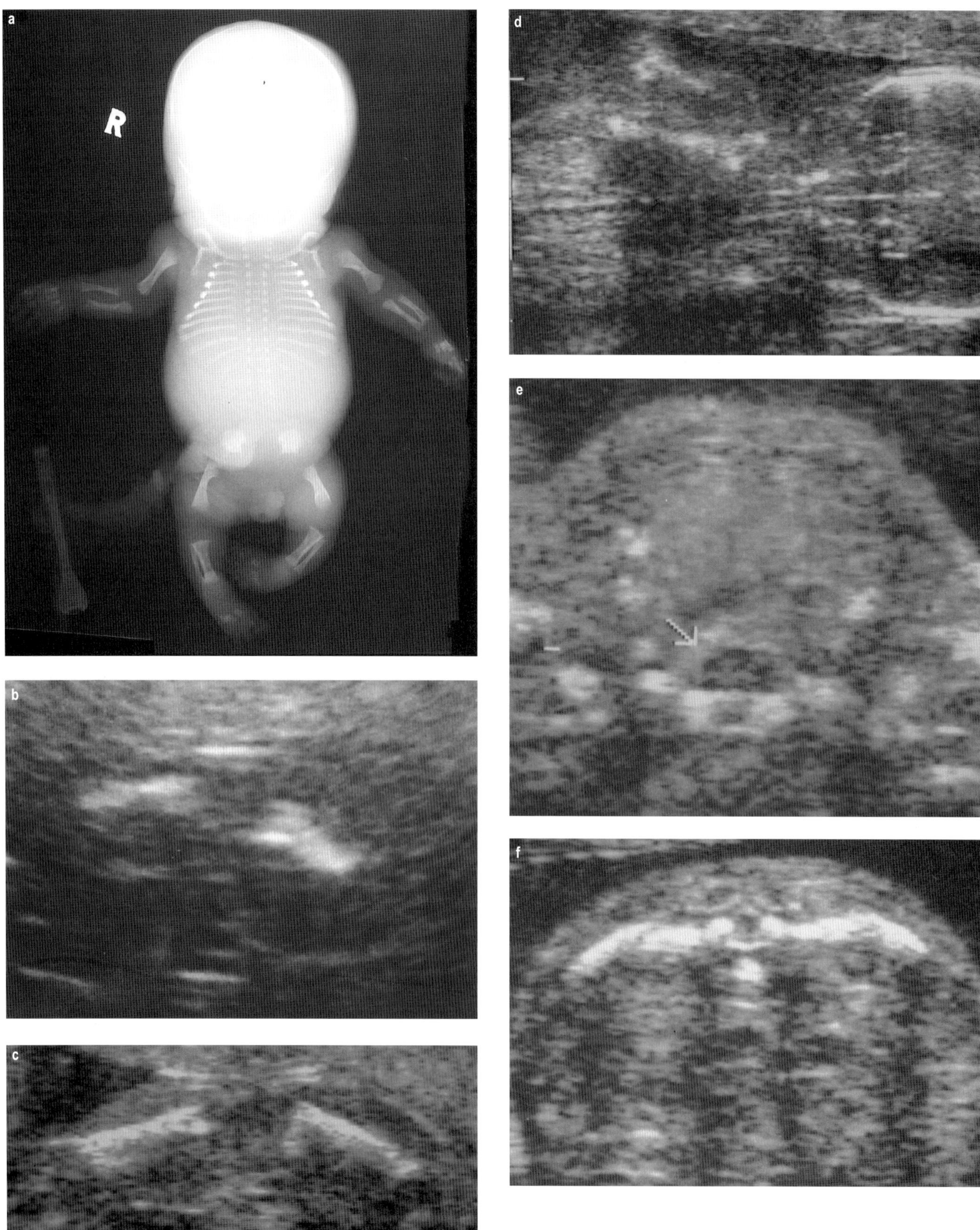

Fig. 36.7 Sonographic findings in achondrogenesis. (a) Radiograph of a fetus with achondrogenesis type II. (b) Very short straight leg bones, showing mesomelic shortening. (c) Very short straight arm bones. (d) Coronal view of the spine showing the 'tram-line appearance' due to hypomineralization of vertebral bodies. (e) Transverse section through a thoracic vertebra demonstrating the hypomineralization of the vertebral body. (f) Transverse section through the lower thorax showing very short ribs. (g) Sagittal view of the cervical spine demonstrating the nuchal edema and hypomineralized cervical spine.

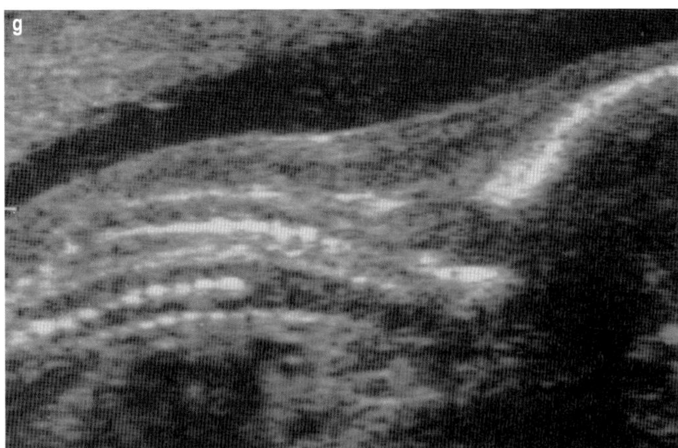

Fig. 36.7 Continued

appearance' (see Fig. 36.10b). The chest can also be small secondary to a short spine as in some of the spondylodysplasias. In these situations, the chest may appear small in a sagittal plane but, when viewed in the axial plane, the ribs appear of normal length and the heart occupies the appropriate proportion of the thoracic cavity. Nomograms of thoracic length are available. The ribs themselves should be examined carefully as they may be short, thick, thin, beaded or irregular in organization or number. Short ribs can be viewed in the axial plane (see Figs 36.7f, 36.9e) and they should be examined in a longitudinal plane to exclude beading which is indicative of fracturing (see Figs 36.8c, 36.9f). Disorganization of the ribs (and spine) may be features of conditions such as Jarcot Levine syndrome (see Fig. 36.4d).

Increased nuchal translucency and oedema

One of the earliest signs of a musculoskeletal problem is an increased nuchal translucency which has been reported in many skeletal dysplasias[21]. Later in pregnancy, this is represented by an increased nuchal fold and generalized skin thickening, as the skin appears to outgrow the bones. In some conditions, frank hydrops can also occur.

Other structures

The rest of the fetal anatomy should be examined carefully as many skeletal dysplasias and genetic syndromes characterized by skeletal anomalies can have abnormalities of the urogenital tract, heart and brain (see Table 36.4).

DESCRIPTION OF INDIVIDUAL CONDITIONS – GENETICS AND SONOGRAPHIC FINDINGS

There are increasing reports of the prenatal detection of a variety of conditions associated with skeletal abnormalities in the literature. A few of those generalized skeletal dysplasias which are seen more commonly, although all are rare, will be described in detail here. In some cases, a definitive diagnosis can be made antenatally following genetic mutation or metabolic analysis but, for the majority, detailed postnatal radiology, and sometimes histopathology, is required in order to make a definitive diagnosis. This is needed in order to counsel parents with regard to recurrence risks and to inform accurate prenatal diagnosis in future pregnancies. However, in a few families, postnatal examination is declined and, in these situations, detailed sonographic information can be the only diagnostic aid available.

Dysplasias associated with hypomineralization

Achondrogenesis type IA
Gene unknown
Autosomal recessive

Achondrogenesis type IB
Gene location 5q31-34
Diastrophic dysplasia sulfate transporter gene (DTDST)
Autosomal recessive

Achondrogenesis type II
Gene location 12q13-14
COL2A1
Autosomal dominant

Achondrogenesis type I (Parenti-Fraccaro type) and type II (Langer-Saldino type) are difficult to distinguish clinically, but postnatal differentiation radiologically after birth is vital as type I is inherited in an autosomal recessive fashion (1:4 recurrence risk), but type II is usually sporadic (low recurrence risk). Type I results from homozygous mutations in the diastrophic dysplasia sulfate transporter gene (DTDST). Achondrogenesis type II (Fig. 36.7a) probably represents the most severe end of the spectrum of the type II collagenopathies which includes hypochondrogenesis, Kniest dysplasia and spondyloepiphyseal dysplasia congenita (SEDC). Defects of type II collagen synthesis have been demonstrated in some cases[22] and, in most cases, are caused by new dominant mutations in the COL2A1 gene. Both conditions result in stillbirth (or neonatal death). Sonographic features include micromelia with very short but straight long bones (Fig. 36.7b,c), a relatively large hypomineralized skull (in type I), a short neck, a short trunk with a protuberant abdomen, hypomineralization of the vertebral bodies (Fig. 36.7d,e) and very short ribs (Fig. 36.7f). Other sonographic features include skin oedema (Fig. 36.7g) and polyhydramnios. Both conditions have a flat nasal bridge with a short nose and anteverted nostrils. Sonographically and radiologically ossification of the skull, spine and pelvis is more deficient in type I than in type II. The long bones are shorter in type I, which has been subdivided into types A (Houston-Harris type) and B (Parenti-Fraccaro type)[23]. Multiple rib fractures and almost complete lack of ossification of the spine are seen in type IA cases.

Hypophosphatasia
Gene locus 1p36.1-p34
Tissue-non-specific alkaline phosphatase gene (TNSALP)
Autosomal recessive

This condition occurs in congenital/infantile, childhood or adult forms correlating with the severity of the reduction in activity of tissue non-specific alkaline phosphatase. All have reduced chondro-osseous mineralization with low levels of alkaline phosphatase in blood, cartilage and bone, together with increased levels of plasma pyridoxal 5′-phosphate and urine phosphoethanoloamine. Measurement of alkaline

Table 36.8 **Features in different categories of osteogenesis imperfecta**

Type of OI	*Gestation at presentation*	*Prenatal features*	*Other postnatal findings*
Type I	Usually postnatal, occasionally 3rd trimester	Occasional fractures late in 3rd trimester	Wormian bones, blue sclera, variable fracturing
Type IIA	>12 weeks	Hypomineralized easily deformable skull, beaded ribs, small chest, very short, crumpled long bones	Lethal
Type IIB	>16 weeks	Mild hypomineralized skull, short and bowed long bones, short flared ribs with occasional beading	Usually perinatally lethal
Type IIC	>12 weeks	As with IIA, but a greater degree of hypomineralization	Lethal
Type III	Around 20 weeks	Bowed leg bones, occasional bowed radius and ulna. Normal skull mineralization, normal chest with very occasional beading. Long bones progressively fall below 5th centile	Early lethality common. Increased fractures, fractured ribs, progressive deformity in survivors
Type IV	From 20 weeks	Long bones often within normal range. Normal skull and chest. Mild bowing of femur and tibia	Variable prognosis. May have rib fractures at birth

phosphatase levels in chorionic villi can be diagnostic[24]. It is the severe neonatal form that is detectable using fetal ultrasound. Affected pregnancies usually result in stillbirth or neonatal death secondary to pulmonary hypoplasia. The severe neonatal form is due to homozygous mutations in the tissue-non-specific alkaline phosphatase gene (TNSALP) and, as such, is inherited in an autosomal recessive fashion with a 1:4 recurrence risk for parents. Sonographic features include a hypomineralized skull, which can assume a globular shape, short and angulated long bones. Unusual bony spurs can occur at the point of the sharply angulated femora[25]. Long bones are also poorly mineralized[26]. Prenatal diagnosis by direct mutational analysis of the TNSALP gene is possible in families at known increased risk where molecular analysis has confirmed a mutation in the TNSALP gene[24,27]. The concentration of phosphoethanolamine can be elevated in the urine of mutation carriers and this can be a useful aid to diagnosis in cases arising de novo in a family.

Osteogenesis imperfecta types IIA, IIB and IIC
Gene locus 17q21.31-q22, 7q22.1
COL1A2 collagen I, alpha-2 polypeptide
COL1A1 collagen I, alpha-1 polypeptide
Autosomal dominant, autosomal recessive, germline mosaicism

Osteogenesis imperfecta (OI) is a disorder of connective tissue that may affect 1–2:10000 individuals. There are several types which result from multiple different mutations in the collagen genes, COL1A1 and COL1A2[28]. The severity of the clinical features is related to the type of mutation and the relative level of expression. Most mutations associated with OI are inherited in a dominant pattern and an autosomal recessive inheritance is very rare but has been described. Most severe cases of OI are caused by new dominant mutations. The recurrence risk after an isolated case is about 5–7% which is thought to be mainly due to somatic/gonadal mosaicism in one of the parents[29,30].

The most commonly used classification is that described by Sillence in 1979[31] (Table 36.8). Type I is the mildest form and usually only presents with fractures occurring after birth. Occasional cases of prenatal detection in the late third trimester have been reported. OI type II refers to a group of severely affected neonates who do present with prenatal sonographic abnormalities and who usually die in the perinatal period. Type II has been further subdivided into subtypes IIA, IIB and IIC according to radiological features. Subtype IIB is characterized by minimal or no rib fractures. The relatively normal chest configuration renders it to be the only form of type II with potential postneonatal survival. Type III is the most severe form which is compatible with life and does present with prenatal shortening and fracturing of the long bones. Type IV is the most diverse group in the classic classification. The more severely affected patients in type IV OI, present with fractures at birth, which can occasionally be detected using prenatal ultrasound. New forms of OI (types V–VII) based on analysis of bone architecture, have been recently added to the classification[28]. Theses types are moderately deforming and, prior to the introduction of the new classification would probably have fallen within the type IV classification.

Type II osteogenesis imperfecta is the severe, usually lethal form which is associated with varying degrees of hypomineralization. Sonographically, types IIA and IIC are difficult to differentiate, although while both types IIA and IIC have hypomineralized skull and facial bones, this is more extreme in IIC (Fig. 36.8a,b). In both types there is continuous beading of the ribs (Fig. 36.8c) indicating multiple fractures. The long bones are broad and crumpled and it can be difficult to

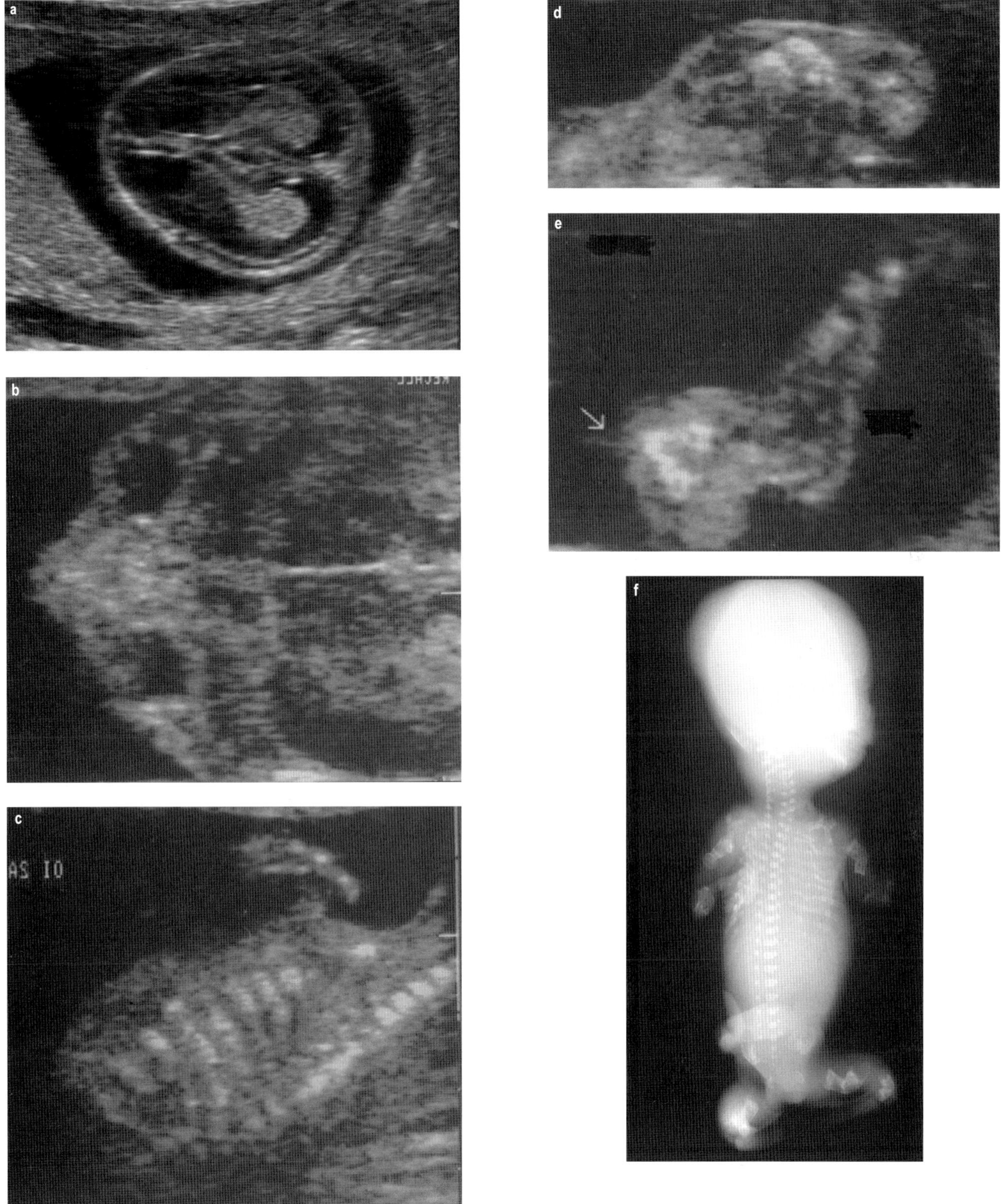

Fig. 36.8 Sonographic findings in the osteogenesis imperfecta types IIA and IIC. (a) Hypomineralized skull. Note the lack of acoustic shadow and clarity of intracranial contents. (b) Hypomineralized facial bones. (c) Beaded ribs. (d) Short crumpled arm bone. (e) Bent distal leg, note the relatively normal length foot with absent mineralization. (f) Radiograph of a fetus with osteogenesis imperfecta type IIC.

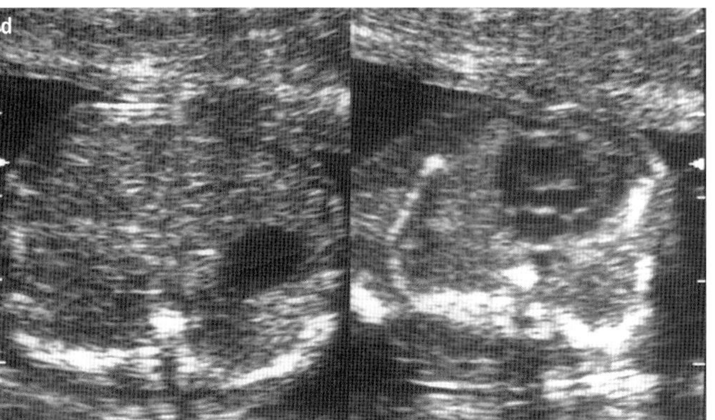

Fig. 36.9 Sonographic findings in osteogenesis imperfecta type IIB (Zahid). (a) View of the skull which does cast an acoustic shadow in the axial plane. (b) The face and frontal bones in this case of OI IIB are mineralized, but note the decreased echoes from the rest of the skull. (c) The sagittal view of the thorax and abdomen shows slight narrowing of the chest. (d) Axial view comparing the size of the thorax and abdomen demonstrating the slightly small chest. (e) In the axial view of the thorax the slightly short ribs with flared ends can be seen. (f) The sagittal view of the ribs shows some beading. (g) The femur is short and angulated. (h) The tibia and fibula are short, but foot length is preserved. (i) The humerus is short and angulated. (j) Fetal femur size chart showing the normal range with measurements from fetuses with OI IIA, IIB, III and IV plotted.

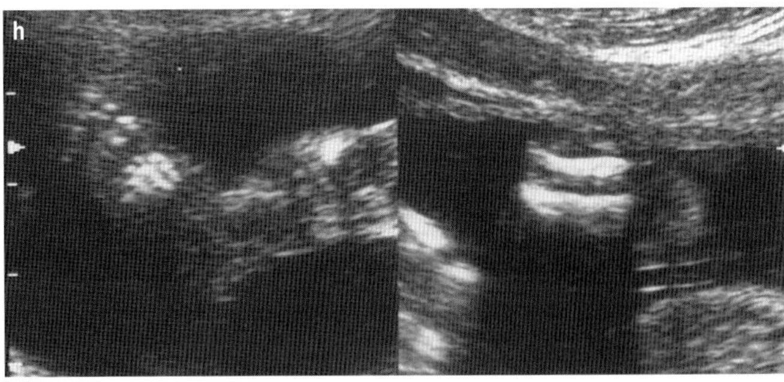

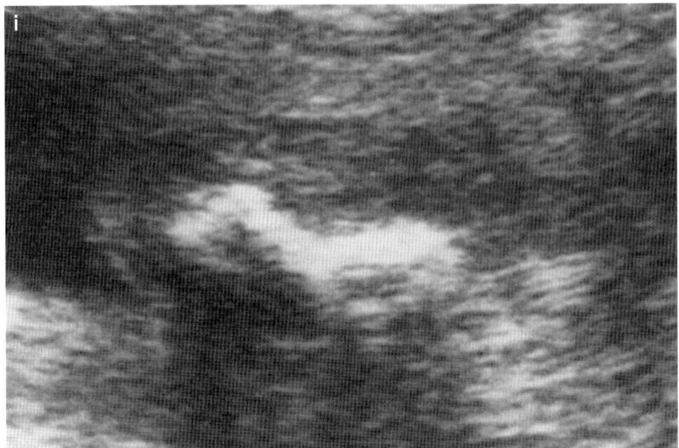

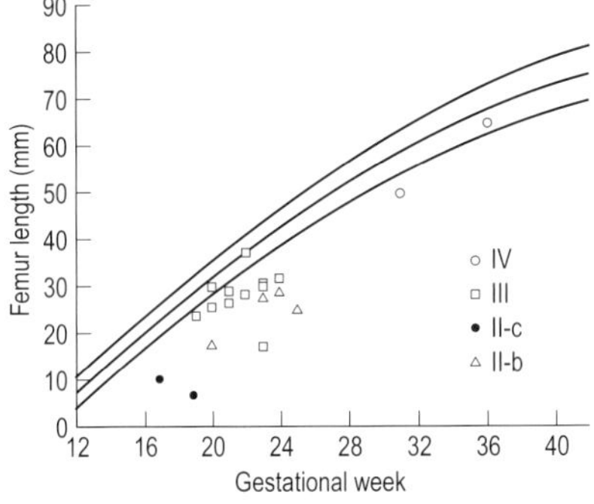

Fig. 36.9 Continued

identify individual bones in the distal limbs (Fig. 36.8d,e). The vertebrae are flattened and hypoplastic and the pelvis is hypoplastic with flattening of the acetabular roofs and iliac crests, but these are features seen more commonly on postnatal radiology (Fig. 36.8f). As with other lethal skeletal dysplasias, an increased nuchal translucency can be an early presenting feature[21,32].

In type IIB, sonographic findings are less severe. The skull can show mild degrees of hypomineralization (Fig. 36.9a,b), but this can be difficult to recognize sonographically. The chest is less obviously affected (see Fig. 36.7c,d) but, in the axial plane, there is a typical configuration with slightly short ribs which flare outwards at the ends (Fig. 36.9e) and rib fractures, while universally present after birth, can be difficult to identify antenatally with beading sometimes obvious (Fig. 36.9f). The long bones are longer and better modeled but show obvious angulation secondary to fracturing (Fig. 36.9g,h,i).

Prenatal diagnosis using molecular and biochemical methods in 129 cases with different types of osteogenesis imperfecta has been described[33]. However, as the genes responsible for this condition are large with many potential mutations and the recurrence risk is generally small, ultrasound is usually the preferred method for prenatal diagnosis in subsequent pregnancies.

Dysplasias associated with a small chest

Achondrogenesis types 1 and 2 – see above
Osteogenesis imperfecta types IIA and IIC – see above

Thanatophoric dysplasia
Gene location 4p16
Fibroblast growth factor receptor gene (FGFR3)
Lethal autosomal dominant, germline mosaicism

This is the most common lethal skeletal dysplasia with an incidence of around approximately 1:20 000. There are two types, I and II. At least 10 mutations in the FGFR3 gene have been shown to cause type 1[34]. Most of these mutations substitute an incorrect amino acid in the fibroblast growth factor receptor 3 protein. The most common mutation is a substitution of the amino acid cysteine for the amino acid arginine at position 248 (Arg248Cys). Other mutations cause the protein to be longer than normal. The mutated receptor is active independent of ligand binding, causing the severe problems with bone growth seen in this condition. Only one mutation has been shown to cause type II thanatophoric dysplasia[34]. This change occurs in a different part of the FGFR3 gene than the mutations that cause type 1. The mutations arise de novo and recurrence risks are very low (<1%) incorporating a small germline mosaicism risk.

Thanatophoric dysplasia is a disorder characterized by short long bones (Fig. 36.10a), with or without bowing, very short ribs, short fingers giving rise to the classical trident hand, platyspondyly and relative macrocephaly with frontal bossing (Fig. 36.10b–g). There are two types, type 1 is the commoner subtype and is distinguished by the presence of curved femora and flattened vertebral bodies (platyspondyly). An unusual head shape, cloverleaf skull, is occasionally seen with type 1 and in virtually all cases of type 2 (Fig. 36.10h–j).

Short ribbed polydactyly syndromes (SRPS)
Gene location unknown
Autosomal recessive inheritance

The short rib polydactyly syndromes comprise a group of lethal skeletal dysplasias all of which have a small thorax secondary to short ribs, short limbs, pre- and postaxial polydactyly and a variety of other visceral anomalies. There are four main categories:

1. SRPS I (Saldino–Noonan type)[70]
2. SRPS II (Majewski)[64, 67]
3. SRPS III (Verma–Naumoff)[68]
4. SRPS IV (Beemer–Langer)[66].

All are inherited in an autosomal recessive fashion and there is considerable phenotypic overlap between the conditions. There are occasional case reports describing their prenatal detection. Sonographic features include an increased nuchal translucency, varying degrees of long bone shortening, a small chest with short ribs, polydactyly and a variety of visceral abnormalities which predominantly include renal dysplasia, bladder outflow obstruction, cardiac and intracerebral anomalies (Fig. 36.11; Table 36.9). Facial clefting is a feature of some of

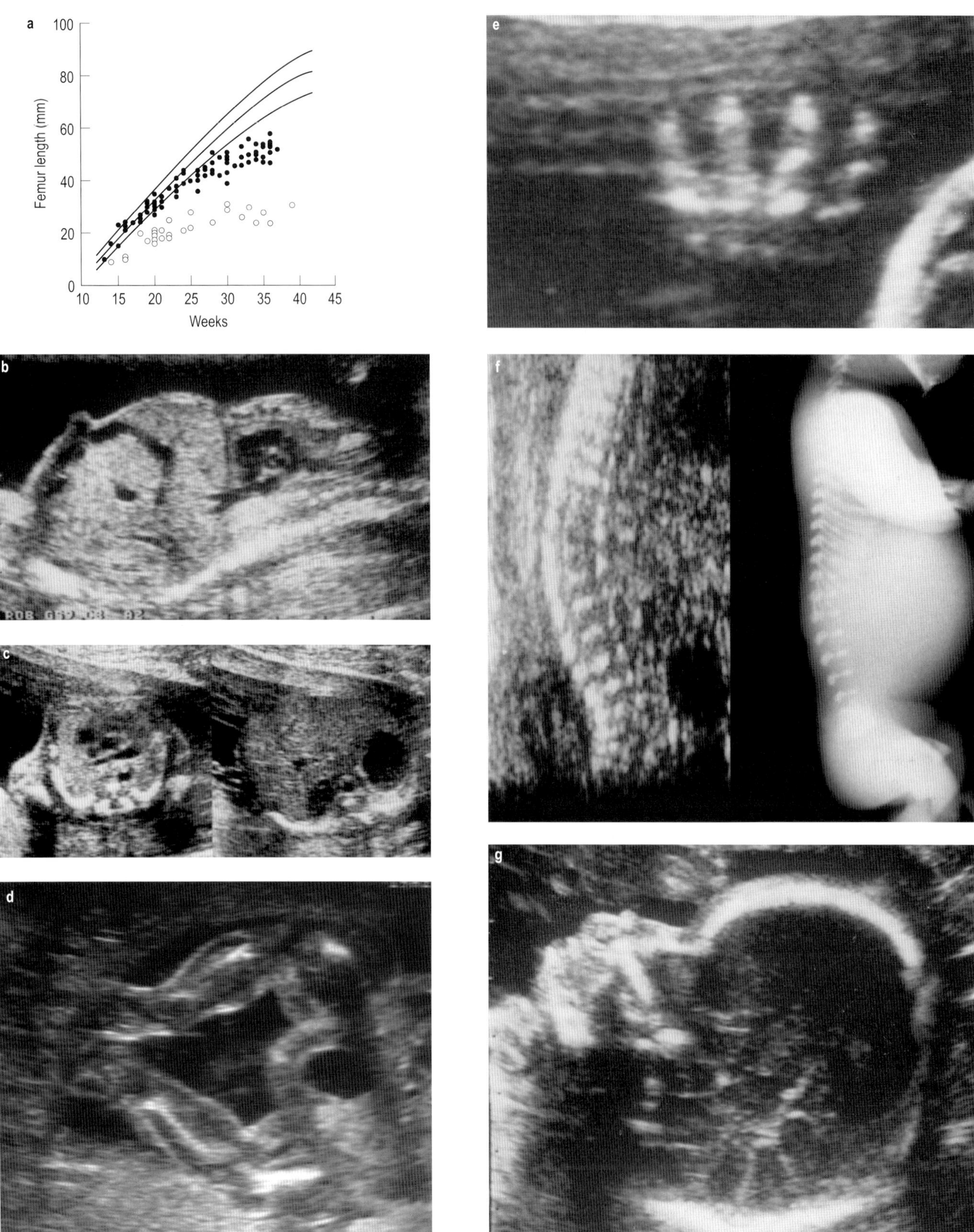

Fig. 36.10 Sonographic findings in thanatophoric dysplasia. (a) Chart of femur length showing the size of the femurs in thanatophoric dysplasia (lighter dots) and achondroplasia (darker dots). (b) Sagittal view of the thorax showing the typical 'champagne cork' appearance. (c) Axial view showing the comparison between the thorax and abdominal circumferences. Note how short the ribs appear in this plane, finishing half way around the thorax such that the heart has no protection from the ribs. (d) View of the short legs in the typical 'frog-like' position. (e) A view of the short fingers showing the 'trident hand appearance'. (f) Sagittal ultrasound and radiological view of the spine demonstrating the marked platyspondyly. (g) Profile at around 22 weeks' showing marked frontal bossing.

Continued.

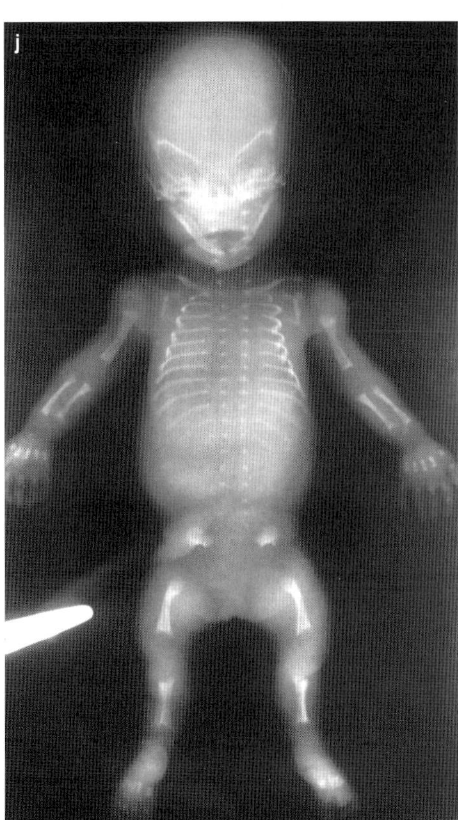

Fig. 36.10 *Continued.* (h)Axial view through the fetal head at 14 weeks, demonstrating early signs of a cloverleaf skull. (i) A cloverleaf skull at 22 weeks. (j) Radiograph of a fetus with thanatophoric dysplasia.

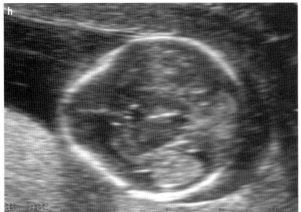

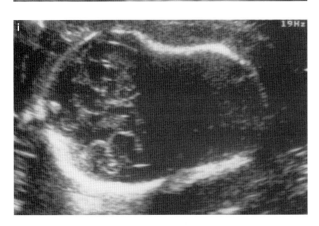

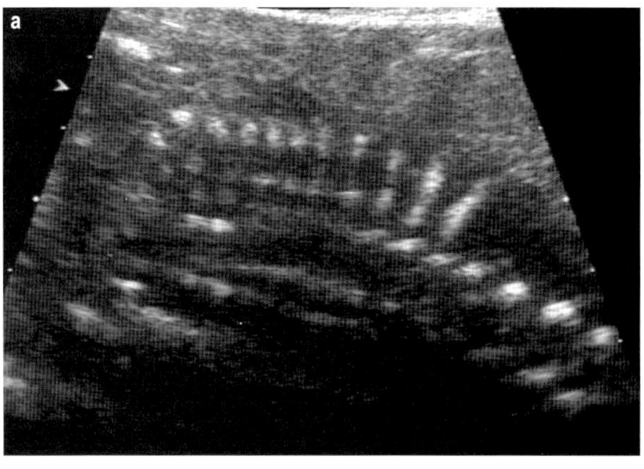

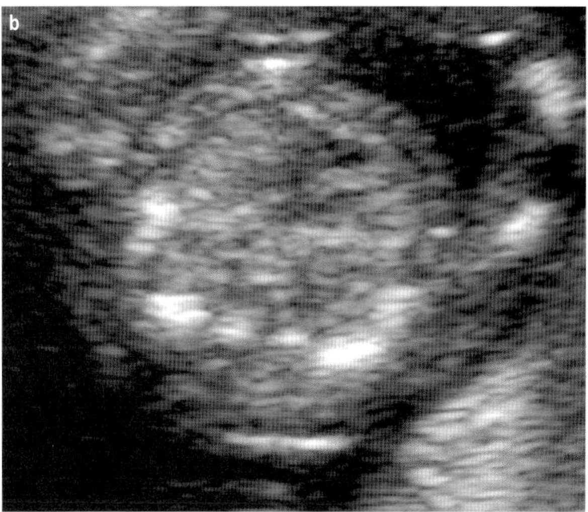

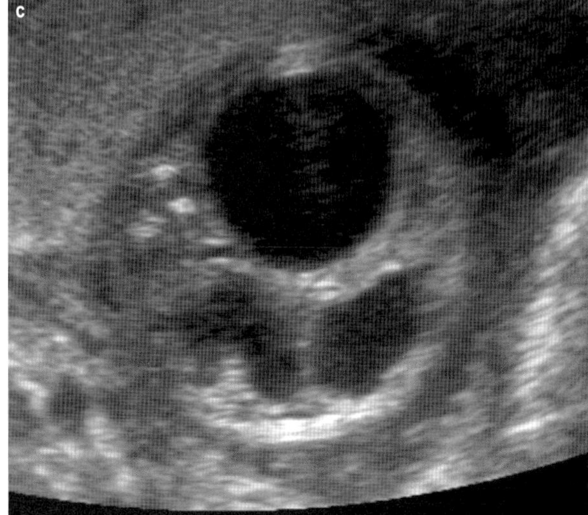

Fig. 36.11 Sonographic findings in short ribbed polydactyly syndromes (SRPS). (a) Longitudinal view through the thorax of a fetus with SRPS demonstrating the extremely short ribs. (b) The thorax of this fetus viewed in the axial plane with the heart appearing to lie virtually outside the thorax. (c) Axial view through the abdomen in this fetus with SRPS and obstructive uropathy.

Table 36.9 **Features that may be sonographically detected in short ribbed polydactyly syndromes**

	Saldino–Noonan	*Majewski*	*Verma–Naumoff*	*Beemer–Langer*
Short ribs	+	+	+	+
Short limbs	+	+	+	+
Bowed limbs				Radius, ulna
Other skeletal anomaly	Hypoplastic/absent fibula, hypoplastic ilia, metaphyseal dysplasia	Hypoplastic or absent tibia, ovoid tibia	Hypoplastic ilia	Talipes, small scapula, hypoplastic ilia
Preaxial polydactyly		Fingers		Fingers, including bifid thumb
Postaxial polydactyly	Fingers and toes	Fingers and toes	Fingers and toes	Fingers
Craniosynostosis				Clover-leaf skull
Macrocephaly		+		+
Hypertelorism				+
Micrognathia		+		
Cleft palate		+	+	+
Midline cleft lip		Midline	Midline	Midline
CNS anomalies		+		+
Ambiguous/absent genitalia	+	+	+	+
Vaginal atresia ± hydrometacolpus	+	+	+	
Cardiac abnormalities	+	+	+	+
Bowel atresias	Anal atresia	+	+	+
Exomphalos				+
Renal dysplasia	Renal cysts	+	+	+
Urinary tract obstruction				+
Edema/hydrops	Ascites	+		Skin edema, ascites

these conditions, for example in Majewski syndrome, a small midline cleft lip may be a distinguishing feature (see Fig. 36.5).

Spondyloepiphyseal dysplasia congenita (SEDC)
Gene locus 12q13.11-q13.2
COL2A1 gene
Autosomal dominant

The incidence of SEDC is around 1:100 000 and is due to mutations in the COL2A1 gene[35]. Affected individuals are very short with a short trunk and marked lordosis. Other complications include myopia, micrognathia, cleft palate and deafness. Prenatally, shortening of the limbs is evident from around 12 weeks' gestation (Fig. 36.12a). Other findings include an increased nuchal translucency, micrognathia, poorly mineralized cervical vertebrae in early pregnancy and a small chest secondary to a short trunk, but normal ribs (Fig. 36.12b,c)[36]. In early pregnancy, the main differential diagnosis is with thanatophoric dysplasia which can be distinguished by screening for mutations in the FGFR3 gene[37]. Later in pregnancy, achondroplasia and acromesomelic dysplasia would be the main differential diagnoses. These may be distinguished from SEDC as this condition does not have relative macrocephaly, frontal bossing or short fingers (Fig. 36.12d).

Jeunes asphyxiating thoracic dystrophy
Gene locus 15q13
Autosomal recessive

This is a rare autosomal recessive condition characterized by variable degrees of rhizomelic shortening of the long bones (Fig. 36.13d) and a small chest with short ribs (Fig. 36.13a,b). Up to 50% of affected individuals have postaxial polydactyly (Fig. 36.13c). Intracerebral anomalies can occasionally occur. Neonatal death from respiratory difficulties secondary to pulmonary hypoplasia is common, occurring in around 70% of cases. Survivors may develop chronic renal failure due to cystic changes and peri-glomerular fibrosis in childhood and also have an increased risk of retinal degeneration, hepatic and pancreatic fibrosis. The limb shortening is usually rhizomelic and the condition might be mistaken for achondroplasia, but the facial contours are normal. Prenatal sonographic findings are

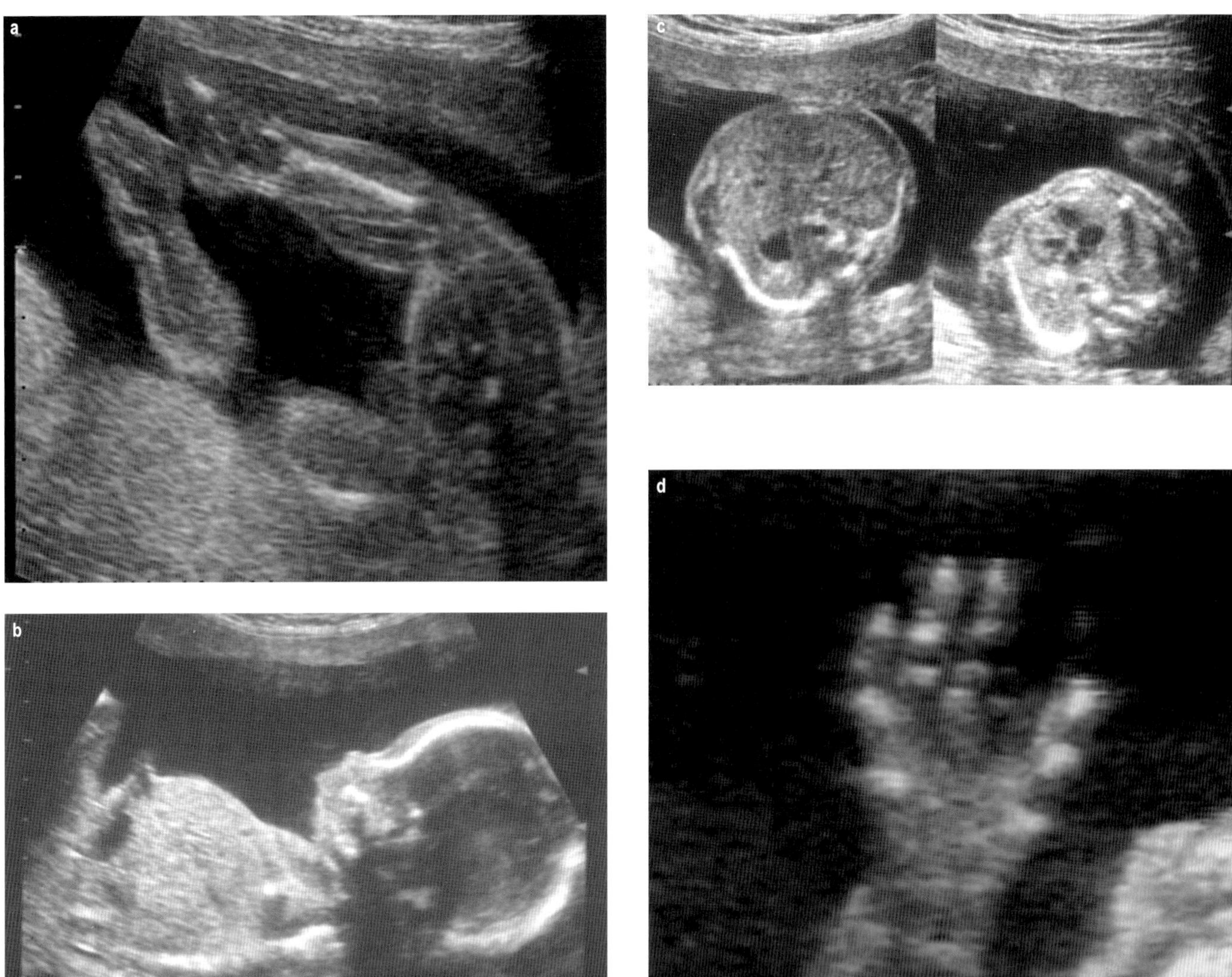

Fig. 36.12 Sonographic findings in spondyloepiphyseal dysplasia congenital (SEDC). (a) Short, straight limbs in SEDC at around 18 weeks. (b) Sagittal view of a fetus with SEDC at 18 weeks demonstrating micrognathia, but no frontal bossing and a short thorax. (c) Axial view through the chest and abdomen at 18 weeks. Note that the chest appears slightly small but the heart only occupies one-third of the chest and the ribs are of normal length. (d) The hand in SEDC with normal length fingers compared with those seen in thanatophoric dysplasia at around the same gestation (see Fig. 36.10e).

variable, but presentation can be from around 16 weeks' gestation with short limbs and a long narrow chest. The main differential diagnosis is Ellis van Creveld syndrome and paternal uniparental disomy for chromosome 14 (UPD14).

Ellis van Creveld syndrome
Gene locus 4p16, 4p16
EVC gene
Autosomal recessive

Ellis-van Creveld syndrome is a rare, autosomal recessive skeletal dysplasia characterized by disproportionate short stature, short limbs, short ribs, postaxial polydactyly, midline cleft or notched upper lip and dysplastic nails and teeth[38,39]. Around 60% of affected individuals have a congenital cardiac defect, often an atrial-ventricular septal defect. Some neonates have respiratory difficulties secondary to the small chest, but this is rarely serious. Sonographic findings include short long bones (Fig. 36.14a), polydactyly in the hands and feet (Fig. 36.14b), a narrow thorax with short ribs with or without a cardiac abnormality (Fig. 36.14c). The differential diagnosis includes Jeunes asphyxiating thoracic dystrophy and other short ribbed polydactyly syndromes, although many of these will have more profound manifestations.

Paternal Uniparental Disomy for chromosome 14
This condition results in a distinctive phenotype which can be recognized and diagnosed antenatally. It typically results in increased nuchal translucency with subsequent small chest size with coat hanger-shaped ribs, anterior abdominal wall defects ranging from marked diastasis recti to exomphalos, polyhydramnios and mild limb contractures. It is most commonly misdiagnosed as Jeunes asphyxiating thoracic dystrophy both pre- and postnatally. The postnatal chest radiograph is diagnostic. Where

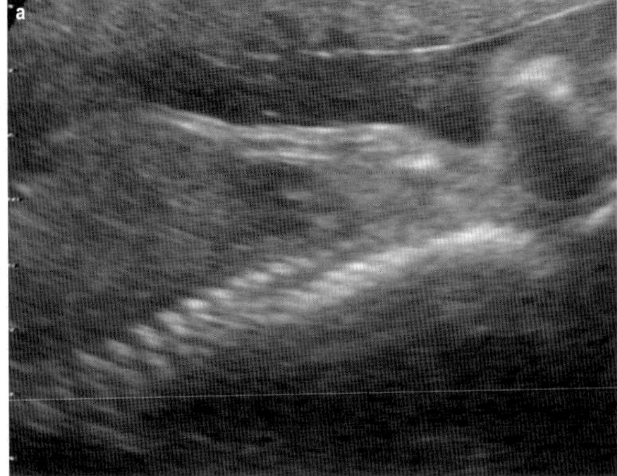

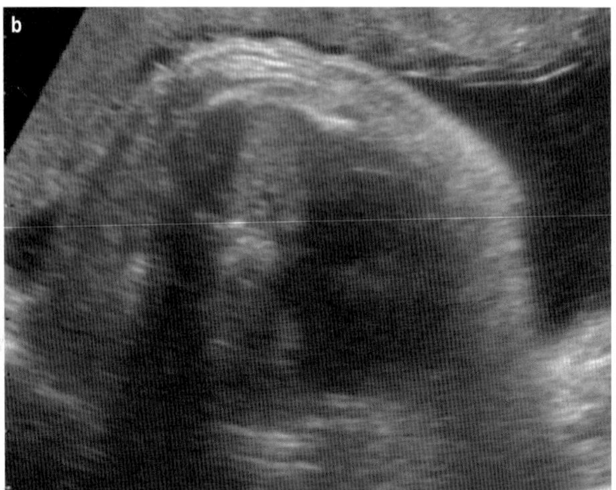

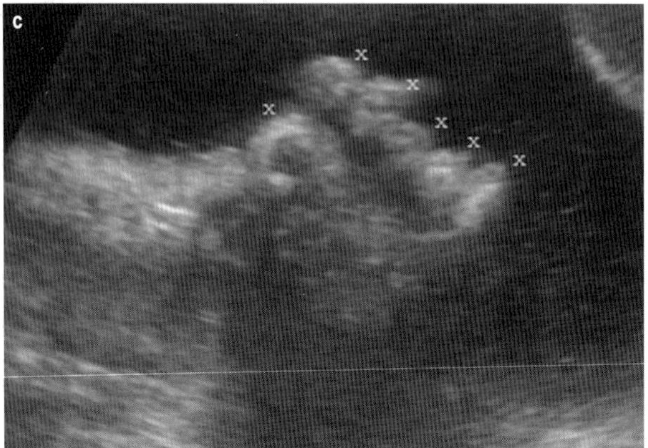

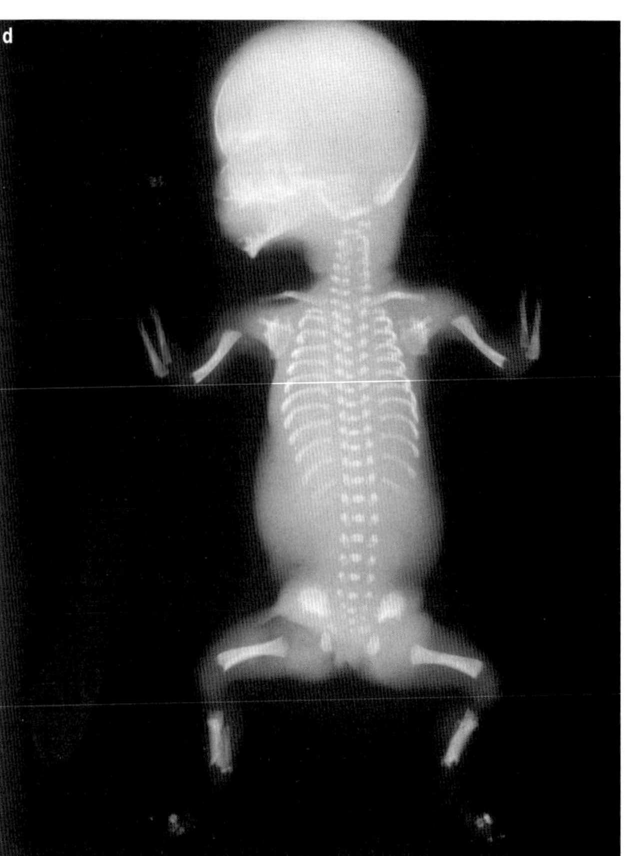

Fig. 36.13 Jeunes asphyxiating thoracic dystrophy. (a) Sagittal view of the thorax demonstrating the narrow chest. (b) Axial view of the thorax demonstrating the short ribs with heart occupying more than one-third of the chest. (c) View of clenched hand with 5 fingers and a thumb (marked by x). (d) Radiograph of a 20-week fetus with Jeunes asphyxiating thoracic dystrophy demonstrating the features, including short but straight limbs.

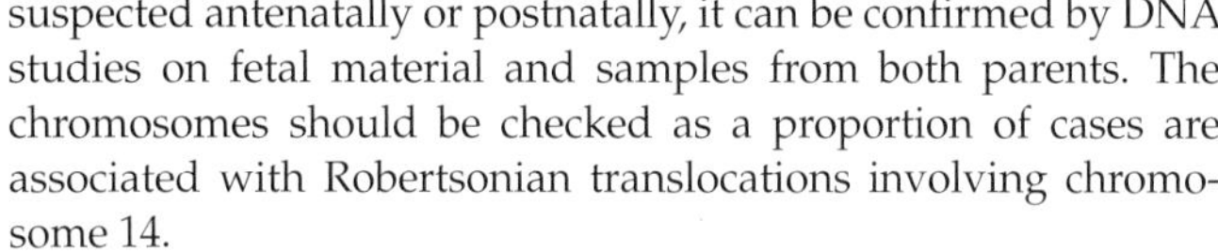

suspected antenatally or postnatally, it can be confirmed by DNA studies on fetal material and samples from both parents. The chromosomes should be checked as a proportion of cases are associated with Robertsonian translocations involving chromosome 14.

Dysplasias associated with bowing of the long bones

Some conditions, such as hypophosphatasia and osteogenesis imperfecta types IIA, B and C, are associated with severe bowing or deformation of the long bones, but others may have less severe degrees (OI III and IV) or be more variable (camptomelic dysplasia) in presentation.

Hypophosphatasia – see above

Osteogenesis imperfecta types IIA, IIB and IIC – see above

Camptomelic dysplasia

Gene locus 17q24.3-q25.1

SOX9 gene

Autosomal dominant

This condition has an incidence around 1:20000. Most cases are due to mutations in the SOX9 gene, an SRY-related gene at 17q23-qter[40], but some are associated with a cytogenetically visible rearrangement of chromosome 17q24 upstream of

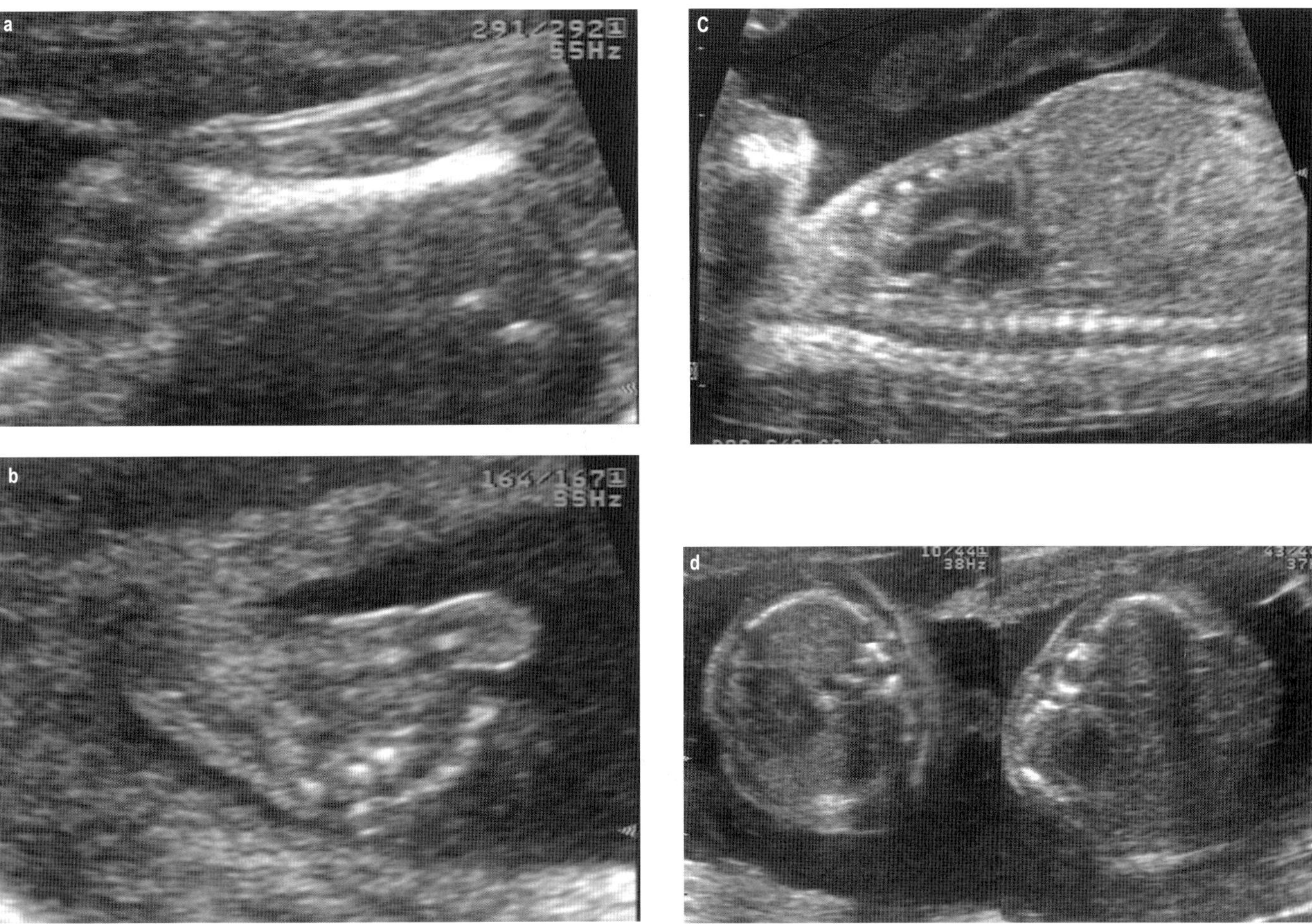

Fig. 36.14 Sonographic findings in Ellis van Creveld syndrome. (a) Short straight femur. (b) Polydactyly of the toes showing 6 toes and a large duplicated great toe. (c) Narrow chest seen in the sagittal plane. (d) Axial view through the thorax and abdomen demonstrating the small chest with short ribs.

SOX9 and a milder clinical phenotype[41]. Perinatal death is common secondary to respiratory problems related to a small chest. Complications in survivors include recurrent apnea, kyphoscoliosis, learning difficulties (mild to moderate), short stature and dislocation of the hip[41]. The main sonographic feature is bowing of the femur and tibia, the arms being unaffected (Fig. 36.15a,b). Other features include a large head, micrognathia, a cleft palate and a flat nasal bridge, with occasional talipes. The chest can be narrow and respiratory distress is common. About a third of cases have cardiac defects (VSD, ASD, Fallot tetralogy) and a third have hydronephrosis, mostly unilateral. Ambiguous genitalia occurs in the majority of cases with an XY karyotype. Confirmation of genetic sex and demonstration of genital ambiguity in male fetuses (Fig. 36.15c) can be diagnostic in the presence of other features described above. Other features, less easily identified on ultrasound include hypoplastic scapulae, narrow iliac wings, a poorly ossified pubis. There may be only 11 pairs of ribs[42].

Osteogenesis imperfecta type III (OI III)
Gene locus 17q21.31-q22, 7q22.1
Type I collagen genes, COL1A1 or COL1A2.
Autosomal dominant (somatic and gonadal mosaicism)[43]

OI III is the most severe form that is compatible with life. It is a rare form characterized by progressive deformation which begins in utero. Individuals may present with multiple fractures at birth and suffer frequent fractures thereafter (Fig. 36.16a)[44]. The skull is normally mineralized but has multiple wormian bones. Patients with type III OI progress to have severely short stature due to spinal compression fractures, deformities of the limbs and disrupted growth plates. Many are wheelchair bound by late childhood[45]. Death in early life was common, but the clinical course may now be amenable to significant amelioration with the use of bisphosphonates[46]. Limb shortening and bowing, particularly in the legs, is usually evident by 20 weeks' gestation (Fig. 36.16b,c,d). Other long bones tend to be on or below the 5th percentile. Some bowing of the arm bones can occasionally be seen. The chest appears normal and often ribs, although thin, do not show beading, although fresh fractures often occur at delivery (Fig. 36.16a,e,f). The head appears normal and casts a reasonable acoustic shadow (Fig. 36.16g).

Osteogenesis imperfecta type IV (OI IV)
Gene locus 17q21.31-q22
Type I collagen genes, COL1A1 or COL1A2

Type IV is the most diverse group in the classic classification. The more severely affected patients in type IV OI, present with fractures at birth, moderate skeletal deformity and a relatively short stature. New forms of OI (types V–VII) based on analysis of

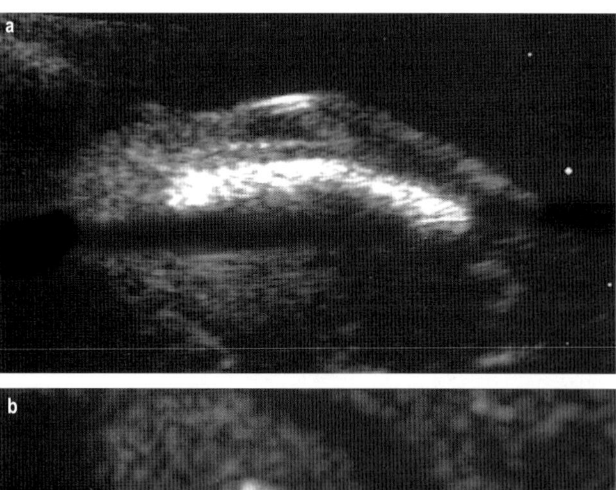

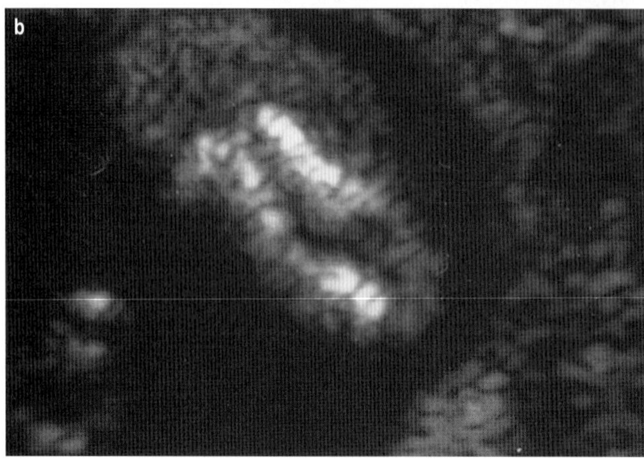

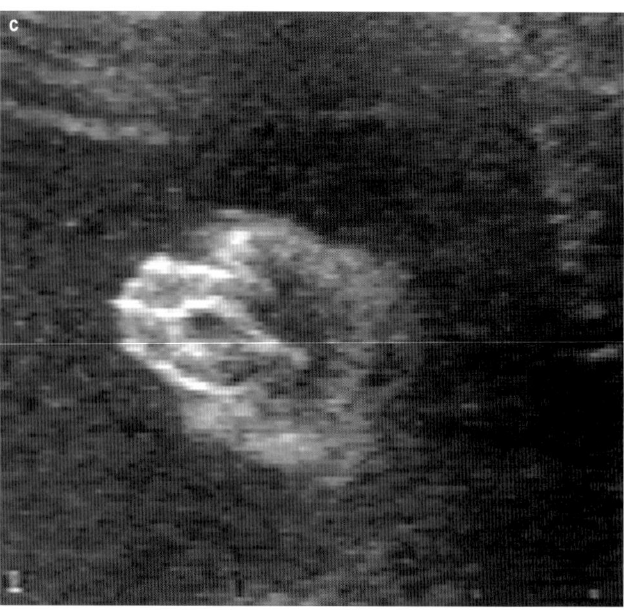

Fig. 36.15 Sonographic findings in camptomelic dysplasia (Jaimimi Patel). (a) Femur showing mid-shaft bowing. (b) Image showing slight bowing of the tibia. (c) Genital ambiguity in a male fetus with camptomelic dysplasia.

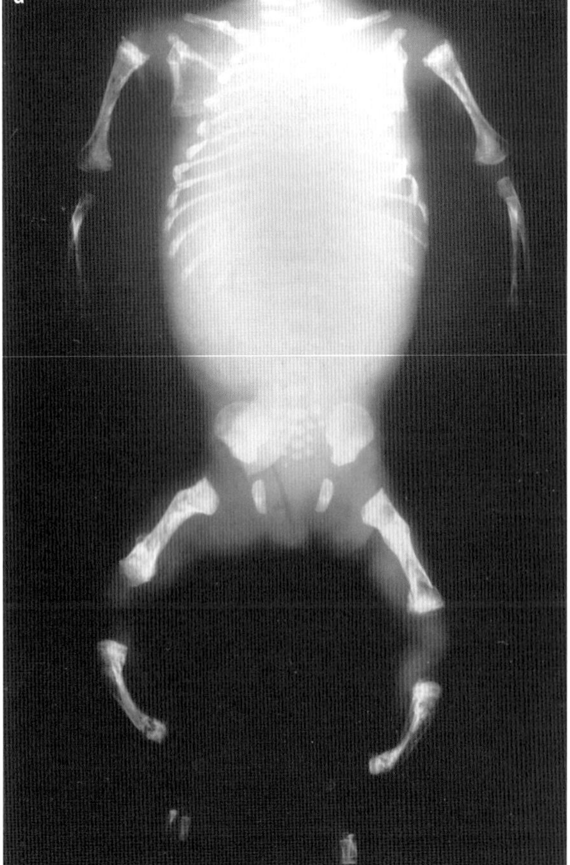

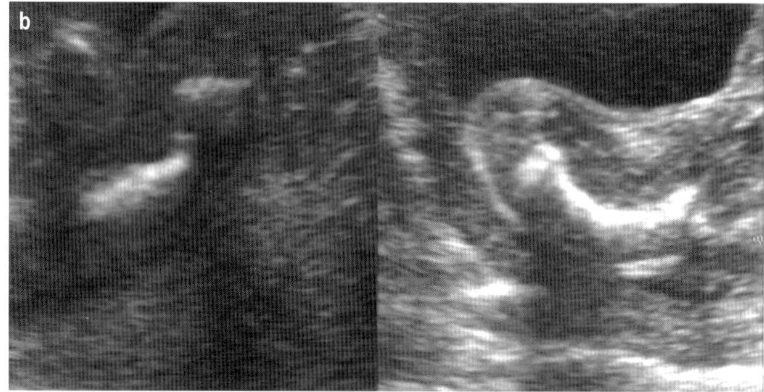

Fig. 36.16 Sonographic findings in osteogenesis imperfecta type III. (a) Radiograph of a fetus with OI III. Note the fresh rib fractures rather than the beading seen in OI II. (b) Note the symmetrical bowing of the femora. (c) Short, bowed lower legs. (d) Short but straight forearm bones. (e) Sagittal view of the thorax and abdomen showing relatively normal proportions. (f) Axial view through the thorax and abdomen demonstrating relatively normal proportions, with the heart occupying an appropriate amount of the thorax. (g) The ribs are thin and slightly irregular, but beading less obvious. (h) The head appears normal and castes a reasonable acoustic shadow.

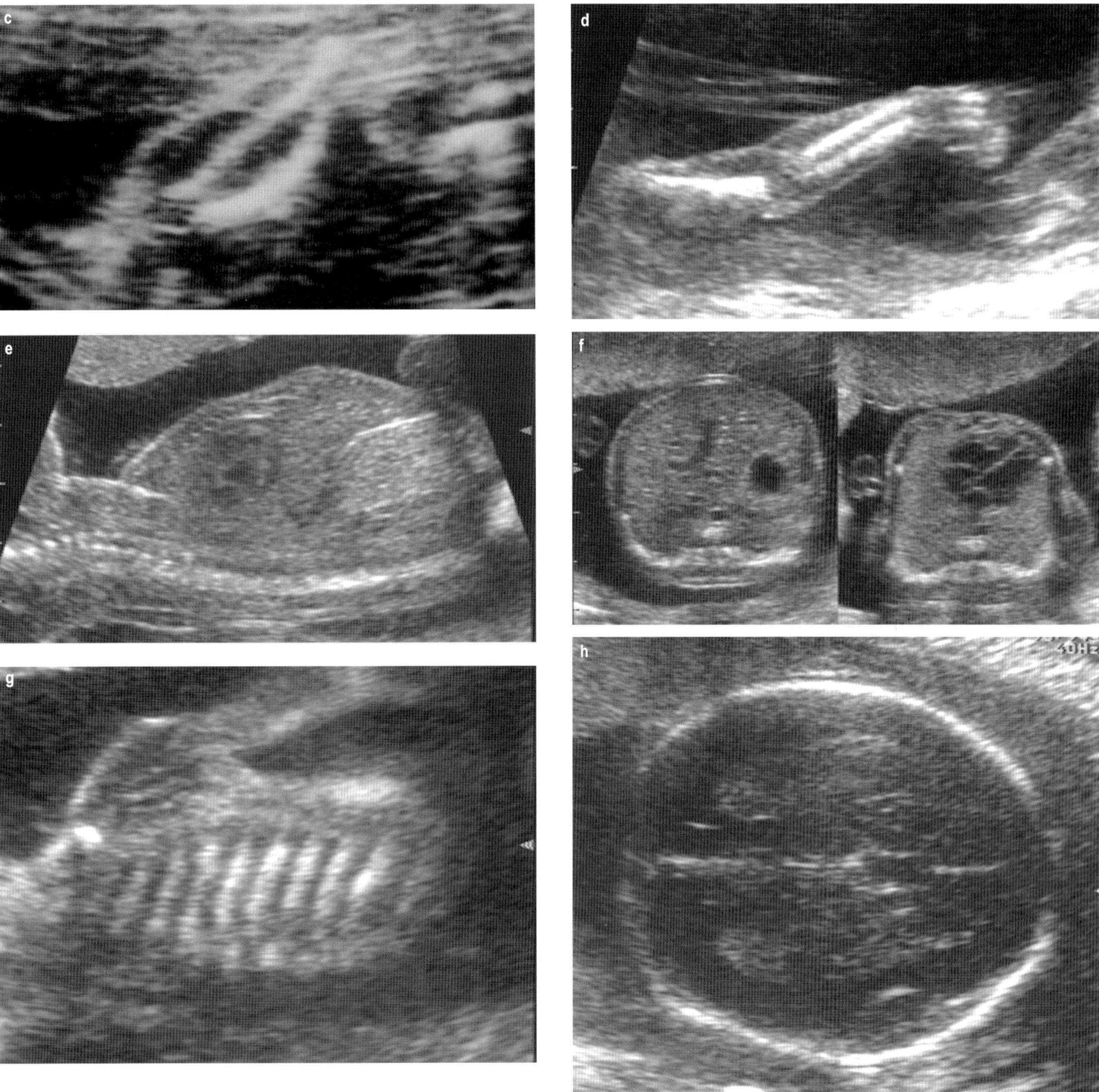

Fig. 36.16 Continued

bone architecture, have been recently added to the classification[47]. These types are moderately deforming and prior to the introduction of the new classification, they would have all fallen into type IV category. Prenatal detection is more difficult. In the author's experience of two cases, long bone length has remained within the normal range throughout pregnancy (Fig. 36.17) and the other feature detectable with prenatal ultrasound was mild symmetrical, bowing of the femora and lower leg bones (Fig. 36.17a–d)[48].

Conditions associated with stippled epiphyses

There are several conditions associated with ectopic calcification around the ephiphyses and in other parts of the skeletal, spine, hands, feet and sternum. The pattern of stippling together with the pattern of limb shortening, degree of symmetry, nasal configuration, fetal sex and other features can give a clue to the underlying etiology and allow for targeted biochemical, cytogenetic or molecular analysis.

Rhizomelic chondrodysplasia punctata

Gene locus

RCDP1 6q22-q24 PEX7 gene encoding the peroxisomal type 2 targeting signal (PTS2) receptor

RCDP2 1q42 acyl-CoA:dihydroxyacetonephosphate acyltransferase (DHAPAT) gene

RCDP3 2q31 alkyldihydroxyacetonephosphate synthase (alkyl-DHAP synthase) gene

Rhizomelic chondropunctata dysplasia is a rare disorder, characterized by rhizomelic shortening of long bones, joint

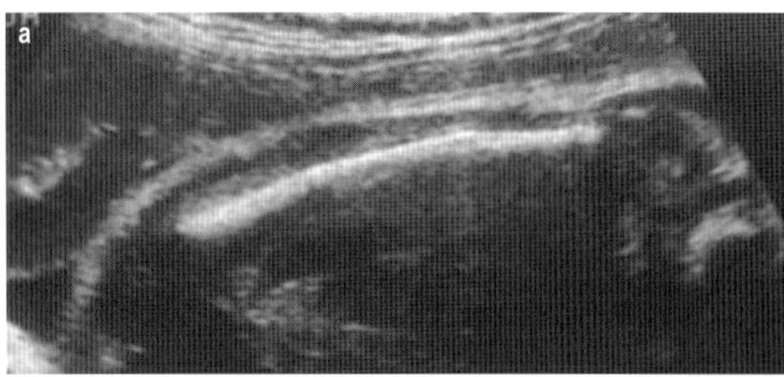

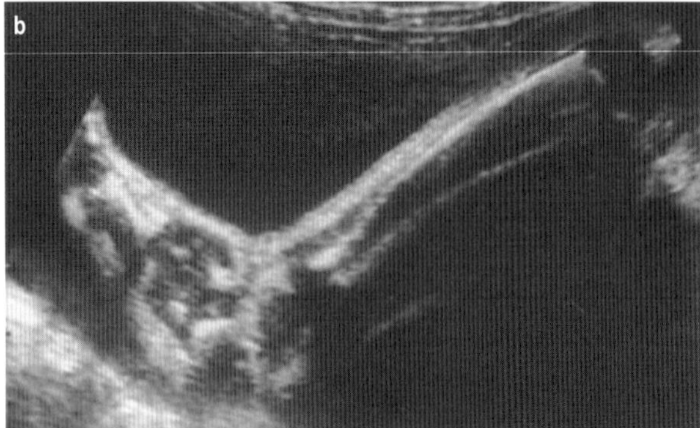

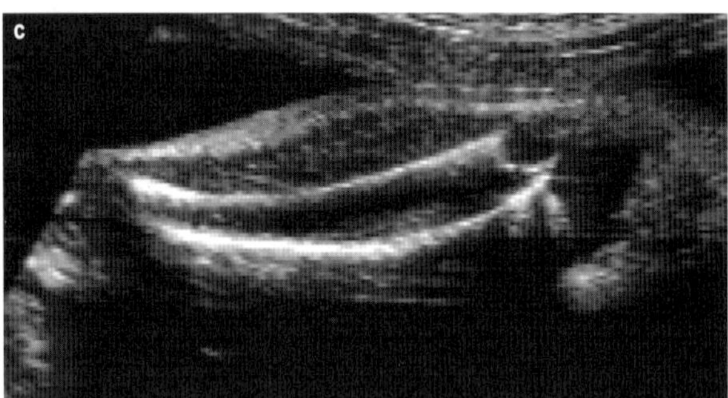

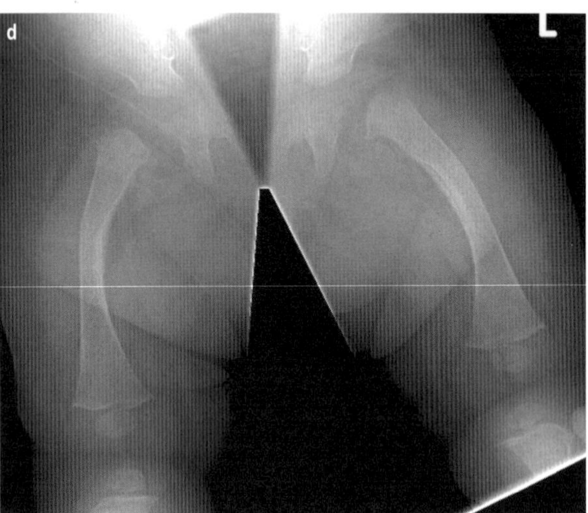

Fig. 36.17 Sonographic findings in osteogenesis imperfecta type IV (Janice Loose). (a) Image of femur showing mild bowing in the proximal one third. (b) Image of lower leg demonstrating minimal bowing of the tibia. (c) Image of lower leg demonstrating minimal bowing of the tibia and fibula. (d) Radiograph showing the bowing of the femora in this neonate.

contractures, nasal hypoplasia, congenital cataracts in about 70% and ichthyosis in 30%. Postnatally, there is progressive microcephaly and severe mental retardation. Many affected individuals die in early childhood, but survivors have shown

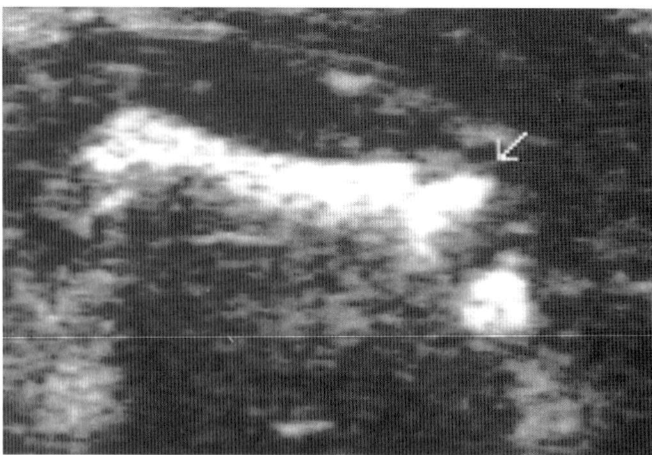

Fig. 36.18 The femur in a fetus with in rhizomelic chondropunctata dysplasia. Note the extra calcification at the epiphysis (arrow).

severe growth and developmental retardation. This condition has a biochemical etiology with defective plasmalogen synthesis and progressive accumulation of phytanic acid. Prenatal diagnosis can be achieved by measuring acyl-CoA:dihydroxyacetone phosphate acyltransferase (DHAP-AT) (specific for RCDP2) in amniotic fluid or chorionic villi[49]. Sonographic features include rhizomelic long bone shortening, ectopic calcification in the hyaline cartilage, epiphyses (Fig. 36.18), pelvis and around the vertebral column, resulting in the appearance of stippled epiphyses and a disorganized spine[50]. Prenatal detection of the cataracts associated with this condition has been reported[51]. Confirmation by enzyme analysis in CVS or skin fibroblasts postnatally is necessary to resolve underlying genetic heterogeneity and allow targeted mutation testing.

Conradi Hünermann
Gene locus Xp11
Emopamil-binding protein (EBP) gene
X-linked dominant

This condition is associated with asymmetric shortening of bones, ichtyosis and other patchy skin changes, areas of alopecia and sparse, coarse hair and occasional cataracts. Intelligence is usually normal. Prenatal sonographic detection has been reported[52]. Sonographic findings included short limbs with epiphyseal stippling and a stippled spine. Affected fetuses are generally, but not exclusively, female. Examination of the mother for cataracts and skin changes that may indicate she is a carrier may be helpful in defining the diagnosis in the affected fetus. Pregnancies at known high risk, where molecular investigations done prior to pregnancy have demonstrated mutations in the EBP gene, may be offered invasive prenatal diagnosis.

X-linked recessive chondrodysplasia punctata
Gene locus Xp22.32
Arylsulfatase E (ARSE) gene[28–37]
X-linked

In this condition males are affected. They have short limbs with stippling of the epiphyses as well as the larynx and trachea (Fig. 36.19a,b) which disappears in early childhood. There can be marked nasal hypoplasia that also improves with age and cataracts can be present in some cases. The condition may arise due to large deletions in Xp22.32 which result in contiguous deletion of the ARSE gene when developmental problems can

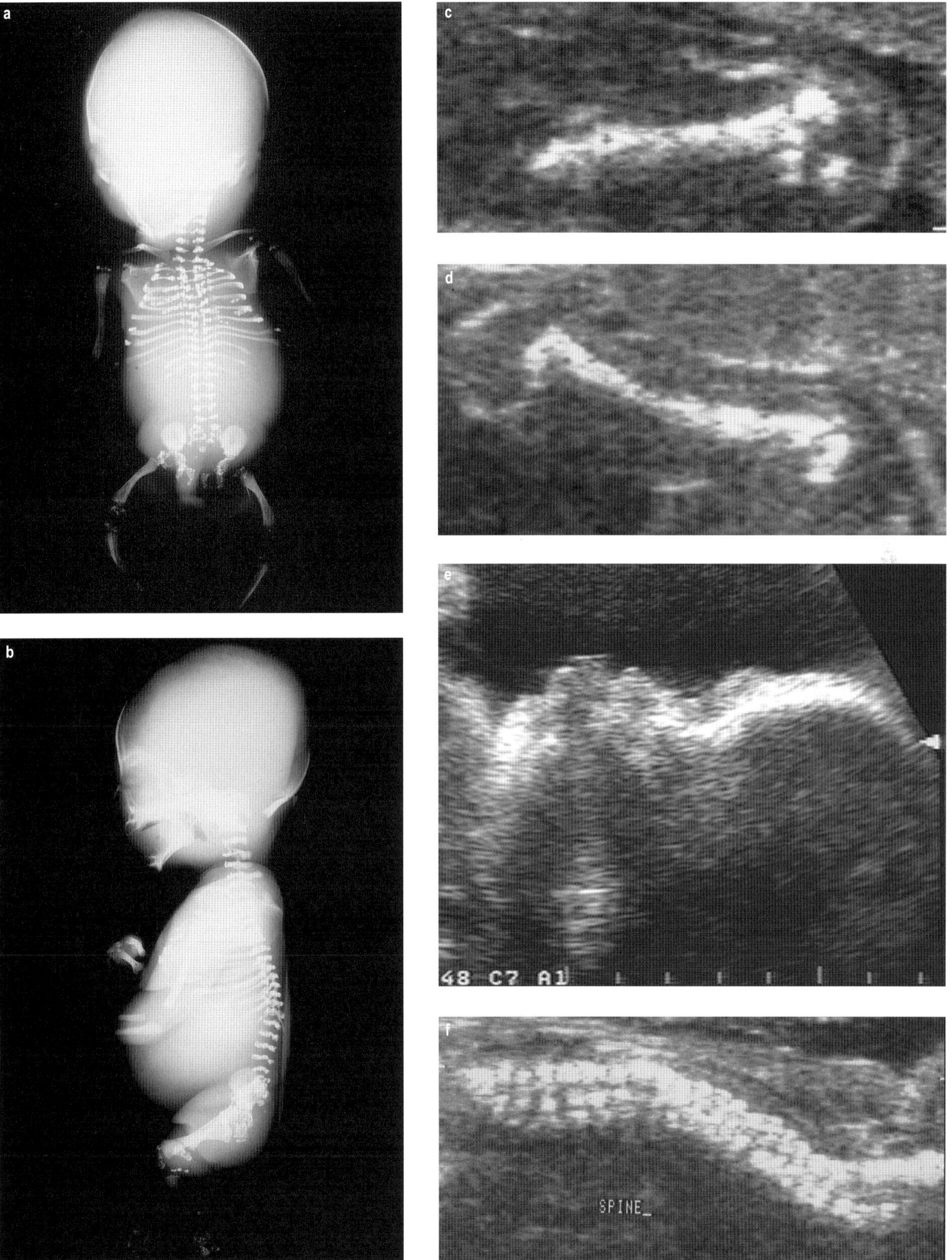

Fig. 36.19 Sonographic findings in X-linked recessive chondropunctata dysplasia. (a) Radiograph of a fetus with X-linked recessive chondropunctata dysplasia showing the extra calcification in the AP (a) and lateral (b) views. (b) Lateral spine radiograph. (c) Ultrasound image of the femur showing the extra calcification at the epiphysis. (d) Ultrasound image of the humerus showing the extra calcification at the epiphysis. (e) Profile demonstrating the depressed nasal bridge. (f) Sagittal view of the spine showing the 'disorganized' appearance due to ectopic calcification.

also ensue, or as a result of smaller deletions or point mutations involving the ARSE gene when additional problems including learning disability are not associated. Female carriers, who are heterozygous for the deletion, tend to have mild short stature, but no radiological stippling. Prenatal sonographic findings include short limbs with epiphyseal stippling (Fig. 36.19c,d), a very depressed nasal bridge and small nose (Fig. 36.19e), stippling of the larynx and trachea and spine (Fig. 36.19f). Testing for contiguous deletions on the X-chromosome is routinely available but, for those without detectable deletions, definitive diagnosis is only possible prenatally following invasive testing and identification of mutations in the ARSE gene in families where the causative mutation has been identified.

Other skeletal dysplasias associated with short straight limbs

Achondroplasia
Gene locus 4p16
Fibroblast growth factor receptor gene 3 (FGFR3)
Autosomal dominant

Achondroplasia (ACH) is the most common non-lethal skeletal dysplasia with an incidence of around 5–15 per 100 000 births. It results from a mutation in the fibroblast growth factor receptor 3 (FGFR3) gene located on 4p16.3[53]. The most common mutation is G→A transition at position 1138, although other disease-causing mutations have also been reported[54]. The majority of cases are sporadic and result from a *de novo* paternal mutation[55]. Prenatal sonographic diagnosis is often not achieved as limb length is preserved until around 22 weeks' gestation. Figure 36.10a shows the growth of the fetal femur in 22 cases compared with normal fetuses. Presentation of *de novo* cases often occurs in the third trimester when the fetus is scanned for some other reason, when short limbs and other features may be evident. These include frontal bossing, short fingers (trident hand) and relative macrocephaly (Fig. 36.20a,b,c). Other features that can occur are a small chest and mild ventriculomegaly. Increased liquor volume or polyhydramnios is an almost universal feature in the third trimester. Other complications such as craniocervical junction compression and spinal cord stenosis may occur in later life[56]. The prenatal diagnosis can be confirmed in de novo cases by screening for mutations in the FGFR3 gene in amniocytes or in free fetal DNA in the maternal blood[57].

Acromesomelic dysplasia
Gene locus 9p21-p12
Natriuretic peptide receptor B gene (NPR2)
Autosomal recessive

Acromesomelic dysplasia is a rare skeletal dysplasia that disproportionately affects the forearms, lower legs, hands and feet. Other characteristics include relative macrocephaly, frontal bossing, bowing of the forearms and a narrow funnel chest. The condition may be obvious at birth, but more frequently becomes evident during the first year of life. Eventual height is below the third percentile. This condition is usually inherited in an autosomal recessive fashion[58] and has been mapped to 9p 13–9q 12 in some families and is inherited in an autosomal recessive fashion[58,59]. Other heterogeneous forms have also been described (e.g. CDMP1/GDF5 gene). The prenatal phenotype is not well

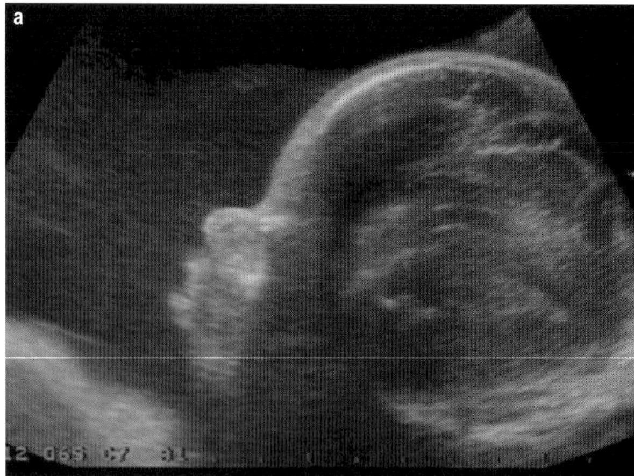

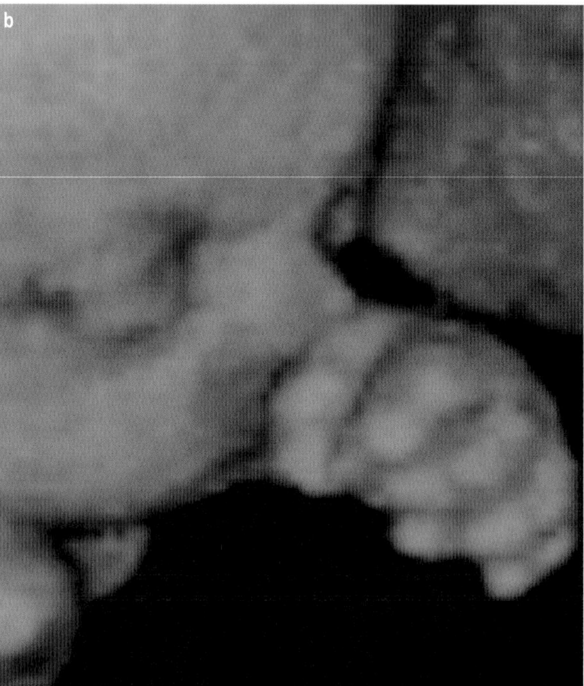

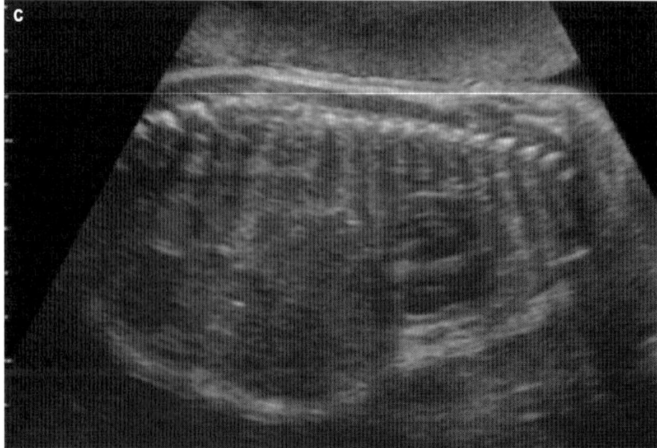

Fig. 36.20 Sonographic findings in achondroplasia. (a) Profile demonstrating the marked frontal bossing. (b) 3D view of the face. (c) View of the thorax demonstrating the narrowing of the chest compared with the abdomen.

described, which is not surprising given the rarity of the condition and the difficulty in coming to a diagnosis even in the postnatal period. The sonographic features are very similar to those seen in achondroplasia, although the pattern of limb shortening in the latter is rhizomelic compared with mesomelic in the former. Relative macrocephaly, frontal bossing, short fingers and a small chest are seen in both conditions (Fig. 36.21a–c) and the gestation at onset of limb shortening appears to be similar, i.e. after 20 weeks. However, it must be remembered that of the two, achondroplasia is by far the most common and thus molecular analysis by screening for mutations in the FGFR3 gene may aid definitive diagnosis.

Diastrophic dysplasia
Gene locus 5q32-q33.1
DTDST gene
Autosomal recessive

This is a severe skeletal dysplasia characterized by variable degrees of rhizomelic shortening of the long bones. Bilateral talipes, micrognathia and the typical 'hitch-hiker' thumbs (Fig. 36.22a) and toes (Fig. 36.22b) are all common findings. Sonographic detection has been reported from 13 weeks using transvaginal ultrasound[60], but the classical features are more likely to be detected slightly later in pregnancy[61].

Kniest dysplasia
Gene map locus 12q13.11-q13.2
COL2A1
Autosomal dominant

The inherited disorders resulting from mutations in COL2A1, the gene for pro α2 collagen (a fibrillar collagen), form a spectrum of phenotypes. These are collectively known as the type II collagenopathies[62], the milder forms of which are Stickler syndrome and familial osteoarthritis. The spectrum includes disorders which range from the lethal or perinatal lethal disorders such as achondrogenesis II and hypochondrogenesis, through to conditions with varying degrees of short stature, which include spondyloepiphyseal dysplasia congenital (SEDC) and Kniest dysplasia. Many of these conditions present prenatally with non-specific limb shortening of varying degrees, but the definitive diagnosis has to await postnatal examination. Even then, while the affected individual can have features typical of a type II collagenopathy with platyspondyly, kyphosis, short limbs, depressed nasal bridge and prominent forehead, definitive radiological classification can be difficult.

Kniest dysplasia is an autosomal dominant condition caused by the defective formation of type II collagen. The phenotype is variable and characterized by a significant degree of disproportionate short stature, a short trunk and small pelvis, kyphoscoliosis, short limbs, with prominent joints and premature osteoarthritis that often restricts movement. Characteristic craniofacial manifestations of Kneist dysplasia include midface hypoplasia, cleft palate, early onset myopia, retinal detachment and hearing loss. This condition is manifest prenatally, although definitive diagnosis will be difficult to achieve. Sonographic findings can be variable. Limb length around 20 weeks was on or just above the 5th percentile in all 4 cases seen by the author, with a tendency to fall further from the centiles as pregnancy progressed. Two cases scanned later in pregnancy appeared to have a small chest, due to a short chest with platyspondyly rather than short ribs, which is of interest as respiratory difficulty in the newborn period is a recognized feature of Kneist

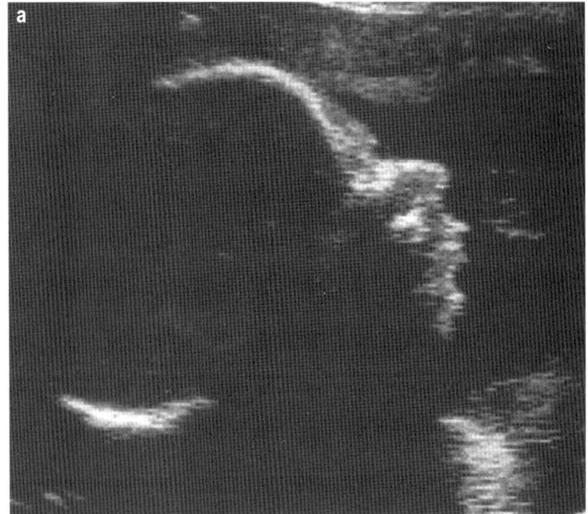

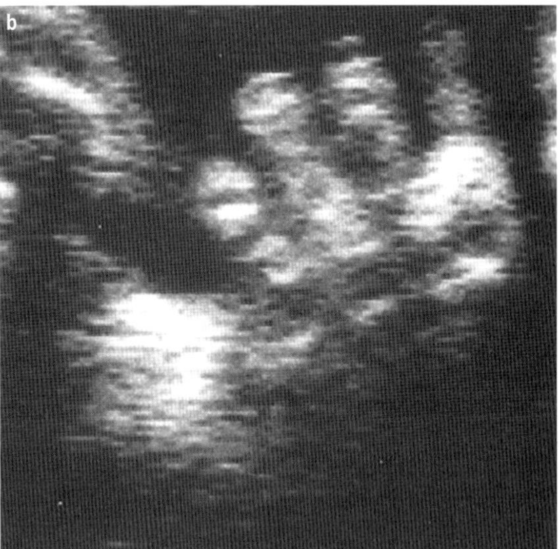

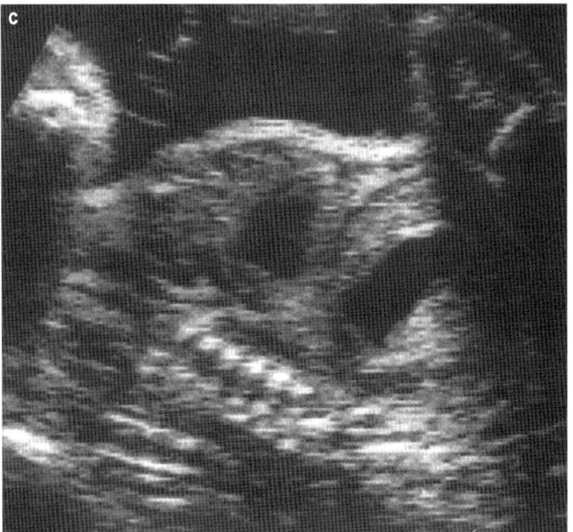

Fig. 36.21 Sonographic findings in acromesomelic dysplasia. (a) Profile showing frontal bossing. (b) Short stubby fingers. (c) Sagittal view through the thorax deomonstrating the relatively narrow chest.

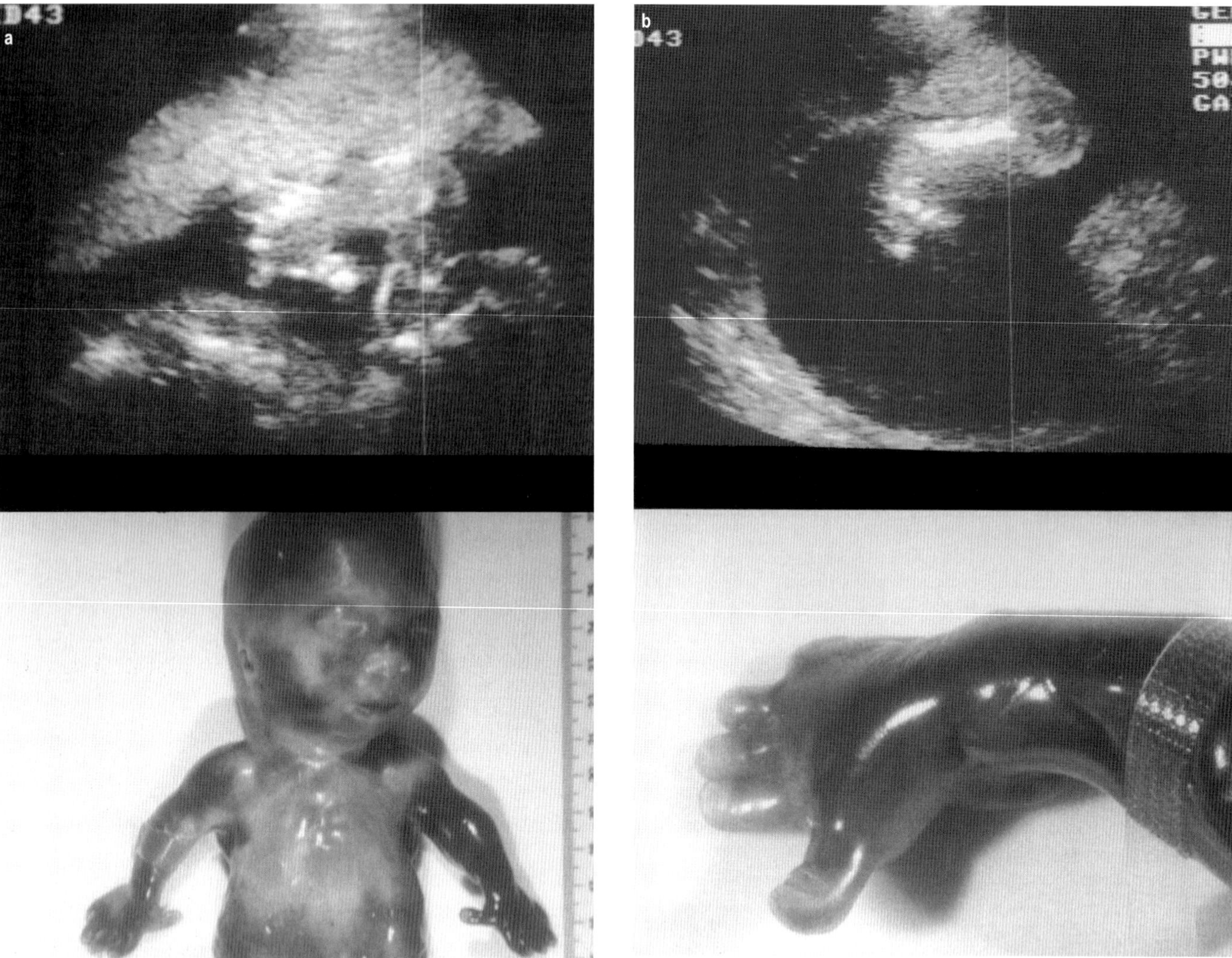

Fig. 36.22 Sonographic findings in diastrophic dysplasia. (a) Hitch-hiker thumbs. (b) Feet demonstrating the talipes and 'hitch-hiker' great toes.

dysplasia. Careful sonographic examination of the limbs can reveal the metaphyseal flaring seen on postnatal radiographs. Other features that may give a clue to the underlying condition include micrognathia, a flat face and mild frontal bossing. The findings can be relatively subtle and definitive diagnosis will have to await postnatal radiology. Mutation analysis of the COLA1 gene in low-risk cases, even if the diagnosis were suspected antenatally, is not feasible at present given the size of the gene and the fact that not all disease causing mutations have been identified.

Limb deficiency or congenital amputations

Conditions associated with forearm defects

Forearm defects including radial club hand, transverse limb defects and hand anomalies may be associated with a variety of etiologies including aneuploidy (particularly trisomy 18), teratogens, genetic syndromes or they may occur as isolated findings. The list of individual conditions is vast with the London Dysmorphology Database listing 204 syndromes, excluding aneuploidy, associated with forearm abnormalities[15]. It is out with the scope of this chapter to go into great detail and the more common of these still rare conditions are given in Table 36.10. It is reasonable to suggest that if the lesion is unilateral and no other abnormalities are seen on ultrasound and fetal growth is normal, it is more likely than not that this is an isolated abnormality. However, detailed fetal echocardiography is to be recommended and the spine should be carefully examined to exclude hemivertebrae. Bilateral lesions, even when apparently isolated, are much more likely to be associated with an underlying genetic syndrome or aneuploidy than unilateral lesions. In a review of 52 fetuses with forearm defects, 21 had bilateral forearm anomalies, four with complete absence of the forearms. Fetuses with bilateral lesions or other abnormalities were more likely to have an underlying genetic or chromosomal pathology (Table 36.11).

Conditions associated with isolated lower limb defects

Femoral anomalies are rarely isolated, the majority being associated with other limb or somatic anomalies which may

Table 36.10 Selected genetic syndromes associated with forearm reduction defects

	Forearms	*Lower limbs*	*Cardiac abnormality*	*Growth*	*Other potential USS findings*	*FH*	*Other diagnostic aids*
Brachmann de Large Syndrome (BDLS)	Asymmetrical and variable forearm reduction, absent fingers or oligodactyly, syndactyly	Small feet	±	IUGR, microcephaly	Diaphragmatic hernia	–	Low PAPP-A
Thrombocytopenia-Absent Radius Syndrome (TAR)	Bilateral radial aplasia, thumbs always present and normal. Ulna hypoplasia	Absent/abnormal tibia, fibula, femur, talipes,	±	Usually normal	Absent/abnormal humeri, flexion deformities	+ (AR)	Fetal platelet count DNA for recently described common rearrangement
Trisomy 18 Trisomy 13	Radial club hand, flexed fingers, polydactyly, absent thumbs	Talipes, rocker bottom feet, polydactyly	+	IUGR	Multiple	–	Fetal karyotype
Holt Oram	Bilateral radial abnormalities of variable severity, absent digits (especially thumb)	Normal	+	Normal		+ (AD)	Examine parents ± X-ray wrists and echocardiography
Fanconi	Hypoplasic thumbs, radial anomalies, polydactyly	Normal	±	IUGR	Cryptorchidism, renal anomalies	+ (AR)	Chromosome breakage studies
Ballergerold	Bilateral radial defects, absent/hypoplastic thumbs	Normal	±	Normal	Intracerebral anomalies, renal anomalies, anal atresia, craniosynostosis	+ (AR)	Genetic consultation
Nager	Bilateral radial defects, absent/hypoplastic thumbs, preaxial polydactyly	Normal, occasional syndactyly of toes	±	Microcephaly,	Micrognathia, cleft lip, absent/ abnormal fibula, renal anomalies	+ (AD)	Genetic consultation
Roberts	Bilateral radial and ulna hypo/aplasia	Hypoplasic or absent lower limb bones	±	Normal	Cleft lip, cystic kidneys	+ (AR)	Fetal karyotype and look for chromosome puffing
VATER (L)	Asymmetrical radial defects	Normal	±	Normal	Hemivertebrae, renal anomalies	–	Polyhydramnios (due to tracheo–esophageal atresia)
Femur-Fibular-Ulna Syndrome (FFU)	Variable degrees of hypoplasia of ulnae, radii and humeri	Asymmetrical bowing/ hypoplasia of lower limbs	–	Normal	Ectrodactyly	–	

Table 36.11 **Outcome in 52 fetuses with forearm defects seen in two tertiary referral units**

Diagnosis	*n*	*Forearm defect*		*Other skeletal anomaly*	*IUGR*	*Other structural*
		uni	*bi*			
Trisomy 18	10	4	6	7	6	16
Other chromosomal	1	–	1	1	–	–
Cornelia de Lange	5	2	3	5	4	3
TAR	2	–	2	2	–	–
Ballergerold	1	–	1	1	1	3
Holt Oram	1	–	1	1	–	1
FFU	2	1	1	2	–	–
Robert's	2	–	2	2	2	2
Gollop	1	–	1	1	–	–
Goldenhar	1	1	–	1	–	1
VATER	2	2	–	–	–	5
Other/ unknown syndrome	12	9	3	12	5	16
Isolated uni	7	7	–	–	1	–
Vascular incident	1	1	–	1	–	1
Lost to follow- up	4	4	–	–	–	–
TOTAL		31	21		18	14

give clues to the underlying diagnosis. If there appears to be isolated shortening of the legs with no bowing and no other abnormalities present, then intrauterine growth retardation and constitutional short stature must be considered in the differential diagnosis (see Fig. 36.3). When bowing is present and the lesion is unilateral, the most likely diagnosis is one of focal hypoplasia, which is at the mild end of the caudal regression spectrum. Of note, in 10 cases with unilateral femoral reduction seen by the author, serial scanning showed that, in most cases, the growth of the affected limb continued at a normal velocity, albeit below the normal centiles (Fig. 36.23). This information is useful in prenatal counseling as it allows the counselor to predict the degree of shortening and, in consultation with orthopedic surgeons, advise the parents as to the likely postnatal management. In the 5 fetuses with bilateral, symmetrical bowing of the femora seen, all had skeletal dysplasias (see Fig. 36.3). In 3 cases, growth of other long bones was initially on the 5th percentile and then fell below this after 20 weeks. These all had osteogenesis imperfecta type III. The remaining two cases had imperfecta type IV. Three fetuses had bilateral asymmetrical femoral and/or lower leg anomalies and, in all cases, this was an isolated finding after birth.

GENERAL COUNSELING AND FOLLOW-UP ISSUES

The finding of a skeletal anomaly at the time of a routine scan should stimulate a detailed examination of the rest of the fetus, paying particular attention to the features listed in Table 36.7. A careful and systematic approach can often lead to the identification of features that narrow the differential diagnosis and suggest other investigations that may be useful (see Table 36.3). Karyotyping should be considered, particularly in the presence of other somatic anomalies or when there appears to be isolated limb shortening. In this latter case, fetal and maternal Doppler examination should be performed as intrauterine growth retardation can present with short limbs. In the majority of cases, consultation with a geneticist and, in all cases with a viable condition, pediatric orthopedic surgeon, can be of great

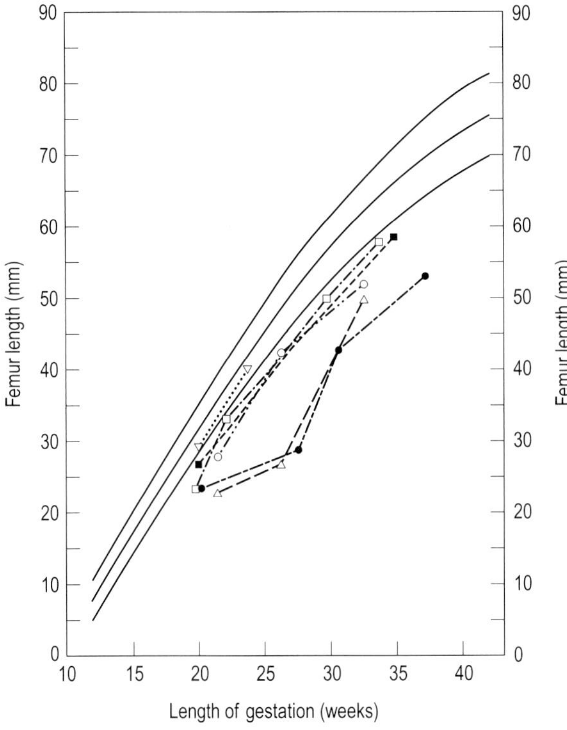

Fig. 36.23 Chart of femur length showing the growth of femurs in fetuses with unilateral isolated lower limb anomalies.

assistance, not just in achieving a diagnosis, but also for informing the parents of likely prognosis and postnatal management. Definitive diagnosis may be possible in some cases prenatally following mutation screening, karyotyping or metabolic testing. A clinical geneticist is usually best placed to advise on the most appropriate tests.

After birth, confirmation of the diagnosis is usually made by expert radiology. In cases ending in fetal or perinatal death, tissue should be stored for DNA analysis. A skin biopsy should be taken in case collagen studies are needed. Survivors are best seen in a multidisciplinary clinic with access to clinical geneticists, orthopedic surgeons, ophthalmologists etc. Many children will require input from other specialists such as cardiologists, nephrologists and audiologists.

CONCLUSIONS

The elucidation of the underlying pathology in a fetus with a skeletal anomaly is challenging, but can be rewarding. It requires careful attention to detail and a team approach. As more genes are identified and molecular technology improves, it will become increasingly possible to come to a definitive diagnosis prenatally and thereby offer accurate prognostic information to the parents.

REFERENCES

1. Brown N, Lumley J, Tickle C, Keene J. *Congenital limb reduction defects. Clues from developmental biology, teratology and epidemiology*. London: HMSO Stationery Office, 1996.
2. Brons JTJ, van der HArten JJ, van Geijn HP. Ultrasonic and radiologic aspects of early ossification in the normal fetus and the fetus affected by skeletal dysplasia. *MD Thesis* 15–33, 1988.
3. Chitty LS, Campbell S, Altman DG. Measurement of the fetal mandible – feasibility and construction of a centile chart. *Prenat Diagn* **13**:749–756, 1993.
4. Altman DG, Chitty LS. Charts of fetal size: 1. Methodology. *Br J Obstet Gynaecol* **101**:29–34, 1994.
5. Chitty LS, Altman DG, Henderson A, Campbell S. Charts of fetal size: 2. Head measurements. *Br J Obstet Gynecol* **101**: 35–43, 1994.
6. Chitty LS, Altman DG, Henderson A, Campbell S. Charts of fetal size: 3. Abdominal circumference. *Br J Obstet Gynaecol* **101**:132–135, 1994.
7. Chitty LS, Altman DG, Henderson A, Campbell S. Charts of fetal size: 4. Femur length. *Br J Obstet Gynaecol* **101**:125–131, 1994.
8. Chitty LS, Altman DG. Charts of fetal size: Limb bones. *Br J Obstet Gynaecol* **109**(8):919–929, 2002.
9. Chitty LS, Altman DG. Charts of fetal size: kidney and renal pelvis measurements. *Prenat Diagn* **23**(11):891–897, 2003.
10. Rosati P, Guariglia L. Transvaginal fetal biometry in early pregnancy. *Early Hum Dev* **49**(2):91–96, 1997.
11. Spranger J. International classification of osteochondrondrodystrophies. The internataional working group on constitutional diseases of bone. *Eur J Pediatr* **151**:407–415, 1992.
12. Superti-Furga A, Bonafe L, Rimoin D. Molecular-pathogenetic classification of genetic disorders of the skeleton. *Am J Med Genet* **106**:282–293, 2002.
13. Hall CM. International nosology and classification of constitutional disorders of bone. *Am J Med Genet* **113**:65–77, 2002.
14. Maron JL, Bianchi DW. Prenatal diagnosis using cell-free nucleic acids in maternal body fluids: a decade of progress. *Am J Med Genet* **145c**:5–17, 2007.
15. Winter RM, Baraitser M. Winter-Baraitser London Medical Databases. Version 1.0, 2006.
16. Martinez-Frias 1994.
17. Vincent A, McConville J, Farrugia ME et al. Antibodies in myasthenia gravis and related disorders. *Ann NY Acad Sci* **998**:324–335, 2003.
18. Upadhyay K, Thomson A, Luckas MJ. Congenital myotonic dystrophy. *Fetal Diagn Ther* **20**(6):512–514, 2005.
19. Esplin MS, Hallam S, Farrington PF, Nelson L, Byrne J, Ward K. Myotonic dystrophy is a significant cause of idiopathic polyhydramnios. *Am J Obstet Gynecol* **179**(4):974–977, 1998.
20. Kozlowski K, Basel D, Beighton P. Chondrodysplasia punctata in siblings and maternal lupus erythematous. *Clin Genet* **66**:545–549, 2004.
21. Makrydimas G, Souka A, Skentou H, Lolis D, Nicolaides K. Osteogenesis imperfecta and other skeletal dysplasias presenting with increased nuchal translucency in the first trimester. *Am J Med Genet* **98**:117–120, 2001.
22. Horton WA, Machado MA, Chou JW, Campbell D. Achondrogenesis type II: abnormalities of extracellular matrix. *Pediatr Res* **22**:324–329, 1987.
23. Kozlowski K, Masel J, Morris L et al. Neonatal death dwarfism. *Fortschr Rontgenstr* **129**:626–633, 1978.
24. Mornet E, Muller F, Ngo S et al. Correlation of alkaline phosphatase (ALP) determination and analysis of the tissue non-specific ALP gene in prenatal diagnosis of severe hypophosphatasia. *Prenat Diagn* **19**(8):755–757, 1999.
25. Sinico M, Levaillant JM, Vergnaud A et al. Specific osseous spurs in a lethal form of hypophosphatasia correlated with 3D prenatal ultrasonographic images. *Prenat Diagn* **27**(3):222–227, 2007.

26. Tongsong T, Pongsatha S. Early prenatal sonographic diagnosis of congenital hypophosphatasia. *Ultrasound Obstet Gynecol* **15**(3):252–255, 2000.
27. Henthorn PS, Whyte MP. Infantile hypophosphatasia: successful prenatal assessment by testing for tissue-non-specific alkaline phosphatase isoenzyme gene mutations. *Prenat Diagn* **15**:1001–1006, 1995.
28. Pollitt R, McMahon R, Nunn J et al. Mutation analysis of COL1A1 and COL1A2 in patients diagnosed with osteogenesis imperfecta type I-IV. *Hum Mutat* **27**(7):716, 2006.
29. Thompson EM, Young ID, Hall CM, Pembrey ME. Recurrence risks and prognosis in severe sporadic osteogenesis imperfecta. *J Med Genet* **24**:390–405, 1987.
30. Cole WG, Dalgleish R. Syndrome of the month. Perinatal lethal osteogenesis imperfecta. *J Med Genet* **32**:284–289, 1995.
31. Sillence DO, Senn A, Danks DM. Genetic heterogeneity in osteogenesis imperfecta. *J Med Genet* **16**:101–116, 1979.
32. Viora E, Sciarrone A, Bastonero S et al. Increased nuchal translucency in the first trimester as a sign of osteogenesis imperfecta. *Am J Med Genet* **109**:336–337, 2002.
33. Pepin M, Atkinson M, Starman BJ, Byers PH. Strategies and outcomes of prenatal diagnosis for osteogenesis imperfecta: a review of biochemical and molecular studies completed in 129 pregnancies. *Prenat Diagn* **17**:559–570, 1997.
34. Tavormina PL, Shiang R, Thompson LM et al. Thanatophoric dysplasia (types I and II) caused by distinct mutations in fibroblast growth factor receptor 3. *Nat Genet* **9**:321–328, 1995.
35. Tiller GE, Rimoin DL, Murray LW, Cohn DH. Tandem duplication within a type II collagen gene (COL2A1) exon in an individual with spondyloepiphyseal dysplasia. *Proc Nat Acad Sci* **87**:3889–3893, 1990.
36. Chitty LS, Tan AW, Nesbit DL, Hall CM, Rodeck CH. Sonographic diagnosis of SEDC and double heterozygote of SEDC and achondroplasia: a report of six pregnancies. *Prenat Diagn* **26**(9):861–865, 2006.
37. Tan AWC, Chitty LS. Early onset skeletal dysplasias: differentiating lethal from non-lethal. *J Obstet Gynaecol* **26**(suppl 1): S62, 2006.
38. Ruiz-Perez V, Ide SE, Strom TM et al. Mutations in a new gene in Ellis-van Creveld syndrome and Weyers acrodental dysostosis. *Nat Genet* **24**: 283–286, 2000.
39. Ruiz-Perez VL, Tompson SW, Blair HJ et al. Mutations in two nonhomologous genes in a head-to-head configuration cause Ellis-van Creveld syndrome. *Am J Hum Genet* **72**:728–732, 2003.
40. Kwok C, Weller PA, Guioli S et al. Mutations in SOX9, the gene responsible for camptomelic dysplasia and autosomal sex reversal. *Am J Hum Genet* **57**: 1028–1036, 1995.
41. Mansour S, Offiah AC, McDowall S, Sim P, Tolmie J, Hall C. The phenotype of survivors of camptomelic dysplasia. *J Med Genet* **39**:597–602, 2002.
42. Mansour S, Hall CM, Pembrey ME, Young ID. A clinical and genetic study of camptomelic dysplasia. *J Med Genet* **32**:415–420, 1995.
43. Lund AM, Nicholls AC, Schwartz M, Skovby F. Parental mosaicism and autosomal dominant mutations causing structural abnormalities of collagen I are frequent in families with osteogenesis imperfecta type III/IV. *Acta Paediatr* **86**:711–718, 1997.
44. Sillence DO, Barlow KK, Cole WG, Dietrich S, Garber AP, Rimoin DL. Osteogenesis imperfecta type III: delineation of the phenotype with reference to genetic heterogeneity. *Am J Med Genet* **23**:821–832, 1986.
45. Engelbert RH, Uiterwaal CS, Gulmans VA, Pruijs H, Helders PJ. Osteogenesis imperfecta in childhood: prognosis for walking. *J Pediatr* **137**: 397–402, 2000.
46. Smith R. Severe osteogenesis imperfecta: new therapeutic options? *Br Med J* **322**:63–64, 2001.
47. Roughley PJ, Rauch F. Glorieux FHOsteogenesis imperfecta – clinical and molecular diversity. *Eur Cell Mater* **30**: 541–577, 2003.
48. Chitty LS, Griffin DR, Weisz , Hall CM. Sonographic diagnosis of osteogenesis imperfecta types III and IV. *J Med Genet* **42**(suppl 1):54, 2005.
49. Steinberg SJ, Elçioglu N, Slade CM et al. Peroxisomal disorders: clinical and biochemical studies in 15 children and prenatal diagnosis in 7 families. *Am J Med Genet* **85**(5):502–510, 1999.
50. Hertzberg BS, Kliewer MA, Decker M, Miller CR, Bowie JD. Antenatal ultrasonographic diagnosis of rhizomelic chondrodysplasia punctata. *J Ultrasound Med* **18**(10):715–718, 1999.
51. Basbug M, Serin IS, Ozcelik B, Gunes T, Akcakus M, Tayyar M. Prenatal ultrasonographic diagnosis of rhizomelic chondrodysplasia punctata by detection of rhizomelic shortening and bilateral cataracts. *Fetal Diagn Ther* **20**(3):171–174, 2005.
52. Pryde PG, Bawle E, Brandt F, Romero R, Treadwell MC, Evans MI. Prenatal diagnosis of nonrhizomelic chondrodysplasia punctata (Conradi-Hünermann syndrome). *Am J Med Genet* **47**(3):426–431, 1993.
53. Rousseau F, Bonaventure J, Legeai-Mallet L et al. Mutations in the gene encoding fibroblast growth factor receptor-3 in achondroplasia. *Nature* **371**:252–254, 1994.
54. Bellus GA, Hefferon TW, Ortiz de Luna RI et al. Achondroplasia is defined by recurrent G380R mutations of FGFR3. *Am J Hum Genet* **56**:368–373, 1995.
55. Wilkin DJ, Szabo JK, Cameron R et al. Mutations in fibroblast growth factor receptor 3 in sporadic cases of achondroplasia occur exclusively on the paternally derived chromosome. *Am J Hum Genet* **63**:711–716, 1998.
56. Hunter AGW, Bankier A, Rogers JG, Sillence D, Scott C, Jr. Medical complications of achondroplasia: a multicentre patient review. *J Med Genet* **35**:705–712, 1998.
57. Li Y, Godelieve C, Page-Christiaens ML, Gille JJP, Holzgreve W, Hahn S. Non-invasive prenatal diagnosis of achondroplasia using size-fractionated cell-free DNA by MALDI-TOF MS assay. *Prenat Diagn* **27**:11–17, 2007.
58. Kant SG, Polinkovsky A, Mundlos S, Zabel B et al. Acromesomelic dysplasic Maroteaux type maps to chromosome 9. *Am J Hum Genet* **63**:155–162, 1988.
59. Faivre L, Le Merrer M, Mégarbané A et al. Exclusion of chromosome 9 helps to identify mild variants of acromesomelic dysplasia Maroteaux type. *J Med Genet* **37**:52–54, 2000.
60. Severi FM, Bocchi C, Sanseverino F, Petraglia F. Prenatal ultrasonographic diagnosis of diastrophic dysplasia at 13 weeks of gestation. *J Matern Fetal Neonatal Med* **13**(4):282–284, 2003.
61. Wax JR, Carpenter M, Smith W et al. Second-trimester sonographic diagnosis of diastrophic dysplasia: report of 2 index cases. *J Ultrasound Med* **22**(8):805–808, 2003.
62. Spranger J, Winterpacht A, Zabel B. The type II collagenopathies: a spectrum of chondrodysplasias. *Eur J Pediatr* **153**: 56–65, 1994.
63. Aughton D et al. reported a male with more classical features of X-linked chondroplasia punctata (CBDX2) who was mosaic for an EBP mutation. (47,XXY males may also survive and manifest), 2003.
64. Chen CP, Chang TY, Tzen CY, Wang W. Second-trimester sonographic detection of short rib-polydactyly syndrome type II (Majewski) following an abnormal maternal serum biochemical screening result. *Prenat Diagn* **23**(4):353–355, 2003.
65. Comstock C, Bronsteen R, Lee W, Vettraino I. Mild hypophosphatasia in utero: bent bones in a family with dental disease. *J Ultrasound Med* **24**(5):707–709, 2005.
66. den Hollander NS, van der Harten HJ, Laudy JA, van de Weg P, Wladimiroff JW. Early transvaginal ultrasonographic diagnosis of Beemer-Langer dysplasia: a

report of two cases. *Ultrasound Obstet Gynecol* **11**(4):298–302, 1998.
67. Elçioglu NH, Hall CM. Diagnostic dilemmas in the short rib-polydactyly syndrome group. *Am J Med Genet.* **111**(4):392–400, 2002.
68. Kumru P, Aka N, Kose G, Vural ZT, Peker O, Kayserili H. Short rib polydactyly syndrome type 3 with absence of fibulae (Verma-Naumoff syndrome). *Fetal Diagn Ther* **20**(5):410–414, 2005.
69. Souka AP, Raymond FL, Mornet E, Geerts L, Nicolaides KH. Hypophosphatasia associated with increased nuchal translucency: a report of two affected pregnancies. *Ultrasound Obstet Gynecol* **20**(3):294–295, 2002.
70. Sridhar S, Kishore R, Thomas N, Jana AK. Short rib polydactyly syndrome-Type I. *Indian J Pediatr* **71**(4):359–361, 2004.

CHAPTER

37 Fetal hydrops

Jon Hyett

KEY POINTS

- This chapter deals with the prenatal diagnosis of hydrops. It discusses the pathophysiology and underlying etiologies of this condition and details appropriate investigations to identify the cause and potential therapies
- Fetal hydrops is a common endpoint for a wide variety of conditions. It demonstrates that normal compensatory mechanisms have failed and is associated with a high rate of mortality
- Hydrops is traditionally described as having an immune or non-immune basis. Effective prophylaxis against Rhesus isoimmunization has led to a decline in the proportion of cases having an immune basis
- Despite the fact that hundreds of conditions have been reported as causing non-immune hydrops, a systematic method of investigation will allow identification of the cause in approximately 80% of cases

INTRODUCTION

Hydrops fetalis describes the excessive accumulation of fluid in at least two serous cavities or body tissues. It is a feature of significant fetal compromise that is associated with high rates of perinatal mortality and neonatal morbidity. Although a large number of underlying etiologies have been described, the condition is still categorized at the most basic level as being immune or non-immune in nature. The introduction of postpartum immunoglobulin prophylaxis for Rhesus-D isoimmunization in the 1970s has led to a significant reduction in the number of cases related to this immunological disorder and, consequently, a relative increase in the prevalence of non-immune disease, estimated at 1 in 2000 pregnancies. Despite the extensive list of potential underlying causes, systematic evaluation should allow the etiology to be recognized in 80% of cases. Once a diagnosis has been made, the prognosis for the fetus becomes clearer, therapeutic intervention may be appropriate and risks to future pregnancies can be considered.

THE DIAGNOSIS OF FETAL HYDROPS

Hydrops is most commonly diagnosed during ultrasound examination of the fetus through the recognition of a collection of fluid in two or more cavities including the abdomen (ascites), thorax (pleural or pericardial effusion) or skin (subcutaneous edema)[1–3]. Although these features may be present at the routine first- or second-trimester scan, they frequently develop with advancing gestation and the indication for ultrasound evaluation may be clinical presentation with decreased fetal movements, a suspicion of polyhydramnios or through maternal illness – such as pre-eclampsia. The pattern of fluid collection varies and may provide a clue as to the underlying etiology – for example the anemic fetus with immune hydrops often develops ascites followed by subcutaneous edema with less significant thoracic collections of fluid, whereas the fetus with a chromosomal abnormality may present with significant subcutaneous edema and a pleural effusion but no, or minimal, ascites[4].

Fetal ascites is recognizable as the echolucent collection of fluid within the abdominal cavity that clearly outlines the visceral contents (Fig. 37.1). While a significant collection of fluid is very obvious, a small rim of fluid confined to the periphery of the abdominal cavity may be more difficult to visualize and a false positive diagnosis can be made if the hypoechogenic features of the muscular layer of the anterior abdominal wall are misinterpreted. Pleural effusions may be unilateral or bilateral, initially forming an echolucent rim of fluid around the margins of the lung but also outlining the mediastinal structures as the effusions become more significant (Fig. 37.2). A small collection of pericardial fluid (<2 mm in depth) is a normal finding

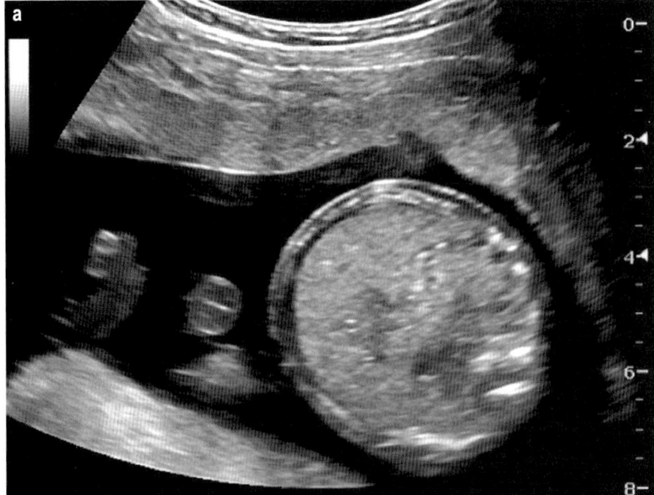

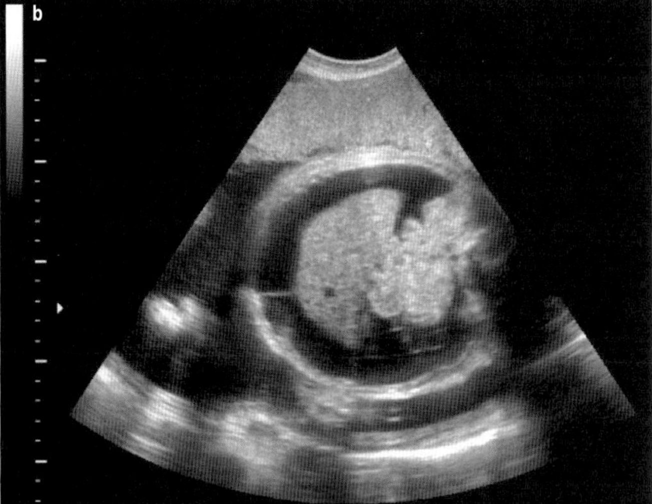

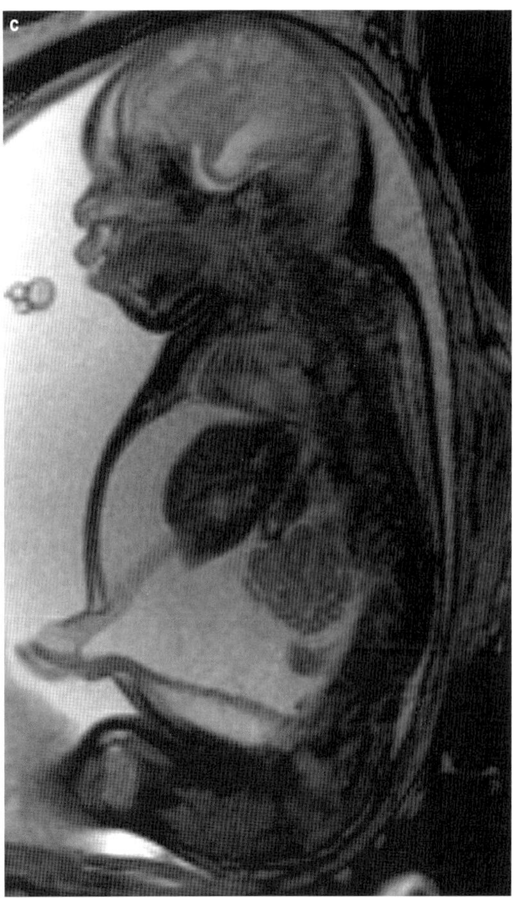

Fig. 37.1 (a,b) Axial sections of the fetal abdomen showing a subtle rim and a moderate collection of fetal ascites respectively; (c) shows the collection of ascites in a sagittal section on fetal MR. This fetus also has significant facial and nuchal skin edema.

during a routine 18–23 week scan, but a more significant echolucent collection is considered to represent a pericardial effusion (Fig. 37.3). Subcutaneous edema may extend throughout the skin tissues, or be confined to the nuchal region (described as increased nuchal translucency in the first trimester and nuchal edema in the second) (Fig. 37.4). On some occasions, the edema will appear to be clearly associated with either an upper or lower body distribution. While it is often most readily visualized in the scalp – contrasting with the bony skull, more care must be taken with assessment over the abdomen – where subcuticular fat may also be thickened.

The placenta may also become edematous and thickened when the fetus is affected by hydrops – and some authors have suggested that significant placental thickening be included as one of the two collections of fluid needed to make a formal diagnosis. A thickness ≥5 cm is considered to be abnormal and the edematous placenta is often described as having a 'ground glass' appearance (Fig. 37.5)[5].

PATHOPHYSIOLOGY

Hydrops describes the collection of (and therefore an imbalance in the production and reabsorption of) interstitial fluid. Extravasation of fluid through the capillary circulation is normally matched by lymphatic return to the vascular space. As a final common pathway, hydrops either results from an increase in the production of interstitial fluid or from an obstruction of lymphatic return.

The factors controlling extravasation of fluid through the capillary wall were first described by Starling 111 years ago and include the hydrostatic pressure within the vessel lumen, the

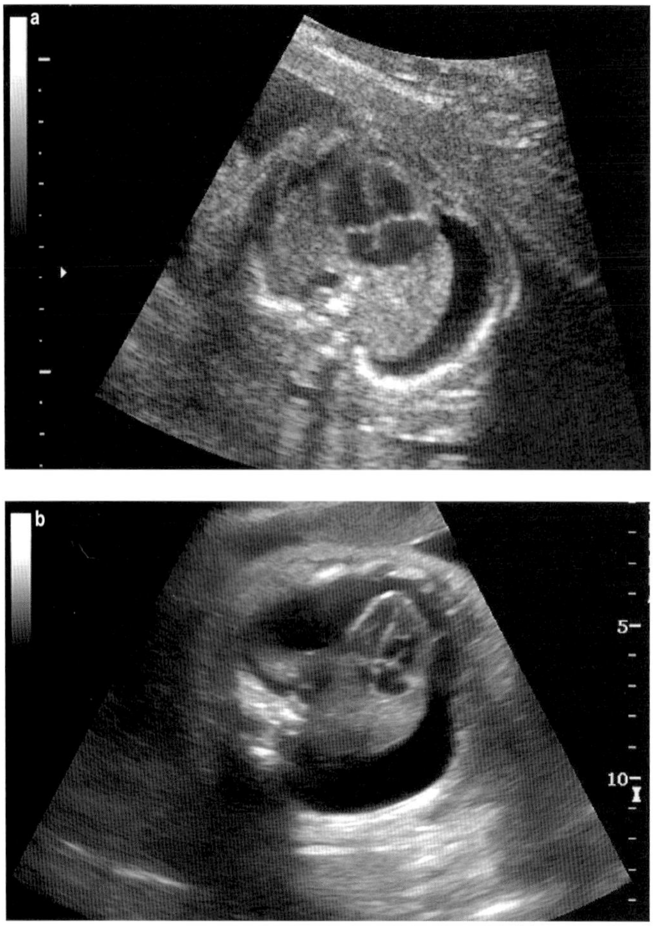

Fig. 37.2 (a) A moderate pleural effusion that is essentially unilateral; (b) this bilateral effusion is more extensive and would be classified as being severe.

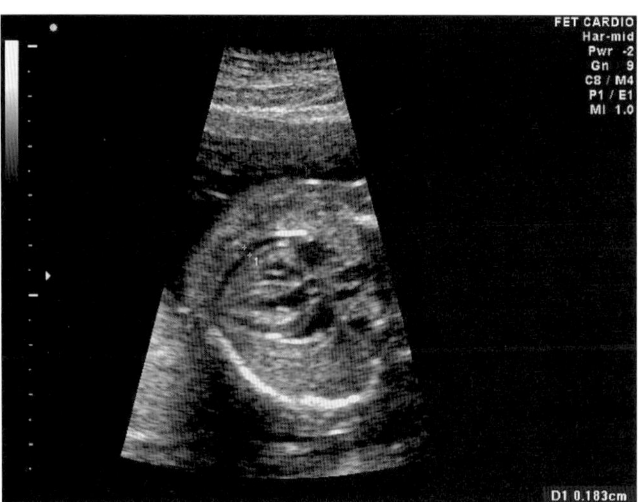

Fig. 37.3 This small (1.8 mm) pericardial effusion lies within normal limits for the 18–20 week scan. Detailed structural examination of the heart is warranted but most clinicians use a cut-off of >2 mm to define a pathological effusion.

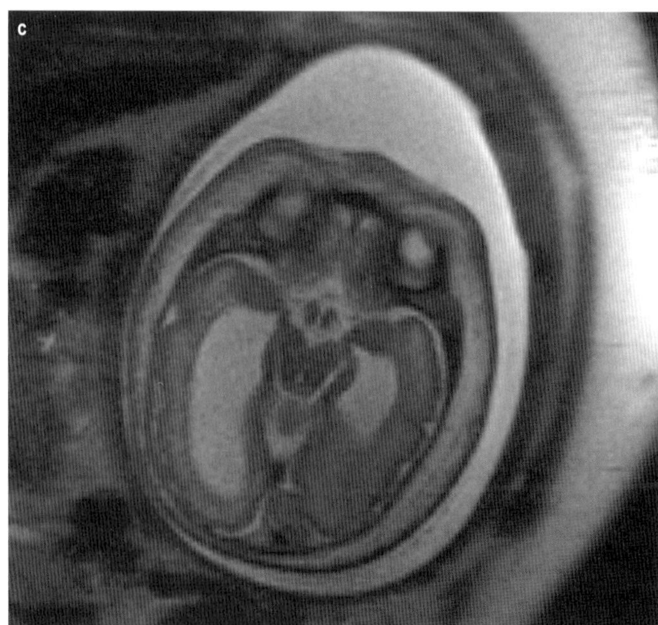

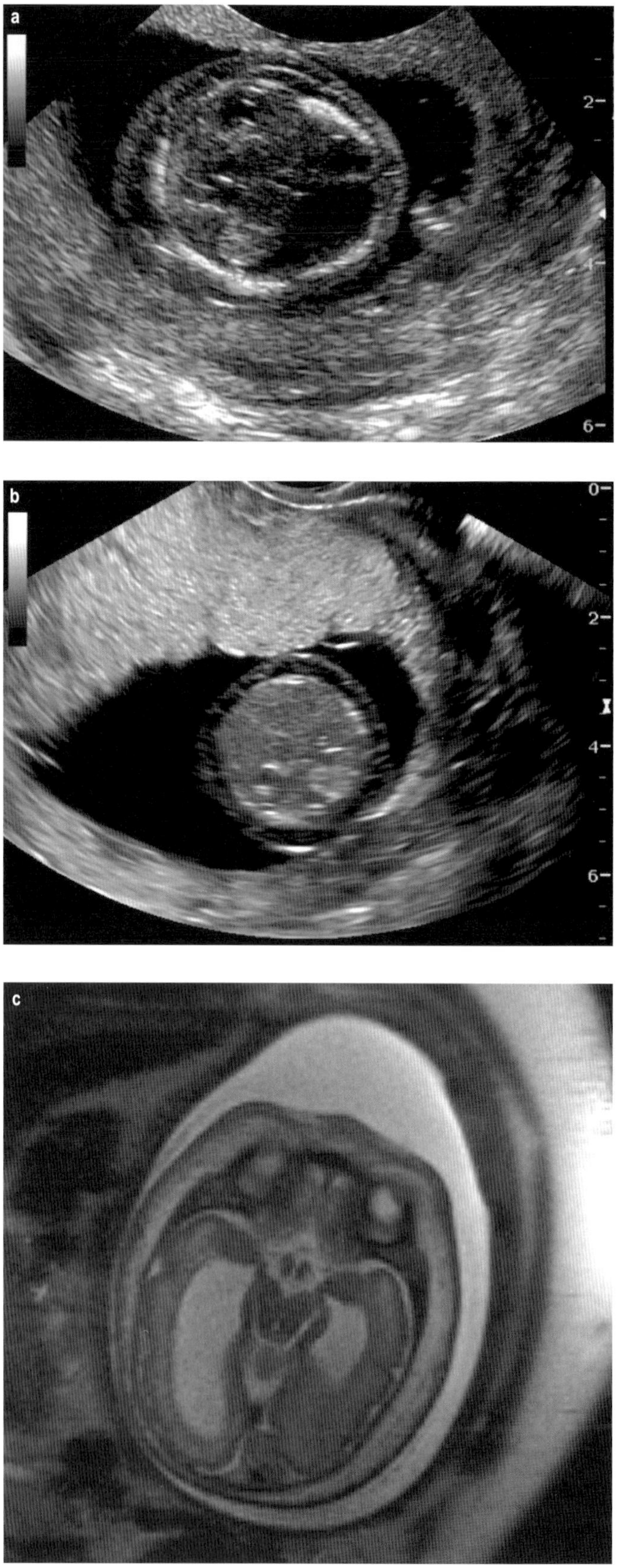

Fig. 37.4 (a,b) Axial sections of the head and abdomen of a first-trimester fetus with significant skin edema; (c) MR image of an axial section of the fetal brain at 33 weeks' gestation showing scalp edema. The MR was performed to investigate further the unilateral ventriculomegaly seen in this fetus presenting with hydrops in the third trimester.

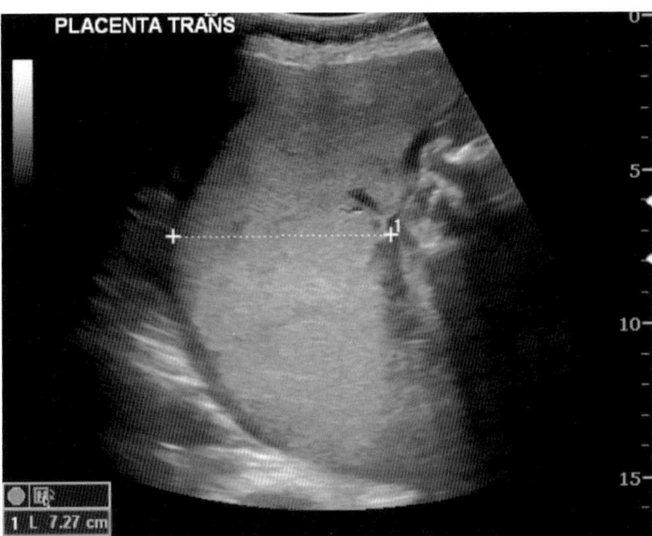

Fig. 37.5 The ground glass appearance of a thickened placenta (>5 cm) seen in association with fetal hydrops.

permeability of the vessel wall and the colloid oncotic pressure of the interstitial space[6]. In comparison to the adult circulation, both water and plasma proteins appear to move more freely across the fetal capillary wall into the interstitial space. As a consequence, there is greater extravasation of fluid for a given pressure gradient and an increased interstitial oncotic pressure that drives less fluid back into the intravascular space. In addition, the interstitial space appears to be more compliant in the fetus, absorbing water with little increase in pressure countering the direction of flow[7]. While lymphatic flow also appears to be significantly increased, the fetus exists in a physiological state that is closer to the limits of tolerance than that seen in the adult circulation[8].

Many of the common cardiovascular conditions associated with hydrops may cause interstitial fluid retention through compensatory mechanisms designed to maintain tissue perfusion. Cardiac output, which is dependent on stroke volume and heart rate, is regulated to maintain delivery of oxygen and other metabolic substrates to the tissues, but compensatory change is limited by the fact that myocardial compliance is relatively poor in the fetus[9]. In these circumstances, organ perfusion may be preserved by increasing local venous pressure, which may lead to the development of hydrops in fetuses with circulatory failure[10,11]. Similarly, cardiac failure is associated with an increase in central venous pressure which will also reduce lymphatic return. A third mechanism underlying interstitial fluid accumulation in fetuses with circulatory failure has been described. In addition to increased venous pressures, compensatory mechanisms preserve perfusion to the brain and heart preferentially. As a consequence, hepatic perfusion and synthesis of albumin and other oncotically active plasma proteins is disrupted and intravenous oncotic pressure falls, further reducing fluid return to the vascular bed[12].

Hydrops is recognized as a common consequence of a multitude of different disease processes and frequently reflects end-stage disease. It appears that many of these cause accumulation of interstitial fluid by a disruption of normal homeostatic mechanisms and that the fetus is prone to these as it has limited means of compensation during development. In the discussion of the underlying etiology of hydrops that follows, there is an attempt to describe the underlying pathophysiology. A better understanding of these complex pathways is needed to develop therapeutic approaches that will reverse this state.

IMMUNE HYDROPS

Immune hydrops describes the process of maternal sensitization to a fetal red blood cell antigen followed by transplacental passage of circulating maternal IgG antibody and fetal red cell hemolysis causing severe fetal anemia. The severity of the hemolytic process is variable and is primarily dependent on the antibody involved and the antibody load. The fetus initially compensates by increasing extramedullary erythropoiesis – which can often be demonstrated sonographically as there is hepatosplenomegaly. In addition to becoming hypoalbuminemic, once the hemoglobin falls <7 g/dl, the fetus fails to maintain tissue oxygenation through an increase in cardiac output and becomes acidotic. Cardiac failure and death can follow within 24–48 hours[13].

Prior to the 1970s, hemolytic disease of the newborn most commonly affected Rhesus-D negative women who had been sensitized to the Rhesus-D antigen through maternofetal hemorrhage in a previous pregnancy (where the fetus was Rhesus-D positive). The introduction of postpartum anti-D immunoglobulin prophylaxis for Rhesus-D negative women has been shown in randomized controlled trials to reduce the risk of alloimmunization in a subsequent pregnancy (relative risk 0.12) and has led to a significant reduction in the prevalence of this disease[14–16]. The detection, investigation and management of red cell alloimmune disease is covered in Chapter 40 and will not be discussed here in any further detail. However, it is important to recognize that, despite the introduction of anti-D prophylaxis, Rhesus-D alloimmunization has continued to be reported in 10 in 10000 births and other antibodies, particularly Rhesus-c, Rhesus-E and Kell, may cause severe hemolytic disease[17–20]. Although the relative prevalence of hydrops due to non-immune disease has increased markedly over the last 30 years, it is important to consider immune disease – by taking an appropriate medical history and testing for the presence of maternal red cell antibodies when trying to define the underlying etiology of this condition.

NON-IMMUNE HYDROPS

Ballantyne first reported that non-immune hydrops was a common end stage for a number of different pathological conditions in 1892[21]. The division between immune and non-immune causes was suggested by Potter in 1943[22]. and, following the success of immunoglobulin prophylaxis for Rhesus alloimmunization, non-immune causes figure in 90% of diagnoses[23]. The publication of the first case reports describing the sonographic signs of fetal hydrops led a number of groups to describe their experiences – demonstrating the difficulties with reaching a diagnosis when these signs are common to so many different etiologies. In 1989, data from 47 series including 804 cases were summarized in an attempt to define appropriate guidelines for prenatal diagnosis and management[24]. Since this time there have been surprisingly few publications detailing experiences with the diagnosis of fetal hydrops and the major series are summarized in Table 37.1[24–30]. Although these studies

Table 37.1 Studies reviewing the underlying aetiology of non-immune fetal hydrops

Author Study details	*N*	*Chromosomal*	*Cardiovascular*	*Thoracic*	*Cystic hygroma*	*Hematological*	*Infection*	*Genetic*	*Twins*	*Other*	*Not defined*
Machin[24] Combines 47 series	731	80 (11%)	164 (22%)	58 (8%)	17 (2%)	124 (17%)	32 (4%)	22 (3%)	64 (9%)	23 (3%)	147 (20%)
Hansmann et al.[25] Fetal series	361	54 (15%)	71 (20%)	23 (6%)	48 (13%)	39 (11%)	11 (3%)	18 (5%)	–	40 (11%)	64 (18%)
McCoy et al.[26] Fetal series	82	13 (16%)	19 (23%)	11 (13%)	–	7 (9%)	–	9 (11%)	5 (6%)	–	18 (22%)
Lallemand et al.[27] Pathology series	94	31 (33%)	13 (14%)	4 (5%)	–	–	15 (16%)	4 (5%)	8 (9%)	10 (11%)	9 (10%)
Ismail et al. [28] Fetal series	55	14 (25%)	5 (9%)	6 (11%)	6 (11%)	–	8 (15%)	2 (4%)	2 (4%)	1 (2%)	11 (20%)
Trainor et al.[29] Neonatal series	28	4 (14%)	4 (14%)	2 (7%)	–	–	1 (4%)	–	–	–	17 (61%)
Abrams et al.[30] Neonatal series	571	45 (8%)	144 (25%)	19 (3%)	10 (2%)	30 (5%)	40 (7%)	26 (5%)	59 (10%)	41 (7%)	157 (27%)
Total	**1972**	**241 (12%)**	**420 (21%)**	**123 (6%)**	**81 (4%)**	**200 (10%)**	**107 (5%)**	**86 (4%)**	**138 (7%)**	**115 (6%)**	**423 (21%)**

are somewhat heterogeneous in nature, it is possible to draw some conclusions about the underlying pathologies seen in non-immune hydrops and these can essentially be categorized into 8 main areas (Table 37.1). The most important among these appears to be fetal cardiovascular anomalies, although two other recent series have demonstrated an extremely high prevalence of chromosomal abnormality in fetuses with non-immune hydrops identified in early pregnancy (<20 weeks)[31,32].

Chromosomal abnormality

Chromosomal abnormalities account for a significant proportion of cases of hydrops, with a prevalence of 11– 33% in second-trimester series (see Table 37.1). The commonest association is with Turner's syndrome – reported in up to 15% of cases[24]. Subcuticular edema is often a major feature of hydrops in fetuses with chromosomal abnormality. In fetuses affected by Turner's syndrome, there is often an extremely large and striking septate cystic hygroma in the posterior aspect of the neck which, if the infant survives, forms a redundant skin fold, or webbing of the neck[33,34]. There is a significant association between 45X, cystic hygroma (or a webbed neck) and coarctation of the aorta and pathological studies have demonstrated obstruction of the jugular lymphatics with a paucity of peripheral lymphatic channels[34,35]. In contrast, the fetal trisomies (21, 18 and 13) are associated with nuchal edema (rather than a septated nuchal lesion) and develop hydrops less frequently, although in the first trimester the finding of increased nuchal translucency is the most effective single marker available for screening for these chromosomal abnormalities[36]. The underlying cardiac defects seen in these fetuses differ to those found in Turner's syndrome and are not necessarily a feature of those fetuses that become hydropic[37]. Once again, there appear to be lymphatic changes, although here there is an increase rather than a reduction in the number of peripheral lymphatic channels[35,38]. Unfortunately, many of the pathological studies detailing the lymphatic development of hydropic fetuses were reported prior to routine fetal karyotyping and our understanding of the underlying pathophysiology remains incomplete. Although a detailed anatomical survey should be completed for any fetus presenting with hydrops, those with chromosomal abnormalities may demonstrate other structural abnormalities which may be suggestive of the underlying etiology. Even in the absence of such features, karyotyping should be offered, and should include a long-term culture as a small proportion of hydropic fetuses have rarer chromosomal rearrangements.

Genetic conditions

In addition to a strong association with chromosomal abnormalities, a significant proportion of fetuses with non-immune hydrops will have an underlying genetic disorder (see Table 37.1). Identifying the underlying etiology is important not only with respect to treatment options but also when considering the risk of recurrence in future pregnancies. Dysmorphic features are difficult to detect prenatally and, consequently, the diagnosis of a genetic syndrome is often very difficult. Involvement of a clinical geneticist at an early stage may improve diagnostic accuracy and prevent omission of relevant investigations. Some syndromes are included in other sections of this chapter due to the nature of the etiology of fetal hydrops. Many others have been documented in isolated case reports but have a low prevalence and are not discussed here. Discussion is limited here to three groups of genetic anomalies that are uncommon but can be diagnosed prenatally with some thought.

A wide variety of skeletal dysplasias with varying phenotypes have been described with hydrops[40]. Shortening of long bones is often the starting point for prenatal diagnosis, although this will be subtle in fetuses with some anomalies, before 24 weeks. Long bones should also be examined for evidence of fractures/poor mineralization and the shape and ossification of other bones, such as the skull, spine and rib cage, should also be carefully assessed[40]. Hydrops is commoner in skeletal anomalies associated with thoracic narrowing, such as thanatophoric dysplasia, Jeune thoracic asphyxiating dystrophy and short rib polydactyly syndrome, and this may be due to increased intrathoracic pressures affecting venous and lymphatic return, although the precise etiology in respect of these disorders remains unclear[24].

Fetuses that have neuromuscular disorders causing paralysis may also present with hydrops and the prognosis in such a case is normally extremely poor[38]. The range of fetal movement can be assessed during ultrasound examination and may help define such an anomaly, although it is often difficult to determine the nature of the underlying condition. Complete investigation includes examination of muscle/skin biopsies and a clinical geneticist and pathologist should be involved to ensure correct samples are taken and forwarded for specialist evaluation[41].

Although inborn errors of metabolism were only noted in 1% of the cases summarized by Machin in 1989, the prevalence now appears to be more widespread, particularly of lysosomal storage diseases, which are described in up to 5–8% of cases of non-immune hydrops (Table 37.2)[24,42,43]. These disorders result in deficiencies or inappropriate accumulation of metabolic substrates followed by hepatic dysfunction. This in turn results in hypoalbuminemia, the significance of which has been discussed previously. Investigation should ideally be performed after discussion with a specialist in metabolic genetics, as this will help to focus attention on disorders that are appropriate to the clinical circumstances and will also ensure that the correct fetal sample (cultured fibroblasts/cultured white cells/fetal serum) is collected.

Cardiovascular abnormalities

Approximately a quarter of the cases of non-immune hydrops seen today have an underlying cardiac or vascular anomaly, the commonest being cardiac arrhythmias (see Chapter 31). Both tachy- and bradyarrhythmias have been associated with fetal hydrops. They have the advantage that a diagnosis can often be made relatively easily and they are frequently amenable to treatment[44]. Supraventricular tachycardia is the commonest tachyarrhythmia seen in fetuses with hydrops. A cardiologist should be involved in treatment, which involves the administration of antiarrhythmic drugs, normally given to the mother, who's own cardiac function needs to be monitored. Fetal mortality is higher in cases where hydrops is present and transplacental passage of drugs will be poor in this circumstance, so direct administration by cordocentesis may be considered[45]. Complete heart block may also cause fetal hydrops, normally once the fetal heart rate has fallen <60 bpm. This bradyarrhythmia may be associated with an underlying structural

Table 37.2 **Hereditary metabolic diseases found in association with non-immune hydrops**

Lysosomal storage diseases	*Non-lysosomal diseases*
Mucopolysaccharidoses: Mucopolysaccharidosis I (Hurler) Mucopolysaccharidosis IVa (Morquio A) Mucopolysaccharidosis VII (β-glucuronidase deficiency)	Glycogenoses: Glycogenosis type IV (Anderson disease)
Oligosaccharidosis: Galactosialidosis Sialidosis GM_1-gangliosidosis	Fatty acid oxidation defects: Long-chain hydroxyacyl CoA dehydrogenase deficiency
Lysosomal transport defects: Sialic acid storage disease	Cholesterol biosynthesis defects: Smith–Lemli–Opitz syndrome 3β-hydroxysterol-Δ^{14}-reductase deficiency
Sphingolipidoses: Gaucher type 2 Niemann– Pick A Niemann– Pick C Lipogranulomatosis (Farber) Wolman	Congenital disorders of glycosylation: CDG Ix
Mucolipidoses: Mucolipidosis II (I-cell disease)	Others: Citric acid cycle defect Hereditary hemochromatosis
Others: Multiple sulfatase deficiency	

From Kooper et al. *Clinica Chimica Acta* **371**:176-182, 2006; © 2006 Elsevier[43]

defect of the heart or with maternal autoimmune disease and the presence of maternal anti-Ro and anti-La antibodies should be assessed[46,47]. It has recently been suggested that maternal therapy with corticosteroids may reduce the risk of disease progression and reduce the risk of heart block in future pregnancies, although the data supporting this are limited to date[48].

Many different types of structural cardiac defects have been associated with fetal hydrops. Although they may not be causative, a mechanism for the development of hydrops can often be described. The fetal circulation is unique in so far as it has three shunts: the ductus venosus, ductus arteriosus and patent foramen ovale, which may play a significant role. For example, an obstructive lesion on the right side of the heart, such as tricuspid or pulmonary atresia, will cause increased right atrial pressure[49]. While a moderate increase in pressure may be compensated for by increased flow across the foramen ovale into the left atrium, in other circumstances the increase in right atrial pressure will lead to increased venous and lymphatic pressure changing the dynamics of capillary drainage, causing fluid retention in the tissues.

Alternatively, obstruction to flow out of the left ventricle or maldevelopment of the left ventricle will prevent left ventricular filling so flow through the foramen ovale, which normally streams oxygenated blood from the right side of the heart to the left side, will be reversed. This will lead to increased right atrial pressure, with subsequent increases in venous and lymphatic pressures beyond. It is not clear why a proportion of fetuses with a left-sided heart lesion that causes obstruction do not develop hydrops, but it has been suggested that, in some circumstances, the right ventricular stroke volume increases, with blood flowing through a dilated ductus venosus, and this reduces the right atrial load.

Hydrops can also develop with some lesions that do not have a typically obstructive picture – an example would be a large atrioventricular defect (AVSD) where valvular regurgitation directed into the right atrium increases venous pressure. In other cases, the mechanism for the development of hydrops is not clear, although it should be remembered that structural defects may be associated with a rhythm abnormality.

Rarer cardiovascular causes of fetal hydrops include fetal or placental arteriovenous shunts that cause a vascular steal and hyperdynamic fetal circulation. Examples include sacrococcygeal teratomas, which may grow rapidly during the second and third trimester with a low resistant arteriovenous shunt developing around the middle sacral artery circulation. A small proportion of these fetuses develop hydrops at a stage where delivery cannot be expedited. In utero ablation of the vascular supply to the tumor has been attempted but, despite this, the pregnancy outcome is generally poor[50]. It has been suggested that the low-resistance arteriovenous shunt also draws blood away from the placenta and this may also cause fetal tissue hypoxia, making the hydrops worse. Similarly, arteriovenous shunts, such as a vein of Galen aneurysm, have been shown to divert cardiac output and disturb the normal perfusion[51]. Placental tumors, such as a chorioangioma, may also cause fetal hydrops and, when a hyperdynamic circulation is suspected, a careful examination of the placenta is mandatory[52].

Table 37.3 **Hematological causes of non-immune hydrops[75]**

Underlying pathophysiology			*Condition*
Excessive erythrocyte loss			
	Hemolysis: Intrinsic	Hemoglobinopathies:	α-thalassemia syndromes
		Erythrocyte enzyme disorders:	Glucose-6-phosphate dehydrogenase Pyruvate kinase Glucosephosphate isomerase
		Erythrocyte membrane disorders:	Abnormalities of spectrin
	Hemolysis: Extrinsic		Kasabach – Merritt syndrome
	Hemorrhage	Fetomaternal hemorrhage Fetal hemorrhage	 Twin-twin transfusion syndrome
Erythrocyte underproduction		Fetal liver/bone marrow replacement anomalies:	Transient myeloproliferative disorder Congenital leukemia
		Red cell aplasia/ dyserythropoiesis:	Blackfan – diamond syndrome Congenital dyserythropoiesis

From Arcasoy MO, Gallagher PG. Hematological disorders and nonimmune hydrops fetalis. *Semin Perinatol* **19**:502–515, 1995. Copyright 1995 WB Saunders Company.

Thoracic abnormalities

A space-occupying lesion within the chest may cause fetal hydrops and this is the primary pathology in a small but significant number of cases (see Table 37.1). Experiments in animal models suggest that an intrathoracic mass causes cardiac compression and an increase in intrathoracic pressure. This results in increased central venous pressure and obstruction of venous and lymphatic return[53]. In some circumstances, the primary lesion may be large pleural effusions due to a lymphatic anomaly, described as a chylothorax, that cause hemodynamic changes and hydrops as a secondary effect. This can be effectively treated by placing an thoracoamniotic shunt to drain the effusion and reverse the hemodynamic effect[54,55]. When the hydropic fetus presents with significant effusions, it is worth considering shunting at an early stage as this may provide both the diagnosis and provide a therapeutic intervention, although it is unclear whether this improves survival[56].

A small number (10–20%) of fetuses affected by congenital cystic adenomatous malformation of the lung have a lesion that is of sufficient size to cause hydrops. Many of these tumors regress with advancing gestation and spontaneous resolution of hydrops has been described[57]. Older series suggested that a finding of hydrops in a fetus with congenital cystic adenomatous malformation of the lung was associated with an extremely poor prognosis and this led to some groups developing techniques for open fetal surgery allowing resection of the affected tissue[58–60]. Hydrops can occur with both macrocystic and microcystic disease, although the former may be more amenable to treatment by drainage of large cysts or placement of a thoracoamniotic shunt, which reduces the risk of maternal morbidity in comparison to an open procedure[56,61].

Other congenital anomalies of the respiratory tract may also cause fetal hydrops, although they are rarer. Pulmonary sequestration describes a non-functional mass of lung tissue that has an arterial supply derived from a systemic artery – frequently the thoracic aorta – which is usually the defining feature from a prenatal perspective. A pulmonary sequestration may cause hydrops either due to a mass effect, as described previously, or due to extravasation of fluid into the thoracic cavity forming a hydrothorax. There are isolated case reports suggesting that, on occasion, these tumors can be successfully treated in utero[62]. Laryngeal or tracheal atresia typically causes lung fluid retention and massive expansion of the lungs will result in fetal hydrops on some occasions. This is an extremely rare anomaly and is immediately recognizable by the presence of bilateral large echogenic lungs causing splinting of the diaphragm and mediastinal compression[63].

Hydrops has been reported in fetuses with diaphragmatic hernia, although this is an unusual finding. In contrast, diaphragmatic eventration is often associated with pleural effusions, and the presence of pleural fluid in a fetus that appears to have a congenital diaphragmatic hernia should raise clinician suspicion for this anomaly[64].

Fetal anemia and hematological abnormalities

Although the proportion of cases of hydrops related to immune disease has decreased, hematological diseases have remained important and are responsible for a significant proportion of non-immune cases (Table 37.3). From the perspective of underlying pathophysiology, the common final pathway is normally fetal anemia, which results either from an increased loss of erythrocytes (by hemolysis or hemorrhage) or from a reduction in red cell synthesis. Anemia may cause hydrops either directly, due to capillary and tissue hypoxia with extravasation of protein or by compensatory mechanisms resulting in high output cardiac failure[65].

The commonest cause of fetal hydrops in Chinese and Southeast Asian pregnancies is related to the hemoglobinopathy α^0-thalassemia. α-Thalassemia describes abnormalities in the α-globin genes, of which there are normally four found on chromosome 16[66]. Deletion of all four α-globin genes results in Hb Bart's disease, which is almost universally fatal in fetal life. The association with fetal hydrops was first described in 1960 and, in Southeast Asia, Hb Bart's has been reported in 60–90% of non-immune cases[67,68]. As no α-globin chains are produced, the fetus combines four γ-globin chains to form the Hb Bart's homotetramer. This form of hemoglobin has such a high affinity for oxygen that delivery fails and there is severe tissue fetal hypoxia. Deletion of 3 α-globin genes, Hb H disease, is generally associated with mild/moderate hemolytic disease and fetal hydrops is relatively rare but has been reported[69]. The diagnosis of α^0-thalassemia, which used to be dependent on analysis of fetal blood, can now be accurately made using molecular techniques, so an amniotic fluid sample (as would be used for karyotyping) is sufficient[69]. From a screening perspective, ultrasound assessment of the cardiothoracic ratio and of placental thickness appear to be highly sensitive as a non-invasive technique[70] (see Chapter 27).

Glucose 6-phosphate dehydrogenase (G6PD) deficiency, an inherited red cell enzyme deficiency, affects almost 10% of the world's population and has, on rare occasions, been associated with non-immune fetal hydrops following maternal ingestion of sulfisoxazole and fava beans respectively[71,72]. Similarly, other red cell enzyme abnormalities, such as deficiencies of the enzymes pyruvate kinase and glucose phosphate isomerase affect ATP production and water/electrolyte homeostasis in red cells which consequently have a shorter half-life and have been reported to cause fetal anemia and hydrops[73,74]. Other disorders causing red cell hemolysis that have been reported to cause fetal hydrops are listed in Table 37.3[75].

Anemia resulting from failed erythropoiesis is most commonly associated with parvovirus infection. Roughly 60% of the population have antibodies to parvovirus and there is an estimated 1–2% risk of seroconversion during pregnancy in endemic periods rising to 10% during epidemics[76]. In a UK study of 190 women found to be IgM positive for parvovirus during pregnancy, 30 (16%) fetal deaths were reported[77]. A second study found that the excess rate of fetal loss (9%) was confined to women infected in the first 20 weeks of pregnancy and that 3% of fetuses infected at 9–20 weeks' gestation became hydropic[78]. Most recent estimates suggest there are 1250 maternal infections of parvovirus in the UK each year, resulting in 59 fetal deaths and 11 cases of fetal hydrops[79]. Death is most commonly associated with severe fetal anemia, as the virus infects erythroid progenitor cells, causing cell lysis of immature red cells[80]. Although this is normally transient, it can be quite profound, affecting the oxygen-carrying capacity of the blood and leading to hydrops as described previously. In addition, parvovirus has a direct affect on the myocardium and hydrops may also result from congestive cardiac failure related to myocarditis[81]. While the long-term outcome for the majority of fetuses exposed to parvovirus appears to be very good, those that develop hydrops have a high (>50%) risk of death and red cell/platelet transfusion is of benefit for support through the aplastic crisis[82,83]. Doppler assessment of the peak velocity of blood flow through the mid-cerebral artery has been shown to be a useful method of screening for fetal anemia and determining when invasive testing and intrauterine transfusion should be performed[84,85]. Despite this, the risk of fetal death remains high – 8/24 (33%) in one series – and there appears to be an increased risk of neurological deficit in survivors (32%)[86].

The synthesis of red cells is also reduced in fetuses that have myeloproliferative disorders and congenital leukemia[87,88]. These conditions are rare and, in many instances, the fetus has an underlying chromosomal abnormality, such as Down's syndrome. Although there may be significant fetal anemia in these circumstances, there may be other underlying etiologies for hydrops, such as lymphatic obstruction, in the presence of chromosomal abnormality[38].

Fetal anemia due to fetomaternal hemorrhage is rare and, in the acute circumstance is likely to lead to fetal death rather than the development of hydrops[89]. Chronic fetal hemorrhage most commonly occurs in twin-twin transfusion syndrome, affecting 10–15% of monochorionic diamniotic twin pregnancies in the second trimester of pregnancy. In this circumstance, hydrops normally affects the recipient twin at a relatively late stage of disease progression – due to fluid overload and high output failure[90]. Hydropic presentation of the smaller donor twin is rare and it is notable that, in one small study of infants with chronic twin-twin transfusion syndrome at this early gestation, the difference in fetal hematocrit was not as significant as that described postnatally[91] (see Chapter 46).

Infectious causes of hydrops fetalis

Maternofetal infection has been described as the underlying cause of non-immune hydrops in 1–8% of cases (see Table 37.1 and Chapter 44)[24,30]. The most common infectious agents are parvovirus B19, cytomegalovirus, syphilis and toxoplasmosis, but many other bacterial and viral infections have also been associated. Parvovirus infection causes an aplastic fetal anemia and this is described in the section on fetal anemia (see above).

Cytomegalovirus and toxoplasmosis may also cause fetal anemia due to their affect on erythroid precursors. Cytomegalovirus infection is also relatively common – with maternal seroconversion seen in 1–2% of pregnancies – and is recognized as being the cause of non-immune hydrops in 1–2% of cases[92,93]. Diagnosis is complicated by the fact that 95% of maternal infections are asymptomatic, but important as maternofetal infection occurs in 50% of cases and the fetus may be affected, with a significant long-term neurological deficit in 10% of these[94]. Additional signs of fetal CMV infection may be seen on ultrasound including microcephaly, ventriculomegaly, intracranial and intrahepatic calcification and growth restriction[95]. Infected fetuses will almost universally excrete virus (>20 weeks' gestation/>6 weeks post infection) and this can be detected in amniotic fluid[96]. In comparison to cytomegalovirus, maternofetal infection with toxoplasmosis is rare[97,98]. Maternal infection with this protozoan leads to a parasitemia and widespread dissemination including transplacental transfer in 30– 40% of cases depending on gestational age[99]. While rates of maternofetal infection increase with advancing gestation, the fetus is more likely to be affected with early infection and it is in this circumstance that hydrops fetalis is normally described. There is limited evidence that medical therapy will lead to resolution of hydrops and a good perinatal outcome[100].

Coxsackie, herpes simplex and adenovirus infections have all been reported in association with fetal hydrops, causing a fetal myocarditis, although this is rare[101]. Similarly, rubella and syphilis may cause hydrops, although these are less likely to be of importance in countries which routinely screen for these conditions antenatally.

CLINICAL EVALUATION OF THE HYDROPIC FETUS

It is important to recognize that hydrops is a sign of disease rather than being a specific anomaly in its own right. From this perspective, there may be no evidence of fetal compromise at the time of the routine 12- or 20-week scan and hydrops may be an incidental finding in the third trimester. The few series that have reported the underlying etiology and outcomes of pregnancies affected by hydrops at <20 weeks' gestation have shown that the prevalence of chromosomal abnormalities is higher in this group[31,32]. Indeed, in terms of screening for chromosomal abnormality in the late first trimester, where nuchal translucency has proven to be the best ultrasound marker, hydrops may be regarded as an extreme end of a spectrum of such fetuses[102]. Early onset of hydrops is also considered to be an indicator of poor prognosis, although there are certainly some fetuses that have significant edema in early pregnancy that continue to have good outcomes[103].

When hydrops is recognized at the 20-week scan, or in the later stages of pregnancy, it is useful to document the extent of fluid retention carefully, so that any improvement or deterioration in fetal condition can be noted during subsequent examination. The examination is not complete without evaluation of the placenta, including measurement of placental thickness and of the amniotic fluid index. A systematic evaluation of fetal anatomy should then be performed to try to define the underlying etiology. Many fetuses with chromosomal abnormality will have multiple structural anomalies or markers of aneuploidy that are visible on scan. If the scan shows no obvious abnormality and previous investigations (such as first-trimester NT assessment or maternal serum biochemistry) have demonstrated a low risk for aneuploidy, then this etiology appears to be unlikely, but cases have been reported and karyotyping should be offered[104].

Fetal structural cardiac defects and arrhythmias are one of the most common causes of hydrops, the latter being amenable to medical therapy in many circumstance[24,30,44]. Specialists in fetal echocardiography will detect the majority of structural defects or rhythm abnormalities and they should be involved in the evaluation of these fetuses. A more extended evaluation of the fetal chest is needed to demonstrate an intrathoracic mass, which may be solid or could merely be a large hydrothorax. A systematic system review will involve measurement of biometry; fetuses with systemic infection are often growth restricted as are fetuses with an underlying genetic disorder. The examination and measurement of long bones should be extended as a comprehensive skeletal survey may show evidence of a skeletal dysplasia. The intracranial anatomy and abdominal viscera should be examined for evidence of structural abnormality and color Doppler is useful for the identification of rare arteriovenous malformations such as an aneurysm of the vein of Galen or an arteriovenous malformation in the liver. Other causes of a hyperdynamic circulation, such as a placental chorioangioma or a sacrococcygeal teratoma, should be excluded at the same time.

The finding of hydrops in one twin of a twin pregnancy is most commonly seen in twin-twin transfusion syndrome. Chorionicity, and therefore the risk of this condition, can be defined with almost 100% accuracy at the 11–14 week scan and monochorionic pregnancies will ideally be enrolled in a program offering a high level of fetal surveillance. In the event that hydrops is seen at presentation (normally at 16–24 weeks' gestation), then the placenta should be examined to determine chorionicity, although this is more difficult at this stage. As hydrops affects the recipient fetus at a relatively late stage in this disease, there should be evidence of significant growth and liquor discrepancy between the two fetuses. In rare circumstances, an acute fetofetal transfusion may occur in the absence of other signs of twin-twin transfusion, and the finding of relatively close cord insertions with a large anastomosis between them supports this diagnosis. If a dichorionic fetus presents with hydrops then the process of investigation used for singleton pregnancies is more relevant.

Suspicion of fetal anemia can be investigated non-invasively by measuring the mid-cerebral artery peak velocity, which will be increased in a hyperdynamic circulation. This test was initially demonstrated to be of value in the assessment of fetuses at risk of Rhesus isoimmunization and has since been shown to be effective at predicting fetal anemia related to other etiologies such as parvovirus. Care should be taken in its application once hydrops has developed, as a reduction in cardiac output may affect cerebral perfusion.

Due to the high prevalence of genetic disease in fetuses with hydrops and the difficulties in defining many of these conditions by ultrasound, it is useful to obtain a detailed family history from the parents. Involvement of a clinical geneticist may make this a more valuable process, as they may recognize dysmorphic features in other family members that are relevant to the case. An example may be the initial presentation of fetal talipes that continues to develop with polyhydramnios, reduced fetal movement and eventual hydrops – a process that can be seen in myotonic dystrophy. This is an autosomal dominant condition with very variable penetrance, but the mother will normally be more mildly affected and this may be detected for the first time at the time of fetal examination.

Further investigation includes amniocentesis, which has been described above in relation to the diagnosis of chromosomal abnormality. Amniotic fluid may also be useful for the diagnosis of fetal infection and for some metabolic syndromes and an extra volume of fluid should be taken for this purpose. DNA can also be extracted from cultured amniocytes and stored for further genetic analysis if/when this is indicated. If fetal anemia is suspected, this can be confirmed by blood sampling. A fetal blood sample can also be used to check for evidence of a hemoglobinopathy (by electrophoresis) and for evidence of red cell dyscrasia (blood film). Viral infection may also cause thrombocytopenia and abnormal liver function and these features can be assessed. Anemia is frequently associated with thrombocytopenia in the hydropic fetus, making cord sampling more hazardous. Blood should be available for transfusion at the time of sampling and, if thrombocytopenia is suspected, it is useful to have platelets available for transfusion as well as red cells.

A maternal blood sample should also be taken at the time of presentation to determine blood group and antibody status, the presence (and therefore risk) of hemoglobinopathy and for evidence of recent maternal infection (of parvovirus, cytomegalovirus, toxoplasmosis or syphilis). A Kleihauer-Betke test may provide evidence of fetomaternal hemorrhage.

A comprehensive and systematic approach to the examination and investigation of the hydropic fetus will allow the underlying etiology to be identified in the majority of cases. This enables the clinician to be more forthcoming about the likely outcome of the pregnancy and the long-term prognosis for the infant as well as being able to discuss therapeutic options in utero. In some circumstances, the fetus will continue to deteriorate and be stillborn. A postmortem will provide valuable information in all cases, confirming the prenatal diagnosis or providing more information to support a diagnosis in others. This then enables the clinician to have a detailed discussion with the parents about the risks of recurrence in a future pregnancy and plan appropriate management for early prenatal diagnosis at that time.

OBSTETRIC MANAGEMENT AND DELIVERY

In addition to the extended investigation and assessment of the hydropic fetus described above, it is important to recognize that this condition, through features such as placentomegaly, may cause significant maternal illness – commonly described as the maternal mirror syndrome[106]. This mimics severe pre-eclampsia and maternal blood pressure, urinary protein and hematological indices should be monitored accordingly. Although the preterm hydropic fetus will have a poorer neonatal outcome that its term equivalent, delivery may, in some circumstances, have to be considered on maternal grounds. Effective treatment of the fetal condition has also been shown to lead to an improvement in maternal disease in several cases[107].

The hydropic fetus is best delivered in an institution with tertiary neonatal facilities and there should be extensive involvement of the neonatal team in the timing of delivery. A recent study reporting the outcome of 30 liveborn infants with non-immune hydrops suggests that the reduced mortality and morbidity generally seen in neonatal care is not reflected in the outcome for hydropic fetuses[108]. Those delivered preterm, with a significant pleural effusion, or with low serum albumin levels, had a poorer outcome[17,109]. The mode of delivery should be determined by individual circumstances, the gestation of pregnancy and the anticipated outcome for the pregnancy. Vaginal delivery may be complicated by the fact that significant polyhydramnios may be associated with an unstable lie and there may be an increased risk of both cord prolapse and placental abruption at the time of rupture of membranes. In addition, in term pregnancies, significant pleural effusions or ascites, or significant generalized edema may splint the thorax and abdomen increasing the risk of shoulder or abdominal dystocia significantly. Indeed, delivery at cesarean section may still be complicated by this factor and drainage of free fluid may both make delivery easier and make neonatal resuscitation easier[110]. Following delivery, there is an increased risk of postpartum hemorrhage due to uterine atony and this should be actively managed.

The majority of hydropic fetuses will require extensive resuscitation at the time of delivery and the neonatal team will usually be in attendance with several experienced doctors and nurses who can manage the various parts of the resuscitation process[111]. It is important that delivery occurs in an environment that allows the neonatal team to work efficiently at stabilizing the infant. Data regarding the long-term outcome for infants that survive fetal hydrops are sparse, but larger datasets are now being reported. This morbidity may be related to the underlying etiology of hydrops or to premature delivery and it is probably important to counsel on this basis rather than using a more global assessment of risk for 'hydropic' fetuses. In a series of 18 hydropic fetuses due to immune disease, there were 16 live births and 2/14 (14%) surviving infants were described as having major neurological sequelae – suggesting that even profoundly anemic fetuses have a high chance (86%) of a normal outcome[112]. In contrast, when fetal anemia was related to parvovirus infection, 5 of 16 (31%) survivors had impaired neurodevelopment which may have been due to central nervous system effects of the viral infection rather than due to fetal anemia and transfusion[86]. Fetal arrhythmias can often be treated successfully, although it is recognized that the hydropic fetus has a higher mortality. In a series of 10 hydropic fetuses presenting with a bradyarrhythmia, none of the 5 survivors had a neurodevelopmental issue[113]. A second series of 11 hydropic fetuses affected by a tachyarrhythmia described neurodevelopmental anomalies in 2 of 9 (22%) survivors[114].

CONCLUSIONS

Fetal hydrops is a common endpoint for a wide variety of conditions. It demonstrates that normal compensatory mechanisms have failed and is associated with a high rate of mortality. The proportion of fetuses that have an immune rather than a non-immune cause has decreased markedly since the introduction of immunoprophylaxis for women at risk of Rhesus-D isoimmunization and routine antenatal screening for blood antibodies. Although a high proportion of fetuses with non-immune hydrops have karyotypic abnormalities, this is also likely to change as effective methods of screening for chromosomal abnormality in early pregnancy become more widespread. A systematic process of investigation for the underlying cause of hydrops will reveal the cause in the majority (80%) of cases. This is often best pursued in a tertiary centre where clinicians from multiple disciplines can contribute to the diagnostic process. Many causes of hydrops are amenable to treatment and fetuses that survive pregnancy and delivery will frequently have a good long-term outcome.

REFERENCES

1. Fleischer AC, Killam AP, Boehm FH et al. Hydrops fetalis: sonographic evaluation and clinical implications. *Radiology* **141**:163–168, 1981.
2. Hutchison AA, Drew JH, Yu VYH, Williams ML, Fortune DW, Beischer NA. Nonimmune hydrops fetalis: a review of 61 cases. *Obstet Gynecol* **59**:347–352, 1982.
3. Mahony BS, Filly RA, Callen PW, Chinn DH, Golbus MS. Severe nonimmune hydrops fetalis: sonographic evaluation. *Radiology* **151**:575–761, 1984.
4. Saltzman DH, Frigoletto FD, Harlow BL, Barss VA, Benacerraf BR. Sonographic evaluation of hydrops fetalis. *Obstet Gynecol* **74**:106–111, 1989.
5. Hoddick WK, Mahony BS, Callen PW, Filly RA. Placental thickness. *J Ultrasound Med* **4**:479–482, 1985.

6. Starling EH. On the absorption of fluids from the connective tissue spaces. *J Physiol* **19**:312–326, 1896.
7. Apkon M. Pathophysiology of hydrops. *Semin Perinatol* **19**:437–446, 1995.
8. Brace RA. Effects of outflow pressure on fetal lymph flow. *Am J Obstet Gynecol* **160**:494–497, 1989.
9. Rudolph AM, Heymann MA, Teramo K, Barrett C, Raiha N. Studies on the circulation of the previable human fetus. *Pediatr Res* **5**:452–465, 1971.
10. Weiner CP. Umbilical pressure measurement in the evaluation of nonimmune hydrops fetalis. *Am J Obstet Gynecol* **168**:817–823, 1993.
11. Johnson P, Sharland G, Allan LD, Tynan MJ, Maxwell DJ. Umbilical venous pressure in nonimmune hydrops fetalis: correlation with cardiac size. *Am J Obstet Gynecol* **167**:1309–1313, 1992.
12. Dunn DG, Hayes P, Breen KJ et al. The liver in congestive heart failure: a review. *Am J Med Sci* **265**:174–189, 1973.
13. Nicolaides KH. Studies on fetal physiology and pathophysiology in rhesus disease. *Semin Perinatol* **13**:328–337, 1989.
14. Hamilton EG. Prevention of Rh isoimmunisation by injection of anti-D antibody. *Obstet Gynecol* **30**:812–815, 1967.
15. Crowther C, Middleton P. Anti-D administration after childbirth for preventing Rhesus alloimmunisation. *Cochrane Database Syst Rev* **2**:CD000021, 2000.
16. Adams MM, Marks JS, Gustafson J, Oakley GP. Rh hemolytic disease of the newborn: using incidence observations to evaluate the use of Rh immune globin. *Am J Public Health* **71**:1031–1035, 1981.
17. Chavez GF, Mulinare J, Edmonds LD. Epidemiology of Rh hemolytic disease of the newborn in the Unites States. *J Am Med Assoc* **265**:3270–3274, 1991.
18. Hackney DN, Knudtson EJ, Rossi KQ, Krugh D, O'Shaughnessy RW. Management of pregnancies complicated by anti-c isoimmunization. *Obstet Gynecol* **103**:24–30, 2004.
19. Moran P, Robson SC, Reid MM. Anti-E in pregnancy. *Br J Obstet Gynaecol* **107**: 1436–1438, 2000.
20. McKenna DS, Nagaraja HN, O'Shaughnessy R. Management of pregnancies complicated by anti-Kell isoimmunization. *Obstet Gynecol* **93**: 667–673, 1999.
21. Ballantyne JW. *The diseases and deformities of the fetus*. Edinburgh: Oliver and Boyd, 1892.
22. Potter EL. Universal edema of fetus unassociated with erythroblastosis. *Am J Obstet Gynecol* **46**:130, 1943.
23. Santolaya J, Alley D, Jaffe R, Warsof SL. Antenatal classification of hydrops fetalis. *Obstet Gynecol* **79**:256–259, 1992.
24. Machin GA. Hydrops revistited: literature review of 1414 cases published in the 1980s. *Am J Med Genet* **34**:366–390, 1989.
25. Hansmann M, Gembruch U, Bald R. New therapeutic aspects in nonimmune hydrops fetalis based on 402 prenatally diagnosed cases. *Fetal Ther* **4**:29–36, 1989.
26. McCoy MC, Katz VL, Gould N, Kuller JA. Nonimmune hydrops after 20 weeks' gestation: review of 10 years' experience with suggestions for management. *Obstet Gynecol* **85**:578–582, 1995.
27. Lallemand AV, Doco-Fenzy M, Gaillard DA. Investigation of nonimmune hydrops fetalis: multidisciplinary studies are necessary for diagnosis – review of 94 cases. *Pediatr Dev Path* **2**:432–439, 1999.
28. Ismail KMK, Martin WL, Ghosh S, Whittle MJ, Kilby MD. Etiology and outcome of hydrops fetalis. *J Mat Fetal Med* **10**:175–181, 2001.
29. Trainor B, Tubman R. The emerging pattern of hydrops fetalis – incidence, aetiology and management. *Ulster Med J* **75**:185–186, 2006.
30. Abrams ME, Meredith KS, Kinnard P, Clark RH. Hydrops fetalis: a retrospective review of cases reported to a large national database and identification of risk factors associated with death. *Pediatrics* **120**:84–89, 2007.
31. Iskaros J, Jauniaux E, Rodeck C. Outcome of nonimmune hydrops fetalis diagnosed during the first half of pregnancy. *Obstet Gynecol* **90**:321–325, 1997.
32. Has R. Non-immune hydrops fetalis in the first trimester: a review of 30 cases. *Clin Exp Obstet Gynecol* **28**:187–190, 2001.
33. Chervenak FA, Isaacson G, Blakemore KJ et al. Fetal cystic hygroma. Cause and natural history. *N Engl J Med* **309**:822–825, 1983.
34. Clark EB. Neck web and congenital heart defects: a pathogenic association in 45 X-O Turner syndrome? *Teratology* **29**: 355–361, 1984.
35. Chitayat D, Kalousek DK, Bamforth JS. Lymphatic abnormalities in fetuses with posterior cervical cystic hygroma. *Am J Med Genet* **33**:352–356, 1989.
36. Nicolaides KH. Nuchal translucency and other first-trimester sonographic markers of chromosomal abnormalities. *Am J Obstet Gynecol* **191**:45–67, 2004.
37. Hyett J, Moscoso G, Nicolaides K. Abnormalities of the heart and great arteries in first trimester chromosomally abnormal fetuses. *Am J Med Genet* **69**: 207–216, 1997.
38. Miyabara S, Sugihara H, Maehara N et al. Significance of cardiovascular malformations in cystic hygroma: a new interpretation of the pathogenesis. *Am J Med Genet* **34**:489–501, 1989.
39. Steiner RD. Hydrops fetalis: role of the geneticist. *Semin Perinatol* **19**:516–524, 1995.
40. Dugoff L, Thieme G, Hobbins JC. Skeletal anomalies. *Clin Perinatol* **27**:979–1005, 2000.
41. Witters I, Moerman P, Fryns JP. Fetal akinesia deformation sequence: a study of 30 consecutive in utero diagnoses. *Am J Med Genet* **113**:23–28, 2002.
42. Jauniaux E, Van Maldergem L, De Munter C et al. Non-immune hydrops fetalis associated with genetic abnormalities. *Obstet Gynecol* **75**:568–572, 1990.
43. Kooper AJA, Janssens PMW, de Groot ANJA et al. Lysosomal stroage diseases in non-immune hydrops fetalis pregnancies. *Clin Chim Acta* **371**:176–182, 2006.
44. Kleinman CS, Nehgme RA. Cardiac arrhythmias in the human fetus. *Pediatr Cardiol* **25**:234–251, 2004.
45. Simpson JM, Sharland GK. Fetal tachycardias: management and outcome of 127 consecutive cases. *Heart* **79**: 576–581, 1998.
46. Jaeggi ET, Hornberger LK, Smallhorn JF, Fouron JC. Prenatal diagnosis of complete atrioventricular block associated with structural heart disease: combined experience of two tertiary care centers and review of the literature. *Ultrasound Obstet Gynecol* **26**:16–21, 2005.
47. Berg C, Geipel A, Kohl T et al. Atrioventricular block detected in fetal life: associated anomalies and potential prognostic markers. *Ultrasound Obstet Gynecol* **26**:4–15, 2005.
48. Costedoat-Chalumeau N, Amoura Z, Villain E, Cohen L, Piette JC. Anti-SSA/Ro antibodies and the heart: more than complete congenital heart block? A review of electrocardiographic and myocardial abnormalities and of treatment options. *Arthritis Res Ther* **7**:69–73, 2005.
49. Moller JH, Lynch RP, Edwards JE. Fetal cardiac failure resulting from congenital anomalies of the heart. *J Pediatr* **68**: 699–703, 1966.
50. Makin EC, Hyett J, Ade-Ajayi N, Patel S, Nicolaides K, Davenport M. Outcome of antenatally diagnosed sacrococcygeal teratomas: single-center experience (1993–2004). *J Pediatr Surg* **41**:388–393, 2006.
51. Doyle NM, Mastrobattista JM, Thapar MK, Lantin-Hermoso MR. Perinatal pseudocoarctation: echocardiographic findings in vein of Galen malformation. *J Ultrasound Med* **24**:93–98, 2005.
52. Russell RT, Carlin A, Ashworth M, Welch CR. Diffuse placental chorioangiomatosis and fetal hydrops. *Fetal Diagn Ther* **22**:183–185, 2007.
53. Rice HE, Estes JM, Hedrick MH, Bealer JF, Harrison MR, Adzick NS. Congenital cystic adenomatoid

malformation: a sheep model of fetal hydrops. *J Pediatr Surg* **29**:692–696, 1994.
54. Rodeck CH, Fisk NM, Fraser DI, Nicolini U. Long-term in utero drainage of fetal hydrothorax. *N Engl J Med* **319**:1135–1138, 1988.
55. Yamamoto M, Insunza A, Carrillo J, Caicedo LA, Paiva E, Ville Y. Intrathoracic pressure in congenital chylothorax: keystone for the rationale of thoracoamniotic shunting? *Fetal Diagn Ther* **22**:169–171, 2007.
56. Knox EM, Kilby MD, Martin WL, Khan KS. In-utero pulmonary drainage in the management of primary hydrothorax and congenital cystic lung lesion: a systematic review. *Ultrasound Obstet Gynecol* **28**:726–734, 2006.
57. Ierullo AM, Ganapathy R, Crowley S, Craxford L, Bhide A, Thilaganathan B. Neonatal outcome of antenatally diagnosed congenital cystic adenomatoid malformations. *Ultrasound Obstet Gynecol* B :150–153, 2005.
58. Adzick NS, Harrison MR, Glick PL et al. Fetal cystic adenomatoid malformation: prenatal diagnosis and natural history. *J Pediatr Surg* **20**:483–488, 1985.
59. Adzick NS, Harrison MR, Flake AW, Howell LJ, Golbus MS, Filly RA. Fetal surgery for cystic adenomatoid malformation of the lung. *J Pediatr Surg* **28**:806–812, 1993.
60. Grethel EJ, Wagner AJ, Clifton MS et al. Fetal intervention for mass lesions and hydrops improves outcome: a 15-year experience. *J Pediatr Surg* **42**:117–123, 2007.
61. Wilson RD, Baxter JK, Johnson MP et al. Thoracoamniotic shunts: fetal treatment of pleural effusions and congenital cystic adenomatoid malformations. *Fetal Diagn Ther* **19**:413–420, 2004.
62. Oepkes D, Devlieger R, Lopriore E, Klumper FJ. Successful ultrasound-guided laser treatment of fetal hydrops caused by pulmonary sequestration. *Ultrasound Obstet Gynecol* **29**:457–459, 2007.
63. Lim FY, Crombleholme TM, Hedrick HL et al. Congenital high airway obstruction syndrome: natural history and management. *J Pediatr Surg* **38**:940–945, 2003.
64. Jeanty C, Nien JK, Espinoza J et al. Pleural and pericardial effusion: a potential ultrasonographic marker for the prenatal differential diagnosis between congenital diaphragmatic eventration and congenital diaphragmatic hernia. *Ultrasound Obstet Gynecol* **29**:378–387, 2007.
65. Bernischke K, Kaufmann P. Erythroblastosis fetalis and hydrops fetalis. In *Pathology of the human placenta*, pp. 421–448. New York: Springer-Verlag, 1995.
66. Chui DH, Waye JS. Hydrops fetalis caused by alpha-thalassemia: an emerging health care problem. *Blood* **91**:2213–2222, 1998.
67. Eng L-I, Hie JB. Hydrops fetalis with a fast moving haemoglobin. *Br Med J* **2**:1649–1650, 1960.
68. Chan V, Chan TK, Liang ST et al. Hydrops fetalis due to an unusual form of HbH disease. *Blood* **66**:224–228, 1985.
69. Basran RK, Patterson M, Walker L et al. Prenatal diagnosis of hemoglobinopathies in Ontario, Canada. *Ann NY Acad Sci* **1054**:507–510, 2005.
70. Leung KY, Liao C, Li QM et al. A new strategy for prenatal diagnosis of homozygous alpha(0)-thalassemia. *Ultrasound Obstet Gynecol* **28**:173–177, 2006.
71. Perkins RP. Hydrops fetalis and stillbirth in a male glucose-6-phosphate dehydrogenase deficient fetus possibly due to maternal ingestion of sulfisoxazole: a case report. *Am J Obstet Gynecol* **111**:379–381, 1971.
72. Mentzer WC, Collier E. Hydrops fetalis associated with erythrocyte G-6-PD deficiency and maternal ingestion of fava beans and ascorbic acid. *J Pediatr* **86**: 565–567, 1975.
73. Gilsanz F, Vega MA, Gomez-Castillo E et al. Fetal anaemia due to pyruvate kinase deficiency. *Arch Dis Child* **69**: 523–524, 1993.
74. Ravindranath Y, Paglia DE, Warrier I et al. Glucose phosphate isomerase deficiency as a cause of hydrops fetalis. *N Engl J Med* **316**:258–261, 1987.
75. Arcasoy MO, Gallagher PG. Hematological disorders and nonimmune hydrops fetalis. *Semin Perinatol* **19**:502–515, 1995.
76. Dembinski J, Eis-Hubinger AM, Maar J, Schild R, Bartmann P. Long term followup of serostatus after maternal parvovirus B19 infection. *Arch Dis Child* **88**:219–221, 2003.
77. Cohen B. Parvovirus B19: an expanding spectrum of disease. *Br Med J* **311**: 1549–1552, 1995.
78. Miller E, Fairley CK, Cohen BJ, Seng C. Immediate and long term outcome of human parvovirus B19 infection in pregnancy. *Br J Obstet Gynecol* **105**: 174–178, 1998.
79. Vyse AJ, Andrews NJ, Hesketh LM, Pebody R. The burden of parvovirus B19 infection in women of childbearing age in England and Wales. *Epidemiol Infect* Feb 12: 1–9 (Epub ahead of print), 2007.
80. Chisaka H, Morita E, Yaegashi N, Sugamura K. Parvovirus B19 and the pathogenesis of anaemia. *Rev Med Virol* **13**:347–359, 2003.
81. Naides SJ, Weiner CP. Antenatal diagnosis and palliative treatment of non-immune hydrops fetalis secondary to fetal parvovirus B19 infection. *Prenat Diagn* **9**:105–114, 1989.
82. Schild RL, Bald R, Plath H, Eis-Hubinger AM, Enders G, Hansmann M. Intrauterine management of fetal parvovirus B19 infection. *Ultrasound Obstet Gynecol* **13**:161–166, 1999.
83. Fairley CK, Smoleniec JS, Caul OE, Miller E. Observational study of effect of intrauterine transfusions on outcome of fetal hydrops after parvovirus B19 infection. *Lancet* **346**:1335–1337, 1995.
84. Delle Chiaie L, Buck G, Grab D, Terinde R. Prediction of fetal anemia with Doppler measurement of the middle cerebral artery peak systolic velocity in pregnancies complicated by maternal blood group alloimmunization or parvovirus B19 infection. *Ultrasound Obstet Gynecol* **18**:232–236, 2001.
85. Hernandez-Andrade E, Scheier M, Dezerega V, Carmo A, Nicolaides KH. Fetal middle cerebral artery peak systolic velocity in the investigation of non-immune hydrops. *Ultrasound Obstet Gynecol* **23**:442–445, 2004.
86. Nagel HTC, de Haan TR, Vandenbussche FPHA, Oepkes D, Walther FJ. Long-term outcome after fetal transfusion for hydrops associated with parvovirus B19 infection. *Obstet Gynecol* **109**:42–47, 2007.
87. Foucar K, Friedman K, Llewellyn A et al. Prenatal diagnosis of transient myeloproliferative disorder via percutaneous umbilical blood sampling. Report of two cases in fetuses affected by Down's syndrome. *Am J Clin Pathol* **97**:584–590, 1992.
88. Donnenfeld AE, Scott SC, Henselder-Kimmel M et al. Prenatally diagnosed non-immune hydrops caused by congenital transient leukaemia. *Prenat Diagn* **14**:721–724, 1994.
89. Giacoia GP. Severe fetomaternal hemorrhage: a review. *Obstet Gynecol Surv* **52**:372–380, 1997.
90. Quintero RA, Morales WJ, Allen MH, Bornick PW, Johnson PK, Kruger M. Staging of twin-twin transfusion syndrome. *J Perinatol* **19**: 550–555, 1999.
91. Saunders NJ, Snijders RJ, Nicolaides KH. Twin-twin transfusion syndrome during the 2nd trimester is associated with small intertwin hemoglobin differences. *Fetal Diagn Ther* **6**:34–36, 1991.
92. Beksac MS, Saygan-Karamursel B, Ustacelebi S et al. Prenatal diagnosis of intrauterine cytomegalovirus infection in a fetus with non-immune hydrops fetalis. *Acta Obstet Gynecol Scand* **80**:762–765, 2001.

93. Lujan-Zilbermann J, Lacson A, Gilbert-Barness E, Pomerance HH. Clinicopathologic conference: newborn with hydrops fetalis caused by CMV infection case report. *Pediatr Pathol Mol Med* **22**:481–494, 2003.
94. Fowler KB, Stagno S, Pass RF, Britt WJ, Boll TJ, Alford CA. The outcome of congenital cytomegalovirus infection in relation to maternal antibody status. *N Engl J Med* **326**:663–667, 1992.
95. Degani S. Sonographic findings in fetal viral infections: a systematic review. *Obstet Gynecol Surv* **61**(5): 329–336, 2006.
96. Enders G, Bander U, Lindemann L, Schalasta G, Daiminger A. Prenatal diagnosis of congenital cytomegalovirus infection in 189 pregnancies with known outcome. *Prenat Diagn* **21**:362–377, 2001.
97. Walpole IR, Hodgen N, Bower C. Congenital toxoplasmosis: a large survey in western Australia. *Med J Aust* **154**:720–724, 1991.
98. Abdel-Fattah SA, Bhat A, Illanes S, Bartha JL, Carrington D. TORCH test for fetal medicine indications: only CMV is necessary in the United Kingdom. *Prenat Diagn* **25**:1028–1031, 2005.
99. Petersen E. Toxoplasmosis. *Semin Fetal Neonat Med* **12**:214–223, 2007.
100. Friedman S, Ford-Jones LE, Toi A, Ryan G, Blaser S, Chitayat D. Congenital toxoplasmosis: prenatal diagnosis, treatment and postnatal outcome. *Prenat Diagn* **19**:330–333, 1999.
101. Barron SD, Pass RF. Infectious causes of hydrops fetalis. *Semin Perinatol* **19**: 493–501, 1995.
102. Nicolaides KH, Azar G, Byrne D, Mansur C, Marks K. Fetal nuchal translucency: ultrasound screening for chromosomal defects in first trimester of pregnancy. *Br Med J* **304**:867–869, 1992.
103. Souka AP, Von Kaisenberg CS, Hyett JA, Sonek JD, Nicolaides KH. Increased nuchal translucency with normal karyotype. *Am J Obstet Gynecol* **192**:1005–1021, 2005.
104. Hojo S, Tsukimori K, Kitade S et al. Prenatal sonographic findings and hematological abnormalities in fetuses with transient abnormal myelopoiesis with Down syndrome. *Prenat Diagn* **27**:507–511, 2007.
105. Hofstaetter C, Hansmann M, Eik-Nes SH, Huhta JC, Luther SL. A cardiovascular profile score in the surveillance of fetal hydrops. *J Matern Fetal Neonatal Med* **19**:407–413, 2006.
106. van Selm M, Kanhai HH, Gravenhorst JB. Maternal hydrops syndrome: a review. *Obstet Gynecol Surv* **46**(12):785–788, 1991.
107. Livingston JC, Malik KM, Crombleholme TM, Lim FY, Sibai BM. Mirror syndrome: a novel approach to therapy with fetal peritoneal amniotic shunt. *Obstet Gynecol* **110** :540–543, 2007.
108. Simpson JH, McDevitt H, Young D, Cameron AD. Severity of non-immune hydrops fetalis at birth continues to predict survival despite advances in perinatal care. *Fetal Diagn Ther* **21**: 380–382, 2006.
109. Huang HR, Tsay PK, Chiang MC, Lien R, Chou YH. Prognostic factors and clinical features in liveborn neonates with hydrops fetalis. *Am J Perinatol* **24**:33–38, 2007.
110. Cardwell MS. Aspiration of fetal pleural effusions or ascites may improve neonatal resuscitation. *South Med J* **89**:177–178, 1996.
111. McMahan MJ, Donovan EF. The delivery room resuscitation of the hydropic neonate. *Semin Perinatol*, **19**: 474–482, 199;.
112. Harper DC, Swingle HM, Weiner CP, Bonthius DJ, Aylward GP, Widness JA. Long-term neurodevelopmental outcome and brain volume after treatment for hydrops fetalis by in utero intravascular transfusion. *Am J Obstet Gynecol* **195**:192–200, 2006.
113. Breur JM, Gooskens RH, Kapusta L et al. Neurological outcome in isolated congenital heart block and hydrops fetalis. *Fetal Diagn Ther* **24**:457–461, 2007.
114. Oudijk MA, Gooskens RH, Stoutenbeek P, De Vries LS, Visser GH, Meijboom EJ. Neurological outcome of children who were treated for fetal tachycardia complicated by hydrops. *Ultrasound Obstet Gynecol* **24**:154–158, 2004.

CHAPTER

38 Fetal tumors

Mark P Johnson and Stephanie Mann

KEY POINTS

- Giant neck masses can obstruct or infiltrate the fetal airway creating a surgical emergency at time of birth. Delivery using the EXIT strategy allows establishment of a stable airway while the infant remains on maternal–placental support
- Cervical and sacral teratoma can place excessive cardiac demands through a vascular steal phenomenon that leads to high output physiology, polyhydramnios and risk of preterm delivery and/or hydrops from cardiac failure and intrauterine death
- Neuroblastoma usually presents as an adrenal mass and requires ongoing prenatal surveillance for complications of mass effect from tumor growth, metastasis, hydrops or onset of maternal pre-eclampsia

INTRODUCTION

The widespread use of prenatal ultrasound has led to the increased recognition of a number of fetal structural malformations that can have a direct impact on perinatal management and fetal outcome. There is no more striking example of this than giant fetal neck masses (Table 38.1) such as cervical teratoma and lymphangioma. These lesions can grow to such large proportions that the fetal airway can become distorted and obstructed. Unsuspected obstructing fetal neck masses often prove fatal because of an inability to secure an airway at time of delivery. They can also cause compression of the esophagus and obstruct the oropharynx resulting in polyhydramnios that leads to severe preterm delivery. Cervical and sacral teratoma can place significant hemodynamic demands on the fetus that can lead to congestive heart failure, spontaneous tumor rupture or hemorrhage into the mass leading to exsanguination, or cause dystocia at time of delivery with high trauma-related morbidity and mortality. Neuroblastomas are sporadically occurring neural crest-derived tumors that, when diagnosed in the prenatal period, generally have a favorable outcome. Serial imaging is necessary for these masses to monitor growth and for the rare occurrence of in utero metastasis. In this chapter, we will explore the prenatal diagnoses, issues of antepartum and intrapartum management and postnatal therapy of these congenital tumors.

Table 38.1 **Differential diagnosis of neck masses**

Branchial cleft cyst
Congenital goiter
Hamartoma
Hemangioma
Laryngocele
Lipoma
Lymphangioma
Neuroblastoma
Neural tube defect*
Parotid tumor
Solid thyroid tumor
Thyroid cyst or thyroglossal duct cyst

*Occipital encephalocele, cervical myelomeningocele

CYSTIC HYGROMA AND LYMPHANGIOMA

Cystic hygroma, or lymphangioma, is a benign malformation comprised of dilated cystic lymphatics that are present at birth and are second only to hemangioma as a cause of soft tissue mass in the newborn[1–3]. They can occur in almost any location, most commonly seen in the soft tissue of the neck, axilla, thorax and lower extremities. Isaacs[3] reported a case series of 97 consecutive lymphangiomas in which 45 occurred in the neck, 22 in the chest wall, 12 in the extremities and 4 involved the abdominal wall. These lesions can vary in size from tiny subepidermal skin cysts to large dilated cystic fluid-filled masses that, when present in the neck, are commonly referred to as a cystic hygroma.

Prenatal sonographic examination in the second trimester identifies a group of fetuses with cystic hygroma in which 60% have associated chromosomal abnormalities, are often associated with other structural malformations and have a high mortality rate[4–6]. Multiple cystic hygroma are usually present at an early gestational age, occupy the posterior triangle of the neck, frequently develop hydrops fetalis and have a high incidence of intrauterine death with rare postnatal survival. In contrast, isolated cystic hygroma generally presents during the latter half of pregnancy and frequently has had a normal screening ultrasound earlier in gestation. The lymphangiomas in these infants are usually located anteriorly or anterior lateral involving the anterior cervical triangle, and have much better survival[7,8].

The lymphatic system develops at the end of the fifth week of gestation. Cystic hygromas involving the neck are thought to arise secondary to failure of the jugular lymph sacs to join the lymphatic system resulting in tiny sac-like structures sprouting from the existing cystic spaces. Lymph-like fluid is secreted into these endothelial-lined cystic spaces causing local dilation and progressive enlargement of the cystic spaces[2,9].

Lymphangiomas diagnosed in utero are commonly seen in association with Turner's syndrome, hydrops, oligohydramnios, single umbilical artery, Noonan syndrome, fetal alcohol syndrome and chromosomal aneuploidy, particularly trisomy 18 and 21[6,9,10]. Cystic hygromas in the presence of a normal karyotype have been associated with Noonan syndrome, multiple pterygium syndrome, polysplenia syndrome, Robert syndrome, or an autosomal recessive trait[11–14]. Cystic hygromas that develop late in gestation appear to be a different entity and are not generally associated with other anomalies or hydrops. Such masses may regress in utero, presumably due to development of collateral lymphatic and venous connections. However, postnatal webbing of the neck and persistent lymphedema of the tops of the hands and feet are characteristic features of Turner's syndrome in which the fetal cystic hygromas have spontaneously resolved.

The prenatal sonographic features of a lymphangioma include fluid-filled cystic spaces divided by fine septa commonly observed in the nuchal region and anterior (Fig. 38.1) and posterior triangle of the neck (Fig. 38.2). They often have a dense midline posterior septum extending from the fetal neck across the full width of the hygroma. This septum appears to be the sonographic equivalent of the nuchal ligament. To differentiate a lymphangioma from other diagnoses, it is important to exclude a bony defect in the skull or cervical spine that would be seen with encephalocele. Cysts that are separated by septa are helpful in distinguishing nuchal edema from a true hygroma. Solid components containing calcifications should be excluded to distinguish lymphangiomas from cystic teratomas. Once a cystic hygroma or lymphangioma is identified, further evaluation should be performed to identify other features such as skin edema, ascites or pleural effusions that might suggest a diagnosis of non-immune hydrops.

The differential diagnosis of cystic neck masses includes nuchal edema, encephalocele or other neural tube defects and cystic teratoma. The distinction between a lymphangioma and cervical teratoma can be extremely difficult. However, teratomas generally have a more complex sonographic appearance with solid as well as cystic components and calcifications within the mass are thought to be diagnostic of teratoma. Fetal

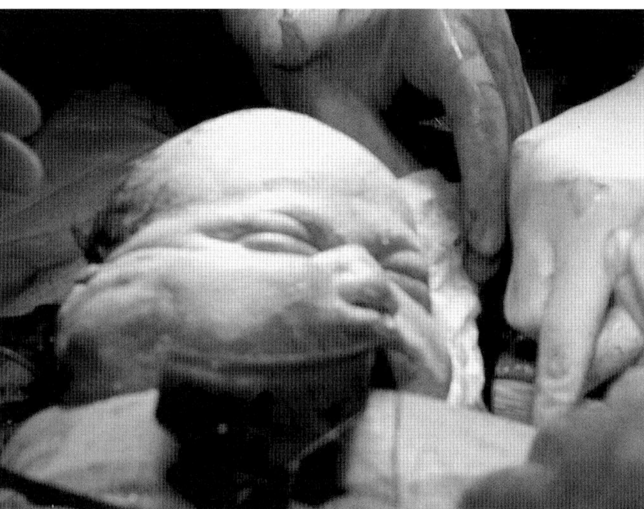

Fig. 38.1 Cystic lymphangioma of the anterior right neck in a fetus undergoing delivery by elective repeat cesarean section.

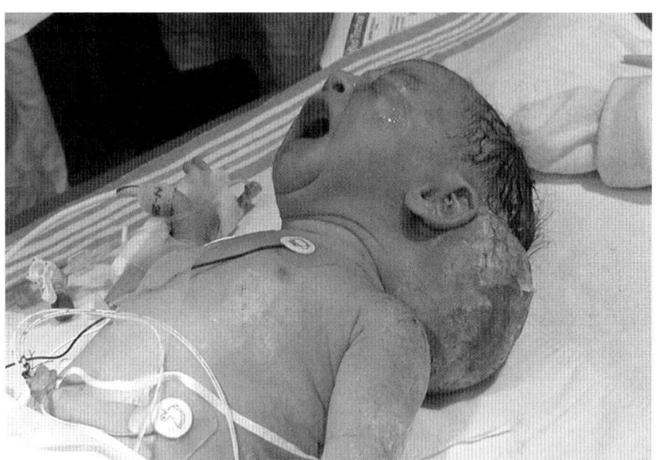

Fig. 38.2 Lymphangioma of the posterior left neck in a newborn.

magnetic resonance imaging (MRI) can be very helpful in distinguishing cystic hygroma from cervical teratomas[15,16]. Nuchal edema generally does not contain septa other than the midline nuchal ligament and are generally only a few millimeters in thickness.

The natural history of prenatally diagnosed cystic hygroma appears to depend on gestational age of diagnosis, location of the lesion and whether or not there are associated chromosomal or additional structural abnormalities. The mortality rate for prenatally diagnosed lymphangiomas prior to 30 weeks of gestation that are posterior in location is extremely high because of the high incidence of non-immune hydrops and associated chromosomal defects. Cystic hygroma associated with non-immune hydrops is almost universally fatal and 80% of these cases are associated with cardiac malformations and chromosomal abnormalities[8]. In a review of 100 prenatally identified fetuses with nuchal thickening or cystic hygroma between 10 and 15 weeks' gestation, Nadel et al.[17] showed that the prognosis correlated with absence of hydrops, no septations within the mass and presence of a normal karyotype. In the absence of an associated genetic syndrome, structural anomaly, abnormal karyotype, or hydrops, isolated cystic hygroma generally carries an excellent prognosis.

Pregnancy management should include a detailed sonographic evaluation to rule out other structural anomalies, phenotypic markers, or evidence of non-immune hydrops. Echocardiography should be performed to rule out structural or functional abnormalities. Amniocentesis is recommended in all cases because of the high incidence of associated chromosomal abnormalities. Because of the risks of airway compromise with larger masses, delivery at a tertiary care center with neonatology and pediatric surgery immediately available at time of delivery is recommended, as it may be difficult to establish a stable airway, bronchoscopy may be required and emergency tracheostomy could be necessary. Delivery planning should include a careful assessment of the fetal airway on ultrasound and ultrafast fetal MRI. Cases in which airway compromise is suspected, should be considered for delivery utilizing the EXIT (ex utero intrapartum treatment) approach in which the infant is partially delivered and an airway established by endotracheal intubation or tracheostomy while the infant remains on maternal–placental perfusion. Large masses can also cause polyhydramnios by obstructing the oropharynx, placing the pregnancy at risk for preterm labor and delivery. In such instances, serial amnioreductions may be necessary to decrease this risk and prolong the gestation.

Prenatally, in utero surgical management for lymphangioma is generally unnecessary other than amnioreduction for polyhydramnios. In utero sclerotherapy with OK-432 at 27 and 28 weeks of gestation has been reported[18]. OK-432 is a lyophilized mixture of low-virulence strain of human *Streptococcus pyogenes* incubated with penicillin G. In this single case, involution of the cystic hygroma was observed such that only a slight skin fold was noted at time of birth. However, there are minimal data on the use of this agent and nothing reported on its potential effects in the developing fetus. Currently, the only fetal procedure indicated for large cystic hygromas is the EXIT approach to delivery.

Once the infant is born, a computed tomography (CT) scan and MRI scan with magnetic resonance angiography should be obtained of the infant's head and neck to confirm the diagnosis of lymphangioma and determine the extent of the lesion. It is particularly important to define whether there is extension into the mediastinum, the floor of the mouth and tongue, or into the trachea. In infants with a large cystic hygroma expected to have an unstable airway, surgical resection should proceed as soon as the diagnostic evaluation is completed. Smaller hygromas that do not compromise the airway can be surgically managed on an elective basis. The histologic nature of lymphangiomas often makes complete resection impossible and therefore the surgical approach is focused on resecting as much of the mass as possible without compromising other vital structures within the neck or oral cavity. Sclerosing agents have been used as an alternative to surgical resection with variable results. Bleomycin (microsphere in oil bleomycin fat emulsion, BLM) has been used with some success[19,20]. After cyst aspiration, injection into the lymphangioma of 0.3–0.6 mg of BLM per kilogram of body weight was utilized. This therapy is contraindicated in infants less than 6 months of age, presence of airway compromise, or mediastinal involvement because of the severe tissue edema that results. Side effects of this therapy include fever, diarrhea, infection, bleeding and vomiting. Long-term complications, such as potential pulmonary fibrosis, are unknown. The sclerosing agent OK-432 has also been utilized in a concentration of 0.1 mg diluted in 10 ml of saline solution as an intracystic injection following cyst aspiration. This therapy reportedly can be repeated 3–4 weeks later if necessary. However, no prospective trials have been performed to confirm the efficacy of this treatment.

As noted earlier, long-term prognosis for cystic hygromas associated with anomalies or non-immune hydrops is quite poor. In cases of isolated cystic hygromas, overall mortality is low. However, complete resection is possible in only 75% and recurrence can occur in up to 10–27% of cases[21]. In cases where only partial resection was possible, recurrence is observed in 50–100% of patients. Significant complications can occur in up to 30% of patients. Neurologic complications can result from injury to the cranial nerves, particularly the facial nerve (VIIth). Injuries to the IXth, Xth, XIth and XIIth cranial nerves have also been reported as well as Horner syndrome, due to injury to the sympathetic chain, and phrenic nerve injury resulting in diaphragmatic paralysis.

CERVICAL TERATOMA

Cervical teratoma is a rare tumor and, as with other teratomas, is composed of tissues derived from all three germ layers. Neural tissue is the most common histologic component, with respiratory epithelium and cartilage also commonly present[22]. Thyroid tissue occurs in 30–40%, but it is unclear whether this represents ectopic thyroid tissue or actual involvement of the thyroid gland[23]. Theories regarding the origin of cervical teratomas include development from totipotential germ cells or abnormal development of a conjoined twin[24]. There is no relationship to maternal age, parity, race or gender of the fetus.

On ultrasound examination, cervical teratomas are typically asymmetric, unilateral, well demarcated and relatively immobile. Most are irregular, multiloculated masses that contain both solid and cystic components (Fig. 38.3). More than half have calcifications present within the solid components and, when identified, are virtually diagnostic of cervical teratoma[25]. These tumors are usually large and bulky, measuring 5 to over 12 cm in diameter. They usually extend to the mastoid process and body of the mandible and can extend superiorly displacing the ear. Inferiorly, they can extend to the clavicle and suprasternal notch, or extend into the mediastinum. Posteriorly, they may extend to the anterior border of the trapezius muscle. Involvement of the oral floor, or involvement of the oral cavity (epinathus) can occur. Mandibular hypoplasia may occur as the direct result of mass effect on the developing mandible. Polyhydramnios will complicate 20–40% of prenatally diagnosed cases due to oropharyngeal or esophageal obstruction as suggested by the associated finding of a small or empty stomach[26]. Cystic hygroma (lymphangioma) is the most likely neck mass to be mistaken prenatally for a cervical teratoma. The similarities in size, sonographic findings, clinical characteristics and location, as well as gestational age at presentation can make differentiation difficult. However, cystic hygromas are typically multiloculated cystic masses with poorly defined borders that infiltrate the normal structures of the neck. Cervical teratomas, in contrast, usually have well-defined borders within the tissues of the neck. Also, cystic hygroma is usually unilateral, more frequently involves the posterior triangle of the neck, and is generally smaller in size. Ultrafast fetal MRI

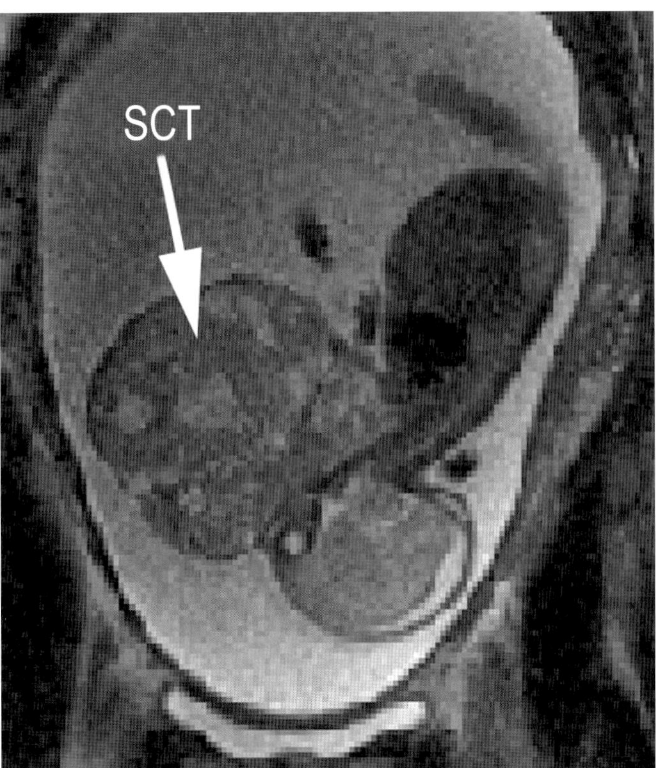

Fig. 38.3 Ultrafast MRI of a fetus with a large cervical teratoma that is invading the oral cavity, facial structures and extending into the thoracic inlet and anterior mediastinum at 24 weeks' gestation.

has been shown to be particularly useful in distinguishing the more solid teratoma from its complex, cystic lymphangioma counterpart.

The vast majority of cervical teratomata in fetuses and infants are benign in contrast to the often malignant form that occurs in adults. However, rare cases of malignancies have occurred in the fetal and infant population[27]. Despite the existence of primitive tissue types within the tumor, and metastases to regional lymph nodes, many infants following complete resection of the teratoma have remained free from recurrence. Such cases suggest that malignant biologic behavior is uncommon in this young population[25].

Prenatal management requires repeated ultrasound examinations to monitor amniotic fluid volume, tumor size and fetal well-being. Stillbirth rates are high due to high output cardiac failure or fetal exsanguination secondary to hemorrhage into the mass or following spontaneous intrauterine rupture. There is a high incidence of preterm labor and preterm delivery that can be due to the increasing uterine size due to polyhydramnios or significant enlargement of the tumor mass. Because of the hyperextension of the fetal neck, there is an increased incidence of malpresentation and dystocia. Cesarean section is recommended because of abnormal fetal position, risk of tumor rupture and risk of significant hemorrhage into the tumor associated with birth-related trauma. Stabilization of the newborn airway at delivery is essential and requires a resuscitation team qualified to obtain a bronchoscopic or surgical airway if orotracheal intubation is unsuccessful. Currently, the fetus with cervical teratoma is best managed by the EXIT procedure that provides time for laryngoscopy, bronchoscopy and even tracheostomy, if necessary, to secure a stable airway[16].

Airway obstruction and respiratory compromise at birth can be life-threatening and account for up to 45% of mortality that is usually associated with the delay in obtaining an airway and an inability to ventilate the infants effectively. Delay results in hypoxia and acidosis and, if delay is greater than five minutes, anoxic injury can occur[28]. Mortality can be as high as 80–100% in untreated infants, regardless of the tumor size, and delay in surgery can result in retention of secretions, atelectasis and pneumonia due to aspiration. Precipitous airway obstruction can also occur due to hemorrhage into the tumor even in asymptomatic newborns. For this reason, orotracheal intubation is indicated for all patients regardless of the presence or absence of symptoms. Mortality decreases between 9 and 17% in infants treated surgically[25].

As these tumors tend to be large, disfiguring masses that displace and surrounded vital structures in the neck, extensive dissection and multiple procedures are often necessary for complete removal of the tumor with acceptable cosmetic and functional results. Infants are at risk of transient or permanent hypothyroidism and hypoparathyroidism. The tumor may completely replace the thyroid gland and tumor resection may result in permanent loss of thyroid function. However, more commonly, thyroid tissue may be preserved but may not be adequately functioning and thyroxine supplementation may be required. Because of the size of these tumors, it is commonly difficult to identify the parathyroid glands, and transient or permanent hypoparathyroidism can occur requiring calcium and vitamin D supplementation. While cervical teratoma is generally a benign tumor, there is the potential for malignant transformation requiring close surveillance for tumor recurrence. Recommendations involve following serum alphafetoprotein levels at 3-month intervals in infancy, and yearly thereafter. CT or MRI scanning twice a year for the first 3 years of life is also suggested.

Cervical teratoma is considered to be a spontaneous malformation such that risk for recurrence in subsequent pregnancies would not be anticipated. However, there has been one report of congenital cervical teratoma occurring in siblings, but no other familial predisposition has been described[29].

EX UTERO INTRAPARTUM TREATMENT (EXIT)

In the fetus with a giant neck mass, the risk of airway compromise at birth is high. The airway may be compressed, occluded or distorted and there may be associated tracheal or laryngomalacia. If a giant neck mass is undiagnosed, or no planning for delivery and airway control is made, the fetus with an obstructed airway may suffer hypoxic brain injury or death. The EXIT procedure was designed to provide time to secure a stable airway while utero placental gas exchange is preserved (Fig. 38.4). The procedure was originally described for delivery of fetuses with diaphragmatic hernia who had undergone in utero tracheal clip application to induce prenatal lung growth. The EXIT procedure involves deep maternal–fetal anesthesia to facilitate uterine relaxation, controlled hysterotomy using fetal surgical techniques, delivery of the fetal head and neck and an establishment of an airway while maintaining fetal placental circulation. After an airway has been established, the baby is delivered and the umbilical cord divided. This technique allows up to 60 minutes of cord perfusion before utero placental gas exchange begins to deteriorate[16]. A variety of procedures can be performed during the EXIT procedure including laryngoscopy, bronchoscopy, oral tracheal intubation, tracheostomy and installation of surfactant.

Recently, additional indications for this approach to delivery have been reported for fetuses with other critical airway or respiratory issues[30]. However, it is critical to obtain as much information about the anatomy of the mass and any other potentially complicating abnormalities in the fetus as part of the preoperative planning for this procedure. We routinely perform ultrafast fetal MRI evaluations of the head, neck and chest to assist in preoperative planning. MRI allows for more global imaging of the mass than ultrasound because of the larger field of view. MRI provides the surgeon with better detail about the size and position of the mass and its relationship to the airway. The ability of improved visualization of the relationship of the mass to the entire airway may help predict which fetuses are at highest risk for airway obstruction.

There are a number of potential risks to the mother who undergoes an EXIT delivery and risks should not be considered similar to a routine cesarean delivery. There is a risk of significant hemorrhage because of uterine atony secondary to the inhalation agents utilized to keep the uterus relaxed. The risk of uterine atony and hemorrhage can be minimized through coordination between the anesthesiologist and surgeon to decrease the concentration of inhalation anesthetic and administration of oxytocin at the time of umbilical cord ligation. The use of a uterine stapling device also decreases blood loss from the hysterotomy. A lower uterine segment hysterotomy is preferred as it allows for the possibility of future vaginal delivery. However, a low anterior placental position, or extremely large neck mass may make lower uterine hysterotomy impossible. A classical hysterotomy may be necessary in these cases, and necessitate cesarean delivery for all future deliveries because of the risk of uterine rupture during labor. Prior to an EXIT procedure, the mother should be carefully counseled about these additional risks.

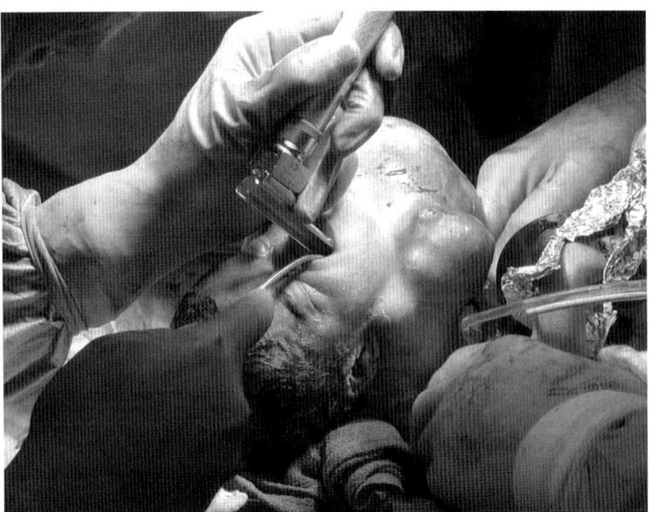

Fig. 38.4 Initial evaluation of the airway in a fetus with an anterior cervical teratoma at time of EXIT delivery.

SACROCOCCYGEAL TERATOMA

Sacrococcygeal teratoma (SCT) has traditionally been defined as a mass composed of tissues from either all three germ layers or multiple foreign tissues lacking an organ specificity. More recently, it has been thought to arise from a totipotential somatic cell originating in Hensen's node, that is a caudal-cell mass in the embryo that appears to escape normal inductive regulation[31]. SCT has been classified by the relative amounts of external and presacral tumor that is present (Table 38.2)[32]. The usefulness of this classification lies in the relationship between stage and timing of diagnosis, ease of resection and malignant potential. Type 1 is evident at birth, is usually easily resected and has a low malignant potential. Similarly, types 2 and 3 are recognized at birth, but resection may be difficult, requiring both an anterior and posterior approach. In type 4, the diagnosis may be delayed until it becomes symptomatic at a later age in infancy. Malignant transformation has frequently occurred by the time a type 4 SCT is diagnosed.

SCT is one of the most common tumors in newborns, however, they remain rare occurring in 1 in 35000 to 1 in 40000 live births. Females are four times more likely to be affected than males, however, malignant changes are more frequently observed in males. The majority of cases are felt to be a sporadic event, with the risk for subsequent recurrence in future pregnancies to be extremely low. However, some forms appeared to be familial with the suggestion of an autosomal dominant inheritance[33].

Prenatally, the most common clinical presentation is uterine size greater than expected for gestational dating that leads to an ultrasound examination. SCTs can grow at an unpredictable rate to extremely large masses. These tumors are generally exophytic (type I) and can extend retroperitoneally displacing pelvic (type II) or abdominal structures (type III) resulting in obstructive hydronephrosis and subsequent renal failure or onset of non-immune hydrops due to obstruction of venous return to the heart. Most SCTs are solid or mixed solid and cystic consisting of randomly arranged irregularly shaped cysts. However, purely cystic SCT has also been prenatally described[34]. Calcifications can be seen on histologic examination, but may not be visible on prenatal ultrasound examination. Most prenatally diagnosed tumors are extremely vascular, as demonstrated with the use of color flow Doppler studies. Polyhydramnios is a frequent finding and the mechanism may be secondary to high output cardiac physiology and renal hyperperfusion. However, oligohydramnios can also occur secondary to bladder displacement

Table 38.2 **Staging and classification of sacrococcygeal teratomas[32]**

Class	*Definition*
Type I	Completely external with no presacral component
Type II	External component with small internal pelvic component
Type III	External component with internal component extending into abdomen
Type IV	Completely internal with no external components

and urethral or ureteral obstruction. Hepatomegaly, placentomegaly and non-immune hydrops can occur and appear to be secondary to high output cardiac failure[35]. Cardiac failure and subsequent hydrops may be due to severe fetal anemia secondary to tumor hemorrhage, however, congestive heart failure is more often due to high output cardiac physiology from arteriovenous shunting within the mass. The presence of severe cardiac compromise and/or hydrops on ultrasound examination suggests impending fetal demise[35,36].

Coexisting malformations occur in 11–30%, primarily involving the cardiac, nervous, gastrointestinal, genitourinary and musculoskeletal systems (Table 38.3)[37]. Given the localized nature of these abnormalities to the tumor mass, the majority of these anomalies are felt to be secondary to tumor growth during fetal development. An increased incidence of chromosomal abnormalities has not been reported in the presence of SCT and, therefore, amniocentesis is generally not recommended in the absence of other indications, unless fetal surgery is contemplated.

Differential diagnosis of SCT includes neural tube defects. Lumbosacral myelomeningoceles invariably demonstrate a dorsal bony spinal defect and have a cystic or semi-cystic rather than a solid appearance and do not contain calcifications. Examination of the fetal brain is helpful as most fetuses with lumbosacral myelomeningocele will have cranial signs such as ventriculomegaly, effacement of posterior fossa (banana sign) and characteristic altered shaped of the skull (lemon sign). Less common entities include neuroblastoma, glioma, hemangioma, neurofibroma, lipoma, or any of 50 rare tumors or malformations reported in the sacrococcygeal region[38]. The antepartum natural history of prenatally diagnosed SCT is not as favorable as that of SCT presenting at birth. The outlined prognostic factors for SCT described in the American Academy of Pediatrics Surgical Section (AAPSS) classification system does not necessarily apply to fetal cases. While the mortality rate for SCT diagnosed in the newborn is at most 5%, the mortality rate for fetal SCT approaches 50%[35,39]. Most SCTs are histologically benign, but malignancy appears to be more common in solid versus complex or cystic tumors. However, the presence of histologically immature tissue does not necessarily signify malignancy[33]. The presence of calcifications is an unreliable indicator of malignant potential as they occur in both benign and malignant tumors. Although there is one reported case of malignant yolk sac differentiation in a fetal SCT, there has not been a case of metastatic teratoma in a neonate with a prenatally diagnosed SCT[39].

Flake et al. reviewed 27 cases of prenatally diagnosed SCT[36]. Five cases were electively terminated and 15 of the remaining 22 died either in utero or shortly after delivery. The majority of cases presented between 24 and 34 weeks of gestation with a uterus that was large for gestational age secondary to severe polyhydramnios. The presence of hydrops and/or polyhydramnios was associated with intrauterine death in all 7 of 7 cases. Bond et al.[35] reported survey data from the International Fetal Medicine and Surgery Society on prenatally diagnosed SCT, confirming a high mortality rate of 52%, and when seen in association with placentomegaly or hydrops, all 15 fetuses died in utero. We have recently reported on the pre- and postnatal outcomes of 30 cases of SCT that included three sets of twins[37]. The mean gestational age at time of presentation was 23.9 weeks and outcomes included 4 elective terminations, 5 in utero fetal demises, 7 neonatal deaths and 14 survivors. Significant obstetrical complications occurred in 81% of the 26 continuing pregnancies with polyhydramnios in 7, oligohydramnios in 4, preterm labor in 13, pre-eclampsia in 4, and HELLP syndrome in one. Fetal interventions included cyst aspiration in 6, amnioreduction in 3, amnioinfusion in 1 and open fetal surgical resection in 4 cases. Indications for cyst aspiration and amnioreduction were maternal discomfort, preterm labor and prevention of tumor rupture at delivery. Although 15 tumors were solid causing risk for cardiac failure, only 4 fetuses met criteria for fetal debulking (Fig. 38.5) based on ultrasound and echocardiographic evidence of impending high output failure and had

Table 38.3 **Anomalies associated with SCT**

Pulmonary hypoplasia
Meconium peritonitis
Rectal stenosis/atresia
Duplex renal collecting system
Hydrocolpus
Renal dysplasia
Hydronephrosis
UPJ obstruction
Urethral atresia/stenosis
Urinary ascites
Urogenital sinus
Clubfoot deformity
Hip dislocation

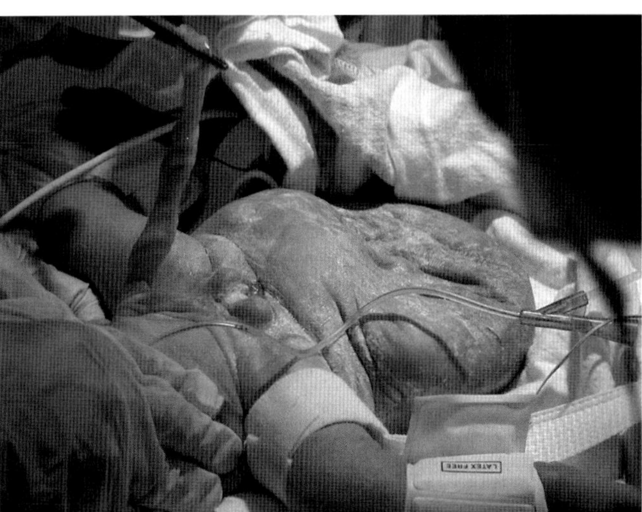

Fig. 38.5 Newborn with a large, mostly cystic SCT that was drained under ultrasound guidance prior to cesarean delivery to reduce the risk of dystocia and tumor rupture. This particular SCT had very prominent cystic components that enlarged such that the mass was significantly larger than the fetus resulting in preterm contractions beginning at 33 weeks. Weekly ultrasound-guided drainage of the dominant cysts (1200–1800 ml) reduced the mass volume and prevented onset of labor during the remainder of the pregnancy.

favorable anatomy at 21, 24, 25 and 26 weeks' gestation. In the fetal resection group, 3 of 4 survived with the mean gestational age at delivery of 29 weeks, mean birth weight of 1.3 kg, and hospital stays ranging from 16 to 34 weeks. Postnatal complications in the fetal surgery group included one neonatal death secondary to premature closure of the ductus arteriosus and subsequent heart failure, an embolic event in one fetus resulting in unilateral renal agenesis and duodenal atresia, chronic lung disease in one infant and tumor recurrence in one child.

Sonographic features of size, AAPSS classification, solid or cystic composition, or presence or absence of calcifications had not been predictive of either fetal survival or future malignant potential. One exception may be the unilocular cystic form that has a relatively favorable prognosis because of the limited vascular and metabolic demands. The growth of the SCT in relationship to the size of the fetus is unpredictable and may increase, decrease or remain stable as gestation proceeds. However, a rapid phase of tumor growth and/or increased vascularity usually precedes the development of placentomegaly and hydrops. Prenatal mortality is due to complications of tumor mass or tumor physiology, unlike postnatal mortality due to malignant degeneration. The tumor mass may cause malpresentation or dystocia resulting in tumor rupture and hemorrhage during delivery. Perhaps the most important benefit of prenatal diagnosis is the prevention of dystocia and the associated risk of tumor rupture or hemorrhage by elective or emergency cesarean section.

The physiologic consequences of fetal SCT depend on the metabolic demands of the tumor, blood flow to the mass and presence and degree of fetal anemia. While originally these tumors were thought to derive their blood supply from the middle sacral artery, we have found they often parasitize blood supply from the internal and external iliac systems. This may represent a vascular 'steal' from the umbilical arterial blood flow to the placenta. An additional confounding factor is the development of fetal anemia from hemorrhage into the tumor. In addition, the external tumor component may rupture as a result of necrosis caused by the tumor outgrowing its blood supply. The vascular steal and/or fetal anemia may contribute to the high output state seen with these tumors. Serial sonographic and echocardiographic examinations often show progressive increase in combined cardiac output and descending aortic flow velocity. Placental blood flow can be significantly decreased by the vascular steal of the tumor mass. Postpartum measurements of umbilical artery blood gases before and after removal of a large SCT have shown that the tumor acts as a large arteriovenous shunt[39].

Prenatal management of SCT should focus on cardiovascular status and development of secondary complications such as hemorrhage into the tumor (seen on ultrasound as an acute change in size and echogenic appearance of the mass), rupture of the external component, or polyhydramnios that can lead to preterm delivery. Weekly sonographic examination should be performed to assess amniotic fluid index, tumor growth, fetal well-being and evidence of early hydrops. Serial echocardiographic evaluations are helpful in detecting changes in high output state that can be reflected by increase combined cardiac output and increased diameter of the inferior vena cava[39]. Particular attention should be focused on increasing cardiac output and associated progressive cardiac dysfunction, increasing placentomegaly or early signs of hydrops such as the development of effusions, skin edema or ascites as these have all been shown to be associated with imminent fetal demise. In addition, these features have been shown to be associated with a high risk for maternal mirror syndrome, a form of severe pre-eclampsia initially described by Nicolay et al.[40] that can result in significant morbidity or mortality. When placentomegaly is recognized sonographically, maternal surveillance for pre-eclampsia should be initiated. Mode of delivery should be determined by the size of the tumor. Vaginal delivery may be possible with some small, mostly cystic tumors where the risk for trauma related hemorrhage is minimal[39]. However, cesarean delivery is recommended to avoid trauma-related hemorrhage or dystocia, particularly when the mass has a significant solid, vascular component and is greater than 5–10 cm in size[39,40]. The size of the tumor may also influence the type of uterine hysterotomy, as a large tumor may warrant a vertical, classical incision, particularly for a preterm infant. Transabdominal aspirations of large cysts within the mass prior to cesarean delivery can decrease overall mass volume to facilitate easier and less traumatic delivery at time of cesarean section (Fig. 38.6).

Because of universally fatal outcomes in fetuses with SCT, placentomegaly and hydrops, in utero mass resection has been attempted in an effort to salvage these pregnancies. The first successful resection of the fetal SCT with long-term survival occurred in a 25 weeks' gestation with a type II SCT that had rapid enlargement and development of polyhydramnios and placentomegaly. This was associated with maternal tachycardia and proteinuria suggesting evolving pre-eclampsia. At surgery, the external portion of the tumor was dissected free of the anus and rectum and the base of the tumor excised with a thick tissue stapling device. The mother and fetus did well with resolution of the placentomegaly and fetal hydrops within 10 days. At 29 weeks' gestation, onset of preterm labor resulted in cesarean delivery. After birth, the female infant underwent resection of the coccyx and surrounding tissues at 2 months of age. At one year of age serum alpha-fetoprotein levels became elevated (22 000 ng/ml) and she developed pleural effusions, lung nodules and a recurrent mass on the buttock from a metastatic yolk sac tumor. She was subsequently treated with chemotherapy and had an excellent response[41].

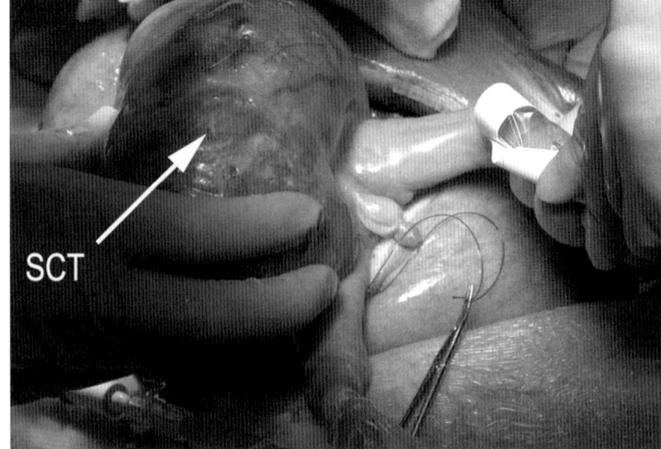

Fig. 38.6 25-week fetus with a large type I SCT associated with early hydrops undergoing in utero mass resection. Note that only the mass, legs and pelvis are delivered through the uterine hysterotomy in an effort to maintain intrauterine volume and reduce the risk of placental dysfunction or separation. A catheter that is connected to an infusion device is placed through the hysterotomy into the uterine cavity to help maintain uterine volume and temperature throughout the procedure.

At time of birth, careful handling and positioning of the infant is important to prevent rupture or exsanguinating hemorrhage into the tumor. Establishment of venous access is essential should hemorrhage into the tumor occur. Initiation of pressor agents, such as dopamine or dobutamine, is helpful to support the heart in its hyperdynamic state. Hemoglobin level should be monitored as transfusion may be necessary immediately after birth because of hemorrhage into the tumor that may not be obvious on external examination of the tumor. Echocardiography should be obtained to assess the cardiac status of the newborn and abdominal bedside ultrasound performed to evaluate the intrapelvic extent of the tumor. If a high output, hyperdynamic state exists, attention should be directed to supporting the newborn's cardiac function with urgent resection of the tumor mass. If there is no high output state, management should focus on the correction of anemia and treatment of any respiratory issues. When stable, additional imaging studies can be obtained to assess the extent of tumor extension within the pelvis and abdomen as part of the preoperative planning.

Long-term outcome in newborns with SCT is generally excellent as these tumors are usually benign but do have premalignant potential. Therefore, follow-up is important and current recommendations are for serum alpha-fetoprotein levels and physical examinations including digital rectal examinations at 3-month intervals. If the original tumors were shown to be functional, AFP levels may be a useful marker for recurrence. If the initial serum AFP was not elevated, then a pelvic ultrasound examination is recommended yearly. Tumor recurrence does not necessarily mean malignancy and such recurrence should be treated as a premalignant lesion and surgically excised. Even with evidence of malignant transformation, results with current chemotherapy have achieved excellent survival rates of 88% with localized disease and 75% even with distant metastases[42].

NEUROBLASTOMA

Neuroblastoma is the most common fetal malignancy[43]. This biologically and clinically heterogeneous tumor is derived from sympathetic ganglion precursor cells of neural crest origin[44]. Fetal neuroblastomas are thought to develop from residual microscopic neuroblastic nodules that do not respond to normal developmental signals[45]. Specifically, the oncogenic events that cause neuroblastomas appear to be related to altered expression of neurotrophic factors and their receptors (i.e. tyrosine kinase (Trk) A and TrkB) that normally regulate terminal differentiation of neural crest cells[46,47]. Cytogenetic abnormalities within the tumor itself including partial trisomies, 17q being the most common[48], chromosomal deletions, e.g. 1p, 11q, and 14q have also been identified and implicated in the pathogenesis of neuroblastomas. The exact contribution of all of these factors to neuroblastoma tumorigenesis remains to be elucidated.

The majority of neuroblastomas are thought to be sporadic and not associated with a specific teratogen, inherited predisposition or congenital anomaly. However, this tumor has been found to occur with increased frequency in genetic syndromes associated with malformations of neural crest derivatives; one example is the congenital central hypoventilation syndrome[49]. There is also a familial form that accounts for 1–2% of neuroblastomas[50–52]. Other than the rare familial form, these tumors usually do not recur in subsequent pregnancies. No preventative measures have been identified; however, there is one large

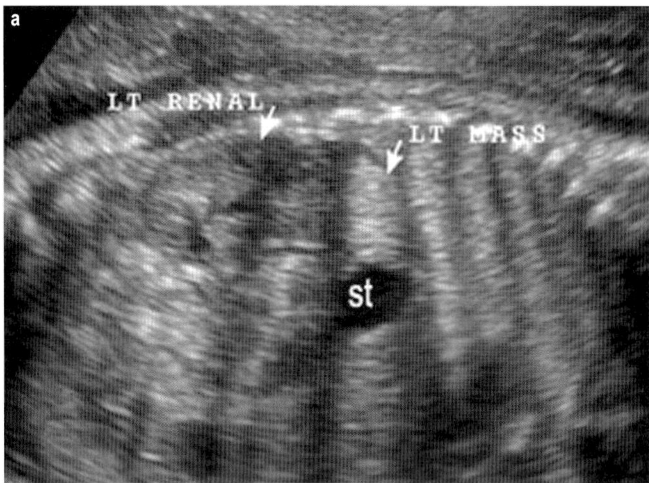

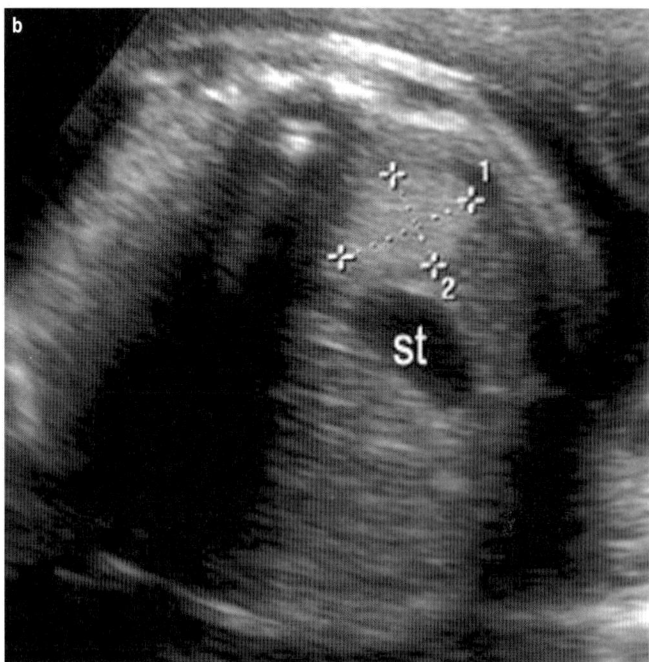

Fig. 38.7 Ultrasound image of a 32-week fetus with neuroblastoma. (a) Sagittal view of homogeneous echogenic mass superior to the kidney in the suprarenal fossa. (b) The well-circumscribed solid mass in suprarenal fossa posterior to the stomach (st).

Canadian population based study that suggests maternal folic acid supplementation may reduce the incidence of perinatal neuroblastoma[53].

As imaging modalities have become more sophisticated, prenatal identification of neuroblastomas has increased. Ninety percent of prenatally diagnosed neuroblastomas are located in the adrenal gland (Fig. 38.7) with the right gland being more commonly affected[54,55]. Occasionally, neuroblastomas are found in the chest[56] or neck[57]. In the majority of prenatally diagnosed neuroblastomas, the ultrasound appearance is cystic with a smaller number being solid or having a mixture of cystic and solid components. Theses tumors are usually well encapsulated and can downwardly displace the ipsilateral kidney. In addition to neuroblastomas, other etiologies of a solid or cystic adrenal mass such as hemorrhage, renal anomalies, or subdiaphragmatic extralobar pulmonary sequestration (systemic vessel originating from the aorta) should be considered in the differential diagnosis[54,58,59]. Therefore, once an adrenal mass is identified on ultrasound, the size, appearance (i.e. cystic versus solid) and blood supply should be evaluated[60]. MRI is also proving to be a useful imaging modality to delineate further the origin and etiology of suprarenal masses diagnosed in the prenatal period[61].

While the majority of fetuses with antenatally detected neuroblastomas have a good outcome, ongoing surveillance is necessary due to the unknown growth pattern of these lesions. The primarily solid masses tend to increase in size, whereas the cystic and complex masses have been observed to remain unchanged, grow or decrease in size[62]. Though spontaneous regression of prenatally diagnosed neuroblastomas has been observed in the neonate after delivery[54,62], this behavior has not been confirmed in utero.

Neuroblastomas can metastasize in utero; the fetal liver is the most common site. Neuroblastomas can also metastasize to the placenta, umbilical cord and chorionic villi[54]. If the metastatic masses are large enough, there can be obstructive effects leading to placental insufficiency, compromised liver function secondary to occlusion of the inferior vena cava, or hydrops[55,63,64]. Hydrops associated with neuroblastoma has been attributed to catecholamine induced fetal tachycardia and/or anemia secondary to tumor infiltration of the bone marrow.

Once the diagnosis of a neuroblastoma has been made, serial antenatal ultrasounds are recommended to monitor the mass size, carefully look for evidence of metastatic lesions and identify the early occurrence of hydrops. Since the majority of neuroblastomas are diagnosed after 32 weeks[50], preterm delivery is rarely indicated. Hence, expectant obstetrical management and postnatal evaluation and management are recommended. Prenatal diagnostic procedures such as cyst aspiration and/or biopsy or amniocentesis for tumor-secreted catecholamines (e.g. vanillylmandelic acid) had been suggested, but currently are not indicated as there are no interventions available at this time even if the in utero diagnosis is confirmed.

The major maternal complication associated with fetal neuroblastoma is pre-eclampsia that results from tumor-secreted catecholamines reaching the maternal circulation[55]. The development of pre-eclampsia may portend a poor neonatal outcome as this hypertensive disorder has been found primarily in metastatic neuroblastomas[55,63]. Other than close monitoring of maternal blood pressure and proteinuria, the presence of an adrenal neuroblastoma should not alter other aspects of prenatal management or impact mode of delivery unless there is a concern for abdominal dystocia due to an increase in tumor size.

Overall, the prognosis for those infants whose neuroblastomas are diagnosed in utero is good as these tumors usually have favorable biologic features, i.e. early stage, high DNA index, negative N-*myc* status and absence of deletion of the chromosome 1p[65,66]. The management of an infant with prenatally diagnosed neuroblastoma will depend upon the stage and biological features of the tumor[66]. After biopsy confirmation of the diagnosis, those infants who are candidates undergo surgical resection which, in most cases, will provide adequate treatment.

Though much information remains to be learned about neuroblastoma, when appropriate prenatal assessment and follow-up is provided, the outcome for fetuses diagnosed with this tumor is quite favorable.

REFERENCES

1. Isaacs H, Jr. Neoplasms in infants: a report of 25 cases. *Pathol Annu* **18**:165–170, 1983.
2. Isaacs H, Jr. *Tumors of the fetus and newborn*. pp. 69–72. Philadelphia: Saunders, 1997.
3. Isaacs H, Jr. *Tumors of the newborn and infant*. St. Louis: Mosby-Year Book, 1991.
4. Cohen MM, Schwartz S, Schwartz MF et al. Antenatal detection of cystic hygroma. *Obstet Gynecol Surg* **44**:481–485, 1989.
5. Romero R, Pilu G, Jeanty P, Ghidini A, Hobbins JC. *Prenatal diagnosis of congenital anomalies*. pp. 115-118. Norwalk, CT: Appleton & Lange, 1988.
6. Welborn JL, Timm NS. Trisomy 21 and cystic hygromas in early gestational age fetuses. *Am J Perinatol* **11**:19–25, 1994.
7. Benacerraf BR, Frigoletto FD. Prenatal sonographic diagnosis of isolated congenital cystic hygroma, unassociated with lymphedema or other morphologic abnormality. *J Ultrasound Med* **6**:63–66, 1987.
8. Langer JC, Fitzgerald PG, Desa D et al. Cervical cystic hygroma in the fetus: clinical spectrum and outcome. *J Pediatr Surg* **25**:58–62, 1990.
9. Chervenak FA, Isaacson G, Blakemore KJ et al. Fetal cystic hygroma: cause and natural history. *N Engl J Med* **309**:822–826, 1983.
10. Pijpers L, Reuss A, Stewart PA et al. Fetal cystic hygroma: prenatal diagnosis and management. *Obstet Gynecol* **72**:223–224, 1988.
11. Chen H, Immken L, Blumberg B, et al. Lethal form of multiple pterygium syndrome. Presented at the 1982 March of Dimes Birth Defects Conference, Atlanta, GA 1982.
12. Graham JM, Stephens TD, Shepard TH. Nuchal cystic hygroma in a fetus with presumed Robert's syndrome. *Am J Med Genet* **15**:163–167, 1983.
13. Zarabi M, Mieckowski GC, Maser J. Cystic hygroma associated with Noonan's syndrome. *J Clin Ultrasound* **11**:398–404, 1983.
14. Zelante L, Perla G, Villani G. Prenatal diagnosis of recurrence of cystic hygroma with normal chromosomes. *Prenat Diagn* **4**:383–386, 1984.
15. Hubbard A, Crombleholme TM, Adzick NS. Prenatal MRI evaluation of giant neck masses in preparation for the fetal EXIT procedure. *Am J Perinatol* **15**:253–257, 1998.
16. Liechty K, Crombleholme TM, Flake AW et al. Intrapartum airway management for giant fetal neck masses: the EXIT procedure (ex utero intrapartum treatment). *Am J Obstet Gynecol* **177**:870–874, 1997.
17. Nadel A, Bromley B, Benacerraf BR. Nuchal thickening or cystic hygromas in the first and early second trimester fetuses: prognosis and outcome. *Obstet Gynecol* **82**:43–48, 1993.
18. Wattori A, Yamada H, Gigino T et al. A case of intrauterine medical treatment for cystic hygroma. *Eur J Obstet Gynecol Reprod* **70**:201–203, 1996.
19. Tanaka K, Inomata Y, Utsunomiya H et al. Sclerosing therapy with bleomycin emulsion for lymphangioma in children. *Pediatr Surg Int* **5**:270–275, 1990.
20. Tanigawa N, Shimomatsuya T, Takahashi K et al. Treatment of cystic hygroma and lymphangioma with the use of bleomycin fat emulsion. *Cancer* **60**:741–749, 1987.
21. Hancock BJ, St-Vil D, Lebs FI et al. Complication of lymphangiomas in children. *J Pediatr Surg* **27**:220–225, 1982.
22. Schoenfeld A, Edelstein T, Joel-Cohen SJ. Prenatal ultrasonic diagnosis of fetal teratoma of the neck. *Br J Radiol* **51**:742–744, 1978.
23. Jordan RB, Gauderer MWL. Cervical teratomas: an analysis, literature review and proposed classification. *J Pediatr Surg* **23**:583–591, 1988.

24. Hitchcock A, Sears RT, O'Neill T. Immature cervical teratoma arising in one fetus of a twin pregnancy. *Acta Obstet Gynecol Scand* **66**:377–379, 1987.
25. Gundry SR, Wesley JR, Klein MD, Barr M, Coran AG. Cervical teratomas in the newborn. *J Pediatr Surg* **18**:382–386, 1983.
26. Rosenfeld CR, Coln CD, Duenhoelter JH. Fetal cervical teratomas as a cause of polyhydramnios. *Pediatrics* **64**:174–179, 1979.
27. Azizkhan RG, Haase GM, Applebaum H et al. Diagnosis, management, and outcome of cervicofacial teratomas in neonates: a children's cancer group study. *J Pediatr Surg* **30**:312–316, 1995.
28. Dawes G. *Fetal and neonatal physiology*. Chicago: Year Book, 1968.
29. Hurlbut HJ, Webb HW, Moseley T. Cervical teratoma in infant siblings. *J Pediatr Surg* **2**:424–426, 1967.
30. Bouchard S, Johnson MP, Flake AW, Howell LJ, Myers LB, Adzick NS. The EXIT procedure: experience and outcome in 31 cases. *J Pediatr Surg* **37**:418–426, 2002.
31. Bale PM. Sacrococcygeal developmental abnormalities and tumors in children. *Perspect Pediatr Pathol* **1**:9–56, 1984.
32. Altman RP, Randolph JG, Lilly JR. Sacrococcygeal teratoma. American Academy of Pediatrics Surgical Section Survey – 1973. *J Pediatr Surg* **9**:389–398, 1974.
33. Gonzalez-Crussi F. Extragonadal teratomas. *Atlas of tumor pathology*, 2nd series, fascicle 18, pp. 50-76. Bethesda: Armed Forces Institute of Pathology, 1983.
34. Seeds JW, Mittelstaedt CA, Cefalo RC, Parker TF. Prenatal diagnosis of sacrococcygeal teratoma: an anechoic caudal mass. *J Clin Ultrasound* **10**:193–195, 1982.
35. Bond SJ, Harrison MR, Schmidt KG et al. Death due to high-output cardiac failure in fetal sacrococcygeal teratoma. *J Pediatr Surg* **25**:1287–1291, 1990.
36. Flake AW, Harrison MR, Adzick NS, Laberge J, Warsof SL. Fetal sacrococcygeal teratoma. *J Pediatr Surg* **21**:563–566, 1986.
37. Hedrick HL, Flake AW, Crombleholme TM et al. Sacrococcygeal teratoma: prenatal assessment, fetal intervention, and outcome. *J Pediatr Surg* **39**:430–438, 2004.
38. Lemire RJ, Beckwith JB. Pathogenesis of congenital tumors and malformations in the sacrococcygeal region. *Teratology* **25**:201–213, 1982.
39. Flake AW. Fetal sacrococcygeal teratoma. *Semin Pediatr Surg* **2**:113–120, 1993.
40. Nicolay KS, Gainey HL. Pseudotoxemic state associated with severe Rh isoimmunization. *Am J Obstet Gynecol* **89**:41–45, 1964.
41. Adzick NS, Crombleholme TM, Morgan MA, Quinn TM. A rapidly growing fetal teratoma. *Lancet* **349**:538, 1997.
42. Misra D, Pritchard J, Drake DP et al. Markedly improved survival in malignant sacrococcygeal teratomas – 16 years' experience. *Curr J Pediatr Surg* **7**:152–157, 1997.
43. Woodward PJ, Sohaey R, Kennedy A, Koeller KK. From the archives of the AFIP: a comprehensive review of fetal tumors with pathologic correlation. *Radiographics* **25**(1):215–242, 2005.
44. Nakagawara A, Ohira M. Comprehensive genomics linking between neural development and cancer: neuroblastoma as a model. *Cancer Lett* **204**(2):213–224, 2004.
45. Nakagawara A. Neural crest development and neuroblastoma: the genetic and biological link. *Progr Brain Res* **146**: 233–242, 2004.
46. Nakagawara A, Arima-Nakagawara M, Scavarda NJ et al. Association between high levels of expression of the TRK gene and favorable outcome in human neuroblastoma. *N Engl J Med* **328**(12): 847–854, 1993.
47. Nakagawara A, Azar CG, Scavarda NJ, Brodeur GM. Expression and function of TRK-B and BDNF in human neuroblastomas. *Molec Cell Biol* **14**(1): 759–767, 1994.
48. Bown N, Cotterill S, Lastowska M et al. Gain of chromosome arm 17q and adverse outcome in patients with neuroblastoma. *N Engl J Med* **340**(25):1954–1961, 1999.
49. McConville C, Reid S, Baskcomb L, Douglas J, Rahman N. PHOX2B analysis in non-syndromic neuroblastoma cases shows novel mutations and genotype-phenotype associations. *Am J Med Genet* **140**(12):1297–1301, 2006.
50. Maris JM, Kyemba SM, Rebbeck TR et al. Familial predisposition to neuroblastoma does not map to chromosome band 1p36. *Cancer Res* **56**(15):3421–3425, 1996.
51. Kushner BH, Gilbert F, Helson L. Familial neuroblastoma. Case reports, literature review, and etiologic considerations. *Cancer* **57**(9):1887–1893, 1986.
52. Arenson EB, Jr, Hutter JJ, Jr, Restuccia RD, Holton CP. Neuroblastoma in father and son. *J Am Med Assoc* **235**(7):727–729, 1976.
53. French AE, Grant R, Weitzman S et al. Folic acid food fortification is associated with a decline in neuroblastoma. *Clin Pharm Therap* **74**(3):288–294, 2003.
54. Acharya S, Jayabose S, Kogan SJ et al. Prenatally diagnosed neuroblastoma. *Cancer* **80**(2):304–310, 1997.
55. Jennings RW, LaQuaglia MP, Leong K, Hendren WH, Adzick NS. Fetal neuroblastoma: prenatal diagnosis and natural history. *J Pediatr Surg* **28**(9): 1168–1174, 1993.
56. de Filippi G, Canestri G, Bosio U, Derchi LE, Coppi M. Thoracic neuroblastoma: antenatal demonstration in a case with unusual post-natal radiographic findings. *Br J Radiol* **59**(703):704–706, 1986.
57. Alvarado CS, London WB, Look AT et al. Natural history and biology of stage A neuroblastoma: a Pediatric Oncology Group Study. *J Pediatr Hematol Oncol* **22**(3):197–205, 2000.
58. Nuchtern JG. Perinatal neuroblastoma. *Sem Pediatr Surg* **15**(1):10–16, 2006.
59. Curtis MR, Mooney DP, Vaccaro TJ et al. Prenatal ultrasound characterization of the suprarenal mass: distinction between neuroblastoma and subdiaphragmatic extralobar pulmonary sequestration. *J Ultrasound Med* **16**(2):75–83, 1997.
60. Goldstein GK, I, Copel JA. The real-time and color Doppler appearance of adrenal neuroblastoma in a third-trimester fetus. *Obstet Gynecol* **83**(5):854–856, 1994.
61. Aslan H, Ozseker B, Gul A. Prenatal sonographic and magnetic resonance imaging diagnosis of cystic neuroblastoma. *Ultrasound Obstet Gynecol* **24**(6):693–694, 2004.
62. Chen CP, Chen SH, Chuang CY et al. Clinical and perinatal sonographic features of congenital adrenal cystic neuroblastoma: a case report with review of the literature. *Ultrasound Obstet Gynecol* **10**(1):68–73, 1997.
63. Crombleholme TM, Murray TA, Harris BH. Diagnosis and management of fetal neuroblastoma. *Curr Opin Obstet Gynecol* **6**(2):199–202, 1994.
64. Kesrouani A, Duchatel F, Seilanian M, Muray JM. Prenatal diagnosis of adrenal neuroblastoma by ultrasound: a report of two cases and review of the literature. *Ultrasound Obstet Gynecol* **13**(6):446–449, 1999.
65. Granata C, Fagnani AM, Gambini C et al. Features and outcome of neuroblastoma detected before birth. *J Pediatr Surg* **35**(1):88–91, 2000.
66. Sauvat F, Sarnacki S, Brisse H et al. Outcome of suprarenal localized masses diagnosed during the perinatal period: a retrospective multicenter study. *Cancer* **94**(9):2474–2480, 2002.

SECTION 8

Diagnosis and management of other fetal conditions

39 Fetal growth and growth restriction 541
Elisabeth Peregrine and Donald Peebles

40 Red cell alloimmunization 559
Charles H Rodeck and Anne Deans

41 Fetal platelet disorders 578
Leendert Porcelijn, Eline SA van den Akker and Humphrey HH Kanhai

42 Treatable fetal endocrine and metabolic disorders 592
Guy Rosner, Shai Ben Shahar, Yuval Yaron and Mark I Evans

43 Early pregnancy failure 602
Jemma Johns and Eric Jauniaux

44 Fetal infections 620
Guillaume Benoist and Yves Ville

45 Amniotic fluid 642
Pamela A Mahon and Karim D Kalache

46 Multiple pregnancy 649
Neelam Engineer and Nick Fisk

47 In utero stem cell transplantation 678
Sicco Scherjon and Elles in't Anker

48 Fetal gene therapy 689
Anna David and Charles H Rodeck

CHAPTER 39

Fetal growth and growth restriction

Elisabeth Peregrine and Donald Peebles

KEY POINTS

- Fetal growth restriction is a major cause of perinatal morbidity and mortality and may be associated with long-term consequences for the infant
- It is essential to distinguish between 'intrauterine growth restriction' or IUGR (failure of the fetus to reach its genetic growth potential) and 'small for gestational age' or SGA (a baby with growth parameters below the 10th centile for gestational age) as the former is the condition associated with an increased perinatal morbidity and mortality. Customized growth charts may improve the accuracy of diagnosing IUGR
- Fetal growth restriction is a heterogeneous condition with many known causes including: maternal disease, malnutrition, drugs and toxins, uteroplacental insufficiency, fetal aneuploidy, fetal abnormality, genomic imprinting and congenital infection
- Once a prenatal diagnosis of IUGR is made using repeated biometric measurements of the fetus, an underlying cause should be sought by assessment of amniotic fluid volume, uterine and fetal Doppler and detailed anatomical survey of the fetus
- The growth-restricted fetus should be monitored by regular assessment of biometry, amniotic fluid volume and fetal Doppler and delivery timed to gain maximum fetal maturity without irreversible fetal damage
- In 'term IUGR' (gestational age greater than 34 weeks), the pregnancy can usually continue until 40 weeks' gestation if the umbilical artery Doppler remains normal
- In 'preterm IUGR', monitoring should increase once there is AED in the umbilical artery Doppler. Delivery should be considered if there is an abnormal ductus venosus Doppler, a grossly abnormal CTG or other signs of fetal compromise such as cardiomegaly

INTRODUCTION

Fetal growth restriction is one of the commonest problems facing both obstetricians and neonatalogists. It frequently presents a dilemma for the obstetrician with regards to management of the pregnancy and delivery. It remains a major cause of perinatal morbidity and mortality and is associated with long-term consequences for the infant.

Fetuses with growth restriction frequently require delivery preterm and, in the immediate neonatal period, encounter problems such as hypothermia, hypoglycemia, pulmonary hemorrhage, encephalopathy and necrotizing enterocolitis. As adults they are at increased risk of heart disease, hypertension and type 2 diabetes.

Many aspects of fetal growth restriction remain unclear: a significant proportion of the infants are not identified before birth and undiagnosed growth restriction is the likely cause of a large proportion of unexplained stillbirths. If an antenatal diagnosis is made, there is no known prevention or therapy except appropriate timing of delivery. Management therefore consists of making the diagnosis, elucidating the underlying cause and appropriate fetal monitoring to allow timely delivery.

A thorough understanding of the pathology of the placenta both in health and disease is essential for a full understanding of the processes of normal fetal growth and fetal growth restriction and for interpretation of the clinical investigations. The pathophysiology is covered in Chapter 7.

DEFINITIONS

Intrauterine growth restriction (IUGR) is defined as the failure of the fetus to achieve its genetic growth potential in utero and implies that one or more of the pathological processes described below are limiting fetal growth.

In contrast, *small for gestational age* (SGA) is defined as a fetus or baby with growth parameters below a defined centile for gestational age (usually the 10th centile). These babies are usually small due to constitutional factors and are usually associated with normal placental function.

There is considerable overlap between these two definitions: an IUGR baby is usually SGA, but not necessarily so and not all SGA babies are IUGR. A distinction between the two is important clinically as they have different causes and implications and often require different management.

Low birth weight (defined by the World Health Organization (WHO) as a birth weight of less than 2500 g) is not useful in this context as it takes no account of gestational age and therefore includes normally grown babies born prematurely.

Uteroplacental insufficiency (UPI) is a term often used to describe the clinical scenario when both uterine and umbilical artery Dopplers are abnormal.

IUGR can be subdivided into *symmetric* and *asymmetric* IUGR depending on whether there is head sparing (asymmetrical) and this maybe helpful in establishing the etiology.

NORMAL FETAL GROWTH

Fetal growth is a complex and dynamic process controlled by many factors in the baby, placenta and mother. Although many of these factors are known, the exact molecular and cellular mechanisms involved in fetal growth are not fully understood.

Fetal size at birth is ultimately determined by the interaction between genetic determinants of fetal size and substrate supply. It is estimated that 40% of the variation in human fetal growth derives from genotype and 60% from environmental factors. This is clearly demonstrated by classic embryo transfer experiments in horses, where pony embryos were transferred into larger thoroughbred mares (P into Tb) and vice versa (Tb into P); Tb into P foals were smaller than Tb in Tb and showed clear evidence of growth restriction, while P in Tb were larger than both P in P and Tb in P offspring[1]. In this example, the pony foal, that on genetic grounds should be smaller than the thoroughbred, ended up being larger when the constraints of a small uterus were removed. Maternal size appeared to influence the area of fetoplacental contact and so the ability to transfer substrate from mother to fetus.

GENETIC CONTROL OF GROWTH

Fetal growth is partly regulated by a complex pattern of genetic signals that affect production of growth factors, transport of substrate across the placenta and into fetal cells and the rate of tissue accretion. The 'parental conflict' theory proposes that the maternal genome harbors genes critical for fetal development while the paternal genome harbors genes critical for extra-embryonic/placental development. The consequences of this are that the maternal genome acts to allocate resources within a litter and over future pregnancies, while the paternal genome is focused on producing fit offspring, possibly at the expense of maternal well-being[2].

An extreme example is provided by experiments in mice where isoparental embryos are created with pronuclei derived from only the father (androgenetic conceptus) or mother (gynogenetic); the former result in overgrowth of extraembryonic tissue but the embryo fails to develop properly (in a similar way to complete hydatidiform moles) while the latter results in a very growth-restricted embryo because the placenta fails to develop properly[3]. One mechanism by which this can occur is genomic imprinting; this is the differential expression of a maternal or paternal gene or chromosome region due to suppressed expression of either the maternal or paternal alleles. It appears to play a major role in the control of fetal growth, with a large proportion of the identified imprinted genes involved in growth regulation[4]. Thus, fetal size and weight at birth are the consequence of the interplay between paternally expressed genes that promote growth and maternally expressed genes that often have a growth suppressant effect. This concept is supported by experimental evidence from gene knockout murine models of paternally or maternally expressed growth factors such as the insulin-like growth factor (IGF) or insulin[5].

ENDOCRINE CONTROL OF GROWTH

The main regulatory mechanism for fetal growth is the IGF system. This includes IGF-1 and IGF-2, the IGF binding proteins (IGFBP) 1–6, IGF receptors 1 and 2 and the IGFBP specific proteases. Fetal insulin is the main regulator of fetal IGF-1 production, which enhances substrate uptake and suppresses catabolism. Fetal serum IGF-1 levels have been correlated with birth weight and lower levels have been observed in IUGR[6]. IGF-2 is the main regulator of embryonic growth in early pregnancy. Its overexpression leads to somatic overgrowth in animals and it may be involved in placental development[6]. Other agents involved in fetal growth regulation are: insulin by its effect on IGF-1 stimulates fat deposition in the fetus; fetal growth hormone and thyroid hormones which have an effect on fetal growth in the third trimester; and placental growth hormone which is involved in placental function and is reduced in IUGR.

An adequate substrate supply to the fetus depends on the integrity of both the placental and the uterine vascular systems. The correct process of implantation, trophoblastic invasion of the maternal spiral arterioles and development of the chorionic villi are all essential for normal fetal growth. The developmental biology of these processes and the defects in them which result in IUGR are discussed in detail in Chapter 7.

MATERNAL CONSTRAINT

Maternal constraint is a set of maternal and uteroplacental processes which act to limit the growth of the fetus. This happens to some extent in all pregnancies but will only have an adverse affect on fetal growth if the constraint is excessive. The constraint may be an inadequate supply to the fetus (maternal size, age, parity, diet and programming) and increased demand (such as in multiple pregnancies which is discussed below).

Maternal size is the primary determinant of fetal size[1] and this fact is of essential evolutionary importance to reduce the risk of obstructed labor and subsequent extinction of the genome. The effect of genomic imprinting is discussed below. Maternal parity has a known effect on birth weight with the firstborn usually being the smallest. The mechanism of this is poorly understood but may relate to the response of the uteroplacental vasculature to first pregnancy. Maternal age (both teenage and greater than 40 years) are associated with SGA, but the mechanisms for these findings are not clear[7,8]. Maternal diet has been thought only to affect fetal growth at extremes of undernutrition, however, recent evidence suggests that, even within the normal range of nutritional intake, subtle changes can affect the pattern of fetal growth[9].

There is increasing evidence that maternal constraint is an important factor in determining the increased risk of adult diseases in those that have IUGR as fetuses. The 'predictive adaptive response' of limited nutritional supply to the fetus leads to a postnatal physiology where fat is laid down, there is relative insulin resistance, reduced muscle mass and reduced nephron number and capillary density. However, now that the majority of humans live well beyond peak reproductive age and in a plentiful nutritional environment postnatally, the consequence of an increase in the lifestyle diseases (type 2 diabetes, heart disease and hypertension) can be predicted[10].

CAUSES OF FETAL GROWTH RESTRICTION

Fetal growth restriction is a heterogeneous condition with many known causes originating in the mother, placenta or fetus. The likely cause varies with the gestational age of the fetus. Early onset IUGR (requiring delivery before 32 weeks' gestation) is much less common than late onset disease and is more likely to be due to congenital infection, aneuploidy or a genetic disorder. The more common late onset IUGR typically presents late in the third trimester and is usually caused by uteroplacental insufficiency.

However, in many cases, a demonstrable association is not apparent and, even if it is, may not necessarily imply a causal link with IUGR. Separate from the causes listed below there are many risk factors for the development of IUGR which include: maternal age above 40 years[8], history of previous IUGR[11] and spontaneous preterm delivery[12].

The well-known causes of IUGR will be considered in turn.

Maternal factors

Maternal disease

Any maternal condition that impairs substrate delivery to the fetus can result in growth restriction. Both chronic hypertension and pre-eclampsia are associated with IUGR and may occur in up to 40% of pregnancies affected by IUGR. Pre-eclampsia is associated with a fourfold increase in the risk of an SGA infant: the worse and earlier the pre-eclampsia, the lower the birth weight[13]. Non-proteinuric hypertension is associated with a less pronounced effect on fetal growth. Maternal antihypertensive therapy does not appear to improve fetal growth. The abnormal implantation and failure of the placental vascular adaptation, which occurs in both IUGR and pre-eclampsia, suggest a similar placental disease. One hypothesis is that both pre-eclampsia and IUGR secondary to placental insufficiency share the same cause but produce different clinical manifestations[14]. However, a recent detailed study of the risk factors and perinatal outcomes for pre-eclampsia and unexplained IUGR suggest that these appear to be independent entities[15].

Maternal autoimmune disease such as systemic lupus erythematosus (SLE) is associated with poor perinatal outcome. The presence of the anti-phospholipid antibody in this condition is associated with a sixfold increase in IUGR[16].

Data on the association between maternal thrombophilia and IUGR are conflicting. A recent systematic review of 10 case-control studies found an association between both factor V Leiden and prothrombin gene variant and IUGR (odds ratios 2.7; CI = 1.3–5.5 and 2.5; CI = 1.3–5.0 respectively)[17]. The link with other thrombophilias is yet to be proven.

Other chronic maternal diseases have also been linked to IUGR, such as renal insufficiency[18], chronic anemia and pre-existing diabetes[19].

Malnutrition

Severe maternal undernutrition can cause IUGR. Studies in families exposed to famine have shown an association and demonstrate an effect with exposure in any trimester. However, restricting nutrients in early pregnancy has a more prolonged effect on the neonate causing IUGR and an adverse effect on long-term postnatal growth[20].

Toxins

Many therapeutic agents used in pregnancy such as chemotherapy agents, phenytoin, beta-blockers and steroids have been implicated in IUGR. A current controversy exists on the safety of repeated doses of antenatal glucocorticoids used to induce fetal lung maturity. The National Institutes of Health Consensus Development Panel discourages multiple courses due to animal and human data, suggesting that they can cause suppression of fetal somatic growth and neurodevelopmental problems[21].

Maternal use of recreational substances has also been associated with IUGR. However, a causal relationship is often difficult to establish due to common confounders. Cigarette smoking in pregnancy has long been associated with SGA infants and may account for up to 40% of IUGR in developed countries[22]. The effect appears to be dependent on the length of exposure throughout gestation and is dose dependent[23]. Women who smoke have a 3.5-fold increased risk of having an SGA infant than non-smokers[24]. Although alcohol consumption in pregnancy per se has not been associated with isolated IUGR, excessive use may result in fetal alcohol syndrome, of which IUGR is a cardinal feature[25]. Cocaine is a potent vasoconstrictor and its use in pregnancy is associated with an adverse fetal and maternal outcome and, after controlling for confounders, has been associated with IUGR[26]. Heroin use may cause IUGR in up to 50% of cases[27].

Placental causes

Uteroplacental insufficiency (UPI) is a clinical term used to describe IUGR associated with abnormal uterine and umbilical artery Dopplers. Although these clinical changes may be seen in several different causes of IUGR, primary UPI is caused by maldevelopment of the uteroplacental vascular system. One component of this is a defect of endovascular trophoblast erosion at the implantation site which may produce an inadequate basal plate. A second component is a failure of interstitial extravillous trophoblastic invasion of the spiral arterioles leading to a failure of local angiogenic and systemic cardiovascular adaptation signals[28]. The maldevelopment of the placenta seen in association with IUGR is discussed in detail in Chapter 7.

Fetal causes

Fetal abnormality

The presence of certain fetal malformations, particularly cardiac defects, anencephaly and abdominal wall defects have been associated with IUGR[29]. In a population-based study, 22% of infants with congenital abnormalities had IUGR. Multiple malformations increased the risk further. A single umbilical artery may be associated with IUGR.

Aneuploidy

Fetal aneuploidy is strongly associated with IUGR. In one high-risk referral center, 20% of all IUGR fetuses had a chromosomal defect. IUGR is frequently seen in trisomy 18 fetuses (90%), commonly with trisomy 13 and less frequently with trisomy 21 (30%). It has also been associated with many autosomal abnormalities such as duplications, deletions and ring chromosomes. The IUGR associated with aneuploidy more commonly presents in the first or second trimester, is symmetrical and is associated with structural abnormalities, normal or increased liquor volume and normal uterine and umbilical artery Dopplers[30]. Conversely, in triploidy the IUGR is asymmetrical.

Genomic imprinting

Uniparental disomy (UPD) is the inheritance of both chromosomes from a single parent and has been associated with IUGR. Confined placental mosaicism, where the karyotype of the placenta is different from the fetus, is thought to arise during a process called trisomic rescue, where the loss of a supernumerary chromosome from a trisomic conceptus leaves two homologues from the same gamete. Confined placental mosaicism is common, occurring in approximately 1–2% of routine chorionic villus samples (CVS) and is a common cause of 'unexplained IUGR', being present in up to 25% of cases[31]. The IUGR observed may be caused by fetal UPD or the presence of a mosaic placenta or both. The higher the proportion of trisomic cells in the placenta, the more severe the likely effects on the fetus. Trisomy 16 is the most common trisomy found in confined placental mosaicism associated with IUGR and is associated with a severe form of IUGR. However, there are several other UPD phenotypes associated with disruption of fetal and postnatal growth. For example Silver-Russell syndrome, caused by maternal UPD of chromosome 7, causes IUGR, reduced postnatal growth and dysmorphic features.

Congenital infection

In utero viral infection with rubella, cytomegalovirus, human immunodeficiency virus and varicella zoster and protozoan infection with malaria and toxoplasma have all been implicated in IUGR. Primary cytomegalovirus (CMV) infection in early pregnancy is the commonest infective cause of IUGR in developed countries, affecting 0.5–2% of all live births[32,33]. World-wide, malaria is by far the most important numerically[34]. The type of growth restriction in congenital infection is typically symmetrical but not necessarily so and may present in any trimester.

MULTIPLE PREGNANCY

Normal growth curves are similar in singleton and twin fetuses until approximately 30–32 weeks' gestation, after which twins tend to lag behind singletons. This is likely to represent the fetal adaptation to shared resources and does not necessarily imply growth compromise. However, IUGR is more frequent in multiple pregnancies, particularly in monochorionic gestations, and will usually manifest as discordant growth. Early discordant growth prior to 30 weeks' gestation is likely to represent twin-to-twin transfusion syndrome[35].

FETAL PHYSIOLOGICAL RESPONSES TO SUBSTRATE DEPRIVATION

Cordocentesis studies in humans have shown that small-for-gestational-age (SGA) fetuses are relatively hypercapnic, hypoxic, hyperlacticemic, acidotic and hypoglycemic compared to appropriate for gestational age fetuses[36,37]. Obviously, the degree of hypoglycemia and hypoxia will vary, depending on the severity of placental dysfunction. The fetus has a well-characterized series of metabolic and hemodynamic responses to reductions in substrate and, in particular, oxygen delivery, that allow short-term survival and continued development of essential organs, such as the heart and brain. Understanding fetal responses to hypoxia is of clinical relevance as they provide the physiological basis for methods of fetal assessment such as fetal heart rate monitoring and Doppler studies.

Hemodynamic responses

Most of the data describing the fetal responses to hypoxia come from experiments in fetal sheep where fetal hypoxemia is achieved by a variety of methods including partial occlusion of the uterine arteries and embolization of the fetoplacental circulation. The fetal response to acute hypoxia is well described[38,39]. There is an initial bradycardia followed by a slow increase in heart rate that returns to or exceeds its control value over the next few minutes. Arterial blood pressure increases and usually remains elevated. Cerebrovascular resistance falls and cerebral blood flow increases, while flow to carcass muscle, kidneys and gut decreases. However, if hypoxemia is maintained, the acute changes in fetal heart rate (FHR) revert to baseline values[40]. These data suggest that, in the context of fetal assessment for fetal growth restriction, FHR will be unchanged during the early stages and the pattern only becomes abnormal as the fetus begins to decompensate; data from sheep and human fetuses support this observation[41,42]. Blood pressure also returns to normal, both in the presence or absence of acidemia, if hypoxemia becomes chronic[40,43]. Hence blood pressure in the chronically hypoxemic, growth restricted sheep fetus is not different from that of normally grown normoxemic fetuses.

In contrast to the minimal changes in fetal heart rate and blood pressure seen in prolonged hypoxemia, the redistribution of cardiac output that occurs in acute hypoxemia in fetal sheep appears to be maintained with prolonged hypoxemia. Blood flow to the brain, heart and adrenal glands was still increased 48 hours after the onset of hypoxemia in fetal sheep, although not at the levels observed with acute hypoxemia[40]. The effect of increasing blood flow to heart, brain and adrenals is to maintain substrate delivery that is critically important for the maintenance of growth and optimal function of these key organs. There is a hierarchy, with oxygen delivery to the heart remaining increased, but cerebral oxygen delivery relatively decreased, after 7 days of prolonged hypoxemia[44]. Detection of substrate deficiency occurs both locally and at central chemoreceptors and is sensitive and rapid – increases in cardiac and cerebral blood flow are apparent within minutes of the onset of hypoxia. Detection of cerebral vasodilation is therefore an early finding in fetal growth restriction, but represents a normal physiological response; it is not surprising that abnormal cerebral blood flow is an extremely sensitive test for the prediction of growth restriction, but that it has poor specificity in the detection of adverse perinatal outcome[45]. There are few experimental data to show whether the changes in blood flow to other organs, such as gut, lungs and kidneys, that are observed during acute hypoxia are maintained during sustained hypoxemia. Forty-eight hours after the onset of moderately severe uterine artery restriction in fetal sheep, both kidney and muscle flow had returned to normal. However, Doppler studies in the growth-restricted human fetus suggest that vascular resistance is increased in a variety of vessels, including the splanchnic, renal and pulmonary circulations[46–48]. The resultant prolonged ischemia is likely to contribute to many of the features associated with growth-restricted fetuses, such as oligohydramnios (a reduction in renal perfusion), necrotizing enterocolitis (reperfusion of chronically ischemic bowel) and even the early failure of femur growth that can be one of the earliest signs of growth restriction (due to reduced carcass blood flow).

In addition to the redistribution of cardiac output, chronic hypoxia can also influence the venous pattern of blood flow and return of blood to the heart. Data from the human fetus suggest that 25–50% of blood returning from the placenta via the umbilical vein (UV) is shunted via the ductus venosus (DV), which connects with the inferior cava near its entrance to the heart[49]. This well-oxygenated blood is preferentially streamed through the foramen ovale into the left atrium and from there towards the cardiac and cerebral circulations. In both animals and humans, the amount of blood flowing through the ductus venosus increases during hypoxia[50,51]. A direct consequence of increased DV shunting is that the proportion of UV flow that passes via the hepatic circulation is reduced; a fall in hepatic perfusion and decreased substrate supply can impair liver function and glycogen synthesis and storage (reflected in a decrease in growth velocity in the abdominal circumference). Not surprisingly, flow velocity is maintained in the ductus venosus even with severe growth restriction[52], however, because the ductus venosus and left atrium are linked by a direct column of blood, increases in left atrial filling pressure, due mainly to impaired ventricular contractility, but also increased afterload, will lead to reduced forward flow in the DV during atrial systole. Decreased or absent flow during atrial systole is a late finding in the hemodynamic response to hypoxia and, because it indicates cardiac compromise, correlates strongly with poor perinatal outcome[52,53].

Metabolic and behavioral responses

One of the ways in which the fetus responds to a reduction in substrate delivery is by reducing growth; indeed, growth restriction appears to be the most important factor in balancing reduced oxygen delivery and consumption. Within hours of acute onset hypoxemia, protein synthesis is decreased in the fetal sheep with a corresponding decrease in overall oxygen consumption of up to 10%[54,55]. Indeed, growth restriction can so successfully reduce oxygen consumption that the arterial oxygen concentration can be maintained or only minimally decreased until substrate delivery is severely restricted[55].

Fetal body and breathing movements are an important source of oxygen consumption in the normal fetus; prevention of body movements by neuromuscular blockade reduces oxygen consumption by 20% in the sheep fetus[56]. It is not therefore surprising that acute hypoxemia in fetal sheep leads to a marked reduction in both fetal breathing and generalized movements[57,58]. However, fetal breathing movements return to normal after several hours[59] and even prolonged substrate deprivation and fetal growth restriction lead to only marginal decreases in fetal breathing movements[60]. Activity in the growth restricted human fetus can be well preserved, even with absent end diastolic flow in the UA, but is decreased in more severely affected fetuses[61,62]. Although these subtle decreases in fetal movement will reduce oxygen consumption and may prolong survival, they are relatively late indicators of fetal compromise and so may be of limited clinical use.

PRENATAL DIAGNOSIS OF FETAL GROWTH RESTRICTION

IUGR versus SGA

The correct prenatal identification of IUGR is crucial to ensure appropriate management and therefore optimal outcome. The challenge is to identify the fetus at risk due to a hostile intrauterine environment and deliver at an appropriate gestation. However, clinicians tend to manage IUGR and SGA in the same way, despite the fact that many of the SGA group will be small but healthy and do not require elective delivery. It is growth restriction rather than just being SGA that is associated with increased perinatal mortality and morbidity. Distinguishing between IUGR and SGA is therefore important to avoid overtreatment and the resulting unnecessary fetal and maternal risk. However, distinguishing between the two diagnoses is often challenging and, in clinical practice, is not always possible. Much of the research on IUGR lumps the two together using the single measurement 'estimated fetal weight' (EFW) as the studied variable and repeated measurements are often required to diagnose IUGR.

Clinical suspicion

Suspected growth restriction may present to the obstetrician and sonographer as a referral for a growth scan in a clinically small fetus or at a routine growth scan in a woman at risk of IUGR (e.g. previous history of SGA or IUGR, maternal disease such as pre-eclampsia, abnormal uterine artery Dopplers, known congenital infection).

In the UK, it is routine obstetric practice clinically to assess fetal growth by measuring the symphysio-fundal height (SFH) at each antenatal visit and to refer on for a sonographic estimation if the SFH varies from the normal range for the gestation[63]. The aim of this practice is to detect the small or large for gestational age fetus. Normal range charts exist for SFH and plotting serial measurements in routine antenatal practice may improve prenatal detection of IUGR[64,65].

Biochemical markers

Routine screening for chromosomal abnormalities using serum markers is currently used in many countries. In the presence of normal chromosomes, several of these markers have been associated with an increased risk of pregnancy complications including IUGR. A raised human chorionic gonadotrophin, alpha-fetoprotein and inhibin and a low pregnancy-associated placental protein A (PAPP-A) and estriol have all been associated with IUGR and other obstetric complications[66]. Their role in screening a high-risk population for both IUGR and pre-eclampsia needs to be investigated further.

Pregnancy dating

The accuracy of pregnancy dating should be checked in all referrals for suspected IUGR. The crown–rump length (CRL) in the first trimester can reliably date a pregnancy to within 5 days and a discrepancy beyond this should prompt correction from the last menstrual period (LMP) dates to ultrasound dating by CRL. Where the LMP is unknown and there are no ultrasound data below 13 weeks' gestation, ultrasound biometry below 20 weeks' gestation can date to within 7–10 days. Dating by ultrasound parameters beyond this gestation is highly inaccurate and should not be used to change LMP dates. Some authors have proposed the use of parameters such as transcerebellar diameter and foot length for pregnancy dating in the third trimester as they are gestational dependent but not affected by IUGR[67,68]. Ratios of ultrasound parameters such as the femur length (FL)/abdominal circumference (AC) ratio may help in distinguishing IUGR from incorrect dates by assessing the degree of subcutaneous fat and muscle loss[69]. Care should be taken when redating a pregnancy as IUGR may present as early as the first trimester in certain etiologies such as aneuploidy.

Biometry

The aim of ultrasound assessment is to diagnosis IUGR and then to establish the underlying cause to aid parental counseling and decision making regarding further management. Prior to the advent of ultrasound, the diagnosis of a small infant was usually only made at delivery. Routine third-trimester ultrasound has not been shown to improve outcome in a low-risk population[70]. However, screening those at particular risk or in whom SGA is suspected clinically would seem appropriate.

Ultrasound allows an assessment of fetal size to be made from biometric measurements; typically these are biparietal diameter (BPD), head circumference (HC), abdominal circumference (AC) and femur length (FL). The fetal weight can be estimated (EFW) by combining these using a pre-determined formula; many such formulae have been proposed using a variety of combinations of fetal measurements. Both EFW and AC alone or in combination with umbilical artery Dopplers have the best sensitivity, specificity and positive and negative predictive values to identify IUGR[71].

There is wide variation in the errors of the EFW methods used to predict birth weight, particularly at the extremes of weight[72]. A recent systematic review found that the formulae proposed by Hadlock[73,74] were the most consistent across studies in the normal clinical population[72]. However, all ultrasound estimates of fetal weight have inherent inaccuracies with large intra- and inter-observer variability[72] and mean absolute errors of up to 6–11% compared with birth weight have been described[75–79]. Specific formulae for premature or very low birth weight fetuses have not been found to be more accurate in estimating birth weight than other standard formulae[80].

An EFW either two standard deviations below the mean or below the 10th centile for gestation raises the suspicion of IUGR. However, only repeated ultrasound measurements can truly distinguish between SGA and IUGR, by demonstrating reduced growth velocity, indicating IUGR.

More recent studies have suggested that other methods of estimating fetal weight by ultrasound may be more accurate. Customized growth charts using the mother's characteristics (ethnicity, age and weight) and obstetric history in combination with ultrasonographic parameters have been proposed to calculate an ideal weight for a specific fetus to improve the accuracy of diagnosing IUGR[81–83]. Gardosi et al. have developed a formula incorporating all of these factors to calculate the 'optimal' weight at each gestation from 24 weeks[84]. These elements have been incorporated into a software program, GROW (gestation-related optimal weight), and this program is freely available from www.gestation.net, but there is a lack of prospective studies addressing efficacy. Others have proposed gender-specific fetal weight calculations[85] and individualized growth assessments based on measurements in the second trimester.[86] However, there is a lack of prospective studies addressing the efficacy of customized growth charts. More accurate weight estimations maybe obtained when the coefficients of the weight estimation function are derived from the population studied and not taken from the literature. Adjusting for these variables has been shown to have a higher sensitivity in distinguishing between IUGR and SGA[87–89] for a lower false positive rate[90]. In future, 3-D ultrasound may enable better estimation of fetal weight by including soft tissue volume[91]. Intra- and inter-observer variability can be minimized by averaging multiple measurements, improving image quality, uniform equipment calibration, careful design of measurement methods, appropriate training and regular audit of measurement quality[72].

If a diagnosis of IUGR is suspected or has been confirmed with repeated measurements, clues to the underlying mechanisms should immediately be sought. The identification of the specific cause of IUGR prior to delivery is essential as it will determine parental counseling, clinical management and pregnancy outcome. A detailed maternal history should be taken including social, obstetric and medical history, prior screening for chromosomal abnormalities and exposure to infection. Screening for pre-eclampsia should continue throughout the pregnancy.

Within the literature, much emphasis has been put on EFW alone. However, in clinical practice, the individual fetal measurements, particularly serial measurements, remain important and in fact are often essential to establishing the underlying cause. Around 75% of all IUGR is asymmetrical with disproportionate fetal measurements (i.e. maintained head growth) (Fig. 39.1). This is most frequently due to uteroplacental insufficiency leading to preferential shunting of blood to the brain. These

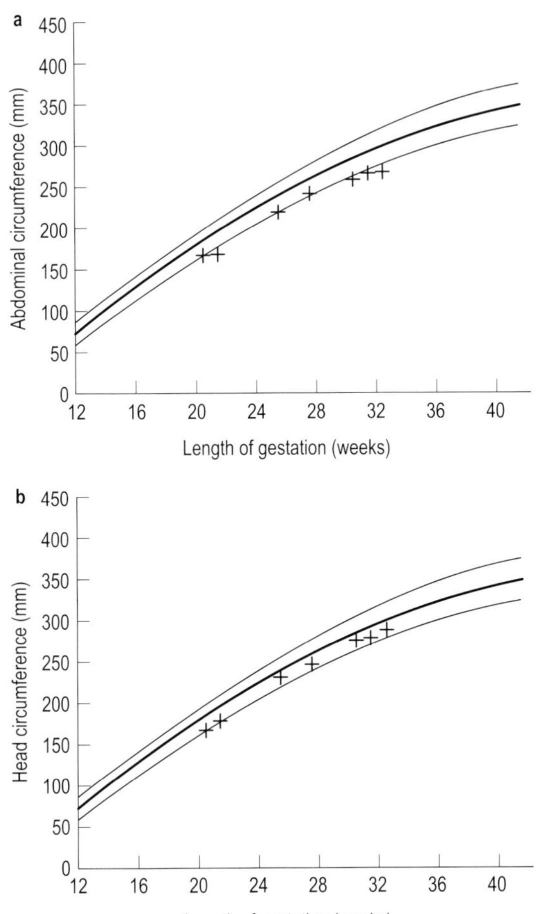

Fig. 39.1 The graphs show growth of the abdominal circumference below the 3rd centile through gestation (a), whereas the head circumference shows growth well within the normal range for gestation (b). This demonstrates asymmetrical growth restriction and was caused by uteroplacental insufficiency.

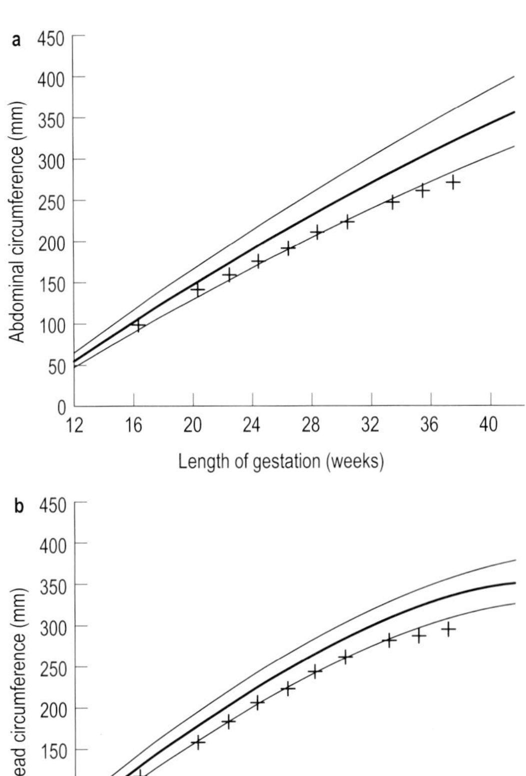

Fig. 39.2 Graphs showing growth of both the abdominal circumference and head circumference below the 3rd centile throughout gestation, demonstrating symmetrical growth restriction.

pregnancies are at a significant risk of severe pre-eclampsia, fetal distress and obstetric intervention compared to symmetrical IUGR. Symmetrical IUGR (i.e. reduced velocity of all fetal biometric parameters) is more frequently caused by an early fetal insult such as maternal smoking, congenital infection or aneuploidy (Fig. 39.2). The sonographic HC to AC ratio may be useful in distinguishing between these entities[92], however, in clinical practice, the individual causes do not always fit into the expected pattern of growth restriction. There is some debate as to whether symmetrical or asymmetrical IUGR is associated with a worse perinatal outcome and data on this are conflicting[92–96].

Amniotic fluid volume

Assessment of amniotic fluid volume is the next stage of any ultrasound examination and may help to determine the underlying cause of IUGR. If, subjectively, the amniotic fluid volume does not appear normal on ultrasound, the volume can be assessed using either the amniotic fluid index or maximum pool depth and normal ranges for gestation exist for both of these[97–99] (see Chapter 45). Maternal and placental causes leading to impaired uteroplacental perfusion are likely to cause reduced amniotic fluid volume (due to reduced fetal kidney perfusion) and fetal causes are likely to be associated with a normal amniotic fluid volume. However, certain chromosomal and structural fetal malformations such as trisomy 18 and duodenal atresia are associated with polyhydramnios.

Occasionally, a referral for suspected IUGR will, in fact, be preterm rupture of membranes (PROM). A detailed maternal history, demonstration of amniotic fluid on speculum examination and as detailed ultrasound examination as possible should help to distinguish this separate diagnosis. PROM may cause fetal measurements to appear small, either due to technical difficulties on ultrasound due to oligohydramnios or as a secondary effect on the fetus of prolonged oligohydramnios, and will be associated with normal uterine and fetal Dopplers.

Karyotyping

The finding of a small baby with or without normal amniotic fluid volume should prompt a detailed anatomical survey of the fetus. The finding of markers of aneuploidy or one or more structural malformations raises the possibility of chromosomal abnormality and should lead to discussion with the parents regarding chromosomal analysis via amniocentesis or chorionic villus sampling. Chromosomal abnormalities may be present in up to 20% of cases of IUGR[30]. Early onset IUGR raises the possibility of aneuploidy further and typically there will be normal or increased amniotic fluid volume and normal or mildly abnormal Dopplers. As previously described, certain structural abnormalities are associated with IUGR. Multiple abnormalities in the presence of normal chromosomes raises the possibility of a genetic syndrome. Confined placental mosaicism would be diagnosed by placental biopsy at CVS (and normal fetal chromosomes confirmed by analysis of the amniotic fluid).

Detection of congenital infection

IUGR caused by congenital infection can present at any gestation but, typically, causes symmetrical IUGR. Maternal viral serology screening should be performed in all cases of IUGR as the presentation is not always typical. Primary CMV is by far the commonest cause and may show the associated signs on ultrasound of ventriculomegaly, microcephaly, hydrops, intracranial calcifications and hyperechogenic bowel. Amniotic fluid analysis for infection can be performed on an amniocentesis sample for chromosome analysis and virus isolation by culture and polymerase chain reaction (PCR) provides a diagnosis of congenital infection with 72% sensitivity and 97.6% specificity[100]. Quantitative PCR on this sample will determine the fetus which is affected by the congenital infection[101,102]. The prenatal diagnosis of congenital infection is discussed in more detail in Chapter 44.

Doppler assessment of the uteroplacental circulation

Doppler studies of the uterine and fetal vessels should be performed in any diagnosed case of SGA or IUGR. These are crucial in distinguishing between the two.

Assessment of the impedance to flow in both uterine arteries provides a measure of possible uteroplacental damage in pregnancies affected by IUGR. Uterine artery Dopplers performed at 23–24 weeks' gestation selects a group at increased risk of IUGR and adverse perinatal outcome[103–105]. The best index to quantify the waveform of the uterine arteries remains controversial. An increased pulsatility index, persistence of an early notch beyond 23 weeks and difference between the left and right uterine artery have all been associated with IUGR, pre-eclampsia and adverse perinatal outcome (Fig. 39.3)[106–108]. A review of routine uterine artery Dopplers in unselected populations showed considerable heterogeneity but showed that abnormal uterine arteries at 24 weeks' gestation identify 20% of those who develop IUGR[109]. However, with few data from randomized trials, its routine use in low-risk populations has not been proven. Uterine artery Doppler does have a role in the assessment of the pregnancy already affected by IUGR as presence of abnormal uterine artery Doppler waveforms suggests a uteroplacental rather than fetal cause for the IUGR.

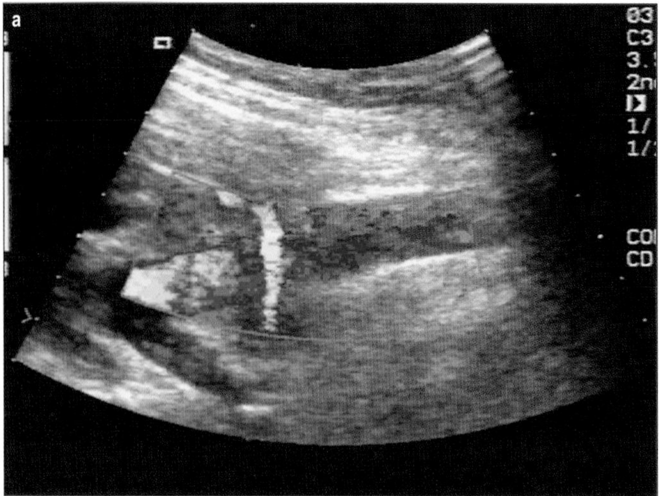

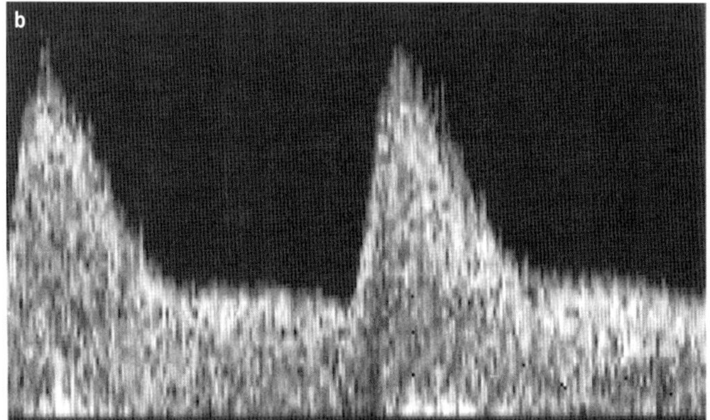

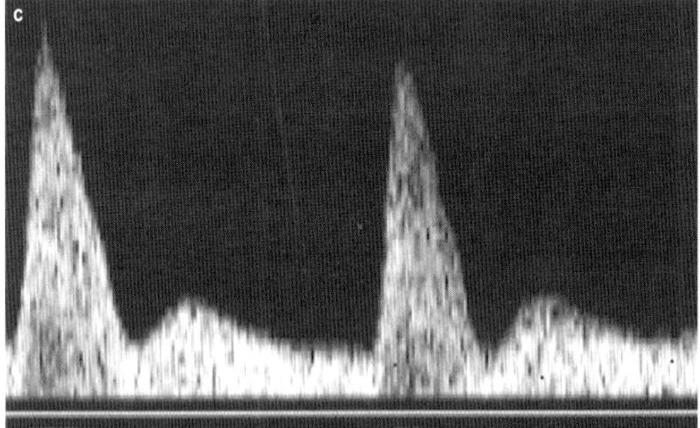

Fig. 39.3 (a) The use of color Doppler to locate the uterine artery crossing the iliac vessels on one side. (b) A normal flow pattern in the uterine artery at 24 weeks' gestation. (c) A high resistance to flow and an early diastolic notch in the uterine artery at the same gestation.

Doppler assessment of the fetoplacental circulation

The vessel that has been studied most intensively is the umbilical artery (UA). Abnormalities of the umbilical artery Doppler waveform, such as an increased pulsatility index (PI), absent end-diastolic flow (AED) or reversed end-diastolic flow (RED) in an SGA fetus, imply a degree of placental insufficiency and identify the small fetus that is at risk (Fig. 39.4)[110–112]. Abnormal UA Doppler indices are associated with fetal acid–base compromise[113] and the use of UA Dopplers in management of the SGA fetus significantly reduces perinatal death and unnecessary preterm delivery in prospective randomized trials[114,115]. The presence of absent or reversed end-diastolic flow in the umbilical

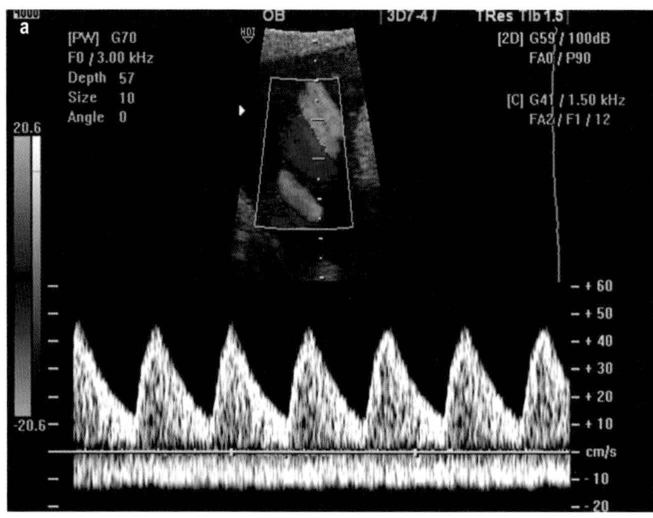

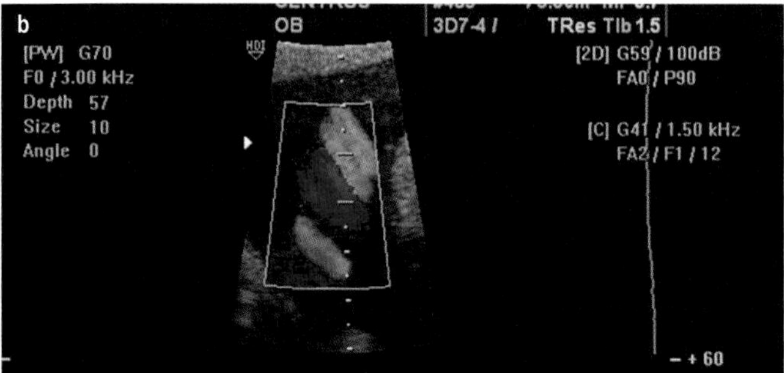

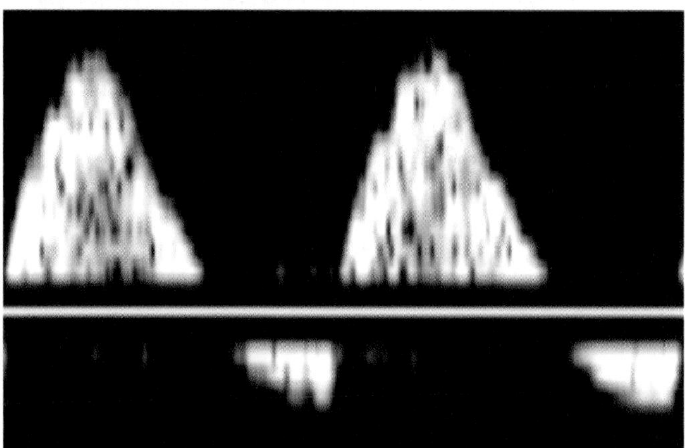

Fig. 39.4 (a) The use of color Doppler to demonstrate normal flow velocity in the umbilical artery. (b) Reversed end diastolic flow in the umbilical artery.

artery is associated with a poor perinatal outcome and high perinatal mortality rate[113,116,117]. In contrast, a small fetus with an EFW below the 10th centile but with normal amniotic fluid volume and umbilical artery Dopplers will rarely have significant morbidity[113–115] and is likely to be a normal small fetus rather than a growth restricted fetus.

Doppler assessment of the middle cerebral artery

While UA Doppler provides information about resistance to flow in the fetoplacental circulation, it is less useful in determining the fetal response and therefore extent of substrate deprivation. Because of the rapid and sustained redistribution of cardiac output observed with the onset of fetal hypoxia (see Fetal Physiological responses section) and the associated fall in cerebrovascular resistance, a reduction in the pulsatility index of the middle cerebral artery Doppler waveform is one of the earlier changes to occur in a hypoxic fetus (Fig. 39.5). Recent data suggest that even fetuses with normal umbilical artery Dopplers but with abnormal middle cerebral artery waveforms have earlier deliveries, more SGA, higher cesarean section rates and increased admission to neonatal units[118,119]. A complete assessment of the mother and fetus as described will allow the diagnosis of IUGR to be made in the majority of cases and will usually allow the underlying cause to be established. Once this has been done, a clear plan of monitoring and decision for delivery can be made and the parents counseled appropriately.

MANAGEMENT OF FETAL GROWTH RESTRICTION

In the majority of cases of growth restriction, the underlying placental dysfunction will require monitoring of the pregnancy by longitudinal assessment of fetal well-being and delivery timed to minimize morbidity and mortality. However, in certain causes of IUGR, an alternative or additional management strategy may be required.

In maternal disease, continual monitoring of the maternal condition will be required alongside fetal monitoring. In many conditions, such as pre-eclampsia, the maternal and fetal condition may deteriorate simultaneously, however, there will be situations where delivery will be required for maternal reasons prior to that of the fetus. In 'unexplained IUGR', the mother is at an increased risk of developing pre-eclampsia and therefore regular maternal monitoring of blood pressure and urinalysis is recommended to ensure prompt diagnosis of pre-eclampsia.

Where the underlying cause of IUGR is thought to be due to a toxin, such as therapeutic drugs or recreational substances, advice should be given to reduce the intake if possible. When smoking is discontinued after the first trimester, the reduction in birth weight is significantly less than when smoking continues throughout gestation[23].

If a fetal structural or chromosomal abnormality is the likely cause of the growth restriction, then appropriate parental counselling is required to ensure they have accurate information regarding the diagnosis, prognosis and possible outcomes. If the fetus has a chromosomal abnormality, it may be appropriate to discuss termination of pregnancy depending on the gestation at diagnosis. As the prognosis is likely to be poor, the alternative option of conservative management, awaiting spontaneous labor and compassionate care of the neonate may be appropriate. In the presence of a fetal structural abnormality, delivery may need to be timed to optimize postnatal care depending on the nature of the abnormality and discussions with the neonatologists will be required. Again, discussion regarding termination of pregnancy may be appropriate.

In congenital infection, antenatal treatment may be required to reduce the risk of transmission to the fetus and the timing of delivery will depend on the severity to which the fetus is affected. This is discussed further in Chapter 44. A meta-analysis of randomized trials has shown that routine administration of

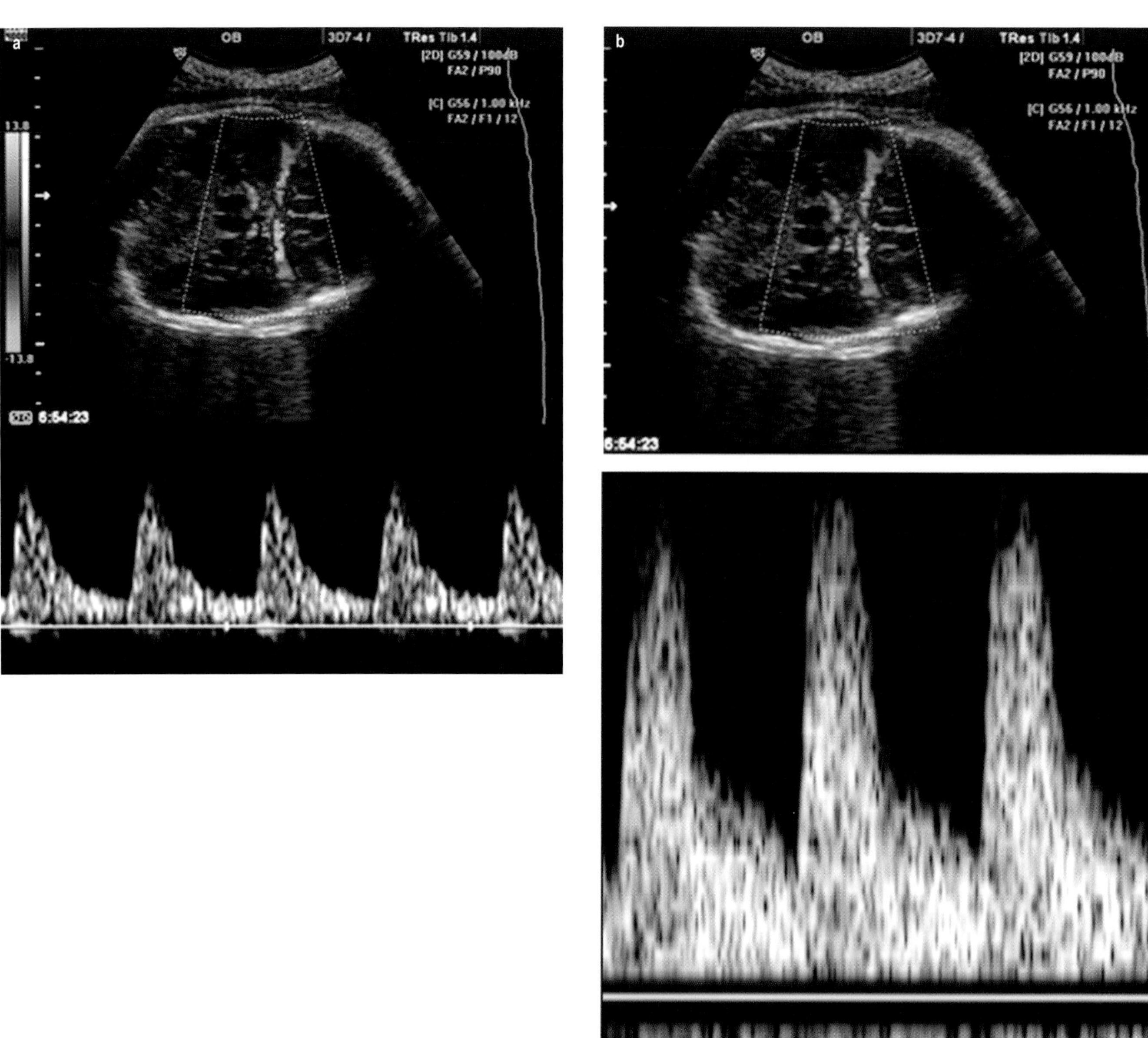

Fig. 39.5 (a) Color Doppler flow in the middle cerebral artery demonstrates a normal waveform. (b) Increased velocity in the middle cerebral artery flow suggesting evidence of redistribution of blood flow to the brain.

antimalarials in pregnancy in endemic areas was associated with a higher birth weight and fewer low birth weight infants[120].

In all other causes and 'unexplained' IUGR, the mainstay of treatment after the diagnosis is made remains antenatal surveillance of the fetus. Various prenatal therapies have been investigated as potentially beneficial in IUGR with little success. Bed rest is frequently recommended in IUGR, presumably with the aim of improving uteroplacental perfusion. There are few data from randomized controlled trials on bed rest as a treatment for IUGR and no evidence of benefit has been found[121]. Moreover, it may cause maternal harm by increasing the risk of thromboembolism. The use of maternal oxygen therapy has also been advocated as a treatment for IUGR, due to the finding that in situations of hypoxemia, such as maternal cyanotic heart disease and at high altitude, the risk of IUGR is increased. However, oxygen therapy has not been proven to be effective at improving fetal growth or perinatal outcome[122] and, in fact, may be harmful[123]. The following have all been investigated as potential prenatal therapies for IUGR but with insufficient data or data confirming no benefit: maternal nutritional supplementation[124], iron and folate supplementation[125], betamimetic drugs[126] and calcium channel blockers[127]. A meta-analysis of the use of low-dose aspirin in IUGR demonstrated a significant reduction in growth restriction[128]. However, a more recent meta-analysis showed no reduction in IUGR or perinatal deaths but a reduction in the risk of preterm birth[129].

Antenatal monitoring of the fetus

In the vulnerable growth-restricted fetus, antenatal surveillance tests are required to assess fetal well-being over time to aid decisions regarding the timing of delivery. The majority of monitoring, such as regular biometry, amniotic fluid volume assessment, cardiotocography (CTG) and biophysical profile (BPP) scoring, evaluate indirect manifestations of the fetal response to impaired oxygenation. In addition, fetal Dopplers provide direct assessment of placental and fetal function by measuring the regional blood flow changes.

As previously discussed, serial ultrasound measurements of the fetus (HC, AC and FL) provide crucial information for the detection of and assessment of the severity of IUGR. The growth velocity of the AC and EFW provide the most useful information. Generally, the measurements should be performed every 2 weeks as changes over a shorter interval are difficult to interpret. The measurements are associated with false positive rates for growth restriction of around 10%[130] and, therefore, a trend over a long period is more accurate and the measurements need to be used in conjunction with other assessments to make appropriate decisions regarding delivery. Multiple measurements by the same operator may help improve accuracy.

Abnormalities of the amniotic fluid volume are highly prevalent in IUGR and amniotic fluid volume monitoring is an essential part of fetal surveillance. Measurement of the amniotic fluid index (AFI) has not been shown to have any advantage over a single deepest pool[131]. In a meta-analysis, an antepartum AFI of 5cm or below was associated with an increased risk of cesarean section for fetal distress and an Apgar score of less than 7 at 5 minutes[132]. Many would recommend weekly AFI in IUGR and more frequent fetal surveillance once oligohydramnios has developed[133], although this will depend on the clinical scenario. Many would advocate delivery if there is a sudden deterioration in the amniotic fluid volume.

The cardiotocograph (CTG) is widely used antenatally and in labor to detect fetal hypoxia. In hypoxia, the fetal heart rate tends to increase and have a lower baseline variation. However, a systematic review of randomized trials comparing antenatal CTG with controls in intermediate and high-risk pregnancies did not demonstrate a reduction in perinatal morbidity and mortality[134]. Despite this, it remains an integral part of our obstetric practice. The CTG provides a short-term assessment of fetal well-being, however, some pathological patterns may not be apparent until a preterminal phase for the fetus. Poor fetal heart rate variability, persistent lack of accelerations and persistent variable or late decelerations may all be a sign of fetal compromise. A grossly abnormal CTG is likely to prompt delivery in the majority of cases at a viable gestation and EFW as it may represent imminent fetal death. More subtle CTG changes are more difficult to interpret and knowledge of the range of normality for a preterm fetus is important. Given that pathological changes in the CTG are seen after abnormal umbilical artery Doppler indices[135], the CTG does not have a proven role in the monitoring of the IUGR fetus. If it is used for antenatal monitoring, its limitations should be recognized. If nothing else it is likely to provide parental reassurance. The frequency of CTG monitoring will be determined by the severity of the IUGR, varying from weekly to twice daily.

The biophysical profile (BPP) score is an assessment of fetal behaviorly ultrasonography (tone, breathing and movements) in combination with amniotic fluid volume and the CTG. A low BPP score has been associated with good diagnostic accuracy in predicting adverse perinatal outcome[136]. Typically, fetal breathing movements are the first to be affected in IUGR, followed by fetal movements and then fetal tone. The superiority of the BPP over simpler forms of assessment, however, has been questioned[137]. In IUGR, it is likely that Doppler changes occur prior to deterioration of the BPP score and therefore it use in growth restriction is limited[138]. However, many would advocate the use of a combination of the BPP score and Doppler in the monitoring of IUGR[138].

Fetal blood sampling can be used to assess fetal hypoxia and acidemia. However, it is invasive and is associated with a risk of fetal death, miscarriage or inducing labor and carries little advantage over Doppler studies[139].

Fetal Doppler

Fetal Doppler studies provide the most accurate non-invasive assessment of placental function in IUGR. The changes described in the umbilical artery Doppler in IUGR are increased PI, AED and RED. Use of umbilical artery Doppler waveforms in IUGR reduce antenatal admissions and unnecessary induction of labor and reduces the risk of perinatal death[140]. In contrast, routine Doppler in low-risk populations does not improve outcome for mother or baby[141]. As the placental function progressively deteriorates, changes in the Doppler indices will be seen. The presence of absent or reversed end-diastolic flow in the umbilical artery Doppler during the second half of pregnancy is associated with an odds ratio of perinatal death of 4.0 and 10.6 respectively (see Fig. 39.4)[142]. Knowledge of UA Doppler helped in the management of the high-risk pregnancy as there is a fivefold increase in the perinatal mortality when the obstetrician did not know the UA Doppler result[143]. It should be remembered that these abnormal umbilical artery waveforms are also associated with other clinical manifestations of placental disease such as pre-eclampsia and these too will lead to progressive fetal hypoxia and ultimately intrauterine death. The UA Doppler is usually performed initially weekly during fetal surveillance but should be more frequent once the waveform is abnormal.

The changes described in the umbilical artery Doppler (increased PI, AED and RED) are all significantly associated with a decrease in the middle cerebral artery (MCA) PI (see Fig. 39.5). As described above, the growth-restricted fetus adapts to hypoxemia over time by redistributing blood flow to the brain. This produces the decreased resistance and increased flow seen in the MCA that represents one of the fetal compensatory responses to hypoxia. There are no randomized controlled trials of sufficient size to confirm the effectiveness of the MCA Doppler in IUGR. However, it is now widely used in combination with the UA Doppler as monitoring once the diagnosis has been made.

Assessment of fetal venous Doppler can provide additional information in the evaluation of the IUGR fetus and reflects the ventricular function of the fetus. The fetal acidosis present in progressive IUGR will compromise cardiac function which will, in turn, cause an increased preload reflected in: absence or reversal of flow during atrial contraction in the ductus venosus, pulsations in the umbilical vein and increased reversed flow during atrial contraction in the inferior vena cava. Analysis of all three vessels is possible, but the ductus venosus has become the most frequently used (Fig. 39.6). Venous Doppler changes reflect a more advanced stage of the placental disease and will usually prompt delivery to prevent intrauterine death. IUGR fetuses with abnormal venous flow in the ductus venosus have

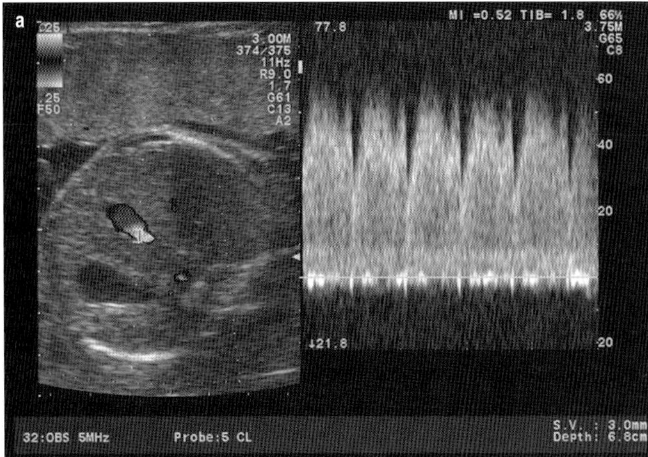

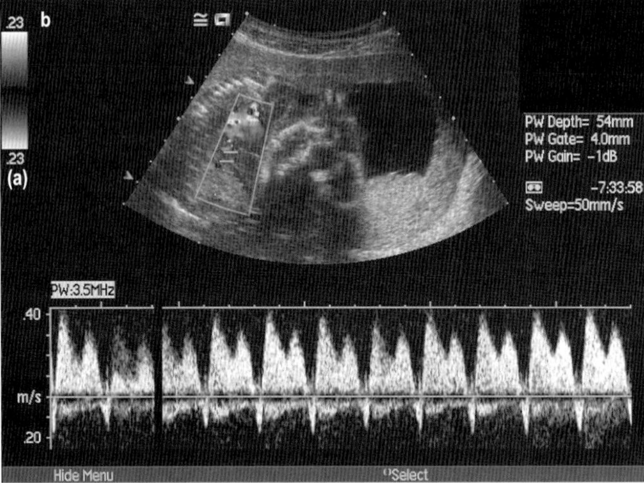

Fig. 39.6 (a) Doppler measurement of flow in the ductus venosus demonstrates a normal waveform in the third trimester.
(b) Measurement in the ductus venosus at 25 weeks' gestation in a fetus with severe early onset growth restriction shows a wave reversal. This pregnancy terminated in intrauterine death at 27 weeks' gestation and the cause was found to be congenital cytomegalovirus.

a worse perinatal outcome than those that have abnormal UA and MCA Dopplers alone[111,144], although there are no randomized trials to demonstrate their effectiveness in improving outcome. In view of this, venous Doppler should be considered in the IUGR fetus that already has changes in the UA and MCA Dopplers.

Monitoring of the IUGR fetus will involve at least one of the methods described above. However, there is a wide variation in the investigations used and disagreement regarding their timing and what combination of changes should prompt delivery[145].

TIMING OF DELIVERY

Although several attempts have been made at fetal therapy in the IUGR fetus (see p. 550), ultimately, delivery remains the mainstay of treatment. In each case, the risk of continued fetal hypoxia in utero (and possible intrauterine death) is balanced against the risks of prematurity. The main factor affecting the decision is the gestational age of the pregnancy. The optimal timing of delivery is likely to be more difficult to decide at earlier gestations[146]. In the very preterm fetus, the ideal scenario would be to allow the pregnancy to continue to gain sufficient fetal maturity until a point just before irreversible fetal damage occurs. Presentation of IUGR at an early gestation and superimposed maternal pathology, such as pre-eclampsia, are associated with a worse perinatal outcome[147,148].

Many would consider preterm and term growth restriction as two separate entities as regarding their management. In late onset or term fetal growth restriction, the IUGR is typically asymmetrical and may be associated with normal UA and uterine artery Dopplers. There is usually reduced amniotic fluid volume and a mature placenta on ultrasound. There are minimal risks of prematurity compared to the risks of fetal hypoxia and so there will be a lower threshold for delivery. At gestations over 34 weeks', AED flow in the UA Doppler is likely to prompt delivery even if all other tests are normal[149]. If all investigations are normal or stable and the fetal growth velocity is normal, then it is reasonable to allow the pregnancy to continue until term. Generally, continuation beyond 40 weeks is unlikely to be of benefit and delivery should be considered at this stage. Fetal growth restriction is likely to be a factor in many cases of 'unexplained' stillbirth particularly at term[150] and, while this does not represent a cause in itself, it is a clinical condition for which diagnosis and prevention is a possibility. Early onset of preterm IUGR is a much less common disease and typically results in fetal death or elective delivery prior to 34 weeks. It is characterized by reduced, absent or reversed end-diastolic flow in the UA and abnormalities of the uterine artery Doppler.

It is impossible to give a prescribed need for delivery for all cases of IUGR as each pregnancy should be considered as individual, however, the following should prompt discussion regarding delivery depending on the gestation and factors described above: no growth over a 2-week period, significant drop in the amniotic fluid volume or anhydramnios, progression from AEDF to REDF in the UA Doppler, gross CTG abnormalities as described above, a BPP of ≤ 4, reversal of flow during atrial contraction in the fetal veins.

Many groups have studied the sequential changes in the tests of fetal well-being, however, as IUGR is a heterogeneous group of disorders with many different causes, each case does not follow the same sequence and timing of changes. Therefore, the management of each case should be individualized given the gestational age, severity of the IUGR, amniotic fluid volume, CTG, Doppler changes, the likely underlying cause, the maternal condition and previous obstetric history. The management and decision to deliver should be discussed with the parents in conjunction with the neonatologists.

Surveillance of the fetus and mother will usually be as an outpatient depending on the maternal condition. If, however, there is deterioration in the fetal condition and intense fetal monitoring is required, then inpatient monitoring may be recommended, particularly once the decision for delivery has been made while awaiting fetal lung maturity after the administration of steroids.

Normal fetal Dopplers

As previously discussed, cesarean section rates, admission to neonatal units, perinatal mortality, cerebral hemorrhage, anemia and hypoglycemia are all significantly lower in the presence of normal UA Dopplers compared to AED or RED flow[142,151]. If the UA Dopplers are normal at presentation in the SGA fetus then this is a good indicator of fetal well-being. Generally, a normal UA Doppler suggests normal placental function and therefore another cause of the SGA other than placental insufficiency should be considered. However, a proportion of these fetuses will turn out to have IUGR of a uteroplacental cause who are diagnosed at an early stage of the disease and therefore continued monitoring with biometry, amniotic fluid volume, CTG and weekly Dopplers is recommended until delivery. If these remain normal, delivery can usually be delayed until term[149]. In fact, if the Dopplers are normal at presentation of the IUGR, they are likely to remain normal. The SGA fetus with normal Dopplers appears to tolerate labor and labor induction well[152].

Abnormal tests of fetal well-being

Hecher et al. studied the sequence of the changes in fetal monitoring of the IUGR fetus and correlated them with neonatal outcome[143]. They found that a reduction in the amniotic fluid index and a rise in the UA PI were the first variables to become abnormal, followed by MCA and aortic Doppler changes, then a decrease in the short-term variation on the CTG and, finally, the ductus venosus and inferior vena cava Doppler. In the preterm cases delivered before 32 weeks, the UA and MCA Dopplers and amniotic fluid index changed, on average, at least four weeks prior to delivery and the ductus venosus and CTG only one week prior to delivery.

Baschat et al. studied predictors of poor neonatal outcome in a prospective study of 604 IUGR infants born at less than 33 weeks' gestation[154]. They found that gestational age was by far the most significant determinant of neonatal survival until 26+6 weeks and a significant contributor to major morbidity until 29+2 weeks' gestation. Beyond this gestational age, the ductus venosus and cord artery pH at delivery predicted neonatal mortality and ductus venosus Doppler alone predicted intact survival. This group found a neonatal mortality rate of 20% in IUGR infants and an intact survival rate of 58%. The study provides data across gestational age and birth weights relevant to aid counseling and management decisions.

There has been some controversy on the management of the IUGR fetus once the UA Doppler shows AED or RED flow. It will depend on the gestational age and other factors. Some would advocate delivery and/or admission to hospital, whereas others would recommend a step up in the surveillance of the pregnancy as an outpatient. The Growth Restriction Intervention Trial (GRIT) was a randomized trial that aimed to address this issue by comparing outcome in women with an IUGR fetus that was delivered early compared with those where delivery was delayed for as long as possible to increase maturity[153]. The GRIT study showed that when the delivery of the IUGR fetus with a normal UA Doppler at a mean gestational age of 32 weeks was delayed for 4 days, there was a fivefold increase in the number of stillbirths and a twofold decrease in neonatal deaths with no overall difference in the perinatal mortality rate. This trial failed to show any clear benefit for either management plan and therefore leaves it open for obstetricians to make the decision on an individual basis. The optimal timing of delivery in severe early IUGR requires a randomized trial with different management protocols and such a trial is underway: the TRUFFLE trial (trial of umbilical and fetal flow in Europe)[155].

Once there is AED in the UA Doppler prior to 32 weeks, the monitoring of the fetus and pregnancy should be more intense and Dopplers should be repeated twice weekly. If there are other markers of compromise such as echogenic bowel, cardiomegaly, increased pulsatility in the ductus venosus or an abnormal CTG, delivery should be considered[143] after the administration of steroids for lung maturity[156]. Delivery will usually be by cesarean section.

INTRAPARTUM MANAGEMENT AND DELIVERY

The mode of delivery will depend primarily on the gestational age but also on the state of the fetus. In the pre-viable fetus, a decision may be made in discussion with the parents for termination of pregnancy by induction of labor if it is felt that the fetus is unlikely to reach a viable weight. In the viable fetus below 32 weeks' gestation, induction of labor is unlikely to be successful and therefore cesarean section is the usual mode of delivery. Beyond 32 weeks, induction of labor can be considered. In the presence of normal UA Dopplers, labor may be tolerated well[157]. Mode of delivery should be individualized depending on the gestational age, state of the fetus, condition of the cervix, maternal condition and previous obstetric history in discussion with the parents and neonatologists. One study has shown that elective cesarean section for IUGR results in lower rates of respiratory distress syndrome, neonatal seizures and death, but these differences did not reach statistical significance[158]. If labor is considered, fetal well-being should be carefully assessed with a low threshold for cesarean section in labor given that many of these fetuses are chronically hypoxic and will not tolerate a further acute hypoxic insult.

The decision to use CTG monitoring depends on whether action will be taken if the trace is abnormal. If cesarean section would be performed for fetal distress, continuous CTG monitoring should be performed in labor in conjunction with appropriate use of fetal scalp blood sampling. Although systematic reviews of randomized trials have found that routine continuous intrapartum CTG monitoring in high- and low-risk populations does not reduce perinatal mortality rates[159], in high-risk pregnancies such as IUGR, there are some observational data that it may be of benefit[160]. Significant oligohydramnios is likely to increase the risk of cord compression and therefore the associated variable decelerations. Cesarean section in labor is therefore more frequent in IUGR.

POSTNATAL MANAGEMENT

In severe IUGR requiring preterm delivery, postnatal follow-up should be arranged with the parents to discuss the outcome of the pregnancy and plans for future pregnancies. In unexplained IUGR, screening for thrombophilias should be considered at least 6–8 weeks post delivery.

PEDIATRIC CONSEQUENCES OF GROWTH RESTRICTION

The growth-restricted neonate is at an increased risk of hypothermia, hypoglycemia, respiratory distress, hypocalcemia, polycythemia, intraventricular hemorrhage and necrotizing enterocolitis during the neonatal period compared to normally grown infants[161] (see Chapter 49). Stillbirth rates are increased in the IUGR fetus at all gestations[162,163] with the overall perinatal mortality rate 8–10 times higher compared to normally grown infants. Careful timing of delivery is important to minimize these risks.

In the medium term, IUGR appears to be associated with an increased risk of poor neurological outcome for the infant. There is an increased risk of cerebral palsy in infants born with IUGR beyond 32 weeks[164]. Below 32 weeks, the effects of prematurity appear to negate the adverse effects of fetal growth restriction[165]. Poor prenatal head growth is particularly associated with a poor outcome[166]. Postnatal growth is usually poor in the growth-restricted infant, however, the majority have demonstrated catch-up growth by 2 years. As adults they are at increased risk of heart disease, hypertension and type 2 diabetes[167].

CONCLUSION

Fetal growth restriction is a major cause of perinatal mortality and morbidity and may have long-term sequelae for the infant. However, the vast majority of small fetuses are healthy and have no increased morbidity and mortality. The challenge is to recognize true IUGR, to determine the underlying cause and optimize monitoring and delivery to minimize the impact on the infant. The decision to deliver will depend on balancing the risks of continued chronic hypoxia and prematurity.

REFERENCES

1. Allen WR, Wilsher S, Turnbull C et al. Influence of maternal size on placental, fetal and postnatal growth in the horse. I. Development in utero. *Reproduction* **123**(3):445–453, 2002.
2. Moore G, Cheung W, Schwarzacher T, Flavell R. BIS 1, a major component of the cereal genome and a tool for studying genomic organization. *Genomics* **10**(2):469–476, 1991.
3. Barton SC, Surani MA, Norris ML. Role of paternal and maternal genomes in mouse development. *Nature* **311**(5984):374–376, 1984.
4. Morison IM, Reeve AE. A catalogue of imprinted genes and parent-of-origin effects in humans and animals. *Hum Mol Genet* **7**(10):1599–1609, 1998.
5. Tycko B, Morison IM. Physiological functions of imprinted genes. *J Cell Physiol* **192**(3):245–258, 2002.
6. Carter AM, Hills F, O'Gorman DB et al. The insulin-like growth factor system in mammalian pregnancy – a workshop report. *Placenta* **25**(Suppl A):S53–S56, 2004.
7. Kirchengast S, Hartmann B. Impact of maternal age and maternal somatic characteristics on newborn size. *Am J Hum Biol* **15**(2):220–228, 2003.
8. Odibo AO, Nelson D, Stamilio DM, Sehdev HM, Macones GA. Advanced maternal age is an independent risk factor for intrauterine growth restriction. *Am J Perinatol* **23**(5):325–328, 2006.
9. Barker M, Robinson S, Osmond C, Barker DJ. Birth weight and body fat distribution in adolescent girls. *Arch Dis Child* **77**(5):381–383, 1997.
10. Gluckman PD, Hanson MA. Maternal constraint of fetal growth and its consequences. *Semin Fetal Neonatal Med* **9**(5):419–425, 2004.
11. Chauhan SP, Magann EF. Screening for fetal growth restriction. *Clin Obstet Gynecol* **49**(2):284–294, 2006.
12. Bukowski R, Gahn D, Denning J, Saade G. Impairment of growth in fetuses destined to deliver preterm. *Am J Obstet Gynecol* **185**(2):463–467, 2001.
13. Odegard RA, Vatten LJ, Nilsen ST, Salvesen KA, Austgulen R. Preeclampsia and fetal growth. *Obstet Gynecol* **96**(6):950–955, 2000.
14. Sibai B, Dekker G, Kupferminc M. Pre-eclampsia. *Lancet* **365**(9461):785–799, 2005.
15. Villar J, Carroli G, Wojdyla D et al. Preeclampsia, gestational hypertension and intrauterine growth restriction, related or independent conditions? *Am J Obstet Gynecol* **194**(4):921–931, 2006.
16. Yasuda M, Takakuwa K, Tokunaga A, Tanaka K. Prospective studies of the association between anticardiolipin antibody and outcome of pregnancy. *Obstet Gynecol* **86**(4 Pt 1):555–559, 1995.
17. Howley HE, Walker M, Rodger MA. A systematic review of the association between factor V Leiden or prothrombin gene variant and intrauterine growth restriction. *Am J Obstet Gynecol* **192**(3):694–708, 2005.
18. Cunningham FG, Cox SM, Harstad TW, Mason RA, Pritchard JA. Chronic renal disease and pregnancy outcome. *Am J Obstet Gynecol* **163**(2):453–459, 1990.
19. Rotmensch S, Liberati M, Luo JS et al. Color Doppler flow patterns and flow velocity waveforms of the intraplacental fetal circulation in growth-retarded fetuses. *Am J Obstet Gynecol* **171**(5): 1257–1264, 1994.
20. Stein Z, Susser M. The Dutch famine, 1944–1945, and the reproductive process. I. Effects or six indices at birth. *Pediatr Res* **9**(2):70–76, 1975.
21. Antenatal corticosteroids revisited: repeat courses – National Institutes of Health Consensus Development Conference Statement, August 17-18, 2000. Obstet Gynecol, 98(1): 144–150, 2001.
22. Kramer MS. Determinants of low birth weight: methodological assessment and meta-analysis. *Bull World Health Org* **65**(5):663–737, 1987.
23. Cliver SP, Goldenberg RL, Cutter GR, Hoffman HJ, Davis RO, Nelson KG. The effect of cigarette smoking on neonatal anthropometric measurements. *Obstet Gynecol* **85**(4):625–630, 1995.
24. Ounsted M, Moar VA, Scott A. Risk factors associated with small-for-dates and large-for-dates infants. *Br J Obstet Gynaecol* **92**(3):226–232, 1985.
25. Sokol RJ, Delaney-Black V, Nordstrom B. Fetal alcohol spectrum disorder. *J Am Med Assoc* **290**(22):2996–2999, 2003.
26. Bada HS, Das A, Bauer CR et al. Gestational cocaine exposure and intrauterine growth: maternal lifestyle study. *Obstet Gynecol* **100**(5 Pt 1):916–924, 2002.
27. Naeye RL, Blanc W, Leblanc W, Khatamee MA. Fetal complications of maternal heroin addiction: abnormal growth, infections, and episodes of stress. *J Pediatr* **83**(6):1055–1061, 1973.
28. Chaddha V, Viero S, Huppertz B, Kingdom J. Developmental biology of the placenta and the origins of placental insufficiency. *Semin Fetal Neonatal Med* **9**(5):357–369, 2004.
29. Khoury MJ, Erickson JD, Cordero JF, McCarthy BJ. Congenital malformations and intrauterine growth retardation: a population study. *Pediatrics* **82**(1):83–90, 1988.
30. Snijders RJ, Sherrod C, Gosden CM, Nicolaides KH. Fetal growth retardation: associated malformations and chromosomal abnormalities. *Am J Obstet Gynecol* **168**(2):547–555, 1993.
31. Wilkins-Haug L, Quade B, Morton CC. Confined placental mosaicism as a risk factor among newborns with fetal growth restriction. *Prenat Diagn* **26**(5):428–432, 2006.
32. Stagno S, Reynolds DW, Tsiantos A, Fuccillo DA, Long W, Alford CA. Comparative serial virologic and

serologic studies of symptomatic and subclinical congenitally and natally acquired cytomegalovirus infections. *J Infect Dis* **132**(5):568–577, 1975.

33. Fowler KB, Stagno S, Pass RF, Britt WJ, Boll TJ, Alford CA. The outcome of congenital cytomegalovirus infection in relation to maternal antibody status. *N Engl J Med* **326**(10):663–667, 1992.
34. Shulman CE, Marshall T, Dorman EK et al. Malaria in pregnancy: adverse effects on haemoglobin levels and birthweight in primigravidae and multigravidae. *Trop Med Int Health* **6**(10):770–778, 2001.
35. Crane JP, Tomich PG, Kopta M. Ultrasonic growth patterns in normal and discordant twins. *Obstet Gynecol* **55**(6):678–683, 1980.
36. Economides DL, Nicolaides KH, Campbell S. Metabolic and endocrine findings in appropriate and small for gestational age fetuses. *J Perinat Med* **19** (1–2):97–105, 1991.
37. Soothill PW, Nicolaides KH, Campbell S. Prenatal asphyxia, hyperlacticaemia, hypoglycaemia, and erythroblastosis in growth retarded fetuses. *Br Med J (Clin Res Ed)* **294**(6579):1051–1053, 1987.
38. Giussani DA, Spencer JA, Moore PJ, Bennet L, Hanson MA. Afferent and efferent components of the cardiovascular reflex responses to acute hypoxia in term fetal sheep. *J Physiol* **461**:431–449, 1993.
39. Hanson MA, Spencer JAD, Rodeck CH. *The circulation (Vol 1): the fetus and neonate, physiology and clinical applications*. Cambridge University Press, 1993.
40. Bocking AD, Gagnon R, White SE, Homan J, Milne KM, Richardson BS. Circulatory responses to prolonged hypoxemia in fetal sheep. *Am J Obstet Gynecol* **159**(6):1418–1424, 1988.
41. Gagnon R, Johnston L, Murotsuki J. Fetal placental embolization in the late-gestation ovine fetus: alterations in umbilical blood flow and fetal heart rate patterns. *Am J Obstet Gynecol* **175**(1): 63–72, 1996.
42. Weiner Z, Farmakides G, Schulman H, Penny B. Central and peripheral hemodynamic changes in fetuses with absent end-diastolic velocity in umbilical artery: correlation with computerized fetal heart rate pattern. *Am J Obstet Gynecol* **170**(2):509–515, 1994.
43. Rurak DW, Richardson BS, Patrick JE, Carmichael L, Homan J. Blood flow and oxygen delivery to fetal organs and tissues during sustained hypoxemia. *Am J Physiol* **258**(5 Pt 2):R1116–R1122, 1990.
44. Davis LE, Hohimer AR. Hemodynamics and organ blood flow in fetal sheep subjected to chronic anemia. *Am J Physiol* **261**(6 Pt 2):R1542–R1548, 1991.
45. Chan FY, Pun TC, Lam P, Lam C, Lee CP, Lam YH. Fetal cerebral Doppler studies as a predictor of perinatal outcome and subsequent neurologic handicap. *Obstet Gynecol* **87**(6):981–988, 1996.
46. Rizzo G, Capponi A, Chaoui R, Taddei F, Arduini D, Romanini C. Blood flow velocity waveforms from peripheral pulmonary arteries in normally grown and growth-retarded fetuses. *Ultrasound Obstet Gynecol* **8**(2):87–92, 1996.
47. Mari G, Abuhamad AZ, Uerpairojkit B, Martinez E, Copel JA. Blood flow velocity waveforms of the abdominal arteries in appropriate- and small-for-gestational-age fetuses. *Ultrasound Obstet Gynecol* **6**(1): 15–18, 1995.
48. Vyas S, Nicolaides KH, Campbell S. Renal artery flow-velocity waveforms in normal and hypoxemic fetuses. *Am J Obstet Gynecol* **161**(1):168–172, 1989.
49. Kiserud T. Hemodynamics of the ductus venosus. *Eur J Obstet Gynecol Reprod Biol* **84**(2):139–147, 1999.
50. Behrman RE, Lees MH, Peterson EN, De Lannoy CW, Seeds AE. Distribution of the circulation in the normal and asphyxiated fetal primate. *Am J Obstet Gynecol* **108**(6):956–969, 1970.
51. Tchirikov M, Rybakowski C, Huneke B, Schroder HJ. Blood flow through the ductus venosus in singleton and multifetal pregnancies and in fetuses with intrauterine growth retardation. *Am J Obstet Gynecol* **178**(5):943–949, 1998.
52. Kiserud T, Eik-Nes SH, Blaas HG, Hellevik LR, Simensen B. Ductus venosus blood velocity and the umbilical circulation in the seriously growth-retarded fetus. *Ultrasound Obstet Gynecol* **4**(2):109–114, 1994.
53. Baschat AA, Gembruch U, Weiner CP, Harman CR. Qualitative venous Doppler waveform analysis improves prediction of critical perinatal outcomes in premature growth-restricted fetuses. *Ultrasound Obstet Gynecol* **22**(3):240–245, 2003.
54. Hooper SB, Bocking AD, White S, Challis JR, Han VK. DNA synthesis is reduced in selected fetal tissues during prolonged hypoxemia. *Am J Physiol* **261**(2 Pt 2):R508–R514, 1991.
55. Richardson BS, Bocking AD. Metabolic and circulatory adaptations to chronic hypoxia in the fetus. *Comp Biochem Physiol A Mol Integr Physiol* **119**(3):717–723, 1998.
56. Rurak DW, Gruber NC. The effect of neuromuscular blockade on oxygen consumption and blood gases in the fetal lamb. *Am J Obstet Gynecol* **145**(2):258–262, 1983.
57. Bocking AD, Harding R. Effects of reduced uterine blood flow on electrocortical activity, breathing, and skeletal muscle activity in fetal sheep. *Am J Obstet Gynecol* **154**(3):655–662, 1986.
58. Natale R, Clewlow F, Dawes GS. Measurement of fetal forelimb movements in the lamb in utero. *Am J Obstet Gynecol* **140**(5):545–551, 1981.
59. Bocking AD, Gagnon R, Milne KM, White SE. Behavioral activity during prolonged hypoxemia in fetal sheep. *J Appl Physiol* **65**(6):2420–2426, 1988.
60. Worthington D, Piercy WN, Smith BT. Effects of reduction of placental size in sheep. *Obstet Gynecol* **58**(2):215–221, 1981.
61. Pillai M, James D. Continuation of normal neurobehavioural development in fetuses with absent umbilical arterial end diastolic velocities. *Br J Obstet Gynaecol* **98**(3):277–281, 1991.
62. Ribbert LS, Nicolaides KH, Visser GH. Prediction of fetal acidaemia in intrauterine growth retardation: comparison of quantified fetal activity with biophysical profile score. *Br J Obstet Gynaecol* **100**(7):653–656, 1993.
63. RCOG, Antenatal care: routine care for the healthy pregnant women, Clinical Guideline, 2003
64. Challis K, Osman NB, Nystrom L, Nordahl G, Bergstrom S. Symphysis-fundal height growth chart of an obstetric cohort of 817 Mozambican women with ultrasound-dated singleton pregnancies. *Trop Med Int Hlth* **7**(8): 678–684, 2002.
65. Gardosi J, Francis A. Controlled trial of fundal height measurement plotted on customised antenatal growth charts. *Br J Obstet Gynaecol* **106**(4):309–317, 1999.
66. Audibert F, Benchimol Y, Benattar C, Champagne C, Frydman R. Prediction of preeclampsia or intrauterine growth restriction by second trimester serum screening and uterine Doppler velocimetry. *Fetal Diagn Ther* **20**(1):48–53, 2005.
67. Goldstein I, Reece EA, Pilu G, Bovicelli L, Hobbins JC. Cerebellar measurements with ultrasonography in the evaluation of fetal growth and development. *Am J Obstet Gynecol* **156**(5):1065–1069, 1987.
68. Reece EA, Goldstein I, Pilu G, Hobbins JC. Fetal cerebellar growth unaffected by intrauterine growth retardation: a new parameter for prenatal diagnosis. *Am J Obstet Gynecol* **157**(3):632–638, 1987.
69. Hadlock FP, Deter RL, Harrist RB, Roecker E, Park SK. A date-independent predictor of intrauterine growth retardation: femur length/abdominal circumference ratio. *Am J Roentgenol* **141**(5):979–984, 1983.
70. Jahn A, Razum O, Berle P. Routine screening for intrauterine growth retardation in Germany: low sensitivity and questionable benefit for diagnosed cases. *Acta Obstet Gynecol Scand* **77**(6): 643–648, 1998.
71. Ott WJ. Diagnosis of intrauterine growth restriction: comparison of ultrasound parameters. *Am J Perinatol* **19**(3):133–137, 2002.

72. Dudley NJ. A systematic review of the ultrasound estimation of fetal weight. *Ultrasound Obstet Gynecol* **25**(1):80–89, 2005.
73. Hadlock FP, Harrist RB, Carpenter RJ, Deter RL, Park SK. Sonographic estimation of fetal weight. The value of femur length in addition to head and abdomen measurements. *Radiology* **150**(2):535–540, 1984.
74. Hadlock FP, Harrist RB, Sharman RS, Deter RL, Park SK. Estimation of fetal weight with the use of head, body, and femur measurements: a prospective study. *Am J Obstet Gynecol* **151**(3):333–337, 1985.
75. Predanic M, Cho A, Ingrid F, Pellettieri J. Ultrasonographic estimation of fetal weight: acquiring accuracy in residency. *J Ultrasound Med* **21**(5):495–500, 2002.
76. Platek DN, Divon MY, Anyaegbunam A, Merkatz IR. Intrapartum ultrasonographic estimates of fetal weight by the house staff. *Am J Obstet Gynecol* **165**(4. Part 1):842–845, 1991.
77. Shamley KT, Landon MB. Accuracy and modifying factors for ultrasonographic determination of fetal weight at term. *Obstet Gynecol* **84**(6):926–930, 1994.
78. Chuang L, Hwang JY, Chang CH, Yu CH, Chang FM. Ultrasound estimation of fetal weight with the use of computerized artificial neural network model. *Ultrasound Med Biol* **28**(8):991–996, 2002.
79. Hanretty KP, Faber BL. Ultrasonographic estimation of fetal weight during labour. *S Af Med J* **73**(3):181–182, 1988.
80. Jouannic JM, Grange G, Goffinet F, Benachi A, Carbrol D. Validity of sonographic formulas for estimating fetal weight below 1,250 g: a series of 119 cases. *Fetal Diagn Ther* **16**(4):254–258, 2001.
81. Gardosi J, Chang A, Kalyan B, Sahota D, Symonds EM. Customised antenatal growth charts. *Lancet* **339** (8788):283–287, 199.
82. Clausson B, Gardosi J, Francis A, Cnattingius S. Perinatal outcome in SGA births defined by customised versus population-based birthweight standards. *Br J Obstet Gynaecol* **108**(8): 830–834, 2001.
83. De Jong CL, Francis A, van Geijn HP, Gardosi J. Customized fetal weight limits for antenatal detection of fetal growth restriction. *Ultrasound Obstet Gynecol* **15**(1):36–40, 2000.
84. Gardosi J. Customized fetal growth standards: rationale and clinical application. *Semin Perinatol* **28**(1):33–40, 2004.
85. Schild RL, Sachs C, Fimmers R, Gembruch U, Hansmann M. Sex-specific fetal weight prediction by ultrasound. *Ultrasound Obstet Gynecol* **23**(1):30–35, 2004.
86. Hata T, Deter RL, Hill RM. Individual growth curve standards in triplets: prediction of third-trimester growth and birth characteristics. *Obstet Gynecol* **78**(3 Pt 1):379–384, 1991.
87. de Jong CL, Gardosi J, Dekker GA, Colenbrander GJ, van Geijn HP. Application of a customised birthweight standard in the assessment of perinatal outcome in a high risk population. *Br J Obstet Gynaecol* **105**(5):531–535, 1998.
88. Sanderson DA, Wilcox MA, Johnson IR. The individualised birthweight ratio: a new method of identifying intrauterine growth retardation. *Br J Obstet Gynaecol* **101**(4):310–314, 1994.
89. Sciscione AC, Gorman R, Callan NA. Adjustment of birth weight standards for maternal and infant characteristics improves the prediction of outcome in the small-for-gestational-age infant. *Am J Obstet Gynecol* **175**(3 Pt 1):544–547, 1996.
90. Mongelli M, Gardosi J. Reduction of false-positive diagnosis of fetal growth restriction by application of customized fetal growth standards. *Obstet Gynecol* **88**(5):844–848, 1996.
91. Schild RL, Fimmers R, Hansmann M. Fetal weight estimation by three-dimensional ultrasound. *Ultrasound Obstet Gynecol* **16**:445–452, 2000.
92. Campbell S, Thoms A. Ultrasound measurement of the fetal head to abdomen circumference ratio in the assessment of growth retardation. *Br J Obstet Gynaecol* **84**(3):165–174, 1977.
93. Villar J, de Onis M, Kestler E, Bolanos F, Cerezo R, Bernedes H. The differential neonatal morbidity of the intrauterine growth retardation syndrome. *Am J Obstet Gynecol* **163**(1 Pt 1):151–157, 1990.
94. Patterson RM, Pouliot MR. Neonatal morphometrics and perinatal outcome: who is growth retarded? *Am J Obstet Gynecol* **157**(3):691–693, 1987.
95. Lockwood CJ, Weiner S. Assessment of fetal growth. *Clin Perinatol* **13**(1):3–35, 1986.
96. Lin CC, Santolaya-Forgas J. Current concepts of fetal growth restriction: part I. Causes, classification, and pathophysiology. *Obstet Gynecol* **92**(6):1044–1055, 1998.
97. Phelan JP, Vernon Smith C, Broussard RN, Small M. Amniotic fluid volume assessment with the four-quadrant technique at 36-42 weeks gestation. *J Reprod Med* **32**(7):540–542, 1987.
98. Moore TR, Cayle JE. The amniotic fluid index in normal human pregnancy. *Am J Obstet Gynecol* **162**(5):1168–1173, 1990.
99. Nwosu EC, Welch CR, Walkinshaw S. Measurement of amniotic fluid volume using maximum pool depth. *Contemp Rev Obstet Gynaecol* **6**:25–30, 1994.
100. Gouarin S, Palmer P, Cointe D et al. Congenital HCMV infection: a collaborative and comparative study of virus detection in amniotic fluid by culture and by PCR. *J Clin Virol* **21**(1): 47–55, 2001.
101. Donner C, Liesnard C, Content J, Busine A, Aderca J, Rodesch F. Prenatal diagnosis of 52 pregnancies at risk for congenital cytomegalovirus infection. *Obstet Gynecol* **82**(4 Pt 1):481–486, 1993.
102. Lazzarotto T, Varani S, Gabrielli L, Spezzacatena P, Landini MP. New advances in the diagnosis of congenital cytomegalovirus infection. *Intervirology* **42**(5-6):390–397, 1999.
103. Albaiges G, Missfelder-Lobos H, Lees C, Parra M, Nicolaides KH. One-stage screening for pregnancy complications by color Doppler assessment of the uterine arteries at 23 weeks' gestation. *Obstet Gynecol* **96**(4):559–564, 2000.
104. Chien PF, Arnott N, Gordon A, Owen P, Khan KS. How useful is uterine artery Doppler flow velocimetry in the prediction of pre-eclampsia, intrauterine growth retardation and perinatal death? An overview. *Br J Obstet Gynaecol* **107**(2):196–208, 2000.
105. Bower S, Schuchter K, Campbell S. Doppler ultrasound screening as part of routine antenatal scanning: prediction of pre-eclampsia and intrauterine growth retardation. *Br J Obstet Gynaecol* **100**(11):989–994, 1993.
106. Campbell S, Pearce JM, Hackett G, Cohen-Overbeek T, Hernandez C. Qualitative assessment of uteroplacental blood flow: early screening test for high-risk pregnancies. *Obstet Gynecol* **68**(5):649–653, 1986.
107. Trudinger BJ, Giles WB, Cook CM. Uteroplacental blood flow velocity-time waveforms in normal and complicated pregnancy. *Br J Obstet Gynaecol* **92**(1): 39–45, 1985.
108. Schulman H, Ducey J, Farmakides G et al. Uterine artery Doppler velocimetry: the significance of divergent systolic/diastolic ratios. *Am J Obstet Gynecol* **157**(6):1539–1542, 1987.
109. Papageorghiou AT, Yu CK, Cicero S, Bower S, Nicolaides KH. Second-trimester uterine artery Doppler screening in unselected populations: a review. *J Matern Fetal Neonatal Med* **12**(2):78–88, 2002.
110. Baschat AA, Gembruch U, Reiss I, Gortner L, Weiner CP, Harman CR. Absent umbilical artery end-diastolic velocity in growth-restricted fetuses: a risk factor for neonatal thrombocytopenia. *Obstet Gynecol* **96**(2):162–166, 2000.
111. Baschat AA, Gembruch U, Reiss I, Gortner L, Weiner CP, Harman CR. Relationship between arterial and venous Doppler and perinatal outcome

in fetal growth restriction. *Ultrasound Obstet Gynecol* **16**(5):407–413, 2000.

112. Baschat AA, Weiner CP. Umbilical artery doppler screening for detection of the small fetus in need of antepartum surveillance. *Am J Obstet Gynecol* **182**(1 Pt 1):154–158, 2000.
113. Nicolaides KH, Bilardo CM, Soothill PW, Campbell S. Absence of end diastolic frequencies in umbilical artery: a sign of fetal hypoxia and acidosis. *Br Med J* **297**(6655):1026–1027, 1988.
114. Alfirevic Z, Neilson JP. Doppler ultrasonography in high-risk pregnancies: systematic review with meta-analysis. *Am J Obstet Gynecol* **172**(5):1379–1387, 1995.
115. Davies JA, Gallivan S, Spencer JA. Randomised controlled trial of Doppler ultrasound screening of placental perfusion during pregnancy. *Lancet* **340**(8831):1299–1303, 1992.
116. Kingdom JC, Burrell SJ, Kaufmann P. Pathology and clinical implications of abnormal umbilical artery Doppler waveforms. *Ultrasound Obstet Gynecol* **9**(4):271–286, 1997.
117. Kingdom JC, Rodeck CH, Kaufmann P. Umbilical artery Doppler – more harm than good? *Br J Obstet Gynaecol* **104**(4):393–396, 1997.
118. Hershkovitz R, Kingdom JC, Geary M, Rodeck CH. Fetal cerebral blood flow redistribution in late gestation: identification of compromise in small fetuses with normal umbilical artery Doppler. *Ultrasound Obstet Gynecol* **15**(3):209–212, 2000.
119. Severi FM, Bocchi C, Visentin A et al. Uterine and fetal cerebral Doppler predict the outcome of third-trimester small-for-gestational age fetuses with normal umbilical artery Doppler. *Ultrasound Obstet Gynecol* **19**(3):225–228, 2002.
120. Garner P, Gulmezoglu AM. Drugs for preventing malaria-related illness in pregnant women and death in the newborn. *Cochrane Database Syst Rev* **1**:CD000169, 2003.
121. Gulmezoglu AM, Hofmeyr GJ. Bed rest in hospital for suspected impaired fetal growth. *Cochrane Database Syst Rev* **2**:CD000034, 2000.
122. Say L, Gulmezoglu AM, Hofmeyr GJ. Maternal oxygen administration for suspected impaired fetal growth. *Cochrane Database Syst Rev* **1**:CD000137, 2003.
123. Harding JE, Owens JA, Robinson JS. Should we try to supplement the growth retarded fetus? A cautionary tale. *Br J Obstet Gynaecol* **99**(9):707–709, 1992.
124. Say L, Gulmezoglu AM, Hofmeyr GJ. Maternal nutrient supplementation for suspected impaired fetal growth. *Cochrane Database Syst Rev* **1**:CD000148, 2003.
125. Mahomed K. Iron and folate supplementation in pregnancy. *Cochrane Database Syst Rev* **2**:CD001135, 2000.
126. Gulmezoglu AM, Hofmeyr GJ. Betamimetics for suspected impaired fetal growth. *Cochrane Database Syst Rev* **4**:CD000036, 2001.
127. Gulmezoglu AM, Hofmeyr GJ. Calcium channel blockers for potential impaired fetal growth. *Cochrane Database Syst Rev* **2**:CD000049, 2000.
128. Leitich H, Egarter C, Husslein P, Kaider A, Schemper M. A meta-analysis of low dose aspirin for the prevention of intrauterine growth retardation. *Br J Obstet Gynaecol* **104**(4):450–459, 1997.
129. Kozer E, Costei AM, Boskovic R, Nulman I, Nikfar S, Koren G. Effects of aspirin consumption during pregnancy on pregnancy outcomes: meta-analysis. *Birth Defects Res B Dev Reprod Toxicol* **68**(1):70–84, 2003.
130. Mongelli M, Ek S, Tambyrajia R. Screening for fetal growth restriction: a mathematical model of the effect of time interval and ultrasound error. *Obstet Gynecol* **92**(6):908–912, 1998.
131. Chauhan SP, Doherty DD, Magann EF, Cahanding F, Moreno F, Klausen JH. Amniotic fluid index vs single deepest pocket technique during modified biophysical profile: a randomized clinical trial. *Am J Obstet Gynecol* **191**(2):661–667, 2004.
132. Chauhan SP, Sanderson M, Hendrix NW, Magann EF, Devoe LD. Perinatal outcome and amniotic fluid index in the antepartum and intrapartum periods: a meta-analysis. *Am J Obstet Gynecol* **181**(6):1473–1478, 1999.
133. Maulik D. Management of fetal growth restriction: an evidence-based approach. *Clin Obstet Gynecol* **49**(2):320–334, 2006.
134. Pattison N, McCowan L. Cardiotocography for antepartum fetal assessment. *Cochrane Database Syst Rev* **2**:CD001068, 2000.
135. Bekedam DJ, Visser GH, van der Zee AG, Snijders RJ, Poelmann-Weesjes G. Abnormal velocity waveforms of the umbilical artery in growth retarded fetuses: relationship to antepartum late heart rate decelerations and outcome. *Early Hum Dev* **24**(1):79–89, 1990.
136. Manning FA, Morrison I, Harman CR, Lange IR, Menticoglou S. Fetal assessment based on fetal biophysical profile scoring: experience in 19,221 referred high-risk pregnancies. II. An analysis of false-negative fetal deaths. *Am J Obstet Gynecol* **157**(4 Pt 1):880–884, 1987.
137. Alfirevic Z, Neilson JP. Biophysical profile for fetal assessment in high risk pregnancies. *Cochrane Database Syst Rev* **2**:CD000038, 2000.
138. Baschat AA. Integrated fetal testing in growth restriction: combining multivessel Doppler and biophysical parameters. *Ultrasound Obstet Gynecol* **21**(1):1–8, 2003.
139. Nicolini U, Nicolaides P, Fisk NM et al. Limited role of fetal blood sampling in prediction of outcome in intrauterine growth retardation. *Lancet* **336**:768–772, 1990.
140. Neilson JP, Alfirevic Z. Doppler ultrasound for fetal assessment in high risk pregnancies. *Cochrane Database Syst Rev* **2**:CD000073, 2000.
141. Bricker L, Neilson JP. Routine doppler ultrasound in pregnancy. *Cochrane Database Syst Rev* **2**:CD001450, 2000.
142. Karsdorp VH, van Vugt JM, van Geijn HP et al. Clinical significance of absent or reversed end diastolic velocity waveforms in umbilical artery. *Lancet* **344**(8938):1664–1668, 1994.
143. Hecher K, Bilardo CM, Stigter RH et al. Monitoring of fetuses with intrauterine growth restriction: a longitudinal study. *Ultrasound Obstet Gynecol* **18**(6):564–570, 2001.
144. Bilardo CM, Wolf H, Stigter RH et al. Relationship between monitoring parameters and perinatal outcome in severe, early intrauterine growth restriction. *Ultrasound Obstet Gynecol* **23**(2):119–125, 2004.
145. When do obstetricians recommend delivery for a high-risk preterm growth-retarded fetus? The GRIT Study Group. Growth Restriction Intervention Trial. *Eur J Obstet Gynecol Reprod Biol* **67**(2):121–126, 1996.
146. Romero R, Kalache KD, Kadar N. Timing the delivery of the preterm severely growth-restricted fetus: venous Doppler, cardiotocography or the biophysical profile? *Ultrasound Obstet Gynecol* **19**(2):118–121, 2002.
147. Arduini D, Rizzo G, Romanini C. The development of abnormal heart rate patterns after absent end-diastolic velocity in umbilical artery: analysis of risk factors. *Am J Obstet Gynecol* **168**(1 Pt 1):43–50, 1993.
148. Forouzan I. Absence of end-diastolic flow velocity in the umbilical artery: a review. *Obstet Gynecol Surv* **50**(3): 219–227, 1995.
149. Royal College of Obstetricians and Gynaecologists. *The investigation and management of the small for gestational age fetus. Guideline no.13.* London: RCOG, 2002.
150. Maternal and child health consortium. *CESDI 8th annual report: Confidential enquiry of stillbirths and deaths in infancy,* 2001.
151. Vyas S, Nicolaides KH, Bower S, Campbell S. Middle cerebral artery flow velocity waveforms in fetal hypoxaemia. *Br J Obstet Gynaecol* **97**(9):797–803, 1990.

152. Soothill PW, Bobrow CS, Holmes R. Small for gestational age is not a diagnosis. *Ultrasound Obstet Gynecol* **13**(4):225–228, 1999.
153. The Growth Restriction Intervention Trial (GRIT). A randomised trial of timed delivery for the compromised preterm fetus: short term outcomes and Bayesian interpretation. *Br J Obstet Gynaecol*, 110(1): 27–32,2003.
154. Baschat AA, Cosmi E, Bilardo CM et al. Predictors of neonatal outcome in early-onset placental dysfunction. *Obstet Gynecol* **109**(2 Pt 1):253–261, 2007.
155. Lees C, Baumgartner H. The TRUFFLE study – a collaborative publicly funded project from concept to reality: how to negotiate an ethical, administrative and funding obstacle course in the European Union. *Ultrasound Obstet Gynecol* **25**(2):105–107, 2005.
156. Royal College of Obstetricians and Gynaecologists. *Antenatal corticosteroid to prevent respiratory distress syndrome. Guideline no. 7*. London: RCOG, 1999.
157. Williams KP, Farquharson DF, Bebbington M et al. Screening for fetal well-being in a high-risk pregnant population comparing the nonstress test with umbilical artery Doppler velocimetry: a randomized controlled clinical trial. *Am J Obstet Gynecol* **188**(5):1366–1371, 2003.
158. Grant A, Glazener CM. Elective caesarean section versus expectant management for delivery of the small baby. *Cochrane Database Syst Rev* **2**:CD000078, 2001.
159. Thacker SB, Stroup D, Chang M. Continuous electronic heart rate monitoring for fetal assessment during labor. *Cochrane Database Syst Rev* **2**:CD000063, 2001.
160. Hornbuckle J, Vail A, Abrams KR, Thornton JG. Bayesian interpretation of trials: the example of intrapartum electronic fetal heart rate monitoring. *Br J Obstet Gynaecol* **107**(1):3–10, 2000.
161. Yu VY, Upadhyay A. Neonatal management of the growth-restricted infant. *Semin Fetal Neonatal Med* **9**(5): 403–409, 2004.
162. Piper JM, Xenakis EM, McFarland M, Elliott BD, Berkus MD, Langer O. Do growth-retarded premature infants have different rates of perinatal morbidity and mortality than appropriately grown premature infants? *Obstet Gynecol* **87**(2):169–174, 1996.
163. Clausson B, Cnattingius S, Axelsson O. Outcomes of post-term births: the role of fetal growth restriction and malformations. *Obstet Gynecol* **94**(5 Pt 1):758–762, 1999.
164. Blair E, Stanley F. Intrauterine growth and spastic cerebral palsy. I. Association with birth weight for gestational age. *Am J Obstet Gynecol* **162**(1):229–237, 1990.
165. Drummond PM, Colver AF. Analysis by gestational age of cerebral palsy in singleton births in north-east England 1970-94. *Paediatr Perinat Epidemiol* **16**(2):172–180, 2002.
166. Strauss RS, Dietz WH. Growth and development of term children born with low birth weight: effects of genetic and environmental factors. *J Pediatr* **133**(1):67–72, 1998.
167. Ozanne SE, Fernandez-Twinn D, Hales CN. Fetal growth and adult diseases. *Semin Perinatol* **28**(1):81–87, 2004.

CHAPTER

40

Red cell alloimmunization

Charles H Rodeck and Anne Deans

This chapter is dedicated to the memory of Dr. Umbrento Nicoline who would have been a co-author

KEY POINTS

- Prevention of RhD alloimmunization is crucial and is highly effective if anti-D immunoglobulin is administered to RhD negative women (without antibodies) both antenatally and postnatally
- The fetus can be RhD genotyped with a high degree of reliability by PCR-based techniques analyzing cell-free fetal DNA in maternal plasma
- Invasive monitoring of fetal anemia has been supplanted by non-invasive measurement by Doppler ultrasound of the peak systolic velocity in the fetal middle cerebral artery
- Intravascular transfusion (IVT) is highly effective treatment for severe cases and, in skilled hands, achieves a 90% healthy survival rate
- Circumstantial evidence suggests that intrahepatic umbilical vein puncture is safer than cord puncture for IVT and that intraperitoneal transfusion is easier and less risky than either route for IVT

INTRODUCTION

Over the last 35 years, the incidence of severe hemolytic disease of the fetus and newborn (HDFN) caused by red cell alloimmunization has dramatically fallen due to the widespread use of prophylactic anti-D immunoglobulin. In 1971, when anti-D immunoglobulin became generally available in the UK to be given to all unsensitized rhesus Rh(D)-negative women after termination of pregnancy or delivery of a rhesus-positive baby, the stillbirth and neonatal death rate attributable to Rh(D) alloimmunization was around 120 per 100 000 births[1]. By 1992, this figure had fallen to 1.3 per 100 000 births[2]. Despite such successes, around 600–700 new Rh(D) immunizations continue to occur each year in the UK[3]. Reasons for failure of immunoprophylaxis include the administration of an insufficient dose of anti-D and failure to give anti-D after potentially sensitizing events. Immunization occurring in the last few weeks of uncomplicated pregnancy is now the single commonest identifiable cause suggesting that antenatal prophylaxis of all Rh(D)-negative women will reduce the maternal immunization rate still further[4]. In North America, where such policy is routinely employed, there has been a more dramatic decline in the number of sensitized Rh(D)-negative women[5]. While Rh(D) alloimmunization remains the most prevalent, there are also a small number of women who develop antibodies to other Rhesus antigens or to atypical antigens, such as Kell (K), Duffy (Fy^a) and Kidd (Jk^a, Jk^b). Fetal and newborn deaths attributable to hemolytic disease due to these antibodies have remained stable at around six cases per year in the UK[2].

The reduction in perinatal deaths due to HDFN has also occurred as a result of the great advances made in neonatal care and in the management of the affected fetus over the last few years. The introduction of high-resolution real-time ultrasound and the development of intravascular fetal blood transfusion, in combination with increasing knowledge of the pathophysiology of the disease process, has meant that, even in severely alloimmunized women, the prognosis can be optimistic.

HISTORY

In 1941, Levine et al. demonstrated that maternal Rh antibodies were responsible for causing erythroblastosis fetalis, a condition characterized by hydrops fetalis, icterus gravis and severe anemia of the newborn[6]. Such ominous features had been recognized for centuries but had only been attributed to a single disease process, together with hepatosplenomegaly and erythroblastosis (increased nucleated red blood cell count), when described in the medical literature in 1932[7]. Soon after this, exchange transfusion was shown to improve the prognosis for affected neonates[8]. It was also discovered that early delivery improved perinatal survival and work by Bevis showed that the severity of the fetal hemolytic disease could be predicted by serial amniocentesis[9]. A major therapeutic breakthrough though came in 1963 when

Liley successfully performed the first intraperitoneal blood transfusions in severely affected fetuses in utero using adult red blood cells[10]. At about the same time, several attempts were made at intravascular transfusion but this required hysterotomy and the fetal and maternal risks were deemed too high. Twenty years later, Rodeck et al. reported a percutaneous technique for intravascular fetal blood transfusion (IVT) using fetoscopy[11]. Refinements of these techniques remain the basis for successful treatment of the severely affected fetus today. Fortunately, most Rh(D)-negative women will never require such intervention due to the work of Clarke's group which led to the development of anti-D immunoglobulin in 1961[12].

MECHANISM OF RED CELL ALLOIMMUNIZATION

Pathophysiology

Red cell membranes contain numerous surface antigens including those of the ABO and Rhesus groups. Maternal IgG red cell antibodies can be raised against most of the blood group specificities following exposure to an adequate quantity of foreign red blood cell antigen, either as a result of transplacental hemorrhage from the fetus to the mother or after heterologous blood transfusion. It has been demonstrated using Kleihauer testing that around 75% of women have fetal red cells in their circulation at some time during pregnancy and delivery, although the number of fetal red cells varies considerably depending on gestation[13]. Anti-A,B antibodies in group O women are the commonest antibodies found in the UK but are very rarely seen to cause significant problems for the fetus or require intrauterine transfusion. For practical purposes anti-Rh(D), anti-c, anti-E and anti-Kell should be considered as the antibodies likely to have the potential to cause moderate to severe HDFN[14]. Other antibodies such as anti-Fy^a (Duffy) and Kidd (Jk^a, Jk^b) rarely cause significant problems.

Initial exposure to foreign red blood cell antigen leads to a weak primary immune response in the mother whereby predominantly IgM is produced after a latent period of some weeks. Since IgM cannot cross the placenta, the fetus is unaffected, although the presence of these antibodies can be detected in maternal blood for up to a year after the primary event, thus indicating maternal sensitization. On subsequent exposure of the mother to similar antigenic red cells (usually in a subsequent pregnancy), her previously primed memory B cells act swiftly to produce IgG antibody. Considerably less antigenic stimulus is required for this secondary response compared to the first exposure and results in much higher antibody titers being produced. Maternal IgG antibodies are actively transported across the placenta via receptors to the Ig Fc portion located on the synctiotrophoblast. IgG immunoglobulin directed against a red cell antigen will bind to fetal red cells that express that antigen, so causing their sequestration. Red cell destruction appears to be mediated by subclasses IgG1 and IgG3 only[15]. IgG-sensitized red cells bind, via the Fc part of the antibody molecule, to Fcγ receptors (FcγR) on mononuclear phagocytes in the fetal reticuloendothelial system so triggering erythrocyte destruction by phagocytosis and/or cytolysis[16]. Three distinct classes of Fcγ receptor have been identified[17]. Recent work shows that, in the fetus, high affinity FcγR1 plays a major role in the IgG anti-D-mediated attachment to, and phagocytosis by, circulating monocytes and splenic mononuclear phagocytes[15]. The latter cells also have high expression of FcγR111 which is primarily involved in target ingestion. Monoclonal antibody to FcγR1 will almost completely inhibit the effector function of fetal or newborn monocytes and markedly reduce that of fetal splenic mononuclear phagocytes in vitro. It is possible that this could be the basis for a new therapeutic intervention for HDFN.

FcγR-mediated phagocytosis by monocytes and macrophages appears to be well developed by the early second trimester, i.e. some time before the onset of even the most severe Rh(D) hemolytic disease at 17–18 weeks[15]. Although placental transfer of maternal IgG has been shown to occur as early as 6–10 weeks' gestation, it is not until later in the second trimester that significant amounts are found in the fetal circulation[18,19]. Before this gestation, there is insufficient maternal anti-D transfer to cause severe fetal red cell hemolysis. By the end of pregnancy, a significantly higher concentration of IgG1 has accumulated in the fetus compared to that found in maternal blood while levels of the other IgG subclasses are similar in both mother and fetus[20]. Sensitized mothers carrying an Rh(D)-positive anemic fetus demonstrate higher maternal levels of IgG1 compared to control pregnancies. In addition, there appears to be a preferential accumulation of IgG1 in those fetuses affected by the hemolytic process along with significantly lower levels of fetal IgG3 than are found in fetuses not at risk of HDFN. When measuring antibody levels in maternal serum for the purpose of predicting the severity of fetal hemolytic disease, the results are not normally corrected to allow for this discrepancy in IgG1 and IgG3 levels between mother and fetus. Furthermore, recent work suggests that the quantitative composition of IgG1 and IgG3 in the maternal serum, as determined by flow cytometry or enzyme-linked immunosorbent assay (ELISA), is important in determining the severity of hemolysis in the fetus[21,22]. Although the IgG3 subclass has a higher potential for inducing phagocytosis and monocyte adherence in vitro, IgG1 has a greater influence on the severity of HDFN in vivo than IgG3. Some laboratory anti-D assays currently in use display higher functional activities with IgG1 + IgG3 Rh(D) antibodies than with purely IgG1 antibodies and may fail to predict severe HDFN where serum antibodies comprise mainly of IgG1 antibodies[23].

Without a program of anti-D prophylaxis, approximately 1% of Rh(D)-negative women will have detectable anti-D in their serum by the end of their first pregnancy with an Rh(D)-positive baby. A further 7–9% of these women will have detectable antibodies 6 months following delivery of that pregnancy and roughly the same number again will develop antibodies during a second pregnancy carrying an Rh(D)-positive fetus; thus around 17% Rh(D)-negative women are immunized by a single Rh(D)-positive pregnancy[24]. ABO incompatibility between the mother and fetus offers a protective effect against alloimmunization because fetal cells entering the maternal circulation are quickly destroyed by maternal ABO antibodies before the Rh(D) antigen can be recognized by the maternal immune system. This reduces the chances of maternal sensitization by around 20%[25]. The risk of Rh(D) alloimmunization during pregnancy increases with advancing gestation because of the increasing incidence of fetomaternal transplacental hemorrhage (TPH) and the likelihood that larger amounts of incompatible red cells will enter the maternal circulation. Using the Kleihauer acid elution technique, it has been shown that, during the first trimester, TPH is rare (3% of pregnancies) and involves only 0.03 ml of fetal blood whereas, in the third trimester, the frequency is as high as 45% of pregnancies with amounts as great as 25 ml recorded[13]. It is important to note that, whereas miscarriage in the first trimester carries a risk of sensitization of less than 1%, surgical termination is associated with a much higher risk in the order of 20–25%. Bleeding in pregnancy, abdominal trauma, fetal blood sampling (FBS), amniocentesis, external cephalic version and chorionic villus sampling (CVS) should be regarded as potentially high-risk situations. Amniocentesis is associated with a 2% risk of maternal sensitization even when performed under ultrasound guidance[26]. CVS carries a higher risk than amniocentesis, possibly as high as 50%, although the amount of fetomaternal hemorrhage that is associated with the procedure is dependent on the operator and technique used[27,28].

Being Rh(D) negative does not mean that the formation of maternal anti-Rh(D) antibodies and subsequent Rh(D) HDFN is inevitable in the event of prophylaxis being unavailable. Some Rh(D)-negative women are poor responders to the Rh(D) antigen while others may produce anti-Rh(D) that has a low potency or poor efficacy at mediating Fc receptor interaction with phagocytic cells. In addition, there is the protective effect of ABO incompatibility and the fact that some women will have partners who are heterozygous for Rh(D) so may deliver Rh(D)-negative babies. When maternal sensitization with anti-RH(D) does occur, it is estimated that around 50% of affected infants will have mild or no anemia, 25–30% of fetuses will have a moderate anemia which will require treatment in the neonatal period, while the remaining 20–25% will develop hydrops, likely to lead to intrauterine death or neonatal death, unless antenatal fetal therapy is undertaken[29].

Hydrops fetalis

Ascites, pericardial and pleural effusions, subcutaneous edema and placentomegaly are the classical sonographic features of hydrops, although the precise mechanism behind their development remains speculative. The affected fetus becomes progressively anemic due to red cell hemolysis and compensates with cardiovascular adjustments and by increasing erythropoiesis. Initially, cardiac output rather than heart rate is increased to maintain tissue oxygenation as a consequence of the fall in peripheral resistance secondary to vasodilatation and decreased blood viscosity[30]. Evidence to support this comes from Doppler blood flow – velocity measurements of the umbilical vein and fetal descending aorta which correlate inversely with the degree of fetal anemia[31,32]. A similar relationship is found between mean blood flow velocities in the middle cerebral artery and fetal hemoglobin (as measured at FBS) which appears to hold true irrespective of the pulsatility index value (PI) or whether there is fetal hypoxemia suggesting that the hyperdynamic circulation is partly as a consequence of decreased blood viscosity[33].

In response to mild or moderate degrees of anemia (fetal hemoglobin deficit of 2–7 g/dl for gestational age), intramedullary hematopoiesis is stimulated through increased erythropoietin production; analysis of fetal blood at this stage reveals an increased fetal reticulocyte count, in the absence of erythroblastosis[34]. Excessive and prolonged hemolysis results in marked erythroid hyperplasia of the bone marrow. As severe anemia develops (hemoglobin deficit >7 g/dl), large areas of extramedullary hematopoiesis are recruited in the liver which is characterized by an erythroblastosis or increased nucleated red blood cell count in fetal blood[35]. Pronounced leukocytosis may be present as a result of increased activity of the reticuloendothelial system. Fetal thrombocytopenia can occur, although levels less

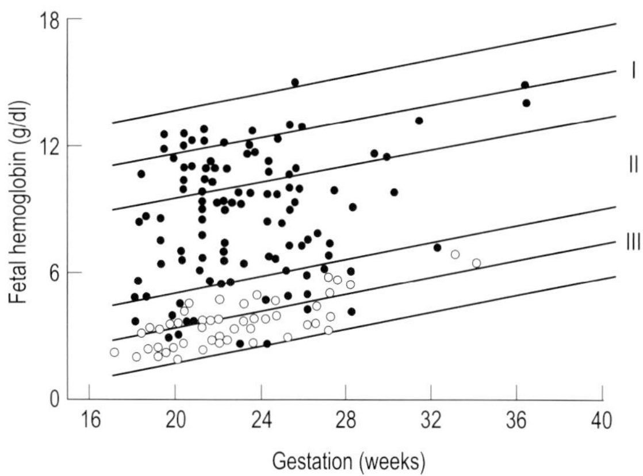

Fig. 40.1 Fetal hemoglobin concentration in Rh-alloimmunized pregnancies with (o) and without (•) fetal hydrops plotted on the normal range: mean and 95% data intervals (from Nicolaides et al.[37] with permission).

than 80 × 10^9 are rare. Occasionally, in a severely hydropic fetus, widespread hemopoietic failure is indicated by a leukopenia and absence of a reticulocytosis or erythroblastosis[36].

Fetal hemoglobin concentration rises with gestational age and hydrops tends to occur at higher hemoglobin levels at later gestations compared to early on in pregnancy (Fig. 40.1)[37]. It is therefore more appropriate to relate severity of fetal disease to the hemoglobin deficit for gestational age rather than to the actual fetal hemoglobin or hematocrit value. The presence of hydrops indicates a fetal hemoglobin deficit ≥7 g/dl which, in the second trimester, means a hematocrit of under 15% or hemoglobin of 4 g/dl or less[34,38]. However, even at these levels, the fetus may not become hydropic. There are several possible explanations for the genesis of hydrops at this degree of anemia including cardiac failure due to myocardial hypoxia, increased capillary permeability caused by chronic tissue hypoxia and decreased colloid oncotic pressure due to hypoproteinemia secondary to liver dysfunction.

It has been suggested that hydrops is secondary to hypoproteinemia caused by disruption of protein synthesis as the liver parenchyma becomes extensively infiltrated by erthyropoietic tissue. This now seems doubtful because, although hypoproteinemia and hypoalbuminemia are found in hydropic fetuses (total protein concentration <3 g/dl, albumin <2 g/dl) together with liver enlargement and significantly elevated liver transaminases, when compared to controls such findings are not unique to the hydropic state and can also be present in severely anemic but non-hydropic fetuses[39–41]. Nicolini et al. have reported that in both hydropic and non-hydropic fetuses aspartate transaminase levels correlate with the erythroblast count indicating liver dysfunction to be a direct result of the fetal anemia rather than a consequence of hydrops[41]. Correction of anemia by transfusion causes fetal transaminases to revert to normal. After the first intrauterine transfusion, rises in fetal γ-glutamyl transpeptidase can be demonstrated to correlate directly with the amount of blood transfused[41]. This appears to be more marked in hydropic fetuses and may indicate portal hypertension following the transfusion of a large blood volume. An alternative hypothesis is that the enlarged erythropoietic tissue causes a mechanical compression of the portal and umbilical veins altering substrate uptake and rate of synthesis[42]. Portal or umbilical hypertension with intrahepatic venous stasis secondary to such compression seems unlikely, though, in view of the hyperdynamic circulation demonstrated by Doppler ultrasound.

The fetus is able to tolerate mild-to-moderate anemia by increasing blood flow to the tissues. However, with progressive anemia, oxygen delivery to the tissues falls and, at a critical level, there is redistribution of blood flow to vital organs such as the brain and heart. Severe anemia causes tissue hypoxia and fetal hemoglobin levels correlate significantly with umbilical artery blood acid–base values[43]. Since hemoglobin is the principal buffer in fetal blood, at a critical level, a metabolic acidemia and hyperlactic acidemia occurs. Soothill et al. have demonstrated that when the fetal hemoglobin drops below 8 g/dl umbilical artery lactate concentrations increase, although umbilical vein hyperlactatemia is not evident until hemoglobin levels of 4 g/dl or under are reached[35]. At this point, placental capacity for lactate clearance appears to be saturated so leading to fetal metabolic acidosis. In this environment, it seems reasonable to postulate that myocardial dysfunction occurs and leads to congestive cardiac failure and fluid retention in a manner similar to myocardial ischemia in the adult.

Hypervolemia related to a high-output cardiac failure has also been put forward as a reason for extravasation of fluids into the tissues. Very high levels of atrial natriuretic factor are found in association with immune hydrops implying an expanded intravascular volume[44]. Increased amniotic fluid volume is a recognized finding preceding the onset of hydrops which raises the possibility that the normoxemic severely anemic fetus is able to compensate by increasing urine production. However, estimations of fetoplacental blood volume before the first intrauterine blood transfusion in both hydropic and non-hydropic fetuses have failed to show any significant difference between the two groups[45]. A more credible theory is that hypoxia and its arterial vasoactive response leads to myocardial insufficiency and relative cardiac failure. Weiner et al. have reported elevated umbilical venous pressure (assumed to be an approximation of fetal central venous pressure) in two fetuses with immune hydrops immediately prior to first intrauterine transfusion while, in the same study, all anemic non-hydropic fetuses had pressure values within the normal range[46]. These elevated levels rapidly corrected within 24 hours of intrauterine transfusion, although the hydrops took longer to resolve. This would support the suggestion that correction of hypoxia by infusion of blood increases the oxygen-carrying capacity of the blood so improving myocardial function. Further evidence comes from pulsed Doppler measurement of ductus venosus blood flow before fetal transfusion which indicates that cardiac preload is increased in severely anemic fetuses, possibly reflecting imminent congestive cardiac failure[47]. Hypoxia may affect not only the cardiac efficiency but also capillary endothelial cells, increasing their permeability to water and colloids.

Genetics

The Rh blood group antigens are carried by a series of at least three very similar but distinct transmembrane proteins scattered across the red cell surface[48]. Two Rhesus antigens have immunologically distinguishable isoforms Cc and Ee, but there is no evidence of an isoform d for the major antigen D. The Rhesus gene locus is located on chromosome 1p34–p36[49]. It consists of two closely linked, highly homologous (96% identical) genes, each 10 exons in length[50]. One gene is designated RHCE

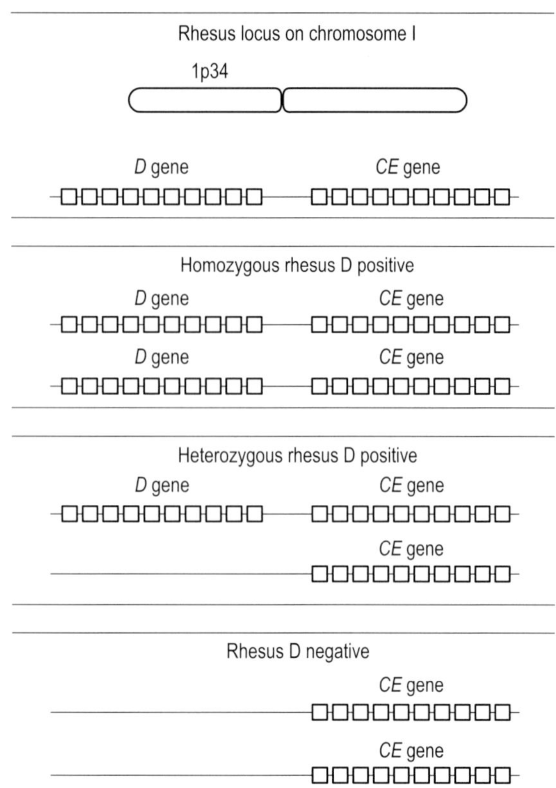

Fig. 40.2 RhD gene locus on chromosome 1

encoding both the Cc and Ee proteins by alternate splicing of a primary transcript, and a second gene, RHD, encodes the major antigen RHD (Fig. 40.2). An individual may be homozygous or heterozygous for Cc,Dd and Ee inheriting one set from each parent with d indicating an absence of the RHD gene. Being serologically Rh(D) negative means the absence of the major D antigen on the red cell surface, either as a result of homozygous absence of Rh(D) gene or partial deletion of exons 7 to 9 or a stop codon exon 5 of the RHD gene[51]. There are as many as 40 other Rh antigens but the RHD epitope is the most immunogenic of the Rh system, followed by Rhc which is more than 20-fold less potent. The use of 'Rhesus negative' or 'Rhesus positive' is best abandoned in favor of the more accurate and precise terms of Rh(D) negative and Rh(D) positive. A few individuals have an abnormality of the D antigen and are termed D^u positive. In some cases, part of the D antigen is missing and these women could form anti-D if exposed to a normal D antigen[52]. There is increasing evidence that they should receive anti-D immunoglobulin in appropriate circumstances[4].

Around 15% of the white Caucasian population are Rh(D) negative, apart from the Basque population where the incidence is as high as 30% giving rise to the hypothesis that the mutation originated there. In the Afro-Caribbean black population, the incidence is around 7–8% and drops to less than 1% in Chinese and Japanese peoples; 56% of Rh(D)-positive whites are heterozygous for the Rh(D) antigen and thus have a 50% chance of an Rh(D)-positive offspring from a partnership with an Rh(D)-negative woman.

The fetal genotype in respect to Rh(D) status was initially determined using a polymerase chain reaction (PCR) method on small amounts of fetal DNA in amniotic fluid and chorionic villus cells[53,54]. However, differences between serological and DNA primer Rh(D) typing also arise because of variations in the structure of the RHD gene. There are examples of individuals who are serologically Rh(D) negative but, because they have retained exon 10 of an internally deleted RHD gene, are typed as Rh(D) positive by PCR, while other individuals are serologically Rh(D) positive but, because they have a partial deletion of the RHD gene or substitution of Cc,Ee sequences into RHD gene exons, they are typed as Rh(D) negative by PCR[51]. Because of the far-reaching implications of incorrect prenatal Rh(D) testing, most groups now use two independent primer sets, designed from different parts of the RHCE and D genes, for instance using one set of primers specific for exons 4 and 5 and another specific for exon 10 of the RHD gene[55].

The DNA amplification technique has several advantages over serological fetal RHD typing which was carried out on erythrocytes obtained by fetal blood sampling (FBS) or chorionic villus sampling (CVS)[56]. It can be performed on amniotic fluid, thus potentially reducing the fetal loss rate associated with FBS and CVS. Amniocentesis carries a lower risk of feto-maternal hemorrhage so there is less likelihood of the test causing an increase in maternal antibody levels and thus worsening fetal anemia[57].

The isolation of fetal cells from the cervix using techniques such as mucus aspiration, endocervical lavage and cytobrush has meant that it may be possible to determine fetal RhD type by this less invasive method in the future[58]. Adinolfi et al. have shown that fetal RHD sequences can be detected in this manner but with insufficient reliability at present to be used in clinical practice[59]. It is now also theoretically possible to offer in vitro fertilization with pre-implantation determination of embryonic Rh(D) type so that only Rh(D)-negative embryos are transferred.

Cell-free fetal DNA (cff DNA) in maternal blood

Fetal DNA was found in maternal blood from as early as 7 weeks in an IVF population[60]. Moreover, cell-free fetal DNA is also seen in maternal plasma from about 7 weeks' gestation[61]. It represents about 3% of total (maternal and fetal) DNA in maternal plasma in early pregnancy, rising to about 6% in late gestation[62–64] (see Chapter 21).

Rh genotyping using this material has become a clinical service in the UK since 2001[65] using real-time PCR to detect the presence of the RHD gene. Out of 359 cases, the International Blood Group Reference Laboratory in Bristol, UK, was able to report results in 347 cases with a near 100% accuracy[66]. High test accuracies have also been reported in France and the Netherlands[67,68]. In a meta-analysis of 37 studies, 16 reported 100% accuracy[69]. A total of 3261 samples were analyzed, 783 of which were alloimmunized. The overall test accuracy was 91.4% and 92% in the alloimmunized samples. In the first trimester, it was 91% but, in the second and third trimesters, 85%. The sensitivity, specificity, PPV and NPV for all studies were 95%, 98%, 99% and 92% respectively.

However, false positive cases do occur usually in people of black African origin. Most whites who are RhD negative have a deletion of the RhD gene. On the other hand, only 18% of RhD negative black Africans have this deletion. Mostly they have one of two variants, the RHD psuedogene (67%) or the RHD-CE-D hybrid gene (15%)[70,71]. These variants are non-functional and behave as RhD negative, although they may test positive on PCR. To overcome this problem, Finning et al.[66] developed a PCR method to amplify certain parts of the RHD gene, thus differentiating it from the pseudo or hybrid genes.

False negative results are due to either a lack of fetal DNA in the maternal circulation (e.g. sampling too early in gestation) or to insufficient sensitivity of the method to detect low amounts of fetal DNA against the background of maternal DNA. In most studies, the SRY gene was used as Y-chromosome-specific marker. Targetting DYS 14 instead of SRY improves the limit of detection 10-fold[72]. These methods, although highly effective in detecting male cff DNA, are obviously not suitable for female fetuses. For females, gender independent markers are necessary. Van der Schoot used a panel of bi-allelic insertion-deletion polymorphisms to detect fetal derived paternally inherited markets[73]. This method, however, is complex and single-allelic base-extension reaction followed by mass spectrometry has also been described[74]. The use of epigenetic markers for feto-maternal DNA differentiation is also promising[75].

This non-invasive approach to fetal RhD genotyping is a major advance. It needs to be centralized in highly experienced laboratories to attain the necessary level of accuracy and to cope with false positives and negatives. In alloimmunized pregnancies it has already proven to be clinically useful – a maternal blood test at 8 or 9 weeks can prevent invasive procedures and multiple follow-up appointments if the fetus is RHD negative. Applying it to all Rh negative women and giving anti-D only to those with RHD negative fetuses may be cost effective[70], but antenatal care routines will have to be changed. Research into these aspects is currently being carried out.

MONITORING A PREGNANCY AT RISK

Routine antenatal management for all women should include first-trimester determination of their ABO blood group and Rhesus status together with a red cell antibody screen. For those women who are Rh(D) positive, it is reasonable to repeat the antibody screen at the beginning of the third trimester to detect red cell antibodies other than anti-Rh(D) that may have developed during the course of the pregnancy. In the UK, it is standard practice to repeat the antibody screen at 28 and 34 weeks' gestation for Rh(D)-negative women who have no relevant previous history and no evidence of sensitization at booking. Nearly a third of women who subsequently have evidence of Rh alloimmunization in a pregnancy do not demonstrate antibodies on initial testing of their blood[76]. Repeated testing is therefore important, although antibodies detected early on are more likely to cause severe fetal disease. Paternal blood group testing and the reduction of maternal surveillance should the partner prove to be Rh(D) negative, is useful as long as there are no doubts regarding paternity.

Once a woman is known to be alloimmunized, several factors can be used to predict the course of the disease. The management of red cell alloimmunization is similar regardless of the inciting antigen, with the exception of Kell which will be discussed later but, for the sake of clarity, we will refer to Rh(D) immunization here.

Previous obstetric history

In the first sensitized pregnancy, the risk of fetal disease is very low with significant fetal anemia and hydrops being unlikely to occur. With subsequent pregnancies, the severity of the fetal disease often becomes progressively worse with onset of fetal anemia at an earlier gestational age. Fetal death or hydrops due to alloimmunization before 18 weeks is exceptionally rare. If hydrops or fetal death has occurred in one pregnancy, then it is likely to occur in subsequent pregnancies carrying an Rh-incompatible fetus if treatment is not undertaken.

Antibody levels

Serial measurement of maternal serum red cell antibody levels has traditionally been an important part of monitoring because of the well-established association between maternal antibody concentration and outcome of pregnancy. Routine antibody testing is by the indirect Coombs' method. This technique involves incubating the patient's serum with red blood cells carrying the antigen against which the patient's antibodies are thought to be directed. Antihuman antiglobulin is then added, which causes agglutination of the red cells if they have absorbed the patient's antibodies. The antibody titer is expressed as a reciprocal of the highest dilution of serum that causes agglutination. Many laboratories now use an automated system that quantifies the concentration of anti-Rh(D). Although this is less subjective and related to an international standard, the most reproducible results are best obtained by testing all samples from one individual in the same laboratory.

Unfortunately, antibody levels do not always correlate well with the severity of fetal disease, probably reflecting the fact that the quality of the antibodies, i.e. the IgG subclass, and number of IgG-bound molecules is important. The trend, e.g. a sudden rise in antibodies, is more significant than the absolute value, especially in more severely affected pregnancies where antibody titers do not distinguish between hydropic and non-hydropic fetuses. However, for those women in their first affected pregnancy, or with only a previous mildly affected pregnancy, maternal hemolytic antibody levels are reasonably reliable and should be measured at 2–4-weekly intervals. MacKenzie et al. have reported from a series of more than 1200 Rh(D) sensitized pregnancies[77]. They demonstrate that, where antibody levels are persistently below 4 IU/ml, this indicates insignificant or, at the most, mild fetal hemolysis and that it is safe to allow the fetus to deliver spontaneously at term. Management of such cases is associated with a less than 5% risk of requiring an exchange transfusion for hyperbilirubinemia. Moreover, the authors found that it was very rare for the cord hemoglobin level to be less than 10 g/dl at birth if the maternal antibody levels had been under 10 IU/ml during the week prior to delivery (only 2 babies out of 800 cases where antibodies demonstrated this pattern), although neonatal exchange transfusion was required for treatment of neonatal hyperbilirubinemia in more than half of this group. It was recommended that invasive testing or delivery (if the pregnancy had reached 36 weeks' gestation) should only be undertaken at antibody levels greater than 10 IU/ml More recently, Nicolaides and Rodeck, in a cross-sectional study of 237 pregnancies with Rhesus alloimmunization between 17 and 38 weeks, found that as long as the maternal anti-D concentration was <15 IU/ml, the fetus was, at the most, mildly anemic (Hb deficit <3 g/dl) on cordocentesis[78]. A sudden rise in antibody levels is often indicative of increasing severity of disease and may require intervention. Laboratories using titers will have a 'critical titer' at which there is a significant risk of fetal hydrops, typically 1:32 dilutions.

A recent retrospective analysis of 120 mothers with anti-c antibodies, of whom 100 gave birth to a c-positive infant, showed that when the level of anti-c was below 7.5 IU/ml then the fetus was unlikely to be seriously affected[79]. However, above this level, prediction of fetal disease was difficult, maternal anti-c levels over 9.5 IU/ml being associated with exchange transfusion in 14 babies but with no treatment or phototherapy in 15 babies. Anti-Kell antibody levels should not be relied upon to determine the degree of fetal anemia as fetal hydrops has been reported at indirect Coombs' titers as low as 1:4[80].

The problem is that, although it is possible to decide upon a 'cut-off' level below which severe fetal disease does not occur, quantification of maternal antibody levels does not accurately predict fetal anemia once this level has been exceeded. A number of workers have investigated the use of in vitro assays, such as the monocyte monolayer assay (MMA), antibody-dependent cell-mediated cytotoxicity assay (ADCC) and monocyte chemiluminescence (CL) test, which measure the ability of the anti-D antibodies to mediate red cell destruction through hemolysis and activation of effector cells. Some have demonstrated that these tests are superior to routine quantification of antibodies by indirect Coombs' when it comes to predicting the severity of HDFN and the need for neonatal exchange transfusion, but similar claims in respect to predicting fetal anemia and determining when to perform invasive testing are not proven[21,81,82].

Ultrasound assessment

Ultrasound assessment of the at-risk fetus is important for detecting fetal hydrops. Weekly ultrasonography is appropriate in high-risk cases. The sonographic features of hydrops fetalis have been well described and include ascites, pericardial and pleural effusions, subcutaneous and scalp edema, polyhydramnios and placentomegaly. There is no standard definition of hydrops and classification in terms of mild, moderate and severe is subjective. A fetus with hydrops will be severely anemic with a hemoglobin deficit of 7 g/dl or more[37]. Even so, the presence or absence of hydrops is still not totally reliable as only two-thirds of fetuses with a hemoglobin this low will demonstrate fetal ascites. The earliest indicators of hydrops include the first signs of fetal ascites, such as the 'bowel halo' sign of free fluid within the peritoneal cavity or the ability to visualize both sides of the fetal bowel, and the presence of fluid within the pericardial space[83].

It is important to be able to identify those fetuses whose condition is deteriorating but who have not yet developed hydrops. Sonographic measurement of parameters such as extrahepatic and intrahepatic umbilical vein diameter, placental thickness, abdominal circumference, intraperitoneal volume and the ratio between the head and abdominal circumference have been investigated as to their usefulness in diagnosing anemia, but have now been shown to be unreliable in predicting fetal hematocrit in the absence of hydrops[84]. On the other hand, measurement of fetal liver length (as measured in a parasagittal plane) and fetal spleen perimeter (measured by tracing round the spleen in the same cross-sectional plane as the fetal stomach) appear to show some potential in evaluating fetal anemia, enlargement of these dimensions reflecting the increased extramedullary erythropoietic mass[85–87]. Reference ranges for these two parameters have been established[88].

Doppler studies

The use of fetal Doppler ultrasound in the evaluation of severe alloimmunization is appealing in view of the correlation between fetal hemoglobin and the increased maximum systolic flow velocities found in various parts of the fetal circulation as a consequence of elevated cardiac output and decreased blood viscosity[89]. There is considerable literature describing various arterial and venous Doppler velocity measurements from fetal vessels such as the umbilical vein, descending thoracic aorta, middle cerebral artery, common carotid artery in relationship to the degree of fetal anemia[31–33,90–93]. Intracardiac Doppler evaluation and demonstration of increased outflow tract velocities provide evidence of increased cardiac work with worsening anemia[94,95].

Fetal middle cerebral artery Doppler

It is the Doppler ultrasound evaluation of the middle cerebral artery (MCA) that has become the most widely used non-invasive method for assessing fetal anemia[96]. The peak systolic velocity (PSV) is measured and compared to the established normal values. Using a cut-off of 1.5 MoM, all fetuses with moderate to severe anemia were identified with a false positive rate of 12% and positive and negative predictive values of 65% and 100% respectively.

The MCA is the direct continuation of the internal carotid artery and runs anterolaterally from the circle of Willis (Fig. 40.3a). The ultrasound image is obtained in the axial plane by sliding caudally from the level of the biparietal diameter. To measure the PSV, the MCA is sampled with a sample volume of 1–2 mm, at the proximal point of the vessel with an insertion angle as close as possible to zero[97] (see Fig. 40.3c). Consistent measurements can be obtained at this point, with good intra- and inter-observer variability, but the peak velocity decreases in the distal regions of the vessel[98].

In one study comparing MCA Doppler with conventional management, i.e. amniocentesis, both were found to be equally accurate[99]. In another, better sensitivity, positive predictive values and larger false positive rates were obtained with MCA Doppler[100]. After 35 weeks' gestation, the false positive rate of MCA PSV increases, reducing its accuracy[101].

In our own practice, we adopted non-invasive techniques 15 years ago, at first as proposed by Oepkes[88], and then MCA PSV. In high-risk patients, with poor past histories and for high antibody levels, weekly measurements are taken. If the MCA PSV rises above 1.5 MoM, it is repeated a week later (unless there are signs of ascites). If it is elevated a second time, preparations are made for intravascular transfusion (IVT). This regimen has had two important consequences: (a) invasive monitoring of red cell alloimmunization using amniocentesis has become obsolete; and (b) transfusions are performed when they are necessary, i.e. unnecessary therapeutic interventions are avoided. We have not used MCA PSV to time subsequent transfusions, as the reliability of this has not yet been demonstrated and scheduling a transfusion program at 2–3 week intervals is highly successful (see below).

Other non-invasive techniques for assessment

Fetal movement counting is of some value and a reported change in the frequency of fetal movements should prompt

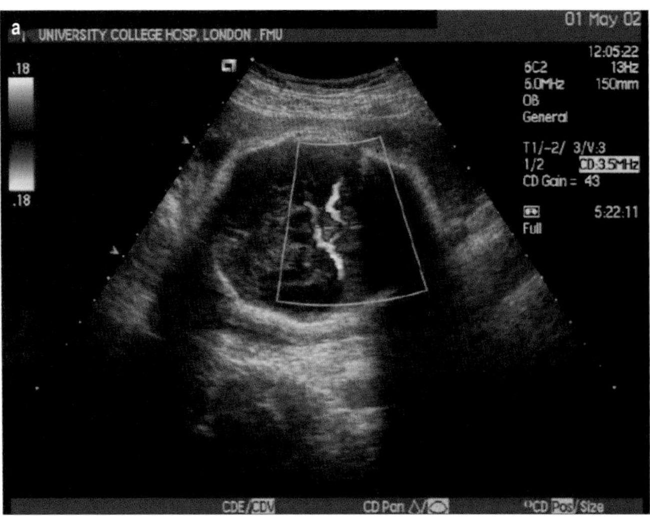

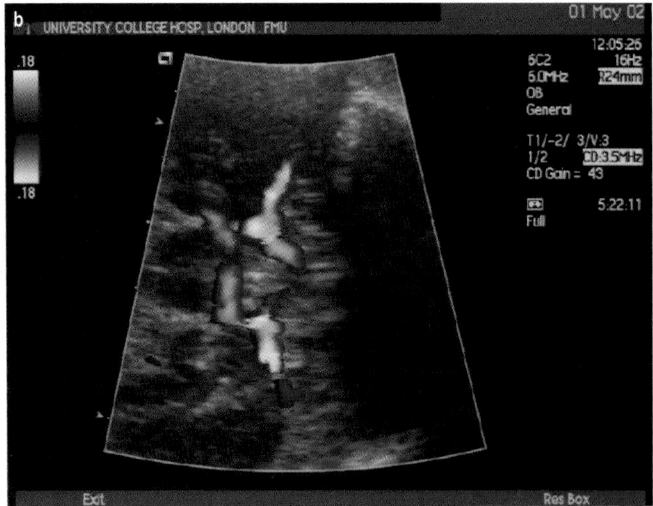

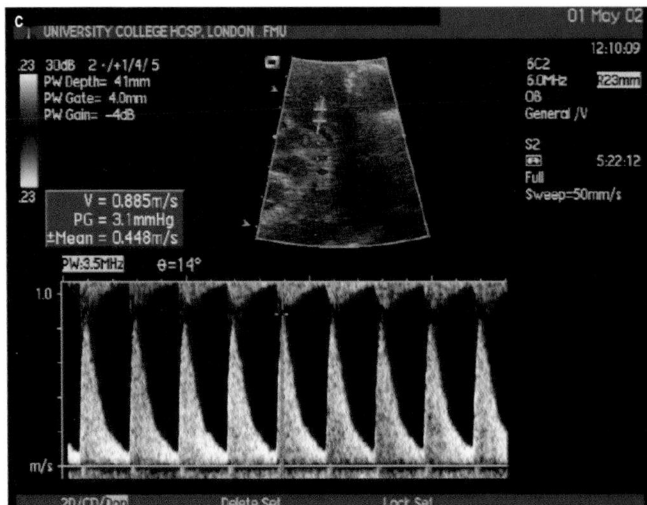

Fig. 40.3 (a) The circle of Willis is imaged by color Doppler at a plane caudal to the transthalamic view. (b) The middle cerebral artery (arrow) originates from the circle of Willis in an anterolateral fashion. (c) The MCA is sampled at the proximal end with an angle as close as possible to zero. The typical MCA Doppler flow waveform is shown.

further investigation. Patients usually observe that fetal movements are less before and increase after a transfusion. A reduction in fetal movements in association with the ultrasound findings of hydrops indicates a severely distressed fetus, although fetal movements have been said to be present until almost the time of death[102,103]. Sporadic or absent breathing movements may also be an ominous sign. Cardiotocographic (CTG) assessment of the fetus is not particularly helpful. A decrease in fetal heart rate (FHR) reactivity and baseline variability may be the first CTG indicators of anemia but these FHR changes, along with CTG abnormalities, such as a sinusoidal pattern or late decelerations, tend only to occur once the fetus is severely compromised and hypoxic[104]. CTG pattern do not appear to allow for accurate prediction of mild-to-moderate fetal anemia[105].

INVASIVE TESTING OF THE FETUS

There are two invasive methods of assessing the degree of fetal anemia: indirectly by spectrophotometric assessment of the amount of bilirubin in the amniotic fluid around the fetus; or directly by hematological studies on a fetal blood sample (FBS). Both are now obsolete but some consideration will be given to them because of their historial and pathophysiological interest.

Amniocentesis

The end product of fetal red cell destruction is bilirubin. Fetal bilirubin has been shown to be raised in fetuses affected with hemolytic anemia[106]. Most bilirubin is removed from the fetus via the placenta, but small amounts enter the amniotic fluid in fetal urine and pulmonary fluid during the second and third trimester and increases in the bilirubin level in amniotic fluid correlate with the degree of fetal red cell destruction[9]. The amniotic bilirubin concentration can be quantified spectrophotometrically by assessing the change in optical density at the wavelength 450 nm[107,108]. This is expressed as the ΔOD_{450} value (Fig. 40.4). Serial amniocentesis tests were performed, with each one potentially worsening maternal sensitization. To reduce the risk of fetomaternal hemorrhage, it was essential to avoid passage of the needle through the placenta by careful ultrasound guidance.

In 1961, Liley devised a system for managing pregnancies complicated by rhesus alloimmunization based on his observation that amniotic fluid ΔOD_{450} values between 27 and 35 weeks' gestation correlated with newborn outcome[107]. The Liley chart was divided into three zones: a lower zone indicating mildly affected or unaffected fetuses, a mid-zone indicating mildly to moderately affected fetuses and an upper zone indicating those who are severely affected and require treatment or delivery (Fig. 40.5). Very high ΔOD_{450} values confidently anticipate hydrops and, from 27 weeks onwards, accuracy of levels in zone 1 at predicting severe hemolysis have been reported as high as 96% and are an indication for intervention by transfusion or delivery[108]. In zone 3, levels were less predictive because of considerable overlap of mildly and severely affected fetuses[109–111]. This was to be expected because ΔOD_{450} values indicated the amount of hemolysis that was occurring and the likely outcome in the untreated fetus rather than the fetal hematopoietic response and resulting hematocrit.

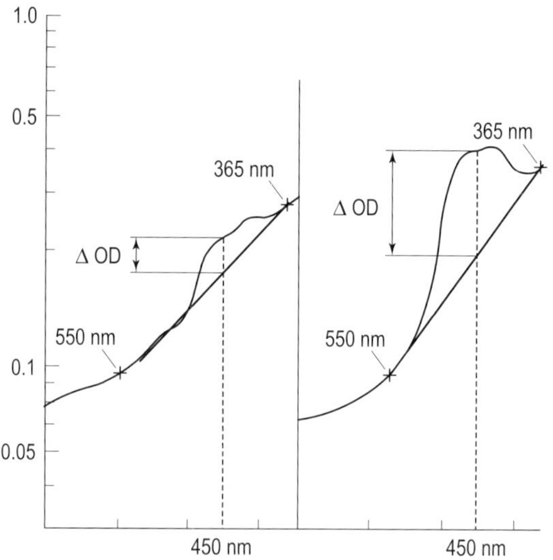

Fig. 40.4 Measurement of ΔOD_{450} at 450 nm, using a baseline drawn between the OD reading at 365 nm and 550 nm. The size of the peak at 450 nm is proportional to the amount of bilirubin present.

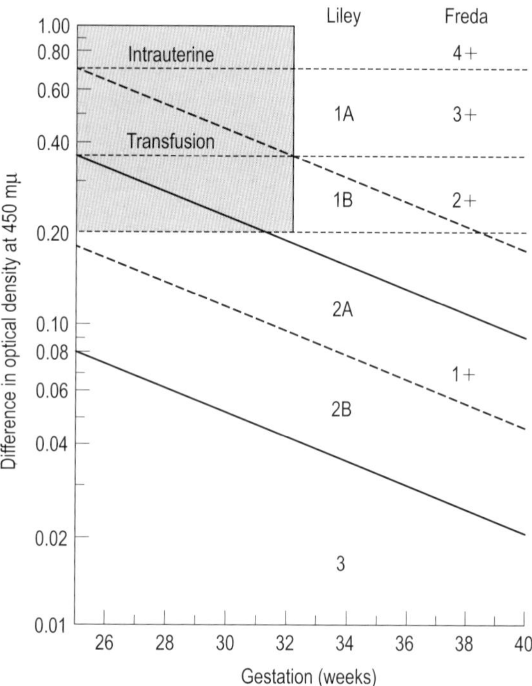

Fig. 40.5 Liley's chart showing ΔOD_{450} values in amniotic fluid against gestational age (Freda's classification is also included).

Confidence in the reliability of serial amniocentesis in the third trimester did not extend to its use in the second trimester. Liley's original work only examined pregnancies beyond 27 weeks. Nicolaides et al. showed that the backward extrapolation of the Liley lines was of little value in accurately separating severely affected from mildly affected fetuses prior to this gestation[112]. A number of modified charts were proposed using data from pregnancies sampled during the mid trimester and these suggested a curvilinear pattern to amniotic bilirubin levels during this time[113,114].

Fetal blood sampling

The obvious advantage of obtaining fetal blood is to measure fetal hemoglobin and hematocrit. The first experimental attempts at FBS were during hysterotomy and were reported in 1973[115]. Subsequently, Rodeck and Campbell demonstrated that pure fetal blood could be reliably obtained from umbilical cord vessels at the placental or fetal insertion using percutaneous fetoscopy[116]. Later FBS became an ultrasound-guided procedure[117]. Depending on fetal position, the umbilical vein was needled either at the placental insertion or in the intrahepatic portion. By having a blood analyzer close at hand, the fetal hematocrit could be obtained within one minute and treatment, by intravascular transfusion, could be given immediately through the same needle. FBS also allowed for measurement of other hematological and biochemical parameters[37,106,118]. Knowledge of the fetal reticuloctye count and direct Coombs' test were helpful in predicting the course of the fetal anemia. The fetal ABO group and Rhesus status could be determined in the event of the fetus proving not to be anemic. FBS is more invasive than amniocentesis and, in the largest reported series (606 cases), the fetal loss rate following FBS by skilled operators was 1.9%, although severely affected fetuses or those at early gestations are at greater risk[119,120]. Complications of FBS included exsanguination, intra-amniotic bleeding, fetal bradycardia, cord tamponade and failure to obtain a sample[119,120]. The degree of alloimmunization was also worsened as fetomaternal hemorrhage occurred in 70% of cases where the placenta was transgressed[121]. The reliability of non-invasive monitoring using the MCA PSV has meant that FBS is now only used as the preliminary step before performing an IVT.

MANAGEMENT

Broadly speaking, red cell alloimmunized women can be grouped into four categories which determine the type of management that they require. For the sake of clarity, Rh(D) will be used but can refer to the other red cell antigens.

1. *Women with a partner who is heterozygous for Rh(D).* They should be offered fetal genotyping by cell-free fetal DNA in maternal plasma when first seen, but not earlier than 12 weeks' gestation. This is also useful if the partner is not available or if paternity is uncertain. If the fetus is Rh(D) negative then no further follow-up is required.
2. *Women with a mild previous history and a homozygous partner, or a known Rh(D)-positive fetus.* Maternal antibody levels are done serially from a base-line in early pregnancy, monthly up to 20 weeks and 2-weekly thereafter. Levels rising above 15 iu/ml or a titer of 1 in 128 or more suggest worsening fetal anemia. MCA PSV measurements are also done 2-weekly starting at 20 weeks. If observations do not rise, delivery is planned for 38–40 weeks. If they rise after 34 weeks, delivery is planned for 36–38 weeks. A consistently high MCA PSV before 34 weeks indicates FBS and transfusion. Rising antibodies with a normal MCA PSV does not require intervention, but further close monitoring (weekly) is mandatory.
3. *Women with a severe previous history and a homozygous partner or a known Rh(D)-positive fetus.* Maternal antibody levels are likely to be high, but should be done serially from a base-line early in the pregnancy. They often rise further, suggesting fetal deterioration. Sometimes, however, they remain the same or even fall. Serial ultrasound is the most important monitoring of the fetus and should begin around 16 weeks to detect exceptionally early hydrops. MCA PSV measurements are started at 20 weeks and done 2-weekly until the velocity rises above 1.5 MoM. It is then done weekly and, if consistently high, IVT is prepared.
4. *Exceptional cases – death of an affected fetus before 20 weeks' gestation.* In these women, fetal blood transfusion will be necessary before 20 weeks' gestation if the fetus is Rh(d) positive. The risks of intravascular transfusion are high before this time (14% procedure related loss) and early intraperitoneal transfusion is preferable.[122]

Intrauterine blood transfusion

The main indication for intrauterine transfusion is now a consistently raised MCA PSV, provided that an FBS shows the fetal hematocrit is low. More rarely a hydropic fetus will require urgent IVT. Either intravascular or intraperitoneal transfusion, or a combination of the two methods, can be performed depending on circumstances and operator preference as will be discussed below.

Background

Fetal intravascular exchange transfusions were first attempted in the 1960s by open cannulation of fetal vessels, such as the femoral artery[123], saphenous vein[124] or chorionic plate vasculature[125], but these techniques required hysterotomy and fetal loss rates were nearly 100%. A more successful and safer technique pioneered at this time was percutaneous intraperitoneal transfusion, first described by Liley in 1963. It remained the only practical method for intrauterine transfusion for the next 20 years[10]. Without the benefit of ultrasound, Liley relied on fluoroscopic screening to position correctly the transfusion needle and catheter in the fetal peritoneal cavity. Urografin was injected into the amniotic cavity and the fetal bowel was visualized using X-rays as the fetus swallowed the contrast medium. Introduction of ultrasound-assisted intraperitoneal transfusion increased survival rates by avoiding the risk of fetal death from traumatic complications, such as damage to intra-abdominal and intrathoracic viscera, which accounted for up to 50% of the total mortality rate[126].

By the early 1980s, intrauterine intraperitoneal blood transfusion was firmly established as a treatment for fetuses identified by amniotic fluid ΔOD_{450} estimation as being severely affected but who were too immature for delivery (i.e. under 32–34 weeks). The outlook for fetuses with hydrops under 26 weeks of gestation, however, remained extremely poor so most centers did not perform transfusions before this gestation[127]. The presence of ascites appeared to prevent adequate absorption of erythrocytes[128]. In order to overcome these problems, Rodeck et al. in 1981 described a technique for intravascular transfusion by needling the umbilical artery under direct fetoscopic vision[11]. With this treatment, the same group reported a survival rate of 84% in 19 fetuses, both hydropic and non-hydropic, who received their first transfusion on or before 25 weeks' gestation, some as early as 19 weeks[129]. They also observed the disappearance of hydrops after IVT. Ultrasound-guided techniques for direct intravascular transfusion into the intrahepatic portion of the umbilical vein[130,131], the umbilical cord at the placental insertion[132] and the heart[133] were reported soon afterwards. Ultrasound-guided needling became established practice, being less invasive and easier to use compared to fetoscopy. Several groups have published their experiences showing that repeated intravascular transfusions from as early as 18 weeks' gestation to up to 36 weeks' gestation are associated with survival rates ranging from 76 to 96%[132,134–137]. Delivery can be delayed until near term (in practice 36–37 weeks) so reducing the need for cesarean section and prolonged, expensive neonatal care.

Pathophysiology

The anemic fetus has a reduced capacity for tissue oxygenation. Compensatory mechanisms such as redistribution of blood flow to vital organs and fall in oxygen delivery to other fetal tissues allow the fetus to maintain normal blood gas and acid–base indices until the hemoglobin falls below 30% of normal (4–6 g/dl depending on gestational age), at which point tissue hypoxia is present[43]. Severe fetal anemia is treated by infusing adult hemoglobin to increase the oxygen-carrying capacity of the blood. After the second or third transfusion, fetal erythropoiesis in suppressed and fetal erythrocytes are completely replaced by adult red blood cells in the fetal circulation.

Infusion of packed cells into anemic non-hypoxic fetuses (hemoglobin >4 g/dl) produces only a slight fall in pH and change in base excess, despite the fact that donor blood is relatively acidic (mean pH 6.76) with a high $P\text{CO}_2$ content, because of the buffering effect of the fetomaternal circulation[138]. Once the fetal circulation contains predominantly adult hemoglobin, fetal umbilical artery blood is more acidotic with a higher base deficit compared to when only fetal hemoglobin is present[139]. In the fetal umbilical venous circulation, $P\text{O}_2$ is around 5 mmHg higher with predominantly adult hemoglobin[139]. This suggests that oxygen delivery to the tissues is better with fetal hemoglobin, most likely to be due to the differences in the oxygen dissociation curves of fetal and adult hemoglobin. The relative acidosis found in association with adult hemoglobin would shift the oxygen dissociation curve to the right and promote oxygen release. The high umbilical venous $P\text{O}_2$ found in association with adult hemoglobin indicates greater oxygen transfer across the placenta. In situations where the fetus has pre-existing acidosis, transfusion could worsen the acidosis and be responsible for the higher rate of adverse outcome seen in such cases. In addition, at low $P\text{O}_2$ levels adult hemoglobin has a smaller reserve and releases less oxygen than fetal hemoglobin in response to the same fall in $P\text{O}_2$ which would be worse in the presence of fetal hypoxia. These phenomena suggest that the risks of labor are higher in the transfused fetus with adult hemoglobin in its circulation.

Intravascular versus intraperitoneal transfusion

Intravascular transfusion (IVT)

Advantages

Intravascular transfusion offers a number of advantages over the intraperitoneal route, including:

- determination of the fetal blood group; the fetus may be Rhesus negative so rendering further investigation unnecessary
- direct assessment of the hematocrit and hemoglobin
- measurement of the pre- and post-transfusion hematocrit
- enables the appropriate amount of blood to be calculated and transfused
- blood is transfused into the fetal circulation, avoiding the lymphatic transport from the peritoneal cavity
- more effective correction of anemia when the fetus is hydropic
- reversal of hydrops in utero
- avoids trauma to fetal intraperitoneal organs
- allows timing of subsequent transfusions and optimum time for delivery by calculation of the fall in hematocrit per day
- treatment can be continued until well into the third trimester, thus avoiding the complications of premature delivery and exchange transfusions at birth.

Technique

Initially a 20-gauge spinal needle is passed under ultrasound guidance to obtain a fetal blood sample in the normal manner. A Teflon-coated needle may be superior[140]. Ideally, three trained personnel are required: an experienced operator who performs the needling of the fetal vasculature and monitors the transfusion throughout by visualization on the ultrasound screen, an assistant who administers the blood and a third person who acts as a 'runner' performing the blood tests and calculations.

Premedication. In general, fetal transfusions are performed as an outpatient procedure and are associated with only minimal maternal discomfort. Although maternal anxiety can usually be allayed by appropriate counseling, very occasionally it may be necessary to administer a premedication. This will also sedate the fetus.

Site for transfusion. Most operators favor the umbilical cord vein at its placental insertion, others the intrahepatic umbilical vein. The umbilical vein is used for a number of reasons. It is wider in diameter than the artery and is more easily targeted. Its use allows the operator to watch the flow of transfused blood sonographically confirming the correct placement of the needle. This helps to avoid the potentially fatal complications of internal dissection of the intima and/or cord tamponade should the needle slip out of the lumen and which occurs more commonly with arterial punctures. If fetal lie and placental position prevents safe access to this site then an alternative approach is to needle the intrahepatic vein. Unlike some, we would not advocate use of a free loop of umbilical cord because of the potential for needle displacement. Cardiac puncture is rarely used because of the potential hazards such as cardiac tamponade, hemopericardium and arrhythmia including asystole[133].

Fetal paralysis. If the fetus moves during an IVT procedure, this can cause needle displacement, hemorrhage or fetal trauma. If the fetus is very active and the placenta is posterior, temporary paralysis may be advisable. Various neuromuscular blocking agents have been used including intramuscular or intravenous pancuronium bromide and curare[141,142].

Volume and rate of transfusion. On gaining access to the fetal circulation, a 1-ml sample of fetal blood is aspirated to determine the fetal hematocrit. A blood analyzer should be adjacent to the procedure room so that the result is obtained within a few seconds, during which time the tip of the needle remains in the fetal vessel. The mean fetal hematocrit and hemoglobin varies with gestation (see Fig. 40.1). If the fetal hematocrit is more than 2 SD below the mean for gestation, in practice below 30%, then an IVT is performed. The needle is first connected to a three-way stop-cock via extension tubing so that the blood transfusion can be administered with minimal chance of disturbing the needle during the procedure (Fig. 40.6). If transfusion is not necessary because the hematocrit is normal, then the needle can be withdrawn and conservative management by non-invasive monitoring be pursued.

The volume of blood transfused is determined by three factors: the pretransfusion fetal hematocrit, the estimated fetoplacental blood volume and the hematocrit of the donor blood. Nomograms have been constructed to provide an estimation of the volume of donor blood required to raise the fetal hematocrit to 40% (Fig. 40.7)[132]. Alternatively, a simple calculation can be performed:

$$\text{Volume to be transfused} = \frac{\text{Desired hematocrit} - \text{Fetal hematocrit}}{\text{Donor hematocrit} - \text{Desired hematocrit}} \times \text{Fetoplacental blood volume}$$

We aim to raise the fetal hematocrit to supraphysiological levels, i.e. to 35–40% in the early mid trimester and to 45–55% later on in pregnancy. Sometimes, a sample of fetal blood is aspirated mid-way during the transfusion to check the fetal hematocrit and to confirm the amount of blood to be further transfused. At the end, a final sample of fetal blood is taken to estimate the post-transfusion fetal hematocrit and for a Kleihauer–Betke test to determine the proportion of adult red blood cells now present in the fetal circulation.

The blood is transfused at a rate of 5–10 ml per minute. During the procedure the flow of blood is continuously visualized on the ultrasound screen to confirm that the needle remains correctly placed and the fetal heart periodically checked for arrhythmias, in particular fetal bradycardia. In our unit, we use a free-hand technique rather than a needle guide so allowing independent movement of the ultrasound transducer.

Donor blood. The blood used should be adult group O RhD-negative blood which has been collected within 24 hours and cross-matched with the maternal blood. It should have been screened for hepatitis B and C, cytomegalovirus and HIV as well as irradiated and washed to remove the white blood cells to avoid 'graft-versus-host'-like complications in the fetus. The blood is packed to a hematocrit of 80–85% to minimize the volume of blood that needs to be transfused.

'Top-up' versus exchange transfusion. Concerns have been voiced that by directly transfusing blood into the fetus without removing any blood, the so-called 'top-up' transfusion, there might be a danger of volume overload and cardiac embarrassment. Some groups have reported a technique of exchange transfusion whereby small amounts of blood are aspirated from the fetus at regular intervals during its blood transfusion

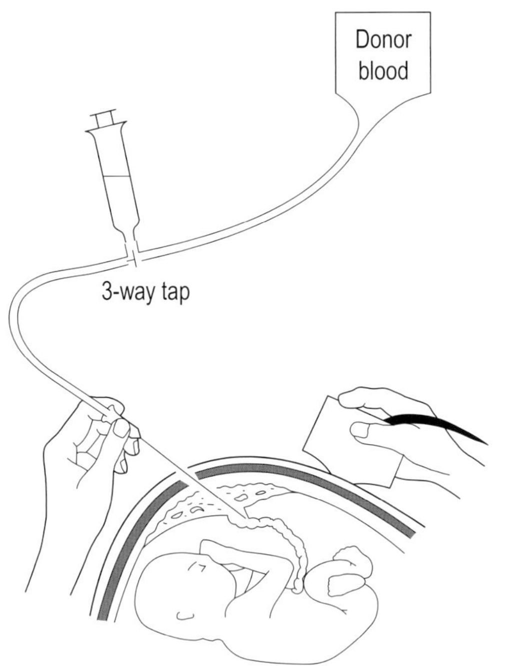

Fig. 40.6 Diagram of fetal blood transfusion into the umbilical vein at the placental cord insertion.

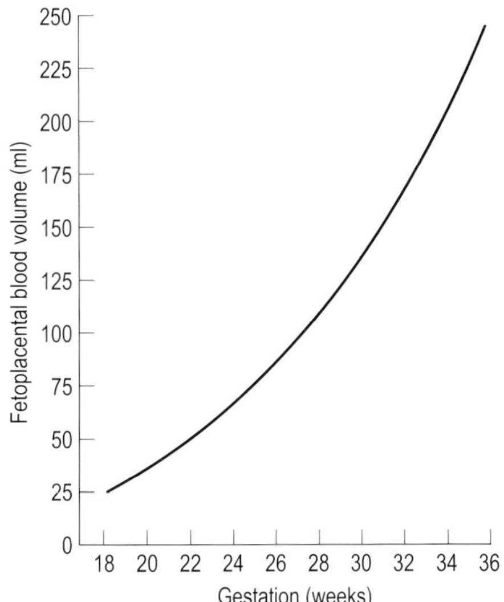

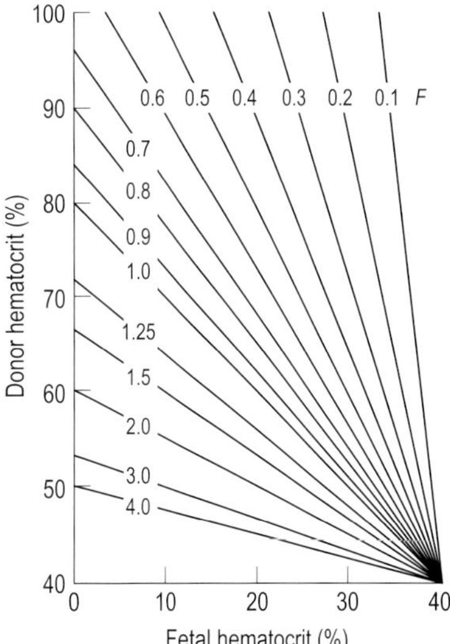

Fig. 40.7 Nomogram for intravascular transfusion. To calculate the volume of donor blood necessary to achieve a fetal hematocrit of 40%, the estimated fetoplacental blood volume (left, e.g. 100 ml at 27 weeks) is multiplied by *F* (right, e.g. 0.8 for a pretransfusion hematocrit of 10% and a donor hematocrit of 80%) (from Nicolaides et al.[37] with permission).

with the intention of preventing hypervolemia, especially in the hydropic fetus whose myocardium may be already overstressed[134,143]. Others suggest that the umbilical venous pressure should be routinely monitored and if the change in pressure exceeds 10 mmHg then blood should be removed and replaced with an equal volume of saline as such changes in pressure are associated with fetal demise[144]. In practice, although umbilical venous pressure can be demonstrated to rise significantly during transfusion (mean increase 4.6 mmHg), the fetus appears to tolerate 'top-up' transfusions of 100–150% of its fetoplacental blood volume[46,133,145]. Pressure increments in the umbilical vein of up to 12 mmHg have been recorded after transfusion without complication[146]. 'Top-up' transfusions have the advantage of being quicker than exchange transfusions, which reduces the risk of needle displacement, bacterial contamination, myometrial stimulation and umbilical vein thrombosis. Fetal blood viscosity is probably a more important consideration than volume infused, particularly at earlier gestations. Post-transfusion fetal blood viscosity tends to be above the 95th centile for gestational age following IVT[147]. Of 19 severely anemic, hydropic fetuses receiving their first intravascular transfusion in the mid trimester, seven (36.8%) died 24–72 hours after transfusion with no evidence of fetal distress associated with the procedure[148]. There were no significant differences in gestational age, in the total blood volume infused or volume transfused as a percentage of total fetoplacental blood volume between survivors and those who died. The only significant difference was in the relative increase in hematocrit. It was 5.5-fold in those who died compared to 3.5-fold in the survivors. Such acute increases in hematocrit represent substantial increases in fetal blood viscosity and confirm our opinion that it is this that leads to fetal demise rather than volume overload.

Timing of subsequent transfusions

The second transfusion should be performed not later than 2 weeks after the first transfusion. In cases of severe anemia or where a small first transfusion has been given, then the second transfusion will need to be performed after one week. The mean fall in hematocrit is around 1% per day but there can be a wide variation (SD 0.44)[149]. This rate of fall is particularly unpredictable during the interval between the first and second transfusions when the percentage of fetal erythrocytes left in the fetal circulation and suppression of erythropoiesis in the fetus after the initial transfusion are variable. The general tendency is for a less marked fall between the second and third transfusion with the exception of a few fetuses who show active erythropoiesis after the first transfusion. In these latter cases, the Kleihauer test indicates that there is an increase in the percentage of fetal erythrocytes at the start of the second transfusion compared to at the end of the first transfusion, thus alerting one to the likelihood that the fall in hematocrit will be higher in the subsequent than the previous interval due to more (fetal) red cells being hemolyzed. After the second and third transfusions, the rate of fall in hematocrit per day is usually very constant for an individual fetus and is usually close to 1%/day. The fetal circulation now contains adult red blood cells almost exclusively (as shown by the Kleihauer test), fetal erythropoiesis is suppressed (fetal reticuloctye count <1%) and fall in hematocrit is due to fetal growth and plasma expansion, not due to hemolysis. The pre- and post-transfusion hematocrit values are plotted on a graph (transfusogram). By calculating the rate of fall during transfusions, one can predict when the next IVT should be scheduled in order to prevent the development of hydrops. This means maintaining the fetal hematocrit above the critical level of one-third of the normal mean for the gestational age (hematocrit 20–25%). Provided post-transfusion hematocrits are above the normal range, the next transfusion can be scheduled in three weeks. Maintaining the longest possible interval between transfusions reduces the overall number needed and reduces risk of procedure-related loss (Fig. 40.8).

Complications. The fetal loss rate per IVT ranges from 0.6 to 4%[149,150]. The risks are greatest before 20 weeks, procedure-related losses being as high as 14% in this group[122]. The most common complication is that of a transient fetal bradycardia which occurs in around 8% of procedures, although this rarely requires delivery of the fetus[137]. Other potentially fatal complications include 'cord accidents', such as cord tamponade resulting from a cord hematoma, intimal dissection of the fetal vessel, umbilical artery spasm, hemorrhage from the puncture site, thromboembolism and overload of the fetal circulation[132,136,137]. 'Cord accidents' do not occur when transfusions are given into the intrahepatic umbilical vein and it has been our strong impression that this is the safer route than cord puncture. Chorioamnionitis, preterm rupture of the membranes and preterm labor can occur but are infrequent. The intravascular route has the potential to cause fetomaternal hemorrhage, particularly if the placenta is traversed, thus worsening the degree of maternal sensitization.

Fetal surveillance. Following administration of an IVT, we recommend monitoring the fetal heart rate by cardiotocography for 1 hour. It should be pointed out that, if the fetus has been given pancuronium bromide during the procedure, the fetal heart rate variability is often poor because there are no fetal movements[151]. The mother should be warned that she may feel no movements for some hours and be given a fetal-movement chart and attend for weekly monitoring by ultrasonography and umbilical artery Doppler waveform assessment until the next transfusion. We also measure the MCA PSV but this does not determine the timing of the next transfusion.

Consequences of transfusion. After in utero transfusion, the fetal circulation will contain adult red blood cells and, after a number of transfusions (usually three), the Kleihauer–Betke test will show that there are virtually no fetal erythrocytes present. Fetal erythropoiesis is then suppressed. At birth, the fetal blood group will be group O RhD negative. It can take several weeks for resumption of erythropoiesis and parents should be warned that 'top-up' blood transfusions may be necessary, anemia developing as the baby grows, and that this should not be regarded as a failure. Regular monthly hemoglobin estimations until 6 months of age are advisable. In the future, exogenous erythropoietin may prove to be effective in preventing late anemia[152]. Babies born after intrauterine transfusion do not appear to have an increased risk of compromise at birth. Normal growth and brain volume and neurological and development outcomes have been reported[153–155].

Rh-alloimmunized fetuses have been shown to have high serum ferritin levels – often above the normal reference range[156]. Serial in utero transfusions are associated with further increase in these levels to concentrations that would be considered to represent iron overload in children. One case of liver disease consistent with iron overload has been reported in an infant after in utero transfusion therapy[157]. It is recommended that serum ferritin levels are monitored in the neonatal and infant period and iron supplementation withheld until levels are within the normal range.

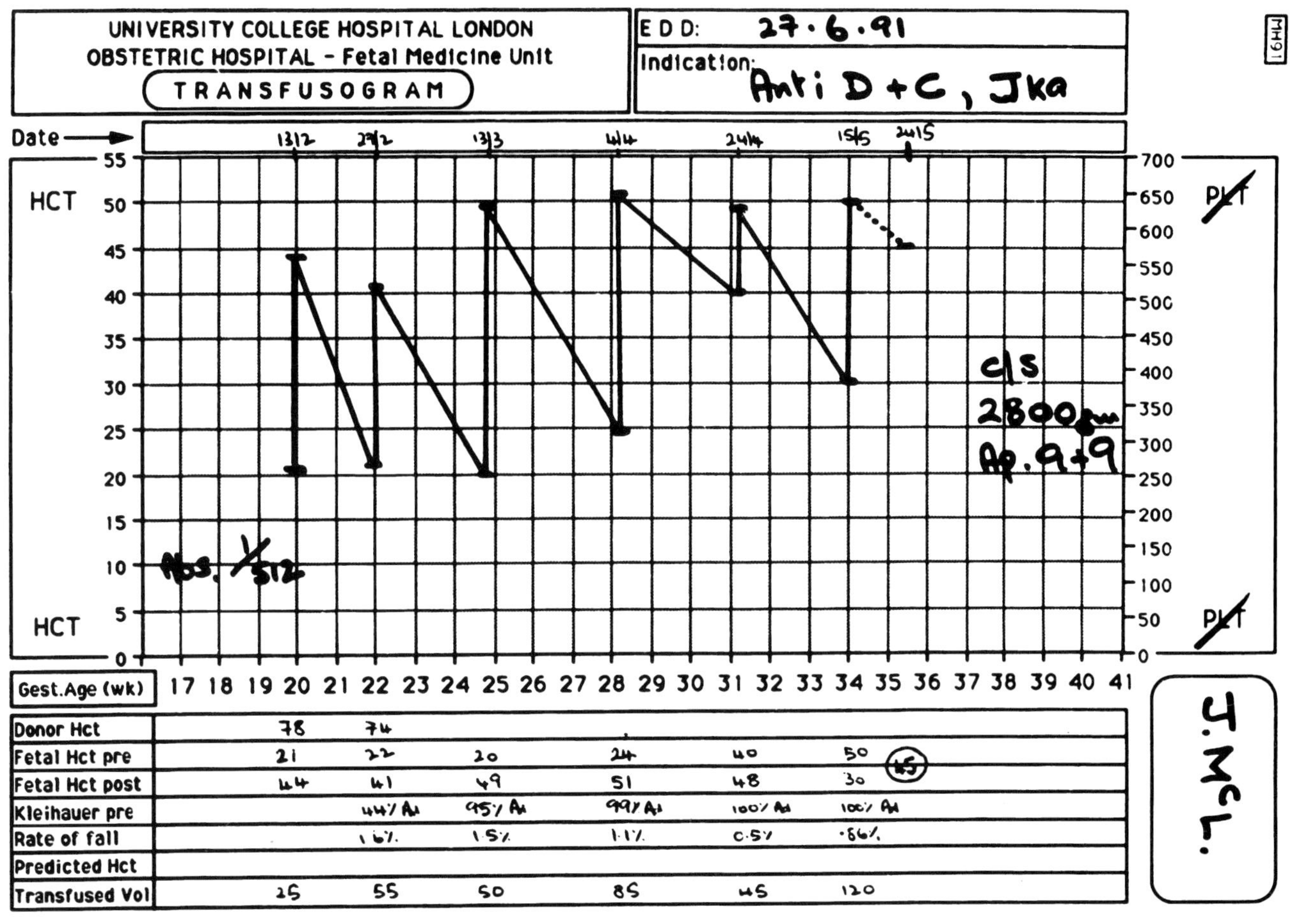

Fig. 40.8 A transfusogram of a patient who had a successful programme of IVTs.

Intraperitoneal transfusion (IPT)

As described earlier, Liley successfully pioneered this method of transfusion over 30 years ago but, since the development of intravascular techniques, many have advocated intravascular transfusion as the treatment of choice[125,137,150]. Intraperitoneal transfusion relies on placing the donor red cells into the peritoneal cavity and absorption into the fetal circulation occurs via the subdiaphragmatic lymphatics and thoracic duct. However, the presence of ascites reduces the efficacy of this process. For this reason, in the hydropic fetus, intravascular transfusion is considerably more successful at reversing hydrops and ensuring survival in the neonatal period. In a case-control study by Harman et al., 18/21 (86%) of hydropic fetuses survived after IVT compared to 10/21 (48%) who had IPT[150]. The situation, however, is less clearcut when considering non-hydropic fetuses as survival rates for both IVT and IPT are in the region of 80–100% when ultrasound is routinely employed.

Advantages

- Method of choice if treatment becomes necessary at very early gestations, under 18 weeks when direct access to the fetal vasculature is difficult and hazardous
- Enables transfusion when fetal lie and position of the placental cord insertion technically precludes access to the fetal circulation
- When combined with IVT, allows an increased blood volume to be given (so lengthening the interval between transfusions) without overloading the fetal circulation
- Should be easier and safer than IVT if IVT skills are not optimal.

Disadvantages

- Not suitable for the hydropic fetus
- Cannot obtain pre- and post-transfusion hemoglobin so have to estimate blood volume to be transfused based on gestational age
- Danger of trauma to fetal abdominal organs, although this has been greatly reduced by the use of ultrasound
- Inadvertent transfusion into fetal bowel, liver or abdominal wall can occur
- Increased intraperitoneal pressure can compromise venous return to the heart resulting in fetal bradycardia.

Technique

The mother is prepared in a similar manner as for IVT. A 20- or 18-gauge spinal needle is inserted into the fetal abdomen under ultrasound guidance. Ideally, the needle should enter the fetal abdominal cavity through the anterior abdominal wall, below the umbilical vein but above the fetal bladder, thus avoiding trauma to the fetal liver which may well be enlarged. To verify that the needle is correctly positioned, the operator should either aspirate ascitic fluid if the fetus is hydropic or, in the absence of ascites, can infuse a bolus of saline solution into the peritoneal cavity while observing the tip of the needle sonographically. Pancuronium bromide can be given intraperitoneally if there is a concern that the fetus may move and dislodge the needle. The needle can then be connected via a three-way tap to the infusion tubing and donor blood administered at a rate of about 10 ml/min, as described for IVT. Throughout the infusion, the tip of the needle is monitored sonographically to observe the flow of blood entering the peritoneal cavity and the fetal heart rate observed in case persistent bradycardia indicates that the transfusion should be discontinued.

The amount of donor blood to be given is calculated using the following empirical formula:

$$(\text{gestation in weeks} - 20) \times 10\,\text{ml}$$

It should be noted that this means that the quantity of blood being infused is related to the gestational age of the fetus rather than the degree of anemia. If a large amount of ascitic fluid is present, this should be removed.

Combined IVT and IVP transfusions

In view of the procedure-related risks for both IVT and IPT techniques, it would clearly be beneficial to maintain the longest possible interval between transfusions. One way to achieve this is to combine both techniques as this permits a high-volume transfusion to be given without overloading the fetal circulation. Animal studies and our own observations indicate that intraperitoneal blood is absorbed over a few days[158]. Data from Nicolini et al., reporting on 31 fetuses who had a total of 99 intrauterine transfusions, of which 59 were combined intravascular and intraperitoneal procedures, showed a significantly longer interval between transfusions when blood was given both intravascularly and into the peritoneal cavity compared to when only intravascular transfusion was given[149]. Although the increase in time interval between the combined IVT–IPT and single IVT technique was only 3 days, the initial hematocrit at subsequent transfusions was a mean of 3.9 g/dl higher with the combined procedure. There is no overall difference in the percentage fall in hematocrit indicating that, effectively, all the intraperitoneal blood is absorbed.

The technique used is the same as for IVT. Enough donor blood is given intravascularly to raise the fetal hematocrit to 40%, as confirmed by a post-transfusion hematocrit. The same spinal needle is then used to perform an IPT, particularly easy if the intrahepatic portion of the umbilical vein has been used[159], with the amount of donor blood transfused intraperitoneally being the same as that amount that would be required intravascularly to raise the hematocrit to 60%.

Outcome of treatment

Over a 2-year period at University College Hospital, London, 46 fetuses underwent 169 intrauterine transfusion of whom 8 (17%) were hydropic at the first transfusion. The fetal loss rate per transfusion was 2.4% and the overall survival rate was 91% (92% for non-hydropic fetuses and 88% for hydropic fetuses). Ten fetuses had their first transfusion at 20 weeks or earlier and, in this group, the survival rate was 80%. There were no losses in those fetuses who had their first transfusion after 24 weeks' gestation. The last transfusion should be performed so that when delivery occurs, ideally 37–38 weeks, the fetal hematocrit is not less than 20–25%.

Other treatments of red cell alloimmunization

A variety of alternative treatments for alloimmunization have been proposed with varying success. Plasmapheresis has been reported as reducing maternal anti-D levels, but there is little evidence that severe fetal disease can be prevented by doing this[160,161]. The technique is costly and time-consuming, involving the removal of large volumes of plasma several times a week, and is not without complications. The use of high-dose intravenous immunoglobulin (IVIG) has been described in two series where pregnancies were complicated by severe Rh alloimmunization[162,163]. Although there is some evidence for its efficacy before 28 weeks' gestation, it does not appear to alleviate the need for IVT. Promethazine, in large doses, has been cited as decreasing red cell phagocytosis and decreasing antibody production, but the evidence for the effectiveness of such treatment remains unproven[164].

Other antigen sensitization

There are numerous minor antigens found in addition to the D antigen on the surface of red blood cells. Antibodies raised to these antigens have become relatively more common in pregnancy as Rh(D) sensitization has become less frequent due to the use of anti-D immunoglobulin prophylaxis. In the majority of cases, sensitization to these minor antigens can be traced back to a blood transfusion which the mother has received. Those antibodies which can cause severe hemolytic disease of the newborn include anti-c, anti-E and anti-Kell. Anti-Fy^a (Duffy) rarely causes more than mild HDFN but, recent data indicate that pregnancies where anti-Fy^a titers are found in excess of 64 are at significant risk of severe anemia[165]. Fetal genotyping may be appropriate where the father is known to be heterozygous and antibody titers are high or rising. Multiple antibodies may be present and can also occur in combination with anti-Rh(D). In a 12-year study in Sweden investigating the prevalence of red cell antibodies, 0.57% of mothers tested in routine antenatal screening had red cell antibodies with 0.24% being clinically significant[166]. Multiple antibodies occurred in 8.2%.

Management of minor antigen sensitivity is, in essence, the same as that undertaken for Rh(D) disease. Regular measurement of maternal antibody titers should be performed throughout the pregnancy and significant rises in antibody titers should lead to further assessment similar to that described for anti-Rh(D) alloimmunization. Non-invasive monitoring of MCA PSV by Doppler ultrasound is most important. Van Dijk et al., reporting on a retrospective study of 418 pregnancies complicated by red cell alloantibodies, showed that at titers of 1 in 16 for anti-c, anti-E and anti-Kell only 4% of newborn required transfusion compared to 20% with anti-D[167]. In the future, assays to measure cytotoxic lysis or phagocytosis may be more helpful. With anti-c levels below 7.5 IU/ml, the fetus is unlikely to be seriously affected; above this, intervention may be necessary[168].

DNA-based RhCcEe genotyping is now possible with cell-free fetal DNA in maternal blood.

Anti-Kell

Around 10% of the population are Kell positive. The vast majority of Kell-negative women who develop Kell antibodies do so as a consequence of receiving a transfusion of Kell-positive blood. Anti-Kell antibodies are usually benign but can cause severe fetal anemia and hydrops in utero. The frequency of affected neonates is 1 in 10 000[169].

Maternal antibody titers are unreliable at predicting whether the fetus is Kell positive (large rises in antibody titers have been reported in the presence of a Kell-negative fetus) or at indicating the severity of fetal disease. Nor do amniotic fluid ΔOD450 levels correlate with the degree of fetal anemia[170,171]. A recent study of 11 fetuses who were anemic due to maternal anti-Kell alloimmunization showed them to have a significantly lower reticulocyte count and reduced erythroblastosis when compared to anemic fetuses (matched for hematocrit, gestational age, hydrops and perinatal outcome) where the mother was alloimmunized to anti-D[172]. These findings suggest that erythroid suppression, rather than hemolysis, is the predominant mechanism in producing fetal anemia secondary to maternal Kell alloimmunization. The authors also found that amniotic fluid bilirubin concentrations correlated poorly with fetal hematocrit which is consistent with reduced hemolysis. Amniocentesis is therefore not helpful in predicting fetal anemia.

Our approach to mothers with anti-Kell sensitization is first to determine the paternal antigen status with regards to Kell. If he is Kell negative, then the fetus should be as well. No further investigation is needed, although serial ultrasound monitoring for hydrops may still be advisable as paternity cannot always be guaranteed. If he is Kell positive, only 3% of such people are homozygous positive so the fetus may still be Kell negative despite the fact that maternal anti-Kell titers are elevated. In these cases, amniotic fluid is used for Kell grouping as this cannot yet be done on maternal blood. If the fetus is Kell positive, serial MCA PSV measurements are performed.

THE FUTURE

Advances in the management of fetal disease caused by red cell alloimmunization has meant that sensitized women, who in the past would have suffered multiple fetal and neonatal losses, can now be optimistic about achieving a successful pregnancy outcome and completing their families. Some couples choose to go through two or even three pregnancies that require serial in utero blood transfusion, although it should not be forgotten that each pregnancy does involve considerable commitment by both parents and medical staff as well as not being completely risk-free for both mother and fetus.

There are further inroads to be made into the antenatal prevention of red cell sensitization: namely, the universal adoption of the routine administration of anti-D immunoglobulin to Rh-negative mothers during the antenatal period and routine assessment of donor–recipient compatibility for atypical red blood cell antigens that could cause alloimmunization when blood transfusion is planned for women of child-bearing age.

There are new therapeutic interventions on the horizon. One possibility is the development of monoclonal antibody therapy directed against the FcγR1 receptor that is so important in mediating the attachment of IgG anti-D to, and phagocytosis by, fetal monocytes during the Rh(D) hemolytic process. Another possibility would be the use of fetal stem cell transfusions from an antigen negative donor, although this has not yet been proved to be successful[173].

As prevention improves, severe cases requiring IVT are becoming increasingly rare. Even subspecialists in tertiary centers are becoming de-skilled and the maintenance of expertise is a challenge that will only be met by still further centralization.

ACKNOWLEDGMENT

The authors are grateful for the assistance of Dr Khalil Abi Nader with the revision of this chapter.

REFERENCES

1. Clarke CA, Whitfield AGW. Deaths from rhesus haemolytic disease in England and Wales in 1977: accuracy of records and assessment of anti-D prophylaxis. *Br Med J* **i**:1665–1669, 1979.
2. Clarke C, Hussey RM. Decline in deaths from Rhesus haemolytic disease of the newborn. *J R Col Physicians Lond* **28**: 310–311, 1994.
3. Tovey LAD. Haemolytic disease of the newborn and its prevention. *Br Med J* **300**:313–316, 1990.
4. Hughes RG, Craig JIO, Murphy WG, Greer IA. Causes and clinical consequences of Rhesus(D) haemolytic disease of the newborn: a study of a Scottish population, 1985–1990. *Br J Obstet Gynaecol* **101**:297–300, 1994.
5. Walker RH, Batton DG, Morrison M. The current rarity of RhD haemolytic disease of the newborn in a community hospital. *Am J Clin Pathol* **100**:340–341, 1993.
6. Levine P, Katrin EM, Burnham L. Isoimmunization in pregnancy: its possible bearing on the etiology of erythroblastosis foetalis. *J Am Med Assoc* **116**:825–830, 1941.
7. Diamond LK, Blackfan KD, Baty JM. Erythroblastosis fetalis and its association with universal edema of the fetus, icterus gravis neonatorum and anemia of the newborn. *J Pediatr* **1**:269–274, 1932.
8. Wallerstein H. Treatment of severe erythroblastosis by simultaneous removal and replacement of the blood of the new born infant. *Science* **103**: 583–584, 1946.
9. Bevis DCA. The antenatal prediction of haemolytic disease of the newborn. *Lancet* **ii**:395–398, 1952.
10. Liley AW. Intrauterine transfusion of the foetus in haemolytic disease. *Br Med J* **2**:1107–1109, 1963.
11. Rodeck CH, Holman CA, Karnicki J, Kemp JR, Whitmore DN, Austin MA. Direct intravascular fetal blood transfusion by fetoscopy in severe rhesus isoimmunization. *Lancet* **i**:625–627, 1981.
12. Finn R, Clarke CA, Donohoe WTA et al. Experimental studies on the prevention of Rh haemolytic disease. *Br Med J* **i**:486–490, 1961.
13. Bowman JM, Pollock JM, Penston LE. Fetomaternal transplacental haemorrhage during pregnancy and after delivery. *Vox Sang* **51**:117–125, 1986.
14. Walker RH, Hartrick MB. Non-ABO clinically significant erythrocyte allo-antibodies in Caucasian obstetric patients. *Transfusion* **31**:52S, 1991.

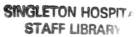

15. Wiener E, Mawas F, Dellow RA, Singh I, Rodeck CH. A major role of class I Fcγ receptors in immunoglobulin G anti-D mediated red blood cell destruction by fetal mononuclear phagocytes. *Obstet Gynecol* **86**:157–162, 1995.
16. Weiner E. The ability of IgG subclasses to cause elimination of targets *in vivo* and to mediate their destruction by phagocytosis/cytolysis *in vitro*. In *The human IgG subclasses*, F Shakib (ed.), pp. 135–160. Oxford: Pergamon Press, 1990.
17. Schreiber AD, Rossman MD, Levinson AI. The immunobiology of human Fc receptors on hemopoietic cells and tissue macrophages. *Clin. Immunol Immunopathol* **62**:566–572, 1992.
18. Chown B. On a search for rhesus antibodies in very young fetuses. *Arch Dis Childh* **30**:237, 1955.
19. Gitlin D. Development and metabolism in the immune globulins. In *Immunological incompetence*, BM Kaga, ER Stiehm (eds). Chicago: Year Book, 1971.
20. Lubenko A, Contreras M, Rodeck CH, Nicolini U, Savage J, Chana H. The transplacental IgG subclass concentrations in pregnancies at risk of haemolytic disease of the newborn. *Vox Sang* **67**: 291–298, 1994.
21. Garner SF, Gorick BD, Lai WY et al. Prediction of the severity of haemolytic disease of the newborn. Quantitative IgG anti-D subclass determinations explain correlation with functional assay results. *Vox Sang* **69**:169–176, 1995.
22. Thomas NC, Shirey RS, Blakemore K, Kickler TS. A quantitative assay for subclassing IgG alloantibodies implicated in hemolytic disease of the newborn. *Vox Sang* **69**:120–125, 1995.
23. Report from nine collaborating laboratories. Results of tests with different cellular bioassays in relation to severity of RhD haemolytic disease. *Vox. Sang.* **60**:225–229, 1991.
24. Mollison PL, Engelfriet CP, Contreras M. *Blood Transfusion in clinical medicine*, 9th edn. Oxford: Blackwell Scientific Publications, 1993.
25. Contreras M, de Silva M. The prevention and management of haemolytic disease of the newborn. *J Roy Soc Med* **87**:256–258, 1994.
26. Bowman JM, Pollack JM. Transplacental fetal hemorrhage after amniocentesis. *Obstet Gynecol* **66**:749–755, 1985.
27. Blakemore KJ, Baumgarten A, Schoenfeld-Dimaio M, Hobbins JC, Mason EA, Mahoney MJ. Rise in maternal serum α-fetoprotein concentration after chorionic villus sampling and the possibility of isoimmunization. *Am J Obstet Gynecol* **155**:988–993, 1986.
28. Rodeck CH, Sheldrake A, Beattie B, Whittle MJ. Maternal serum alpha-fetoprotein after placental damage in chorionic villous sampling. *Lancet* **341**:500, 1993.
29. Nicolaides KH, Rodeck CH. Rhesus disease: the model for fetal therapy. *Br J Hos. Med.* **34**:141–148, 1985.
30. Huikeshoven FJ, Hope ID, Power GG, Gilbert RD, Longo LD. A comparison of sheep and human fetal oxygen delivery systems with the use of mathematical model. *Am J Obstet Gynecol* **151**:449–455, 1988.
31. Kirkinen P, Jouppila P, Eik-Nes S. Umbilical vein blood flow in rhesus-isoimmunization. *Br J Obstet Gynaecol* **90**:640–644, 1983.
32. Rightmire DA, Nicolaides KH, Rodeck CH, Campbell S. Midtrimester fetal blood velocities in Rh isoimmunisation: relationship to gestational age and to fetal haematocrit. *Obstet Gynecol* **68**:233–236, 1986.
33. Vyas S, Nicolaides KH, Campbell S. Doppler examination of the middle cerebral artery in anaemic fetuses. *Am J Obstet Gynecol* **162**:1066–1068, 1990.
34. Nicolaides KH, Thilaganathan B, Rodeck CH, Mibashan RS. Erythroblastosis and reticulocytosis in anemic fetuses. *Am J Obstet Gynecol* **159**:1063–1065, 1988.
35. Soothill PW, Nicolaides KH, Rodeck CH, Clewell WH, Lindridge J. Relationship of fetal hemoglobin and oxygen content to lactate concentration in Rh isoimmunized pregnancies. *Obstet Gynecol* **69**:268–270, 1987.
36. Rodeck CH, Santolaya J, Nicolini U. The fetus with immune hydrops. In *The unborn patient – prenatal diagnosis and treatment*, MR Harrison, MS Golbus, RA Filley (eds). Philadelphia: WB Saunders, 1991.
37. Nicolaides KH, Soothill PW, Clewell WH, Rodeck CH, Mibashan RS, Campbell S. Fetal haemoglobin measurement in the assessment of red cell isoimmunisation. *Lancet* **i**:1073–1075, 1988.
38. Nicolaides KH, Rodeck CH, Millar DS, Mibashan RS. Fetal haematology in rhesus isoimmunization. *Br Med J* **290**:661–663, 1985.
39. Nicolaides KH, Warenski JC, Rodeck CH. The relationship of fetal plasma protein concentration and hemoglobin level in the development of hydrops in rhesus isoimmunization. *Am J Obstet Gynecol* **152**:341–344, 1985.
40. Roberts A, Mitchell J, Pattison NS. Fetal liver length in normal and isoimmunized pregnancies. *Am J Obstet Gynecol* **161**: 42–46, 1989.
41. Nicolini U, Nicolaidis P, Tannirandorin Y, Fisk NM, Nasrat H, Rodeck CH. Fetal liver dysfunction in Rh alloimmunization. *Br J Obstet Gynaecol* **98**:287–293, 1991.
42. Bowman JM. The management of Rh isoimmunization. *Obstet Gynecol* **53**:1, 1978.
43. Soothill PW, Nicolaides KH, Rodeck CH. Effect of anaemia on fetal acid–base status. *Br J Obstet Gynaecol* **84**:880–883, 1987.
44. Robillard JE, Weiner CP. Atrial natriuretic factor in the human fetus – effect of volume expansion. *J Pediatr* **113**:552–555, 1988.
45. Nicolaides KH, Clewell WH, Rodeck CH. Measurement of fetoplacental blood volume in erythroblastosis fetalis. *Am J Obstet Gynecol* **157**:60, 1987.
46. Weiner CP, Pelzer GD, Heilskoy J, Wenstrom KD, Williamson RA. The effect of intravascular transfusion on umbilical venous pressure in anemic fetuses with and without hydrops. *Am J Obstet Gynecol* **161**:1498–1501, 1989.
47. Oepkes D, Vandenbussche FP, Van Bel F, Kanhai HH. Fetal ductus venosus blood flow velocities before and after transfusion in red-cell alloimmunized pregnancies. *Obstet Gynecol* **82**:237–241, 1993.
48. Blanchard D, Bloy C, Hermand P et al. Two-dimensional idopeptide mapping demonstrated that erythrocyte RhD, c, and E polypeptides are structurally homologous but nonidentical. *Blood* **72**:1424–1427, 1988.
49. Cherif-Zahar B, Mattei MG, Le Van Kim C, Bailly P, Cartron JP, Colin Y. Localization of the human Rh blood group gene structure to chromosome region 1p34–1p36 by *in situ* hybridization. *Hum Genet* **86**:398–400, 1991.
50. Colin Y, Cherif-Zahar B, Le Van Kim C, Raynal V, Van Huffel V, Cartron JP. Genetic basis of the RhD-positive and RhD-negative blood group polymorphism as determined by Southern analysis. *Blood* **78**:2747–2752, 1991.
51. Carritt B, Steers FJ, Avent ND. Prenatal determination of fetal RhD type. *N Engl J Med* **344**:205–206, 1994.
52. Lacey PA, Caskey CR, Werner DJ, Moulds JJ. Fatal haemolytic disease of the newborn due to anti-D in an Rh-positive Du variant mother. *Transfusion* **23**:91–94, 1983.
53. Bennett PR, Le Van Kim C, Colin Y et al. Prenatal determination of fetal RhD type by DNA amplification. *N Engl J Med* **329**:607–610, 1993.
54. Lighten A, Overton T, Sepulveda W, Warwick RM, Fisk NM, Bennett PR. Accuracy of prenatal determination of RhD type status by polymerase chain reaction using amniotic cell in RhD-negative women. *Am J Obstet Gynecol* **173**:1182–1185, 1995.
55. Rossiter JP, Blakemore KJ, Kickler TS et al. The use of polymerase chain reaction to determine fetal RhD status. *Am J Obstet Gynecol* **171**:1047–1051, 1994.
56. Spence WC, Maddalena A, Demers DB, Bick DP. Molecular analysis of the RhD genotype in fetuses at risk for RhD hemolytic disease. *Obstet Gynecol* **85**: 296–298, 1995.

57. Bowell PJ, Selinger M, Ferguson J, Giles J, MacKenzie IZ. Antenatal fetal blood sampling for the management of alloimmunized pregnancies: effect on maternal anti-D potency levels. *Br J Obstet Gynaecol* **95**:759–764, 1988.
58. Rodeck C, Tutschek B, Sherlock J, Kingdom J. Methods for the transcervical collection of fetal cells during the first trimester of pregnancy. *Prenat Diagn* **15**:933–942, 1995.
59. Adinolfi M, Sherlock J, Kemp T et al. Prenatal detection of fetal RhD DNA sequences in transcervical samples. *Lancet* **345**:318, 1995.
60. Thomas MR, Tutschek B, Frost A et al. The time of appearance and disappearance of fetal DNA from the maternal circulation. *Prenat Diagn* **15**:641–646, 1995.
61. Lo YMD, Corbetta N, Chamberlain PR, Sargent JL. Presence of fetal DNA in maternal plasma and serum. *Lancet* **350**: 485–487, 1997.
62. Lo YMD, Tein MSC, Lau TR et al. Quantitative analysis of fetal DNA in maternal plasma and serum – implications for non-invasive prenatal diagnosis. *Am J Hum Genet* **62**:768–775, 1998.
63. Bianchi DW. Fetal DNA in maternal plasma – the plot thickens and the placental barrier thing. *Am J Hum Genet* **62**:763–764, 1998.
64. Maron JL, Bianchi DW. Prenatal diagnosis, using cell-free nucleic acids in maternal body fluids – a decade of progress. *Am J Med Genet* **145**:5–17, 2007.
65. Finning K, Martin P, Daniels G. A clinical service in the UK to predict fetal Rh(Rhesus)D blood group using free fetal DNA in maternal plasma. *Ann NY Acad Sci* **1022**:119–123, 2004.
66. Finning K, Martin P, Soothill PW, Avent N. Prediction of fetal D status from maternal plasma – introduction of a new non-invasive fetal RHD genotyping service. *Transfusion* **42**:1079–1085, 2002.
67. Gautier E, Benachi A, Giovangrande Y et al. Fetal RhD genotyping by maternal serum analysis – a two year experience. *Am J Obstet Gynecol* **192**:666–669, 2005.
68. Van der Schoot CE, Soussam AA, Dee R, Bousel GJ, de Haas M. Screening for foetal RhD-genotype by plasma PCR in all D-negative pregnant women is feasible. *Vox Sang* **87**(suppl 3):S2–S16, 2004.
69. Geifman-Holtzman O, Grotegant C, Gaughan J. Diagnostic accuracy of non-invasive fetal Rh genotyping from maternal blood – a meta-analysis. *Am J Obstet Gynecol* **195**:1163–1173, 2006.
70. Daniels G, Finning K, Martin P, Soothill P. Fetal blood group genotyping from DNA from maternal plasma – an important advance in the management and prevention of haemolytic disease of the fetus and newborn. *Vox Sang* **87**:225–325, 2004.
71. Bianchi DW, Avent N, Costa JM, Van der Schoot CE. Non-invasive prenatal diagnosis of fetal rhesus D – ready for prime time. *Obstet Gynaecol* **106**:841–844, 2005.
72. Zimmermann BG, Holzgreve W, Avent N, Hahn S. Optimised real-time quantitative PCR measurement of male fetal DNA in maternal plasma. *Ann NY Acad Sci* **1075**:347–349, 2004.
73. Page-Christiaens GC, Bossers B, Van der Schoot CE, DE Haas M. Use of bi-allelic insertion/deletion polymorphisms as a positive control for fetal genotyping in maternal blood: first clinical experience. *Ann NY Acad Sci* **1075**:123–129, 2006.
74. Ding C, Chin RWK, Lan TK et al. MS analysis of single-nucleotide differences in circulating nucleic acids: application to noninvasive prenatal diagnosis. *Proc Natl Acad Sci* **101**(29):10762–10767, 2004.
75. Chim SSC, Tong YK, Chiu RWK et al. Detection of the placental epigenetic signature of the maspin gene in maternal plasma. *Proc Natl Acad Sci USA* **102**: 14753–14758, 2005.
76. Bowell PJ, Allen DL, Entwistle CC. Blood group antibody screening tests during pregnancy. *Br J Obstet Gynaecol* **93**: 1038–1043, 1986.
77. MacKenzie IZ, Selinger M, Bowell PJ. Management of red cell isoimmunization in the 1990s. In *Progress in obstetrics and gynaecology*, J Studd (ed.), vol. 9. Edinburgh: Churchill Livingstone, 1991.
78. Nicolaides KH, Rodeck CH. Maternal serum anti-D antibody concentration and assessment of rhesus isoimmunisation. *Br Med J* **304**:1155–1156, 1992.
79. Kozlowski CL, Lee D, Shwe KH, Love EM. Quantification of anti-c in haemolytic disease of the newborn. *Transfus Med* **5**:37–42, 1995.
80. Bowman JM, Pollock JM, Manning FA, Harman CR, Menticoglou S. Maternal Kell blood group alloimmunization. *Obstet Gynecol* **79**:239–244, 1992.
81. Noble AL, Poole GD, Anderson N, Lucas GF, Hadley AG. Predicting the severity of haemolytic disease of the newborn: an assessment of the clinical usefulness of the chemiluminescence test. *Br J Haematol* **90**:718–720, 1995.
82. Moise KJ, Perkins JT, Sosler SD et al. The predictive value of maternal serum testing for detection of fetal anemia in red blood cell alloimmunization. *Am J Obstet Gynecol* **172**:1003–1009, 1995.
83. Benacerraf BR, Frigoletto FD. Sonographic sign for the detection of early fetal ascites in the management of severe isoimmune disease without intrauterine transfusion. *Am J Obstet Gynecol* **152**:1039–1041, 1985.
84. Nicolaides KH, Fontanarosa M, Gabbe SG, Rodeck CH. Failure of ultrasonographic parameters to predict the severity of fetal anaemia in rhesus isoimmunization. *Am J Obstet Gynecol* **158**:920–926, 1988.
85. Vintzileos AM, Campbell WA, Storlazzi E, Mirochnick MH, Escoto DT, Nochimson DJ. Fetal liver ultrasound measurements in isoimmunized pregnancies. *Obstet Gynecol* **68**:162–167, 1986.
86. Roberts AB, Mitchell JM, Pattison NS. Fetal liver length in normal and isoimmunized pregnancies. *Am J Obstet Gynecol* **161**:42–46, 1989.
87. Oepkes D, Meerman RH, Vandenbussche FPHA, van Kamp IL, Kok FG, Kanhai HHH. Ultrasonographic fetal spleen measurements in red blood cell alloimmunized pregnancies. *Am J Obstet Gynecol* **169**:121–128, 1993.
88. Oepkes D. Ultrasonography and Doppler in the management of red cell alloimmunized pregnancies. MD thesis University of Leiden, 1993.
89. Fan FC, Chan RY, Schuessler GB, Chien S. Effects of heamatocrit variations on regional haemodynamics and oxygen transport in the dog. *Am J Physiol* **238**:H545–H552, 1980.
90. Nicolaides KH, Bilardo CM, Campbell S. Prediction of fetal anaemia by measurement of the mean blood velocities in the fetal aorta. *Am J Obstet Gynecol* **162**:209–212, 1990.
91. Oepkes D, Brand R, Vandenbussche FP, Meerman RH, Kanhai HHH. The use of ultrasonography and Doppler in the prediction of fetal haemolytic anaemia: a multivariant analysis. *Br J Obstet Gynaecol* **101**:680–684, 1994.
92. Hecher K, Snijders R, Campbell S, Nicolaides KH. Fetal venous, arterial and intracardiac blood flows in red cell isoimmunization. *Obstet Gynecol* **85**: 122–128, 1995.
93. Steiner H, Schaffer H, Spitzer D, Batka M, Graf AH, Staudach A. The relationship between peak velocity in the fetal descending aorta and hematocrit in rhesus isoimmunisation. *Obstet Gynecol* **85**:659–662, 1995.
94. Copel JA, Grannum PA, Green JJ. Fetal cardiac output in the isoimmunized pregnancy: a pulsed Doppler–echocardiographic study of patients undergoing intravascular transfusion. *Am J Obstet Gynecol* **161**:361–365, 1989.
95. Oepkes D, Vandenbussche FP, Van Bel F, Kanhai HHH. Fetal ductus venosus blood flow velocities before and after transfusion in red cell alloimmunized pregnancies. *Obstet Gynecol* **82**:237–241, 1993.
96. Mari G, Deter RL, Carpenter RL, et al. Non-invasive diagnosis by Doppler ultrasonography of fetal anaemia due to red call alloimmunisation. *N Eng J Med* **342**:9–14, 2000.
97. Imbar T, Lev-Sagie A, Cohen S, Yanai N, Yagal S. Diagnosis, surveillance and treatment of the anaemic fetus using middle cerebral artery peak systolic velocity measurement. A review. *Prenat Diagn* **26**:45–51, 2006.

98. Mari G, Andrignolo A, Abuhamad AZ et al. Diagnosis of fetal anaemia with Doppler ultrasound in the pregnancy complicated by maternal blood immunization. *Ultrasound Obstet Gynecol* 5:400–405, 1995.
99. Bullock R, Martin WL, Comerasamy A, Kilby MD. Prediction of fetal anaemia in pregnancies with red cell alloimmunisation – comparison of middle cerebral artery peak systolic velocity and amniotic fluid OD450. *Ultrasound Obstet Gynecol* **25**:331–334, 2005.
100. Pereira L, Jenkins TM, Berghella V. Conventional management of maternal red cell alloimmunisation compared with management by Doppler assessment of middle cerebral artery peak systolic velocity. *Am J Obstet Gynecol* **189**:1002–1006, 2003.
101. Zimmerman R, Durig P, Carpenter R et al. Longitudinal measurement of the peak systolic velocity in the fetal middle cerebral artery for monitoring pregnancies complicated by red cell alloimmunisation – a prospective multi-center trial with intention to treat. *Br J Obstet Gynaecol* **109**:746–752, 2002.
102. Gordon H. The diagnosis of hydrops fetalis. *Clin Obstet Gynecol* **14**:548–560, 1971.
103. Sadovsky E, Laufer N, Beyth Y. The role of fetal movements: assessment in cases of severe Rh immunized patients. *Acta Obstet Gynecol Scand* **58**:313–316, 1979.
104. Visser G. Antepartum sinusoidal and decelerative heart rate patterns in Rh disease. *Am J Obstet Gynecol* **143**: 538–544, 1982.
105. Nicolaides KH, Sadovsky G, Cetin E. Fetal heart rate patterns on red blood cell isoimmunized pregnancies. *Am J Obstet Gynecol* **161**:351–356, 1989.
106. Weiner CP. Human fetal bilirubin and fetal hemolytic disease. *Am J Obstet Gynecol* **116**:1449–1454, 1992.
107. Liley AW. Liquor amnii analysis in the management of the pregnancy complicated by rhesus sensitization. *Am J Obstet Gynecol* **82**:1359–1370, 1961.
108. Bowman JM, Pollock JM. Amniotic fluid spectrophotometry and early delivery in the management of erythroblastosis fetalis. *Pediatrics* **35**:815–820, 1965.
109. Pridmore BR, Robertson EG, Walker W. Liquor bilirubin levels and false prediction of severity in rhesus haemolytic disease. *Br Med J* **iii**:136–139, 1972.
110. Fairweather DVI, Whyley GA, Millar MD. Six years experience of the prediction of severity in rhesus haemolytic disease. *Br J Obstet Gynaecol* **83**:698–706, 1976.
111. MacKenzie IZ, Bowell PJ, Castle BM, Selinger M, Ferguson JF. Serial fetal blood sampling for the management of pregnancies complicated by severe rhesus(D) isoimmunization. *Br J Obstet Gynaecol* **95**:753–758, 1988.
112. Nicolaides KH, Rodeck CH, Mibashan RS, Kemp JR. Have Liley charts outlived their usefulness? *Am J Obstet Gynecol* **155**:90–94, 1986.
113. Queenan JT, Tomai TP, Ural SH, King JC. Deviation in the amniotic fluid optical density at a wave length of 450 nm in Rh-immunized pregnancies from 14–40 weeks gestation: a proposal for clinical management. *Am J Obstet Gynecol* **168**:1370–1376, 1993.
114. Whitfield CR. A three-year assessment of an action-line method of timing intervention in Rhesus isoimmunization. *Am J Obstet Gynecol* **108**:1239–1244, 1970.
115. Valenti C. Antenatal detection of haemoglobinopathies. A preliminary report. *Am J Obstet Gynecol* **115**: 851–853, 1973.
116. Rodeck CH, Campbell S. Sampling pure fetal blood by fetoscopy in second trimester of pregnancy. *Br J Med* **ii**: 728–730, 1978.
117. Daffos F, Capella-Pavlovsky M, Forestier F. A new procedure for fetal blood sampling *in utero*. *Prenat Diagn* **3**:271–274, 1983.
118. Nicolaides KH, Thilaganathan B, Mibashan RS. Cordocentesis in the investigation of fetal erythropoiesis. *Am J Obstet Gynecol* **161**:1197–2000, 1989.
119. Daffos F, Capella-Pavlovsky M, Forestier F. Fetal blood sampling during pregnancy with the use of a needle guided by ultrasound a study of 606 consecutive cases. *Am J Obstet Gynecol* **153**:655–660, 1985.
120. Weiner CP. Cordocentesis for diagnostic indications: two years' experience. *Obstet Gynecol* **70**:664–667, 1987.
121. Nicolini U, Kochenour NK, Greco P et al. Consequences of fetomaternal haemorrhage after intrauterine transfusion. *Br Med J* **297**:1379–1381, 1988.
122. Vaughan JI, Rodeck CH. Interventional procedures. In *Ultrasound in obstetrics and gynaecology*, K Dewbury, H Meire, D Cosgrove (eds). Edinburgh: Churchill Livingstone, 1993.
123. Freda VJ, Adamsons K. Exchange transfusion *in utero*. *Am J Obstet Gynecol* **89**:817–821, 1964.
124. Asensio SH, Figueroa-Longo JG, Pelegrina IA. Intrauterine exchange transfusion. *Am J Obstet Gynecol* **95**: 1129–1133, 1966.
125. Seelen J, Van Kessel H, Eskes T et al. A new method of exchange transfusion *in utero*. Cannulation of vessels on the fetal side of the human placenta. *Am J Obstet Gynecol* **95**:872–876, 1966.
126. Harman CR, Manning FA, Bowman JM, Lange IR. Severe Rh-disease – poor outcome is not inevitable. *Am J Obstet Gynecol* **145**:823–829, 1983.
127. Frigoletto FD, Umansky I, Birnholtz J et al. Intrauterine transfusion in 365 fetuses during 15 years. *Am J Obstet Gynecol* **139**:781–790, 1981.
128. Lewis M, Bowman JM, Pollock J, Lowen B. Absorption of red cells from the peritoneal cavity of an hydropic twin. *Transfusion* **13**:37–40, 1973.
129. Rodeck CH, Nicolaides KH, Warsof SL, Fysh WJ, Gamsu HR, Kemp JR. The management of severe rhesus isoimmunization by fetoscopic intravascular transfusions. *Am J Obstet Gynecol* **150**:769–774, 1984.
130. Bang J, Bock JE, Trolle D. Ultrasound-guided fetal intravascular transfusion for severe rhesus haemolytic disease. *Br Med J* **284**:373–374, 1982.
131. de Crespigny LC, Robinson HP, Quinn M, Doyle L, Ross A, Cauchi M. Ultrasound-guided fetal blood transfusion for severe rhesus isoimmunization. *Obstet Gynecol* **66**:529–532, 1985.
132. Nicolaides KH, Soothill PW, Rodeck CH, Clewell W. Rh disease: intravascular fetal blood transfusion by cordocentesis. *Fetal Ther* **1**:185–192, 1986.
133. Westgren M, Selbing A, Stangenberg M. Fetal intracardiac transfusions in patients with severe rhesus isoimmunization. *Br Med J* **298**:885–886, 1988.
134. Berkowitz RL, Chitkara U, Wilkins IA, Lynch L, Plosker H, Bernstein HH. Intravascular monitoring and management of erythroblastosis fetalis. *Am J Obstet Gynecol* **158**: 783–795, 1988.
135. Sampson AJ, Permezel M, Doyle LW, de Crespigny L, Ngu A, Robinson H. Ultrasound-guided fetal intravascular transfusions for severe eythroblastosis, 1984–1993. *Aust NZ J Obstet Gynecol* **34**(2):125–130, 1994.
136. Poissonnier HM, Brossard Y, Demedeiros N et al. Two hundred intrauterine exchange transfusions in severe blood incompatibilities. *Am J Obstet Gynecol* **161**:709–713, 1989.
137. Weiner CP, Williamson RA, Wenstrom KD et al. Management of fetal hemolytic disease by cordocentesis. II. Outcome of treatment. *Am J Obstet Gynecol* **165**:1302–1307, 1991.
138. Nicolini U, Santolaya J, Fisk NM et al. Changes in fetal acid–base status during intravascular transfusion. *Arch Dis Childh* **63**:710–714, 1988.
139. Soothill PW, Nicolaides KH, Rodeck CH, Bellingham AJ. The effect of replacing fetal with adult haemoglobin on blood gas and acid/base parameters in human fetuses. *Am J Obstet Gynecol* **158**:66–69, 1988.
140. Welch CR, Talbert DG, Warwick RM, Letsky EA, Rodeck CH. Needle modifications for invasive fetal procedures. *Obstet Gynecol* **85**: 113–117, 1995.
141. Moise KJ, Deter RL, Kirshon B, Karolina A, Patton DE, Carpenter RJ.

Intravenous pancuronium bromide for fetal neuromuscular blockade during intravascular transfusion for red-cell alloimmunization. *Obstet Gynecol* **74**:905–908, 1989.

142. de Crespigny LC, Robinson HP, Ross AW, Quinn M. Curarisation of fetus for intrauterine procedures. *Lancet* **i**:1164, 1985.
143. Ronkin S, Chayen B, Wapner RJ et al. Intravascular exchange and bolus transfusion in the severely isoimmunized fetus. *Am J Obstet Gynecol* **160**:407–411, 1989.
144. Hallak M, Moise KJ, Hesketh DE, Cano LE, Carpenter RJ. Intravascular transfusion of fetuses with rhesus incompatibility: prediction of fetal outcome by changes in umbilical venous pressure. *Obstet Gynecol* **80**:286–290, 1992.
145. Nicolini U, Rodeck CH. A proposed scheme for planning intrauterine transfusion in patients with severe Rh-immunization. *J Obstet Gynecol* **9**:162–163, 1988.
146. Nicolini U, Talbert DG, Fisk NM, Rodeck CH. Pathophysiology of pressure changes during intrauterine transfusion. *Am J Obstet Gynecol* **160**:1139–1145, 1989.
147. Welch R, Rampling MW, Anwar A, Talbert DG, Rodeck CH. Changes in hemorheology with fetal intravascular transfusion. *Am J Obstet Gynecol* **170**:726–732, 1994.
148. Radunovic N, Lockwood CJ, Alvarez M, Plecas D, Chitkara U, Berkowitz RL. The severely anaemic and hydropic isoimmune fetus: changes in fetal haematocrit associated with intrauterine death. *Obstet Gynecol* **79**:390–393, 1992.
149. Nicolini U, Kochenour NK, Greco P, Letsky E, Rodeck CH. When to perform the next intra-uterine transfusion in patients with Rh allo-immunization: combined intravascular and intraperitoneal transfusion allows longer intervals. *Fetal Therapy* **4**:14–20, 1989.
150. Harman CR, Bowman JM, Manning FA, Menticoglou SM. Intrauterine transfusion – intraperitoneal versus intravascular approach: a case control comparison. *Am J Obstet Gynecol* **162**:1053–1059, 1990.
151. Spencer JAD, Ryan G, Ronderos-Dumit D, Nicolini U, Rodeck CH. The effect of neuromuscular blockade on human fetal heart rate and its variation. *Br J Obstet Gynaecol* **101**:121–124, 1994.
152. Scaradavou A, Inglis S, Peterson P, Dunne J, Chervenak F, Bussel J. Suppression of erythropoiesis by intrauterine transfusions in hemolytic disease of the newborn: use of erythropoietin to treat the late anaemia. *J Pediatr* **123**:279–284, 1993.
153. Roberts A, Grannum P, Belanger K, Pattison N, Hobbins J. Fetal growth and birthweight in isoimmunized pregnancies after intravenous intrauterine transfusion. *Fetal Diagn Ther* **8**:407–411, 1993.
154. Doyle LW, Kelley EA, Rickards AJ, Ford GW, Callanan C. Sensorineural outcome at 2 years for survivors of erythroblastosis treated with fetal intravascular transfusions. *Obstet Gynecol* **81**:931–935, 1993.
155. Harper DC, Swingle HM, Weiner CP, Borthius DJ, Ryleward GP, Widness JA. Long-term neurodevelopmental outcome and brain volumes of this treatment for hydrops fetalis by in vitro intravascular transfusion. *Am J Obstet Gynecol Med* **195**:192–200, 2006.
156. Nasrat HA, Nicolini U, Nicolaidis P, Letsky EA, Gau G, Rodeck CH. The effect of intrauterine intravascular blood transfusion on iron metabolism in fetuses with Rh alloimmunization. *Obstet Gynecol* **77**:558–562, 1991.
157. Lasker MR, Eddleman K, Toor AH. Neonatal hepatitis and excessive hepatic iron deposition following intrauterine blood transfusion. *Am J Perinatol* **12**: 14–17, 1995.
158. Harman CR, Biehl DR, Pollock JM. Intrauterine transfusion: kinetics of absorption of donor cells in fetal lambs. *Am J Obstet Gynecol* **145**:830–836, 1983.
159. Nicolini U, Nicolaidis P, Fisk NM, Tannirandorn Y, Rodeck CH. Fetal blood sampling from the intrahepatic vein: analysis of safety and clinical experience with 214 procedures. *Obstet Gynecol* **76**:47–53, 1990.
160. Graham-Pole J, Barr W, Willoughby ML. Continuous-flow plasmapheresis in management of severe rhesus disease. *Br J Med* **i**:1185–1188, 1977.
161. Erkkola R, Ekblad U, Piiroinen O et al. Plasma exchange and intrauterine transfusion in the management of severe rhesus isoimmunization. *Int J Feto-Maternal Med* **2**:11–14, 1989.
162. Chitkara U, Bussel J, Alvarez M, Lynch L, Meisel RL, Berkowitz RL. High dose gamma globulin: does it have a role in the treatment of severe erythroblastosis fetalis? *Obstet Gynecol* **76**:703–708, 1990.
163. Margulies M, Voto LS, Mathet E, Margulies M. High dose intravenous IgG for the treatment of severe Rhesus alloimmunization. *Vox Sang* **61**:181–189, 1991.
164. Charles AG, Blumenthal LS. Promethazine hydrochloride therapy in severely Rh-sensitised pregnancies. *Obstet Gynecol* **60**:627–630, 1982.
165. Goodrick MJ, Hadley AG, Poole G. Haemolytic disease of the fetus and newborn due to anti-Fy[a] and the potential clinical value of Duffy genotyping in pregnancies at risk. *Transfus Med* **7**:301–304, 1997.
166. Fillbey D, Hanson U, Wesstrom G. The prevalence of red cell antibodies in pregnancy correlated to the outcome of the newborn: a 12 year study in central Sweden. *Acta Obstet Gynaecol Scand* **74**:686–692, 1995.
167. van Dijk BA, Dororen MC, Overbeeke MA. Red cell antibodies in pregnancy: there is no 'critical' titre. *Transfus Med* **5**:199–202, 1995.
168. Kozlowski CL, Lee D, Shwe KH, Love EM. Quantification of anti-c in haemolytic disease of the newborn. *Transfus Med* **5**:37–42, 1995.
169. Tovey LAD. Haemolytic disease of the new born – the changing scene. *Br J Obstet Gynaecol* **93**:960–966, 1986.
170. Copel JA, Scioscia A, Grannum PA et al. Percutaneous umbilical blood sampling in the management of Kell immunisation. *Obstet Gynecol* **67**: 288–290, 1986.
171. Leggat HM, Gibson JM, Barron SL, Reid MM. Anti-Kell in pregnancy. *Br J Obstet Gynaecol* **98**:162–165, 1991.
172. Vaughan JL, Warwick R, Letsky E, Nicolini U, Rodeck CH, Fisk NM. Erythropoietic suppression in fetal anaemia because of Kell alloimmunisation. *Am J Obstet Gynecol* **171**:247–252, 1995.
173. Linch DC, Rodeck CH, Nicolaides KH, Jones HM, Brent L. Attempted bone marrow transplantation in a 17 week fetus. *Lancet* **i**:1402–1405, 1986.

CHAPTER

41 Fetal platelet disorders

Leendert Porcelijn, Eline SA van den Akker and Humphrey HH Kanhai

KEY POINTS

- Thrombocytopenia of the fetus/newborn may lead to intracranial hemorrhage (ICH), resulting in severe morbidity or death
- Frequent causes of fetal thrombocytopenia are either caused by autoimmune thrombocytopenia (ITP) or alloimmunization of the mother (FNAIT)
- ITP:
  - Leads to severe neonatal thrombocytopenia in approximately 20% of the cases
  - Fetal bleed in ITP is not documented
  - Platelet counts of a second newborn correlate well with that of the sibling
  - Cesarean section is recommended only for obstetric reason
- FNAIT:
  - ≥50% of ICH occur in utero
  - as in ITP, serological tests are not sensitive enough to predict the severity of fetal thrombocytopenia
  - although fetal blood sampling is reliable for diagnosis of thrombocytopenia, its routine use is discouraged because the high risk of iatrogenic morbidity and pregnancy loss
  - weekly high-dose intravenous immunoglobulins to the mother is effective for preventing ICH in the fetus and newborn in a substantial proportion of cases
  - the management of FNAIT should be undertaken in or in collaboration with an experienced center

INTRODUCTION

Fetal thrombocytopenia is both a rare and potentially devastating condition. In contrast to thrombocytopenia in newborns, the exact frequency of the condition in fetuses is unknown. The incidence of thrombocytopenia ($<150 \times 10^9$/l) in all newborns is 1–4%. However, due to absence of clinical signs, it is often not noted. Thrombocytopenia with an immunological origin is encountered[1–5] in 0.3% of the newborns.

Most patients at risk of a fetal platelet disorder are identified only after a baby is born with a low platelet count. In order to institute proper management in the next pregnancy, it is vital to identify the cause of the thrombocytopenia.

NON-IMMUNE CAUSES FOR FETAL/NEONATAL THROMBOCYTOPENIA

Although the mechanism of fetal/neonatal thrombocytopenia is often unclear it seems that impaired megakaryocytopoiesis is a major cause[6].

Non-immune pathological conditions associated with fetal/neonatal thrombocytopenia include preterm birth, severe intrauterine growth restriction, asphyxia, congenital malformations (TAR syndrome, trisomy 21), congenital infection and rare cases of amegakaryocytosis or Bernard Soulier syndrome (thrombasthenia caused by congenital glycoprotein Ib/V/IX deficiency resulting in thrombocytopenia and giant platelets) (Table 41.1).

Table 41.1 **Causes of fetal and early neonatal (<72h old) thrombocytopenia**

Alloimmune thrombocytopenia
Congenital infections (CMV, syphilis, parvovirus, toxoplasmosis, rubella, HIV)
Maternal autoimmune diseases (ITP, SLE)
Severe fetal hemolytic disease due to red cell alloimmunization
Placental insufficiency (pre-eclampsia, IUGR, diabetes)
Asphyxia
Perinatal infection (GBS, *E. coli*, *Listeria*)
Disseminated intravascular coagulation (DIC)
Thrombosis (renal vein, aortic)
Congenital syndromes (TAR, Wiskott-Aldrich, Kasabach-Meritt, Amegakaryocytosis, trisomy 13, 18, 21, triploidy)
Metabolic disorder
Hepatomegaly/splenomegaly

CMV = Cytomegalovirus; ITP = idiopathic thrombocytopenic purpura; SLE = systemic lupus erythematosus; TAR = thrombocytopenia with absent radii; IUGR = intrauterine growth restriction; GBS = group B streptococcus; DIC = disseminated intravascular coagulation

In this chapter, immune thrombocytopenia, being the most frequent cause of fetal platelet disorders, will be discussed. Since severely affected fetuses are predominantly born to mothers with alloimmune platelet antibodies[2], this condition will be described in greater detail.

IMMUNE CAUSES FOR FETAL/NEONATAL THROMBOCYTOPENIA

Fetal or neonatal alloimmune thrombocytopenia (FNAIT) (also known as alloimmune thrombocytopenia (AITP) or neonatal alloimmune thrombocytopenia [NAIT]) and autoimmune thrombocytopenia (also known as idiopathic thrombocytopenic purpura (ITP), isoimmune thrombocytopenia (ITP) or Morbus Werlhoff) are immune-mediated thrombocytopenias. Also, a small proportion of cases with severe red blood cell alloimmunization are associated with thrombocytopenia in the fetus/newborn. In these cases, the mechanism causing thrombocytopenia is not known.

In the last 15 years, the knowledge about several aspects of immune-mediated thrombocytopenia has grown substantially. The value of the different tests for each disorder has become clear and thus resolving most of the serological problems. The molecular genetics and the exact position on the glycoproteins of most of the important antigens are known (Table 41.2).

AUTOIMMUNE OR IDIOPATHIC THROMBOCYTOPENIA (ITP)

ITP in the mother is defined as thrombocytopenic purpura without responsible exogenous factors or causal disorders. Two different forms of ITP can be distinguished: the acute and the chronic form. Acute ITP is mainly a disorder of children and can be described as a cross-reactivity between viral antigens and platelet antigens. It is mostly preceded by a symptomatic viral infection, with a higher incidence in the autumn and winter. The thrombocytopenia in the acute form resolves within weeks or months, but can last for as long as one year. Chronic ITP is an autoimmune disorder, mostly seen in adults, without any seasonal preference, with an incidence of 1–10/100 000[7–9]. The symptoms are variable, from purpura and mucosal bleedings to being non-existent. Severe bleedings are rare. As ITP is relatively common in women of childbearing age, it is frequently found by routine testing during pregnancy (0.14%) and accounts for 3% of cases of maternal thrombocytopenia at delivery[10].

ITP is an autoimmune process, which means that the patient (the mother) produces antibodies against platelet surface glycoproteins. The disease can occur in isolation or associated with other organ-specific or generalized autoimmune disorders. With the development of antibody detection methods, the idiopathic aspect of this disorder could be replaced by autoantibody mediated platelet destruction disorder for the majority (approximately 70%, see below) of cases. In the large majority of the chronic ITP patients, the autoantibodies are of the IgG class[11]. Most antibodies are bound to platelets, whereas in a minority of patients free circulating antibodies are also detectable.

Natural history

In 95% of pregnant women, the platelet count is between 100 and $150 \times 10^9/l$[2,12]. Thrombocytopenia below $100 \times 10^9/l$ occurs in 1–2% of pregnant women[2]. The most common cause is gestational thrombocytopenia, which has an overall frequency of 5–8%. Also pre-eclampsia, HIV (human immunodeficiency virus), or rarer causes, such as von Willebrand's disease type IIB[13] and underlying systemic diseases such as systemic lupus erythematosus (SLE), antiphospholipid syndrome, thyroid dysfunction and hematological disease can cause maternal thrombocytopenia during gestation but do not cause fetal/neonatal thrombocytopenia and must be excluded.

ITP is more a problem for the mothers than for the fetuses. The clinical symptoms in ITP mothers can vary from none or slight to severe hemorrhagic diathesis. Hemorrhage due to thrombocytopenia is unlikely if the platelet count is $>50 \times 10^9/l$[14]. Severe maternal thrombocytopenia ($<30 \times 10^9/l$) is a risk for spontaneous bleeding antenatally as well as at delivery and requires treatment. A platelet count $>80 \times 109/l$ is usually considered to be safe to perform epidural analgesia[15,16].

ITP in pregnancy may cause neonatal thrombocytopenia. The antibodies, mostly of the IgG class, can pass the placenta, bind to the fetal platelets and cause fetal thrombocytopenia. The reported incidence of severe neonatal thrombocytopenia ($<50 \times 10^9/l$) in ITP mothers varies between 10 and 30%[14,17]. The nadir of the platelet count in the affected newborn mostly occurs within 7 days after birth[18]. Unfortunately, there are no reliable predictive parameters for the severity of the neonatal thrombocytopenia caused by the maternal platelet autoantibodies. No correlation exists between the platelet count in the mother and in her child. Also the platelet-associated immunoglobulin G level does not predict the fetal platelet count[19,20]. A maternal history of splenectomy may be associated with

Table 41.2 **Human platelet antigens**[66]

System	*Antigen*	*Original names*	*Glycoprotein*	*Nucleotide change*	*Amino acid change*	*CD*
HPA-1	HPA-1a	Zw^a, Pl^{A1}	GPIIIa	T176	Leu_{33}	CD61
	HPA-1b	Zw^b, Pl^{A2}		C176	Pro_{33}	
HPA-2	HPA-2a	Ko^b	GPIbα	C482	Thr_{145}	CD42b
	HPA-2b	Ko^a, Sib^a		T482	Met_{145}	
HPA-3	HPA-3a	Bak^a, Lek^a	GPIIb	T2621	Ile_{843}	CD41
	HPA-3b	Bak^b		G2621	Ser_{843}	
HPA-4	HPA-4a	Yuk^b, Pen^a	GPIIIa	G506	Arg_{143}	CD61
	HPA-4b	Yuk^a, Pen^b		A506	Gln_{143}	
HPA-5	HPA-5a	Br^b, Zav^b	GPIa	G1600	Glu_{505}	CD49b
	HPA-5b	Br^a, Zav^a, Hc^a		A1600	Lys_{505}	
	HPA-6bw	Ca^a, Tu^a	GPIIIa	1544G > A	Gln489Arg	CD61
	HPA-7bw	Mo^a	GPIIIa	1297C > G	Ala407Pro	CD61
	HPA-8bw	Sr^a	GPIIIa	1984C > T	Cys636Arg	CD61
	HPA-9bw	Max^a	GPIIb	2602G > A	Met837Val	CD41
	HPA-10bw	La^a	GPIIIa	263G > A	Gln62Arg	CD61
	HPA-11bw	Gro^a	GPIIIa	1976G > A	His633Arg	CD61
	HPA-12bw	Iy^a	GPIbβ	119G > A	Glu15Gly	CD42c
	HPA-13bw	Sit^a	GPIa	2483C > T	Met799Thr	CD49b
	HPA-14bw	Oe^a	GPIIIa	1909_1911 Del AAG	Del Lys_{611}	CD61
HPA-15	HPA-15a	Gov^b	CD109	C2108	Ser_{703}	CD109
	HPA-15b	Gov^a		A2108	Tyr_{703}	
	HPA-16bw	Duv^a	GPIIIa	497C > T	Thr140Ile	CD61
		Va^a	GPIIb/IIIa			
		Mou^a	Unknown			

a low newborn platelet count[16,20,21]. There is one report that a specific maternal HLA type (DRB3*) is protective for the occurrence of thrombocytopenia in the newborn[22]. The strongest correlation found so far is with both the early and nadir neonatal platelet counts of the newborns with those of the prior siblings[14,18]. In the neonate, the clinical symptoms can vary from slight to severe hemorrhagic diathesis. The reported incidence of intracranial hemorrhage in the newborn is low and varies between 0 and 1.2%[2,23,24]. In reviews of large series of patients no cases of severe in utero bleeding have been documented[18,25].

Diagnosis

The diagnostic evaluation of ITP, based principally on medical history, physical examination and investigation of the peripheral blood is based on the exclusion of other causes of thrombocytopenia[21]. Along with thrombocytopenia, an elevated mean platelet volume as a sign of increased platelet production can be present. Normal or elevated megakaryocytic numbers are found in the bone marrow. It is possible to distinguish platelet production disorders from platelet destruction disorders, by measuring the plasma thrombopoietin (TPO) level in the thrombocytopenic patient. TPO levels in ITP patients are normal or only slightly elevated, contrasting with the elevated levels in patients with platelet production disorders[26–29].

Unfortunately, the sensitivity of the available serological techniques for the detection of platelet autoantibodies is not very high. The platelet immunofluorescence test (PIFT) based on the detection of platelet-bound antibodies on whole platelets is one of the first techniques used with a sensitivity for ITP patients of 70%[11,30,31]. A positive reaction in the PIFT is defined as being >1000 molecules of IgG bound to a platelet, whereas >450 molecules of IgG bound can already cause platelet destruction. ITP without detectable platelet autoantibodies can also be due to a T-cell-mediated destruction mechanism without antibodies present. Olsson et al. recently found platelet lysis by T cells from patients with active ITP[32]. It might well be that, in some patients, T-cell-mediated platelet destruction is the main mechanism explaining a percentage of patients without measurable platelet autoantibodies. This, of course, is important for the diagnosis and management of ITP patients, but the consequences for the neonate are probably limited as it is the IgG fraction that crosses the placenta causing neonatal thrombocytopenia. The specificity of the PIFT is low[33]. Probably the binding of immune complexes and the presence of anti-HLA antibodies are the main reasons for the low specificity of the PIFT.

In cases sent in for serological evaluation of FNAIT, we perform a direct PIFT to detect maternal platelet-bound autoantibodies, an indirect PIFT to detect antibodies in the serum and we make an eluate to rule out false-positive reactions due to the binding of immune complexes. When testing the eluate in the indirect PIFT with fixated donor platelets, immune complexes are not able to bind. To differentiate platelet autoantibodies from anti-HLA antibodies we use chloroquine-treated donor platelets. With chloroquine treatment, the β_2-microglobulin part of the HLA antigens is removed, causing the 44-kDa band (carrying all HLA-class I antigens) to unfold and so preventing the binding of anti-HLA antibodies.

Platelet autoantibodies are mostly directed against the glycoproteins (GP) IIb/IIIa, Ib/IX and V[34–37]. Therefore, more recent techniques are platelet glycoprotein-specific assays, modeled on the monoclonal antibody immobilization of platelet antigens assay (MAIPA)[38–40]. The specificity of these techniques seems to be higher, 80–90% but at the expense of a lower sensitivity, 40–70%[41–45]. Other antibody specificities than the glycoproteins tested or inhibition of antibody binding by MoAb binding on the same epitope might be part of the reason for this low sensitivity.

Management

ITP is not a reason to discourage pregnancy, except for those women with severe thrombocytopenia despite high doses of corticosteroids and after splenectomy. It is wise to evaluate the degree of ITP and optimize treatment before planning pregnancy in order to be able to recognize the need for splenectomy before pregnancy. Although pregnancy seems not to influence the natural course of ITP, the platelet counts in pregnant women with ITP tend to decrease, reaching their nadir during the third trimester[2].

For pregnant patients with severe thrombocytopenia, corticosteroids are the first-choice therapy. In the rare cases resistant to corticosteroid therapy, intravenous immunoglobulins, plasmapheresis or even splenectomy may be considered. A maternal platelet count above 30×10^9/l , in the absence of spontaneous bleeding, is considered safe for vaginal delivery[46]. A platelet count of the mother $>50 \times 10^9$/l is considered safe for both vaginal and cesarean delivery. A platelet count $>80 \times 10^9$/l is recommended if epidural anesthesia is planned[15,16]. Platelet transfusions are given to ITP mothers with very low platelet counts ($<20 \times 10^9$/l) and at risk for major hemorrhages (e.g. during parturition). There is no evidence that maternal therapy with, for example, corticosteroids or immunoglobulins leads to an increase of the fetal/neonatal platelet count.

Initially, the management of labor and delivery in ITP patients was based on the fear of intracranial hemorrhage (ICH) in the thrombocytopenic neonate, secondary to vaginal birth trauma. Therefore cesarean delivery was preferred when the fetus was found to have a platelet count of $<50 \times 10^9$/l following fetal scalp blood sampling or cordocentesis. Fetal scalp or breech blood sampling during labor is cumbersome for the woman and appeared to yield falsely low counts in a substantial proportion of cases[47]. Predelivery cordocentesis produces a reliable fetal platelet count but has a significant risk of fetal loss and severe morbidity. In addition, platelet counts may decrease in the time interval between cordocentesis and delivery[25]. These arguments, in combination with the low incidence of perinatal bleeding and the fact that the route of delivery (vaginal or cesarean section) does not seem to affect the incidence of ICH[48], lead to the following recommendations for management in pregnancy, predelivery and during delivery (Fig. 41.1). Fetal blood sampling by either scalp puncture or cordocentesis is not indicated as a routine procedure in ITP patients. Nowadays, it is widely accepted that cesarean section in ITP patients should only be performed for obstetric indications.

FETAL AND NEONATAL ALLOIMMUNE THROMBOCYTOPENIA (FNAIT)

Fetal and neonatal alloimmune thrombocytopenia occurring in approximately 1:1500 random fetuses/newborns[49–55] is the result of a disease process in which the mother produces an antibody-mediated response against a platelet-specific antigen present on the fetal but not on her own platelets. In the last decades, advances in immunology, molecular biology, fetal ultrasound and fetal therapy, have resulted in substantial progress in the diagnosis and management of FNAIT.

Platelet alloantigens

The identified platelet-specific alloantigens are located on the glycoprotein structures IIb/IIIa, Ib/IX, Ia/IIa and CD109 on the platelet membrane (see Table 41.2). These glycoproteins play an important role in platelet adhesion and aggregation by serving as receptors for specific ligands (Table 41.3).

Platelets also share antigens with other blood cells such as the human leukocyte antigens (HLA)-A, -B and -C and the red cell antigens, ABH, Lewis, I, i and P[56–61]. The presence of human leukocyte antigens (HLA class I) on platelets is partly due to adsorption of HLA antigens from plasma. Although some of the red cell antigens and most of the HLA class antigens can evoke an alloantibody response, their role in FNAIT is controversial. HLA antibodies are not believed to enter the fetal circulation because they are adsorbed onto placental tissues[62–65]. A severe fetal-maternal ABO immunization with high levels of IgG anti-A or anti-B is known to cause not only fetal/neonatal red blood cell destruction but also platelet destruction, depending on the anti-A or -B IgG titer and the A- or B-antigen expression on the fetal/neonatal red blood cells and platelets.

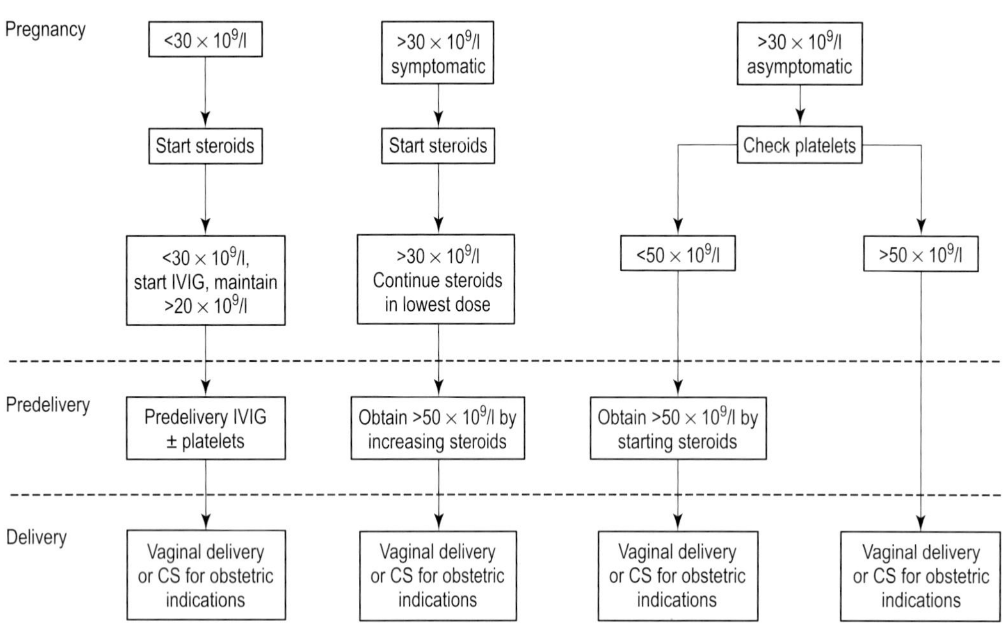

Fig. 41.1 ITP: Recommendations for management in pregnancy and during delivery, depending on maternal platelet count. (CS-cesarean section.)

Table 41.3 **Platelet membrane adhesive glycoproteins**

Family/ subfamily	*Member*	*CD*	*Ligands*
Integrins VLA	GPIa/IIa (VLA-2, α_2, β_1)	CD49b/29	Col
	GPIc/IIa (VLA-5, α_5 β_1)	CD49e/29	Fn
	GPIc′ IIa (VLA-6, α_6 β_1)	CD49f/29	Lm
Cytoadhesion	GPIIb/IIIa (αIIbβ_3)	CD41/61	Fb, Fn, vWF, Vn
	VNR ($\alpha^V\beta_3$)	CD51/61	Fb, Fn, vWF, Vn, Tsp
Leucine-rich glycoproteins	GPIbα	CD42b	vWF
	GPIbβ	CD42a	
	GPIX	CD42c	
	GP V	CD42d	

CD = cluster designation; Col = collagen; Lm = laminin; Fb = fibrinogen; Fn = fibronectin; GP = glycoprotein; Tsp = thrombospondin; VLA = very late antigen; Vn = vitronectin; VNR = vitronectin receptor; vWF = von Willebrand factor

The specific human platelet antigens (HPA) defined so far are all known to be able to cause FNAIT and are shown in Table 41.2. This table lists also the glycoproteins (GP) upon which the antigens are located, the position of the genetic single nucleotide polymorphism and the amino acid change[66]. For example, as first described in 1989 by Newman et al.[67], a polymorphism (T ↔ C) at base 176 of platelet GPIIIa DNA resulted in an amino acid change leucine ↔ proline on amino acid position 33, which is responsible for the HPA-1a or HPA-1b phenotype. More information about HPA genetics and allele frequencies can be found on www.ebi.ac.uk/ipd/hpa.

Although it was originally thought that these specific antigens could only be found on platelets and platelet precursors, it is shown that the GPIIIa structures, with the alloantigen systems HPA-1 and HPA-4, are also expressed by endothelial cells, vascular smooth muscle cells and foreskin fibroblasts and that the GPIa/IIa structures with HPA-5 are also expressed on endothelial cells and activated T lymphocytes[68–72]. The proportion of individuals belonging to a particular platelet antigen type varies according to the race involved. Some of these differences in frequencies of HPA alloantigens in different populations are shown in Table 41.4[73–78]. Remarkable differences in antigen frequencies for the different populations may be found. First, Caucasians, compared to other populations, have a relatively low (97.9%) frequency of the HPA-1a antigen. In Caucasians FNAIT is mostly caused by alloimmunization against HPA-1a[79–81] (Table 41.5).

A second important difference is the relatively high number of Orientals that are positive for the HPA-4b antigen and low number that are negative for HPA-1a. Because of this, FNAIT in the Oriental populations is less often caused by alloimmunization against HPA-1a and more often by alloimmunization against HPA-4b. HPA-4b is not found in Caucasians.

Nomenclature

Several different names for platelet alloantigen systems have been proposed in the past. The first platelet antigen system, which was discovered in 1959 by Van Loghem et al.[82], was named Zw after the two first letters of the patient's family name. Zw^a was discovered first and later the allelic antigen Zw.^{b} In 1964, Shulman et al.[83] described PL^{A1}, which appeared to be identical to Zw^a. They proposed to change the symbol Zw into PL, a more uniform platelet antigen symbol. Thus the two alleles were named PL^{A1} and PL^{A2}, a nomenclature still often used by Americans. The International Platelet Antigen Working Party suggested another nomenclature[84]. In Table 41.2, this nomenclature of the human platelet alloantigens (HPA) is depicted together with the alternative nomenclature.

Table 41.4 **Human platelet alloantigen frequencies**

Antigens	*Percentage frequency*				
	Caucasians	*Japanese*	*Koreans*	*Blacks*	*Chinese Han*
HPA-1a	97.9	>99.9	99.5	99.9	>99.9
HPA-1b	28.6	3.7	2.0	16.0	1.2
HPA-2a	>99.9	n.t.	99.0	97.0	99.9
HPA-2b	13.2	25.4	14.0	33.0	9.6
HPA-3a	80.9	78.9	82.5	85.0	83.1
HPA-3b	69.8	70.7	71.5	60.0	64.2
HPA-4a	>99.9	99.9	>99.9	100.0	>99.9
HPA-4b	0.0	1.7	2.0	0.0	0.9
HPA-5a	99.0	n.t.	>99.9	96.0	99.9
HPA-5b	19.7	n.t.	4.5	38.0	2.7

n.t. = not tested

Table 41.5 **Antibodies involved in FNAIT in Caucasians**

Authors	*Number of patients*	*Antibodies detected*
Mueller-Eckhardt et al. (1989)[80]	106	90% anti HPA-1a 8% anti HPA-5b 0.8% anti HPA-1b 0.8% anti HPA-3a 0.8% combination anti HPA-1a + 5b 0.8% anti B
Porcelijn et al. (2004)[81]	217	73.7% anti HPA-1a 1.4% anti HPA-1b 4.6% anti HPA-3a 0.9% anti HPA-5a 14.7% anti HPA-5b 0.5% anti HPA-15a 0.5% anti HPA-15b 1.5% anti Priv.Ag 2.8% anti A or anti B
Davoren et al. (2004)[79]	1162	79% anti HPA-1a 4% anti HPA-1b 0.1% anti HPA-2b 2% anti HPA-3a 0.8% anti HPA-3b 0.1% anti HPA-4a 0.1% anti HPA-4b 1% anti HPA-5a 9% anti HPA-5b 0.1% anti HPA-6bw 3.1% combinations (most HPA-1a + 5b) 0.4% anti GPIV (CD36)

The present nomenclature is based on the chronological numbering of alloantibodies in the order of their discovery. The letters 'a' or 'b' are assigned to the high-frequency and low-frequency allele respectively. A 'W' is used to mark an HPA system of which only one allele has been identified so far. Until now, 12 HPA antigens belonging to one of the six HPA systems (HPA systems 1, 2, 3, 4, 5 and 15), 10 low-frequency antigens assigned an HPA number and two (Va^a and Mou^a) antigens of which the genetic basis has not yet been determined are known (see Table 41.2)[66].

Platelet alloantibodies

The immune response to alloantigens is mediated by HLA class II molecules. Antigen-presenting cells (APC) such as dendritic cells, macrophages and B lymphocytes, process the antigens into small peptides, which are presented by the HLA-class-II antigens on their surface. CD4-positive T-helper lymphocytes can recognize the peptide–HLA complex, leading to the activation of the T cell. Activated T cells then interact with B lymphocytes, initiating antibody production[85–89].

About 10% of HPA-1a negative women develop anti-HPA-1a antibodies[49,50,52–54,55,90].

This is associated with certain HLA antigens. The strongest association is with HLA DR52a (DRB3*0101 in the most recent nomenclature). At least 80% of mothers who developed anti-HPA-1a antibodies were HLA DR52a positive[91–97]. HLA-B8 and HLA-DR3 are also positively correlated with the development of anti-HPA-1a antibodies[63,92,96,98–101]. Of interest is that in (rare) cases of HPA-1b alloimmunization, no particular HLA type seems to be involved. Thus, HLA restriction seems to play a role in enhancement of the immune response.

Since 1953, when Harrington et al.[102] suggested an alloimmune etiology for FNAIT and 1959 when Van Loghem et al.[82] described the first case together with the Zw system, 24 different platelet-specific alloantigens and alloantibodies have been discovered. Most of these alloantigens were discovered after antibody detection during laboratory tests performed for neonatal thrombocytopenia. These antibodies were always of the IgG class and thus capable of crossing the placenta. In Caucasians, anti-HPA-1a is responsible for the majority (75–95%) of cases of FNAIT[79,80,81,103–105] (see Table 41.4). This is a striking finding if we consider that only about 2% of the pregnant (Caucasian) women are negative for HPA-1a (see Table 41.4). Only about 5–25% of FNAIT is caused by other anti-HPA antibodies, most frequently anti HPA-5b, anti HPA-3a and anti HPA-1b (see Table 41.5).

As discussed earlier, in the Japanese population, the incidence of FNAIT caused by anti HPA-1a is very rare, whereas anti-HPA 4b and anti HPA-5b are involved in a substantial number of cases[106–108].

Incidence of FNAIT

The reported incidence of FNAIT in the literature varies widely. Using data from all published prospective studies, Turner et al. estimated the overall incidence of FNAIT due to anti-HPA-1a to be 1 in 1163 live births and the incidence of severe thrombocytopenia ($<50 \times 10^9/l$) to be 1 in 1695[55]. Intracranial hemorrhage in the neonates approximates 1:37 000 births[49–55].

It is generally accepted that FNAIT is likely to be underdiagnosed, with only 37% of cases of severe FNAIT detected in the absence of screening programs. Davoren et al. estimated that only 7% of expected cases are detected clinically[53,109].

At the moment, FNAIT is only recognized and can be treated in the next pregnancy after bleeding has occurred or severe thrombocytopenia was detected by chance. Pros and cons for FNAIT screening in the first pregnancy have been discussed for several years[51,55,110,111,112] and include the following. First, screening can be effective given the fact that, in Caucasians, 75% of FNAIT cases are caused by HPA-1a antibodies. Second, the positive predictive value of HPA-1a antibody screening is less than 50% and thus a more specific screening assay is necessary to predict severe thrombocytopenia in the fetus/newborn. Third, currently, the predictive value of maternal HPA-1a antibody concentrations for severe thrombocytopenia is unclear. Fourth, given the fact that there is still debate on the optimal management of FNAIT, routine screening may lead to unnecessary medical interventions in pregnancy.

Untreated newborns with FNAIT are reported to be affected by ICH in 7–26% of cases, of which approximately 50% occurs in utero[80,104,105,113–119]. In a review, Spencer and Burrows reported that even 80% of ICH due to FNAIT occurred in utero, with 14% occurring before 20 weeks and a further 28% occurring before 30 weeks[119]. Therefore, FNAIT should be considered as the most likely cause in any type of ICH which is discovered in the fetus. In Caucasians, HPA-1a immunization is the most frequent cause of ICH in FNAIT cases.

Natural history and pathophysiology

FNAIT is considered the platelet equivalent of hemolytic disease of the newborn. However, in contrast to red cell alloimmunization, FNAIT occurs in the first pregnancy in over 50% of cases[80].

HPA antigens are already expressed on fetal platelets in the first trimester. Once the mother has produced HPA antibodies, these specific IgG antibodies are able to cross the placenta and cause platelet destruction in the fetus. Unfortunately, there is a lack of a reliable correlation between the maternal antibody levels and the severity of FNAIT[120–122]. However, some recent studies indicate a higher risk of severe FNAIT with high antibody levels[121–123]. Determination of IgG subclasses involved, particularly IgG3, has been suggested to be of value to identify a high-risk group[124]. Thus far, no laboratory test is available for reliable selection of pregnancies truly at risk for severe FNAIT.

Although thrombocytopenia is commonly defined as a platelet count below $150 \times 10^9/l$, clinical symptoms are only likely to occur when the platelet count drops to below $50 \times 10^9/l$[125]. The most feared complication of a low platelet count in the fetus or the neonate is intracranial hemorrhage (ICH).

The role of the delivery or mode of delivery in the development of ICH is unclear. There is a lack of evidence that a cesarean section has any protective effect. A recent study from our group showed that vaginal delivery may be a safe option even in FNAIT cases with a low platelet count[126].

The recurrence rate of FNAIT in subsequent, incompatible pregnancies is high and varies from 75 to 90%[80,114,115,117,120,127]. Bussel et al. found that in 50% of their cases with affected siblings the initial platelet count at cordocentesis, performed between 20 and 28 weeks, was $\leq 20 \times 10^9/l$[128]. There are a few observations of worsening FNAIT with successive pregnancies, resulting in a progressively earlier occurrence of ICH[129–131].

However, in the majority of cases with a prior thrombocytopenic sibling with an ICH, neither the prevalence nor the time of occurrence of ICH is precisely known. This implies that, in cases where the previous infant was thrombocytopenic but without signs of hemorrhage, an assessment of the risk of ICH in utero in a subsequent pregnancy is difficult to make.

DIAGNOSIS

Laboratory analysis

Maternal HPA antibody screening during pregnancy is not performed routinely and therefore an affected first child in a family is usually totally unexpected. Depending on the clinical situation and the platelet count of the newborn, acute treatment with intravenous immunoglobulin and platelet transfusions may be necessary. The laboratory protocol and the donor management must be supportive; meaning that first serology results (HPA-1a typing mother and first cross match between maternal serum and paternal platelets) should be ready within 3 to 4 hours and correctly typed donor platelets (negative for the antigen involved) should be available as soon as possible.

HPA pheno- or genotyping

Cito HPA-1a phenotyping of the mother is essential to advise the antigen typing of donor platelets. Several ELISA techniques are available[132–134]. In urgent cases, we use the monoclonal antibody solid phase platelet antibody test (MASPAT, Sanquin Amsterdam) for maternal HPA-1a typing and a cross match of maternal serum with paternal platelets, giving results within 2 hours.

HPA genotyping has become available as a routine laboratory technique and can be used to identify HPA incompatibilities between mother and child. Several techniques are known of which the polymerase chain reaction with sequence-specific primers (PCR-SSP) and lately the Taqman-technology-based allelic discrimination assays are most used[135–141]. In our laboratory, we genotype mother, father and child for HPA-1, -2, -3, -5 and -15 by Taqman-technology.

Genotyping favors phenotyping because no platelets and specific antisera are necessary. Furthermore, paternal heterozygosity can be easily determined and used to predict the risk of FNAIT in the next pregnancy.

New microarray technologies[142] will support routine genotyping of all known HPAs which allows detection of incompatibilities for low-frequency antigens and increases the sensitivity for the detection of antibodies against low-frequency antigens[143].

HPA antibodies (platelet-specific alloantibodies)

For the detection of platelet-specific antibodies (anti-HPAs), it is necessary to use techniques in which the presence of antibodies can be tested with isolated GP complexes. Since, there are only a limited number of copies of the glycoprotein Ia/IIa complexes which carry the HPA-5 system on the platelet membrane, techniques based on antibody binding to whole platelets are not sensitive enough, especially not for the clinically important HPA-5b antibodies[144].

The breakthrough in HPA antibody detection was the monoclonal antibody-specific immobilization of platelet antigens assay (MAIPA) described by Kiefel et al. in 1987[145]. This complex assay is based on a sandwich ELISA technique and has become possible by the development of glycoprotein-specific monoclonal antibodies[145]. Recent modifications made it possible to perform the MAIPA within one day[146,147]. Still it is a complex technique and requires well-skilled technicians and panels of (frozen) typed platelets.

Several solid phase (microtiterplate) techniques have been developed based on the MAIPA, with the important GPs already isolated and bound on the microtiterplate well. These techniques require fewer laboratory skills and can be performed within 4 hours. Therefore, many laboratories use these techniques but, unfortunately, the sensitivity (70–75%) and the specificity (85%) is less than the MAIPA (both sensitivity and specificity >90%) and these techniques should only be used by experienced laboratories with knowledge of their limitations. Over-dependence on such kits or their use by inexperienced users may lead to failure to detect clinically significant antibodies[148–150].

Donor HPA genotyping

Depending on the clinical situation and the platelet count, acute platelet transfusions may be necessary. In the Netherlands, a sufficient number of donors are genotyped to guarantee continuous availability (within 2 hours) of HPA-1a- and -5b-negative platelets. Donors with this HPA typing (approximately 1.7% of the Caucasian population) are asked to donate via platelet aphaeresis at a regular base. HPA-1a- and -5b-negative platelets are the correct choice for approximately 90% of the FNAIT neonates (75% anti HPA-1a and 15% anti HPA-5b). For large-scale HPA genotyping, we developed a fully automated HPA-1, -2, -3, -5, -15 genotyping assay based on DNA isolation with a MagNa Pure LC DNA isolation robot and typing with Taqman-technology-based allelic discrimination assays.

Neonatal plasma thrombopoietin (Tpo) measurement

Regulation of platelet production strongly depends on the free plasma thrombopoietin (Tpo) levels[151–156]. Tpo, mainly produced in the liver at a constant level, binds to the mpl-receptors on $CD34^+$ stem cells, megakaryocytes and platelets. Measurement of plasma Tpo levels is useful to discriminate thrombocytopenia caused by megakaryocyte and platelet production failure (highly elevated Tpo levels) from thrombocytopenia caused by elevated platelet destruction as in autoimmune (ITP) and fetal and neonatal alloimmune (FNAIT) thrombocytopenia (normal or only slightly elevated Tpo levels[26,27,29,31,157,158]). In a retrospective study, we analyzed the Tpo levels in different groups of patients with neonatal thrombocytopenia and compared them with a control group of healthy neonates. We observed that neonatal thrombocytopenia due to congenital CMV infections, severe asphyxia or dysmaturity correlates with high plasma Tpo levels, strongly indicating that the thrombocytopenia is caused by decreased platelet production because of BM suppression. At present, we measure plasma Tpo levels together with the routine serology tests for thrombocytopenic neonates referred to our laboratory for suspected FNAIT.

Summary of laboratory analysis

In our laboratory, the following procedures are performed when FNAIT is expected to be the cause of neonatal thrombocytopenia:

- Immediate HPA-1a phenotyping test results available <2 hours *(to advise for antigen typing of donor platelets)*
- HPA-1a, -1b, -2a, -2b, -3a, -3b, -5a, -5b, -15a and -15b genotyping of mother, father and neonate *(to screen for HPA incompatibilities)*
- Cross-matching of untreated and cloroquine-treated paternal platelets with maternal serum in the PIFT and in the MAIPA
- Results of first cross match in the monoclonal antibody solid phase platelet antibody test (MASPAT, Sanquin, Amsterdam) available <2 hours *(to screen for HPA and private platelet alloantibodies)*
- Screening for anti-HPA antibodies in the maternal serum with typed donor platelets in the PIFT and in the MAIPA (results, with first indication what antibody is present, within 7 hours)
- Identification of HPA antibodies in the MAIPA (result next day)
- Testing for autoantibodies on maternal platelets, in the maternal serum and in an eluate made of maternal platelets in the PIFT (result within 7 hours)
- Testing for autoantibodies on the paternal platelets (this can cause false-positive reactions in the cross matches) in the PIFT (result within 7 hours)
- Measurement of neonatal plasma thrombopoietin level (to find indications for platelet production or destruction defects).

Antenatal management

In contrast to the management of the neonate, there is divergence of opinion about the antenatal management of FNAIT.

The management of FNAIT in the neonate is straightforward and includes intravenous immunoglobulin (IVIG) administration and (if necessary) transfusion of matched donor platelets.

For the antenatal management, it is important to know whether the father is homozygous or heterozygous for the offending antigen. In case of heterozygosity of the father, it might be useful to perform genotyping of the fetus. Although this is possible by using either chorionic villi or amniocytes, by the polymerase chain reaction (PCR), amniocentesis in second trimester is preferable because of its lower risk of boosting antibodies. Recently, methods were being developed to assess the fetal HPA type using free fetal DNA in maternal plasma. When the fetus is positive for the offending antigen, the pregnancy should be managed in or in collaboration with a specialized fetal center.

As no routine screening is performed, FNAIT is mostly only recognized after an affected sibling. The antenatal management protocols in FNAIT are aimed to prevent ICH. Unfortunately, monitoring anti-HPA antibodies by titration and quantification does not accurately predict the severity of fetal thrombocytopenia. However, recent studies indicate that it might be helpful in predicting the severity of fetal thrombocytopenia[112,120,121,159,160]. In order to diagnose fetal thrombocytopenia as early as possible, various centers have designed protocols for routine fetal blood sampling beginning as early as 20 weeks[161–165]. In cases of fetal thrombocytopenia and platelet transfusion, the procedure is generally repeated frequently given the fact that the half-life of transfused platelets is only 5 days. Although cordocentesis is a reliable tool for direct monitoring of the fetal thrombocytopenia, the cumulative procedure-related risk for fetal loss is high and approximates 6% per pregnancy[163,166].

Currently, most centers have adopted the use of weekly high-dose maternal IVIG. A few centers use corticosteroids as first-line treatment. Although corticosteroids do not enhance the effect of IVIG[116,164] combinations of these options are also in use. Bussel et al. were the first who reported in 1988 that weekly maternal IVIG (1.0 g/kg maternal weight) was effective at elevating the fetal platelet count[114]. Later studies showed that not all fetuses showed a substantial increase in platelet count with this treatment. The reported response rate in the literature varies between 30% and 85%. In addition, observational studies suggested that IVIG reduced the risk of ICH even in non-responders to IVIG[104,167,169,170].

The mechanism of action of IVIG in FNAIT is still unclear. Possible explanations include the following. First, in the maternal circulation, the IVIG will dilute the anti-HPA antibodies, resulting in a lower proportion of anti-HPA antibodies among the IgG transferred via the Fc-receptors in the placenta. Secondly, in the placenta, IVIG may block the placenta receptor (Fc-R) and decrease the placental transmission of maternal antibodies including anti-HPA-antibodies. Thirdly, in the fetus, IVIG may block the Fc-receptors on the macrophages and prohibit the destruction of antibody-covered platelets. Recently, Ni et al. presented a murine model of FNAIT, measuring response to IVIG therapy[171]. This model demonstrates that maternal IVIG administration has multiple effects on the amelioration of FNAIT, including decreased maternal antiplatelet antibody, decreased fetal platelet clearance, reduced bleeding disorders and increased fetal survival[171].

Further cost-effectiveness analysis, performed by Thung et al., comparing non-invasive empiric intravenous immunoglobulin with invasive fetal treatment, showed that non-invasive

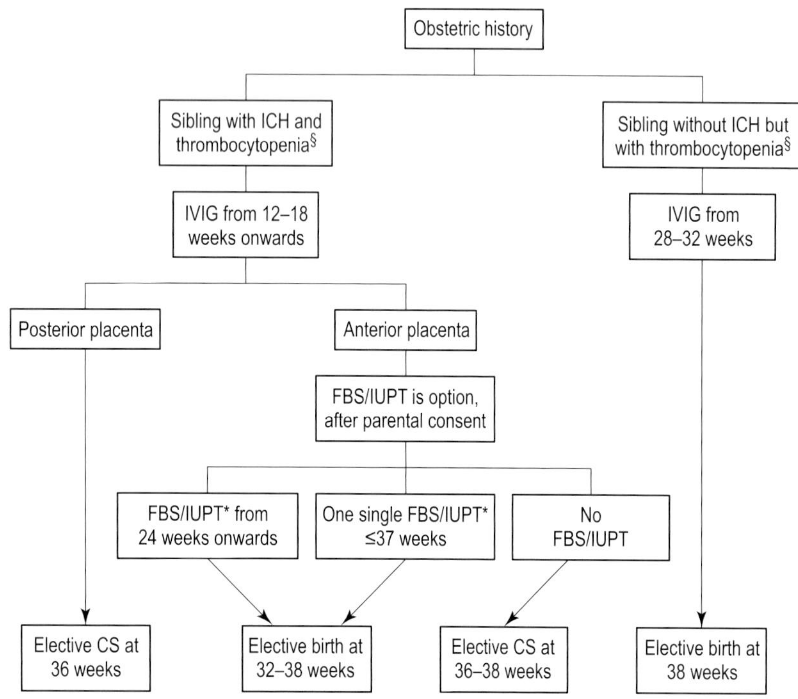

Fig. 41.2 FNAIT: Recommendations for management in pregnancy and delivery, depending on the obstetric history and in case the fetus is positive for the offending antigen.

IVIG is a cost-effective strategy when the rate of perinatal ICH is less than 28%[172].

Follow-up studies of FNAIT infants, treated antenatally with IVIG in a dose of 1 g/kg/week, show that the developmental and behavioral outcome are equal or even better compared to untreated infants[173–175]. The results of the study by Ward et al. suggest this positive effect regards all antenatal treatment modes[175].

In the antenatal management of FNAIT, it is important to realize that the majority of at-risk patients are those having a sibling with a history of severe thrombocytopenia but without internal bleeding. The risk of ICH in this category of patients is low and approximates the risk of fetal loss of invasive management. Therefore, a non-invasive approach is preferable in this category of patients. Considering that the large majority of ICH in these patients occurs later in pregnancy and the high cost of IVIG, treatment of FNAIT pregnancies without a history of ICH may be started between 28 and 32 weeks (Fig. 41.2). A completely non-invasive approach with IVIG treatment in 52 patients resulted in healthy infants, born at term[170]. In pregnancies with a previous sibling with an ICH, IVIG should be started at 12–18 weeks. To evaluate the response a cordocentesis can be performed at 24–28 weeks. In cases when the anticipated risk of the procedure is high (e.g. less experienced center or a posteriorly located cord insertion), IVIG should be continued until delivery without cordocentesis. Recently, we published our results with this less invasive approach in 7 pregnancies with a prior sibling with ICH[169]. IVIG (1 g/kg/week) was administered from a median of 16 weeks (range 16–29 weeks) without initial and follow-up cordocentesis. Although all neonates had a birth platelet count of less than $50 \times 10^9/l$, none of them showed signs of internal or external bleeding. Our results demonstrate that the primary goal in the management of pregnancies at risk for FNAIT is the prevention of severe bleeding complications and not thrombocytopenia per se. In the very rare case, a patient with a history of early antenatal ICH might benefit from a more aggressive approach (e.g. high-dose IVIG, followed by repeated cordocentesis and rescue high-dose corticosteroids).

In FNAIT patients, safety precautions may lower the risk of hemorrhage at fetal blood sampling. At the Leiden University Medical Centre (LUMC), the protocol for cordocentesis includes the following:

1. Cordocenteses in FNAIT pregnancies are performed by the most experienced members of the fetal medicine unit
2. Using a cell counter in the operating room, platelet count and histogram are obtained within 2 minutes
3. Before each cordocentesis, compatible platelets are collected and infused during the procedure, if necessary, to achieve a platelet count of $>100 \times 10^9/l$.

CONCLUSION

ITP and FNAIT are the most frequent causes of fetal and neonatal platelet disorders. In ITP patients, the low risk for perinatal ICH does not justify routine invasive fetal testing. Antenatal therapy is only instituted for maternal reasons. There is no evidence that maternal therapy leads to an increase of the fetal/neonatal platelet count. Platelet counts of second newborns correlate well with those of their siblings. At present, cesarean section is recommended only for obstetric reasons.

In contrast to ITP patients, in FNAIT patients, the treatment is aimed to prevent fetal and neonatal ICH. FNAITP occurs in approximately 1:1500 random fetuses/newborns. Because screening is not widely used yet, therapy can only be started after an affected sibling. Antenatal management depends on the obstetric history.

It is generally accepted that pregnant women who have previously given birth to an infant with an ICH have a high recurrent risk. Both invasive and non-invasive strategies are used in order to prevent ICH in these fetuses. There is controversy about the risk for ICH in those fetuses that have a thrombocytopenic sibling without an ICH. There is growing evidence that the use of fetal blood sampling in the management of pregnancies complicated by FNAIT, does more harm than good. A non-invasive strategy using only treatment with intravenous immunoglobulins should be the antenatal management in these cases.

Because of both its rarity and seriousness, the treatment of this disorder should be undertaken in, or in collaboration with, a center experienced in invasive fetal procedures and with expert laboratory and blood-bank back-up. Since FNAIT is a potentially devastating but rare disease, rapid advances in our insights to improve management can only be made by multicenter collaboration. We therefore encourage all colleagues caring for these patients to consider participating in international trials and registries.

Results from laboratory, epidemiological and clinical research on the course of the disease are still necessary to optimize the management.

REFERENCES

1. Dreyfus M, Kaplan C, Verdy E et al. Immune Thrombocytopenia Working Group. Frequency of immune thrombocytopenia in newborns: a prospective study. *Blood* **89**(12):4402–4406, 1997.
2. Burrows RF, Kelton JG. Fetal thrombocytopenia and its relation to maternal thrombocytopenia. *N Engl J Med* **329**(20):1463–1466, 1993.
3. Roberts I, Murray NA. Neonatal thrombocytopenia: causes and management. *Arch Dis Child Fetal Neonatal Ed* **88**(5):F359–f364, 2003.
4. Sainio S, Jarvenpaa AL, Renlund M et al. Thrombocytopenia in term infants: a population-based study. *Obstet Gynecol* **95**(3):441–446, 2000.
5. de Moerloose P, Boehlen F, Extermann P et al. Neonatal thrombocytopenia: incidence and characterization of maternal antiplatelet antibodies by MAIPA assay. *Br J Haematol* **100**:735–740, 1998.
6. Murray NA, Roberts IA. Circulating megakaryocytes and their progenitors in early thrombocytopenia in preterm neonates. *Pediatr Res* **40**(1):112–119, 1996.
7. Frederiksen H, Schmidt K. The incidence of idiopathic thrombocytopenic purpura in adults increases with age. *Blood* **94**(3):909–913, 1999.
8. Neylon AN, Saunders PWG, Howard MR et al. Clinically significant newly diagnosed presenting autoimmune thrombocytopenic pupura in adults: a prospective study of a population-based cohort of 245 patients. *Br J Haem* **122**:966–974, 2003.
9. George JN, el Harake MA, Aster RH. Thrombocytopenia due to enhanced

platelet destruction by immunologic mechanisms. In *Williams Hematology*, MAE Beutler, BS Lichtmann, TJ Kipps Coller (eds), p. 1315. New York: McGraw-Hill, 1995.

10. Crowther MA, Burrows RF, Ginsberg J et al. Thrombocytopenia in pregnancy: diagnosis, pathogenesis and management. *Blood Rev* **10**(1):8–16, 1996.
11. Von dem Borne AEGK, Helmerhorst EM, Leeuwen EF et al. Autoimmune thrombocytopenia: detection of platelet autoantibodies with the suspension immunofluorescence test. *Br J Haematol* **45**:319–327, 1989.
12. Burrows RF, Kelton JG. Thrombocytopenia at delivery: a prospective survey of 6715 deliveries. *Am J Obstet Gynecol* **162**(3):731–734, 1990.
13. Giles AR, Hoogendoorn H, Benford K. Type IIB von Willebrand's disease presenting as thrombocytopenia during pregnancy. *Br J Haematol* **67**(3):349–353, 1987.
14. Samuels P, Bussel JB, Braitman LE et al. Estimation of the risk of thrombocytopenia in the offspring of pregnant women with presumed immune thrombocytopenia purpura. *N Engl J Med* **323**(4):229–235, 1990.
15. Beilin Y, Zahn J, Comerford M. Safe epidural analgesia in thirty parturients with plateletcounts between 69,000 and 98,000 mm^{-3}. *Anasth Analg* **85**:385–388, 1997.
16. British Committee for Standards in Haematology General Haematology Task Force. Guidelines for the investigation and management of idiopathic thrombocytopenic purpura in adults, children and pregnancy. *Br J Haematol* **120**:274–296, 2003.
17. Burrows RF, Kelton JG. Pregnancy in patients with idiopathic thrombocytopenic purpura: assessing the risks for the infant at delivery. *Obstet Gynecol Surv* **48**(12):781–788, 1993.
18. Christiaens GCML, Nieuwenhuis K, Bussel JB. Comparison of platelet counts in first and second newborns of mothers with immune thrombocytopenic purpura. *Obstet Gynecol* **90**:546–552, 1998.
19. Scott JR, Rote NS, Cruikshank DP. Antiplatelet antibodies and platelet counts in pregnancies complicated by autoimmune thrombocytopenia. *Am J Obstet Gynecol* **145**:932, 1983.
20. Kaplan C, Daffos F, Forestier F et al. Fetal platelet counts in thrombocytopenic pregnancy. *Lancet* **336**:979–982, 1990.
21. George JN, Woolf SH, Raskob GE et al. Idiopathic thrombocytopenic purpura: a practice guideline developed by explicit methods for the American Society of Hematology. *Blood* **88**:3–40, 1996.
22. Gandemer V, Kaplan C, Quelvennec E et al. Pregnancy-associated autoimmune neonatal thrombocytopenia: role of maternal HLA genotype. *Br J Haematol* **104**:878–885, 1999.
23. Bussel JB, McFarland JG, Berkowitz RL. Antenatal management of fetal alloimmune and autoimmune thrombocytopenia. *Transfus Med Rev* **4**:149–162, 1990.
24. Bussel J, Kaplan C, McFarland J. Recommendations for the evaluation and treatment of neonatal autoimmune and alloimmune thrombocytopenia. *Thromb Haemost* **65**:631–634, 1991.
25. Berry SM, Leonardi MR, Wolfe HM et al. Maternal thrombocytopenia: predicting neonatal thrombocytopenia with cordocentesis. *J Reprod Med* **42**:276–280, 1997.
26. Emmons RV, Reid DM, Cohen RL et al. Human thrombopoietin levels are high when thrombocytopenia is due to megakaryocyte deficiency and low when due to increased platelet destruction. *Blood* **87**:4068–4071, 1996.
27. Kosugi S, Kurata Y, Tomiyama Y et al. Circulating thrombopoietin level in chronic immune thrombocytopenic purpura. *Br J Haematol* **93**:704–706, 1996.
28. Porcelijn L, Folman CC, Bossers B et al. The diagnostic value of thrombopoietin level measurements in thrombocytopenia. *Thromb Haemost* **79**:1101–1105, 1998.
29. Tahara T, Usuki K, Sato H et al. A sensitive sandwich ELISA for measuring thrombopoietin in human serum: serum thrombopoietin levels in healthy volunteers and in patients with haemopoietic disorders. *Br J Haematol* **93**:783–788, 1996.
30. von dem Borne AEGK, Verheugt FWA, Oosterhof F et al. A simple immunofluorescence test for the detection of platelet antibodies. *Br J Haematol* **39**:195–207, 1978.
31. Porcelijn L, Huiskes E, von dem Borne AEGK. Glycoprotein V plays an important role in ITP. Unpublished data, 1998.
32. Olsson B, Andersson PO, Jernas M et al. T-cell-mediated cytotoxicity toward platelets in chronic idiopathic thrombocytopenic purpura. *Nat Med* **9**(9):1123–1124, 2003.
33. Mueller-Eckhardt C, Kayser W, Mersch-Baumert K et al. The clinical significance of platelet-associated IgG: a study on 298 patients with various disorders. *Br J Haematol* **46**(1):123–131, 1980.
34. van Leeuwen EF, van der Ven JT, Engelfriet CP et al. Specificity of autoantibodies in autoimmune thrombocytopenia. *Blood* **59**(1):23–26, 1982.
35. Kiefel V, Freitag E, Kroll H et al. Platelet autoantibodies (IgG, IgM, IgA) against glycoproteins IIb/IIIa and Ib/IX in patients with thrombocytopenia. *Ann Hematol* **72**(4):280–285, 1996.
36. Berchtold P, Wenger M. Autoantibodies against platelet glycoproteins in autoimmune thrombocytopenic purpura: their clinical significance and response to treatment. *Blood* **81**(5):1246–1250, 1993.
37. Joutsi-Korhonen L, Javela K, Hormila P et al. Glycoprotein V-specific platelet-associated antibodies in thrombocytopenic patients. *Clin Lab Haematol* **23**(5):307–312, 2001.
38. Meyer O, Agaylan A, Bombard S et al. A novel antigen-specific capture assay for the detection of platelet antibodies and HPA-1a phenotyping. *Vox Sang* **91**(4): 324–330, 2006.
39. Tomer A. Flow cytometry for the diagnosis of autoimmune thrombocytopenia. *Curr Hematol Rep* **5**(1):64–69, 2006.
40. Fabris F, Scandellari R, Ruzzon E et al. Platelet-associated autoantibodies as detected by a solid-phase modified antigen capture ELISA test (MACE) are a useful prognostic factor in idiopathic thrombocytopenic purpura. *Blood* **103**(12):4562–4564, 2004.
41. Berchtold P, Muller D, Beardsley D et al. International study to compare antigen-specific methods used for the measurement of antiplatelet autoantibodies. *Br J Haematol* **96**(3): 477–483, 1997.
42. Davoren A, Bussel J, Curtis BR et al. Prospective evaluation of a new platelet glycoprotein (GP)-specific assay (PakAuto) in the diagnosis of autoimmune thrombocytopenia (AITP). *Am J Hematol* **78**(3):193–197, 2005.
43. Joutsi L, Kekomaki R. Comparison of the direct platelet immunofluorescence test (direct PIFT) with a modified direct monoclonal antibody-specific immobilization of platelet antigens (direct MAIPA) in detection of platelet-associated IgG. *Br J Haematol* **96**:204–209, 1997.
44. Lin JS, Lyou JY, Chen YJ et al. Screening for platelet antibodies in adult idiopathic thrombocytopenic purpura: a comparative study using solid phase red cell adherence assay and flow cytometry. *J Chin Med Assoc* **69**(12):569–574, 2006.
45. McMillan R. Antiplatelet antibodies in chronic adult immune thrombocytopenic purpura: assays and epitopes. *J Pediatr Hematol Oncol* **25**(Suppl 1):S57–s61, 2003.
46. George JN, Woolf SH, Raskob GE et al. Idiopathic thrombocytopenic purpura: a practice guideline developed by explicit methods for the American Society of Hematology. *Blood* **88**:3–40, 1996.
47. Christiaens GCML, Helmerhorst FM. Validity of intrapartum diagnosis of fetal thrombocytopenia. *Am J Obstet Gynecol* **157**:864–865, 1987.
48. Kagan R, Laros RK, Jr. Immune thrombocytopenia. *Clin Obstet Gynecol* **26**:537–540, 1983.

49. Blanchette VS, Chen L, de Friedberg ZS et al. Alloimmunization to the PlA1 platelet antigen: results of a prospective study. *Br J Haematol* **74**(2):209–215, 1990.
50. Durand-Zaleski I, Schlegel N, Blum-Boisgard C et al. Screening primiparous women and newborns for fetal/neonatal alloimmune thrombocytopenia: a prospective comparison of effectiveness and costs. *Am J Perinatol* **13**(7):423–431, 1996.
51. Williamson LM, Hackett GA, Rennie JM et al. The natural history of fetomaternal alloimmunization to the platelet-specific antigen HPA-1a (PL^{A1}, Zw^{a}) as determined by antenatal screening. *Blood* **92**:2280–2287, 1995.
52. Maslanka K, Guz K, Zupanska B. Antenatal screening of unselected pregnant women for HPA-1a antigen, antibody and alloimmune hrombocytopenia. *Vox Sang* **85**(4):326–327, 2003.
53. Davoren A, McParland P, Crowley J et al. Antenatal screening for human platelet antigen-1a: results of a prospective study at a large maternity hospital in Ireland. *Br J Obstet Gynaecol* **110**(5):492–496, 2003.
54. Kjeldsen-Kraghl J, Killie MK, Aune B et al. An intervention program for reducing morbidity and mortality associated with neonatal alloimmune thrombocytopenic purpura. 8th European Symposium on platelet and granulocyte immunobiology. Rust, 2004.
55. Turner ML, Bessos H, Fagge T et al. Prospective epidemiologic study of the outcome and cost-effectiveness of antenatal screening to detect neonatal alloimmune thrombocytopenia due to anti-HPA-1a. *Transfusion* **45**(12):1945–1956, 2005.
56. Lalezari P, Murphy GB. Cold reacting leukocyte agglutinins and their significance. In *Histocomp Testing*, ES Curtoni, PL Mattiuz, RM Tosi (eds), p. 421. Copenhagen: Munksgaard, 1967.
57. Shumak KH, Rachkewich RA, Crookston MC et al. Antigens of the Ii system on lymphocytes. *Nature (New Biol)* **231**:148, 1971.
58. Dunstan RA, Simpson MB. Heterogeneous distribution of antigens on human platelets demonstrated by fluorescence flow cytometry. *Br J Haematol* **61**:603–609, 1985.
59. Dunstan RA, Simpson MB, Knowles RW et al. The origin of ABH antigens on human platelets. *Blood* **65**:615–619, 1985.
60. Kools A, Collins J, Aster RH. Studies of the ABO antigens of human platelets (abstract). *Transfusion* **21**:615–616, 1981.
61. Kelton JG, Hamid C, Aker S et al. The amount of blood group A substance on platelets is proportional to the amount in the plasma. *Blood* **59**:980–985, 1982.
62. Taaning E, Skibsted L. The frequency of platelet alloanti-bodies in pregnant women and the occurrence and management of neonatal alloimmune thrombocytopenia purpura. *Obstet Gynecol Surv* **45**:521–525, 1990.
63. Sternbach MS, Malette M, Nadon F. Severe alloimmune neonatal thrombocytopenia due to specific HLA antibodies. *Curr Stud Hematol Blood Transfus* **59**:97–103, 1986.
64. Skacel PO, Contreras M. Neonatal thrombocytopenia. *Blood Rev* **3**:174–179, 1989.
65. Sharon R, Amar A. Maternal anti-HLA antibodies and neonatal thrombocytopenia. *Lancet* i:1313, 1981.
66. Metcalfe P, Watkins NA, Ouwehand WH et al. Nomenclature of human platelet antigens. *Vox Sang* **85**(3):240–245, 2003.
67. Newman PJ, Derbes RS, Aster RH. The human platelet alloantigens, Pl^{A1} and Pl^{A2}, are associated with a $leucine^{33}$/$proline^{33}$ amino acid polymorphism in membrane glycoprotein IIIa, and are distinguishable by DNA typing. *J Clin Invest* **83**:1778–1781, 1989.
68. Ginsberg MH, Loftus JC, Plow EF. Cytoadhesins, integrins and platelets. *Thromb Haemos* **59**:1–6, 1988.
69. Giltay JC, Brinkman HJM, Modderman PW. Human vascular endothelial cells express a membrane protein complex immuno-chemically indistinguishable from the platelet VLA-2 (glycoprotein Ia–IIa) complex. *Blood* **73**:1235–1241, 1989.
70. McEver RP, Beckstead JM, Moore KL. GMP-140, a platelet alpha-granule membrane protein, is also synthesized by vascular endothelial cells and is localized in Weibel-Palade bodies. *J Clin Invest* **84**:92–99, 1989.
71. Sugiyama T, Pidard D, Wautier MP et al. Comparative immunochemical analysis of membrane proteins from human platelets and endothelial cells. *Nouv Rev Fr Hematol* **32**:199–205, 1990.
72. Zhong CH, Jacques PC. Are megakaryocytes and endothelial cells sisters? *J Lab Clin Med* **121**:821–825, 1993.
73. Williamson LM, Lubenko A, Hadfield R et al. Large-scale genotyping of platelet donors for the platelet-specific alloantigens HPA-1, 2 and 3. *Br J Haematol* **84**:7, 1993.
74. Kim HO, Jin Y, Kickler TS et al. Gene frequencies of the five major human platelet antigens in African American, white, and Korean populations. *Transfusion* **35**:863–837, 1995.
75. Urwijitaroon Y, Barusrux S, Romphruk A et al. Frequency of human platelet antigens among blood donors in northeastern Thailand. *Transfusion* **35**: 868–870, 1995.
76. Simsek S, Faber NM, Bleeker PM et al. Determination of human platelet antigen frequencies in the Dutch population by immunophenotyping and DNA (allele-specific restriction enzyme) analysis. *Blood* **81**:835–840, 1993.
77. Feng ML, Liu DZ, Shen W et al. Establishment of an HPA-1- to -16-typed platelet donor registry in China. *Transfus Med* **16**(5):369–374, 2006.
78. Seo DH, Park SS, Kim DW et al. Gene frequencies of eight human platelet-specific antigens in Koreans. *Transfus Med* **8**(2):129–132, 1998.
79. Davoren A, Curtis BR, Aster RH et al. Human platelet antigen-specific alloantibodies implicated in 1162 cases of neonatal alloimmune thrombocytopenia. *Transfusion* **44**(8):1220–1225, 2004.
80. Mueller-Eckhardt C, Kiefel V, Grubert A et al. 348 cases of suspected neonatal alloimmune thrombocytopenia. *Lancet* **1**:363–366, 1989.
81. Porcelijn I, Huiskes E, von dem Borne AEGK. Antibodies involved in NAIT. Unpublished data, 2004.
82. van Loghem JJ, Dorfmeijer H, van der Hart M et al. Serological and genetical studies on a platelet antigen (Zw). *Vox Sang* **4**:161–169, 1959.
83. Shulman NR, Nader VJ, Hiller MC et al. Platelet and leucocyte isoantigens and their antibodies. Serologic and clinical studies. *Progr Haematol* **4**:222, 1964.
84. von dem Borne AEGK, Decary F. ICSH/ISBT Working Party on Platelet Serology. Nomenclature of platelet-specific antigens. *Vox Sang* **58**:176, 1990.
85. Lanzavecchia A. Clonal sketches of the immune response. *EMBO J* **7**:2945–2951, 1988.
86. Rudensky AY, Preston-Hurlburt P, Hong SC et al. Sequence analysis of peptide bound to MHC class II molecules. *Nature* **353**:622–627, 1991.
87. Marrack P, Kappler J. The T cell receptor. *Science* **238**:1073–1079, 1987.
88. Trowsdale J, Ragoussis J, Campbell RD. Map of the human MHC. *Immunol Today* **12**:443–446, 1991.
89. Tsuji K. *Proceedings of the Eleventh International Histocompatibility Workshop and Conference* held in Tokyo, Japan, pp. 1167–1168. Oxford: Oxford University Press, 1992.
90. Williamson LM, Hackett G, Rennie J et al. The natural history of fetomaternal alloimmunization to the platelet-specific antigen HPA-1a (PlA1, Zwa) as determined by antenatal screening. *Br J Haematol* **92**:2280–2287, 1998.
91. De Waal LP, van Dalen CM, Engelfriet CP et al. Alloimmunization against the platelet-specific Zw (a) antigen, resulting in neonatal alloimmune thrombocytopenia or posttransfusion purpura, is associated with the supertypic DRw52 antigen including DR3 and DRw6. *Human Immunol* **17**:45–53, 1986.
92. Valentin N, Vergracht A, Bignon JD et al. HLA-DRw52a is involved in alloimmunization against PL-A1 antigen. *Human Immunol* **27**:73–79, 1990.
93. Reznikoff-Etievant MF, Kaplan C, Muller JY et al. Allo-immune thrombocytopenias, definition of a group at risk; a prospective study. *Curr Stud Hematol Blood Transf* **55**:119–124, 1988.

94. L'Abbé D, Tremblay L, Goldman M et al. Alloimmunization to platelet antigen HPA-1a (Zwa) association with HLA-DRw52a is not 100%. *Transf Med* **2**:251, 1992.
95. Taaning E. HLA antigens and maternal antibodies in alloimmune neonatal thrombocytopenia. *Tiss Antigens* **21**: 351–359, 1983.
96. Mueller-Eckhardt C, Mueller-Eckhardt G, Willen Ohff H et al. Immunogenicity of an immune response to human platelet antigen Zw (a) is strongly associated with HLA-B8 and DR3. *Tiss Antigens* **26**:71–76, 1985.
97. Mueller-Eckhardt G, Mueller-Eckhardt C. Alloimmunization against the platelet specific Zw (a) antigen associated with HLA-DRw52 and/or DRw6? *Human Immunol* **18**:181–182, 1987.
98. Reznikoff-Etievant MF, Dangu C, Lobet R. HLA-B8 antigens and anti-PL (A1) alloimmunisation. *Tiss Antigens* **18**: 66–68, 1981.
99. L'Abbé D, Tremblay L, Filion M et al. Alloimmunization to platelet antigen HPA-1a (PL-A1) is strongly associated with both HLA-DRB3* 0101 and HLA-DQB1*0201. *Human Immunol* **34**:107–114, 1992.
100. Reznikoff-Etievant MF, Muller JY, Julien F et al. An immune response gene linked to HLA in man. *Tiss Antigens* **22**:312–313, 1983.
101. Reznikoff-Etievant MF, Muller JY, Kaplan C et al. L'immunisation contre l'antigène plaquettaire zw (a) (PL (A1)): groupe è risque, prévention des complications a propos de 132 cas. *Path Biol* **341**:783–787, 1986.
102. Harrington WJ, Sprague CC, Minnich V et al. Immunologic mechanisms in idiopathic and neonatal thrombocytopenic purpura. *Ann Intern Med* **38**:433–469, 1953.
103. Reznikoff-Etievant MF. Management of alloimmune neonatal and antenatal thrombocytopenia. *Vox Sang* **55**:193–201, 1988.
104. Bussel JB, Berkowitz RL, Lynch L et al. Antenatal management of alloimmune thrombocytopenia with intravenous gamma-globulin: a randomized trial of the addition of low-dose steroid to intravenous gamma-globulin. *Am J Obstet Gynecol* **174**:1414–1423, 1996.
105. Kuijpers RWAM. Neonatal alloimmune thrombocytopenia: relation between serological parameters and clinical picture. Thesis: Maastricht University, 1993.
106. Ohto H, Miura S, Ariga H et al. The natural history of maternal immunization against foetal platelet alloantigens. *Transfus Med* **14**(6):399–408, 2004.
107. Shibata Y, Miyaji T, Ickikawa Y et al. A new platelet antigen system, Yuk (a)/ Yuk (b). *Vox Sang* **51**:334–336, 1986.
108. Shibata Y, Matsuda I, Miyaji T et al. A new platelet antigen involved in two cases of neonatal alloimmune thrombocytopenia. *Vox Sang* **50**:177–180, 1986.
109. Davoren A, McParland P, Barnes CA et al. Neonatal alloimmune thrombocytopenia in the Irish population: a discrepancy between observed and expected cases. *J Clin Pathol* **55**(4):289–292, 2002.
110. Murphy MF, Williamson LM, Urbaniak SJ. Antenatal screening for fetomaternal alloimmune thrombocytopenia: should we be doing it? *Vox Sang* **83**(Suppl 1):409–416, 2002.
111. Killie MK, Kjeldsen-Kragh, J, Husebekk A et al. Cost-effectiveness of antenatal screening for neonatal alloimmune thrombocytopenia. *Br J Obstet Gynaecol* online early article, 2007.
112. Bertrand C, Martageix C, Jallu V et al. Predictive value of sequential anti-HPA-1a antibody concentrations for the severity of fetal alloimmune thrombocytopenia. *J Thromb Haemost* **4**(3):628–637, 2006.
113. Herman JH, Jumbelic MI, Ancona RJ et al. In utero cerebral hemorrhage in alloimmune thrombocytopenia. *Am J Pediatr Hemotol Oncol* **8**:312–317, 1986.
114. Bussel JB, Richard MD, Berkowitz L et al. Antenatal treatment of neonatal alloimmune thrombocytopenia. *N Engl J Med* **319**:1374–1378, 1988.
115. Muller JY, Reznikoff-Etievant MF, Patereau C et al. Thrombopénies néo-natales allo-immunes étude clinique et biologique de 84 cas. *Presse Méd* **14**: 83–86, 1985.
116. Bussel JB. Neonatal alloimmune thrombocytopenia (NAITP): a prospective case accumulation study. *Pediatr Res* **23**:337A, 1988.
117. Kaplan C, Morel-Kopp MC, Kroll H et al. HPA-5b (Bra) neonatal alloimmune throbocytopenia: clinical and immunological analysis of 39 cases. *Br J Haematol* **78**:425–429, 1991.
118. Sharif U, Kuban K. Prenatal intracranial hemorrhage and neurologic complications in alloimmune thrombocytopenia. *J Child Neurol* **16**(11):838–842, 2001.
119. Spencer JA, Burrows RF. Feto-maternal alloimmune thrombocytopenia: a literature review and statistical analysis. *Aust NZ J Obstet Gynaecol* **41**:45–45, 2001.
120. Kaplan C, Daffos F, Forestier F et al. Management of alloimmune thrombocytopenia: antenatal diagnosis and in utero transfusion of maternal platelets. *Blood* **72**:340–343, 1988.
121. Proulx C, Filion MM, Goldman M et al. Analysis of immunoglobulin class IgG subclass and titre of HPA-1a antibodies in alloimmunized mothers giving birth to babies with or without neonatal alloimmune thrombocytopenia. *Br J Haematol* **87**:813–817, 1994.
122. Metcalfe P, Allen D, Chapman J et al. Interlaboratory variation in the detection of clinically significant alloantibodies against human platelet alloantigens. *Br J Haematol* **97**(1):204–207, 1997.
123. Jaegtvik S, Husebekk A, Aune B et al. Neonatal alloimmune thrombocytopenia due to anti-HPA 1a antibodies: the level of maternal antibodies predicts the severity of thrombocytopenia in the newborn. *Br J Obstet Gynaecol* **107**(5):691–694, 2000.
124. Mawas F, Wiener E, Williamson LM et al. Immunoglobulin G subclasses of anti-human platelet antigen 1a in maternal sera: relation to the severity of neonatal alloimmune thrombocytopenia. *Eur J Hematol* **59**:287–292, 1997.
125. Jhawar BS, Ranger A, Steven D et al. Risk factors for intracranial hemorrhage among full-term infants: a case-control study. *Neurosurgery* **52**(3):581–590, 2003.
126. Van den Akker ESA, Oepkes D, Brand A et al. Vaginal delivery for fetuses at risk of alloimmune thrombocytopenia? *Br J Obstet Gynaecol* **113**:781–783, 2006.
127. Montemagno R, Soothill PW, Scarelli M et al. Detection of alloimmune thrombocytopenia as a cause of isolated hydrocephalus by fetal blood sampling. *Lancet* **343**:1300–1301, 1994.
128. Bussel JB, Zabusky MR, Berkowitz RL et al. Fetal alloimmune thrombocytopenia. *N Engl J Med* **337**:22–24, 1997.
129. Murphy MF, Metcalfe P, Waters AH et al. Antenatal management of severe feto-maternal alloimmune thrombocytopenia: HLA incompatibility may affect responses to fetal platelet transfusions. *Blood* **81**:2174–2179, 1993.
130. de Vries LS, Connell J, Bydder GM et al. Recurrent intracranial haemorrhages in utero in an infant with alloimmune thrombocytopenia. Case report. *Br J Obstet Gynaecol* **95**:299–302, 1988.
131. Khouzami AN, Kickler TS, Callan NA et al. Devastating sequelae of alloimmune thrombocytopenia: an entity that deserves more attention. *J Maternal Fetal Med* **5**:137–141, 1996.
132. Sorel N, Brabant S, Christiaens L et al. A rapid and specific whole blood HPA-1 phenotyping by flow cytometry using two commercialized monoclonal antibodies directed against GP IIIa and GP IIb-IIIa complexes. *Br J Haematol* **124**(2):221–223, 2004.
133. Garner SF, Smethurst PA, Merieux Y et al. A rapid one-stage whole-blood HPA-1a phenotyping assay using a recombinant monoclonal IgG1 anti-HPA-1a. *Br J Haematol* **108**(2):440–447, 2000.
134. Bessos H, Hofner M, Salamat A et al. An international trial demonstrates suitability of a newly developed whole-blood ELISA kit for multicentre platelet HPA-1 phenotyping. *Vox Sang* **77**(2): 103–106, 1999.
135. Skogen B, Bellissimo DB, Hessner MJ et al. Rapid determination of platelet alloantigen genotypes by polymerase

chain reaction using allele-specific primers. *Transfusion* **34**(11):955–960, 1994.
136. Tanaka S, Taniue A, Nagao N et al. Simultaneous DNA typing of human platelet antigens 2, 3 and 4 by an allele-specific PCR method. *Vox Sang* **68**(4):225–230, 1995.
137. Kluter H, Fehlau K, Panzer S et al. Rapid typing for human platelet antigen systems-1, -2, -3 and -5 by PCR amplification with sequence-specific primers. *Vox Sang* **71**(2):121–125, 1996.
138. Livak KJ. Allelic discrimination using fluorogenic probes and the 5′ nuclease assay. *Genet Anal* **14**(5-6):143–149, 1999.
139. Ranade K, Chang MS, Ting CT et al. High-throughput genotyping with single nucleotide polymorphisms. *Genome Res* **11**(7):1262–1268, 2001.
140. Syvanen AC. Accessing genetic variation: genotyping single nucleotide polymorphisms. *Nat Rev Genet* **2**(12):930–942, 2001.
141. Ficko T, Galvani V, Ruprecht R et al. Real-time PCR genotyping of human platelet alloantigens HPA-1, HPA-2, HPA-3 and HPA-5 is superior to the standard PCR-SSP method. *Transfus Med* **14**(6):425–432, 2004.
142. Beiboer SH, Wieringa-Jelsma T, Maaskant-Van Wijk PA et al. Transfusion. Rapid genotyping of blood group antigens by multiplex polymerase chain reaction and DNA microarray hybridization. *Transfusion* **45**(5):667–679, 2005.
143. Kaplan C, Porcelijn L, Vanlieferinghen P et al. Anti-HPA-9bw (Maxa) fetomaternal alloimmunization, a clinically severe neonatal thrombocytopenia: difficulties in diagnosis and therapy and report on eight families. *Transfusion* **45**(11):1799–1803, 2005.
144. Santoso S, Kiefel V, Mueller-Eckhardt C. Immunochemical characterization of the new platelet alloantigen system Bra/Brb. *Br J Haematol* **72**(2):91–198, 1989.
145. Kiefel V, Santoso S, Weisheit M. Monoclonal antibody-specific immobilization of platelet antigens (MAIPA): a new tool for the identification of platelet reactive antibodies. *Blood* **70**:1722–1726, 1987.
146. Campbell KA, Mushens R, Ouwehand WH et al. Selection of optimal glycoprotein capture antibodies in a rapid monoclonal antibody immobilisation of platelet antigen (MAIPA) assay. (Poster) 8th European Symposium on platelet and granulocyte immunobiology. Rust, 2004.
147. Ruiter M, Onderwater L, Huiskes E et al. MAIPA in one day modification of the standard MAIPA. (Poster) NVB symposium transfusion medicine. Ede, 2005.
148. Lucas GF, Rogers SE. Evaluation of an enzyme-linked immunosorbent assay kit (GTI PakPlus) for the detection of antibodies against human platelet antigens. *Transfus Med* **9**(1):63–67, 1999.
149. Lucas GF, Rogers SE. Evaluation of an enzyme-linked immunosorbent assay kit (GTI PakPlus(R)) for the detection of antibodies against human platelet antigens. *Transfus Med* **9**(4):385–386, 1999.
150. Allen D, Murphy MF. Comment on: Transfus Med. 1999 Mar 9(1):63–7. Evaluation of an enzyme-linked immunosorbent assay kit (GTI PakPlus) for the detection of antibodies against human platelet antigens. *Transfus Med* **9**(4):384–386, 1999.
151. Kaushansky K. Thrombopoietin. *N Engl J Med* **339**:746–754, 1998.
152. Debili N, Wendling F, Cosman D et al. The Mpl receptor is expressed in the megakaryocytic lineage from late progenitors to platelets. *Blood* **85**: 391–401, 1995.
153. Broudy VC, Lin NL, Sabath DF et al. Human platelets display high affinity receptors for thrombopoietin. *Blood* **89**:1896–1904, 1997.
154. Folman CC, de Jong SCM, de Haas M et al. Analysis of the kinetics of thrombopoietin uptake during platelet transfusion. *Transfusion* **41**:517–521, 2001.
155. Fielder PJ, Hass P, Nagel M et al. Human platelets as a model for the binding and degradation of thrombopoietin. *Blood* **89**:2782–2788, 1997.
156. Li J, Xia Y, Kuter DJ. Interaction of thrombopoietin with the platelet c-mpl receptor in plasma: binding, internalization, stability and pharmacokinetics. *Br J Haematol* **106**: 345–356, 1999.
157. Folman CC, von dem Borne AE, Rensink IH et al. Sensitive measurement of thrombopoietin by a monoclonal antibody based sandwich enzyme-linked immunosorbent assay. *Thromb Haemost* **78**:1262–1267, 1997.
158. Porcelijn L, Folman CC, de Haas M et al. Fetal and neonatal thrombopoietin levels in alloimmune thrombocytopenia. *Pediatr Res* **52**(1):105–108, 2002.
159. Killie MK, Kjeldsen-Kragh J, Skogen B et al. Maternal anti-HPA 1a antibody level as predictive value in Neonatal alloimmune thrombocytopenic purpura (NAITP) (abstract). *Blood* **104**:2072, 2004.
160. Killie MK, Husebekk A, Kaplan C et al. Maternal human platelet antigen-1a antibody level correlates with the platelet count in the newborns: a retrospective study. *Transfusion* **47**(1):55–58, 2007.
161. Lynch L, Bussel JB, McFarland JG et al. Antenatal treatment of alloimmune thrombocytopenia. *Obstet Gynecol* **80**: 67–71, 1992.
162. Kelsey HC, Rodeck CH. Prenatal management of fetal alloimmune thrombocytopenia. International Forum. *Vox Sang* **65**:183–184, 1993.
163. Birchall JE, Murphy MF, Kaplan C et al. European collaborative study of the antenatal management of feto-maternal alloimmune thrombocytopenia. *Br J Haematol* **122**:275–288, 2003.
164. Berkowitz RL, Kolb EA, McFarland JG et al. Parallel randomized trials of risk-based therapy for fetal alloimmune thrombocytopenia. *Obstet Gynecol* **107**:91–96, 2006.
165. Berkowitz RL, Bussel JB, McFarland JG. Alloimmune thrombocytopenia: state of the art 2006. *Am J Obstet Gynecol* **195**:907–913, 2006.
166. Overton TG, Duncan KR, Jolly M et al. Serial aggressive platelet transfusion for fetal alloimmune thrombocytopenia: platelet dynamics and perinatal outcome. *Am J Obstet Gynecol* **186**:826–831, 2002.
167. Wenstrom KD, Weiner CP, Williamson RA. Antenatal treatment of fetal alloimmune thrombocytopenia. *Obstet Gynecol* **80**:433–435, 1992.
168. Radder CM, Brand A, Kanhai HHH. A less invasive treatment strategy to prevent intracranial hemorrhage in fetal and neonatal alloimmune thrombocytopenia. *Am J Obstet Gynecol* **185**:683–688, 2001.
169. Kanhai HHH, van den Akker ESA, Walther FJ et al. Intravenous immunoglobulins without initial and follow-up cordocentesis in alloimmune fetal and neonatal thrombocytopenia at high risk for intracranial hemorrhage. *Fetal Diagn Ther* **21**:55–60, 2006.
170. Van den Akker E, Oepkes D, Lopriore E et al. Noninvasive antenatal management of fetal and neonatal alloimmune thrombocytopenia: safe and effective. *Br J Obstet Gynaecol* **114**:469–473, 2007.
171. Ni H, Chen P, Spring CM, Sayeh E et al. A novel murine model of fetal and neonatal alloimmune thrombocytopenia: response to intravenous IgG therapy. *Blood* **107**:2976–2983, 2006.
172. Thung SF, Grobman WA. The cost effectiveness of empiric intravenous immunoglobulin for the antepartum treatment of fetal and neonatal alloimmune thrombocytopenia. *Am J Obstet Gynecol* **193**(3 Pt 2):1094-1099, 200;.
173. Radder CM, Roelen DL, Van de Meer-Prins EM et al. The immunologic profile of infants born after maternal immunoglobulin treatment and intrauterine platelet transfusions for fetal/neonatal alloimmune thrombocytopenia. *Am J Obstet Gynecol* **191**:815–820, 2004.
174. Radder CM, de Haan MJJ, Brand A et al. Follow up of children after antenatal treatment for alloimmune thrombocytopenia. *Early Hum Dev* **80**:65–76, 2004.
175. Ward MJ, Pauliny J, Lipper EG, Bussel JB. Long-term effects of fetal and neonatal alloimmune thrombocytopenia and its antenatal treatment on the medical and developmental outcomes of affected children. *Am J Perinatol* **23**(8):487–492, 2006.

CHAPTER

42 Treatable fetal endocrine and metabolic disorders

Guy Rosner, Shai Ben Shahar, Yuval Yaron and Mark I Evans

KEY POINTS

- This chapter deals with fetal metabolic and endocrine disorders that may be treated pharmacologically. In addition, the use of folic acid supplementation for the prevention of neural tube defects is discussed
- Endocrine disorders are discussed including congenital adrenal hperplasia (CAH), hypothyroidism and hyperthyroidism, as well as modalities for fetal pharmacologic therapy
- Several inborn errors of metabolism are discussed, such as methylmalonic acidemia, multiple carboxylase deficiency, Smith–Lemli–Optiz syndrome and galactosemia. Pharmacologic and nutritional approaches are discussed
- Multifactorial disorders, chiefly neural tube defects and their prevention by folic acid supplementation, are discussed

INTRODUCTION

The diagnostic armamentarium of prenatal diagnosis has continued to grow rapidly over the past two decades. The number of conditions amenable to early diagnosis has increased geometrically and it is likely to continue on a geometric rise. Such possibilities have enhanced patients' reproductive choices including safer and earlier termination of pregnancy when chosen by the parents and increasing options for limited treatments in utero. However, some metabolic and endocrine disorders, such as congenital adrenal hyperplasia and cardiac arrhythmias, may also be amenable to pharmacological interventions[1,2]. The use of folic acid supplementation for the prevention of neural tube defects has numerically been the single most successful active pharmacologic therapy preventing, by estimation, literally thousands of babies suffering with the sequelae of neural tube defects. Surgical and genetic approaches are discussed elsewhere.

ENDOCRINE DISORDERS

Congenital adrenal hyperplasia

Treatment of congenital adrenal hyperplasia (CAH) during fetal life is the classic example of the pharmacological prevention of a birth defect. CAH actually comprises a group of metabolic disorders all of which include enzymatic defects in the steroidogenic pathway. Cortisol production is diminished because of the enzymatic abnormalities and there is a compensatory increase in adrenocorticotrophic hormone (ACTH) secretion, which leads to overproduction of the steroid precursors in the adrenal cortex – hence the adrenal hyperplasia.

All forms are inherited in an autosomal recessive manner with the phenotype of each form determined by the severity of the cortisol deficiency and the nature of the steroid precursors. The most common abnormality, responsible for >90% of patients with CAH, is caused by a deficiency of the 21–hydroxylase (21–OH) enzyme. Other, but rare, causes for CAH, include deficiencies in 11β-hydroxylase, 17α-hydroxylase, and 3β-hydroxysteroid-dehydrogenase. Diminished 21–OH activity results in accumulation of 17–hydroxyprogesterone (17–OHP) as a result of its decreased conversion to 11–deoxycorticosterone. The excess 17–OHP is then converted via androstenedione to androgens, the levels of which increase by as much as several hundred-fold (Fig. 42.1). The excess androgens cause virilization of the undifferentiated female external genitalia. The degree of virilization may vary from mild clitoral hypertrophy to complete formation of a phallus and scrotum. In contrast, genital development in male fetuses is normal. The excess androgens cause postnatal virilization in both genders and may manifest in precocious puberty.

The 'classical' form of CAH involves a severe enzyme deficiency or even a complete block of enzymatic activity, which is associated in two-thirds to three-quarters with salt loss that may be life-threatening. The classical form is easy to recognize in female newborns but may be overlooked in males which may present at a later stage with severe dehydration and even demise. The estimated incidence of classical CAH varies by populations enormously from perhaps 1:5000 to 1:60 000,

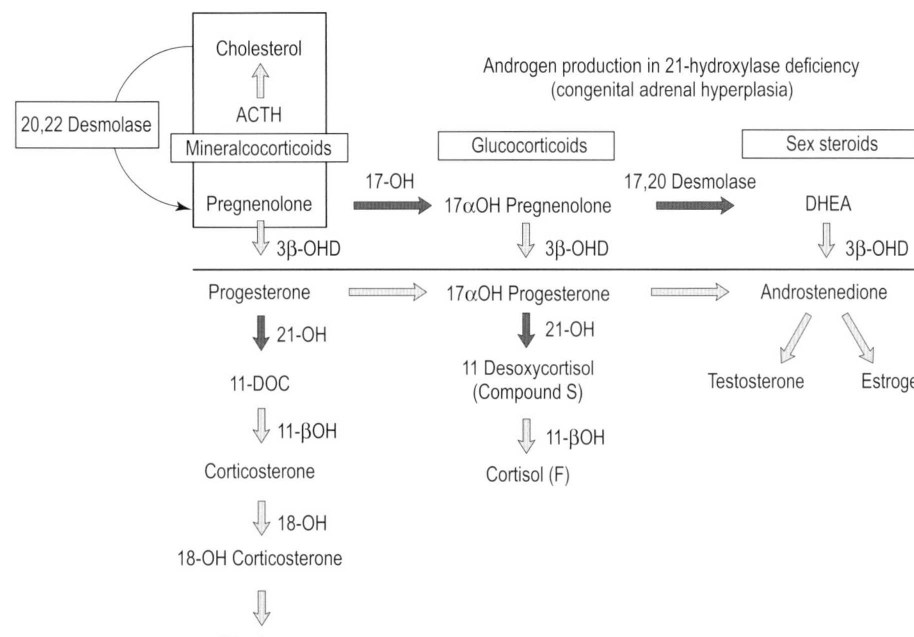

Fig. 42.1 Steroidogenic pathway. Conversion from cholesterol to cortisol is vulnerable to enzymatic errors. Blockage at 21 hydroxylase leads to over production of 17 hydroxyprogesterone which ultimately leads to excess androgens that produce masculinization of the external genitalia.

depending on the ethnic background. The 'non-classical' attenuated form of 21–OH deficiency results in partial blockade of the enzymatic activity and is usually clinically apparent as simple virilization in women only later in life. It is estimated to occur in ≈3.5% in Ashkenazi Jews and ≈2% in Hispanics[3]. The gene for 21OH is *CYP21A2*, located on the RCCX module, which happens to be a chromosomal region highly prone to genetic recombination events resulting in a wide variety of complex rearrangements[4]. *CYP21A2* is mapped to chromosome 6p21.3, and currently more than 100 disease-causing mutations have been described[5], allowing direct prenatal mutation analysis.

Two decades ago, diagnosis of CAH was made by the finding of elevated levels of 17–OHP in amniotic fluid. With the development of chorionic villus sampling (CVS) in the 1980s, linkage-based molecular diagnosis in the first trimester became available. Since discovery and mapping of the gene, direct DNA mutation analysis has become the routine approach. It is estimated that approximately 95–98% of the mutations causing 21OHD have been identified through a combination of molecular genetic techniques making CVS, rather than amniocentesis, the preferred diagnostic method in use[5]. However, when amniocentesis is used as an alternative, the supernatant is used for hormonal measurement and the cells are cultured to obtain a genotype through DNA analysis. Preimplantation genetic diagnosis (PGD), which identifies genetic abnormalities in preimplantation embryos prior to embryo transfer, has not been utilized yet in congenital adrenal hyperplasia, but probably will in the near future.

The fetal adrenal gland can be pharmacologically suppressed by maternal replacement doses of dexamethasone[6]. The suppression can prevent masculinization of affected female fetuses in couples that are carriers of classical CAH (fetuses at risk for non-classical CAH do not require any prenatal treatment). In the first attempt to prevent female genital birth defects in 1982, Evans et al. administered dexamethasone to a carrier mother beginning at 10 weeks of gestation[6]. Serial maternal estriol and cortisol levels indicated that adrenal gland suppression had been achieved. The female fetus was born at 39 weeks' gestation with normal external genitalia. Forrest and David then employed a similar protocol beginning at 9 weeks' gestation to treat several fetuses at risk for CAH[7]. Female fetuses subsequently confirmed to be affected with severe CAH were spared masculinization of the external genitalia. Several hundred pregnant women and their fetuses have since been treated with prevention of masculinization in more than 85% of affected females[8].

Since the differentiation of the external genitalia begins at about 7 weeks of gestation, diagnosis by amniocentesis or even CVS comes far too late to prevent masculinization. Thus for carrier parents at risk of having an affected fetus, pharmacological therapy has to be initiated prior to diagnosis, usually at the sixth or seventh week of gestation. This implies that therapy needs to be administered to all patients at risk despite the fact that the chance of an affected female fetus for carrier parents is only 1 in 8 (i.e. 1/4 affected × 1/2 female). Direct DNA diagnosis may then be performed by CVS in the first trimester. Thus, for 7 out of 8 of patients, therapy can be discontinued as soon as the diagnosis of male sex is made or if CAH is ruled out. However, if the fetus is indeed found to be an affected female, then therapy is continued throughout gestation. Stress-dose corticosteroids should be given to the mother during labor and tapered gradually postpartum. If, however, the fetus is a male, or is unaffected, then therapy can be discontinued at the time of diagnosis.

No consistent untoward effects on fetuses have been reported, as in follow-up studies of prenatally treated children where pre- and postnatal growth has been normal[8]. However, concern has risen as several adverse events like corpus callosum agenesis, hydrocephalus, failure to thrive and mental retardation were reported prenatally in treated children, though without any obvious causal relationship[9,10]. Importantly, animal studies which found adverse effects cognitively and somatically in animals exposed perinatally to corticosteroids are inaccurate to interpret into human studies as dexamethasone doses used were high in contrast to the low dosage used in humans[11]. A Swedish study published recently assessed cognitive skills in 26 children who were treated with corticosteroids prenatally and found prenatal dexamethasone treatment to be associated with long-term effects on verbal working memory, but without an affect on major cognitive measures like IQ, learning and long-term memory[11]. Regarding therapy risks in the pregnant mother, one can expect greater weight gain, edema and striae, but no increased risk of hypertension or gestational diabetes[8]. Inclusion criteria of the European Society for Pediatric Endocrinology and Wilkins Pediatric Endocrine Society[12] for prenatal treatment of CAH include:

1. a previously affected sibling or first-degree relative with known mutation causing classical CAH proven by DNA analysis
2. reasonable expectation that the father is the same as the proband's
3. availability of rapid and quality genetic analysis
4. therapy started less than 9 weeks following the last menstrual period (LMP)
5. lack of intent for therapeutic abortion
6. reasonable expectation of patient's compliance.

There is an agreement that the treatment requires a professional team that includes an expert high-risk obstetrician, a pediatric endocrinologist, genetic counselor and a molecular genetic laboratory.

Thyroid disorders

Hypothyroidism

Congenital hypothyroidism affects about 1:3000 to 1:4000 infants[13]. About 85% of the cases are the result of thyroid dysgenesis, a heterogeneous group of developmental defects characterized by inadequate amount of thyroid tissue. Congenital hypothyroidism is only rarely associated with errors of thyroid hormone synthesis, thyroid stimulating hormone (TSH) insensitivity, or absence of the pituitary gland. Fetal hypothyroidism may not necessarily manifest in a goiter before birth since maternal thyroid hormones may cross the placenta. Congenital hypothyroidism presenting with a goiter can be found in only about 10–15% of cases, with an estimated prevalence of 1:30 000-1:50 000 live births[14].

Fetal goiterous hypothyroidism is caused in most instances by maternal exposure to thyrostatic agents used to treat maternal hyperthyroidism[15]. The most common agents include propylthiouracil (PTU), the inadvertent use of radioactive I^{131} in the pregnant women, or iodide exposure. Maternal ingestion of amiodarone or lithium may also cause hypothyroidism in the fetus. Finally, fetal hypothyroidism may result from transplacental passage of maternal blocking antibodies (known as TBIAb or TBII) or rarely due to rare defects in fetal thyroid hormone biosynthesis[13].

Fetal goiterous hypothyroidism may lead to severe fetal and neonatal consequences. An enlarged goiter may cause esophageal obstruction, which may lead to polyhydramnios, which may result in preterm delivery or premature rupture of membranes. Rarely, a goiter may even lead to high-output heart failure due to high vascular flow in the goiter[16]. A large fetal goiter can cause extension of the fetal neck leading to dystocia. The effects of the fetal hypothyroidism itself may be devastating. Without treatment, postnatal growth delay and severe mental retardation may ensue. Even with immediate diagnosis and treatment at birth, long-term follow-up of children with congenital hypothyroidism has demonstrated that they have lower scores on perceptual-motor, visuospatial and language tests[17].

In suspicious cases, an extensive maternal and family history should be obtained. In patients with a positive history, maternal thyroid hormone levels, as well as blocking immunoglobulin levels should be measured. In addition, all women with a history of any thyroid disease (both hypothyroidism and hyperthyroidism) are advised to have monthly fetal ultrasound scans to screen for fetal goiter, polyhydramnios or fetal tachycardia[17].

Rarely, fetal goiterous hypothyroidism may be identified by a routine ultrasound performed due to increased uterine size caused by polyhydramnios secondary to esophageal obstruction and impaired swallowing. Sometimes, a fetal goiter may incidentally be discovered on a routine scan. Before the advent of cordocentesis, amniotic fluid levels of TSH and FT4 were used as potential indicators of fetal thyroid function. However, these proved to be inconsistent[18]. With cordocentesis, fetal thyroid status can be directly and accurately evaluated; fetal response to therapy can therefore be reliably measured using available appropriate nomograms for fetal serum levels of free T4, total T4, free T3, total T3 and TSH[19,20]. In utero treatment was initially suggested by Van Herle et al. using intramuscular injection of levothyroxine sodium[21]. Subsequent studies, however, have indicated that intra-amniotic (IA) administration of thyroxine may be superior and can lead to resolution of the polyhydramnios as well. The dose of the injected drug may be refined using the fetal thyroid profile in the amniotic fluid and the thyroid size[22]. The doses commonly used for treatment range from 200 to 500 mg IA every week[23]. With this regimen, fetal goiters have been shown to regress, the hyperextension of the fetal head has been shown to resolve and fetal and newborn TSH levels have normalized[22].

Hyperthyroidism

Neonatal hyperthyroidism is rare with an incidence of 1:4000 to 1:40 000/live births[14]. Fetal thyrotoxic goiter is usually secondary to maternal autoimmune disease, principally Graves' disease or Hashimoto's thyroiditis. As many as 12% of infants of mothers with a known history of Graves' disease are affected with neonatal thyrotoxicosis, which may occur even if the mother is euthyroid[23]. As with hypothyroidism, inherent to the underlying mechanism is the transplacental passage of maternal IgG antibodies. In this case, the antibodies, known as TSAb or (TSI), are predominantly directed against the TSH receptor.

Usually, the investigation of fetal hyperthyroidism begins only after the discovery of fetal goiter. Often, the goiter is diagnosed on ultrasound in patients referred due to elevated thyroid stimulating antibodies. In some cases, fetal goiters are realized serendipitously on routine ultrasonography. Others may be discovered in patients referred for scan because of polyhydramnios. Beside the risks related to the goiter itself, untreated fetal hyperthyroidism may be associated with a mortality rate of 12–25% due to high-output cardiac failure[24]. Once a fetal goiter is identified, biochemical evaluation is indicated. Historically, amniotic fluid levels of TSH and FT4 were used as potential indicators of fetal thyroid function. These, however, proved inconsistent in that amniotic fluid levels of these hormones do not always correlate with their serum levels. Some controversy still exists regarding their use, however, they may be of some benefit in centers that do not have available cordocentesis[25]. As previously stated, cordocentesis allows reliable assessment of fetal thyroid status TSH[26,27] and treatment can be planned accordingly.

Once the diagnosis of fetal hyperthyroidism is confirmed, fetal treatment should be initiated. Authors have attempted treating fetal hyperthyroidism with maternally administered antithyroid drugs. Porreco has reported maternal treatment of fetal thyrotoxicosis with PTU, which led to a good outcome[28]. The initial dose used was 100 mg PO three times a day, which was later decreased to 50 mg PO three times a day. Wenstrom et al. described a favorable outcome using maternal methimazole to treat fetal hyperthyroidism in a patient who could not tolerate PTU failure[24]. Hatjis[29] also treated fetal goiterous hyperthyroidism with a maternal dose of 300 mg PTU. This patient, however, required supplemental synthroid to remain euthyroid. There was good fetal outcome in this case as well.

INBORN ERRORS OF METABOLISM

Methylmalonic acidemia

The methylmalonic acidemias (MMA) are a group of enzyme-deficiency diseases inherited in an autosomal recessive manner resulting from one of several genetically distinct etiologies. Some cases are caused by mutations in the gene encoding methylmalonyl-coenzyme A mutase while others are due to a defect that reduces the biosynthesis of adenosylcobalamin from B12. The disease is characterized by a wide clinical spectrum ranging from a benign condition to a fatal neonatal disease. In the severe form, MMA is characterized by severe metabolic acidosis, developmental delay and biochemical abnormalities that include methylmalonic aciduria, long chain ketonuria and intermittent hyperglycinemia. Patients with defects in adenosylcobalamin biosynthesis may respond to administration of large doses of B12, which may enhance the amount of active holoenzyme (mutase apoenzyme plus adenosylcobalamin). A proposed mechanism for the neurological abnormalities observed in methylmalonic acidemia was suggested by a group of Brazilian investigators[30] who administered methylmalonic acid to rats during the first month of their life. A significant diminution of myelin content and of ganglioside N-acetylneuraminic acid was noted in the cerebrum. There seems to be a lack of consensus on the most reliable method by which to conduct investigation for pregnancies at risk for methylmalonic acidemia as well as for other inborn errors of cobalamin metabolism. Morel et al. have published their experience in prenatal diagnosis of 117 high-risk pregnancies for these disorders[31]. Diagnosis was made from either cultured chorionic villus cells (CCVC) or by cultured amniocytes (CA). There was one false negative and one false positive result with CCVC, and two cases with elevated amniotic fluid levels of MMA at CA later on appeared to be false positive results. Based on their experience, the authors concluded that combining two independent methods for prenatal diagnosis is recommended and that CA studies appear more reliable than CCVC studies.

Reports of prenatal treatment in such disorders are somehow lacking. In the next paragraph, we briefly bring some of the published experience.

More than 20 years ago, Ampola and colleagues were the first to attempt prenatal diagnosis and treatment of a B12-responsive variant of MMA[32]. They followed the pregnancy of a patient who had previously suffered the loss of a child to severe acidosis and dehydration at the age of 3 months. The diagnosis of MMA was made posthumously by chemical analysis of blood and urine. In the subsequent pregnancy, amniocentesis at 19 weeks revealed elevated methylmalonic acid in the amniotic fluid. Cultured amniocytes also demonstrated defective propionate oxidation and undetectable levels of adenosylcobalamin. When adenosylcobalamin was added, normal succinate oxidation and methylmalonyl-coenzyme A mutase activity were noted. These studies established that the fetus also suffered from MMA apparently due to deficient synthesis of adenosylcobalamin. It was already been known that fetal MMA is associated with increased methylmalonic acid excretion in the maternal urine. Indeed, Ampola et al. documented increased methylmalonic acidemia in maternal urine at 23 and 25 weeks' gestation. Late in the pregnancy, cyanocobalamin (10 mg/day) was orally administered to the mother in divided doses. The treatment only marginally altered the maternal serum B12 level. However, there was a slight reduction of maternal urinary methylmalonic acid excretion that remained several fold above normal. At approximately 34 weeks' gestation, 5 mg of cyanocobalamin per day was administered intramuscularly. The maternal serum B12 level then rose gradually to more than sixfold above normal and was accompanied by a progressive decrease in urinary methylmalonic acid excretion. Maternal urinary methylmalonate was only slightly above the normal range when delivery occurred at 41 weeks. Amniotic fluid methylmalonic acid concentrations were three times the normal mean at 19 menstrual weeks and four times the normal mean at term, despite prenatal treatment. Postnatally, the diagnosis of methylmalonic acidemia was confirmed. The infant suffered no acute neonatal complications and had an extremely high serum B12 level. Long-term postnatal management involved protein restriction; however, no continuous B12 treatment was required. In this instance, prenatal treatment certainly improved the fetal and, secondarily, the maternal biochemistry. Whether there was any significant clinical benefit to the fetus by in utero treatment cannot be assessed adequately. It seems likely that reducing the fetal burden of methylmalonic acid should have some beneficial effect on fetal development and could reduce the risks in the neonatal period.

Andersson et al.[33] followed a cohort of eight children with MMA for 5.7 years. Congenital malformations were described, reinforcing the deleterious effects of prenatally abnormal cyanocobalamin metabolism. Growth was significantly improved in most cases after initiation of therapy postnatally and, in one case, microcephaly resolved. However, developmental delay of variable severity was always present regardless of treatment onset. These data suggest that prenatal therapy of MMA may be effective and perhaps ameliorate some of the prenatal effects. Evans et al. have documented the changing dose requirements necessary over the course of pregnancy to maintain adequate levels of B12. They sequentially followed maternal plasma and urine levels in a prenatal treated pregnancy[34]. Data such as these suggest that modulation of maternal–fetal pharmacological interchange of therapeutic drugs will be difficult to control precisely.

Multiple carboxylase deficiency

Biotin-responsive multiple carboxylase deficiency is an inborn error of metabolism caused by diminished activity of the mitochondrial biotin-dependent enzymes (pyruvate carboxylase, propionyl-coenzyme A carboxylase and α-methylcrotonyl-coenzyme A carboxylase). The condition may arise from mutations in the holocarboxilase synthetase gene (HCS) mapped to chromosome 21q22.1 or the biotinidase gene localized to chromosome 3p25[35–39]. Affected patients present as newborns or in early childhood with dermatitis, severe metabolic acidosis and a characteristic pattern of organic acid excretion. It has been demonstrated that metabolism in patients or in their cultured cells can be restored toward normal levels by biotin supplementation. Prenatal diagnosis can be made by demonstration of elevated levels of typical organic acids (3-hydroxyisovalerate, methylcitrate) in the amniotic fluid or in the chorionic villi. However, the existence of a mild form of HCS deficiency can complicate prenatal diagnosis as organic acid levels in amniotic fluid might be normal[40]. Therefore, prenatal diagnosis must be performed by enzyme assay in cultured fetal cells in biotin-restricted medium. When the disease-causing mutation is known, direct DNA sequencing of chorionic villus sample is the preferred choice as was demonstrated by the report of Malvagia et al.[41].

Roth and colleagues treated a fetus without the benefit of prenatal diagnosis in a case in which two previous siblings had died of multiple carboxylase deficiency[42]. The first had died within 3 days of birth and, in the second, the diagnosis of biotin-responsive carboxylase deficiency was made posthumously. Since the mother was first seen at 34 weeks' gestation, prenatal diagnosis was not attempted. Because of severe neonatal manifestations in previous offspring and due to the probable harmlessness of biotin, oral administration was begun at a dose of 10 mg/day. There were no apparent untoward effects; maternal urinary biotin excretion increased by a factor of approximately 100 during biotin administration. Non-identical twins were subsequently delivered at term. Cord blood and urinary organic acid profiles were normal and cord blood biotin concentrations were four to seven times greater than normal. The neonatal course for both twins was unremarkable. Subsequent study of the cultured fibroblasts of both twins indicated that the cells of twin B (but not of twin A) had virtually complete deficiency of all three carboxylase activities. Genetic complementation studies confirmed that, despite the normal clinical presentation during the newborn period, twin B was homozygous for the disease mutation.

Packman and colleagues have also reported prenatal diagnosis and treatment of biotin-responsive multiple carboxylase deficiency for a mother who had previously given birth to a male with the neonatal-onset form of this disease[43]. In the subsequent pregnancy, maternal urine organic acid profiles were normal. Carboxylase activities were assayed in cultured amniotic fluid cells obtained by amniocentesis at 17 weeks. In a biotin-restricted medium, the amniotic cells demonstrated the characteristic severe reduction in carboxylase activities. Since these initial reports of prenatal administration of biotin to fetuses affected with this disorder, other cases that have been published[40,44] provide further compelling evidence that biotin administration antenatally is effectively taken up by the fetus and prevents functional deficiency of the carboxylases in an affected newborn. No toxicity from treatment was observed. However, because experience with this treatment is confined to a small number of cases, it is reasonabe to carry out prenatal diagnosis and only then to initiate treatment with biotin in any affected fetus.

Smith–Lemli–Optiz Syndrome (SLOS)

Smith–Lemli–Optiz syndrome (SLOS) is a dysmorphological syndrome first reported in 1964[45] but has since been found to be an autosomal recessive disorder of endogenous cholesterol biosynthesis caused by deficiency of 7-dehydrocholesterol reductase (DHCR7)[46].

Features include characteristic facies, growth and mental retardation, and anomalies of the heart, kidneys, central nervous system and limbs. Cleft palate, postaxial polydactyly, 2-3 syndactyly of the toes and cataracts are often seen in affected patients. The 2-3 syndactyly of the toes is very specific for this disorder and is seen in >90% of affected patients. Affected patients typically present with a narrow forehead, ptosis, anteverted nares, low-set ears and micrognathia.

Males may present with ambiguous genitalia. In contrast with CAH, patients with SLOS are deficient in cholesterol and therefore lack steroid precursors. This leads to lack of androgens that results in under-masculinization of the male genitalia. Patients with the severe form of the syndrome present not only with these dysmorphological findings but also with a high rate of neonatal mortality[47]. The incidence of SLOS is estimated to be 1:20 000–1:40 000 live births[48] and it appears to be most common in Caucasians population of North European origin, with an estimated carrier frequency of 1:70[49]. In 1993, the etiology of SLOS was discovered to be an inborn error of cholesterol biosynthesis due to a deficiency of the enzyme dehydrocholesterol-Δ^7reductase[48,50–52]. The gene for 7-dehydrocholesterol-Δ^7reductase has been localized to chromosome 11q12-13[52].

As a result of this enzymatic defect, there is a characteristic biochemical pattern of reduced cholesterol levels and elevated 7 and 8 dehydrocholesterol levels (7-DHC and 8-DHC respectively) in all body fluids and tissues including red blood cells, fibroblasts, amniotic fluid and chorionic villi. The values observed in affected patients may be extremely variable. The diagnosis is made primarily by the presence of the cholesterol precursor, 7-DHC, and not by the deficiency of cholesterol. The level of 7-DHC in affected patients is 100 to 1000 times normal. Unaffected individuals have levels of 7-DHC and 8-DHC of less than 1 mg/dl, whereas patients with SLOS have levels of 7 to 20 or greater. Clinical manifestations correlate with cholesterol levels. Severely affected patients have very low levels (usually <10–15 mg/dl), while those with more mild manifestations may present with levels of 40–70 mg/dl. Prenatal diagnosis of SLOS has been available since 1994 by either amniocentesis or chorionic villus sampling[53–55].

With the identification of the affected gene, DHCR7, it became possible to perform a prenatal molecular diagnosis of mutations. Wave et al. have shown that mutation analysis for SLOS is a rapid and reliable method for prenatal diagnosis and provides an alternative to specialized biochemical tests for elevated 7DHC in amniotic fluid or CVS[46].

Since the identification of the cholesterol metabolic defect in SLOS, a treatment protocol has been attempted providing exogenous cholesterol. This form of therapy has now been provided to many patients with SLOS for the past several years in many centers in the USA and internationally[50–52], with the goal of raising cholesterol levels and decreasing the precursors, 7-DHC and 8-DHC. It has been shown that dietary cholesterol supplementation can restore a normal growth pattern in children and adolescents with SLOS, alleviate behavioral abnormalities and improve general health[56–59].

Fetal therapy strategies may theoretically include providing cholesterol to the mother or to the fetus. The former, however, is not possible because cholesterol does not cross the placenta well in the second trimester and there is lack of evidence that it crosses the placenta in the third trimester. Moreover, cholesterol is available only in a crystalline form that cannot be given intravenously or intramuscularly. Furthermore, it is impractical to inject cholesterol into the amniotic fluid because it would precipitate. However, cholesterol can be given to the fetus by giving fresh frozen plasma in the form of LDL-cholesterol. The group at Tufts University has attempted treatment antenatally in several affected fetuses. In cases where treatment was started late in pregnancy, the results were inconclusive. Although few descriptions of fetal therapy for SLOS exist, the latest report of antenatal treatment comes from that same group of investigators[60]. Therapy was begun at 34 weeks of gestation and resulted in increased fetal cholesterol levels and red blood cell mean corpuscular volume with subtle improvement in fetal growth, as assessed by consequent fetal weight plots. However, no significant change in 7-DHC and 8-DHC levels was observed, further emphasizing the inconclusiveness of that treatment. However, the main point is that since significant development of the central nervous system and myelination occurs prior to birth, it is a reasonable to assume that providing cholesterol to the fetus, as early as possible, would result in the most clinical benefit.

Galactosemia

Galactosemia is an inborn error of metabolism caused by diminished activity of the enzyme galactose-1-phosphate uridyltransferase (GALT). It is inherited in an autosomal recessive manner and results in cataracts, growth deficiency and ovarian failure. Clinical symptoms appear in the neonatal period and can be largely ameliorated by elimination of galactose from the diet. Cellular damage in galactosemia is thought to be mediated by accumulation of galactose-l-phosphate intracellularly and of galactitol in the lens. The *GALT* gene, localized to chromosome 9p13, is the only known gene to be associated with galactosemia. Several disease-causing mutations are commonly encountered in classical galactosemia, the most frequently observed is the Q188R classical mutation. Mutational analysis is available usefully for the six classical galactosemia alleles (Q188R, S135L, K285N, L195P, Y209C, F171S) and for the N314D Durate variant mutation[61]. In cases in which disease-causing mutations are not identified (as observed in 10–29% of classic galactosemia), GALT sequence analysis may be performed to detect private mutations. Galactosemia can be diagnosed prenatally by study of cultured amniocytes and chorionic villi.

There are suggestions that even the early postnatal treatment of galactosemic individuals with a low-galactose diet may not be sufficient to ensure normal development. Some have speculated that prenatal damage to galactosemic fetuses could contribute to subsequent abnormal neurological development and to lens cataract formation. Furthermore, it has been recognized that female galactosemics, even when treated from birth with galactose deprivation, have a high frequency of primary or secondary amenorrhea because of ovarian failure. This is because oocytes have already been damaged irreversibly long before birth. There also may be some subtle abnormalities of male gonadal function.

Exposure to a high-galactose diet has been considered to represent an animal model for human galactosemia. Chen and colleagues have observed a reduction in the oocyte content of rat ovaries after prenatal exposure to a 50% galactose diet[62]. No analogous alterations in the testes were observed in prenatally treated males. Experiments in rats suggest that toxicity to the female gonads from galactose or its metabolites is most obvious during the premeiotic stages of ovarian development. Impaired germ cell migration leading to the development of gonads with deficient initial pools of germ cells was proposed as the causal link between galactosemia and premature ovarian failure[63].

These observations in animals and human beings have led to speculation that galactose restriction during pregnancy may be desirable if the fetus is affected with galactosemia. In the human female, ovarian meiosis begins at 12 and is complete by 28 menstrual weeks. Thus, ovarian damage, and perhaps neurological or lens abnormalities, might occur prior to the usual time when prenatal diagnosis by amniocentesis can be accomplished. Thus, anticipatory treatment in pregnancies at risk for having a galactosemic fetus might best be initiated very early in gestation or even preconceptually.

Despite these experiments and speculations, we are unaware of studies that adequately assess the impact of prenatal administration of a low-galactose diet to galactosemic infants. For obvious reasons, such data, especially controlled, will be difficult to obtain. Nevertheless, prenatal galactose restriction is probably desirable in galactosemia and should be harmless. There is little reason to suppose that galactose restriction would have adverse consequences, since galactosemic and normal fetuses are both capable of some endogenous galactose synthesis.

MULTIFACTORIAL DISORDERS

Neural tube defects

Neural tube defects (NTDs) are malformations secondary to abnormal neural tube closure between the third and fourth weeks of gestational age. The etiology is complex and imperfectly understood with both genetic and environmental factors involved. Animal studies suggest that NTDs can arise from a variety of vitamin or mineral deficiencies. There are historical data in humans suggesting increased NTD frequencies in subjects with poor dietary histories or with intestinal bypasses. Biochemical evidence of suboptimal nutrition is present in some women bearing infants with NTDs. Analysis of recurrence patterns within families and of twin–twin concordance data provides evidence of a genetic influence in non-syndromal cases, although factors such as socioeconomic status, geographic area, occupational exposure and maternal use of antiepileptic drugs are also associated with variations in the incidence of NTDs[64]. In 1980, Smithells et al. suggested that vitamin supplementation containing 0.36 mg folate can reduce the frequency of NTD recurrence by sevenfold in women with one or more prior affected children[65,66]. For almost a decade, there was a great deal of controversy regarding the benefit of folate supplementation for the prevention of NTDs[67–70].

Finally, in 1991, a randomized double-blinded trial designed by the MRC Vitamin Study Research Group demonstrated that preconceptual folate reduces the risk of recurrence in high-risk patients[71]. Subsequently, it was shown that preparations containing folate and other vitamins also reduce the occurrence of first time NTDs[72]. In response to these findings, guidelines were issued calling for consumption of 4.0 mg/day folic acid by women with a prior child affected with a NTD, for at least 1 month prior to conception through the first 3 months of pregnancy. In addition, 0.4 mg/day folic acid is recommended to all women planning a pregnancy to be taken preconceptually. The data on NTD recurrence prevention are now very well established and became routine for high-risk cases. As of January 1998, the United States Food and Drug Administration have mandated that breads and grains be supplemented with folic acid. The impact of food fortification with folic acid on NTDs birth prevalence during the years 1990–1999 was evaluated by assessing birth certificate reports before and after mandatory fortification[73]. It was found that the birth prevalence of NTDs reported decreased by 19%. It is important to note that the continuing decline in NTDs rates are estimated to be due to the introduction and increased utilization of prenatal diagnosis in addition to the recommendations for multivitamin use in women of childbearing age and the population-wide increases in blood folate levels since food fortification was mandated[74]. In 2004, Evans et al. have shown a nearly 30% drop in high maternal serum alpha-fetoprotein (MSAFP) values in the USA comparing 2000 values versus 1997 before the introduction of folic acid supplementation[75].

Folate plays a central part in embryonic and fetal development because of its role in nucleic acid synthesis, mandatory for the widespread cell division that takes place during embryogenesis. Folate deficiency can occur because of low dietary folate intake or because of increased metabolic requirement as seen in particular genetic alterations such as the polymorphism of the thermolabile enzyme methyltetrahydrofolate reductase (MTHFR). A metabolic effect of folate deficiency is homocysteine elevation in blood. As mentioned, the thermolabile variant of MTHFR, 677TT, is a known risk factor for NTDs. However, evidence regarding a second polymorphism in the same gene, 1298A→C, does not support its role in NTDs[76]. Additionally, numerous studies analyzing MTHFR variants have resulted in positive associations with increased NTD risk only in certain populations, suggesting that these variants are not large contributors to the etiology of NTDs[77]. Therefore, it seems less likely to advise parents prospectively to test for MTHFR variants. Reinforcement to the assumption that additional candidate genes other than MTHFR may be responsible for an increase risk to NTDs comes from the NTD collaborative group of Duke University[78]. One hundred and seventy-five American Caucasian NTD patients and their families were examined for the thermolabile variant of MTHFR. Although a significant association has been found comparing patients and controls, no such association was found in patients' parents. Two other key enzymes in the metabolic pathway of homocysteine are methionine synthase (MTR) and methionine synthase reductase (MTRR). Recently reported, MTR and a specific (A66G) MTRR polymorphism have been found to be associated with increased risk for NTDs. Interestingly, the NTDs' risk was not influenced by maternal preconception folic acid intake at doses of 0.4 mg/day. However, due to limited sample size further studies are needed in order to draw meaningful inferences[79]. Other candidate genes suggested as risk factor for NTDs (mainly spina bifida), are polymorphisms in the mitochondrial membrane transporter gene UCP2[80]. Despite previous studies suggesting zinc deficiency to play a role in the etiology of NTDs[81,82], further studies found this observation inconclusive[83,84]. Methionine deficiency might be involved in NTDs as 30–55% reduction in the risk of having NTD associated pregnancy was reported when methionine intake was greater than the lowest quartile of intake, with further reduction in risk with greater methionine intake[85]. In conclusion, preconception folic acid intake as a sole vitamin or as multivitamin supplementation reduces the risk of recurrence and first time NTDs. Additionally, folic acid-multivitamin supplementation reduces the occurrence of other congenital anomalies such as those seen in the urinary tract and cardiovascular systems, and anomalies involving the limbs and face (orofacial clefting). Recently, Ray et al.[86] evaluated whether low maternal vitamin B12 status may be a risk factor for NTDs. They found that there was almost a tripling in the risk for NTD in the presence of low maternal B12 status, measured by holoTC. However, it is yet too early to recommend adding synthetic B12 to current recommendations for periconceptional folic acid tablet supplements or folic-acid-fortified foods, and this issue definitely should be investigated in the coming years.

An interesting hypothesis was raised suggesting that bioavailability of nutrients to the fetus might be compromised in NTD-affected pregnancies. It is possible that, for example, maternal *Helicobacter pylori* infection could cause nutrient loss to the fetus, as folate, B12 and ferritin are depleted in *H. pylori* infection and these same deficiencies are related to NTD risk. Felkner et al.[87] found that *H. pylori* seropositivity was modestly associated with NTD-affected pregnancies (OR 1.4), while ORs of 2.0 or greater were seen in women younger than age 25 and with less than 7 years' education. Further research in this field is warranted.

PHARMACOLOGIC AND NUTRITIONAL APPROACHES

It might be appropriate to consider suppressing excessive cholesterol production prenatally in severe hypercholesterolemia when a safe and effective agent for accomplishing this becomes available (although there is no clear evidence for hypercholesterolemic prenatal damage). If cysteamine or related agents were to prove an effective treatment for lethal variants of cystinosis, prenatal therapy might be considered, because excessive and possibly harmful cystine accumulation is evident even in cystinotic fetuses. Cysteamine levels have been detected in chorionic villi and significant elevations even at 10 weeks' gestation have been hypothesized. Inhibitors of gamma-glutamyl transpeptidase, if safe, would elevate intracellular glutathione levels and inhibit oxoproline production in glutathione synthase deficiency, thereby averting the characteristic neonatal acidosis. In theory, it would be desirable to minimize copper accumulation in Wilson disease as early as possible. If and when reliable prenatal diagnosis of Wilson disease is possible, cautious administration of penicillamine prenatally might be considered. This would be a double-edged sword, however, as the teratogenic potential of penicillamine would demand careful evaluation. Batshaw and colleagues[88] have treated certain urea cycle defects by administering arginine and benzoate. Since hyperammonemia in some of these entities develops very acutely after birth, it might be desirable to consider pretreating the fetus with these compounds just prior to or during labor to minimize postnatal hyperammonemia. Conversely, it may be desirable to consider drug avoidance as an approach to fetal treatment. For example, fetuses with glucose-6-phosphate dehydrogenase deficiency are sensitive to a variety of drugs that induce hemolysis. It would probably be appropriate to avoid administering such agents to women carrying or known to be at risk for carrying fetuses deficient in glucose-6-phosphate dehydrogenase.

Umbilical cord catheterization under ultrasound guidance may lead to the development of other types of fetal treatment[89]. Systems, such as gene replacement, are being developed for certain lysosomal storage disorders. Progress is being made in postnatal experimental models on administration of thymic cells for certain immune deficiency states, bone marrow transplantation for a variety of genetic disorders, and gene transfer. The development of better and earlier techniques for prenatal treatment will be complex, especially with regard to gene transfer; but progress will be made and access to the fetal vasculature may be required for these methods to have a chance for success.

Bone marrow transplantation or thymic cell infusion is actually only a specialized example of organ transplantation. In the future, fetal organ transplantation may become possible and may open many prospects for surgical treatment of certain biochemical genetic disorders.

One can also speculate about the therapeutic possibilities involving compounds administered directly into the amniotic fluid or into the fetal intestinal tract. It might be possible, for example, to administer thyroid hormone in this fashion or to prevent meconium ileus in cystic fibrosis by instilling not yet determined enzymes into the fetal intestinal tract.

CONCLUSION

While a multitude of metabolic disorders exist, prenatal treatment for most has never been attempted or considered. The discovery of new disease associated genes and prenatal carrier testing may, in the future, allow preconceptual carrier detection, without the tragedy of first having an affected child. This may provide targeted therapy in families who chose to continue the pregnancy and offer the prospect of improved outcome by ameliorating at least some of the prenatal deleterious effects of the metabolic disease.

REFERENCES

1. Hume RF. Fetal pharmacologic therapy for mendelian disorders. In *Prenatal diagnosis*, MI Evans, MP Johnson, Y Yaron, A Drugan (eds), pp. 633–640. New York: McGraw Hill Publishing Co., 2006.
2. Johnson MP, Evans MI, Quintero RA, Flake AW. In utero therapy of the fetus. In *Principles and practice of medical therapy in pregnancy*, 3rd edn, N Gleisher, L Buttino, Jr, U Elkayam et al (eds). Norwalk: Appleton & Lange Publishing Co, 1998.
3. Speiser PW, Dupont B, Rubinstein P, Piazza A, Kastelan A, New MI. High frequency of nonclassical steroid 21-hydroxylase deficiency. *Am J Hum Genet* **37**:650–656, 1985.
4. Concalves J, Friaes A, Moura L. Congenital adrenal hyperplasia: focus on the molecular basis of 21-hydroxylase deficiency. *Expert Rev Mol Med* **9**:1–23, 2007.
5. Nimkarn S, Mew M. Prenatal diagnosis and treatment of congenital adrenal hyperplasia. *Pediatr Endocrinol Rev* **4**(2):99–105, 2006.
6. Evans MI, Chrousos GP, Mann DL et al. Pharmacologic suppression of the fetal adrenal gland in utero: attempted prevention of abnormal external genital masculinization in suspected congenital adrenal hyperplasia. *J Am Med Assoc* **253**:1015, 1985.
7. Forrest M, David M. Prenatal treatment of congenital adrenal hyperplasia due to 21-hydroxylase deficiency. 7th International Congress of Endocrinology, Abstract y11, Quebec, Canada, 1984.
8. New MI, Carlson A, Obeid J et al. Prenatal diagnosis for congenital adrenal hyperplasia in 532 pregnancies. *Clin Endocrinol Metab* **86**:5651–5657, 2001.
9. Forest MG, Dorr HG. Prenatal treatment of congenital adrenal hyperplasia (CAH) due to 21-hydroxylase deficiency: European experience in 223 pregnancies at risk. *Pediatr Res* **33**:S3, 1993.
10. Lajic S, Wedell A, Bui TH, Ritzen EM, Holst M. Long-term somatic follow-up of prenatally treated children with congenital adrenal hyperplasia. *J Clin Endocrinol Metab* **83**:3872–3880, 1998.
11. Hirvikovsky T, Nordenstrom A, Lindholm T et al. Cognitive functions in children at risk for congenital adrenal hyperplasia treated prenatally with dexamethasone. *J Clin Endocrinol Metab* **92**(2):542–548, 2007.
12. Clayton PE, Miller WL, Oberfield SE et al. ESPE/ LWPES CAH Working Group. Consensus statement on 21-hydroxylase deficiency from the European Society for Paediatric Endocrinology and the Lawson Wilkins Pediatric Endocrine Society. *Horm Res* **58**:188–195, 2002.
13. Fisher DA, Klein AH. Thyroid development and disorders of thyroid function in the newborn. *N Engl J Med* **304**:702–712, 1981.
14. Fisher DA. Neonatal thyroid disease of women with autoimmune thyroid disease. *Thyroid Today* **9**:1–7, 1986.
15. Volumenie JL, Polak M, Guibourdenche J et al. Management of fetal thyroid goitres: a report of 11 cases in a single perinatal unit. *Prenat Diagn* **20**:799, 2000.
16. Morine M, Takeda T, Minekawa R et al. Antenatal diagnosis and treatment of a case of fetal goitrous hypothyroidism associated with high-output cardiac failure. *Ultrasound Obstet Gynecol* **19**:506–509, 2002.
17. Rovet J, Ehrlich R, Sorbara D. Intellectual outcome in children with fetal hypothyroidism. *J Pediatr* **110**:700–704, 1987.
18. Sack J, Fisher DA, Hobel CJ, Lam R. Thyroxine in human amniotic fluid. *J Pediatr* **87**:364–368, 1975.
19. Thorpe-Beeston JG, Nicolaides KH, McGregor AM. Fetal thyroid function. *Thyroid* **2**:207–217, 1992.
20. Ballabio M, Nicolini U, Jowett T, Ruiz de Elvira MC, Ekins RP, Rodeck CH. Maturation of thyroid function in normal human fetuses. *Clin Endocrinol* **31**:565–571, 1989.
21. Van Herle AJ, Young RT, Fisher DA, Uller RP, Brinkman CR, III. Intra-uterine treatment of a hypothyroid fetus. *J Clin Endocrinol. Metab* **40**:474–477, 1973.
22. Gruner C, Kollert A, Wildt L, Dorr HG, Beinder E, Lang N. Intrauterine treatment of fetal goitrous hypothyroidism controlled by determination of thyroid-stimulating hormone in fetal serum: a case report and review of the literature. *Fetal Diagn Ther* **16**:47–51, 2001.
23. Bruinse HW, Vermeulen-Meiners C, Wit JM. Fetal treatment for thyrotoxicosis in non-thyrotoxic pregnant women. *Fetal Ther* **3**(3):152–157, 1988.
24. Wenstrom KD, Weiner CP, Williamson RA, Grant SS. Prenatal diagnosis of fetal

hyperthyroidism using funipuncture. *Obstet Gynecol* **76**:513–517, 1990.
25. Sack J, Fisher DA, Hobel CJ, Lam R. Thyroxine in human amniotic fluid. *J Pediatr* **87**:364–368, 1975.
26. Thorpe-Beeston JG, Nicolaides KH, McGregor AM. Fetal thyroid function. *Thyroid* **2**:207–217, 1992.
27. Ballabio M, Nicolini U, Jowett T, Ruiz de Elvira MC, Ekins RP, Rodeck CH. Maturation of thyroid function in normal human fetuses. *Clin Endocrinol* **31**:565–571, 1989.
28. Porreco RP, Bloch CA. Fetal blood sampling in the management of intrauterine thyrotoxicosis. *Obstet Gynecol* **76**:509–512, 1990.
29. Hatjis CG. Diagnosis and successful treatment of fetal goitrous hyperthyroidism caused by maternal Graves' disease. *Obstet Gynecol* **81**(5(Pt2)):837–839, 1993.
30. Brusque A, Rotta L, Pettenuzzo LF et al. Chronic postnatal administration of methylmalonic acid provokes a decrease of myelin content and ganglioside N-acetylneuraminic acid concentration in cerebrum of young rats. *Braz J Med Biol Res* **34**:227–231, 2001.
31. Morel CF, Watkins D, Scott P, Rinaldo P, Rosenblatt DS. Prenatal diagnosis for methymalonic academia and inborn errors of vitamin B12 metabolism and transport. *Molec Genet Metab* **86**:160–171, 2005.
32. Ampola MG, Mahoney MI, Nakamura E et al. Prenatal therapy of a patient with vitamin B responsive methylmalonic acidemia. *N Engl J Med* **293**:313, 1975.
33. Andersson HC, Marble M, Shapira E. Long term outcome in treated combined methylmalonic acidemia and homocysteinemia. *Genet Med* **1**:146–150, 1999.
34. Evans MI, Duquette DA, Rinaldo P et al. Modulation of B12 dosage and response in fetal treatment of methylmalonic aciduria (MMA): titration of treatment dose to serum and urine MMA. *Fet Diagn Ther* **12**:21–23, 1997.
35. Leon Del Rio A, Leclerc D, Gravel RA. Isolation of a cDNA encoding human holocarboxylase synthetase by functional complementation of a biotinauxotroph of *E.coli*. *Proc Natl Acad Sci USA* **92**:4626–4630, 1995.
36. Suzuki Y, Akoi Y, Ishida Y et al. Isolation and characterization of mutations in the holocarboxylase synthetase cDNA. *Nat Genet* **8**:122, 1994.
37. Akoi Y, Suzuki Y, Sakamoto O et al. Molecular analysis of holocarboxylase synthetase deficiency: a missense mutation and a single base deletion are predominant in Japanese patients. *Biochim Biophys Acta* **1272**:168, 1995.
38. Dupuis L, Leon-Del-Rio A, Leclerc D et al. Clustering of mutations in the biotin-binding region of holocarboxilase synthetase in biotin responsive multiple carboxylase deficiency. *Hum Mol Genet* **5**:1011–1016, 1996.
39. Popmponio RJ, Hymes J, Reynolds TR et al. Mutation in the human biotinidase gene that cause profound biothinidase deficiency in symptomatic children: molecular, biochemical, and clinical analysis. *Pediatr Res* **42**:840–848, 1997.
40. Suormala T, Fowler B, Jakobs C et al. Late onset holocarboxylase synthetase deficiency: pre- and post-natal diagnosis and evaluation of effectiveness of antenatal biotin therapy. *Eur J Pediatr* **157**:570–575, 1998.
41. Malvagia S, Morrone A, Pasquini E et al. First prenatal molecular diagnosis in a family with holocarboxylase synthetase deficiency. *Prenat Diagn* **25**:1117–1119, 2005.
42. Roth KS, Yang W, Allen L et al. Prenatal administration of biotin: biotin responsive multiple carboxylase deficiency. *Pediatr Res* **16**:126, 1982.
43. Packman S, Cowan Mj, Golbus MS et al. Prenatal treatment of biotin responsive multiple carboxylase deficiency. *Lancet* **1**:1435, 1982.
44. Thuy LP, Jurecki E, Nemzer L et al. Prenatal diagnosis of holocarboxylase synthetase deficiency by assay of the enzyme in chorionic villus material followed by prenatal treatment. *Clin Chim Acta* **284**:59–68, 1999.
45. Smith DW, Lemli L, Opitz JM. A newly recognized syndrome of multiple congenital anomalies. *J Pediatr* **64**:210–217, 1964.
46. Waye JS, Eng B. Nowaczyk MJ Prenatal diagnosis of Smith-Lemli-Opitz syndrome (SLOS) by DHCR7 mutation analysis. *Prenat Diagn* **27**(7):638–640, 2007.
47. Curry CJR, Carey JC, Holland JS. Smith-Lemli-Opitz syndrome – type II: multiple congenital anomalies with male pseudohermaphroditism and frequent early lethality. *Am J Med Genet* **26**:45–57, 1987.
48. Opitz JM. RSH-SLO ('Smith-Lemli-Opitz') syndrome: historical, genetic, and development considerations. *Am J Med Genet* **50**:344–346, 1994.
49. Kelley RI. A new face for an old syndrome. *Am J Med Genet* **65**:251–256, 1997.
50. Kelley RI. Diagnosis of Smith-Lemli-Opitz syndrome by gas chromatography/mass spectrometry of 7-dehydrocholesterol in plasma, amniotic fluid and cultured skin fibroblasts. *Clin Chim Acta* **236**:45–58, 1995.
51. Tint GS, Irons M, Elias E et al. Defective cholesterol biosynthesis associated with the Smith-Lemli-Opitz syndrome. *N Engl J Med* **330**:107–113, 1994.
52. Waterham HR, Wijburg FA, Hennekam RCM et al. Smith-Lemli-Opitz is caused by mutations in the 7-dehydrocholesterol reductase gene. *Am J Hum Genet* **63**:329–338, 1998.
53. Johnson JA, Aughton DJ, Comstock CH et al. Prenatal diagnosis of Smith-Lemli-Opitz syndrome, type II. *Am J Med Genet* **49**(2):240–243, 1994.
54. Hobbins JC, Jones OW, Gottesfeld MD, Persutte W. Transvaginal ultrasonography and transabdominal embryoscopy in the first-trimester diagnosis of Smith-Lemli-Opitz syndrome, type II. *Am J Obstet Gynecol* **171**:546–549, 1994.
55. Sharp P, Haan E, Fletcher JM, Khong TY, Carey WF. First trimester diagnosis of Smith-Lemli-Opitz syndrome. *Prenat Diagn* **17**:4:355–:4361, 1997.
56. Irons M, Elias E, Tint GS et al. Abnormal cholesterol metabolism in the Smith-Lemli-Opitz syndrome: report of clinical and biochemical findings in 4 patients and treatment in 1 patient. *Am J Med Genet* **50**:347–352, 1994.
57. Irons M, Elias ER, Abuelo D et al. Treatment of Smith-Lemli-Opitz syndrome: results of a multicenter trial. *Am J Med Genet* **68**:311–314, 1997.
58. Elias ER, Irons MB, Hurley AD, Tint GS, Salen G. Clinical effects of cholesterol supplementation in six patients with the Smith-Lemli-Opitz syndrome (SLOS). *Am J Med Genet* **68**:305–310, 1997.
59. Nowaczyk MJM, Whelan DT, Heshka TW, Hill R. Smith-Lemli-Opitz syndrome: a treatable inherited error of metabolism causing mental retardation. *Can Med Assoc J* **161**(2):165–170, 1999.
60. Irons MR, Nores J, Stewart TL et al. Antenatal therapy of Smith-Lemli-Opitz syndrome. *Fetal Diagn Ther* **14**:133–137, 1999.
61. Elsas LJ. Prenatal diagnosis of galactos-1-phosphate uridyltransferase (GALT) deficient galactosemia. *Prenat Diagn* **21**:302–303, 2001.
62. Chen YT, Mattis'on DR, Feigenbaum L et al. Reduction in oocvte number following prenatal exposure to a high galactose diet. *Science* **314**:1145, 1981.
63. Bandyopadhyay S, Chakrabarti J, Banerjee S et al. Prenatal exposure to high galactose adversely affects initial gonadal pool of germ cells in rats. *Hum Reprod* **18**:276–282, 2003.
64. Frey L, Hauser WA. Epidemiology of neural tube defects. *Epilepsia* **44**(Suppl 3):4–13, 2003.
65. Smithells RW, Sheppard S, Schorah CJ et al. Possible prevention of neural tube defects by preconceptual vitamin supplementation. *Lancet* **1**:399-340, 1980.
66. Smithells RW, Nevin NC, Seller MJ et al. Further experience of vitamin supplementation for prevention of neural tube defect recurrences. *Lancet* **1**:1027, 1983.
67. Younis JS, Granat M. Insufficient transplacental digoxin transfer in severe

hydrops fetalis. *Am J Obstet Gynecol* **157**:1268, 1987.
68. Mills JL, Rhoads GG, Simpson JL et al. The absence of a relation between the periconceptional use of vitamins and neural-tube defects. *N Engl J Med* **321**:430, 1989.
69. Mulinare J, Cordero JF, Erickson JD, Berry RJ. Periconceptional use of multivitamins and the occurrence of neural tube defects. *J Am Med Assoc* **260**:3141, 1988.
70. Schulman JD. Treatment of the embryo and the fetus in the first trimester: current status and future prospects. *Am J Med Genet* **35**:197, 1990.
71. MRC Vitamin Study Research Group. Prevention of neural tube defects: results of the MRC vitamin study. *Lancet* **338**:132–137, 1991.
72. Czeizel AE, Dudas I. Prevention of the first occurrence of neural-tube defects by preconceptional vitamin supplementation. *N Engl J Med* **327**:1832–1835, 1992.
73. Honein MA, Paulozzi LJ, Mathews TJ, Erickaon JD, Wong LY. Impact of folic acid fortification of the US food supply on the occurrence of neural tube defects. *J Am Med Assoc* **285**:2981–2986, 2001.
74. Olney RS, Mulinare J. Trends in neural tube defect prevalence, folic acid fortification, and vitamin supplement use. *Semin Perinatol* **26**:277–285, 2002.
75. Evans MI, Llurba E, Landsberger EJ, Dvorin E, Huang X, Harrison HH. Impact of folic acid supplementation in the United States: markedly diminished high maternal serum AFPs. *Obstet Gynecol* **103**:474–479, 2004.
76. Parle-McDermott A, Mills JL, Kirke PN et al. Analysis of MTHFR 1298A → C and 677 C→T polymorphisms as risk factor neural tube defects. *J Hum Genet* **48**: 190–193, 2003.
77. Finnell RH, Shaw GM, Lammer EJ, Volcik KA. Does prenatal screening for 5,10-methylenetetrahydrofolate reductase (MTHFR) mutations in high-risk neural tube defect pregnancies make sense? *Genet Test* **6**:47–52, 2002.
78. Rampersaud E, Melvin EC, Siegel D et al. Updated investigations of the role of methylenetetrahydrofolate reductase in human neural tube defects. *Clin Genet* **63**:210–214, 2003.
79. Zhu H, Wicker NJ, Shaw GM et al. Homocysteine remethylation enzyme polymorphisms and increased risks for neural tube defects. *Mol Genet Metab* **78**:216–221, 2003.
80. Volocik KA, Shaw GM, Zhu H et al. Risk factors for neural tube defects: associations between uncoupling protein 2 polymorphisms and spina bifida. *Birth Defects Res Part A Clin Mol Teratol* **67**:158–161, 2003.
81. Sever LE. Zinc deficiency in man. *Lancet* **1**:887, 1973.
82. McMichael AJ, Dreosti IE, Gibson GT. A prospective study of serial maternal serum zinc levels and pregnancy outcome. *Early Hum Dev* **7**:59-69, 198.
83. Stoll C, Dott B, Alembik Y, Koehl C. Maternal trace elements, vitamin B12, vitamin A, folic acid, and fetal malformations. *Rep Toxicol* **13**:53–57, 1999.
84. Hambidge M, Hackshaw A, Wald N. Neural tube defects and serum zinc. *Br J Obstet Gynecol* **100**:746–749, 1993.
85. Shoob HD, Sargent RG, Thompson SJ et al. Dietary methionine is involved in the etiology of neural defect-affected pregnancies in humans. *J Nutr* **131**:2653–2658, 2001.
86. Ray JG, Wyatt PR, Thompson MD et al. Vitamin B12 and the risk of neural tube defects in a folic-acid-fortified population. *Epidemiology* **18**(3):362–366, 2007.
87. Felkner M, Suarez L, Liszka B, Brender JD, Canfield M. Neural tube defects, micronutrient deficiencies, and Helicobacter pylori: a new hypothesis. *Birth Defects Res A Clin Mol Teratol* **79**(8):617–621, 2007.
88. Batshaw M, Brusilow S, Waber L et al. Treatment of inborn errors of urea synthesis: activation of alternative pathways of waste nitrogen synthesis and excretion. *N Engl J Med* **306**:1387, 1982.
89. Weiner C. Cordocentesis. In *Prenatal diagnosis*, MI Evans, MP Johnson, Y Yaron, A Drugan (eds), pp. 443–448. New York: McGraw Hill Publishing Co, 2006.

CHAPTER

43 Early pregnancy failure

Jemma Johns and Eric Jauniaux

KEY POINTS

- Spontaneous miscarriage is the commonest complication of pregnancy, affecting 10–20% of clinically recognized pregnancies
- Greater than 50% of early pregnancy failures are associated with a chromosomal defect
- Other causes include endocrine diseases and maternal illness, anatomical abnormalities of the female genital tract, infections, immune factors, thrombophilias and environmental toxins
- Trophoblastic cells from the cytotrophoblastic shell form plugs in the endometrial arteries in the early part of pregnancy and blood flow in the intervillous space is sluggish, only becoming significant later in the first trimester. There is good evidence that early pregnancy failure is associated with defective development of the placental bed
- Histological examination of early products of conception will identify about 60–70% of molar pregnancies
- Use of appropriate terminology to describe clinical and ultrasound findings in early pregnancy failure is essential and the use of obsolete terms such as blighted ovum, anembryonic sac and trophoblastic bleeding should be abandoned
- The incidence of miscarriage in women presenting with first-trimester threatened miscarriage is increased, particularly when bleeding occurs before 8 weeks
- Threatened miscarriage has been associated with longer-term adverse pregnancy outcomes, including preterm labor, preterm pre-labor rupture of the membranes and low birth weight
- There is limited information on the feasibility of screening for anomalies at 11–14 weeks
- The success of expectant management of miscarriage is variable, with a completion rate of 80–96% within 2 weeks in women with incomplete miscarriage and a low complication rate
- There are clear advantages of a dedicated Early Pregnancy Unit

INTRODUCTION

Spontaneous miscarriage is the commonest complication of pregnancy, affecting 10–20% of clinically recognized pregnancies[1–3]. The diagnosis of a specific anomaly in cases of early spontaneous miscarriage could have important epidemiological value, helping to elucidate causation in some early pregnancy failures. Recent advances in prenatal diagnosis during the last decade have seen the development and implementation of preimplantation genetic diagnosis (PGD), population screening for fetal aneuploidy and technical advances in ultrasound equipment, enabling the diagnosis of major fetal abnormalities in the first trimester that historically were not diagnosed until the mid-trimester of pregnancy.

As the availability of new and improved prenatal diagnostic techniques increases, so does the emotional impact on the couple of early pregnancy failure or abnormality. In this chapter, we will present the most recent data and advanced techniques available for the investigation, diagnosis and management of early pregnancy failure. We include sections on the clinical diagnosis of first-trimester miscarriage, diagnosis of fetal abnormality and aneuploidy in the first trimester, the pathological examination of the specimen and on the management options available.

INCIDENCE OF PREGNANCY LOSS IN HUMANS

It has been estimated that about 60% of all fertilized ova are lost before the end of the first trimester is reached[4]. Most of them are lost during the first month after the last menstrual period and are often not recognized as pregnancies, particularly if they occur around the time of an expected menstrual period.

During the first month of gestation

Pregnancy loss rates during the first three cycles in fertile couples trying to conceive have been found to be 31%, 40% of which were detectable by urine human chorionic gonadotrophin (hCG) alone with no detectable ultrasound signs of pregnancy[5].

After the first month of gestation

The rate of pregnancy loss is known to decrease with gestational age (Table 43.1). The precise incidence of early pregnancy failure (EPF) at different periods of gestation has been more clearly defined with the routine use of transvaginal ultrasound. In a prospective study of 232 women with positive urinary pregnancy tests and no antecedent history of vaginal bleeding, pregnancy loss was virtually complete by the end of the embryonic period (70 days after the onset of the last menstrual period)[6]. Once a gestational sac has been documented on scan, subsequent loss of viability in the embryonic period is still around 11.5%. If an embryo has developed up to 5 mm, subsequent loss of viability still occurs in 7.2%. Loss rates drop rapidly after that to 3.3% for embryos of 6–10 mm and to 0.5% for embryos over 10 mm. No pregnancies were lost between 8.5 and 14 menstrual weeks. The fetal loss rate after 14 weeks was 2%. The ultrasound screening of a large group of women with pregnancies between 10 and 13 weeks' gestation has confirmed that the prevalence of EPL at the end of first trimester is around 2–3%[7].

THE ETIOLOGY OF EPF

Although EPF is a common disorder, very little is known about its pathological basis. Epidemiological studies are fraught with pitfalls and often reflect the widespread medical belief that there is little to gain from the investigation of an isolated first-trimester miscarriage. It is only after three similar pregnancy losses or when the miscarriage occurs after 12 weeks that a detailed investigation is undertaken.

Recurrent miscarriage (RM) is traditionally defined as three or more consecutive miscarriages occurring before 20 weeks post-menstruation[8,9]. Around 1% of fertile couples will experience recurrent early pregnancy failures[8].

Greater than 50% of early pregnancy failures are associated with a chromosomal defect of the conceptus[10] and that frequency of abnormal chromosomal complement increases when the embryonic demise occurs earlier in gestation[11,12]. The risk of a chromosomal abnormality is well recognized to be associated with increasing maternal age[13]. The role of abnormal karyotype in repeated miscarriage is less clear and there is good evidence that there is a higher rate of subsequent miscarriage in women who have miscarried a fetus with a normal karyotype[14,15] and that women with recurrent miscarriage have a higher number of chromosomally normal miscarriages when compared with controls[16].

Other causes of EPF include endocrine diseases and maternal illness, anatomical abnormalities of the female genital tract, infections, immune factors, thrombophilias and environmental toxins. None of these etiologies can quantitatively be shown to cause more than a small percentage of pregnancy losses.

Table 43.1 **Incidence of early pregnancy failure (EPF)**

*Variable**	*Percentage*
Total loss of conceptions	50–70
Total clinical miscarriages	25–30
Before 6 weeks' gestation	18
Between 6 and 9 weeks' gestation	4
After 9 weeks' gestation	3
EPF in primigravidas	6–10
Risk of EPF after three miscarriages	25–30
Risk of EPF of 40-year-old women	30–40
Ectopic pregnancies per live births	1–2

Chromosomal abnormalities

Chorionic villus sampling at the time of ultrasound diagnosis of fetal demise, indicates an even higher frequency of chromosomal abnormalities with values ranging between 65 and 90%[17,18]. Autosomal trisomies are the most common with an incidence of 30–43%, followed by triploidies and monosomy X[10,17,19]. All possible autosomal trisomies have been described in cytogenetically abnormal miscarriages except trisomy 1 which has only been reported in an eight-cell embryo[20]. Triploidy and tetraploidy are frequent but are extremely lethal chromosomal abnormalities and are therefore rarely found in late miscarriages. Triploid conceptions may result from fertilization of a haploid ovum by either a single sperm that undergoes reduplication, or two sperm (diandry) or are due to a double maternal contribution when the ovum fails to undergo the first or second meiotic division before fertilization (digyny). A supernumerary paternal haploid set is thus imparted to the ovum, giving a total of 69 chromosomes with three possible sex chromosome permutations of XXX, XXY and XYY[19].

The frequency of most trisomies is influenced by maternal age at any gestation suggesting that autosomal trisomies are predictably more likely to arise cytologically in maternal than paternal meiosis (90%)[21]. This is true for trisomy 21 and for all the acrocentric chromosomes. In particular, trisomy 16 is exclusively attributable to errors in maternal meiosis I, whereas trisomy 18 usually arises at maternal meiosis II[22–24].

Chromosomal complements of successive miscarriages in a given family are more likely to be either recurrently normal or recurrently abnormal. If the complement of the first miscarriage is abnormal, the chromosomal complement of the subsequent one will be abnormal in up to 80% of the cases and the recurrent abnormality is usually a trisomy[24]. This can be supported by the observation that the risk of liveborn trisomy 21 following an aneuploid abortus is about 1–2% compared to 1 in 800 in the general population[24,25].

Structural chromosomal rearrangements, such as translocation or inversions, are present in only 1.5% of abortuses in the general population but are a significant cause of repetitive spontaneous miscarriages. Translocations are observed in about 5% of couples experiencing repeated losses[26,27]. Individuals with balanced translocations are phenotypically normal, but miscarriages or abnormal liveborns may show chromosomal duplications or deficiencies as a result of normal meiotic segregation. The reproductive risk conferred by chromosome rearrangements is dependent on the type of rearrangement and whether it is carried by the woman or her male partner[28]. About 60% of the translocations detected are reciprocal; 40% are Robertsonian. Females are twice as likely as males to show a balanced translocation.

Maternal age

Maternal age and number of previous miscarriages are independent risk factors for early pregnancy failure. Primigravidas and women with a history of exclusively successful pregnancies have an overall pregnancy loss rate of 5 and 4% respectively, whereas women with exclusively unsuccessful pregnancies have a miscarriage rate of as high as 24%[3]. Maternal age at conception has been found to be an independent risk factor for early pregnancy failure[29]. The risk of spontaneous miscarriage aged 20–24 years is 9% and increases to 74% in women aged 45 years or more. This increase is largely related to the increasing number of aneuploid conceptions with increasing maternal age.

Medical and endocrine disorders

Chronic maternal diseases can affect reproduction via a reduction in fertility and implantation, by impairment of placental function resulting in miscarriage or growth restriction, or via the drugs used to treat the disease, for example antiepileptic drugs. In general, however, maternal disease appears to have a limited impact on the early embryo unless illness is severe, possibly as a result of its 'protected' status in the early first trimester.

An exception to this appears to be maternal diabetes. Congenital abnormalities are 2–3 times more common in infants of diabetic mothers compared with normal controls[30]. Miscarriage rates are also increased in type 1 diabetes[31,32]. Diabetic embryopathy has been associated with increased levels of oxidative stress[33,34] and vitamin C and E supplementation of diabetic rats has been shown to reduce the incidence of malformations[35,36]. Raised glucose levels have also been found to disturb the expression of regulatory genes in embryonic development and cell-cycle progression leading to premature cell death in animal models[37]. When this occurs at the preimplantation stage, spontaneous miscarriage and congenital abnormalities occur. At the post-implantation stage, alterations in gene expression result in neural tube, musculoskeletal and cardiac defects.

Recent studies have suggested a relationship between EPF and polycystic ovarian syndrome (PCOS) associated with increased insulin resistance[38]. A recent study has suggested that the spontaneous miscarriage rate in women with insulin resistance undergoing assisted conception techniques is as high as 18%[39]. Treatment of these women in pregnancy with metformin in an attempt to reduce the rate of adverse pregnancy outcomes including EPF is still debated and evidence from large scale studies is lacking[40]. It has also been suggested that hypersecretion of luteinizing hormone (LH) may be associated with a higher rate of pregnancy loss. Unfortunately, suppression of high LH levels with gonadotrophin-releasing hormone analogues combined with human menopausal gonadotrophin stimulation is ineffective in improving the pregnancy outcome in these women[41]. Obesity is associated with a statistically significant increased risk of first-trimester and recurrent miscarriage[42] and several studies have shown that the association between polycystic ovarian syndrome and recurrent miscarriage could be secondary to the association between obesity and miscarriage[43].

Hyperprolactinemia has been associated with an increase in miscarriage rates with treatment using bromocriptine producing a reduction in the pregnancy loss rates with no adverse effect on fetal development[44]. There have been several reports suggesting that there is an increased rate of EPF in women with thyroid autoantibodies[45] and that treating these women to reduce the thyroid stimulating hormone (TSH) level has reduced the early pregnancy failure rate[45]. Again, however, information from large randomized controlled trials (RCTs) is lacking.

Anatomical abnormalities

Leiomyomas, uterine septa or endometrial adhesions have all been reported to interfere with implantation or with early embryonic development, but their impact in the incidence of EPF is uncertain. Uterine anomalies such as fibroids are common and their role in EPF is unclear, although there is some evidence suggesting a reduction in the rate of EPF after myomectomy[46]. Relatively few women with congenital or acquired uterine anatomical anomalies develop symptoms requiring medical or surgical therapy. Women with subseptate uteri have been shown to have an increased incidence of EPF when compared to women with normal 3D ultrasound findings[47]. Women with an arcuate uterus were found to have an increased incidence of second-trimester loss. Small studies do suggest an improvement in pregnancy outcome after hysteroscopic septoplasty, however, large randomized studies are lacking[48].

Infections

Infections such as cytomegalovirus, toxoplasmosis, rubella and herpes simplex are well-recognized causes of late fetal loss, however, an association with EPF has yet to be demonstrated. Among the many infections reported to have been associated with early spontaneous miscarriage are *Salmonella typhi*, malaria, *Brucella*, *Mycoplasma hominis*, *Chlamydia trachomatis* and *Ureaplasma urealyticum*. Transplacental infection doubtless occurs with each of these, and sporadic losses could be caused theoretically by any. Prospective epidemiological surveys suggest, however, that the attributable risk of infection in first-trimester spontaneous miscarriage is small[49]. The most frequently investigated infection associated with pregnancy loss is bacterial vaginosis (BV) and first-trimester detection of BV has been associated with mid-trimester loss and preterm labor[50], although trials examining intervention to reduce the rate of preterm labor in such cases have been contradictory. The role of BV in EPF still remains unclear[51,52].

Immune factors

The role of immune factors in pregnancy loss remains controversial. It centers around the maternal immune response to fetal antigens. Current interest surrounds the role of natural killer (NK) cells in reproduction. Natural killer cells are believed to play a role in trophoblast invasion as they are present in the uterine decidua and have been found to be present in higher levels in the decidua of women with early recurrent miscarriage[53,54]. Further research is required before a definite link can be made between NK cells and EPF and, at present, there does not appear to be a role for screening women for increased NK activity other than in the confines of research studies.

Antiphospholipid syndrome and thrombophilias

Antiphospholipid syndrome (APLS) is detected in 15% of women with recurrent miscarriage[55] and is responsible for a 90% miscarriage rate in untreated women. It is defined as the presence in maternal serum of antiphospholipid antibodies with clinical manifestation of significant obstetric morbidity and vascular thrombosis[56]. The two main antibodies responsible are anti-cardiolipin and lupus anticoagulant, although there are many more. Treatment of women with APLS and recurrent pregnancy loss with aspirin and heparin in pregnancy has been shown to reduce the pregnancy loss rate by up to 54%[57].

There are several inherited thrombophilias associated with an increased risk of recurrent thromboembolism in pregnancy or the puerperium, the commonest being factor V Leiden mutation (resulting in activated protein C resistance and present in about 5% of the UK population), the prothrombin gene mutation (leading to raised prothrombin levels and present in approximately 2% of the UK population) and the methylenetetrahydrofolate reductase gene mutation (MTHFR). In addition to their association with thromboembolic disorders, factor V Leiden and the prothrombin gene mutation have been associated with recurrent EPF[58].

Drugs and toxins

The use of medicinal drugs in pregnancy remains controversial, with many drugs in use having limited safety profiles. The placenta is not a complete barrier to the transfer of drugs and active transporters have been identified in the trophoblast that transfer drugs across from the maternal to the fetal compartment[59]. The transfer of several drugs has been examined in early pregnancy[60], demonstrating rapid transfer and accumulation within the first-trimester embryo[61,62]. The placenta also contains drug metabolizing enzymes which further alter the rate of drug transfer and drug activity in the fetus[59], with a possible detoxification role in some cases. Several major drug groups have been associated with congenital abnormalities or growth restriction, but their effect on very early embryogenesis is uncertain and they will not be discussed in detail here. In many cases, the risks of therapeutic drug use may well outweigh the fetal risks and their use may be indicated once the period of organogenesis is completed. The treatment of the mother with drugs for 'fetal therapy' is also well recognized; the most well-researched and recognized form being the use of prophylactic folic acid in the prevention of neural tube defects[63,64]. Low levels of folic acid in pregnancy have also been associated with a number of adverse pregnancy outcomes including spontaneous miscarriage, abruption, pre-eclampsia and fetal growth restriction[65–67]. Folic acid has been shown to be concentrated in the exocelomic space in early pregnancy and the folic acid receptor has been found in the secondary yolk sac suggesting active uptake and use from very early gestation[68]. The interplay between low folic acid intake in pregnancy and abnormally high levels of homocysteine and homozygosity for the heat labile methylenetetrahydrofolate reductase (MTHFR) gene are believed to be the pathophysiological mechanism for many of these adverse outcomes[66,67].

Recreational drug use in pregnancy is difficult to quantify, however, a national survey in England and Wales revealed that 11% of registered drug users had given birth in 1993, representing an estimated 568 deliveries[69]. The effect of drug use on pregnancy outcome is difficult to quantify as the outcomes are often confounded by maternal malnourishment, anemia, smoking and alcohol consumption and drug use is associated with inadequate or no antenatal care in many cases. Heroin and methadone use in pregnancy is associated with an increased perinatal mortality rate and the neonatal abstinence syndrome, but there is no evidence for an increased congenital abnormality or miscarriage rate over and above that associated with the above confounders. Cocaine has been shown to be independently associated with spontaneous miscarriage[70]. It is a potent vasoconstrictor, resulting in vasoconstriction of uterine, placental and umbilical vessels[71], resulting in miscarriage, congenital abnormality, abruption, growth restriction and stillbirth depending on the timing and the degree of the insult[72]. Cocaine use has been associated with congenital abnormalities such as hydronephrosis, hypospadias[73] and cardiac abnormalities[74] and with abnormalities associated with vascular disruption[75] such as limb reduction defects and intestinal atresias. Benzodiazepines readily cross the placenta from early pregnancy[62] and their use in pregnancy has been associated with an increased incidence of cleft palate[76]. Amphetamines, probably also via vasoconstriction, have been associated with miscarriage, abruption and growth restriction[77]. There has been no proven link between marijuana use and adverse pregnancy outcome over and above that associated with tobacco consumption[78]. Using maternal hair samples, the incidence of peri-conceptional recreational drug use has been found to be high (18%) in women with a fetus affected by gastroschisis, possibly explaining the recent increased incidence of this anomaly in young women[79].

Data regarding the effect of caffeine on pregnancy outcome and on miscarriage in particular are varied. Studies are often small and retrospective, with little or poor control for confounding factors such as smoking and alcohol use. There is some evidence that caffeine consumption may be associated with an increased risk of spontaneous early pregnancy failure, with increased risk associated with heavier ingestion, however, data remain inconclusive[80,81]. It is well known that excessive alcohol consumption in pregnancy can lead to the development of the fetal alcohol syndrome (FAS)[82], a spectrum of disorders, one of the mechanisms for which has recently been postulated to be apoptosis from oxidative damage[83] or activation of the caspase-3 pathway[84]. It is thought that alcohol is concentrated in the lipid membranes of cells and that it impairs the activity of membrane channels[83]. In vitro work on animal models has found low levels of antioxidants, an exaggerated response to pro-oxidant stimuli and evidence of mitochondrially mediated cell death in fetuses exposed to alcohol in utero[85,86]. A review of experimental data suggests that antioxidant use in pregnancy may reduce the risk of alcohol-induced damage[83]. The effect of alcohol on early embryonic development is difficult to quantify, but is potentially very important, as up to 60% of women who consume alcohol are unaware of their pregnancy until the fourth week post-conception[87].

Cigarette smoking has been shown to increase the risk of spontaneous miscarriage when compared with non-smoking controls[70,88–95]. Cigarette smoke is known to be a potent inducer of reactive oxygen species and increases the risk of preterm rupture of the membranes 2- to 4-fold compared with non-smokers[96]and cotinine has been shown to accumulate in the first-trimester fetal compartments from as early as 7 weeks' gestation[97]. Smoking is associated with congenital anomalies such as orofacial clefts[98,99], limb reduction defects[100], the Poland Sequence[101] and urogenital anomalies[102] and also with fetal growth restriction[94], oligohydramnios, stillbirth[103] and abruption and placenta previa[104]. Levels of folic acid have been found to be lower in women who smoke[68], possibly accounting for the increased incidence of adverse pregnancy outcome and congenital abnormality in this group[105] and women who smoke may well benefit from higher prophylactic doses of folic acid prior to conception. Fetal plasma levels of essential amino acids have also been shown to be lower in smokers than non-smokers in early pregnancy, suggesting a direct effect of maternal smoking on trophoblastic transfer and synthesis[106]. Passive smoking has also been associated with an increased risk of adverse pregnancy outcome and cotinine concentrations comparable to those of smokers have been found in the exocelomic fluid in the pregnancies of passive smokers[97].

Assessment of the effect of environmental toxins on pregnancy outcome in humans is hampered by the presence of multiple confounders such as smoking and alcohol. Many studies have attempted to examine the effects of exposure to heavy metals, ionizing radiation and organic solvents on miscarriage and congenital abnormality rates, but studies are often small and methodologically flawed. Air carrier personnel are exposed to ionizing radiation from galactic cosmic rays, and concern has been raised over the safety of pregnant air staff. The Federal Aviation Administration has issued radiation exposure limits for pregnant staff. It is unlikely that even a frequent air traveler will be exposed to high enough levels of radiation to be at increased risk and there is no evidence for a risk associated with air travel in pregnancy other than that associated with deep venous thrombosis[107]. There has been some suggestion that there may be a link between dental amalgam (mercury toxicity) and miscarriage or congenital anomalies. The amount of mercury vapor released into the circulation from dental amalgam is small and unlikely to reach teratogenic levels[108].

Iatrogenic causes

Procedures such as chorionic villus sampling (CVS) and amniocentesis, used to obtain a fetal karyotype, in prenatal diagnosis each carry a risk of fetal loss. CVS, performed before 14 weeks' gestation, carries an excess risk over amniocentesis, performed after 16 weeks, of up to 3%[109] compared to 1%[110]. A Cochrane meta-analysis did suggest that transcervical CVS in the first trimester was, however, associated with a significantly increased risk of pregnancy loss over second-trimester amniocentesis[111]. More recent data suggest, however, that with increasing experience that has inevitably occurred over the last decade, the procedure-related risks have reduced and that there is little difference between the risk from first-trimester transabdominal CVS and second-trimester amniocentesis, with the additional risk of pregnancy loss being in the order of 0.5–2%[112–114]. Early amniocentesis has been associated with an increase in unintended pregnancy loss and equinovarus compared with CVS[113]. As the availability and demand for first-trimester prenatal diagnosis is increasing rapidly, especially among women of advanced maternal age, the impact of invasive techniques is also increasing. The procedure-related accident is obviously related to the type of equipment used and operator experience and, in particular, to the number of attempts needed to obtain a sufficient villus sample. This particular factor is rarely considered in epidemiological studies or in economic evaluation of the benefits and costs of prenatal diagnosis.

ROLE OF HISTOPATHOLOGICAL ANALYSIS IN EARLY PREGNANCY FAILURE

Diagnosing the cause of an EPF

Consideration of the pathology of EPF has often led to the conclusion that morphololological studies have relatively little to offer to our understanding of the etiology or pathogenesis of EPF. However, the histopathological investigation of a first-trimester conceptus is particularly difficult, not only because of the limited amount of material available, but also because the specimens are often fragmented or macerated. Around one-half of early spontaneous miscarriage specimens contain no embryonic or fetal part and about 12% consist of maternal decidua only[115] and there is a suggestion that routine histology provides no additional useful clinical information[116]. The rationale for routinely sending products of conception for histopathological analysis is currently solely to exclude molar pregnancy and looks likely to remain limited to this.

Studying the pathophysiology of EPF

After implantation, the embryo is completely surrounded by proliferative cytotrophoblast cells. Subsequently extravillous trophoblast (EVT) invades into the decidual and myometrial layers where it surrounds and invades the maternal spiral arteries[117]. This results in transformation of the arteries, with a loss of the musculoelastic structure of the vessel walls and an increase in vessel diameter converting them into low-resistance, high-capacitance vessels[118]. Traditional teaching is that maternal blood circulates in the intervillous space from a very early stage in placental development[119]. The primitive uteroplacental circulation has always been thought to begin within the first 2 weeks after conception, with functioning primary chorionic villi present by the third week (Fig. 43.1b). More recent work has suggested, however, that trophoblastic cells from the cytotrophoblastic shell form plugs in the endometrial arteries in the early part of pregnancy[120] and that blood flow in the intervillous space is sluggish in early pregnancy[121], only becoming significant later in the first trimester (Fig. 43.1a). This work has been further supported by Doppler ultrasound, anatomical and hysteroscopic studies in early pregnancy, examining blood flow in the intervillous space (IVS)[122–126], confirming that there is minimal flow before approximately 11 weeks'

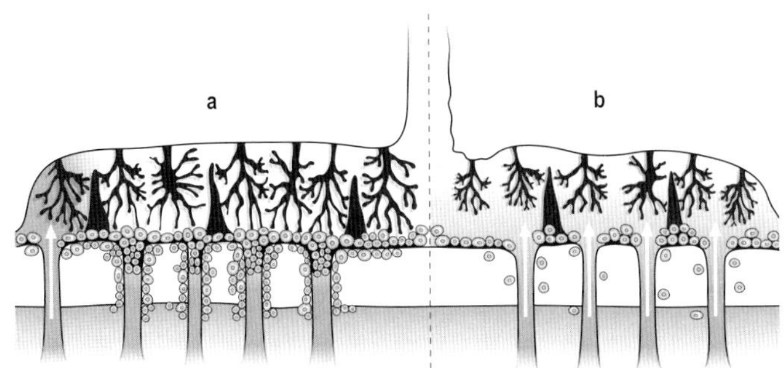

Fig. 43.1 Diagram representing placentation in normal first-trimester pregnancy (a) and miscarriage (b). Note trophoblast plugging of maternal spiral arteries and trophoblast invasion of the decidua and superficial myometrium in the central area of the normally developing placenta (a). By contrast, in the miscarriage (b) there is a shallow trophoblastic invasion and the plugs are loose allowing premature entry of maternal blood (arrows).

gestation. It has also been shown that greater trophoblast invasion of the spiral arteries occurs in the central region of the placental bed[127] suggesting that the plugs are more extensive and complete in this area. Recent studies have confirmed that dissipation of the plugs occurs first at the periphery of the placenta in the majority of normal pregnancies[128]. This flow of blood in the intervillous space at the periphery of the placenta, and subsequent 'physiological' oxidative stress, has been suggested as the trigger responsible for the development of the placental membranes or 'chorion laeve' in human pregnancy[129].

There is good evidence that early pregnancy failure is associated with defective development of the placental bed[130,131]. Placental bed tissue shows defective trophoblast invasion, with limited maternal arterial 'transformation' in women with missed miscarriages in both the first and second trimester[131]. These findings have been confirmed in a larger study[132] where spontaneous miscarriage specimens were associated with a thinner discontinuous trophoblastic shell and defective intravascular trophoblastic plugs.

In normal early pregnancy, maternal blood flow starts at the periphery of the placenta, possibly where plugging by the trophoblast is less complete. In missed miscarriage, this process appears to be reversed with flow in the IVS being more commonly seen in the central region of the placenta (see Fig. 43.1b). A study of miscarriage specimens from women with antiphospholipid syndrome has also shown that the normal endovascular trophoblastic plugging described above could only be identified in 23% of cases compared to 75% of normal controls[133]. These findings appeared to be in agreement with early work on placental development[117,127] which showed that trophoblastic migration and morphological changes in the uteroplacental arteries are more extensive in the central area of the placental bed, with invasion starting at the center of the implantation site and extending to the periphery in an annular pattern; trophoblast invasion of the endometrial arteries is also most extensive, i.e. deep in the central regions[127].

Impairment of the trophoblast shell in abnormal early pregnancy with premature onset of the maternal circulation, such as in threatened miscarriage, could well result in oxidative damage to the developing placenta and embryo, resulting in miscarriage. Lesser degrees of impairment of early placental or membrane development with influx of oxygenated maternal blood may result in a chronic state of oxidative stress resulting from inflammation and the presence of substances which form free radicals (such as free ferrous ions), resulting in later complications of pregnancy such as pre-eclamptic toxemia (PET), preterm pre-labor rupture of the membranes (PPROM), fetal growth restriction (FGR) and preterm labor.

Screening for gestational trophoblastic disorders (GTD)

The diagnosis of partial mole is initially based on the ultrasound appearance of the placenta in utero or gross examination of the placenta at delivery during the second or third trimester of pregnancy. In the UK, spontaneous miscarriages are routinely sent for histopathological analysis to exclude molar pregnancy. Histological examination of early products of conception will identify about 60–70% of molar pregnancies[134]. The distinction between complete hydatidiform mole (CHM) and partial hydatidiform mole (PHM) was made in the late 1970s on the basis of gross morphological, histological and cytogenetic criteria in second- and third-trimester pregnancies[135,136]. The complete or classical hydatidiform mole has been defined as a conceptus with a placenta showing generalized swelling of the villi and diffuse trophoblastic hyperplasia, in the absence of an ascertainable fetus[137]. The PHM has been characterized by focal trophoblastic hyperplasia with focal villous hydrops and identifiable embryonic or fetal tissue. The clinicopathologic picture of the two molar syndromes overlap to a degree since both the phenotype and natural history of the PHM seem to represent a mild, bland version of those of the CHM[138].

Morphological features, including villous size and proliferative activity of trophoblast, change with gestation and need to be taken into account when examining specimens of varying gestations[139]. Difficulties arise when determining between PHM, CHM and hydropic abortion (HA), particularly when there is prolonged postmortem retention in utero in missed miscarriage for example[134] and where there are focal hydropic changes found in aneuploidies. It has been suggested that PHM in the first trimester are frequently missed on ultrasound and that pathological examination should remain the mainstay of diagnosis[140]. As diandric triploidies are much more common in the first trimester, a large group of women at risk of persistent GTD theoretically escape detection and, if treatment is required, it would only be started at a later stage of the disease. The use of standardized criteria for detection by microscopic examination is both accurate and reproducible and should play a pivotal role in screening women at risk of persistent GTD.

CLINICAL ASSESSMENT OF EPL AND TERMINOLOGY

The use of transvaginal sonography has clearly revolutionized the management of early pregnancy problems. The development of highly sensitive urinary hCG assays and greater awareness of early pregnancy ultrasound among healthcare professionals and women alike has resulted in ever earlier presentation. This has led to an increase in the number of inconclusive scans and, as a result, an increase in the requirement for repeat assessments to determine both pregnancy location and viability. Knowledge of the ultrasound appearances of normal early pregnancy development and a good understanding of its pitfalls are essential for the diagnosis and management of early pregnancy failure.

Use of appropriate terminology to describe clinical and ultrasound findings in early pregnancy failure is also essential, and the use of obsolete terms such as blighted ovum, anembryonic sac and trophoblastic bleeding should be abandoned (Table 43.2). Such descriptions are of limited clinical usefulness and have no histopathological correlates and have therefore been replaced by more ultrasound-based terminology[141] (Table 43.3).

THE ROLE OF ENDOCRINOLOGY

Many maternal serum markers have been investigated in attempts to predict the outcome of pregnancy in the first trimester and, in particular, the likelihood of subsequent miscarriage, with varying degrees of success. Many of these studies looked at multiple markers and were conducted after embryonic demise had already occurred[142,143]. Maternal serum markers, combined with ultrasound parameters, maternal age, smoking habits, obstetric history and the occurrence of vaginal bleeding have all been combined in multivariate analyses, with mixed results[144,145]. First-trimester human chorionic gonadotrophin (hCG) and, more recently, progesterone remain the only consistent markers of early pregnancy failure[143,146], but their predictive value is low[147]. As a clinical predictive tool, measurement of these compounds is unnecessary if a viable pregnancy can be demonstrated by ultrasound.

Other placental hormones have been tested at an experimental level. Several studies have investigated inhibin A and activin A in early pregnancy failure and maternal serum (MS) concentrations of inhibin A have been found to be lower in miscarriages when compared with gestation matched control pregnancies[148–150]. A recent study on asymptomatic women with ongoing pregnancies showed that MS levels of inhibin A, pro-α C and hCG were significantly lower in women who subsequently suffered a first-trimester miscarriage compared with controls, but that it was less useful than hCG or progesterone[150]. Preliminary work on women with a history of recurrent miscarriages has shown that inhibin A levels are lower in women who go on to miscarry[151,152] and that inhibin may predict those women who are destined to miscarry after in vitro fertilzation (IVF)[153], but studies are small and larger studies are needed to confirm this observation. A recent study found inhibin A levels four times lower in pregnancies destined to miscarry and that these levels correlated with MShCG levels[151]. Inhibin A has been used to assess the likelihood of miscarriage in early pregnancies, where viability is uncertain, or after IVF prior to the onset of clinical symptoms. Overall, inhibin A levels, although decreased in early spontaneous miscarriage, appear to add little to progesterone and hCG measurements for the prediction of miscarriage in asymptomatic women.

Table 43.2 **RCOG recommended terminology in early pregnancy failure[141]**

Previous term	*Recommended term*
Spontaneous abortion	Miscarriage
Threatened abortion	Threatened miscarriage
Inevitable abortion	Inevitable miscarriage
Incomplete abortion	Incomplete miscarriage
Complete abortion	Complete miscarriage
Missed abortion/anembryonic pregnancy/blighted ovum	Missed miscarriage/early fetal demise/delayed miscarriage/ silent miscarriage
Septic abortion	Miscarriage with infection
Recurrent abortion	Recurrent miscarriage

CLINICAL AND ULTRASOUND CRITERIA USED TO DIAGNOSE EPF

Gestational sac size

The deciduo-placental interface and the exocelomic cavity (ECC) are the first sonographic evidence of a pregnancy that can be visualized with transvaginal ultrasound from around 4.4–4.6

Table 43.3 **Ultrasound and clinical correlates in early pregnancy failure**

Diagnosis	*Ultrasound appearance*	*Clinical presentation*
Complete miscarriage[141]	Endometrial thickness <15 mm[232] No evidence of RPOC	Cessation of vaginal bleeding and abdominal pain
Incomplete miscarriage[141]	Any endometrial thickness Heterogeneous tissues (±sac) distorting midline endometrial echo[232]	± Bleeding and/or abdominal pain
Delayed miscarriage[141] (previously anembryonic/missed)	Gestational sac diameter ⩾20 mm with no fetal pole or yolk sac (or <20 mm with no change 7 days apart) *or* Fetal pole >6 mm with no FHA (or <6 mm with no change 7 days apart)[232]	Minimal vaginal bleeding or pain Loss of pregnancy symptoms
Intrauterine hematoma[201]	Crescent shaped echo-free areas between the chorionic membrane and the myometrium[201]	± Vaginal bleeding

FHA = fetal heart activity; RPOC = retained products of conception menstrual weeks (32–34 days) when they reach together a size of 2–4 mm. In normal intrauterine pregnancies between the 5th and 6th weeks, the gestational sac grows at a rate of approximately 1 mm/day in mean diameter[154]. Gestational sac growth has been documented on serial ultrasound examinations to be slower in women who subsequently miscarry[155], however, it has long been recognized that there is wide scatter in gestational sac volume measurements in 'normal' early pregnancy[156].

Once a gestational sac has been documented on ultrasound, subsequent loss of viability in the embryonic period remains around 11%[157]. A smaller than expected gestational sac can be a predictor of poor pregnancy outcome, both alone and in combination with other parameters, even in the presence of embryonic cardiac activity[145,158–161]. Unfortunately, the predictive value of a smaller than expected GSD in isolation is variable and highly dependent upon other presenting factors. Interpretation of pregnancy outcome data for any variable in early pregnancy is hampered by significant differences in study design and entry criteria.

Table 43.4 demonstrates how published study populations vary, including low-risk asymptomatic women, women with threatened miscarriage and women undergoing assisted conception techniques. Demographic data are often not accounted for and clearly these data should not be directly compared, and findings should not be applied to all populations. Overall multivariate analyses appear to provide the most sensitive predictors of pregnancy outcome and GSD features strongly in combination with one or two other parameters in all of these models[144,160]. Small gestation sac size can also be associated with chromosomal abnormality. Triploidy and trisomy 16 are more often associated with a small chorionic sac before 9 weeks of gestation than other chromosomal abnormalities[128,159].

Crown–rump length

The now classical study by Robinson and Fleming on crown–rump length (CRL) is still the main reference for the assessment of gestational age in early pregnancy (Fig. 43.2)[162]. Because transvaginal sonography provides superior resolution and more accurate identification of the embryonic structures than abdominal ultrasound, new charts have been developed for the period of gestation before 7 weeks[163]. If an embryo has developed up to 5 mm in length, subsequent loss of viability occurs in 7.2%[157]. Loss rates drop to 3.3% for embryos of 6–10 mm and to 0.5% for embryos over 10 mm[157]. There is conflicting evidence for an association between early growth restriction, as defined by a deficit between the CRL and that predicted by the last menstrual period (LMP) and karyotypic abnormalities[164–167]. A smaller than expected CRL has, however, been associated with subsequent miscarriage[168].

Table 43.4 **Studies comparing gestational sac size with pregnancy outcome**

Authors	*Year*	*Study type*	*Entry criteria*	*Parameters*	*N*	*Outcome*
Robinson[156]	1975	Prospective	6–13 weeks	GSV	319	Small GSV useful in diagnosis of anembryonic pregnancies
Nyberg et al[155]	1987	Prospective	No demonstrable embryo	GSD growth	83	Growth ≤0.6 mm/day is abnormal
Bromley et al[158]	1991	Prospective case control	Normal FHR	MSD-CRL <5 mm	68	Small MSD – 94% mc rate Normal MSD – 8% mc rate
Dickey et al[159]	1994	Prospective case control	Subfertile population	GSD	700	GSD >50th centile predicts normal outcome in 90–95%
Makrydimas et al[145]	2003	Prospective	6–10 weeks low-risk population	GSD, FHR, CRL	866	Small GSD – significant independent contribution
Falco et al[161]	2003	Prospective cohort	Threatened miscarriage GSD < 16 mm, no embryo	GSD	50	>90% mc if GSD < 1.34 SD
Choong et al[144]	2003	Prospective cross-sectional	Subfertile population	CRL, MSD MSD-CRL	322	MSD-CRL low predictive value Multivariate model gave best results
Elson et al[160]	2003	Prospective observational	No demonstrable embryo	Demographic data MSD, serum markers	200	GSD – overlap between viable and non-viable pregnancies Age, progesterone and GSD: diagnostic of viable pregnancy – sensitivity 99.2%, specificity 70.7%

GSV = Gestational sac volume; GSD = gestational sac diameter; MSD = mean sac diameter; CRL = crown–rump length; LMP = last menstrual period; FHR = fetal heart rate; MC = miscarriage

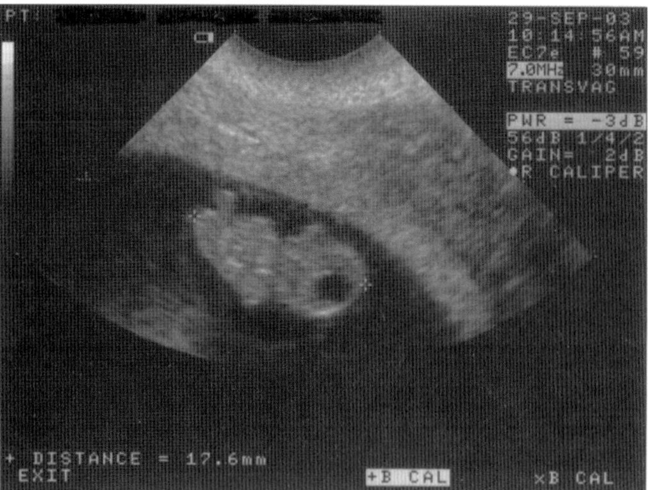

Fig. 43.2 Transvaginal ultrasound scan showing an 8-week fetus demonstrating the crown–rump length measurement.

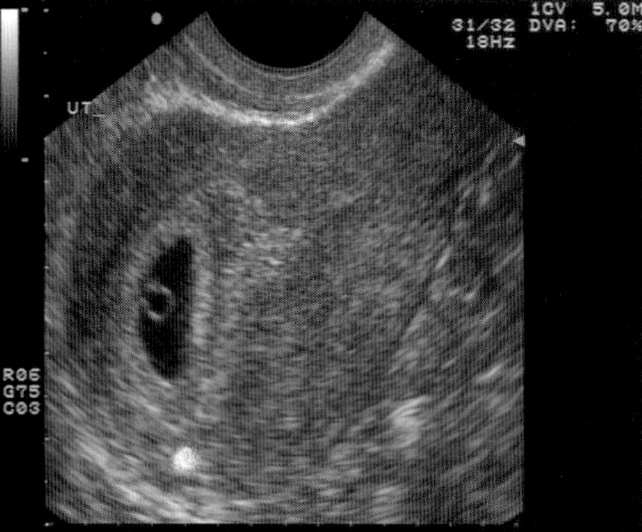

Fig. 43.3 Transvaginal ultrasound scan of a pregnancy sac at 5 weeks' gestation showing a small embryo adjacent to a secondary yolk sac (arrow). No cardiac activity could be detected at this stage.

Mean gestational sac diameter to crown–rump length ratios have also been used to predict pregnancy outcome with varying degrees of accuracy[144,158]. Unfortunately, this technique, as for GSD measurements is of limited clinical usefulness in isolation.

Secondary yolk sac

The first structure to be seen inside the gestational sac, before the embryo itself, is the secondary yolk sac (SYS) which can observed from the beginning of the 5th week of gestation or when the gestational sac reaches 10 mm in diameter (Fig. 43.3)[169]. The SYS diameter increases slightly between 6 and 10 weeks of gestation and then decreases[169]. The comparison of ultrasound features with morphological findings indicates that when the SYS reaches its maximum sonographic size, it already shows important degenerative changes[169]. This suggests that the disappearance of the SYS in normal pregnancies is a spontaneous event in embryonic development rather than the result of mechanical compression by the expanding amniotic cavity. The predictive value of SYS measurements in determining the outcome of an early pregnancy is limited[170–173]. Most pregnancies which miscarry during the third month of pregnancy have normal SYS measurements at their initial scan before 8 weeks of gestation[169]. It is usually the yolk sac that is found to persist inside the gestational sac after embryonic demise[174]. This would suggest that variations in SYS size and sonographic appearance in most abnormal pregnancies are probably the consequence of poor embryonic development or embryonic death rather than being the primary cause of early pregnancy failure.

Fetal heart pulsation

Extensive research has been published, examining the predictive value of fetal heart activity on pregnancy outcome. Studies can be broadly divided into those examining fetal loss after confirmed fetal cardiac activity and those examining fetal heart rate (FHR) in relation to outcome. Fetal heart activity is the earliest proof of a viable pregnancy and it has been documented in utero by transvaginal sonography as early as 36 days' menstrual age, approximately at the time when the heart tube starts to beat[175]. Theoretically, cardiac activity should always be evident when the embryo is over 2 mm[176]. However, in around 5–10% of embryos between 2 and 4 mm, it cannot be demonstrated, although the corresponding pregnancies will have a normal outcome[177,178]. From 5–9 weeks of gestation, there is a rapid increase in the mean heart rate from 110 to 175 beats per minutes (bpm). The heart rate then gradually decreases to around 160–170 bpm[175,179–183].

Abnormal developmental pattern of FHR and/or bradycardia has been associated with subsequent miscarriage[175,184–188]. In particular, a slow FHR at 6–8 weeks appears to be associated with subsequent fetal demise[179,186]. A single observation of an abnormally slow heart rate does not necessarily indicate subsequent embryonic death, but a continuous decline of embryonic heart activity is inevitably associated with miscarriage. In women with recurrent spontaneous miscarriage (defined as 3 or more consecutive losses in the first trimester), there has been much debate regarding whether there is an increased likelihood that fetal heart pulsations will be seen on transvaginal sonography when compared with idiopathic spontaneous miscarriages[189], suggesting a different pathophysiology leading to pregnancy loss in these cases. Evidence would suggest, however, that fetal loss patterns are no different between these groups[190].

Threatened miscarriage

Threatened miscarriage is defined as painless vaginal bleeding with a viable pregnancy occurring any time between implantation and 24 weeks' gestation and occurs in 15–20% of ongoing pregnancies[191] and is generally a clinical diagnosis. It is the commonest reason (along with suspected ectopic pregnancy) for emergency gynecology general practitioner referrals. The incidence of miscarriage in women presenting with first-trimester threatened miscarriage is increased[192–195], particularly when the bleeding occurs before 8 weeks[196]. If the pregnancy continues, threatened miscarriage has been associated with longer-term adverse pregnancy outcomes including preterm labor[192,194,197], preterm pre-labor rupture of the membranes[194,197] and low birth weight[198].

Incomplete miscarriage

An incomplete miscarriage is defined as partial expulsion of the products of conception with continued vaginal bleeding. Products of conception can usually be identified in the uterine cavity on transvaginal ultrasound and the ultrasound features are described in Table 43.3. The sonographic appearance of incomplete miscarriage is of thick irregular echoes in the midline of the uterine cavity (Figs 43.4 and 43.5). However, this is often not diagnostic of retained products as blood clots may look remarkably similar on scan. Conversely, the finding of a well-defined regular endometrial line can effectively exclude this diagnosis. The reliability of ultrasonography in the detection of complete miscarriage is high, enabling correct identification in 98% of patients with an empty uterus (complete miscarriage) and 69% of patients with retained products[199].

Missed miscarriage

The term missed miscarriage is also known as early fetal demise, delayed miscarriage and silent miscarriage, terms that have replaced the traditional 'anembryonic pregnancy' and 'blighted ovum'. Essentially, the term describes either an empty gestational sac measuring greater than 20 mm in mean diameter, or a sac containing a non-viable fetus of greater than 6 mm crown–rump length (CRL) with minimal clinical symptoms (Fig. 43.6)[141].

Other sonographic features

The shape of the gestational sac, the echogenicity of the placenta, the thickness of the trophoblast[200] and the presence of an

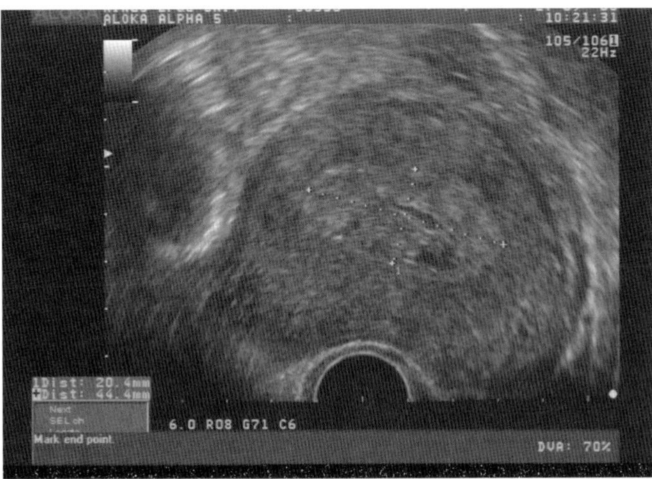

Fig. 43.4 Transvaginal ultrasound image of retained products of conception (calipers).

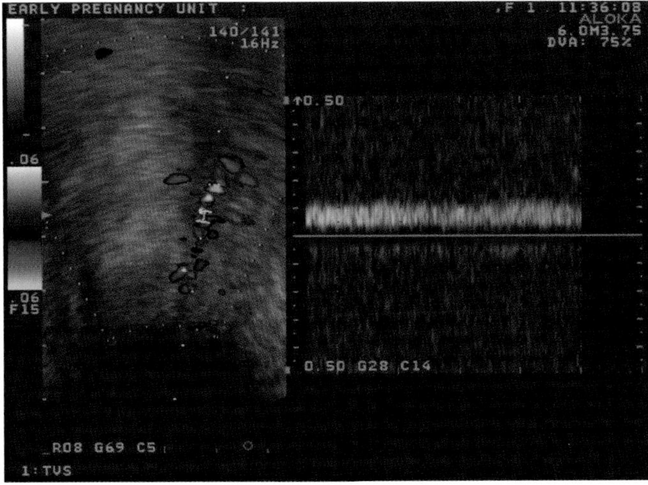

Fig. 43.5 Color Doppler image of retained products of conception.

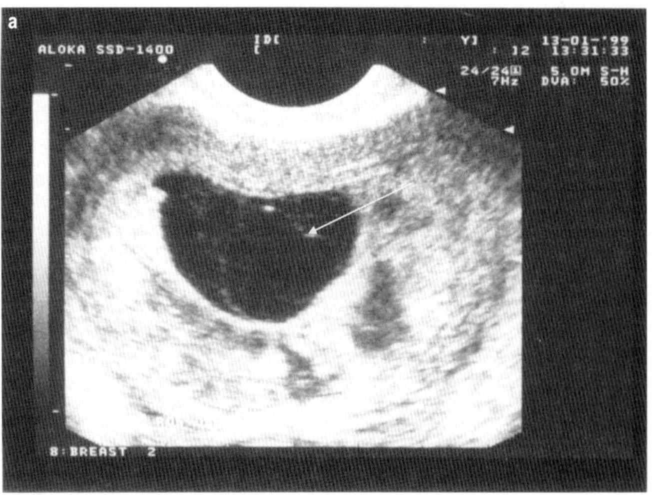

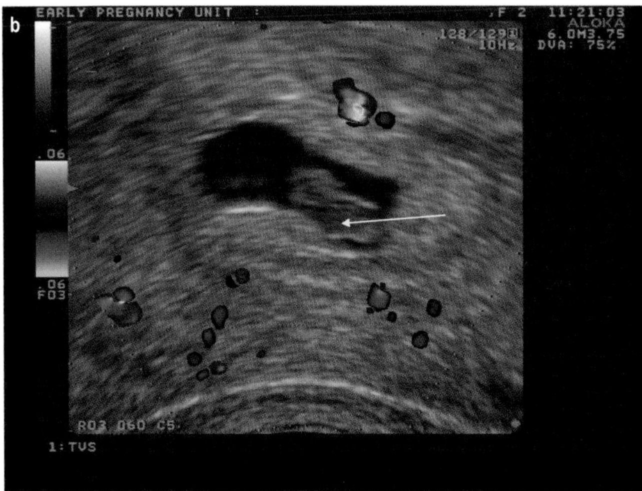

Fig. 43.6 Transvaginal images of missed miscarriages at 8 weeks' gestation; (a) represents an empty sac with a dilated amniotic sac (arrow); (b) shows an embryonic pole (arrow) with no fetal heart activity as demonstrated by color Doppler.

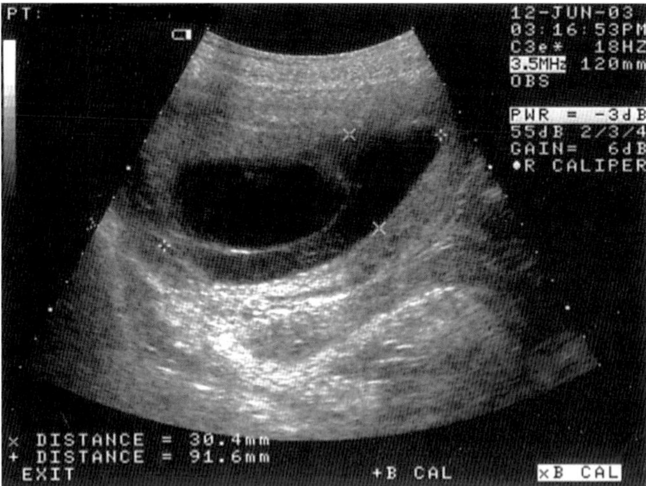

Fig. 43.7 Transvaginal image of an intrauterine hematoma (calipers) at 9 weeks' gestation in a viable pregnancy.

intrauterine hematoma have all been proposed as sonographic markers associated with early spontaneous miscarriage. Many of these studies, however, often highlight problems with experimental design rather than providing unequivocal answers.

Intrauterine hematomas (IUH) are crescent-shaped echo-free areas between the chorionic membrane and the myometrium (Fig. 43.7)[201]. Understanding of the resolution of these hematomas and the prognostic relevance of this ultrasound finding are limited. Many authors have previously focused on an association between the size of the hematoma and subsequent obstetric complications[192,196,201]. Overall, the presence of an IUH has been associated with a 4–33% rate of miscarriage depending on the gestational age at which the complication was described[202]. Vaginal bleeding in very early pregnancy, i.e. before 6 weeks of gestation does not seem to be associated with any immediate or long-term consequences[203]. Conversely, threatened miscarriage symptoms at 7–12 weeks, even in the presence of detectable fetal cardiac activity, is not only associated with a 5–10% miscarriage rate before 14 weeks of gestation, but also with adverse pregnancy outcome at later gestations[195,197,204]. In particular, women with bleeding in the second half of the first trimester are at higher risk of PPROM and preterm labor (PTL). These risks are independent of the presence or absence of an IUH on the initial ultrasound examination and would suggest that threatened miscarriage in the first trimester is a risk factor for adverse pregnancy outcome regardless of the ultrasound findings.

Color Doppler imaging

The ability of transvaginal color Doppler to detect flow velocity waveforms from small vessels, such as the terminal part of the uteroplacental circulation, has given rise to much enthusiasm from clinicians interested in predicting early and late pregnancy complications related to an abnormal placentation. Overall, the predictive value of Doppler measurements of resistance to blood flow in early pregnancy is limited[205,206]. All Doppler studies in the first trimester have failed to demonstrate abnormal blood flow indices in the uteroplacental circulation of pregnancies that subsequently ended in miscarriage[207,208]. Histological assessment of decidual endovascular trophoblast invasion in first-trimester pregnancies about to undergo therapeutic evacuation, with low- and high-resistance umbilical artery (UA) Dopplers has shown that, although the proportion of vessels invaded is increased in women with low-resistance Dopplers, invasion is normal in both groups[209]. A comparison of uterine and intraplacental blood flow velocity waveforms with pathological features in missed miscarriages and normal pregnancies has shown that in the former, the mean pulsatility index (PI) is higher and the intervillous flow premature and increased. These findings are associated with abnormal placentation and dislocation of the trophoblastic shell and are only found when the process of miscarriage is established and irreversible[129,210].

3-dimensional (3D) ultrasound

The emergence of 3D ultrasound in obstetrics provided an opportunity to revisit previously abandoned or disregarded obstetric ultrasound parameters, particularly in early pregnancy. 3D assessment of gestational sac volume in the first trimester has been found to be a sensitive indicator of pregnancy outcome, with a smaller than expected gestational sac volume being predictive of failing early pregnancy[211,212]. It has not, however, proved useful in determining the outcome of expectant management or predicting the success of medical treatment and appears to add little to the diagnostic or prognostic value of 2D imaging[213].

Ultrasound in the prediction of early pregnancy failure

All of the above parameters have been investigated both singly and in combination, in attempts to predict those pregnancies that will result in miscarriage. Ultrasound parameters combined with maternal serum hormone levels, maternal age, smoking habits, obstetric history and the occurrence of vaginal bleeding have all been combined in multivariate analyses, with mixed results[144,145]. Ultimately, the fact remains that the vast majority of early pregnancies where the viability or likely outcome of the pregnancy is uncertain, will require careful counseling and timely follow-up, with limited use in clinical practice of a 'chance of a successful outcome'. Such predictors will, however, provide healthcare professionals with a tool with which to determine the timing of such follow-up and enable more appropriate counseling with regard to possible short- and long-term outcomes.

FIRST-TRIMESTER MARKERS OF ANEUPLOIDY

Advances in ultrasound technology and the introduction of early screening for aneuploidies have enabled earlier investigation of pregnancies between 11 and 14 weeks of gestation in large populations. This has led to a rapid increase in published data on the detection of fetal anomalies at 11–14 weeks. Most of these data have been provided by specialized centers with considerable experience in fetal anomaly scanning. However, there is still limited information on the feasibility and limitations of

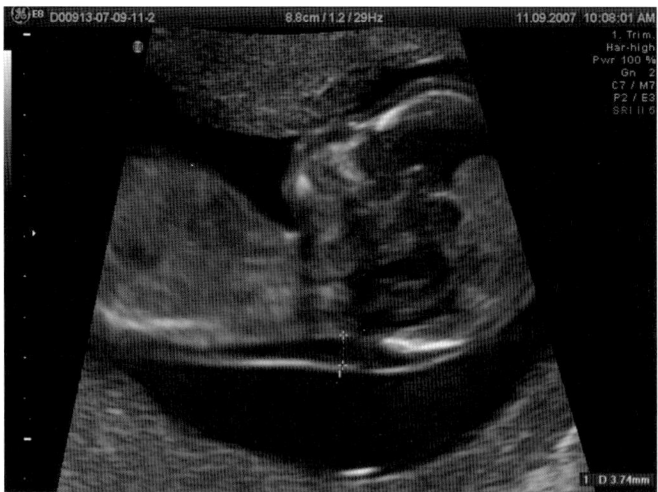

Fig. 43.8 Increased nuchal translucency thickness and generalized skin edema in an 11-week fetus with trisomy 21. Courtesy of Dr. Pranaus Pandya.

the screening of these anomalies at 11–14 weeks as compared to the now classical mid-gestation screening. The introduction of nuchal translucency measurement for the early screening for aneuploidies has resulted in large populations, first in Europe and subsequently in the USA[214,215], to be scanned by specialists in prenatal diagnosis at 11–14 weeks of gestation. There are several differences between first- and mid-trimester scanning for fetal anomalies, the size of the fetus before 12 weeks being the limiting factor due to the resolution of the ultrasound equipment (1 mm). Furthermore many fetal anomalies develop at the end of organogenesis over a variable period of time and many anomalies may not be apparent before the end of the first trimester, such as the agenesis of the corpus callosum. Some anomalies have sonographic features which are different than those usually seen during the routine mid-trimester anomalies scan (e.g. anencephaly). By contrast, normal fetal developmental features, such as the midgut herniation have the same features as the pathological exomphalos and thus the confirmation of the exact gestational age is crucial for such early diagnosis. Finally, dynamic changes in severity and sonographic appearance of abnormalities with advancing gestation cannot be evaluated by a single scan at 11–14 weeks. Widespread population screening for fetal aneuploidy has now been introduced in most centers in the UK. As a result of this, there is increasing interest in the predictive value of very early ultrasound markers of aneuploidy in pregnancies reaching the end of first trimester (Fig. 43.8). This may be of particular interest as aneuploidies are strongly associated with a high incidence of late pregnancy loss.

THE MANAGEMENT OF EARLY PREGNANCY FAILURE

The routine use of transvaginal ultrasound in the investigation and diagnosis of early pregnancy problems, has also led to improvements in the management of early pregnancy failure. Improved access to Early Pregnancy Units and increasing awareness among women of their choices in the management of early pregnancy problems has led to an increasing demand for more conservative management of early miscarriage.

Expectant management

Up to 70% of women will choose expectant management of miscarriage if given the choice[216]. The diagnosis of a complete miscarriage is generally accepted as an endometrial thickness <15 mm with no evidence of retained products of conception[217] and transvaginal sonography is a sensitive tool for detecting residual trophoblastic tissue[218]. The finding of blood flow in the intervillous space in cases of first-trimester miscarriage using color Doppler also appears to be useful in the prediction of success of expectant management. Miscarriages with blood flow within the intervillous space are up to four times more likely to complete with expectant management[219].

The success of expectant management is variable across studies, with a completion rate of 80–96% within 2 weeks in women with incomplete miscarriage and a low complication rate[216,220]. Completion rates are lower in missed miscarriages (59–62%)[216,220] and 'anembryonic pregnancies' (52%)[216] at 2 weeks and it is generally accepted that the likelihood of completion after this is low and evacuation of the uterus (ERPC) should be offered. In cases of incomplete miscarriage, where completion rates are high, it has been shown that other ultrasound parameters such as endometrial thickness and the presence or absence of a gestational sac did not add any further information to the likely outcome[221]. Expectant management of miscarriage, using ultrasound parameters to determine eligibility could significantly reduce the number of unnecessary ERPCs, depending on the criteria used.

Surgical management

Evacuation of retained products of conception (ERPC) is an extremely common procedure in the UK and is commonly performed by junior doctors in the 'out-of-hours' setting. Vacuum aspiration of products of conception is the method of choice and is recommended by the RCOG[141], as it is associated with reduced blood loss and shorter duration of operation. The risks associated with ERPC are perceived to be small, but serious morbidity occurs with an incidence of 2.1%[222], with a mortality of 0.5/100 000[223]. Complications include: uterine perforation, cervical tears, damage to internal organs, intrauterine adhesions and hemorrhage. Some of these complications are prevented by cervical preparation and the use of ultrasound guidance. Prostaglandin analogue administration (e.g. gemeprost and misoprostol) is well recognized to reduce the trauma associated with termination of pregnancy, however, no data exist for its efficacy prior to ERPC. It would seem sensible to use when a difficult cervical dilatation is anticipated.

Medical management

This has been made possible with the introduction of prostaglandins into gynecological practice and has led to improved choice for women in the management of miscarriage[224] with up to 20% preferring medical management[225], Various methods using different types of prostaglandin analogue, route of administration (vaginal or oral in the case of misoprostol) and with or without the use of mifepristone (an antiprogestagenic agent also known as RU486), with success rates varying from 13 to 96%[225–229]. Unfortunately, the lack of a standardized dose and route of administration of prostaglandins in the first trimester means that many units have failed to implement management protocols that include the use of medical management of first-trimester miscarriage, despite obvious cost savings and potential decreased risks to women. At the present time this appears unlikely to change.

THE ROLE OF THE EARLY PREGNANCY UNIT

Early pregnancy units (EPUs) are dedicated units for the assessment, diagnosis, treatment, psychological support and counseling of patients with early pregnancy complications. It has been shown that an EPU offers improved quality of care and produces considerable savings in financial and staff resources.[229,230] The clear advantages of a dedicated EPU include: easy open access to medical facilities with quicker diagnosis and treatment options, improved patient satisfaction, a reduction in the number and duration of inpatient admissions, structured training for junior doctors and appropriate counseling and follow-up of women who require support.

REFERENCES

1. Alberman E. Spontaneous abortion: epidemiology. In *Spontaneous abortion: diagnosis and treatment*, S Stabile, JG Grudzinskas, T Chard (eds), pp. 9–30. London: Springer-Verlag, 1992.
2. Miller JF, Williamson E, Glue J, Gordon YB, Grudzinskas JG, Sykes A. Fetal loss after implantation: a prospective study. *Lancet* **1**:554–556, 1980.
3. Regan L, Braude PR, Trembath PL. Influence of past reproductive performance on risk of spontaneous abortion. *Br Med J* **299**:541–545, 1989.
4. Edmonds DK, Lindsay KS, Miller JF, Williamson E, Wood P. Early embryonic mortality in woman. *Fertil Steril* **38**:447–453, 1982.
5. Zinaman MJ, Clegg ED, Brown CC, O'Connor J, Selevan SG. Estimates of human fertility and pregnancy loss. *Fertil Steril* **65**(3):503–509, 1996.
6. Goldstein SR. Embryonic death in early pregnancy: a new look at the first trimester. *Obstet Gynecol* **84**:294–297, 1994.
7. Pandya PP, Snijders RJ, Psara N, Hibert L, Nicolaides K. The prevalence of non-viable pregnancy at 10-13 weeks of gestation. *Ultrasound Obstet Gynecol* **7**:170–173, 1996.
8. Berry CW, Brambati B, Eskes TKAB et al. The Euro-Team Early Pregnancy (ETEP) protocol for recurrent miscarriage. *Hum Reprod* **10**:1516–1520, 1995.
9. Stirrat GM. Recurrent miscarriage: I. Definitions and epidemiology. *Lancet* **336**:673–675, 1990.
10. Simpson JL, Bombard AT. Chromosomal abnormalities in spontaneous abortion: frequency, pathology and genetic counselling. In *Spontaneous abortion*, K Edmonds, MJ Bennett (eds), pp. 51–76. London: Blackwell, 1987.
11. Barnea E. Epidemiology, etiology of early pregnancy disorders. In *The first twelve weeks of gestation*, E Barnea, J Hustin, E Jauniaux (eds), pp. 263–279. Heidelberg: Springer-Verlag, 1992.
12. Edwards RG. Causes of early embryonic loss in human pregnancy. *Hum Reprod* **1**(3):185–198, 1986.
13. Warburton D, Fraser FC. Spontaneous abortion risks in man: data from reproductive histories collected in a medical genetics unit. *Hum Genet* **16**:1–25, 1964.
14. Boue J, Boue A, Lazar P. Retrospective and prospective epidemiological studies of 1500 karyotyped spontaneous human abortions. *Teratology* **12**:11–26, 1975.
15. Lauristen JG. Aetiology of spontaneous abortion: a cytogenetic and epidemiological study of 288 cases. *Acta Obstet Gynecol Scand* **52**:S1, 1976.
16. Strobino BA, Pantel-Silverman J. First-trimester vaginal bleeding and the loss of chromosomally normal and abnormal conceptions. *Am J Obstet Gynecol* **157**: 1150–1154, 1987.
17. Greenwold N, Jauniaux ER, Gulbis B, Hempstock J, Gervy C, Burton GJ. Relationship among maternal serum endocrinology, placental karyotype and intervillous circulation in early pregnancy failure. *Fertil Steril* **79**(6):1373, 2003.
18. Sorokin Y, Johnson MP, Uhlman WR et al. Postmortem chorionic villus sampling: correlation of cytogenetic and ultrasound findings. *Am J Med Genet* **39**(3):314–316, 1991.
19. Jauniaux E, Brown R, Snijders JM, Noble P, Nicolaides KH. Early prenatal diagnosis of triploidy. *Am J Obstet Gynecol* **176**(3):550–554, 1997.
20. Watt JL, Templeton AA, Messinis I, Bell L, Cunningham P, Duncan RO. Trisomy 1 in an eight cell human pre-embryo. *J Med Genet* **24**(1):60–64, 1987.
21. Zaragoza MV, Jacobs PA, James RS. Non-disjunction of human acrocentric chromosomes: studies of 432 trisomic fetuses and liveborns. *Hum Genet* **19**(4):411–417, 1994.
22. Delhanty JDA, Handyside AH. The origin of genetic defects in the human and their detection in the preimplantation embryo. *Hum Reprod Update* **1**(3):201–215, 1995.
23. Fisher JM, Harvey JF, Morton NE, Jacobs PA. Trisomy 18: studies of the parent and cell division of origin and the effect of aberrant recombination or non-disjunction. *Am J Hum Genet* **56**(3):669–675, 1995.
24. Warburton D, Kline J, Stein Z, Hutzler M, Chin A, Hassold T. Does the karyotype of a spontaneous abortion predict the karyotype of a subsequent abortion? Evidence from 273 women with two karyotyped spontaneous abortions. *Am J Hum Genet* **41**(3):465–483, 1987.
25. Alberman E. The abortus as a predictor of future trisomy 21. In *Trisomy 21 Down's Syndrome*, FF De la Cruz, PS Gerald (eds), pp. 69–78. Baltimore: University Park Press, 1981.
26. De Braekeleer M, Dao TN. Cytogenetic studies in couples experiencing repeated pregnancy losses. *Hum Reprod* **5**(5): 519–528, 1990.
27. Stephenson MD. Frequency of factors associated with habitual abortion in 197 couples. *Fertil Steril* **66**(1):24–29, 1996.
28. Munne S, Escudero T, Sandlinas M, Sable D, Cohen J. Gamete segregation in female carriers of Robertsonian translocations. *Cytogenet Cell Genet* **90**:303–308, 2000.
29. Nybo Andersen AM, Wohlfahrt J, Christens P, Olsen J, Melybye M. Maternal age and fetal loss: population based register linkage study. *Br Med J* **320**(7215):1708–1712, 2000.
30. Wiznitzer A, Furman B, Mazor M, Reece EA. The role of prostanoids in the development of diabetic embryopathy. *Sem Reprod Endocrinol* **17**:175–181, 2004.
31. Temple R, Aldridge V, Greenwood R, Heyburn P, Sampson M, Stanley K. Association between outcome of pregnancy and glycaemic control in early pregnancy in type 1 diabetes: population

based study. *Br Med J* **325**(7375): 1275–1276, 2002.
32. Penney GC, Mair G, Pearson DW Scottish Diabetes in Pregnancy Group. Outcomes of pregnancies in women with type 1 diabetes in Scotland: a national population based study. *Br J Obstet Gynaecol* **110**(3):315–318, 2003.
33. Reece EA, Homko CJ, Wu YK. Multifactorial basis of the syndrome of diabetic embryopathy. *Teratology* **54**:171–182, 1996.
34. Eriksson UJ. The pathogenesis of congenital malformations in diabetic pregnancy. *Diabetes Metab Rev* **11**:63–82, 1995.
35. Cederberg J, Siman CM, Eriksson UJ. Combined treatment with vitamin E and vitamin C decreases oxidative stress and improves fetal outcome in experimental diabetic pregnancy. *Pediatr Res* **49**(6): 742–743, 2001.
36. Siman CM, Eriksson UJ. Vitamin E decreases the occurrence of malformations in the offspring of diabetic rats. *Diabetes* **46**(6):1054–1061, 1997.
37. Moley K. Hypergylcaemia and apoptosis: mechanisms for congenital malformations and pregnancy loss in diabetic women. *Trends Endocrinol Metab* **12**(2):78, 2001.
38. Craig LB, Ke RW, Kutteh WH. Increased prevalence of insulin resistance in women with a history of recurrent pregnancy loss. *Fertil Steril* **78**(3):487–490, 2002.
39. Tian L, Shen H, Lu Q, Norman RJ, Wang J. Insulin resistance increases the risk of spontaneous abortion following assisted reproduction technology treatment. *J Clin Endocrinol Metab* **92**:1430–1433 2007.
40. Hart R, Norman R. Polycystic ovarian syndrome – prognosis and outcomes. *Best Pract Res Clin Obst Gynaecol* **20**(5): 751–778, 2006.
41. Regan L, Owen EJ, Jacobs HS. Hypersecretion of luteinising hormone, infertility and miscarriage. *Lancet* **336**:1141–1143, 1990.
42. Lashen H, Fear K, Sturdee DW. Obesity is associated with increased risk of first trimester and recurrent miscarriage: matched case-control study. *Hum Reprod* **19**:1644–1646, 2004.
43. Bellver J, Rossal LP, Bosch E et al. Obesity and the risk of spontaneous abortion after oocyte donation. *Fertil Steril* **79**(5): 1136–1140, 2003.
44. Hirahara F, Andoh N, Sawai K, Hirabuki T, Uemura T, Minaguchi H. Hyperprolactinemic recurrent miscarriage and results of randomized bromocriptine treatment trials. *Fertil Steril* **70**(2):246–252, 1998.
45. Stagnaro-Green A, Glinoer D. Thyroid autoimmunity and the risk of miscarriage. *Best Pract Res Clin Endocrinol Metab* **18**(2):167–181, 2004.
46. Bajekal N, Li TC. Fibroids, infertility and pregnancy wastage. *Hum Reprod Update* **6**(6):614–620, 2000.
47. Woelfer B, Salim R, Bannerjee S, Elson J, Regan L, Jurkovic D. Reproductive outcomes in women with congenital uterine anomalies detected by three-dimensional ultrasound screening. *Obstet Gynecol* **98**(6):1099–1103, 2001.
48. Kupesic S. Clinical implications of sonographic detection of uterine anomalies for reproductive outcome. *Ultrasound Obstet Gynecol* **18**:387–400, 2001.
49. Simpson JL, Mills JL, Kim H et al. Infectious processes: an infrequent cause of first trimester spontaneous abortions. Hum Reprod 3:668–672, 1996.
50. Hay PE, Lamont RF, Taylor-Robinson D, Morgan DJ, Ison C, Pearson J. Abnormal bacterial colonisation of the genital tract and subsequent preterm delivery and late miscarriage. *Br Med J* **308**:295–298, 1994.
51. Ralph SG, Rutherford AJ, Wilson JD. Influence of bacterial vaginosis on conception and miscarriage in the first trimester: cohort study. *Br Med J* **319**: 220–223, 1999.
52. Llahi-Camp J, Rai R, Ison C, Regan L, Taylor-Robinson D. Association of bacterial vaginosis with a history of second trimester miscarriage. *Hum Reprod* **11**:1575–1578, 1996.
53. Clifford K, Flanagan AM, Regan L. Endometrial CD56+ natural killer cells in women with recurrent miscarriage: a histomorphometric study. *Hum Reprod* **14**(11):2727–2730, 1999.
54. Quenby S, Bates M, Doig T et al. Pre-implantation endometrial leukocytes in women with recurrent miscarriage. *Hum Reprod* **14**(9):2386–2391, 1999.
55. Rai R, Regan L. Recurrent miscarriage. *Lancet* **368**(9535):601–611, 2006.
56. Wilson WA, Gharavi AE, Piette JC. International classification criteria for antiphospholipid syndrome: synopsis of a post-conference workshop held at the Ninth International (Tours) aPL Symposium. *Lupus* **10**:457–460, 2001.
57. Empson M, Lassere M, Craig JC, Scott JR. Recurrent pregnancy loss with antiphospholipid antibody: a systematic review of therapeutic trials. *Obstet Gynecol* **99**(1):135–144, 2002.
58. Kovalevsky G, Gracia CR, Berlin JA, Sammel MD, Barnhart KT. Evaluation of the association between hereditary thrombophilias and recurrent pregnancy loss: a meta-analysis. *Arch Intern Med* **164**(5):558–560, 2004.
59. Syme MR, Paxton JW, Keelan JA. Drug transfer and metabolism by the human placenta. *Clin Pharmacokinet* **43**(8): 487–514, 2004.
60. Jauniaux E, Lees C, Jurkovic D, Campbell S, Gulbis B. Transfer of inulin across the first trimester human placenta. *Am J Obstet Gynecol* **176**(1 Pt 1):33–36, 1997.
61. Cooper J, Jauniaux E, Gulbis B, Quick D, Bromley L. Placental transfer of fentanyl in early human pregnancy and its detection in fetal brain. *Br J Anaesth* **82**(6):929–931, 1999.
62. Jauniaux E, Jurkovic D, Lees C, Campbell S, Gulbis B. *In-vivo* study of diazepam transfer across the first trimester human placenta. *Hum Reprod* **11**(4):889–892, 1996.
63. Czeizel AE, Dudas I. Prevention of the first occurrence of neural tube defects by periconceptual vitamin supplementation. *N Engl J Med* **327**:1832–1835, 1992.
64. Milunsky A, Jick H, Jick SS, MacLaughlin DS, Rothman KJ, Willett W. Multivitamin/folic acid supplementation in early pregnancy reduces the prevalence of neural tube defects. *J Am Med Assoc* **262**:2847–2852, 1989.
65. George L, Mills JL, Johansson ALV et al. Plasma folate levels and risk of spontaneous abortion. *J Am Med Assoc* **288**(15):1867, 2002.
66. Scholl TO, Johnson WG. Folic acid: influence on the outcome of pregnancy. *Am J Clin Nutr* **71**(suppl):1295S–1303S, 2000.
67. Ray JG, Laskin CA. Folic acid and homocysteine metabolic defects and the risk of placental abruption, pre-eclampsia and spontaneous pregnancy loss: a systematic review. *Placenta* **20**:519–529, 1999.
68. Jauniaux E, Johns J, Gulbis B, Spasik-Boskovic O, Burton GJ. Transfer of folic acid inside the first-trimester gestational sac and the effect of maternal smoking. *Am J Obstet Gynecol* **197**(58):e1–e58, 2007.
69. Morrison C, Siney C. Maternity services for drug misusers in England and Wales: a national survey. *Hlth Trends* **27**:1, 1995.
70. Ness RB, Grisso JA, Hirschinger N et al. Cocaine and tobacco use and the risk of spontaneous abortion. *N Engl J Med* **340**(5):333, 1999.
71. Woods JR, Plessinger MA, Clarke XE. Effect of cocaine on uterine blood flow and fetal oxygenation. *J Am Med Assoc* **257**:957–961, 1987.
72. Plessinger MA, Wood JR, Jr. Maternal, placental and fetal pathophysiology of cocaine exposure during pregnancy. *Clin Obstet Gynecol* **36**(2):267–278, 1993.
73. Buchler BA, Conover B, Andres RL. Teratogenic potential of cocaine. *Semin Perinatol* **20**(2):93–98, 1996.
74. Offidani C, Pomani F, Caruso A, Ferrazzani S, Chiarotti M, Fiori A. Cocaine during pregnancy: a critical review of the literature. *Minerva Gynecol* **47**(9):381–390, 1995.
75. Hoyme HE, Jones KL, Dixon SD et al. Prenatal cocaine exposure and fetal vascular disruption. *Pediatrics* **85**:743–747, 1990.
76. Dolovich LR, Addis A, Vaillancourt JMR, Power B, Einarson TR. Benzodiazepine

use in pregnancy and major malformations or oral cleft: meta-analysis of cohort and case-control studies. *Br Med J* **317**:839–843, 1998.

77. Oro AS, Dixon SD. Perinatal cocaine and methamphetamine exposure: maternal and neonatal correlates. *J Pediatr* **111**: 571–578, 1987.
78. English DR, Hulse GK, Milne E, Holman CD, Bower CI. Maternal cannabis use and birth weight: a meta-analysis. *Addiction* **92**:1553–1560, 1997.
79. Morrison JJ, Chitty LS, Peebles D, Rodeck CH. Recreational drugs and fetal gastroschisis: maternal hair analysis in the peri-conceptional period and during pregnancy. *Br J Obstet Gynaecol* **112**(8):1022–1025, 2005.
80. Signorello LB, McLaughlin JK. Maternal caffeine consumption and spontaneous abortion: a review of the epidemiological evidence. *Epidemiology* **15**(2):646, 2004.
81. Golding J. Reproduction and caffeine consumption. *Early Hum Dev* **43**(1): 1–14, 1995.
82. Jones KL, Smith DW, Ulleland CL, Streissguth P. Pattern of malformations in offspring of chronic alcoholic mothers. *Lancet* **9**(1):1267–1271, 1973.
83. Cohen-Kerem R, Koren G. Antioxidants and fetal protection against ethanol teratogenicity I: Review of the experimental data and implications to humans. *Neurotoxicol Teratol* **25**:1–9, 2003.
84. Goodlett CR, Horn KH, Zhou FC. Alcohol teratogenesis: mechanism of damage and strategies for intervention. *Exp Biol Med* **230**(6):394–406, 2005.
85. Henderson GI, Chen JJ, Schenker S. Ethanol, oxidative stress, reactive aldehydes and the fetus. *Front Biosci* **15**(4):D541–D550, 1999.
86. Ramachandran V, Perez A, Chen J, Senthil D, Schenker S, Henderson GI. In utero ethanol exposure causes mitochondrial dysfunction, which can result in apoptotic cell death in fetal brain: a potential role for 4-hydroxynonenal. *Alcohol Clin Exp Res* **25**(6):862–871, 2001.
87. Floyd RL, Decoufle DW, Hungerford DW. Alcohol use prior to pregnancy recognition. *Am J Prev Med* **17**:101–107, 1999.
88. Ananth CV, Savitz DA, Luther ER. Maternal cigarette smoking as a risk factor for placental abruption, placenta previa and uterine bleeding in pregnancy. *Am J Epidemiol* **144**:881–889, 1996.
89. Cnattingius S, Axelsson O, Eklund G, Lindmark G. Smoking, maternal age and fetal growth. *Obstet Gynecol* **66**(4):449–452, 1985.
90. Economides D, Braithwaite J. Smoking, pregnancy and the fetus. *J R Soc Health* **114**(4):198–201, 1994.
91. Andres RL. The association of cigarette smoking with placenta previa and abruptio placentae. *Semin Perinatol* **20**(2):154–159, 1996.
92. Wang X, Tager IB, Van Vunakis H, Speizer FE, Hanrahan JP. Maternal smoking during pregnancy, urine cotinine concentrations, and birth outcomes. A prospective cohort study. *Int J Epidemiol* **26**(5):978–988, 1997.
93. Chatenoud L, Parazzini F, Di Cintio E et al. Paternal and maternal smoking habits before conception and during the first trimester: relation to spontaneous abortion. *Ann Epidemiol* **8**:520–526, 1998.
94. Royal College of Physicians. *Smoking and the young*. London: Royal College of Physicians, 1992.
95. Armstrong BG, McDonald AD, Sloan M. Cigarette, alcohol and coffee consumption and spontaneous abortion. *Am J Pub Hlth* **82**:85–87, 1992.
96. Harger JH, Hsing AW, Tuomala RE et al. Risk factors for preterm premature rupture of fetal membranes: a multicentre case-control study. *Am J Obstet Gynecol* **163**:130–137, 1990.
97. Jauniaux E, Gulbis B, Acharya G, Thiry P, Rodeck C. Maternal tobacco exposure and cotinine levels in fetal fluids in the first half of pregnancy. *Obstet Gynecol* **93**(1):25–29, 1999.
98. Hwang SJ, Beaty TH, Panny SR et al. Association study of transforming growth factor alpha (TGF-alpha) Tag 1 polymorphism and oral clefts: indication of gene-environment interaction in a population based sample of infants with birth defects. *Am J Epidemiol* **141**(629):636, 1995.
99. Beaty TH, Maestri NE, Hetmanski JB et al. Testing for interaction between maternal smoking and TGFA genotype and oral cleft cases born in Maryland 1992–1996. *Cleft Palate Craniofac J* **34**(5):447–454, 1997.
100. Czeizel AE, Kodaj I, Lenz W. Smoking during pregnancy and congenital limb deficiency. *Br Med J* **308**:1473–1476, 1994.
101. Martinez-Friaz ML, Czeizel AE, Rodriguez-Pinilla E, Bermejo E. Smoking during pregnancy and Poland sequence: results of a population based registry and a case-control registry. *Teratology* **59**(35):38, 1999.
102. Kallen K. Maternal smoking and urinary organ malformations. *Int J Epidemiol* **26**:571–574, 1997.
103. Kleinman JC, Pierre MB Jr, Madans JH, Land GH, Schramm WF. The effects of maternal smoking on fetal and infant mortality. *Am J Epidemiol* **127**(2):274–282, 1988.
104. Naeye RL. Abruptio placentae and placenta previa: frequency, perinatal mortality and cigarette smoking. *Obstet Gynecol* **55**:701–704, 1980.
105. McDonald SD, Perkins SL, Jodouin CA, Walker MC. Folate levels in pregnant women who smoke: an important gene/environment interaction. *Am J Obstet Gynecol* **187**:620–625, 2002.
106. Jauniaux E, Gulbis B, Acharya G, Gerlo E. Fetal amnio acid and enzyme levels with maternal smoking. *Obstet Gynecol* **93**:680–683, 1999.
107. Friedberg W, Copeland K, Duke FE, O'Brien K, 3rd, Darden EB, Jr. Radiation exposure during air travel: guidance provided by the Federal Aviation Administration for air carrier crews. *Health Phys* **79**(5):591–595, 2000.
108. Larsson KS. Teratological aspects of dental amalgam. *Adv Dent Res* **6**: 114–119, 1992.
109. Caughey AB, Hopkins LM, Norton ME. Chorionic villus sampling compared with amniocentesis and the difference in the rate of pregnancy loss. *Obstet Gynecol* **108**(3 Pt 1):612–616, 2006.
110. Jauniaux E. A comparison of chorionic villus sampling and amniocentesis for prenatal diagnosis in early pregnancy. In *Screening for Down's syndrome in the first trimester*, JG Grudzinskas, RHT Ward (eds), pp. 259–269. London: RCOG Press, 1997.
111. Alfirevic Z, Sundberg K, Brigham SA. Amniocentesis and chorionic villus sampling for prenatal diagnosis. *Cochrane Database Syst Rev* **3**(CD003252), 2003.
112. Evans MI, Wapner RJ. Invasive prenatal diagnostic procedures 2005. *Semin Perinatol* **29**(4):215–218, 2005.
113. Philip J, Silver RK, Wilson RD et al. Late first-trimester invasive prenatal diagnosis: results of an international randomized trial. *Obstet Gynecol* **103**(6):1164–1173, 2004.
114. Borrell A, Fortuny A, Lazaro L et al. First-trimester transcervical chorionic villus sampling by biopsy forceps versus mid-trimester amniocentesis: a randomised controlled trial project. *Prenat Diagn* **19**(12):1138–1142, 1999.
115. Kalousek DK. Anatomic and chromosome anomalies in specimens of early spontaneous abortion: seven-year experience. *Birth Defects Orig Artic Ser* **23**(1):153–168, 1987.
116. Heath V, Chadwick V, Cooke I, Manek S, MacKenzie IZ. Should tissue from pregnancy termination and uterine evacuation routinely be examined histologically? *Br J Obstet Gynaecol* **107**:727–730, 2000.
117. Pijnenborg R, Bland JM, Robertson WB, Brosens I. Uteroplacental arterial changes related to interstitial trophoblast migration in early human pregnancy. *Placenta* **4**:397–414, 1983.
118. Brosens I, Robertson WB, Dixon HG. The physiological response of the vessels of the placental bed to normal pregnancy. *J Pathol Bacteriol* **93**:569–579, 1967.
119. Larsen WJ. *Human embryology*, 2nd edn. New York: Churchill Livingstone, 1997.

120. Hustin J, Schaaps JP, Lambotte R. Anatomical studies of the utero-placental vascularisation in the first trimester of pregnancy. *Troph Res* **3**:49–60, 1988.
121. Burton GJ, Jauniaux ER, Watson AL. Maternal arterial connections to the placental intervillous space during the first trimester of pregnancy: The Boyd Collection revisited. *Am J Obstet Gynecol* **181**:718–724, 1999.
122. Jauniaux E, Jurkovic D, Campbell S. In vivo investigations of anatomy and physiology of early human placental circulations. *Ultrasound Obstet Gynecol* **1**:435–445, 1991.
123. Hustin J, Schaaps JP. Echographic and anatomic studies of the maternotrophoblastic border during the first trimester of pregnancy. *Am J Obstet Gynecol* **157**:162–168, 1987.
124. Jaffe R, Woods JR. Colour Doppler imaging and in vivo assessment of the anatomy and physiology of early uteroplacental circulation. *Fertil Steril* **60**(2):293–297, 2004.
125. Schaaps JP, Hustin J. In vivo aspects of the maternal-trophoblastic border during the first trimester of gestation. *Troph Research* **3**:39–48, 1988.
126. Jauniaux E, Zaidi J, Jurkovic D, Campbell S, Hustin J. Comparison of colour Doppler features and pathological findings in complicated early pregnancy. *Hum Reprod* **9**(12): 2432–2437, 1994.
127. Pijnenborg R, Bland JM, Robertson WB, Dixon G, Brosens I. The pattern of interstitial invasion of the myometrium in early human pregnancy. *Placenta* **2**:303–316, 1981.
128. Jauniaux E, Greenwold N, Hempstock J, Burton GJ. Comparison of ultrasonographic and Doppler mapping of the intervillous circulation in normal and abnormal early pregnancies. *Fertil Steril* **79**(1): 100–1066, 2003.
129. Jauniaux E, Hempstock J, Greenwold N, Burton GJ. Trophoblastic oxidative stress in relation to temporal and regional differences in maternal placental blood flow in normal and abnormal early pregnancies. *Am J Pathol* **162**(1): 115–125, 2003.
130. Robertson WB, Brosens I, Landells WN. Abnormal placentation. *Obstet Gynecol Annu* **14**:411–426, 1985.
131. Khong TY, Liddell HS, Robertson WB. Defective haemochorial placentation as a cause of miscarriage: a preliminary study. *Br J Obstet Gynaecol* **94**:649–655, 1987.
132. Hustin J, Jauniaux ER, Schapps JP. Histological study of the materno-embryonic interface in spontaneous abortion. *Placenta* **11**:477–486, 1990.
133. Sebire N, Fox H, Backos M, Rai R, Paterson C, Regan L. Defective endovascular trophoblast invasion in primary antiphospholipid antibody syndrome – associated early pregnancy failure. *Hum Reprod* **17**(4):1067–1071, 2002.
134. Jauniaux E, Kadri R, Hustin J. Partial mole and triploidy: screening patients with first trimester spontaneous abortion. *Obstet Gynecol* **88**:616–619, 1996.
135. Szulman AE, Surti U. The syndromes of hydatidiform mole. I. Cytogenetic and morphologic correlations. *Am J Obstet Gynecol* **131**:665–671, 1978.
136. Szulman AE, Surti U. The syndromes of hydatidiform mole. II. Morphologic evolution of complete and partial mole. *Am J Obstet Gynecol* **132**:20–27, 1978.
137. Fox H. Differential diagnosis of hydatidiform mole. *Gen Diagn Pathol* **143**(2–3):117–125, 1997.
138. Jauniaux E. Partial moles: from postnatal to prenatal diagnosis. *Placenta* **20**:379–388, 1999.
139. Paradinas FJ. The histological diagnosis of hydatidiform moles. *Curr Diag Pathol* **1**:24–31, 1994.
140. Fukunaga M. Early partial hydatidiform mole: prevalence, histopathology, DNA ploidy and persistence rate. *Virchows Arch* **437**:180–184, 2000.
141. RCOG Guidelines and Audit Committee. The management of early pregnancy failure. Green-top Guideline (25), 1997.
142. Johnson MR, Riddle AF, Sharma V, Collins WP, Nicolaides KH, Grudzinskas JG. Placental and ovarian hormones in anembryonic pregnancy. *Hum Reprod* **8**(112):115, 1993.
143. Dumps P, Meisser A, Pons D et al. Accuracy of single measurement of pregnancy associated plasma protein-A, human chorionic gonadotrophin and progesterone in the diagnosis of early pregnancy failure. *Eur J Obstet Gynecol Reprod Biol* **100**:174–180, 2002.
144. Choong S, Rombauts L, Ugoni A, Meagher S. Ultrasound prediction of risk of spontaneous miscarriage in live embryos from assisted conception. *Ultrasound Obstet Gynecol* **22**(6):571–577, 2003.
145. Makrydimas G, Sebire N, Lolis D, Vlassis N, Nicolaides KH. Fetal loss following ultrasound diagnosis of a live fetus at 6–10 weeks of gestation. *Ultrasound Obstet Gynecol* **22**(4): 368–372, 2003.
146. Banerjee S, Aslam N, Woelfer B, Lawrence A, Elson J, Jurkovic D. Expectant management of early pregnancies of unknown location: a prospective evaluation of methods to predict spontaneous resolution of pregnancy. *Br J Obstet Gynaecol* **108**: 158–160, 2001.
147. Lower AM, Yovich JL. The value of serum levels of oestradiol, progesterone and β-human chorionic gonadotrophin in the prediction of early pregnancy failure. *Hum Reprod* **7**(5):711–717, 1992.
148. Muttukrishna S, Jauniaux E, Greenwold N et al. Circulating levels of inhibin A, activin A and follistatin in missed and recurrent miscarriages. *Hum Reprod* **17**(12):3072–3078, 2003.
149. Luisi S, Florio P, D'Antona D et al. Maternal serum inhibin A levels are a marker of a viable trophoblast in incomplete and complete miscarriages. *Eur J Endocrinol* **148**:233–236, 2003.
150. Wallace EM, Marjono B, Tyzack K, Tong S. First trimester levels of inhibins and activin A in normal and failing pregnancies. *Clin Endocrinol* **60**(4): 484–490, 2004.
151. Muttukrishna S, Jauniaux E, Greenwold N et al. Levels of inhibin A, activin A and follistatin in missed and recurrent miscarriages. *Hum Reprod* **17**:3072–3078, 2002.
152. Al-Azemi M, Ledger WL, Diejomaoh M, Mousa M, Makhseed M, Omu A. Measurement of inhibin A and inhibin pro-αc in early pregnancy and their role in the prediction of pregnancy outcome in patients with recurrent pregnancy loss. *Fertil Steril* **80**(6): 1473–1479, 2003.
153. Treetampinich C, O'Connor AE, MacLachlan V, Groome NP, de Kretser D. Maternal serum inhibin-A concentrations in early pregnancy after IVF and embryo transfer reflect the corpus luteum contribution and pregnancy outcome. *Hum Reprod* **15**:2028–2032, 2000.
154. Jauniaux ER, Jurkovic D. The role of ultrasound in abnormal early pregnancy. In *Problems in early pregnancy advances in diagnosis and management*, JG Grudzinskas, PMS O'Brien (eds), p. 137. London: RCOG Press, 1997.
155. Nyberg DA, Mack LA, Laing FC, Patten RM. Distinguishing normal from abnormal gestational sac growth in early pregnancy. *J Ultrasound Med* **6**(1):23–27, 1987.
156. Robinson HP. 'Gestational sac' volumes as determined by sonar in the first trimester of pregnancy. *Br J Obstet Gynecol* **82**(2):100–107, 1975.
157. Goldstein SR. Embryonic death in early pregnancy: a new look at the first trimester. *Obstet Gynecol* **84**(2):294–297, 81994.
159. Bromley B, Harlow BL, Laboda LA, Benacerraf BR. Small sac size in the first trimester: a predictor of poor fetal outcome. *Radiology* **178**:375, 1991.
159. Dickey RP, Grasser R, Olar TT et al. Relationship of initial chorionic sac diameter and abortion and abortus karyotype based on new growth curves for the 16th to 49th post-ovulation day. *Hum Reprod* **9**:559–565, 1994.

160. Elson J, Salim R, Tailor A, Banerjee S, Zosmer N, Jurkovic D. Prediction of early pregnancy viability in the absence of an ultrasonically detectable embryo. *Ultrasound Obstet Gynecol* **21**(1):57–61, 2003.
161. Falco P, Zagonari S, Gabrielli S, Bevini M, Pilu G, Bovicelli L. Sonography of pregnancies with first trimester bleeding and a small intrauterine gestational sac without a demonstrable embryo. *Ultrasound Obstet Gynecol* **21**(1):62–65, 2003.
162. Robinson HP, Fleming JEE. A critical evaluation of sonar 'crown rump length' measurements. *Br J Obstet Gynecol* **82**:702–710, 1975.
163. Hadlock FP, Shah YP KDLJ. Fetal crown-rump length: re-evaluation of relation to menstrual age (5–18 weeks) with high resolution real time US. *Radiology* **182**(2):501–505, 1992.
164. Bahado-Singh , Lynch L, Deren O et al. First-trimester growth restriction and fetal aneuploidy: the effect of type of aneuploidy and gestational age. *Am J Obstet Gynecol* **176**(5):976–980, 1997.
165. Drugan A, Johnson MP, Isada NB et al. The smaller than expected first trimester fetus is at increased risk for chromosome anomalies. *Am J Obstet Gynecol* **167**(6):1525–1528, 1992.
166. Benacerraf BR. Intrauterine growth restriction in the first trimester associated with triploidy. *J Ultrasound Med* **7**(3):153–154, 1988.
167. Goldstein SR, Kerenyi T, Scher J, Papp C. Correlation between karyotype and ultrasound findings in patients with failed early pregnancy. *Ultrasound Obstet Gynecol* **8**(5):314–317, 1996.
168. Reljic M. The significance of crown-rump length measurement for predicting adverse pregnancy outcome of threatened abortion. *Ultrasound Obstet Gynecol* **17**(6):510–512, 2004.
169. Jauniaux E, Jurkovic D, Henriet Y, Rodesch F, Hustin J. Development of the secondary human yolk sac: correlation of sonographic and anatomic features. *Hum Reprod* **6**:1160–1166, 1991.
170. Reece EA, Scioscia AL, Pinter E et al. Prognostic significance of the human yolk sac assessed by ultrasonography. *Am J Obstet Gynecol* **159**(5):1191–1194, 1988.
171. Lindsay DJ, Lovett IS, Lyons EA et al. Yolk sac diameter and shape at endovaginal US: predictors of pregnancy outcome in the first trimester. *Radiology* **183**(1):115–118, 1992.
172. Stampone C, Nicotra M, Muttinelli C, Cosmi EV. Transvaginal sonography of the yolk sac in normal and abnormal pregnancy. *J Clin Ultrasound* **24**(1):3–9, 1996.
173. Kucuk T, Duru NK, Yenen MC, Dede M, Ergun A, Baser I. Yolk sac size and shape as predictors of poor pregnancy outcome. *J Perinat Med* **27**(4):316–320, 1999.
174. Jauniaux E, Gulbis B, Jurkovic D, Gavriil P, Campbell S. The origin of alpha-fetoprotein in first trimester anembryonic pregnancies. *Am J Obstet Gynecol* **173**:1749–1753, 1995.
175. Tezuka N, Sato S, Kanasugi H, Hiroi M. Embryonic heart rates: development in early first trimester and clinical evaluation. *Gynecol Obstet Invest* **32**(4):210–212, 1991.
176. Levi CS, Lyons EA, Zheng XH, Lindsay DJ, Holt SC. Endovaginal US: demonstration of cardiac activity in embryo's of less than 5.0 mm in crown-rump length. *Radiology* **176**:71–74, 1990.
177. Goldstein SR. Significance of cardiac activity on endovaginal ultrasound in very early embryos. *Obstet Gynecol* **80**:670–672, 1992.
178. Brown DL, Emerson DS, Felker RE, Cartier MS, Smith WC. Diagnosis of early embryonic demise by endovaginal sonography. *J Ultrasound Med* **9**(11): 631–636, 1990.
179. Stefos TI, Lolis DE, Sotiriadis AJ, Ziakas GV. Embryonic heart rate in early pregnancy. *J Clin Ultrasound* **26**(1):33–36, 1998.
180. van Heeswijk M, Nijhuis JG, Hollanders HM. Fetal heart rate in early pregnancy. *Early Hum Dev* **22**(3):151–156, 1990.
181. Achiron R, Tadmore O, Mashiach S. Heart rate as a predictor of first-trimester spontaneous abortion after ultrasound proven viability. *Obstet Gynecol* **78**(3 Pt 1):330–334, 1991.
182. Coulam CB, Britten S, Soenksen DM. Early (34–56 days from last menstrual period) ultrasonographic measurements in normal pregnancies. *Hum Reprod* **11**(8):1771–1774, 1996.
183. Yapar EG, Ekici E, Gokmen O. First trimester fetal heart rate measurements by transvaginal ultrasound combined with pulsed Doppler: an evaluation of 1331 cases. *Eur J Obstet Gynecol Reprod Biol* **60**(2):133–137, 1995.
184. May DA, Sturtevant NV. Embryonal heart rate as a predictor of pregnancy outcome: a prospective analysis. *J Ultrasound Med* **10**:591–593, 1991.
185. Merchiers EH, Dhont M, De Sutter P, Beghin CJ, Vanderkerckhove DA. Predictive value of early embryonic cardiac activity for pregnancy outcome. *Am J Obstet Gynecol* **165**:11–14, 1991.
186. Benson CB, Doubilet PM. Slow embryonic heart rate in early first trimester: indicator of poor pregnancy outcome. *Radiology* **192**(2):343–344, 1994.
187. Chittacharoen A, Herabutya Y. Slow fetal heart rate may predict pregnancy outcome in first-trimester threatened abortion. *Fertil Steril* **82**(1):227–229, 2004.
188. Qasim SM, Sachdev R, Trias A, Senkowski K, Kemmann E. The predictive value of first-trimester embryonic heart rates in infertility patients. *Obstet Gynecol* **89**(6): 934–936, 1997.
189. Goto S. Ultrasonographic detection of a live fetus in recurrent spontaneous abortion during the first trimester. *Hum Reprod* **8**(4):627–630, 1993.
190. Brigham SA, Conlon C, Farquharson RG. A longitudinal study of pregnancy outcome following idiopathic recurrent miscarriage. *Hum Reprod* **14**(11):2868–2871, 2002.
191. Farrell T, Owen P. The significance of extrachorionic membrane separation in threatened miscarriage. *Br J Obstet Gynecol* **103**:926–928, 1996.
192. Ball RH, Ade CM, Schoenborn JA, Crane JP. The clinical significance of ultrasonographically detected subchorionic hemorrhages. *Am J Obstet Gynecol* **174**:996–1002, 1996.
193. Borlum KG, Thomsen A, Clausen I, Eriksen G. Long-term prognosis of pregnancies in women with intrauterine hematomas. *Obstet Gynecol* **74**(2): 231–233, 1989.
194. Johns J, Jauniaux E. Threatened miscarriage as a predictor of obstetric outcome. *Obstet Gynecol* **107**(4): 845–850, 2006.
195. Tongsong T, Srisomboon J, Wanapirak C, Sirichotiyakul S, Pongsatha S, Porisuthikul T. Pregnancy outcome of threatened abortion with demonstrable fetal cardiac activity: a cohort study. *J Obstet Gynaecol Tokyo* **21**(4):331–335, 1995.
196. Bennett GL, Bromley B, Lieberman E, Benacerraf BR. Subchorionic haemorrhage in first trimester pregnancies: prediction of pregnancy outcome with sonography. *Radiology* **200**:803–806, 1996.
197. Weiss JL, Malone FD, Vidaver J et al. Threatened abortion: a risk factor for poor pregnancy outcome, a population-based screening study. *Am J Obstet Gynecol* **190**(3):745–750, 2004.
198. Baztofin JH, Fielding WL, Friedman EA. Effect of vaginal bleeding in early pregnancy outcome. *Obstet Gynecol* **63**(4):515–518, 1984.
199. Rulin MC, Bornstein SG, Campbell JD. The reliability of ultrasonography in the management of spontaneous abortion, clinically thought to be complete: a prospective study. *Am J Obstet Gynecol* **168**(1 Pt 1):12–15, 1993.
200. Bajo J, Moreno-Calvo FJ, Martinez-Cortes L, Haya FJ, Rayward J. Is trophoblastic thickness at the embryonic implantation site a new sign of negative evolution in first trimester pregnancy? *Hum Reprod* **15**(7):1629–1631, 2004.

201. Mantoni M, Fog Pedersen J. Intrauterine haematoma – an ultrasonic study of threatened abortion. *Br J Obstet Gynecol* **88**:47–51, 1981.
202. Pearlstone M, Baxi L. Subchorionic haematoma: a review. *Obstet Gynecol Surv* **48**(2):65–68, 1993.
203. Harville EW, Wilcox AJ, Baird DD, Weinberg CR. Vaginal bleeding in very early pregnancy. *Hum Reprod* **18**(9):1944, 2003.
204. Johns J, Hyett J, Jauniaux E. Obstetric outcome after threatened miscarriage with and without a hematoma on ultrasound. *Obstet Gynecol* **102**:483–487, 2003.
205. Pellizzari P, Pozzan C, Marchiori S, Zen T, Gangemi M. Assessment of uterine artery blood flow in normal first trimester pregnancies and in those complicated by uterine bleeding. *Ultrasound Obstet Gynecol* **19**(4):366–370, 2002.
206. Frates MC, Doubilet PM, Brown DL et al. Role of Doppler ultrasonography in the prediction of pregnancy outcome in women with recurrent spontaneous abortion. *J Ultrasound Med* **15**(8):557–562, 1996.
207. Makikallio K, Tekay A, Jouppila P. Effects of bleeding on uteroplacental, umbilicoplacental and yolk-sac haemodynamics in early pregnancy. *Ultrasound Obstet Gynecol* **18**:352–356, 2001.
208. Alcazar JL, Ruiz-Perez ML. Uteroplacental circulation in patients with first trimester threatened abortion. *Fertil Steril* **73**(1):130–135, 2000.
209. Prefumo F, Sebire N, Thilaganathan B. Decreased endovascular trophoblast invasion in first trimester pregnancies with high resistance uterine artery Doppler indices. *Hum Reprod* **19**(1): 206–209, 2004.
210. Jauniaux E, Jurkovic D, Campbell S. Current topic: in vivo investigation of the placental circulations by Doppler echography. *Placenta* **16**:323–331, 1995.
211. Babinszki A, Nyari T, Jordan S, Nasseri A, Mukherjee T, Copperman AB. Three dimensional measurement of gestational and yolk sac volumes as predictors of pregnancy outcome in the first trimester. *Am J Perinatol* **18**: 203–212, 2001.
212. Steiner H, Gregg AR, Bogner G, Graf AH, Weiner CP, Staudach A. First trimester three dimensional ultrasound volumetry of the gestational sac. *Arch Gynecol Obstet* **255**(4):165–170, 1994.
213. Acharya G, Morgan H. First-trimester, three-dimensional transvaginal ultrasound volumetry in normal pregnancies and spontaneous miscarriages. *Ultrasound Obstet Gynecol* **19**(6):575–579, 2002.
214. Wapner R, Thom E, Simpson JL et al. First-trimester screening for trisomies 21 and 18. *N Engl J Med* **349**(15):1405–1413, 2003.
215. Nicolaides KH, Sebire NJ, Snijders RJ. Down's syndrome screening with nuchal translucency. *Lancet* **349**(9049):438, 1997.
216. Luise C, Jermy K, May C, Costello G, Collins WP, Bourne T. Outcome of expectant management of spontaneous first trimester miscarriage: observational study. *Br Med J* **324**:873–875, 2002.
217. Nielsen S, Hahlin M. Expectant management of first-trimester spontaneous abortion. *Lancet* **345**(8942):84–86, 1995.
218. Alcazar JL, Baldonado C, Laparte C. The reliability of transvaginal ultrasonography to detect retained tissue after spontaneous first-trimester abortion, clinically thought to be complete. *Ultrasound Obstet Gynecol* **6**(2):126–129, 1995.
219. Schwarzler P, Holden D, Nielsen S, Hahlin M, Sladkevicius P, Bourne T. The conservative management of first trimester miscarriages and the use of colour Doppler sonography for patient selection. *Hum Reprod* **14**:1341–1345, 1999.
220. Sairam S, Khare M, Michalidis G, Thilaganathan B. The role of ultrasound in the expectant management of early pregnancy failure. *Ultrasound Obstet Gynecol* **17**(506):509, 2001.
221. Luise C, Jermy K, Collons WP, Bourne T. Expectant management of incomplete, spontaneous first trimester miscarriage: outcome according to initial ultrasound criteria and value of follow-up visits. *Ultrasound Obstet Gynecol* **19**(6):580–582, 2002.
222. Joint Study of the Royal College of General Practitioners and the Royal College of Obstetricians and Gynaecologists. Induced abortion operations and their early sequelae. *J R Coll Gen Pract* **35**:175–180, 1985.
223. Lawson HW, Frye A, Atrash HK, Smith JC, Shulman HB, Ramick M. Abortion mortality, United States, 1972 through 1987. *Am J Obstet Gynecol* **171**:1365–1372, 1994.
224. Winikoff B. Pregnancy failure and misoprostol: time for a change. *N Engl J Med* **353**:834–836, 2005.
225. El-Refaey H, Hinshaw K, Henshaw R, Smith N, Templeton A. Medical management of missed abortion and anembryonic pregnancy. *Br Med J* **305**:1399, 1992.
226. de Jonge ETM, Makin JD, Manefeldt E, De Wet GH, Pattinson RC. Randomised clinical trial of medical evacuation and surgical curettage for incomplete miscarriage. *Br Med J* **311**(7006):662, 1995.
227. Demetroulis C, Saridogan E, Kunde D, Naftalin AA. A prospective randomised control trial comparing medical and surgical treatment for early pregnancy failure. *Hum Reprod* **16**(2):365–369, 2001.
228. Henshaw R, Cooper K, El-Refaey H, Smith NC, Templeton A. Medical management of miscarriage: non-surgical uterine evacuation of incomplete and inevitable spontaneous abortion. *Br Med J* **306**:894–895, 1993.
229. Nielsen S, Hahlin M, Platz-Christensen J. Unsuccessful treatment of missed abortion with a combination of an antiprogesterone and a prostaglandin E1 analogue. *Br J Obstetr Gynaecol* **104**: 1094–1096, 1997.
230. Bigrigg MA, Read MD. Management of women referred to early pregnancy assessment unit: care and cost effectiveness. *Br Med J* **302**(6776): 577–579, 1992.
231. Hunter M. Providing information and support. In *Counselling in obstetrics and gynaecology*, M Hunter (ed.), pp. 87–104. London: British Psychological Society, 1994.
232. RCR/RCOG Working Party. *Early pregnancy assessment*. London: RCOG Press, 1996.

CHAPTER

44 Fetal infections

Guillaume Benoist and Yves Ville

KEY POINTS

- Virology, pathogenicity, epidemiology and transmission of the viral infections cytomegalovirus (CMV), parvovirus B19, rubella and varicella-zoster are explored, as well as for toxoplasmosis and syphilis
- Maternal and congenital infection with each of these and their clinical manifestations, diagnosis and management are also examined in detail

CYTOMEGALOVIRUS (CMV)

The virus and its pathogenicity

Virology

The cytomegalovirus (CMV) or Herpesvirus 5 is a member of the Herpetoviridae family. It is the largest of this family. Its genome is made of a double-stranded DNA core of 200 kilobases pairs which encodes for 250 open reading frames (ORF) and over 35 structural proteins and glycoproteins. Human CMV is highly species-specific and humans are its only reservoir. Several strains have been described based on genomic definition, hence possibly explaining reinfections. Like other members of the Herpesvirus group, CMV remains latent in the salivary glands after acute infection. Reactivation can occur during latent infection.

Serologic testing can neither differentiate between different strains of CMV, nor between reactivations and reinfections.

Pathogenesis

The virus is acquired at mucosal sites (community exposure) or by blood-borne transmission (blood transfusion or transplantation). In community exposure, cell-free virus is transmitted by contact with saliva or genital tract secretion. Cell-free virus was retrieved from breast milk. Cell-mediated spread of the virus begins after a replication phase. The main cells infected by CMV are the endothelial cells and the polymorphic nuclear leukocytes (PMLs). The dissemination of the virus is then hematogenous. This viremic phase can be diagnosed by laboratory testing. The secondary sites of replication involved are the spleen and the liver. Dissemination and replication is not completely controlled by host immunity.

Epidemiology and transmission

Transmission of the virus occurs by direct or indirect person-to-person contact, via urine, oropharyngeal, cervical and vaginal secretions, semen, milk, tears, blood products or organ transplants. This is due to prolonged shedding of the virus after primary infection. CMV infection is not very contagious and requires intimate contact.

CMV infection is endemic and has no seasonal variation. It is spread world-wide. The patterns of seropositivity in the population vary greatly with geographic, ethnic and socioeconomic conditions. The prevalence of specific antibodies to CMV increases with age and in lower socioeconomic strata of developed countries as well as in developing countries. Seroprevalence among women of childbearing age also varies accordingly with these epidemiologic factors. Several reports indicate that the seropositivity ranges from 50 to 85% in the USA and in Western Europe.

Incidence of CMV primary infection in pregnancy also varies with socioeconomic conditions, from around 2% per year in developed countries and up to 6% in developing countries[1].

Congenital infection is the result of transplacental transmission. In the USA, around 1% of all newborns are infected when screened at birth. Nevertheless, this rate varies greatly among geographic regions and in correlation with seropositivity rates[1]. The rate of transplacental transmission varies with the type of maternal infection between 30 and 50% for primary infections and 2 and 3% for non-primary infections[1–3].

Congenital infections are mainly due to primary infections but several reports show a possible fetal transmission after reinfection with another strain of the virus or after reactivation of a latent infection[1,4–6]. Irrespective of the type of maternal infection, the rate of maternal–fetal transmission is considered to be low (around 2% as reported by Stagno and al.)[1].

Maternal infection

Clinical manifestations

Clinical symptoms and non-specific biological markers are more often present in primary infection than in recurrent infection. Most primary infections in immunocompetent hosts are nevertheless subclinical. Nigro et al. reported fever in 42.1% of primary infection and 17.1% of recurrent infection with $P > 0.01$, asthenia (31.4% and 11.4%, $P < 0.001$), myalgia (21.5% and 6.7%, $P < 0.001$), rhino-pharyngo-tracheo-bronchitis (42.1% and 29.5%, $P = 0.089$) and 'flu-like syndrome defined as the simultaneous occurrence of fever and at least one of these signs (24.5% and 9.5%, $P < 0.001$), lymphocytosis ≥40% (39.2% and 5.7%, $P < 0.001$), increased aminotransferases blood levels (one or both >40 iu/l) (35.3% and 3.9%, $P < 0.001$). Platelet count was significantly lower in primary infection but within normal range[7].

Laboratory diagnosis

The diagnosis of primary infection can be easily comfirmed by documenting seroconversion (i.e. de novo appearance of virus-specific IgG antibodies in a pregnant woman who was seronegative before the onset of pregnancy). Nevertheless, without a screening program adopted by public health authorities where seronegative women would be prospectively monitored during their pregnancy, this remains a rare situation. More often, serological testing is performed when contamination is suspected with maternal clinical symptoms, or when ultrasound fetal abnormalities are visualized. In this context, the presence of IgG leads to assessment of the type of CMV infection (past, primary or recurrent infection), and to date the time of maternal primary infection as precisely as possible. IgM and IgG avidity assays have been developed for these purposes.

IgM antibody response begins in the first days after maternal contamination reaching a peak in the first month after maternal contamination. High to medium levels of IgM antibodies can therefore be detected during the first 1–3 months after the onset of infection after which the titers start declining. Revello et al. reported that among 9 immunocompetent individuals, 4 became negative for IgM within 6 months, 3 within 12 months and 2 remained positive for more than a year[8].

IgG avidity is indicative of the low functional affinity of the recently produced IgG class antibody. Early after primary infection, antibodies show a low avidity to the antigen, but progressively mature to acquire higher avidity. This characteristic is used at the diagnostic level to discriminate between recent and over 3 months old primary infections. From the publication of Mace et al., avidity index (AI) >70% reflects primary infection >3 months, and AI <30% is highly suggestive of a recent primary infection (<3 months). AI between 30 and 70% is more difficult to interpret. This method is only applicable when IgG levels are not too low[9]. Nevertheless, one limitation of IgG AI testing is the lack of standardization. The best published results reported 100% negative predictive value for a moderate to high IgG avidity index obtained before the 18th week of gestation, and a negative predictive value dropping to 91% when performed between 21 and 23 weeks' gestation[10,11]. Overall, Mace et al. reported that dating maternal primary infection using IgG AI associated with IgM antibody detection failed to date the onset of infection in only 1% of their cases[9].

After primary infection, the virus and viral products can be recovered from various fluid products. However, viral shedding from these sites can occur after recurrences as well. It has also been shown that detection of CMV in blood is diagnostic of primary infection in immunocompetent individuals whereas, in immunocompromised patients, it is indicative of either primary or non-primary infection[12].

Quantification of viremia (i.e. infectious CMV particles in blood, evaluated by culture or rapid shell vial method), antigenemia (i.e. pp65-positive peripheral blood leukocytes), quantification of leukoDNAnemia (CMV DNA in whole blood), leukocytes or plasma, and more recently RNAnemia (CMV mRNA) are available. Revello et al. reported the diagnostic ability of these methods in 52 immunocompetent individuals comprising 40 pregnant women[12]. Antigenemia was detected in 57.1%, 25% and 0% of the patients examined at 1, 2 and 3 months after onset of infection respectively; viremia was detected in 26.3% of cases during the first month only; leukoDNAemia in 100%, 89.5% and 27.3% at each of the 3 first months, 26.6% were still positive at between 4 and 6 months, but none were positive after 6 months. At the same time, none of the patients with recurrent infection was positive with these tests. These results provide a helpful method for dating maternal infection.

Congenital infection

Description of congenital CMV infection

Approximately 10% of the congenitally infected newborns have signs and symptoms at birth. Half of them present the typical cytomegalic inclusion disease (CID) with a high mortality rate. The other half present with atypical symptoms. Of the 90% who are asymptomatic, infection is demonstrated by the presence of the virus in their urine during the first weeks of life.

Symptomatic infected newborns are defined as presenting at least one of the following abnormalities: prematurity, growth restriction, petechiae, jaundice, hepatosplenomegaly, purpura, neurological findings (microcephaly, hypotonia, seizures), elevated alanine aminotransferases levels (>80 UI/l), thrombocytopenia, conjugated hyperbilirubinemia, hemolysis and increased cerebrospinal fluid proteins[13].

Long-term follow-up of these children established the occurrence of at least one sequela in 90% of the subjects in this subgroup. These complications were: psychomotor delay 70%, sensorineural hearing loss 50%, ocular abnormalities (mainly chorioretinitis) 54%. Death due to congenital CMV infection was estimated to occur in around 6%.

The best predictor for adverse neurodevelopmental outcome in these infants is the presence of intracranial abnormalities on computed tomography (CT) within the first month of life[14]. These abnormalities were also associated with sensorineural hearing loss (SNHL) at birth or with deterioration of audiometric status during the first months of life.

Among asymptomatic neonates, who are known to have a better long-term prognosis than symptomatic ones, 10–15% will still develop sequelae, more often during the first 2 years of life. These sequelae include SNHL in 7%, chorioretinis in 2%, intellectual deficit in 4% and microcephaly in 2%[15–19]. SNHL is the most frequent deficit related to congenital CMV infection in asymptomatic neonates. Fowler and al. have reported that 50% of the audiometric deficits were bilateral, 50% worsened during the first years of life and, in 18%, the audiologic deficit was diagnosed on average only at 27 months. CMV congenital infection could be the cause of one third of all SNHL in childhood.

Prenatal diagnosis

Screening programs have not been adopted by public health authorities in the vast majority of developed countries. Therefore, abnormal ultrasound findings related to CMV congenital infection are more likely to be diagnosed by systematic ultrasound examination rather than by follow-up in maternal seroconversion. This may also explain why severe abnormalities are described more often than subtle findings.

Ultrasound diagnosis

Knowledge of the natural history of the infection is essential to understand which ultrasound features are likely to be apparent and justify invasive prenatal diagnosis. It is also important to remember that the appearance of abnormal sonographic findings and evidence of maternal infection may be separated by several weeks[8]. In primary infections, around 25–50% of the infected fetuses can be diagnosed by ultrasound examination. This is more likely to reflect the proportion of papers published on this particular aspect than the performance of ultrasound as a screening test[20]. In the literature, description of fetal CMV infection ultrasound features are twofold: gross abnormalities leading to the diagnosis of fetal CMV infection, and subtle findings discovered after thorough serial ultrasound examination of fetuses at high risk once vertical transmission of the virus has been shown. This at least partly explains why the performance of ultrasound as a screening test could not be demonstrated in a low-risk population.

Ultrasound (US) findings are summarized in Table 44.1. Case reports or series of gross abnormalities mainly picked up

Table 44.1 **Fetal abnormalities diagnosed in utero by ultrasound examination as reported in 7 series in the literature from 2000**

	Enders 2001[31]	*Liesnard 2000*[28]	*Lipitz 2002*[39]	*Azam 2001*[48]	*Picone 2004*[41]	*Guerra 2000*[29]	*Gouarin 2002*[40]	*Total*
Number of congenital CMV infections*	57	55	51	26	42	16	30	277
Overall ultrasound findings	39	14	11	5	26	6	15	116 (42%)
IUGR**	12	6	6	0	10	1	10	45 (16%)
Hydrops	4	0	2	0	2	0	0	8 (3%)
Ascites	15	0	0	2	2	0	1	20 (7%)
Pericardial effusion	3	0	0	0	1	0	0	4 (1%)
Pleural effusion	0	0	1	0	0	0	0	1 (<1%)
Skin edema	2	0	0	0	0	0	0	2 (<1%)
Hyperechogenic bowel	2	8	3	1	14	2	6	36 (13%)
Hepatomegaly/splenomegaly	3	1	0	1	3	0	0	8 (3%)
Liver calcifications	0	1	1	0	0	0	0	2 (<1%)
Placentomegaly	2	0	0	1	2	0	0	5 (2%)
Oligohydramnios/anhydramnios	6	1	4	0	4	0	0	15 (5%)
Polyhydramnios	1	1	1	0	1	0	0	4 (1%)
Other findings***	8	0	0	0	0	0	0	8 (3%)
Microcephaly	11	2	0	1	6	0	5	25 (9%)
Hydrocephaly	9	2	0	0	0	0	2	13 (5%)
Ventriculomegaly	7	1	4	1	14	4	4	35 (13%)
Brain structure abnormalities****	10	1	3	0	13	0	9	36 (13%)

*Congenital CMV infection proved in urine at birth or after examination of fetuses after termination of pregnancy.

**IUGR: intrauterine growth restriction.

***Other findings: asymmetry of cardiac ventricles, cardiomyopathy, small lungs, hyperechogenic abdominal tumor, abnormal head shape, no fetal movements, and short limbs.

****Brain structure abnormalities: brain calcifications, periventricular echogenicity, porencephaly, lissencephaly, subependimal cysts, choroid plexus cysts, cystic structure in cerebellum, agenesis of cerebellar vermis, cerebellar hypoplasia on fetal ventriculomegaly or hydrocephalus, either obstructive (aquaductal stenosis), or a vacuo with or without microcephaly, posterior fossa cysts, cerebellar hypoplasia, severe intrauterine growth restriction or even hydrops fetalis[21]. Cases diagnosed as a consequence of maternal seroconversion followed by serial fetal US examination often lead to diagnosis of more subtle findings, mainly extracerebral, including hyperechogenic bowel and oligohydramnios. Hyperechogenic bowel grade 2 is often a transient finding. However, in a series comprising 175 fetuses with hyperechogenic bowel, only one case was related to CMV infection[22]. It is the expression of viral enterocolitis and can be expressed as meconium ileus or peritonitis in the presence of ascites[23]. Oligohydramnios is more often reported than polyhydramnios and, considering the affinity of the CMV for the kidney, it can be seen as the expression of a fetal nephritis. The fetal heart can also be affected showing cardiomegaly with a thick myocardium which may contain punctuate calcifications. As a functional consequence, Drose et al. have also described tachyarrhythmia[24]. This is a rare finding that could lead to the development of fetal hydrops. Generalized edema and ascites may also suggest anemia-related hydrops due to the combined effect of liver failure and marrow infection. This spectacular presentation has also proven eventually to be transient with both ultrasound and biological normalization at follow-up[25]. Mild or unilateral ventriculomegaly, increased pericerebral spaces, echogenic vessels in the fetal thalami and basal ganglia or punctuate echogenicities in the periventricular area are subtle findings, especially if they are isolated and are therefore likely to slip through non-oriented ultrasound screening. The development of fetal magnetic resonance imaging (MRI) has become an asset in the assessment of infected fetuses[26–28]. MRI, using both T1 and T2 sequences, could help define the onset of fetal infection. Lissencephaly may reflect injury before 16 or 18 weeks, whereas polymicrogyria is likely to follow injury at 18–24 weeks and cases with normal gyral patterns would have probably been injured during the third trimester showing diffuse heterogeneity within the white matter[26].

Laboratory diagnosis

Diagnosis of fetal infection is made by finding the virus or the viral DNA in the fetal compartment. CMV can be detected in the amniotic fluid by conventional viral isolation, rapid culture or molecular assays. Virus isolation has a high specificity but has a lower sensitivity than polymerase chain reaction (PCR). In recent years, PCR has been established as a reliable technique in reference laboratories. Various PCR assays have been described with multiple modalities including single step, nested, nested modified by the use of higher volume or multiples aliquots, and the most recent real time PCR. The efficacy of these methods has been evaluated in several studies and is dependent on the virological method used (nested, one round or real time PCR): sensitivity and specificity range between 75 and 100% and between 67.3% and 100% respectively[8,29–32]. The false negative results reported were explained in most cases by inappropriate timing of amniocentesis. Following seroconversion or reactivation, the process leading to CMV excretion in the fetal urine will take an average of 6–8 weeks and this interval should be recognized in order to avoid false-negative prenatal diagnosis[8]. Amniocentesis should also be performed once fetal micturation is well established and therefore not before 22 weeks. When the conditions of sampling are ideal[33], the sensitivity of prenatal diagnosis by PCR has been reported to be close to 100%. False-positive PCR results have also been reported when the neonate was not infected, these false-positive diagnoses may be explained by contamination of the AF with maternal blood during amniocentesis if the mother had a positive CMV DNAemia at the time of sampling. Indeed, Revello et al. showed that CMV DNA may be recovered in the blood of nearly 50% of immunocompetent patients up to 3 months after CMV primary infection[34]. Another explanation could be laboratory contamination occurring during PCR testing. Indeed, in some of these studies a nested CMV PCR was used, which is known to be a very sensitive technique but at high risk of contamination. Generalization of semi-automated real time PCR might help to overcome the risk of contamination and achieve quasi-absolute specificity for prenatal diagnosis of CMV infection.

Prognostic factors during prenatal period

Currently, the association of positive DNA detection in amniotic fluid and the presence of cerebral abnormalities on ultrasound are considered to be sufficient to accept women's request for termination of the pregnancy. However, the individual prognostic value of ultrasound findings is very difficult to establish because termination of pregnancy prevents follow-up of these infants. Frequent ultrasound abnormalities, such as hyperechogenic bowel or fetal growth restriction, do not appear to be consistently associated with a poor outcome (Table 44.2). The only well-recognized prognostic factor of a poor outcome during childhood is fetal brain abnormalities on fetal ultrasound examination.

The influence of gestational age at maternal infection on the prognosis of fetal infection has been debated over many years but recent data have shed some new light on that topic. Several previous studies suggested that the prognosis could be worse when maternal infection occurs during the first trimester[2,29,35,36]. Nevertheless, fetal infection occurring in the third trimester can also carry a poor neurological outcome[37].

Primary infections were thought to cause more damage than recurrences in women with detectable IgG before pregnancy[32,38–40]. Unlike preconceptional immunity against rubella or toxoplasmosis, preconceptional immunity against CMV provides only partial protection against intrauterine transmission of the virus to the fetus. Although vertical transmission rates vary significantly between primary and non-primary infections (30–50% versus 2–3%)[1–3], it seems that the prognosis of infected fetuses could be similar in primary and in non-primary maternal infections.

Maternal factors predictive of fetal outcome are still poorly elucidated. It seems that neither the presence of clinical symptoms during primary infection, nor virological parameters in the mother are associated with a higher transmission rate of the virus to the fetus[34].

The recent progress in quantitative PCR technology, particularly the development of real time PCR, has allowed evaluation of the clinical significance of CMV viral load in amniotic fluid[33,41,42]. Three studies have compared viral load levels in amniotic fluid between groups of symptomatic and asymptomatic fetuses. In these three studies the median viral loads were higher in the amniotic fluid of symptomatic fetuses than in the amniotic fluid of asymptomatic fetuses, however, this difference reached statistical significance in only one study[41].

Table 44.2 **Outcome at follow-up in relation to antenatal ultrasound findings in CMV congenitally infected newborns reported in six series from 2000**

Reference	*CMV-infected newborns with US abnormalities in utero (n)*	*Prenatal ultrasound abnormalities*	*Outcome at follow-up*
Liesnard et al. 2000[29]	5	HB	Normal at 6 months
		Moderate FGR, oligohydramnios	Normal at 3 years
		Microcephaly, CNS abnormalities, HB	Mental retardation, development retardation
		FGR moderate	Normal at 3 years
		FGR, HMG-SMG, HB	Normal at 13 months
Lipitz et al. 2002[40]	2	FGR, VMG	Birth: cerebral palsy, SNHL
		HB	Birth: normal
Azam et al. 2001[49]	2	Hydrops	Neonatal death
		PV calcifications	50 months: SNHL bilateral
Gouarin et al. 2002[41]	2	FGR	Birth: normal
		FGR	Birth: normal
Picone et al. 2004[42]	4	HB, VMG	Birth: normal
		FGR	Birth: normal
		HB	Birth: normal
		Cerebral calcifications, VMG	Birth: normal
Guerra et al 2000[30]	2	VMG	Birth: VMG resolved in utero, hepatitis
		VMG, HB	Birth: severe VMG, cerebral calcifications. HMG–SMG

HB = hyperechogenic bowel; FGR = fetal growth restriction; CNS = central nervous system; HMG–SMG = hepatomegaly–splenomegaly; VMG = ventriculomegaly; PV = periventricular; SNHL = sensorineural hearing loss

Very few data are available on the prognostic value of fetal blood viral load with only one study published to date[43]. In this study, antigenemia, viremia and DNAemia were found to be higher in fetuses with abnormalities than in asymptomatic fetuses, but the difference was significant only for antigenemia. However, negative PCR was only found in asymptomatic patients and very high blood viral loads were recovered only in symptomatic fetuses. In a recent study of infected neonates, it was reported that the mean values of neonatal blood viral load were statistically higher in newborns that developed sequelae than in those who did not and that approximately 70% of sequelae were found in newborns with a qPCR higher than 10 000 copies per 10^5 PMNLs[44]. Fetal blood viral load is an important potential prognostic factor and further studies are warranted to evaluate its predictive value.

The influence of CMV strains on the biological properties of the virus and particularly on the outcome of congenital infection is a topic of current interest, but the use of viral sequence information has failed to predict outcome[45].

The value of biochemical and hematological parameters in fetal blood are still poorly studied. The results are unclear and the only interesting parameter that could be identified is thrombocytopenia[14].

Recently, fetal gender of infected fetuses has been retrospectively studied. The proportion of females with brain abnormalities was statistically different from that of males (62/258 infected fetuses: 24% versus 30/251: 12%, $P = 0.004$). The risk of abnormal brain development in infected fetuses was twice as high in females as in males (OR = 2, [1.26–3.21])[46].

Management

Termination of pregnancy

Identification of prenatal prognostic factors other than brain ultrasound abnormalities is missing. Termination of pregnancy is therefore probably often performed in fetuses that would have developed into asymptomatic infants.

Antiviral treatment

A number of antiviral drugs are active against CMV and the three licensed anti-CMV drugs (ganciclovir, cidofovir and foscarnet) are being used successfully in immunocompromised patients. However, their potential teratogenic effects and their well-known toxicity do not support their use in pregnancy. Anti-CMV compounds are currently at different stages of development, several of these compounds are very promising in terms of efficacy and lack of toxicity. To date, preliminary results on treatment of CMV congenital infection during pregnancy are available from two studies with promising results. Nigro et al. have recently published the retrospective results of a non-randomized clinical trial using intravenous CMV hyperimmune globulin (HIG) for CMV maternal primary infection[47]. Jacquemard et al. have recently shown the pharmacological efficacity of valaciclovir (VACV) in a pilot study in 21 cases of CMV congenital infections with ultrasound abnormalities[48].

No vaccine is currently available.

FETAL PARVOVIRUS B19 INFECTION

The virus and its pathogenicity

The taxonomy of the Parvoviridae family includes the Densovirinae (insect viruses) and the Parvovirinae (vertebral viruses) which is composed of three genera (Dependovirus, Parvovirus and Erythrovirus). Parvovirus B19 is classified as an Erythrovirus. Parvovirus B19 is the only Parvovirus which can cause human disease. It is a non-enveloped virus with an icosahedric capsid and its genome is a single-stranded DNA of about 5594 nucleotides which mainly encodes for three major proteins: two structural proteins (VP1 and VP2) that make up the viral capsid and one non-structural protein (NS1) which seems to be involved in viral replication.

The primary target for Parvovirus B19 appears to be erythroid precursor cells. Host cell receptor is the globoside or P-antigen (a blood group antigen), a glycosphingolipid, therefore patients without this antigen on their red blood cells are naturally protected against Parvovirus B19 infection[50]. Globoside is situated on the surface of erythrocyte progenitor cells (erythroblasts), but also on that of other cells such as endothelial cells, fetal myocardial cells, placental cells, mature erythrocytes and megakaryocytes[51]. Nevertheless, the presence of this receptor is not sufficient for the virus to penetrate into the cells, for which a co-receptor is required. Inside the host cells, Parvovirus B19 replicates and induces apoptosis and toxic cell injury.

Epidemiology and transmission

Parvovirus B19 infection occurs world-wide and the characteristics of the disease (signs and symptoms) are constant. Neither antigenic nor specific viral genotypes are related to the forms of the disease. Transmission of the virus continues throughout the year with winter and spring outbreaks. Seroprevalence of Parvovirus B19 infection increases with age. In children younger than 5 years, the prevalence of IgG antibodies is less than 5%, increasing to reach a median of 45% in young adults[52] and more than 85% in the geriatric population[53]. Some studies have shown a greater risk of Parvovirus B19 infection in women[54]. Seroprevalence is higher in the white populations[55]. The global incidence of Parvovirus B19 infection has been reported to be 1 to 2 per 10 000 individuals. In childbearing age women, risk factors for seroconversion are: elementary school workers, contact with 5–11-year-old children at home and 5–18-year-old children at work, and women under 30 years of age[55]. Overall, it can be estimated that 1–2% of seronegative women at the onset of pregnancy would become infected during pregnancy in endemic periods and >10% in epidemic periods[54,56–58]. A prospective evaluation of 618 pregnant women exposed to Parvovirus B19 in an endemic period was performed by Harger et al.[59]. In this study, the only significant risk factor that was found was exposure to Parvovirus B19 in their own children. Other studies have found an increased risk for Parvovirus B19 infections in elementary school teachers and day-care workers[60,61].

Infection with Parvovirus B19 usually occurs through contact with respiratory droplets, but Parvovirus B19 can also be transmitted by blood and blood-derived products and can be transmitted vertically from mother to fetus[62]. No vertical transmission has been described if the mother is immune at the time of exposure. Presence of IgG antibodies gives a life-long protection against re-infection with Parvovirus B19.

Maternal infection

Clinical manifestations

In healthy individuals, infection is usually asymptomatic. Erythema infectiosum (fifth disease) is the most common clinical manifestation during childhood[63]. It is characterized by a rash consisting of maculae that undergo central fading over in 1–4 days mainly on the trunk and limbs. These are the result of the deposition of immune complexes within the skin. Symptoms such as erythema infectiosum, mild fever, arthralgia and headache start approximately 10–14 days after contamination and in about 50% of infected women.

Arthralgia and arthritis[63,64] are common in the adult form of the infection. It affects females more often than males (60% versus 30%) and children (10%). Others possible features include: thrombocytopenia[65], meningoencephalitis[66,67], hepatitis, myocarditis and vasculitis[68].

Immunocompromised hosts can also present transient aplastic crisis, chronic red blood cell aplasia and virus-associated hematophagocytic syndrome[69].

Symptoms reported by pregnant women are non-specific and serologic confirmation is required. The typical symptoms of the disease are rarely present in pregnant women. The most characteristic symptom is symmetrical arthralgia, sometimes arthritis often involving small joints of the hands, wrists and feet. The proportion of asymptomatic women is around 30%[70].

Laboratory diagnosis

Specific IgM, IgG and IgA immunoglobulins are produced following infection. Specific IgM are the first antibodies to rise around 10 days post infection. They peak sharply at 10–14 days and then decrease over 2–3 months.

Specific IgG rise considerably more slowly about 3 weeks post infection to reach a plateau at around 4 weeks after infection. They probably last for life. Maternal serum should be tested when there is evidence of maternal exposure or clinical symptoms of Parvovirus B19 infection. A booking sample with positive IgG but negative IgM indicates previous maternal infection. The presence of IgM indicates that a recent maternal infection has occurred regardless of IgG antibody levels. The absence of IgG associated with IgM indicates a very recent infection. Nevertheless, it is important to remember that, after a recent contact, there will be a window of 7 days, during which both IgG and IgM will remain negative. The absence of maternal infection can then only be confirmed by a further blood sample. Furthermore, at the time of clinically overt hydrops fetalis, IgM levels may already have become undetectable. In these cases, PCR analysis of the same blood sample will be informative.

Fetal infection

Description of congenital infection

Vertical transmission occurs in approximately one third of the cases of maternal infection[71]. Fetal infection with parvovirus B19 is associated with intrauterine fetal death (IUFD), non-immune hydrops fetalis (NIHF) and, less often, brain anomalies. Fetal infection can also be asymptomatic[72]. Fetal manifestations due to parvovirus B19 are summarized in Table 44.3.

The consequences of fetal infection are not uniform throughout the pregnancy. Non-immune hydrops fetalis develops following maternal infection mainly in the first half of the pregnancy. The rate of NIHF following primary infection is around 30–40% before 20 weeks and decreases to 3–10% following infections thereafter. Overall, the risk of adverse fetal outcome when fetal infection is proven is of approximately 10%[81,82].

Cases of intrauterine fetal death have been described mainly at around 20–24 weeks of gestation, but as early as 10 weeks and as late as 41 weeks[70,82,83]. Furthermore, intrauterine fetal death could occur without hydrops fetalis[83]. NIHF is mainly related to severe anemia, which can also lead to high output cardiogenic heart failure. NIHF is more frequent during the hepatic stage (8–20 weeks of gestation) of the hematopoietic activity when the half-life of erythrocytes is shorter than later during the bone marrow and splenic hematopoietic stages[51]. The proportion of all NIHF due to Parvovirus B19 infection is around 10–15%. In a series of 50 cases, 4 were related to Parvovirus B19 infection[84]. Its occurrence is 3.9% after maternal infection throughout pregnancy, with a maximum of 7.1% when infection occurred between 13 and 20 weeks of gestational age. The incidence of Parvovirus B19 infection-associated hydrops fetalis peaks at between 17 and 24 weeks of gestation[62]. The interval between maternal Parvovirus B19 parvovirus infection and the development of NIHF ranges from 2 to 6 weeks[85]. In 539 cases reported by Soothill et al., 30% preceded intrauterine fetal death and 34% resolved spontaneously whereas 29% resolved after intrauterine transfusion and 6% died despite intrauterine transfusion[86]. Hydrops fetalis is diagnosed by ultrasound with the association of marked ascites, cardiomegaly and pericardial effusion and, in advanced stages, generalized edema and thick hydropic placenta. Hydrops related to anemia usually presents with tense ascites, as well as thin-walled cardiomegaly. Pleural effusion is a late finding in anemia-related hydrops. Amniotic fluid volume may be normal or even decreased; polyhydramnios is rare. Rarely, maternal symptoms of 'mirror-hydrops' or 'Ballantyne's syndrome' happen secondary to lysis of the hydropic villi of the placenta and is responsible for maternal pre-eclampsia-like syndrome with edema, hypertension, proteinuria and mild anemia[87].

Table 44.3 **Ultrasound abnormalities on fetuses infected by Parvovirus B19**

Cardiac system	Increased cardiac biventricular outer diameter[73] Myocarditis
Non-immune hydrops fetalis	Pleural effusion Pericardial effusion Ascites Abdominal wall edema Bilateral hydroceles Amniotic fluid disorder
Brain abnormalities*	Hydrocephalus[74] Microcephaly Intracranial calcifications
Gastrointestinal system	Fetal liver calcifications[75] Meconium peritonitis[76,77]
Other findings	Sporadic cases of contractures[78] Increased nuchal translucency[79] Intrauterine growth restriction[80]

*Following brain hemorrhage

The involvement of the fetal heart can be limited to dilatation of the cardiac chambers related to anemia and hydrops, or present as a hypertrophic cardiomyopathy or myocarditis that can also develop autonomously after spontaneous resolution of the NIHF[88].

Fetal Parvovirus B19 infection has also been associated with pediatric stroke[89], neonatal encephalitis/meningitis[90] with perivascular calcifications in the fetal cerebral cortex, basal ganglia, thalamus and germinal layers[90], meconium peritonitis[91], fetal liver calcifications[75], eye abnormalities such as corneal opacification and aphakic eyes[92]. Structural defects (cleft lip and palate, micrognathia, arthrogryposis, hypospadias) reported are likely to be coincidental findings[71,93]. Hyperechogenic bowel is likely to reflect resolving ascites. During a large community-wide outbreak of Parvovirus B19 infection, there was no increase in congenital malformation rates compared with the period preceding and following the epidemic, which may lead to the conclusion that the association of birth defects could be fortuitous or the consequence of anemia-related hypoxia or thrombocytopenia-related hemorrhage[94].

Prenatal diagnosis

After serological confirmation of maternal infection, fetal ultrasound examination should be performed to exclude the presence of fetal anemia and hydrops. However, in most cases, hydrops fetalis is a coincidental finding during routine ultrasound examination. In these cases, fetal anemia should be suspected when the middle cerebral artery shows increased peak-systolic velocities[95,96]. These changes in blood flow are the result of increased cardiac output and decreased viscosity of fetal blood[97]. The prediction of fetal anemia by MCA-PSV measurements also allows the severity of the anemia to be evaluated. Values of 2 MOM or above should indicate the need for fetal blood sampling and intrauterine transfusion. Severe NIHF together with normal MCA-PSV in Parvovirus B19 infection indicates either spontaneous resolution of the fetal anemia or progressive and autonomous myocarditis. The virus or its genome can be isolated in amniotic fluid or in fetal blood.

Nucleic acid amplification by PCR is extremely sensitive. This can also be applied in pregnant women lacking an adequate antibody-mediated immune response, immunocompromised or immunosuppressed in whom serological testing for Parvovirus B19 parvovirus is unreliable[98]. Detection of Parvovirus B19 specific IgM in fetal blood has a significantly lower sensitivity than PCR[99,100].

Management options

Intrauterine transfusion (IUT)

Management of Parvovirus B19 infection with IUT can correct fetal anemia and is likely to reduce significantly perinatal mortality associated with Parvovirus B19 infection. It should be restricted to cases with MCA-PSV >2 MOM in which the levels of hemoglobin are under 9 g/dl as confirmed by fetal blood sampling. Timely IUT of anemic fetuses with severe hydrops reduces the risk of fetal death[100–103]. In most cases, one transfusion is sufficient for fetal recovery and high reticulocyte levels indicate that anemia is being corrected spontaneously. Hydropic changes can take up several weeks to resolve and MCA-PSV should be used to evaluate the correction of fetal anemia[96,104,105]. Children who survive a successful IUT for Parvovirus B19-induced fetal anemia and hydrops fetalis have a good neurodevelopmental prognosis[56]. However, severe and prolonged fetal anemia is accompanied by thrombocytopenia that can lead to intraventricular brain hemorrhage.

Management of intrauterine infection

Pregnant women, who have been exposed to Parvovirus B19 infection, or those developing symptoms compatible with Parvovirus B19 infection, should be assessed by serological testing. Seronegative women should be re-tested 2 weeks later. They can be reassured in the absence of seroconversion. In cases with primary infection, serial ultrasound examination including MCA-PSV measurements should be performed every fortnight up until 12 weeks after exposure.

Prevention

General measures

Serological testing is recommended when there is a Parvovirus B19 infection outbreak in infants in nurseries and schools. These cases should be clearly reported to enable pregnant women to be tested and avoid exposure.

Vaccination

Recently, Ballou et al. described a recombinant parvovirus Parvovirus B19 vaccine composed of VP1 and VP2 capsid proteins, which proved to be immunogenic and safe to use in human volunteers[106]. Vaccination of non-immune pregnant women could be a highly effective method to prevent fetal infection with Parvovirus B19, but the cost-effectiveness of this strategy in the general population remains to be determined[106].

FETAL RUBELLA INFECTION

The virus and its pathogenicity

Virology

The rubella virus is an RNA virus, classified as a Togavirus, genus Rubivirus. It is a world-wide human disease without any animal reservoir.

Pathogenesis

This virus spreads by means of airborne transmission or droplets shed from respiratory secretions from 7 days before to 5–7 days or more after the onset of the cutaneous eruption. The mean incubation time is 2 weeks. Viremia occurs 5–7 days after exposure. Transplacental hematogenous transmission can occur during this phase. The immune response is induced by two glycoproteins E1 and E2 of the viral envelope.

Epidemiology and transmission

Rubella is a moderately contagious world-wide disease. Before the development of vaccination programs, epidemics used to occur every 6–9 years. Infections occur mostly in late winter and early spring. Since the introduction of systematic vaccination in childhood, epidemiologic characteristics have changed. The number of cases of congenital infection has drastically decreased. The national congenital rubella syndrome registry, which carries out the congenital rubella syndrome surveillance, has reported 121 cases between 1990 and 2001 in the USA. A large part of these cases were diagnosed in unvaccinated immigrant women.

Maternal infection

Clinical manifestations

Rubella is usually a mild disease. Complications are rare. Nevertheless, clinical illness is more severe in adults and in newborns who are not protected by maternal antibodies when mothers are infected soon after delivery.

A characteristic rash appears and lasts for 1–5 days, extending from the face passing down through the body to the feet, after an incubation period of 14–21 days (mean 17 days). In adults, this rash is often pruriginous and preceded by fever, headache, conjunctivitis, malaise, coryza, lymphadenopathy and dyspnea. Arthralgia and, sometimes, frank arthritis may develop after the rash fades away. These symptoms have been reported in up to 70% of infected women.

Thrombocytopenia, encephalitis, myocarditis, Guillain-Barré syndrome, optic neuritis are rare complications also reported in maternal rubella.

Laboratory diagnosis

Laboratory diagnosis is essential because inapparent or subclinical diseases are common (around half of the cases). Furthermore, other viral eruptions can mimic rubella.

Acute rubella infection is characterized by the appearance of IgG and IgM.

IgM antibodies are most consistently detectable 5–10 days after the onset of the rash, rise rapidly to peak at around 20 days and decline thereafter until disappearance after 50–70 days. In a few patients, IgM remain detectable for up to one year. This rare eventuality provides an important diagnostic role for IgM detection in recent primary infections compared with reinfections.

IgG antibodies can be measured by several methods, but enzyme-linked immunoabsorbent assays (ELISA) are most commonly used. IgG becomes detectable within 5–15 days after rash onset. The titers rapidly increase to peak at 30 days and then gradually decline over a period of years to constant titers.

When dating the infection is difficult, testing avidity of IgG antibodies is helpful. Primary infection is associated with low IgG avidity. The technique used should be taken into account because the kinetics of the antibodies can vary with the technique used.

Fetal infection

Rubella congenital syndrome

Congenital rubella can cause miscarriage, or stillbirth, but can also be asymptomatic. Between these two extremes, the spectrum of congenital anomalies, first described in 1941, is wide, including: heart defects, eye defects and hearing abnormalities (Table 44.4).

The cardiac features of fetal rubella infection include patent ductus arteriosus, pulmonary artery stenosis and pulmonary valvular stenosis. Other rare manifestations have been described: coarctation of aortic isthmus, interventricular septal defect and interauricular septal defects.

Neurosensory hearing loss is the most frequent feature of congenital rubella syndrome occurring in at least 80% of infected infants. It can be uni- or bilateral and ranges from mild to severe.

Table 44.4 **Fetal abnormalities related to congenital rubella infection**

Cardiac system	Atrial septal defects
	Ventricular septal defects
	Pulmonic arterial hypoplasia[116]
	Patent ductus arteriosus[116]
	Coarctation of aortic isthmus[116]
	Aortic regurgitation[117]
Ocular system	Cataract[118]
	Microphthalmia[107]
Central nervous system	Microcephaly[110]
	Intracranial calcifications[109]
	Subependymal pseudocysts
Other abnormalities	Hepatomegaly
	Splenomegaly
	Renal disorders[119]
	Hyperechogenic bowel
	Meconium peritonitis[120]
	Hypospadias[119]
	Growth restriction[121]

Eye defects due to rubella infection are described as a 'salt and pepper' retinopathy caused by abnormal growth of the pigmentary layer of the retina[107], cataract[108], microphthalmia[107,109] which often accompanies cataract and, more rarely, primary glaucoma[109]. These defects can be diagnosed early after birth. Other ocular manifestations can have a late onset including abnormalities of the anterior chamber of the eye.

Others abnormalities can be related to rubella infection: intrauterine growth restriction[110], encephalitis, neurological abnormalities including microcephaly[110] and mental retardation, thrombocytopenia[111], hepatosplenomegaly[112], obstructive jaundice[112] and radiographic changes of the long bones[107].

Very late onset complications have also been attributed to the virus including diabetes mellitus[113], growth hormone deficiency[114] and thyroid dysfunction[113,115].

Fetal rubella syndrome

The most important factor which influences transplacental transmission rate and severity of fetal infection is gestational age at which maternal infection occurs.

The risks of fetal infection and congenital abnormalities decrease with gestation. However, fetal infection can occur at any time during pregnancy. This has been extensively reported by Miller and al.[122]. This rate decreases from 81% before 12 weeks' gestation, 67% between 13 and 14, 25% between 23 and 26, to increase up to 35% between 27 and 30, 60% between 31 and 36 and 100% after 36 weeks' gestation. Periconceptional infection, until 11 days after the last menstruation period was not associated with any risk of fetal infection[123].

The assessment of risk of congenital defects is dependent upon the methodology of investigation, because most infants infected after the first trimester are grossly asymptomatic at birth. Serologic testing for these children is required for precise evaluation of congenital infection. Furthermore, long-term follow-up is needed to evaluate the rate of sequelae attributable to rubella infection.

Peckham and al. reported that the overall incidence of defects in 218 children evaluated when they were at least 2 years of age[124] was 23%, including 52% of them after infection before 8 weeks' gestation, 36% at 9–12 weeks, 10% at 13–20 weeks, and no defect could be attributed to maternal infections occurring after 20 weeks' gestation.

Sever and al. reported 128 cases of proven rubella at different gestational ages: 29 mothers had rubella at or before 14 weeks and 38% of their infants had sequelae; 55 maternal infections between 15 and 28 weeks and 20% of their infants had sequelae. No cases with congenital rubella syndrome were observed when maternal infection occurred after 20 weeks of gestation[125,126].

Miller et al. have shown that none of 102 infants had rubella congenital syndrome when rubella was contracted after 18 weeks of gestation, although 85% of the children whose mothers were infected at or before 12 weeks and 25% between 13 and 18 weeks' gestation were symptomatic[122].

Prenatal diagnosis

Because a proven maternal case of rubella during pregnancy is not always associated with a vertical transmission and a fetal infection is not always indicative of fetal defects, prenatal diagnosis is important to distinguish the cases where the fetus is involved.

Fetal infection can be proven by direct isolation of the virus or genome by PCR in amniotic fluid sampled by amniocentesis at least 6–8 weeks after maternal infection to avoid false negative results. This should be done in association with a targeted ultrasound examination[127,128].

A prognosis can be made by considering the timing of maternal infection, virological diagnosis of fetal infection and associated ultrasound findings.

Management options

Maternal administration of large doses of immune globulin in women exposed to rubella during pregnancy has been proposed[129–131]. This treatment does not prevent fetal infection.

Prevention

Three rubella vaccines were introduced in the USA in 1969. In 1979, the RA27/3 (human diploid fibroblast) strain was introduced that replaced the other three vaccines. It is based on a live, attenuated, non-transmissible virus. It is safe and effective in over 95% of vaccinated patients who develop long-term immunity after a single dose. Side effects include arthralgia or arthritis in about 25% of the cases. The Vaccine In Pregnancy (VIP) registry collected cases of women exposed within 3 months prior to conception and up to term until 1988. No congenital rubella syndrome has been reported after exposure to this vaccine during pregnancy. Three children, however, demonstrated serological evidence of congenital infection with rubella, but none of the three had malformations. Nevertheless, the vaccine is still contraindicated in pregnancy. Effective contraception is recommended around the time of vaccination. In October 2001, the Federal Center for Disease Control and Prevention changed recommendations on delaying pregnancy after receiving the rubella vaccine, reducing it from 3 to 1 month.

CHICKENPOX-ZOSTER VIRUS

The virus and its pathogenicity

Virology

Chickenpox (i.e. varicella) is the acute form of the disease caused by varicella-zoster virus (VZV) and zoster is the representation of the reactivation of the same virus. VZV (Herpesvirus varicellae) is a member of the herpesvirus family that carry a DNA genome.

Pathogenesis

The oropharynx is the site of entry and of initial viral replication. The virus is airborne spread from cutaneous vesicles and by respiratory droplets from patients with varicella or zoster. After the initial replication phase, the virus reaches the local lymph nodes and spreads by transient viremia towards the viscera. A second replication phase is followed by a second and more intense viremia with a cutaneous rash. Crusting and scabbing of the vesicles represent the typical features of the chickenpox rash that occurs following cell-mediated immunity activation. Varicella is most contagious at the time of onset of the rash and for one to 2 days afterwards. After clinical recovery, the patient is not contagious and the latency phase begins. Zoster occurs in persons who have previously had chickenpox. This vesicular infection is generally confined in the dermatome of the ganglia where the VZV was in latency. The virus travels down the axon and then reaches the skin supplied by that nerve. Occasionally, a disseminated zoster can occur, particularly in immunocompromised patients, probably due to a transient viremia.

Epidemiology

Chickenpox ranks as one of the most contagious infectious diseases during childhood. Urbanization contributes to the occurrence of the disease at younger ages, particularly in schools, with a world-wide distribution. The incidence of varicella has decreased in developed countries following the development of vaccination campaigns. Between 70 and 80% of young American adults report a history of varicella[132]. Based on serological studies, it appears that less than 25% of adults with no history of chickenpox are susceptible to an acute disease[133]. In pregnancy, the virus may be transmitted across the placenta resulting in neonatal or fetal chickenpox. Balduci et al. have estimated the incidence of varicella to be around 7/10000 pregnancies[134].

Maternal infection

Clinical symptoms

The usual incubation time is 10–21 days. Chickenpox is then heralded by the simultaneous occurrence of fever and rash. In adults, the eruption is often preceded by prodromal fever by 2 or 3 days. The rash begins typically on the face or scalp and spreads rapidly to the trunk but sparing the extremities. Lesions are characterized by typical evolution from red macules to vesicles, pustules and eventually crusts. All stages of the lesions can be visualized simultaneously in the same anatomical region. Several crops can develop in a period of 5 days. Sometimes mucosal lesions may develop in the mouth or on the vulva. Residual scarring is rare. Severity of the rash ranges from several lesions to thousand, especially in adults.

Chickenpox pneumonia is the most severe complication of varicella and develops in about 15% of adults. Radiological evidence of pneumonia has been found in 16% of a series of 110 cases[135]. The onset of pneumonia is 2–4 days and up to10 days after the appearance of the rash. Dyspnea occurs in 70% of cases and can be accompanied by cyanosis, chest pain, hemoptysis and bronchitic rales. The mortality rate has been reported to be of up to 10% but this includes immunosuppressed individuals.

Specifics of chickenpox in pregnant women are determined by the severity of the clinical picture and the number of lesions as this is the case for all adults. Nevertheless, the severity is due to the higher incidence of pneumonia during pregnancy.

Laboratory diagnosis

In cases with widespread typical vesicular exanthema and a history of recent exposure, the diagnosis is made clinically. Laboratory diagnosis can be achieved by demonstrating VZV antigen by immunofluorescence[136] and VZV DNA by PCR in skin lesions[137,138]. The virus can also be isolated from vesicular fluid.

VZV infections show at least a fourfold increase in specific antibody titers by using a sensitive test as FAMA or ELISA. The presence of IgM suggests a recent infection. The persistence of VZV antibodies beyond the age of 8 months is suggestive of intrauterine varicella.

Congenital infection

Congenital varicella syndrome

The congenital syndrome typically consists of a combination of skin lesions made of scars and skin loss together with eye abnormalities including cataract and microphthalmia, or chorioretinis, limb deformities (including hypoplasia, equinovarus, absent digits), neurological abnormalities (including cortical atrophy, mental retardation, microcephaly, seizures, limb paresis), abnormalities of the intestinal tract and of the urinary tract, prematurity, low birth weight and zoster in infancy[139–142].

Table 44.5 **Ultrasound abnormalities related to varicella infection of the fetus**

Cerebral anomalies[149–153]	Ventriculomegaly Hydrocephalus Microcephaly Polymicrogyria Porencephaly
Ophthalmologic anomalies	Congenital cataract Microphthalmia
Musculoskeletal anomalies[142,148]	Limb contractures Hypoplasia
Other findings	Intestinal echogenic foci Hepatic echogenic foci Hydrops Polyhydramnios Growth restriction

Risk of fetal varicella syndrome

Enders et al. reported the results of a prospective study of 1373 women with varicella and 366 with zoster during their pregnancy. Among the first group, they reported defects attributable to congenital varicella syndrome in 0.4% for infections between 0 and 12 weeks, 2% at between 13 and 20 weeks of gestation. The overall rate of congenital defects was 0.7%[142]. In another large prospective study performed in the USA comprising 347 cases of maternal varicella, the rate of congenital infection was 1.3%[143]. These two studies underline the rarity of the syndrome and, in 1994, Enders and al. concluded: 'although the risk of congenital varicella syndrome is small, the outcome for the affected infant is so serious that a reliable method of prenatal diagnosis would be valuable. In the long term, prevention of maternal varicella would be an option if a safe and effective vaccine were to become routinely available'.

The timing of maternal infection plays a major role in the severity of fetal damage. Most of reported cases of congenital varicella syndrome follow maternal infections that occurred during the first trimester or at the onset of the second trimester. Nevertheless, several publications have reported severe defects in fetuses following maternal chickenpox after the 20th week of gestation[143–146]. The most common risk to infants when VZV is transmitted to the fetus after the 20th week is zoster during early childhood.

Prenatal diagnosis of fetal infection

Targeted ultrasound examination can visualize some of the features of varicella-related embryopathy involving several organs with variable severity. A latency period of 5–19 weeks between maternal infection and sonographic detection of the first fetal anomalies has been reported in serial assessment of high-risk fetuses[147].

Common sonographic findings include intestinal and hepatic echogenic foci and hydrops, musculoskeletal, cerebral and ocular anomalies. Growth restriction and polyhydramnios have also been reported. Skin lesions following a dermatomal distribution are typical of varicella embryopathy but are not always present and usually not identifiable by ultrasound examination. Musculoskeletal anomalies may be related to scar formation and lead to limb contractures and hypoplasia which are accessible to ultrasound examination[142,148]. Cerebral anomalies documented with ultrasound include ventriculomegaly, hydrocephalus[149,150], microcephaly with polymicrogyria, and porencephaly[151–153]. Congenital cataract and microphthalmia are the most common ocular lesions. Hyperechoic foci within the fetal liver have been identified as calcifications at autopsy[148,154].

Ultrasound abnormalities related to varicella infection of the fetus are summarized in the Table 44.5.

Prenatal diagnosis can be made by amplification of the VZV genome by PCR in amniotic fluid. Mouly and al. reported the results of amniocentesis and PCR performed in 107 women who had developed clinical varicella before 24 weeks of gestation. Nine of 107 (8.4%) were positive by polymerase chain reaction, but only 2 of these (1.8%) were positive in cell culture. PCR is therefore the method of choice for diagnosis[142].

Perinatal infection

This is defined by the occurrence of varicella in neonates within 10 days from birth. It is due to maternal infection near term where chickenpox develops in 24–50% of the neonates[155–160]. The interval between the onset of maternal rash and that of neonatal infection is 9–15 days. When delivery occurs within 10 days of the onset of maternal clinical infection, maternal IgG cannot develop and cross the placenta to protect the fetus/neonate. Neonatal chickenpox is lethal in up to 30% of the cases[159].

Management options

VZV infection during pregnancy and more than 10 days before delivery

When maternal chickenpox is suspected, serological testing should be performed. A positive test rules out acute infection.

When the mother is seronegative at the time of sampling, two management options are possible:

1. Ultrasound serial examination alone can rule out severe fetal infections but misses asymptomatic vertical transmission of the virus to the fetus.
2. Amniocentesis can be performed to diagnose all fetal infections. However, fetal transmission will only occur in less than 5% of the cases.

If PCR is positive in the amniotic fluid, targeted ultrasound examination should then be performed every fortnight. MRI can also be informative in assessing the fetal brain.

When maternal infection occurs after 20 weeks of gestation, prenatal diagnosis is not recommended because fetal varicella syndrome has not been reported after 20 weeks[161].

Pregnant women with VZV infection near term and less than 10 days before delivery

When maternal eruption occurs within 10 days before delivery, every attempt should be made to delay delivery until maternal IgG have time to be produced and cross the placenta.

Antiviral treatment for maternal infection

Pregnant women who develop varicella should be treated with oral acyclovir and followed up carefully. Those with pneumonia should be admitted and treated with intravenous antiviral agent. Acyclovir is more effective when administrated within one day after the onset of varicella and it shortens the course of illness by about one day[162].

Passive immunization for infants after possible perinatal infection

Pooled immunoglobulins can attenuate the symptoms without preventing chickenpox when administrated to contact persons within 72 hours of exposure[163]. For infants born between 2 and 4 days after maternal eruption, the use of zoster immunoglobulins could decrease the risk and severity of the neonatal disease in one uncontrolled study[160]. It is also recommended to administer VZV immunoglobulins to infants of mothers who develop varicella within 5 days of delivery within 2 days after delivery[164]. Doses of 125 UI (1.25 ml or one vial)[164] have been given intramuscularly as early as possible after delivery.

Infected mothers and infants should be isolated from maternity and neonatal units in order to avoid spreading the infection.

Prevention

Active immunization against VZV is obtained by a live-attenuated vaccine. This vaccine was approved by the CDC in 1996. The vaccine protects against varicella in about 85% of cases. A mild and transient rash may occur about 1 month after immunization. A possible spread of the vaccine-type strain to non-immunized individuals at the time of this rash is possible. Nevertheless, in all cases reported, iatrogenic cases of varicella were mildly symptomatic. Vaccine indications in the USA are for susceptible women of childbearing age at least 3 months before conception.

FETAL TOXOPLASMOSIS

The parasite and its pathogenicity

Toxoplasma gondii is an intracellular protozoan that belongs to the phylum *Apicomplexa*, subclass *Coccidian*. It can take several different forms: the oocyst; the tachyzoite; and the cyst.

Oocysts

Members of the cat family are definitive hosts of *T. gondii*; replication of the parasite occurs in the intestine of the cat, resulting in the production of oocysts and shedding of million of oocysts in the feces for 7–21 days during acute infection. After sporulation, which takes place within 1–21 days, oocysts containing sporozoites are infective when ingested by mammals, including humans and give rise to the tachyzoite stage.

Tachyzoites

Tachyzoites enter all nucleated cells by active penetration and form a cytoplasmic vacuole. After repeated replications, host cells are disrupted leading to cell death, invasion of neighboring cells and dissemination of the tachyzoites in the bloodstream. The wide spread of tachyzoites infects many tissues, including the CNS, eyes, skeletal and cardiac muscles, as well as placenta. A strong local inflammatory response and tissue destruction are responsible for the clinical manifestations of the disease. The immune response causes the transformation from tachyzoites into bradyzoites and cyst formation.

Cysts

Bradyzoites persist in the host for life inside cysts. They are morphologically identical to tachyzoites but multiply slowly, express stage-specific molecules and are functionally different. Tissue cysts contain hundreds of thousands of bradyzoites and form within the host cells in brain as well as skeletal and cardiac muscles. Bradyzoites can be released from cysts, transform back into tachyzoites and cause recurrences of infection in immunocompromised patients. Cysts are infective stages for both intermediate and definitive hosts.

Epidemiology

Transmission

Humans can be infected with *T. gondii by* ingestion or handling of undercooked or raw meat (mainly pork and lamb) containing cysts as well as water or food containing oocysts excreted in the feces of infected cats. Most individuals are infected inadvertently, thus the specific route of transmission cannot usually be established. Variations in the seroprevalence of *T. gondii* seem to correlate with nutrition and hygiene habits of a population. This finding supports that the oral route is the major source of infection. Epidemics of toxoplasmosis in humans and in sheep are attributed to the exposure to infected cats and demonstrate the important role of oocyst excretion by cats in the propagation of the infection. Transmission during direct human-to-human transmission other than from mother to fetus has not been recorded and transmission by breastfeeding is still controversial[165,166].

Seroprevalence

Seroprevalence for *T. gondii* infection increases with age and does not vary significantly between males and females. It is lower in cold regions as well as in hot and arid areas. Seroprevalence ranges from 20% to 75% among countries[167]. The prevalence of *T. gondii* antibodies has been steadily falling in various countries over the last few decades. In the USA, the overall seroprevalence is 22.5%[168] and only 15% among women of childbearing age. Incidence of congenital infection is 2–3 infants per 1000 live births in France, markedly higher than in the USA where the incidence is of 1/1000 to 1/ 10000.

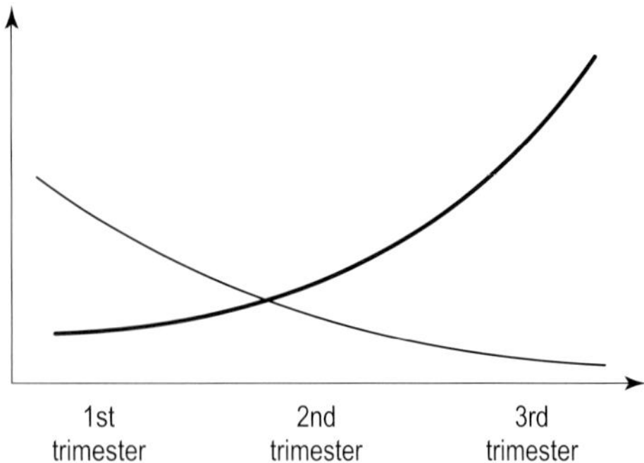

Fig. 44.1 Schematic representation of the severity of the effect on the fetus (thin line) and of the vertical transmission (thick line) of toxoplamosis depending on the trimester of maternal seroconversion.

Maternal infection

Clinical signs

Since more than 90% of primary infections in immunocompetent individuals are asymptomatic, the diagnosis of maternal infection is difficult. In the remaining 10%, clinical symptoms include mononucleosis-like illness with low-grade fever, headache and cervical lymphadenopathy. Other manifestations are rare: encephalitis, myocarditis, hepatitis, pneumonia.

In asymptomatic women, the diagnosis is made by laboratory analysis.

Laboratory diagnosis

Primary infection during pregnancy is diagnosed by seroconversion. IgM and IgG are detected by immunofluorescence antibody tests, enzyme-linked immune filtration assay, immunoabsorbent agglutination assay or other methods[169]. IgG become detectable 1–2 weeks after infection and remain elevated indefinitely. IgM become detectable within the first days and rapidly increase reaching a peak and remain elevated for 2–3 months before decreasing. Elevated IgM have to be interpreted with caution, because it has been shown that 27% of women remain positive for IgM for more than 2 years[170]. Seroconversion is defined as the appearance of specific IgM followed by that of IgG during the pregnancy. Only seroconversions place a fetus at risk for developing congenital toxoplasmosis.

Fetal infection

Risk and consequences of fetal infection

The incidence and severity of the infection depend upon gestational age at the time of maternal infection. The earlier the transplacental passage of the parasite, the more severe the symptoms and the prognosis[171,172]. The risk of fetal infection is multifactorial, depending on the timing of maternal infection, immune reaction of the mother during parasitemia, the parasite load and virulence of the strain involved[167].

The probability of fetal infection is only 1% when primary maternal infection occurs during the preconception period, but increases as pregnancy progresses; infection acquired during the first trimester by women untreated with anti-*T. gondii* drugs results in congenital infection in 10–25% of cases. For infections occurring during the second and third trimesters, the incidence of fetal infection ranges between 30 and 54% and 60 and 65%, respectively[173].

Foulon et al. reported that, when maternal infection occurs before the fifth gestational week, the transmission rate is less than 5%, while this rises up to more than 80% at the end of the pregnancy[174]. The consequences are more severe when fetal infection occurs early in pregnancy. It is associated with miscarriages, severe disease, intrauterine growth retardation or preterm birth.

The highest incidence of severe abnormalities at birth is seen in children whose mothers have acquired primary infection between 10 and 24 weeks of gestation[175] (Fig. 44.1). Hohlfeld et al. have reported that 77.9% of the infected fetuses who had ultrasound abnormalities after maternal infection at the first trimester, 20.4% after infection at the second trimester and no infected fetuses had ultrasound abnormalities when infection occurred at the third trimester[172].

Description of congenital toxoplasmosis syndrome

Approximately 15% of congenitally infected newborns will be symptomatic at birth. The classical triad including hydrocephalus, chorioretinitis and intracranial calcifications is found in less than 10% of cases. Other clinical manifestations are not specific symptoms: maculo-papular rash, generalized lymphadenopathy, hepatomegaly, splenomegaly, anemia, hyperbilirubinanemia and thrombocytopenia[176].

Around 85% of infected infants are asymptomatic at birth. Nevertheless, a large proportion of these children develop sequelae with visual impairment, mental and cognitive abnormalities of variable severity, seizures or learning difficulties only after several months or years. Guerina et al. reported that 40% of the asymptomatic infants will show abnormalities on cranial imaging and ophthalmologic investigations[177].

Vutova et al. investigated eye manifestations in congenital toxoplasmosis in 38 infants and children[178]. The most frequent finding was chorioretinitis with characteristic retinal infiltrates (92%), and this was associated with other ocular lesions in 71% of the cases. The second most common finding was microphthalmia with strabismus. Other ocular lesions included iridocyclitis, cataract, glaucoma and visual loss.

Wallon et al. reported the clinical evolution of ocular lesions and final visual function in a prospective cohort of 327 congenitally infected children in France[179]. The children were identified by maternal prenatal screening and monitored for up to 14 years. After 6 years, 79 (24%) children showed at least one retinochoroidal lesion. In 23 of them, additional lesions were diagnosed within 10 years, mainly in a previously unaffected location. Normal vision was found in about two-thirds of the children with lesions of one eye, in half of the children with lesions in both eyes and none had bilateral visual impairment. Most mothers (84%) had been treated in utero and a combination of pyrimethamine and sulfadiazine had also been given to all children in 38% prior to and in 72% after birth. Late-onset retinal lesions and relapse can occur many years after birth, but the overall visual prognosis of congenital toxoplasmosis seems acceptable when the infection is identified early and treated appropriately. Early diagnosis and treatment are believed to reduce the risk of sequelae[180].

If toxoplasmosis is suspected at the time of birth, diagnostic work-up includes ophthalmologic, auditory and neurological examinations, lumbar puncture and brain imaging[176]. Other laboratory tests include full blood count (CBC), liver function tests and specific *T. gondii* diagnostic tests. The diagnosis of congenital toxoplasmosis can be made by the detection of IgM or IgA antibodies to *T. gondii* in the neonate with a high sensitivity. In addition, amplification of *T. gondii* DNA by PCR is almost 100% sensitive and can be detected in various body fluids of a congenitally infected neonate[169].

Prenatal diagnosis

Prenatal diagnosis of fetal infection is therefore mainly based on PCR amplification of the *Toxoplasma gondii* genome in amniotic fluid or in fetal blood, inoculation of amniotic fluid and/or fetal blood into mice and/or tissue culture[181], as well as on serial detailed fetal ultrasound examination[172,182].

Antsaklis et al. reported the sensitivity, specificity, positive and negative predictive values of the different diagnostic methods. These were of 61.1%, 98.6%, 91.6%, 91.13% and 83.3%, 100%, 100%, 97.1% Se, Sp, PPV and NPV of mouse inoculation and PCR assay respectively. Cordocentesis had no diagnostic value. The combination of the techniques led to 100% Specificity and positive predictive value (PPV)[183]. Furthermore, amniocentesis is easier and safer to perform than cordocentesis.

Infected fetuses should undergo serial targeted ultrasound examination. The most common findings have been described by Hohfeld et al. in 89 cases of fetal infection. Among these infected fetuses, 32 had ultrasound anomalies including 25 cases with ventriculomegaly, more often bilateral and symmetrical, starting in the occipital region before extending to the entire lateral ventricle, 6 cases of intracranial calcification, 11 cases with increased placental thickness, 2 with placental calcifications, 4 cases with liver calcifications as well as hepatomegaly, ascites in 5 cases, pericardial effusions in 2, as well as pleural effusion in 1 case. The presence of one sign was reported in 13 cases, two signs or more were reported in the other 14 cases. Neither intrauterine growth retardation nor microcephaly was observed[184].

Ultrasound fetal abnormalities related to toxoplasmosis infection are reported in Table 44.6.

Table 44.6 **Fetal abnormalities related to fetal infection with toxoplasmosis**

Cerebral signs	Microcephaly[185] Ventricular dilatation, hydrocephaly[172] Intracranial calcifications[172] Brain atrophy[185] Hydranencephaly[185]
Placenta	Increased placental thickness[172] Calcifications[172]
Other findings	Liver calcifications[172] Ascites[186,187] Pericardial effusions[172] Pleural effusions[172] Hepatomegaly[172] Hyperechogenic bowel Intrauterine growth restriction

Treatment

After confirmation of the diagnosis of maternal seroconversion, treatment is often initiated in a reference center, following specialized counseling. Treatment is usually indicated during pregnancy for both symptomatic and asymptomatic maternal disease with or without congenital infection, although this was not proven to be useful[188]. Indeed, if maternal infection is diagnosed, it is not known if antenatal treatment is effective as shown in the European cohort trial comprising of 1208 infected pregnant women, which failed to detect any difference in the risk of congenital infection with treatment or not[188].

The combination of pyrimethamine (25–100 mg/day × 3–4 weeks), sulfadiazine (1–1.5 g qid × 3–4 weeks) and folinic acid (leucovorin, 10–25 mg with each dose of pyrimethamine, to avoid bone marrow suppression) is the treatment protocol recommended by the WHO and the CDC[189].

In other countries in Europe, Asia or South Africa, spiramycin (3 g/day × 3 weeks) and sometimes clindamycin is recommended to prevent transplacental infection. In the USA, spiramycin is currently not approved by the FDA but is available as an investigational drug, requiring special approval.

Reference association comprising pyrimethamine and sulfadiazine to prevent fetal infection is contraindicated during the first trimester of pregnancy due to its potential teratogenicity, and sulfadiazine should be used alone in the first trimester. However, both drugs should be used when the mother is immunocompromised or if the disease is disseminated.

Nevertheless, it is necessary to remember the heterogeneity of the studies published for the evaluation of these treatments. Methodologies used were very different[169]. Wallon et al.[190] reviewed studies comparing treated and untreated concurrent groups of pregnant women with proven or likely acute toxoplasmosis. Outcomes were reported in the offspring. The results showed treatment to be effective in five studies but ineffective in four[191–197]. Further large-scale, carefully controlled studies are necessary in order to clarify this controversial issue.

Prevention

Primary prevention

Primary prevention is based on education programs that have been developed to avoid maternal primary infection during pregnancy. Such educational programs aim at avoiding exposure to the parasite by better culinary and hygienic practical guidelines. Nevertheless, consequences of these methods have not been evaluated by any appropriate study of the incidence of congenital infection before and after the initiation of public health programs.

Development of a vaccine to prevent human disease by active immunization as well as that of animals is necessary. Several antigens are being studied for the development of effective and safe vaccines, mainly SAG1, a surface antigen expressed on tachyzoites[198,199].

Secondary prevention

Secondary prevention is based on routine serological screening of the pregnant women throughout their pregnancy. Modalities of the serologic follow-up vary between countries from 3 times to up to each month as established in France. Screening should begin prior to conception and followed up until seroconversion in seronegative women. Treatment is recommended if one of the tests suggests definite or likely primary maternal infection. The efficacy of spiramycin is further questioned by the interval between the onset of treatment and maternal infection even with monthly screening[188,194].

FETAL SYPHYLIS INFECTION

Bacteriology and pathogenesis

Bacteriology

Treponema pallidum (TP) is a member of the Spirochaetales. There are three other Treponema pathogens (*Treponema pertenue* (yaws), *Treponema carateum* (pinta), and *Treponema endemicum* (endemic syphilis, or bejel)). Only *Treponema pertenue* and *T. palllidum* are able to cause congenital infection. Treponemes are small gram-negative bacteria which can only be visualized by dark-field or phase-contrast microscopy. *T. pallidum* contains a single circular chromosome that has been entirely sequenced.

Pathogenesis

When introduced into the skin or mucosal tissues, the pathogen attaches to a receptor(s) on the host cell surface and subsequently multiplies locally and spreads through the perivascular lymphatic system and into the systemic circulation. It then disseminates widely before any lesion becomes clinically apparent. During the 3-week incubation period (range 10–90 days), there is an intense local inflammatory response, which creates the chancre, together with cellular proliferation in regional lymph nodes when the immune response is unable to eradicate fully the infection, over 2–10 weeks, local replication leads to dissemination in the skin, mucosal membranes, as well as in the central nervous system. The secondary immune response is similar to the primary one with the development of venereal warts in response to the presence of spirochetes. Irrespective of therapy, secondary syphilis will resolve with a phase of relative immunological control. At this stage, viable pathogens remain in low numbers. Around 60% of the cases will remain asymptomatic and latent. Progression of the disease to the tertiary phase, sometimes after several years will continue in 40% of cases. Tertiary syphilis can involve any organ system and the typical lesions are gummas (focal areas of non-suppurative inflammatory necrosis surrounded by fibrotic scarring).

Congenital syphilis occurs when T. *pallidum* crosses the placenta or at the time of birth by direct contact. Transplacental transmission during maternal spirochetemia can occur from as early as 9–10 weeks of gestation onwards. Vertical transmission occurs more frequently during primary or secondary syphilis than with latent disease. The risk decreases after 4 years, even when untreated. Intrauterine transmission causes wide dissemination of the organism in the fetus. The organs most severely affected include bone, brain, liver, lung and the skeleton. Early infection can lead to spontaneous abortion.

Untreated congenital syphilis can progress through the same stages as postnatally acquired syphilis.

Epidemiology and transmission

Humans are the sole natural hosts of syphilis. The main mode of contamination is by sexual contact. The risk of infection is of approximately 30% per sexual contact with an infected partner. Acquisition via non-sexual contact has also been reported including contact with infected lesions in healthcare workers and in laboratory workers who handle infected animals. A newborn can be infected by transplacental passage of *T. pallidum* from an infected untreated or insufficiently treated mother, or at the time of birth through an infected birth canal.

Epidemiological features of this infection have changed with the introduction of penicillin which enabled a drastic reduction in the number of cases. However, a resurgent wave occurred in the 1980s in the USA, mainly linked with drug abuse. With wider screening practices, a decrease was also obtained from the 1990s, mainly linked with the prevention program for HIV. In 1997, the rate of 3.2 cases per 100 000 individuals was reported. Syphilis is more common among men, mainly homosexual and varies between populations and geographical regions. World-wide, the disease is a major public health problem, mainly in Eastern Europe and in the developing countries in Africa and America.

Recognized risk factors include poverty, crack cocaine use, prostitution and HIV infection. Gestational syphilis has well-established risk factors: unmarried mothers, teenage mothers, absence of prenatal care, illicit drug abuse by the mother or sexual partner, multiple sexual partners, low socioeconomic environment, racial/ethnic minority group. In 2002, among 451 cases reported by the CDC, 74% of the cases of fetal infection followed absence of treatment and, in 30% of the cases, there was inappropriate prenatal care.

Maternal infection

Clinical manifestations

The clinical picture is not altered by pregnancy[200]. The primary stage, illustrated by the chancre, is often unrecognized due to its location. The primary lesion appears about 3 weeks after exposure. It is a painless, ulcerated chancre with a raised border and thick base, which persists for 2–8 weeks. Painless adenopathy may also be present. Only 5–10% of all diagnoses are made upon clinical manifestations. Thus, the diagnosis is mainly based on serologic testing. The secondary disseminated stage occurs 4–10 weeks after the first primary lesion. It consists of condyloma latum and a disseminated maculopapular rash involving the palms and soles. Lymphadenopathy, weight loss, fever, anorexia, headache, arthralgia can precede or accompany skin manifestations. Complications include: hepatitis, glomerulonephritis, nephrotic syndrome, osteitis, meningitis and iritis.

This stage resolves spontaneously in 2–6 weeks when the patient enters the asymptomatic, latent stage of syphilis. The diagnosis can be made only by serologic testing. This latent stage can be separated into two phases: early (1 year or less than onset of infection) and late (more than 1 year).

Without treatment, one-third of the cases will develop tertiary syphilis, characterized by lesions involving the cardiovascular, central nervous or musculoskeletal systems as well as other organs.

Laboratory diagnosis

Treponema pallidum (TP) cannot be easily cultivated in vitro and a wide variety of diagnostic tests have been developed.

They can be divided into three broad categories:

1. Direct detection

In clinical practice, darkfield examination is the only technique performed. This is useful for rapid diagnosis, but it requires trained personnel. It consists of inoculation of TP into a rabbit. The animal is examined serially over 3 months for clinical symptoms of syphilis and treponemal tests. If the rabbit develops illness, examination under darkfield microscopy is performed to confirm syphilis. This procedure is only performed in research laboratories. The sensitivity of RIT (rabbit infectivity test) approaches 100%. Polymerase chain reaction (PCR) is rapidly becoming a useful test in clinical settings. Sanchez and al. reported a 71% sensitivity and a 100% specificity on neonatal serum and cerebrospinal fluid relative to RIT[201].

2. Non-treponemal tests

Non-treponemal serologies detect antibodies against the cardiolipin antigen released by damaged host cells. Two tests are available: the Venereal Disease Research Laboratory (VDRL) and the Rapid Plasma Reagin (RPR). They are inexpensive, easy to perform and widely available, making them excellent screening tests. VDRL test is the only non-treponemal test available for the diagnosis of neurosyphilis. False-positive non-treponemal tests have been described, but titers are usually low: viral and bacterial infection, other spirochetal infections, immunization, heroin use, malignancy, chronic illnesses, autoimmune and connective tissue disorders, aging and, sometimes, the pregnancy itself. False-negative tests have been reported with large amounts of antibodies which could inhibit the reaction. Serial dilutions can overcome this phenomenon. Secondary to the limitations of non-treponemal tests, a positive result should always be confirmed with a treponemal test.

3. Treponemal antibody tests

The treponemal tests detect antibodies directed specifically against *T. pallidum*. The two most commonly used are the fluorescent treponemal antibody absorption (FTA-Abs) test and the microhemagglutination assay for anti-*T. pallidum* (MHA-TP) antibodies.

These tests are more expensive and technically more difficult to perform and so are not useful for screening. Furthermore, they cannot be quantitated and are not useful for follow-up after treatment. A positive treponemal test combined with a positive non-treponemal test is very sensitive and specific for syphilis. All are positive within 4 weeks of the chancre's appearance. However, they may be negative at the time the chancre first appears when only the darkfield examination can make the diagnosis.

Fetal manifestations

Vertical transmission

Fetal syphilis is associated with spontaneous abortion, intrauterine fetal death and neonatal demise, as well as preterm delivery. Placental passage of the spirochetes occurs throughout gestation, but fetal clinical manifestations require immunocompetence which only occurs from 16 weeks onwards. It was thought that the inability of TP to cross the placenta was due to the thickness of Langhans' cytotrophoblast layer[202]. However, Harter el al. described histological identification of spirochetes in fetal tissues after spontaneous abortion as early as 9–10 weeks' gestation[203]. First-trimester passage of TP was further proved by Nathan et al. in 1997, using RIT and PCR on amniotic fluid[204].

Vertical transmission rates have been estimated to be 29% (3% stillbirths and 26% livebirths) with untreated primary syphilis at delivery, 59% (20%, 39%) with untreated secondary syphilis, 50% (17%, 33%) with early latent and 13% (5%, 8%) with late latent syphilis[202]. Transmission is more likely when the parasite load is high. A co-infection with HIV seems to increase the likelihood of fetal infection.

Description of congenital syphilis[205]

Neonates affected by TP may present with manifestations divided into early signs (appearing during the first 2 years of life) and late signs (thoses appearing later over the first decades of life). Early signs comprise: hepatosplenomegaly but also generalized lymphadenopathy, hematological abnormalities (anemia, leukocytosis and leukopenia, thrombocytopenia), dermatological anomalies (jaundice, rhinitis, maculopapular eruption, mucous patches), bone lesions on X-ray include diaphyseal periostitis, metaphyseal osteochondritis, renal manifestations, CNS anomalies, ocular manifestations and growth retardation.

Late congenital syphilis is characterized by signs occurring in around 40% of untreated survivors. Many of these features are not reversible at this stage, despite a late onset antibiotic treatment. These manifestations are mainly: dental abnormalities, cartilage destructions and bone deformities, eye involvement, eighth nerve deafness. These three main features constitute the Hutchinson triad.

Prenatal diagnosis

Fetal infection can be suspected when abnormalities are observed on ultrasound examination. These abnormalities are summarized in Table 44.7. Nevertheless, these abnormalities are not specific and are only suggestive of infectious disease. Laboratory methods are always needed to confirm the diagnosis.

Table 44.7 **Fetal ultrasound abnormalities in congenital syphilis**

Hydrops fetalis[208]
Placental thickening[209]
Polyhydramnios[206]
Ascites[206,210]
Subcutanous edema[206]
Hepatomegaly[208]
Splenomegaly
Hyperechogenic or dilatated small bowel[211]
Intrauterine fetal death[210]

Serological testing of cord blood specimens may be performed, but is sometimes difficult to interpret. The titers of non-treponemal tests should be at least fourfold those in maternal blood to confirm a significant fetal IgG production. Indeed, the difficulty of the interpretation of the serological tests stems largely from the inability to distinguish the humoral response of the mother, whose IgG antibodies pass through the placenta, from the specific antibody response of the infant. Due to these difficulties, PCR method has been developed and its results have been shown to be similar results for sensitivity and specificity when compared with RIT, on amniotic fluid samples[201].

Non-specific biochemical and hematologic parameters have also been proved to be modified by fetal syphilis: increased GGT[206], anemia, thrombocytopenia, leukopenia, leukocytosis[207].

Hollier et al. have suggested a continuum of the fetal syphilis infection beginning from fetal hepatic dysfunction and thickening of the placenta, followed by hematologous dysfunction, until isolated ascites or hydrops fetalis[206].

Treatment

The US Centers for Disease Control (CDC) recommend that patients with recent syphilis (primary, secondary or latent syphilis of less than 1 year's duration) receive benzathine penicillin G, 2.4 million units IM in a single dose.

Patients with older active syphilis or with HIV infection should receive 7.2 million units benzathine penicillin G as 2.4 million units IM weekly for 3 consecutive weeks.

Patients with CNS infection require intravenous penicillin for 10–14 days.

The CDC guidelines recommend a serial serologic follow-up after treatment, by quantitative non-treponemal serology. A fourfold decrease in IgG titers indicates a successful treatment. It is expected by 6–12 months for primary and secondary syphilis, 12–24 months for early latent syphilis and greater than 24 months for late latent stage. Pregnancy has been associated with a slower decrease in titers[212].

Penicillin-allergic patients should undergo desensitization prior to treatment. Drug-abuse and lack of or late prenatal care, or failure to complete treatment and obtain follow-up are important risk factors for congenital disease.

McFarlin et al. noted that there was no difference in the rates of congenital infections among women with a disease of less than 1-year if the treatment was one dose or three doses of benzathine penicillin (26.7% versus 30%)[213]. Inadequate therapy or dose regimen also contributes to the development of a congenital disease.

The Jarisch-Herxheimer reaction is common during treatment in adults. It consists of the association of chills, fever, malaise, hypotension, tachycardia, tachypnoea, accentuation of cutaneous lesions and leukocytosis. It is more frequent in the second stage of the infection and could be related to the release of lipoproteins membrane stimulating a pro-inflammatory response. In pregnant women, it happens in around 40% of cases[214] and it is associated with preterm delivery and/or fetal distress. It is in relation with prostaglandins release. No preventive therapy is available.

Prevention

Congenital syphilis is a preventable disease. High-risk women should undergo at least one serology screening test in the first trimester to be repeated at the beginning of the third trimester and at the time of delivery[200,215,216].

REFERENCES

1. Stagno S, Pass RF, Dworsky ME, Alford CA, Jr. Maternal cytomegalovirus infection and perinatal transmission. *Clin Obstet Gynecol* **25**(3):563–576, 1982.
2. Stagno S, Pass RF, Cloud G et al. Primary cytomegalovirus infection in pregnancy. Incidence, transmission to fetus, and clinical outcome. *J Am Med Assoc* **256**(14):1904–1908, 1986.
3. Yow MD, Williamson DW, Leeds LJ et al. Epidemiologic characteristics of cytomegalovirus infection in mothers and their infants. *Am J Obstet Gynecol* **158**(5):1189–1195, 1988.
4. Stagno S, Reynolds DW, Huang ES, Thames SD, Smith RJ, Alford CA. Congenital cytomegalovirus infection. *N Engl J Med* **296**(22):1254–1258, 1977.
5. Schopfer K, Lauber E, Krech U. Congenital cytomegalovirus infection in newborn infants of mothers infected before pregnancy. *Arch Dis Child* **53**(7):536–539, 1978.
6. Boppana SB, Rivera LB, Fowler KB, Mach M, Britt WJ. Intrauterine transmission of cytomegalovirus to infants of women with preconceptional immunity. *N Engl J Med* **344**(18):1366–3771, 2001.
7. Nigro G, Anceschi MM, Cosmi EV. Clinical manifestations and abnormal laboratory findings in pregnant women with primary cytomegalovirus infection. *Br J Obstet Gynaecol* **110**(6):572–577, 2003.
8. Revello MG, Gerna G. Diagnosis and management of human cytomegalovirus infection in the mother, fetus, and newborn infant. *Clin Microbiol Rev* **15**(4):680–715, 2002.
9. Mace M, Sissoeff L, Rudent A, Grangeot-Keros L. A serological testing algorithm for the diagnosis of primary CMV infection in pregnant women. *Prenat Diagn* **24**(11):861–863, 2004.
10. Maine GT, Lazzarotto T, Landini MP. New developments in the diagnosis of maternal and congenital CMV infection. *Expert Rev Mol Diagn* **1**(1):19–29, 2001.
11. Lazzarotto T, Spezzacatena P, Varani S et al. Anticytomegalovirus (anti-CMV)

immunoglobulin G avidity in identification of pregnant women at risk of transmitting congenital CMV infection. *Clin Diagn Lab Immunol* **6**(1):127–129, 1999.
12. Revello MG, Zavattoni M, Sarasini A, Percivalle E, Simoncini L, Gerna G. Human cytomegalovirus in blood of immunocompetent persons during primary infection: prognostic implications for pregnancy. *J Infect Dis* **177**(5): 1170–1175, 1998.
13. Boppana SB, Pass RF, Britt WJ, Stagno S, Alford CA. Symptomatic congenital cytomegalovirus infection: neonatal morbidity and mortality. *Pediatr Infect Dis J* **11**(2):93–99, 1992.
14. Boppana SB, Fowler KB, Vaid Y et al. Neuroradiographic findings in the newborn period and long-term outcome in children with symptomatic congenital cytomegalovirus infection. *Pediatrics* **99**(3):409–414, 1997.
15. Kumar ML, Nankervis GA, Gold E. Inapparent congenital cytomegalovirus infection. A follow-up study. *N Engl J Med* **288**(26):1370–1372, 1973.
16. Saigal S, Lunyk O, Larke RP, Chernesky MA. The outcome in children with congenital cytomegalovirus infection: a longitudinal follow-up study. *Am J Dis Child* **136**(10):896–901, 1982.
17. Melish ME, Hanshaw JB. Congenital cytomegalovirus infection: developmental progress of infants detected by routine screening. *Am J Dis Child* **126**(2):190–194, 1973.
18. Fowler KB, McCollister FP, Dahle AJ, Boppana S, Britt WJ, Pass RF. Progressive and fluctuating sensorineural hearing loss in children with asymptomatic congenital cytomegalovirus infection. *J Pediatr* **130**(4):624–630, 1997.
19. Noyola DE, Demmler GJ, Williamson WD et al. Cytomegalovirus urinary excretion and long term outcome in children with congenital cytomegalovirus infection. Congenital CMV Longitudinal Study Group. *Pediatr Infect Dis J* **19**(6):505–510, 2000.
20. Ville Y. The megalovirus. *Ultrasound Obstet Gynecol* **12**(3):151–153, 1998.
21. Lange I, Rodeck CH, Morgan-Capner P, Simmons A, Kangro HO. Prenatal serological diagnosis of intrauterine cytomegalo-virus infection. *Br Med J* **284**:1673–1674, 1982.
22. Al-Kouatly HB, Chasen ST, Streltzoff J, Chervenak FA. The clinical significance of fetal echogenic bowel. *Am J Obstet Gynecol* **185**(5):1035–1038, 2001.
23. Dechelotte PJ, Bouvier RJ, Vanlieferinghen PC, Lemery DJ. Pseudo-meconium ileus due to cytomegalovirus infection: a report of three cases. *Pediatr Pathol* **12**(1):73–82, 1992.
24. Drose JA, Dennis MA, Thickman D. Infection in utero: US findings in 19 cases. *Radiology* **178**(2):369–374, 1991.
25. Watt-Morse MLLS, Hill LM. The natural history of cytomegalovirus infection as assessed by serial ultrasound and fetal blood sampling: a case report. *Prenat Diagn* **15**(6):567–570, 1995.
26. Barkovich AJ, Lindan CE. Congenital cytomegalovirus infection of the brain: imaging analysis and embryologic considerations. *Am J Neuroradiol* **15**(4): 703–715, 1994.
27. Soussotte C, Maugey-Laulom B, Carles D, Diard F. Contribution of transvaginal ultrasonography and fetal cerebral MRI in a case of congenital cytomegalovirus infection. *Fetal Diagn Ther* **15**(4):219–223, 2000.
28. Malinger G, Lev D, Zahalka N et al. Fetal cytomegalovirus infection of the brain: the spectrum of sonographic findings. *Am J Neuroradiol* **24**(1):28–32, 2003.
29. Liesnard C, Donner C, Brancart F, Gosselin F, Delforge ML, Rodesch F. Prenatal diagnosis of congenital cytomegalovirus infection: prospective study of 237 pregnancies at risk. *Obstet Gynecol* **95**(6 Pt 1):881–888, 2000.
30. Guerra B, Lazzarotto T, Quarta S et al. Prenatal diagnosis of symptomatic congenital cytomegalovirus infection. *Am J Obstet Gynecol* **183**(2):476–482, 2000.
31. Lazzarotto T, Varani S, Guerra B, Nicolosi A, Lanari M, Landini MP. Prenatal indicators of congenital cytomegalovirus infection. *J Pediatr* **137**(1):90–95, 2000.
32. Enders G, Bader U, Lindemann L, Schalasta G, Daiminger A. Prenatal diagnosis of congenital cytomegalovirus infection in 189 pregnancies with known outcome. *Prenat Diagn* **21**(5):362–377, 2001.
33. Revello MG, Zavattoni M, Furione M, Baldanti F, Gerna G. Quantification of human cytomegalovirus DNA in amniotic fluid of mothers of congenitally infected fetuses. *J Clin Microbiol* **37**(10):3350–3352, 1999.
34. Revello MGZM, Sarasini A, Percivalle E, Simoncini L, Gerna G. Human cytomegalovirus in blood of immunocompetent persons during primary infection: prognosis implications for pregnancy. *J Infect Dis* **177**(5): 1170–1175, 1998.
35. Ahlfors K, Forsgren M, Ivarsson SA, Harris S, Svanberg L. Congenital cytomegalovirus infection: on the relation between type and time of maternal infection and infant's symptoms. *Scand J Infect Dis* **15**(2):129–138, 1983.
36. Pass RF, Fowler KB, Boppana SB, Britt WJ, Stagno S. Congenital cytomegalovirus infection following first trimester maternal infection: symptoms at birth and outcome. *J Clin Virol* **35**(2):216–220, 2006.
37. Steinlin MI, Nadal D, Eich GF, Martin E, Boltshauser EJ. Late intrauterine cytomegalovirus infection: clinical and neuroimaging findings. *Pediatr Neurol* **15**(3):249–253, 1996.
38. Ahlfors K, Ivarsson SA, Harris S et al. Congenital cytomegalovirus infection and disease in Sweden and the relative importance of primary and secondary maternal infections: preliminary findings from a prospective study. *Scand J Infect Dis* **16**(2):129–137, 1984.
39. Fowler KB, Stagno S, Pass RF, Britt WJ, Boll TJ, Alford CA. The outcome of congenital cytomegalovirus infection in relation to maternal antibody status. *N Engl J Med* **326**(10):663–667, 1992.
40. Lipitz S, Achiron R, Zalel Y, Mendelson E, Tepperberg M, Gamzu R. Outcome of pregnancies with vertical transmission of primary cytomegalovirus infection. *Obstet Gynecol* **100**(3):428–433, 2002.
41. Gouarin S, Gault E, Vabret A et al. Real-time PCR quantification of human cytomegalovirus DNA in amniotic fluid samples from mothers with primary infection. *J Clin Microbiol* **40**(5):1767–1772, 2002.
42. Picone O, Costa JM, Leruez-Ville M, Ernault P, Olivi M, Ville Y. Cytomegalovirus (CMV) glycoprotein B genotype and CMV DNA load in the amniotic fluid of infected fetuses. *Prenat Diagn* **24**(12):1001–1006, 2004.
43. Revello MG, Zavattoni M, Baldanti F, Sarasini A, Paolucci S, Gerna G. Diagnostic and prognostic value of human cytomegalovirus load and IgM antibody in blood of congenitally infected newborns. *J Clin Virol* **14**(1):57–66, 1999.
44. Lanari M, Lazzarotto T, Venturi V et al. Neonatal cytomegalovirus blood load and risk of sequelae in symptomatic and asymptomatic congenitally infected newborns. *Pediatrics* **117**(1):E76–E83, 2006.
45. Rasmussen L, Geissler A, Winters M. Inter- and intragenic variations complicate the molecular epidemiology of human cytomegalovirus. *J Infect Dis* **187**(5): 809–819, 2003.
46. Picone O, Costa JM, Dejean A, Ville Y. Is fetal gender a risk factor for severe congenital cytomegalovirus infection? *Prenat Diagn* **25**(1):34–38, 2005.
47. Nigro G, Adler SP, La Torre R, Best AM. Passive immunization during pregnancy for congenital cytomegalovirus infection. *N Engl J Med* **353**(13):1350–1362, 2005.
48. Jacquemard FYM, Costa JM, Romand S, Jacz-Aigrain E, Daffos F, Ville Y. Maternal administration of valaciclovir in symptomatic intrauterine Cytomegalovirus infection. Br J Obstet Gynaecol in press, 2007.
49. Azam AZ, Vial Y, Fawer CL, Zufferey J, Hohlfeld P. Prenatal diagnosis of congenital cytomegalovirus infection. *Obstet Gynecol* **97**(3):443–448, 2001.
50. Brown KE, Hibbs JR, Gallinella G et al. Resistance to parvovirus B19 infection due to lack of virus receptor (erythrocyte P antigen). *N Engl J Med* **330**(17): 1192–1196, 1994.

51. Chisaka H, Morita E, Yaegashi N, Sugamura K. Parvovirus B19 and the pathogenesis of anaemia. *Rev Med Virol* **13**(6):347–359, 2003.
52. Koch WC, Adler SP. Human parvovirus B19 infections in women of childbearing age and within families. *Pediatr Infect Dis J* **8**(2):83–87, 1989.
53. Heegaard ED, Brown KE. Human parvovirus B19. *Clin Microbiol Rev* **15**(3):485–505, 2002.
54. Nascimento JP, Buckley MM, Brown KE, Cohen BJ. The prevalence of antibody to human parvovirus B19 in Rio de Janeiro, Brazil. *Rev Inst Med Trop Sao Paulo* **32**(1):41–45, 1990.
55. Adler SP, Manganello AM, Koch WC, Hempfling SH, Best AM. Risk of human parvovirus B19 infections among school and hospital employees during endemic periods. *J Infect Dis* **168**(2):361–368, 1993.
56. Dembinski J, Eis-Hubinger AM, Maar J, Schild R, Bartmann P. Long term follow up of serostatus after maternofetal parvovirus B19 infection. *Arch Dis Child* **88**(3):219–221, 2003.
57. Trotta M, Azzi A, Meli M et al. Intrauterine parvovirus B19 infection: early prenatal diagnosis is possible. *Int J Infect Dis* **8**(2):130–131, 2004.
58. Valeur-Jensen AK, Pedersen CB, Westergaard T et al. Risk factors for parvovirus B19 infection in pregnancy. *J Am Med Assoc* **281**(12):1099–1105, 1999.
59. Harger JH, Adler SP, Koch WC, Harger GF. Prospective evaluation of 618 pregnant women exposed to parvovirus B19: risks and symptoms. *Obstet Gynecol* **91**(3):413–420, 1998.
60. Cartter ML, Farley TA, Rosengren S et al. Occupational risk factors for infection with parvovirus B19 among pregnant women. *J Infect Dis* **163**(2):282–285, 1991.
61. Gillespie SM, Cartter ML, Asch S et al. Occupational risk of human parvovirus B19 infection for school and day-care personnel during an outbreak of erythema infectiosum. *J Am Med Assoc* **263**(15): 2061–2065, 1990.
62. Enders M, Weidner A, Zoellner I, Searle K, Enders G. Fetal morbidity and mortality after acute human parvovirus B19 infection in pregnancy: prospective evaluation of 1018 cases. *Prenat Diagn* **24**(7):513–518, 2004.
63. Ager EA, Chin TD, Poland JD. Epidemic erythema infectiosum. *N Engl J Med* **275**(24):1326–1331, 1966.
64. Anderson MJ, Lewis E, Kidd IM, Hall SM, Cohen BJ. An outbreak of erythema infectiosum associated with human parvovirus infection. *J Hyg (Lond)* **93**(1):85–93, 1984.
65. Saarinen UM, Chorba TL, Tattersall P et al. Human parvovirus B19-induced epidemic acute red cell aplasia in patients with hereditary hemolytic anemia. *Blood* **67**(5):1411–1417, 1986.
66. Brass C, Elliott LM, Stevens DA. Academy rash: a probable epidemic of erythema infectiosum ('fifth disease'). *J Am Med Assoc* **248**(5):568–572, 1982.
67. Tsuji A, Uchida N, Asamura S, Matsunaga Y, Yamazaki S. Aseptic meningitis with erythema infectiosum. *Eur J Pediatr* **149**(6):449–450, 1990.
68. Seishima M, Kanoh H, Izumi T. The spectrum of cutaneous eruptions in 22 patients with isolated serological evidence of infection by parvovirus B19. *Arch Dermatol* **135**(12):1556–1557, 1999.
69. Muir K, Todd WT, Watson WH, Fitzsimons E. Viral-associated haemophagocytosis with parvovirus-B19-related pancytopenia. *Lancet* **339**(8802):1139–1140, 1992.
70. Gratacos E, Torres PJ, Vidal J et al. The incidence of human parvovirus B19 infection during pregnancy and its impact on perinatal outcome. *J Infect Dis* **171**(5):1360–1363, 1995.
71. Prospective study of human parvovirus (B19) infection in pregnancy. Public Health Laboratory Service Working Party on Fifth Disease. *Br Med J* **300**(6733): 1166–1170, 1990.
72. Koch WC, Adler SP, Harger J. Intrauterine parvovirus B19 infection may cause an asymptomatic or recurrent postnatal infection. *Pediatr Infect Dis J* **12**(9):747–750, 1993.
73. Sheikh AU, Ernest JM, O'Shea M. Long-term outcome in fetal hydrops from parvovirus B19 infection. *Am J Obstet Gynecol* **167**(2):337–341, 1992.
74. Katz VL, McCoy MC, Kuller JA, Hansen WF. An association between fetal parvovirus B19 infection and fetal anomalies: a report of two cases. *Am J Perinatol* **13**(1):43–45, 1996.
75. Simchen MJ, Toi A, Bona M, Alkazaleh F, Ryan G, Chitayat D. Fetal hepatic calcifications: prenatal diagnosis and outcome. *Am J Obstet Gynecol* **187**(6): 1617–1622, 2002.
76. Zerbini M, Gentilomi GA, Gallinella G et al. Intra-uterine parvovirus B19 infection and meconium peritonitis. *Prenat Diagn* **18**(6):599–606, 1998.
77. Miniero R, Dalponte S, Linari A, Saracco P, Testa A, Musiani M. Severe Shwachman-Diamond syndrome and invasive parvovirus B19 infection. *Pediatr Hematol Oncol* **13**(6):555–561, 1996.
78. Weiner CP, Grose CF, Naides SJ. Diagnosis of fetal infection in the patient with an ultrasonographically detected abnormality but a negative clinical history. *Am J Obstet Gynecol* **168**(1 Pt 1): 6–11, 1993.
79. Smulian JC, Egan JF, Rodis JF. Fetal hydrops in the first trimester associated with maternal parvovirus infection. *J Clin Ultrasound* **26**(6):314–316, 1998.
80. Brandenburg H, Los FJ, Cohen-Overbeek TE. A case of early intrauterine parvovirus B19 infection. *Prenat Diagn* **16**(1):75–77, 1996.
81. Chisaka H, Morita E, Tada K, Yaegashi N, Okamura K, Sugamura K. Establishment of multifunctional monoclonal antibody to the nonstructural protein, NS1, of human parvovirus B19. *J Infect* **47**(3): 236–242, 2003.
82. Norbeck O, Papadogiannakis N, Petersson K, Hirbod T, Broliden K, Tolfvenstam T. Revised clinical presentation of parvovirus B19-associated intrauterine fetal death. *Clin Infect Dis* **35**(9):1032–1038, 2002.
83. Tolfvenstam T, Papadogiannakis N, Norbeck O, Petersson K, Broliden K. Frequency of human parvovirus B19 infection in intrauterine fetal death. *Lancet* **357**(9267):1494–1497, 2001.
84. Porter HJ, Khong TY, Evans MF, Chan VT, Fleming KA. Parvovirus as a cause of hydrops fetalis: detection by in situ DNA hybridisation. *J Clin Pathol* **41**(4):381–383, 1988.
85. Yaegashi N, Niinuma T, Chisaka H et al. The incidence of, and factors leading to, parvovirus B19-related hydrops fetalis following maternal infection: report of 10 cases and meta-analysis. *J Infect* **37**(1): 28–35, 1998.
86. Soothill P. Intrauterine blood transfusion for non-immune hydrops fetalis due to parvovirus B19 infection. *Lancet* **336**(8707):121–122, 1990.
87. Proust S, Philippe HJ, Paumier A, Joubert M, Boog G, Winer N. [Mirror pre-eclampsia: Ballantyne's syndrome. Two cases]. *J Gynecol Obstet Biol Reprod (Paris)* **35**(3):270–274, 2006.
88. von Kaisenberg CS, Bender G, Scheewe J et al. A case of fetal parvovirus B19 myocarditis, terminal cardiac heart failure, and perinatal heart transplantation. *Fetal Diagn Therm* **16**(6):427–432, 2001.
89. Craze JL, Salisbury AJ, Pike MG. Prenatal stroke associated with maternal parvovirus infection. *Dev Med Child Neurol* **38**(1):84–85, 1996.
90. Isumi H, Nunoue T, Nishida A, Takashima S. Fetal brain infection with human parvovirus B19. *Pediatr Neurol* **21**(3):661–663, 1999.
91. Zerbini M, Musiani M, Gentilomi G et al. Symptomatic parvovirus B19 infection of one fetus in a twin pregnancy. *Clin Infect Dis* **17**(2):262–263, 1993.
92. Plachouras N, Stefanidis K, Andronikou S, Lolis D. Severe nonimmune hydrops fetalis and congenital corneal opacification secondary to human parvovirus B19 infection: a case report. *J Reprod Med* **44**(4):377–380, 1999.
93. Tiessen RG, van Elsacker-Niele AM, Vermeij-Keers C, Oepkes D, van Roosmalen J, Gorsira MC. A fetus with a parvovirus B19 infection and congenital anomalies. *Prenat Diagn* **14**(3):173–176, 1994.

94. Rodis JF, Rodner C, Hansen AA et al. Long-term outcome of children following maternal human parvovirus B19 infection. *Obstet Gynecol* **91**(1): 125–128, 1998.
95. Mari G, Detti L, Oz U, Zimmerman R, Duerig P, Stefos T. Accurate prediction of fetal hemoglobin by Doppler ultrasonography. *Obstet Gynecol* **99**(4):589–593, 2002.
96. Cosmi E, Mari G, Delle Chiaie L et al. Noninvasive diagnosis by Doppler ultrasonography of fetal anemia resulting from parvovirus infection. *Am J Obstet Gynecol* **187**(5):1290–1293, 2002.
97. Mari G, Deter RL, Carpenter RL et al. Noninvasive diagnosis by Doppler ultrasonography of fetal anemia due to maternal red-cell alloimmunization. Collaborative Group for Doppler Assessment of the Blood Velocity in Anemic Fetuses. *N Engl J Med* **342**(1): 9–14, 2000.
98. Jordan JA, Huff D, DeLoia JA. Placental cellular immune response in women infected with human parvovirus B19 during pregnancy. *Clin Diagn Lab Immunol* **8**(2):288–292, 2001.
99. Beersma MF, Claas EC, Sopaheluakan T, Kroes AC. Parvovirus B19 viral loads in relation to VP1 and VP2 antibody responses in diagnostic blood samples. *J Clin Virol* **34**(1):71–75, 2005.
100. Enders M, Schalasta G, Baisch C et al. Human parvovirus B19 infection during pregnancy – value of modern molecular and serological diagnostics. *J Clin Virol* **35**(4):400–406, 2006.
101. Fairley CK, Smoleniec JS, Caul OE, Miller E. Observational study of effect of intrauterine transfusions on outcome of fetal hydrops after parvovirus B19 infection. *Lancet* **46**(8986):1335–1337, 1995.
102. Rodis JF, Borgida AF, Wilson M, et al. Management of parvovirus infection in pregnancy and outcomes of hydrops: a survey of members of the Society of Perinatal Obstetricians. *Am J Obstet Gynecol*, **179**(4):985–988, 19988.
103. Schild RL, Plath H, Thomas P, Schulte-Wissermann H, Eis-Hubinger AM, Hansmann M. Fetal parvovirus B19 infection and meconium peritonitis. *Fetal Diagn Ther* **13**(1):15–18, 1998.
104. Hernandez-Andrade E, Scheier M, Dezerega V, Carmo A, Nicolaides KH. Fetal middle cerebral artery peak systolic velocity in the investigation of non-immune hydrops. *Ultrasound Obstet Gynecol* **23**(5):442–445, 2004.
105. Odibo AO, Campbell WA, Feldman D et al. Resolution of human parvovirus B19-induced nonimmune hydrops after intrauterine transfusion. *J Ultrasound Med* **17**(9):547–550, 1998.
106. Ballou WR, Reed JL, Noble W, Young NS, Koenig S. Safety and immunogenicity of a recombinant parvovirus B19 vaccine formulated with MF59C.1. *J Infect Dis* **187**(4):675–678, 2003.
107. Connolly JH, Hutchinson WM, Allen IV et al. Carotid artery thrombosis, encephalitis, myelitis and optic neuritis associated with rubella virus infections. *Brain* **98**(4):583–594, 1975.
108. Sharan S, Sharma S, Billson FA. Congenital rubella cataract: a timely reminder in the new millennium? *Clin Experiment Ophthalmol* **34**(1):83–84, 2006.
109. Rowen M, Singer MJ, Moran ET. Intracranial calcification in the congenital rubella syndrome. *Am J Roentgenol Radium Ther Nucl Med* **115**(1):86–91, 1972.
110. Preblud SR, Gross F, Halsey NA, Hinman AR, Herrmann KL, Koplan JP. Assessment of susceptibility to measles and rubella. *J Am Med Assoc* **247**(8): 1134–1137, 1982.
111. Choutet P, Binet CH, Goudeau A, Perrotin D, Ginies G, Lamisse F. Bone-marrow aplasia and primary rubella infection. *Lancet* **2**(8149):966–967, 1979.
112. Klein HZ, Markarian M. Dermal erythropoiesis in congenital rubella. Description of an infected newborn who had purpura associated with marked extramedullary erythropoiesis in the skin and elsewhere. *Clin Pediatr (Phila)* **8**(10):604–607, 1969.
113. Floret D, Rosenberg D, Hage GN, Monnet P. Hyperthyroidism, diabetes mellitus and the congenital rubella syndrome. *Acta Paediatr Scand* **69**(2): 259–261, 1980.
114. Preece MA, Kearney PJ, Marshall WC. Growth-hormone deficiency in congenital rubella. *Lancet* **2**(8043): 842–844, 1977.
115. Clarke WL, Shaver KA, Bright GM, Rogol AD, Nance WE. Autoimmunity in congenital rubella syndrome. *J Pediatr* **104**(3):370–373, 1984.
116. Walls WL, Altman DH, Gair DR, Litt RE. Roentgenological findings in congenital rubella. *Clin Pediatr (Phila)* **4**(12):704–708, 1965.
117. Wui ET, Ling LH, Yang H. Severe aortic regurgitation: an exceptional cardiac manifestation of congenital rubella syndrome. *Int J Cardiol* **113**(2):e46–e47, 2006.
118. Malathi J, Therese KL, Madhavan HN. The association of rubella virus in congenital cataract – a hospital-based study in India. *J Clin Virol* **23**(1–2):25–29, 2001.
119. Kaplan GW, McLaughlin AP. Urogenital anomalies and congenital rubella syndrome. *Urology* **2**(2):148–152, 1973.
120. Radner M, Vergesslich KA, Weninger M, Eilenberger M, Ponhold W, Pollak A. Meconium peritonitis: a new finding in rubella syndrome. *J Clin Ultrasound* **21**(5):346–349, 1993.
121. Ueda K, Hisanaga S, Nishida Y, Shepard TH. Low-birth-weight and congenital rubella syndrome: effect of gestational age at time of maternal rubella infection. *Clin Pediatr (Phila)* **20**(11):730–733, 1981.
122. Miller E, Cradock-Watson JE, Pollock TM. Consequences of confirmed maternal rubella at successive stages of pregnancy. *Lancet* **2**(8302):781–784, 1982.
123. Enders G, Nickerl-Pacher U, Miller E, Cradock-Watson JE. Outcome of confirmed periconceptional maternal rubella. *Lancet* **1**(8600):1445–14447, 1988.
124. Peckham C. Congenital rubella in the United Kingdom before 1970: the prevaccine era. *Rev Infect Dis* **7**(Suppl 1):S11–s16, 1985.
125. Sever JL, Hardy JB, Nelson KB, Gilkeson MR. Rubella in the collaborative perinatal research study. II. Clinical and laboratory findings in children through 3 years of age. *Am J Dis Child* **118**(1): 123–132, 1969.
126. Sever JL, Nelson KB, Gilkeson MR. Rubella epidemic, 1964: effect on 6,000 pregnancies. *Am J Dis Child* **110**(4): 395–407, 1965.
127. Kobayashi K, Tajima M, Toishi S, Fujimori K, Suzuki Y, Udagawa H. Fetal growth restriction associated with measles virus infection during pregnancy. *J Perinat Med* **33**(1):67–68, 2005.
128. Chiba ME, Saito M, Suzuki N, Honda Y, Yaegashi N. Measles infection in pregnancy. *J Infect* **47**(1):40–44, 2003.
129. McDonald JC, Peckham CS. Gammaglobulin in prevention of rubella and congenital defect: a study of 30,000 pregnancies. *Br Med J* **3**(566):633–637, 1967.
130. McCallin PF, Fuccillo DA, Ley AC, Gilkeson MR, Traub RG, Sever JL. Gammaglobulin as prophylaxis against rubella-induced congenital anomalies. *Obstet Gynecol* **39**(2):185–189, 1972.
131. Brody JA, Sever JL, Schiff GM. Prevention of rubella by gamma globulin during an epidemic in Barrow, Alaska, in 1964. *N Engl J Med* **272**: 127–129, 1965.
132. Preblud SR, D'Angelo LJ. Chickenpox in the United States, 1972–1977. *J Infect Dis* **140**(2):257–260, 1979.
133. LaRussa P, Steinberg SP, Seeman MD, Gershon AA. Determination of immunity to varicella-zoster virus by means of an intradermal skin test. *J Infect Dis* **152**(5):869–875, 1985.
134. Balducci J, Rodis JF, Rosengren S, Vintzileos AM, Spivey G, Vosseller C. Pregnancy outcome following first-trimester varicella infection. *Obstet Gynecol* **79**(1):5–6, 1992.
135. Weber DM, Pellecchia JA. Varicella pneumonia: study of prevalence in adult men. *J Am Med Assoc* **192**:572–573, 1965.
136. Rawlinson WD, Dwyer DE, Gibbons VL, Cunningham AL. Rapid diagnosis of

varicella-zoster virus infection with a monoclonal antibody based direct immunofluorescence technique. *J Virol Methods* **23**(1):13–18, 1989.
137. Koropchak CM, Graham G, Palmer J et al. Investigation of varicella-zoster virus infection by polymerase chain reaction in the immunocompetent host with acute varicella. *J Infect Dis* **163**(5):1016–1022, 1991.
138. Koropchak CM, Graham G, Palmer J et al. Investigation of varicella-zoster virus infection by polymerase chain reaction in the immunocompetent host with acute varicella. *J Infect Dis* **165**(1):188, 1992.
139. Siegel M. Congenital malformations following chickenpox, measles, mumps, and hepatitis: results of a cohort study. *J Am Med Assoc* **226**(13):1521–1524, 1973.
140. Brunell PA, Kotchmar GS, Jr. Zoster in infancy: failure to maintain virus latency following intrauterine infection. *J Pediatr* **98**(1):71–73, 1981.
141. Paryani SG, Arvin AM. Intrauterine infection with varicella-zoster virus after maternal varicella, N Engl J Med, 1986; 314(24): 1542–1156
142. Enders G, Miller E, Cradock-Watson J, Bolley I, Ridehalgh M. Consequences of varicella and herpes zoster in pregnancy: prospective study of 1739 cases. *Lancet* **343**(8912):1548–1551, 1994.
143. Harger JH, Ernest JM, Thurnau GR et al. Frequency of congenital varicella syndrome in a prospective cohort of 347 pregnant women. *Obstet Gynecol* **100**(2):260–265, 2002.
144. Michie CA, Acolet D, Charlton R et al. Varicella-zoster contracted in the second trimester of pregnancy. *Pediatr Infect Dis J* **11**(12):1050–1053, 1992.
145. Palmer CG, Pauli RM. Intrauterine varicella infection. *J Pediatr* **112**(3): 506–507, 1988.
146. Bai PV, John TJ. Congenital skin ulcers following varicella in late pregnancy. *J Pediatr* **94**(1):65–67, 1979.
147. Pretorius DH, Hayward I, Jones KL, Stamm E. Sonographic evaluation of pregnancies with maternal varicella infection. *J Ultrasound Med* **11**(9):459–463, 1992.
148. Mouly F, Mirlesse V, Meritet JF et al. Prenatal diagnosis of fetal varicella-zoster virus infection with polymerase chain reaction of amniotic fluid in 107 cases. *Am J Obstet Gynecol* **177**(4):894–898, 1997.
149. Cuthbertson G, Weiner CP, Giller RH, Grose C. Prenatal diagnosis of second-trimester congenital varicella syndrome by virus-specific immunoglobulin M. *J Pediatr* **111**(4):592–595, 1987.
150. Scharf A, Scherr O, Enders G, Helftenbein E. Virus detection in the fetal tissue of a premature delivery with a congenital varicella syndrome: a case report. *J Perinat Med* **18**(4):317–322, 1990.
151. Petignat P, Vial Y, Laurini R, Hohlfeld P. Fetal varicella-herpes zoster syndrome in early pregnancy: ultrasonographic and morphological correlation. *Prenat Diagn* **21**(2):121–124, 2001.
152. Hofmeyr GJ, Moolla S, Lawrie T. Prenatal sonographic diagnosis of congenital varicella infection: a case report. *Prenat Diagn* **16**(12):1148–1151, 1996.
153. Ong CL, Daniel ML. Antenatal diagnosis of a porencephalic cyst in congenital varicella-zoster virus infection. *Pediatr Radiol* **28**(2):94, 1998.
154. Da Silva O, Hammerberg O, Chance GW. Fetal varicella syndrome. *Pediatr Infect Dis J* **9**(11):854–855, 1990.
155. Newman CG. Perinatal varicella. *Lancet* **2**(7423):1159–1161, 1965.
156. Pearson HE. Parturition varicella-zoster. *Obstet Gynecol* **23**:21–27, 1964.
157. Brunell PA. Varicella-zoster infections in pregnancy. *J Am Med Assoc* **199**(5):315–317, 1967.
158. Siegel M, Fuerst HT. Low birth weight and maternal virus diseases: a prospective study of rubella, measles, mumps, chickenpox, and hepatitis. *J Am Med Assoc* **197**(9):680–684, 1966.
159. Meyers JD. Congenital varicella in term infants: risk reconsidered. *J Infect Dis* **129**(2):215–217, 1974.
160. Hanngren K, Grandien M, Granstrom G. Effect of zoster immunoglobulin for varicella prophylaxis in the newborn. *Scand J Infect Dis* **17**(4):343–347, 1985.
161. Koren G. Risk of varicella infection during late pregnancy. *Can Fam Physician* **49**:1445–1446, 2003.
162. Dunkle LM, Arvin AM, Whitley RJ et al. A controlled trial of acyclovir for chickenpox in normal children. *N Engl J Med* **325**(22):1539–1544, 1991.
163. Brunell PA, Ross A, Miller LH, Kuo B. Prevention of varicella by zoster immune globulin. *N Engl J Med* **280**(22):1191–1194, 1969.
164. C.D.C. Prevention of varicella: recommendations of the Advisory Committee on Immunization Practices (ACIP). *Morb Mortal Wkly Rep* **45**:1, 1996.
165. Bonametti AM, Passos JN, Koga da Silva EM, Macedo ZS. Probable transmission of acute toxoplasmosis through breast feeding. *J Trop Pediatr* **43**(2):116, 1997.
166. Langer H. Repeated congenital infection with toxoplasma gondii. *Obstet Gynecol* **21**:318–329, 1963.
167. Tenter AM, Heckeroth AR, Weiss LM. Toxoplasma gondii: from animals to humans. *Int J Parasitol* **30**(12–13): 1217–1258, 2000.
168. Jones JL, Kruszon-Moran D, Wilson M, McQuillan G, Navin T, McAuley JB. Toxoplasma gondii infection in the United States: seroprevalence and risk factors. *Am J Epidemiol* **154**(4):357–365, 2001.
169. Montoya JG, Liesenfeld O. Toxoplasmosis. *Lancet* **363**(9425): 1965–1976, 2004.
170. Gras L, Gilbert RE, Wallon M, Peyron F, Cortina-Borja M. Duration of the IgM response in women acquiring Toxoplasma gondii during pregnancy: implications for clinical practice and cross-sectional incidence studies. *Epidemiol Infect* **132**(3):541–548, 2004.
171. Boyer KM. Diagnosis and treatment of congenital toxoplasmosis. *Adv Pediatr Infect Dis* **11**:449–467, 1996.
172. Hohlfeld P, Daffos F, Thulliez P et al. Fetal toxoplasmosis: outcome of pregnancy and infant follow-up after in utero treatment. *J Pediatr* **115**(5 Pt 1): 765–769, 1989.
173. Lynfield R, Guerina NG. Toxoplasmosis. *Pediatr Rev* **18**(3):75–83, 1997.
174. Foulon W, Pinon JM, Stray-Pedersen B et al. Prenatal diagnosis of congenital toxoplasmosis: a multicenter evaluation of different diagnostic parameters. *Am J Obstet Gynecol* **181**(4):843–847, 1999.
175. Remington J. Toxoplasmosis. In *Infectious diseases of the fetus and newborn infant*, JS Remington (ed.), pp. 89–195. Philadelphia: WD Saunders, 1990.
176. Swisher CN, Boyer K, McLeod R. Congenital toxoplasmosis: The Toxoplasmosis Study Group. *Semin Pediatr Neurol* **1**(1):4–25, 1994.
177. Guerina NG, Hsu HW, Meissner HC et al. Neonatal serologic screening and early treatment for congenital Toxoplasma gondii infection: The New England Regional Toxoplasma Working Group. *N Engl J Med* **330**(26):1858–1863, 1994.
178. Vutova K, Peicheva Z, Popova A, Markova V, Mincheva N, Todorov T. Congenital toxoplasmosis: eye manifestations in infants and children. *Ann Trop Paediatr* **22**(3):213–218, 2002.
179. Wallon M, Kodjikian L, Binquet C et al. Long-term ocular prognosis in 327 children with congenital toxoplasmosis. *Pediatrics* **113**(6):1567–1572, 2004.
180. Wilson CB, Remington JS. What can be done to prevent congenital toxoplasmosis? *Am J Obstet Gynecol* **138**(4):357–363, 1980.
181. Daffos F, Forestier F, Capella-Pavlovsky M et al. Prenatal management of 746 pregnancies at risk for congenital toxoplasmosis. *N Engl J Med* **318**(5): 271–275, 1988.
182. Hohlfeld P, Daffos F, Costa JM, Thulliez P, Forestier F, Vidaud M. Prenatal diagnosis of congenital toxoplasmosis with a polymerase-chain-reaction test on amniotic fluid. *N Engl J Med* **331**(11): 695–699, 1994.
183. Antsaklis A, Daskalakis G, Papantoniou N, Mentis A, Michalas S. Prenatal

diagnosis of congenital toxoplasmosis. *Prenat Diagn* **22**(12):1107–1111, 2002.

184. Hohlfeld P, MacAleese J, Capella-Pavlovski M et al. Fetal toxoplasmosis: ultrasonographic signs. *Ultrasound Obstet Gynecol* **1**(4):241–244, 1991.
185. Becker LE. Infections of the developing brain. *Am J Neuroradiol* **13**(2):537–549, 1992.
186. Blaakaer J. Ultrasonic diagnosis of fetal ascites and toxoplasmosis. *Acta Obstet Gynecol Scand* **65**(6):653–654, 1986.
187. Vanhaesebrouck P, De Wit M, Smets K, De Praeter C, Leroy JG. Congenital toxoplasmosis presenting as massive neonatal ascites. *Helv Paediatr Acta* **43**(1–2):97–101, 1988.
188. Gilbert R, Gras L. Effect of timing and type of treatment on the risk of mother to child transmission of Toxoplasma gondii. *Br J Obstet Gynaecol* **110**(2):112–120, 2003.
189. WHO model prescribing information: Drugs used in parasitic diseases. Geneva: World Health Organization, 1995.
190. Wallon M, Liou C, Garner P, Peyron F. Congenital toxoplasmosis: systematic review of evidence of efficacy of treatment in pregnancy. *Br Med J* **318**(7197):1511–1514, 1999.
191. Gras L, Gilbert RE, Ades AE, Dunn DT. Effect of prenatal treatment on the risk of intracranial and ocular lesions in children with congenital toxoplasmosis. *Int J Epidemiol* **30**(6):1309–1313, 2001.
192. Gratzl R, Sodeck G, Platzer P et al. Treatment of toxoplasmosis in pregnancy: concentrations of spiramycin and neospiramycin in maternal serum and amniotic fluid. *Eur J Clin Microbiol Infect Dis* **21**(1):12–16, 2002.
193. Neto EC, Rubin R, Schulte J, Giugliani R. Newborn screening for congenital infectious diseases. *Emerg Infect Dis* **10**(6):1068–1073, 2004.
194. Gilbert RE, Gras L, Wallon M, Peyron F, Ades AE, Dunn DT. Effect of prenatal treatment on mother to child transmission of Toxoplasma gondii: retrospective cohort study of 554 mother–child pairs in Lyon, France. *Int J Epidemiol* **30**(6):1303–1308, 2001.
195. Gilbert R, Dunn D, Wallon M et al. Ecological comparison of the risks of mother-to-child transmission and clinical manifestations of congenital toxoplasmosis according to prenatal treatment protocol. *Epidemiol Infect* **127**(1):113–120, 2001.
196. Bessieres MH, Berrebi A, Rolland M et al. Neonatal screening for congenital toxoplasmosis in a cohort of 165 women infected during pregnancy and influence of in utero treatment on the results of neonatal tests. *Eur J Obstet Gynecol Reprod Biol* **94**(1):37–45, 2001.
197. Foulon W, Naessens A, Ho-Yen D. Prevention of congenital toxoplasmosis. *J Perinat Med* **28**(5):337–345, 2000.
198. Bhopale GM. Development of a vaccine for toxoplasmosis: current status. *Microbes Infect* **5**(5):457–462, 2003.
199. Buxton D, Innes EA. A commercial vaccine for ovine toxoplasmosis. *Parasitology* **110**(Suppl):S11–s16, 1995.
200. Wendel GD. Gestational and congenital syphilis. *Clin Perinatol* **15**(2):287–303, 1988.
201. Sanchez PJ, Wendel GD, Jr, Grimprel E et al. Evaluation of molecular methodologies and rabbit infectivity testing for the diagnosis of congenital syphilis and neonatal central nervous system invasion by Treponema pallidum. *J Infect Dis* **167**(1):148–157, 1993.
202. Remington J. *Syphilis. Infectious diseases of the fetus and newborn infant*, pp. 545–580. Philadelphia: Elsevier Saunders, 2006.
203. Harter C, Benirschke K. Fetal syphilis in the first trimester. *Am J Obstet Gynecol* **124**(7):705–711, 1976.
204. Nathan L, Bohman VR, Sanchez PJ, Leos NK, Twickler DM, Wendel GD, Jr. In utero infection with Treponema pallidum in early pregnancy. *Prenat Diagn* **17**(2):119–123, 1997.
205. Woods CR. Syphilis in children: congenital and acquired. *Semin Pediatr Infect Dis* **16**(4):245–257, 2005.
206. Hollier LM, Harstad TW, Sanchez PJ, Twickler DM, Wendel GD, Jr. Fetal syphilis: clinical and laboratory characteristics. *Obstet Gynecol* **97**(6): 947–953, 2001.
207. Whitaker JA, Sartain P, Shaheedy M. Hematological aspects of congenital syphilis. *J Pediatr* **66**:629–636, 1965.
208. Nathan L, Twickler DM, Peters MT, Sanchez PJ, Wendel GD, Jr. Fetal syphilis: correlation of sonographic findings and rabbit infectivity testing of amniotic fluid. *J Ultrasound Med* **12**(2):97–101, 1993.
209. Hill LM, Maloney JB. An unusual constellation of sonographic findings associated with congenital syphilis. *Obstet Gynecol* **78**(5 Pt 2):895–897, 1991.
210. Zelop C, Benacerraf BR. The causes and natural history of fetal ascites. *Prenat Diagn* **14**(10):941–946, 1994.
211. Satin AJ, Twickler DM, Wendel GD, Jr. Congenital syphilis associated with dilation of fetal small bowel: a case report. *J Ultrasound Med* **11**(1):49–52, 1992.
212. Sanchez PJ, Wendel GD. Syphilis in pregnancy. *Clin Perinatol* **24**(1):71–90, 1997.
213. McFarlin BL, Bottoms SF, Dock BS, Isada NB. Epidemic syphilis: maternal factors associated with congenital infection. *Am J Obstet Gynecol* **170**(2):535–540, 1994.
214. Klein VR, Cox SM, Mitchell MD, Wendel GD, Jr. The Jarisch–Herxheimer reaction complicating syphilotherapy in pregnancy. *Obstet Gynecol* **75**(3 Pt 1): 375–380, 1990.
215. Sanchez PJ, Wendel GD, Norgard MV. Congenital syphilis associated with negative results of maternal serologic tests at delivery. *Am J Dis Child* **145**(9):967–969, 1991.
216. Coles FB, Hipp SS, Silberstein GS, Chen JH. Congenital syphilis surveillance in upstate New York, 1989–1992: implications for prevention and clinical management. *J Infect Dis* **171**(3):732–735, 1995.

CHAPTER

45 Amniotic fluid

Pamela A Mahon and Karim D Kalache

KEY POINTS

- This chapter deals with the mechanisms responsible for amniotic fluid production and with the sonographic assessment of amniotic volume at different gestational ages
- Deficient amniotic fluid (oligohydramnios) or an excess (polyhydramnios) are frequently the first clues to an underlying fetal abnormality or maternal disease state
- Amniotic fluid volume abnormalities can be assessed subjectively by visual interpretation without sonographic measurements
- The use of an objective measure (amniotic fluid index) is considered best practice solely in patients with an abnormal subjective evaluation, at increased risk of pregnancy complications and in all patients examined in the third trimester

INTRODUCTION

Sonographers and sonologists providing maternity care often face a scenario in which the patient is noted to have deficient amniotic fluid (oligohydramnios) or an excess (polyhydramnios). Both conditions are associated with increased perinatal morbidity and mortality[1,2]. Thus, a basic understanding of the mechanisms responsible for amniotic fluid production and knowledge of accurate assessment of amniotic volume at different gestational ages are fundamental to the appropriate management of pregnancies complicated by amniotic fluid volume disorders.

AMNIOTIC FLUID

Amniotic fluid serves as a reservoir of fluid and nutrients for the fetus, provides mechanical cushioning to the fetus and the umbilical cord and has antibacterial properties that provide some protection from infection. In addition, it facilitates normal growth and maturation of the fetal lungs, musculoskeletal and gastrointestinal systems, by providing the necessary fluid, space and growth factors[3].

Mechanisms that regulate amniotic fluid volume are still not completely understood. Before 6 weeks of gestation, there are two fluid sacs that surround the embryo, the amniotic sac containing amniotic fluid and the extracelomic space containing celomic fluid. The composition of celomic fluid is similar to maternal plasma and different from amniotic fluid[4], suggesting that maternal plasma may be its source. Maximum celomic fluid volume is achieved around the 10th week of development and decreases until 12–14 weeks of development when it completely disappears as the amniotic and chorionic membranes fuse. It is likely that solutes and fluid from the exocelomic cavity cross the amniotic membrane into the amniotic fluid and that celomic fluid is an early source of amniotic fluid. Jauniaux et al.[5] provided evidence of this flow system at approximately 9 weeks of pregnancy using inulin, which is an inert substance that can cross from the maternal circulation to the extracelomic space. They showed that inulin can pass into the amniotic cavity where it accumulates. By 7 weeks, as the placenta and fetal vessels develop, maternal plasma passes across the placenta to the fetus and across the fetal skin, which has not yet become keratinized, and the surface of the amnion, placenta and umbilical cord to the amniotic fluid. At about the 10th week of pregnancy, embryonic organs commence excretion which contributes to amniotic fluid accumulation. By 22–24 weeks, the fetal skin is fully keratinized and amniotic fluid volume is determined by the rate of fetal urine excretion and the secretion of pulmonary fluid. Removal is predominantly accomplished by fetal swallowing and transfer through the amniotic membranes[3].

Brace and Wolf[6] reviewed the literature pertaining to the practical assessment of this process and compiled 705 measurements of amniotic fluid between 8 and 43 weeks of gestation. All of the calculations were either by a dye-dilution technique or by direct measurement at hysterotomy. They reported that amniotic fluid volume increased progressively until 33 weeks of gestation when it was shown to plateau.

METHODS OF AMNIOTIC FLUID VOLUME ASSESSMENT

Normal amniotic fluid volume, oligohydramnios or polyhydramnios can be assessed subjectively by visual interpretation

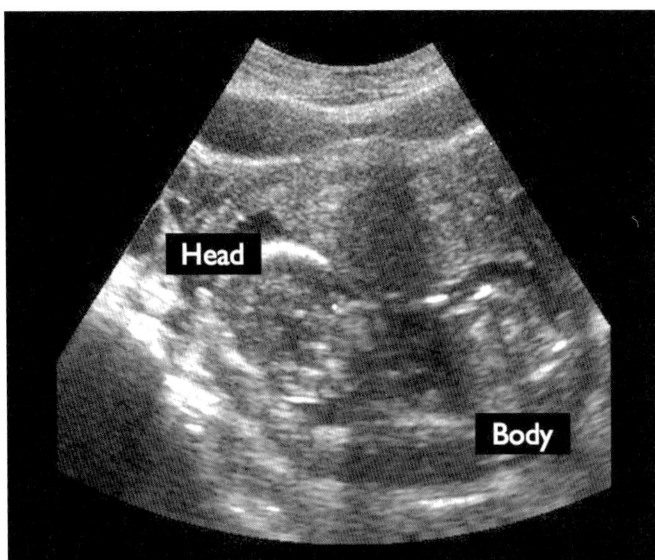

Fig. 45.1 Scan appearance of oligohydramnios. Note the fetal crowding and reduced amniotic fluid pockets.

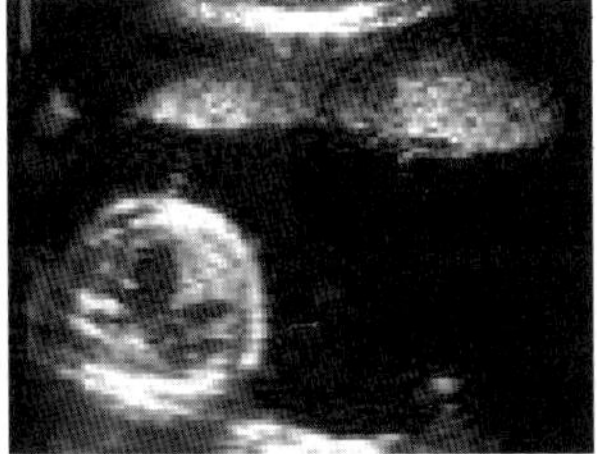

Fig. 45.2 Scan appearance of polyhydramnios in a fetus with left-sided congenital diaphragmatic hernia at 24 weeks' gestation. Note the increased fluid allowing free fetal movement.

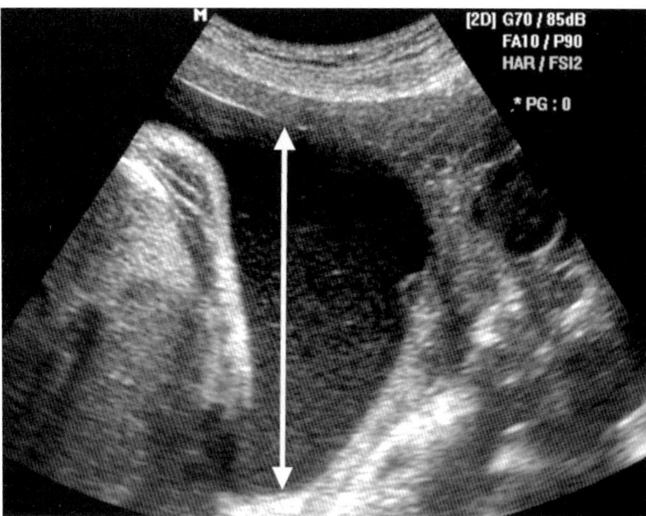

Fig. 45.3 To obtain the best measurement of a single deepest pool of amniotic fluid, a subjective assessment of the fluid is made by the operator in choosing the greatest pocket of amniotic fluid. A vertical measurement is then made from the inner edge of the anterior uterine cavity to the interior edge of the posterior part of the uterine cavity. This measurement should not pass through fetal parts or umbilical cord.

without the need for sonographic measurements by experienced operators[7]. In practice, the appearance of fetal crowding and an obvious absence of fluid pockets throughout the uterine cavity (Fig. 45.1) is used to define oligohydramnios. An increase in the amount of fluid surrounding the fetus, which allows the fetus to move freely (Fig. 45.2) is traditionally termed hydramnios, or polyhydramnios where the increase exceeds a defined value, a subject of debate between various centers. Good intra-observer and inter-observer agreement between subjective assessment and measurement of the single largest pocket determination of amniotic fluid volume have been reported[8]. However, subjective assessment of amniotic fluid volume will not allow comparison of results from serial examinations as the fetal condition changes.

Over the past 25 years, a number of investigators have created models to standardize the measurement of amniotic fluid volume. The importance of having a consistent definition for quantitative assessment of fetal condition in prenatal diagnosis cannot be overemphasized. A review of the pertinent literature shows, however, that at various times, many different definitions for abnormal amniotic fluid volume have been used. Manning et al.[9] proposed to measure the single deepest pocket of amniotic fluid free of fetal extremities and umbilical cord to assess amniotic fluid volume (Fig. 45.3). Qualitative amniotic fluid volume was first termed normal if at least one pocket of amniotic fluid measuring 1 cm in its broadest diameter was identified[10]. This definition was found to be too restrictive and normal amniotic fluid was redefined by the same group using two further definitions including the 1 × 1-cm pocket[11] and the 2 × 1-cm pocket[12]. The 2 × 2-cm pocket technique appears to be a new measurement. Again, the reference cited by ACOG for this technique is Manning et al's 1990 publication[13], which used a 2 × 1-cm pocket to define adequate amniotic volume. Furthermore, it is unclear from the literature how often and how useful this measurement has been used to define sensitively low amniotic fluid volumes.

The amniotic fluid index (AFI) was proposed as a means to evaluate more quantitatively amniotic fluid volume throughout the uterine cavity at 36–42 weeks of gestation (Fig. 45.4). It was hoped that this could aid prediction of a poor pregnancy outcome or the success of external cephalic versions[14]. This method sums the maximum vertical pocket of amniotic fluid in each quadrant of the uterus not containing cord or fetal extremities (Fig. 45.4). Using this technique, oligohydramnios is either defined as an amniotic fluid index <5.0 cm[15] or below the 5th percentile for gestational age[16]. The test is reproducible, with inter-observer and intra-observer variations of 10–15% or 1–2 cm in pregnancies with normal AFI. The margin of error is less in patients with decreased amounts of amniotic fluid. Color Doppler is helpful when evaluating low AFIs[17].

In clinical practice, ultrasound estimation of amniotic fluid volume is used in conjunction with other sonographic assessments, such as biometry for estimated fetal weight, anatomical survey and Doppler studies, to provide useful information for managing complicated pregnancies. Subjective assessment of amniotic fluid volume in all ultrasound examinations and the use of an objective measure if the subjective evaluation is abnormal, is considered best practice in patients at increased risk of pregnancy complications, and in all patients examined in the third trimester.

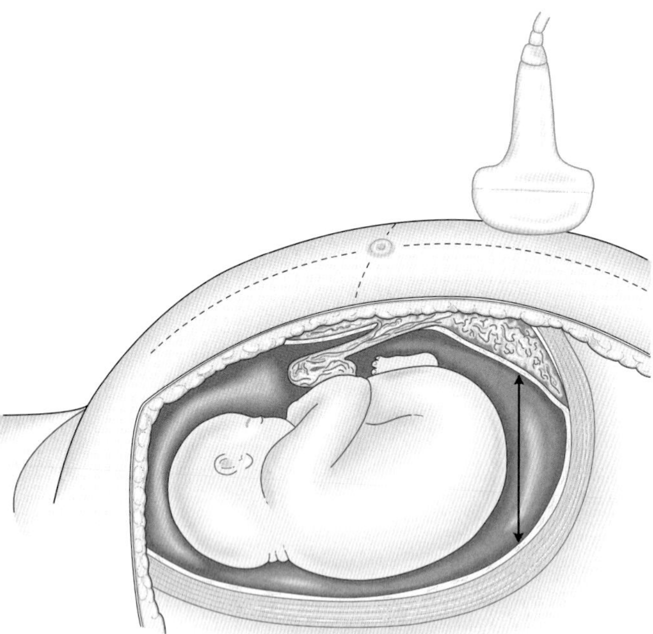

Fig. 45.4 The amniotic fluid index (AFI) measurement is calculated by first dividing the uterus into four quadrants using the linea nigra for the right and left divisions and the umbilicus for the upper and lower quadrants. The maximum vertical amniotic fluid pocket diameter in each quadrant not containing cord or fetal extremities is measured in centimeters. The sum of these measurements in centimeters is the AFI. Measurements may be artificially increased if the transducer is not maintained perpendicular to the floor. Excessive pressure on the maternal abdomen with the transducer may lead to an artificially reduced measurement.

Many studies have shown that the AFI method and the 2 × 2-cm pocket have equal diagnostic accuracies. The 2 × 2-cm technique may be a better means of assessing the amniotic fluid volume in twin gestations and in pregnancies at an early gestational age. Some study results have shown that the AFI has greater sensitivity and a higher predictive value than the 2 × 2-cm technique in diagnosing abnormally high and low amniotic fluid volumes. Currently, most obstetricians prefer to assess a broader area of the uterine cavity by using the AFI because the single measurement of the 2 × 2-cm technique does not allow for an asymmetric fetal position in the uterus.

Three-dimensional ultrasound determination of amniotic fluid volume offers the opportunity to quantify accurately the volume of amniotic fluid pockets and significant correlations between three-dimensional amniotic fluid volumes and AFI ($r = 0.9$, $P < 0.001$) on one side and two-dimensional area ($r = 0.86$, $P < 0.001$) on the other side have been reported[18].

OLIGOHYDRAMNIOS

Oligohydramnios is typically diagnosed by ultrasound examination either in the second trimester at the time of the anomaly scan or later in pregnancy following an ultrasound evaluation for decreased fetal movement or lag in sequential fundal height measurements.

Etiology

Oligohydramnios is secondary to either a loss of fluid or a decrease in fetal urine production or excretion. Etiology is directly related to gestational age at presentation.

Oligohydramnios diagnosed by ultrasound examination in the second trimester at the time of the anomaly scan is commonly caused by *preterm premature rupture of the membranes* (PPROM). Second-trimester PPROM that is associated with oligohydramnios has a particularly poor prognosis with an approximate survival rate of 10%[19]. The earlier in pregnancy that oligohydramnios occurs, the poorer the prognosis. Fetal mortality rates as high as 80–90% have been reported with oligohydramnios diagnosed in the second trimester. Most of this mortality is a result of pulmonary hypoplasia secondary to PPROM before 22 weeks of gestation. The presence of amniotic fluid is required for terminal alveolar development and a reduction in amniotic fluid pressure as a result of oligohydramnios results in a net egress of fluid from the lungs, which can result in pulmonary hypoplasia[20]. Facial and skeletal deformities can occur later and are due to the restriction of fetal movement with oligohydramnios.

Oligohydramnios is a frequent finding in pregnancies involving *intrauterine growth restriction* (IUGR). Historically, the association between intrauterine growth restriction and oligohydramnios has been attributed to decreased fetal urine production. Chronic hypoxia in IUGR results in shunting of fetal blood away from the kidneys to more vital organs. This is associated with decreased renal perfusion, which prevents the formation of urine. However, animal studies have not found that hypoxemia significantly effects urine formation[21]. There is a direct relationship between decreased amniotic fluid volume and the prevalence of IUGR. When a single pocket of amniotic fluid is >2 cm, between 1 and 2 cm and <1 cm, the prevalence of intrauterine growth restriction is 5%, 20% and 37%, respectively[22] (see Chapter 39).

The cause of decreased amniotic fluid volume in post-term pregnancies is unknown. The decreased efficiency of placental function has been proposed as a cause, but this has never been confirmed histologically. Decreased fetal renal blood flow and decreased fetal urine production have been demonstrated beyond 42 weeks in pregnancies involving oligohydramnios. Nevertheless, amniotic fluid volume is considered as an important predictor of fetal well-being in pregnancies beyond 40 weeks and *post-term pregnancies*. Although induction of labor in post-term patients with oligohydramnios (AFI <5 cm or no vertical pocket >2 cm) is considered the standard of care, adherence to this practice clearly results in subsequent increase in labor complications and the incidence of operative delivery potentially without significantly improving outcome[23]. Some researchers concluded that isolated oligohydramnios in patients with appropriate fetal size for gestational age, in the absence of maternal disease, may not be a marker of fetal compromise and induction of labor may therefore not be warranted in most cases[24]. A majority of post-term fetuses, however, are neither immature nor hypoxic and will have a benign perinatal course[25].

The majority of congenital anomalies associated with oligohydramnios involve those associated with congenital absence of functional renal tissue or obstructive uropathy (see Chapter 35). Bilateral renal agenesis can result in oligohydramnios and transvaginal sonography[26] with color or power Doppler[27] can be used to confirm the presence or absence of the kidneys and

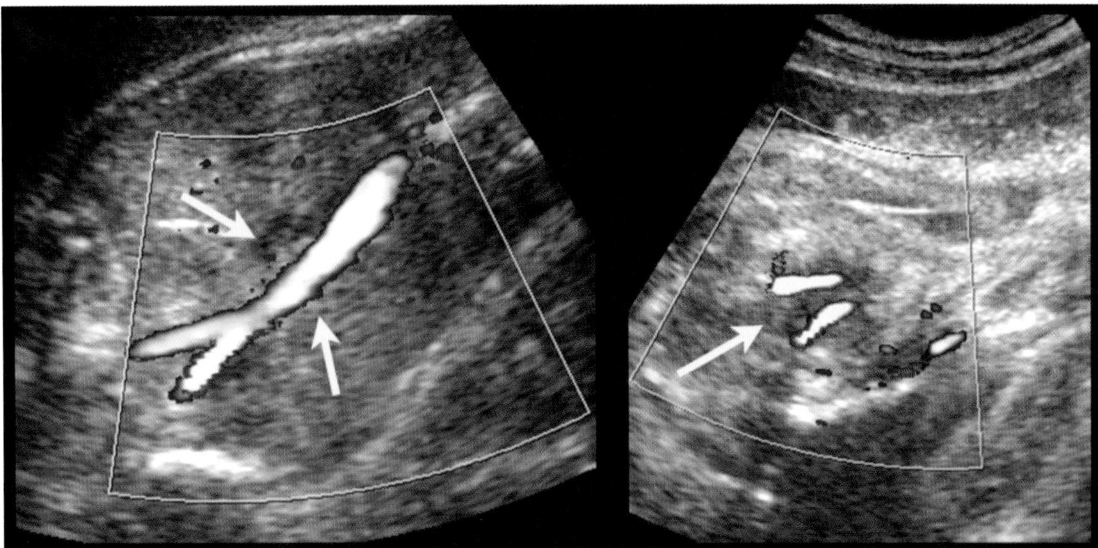

Fig. 45.5 Oligohydramnios due to bilateral renal agenesis. Color Doppler of the aorta shows absent renal arteries in the left picture, and an empty bladder between the intra-abdominal unbilical arteries on the right.

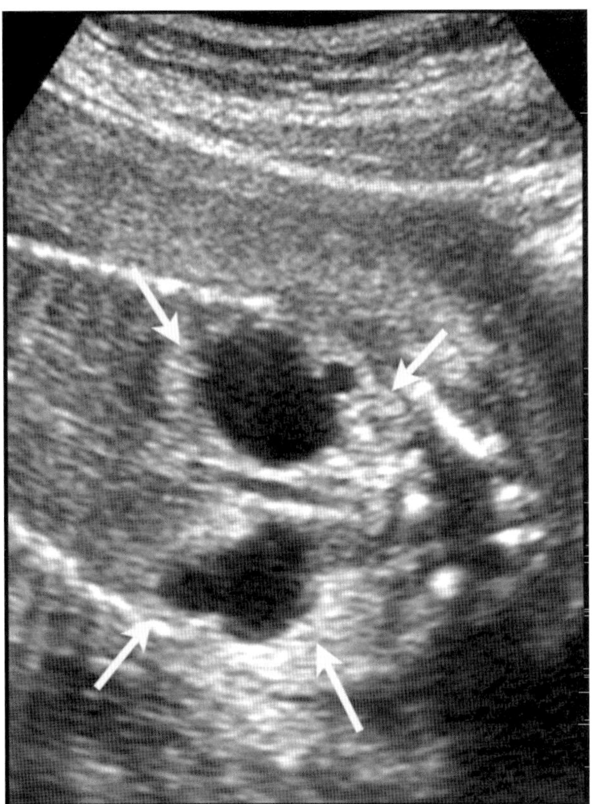

Fig. 45.6 Bilateral fetal hydronephrosis associated with posterior urethral valves and oligohydramnios, due to poor urine output.

renal arteries, respectively (Fig. 45.5). Oligohydramnios can also occur in fetuses with multicystic dysplastic kidneys or posterior urethral valves as urine excretion is interrupted (Fig. 45.6). Karyotypic abnormality should be investigated in the presence of oligohydramnios associated with early symmetric IUGR[28].

Management

The obstetrical management of oligohydramnios is determined by its etiology and the gestational age at presentation. A careful assessment of both the mother and fetus is necessary. Antibiotics and corticosteroids may be utilized with preterm premature rupture of the membranes at a gestational age of <32 weeks[29]. Vesicoamniotic shunts may be used to divert fetal urine to the amniotic fluid cavity in fetuses with obstructive uropathy. Findings from human and animal studies suggest that the amniotic fluid volume will return to normal preventing or at least ameliorating pulmonary hypoplasia. Attempts to achieve this in oligohydramnios of unknown etiology by replacement of amniotic fluid by saline infusions have not been successful[30]. Intrauterine growth restriction is managed with appropriate antepartum testing and determining the optimal time for delivery. It should be remembered that isolated third-trimester oligohydramnios is not necessarily associated with poor perinatal outcome[29]. Before term, expectant management is often the most appropriate course of action, depending on maternal and fetal condition. At term, delivery is often the most appropriate management. However, with reassuring fetal testing, delivery may be safely delayed on the basis of the parity and the inducibility of the mother's cervix. After term, oligohydramnios is considered an indication for delivery in a post-term pregnancy. However, studies have not shown a difference in perinatal outcomes.

POLYHYDRAMNIOS

A largest vertical pocket exceeding 8 cm or an amniotic fluid index exceeding 18 cm, 24 cm or the 95th percentile for the corresponding gestational age have been used to define polyhydramnios. Common reasons for obtaining an AFI in a woman with a low-risk pregnancy include evaluation for fundal height measurements discordant with gestational age, with or without abdominal discomfort. On physical examination, the distended abdomen is tense and tender, and fetal parts are difficult to

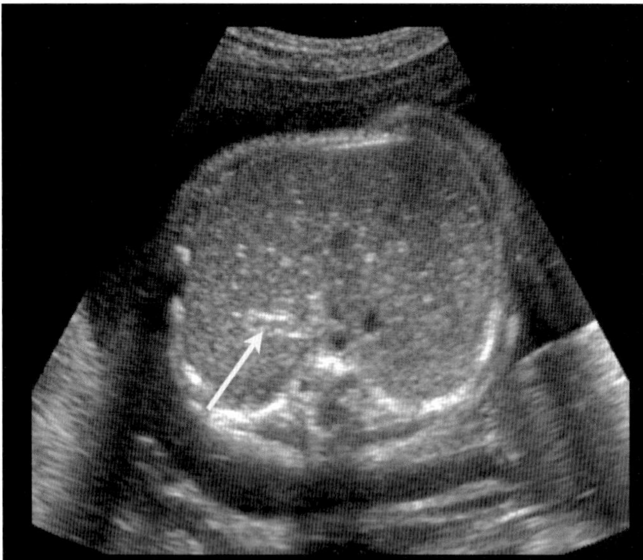

Fig. 45.7 Ultrasound shows polyhydramnios and a persistent small stomach (arrow) in a fetus with esophageal atresia and tracheoesophageal fistula. The amount of polyhydramnios progressively increased throughout the pregnancy.

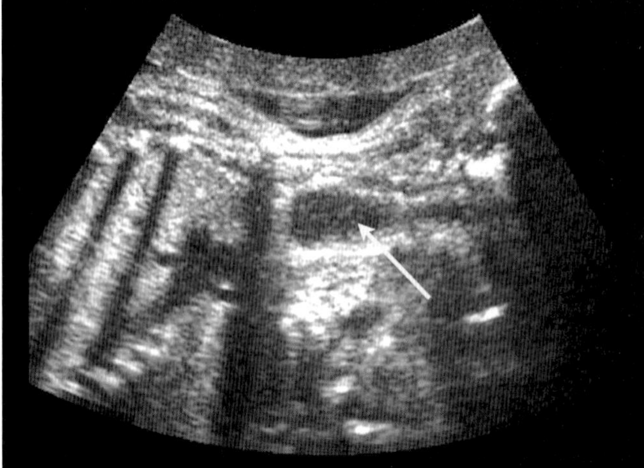

Fig. 45.8 Longitudinal scan section showing an amniotic fluid collection in the fetal esophagus (arrow) in esophageal atresia, associated with polyhydramnios.

palpate. The patient may also report excessive fetal movement, which is a result of increased freedom of fetal limbs.

Etiology

Evaluation of the fetus by thorough, targeted anatomic ultrasonography is the cornerstone of determining a diagnosis and cause when polyhydramnios is suspected. Hence, the presence of polyhydramnios should prompt a search for fetal structural defects that interfere with fetal swallowing such as gastrointestinal obstruction due to oesophageal atresia (Figs 45.7 and 45.8) or duodenal atresia[31,32] (Fig. 45.9). Polyhydramnios can be caused by impaired absorption of amniotic fluid due to extrinsic obstruction of the gastrointestinal tract, perhaps due to congenital diaphragmatic hernia, or masses within the thorax and

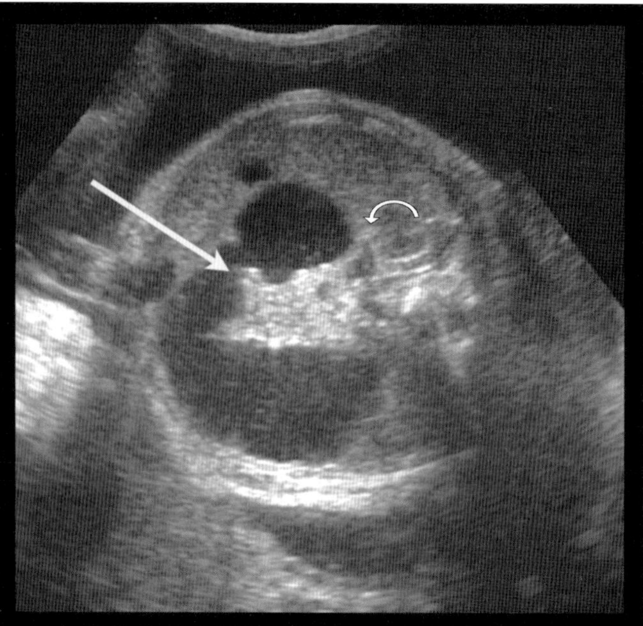

Fig. 45.9 The typical appearance of duodenal atresia seen on a transverse section of fetal abdomen. This view shows the classic 'double bubble' sign of a distended stomach on one side of the phylorus (arrow) and distended duodenum (curved arrow), accompanied by polyhydramnios.

mediastinum. The combination of intrauterine growth restriction and polyhydramnios can suggest the condition of trisomy 18, especially if there is abnormal hand positioning[33]. Other aneuploidies have also been associated with polyhydramnios, most commonly trisomy 21. The differential diagnosis for cases of polyhydramnios in the absence of a structural fetal anomaly or hydrops is limited. Undiagnosed maternal diabetes may be the causative factor and approximately 15–25% of cases of recurrent polyhydramnios are associated with diabetes mellitus[34]. It is not clear whether polyhydramnios in diabetic women is caused by fetal glucosuria or other mechanisms, but poor glycemic control and large fetal size correlate with greater increases in amniotic fluid volume[35]. A maternal glucose tolerance test should be undertaken and, if abnormal, treatment should reduce the excess amniotic fluid volume.

Acute polyhydramnios occurs when amniotic fluid rapidly accumulates, producing severe symptoms in the mother. Clinically, the size of the fundus increases rapidly at a rate of more than 1 cm per day. Acute polyhydramnios rarely occurs in high-output cardiac failure which might be related to fetal anemia caused by alloimmunization, parvovirus infection, fetomaternal hemorrhage, alpha-thalassemia or glucose-6-phosphatase deficiency. More often, it is found in cases of severe twin–twin transfusion syndrome. The stuck twin (donor) will be located at the periphery of the uterine cavity and this fetus may escape initial detection by those less experienced with ultrasound (Fig. 45.10, and see Chapter 46).

When no other cause of polyhydramnios can be identified it is termed idiopathic. A newly evolving area of amniotic fluid volume regulation concerns alterations in the intramembranous pathway. Under normal conditions, the intramembranous pathway is responsible for 400 ml fluid transfer per day at term from the amniotic cavity across the fetal membranes into the fetal circulation[36]. It has been proposed that acute idiopathic polyhydramnios

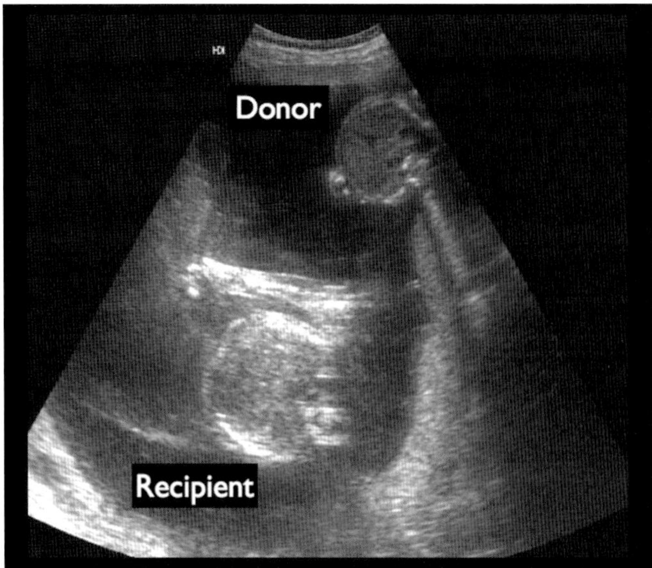

Fig. 45.10 A case of severe twin–twin transfusion syndrome, the donor (stuck twin) is located at the periphery of the uterine cavity. It is apparently surrounded by increased amniotic fluid in the sac of the recipient.

may, in some cases, be due to a functional deficit in the chorionic receptors for prolactin[37]. Prolactin has been shown to increase fluid transport out of the amniotic cavity[38]. Another study had shown that pregnant knockout mice deficient in aquaporin 1 protein had a greater volume of amniotic fluid than their wild-type and heterozygote counterparts[39].

Management

Polyhydramnios has been associated with an increased risk of several obstetric complications related to uterine over-distention. These include preterm labor, rupture of membranes, placental abruption, umbilical cord prolapse and post-partum uterine atony. The risk of these complications varies according to the severity and underlying etiology of the excessive fluid accumulation[2,40]. For most cases of polyhydramnios, no intervention or aggressive therapy is indicated. However, based on the degree of excess amniotic fluid, the pregnancy may be at risk for maternal respiratory restriction. In this situation, indomethacin, a non-steroidal anti-inflammatory agent which works by reducing fetal urine and lung liquid production[41,42], should be considered. In a study of 57 patients with polyhydramnios, indomethacin reduced amniotic fluid in more than 90% of cases[43]. However, indomethacin should not be used in twin–transfusion syndrome or after 34 weeks of gestation as the risk of complications increases in these settings[44]. One complication of indomethacin therapy is the constriction of ductus arteriosus which increases the right ventricular afterload pressure, produces right ventricular dilatation and tricuspid regurgitation. Premature closure of the ductus arteriosus has been attributed to the development of pulmonary hypertension, fetal pleural effusion, hydrops fetalis and persistent fetal circulation. It was shown that pulsed Doppler ultrasound can be used to detect constriction of the fetal ductus arteriosus with a peak systolic velocity of >140 cm/s[45]. If the patient develops evidence of respiratory embarrassment or excessive uterine activity during the prenatal course, therapeutic options include serial amniodrainage, when indomethacin is contraindicated. There is no consensus concerning how much fluid to remove, how rapidly to remove the fluid, the use of tocolytic medications, or the use of antibiotics. A reasonable guideline is to remove the fluid no faster than 1000 ml over 20 minutes and not to remove more than 3–4 liters at one time. The overall complication rate with this procedure is 1.5%[46] and can include initiation of preterm labor, premature rupture of membranes, chorioamnionitis and placental abruption. Patients can develop symptoms such as preterm labor or respiratory compromise, which in turn dictate when a repeat procedure is necessary.

REFERENCES

1. Casey BM, McIntire DD, Bloom SL et al. Pregnancy outcomes after antepartum diagnosis of oligohydramnios at or beyond 34 weeks' gestation. *Am J Obstet Gynecol* **182**:909–912, 2000.
2. Golan A, Wolman I, Sagi J, Yovel I, David MP. Persistence of polyhydramnios during pregnancy – its significance and correlation with maternal and fetal complications. *Gynecol Obstet Invest* **37**:18–20, 1994.
3. Brace RA. Physiology of amniotic fluid volume regulation. *Clin Obstet Gynecol* **40**:280 289, 1997.
4. Campbell J, Wathen N, Macintosh M, Cass P, Chard T, Mainwaring Burton R. Biochemical composition of amniotic fluid and extraembryonic coelomic fluid in the first trimester of pregnancy. *Br J Obstet Gynaecol* **99**:563–565, 1992.
5. Jauniaux E, Lees C, Jurkovic D, Campbell S, Gulbis B. Transfer of inulin across the first-trimester human placenta. *Am J Obstet Gynecol* **176**:33–36, 1997.
6. Brace RA, Wolf EJ. Normal amniotic fluid volume changes throughout pregnancy. *Am J Obstet Gynecol* **161**:382–388, 1989.
7. Magann EF, Perry KG, Jr, Chauhan SP, Anfanger PJ, Whitworth NS, Morrison JC. The accuracy of ultrasound evaluation of amniotic fluid volume in singleton pregnancies: the effect of operator experience and ultrasound interpretative technique. *J Clin Ultrasound* **25**:249–253, 1997.
8. Goldstein RB, Filly RA. Sonographic estimation of amniotic fluid volume. Subjective assessment versus pocket measurements. *J Ultrasound Med* **7**:363–369, 1988.
9. Manning FA, Hill LM, Platt LD. Qualitative amniotic fluid volume determination by ultrasound: antepartum detection of intrauterine growth retardation. *Am J Obstet Gynecol* **139**:254–258, 1981.
10. Manning FA, Platt LD, Sipos L. Antepartum fetal evaluation: development of a fetal biophysical profile. *Am J Obstet Gynecol* **136**:787–795, 1980.
11. Manning FA, Baskett TF, Morrison I, Lange I. Fetal biophysical profile scoring: a prospective study in 1,184 high-risk patients. *Am J Obstet Gynecol* **140**:289–294, 1981.
12. Manning FA, Morrison I, Harman CR, Lange IR, Menticoglou S. Fetal assessment based on fetal biophysical profile scoring: experience in 19,221 referred high-risk pregnancies. II. An analysis of false-negative fetal deaths. *Am J Obstet Gynecol* **157**:880–884, 1987.
13. Manning FA, Harman CR, Morrison I, Menticoglou SM, Lange IR, Johnson JM. Fetal assessment based on fetal biophysical profile scoring. IV. An analysis of perinatal morbidity and mortality. *Am J Obstet Gynecol* **162**:703–709, 1990.
14. Phelan JP, Smith CV, Broussard P, Small M. Amniotic fluid volume assessment with the four-quadrant technique at 36-42 weeks' gestation. *J Reprod Med* **32**:540–542, 1987.

15. Rutherford SE, Phelan JP, Smith CV, Jacobs N. The four-quadrant assessment of amniotic fluid volume: an adjunct to antepartum fetal heart rate testing. *Obstet Gynecol* **70**:353–356, 1987.
16. Moore TR, Cayle JE. The amniotic fluid index in normal human pregnancy. *Am J Obstet Gynecol* **162**:1168–1173, 1990.
17. Bianco A, Rosen T, Kuczynski E, Tetrokalashvili M, Lockwood CJ. Measurement of the amniotic fluid index with and without color Doppler. *J Perinat Med* **27**:245–249, 1999.
18. Grover J, Mentakis EA, Ross MG. Three-dimensional method for determination of amniotic fluid volume in intrauterine pockets. *Obstet Gynecol* **90**:1007–1010, 1997.
19. Shipp TD, Bromley B, Pauker S, Frigoletto FD, Jr, Benacerraf BR. Outcome of singleton pregnancies with severe oligohydramnios in the second and third trimesters. *Ultrasound Obstet Gynecol* **7**:108–113, 1996.
20. Nicolini U, Fisk NM, Rodeck CH, Talbert DG, Wigglesworth JS. Low amniotic pressure in oligohydramnios – is this the cause of pulmonary hypoplasia? *Am J Obstet Gynecol* **161**:1098–1101, 1989.
21. Cock ML, McCrabb GJ, Wlodek ME, Harding R. Effects of prolonged hypoxemia on fetal renal function and amniotic fluid volume in sheep. *Am J Obstet Gynecol* **176**:320–326, 1997.
22. Chamberlain PF, Manning FA, Morrison I, Harman CR, Lange IR. Ultrasound evaluation of amniotic fluid volume. I. The relationship of marginal and decreased amniotic fluid volumes to perinatal outcome. *Am J Obstet Gynecol* **150**:245–249, 1984.
23. Alfirevic Z, Luckas M, Walkinshaw SA, McFarlane M, Curran R. A randomised comparison between amniotic fluid index and maximum pool depth in the monitoring of post-term pregnancy. *Br J Obstet Gynaecol* **104**:207–211, 1997.
24. Conway DL, Adkins WB, Schroeder B, Langer O. Isolated oligohydramnios in the term pregnancy: is it a clinical entity? *J Matern Fetal Med* **7**:197–200, 1998.
25. Shime J, Gare DJ, Andrews J, Bertrand M, Salgado J, Whillans G. Prolonged pregnancy: surveillance of the fetus and the neonate and the course of labor and delivery. *Am J Obstet Gynecol* **148**:547–552, 1984.
26. Hill LM, Rivello D. Role of transvaginal sonography in the diagnosis of bilateral renal agenesis. *Am J Perinatol* **8**:395–397, 1991.
27. DeVore GR. The value of color Doppler sonography in the diagnosis of renal agenesis. *J Ultrasound Med* **14**:443–449, 1995.
28. Nicolaides KH, Rodeck CH, Gosden CM. Rapid karyotyping in non-lethal fetal malformations. *Lancet* **1**:283–287, 1986.
29. Vermillion ST, Soper DE, Bland ML, Newman RB. Effectiveness of antenatal corticosteroid administration after preterm premature rupture of the membranes. *Am J Obstet Gynecol* **183**: 925–929, 2000.
30. Fisk NM, Ronderos-Dumit D, Soliani A, Nicolini U, Vaughan J, Rodeck CH. Diagnostic and therapeutic transabdominal amnioinfusion in oligohydramnios. *Obstet Gynecol* **78**: 270–278, 1991.
31. Ben-Chetrit A, Hochner-Celnikier D, Ron M, Yagel S. Hydramnios in the third trimester of pregnancy: a change in the distribution of accompanying fetal anomalies as a result of early ultrasonographic prenatal diagnosis. *Am J Obstet Gynecol* **162**:1344–1345, 1990.
32. Stoll CG, Roth MP, Dott B, Alembik Y. Study of 290 cases of polyhydramnios and congenital malformations in a series of 225,669 consecutive births. *Community Genet* **2**:36–42, 1999.
33. Dashe JS, McIntire DD, Ramus RM, Santos-Ramos R, Twickler DM. Hydramnios: anomaly prevalence and sonographic detection. *Obstet Gynecol* **100**:134–139, 2002.
34. Golan A, Wolman I, Saller Y, David MP. Hydramnios in singleton pregnancy: sonographic prevalence and etiology. *Gynecol Obstet Invest* **35**:91–93, 1993.
35. Vink JY, Poggi SH, Ghidini A, Spong CY. Amniotic fluid index and birth weight: is there a relationship in diabetics with poor glycemic control? *Am J Obstet Gynecol* **195**:848–850, 2006.
36. Mann SE, Nijland MJ, Ross MG. Mathematic modeling of human amniotic fluid dynamics. *Am J Obstet Gynecol* **175**:937–944, 1996.
37. De Santis M, Cavaliere AF, Noia G, Masini L, Menini E, Caruso A. Acute recurrent polyhydramnios and amniotic prolactin. *Prenat Diagn* **20**:347–348, 2000.
38. Josimovich JB, Archer DF. The role of lactogenic hormones in the pregnant woman and the fetus. *Am J Obstet Gynecol* **129**:777–780, 1977.
39. Mann SE, Ricke EA, Torres EA, Taylor RN. A novel model of polyhydramnios: amniotic fluid volume is increased in aquaporin 1 knockout mice. *Am J Obstet Gynecol* **192**:2041–2044, 2005. discussion 2044–2046.
40. Smith CV, Plambeck RD, Rayburn WF, Albaugh KJ. Relation of mild idiopathic polyhydramnios to perinatal outcome. *Obstet Gynecol* **79**:387–389, 1992.
41. Cabrol D, Landesman R, Muller J, Uzan M, Sureau C, Saxena BB. Treatment of polyhydramnios with prostaglandin synthetase inhibitor (indomethacin). *Am J Obstet Gynecol* **157**:422–426, 1987.
42. Kirshon B, Mari G, Moise KJ, Jr. Indomethacin therapy in the treatment of symptomatic polyhydramnios. *Obstet Gynecol* **75**:202–205, 1990.
43. Moise KJ, Jr. Indomethacin therapy in the treatment of symptomatic polyhydramnios. *Clin Obstet Gynecol* **34**:310–318, 1991.
44. Kirshon B, Mari G, Moise KJ, Jr, Wasserstrum N. Effect of indomethacin on the fetal ductus arteriosus during treatment of symptomatic polyhydramnios. *J Reprod Med* **35**:529–532, 1990.
45. Huhta JC, Moise KJ, Fisher DJ, Sharif DS, Wasserstrum N, Martin C. Detection and quantitation of constriction of the fetal ductus arteriosus by Doppler echocardiography. *Circulation* **75**:406–412, 1987.
46. Leung WC, Jouannic JM, Hyett J, Rodeck C, Jauniaux E. Procedure-related complications of rapid amniodrainage in the treatment of polyhydramnios. *Ultrasound Obstet Gynecol* **23**:154–158, 2004.

CHAPTER 46

Multiple pregnancy

Neelam Engineer and Nicholas Fisk

KEY POINTS

- Early diagnosis and referral of complicated multiple pregnancies are integral to effective care
- Invasive diagnostic tests should be performed in fetal medicine units where the option of selective termination is available
- While MFPR prolongs gestation and improves outcome for continuing fetus(es) in higher order multiples, its effect on miscarriage risk in trichorionic triplets remains unclear
- Fetoscopic laser ablation is the preferred treatment for severe TTTS, although optimal treatment of early stage disease with high spontaneous resolution rates is unclear
- Survivors after single fetal demise of MC twins should have regular ultrasound surveillance and an MRI scan 2–3 weeks after co-twin death
- Due to the increased risk of stillbirth in the mid- and late third trimester, elective delivery prior to term should be considered in presence of complications in MC twins
- While bipolar cord occlusion is an established method for selective feticide between 18–26 weeks' gestation, radiofrequency ablation is emerging as a promising method for selective termination in complicated midtrimester MC pregnancies

INTRODUCTION

Recent decades have seen an unprecedented epidemic of multiple pregnancies, the result principally of assisted reproductive techniques (ART). Although the exponential growth in higher order multiple pregnancies has been recently reversed with restrictive embryo transfer policies, twinning now occurs in 14.7 per 1000 live births compared to 9.6 in 1980[1,2]. Nevertheless, triplet pregnancies continue to occur at a rate of 0.22 per 1000 livebirths, partly attributable to monozygotic twinning (MZ) in ART cycles and partly to spontaneous conception in women of advanced maternal age[2,3]. Multiple pregnancy thus accounts for a significant workload in all fetal medicine units. This reflects the requirement for precise and early chorionicity assessment, recognition of the disproportionate increase in risks associated with monochorionic (MC) pregnancies, the development of successful fetal treatment procedures and the need for streamlined obstetric management of multiple pregnancies.

Perinatal disease burden

World-wide, adverse perinatal outcomes associated with multiple pregnancies remain substantial. These are attributable to prematurity, low birth weight, discordant growth restriction and complications unique to MC pregnancies, including acute transfusion, chronic twin-to-twin transfusion syndrome (TTTS) and monoamniotic (MA) twins. Maternal complications such as antepartum hemorrhage and pre-eclampsia also contribute[4].

The risk of perinatal death is 3 to 6 times higher for twins and approximately 9 times higher for triplets compared with singletons[1]. The corresponding perinatal mortality rates are 14.8 per 1000 live births for twins, 51.8 for triplets compared with 5.4 for singletons[5]. National data from Australia in 2001 show that multiple birth is the biggest single mediator of neonatal death, outnumbering deaths from placental abruption and hemorrhage, respiratory distress or heart defects[6].

Recent data from a large Dutch cohort of twin pregnancies (n = 1407) show that perinatal mortality (>20 weeks of gestation) is significantly higher in MC (11.6%) compared to dichorionic (DC) twins (5%)[7]. After 32 weeks, MC twins have up to an 8-fold increased risk of intrauterine fetal death (IUFD). Despite intensive fetal surveillance, structurally normal monochorionic diamniotic (MCDA) twins with appropriate growth and no TTTS remain at high risk of unexpected IUFD, with a prospective risk of 1/23 pregnancies (95% CI 1/11 to 1/63)[8]. Consistent with this observation, another cohort study demonstrated a prospective risk of stillbirth of 2.0% in 'apparently normal' MC twins after 34 weeks compared to 0.4% in DC twins[9]. Among survivors, neonatal complications such as necrotizing enterocolitis are more frequent (OR: 1.2, 95% CI 2.0–8.4) in MC compared with DC twins[7]. Indeed, these complications of monochorionicity in triplets result in dichorionic triamniotics (DCTA) carrying an 8-fold higher risk of perinatal loss rate than trichorionic triamniotic triplets (TCTA) (OR: 7.9; 95% CI 4.4–14.0)[10].

At least 50% of twins and 90% of triplet babies are born preterm with low birth weight[5]. On an average, twins are nearly 1 kg lighter than singletons (2.3 compared with 3.3 kg) while each triplet weighs about 1.7 kg[2]. Cerebral palsy remains a major contributor to perinatal morbidity in survivors and is 4 times higher for twins and 18 times higher for triplets than for singleton babies[11]. The increased risk of neonatal morbidity from respiratory distress syndrome, necrotizing enterocolitis and intraventricular hemorrhage appears to be similar in triplets, twins and singletons when adjusted for birth weight and gestation, confirming that the main risk in twins and higher order births is being preterm or low birth weight rather than any direct consequence of multiplicity[12].

Chorionicity

Determination of chorionicity is important clinically because of the substantial and increasingly treatable complications of MC multiples and hence an increased need for fetal surveillance. Assessment of chorionicity is also essential for prenatal diagnosis, genetic counseling and planning interventional procedures, particularly in twin pregnancies discordant for fetal structural or chromosomal anomalies and/or growth restriction.

First trimester

Chorionicity is optimally determined in the first trimester. The earliest gestation for determining chorionicity is 5 weeks, for fetal number 6 weeks and for amnionicity 8 weeks. For DC placentation, the presence of two separate placental masses or a single placenta with a 'twin peak' or 'lambda' sign have the highest sensitivity and specificity of 97% to 100% in first trimester[13–16]. Rarely, an MC placenta that is bilobed or has a succenturiate lobe may suggest the misleading appearance of being separate and thus DC placentae, but it is the septum and not the placental count that is the key to reliable chorionicity at this gestation. Monochorionicity is predicted with near perfect (98–100%) accuracy by the presence of a wispy thin membrane with no intervening layer of chorion (the so-called 'T' sign), which diverges with no intervening chorion to reveal a single extraembryonic celom[17].

Second trimester

Diagnosis in early second trimester is similarly made on septal appearance, i.e. the presence or absence of the DC 'lambda' or the MC 'T' sign. Later, identification of discordant fetal gender indicates definitive dichorionicity. In cases where there is only one placental mass and fetuses with concordant sex, assessment of chorionicity depends on other ultrasound features. Detection of an artery-to-artery anastomosis (AAA) confirms monochorionicity, but this can be difficult in early to midgestation and some MC will not have one present.

From the later second trimester, the lambda sign becomes less reliable as it may disappear in up to 7% of DC pregnancies as the chorion frondosum regresses[18]. Hence, its absence does not exclude dichorionicity[17]. Some investigators have suggested measuring thickness of the intertwin membrane using 2D and 3D multiplanar ultrasound[19]. Between 20 and 35 weeks' gestation in DC pregnancies, the mean measurement is approximately 2.4 mm whereas in MC twins mean thickness is 1.4 mm[19]. However, the large standard deviations (up to 0.7 mm) and high inter- and intra-operator variability preclude accurate distinction on this basis[18].

Third trimester

Determination in late pregnancy is less reliable due to compromised views, discordance in amniotic fluid and overcrowding of fetal parts. Attempts in the third trimester, like the midtrimester, comprise a composite of ultrasonographic criteria including fetal sex, number of placentae, presence of an AAA and qualitative membrane thickness.

Prenatal determination of zygosity

Zygosity can be determined in many cases antenatally based on placentation and fetal gender. All MC twins are obligately MZ, while discordant sex indicates definitive dizygosity. For like sex DC pregnancies, most are dizygous, but around 20% will be monozygous[20]. There is only rarely indication in this group for DNA fingerprinting on separately sourced fetal samples.

PRENATAL DIAGNOSIS

Aneuploidy screening

The methods used for aneuploidy screening are similar to singletons and include various combinations of maternal age, first trimester nuchal translucency and first or midtrimester serum markers. In general, however, screening is complicated by zygosity and discordant aneuploidy, so accuracy rates are suboptimal compared to singletons. Screen positive results may have considerable implications for parents, so it is important they be counseled about the complexities in advance.

Risk of aneuploidy based on zygosity

Zygosity not chorionicity mediates the risk of chromosomal abnormalities in multiple pregnancy. MZ twins are almost always genetically identical and of same sex. Hence, the risk of aneuploidy for each fetus in MZ twinning is similar to that in singleton pregnancies with fetuses usually both affected or both normal. Rarely, postzygotic mitotic errors can result in heterokaryotypic twins with chromosomal discordance[21]. These are extremely rare in the absence of fetal anomalies and are not taken into consideration when calculating aneuploidy risk.

Dizygotic (DZ) twins are genetically distinct like siblings and thus aneuploidy when present, is usually discordant. Each twin has an independent risk and the maternal age-related risk is considered the same as in singletons. As a result, the chance of at least one fetus in a DZ twin pregnancy being affected by chromosomal defect is broadly twice as high as that for women of same age with a singleton fetus[22]. However, conventional risk estimation methods are imprecise and fail to account for the lower observed frequency of Down's syndrome in twin pregnancies[23].

Serum biochemistry

In twin pregnancies, conventional second-trimester serum screening tests are not as reliable as in singleton pregnancies and do not provide a fetus specific risk. Investigators have suggested calculating a 'pseudorisk' using the biochemical markers (alpha-fetoprotein (AFP), human chorionic gonadotrophin (hCG) and estriol) for twins similar to singletons, albeit with a lower sensitivity of 51–73% for 5% false positive rate (FPR)[24]. However, these mathematical models assume equal contribution from each fetus, whereas most aneuploidy is likely to be discordant. Another problem is the lack of data available to determine the distribution of markers in twins concordant or discordant for trisomy 21. Thus they work reasonably for the rarer MC but not as well for the more common DC twins with the greater anueploidy risk[25]. As a result, biochemical screening alone has not been widely accepted[26,27].

Nuchal translucency

Although nuchal translucency (NT) is no longer practiced in singletons in isolation due to its high false positive rate, its advantage in twins is that it is fetally specific. Thus, in DC twin pregnacies, the detection rate (75–80%) and FPR (5% per fetus or 10% per pregnancy) for trisomy 21 are similar to those in singleton pregnancies[28]. However, the risk for each fetus is calculated independently using published NT values for singletons and, as with biochemical testing, may thus be an overestimate given the lower risk of Down's syndrome in twin pregnancies. One group has suggested that the overall pregnancy specific risk is summed on the basis of NT[29].

For MC twins, the NT measurements are averaged to calculate a single risk estimate for the entire pregnancy. However, the FPR of NT screening (13% per pregnancy) is much higher than in DC twins, probably because increased NT may reflect early manifestations of transfusional imbalance such as those destined to develop twin-to-twin transfusion syndrome (TTTS) or which have discordant major fetal cardiac or structural anomaly[30–33]. Discordant NT is at least twice as prevalent as in DC twins. It has been advocated as a tool to predict TTTS, albeit with low sensitivity and positive predictive value of only 30%[34].

Risk assessment using NT is currently the only reliable fetally-specific screening tool for higher order multiple pregnancies and studies have shown mean NT thicknesses in these pregnancies to be comparable to singletons[35]. However, in those with an MC set, increased NT may represent signs of early TTTS. Nevertheless, NT risk assessment enables targeted fetal karyotyping and therapeutic interventions including accurate selection of lowest risk fetus(es) to retain at multifetal pregnancy reduction (MFPR).

Combined NT and serum screening

Combining first-trimester NT with serum markers (free beta-hCG and pregnancy-associated placental protein A (PAPP-A)) has been shown to perform better in twin pregnancies than either NT or serum markers alone[26,29,36]. The Fetal Medicine Foundation recommends using the larger rather than the average of the two crown–rump lengths (CRLs) because of the possibility of early onset growth restriction[37]. For DC twins, a pregnancy specific 'pseudorisk' is obtained by 'summing' the risk for each fetus on the basis of the individual NT measurements and then multiplied by the likelihood ratio (LR) derived from the serum markers. However, for MC twins, the two fetus' specific NT measurements are 'averaged' and then multiplied by the LR obtained from serum markers, which then generates a single risk estimate. Overall, for a 5% false positive rate, NT alone, first-trimester combined test, and integrated tests will yield 69%, 72% and 80% detection rates respectively (Table 46.1)[29]. As with singletons, the integrated test is more accurate than the combined, but both have inferior detection rates to that seen in singleton pregnancies.

Table 46.1 **Estimated Down's syndrome screening performance in twin pregnancies according to test used and chorionicity (all tests include maternal age)**

Detection rate/ sensitivity	*Combined test (%)*	*Integrated test (%)*
Monochorionic twins	84	93
Dichorionic twins	70	78
All twins	72	80
Singletons	85	95

Detection rates for a 5% false positive rate after Wald et al. 2003[29]

First-trimester combined test, however, has its limitations:

1. Both free beta-hCG and PAPP-A levels may be confounded by the presence of an unaffected fetus.
2. The results of serum markers are cumbersome to interpret as serum biochemistry relates to the pregnancy while each NT measurement is fetus specific.
3. The 20% of DC pregnancies that are actually monozygous will incorrectly have their risks calculated by the summing rather than the averaging method.
4. Free beta-hCG and PAPP-A levels have been reported to differ between MC and DC twins[38].

Nevertheless, new data show that the distribution of PAPP-A in MC twins is lower than that in DC twins (1.8 versus 2.3 multiples of the median (MoM)) and that recalculation using a correction factor for monochorionicity will improve the accuracy of individual patient specific risk. For free beta-hCG, the difference is not significant (2.0 versus 2.0 MoM) and the observed MoM can be divided by a factor of 2 when adjusting for MC twins[39]. In light of this information and studies supporting improved efficacy of combined screening, the National Screening Committee in the UK has now implemented the policy of first-trimester combined testing for all twin pregnancies.

Invasive prenatal diagnosis

Invasive fetal karyotyping in multiple pregnancies presents a number of distinct challenges compared with singletons. On the one hand, women with multiple pregnancies are at greater risk of aneuploidy due to their age, while on the other they have often conceived after lengthy periods of infertility and thus are most reluctant to countenance any risk of procedure-related miscarriage. Further, in the event of an abnormal result, there is a range of difficult management options, particularly those entailing selective feticide, which may pit parental interests in one fetus against those in the other.

Principles

The indications for invasive fetal testing in multiple pregnancies are similar to singleton pregnancies and include increased aneuploidy risk, discordant structural abnormalities, previous pregnancy affected with a chromosomal abnormality and family history of monogenic disorders. The multiple specific principles listed below should be followed as standard, as failure to sample or label correctly may result in the potentially disastrous consequence of terminating the wrong fetus.

1. Prior determination of chorionicity
2. Detailed ultrasound to determine fetal gender and position, placental site, cord and septal insertions with diagrammatic documentation in the case notes
3. Meticulous labeling of the samples based on above ultrasound features with documentation detailing the needle insertion sites and labeled samples, for example, Twin A (posterior upper maternal right) with lower velamentous cord insertion into left posterolateral placenta and Twin B (anterior maternal left) with left central cord insertion into anterofundal placenta
4. Best practice is for the operator performing invasive testing to be the one performing any subsequent selective termination, although this is not always practicable or necessary if the above guidance is followed

Amniocentesis

Amniocentesis is the gold standard for fetal karotyping in both DC and MC twin pregnancies. Usually, both twin sacs are sampled and this may be achieved by a single or double technique. We advocate the standard double needle technique in which each sac is tapped individually in succession following the general principles as outlined above. In the single needle technique, the proximal sac is sampled and then the same needle advanced through that sac into the second sac[28]. Its advantage is fewer needle insertions; multiple insertions in singleton pregnancies have been associated with a higher chance of procedure-related miscarriage, although this may not necessarily apply to two straightforward intentional insertions in twins. However, the disadvantage is a higher risk of fetal cell contamination. Also tenting of the septum during the procedure can prevent entry into the second sac. The injection of foreign substances to distinguish

Table 46.2 **Pregnancy loss rates following amniocentesis in twin pregnancies in cohort and case control studies**

Study	*Case control study Y/N*	*Study group*	*Miscarriage (%) prior to 20 weeks*	*Total fetal loss (%) up to 28 weeks*	*Control group*	*Miscarriage rate (%)*	*Comments*
Pruggmayer 1992[247]	N	529	2.3	3.7	–	–	Dual tap technique
Sebire 1996[40]	N	176	1.1	2.3	–		Single needle technique
Horger 2001[248]	N	71	5.6	7.6	–	–	
Antsaklis 2002[249]	N	335	4.1	8.7	–	–	Dual tap technique
Ghidini 1993[250]	Y	101	0	3.5	108	3.2	Control twins
Yukobowich 2001[41]	Y	476	2.7	2.7	477	0.6	Two control groups: twins without amniocentesis (shown) and 489 singletons: 0.6% miscarriage rate
Toth Pal 2004[251]	Y	175	3.9	–	300	2.4	Control twins
Millaire 2006[42]	Y	132	3.0	–	248	0.8	Control twins
No/total number of pregnancies studied			**x/1995**	**y/1688**		**z/1133**	
Total loss rate (%)			**3.2**	**4.7**		**1.7**	
95% CI (Confidence Interval)			**1.9–4.5**	**1.9–7.6**		**0.0–3.7**	

the sacs is no longer recommended, as methylene blue is associated with risk of intestinal atresia and fetal death and indigo carmine dye is similarly contraindicated due to its vasoconstrictive effects.

Early studies reported pregnancy loss rates similar to those for singletons[40]. However, more recent evidence suggests that the risk of fetal loss in twins within 4 weeks of amniocentesis is higher (2.7%) than that of exposed singletons (0.6%) or unexposed twins (0.6%)[41]. Further, in a meta-analysis of 2026 women with twin pregnancies, compared with women unexposed to the procedure, amniocentesis increased the risk of fetal loss prior to 24 weeks' gestation (odds ratio 2.4, 95% CI, 1.2–4.7) with an additional risk of one adverse outcome for every 64 amniocenteses[42]. Table 46.2 illustrates the results of amniocentesis in twin pregnancies reported by various investigators.

Chorionic villus sampling

Chorionic villus sampling (CVS) in multiple pregnancies provides the advantage of earlier diagnosis of aneuploidy, enables a more straightforward template for enzyme and DNA studies and affords the option of earlier termination of pregnancy as in singletons. Specifically, it may allow selection of affected fetus(es) in MFPR, although this is rarely important with NT based screening[43]. In twins, the procedure-related loss rates of approximately 2.8% prior to 20 weeks' gestation are similar to amniocentesis[44]. However, a major concern is the possibility of either sampling the same twin twice or contamination of one sample with villi from the second. Contamination rates inferred from inaccurate assignment of gender of up to 5% have been reported (Table 46.3). In an effort to reduce this rate, various techniques have been advocated including a combined transabdominal approach for the upper and transcervical for the lower placenta, sampling in the portion between the umbilical cord insertion and free edge of the placenta or at the margin of a placenta in a DC fused placentation[45]. We are aware of at least one case of missed trisomy 21 using such approaches. For surety, DNA polymorphism studies have been recommended in cases of concordant sex DC twins to distinguish the genotypes. However, this would involve confirmatory amniocentesis with its attendant additional risk in the 20% of like sex DC twins that are MZ.

Choice of procedure for karyotyping

Dichorionic twins

Over the years, there has been controversy as to whether CVS is contraindicated in DC twins. Due to problems with contamination, some investigators suggest restricting CVS to high-risk cases such as monogenic diseases or an aneuploidy risk >1 in 50. The actual risk of contamination (2.2%) is likely to be twice as high as that published since the literature is confined to discordant sex twins[44]. Any benefits of CVS in our view are outweighed by the potentially disastrous consequence of misdiagnosis due to contamination, with subsequent termination of a euploid fetus or wrongful birth of a fetus with trisomy 21.

Table 46.3 **Chorionic villus sampling complications in twin pregnancy**

Study group	*Study type*	*Number recruited*	*Transabdominal (TA)/transcervical (TC)*	*Sampling error rate (%)*	*Loss <24 weeks (%)*	*Total loss rate (%)**	*Comments*
Pergament 1992[252]	Retrospective cohort	128	TA & TC	4.6	2.3	4.9	Includes 3 triplets 6 cell contamination
Wapner 1993[253]	Prospective cohort	161	TA & TC	1.8	3.2	4.8	Twin pregnancies 3 cell contamination
Van den Berg 1999[254]	Retrospective cohort	167	TA	0.6	–	–	Includes 4 triplets
De Catte 2000[255]	Prospective cohort	262	TA & TC	1.9	3.1	5.5	Twin pregnancies 2 sampling error 3 contamination
Antsaklis 2002[249]	Retrospective cohort	44	TA	0	4.5	10.2	Twin pregnancies
No/total number of pregnancies studied				**x/762**	**y/595**	**z/595**	
Mean rate (%)				**2.2**	**3.2**	**6.3**	
95% CI				**0.0–4.9**	**1.8–4.7**	**2.2–10.4**	

*Total loss rate includes abortion, stillbirth and neonatal deaths

For these reasons, amniocentesis should be the preferred option of fetal karyotyping in DC twins.

Monochorionic twins
As both fetuses originate from the same zygote, it is acceptable practice to sample only one fetus by amniocentesis or CVS. There are, however rare cases of heterokaryotypic MC twins[21]. For this reason, double technique amniocentesis of both amniotic sacs is advocated if MC twins are discordant for structural anomalies, NT or growth.

Higher order multiple pregnancies
Due to the higher risk of fetal cell contamination and failure to sample each sac with CVS, amniocentesis is again the preferred option for prenatal diagnosis.

Late karyotyping

The risk of procedure-related fetal loss in both singletons and twins may be minimized by delaying amniocentesis in the third trimester, but is only relevant in those jurisdictions in which late termination of pregnancy is permitted. Although there is small risk of preterm delivery, the risks to the fetus from preterm birth are minimal when invasive testing is performed at or after 32 weeks. In twins, late fetal karyotyping carries an additional advantage of avoiding loss of an unaffected co-twin from earlier selective fetocide if twins are discordant for anomaly.

Fetal blood sampling

Fetal blood sampling is occasionally indicated in cases such as fetal anemia, hydrops, thrombocytopenia and congenital infections and rarely to perform zygosity studies. Fetal blood sampling may be performed using a 22-g needle via intra-umbilical, intrahepatic vein or intracardiac route as for singletons, but the procedure-related loss rate is almost 4 times higher than in singletons (8.2% versus 2.5%)[46]. Fetal blood sampling via intrahepatic vein of each has the advantage of obviating sampling errors.

COMPLICATIONS SPECIFIC TO MONOCHORIONIC PREGNANCIES

The fetal complications that occur exclusively in monochorionic twin pregnancies are twin-to-twin transfusion syndrome (TTTS), twin reversed arterial perfusion (TRAP) sequence, MA twins and conjoined twins.

Twin-to-twin transfusion syndrome

TTTS occurs in 15% of MC twin pregnancies which overall is about 1 in 2000 pregnancies. It typically manifests in midtrimester and rarely in the early third trimester. If untreated, the condition is associated with an 80% perinatal mortality and a 15–20% risk of brain injury in survivors[47].

Diagnosis

This is by ultrasound and there is no role for discredited older definitions involving birth weight or hemoglobin discordancy. In the first trimester, increased NT measurement may be the first marker of TTTS in a minority of cases[34]. Subsequent 2-weekly scans are recommended to assess amniotic fluid volume, fetal growth, ideally with Doppler studies, and bladder size. Marked discordance in amniotic fluid volume between the donor and the recipient fetus may result in the intertwin membrane becoming closely adherent to the donor twin giving the 'stuck twin' appearance. TTTS can be mistaken for MA twin pregnancy if the intertwin membrane is not clearly visible.

Hypervolemia in the recipient and hypovolemia in the donor twin are the basis for the polyuric-polyhydramnios and oliguric-oligohydramnios sequence. A staging system has been described by Quintero et al.[48]:

Stage I	Mildest form with amniotic fluid discordance Polyhydramnios with DVP >8 cm in recipient and oligohydramnios with DVP <2 cm with bladder still visible in donor
Stage II	Above features with lack of visible bladder in donor
Stage III	Critically abnormal Dopplers in either twin: absent or reversed end diastolic flow in donor umbilical artery or reversed ductus venosus flow or pulsatile umbilical venous flow in the recipient ± TTTS cardiomyopathy (atrioventricular valvular incompetence, ventricular hypertrophy and dysfunction)
Stage IV	Ascites or frank hydrops in either recipient or donor
Stage V	Consequent single or double twin death (this category is rarely used as the disease process is by then over)

The above classification is useful for describing the condition in a consistent manner but it does not always denote a logical order of disease progression. It is only loosely linked with prognosis and thus may influence counseling regarding treatment options. Generally, prognosis is better in early TTTS (stages I and II) which may be attributed to a milder form of disease and later presentation (21–24 weeks) compared with advanced disease (stages III–V) which usually presents earlier at 16–20 weeks, and be associated with less favorable prognosis[49–51]. Studies of its predictive value have produced conflicting results and are beset by the treatment paradox[52].

Pathophysiology of TTTS

Placental architecture
All MC placentas have vascular anastomoses classified as artery to artery (AAA), vein to vein (VVA) and artery to vein (AVA).

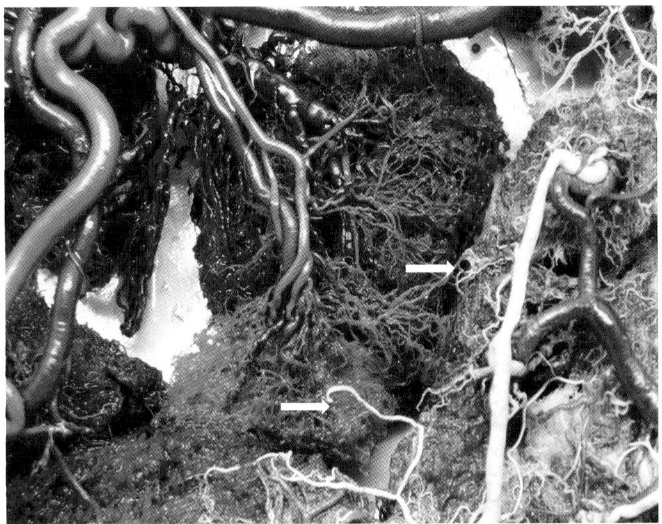

Fig. 46.1 Placental casting of vessels demonstrating hidden anastomoses (arrows).

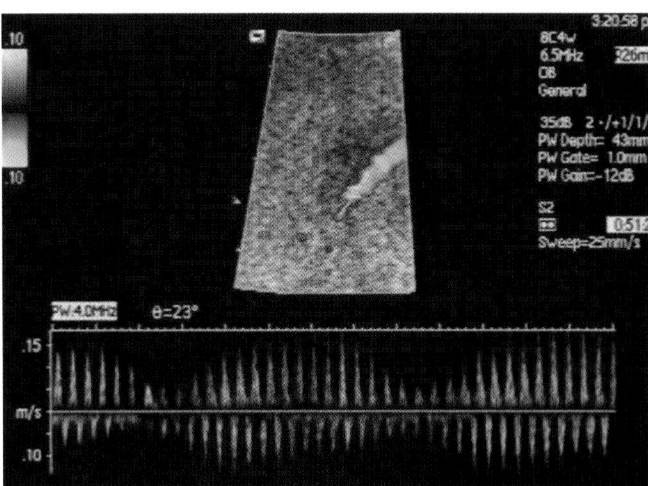

Fig. 46.2 Color Doppler of an artery-to-artery anastomosis demonstrating characteristic bidirectional flow confirming monochorionicity.

AVAs are deep and consist of a chorionic artery from one twin burrowing into the placental tissue to supply an underlying cotyledon with the draining chorionic vein running to the co-twin[53]. They promote only unidirectional flow and hence have a tendency to cause imbalance between the twins which, if uncompensated, may lead to TTTS. Superficial anastomoses are AAA and VVA that are visible branches on the surface of the chorionic plate directly connecting the arteries and veins of the two fetal circulations. Their primary function is rapid compensation for inter-twin hemodynamic imbalance. They often mediate bidirectional flow with the direction of net transfusion dependent on pressure gradients between the twins. Postnatal placental injection studies confirm that almost all MC placentas contain vascular anastomoses[53,54].

Using ex-vivo injection methods on MC placentas, Denbow et al. showed that almost all MC placenta had AVA and 70% also had AAA (Fig. 46.1). In those with absent AAA, 78% developed TTTS. It appears that the lack of superficial anastomoses may predispose to circulatory imbalance that results in uncorrected hypervolemia in one twin[54,55]. These observations are supported by in vivo fetoscopic observation that AVA were found in all MC placentas with TTTS with a preponderance of blood flow towards the recipient[56]. Further, computer modeling confirms that unbalanced AVAs in the absence of superficial anastomoses predispose to development of TTTS[57].

An AAA can be visualized antenatally using color Doppler as early as 12 weeks of gestation in up to 85% of cases. They are seen as arterial vessels on the chorionic plate between the two cord insertions with a characteristic speckled appearance on color Doppler indicating bidirectional flow[55,58] (Fig. 46.2). Detection of an AAA confers a four- to fivefold reduction in the risk of TTTS[55]. Both ex-vivo and fetoscopic studies show that an AAA is present in about a quarter to a third of cases of TTTS[54,56]. When TTTS occurs in the presence of an AAA, it is associated with a better perinatal outcome compared with absent AAA. Nevertheless, in advanced stage TTTS, the presence of an AAA may be detrimental as, when intrauterine death occurs, an AAA may facilitate rapid hemodynamic imbalance leading to acute hypotension in the survivor predisposing to cerebral injury or co-twin demise[59,60]. Ablating an AAA at fetoscopic surgery theoretically may worsen the TTTS, but there is general agreement that they are best ablated at the time of any laser-procedure to reduce the sequelae of laser related fetal loss.

Fetal systemic response

Recent studies have shed insight into the mechanisms of fetal cardiovascular and renal disturbances associated with TTTS. Atrial distension with the recipient's circulatory system stimulates release of atrial natriuretic peptide (ANP) and suppresses antidiuretic hormone resulting in polyuria[61]. Chronic underperfusion in the donor induces degenerative changes in the renal parenchyma and apoptotic changes in renal tubules which may result in renal atrophy and neonatal renal failure[62].

Recipient hypervolemia induces cardiac overload manifesting as biventricular hypertrophy and reduced ventricular function with abnormal venous Dopplers or tricuspid regurgitation. This is exacerbated by release of vascular modulating agents such as endothelin-1[63].

Discordant renin-angiotensin system (RAS) with activation in the donor's kidneys secondary to hypoperfusion and down-regulation in the recipient's kidneys has been implicated in the pathophysiology of TTTS[64,65]. As the recipient's kidneys show features of hypertensive microangiopathy consistent with high levels of circulating RAS mediators, it was proposed that renin might be transfused from the donor into the recipient via placental anastomoses[64]. However, this seems unlikely as angiotensin II activated by renin has a short half-life (<4 mins) and chronic transfusional flows are inadequate to account for the high levels of RAS mediators in the recipient[66]. A recent study demonstrates that both donor and recipient fetuses in chronic TTTS are, in fact, exposed to high levels of circulating renin and angiotensin II and that the placenta is the major source of RAS mediators in the recipient which explains its systemic overload and hypertension both in utero and neonatally[67].

In the donor, abnormal arterial Dopplers, particularly in advanced stage disease, have been attributed to TTTS-related placental vascular dysfunction rather than abnormal placentation. This is evidenced by return of previously absent end diastolic flow in the surviving ex-donor after cord occlusion for stage III–IV TTTS[49,68,69]. This is one of the rationales behind choosing the recipient if selective feticide is indicated in advanced stage TTTS[70].

Echocardiographic features

Cardiovascular dysfunction is common in recipient twins and is associated with fetal demise with subsequent risk of co-twin demise or neurological injury. The overall prevalence of congenital heart disease in TTTS is 6.9%, versus 2.3% in uncomplicated MCDA twins[71]. Echocardiography may assist in determining TTTS stage and thus prognosis with treatment. Cardiovascular compromise ranges from mild ventricular dilatation, hypertrophy, tricuspid regurgitation, through to right ventricular outflow tract obstruction, pulmonary valvular stenosis and severe cardiomegaly with congestive cardiac failure. Usually, the right ventricle is first affected with mild myocardial hypertrophy. Moderate to severe tricuspid and mitral regurgitation is seen in up to 71% of advanced stage TTTS[72]. Acquired right ventricular outflow tract, secondary to muscular or valvular obstruction has been reported in 10% of recipients[73] which may require balloon valvuloplasty postnatally. Postnatally, 3% of neonates affected by TTTS, but with structurally normal hearts, manifest with severe persistent pulmonary hypertension requiring treatment by inhaled nitric oxide[74].

TTTS may adversely affect long-term vascular function in survivors, which may persist in childhood and adult life. Gardiner et al. demonstrated altered arterial distensibility in the donor twin in infancy and early childhood, which was not seen in controlled TTTS twin pairs subjected to laser treatment in utero. This was the first evidence to suggest that aberrant fetal vascular programming may be reversible in humans[75].

Treatment of TTTS

The rationale for treatment is that untreated TTTS has high perinatal morbidity and mortality. Polyhydramnios and uterine distension may result in miscarriage, preterm premature rupture of membranes (PPROM) or preterm delivery. Advanced stage TTTS may progress to cardiac failure with hydrops in the recipient or chronic hypoperfusion of the donor, leading to IUFD of either fetus with the attendant sequelae of single fetal demise. The current modalities of treatment include fetoscopic laser coagulation of vascular anastomoses, amnioreduction with or without septostomy, delivery and selective feticide by cord occlusion.

Laser ablation

Since the Eurofetus randomized trial[76] demonstrating higher survival after fetoscopic laser (76% of at least one twin) compared with serial amnioreduction (56%), endoscopic laser ablation of anastomotic vessels is considered first-line treatment for advanced stage TTTS. This procedure can be performed under either regional or local anesthesia. The technique involves introducing a trocar transabdominally and then 2.0 mm fetoscope to approach the vascular eqautor ideally at near right angles to the chorionic plate. A 400–600 μm laser fiber is then guided alongside the fetoscope and vascular anastomoses are identified and ablated, thus converting an MC placenta into 2 independent circulations (Fig. 46.3).

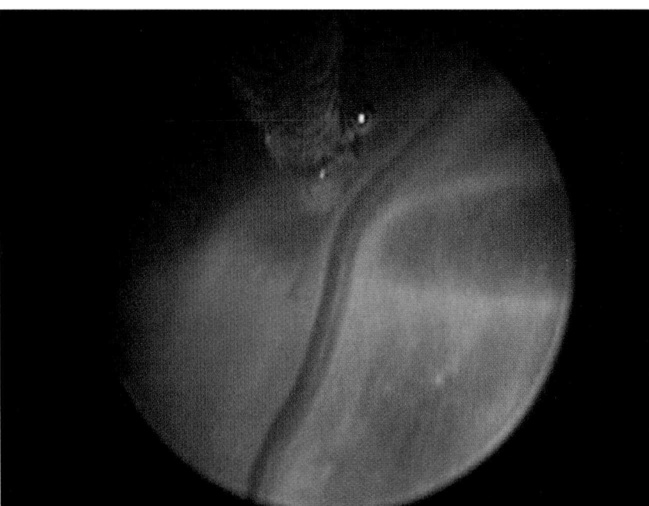

Fig. 46.3 Laser ablation of an AVA during fetoscopic procedure for treatment of TTTS. Arteries have darker color due to deoxgyenated blood.

However, it is not always possible to divide the fetal circulations precisely due to the complexity of placental angioarchitecture and technical limitations of the procedure, including placental accessibility, fetal position in relation to cord insertion and the integrity of the intertwin membrane. Various methods including non-selective, selective and a combination of both have thus been advocated. While the non-selective laser approach aims to ablate all vessels crossing the placental equator, selective laser ablation involves obliteration only of AVAs on the chorionic plate. At fetoscopy, vessels are identified by tracing them from their cord origins, with arteries seen crossing over veins with a darker red color than veins owing to lower oxygen saturation in circulating fetal blood. All AVAs, including those in reverse direction from recipient to donor, are ablated as unbalanced anastomoses may alter net unidirectional flow resulting in IUFD of either twin.

The selective approach was introduced to reduce the high immediate procedure-related loss rates initially reported with laser[77] and cohort studies produce some evidence of better outcome[78,79]. Supporting evidence comes from a recent study that reports significantly better results for postnatal survival of at least one twin and both twins at 28 days in highly selective laser cases (n = 183, 80% and 46% respectively) compared with a low selective laser group (n = 104, 65% and 34% respectively)[80]. Although there was no difference in survival of the recipient (63% versus 58% respectively), survival of the donor was significantly higher with highly selective laser (63% versus 41% for low selective group)[80].

Notwithstanding this, the non-selective versus selective controversy is far from resolved, as a high incidence or persistent and reverse transfusion[77,81] has been reported in which missed anastomoses are implicated. Residual anastomoses can be found in 33% of all placentas examined after laser ablation[82] for which explanations include:

1. anastomoses missed during fetoscopy
2. too selective procedures
3. revascularization of previously ablated vessels
4. new collateral circulation through previously collapsed vessels following release of polyhydramniotic pressure.

Recurrences have been attributed to missing large anastomoses during non-selective procedures while reverse feto-fetal transfusion from recipient to donor due to missed small vessels in selective procedures[80,82,83].

Numerous technical challenges can arise during fetoscopic surgery. An anterior placenta can prevent adequate visualization of AVAs on the chorionic plate. Most endoscopists use a lateral entry with curved introducer to achieve reasonable views. Maternal anesthesia, such as epidural, reduces maternal discomfort and facilitates manipulation and thus visualization of anteriorly situated AVAs[79]. Other approaches include using an additional port with a side-firing laser, as flexible scopes even with the available optics still give inferior visual quality. The available data suggest equally good results with anterior as posterior placenta. However, few placentas are entirely anteriorly situated and such a situation remains a challenge. Previous amnioreduction or septostomy may occasionally hinder access to the chorionic plate due to chorioamniotic separation or blood staining of liquor. Active intra-amniotic bleeding secondary to inadvertent vessel puncture or placental trauma can reduce visibility requiring amnio-exchange, which further lengthens the procedure duration.

IUFD may occur one or several weeks following laser ablation. In the first 6 days after laser ablation, single IUFD and double IUFD may occur in 13–33% and 3–22% respectively[76,78,84]. Single deaths within 24 hours of procedure were reported in early series in up to 60% of cases and within a week in 75% of cases[85]. Associated risk factors for fetal demise include critically abnormal Dopplers pre-procedure or in the postoperative period, absent or reversed end diastolic flow 24 hours after laser treatment[55,68,69,85]. Prognosis for the survivor is reported to be better when the recipient rather than donor dies. Laser ablation of AVAs should in fact protect the survivor from acute agonal transfusion and its neurological sequelae.

Prognosis after laser surgery is dependent upon several factors including intrauterine growth restriction (IUGR), procedure-related fetal demise, residual anemia and persistence or reversal of TTTS[81,86]. PPROM (10%), abruption (1–2%) chorioamnionitis and preterm labour are additional complications inherent in invasive procedures. Preoperative measurement of cervix has been suggested to predict risk of preterm delivery[87]. This does not seem an acute effect as correction of polyhydramnios does not reverse pre-procedural cervical shortening[88]. Rarely, aplasia cutis and limb necrosis secondary to vascular accidents have been reported following laser surgery[89,90].

Late fetal complications presenting at least 7 days after laser ablation include IUFD (1–7%), recurrence of TTTS (14%)[83] and reverse TTTS (5%)[81]. Reversal of donor-recipient phenotype is associated with presence of multiple anastomoses in either direction but may also occur in association with underlying aneuploidy or genetic syndrome[81]. Isolated discordant hemoglobin levels with anemia in previously known recipient[91], as assessed by Middle Cerebral Artery Peak Systolic Velocity (MCA PSV) and fetal blood sampling, has been reported in 13% of cases and is attributed to persistent unidirectional feto–fetal blood transfusion[83]. These complications emphasize the need for continued weekly surveillance by serial ultrasound and Doppler examinations for at least 4 weeks following laser treatment.

Amnioreduction

Serial amnioreduction was introduced as a palliative or temporizing procedure to relieve maternal discomfort and reduce the risk of preterm delivery. Initial studies in TTTS suggested that it prolonged gestation and, in some cases, improved fetal condition. Normalization of intra-amniotic volume has been shown to improve uterine blood flow[92], while alleviating pressure on chorionic plate vessels theortically re-opening compensatory superficial anastomoses, and improve renal perfusion in the donor[93]. Uterine overdistension in relation to the degree of excess amniotic fluid[94] results in mechanical strain on the myometrium and activates a pressor-sensitive system capable of initiating uterine contractility and preterm labor[95,96]. Based on pressure volume relationships, an amniotic fluid index (AFI) of 40–45 cm or deepest pool of 12 cm has been advocated as indication for intervention[94]. Although a single procedure is adequate in around a fifth of cases[97], repeat procedures are usually necessary (median n = 2, range 1–23 in the Australian and New Zealand Registry)[98]. The results of the international amnioreduction registry (n = 223) showed an overall perinatal survival of 78% at birth and 60% at 4 weeks[98,99]. This and data from the Australian and New Zealand registry[96] suggest that amnioreduction works reasonably well in cases with late onset mild disease with normal fetal arterial Dopplers and absence of hydrops. On the other hand, as amnioreduction does not address the underlying transfusional process, it is unlikely to benefit advanced stage disease[100,101] as evidenced by the lower success rate in the Eurofetus trial. Overall, the incidence of procedure-related risks of amnioreduction including PPROM (about 6%), chorioamnionitis and abruption are low[99]. However, neurological morbidity remains a major concern and has been correlated with the number of amnioreductions (>2) and birth weight (<1000 g)[102], as detailed in the neurological injury section.

Microseptostomy

This aims is to equilibrate amniotic fluid volume based on two observations, that TTTS is extremely rare in MA twins and that TTTS anecdotally improves when the septum is inadvertently breached at amnioreduction. A 22-G needle is used to puncture the intertwin membrane under ultrasound control. In a randomized control trial (RCT) comparing amnioreduction with septostomy for TTTS presenting before 24 weeks, the rate of survival of at least 1 twin was similar in both groups (78% versus 80% respectively)[97]. However, septostomy had the advantage of more often requiring only a single procedure. A recent study suggests favorable outcome when septostomy is performed along with amnioreduction[103] and also reduction in further interventions in early stage disease[104].

While the benefit of such treatment is minor, there are occasional disadvantages, as septostomy may rarely impede subsequent laser therapy or even cord occlusion by obscuring the view or approach for subsequent procedures due to chorioamniotic separation; it also carries a theoretical risk of intertwin cord entanglement through extension of the defect in the dividing membrane[86].

Choice of procedure for treatment of TTTS

Although amnioreduction and septostomy are associated with survival rates of 60–65% in the major studies[97], they do not treat the underlying disease. In 2004, the Eurofetus randomized trial showed fetoscopic laser ablation to result in higher survival (76% versus 56% for amnioreduction for at least one survivor) and improved neurological outcome for all stages of TTTS (6% versus 14% respectively)[76]. A systematic review included cohort studies to support laser as more effective with less perinatal morbidity and mortality compared to amnioreduction[105].

In contrast, the NIH multicenter RCT comparing selective laser prior to 24 weeks' gestation with amnioreduction failed to determine the best treatment modality, with 65% versus 75% for at least one survival respectively. Differences in case selection and varying skill or experience of the operators, as well as small numbers (20 in each arm) have been cited as possible explanations for the poorer results in the laser group of this study. Although the Eurofetus trial was the first randomized trial to establish benefit from any invasive fetal treatment, it was a pity that the fetal medicine community was unable to embrace the importance of a further trial. Table 46.4 details the results of fetoscopic laser ablation from the available large studies.

Laser is usually not advocated after 26 weeks' gestation because of technical difficulties in accessing the chorionic plate due to larger fetal size, the increased risk of intra-amniotic bleeding from larger vessels and the availability of delivery as a alternative strategy. However, a recent study of 21 cases of TTTS diagnosed and treated after 26 weeks' gestation reported longer intervals between treatment to delivery in 10 cases treated by laser ablation (31 days) compared with 11 of amnioreduction (9 days). In addition, the incidence of major neonatal morbidity and mortality was higher after amnioreduction (27% and 14% versus 0 and 0% for laser ablation)[106]. Some caution is required due to possible selection bias and small numbers, but these data provide a promising platform for further attempts at laser ablation in the third trimester[107]. Delivery is a definite option after viability, albeit associated with risks of prematurity superimposed on an already compromised fetal condition.

Stage I disease

Although laser ablation is the treatment of choice for advanced stage TTTS, the best therapeutic option of treatment of early stage disease remains controversial as laser-related fetal losses[85] need to be balanced against relatively favorable outcomes with more conservative approaches. In the Eurofetus RCT, only a small number of patients with stage I disease were included and re-analysis of older observational cohorts[51,101] suggests that survival may be comparable if not higher with amnioreduction than laser in early stage disease[108,109]. Additional arguments in favor of a non-laser approach to early stage disease include its high rate of non-progression, which is supported by a recent retrospective analysis where over 70% of stage I TTTS remained stable or regressed with an 80% double survival rate. However, cases that progress had poor double survival, even though laser was available to treat advancing disease. The disadvantages to a non-laser approach to stage I disease include disease progressing too rapidly to arrange definitive treatment, or complications of prior amnioreduction technically impairing later laser treatment[110]. The 2008 Cochrane review, taking into consideration the above controversies, has recommended a randomized evaluation of various interventions and their effects on stage I disease[111].

Neurological brain injury

Neurological injury to either twin remains a major cause of perinatal morbidity in TTTS. The possible mechanisms of cerebral injury include those related to prematurity, insults incurred as a result of chronic TTTS or its in-utero treatment and agonal transfusion following a single IUFD. Both the recipient and donor twin are equally at risk for adverse neurodevelopmental outcome[112–114]. Major cerebral lesions include intraventricular hemorrhage with parenchymal involvement, ventriculomegaly, multicystic encephalomalacia, porencephaly, diffuse cystic white matter disease and polymicrogyria[112,115].

However, it is important to differentiate antenatally acquired lesions as a consequence of TTTS from those that are common in preterm infants. Cranial scans on preterm infants can frequently show lesions (35% of preterm TTTS survivors in one study), such as mild ventriculomegaly, subependymal pseudocysts, basal ganglia echogenicity or lenticulostriate vasculopathy, that are not necessarily associated with long-term impairment[116].

In antenatally acquired lesions, polycythemia and vascular stasis in the recipient and anemia and hypertension in the donor are contributory mediators. Severe cerebral lesions in expectantly managed cases have been reported to be higher than those treated by laser ablation or amnioreduction. In a recent retrospective review of 299 cases of TTTS, 5.4% had cerebral abnormalities following laser ablation, 13.6% following amnioreduction and 21.4% following expectant management[117]. Possible explanations include acute changes in blood pressure in the twins leading to acute temporary high flow insults in those with amnioreduction and incomplete ablation of anatomoses following laser ablation. However, the reduction in incidence of cerebral lesions with the latter has been attributed to delivery at a later gestation while, in cases with complete ablation of anastomosis, the survivor is protected from agonal transfusion and subsequent ischemic injury in event of death of co-twin[117].

The true incidence of long-term neurodevelopmental impairment in TTTS survivors is difficult to ascertain due to paucity of formal studies and of control groups in published data. Minor neurologic deficits include mild spasticity or developmental delay while major handicap includes severe cerebral palsy with hemiparesis or quadriplegia, severe mental and psychomotor delay and deafness. The reported incidence of neurologic deficit following laser ablation ranges from 6 to 17%[47,113,118] and 22 to 26% following amnioreduction[102,112,119]. In one study, long-term follow-up at a median of 3 years of age following laser ablation showed the majority (87%) of children as normally developed, 7% with minor abnormalities and the remaining 6% with major handicap[113], although others suggest higher rates of major sequelae of 11–13%[114,118].

Fetal magnetic resonance imaging (MRI) is increasingly used as an adjunct to ultrasound in the detection of hypoxic–ischemic parenchymal lesions and cortical abnormalities that occur as a result of TTTS[120,121] and has proved reliable when performed from 28 weeks onwards[117]. Ischemic parenchymal injuries are seen on fetal MR imaging as focal or diffuse areas of increased T2 signal intensity in the germinal matrix, cerebral white matter and cortex[122]. Such brain lesions are best visualized if fetal MR imaging is performed 2–3 weeks after the presumed insult or after invasive treatment.

TRAP sequence

The TRAP (twin reversed arterial perfusion) sequence, previously known as acardiac malformation, occurs in 1 in 35 000 pregnancies and accounts for 1% of MC twin pregnancies[123]. The mechanism of this extreme abnormality involves:

1. monochorial placentation with a large AAA between the two fetal circulations

Table 46.4 **Outcome of fetoscopic laser treatment in TTTS (selected studies: recruited number >50 with perinatal outcome)**

Study group	*Study type*	*Number recruited*	*Technique*	*At least 1 survivor N (%)*	*Double survivor N (%)*	*Neurological sequelae N (% among survivors)*	*Miscarriage <24 weeks N (% pregnancies)*	*Laser to delivery interval (weeks)*	*Perinatal survival No of fetuses (%)*
Ville 1998[256]	Prospective cohort	132	Non-selective	97 (73)	47 (36)	6 (4.2)	13 (9.8)	n/a	144 (55)
Hecher 2000[84]	Comparative Laser vs amnioreduction	200	Selective	161 (80)	100 (50)	10 (3.8)	21 (10)	12.9	261 (65)
Quintero 2003[101]	Retrospective	95	Selective	79 (83)	43 (45)	4 (3.3)	8 (8.4)	10.3	122 (64)
Senat 2004[76]	Randomized controlled trial	72	Selective	55 (82)	26 (36)	8 (9.9)	8 (11)	n/a	81 (57)
Yamamoto 2005[50]	Retrospective cohort	175	Selective	128 (73)	61 (35)	n/a	12 (6.8)	n/a	189 (54)
Huber 2006[257]	Prospective cohort	200	Selective	167 (84)	119 (60)	n/a	7 (3.5)	13	286 (72)
Ierullo 2007[258]	Prospective cohort	77	Vascular equator coagulation	57 (74)	31 (40)	n/a	5 (6.5)	9	88 (57)
Middeldorp 2007[107]	Prospective cohort	100	Selective	81 (81)	58 (58)	n/a	8 (8)	n/a	139 (69)
No/total number of pregnancies studied				**825/1051**	**485/1051**	**28/608**	**82/1051**	**x/572**	**1310/2102**
Mean rate (%)				**78.7**	**45**	**5.3**	**8**	**11.6 weeks**	**61.6**
95% CI				**74.8–82.6**	**36.6–53.4**	**2.8–11.1**	**5.9–10.0**	**8.1–14.4**	**55.9–67.3**

2. discordant growth or early fetal demise of one twin allowing for rescue perfusion and thus continued growth of this twin (termed 'perfused' twin) in a paradoxical retrograde fashion by the structurally normal co-twin ('pump' twin) through the AAA[124,125]
3. cardiac atrophy in the perfused fetus[126].

Low pressure deoxygenated blood flows from the pump twin's umbilical artery via the AAA in the placental bed retrogradely into the perfused twin's umbilical arteries to the iliac vessels, thus perfusing the lower part of the body to a far greater extent than the upper part. The result is a spectrum of malformations, reduction anomalies of previously existing tissues and incomplete morphogenesis of tissues primarily in the upper body. The pump twin may become compromised and is at risk of congestive cardiac failure due to continued growth of the perfused twin and the overall volume of parasitic tissue needing to be perfused by the normal heart.

Sonographic assessment

The acardiac twin typically appears as an amorphous mass with tissue edema, deformed lower limbs, rudimentary or absent upper limbs and head and a two-vessel cord. Polyhydramnios in the acardiac twin's sac indicates presence of functional renal tissue[127]. The pump twin may have cardiomegaly, polyhydramnios, hydrops and pleural and pericardial effusions[124].

TRAP sequence can be diagnosed as early as 9 weeks' gestation but may be mistaken for a missed twin. In the second trimester, a history of continued growth of a 'presumed dead' twin on subsequent scans should alert one to the diagnosis. Although cardiac pulsations are as a rule absent, rare cases of monoventricular heart with pulsations have been reported. Definitive diagnosis can be established by demonstrating the TRAP sequence using color flow Doppler to show the paradoxical direction of arterial flow towards the acardiac twin.

Perinatal complications

Polyhydramnios resulting in preterm delivery can occur in up to 50% of these cases. The normal pump twin is also at risk of cardiac failure and fetal hydrops (28%) and intrauterine demise (25%)[127]. Adverse perinatal outcome is associated with increased acardiac:pump twin weight or AC ratio (>70%)[128]. Poor prognostic features in the pump twin include tricuspid regurgitation, cardiac failure, hydrops, abnormal venous Dopplers or fetal anemia[129].

Treatment

Antenatal management is aimed at reducing the risk of preterm delivery from polyhydramnios and intrauterine death of the pump twin secondary to congestive cardiac failure. Sonographic surveillance includes monitoring its growth, Dopplers and cardiac status. Antenatal intervention is indicated when signs of cardiac compromise occur in the pump twin. Given the poor prognosis associated with cardiac failure and polyhydramnios and the technical difficulties in treatment in late gestation, prophylactic intervention is increasingly advocated, i.e. when acardiac:pump twin ratio exceeds 50%[129], with urgent intervention recommended when this ratio exceeds 70%[130,131].

Pharmacological methods of treating cardiac failure with inotropes and polyhydramnios with indomethacin are no longer used due to the development of definitive intervention techniques to interrupt transfusional flow to the TRAP twin. These include ultrasound or fetoscopic guided occlusion of the acardiac twin's cord or its main intra-abdominal vessels[132,129,133]. Technical difficulties occasionally arise during external cord procedures in the presence of short, thin or hydropic cords. Similarly, intrafetal ablative techniques may fail when there is significant flow or large intra-abdominal vessels within the acardiac structure. Treatment is rarely indicated in late midtrimester after 25 weeks when a temporizing approach with amnioreduction and early delivery may be preferable.

Radiofrequency ablation (RFA) of intra-abdominal vessels is emerging as the procedure of choice for TRAP sequence. It is relatively simple compared to other cord occlusive methods and probably safer than interstitial laser. Tines extending from the tip of the needle anchor the ablative device in the region of the intraumbilical vessels (Fig. 46.4). One sizable series reported a survival rate with RFA between 18 and 24 weeks in TRAP of 86% with a mean gestation at delivery of 34.6 weeks[134]. Long-term follow-up data on neurological outcome in surviving pump twins is awaited. Selective termination procedures for TRAP sequence are described in more detail later in this chapter.

Monoamniotic twin pregnancy

Monoamniotic (MA) twin pregnancies represent approximately 2–5% of all MC twins (1 in 10000 pregnancies). Previously, MA twinning was associated with a high perinatal mortality rate of 30–70%, due primarily to cord entanglement[135]. In the last decade, this risk has been reduced to 10–12% due to regular fetal surveillance and elective delivery[136].

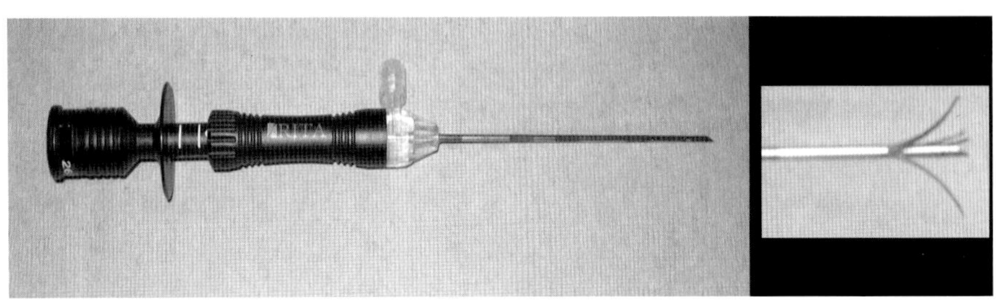

Fig. 46.4 Radiofrequency ablation needle with tines deployed (insert).

Sonographic assessment

High-resolution ultrasound has increased the frequency of first-trimester detection of MA twins. Diagnosis is made by visualization of two separate fetuses with no clear dividing membrane and a single yolk sac. Visualization of two yolk sacs does not necessarily exclude an MA pregnancy as the number of yolk sacs depends on the time of splitting of the germinal disk. When there are two yolk sacs and no dividing membrane before 9 weeks' gestation, a repeat scan must be performed at a later stage as the intertwin membrane in a MCDA twin pregnancy may not easily be seen in early pregnancy.

From the late first trimester onwards, the presence of a single placenta, absent intertwin membrane, same-sex freely moving non-stuck twins in normal amniotic fluid volume support the diagnosis. A pathgnomonic feature of MA twins is the presence of cord entanglement, which can be demonstrated from 10 weeks onwards by insonating a common mass of cord vessels between the two fetuses with color flow Doppler (Fig. 46.5). Two distinct arterial waveform patterns with different heart rates can be discerned in the same direction within the same-pulsed wave sampling gate[137,138].

Perinatal complications

Cord knots, tightening of entanglement and single or double twin deaths are the most common complications. Cord entanglement has been reported in over 70% of MA twins with greater than 50% of deaths attributed to this complication. However, cord entanglement seems almost ubiqitous in the first trimester if looked for, which is not surprising given the relative abundance of amniotic fluid at this stage, allowing relatively unrestricted fetal movements. Thus, entanglement itself is rarely the problem. Doppler waveforms suggestive of tightening of cord entanglement or knotting include a diastolic notch, elevated systolic/diastolic ratio or absent end diastolic flow in the umbilical artery or umbilical venous pulsations[139,140].

Other complications associated with MA twins include congenital anomalies[141], TRAP, anencephaly and congenital cardiac defects. The presence of fetal anomalies almost doubles the perinatal mortality rate[142]. Hence, a detailed anatomy scan of both twins is imperative[143].

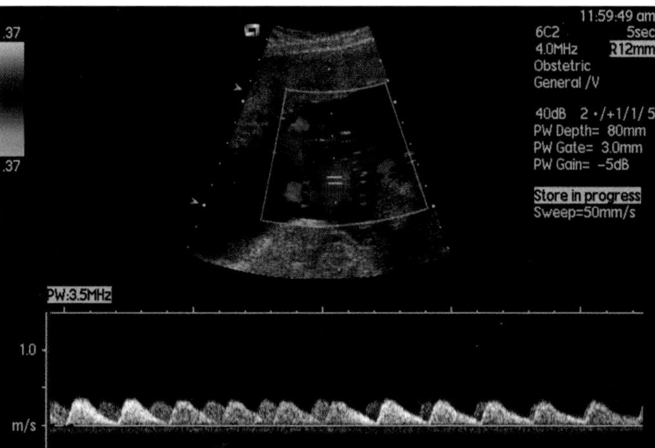

Fig. 46.5 Color Doppler demonstrating cord entanglement and waveform showing two different heart rates in a monoamniotic twin pregnancy.

Although TTTS syndrome occurs in 15% of MCDA pregnancies, it is rare in MA twins (3%)[144]. This reflects their ubiquitous arterioarterial anastomoses, which protect against the development of TTTS. Further, due to absence of the intertwin septum, the amniotic fluid volume equilibrates allowing the donor to swallow any excess amniotic fluid volume. TTTS cannot be diagnosed on the basis of discordant amniotic fluid volume, so suggestive signs in MA twins include polyhydramnios, fetal growth discordance and discordant bladder volumes. MA twins appear to have a lower incidence of growth restriction than diamniotic twins, again arguably due to the greater anastomotic sharing.

Obstetric management

The main focus of antenatal management is prevention of fetal demise and optimal timing of delivery.

Antenatal fetal surveillance

This includes serial fortnightly scans to assess fetal growth, liquor volume and Dopplers. Expectant inpatient management from 25 weeks' gestation with twice daily cardiotocographs (CTGs) and frequent ultrasound monitoring has been recommended, but is contentious. Not only is there no evidence that close fetal surveillance improves fetal outcome, but there is significant risk of iatrogenic preterm delivery, especially as CTGs prior to 28 weeks contain more fetal heart rate decelerations than accelerations[145].

Medical amnioreduction

Our group hypothesized that unrestricted fetal movements due to the absent septum and relatively generous amniotic fluid volume increase the risk of tightening of cord entanglement and that medical amnioreduction using sulindac[146], a non-selective prostaglandin H synthase inhibitor, may splint fetal movements by creating borderline oligohydramnios thus reducing the risk of cord-related complications. Pasquini et al. reported no perinatal deaths in 20 MA pregnancies treated with sulindac 200 mg twice daily from 20 until 32 weeks. The mean AFI reduced by 40% from 21 cm at 20 weeks to 12.4 cm at 32 weeks' gestation and fetal lie remained more stable compared to MCDA controls[147]. Sulindac has a superior profile than indomethacin in terms of COX-2 selectivity and patient tolerance and does not appear to cause ductal constriction before 32 weeks, thus enabling long-term use in pregnancy. Given the rarity of the disease and thus the logistic barriers to conducting a randomized controlled trial, this seems a reasonable interim approach pending confirmatory cohort data.

Conjoined twins

The incidence is approximately 1 in 50 000 live births. Conjoined twinning is a random event resulting from incomplete division of the single blastocyst between 13 and 15 days post conception. An alternative theory suggests it instead originates from the secondary union of two separate embryonic disks[148]. About 75% of conjoined twins are female. Approximately 40% of conjoined twins are stillborn and more than 50% of those born alive die during the neonatal period[149].

Conjoined twins have been classified based on the fused anatomic region (with suffix 'pagus' meaning fixed or fastened). The type of fusion determines the degree to which the internal organs are shared. A newer classification has been proposed on the basis of likely three-dimensional relationships between the two fetal body plans during early embryogenesis[149]. There is a high incidence of congenital anomalies, 60–70% of which involve structural abnormalities not associated with the area of fusion. Neural tube defects, orofacial clefts and cardiac anomalies predominate[150].

Sonographic assessment

In early pregnancy, when transvaginal ultrasound may facilitate diagnosis, the typical picture is that of an MA twin pregnancy with a single yolk sac alongside two embryonic poles. After 8 weeks, increasing fetal activity helps differentiate normal MA from conjoined twins. Increased NT and subcutaneous edema may be noted in thoracopagus twins.

In the second trimester, the sonographic features comprise lack of a separating membrane, inability to demonstrate completely separate fetal bodies, with both heads persistently at the same level with no change in their relative position. Depending on the type of fusion, backward flexion of the cervical and upper thoracic spine may be present. There may be more than three vessels where the umbilical cord is single. Doppler waveforms of the umbilical artery show a characteristic 'double layer' spectral pattern reflecting two separate arterial supplies within the same umbilical cord which is considered diagnostic of conjoined twins[151]. Fetal echocardiography is indicated due to the high incidence of cardiac anomalies. 3D ultrasound may serve as an adjunct to demonstrate the extent of fusion[152]. In addition, prenatal MRI, particularly in the third trimester can provide additional information in planning for delivery and postnatal surgery. MRI can be superior to ultrasound in cases of maternal obesity or oligohydramnios and also produces 3D reconstructed images in any plane[153]. Postnatal MRI is important particularly in craniopagus to assess cortical fusion and in thoracopagus, to evaluate intracardiac anatomy, blood flow and ventricular wall motion[153].

Management

The option of termination of pregnancy should be discussed. The prognosis for the twins depends upon the extent of fusion and the presence of separate organs. Twins with cerebral or cardiac fusion have poor prognosis[154]. Antenatal pediatric surgical consultation with the national center with expertise in conjoined twins is valued and, while the majority of parents decide on termination, those who continue may do so with the understanding of the need for major surgical separation and reconstruction and its associated short- and long-term morbidity.

After defining the extent of fusion and associated anomalies, serial scans are required to monitor fetal growth and liquor volume. In the third trimester, polyhydramnios complicates 50%, for which amnioreduction or sulindac may occasionally be indicated. Cesarean section needs to be classical to effect delivery of viable twins.

Postnatally, detailed MRI and CT imaging with a multidisciplinary team approach involving pediatric surgeons specialized in separation procedures is warranted. In addition, psychiatric, social services, physiotherapy, rehabilitation and nursing support are necessary. Conjoined twins fall into three management categories:

1. inoperable cases
2. operable but warrant emergency separation due to cardiac instability
3. planned elective separation.

Emergency separation carries a high mortality of 71%. In contrast, elective separation, usually planned between 2 to 4 months of age, is safer and has a survival rate of up to 80%[155].

COMPLICATIONS COMMON TO BOTH MONOCHORIONIC AND DICHORIONIC PREGNANCIES

Discordant fetal anomalies

Discordant abnormalities account for 85% of anomalous twin pregnancies[156]. Concordant anomalies, in which both twins have anomalies, are rare in DZ twins but account for 18% in MZ twins[157]. In the latter, discordant anomalies may be a consequence of asymmetric splitting of the cell mass, development of more than one organizer axis termed 'co-dominant axis theory', and/or impaired organogenesis secondary to hemodynamic imbalance due to vascular anastomoses[158]. In contrast, the risk of aneuploidy in MC twins is not increased.

The type of anomalies can be classified as:

1. those related to midline or laterality defects include neural tube defects and facial clefts, holoprosencephaly, cardiac and anterior abdominal wall defects
2. anomalies caused by hemodynamic imbalance including encephalomalacic brain lesions, pulmonary stenosis, renal agenesis, limb reductions defects, aplasia cutis and intestinal atresia
3. congenital malformations unique to MC twins include conjoined twins, acardiac twins and fetus-in fetu[159].

The overall risk of cardiac abnormalities is increased several fold, particularly in MC twins regardless of the presence of TTTS (RR, 9.2, 95%CI, 5.5–15.3)[160]. Ventricular septal defects are the most common in MC twins[161] while atrial septal defects and pulmonary stenosis occur in 7% of fetuses affected by TTTS[71]. In contrast, discordant structural heart defects in DZ twins include the more classic structural abnormalities of hypoplastic heart syndrome and atrioventricular defects.

Management

The options include expectant management, selective feticide and termination of the whole pregnancy. Selective feticide carries risks to the co-twin, so is often only accepted by the parents for anomalies likely to survive or to pose a risk to the co-twin in utero. Although expectant management is a reasonable option for DC twins discordant for lethal anomalies, studies suggest that the presence of a major anomaly, such as anencephaly or lethal trisomy, increases the likelihood of preterm delivery[162,163] and hence selective feticide may be considered on obstetric grounds. Management of discordant anomalies in MC twins is more complex as spontaneous IUFD of the anomalous twin may result in demise or hypoxic-ischemic organ injury in the surviving co-twin. Selective feticide procedures are discussed in detail later in this chapter.

Discordant fetal growth

Discordancy in growth may be quantified as a percentage of the larger fetus's weight (A − B) × 100/A, where A is the weight of the heavier and B the weight of the lighter fetus. This may be mild (<15%), moderate (15–25%) or severe (>25%). Overall, about 20% of twins are mildly discordant and 5% severely discordant[164]. The incidence of severe discordance is higher in MC (20.2%) than in DC twins (7.6%) (OR: 3.1, 95% CI,1.5–6.3)[165]. In triplets, severe discordancy affects about 34%[166] and more commonly affects primiparous women[167].

Etiology of discordant growth

Placental dysfunction, single gene disorders, poor implantation site, chromosomal abnormalities, velamentous cord insertion and single umbilical artery[165] are associated with discordant growth in both DC and MC twins as in singletons. However, in MC twins, TTTS is a major additional cause of discordant growth.

Screening for growth discordancy

Prediction

Twin pregnancies with discordant fetal CRLs at 11–14 weeks' gestation of ≥10 mm have been shown to be at increased risk for growth delay in one twin and birth weight discordancy[168], which supports the use of first-trimester ultrasound as a screening tool to identify those 'at risk'. Uterine artery Dopplers are less useful than in singletons to screen for placental insufficiency as the uterine circulation is of lower resistance in multiple pregnancies and only rarely elevated[169]. Further, uterine artery resistance indices with one on either side are not specific for any particular twin's placenta, and defective trophoblastic invasion in one placenta may be attenuated by the normal process of implantation of the co-twin's placenta[170].

Growth surveillance

There remains some controversy regarding the best ultrasonographic parameter to quantify discordant growth. Estimated fetal weight (EFW) has been reported to have higher sensitivity but lower positive predictive value (PPV) (93% and 72%) when compared to intra-pair AC difference of 20 mm (83% sensitivity and PPV) for the detection of twin growth discordancy[171]. Proponents of the AC ratio suggest that this parameter can be measured throughout pregnancy with AC ratio of 0.93 having a sensitivity and specificity of 61% and 84% respectively. However, % discrepancy in EFW remains the most widely used parameter in monitoring twin growth.

Longitudinal studies show that fetal growth velocity tapers off after 32–34 weeks' gestation in twins and this been proposed as an adaptive phenomenon[172]. Regardless of chorionicity, fetuses grow at a steady rate as in singleton pregnancies until at least 32 weeks' gestation. Most centers do not use twin charts as advocated by some, on the basis that (i) the growth potential of a twin is the same biologically as a singleton, (ii) growth velocity and fetal well-being indices matter more than absolute size.

Doppler surveillance of discordant growth

Doppler surveillance uses the same tools as in singleton pregnancies: middle cerebral artery, umbilical artery and ductus venosus waveforms. Fetal compromise in MC twins may follow a different pattern of progression from DC twins. Latency of absent end diastolic flow (AEDF) lasts longer, up to 12 weeks (median latency: 7–153 days) when compared with DC twins (30 days) and singletons (11 days)[173]. This is due to earlier gestation of presentation of AEDF in MC fetuses (21 weeks) compared to both singleton and DC fetuses (27 weeks). The presence of placental anastomoses, particularly AAA, may contribute to longer latency as well as maintaining nutrition and thus growth along centile lines[54].

Umbilical artery Doppler flow may show cyclical absent/reversed EDF (cyclic AREDF), as demonstrated in 20% of growth-restricted twins[174,175,176]. This transmitted pattern is felt to occur due to retrograde transmission of cyclical pressure changes from a large AAA to the umbilical artery waveform in the smaller MC twin, where it manifests as fluctuating end diastolic flow. Cyclic AREDF therefore should functionally be interpreted as absent end diastolic flow. Cyclic AREDF can be present from the early second trimester and remain unchanged for many weeks or until delivery[177,176]. Although some investigators suggest that cyclic AREDF is associated with worse prognosis than persistent AEDF[178], this is likely to be the result of a management approach that did not recognize its signficance as a form of AEDF.

Fetal risks

In addition to the usual risks of low birth weight (LBW) in singletons, the larger twin is at risk of respiratory distress syndrome as a result of premature delivery and in MC pregnancies, a greater risk of cerebral injury or IUFD in the event of the demise of the growth-restricted fetus. Severely discordant MC twins have a higher perinatal morbidity including preterm delivery before 30 weeks of gestation and longer duration of neonatal unit stay (>10 days) than DC twins[165]. The reported incidence of IUFD in the growth-restricted twin is between 14 and 25%[179,180]. Neuromorbidity in the larger twin including cerebral palsy, intraventricular hemorrhage and periventricular leukomalacia has been reported to be high even in the absence of single IUFD, compared to the smaller twin (20.5% versus 2.8% respectively) and has been attributed to antenatal ischemic events due to large AAAs[180].

Management of discordant growth

Dichorionic twins

Management comprises weekly fetal surveillance with fetal arterial and venous Dopplers, amniotic fluid volume and fortnightly growth assessment. More frequent Doppler studies are indicated when absent or reverse EDF is noted. The timing of delivery is a balance between the risk of iatrogenic prematurity to the healthy co-twin and risk of further decompensation of the growth-restricted fetus. Abnormal umbilical artery (AREDF) or pulsatile venous Dopplers after 28 weeks' gestation with a potentially viable weight (>700 g) or maternal complications including severe pre-eclampsia may be indications for delivery. As in singleton IUGR, prophylactic steroids followed, when the venous Dopplers deteriorate, by cesarean delivery to avoid intrapartum complications is favored over delaying delivery until CTG abnormalities.

Monochorionic twins

Spontaneous IUFD of the growth-restricted fetus jeopardizes the outcome for the healthy co-twin, so intervention is indicated earlier in MC compared to DC twins. Management dilemmas arise when severe discordancy is diagnosed prior to 28 weeks and the smaller twin has pre-viable weight and pre-terminal Dopplers, such that intervention would be solely indicated to protect the larger not the smaller fetus. Here cord occlusion remains a valid pre-emptive intervention in the second trimester to ensure intact survival of the healthy co-twin. Ethical complexities and parental anxiety may arise when faced with the option of selective feticide versus exposing a healthy co-twin to the risks of iatrogenic prematurity. However, if the fetal well-being is not critical and remains stable, elective preterm delivery by cesarean section at 32 weeks' gestation is uncontroversial.

Single intrauterine fetal death

Fetuses of a multiple pregnancy are at higher risk of dying in utero than singletons. In the first trimester, the prevalence of single fetal demise between 10 and 14 weeks' gestation is reportedly 4% for DC twins but less than 1% for MC twins[181]. In contrast, in the second and third trimesters, single IUFD complicates 0.5–2% of DC twins[182] and 6% of MC twin pregnancies[183–185]. The rarity of diagnosis of single IUFD in early MC twins suggests that single deaths soon result in double deaths. In higher order multiple pregnancies, the incidence of single IUFD is higher (4.3–17%) due to the increased number of fetuses[186]. The risk of adverse outcomes in the surviving co-twin is also higher in MC compared with DC pregnancies. Complications range from preterm delivery, co–twin demise to neurological injury in the surviving co-twin. Management of these pregnancies presents an obstetrical dilemma as there are inconsistencies in current data regarding the optimal frequency of antenatal surveillance, timing of pre-emptive delivery and investigations to monitor the surviving co-twin.

Factors determining outcome for the surviving co-twin

The factors determining the outcome for the surviving co-twin are chorionicity, gestation at the time of single IUFD and gestational age at delivery.

Chorionicity

Poor perinatal outcome is attributed to placental vascular communications between the MC twins, which allows transfer of blood, such that the surviving co-twin suffers an episode of acute hemodynamic imbalance with hypoperfusion at the time of demise of the other twin, which may result in neurological injury or death of the co-twin (hemodynamic imbalance or agonal transfusion theory)[20,187]. There are no data to support older mechanistic theories of thromboplastic material from the dead twin transfused into the survivor's circulation, resulting in disseminated intravascular coagulation[173,188].

Gestational age

First-trimester single fetal loss usually leads to co-twin demise in MC twins so is less likely to result in severe neurological morbidity. However, second- and third-trimester fetal losses are associated with higher risk of neurological handicap as well as co-twin demise. Gestational age at delivery determines the risk to the survivor. The overall risk of preterm delivery before 34 weeks' gestation (including iatrogenic and spontaneous) following a single fetal death reported in a systematic review was 65% and MC twins were at higher risk than DC twins (68% versus 57% respectively)[189].

Complications of single fetal death

Multiorgan and neurological injury

Morbidity in the surviving MC co-twin is reported to be 10-fold greater than in DC co-twin survivors[190]. Damage is predominantly to the brain (18% in MC twins and 1% in DC twins), although there are reports of multiorgan damage including pulmonary, hepatic or splenic infarcts, intestinal atresia, limb reduction, renal necrosis and rarely aplasia cutis[189,191]. For twin pregnancies overall, the recent systematic review derived a risk of 9% (95% CI 6–13%) for neurological abnormality[192].

Gestational age at the time of IUFD influences the extent and type of fetal brain injury. Single IUFD in the second trimester can lead to periventricular leukomalacia, multicystic encephalomalacia (cystic lesions in the areas supplied by the anterior and middle cerebral arteries) or germinal matrix hemorrhage which can extend into the lateral ventricles and cerebral parenchyma. In late third trimester, subcortical leukomalacia, basal ganglia damage or lenticulostriate vasculopathy may develop[117]. Secondary sequelae visible on ultrasound comprise porencephalic cysts, ventriculomegaly, cerebral atrophy and cerebellar or cerebral brain infarcts with multicystic encephalomalacia visible from 1 to 4 weeks after the event.

Co-twin demise

The death of one fetus in an MC twin pair substantially increases the risk of co-twin demise mainly in utero, or if recent, also in the early neonatal period[193]. A recent systematic review reported that surviving MC twin fetuses have a six times higher risk of IUFD (12%) following single fetal demise after 20 weeks' gestation than initially surviving DC twins (4%, OR 6.0, 95% CI 1.8-19.8)[192].

Maternal risks

Occasional reports of maternal coagulopathy in the older literature remain unsubstantiated and thus should not influence clinical management. Psychological trauma may be substantial after loss of one fetus, especially where management is expectant and the pregnancy continues, due to concerns over the well-being of the surviving fetus(es).

Management

The management of a multiple pregnancy following a single IUFD depends on chorionicity, gestational age and thus expected lung maturity, and underlying and/or resultant fetal or maternal complications.

Dichorionic twins

In the absence of maternal complications such as pre-eclampsia or abruption or intrinsic fetal pathology like growth restriction, DC twin pregnancies can be managed expectantly until 37 weeks' gestation. Antenatal surveillance includes fortnightly fetal growth and Doppler studies. Prophylactic steroids may be administered if indicated on the basis of gestational age and risk of preterm delivery.

Monochorionic twins

Until recently, there has been little consensus on the optimal care of the surviving MC co-twin. Since accurate estimation of the time of fetal demise may not always be possible, the initial step involves an assessment of the well-being of the surviving fetus followed by later investigation for neurological injury. There is no evidence that immediate delivery protects the survivor and, in fact, it may aggravate the risks due to iatrogenic prematurity[145].

Serial ultrasonography with Doppler studies of MCA is used to assess fetal well-being and anemia. MCA PSV is a non-specific sign of fetal anemia and, in this scenario, has been reported to have 90% sensitivity and specificity for moderate to severe fetal anemia following single IUFD[194]. Intrauterine rescue transfusion within 24 hours of fetal demise has been attempted to correct fetal anemia and hypovolemia and thus prevent co-twin fetal death, but does not appear to prevent brain injury; in fact it may lead to increased survival of otherwise profoundly handicapped survivors[60,195]. Thus, the main role of MCA Doppler in this setting seems to be that normal values exclude a major risk of brain injury, although further data are required to substantiate this[60,194]. After viability, CTGs may complement other tests of fetal well-being to ensure against impending co-twin death.

Sonographically, there can be considerable latency of up to 3–4 weeks between the time of fetal death and clear visualization of cerebral lesions, which is consistent with the known temporal evolution of neonatal brain injury after late intrauterine or early neonatal insults[60,196]. Notwithstanding this, subtle signs on fetal brain ultrasound have been reported within a few days of the insult[197]. Fetal MRI is complementary to ultrasound in diagnosis of transfusional lesions, but it may allow earlier detection of lesions, which is important when management options may be limited, such as approaching the late third trimester, or national limits in some countries for offering termination of pregnancy. The optimal time to perform fetal MRI is unclear, however, as cavitating lesions appear 2 or more weeks after the initial insult and with brain atrophy occurring later; a fetal MRI is thus scheduled in most units 2–3 weeks after the single IUFD. If fetal death occurred early in the second trimester, a repeat MRI may be performed at 30–34 weeks to evaluate cortical development[115,198]. Where lesions are detected, these are likely to be gross and thus associated with substantial risk of physical or mental handicap in survivors. Late termination of pregnancy is a mainstream management option for such cases in jurisdictions where this is sanctioned. Indeed, a window to allow detection of brain lesions can be a justification for continuing rather than delivering the pregnancy in the mid to late third trimester.

Weekly surveillance with growth or Doppler scans may provide reassurance to the parents regarding fetal well-being. In the absence of imaging evidence of fetal brain injury, elective delivery by cesarean section on reaching term is a reasonable option, although vaginal delivery is advocated by some authors.

Management prior to single fetal death

Prevention of co-twin sequelae in MC twins requires intervention before the first intrauterine death. Impending fetal demise of the index twin may be predicted by critically abnormal arterial and venous Dopplers or post-viability by a preterminal CTG. Under such circumstances in MC multiples only, pre-emptive bipolar cord occlusion of the affected twin may be considered before 26 weeks' gestation to prevent neurologic injury to the survivor. However, after 26–28 weeks' gestation, preterm delivery is an option to salvage one or both twins.

REDUCTION

Selective fetal reduction or feticide is usually performed at a later gestation than non-selective multifetal pregnancy reduction and carries an increased risk of miscarriage. Data from the international registry on selective termination for structural or chromosomal anomalies[43] (n = 402) reveal a higher rate of miscarriage before 24 weeks' gestation when triplets were reduced to twins (13%) compared with twins to singletons (7.1%). Further, there was a non-significant trend for the rate of miscarriage to be higher with advancing gestation: 5.4% at 9–12 weeks, 8.7% at 13–18 weeks, 6.8% at 19–24 weeks and 9.1% after 25 weeks. Further, data from the largest single center experience of 200 selective terminations showed a lower loss rate prior to 24 weeks' gestation (4%), even lower when twins were reduced to singletons (2.4%), underlying the importance of operator experience[199].

Selective feticide in dichorionic twins

Intracardiac potassium chloride injection using a 20-G needle under ultrasound guidance is the preferred method in DC pregnancies. Intrafunic KCL injection warrants caution as the wrong cord may be erroneously injected. Correctly targeting a structurally abnormal fetus is straightforward, but an aneuploid fetus without associated defects may be sonographically indistinguishable from a same sex euploid co-twin. Hence, it is imperative to differentiate precisely each twin based on detailed documentation of fetoplacental locations and sample labeling during the prenatal diagnostic procedure in order to avoid terminating the wrong fetus. Based on reports from the international registry, the rate of preterm delivery following intracardiac potassium chloride is relatively low: 12% before 33 weeks and 6% before 28 weeks' gestation[43].

Vascular occlusion in monochorionic twins

The indications for selective fetal reduction in MC twins include TRAP sequence, severe discordant fetal growth restriction, discordant fetal anomalies, heterokaryotypic chromosomal abnormality and severe TTTS in cases where laser therapy is not the preferred treatment.

Techniques

Selective feticide using intracardiac potassium chloride is contraindicated in MC twins because of the risk of interfetal agonal transfusion at the time of fetal demise with its attendant co-twin sequalae.[43] Techniques for selective feticide include mechanical cord ligation, bipolar cord occlusion and laser coagulation of umbilical cord, radiofrequency ablation and interstitial laser. These procedures can be performed either under light sedation and local anesthesia or under epidural analgesia.

Procedures described in the late 1980s and early 1990s involving either injection of sclerosing agents, such as ethanol or cyanoacrylate-based sclerosants, or embolization using thrombogenic coils have been associated with a high rate of technical failure[200] and are no longer in use.

Cord occlusion

Umbilical cord occlusion of the selected fetus for termination can be effectively achieved using any of the three methods described below. Most were originally developed on acardiac fetuses.

Bipolar cord occlusion

This is the most common method, performed between 17 and 25 weeks' gestation where the maximum cord diameter is less than 15–18 mm. Under ultrasound guidance, a 2.7 to 3.3 mm port is inserted into the sac of the affected fetus before inserting 2.0–3.0 mm bipolar forceps with a maximum blade opening width of around 15 mm (Storz etc, or Everest Medical, Minneapolis, USA). The cord is grasped with the forceps at an appropriate place to ensure correct identification and coagulated several times at 30–50 W. The energy is applied for approximately 60 seconds for several exposures at three separate sites in order to ensure complete occlusion. Appearance of steam bubbles or interference of color flow on Doppler are indicative of local heat production and hence tissue coagulation between the flow. Cessation of blood flow distal to the occlusion is checked with color Doppler after each application by loosening the cord within the forceps jaws.

Bipolar cord diathermy has the advantage of simultaneously obliterating the umbilical arteries and vein causing acute cessation of flow and thus obviating hemodynamic changes in the co-twin. Further, it is simpler than other cord occlusive methods, requires relatively inexpensive instruments and can be performed through a single port. It can be performed when fetoscopy is difficult as with blood-stained liquor or in cases of repeat interventions leading to membranous separation. However, amnioinfusion may sometimes be necessary to allow space for intrauterine manipulation and/or improve ultrasonic visualization of the cord target.

Although bipolar cord occlusion has been practiced for a decade, only one study (n = 87) has been reported to date with more than 50 cases. The perinatal survival rate of 84% is encouraging[201]. However, PPROM remains the most common complication with an incidence of 20%[201].

Laser coagulation

Fetoscopic laser coagulation of the umbilical cord may be carried out between 16 and 20 weeks. The procedure is performed via a 1.9- to 2.0-mm fetoscope inserted into the sac of the affected fetus. A 400- or 600-μm Nd:YAG (neodymium-doped yttrium aluminum garnet) laser fiber coagulates the umbilical cord vessels under direct vision. A major drawback of this technique is its higher rate of failure with larger or edematous cord at later gestations, limiting its use to before 20 weeks[90,202]. Another is a 40% risk of iatrogenic PPROM before 32 weeks' gestation[90]. Further, blood staining of liquor during any fetoscopic procedure, in this case due to rupture of vessels, can reduce visibility necessitating amnioexchange. This approach is not recommended because in half of 55 cases in one series, failure to achieve cessation of flow with laser alone required additional cord diathermy[201].

Umbilical cord ligation

Simple suture ligation of the umbilical cord is an attractive option after 26 weeks' gestation when the umbilical cord is too large for bipolar forceps to grasp[203]. Ultrasound-guided ligation via a single port is easier than cord ligation under fetoscopic visualization, as the latter involves insertion of multiple uterine ports and thus more risk of iatrogenic PPROM[204].

A 3-mm port is first inserted into the amniotic sac of the affected fetus near a free loop of umbilical cord and one looped end of suture introduced via the port using a 2-mm forceps (Karl Storz, Germany). The suture is then guided past one side of the free loop of cord and released behind the cord. We prefer PDS to Vicryl, as it is less likely to snap under tension when wet. The grasper is then withdrawn to above the cord and directed down on the other side to grasp the loop of Vicryl, securing the cord. The looped end is withdrawn and an extracorporeal knot is tied and pushed down the port using a knot pusher in a technique similar to laparoscopic knot tying. The knot is tightened until no flow is seen on color Doppler taking care to avoid undue pulling on the cord. Double or triple ligation of the cord ensures complete occlusion of the umbilical vessels.

Intrafetal ablation

The intrafetal approach is the preferred method in MC twins complicated by TRAP sequence, but can also be used for MFPR in MC twins or selective feticide in early onset TTTS. It involves targeting the intra-abdominal umbilical or aortopelvic vessels visualized on color Doppler ultrasound. Intrafetal ablation can be achieved by monopolar thermocoagulation, interstitial laser and radiofrequency energy. Intrafetal ablation has been associated with later median gestational age at delivery when compared to whole cord techniques (37 versus 32 weeks), lower failure rate (13 versus 35%) and lower rate of preterm delivery (23% versus 58%) along with a higher technical success rate (77% versus 50%)[129].

Radiofrequency ablation (RFA)

This is a promising new technique for selective reduction in TRAP sequence[131,202] and MFPR in MC twins[134,205,206]. It has also been used for MC twins discordant for fetal abnormalities[207,208]. The method between 14 and 27 weeks[209] involves use of a 14–17-G RFA needle with deployable electrodes known as tines[134] and a radiofrequency generator which produces high energy radiowaves to induce vessel coagulation (Fig. 46.6). The needle is positioned within the fetal abdomen as for interstitial laser and after advancing the tines, RFA energy is applied until the impedance meter indicates satisfactory tissue coagulation and color Doppler indicates cessation of blood flow, usually after around 3 minutes (Fig. 46.7). The preliminary results are encouraging with one series reporting an 86% survival rate (92% in MCDA) and low risk of membrane rupture[134] presumably because the needle diameter is only 14–17 G with no insertion port needed.

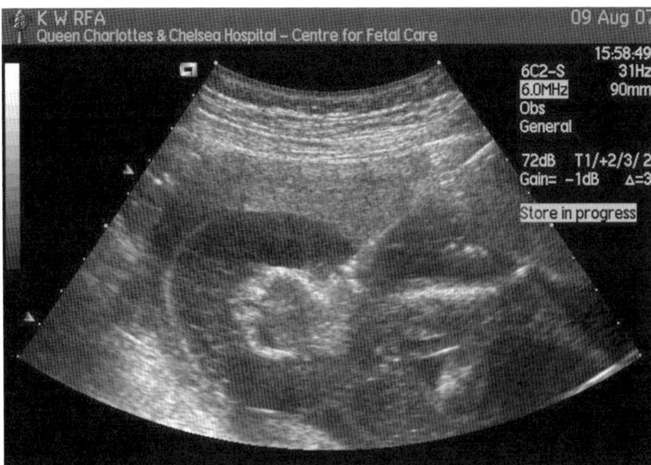

Fig. 46.6 Ultrasound image of RFA needle within the TRAP twin.

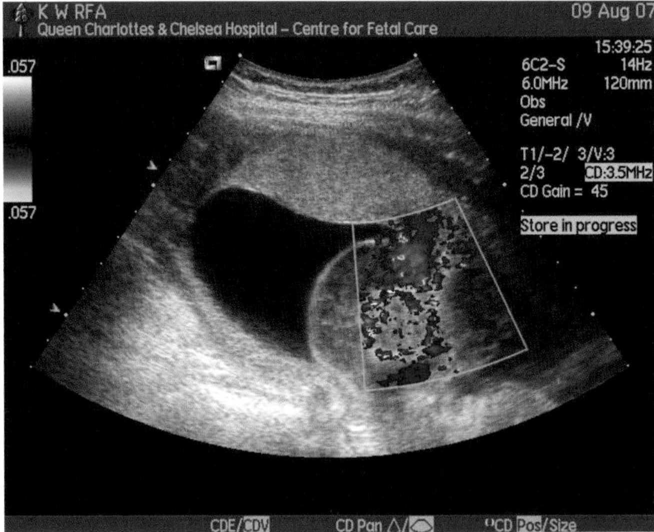

Fig. 46.7 Color Doppler showing disturbance upon deploying radiofrequency energy during intrafetal ablation of TRAP twin.

Interstitial laser ablation

This procedure is performed earlier in gestation, up to 17–20 weeks. Jolly et al. first described interstitial laser to obviate the risks of iatrogenic cord rupture in a free loop of cord, and used a 17-G needle[210] positioned near the intrahepatic vein and intra-abdominal umbilical vessels under color guidance. A 400- or 600-μm laser fiber is then passed down the lumen of the needle until seen protruding ca. 4 mm beyond the needle tip on scan. The vessels are coagulated commencing with spurts of 20 W with 10-W increments up to a maximum of 50 W until no color flow is seen. The only series showed that in 30 pregnancies treated at a median of 15 weeks, the procedure-related unintended fetal loss rate was 10% per pregnancy, but perinatal survival was only 68% in non-reduced fetuses[211].

Monopolar thermocoagulation

Monopolar diathermy involves a 1-mm diameter wire electrode insulated with polytetrafluroethylene along its length inserted via an 18-G needle into the intrafetal umbilical or aortopelvic vessels connected to a monopolar diathermy generator[212]. Although the procedure is simple and can be performed under local anesthesia, there is a potential risk of thermal injury along the path of the needle with resultant damage to the uterus and fetal membranes. Current experience is limited to case reports of selective reduction of TRAP or anomalous fetuses before 14 weeks of gestation[212,213] and with increasing experience of RFA, thermocoagulation is likely to become obsolete.

Selective feticide in monoamniotic twins

Discordant anomalies complicating MA twin pregnancies carry increased risk to both twins. Selective reduction using either umbilical cord occlusion or fetoscopic vessel ablation with cord ligation are options but can be technically challenging due to difficulty identifying the abnormal twin's cord within an entangled cord mass[214]. This can be overcome, albeit with some technical difficulty, by targeting the umbilical cord close to the affected fetus's abdomen. Intrafetal ablation using RFA prior to 24 weeks' gestation is an alternative but limited experience in non-acardiac fetuses suggests higher loss rates of up to one third[206]. Termination of the whole pregnancy is another option in cases with severe anomalies.

To avoid subsequent cord entanglement and the related risk of demise of the survivor, investigators have suggested transection of the umbilical cord[215,216] but this is challenging and prolongs the operating time and it is not clear whether it warrants the additional procedure-related risk.

Elective late feticide

The timing of selective feticide depends on the gestation at diagnosis of fetal abnormality or severe discordant growth. When a second-trimester diagnosis is made, clinicians may opt to offer selective feticide in the early third trimester to obviate procedure-related risks for the surviving co-twin such as miscarriage or amniorrhexis. The rationale is analagous to that of elective late karyotyping. Indeed, late selective feticide may be a consequence of late karyotyping in twins, this package minimizing the early gestational risks of both procedures in concert.

Although appropriate for DC twins undergoing the potassium chloride procedure, caution is required with vaso-occlusive techniques in MC twins. This is because after 26 weeks, the options for feticide in MC twins are limited technically by the size of the cord and its blood flow, with ultrasound-guided cord ligation arguably the only practical option.

Parents contemplating this option must be counseled regarding the possibility of spontaneous preterm labor prior to feticide and thus the risk of unintended birth of a baby with long-term physical or mental handicap. Further, as discussed with late karyotyping, late elective feticide is only appropriate in jurisdictions that allow termination after viability.

HIGHER ORDER MULTIPLE PREGNANCIES

Perinatal outcome is significantly compromised in higher order multiple pregnancies, chiefly as a result of preterm delivery and low birth weight. Apart from mortality, survivors have an increased risk of long-term disabilities such as cerebral palsy, developmental delay and visual impairment. The Western Australian cerebral palsy register estimated the risk of a cerebral palsy-affected child to be 47 times higher for a woman with a triplet pregnancy and 8–12 times higher with a twin pregnancy when compared to a singleton[217,218]. In a retrospective cohort study of 94 triplets, 34% of surviving triplets suffered neurological handicap in the form of cerebral palsy or cerebral dysfunction manifesting as hyperkinetic syndrome, visual, auditory or speech difficulties[219]. Further evidence comes from a European multicenter study which reported 4 times the incidence of cerebral palsy in multiple pregnancies compared to singletons (7.6 versus 1.6 per 1000 live births, RR 4.4; 95% CI, 3.6–4.9)[220]. Figure 46.8 illustrates the published rates of cerebral palsy among infant survivors of singleton, twin and triplet pregnancies.

High order multiples have considerably increased maternal risks with pregnancy-associated hypertension (adjusted odds ratio: 2.8 in triplets versus 2.3 in twins) diabetes (2.0 versus 1.2), incompetent cervix (18.6 versus 3.5), requirement for tocolysis (13.5 versus 4.5) and bleeding in labor and delivery (2.8 versus 1.9)[221]. In addition to increased risk of maternal depression, women with iatrogenic multiple births were more than 3 times likely to have difficulties meeting basic material needs and also twice likely to have lower quality of life and increased social stigma than those with singleton births (Fig. 46.9)[222].

MFPR or non-selective fetal reduction was developed about two decades ago in an attempt to reduce the adverse sequalae associated with multiple pregnancies[223–225] This procedure has since evolved over time reflecting modifications in ART, patient attitudes and practice among fetal medicine specialists[226].

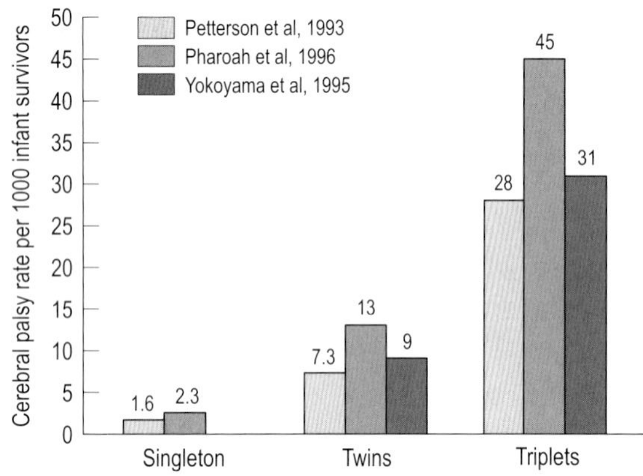

Fig. 46.8 Published rates of cerebral palsy in singletons, twins and triplets. Reproduced from Wimalasundera et al. 2003[218] with permission.

Multifetal pregnancy reduction

MFPR is optimally scheduled between 11 and 14 weeks' gestation for two reasons: to allow sufficient time for the risk of spontaneous first-trimester reduction to have passed and to facilitate selection of fetuses using increased nuchal translucency or a scan for gross structural anomalies. The procedure is performed using a transabdominal approach with intracardiac potassium chloride injected into the targeted fetus(es) via a 20-G needle. The fetus away from the cervix is selected for reduction to reduce the risk of ascending infection in retained dead tissue. The older transvaginal approach was associated with higher miscarriage risk (12% versus 5.4% for transabdominal). Although pregnancy outcomes are similar if CVS is performed prior to fetal reduction, this is now rarely necessary given the availability of NT screening together with the recognition that Down's syndrome is comparatively infrequent in continuing twins[227,228].

Reduction of triplets and quadruplets to twins

The 2001 collaborative data demonstrated that the perinatal outcome of triplets and quadruplets reduced to twins approaches that of spontaneous twins[223,229] with pregnancy loss rates (<24 weeks' gestation) in reduced triplets of only 4.4% and reduced quadruplets of 6.6%. The rates of preterm delivery before were highest with those left as triplets (25%) followed by twins (8.5%) and lowest with singletons (3.9%)[229]. In a smaller series of European cohort (n = 313), the risk of miscarriage also correlated with the finishing number of fetuses with rates of 8.2% and 8.9% for triplets reduced to twins and quadruplets reduced to twins respectively, with increased losses when triplets were reduced to singletons (14.3%)[230].

Unreduced triplets versus reduced triplets

Although there is universal agreement that perinatal outcome improves with reduction of quadruplets and higher order multiples, there remains controversy about the outcome of reduced versus unreduced triplets. In part this reflects reasonable perinatal outcomes for the majority of trichorionic triplets managed expectantly. Further, there is no major difference in outcome between neonates born at 34 versus 32 weeks, the difference between reduced remaining twins versus unreduced triplets[231].

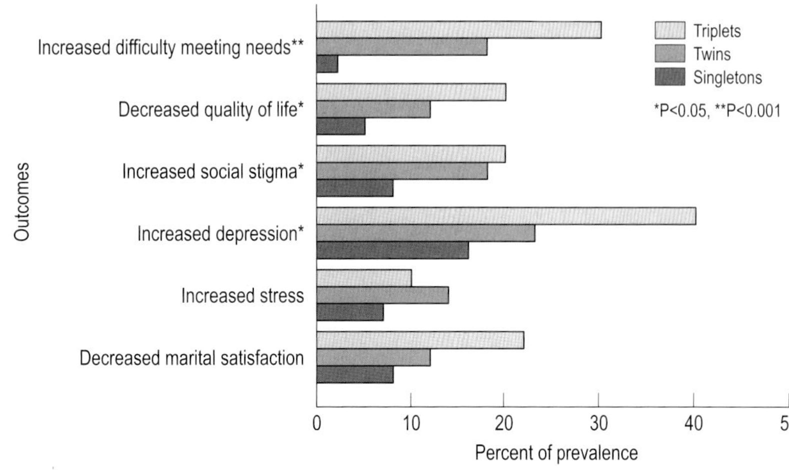

Fig. 46.9 Prevalence (%) in outcomes by multiplicity in full-term births. $^*P < 0.05$. Reproduced from Ellison et al. 2005[222] with permission.

In part this reflects the understandable lack of randomized trials, with interpretation of data from the available observational cohorts hampered by poorly described control cohorts with loose entry criteria, by improvement in expectant outcomes with time and by better results of MFPR with increasing experience. The real controversy concerns miscarriage rates, as MFPR reduces the rate through continuing with a reduced fetal number, but increases the rate through exposure to an invasive procedure.

In this light, one recent meta-analysis of 14 studies (2641 cases) of reduced triplet pregnancies and 17 of unreduced triplets (1041 cases) suggested that there was a non-significant reduction in pregnancy loss prior to 24 weeks' gestation when triplets were reduced to twins compared with unreduced triplets (5.7% versus 7.5%, odds ratio 0.7 95% CI 0.5–1.0). Further, the preterm delivery rate before 28 and 32 weeks' gestation was lower in the reduced group compared with unreduced triplets (4% and 9% versus 10% and 25% respectively), resulting in a reduction in perinatal mortality rate in the reduced group (43/1000 versus 110/1000 live births)[232]. However in contrast, a large single-center series of triplet pregnancies comparing reduced (n = 180) with unreduced trichorionic triplets (n = 185)[233,234] showed that the rate of miscarriage was higher in the reduced compared with non-reduced group (8.3% versus 4.9%, odds ratio 1.7, 95% CI 0.7–3.9). Nevertheless, the early preterm delivery rate was lower in the reduced group (9.7% versus 23.9%) similar to the earlier meta-analysis[232]. The same authors then did their own systematic review of six studies (including their own data above), to substantiate an increased miscarriage risk (8.1% versus 4.4%, RR: 1.8, 95% CI 1.1–3.2, $P = 0.04$) in reduced triplets when compared with non-reduced triplets. The investigators estimated that seven reductions needed to be performed to prevent one early preterm delivery, while the number of reductions to cause one miscarriage was 26[234]. The discrepancy in pregnancy loss rates before 24 weeks in the two meta-analyses may reflect differing stringency of inclusion criteria, as well as the inclusion of the large Papageorghiou study in the later review. However, the later review was less stringent, incorporating studies that included non-trichorionic triplets.

Thus, current statistics on which to counsel women are uncertain and based on weaker observational data. Although randomized controlled trials would be desirable, these are unlikely to happen and, in any case, the incidence of triplet pregnancies is declining in many countries with increasing proscription of three and even one embryo transfers. In the interim, it can be concluded that reduction of triplets to twins reduces the early preterm delivery rate towards that in unreduced twins, which would be expected to be associated with an improvement in short- and long-term perinatal outcomes. Every woman with triplets should be offered reduction, but this can be a very difficult decision for couples with 'precious' pregnancies after years of infertility. Whether the miscarriage rate is or is not increased by reduction is unclear, so parental preferences and social factors are of increasing importance in this difficult area of prenatal counseling.

Reduction to singletons

Previously, MFM (Maternal Fetal Medicine) specialists were reluctant to offer elective reduction to a singleton pregnancy, largely based on the greater risk of miscarriage the more fetuses are reduced, but also an acceptance of reasonable perinatal outcome in twins[235]. However, recent trends in MFPR suggest a change in practice and patient attitudes with approximately 40% of patients in a large single center study opting for reduction to a singleton compared to 11.8% in a previous study performed by the same group[226]. This shift has been attributed to increased awareness among patients of greater perinatal morbidity and mortality in twins compared to singletons and also reduction of the MC twin pairs conceived following blastocyst transfer. Reduction to a singleton pregnancy is associated with lower rate of preterm delivery (11%) and neonatal death (0.6%) when compared to reduction to twins (64% and 3.4% respectively), although the miscarriage rate (6.5% versus 1.9%) is higher as expected, attributed in part to the presence of more residual dead tissue[236]. In terms of patient attitudes, a survey of patients attending a Canadian fertility clinic reported about 60% expressing desire for singleton pregnancy[237] which is in sharp contrast to the recent European study where more (58.7%) preferred having twins to having one child at a time (37.9%)[238]. Any decision to opt for reduction to singleton should be individualized taking into account the woman's age, parental choices and chorionicity.

Ethical dimensions of MFPR

One dimension balances intentional sacrifice of the lives of otherwise healthy fetuses against the reduction in morbidity of the surviving fetuses. Notwithstanding this, nearly 30 million pregnancies globally undergo termination of pregnancy for socioeconomic indications, which is accepted as an important public health measure. Nevertheless, infertile couples who conceive after a protracted period of infertility treatment can be emotionally challenged when faced with the dilemma of MFPR. Between 30 and 70% of women undergoing MFPR had acute feelings of anxiety, stress and emotional trauma[239,240] and, in one study, about one-third thought it was tantamount to a violent death[241]. Almost half of MFPR patients find decision making very difficult[242]. Negative feelings may still be expressed after delivery mainly in the form of guilt, regret and grief for the lost child[243]. Notwithstanding this, the woman's autonomy must be respected in any decision making. In practice, patients should be counseled prior to initiating fertility treatment regarding the maternal and perinatal outcome of higher order multiples and the option of MFPR. The goal remains prevention through more responsible fertility practices and there is evidence that MFPR is declining in frequency.

Monochorionic higher order multiples

An MC pair is reported to occur in 28–50% of higher order multiple pregnancies[244,245] up to 44% of which are conceived spontaneously[246]. These pregnancies are at higher risk of perinatal complications than their corresponding polychorionic controls including TTTS, fetal growth restriction (33% versus 25%), single fetal death (8.8% versus 1.5%, $P < 0.01$), PPROM and preterm labor before 32 weeks (47% versus 32%)[10,246]. Management is thus a dilemma. On the one hand, the increase in perinatal risks argues for an active approach, but on the other hand, reduction to twins involves leaving an MC pair with increased risks which is counterintuitive, or reducing both MC twins which increases miscarriage risk due to the greater number reduced, or some occlusive form of feticide in one of the MC pair, the results of which are considerably poorer in terms of outcome than KCL methods in DC pairs. Although the data are poor, suboptimal results with interstital laser in MC twins[211] suggest that the preferable option instead is reduction of the whole MC pair by intracardiac injection of potassium chloride. This is the least invasive, obviates any transfusional risk in albeit the remaining only singeton. Despite the high rate of procedure-related complications as a consequence of twice the retained fetoplacental tissue mass[234] or ruptured membranes, pregnancy outcome is quite reasonable with live birth rates of 93%[245]. A major reduction in the high rate of preterm labor seen in conservatively managed DC triplets (63%) with reduction to a singleton further supports reduction of the MC component as the preferred strategy for MFPR[246].

CONCLUSIONS

The epidemic of multiple pregnancies secondary to changing demographics and fertility practice remains of major concern to clinicians world-wide because of their high rate of complications and contribution to preventable perinatal disease burden.

Because MC compared to DC twin pregnancies have three-to fivefold increased perinatal morbidity and mortality, early determination of chorionicity underpins management, including prenatal screening, diagnosis, counseling and intervention for discordant fetal anomalies and growth restriction. Nuchal translucency ideally with concomitant biochemistry is the fetal-specific method of choice for risk estimation for aneuploidy in twins. Both CVS and amniocentesis are associated with higher risks of pregnancy loss compared with singletons, while the high risk of sample contamination at CVS renders amniocentesis the preferred diagnostic procedure. High order multiple pregnancies substantially increase obstetric and perinatal complications not to mention parental coping issues. MFPR is offered to reduce perinatal risks, with outcomes in pregnancies reduced to twins approaching that of spontaneous twins.

Recent progress in the treament of complications specific to MC twins includes fetoscopic laser for TTTS, vascular occlusion for TRAP and medical amnioreduction in MA twins. For TTTS, laser ablation of anastomotic vessels has been shown to improve survival and short-term neurologic morbidity compared with amnioreduction, although the optimal management of early stage TTTS, which may resolve spontaneously, remains unclear. Discordant MC growth restriction that progresses to single IUFD exposes the appropriately grown co-twin to risk of sudden death and injury, which may be obviated by pre-emptive cord occlusion and/or timely delivery. Improved results in MA twins through maternal sulindac and elective abdominal delivery at 32 weeks along with the rarity of TTTS, suggest that MA twins paradoxically now have a better outcome than MCDA twins. Because intracardiac KCL used for selective feticide in DC twins is contraindicated in MC, vaso-occlusive techniques including bipolar cord occlusion or radiofrequency ablation are preferred options for this indication and for twin reversed arteral perfusion sequence. Notwithstanding substantial progress over the last decade, future studies to evaluate long-term neurodevelopmental outcomes following fetal therapy are required to optimize management and informed counseling of women with complicated multiple pregnancies.

REFERENCES

1. Kurinczuk J. Epidemiology of multiple pregnancy: changing effects of assisted conception. In *Multiple pregnancy*, MBP Kilby, H Critchley, D Field (eds), pp. 1–28. London: RCOG Press, 2006.
2. Martin JAHB, Sutton PD, Ventura SJ, Menacker F, Kirmeyer S. Births: final data for 2004. *National Vital Statistics Reports* **55**(1):26, 2006.
3. Schachter M, Raziel A, Friedler S, Strassburger D, Bern O, Ron-El R. Monozygotic twinning after assisted reproductive techniques: a phenomenon independent of micromanipulation. *Hum Reprod* **16**(6):1264–1269, 2001.
4. Allan M. Factors affecting developmental outcomes. In *Multiple pregnancy: epidemiology, gestation and perinatal outcome*, LGPE Keith, DM Keith, B Like (eds), pp. 599–612. New York: The Parthenon Publishing Group, 1995.
5. One child at a time: reducing multiple births after IVF. Report of the Expert Group on Multiple Births after IVF 24, 2006.
6. Australian Institute of Health and Welfare bulletin 21 Australia's babies: their health and wellbeing: www.npsu.unsw.edu.au/Publications, 2004.
7. Hack KE, Derks JB, Elias SG et al. Increased perinatal mortality and morbidity in monochorionic versus dichorionic twin pregnancies: clinical implications of a large Dutch cohort study. *Br J Obstet Gynaecol* **115**(1):58–67, 2008.
8. Barigye O, Pasquini L, Galea P, Chambers H, Chappell L, Fisk NM. High risk of unexpected late fetal death in monochorionic twins despite intensive ultrasound surveillance: a cohort study. *PLoS Med* **2**(6):e172, 2005.
9. Lee YM, Wylie BJ, Simpson LL, D'Alton ME. Twin chorionicity and the risk of stillbirth. *Obstet Gynecol* **111**(2):301–308, 2008.
10. Bajoria R, Ward SB, Adegbite AL. Com-parative study of perinatal outcome of dichorionic and trichorionic iatrogenic triplets. *Am J Obstet Gynecol* **194**(2):415–424, 2006.
11. Blickstein I. Epidemiology of cerebral palsy in multiple pregnancies. In *Mutlipe pregnancy*, MBP Kilby, H Critchley, D Field (eds). London: RCOG Press, 2006.
12. Wolf EJ, Vintzileos AM, Rosenkrantz TS, Rodis JF, Lettieri L, Mallozzi A. A comparison of pre-discharge survival and morbidity in singleton and twin very low birth weight infants. *Obstet Gynecol* **80** (3 Pt 1):436–439, 1992.
13. Hertzberg BS, Kurtz AB, Choi HY et al. Significance of membrane thickness in the sonographic evaluation of twin gestations. *Am J Roentgenol* **148**(1):151–153, 1987.
14. Mahony BS, Filly RA, Callen PW. Amnionicity and chorionicity in twin pregnancies: prediction using ultrasound. *Radiology* **155**(1):205–209, 1985.
15. Barss VA, Benacerraf BR, Frigoletto FD, Jr. Ultrasonographic determination of chorion type in twin gestation. *Obstet Gynecol* **66**(6):779–783, 1985.
16. Winn HN, Gabrielli S, Reece EA, Roberts JA, Salafia C, Hobbins JC. Ultrasonographic criteria for the prenatal diagnosis of placental chorionicity in twin gestations. *Am J Obstet Gynecol* **161**(6 Pt 1):1540–1542, 1989.
17. Wood SL, St Onge R, Connors G, Elliot PD. Evaluation of the twin peak or lambda sign in determining chorionicity in multiple pregnancy. *Obstet Gynecol* **88**(1):6–9, 1996.
18. Stagiannis KD, Sepulveda W, Southwell D, Price DA, Fisk NM. Ultrasonographic measurement of the dividing membrane in twin pregnancy during the second and third trimesters: a reproducibility study. *Am J Obstet Gynecol* **173**(5):1546–1550, 1995.

19. Senat MV, Quarello E, Levaillant JM, Buonumano A, Boulvain M, Frydman R. Determining chorionicity in twin gestations: three-dimensional (3D) multiplanar sonographic measurement of intra-amniotic membrane thickness. *Ultrasound Obstet Gynecol* **28**(5):665–669, 2006.
20. Bajoria R, Kingdom J. The case for routine determination of chorionicity and zygosity in multiple pregnancy. *Prenat Diagn* **17**(13):1207–1225, 1997.
21. Lewi L, Blickstein I, Van Schoubroeck D et al. Diagnosis and management of heterokaryotypic monochorionic twins. *Am J Med Genet A* **140**(3):272–275, 2006.
22. Jenkins TM, Wapner RJ. The challenge of prenatal diagnosis in twin pregnancies. *Curr Opin Obstet Gynecol* **12**(2):87–92, 2000.
23. Cuckle H. Down's syndrome screening in twins. *J Med Screen* **5**(1):3–4, 1998.
24. Wald N, Cuckle H, Wu TS, George L. Maternal serum unconjugated oestriol and human chorionic gonadotrophin levels in twin pregnancies: implications for screening for Down's syndrome. *Br J Obstet Gynaecol* **98**(9):905–908, 1991.
25. Odibo AO, Elkousy MH, Ural SH, Driscoll DA, Mennuti MT, Macones GA. Screening for aneuploidy in twin pregnancies: maternal age- and race-specific risk assessment between 9–14 weeks. *Twin Res* **6**(4):251–256, 2003.
26. Spencer K. Screening for trisomy 21 in twin pregnancies in the first trimester using free beta-hCG and PAPP-A, combined with fetal nuchal translucency thickness. *Prenat Diagn* **20**(2):91–95, 2000.
27. Niemimaa M, Suonpaa M, Heinonen S, Seppala M, Bloigu R, Ryynanen M. Maternal serum human chorionic gonadotrophin and pregnancy-associated plasma protein A in twin pregnancies in the first trimester. *Prenat Diagn* **22**(3): 183–185, 2002.
28. Sebire NJ, Snijders RJ, Hughes K, Sepulveda W, Nicolaides KH. Screening for trisomy 21 in twin pregnancies by maternal age and fetal nuchal translucency thickness at 10–14 weeks of gestation. *Br J Obstet Gynaecol* **103**(10): 999–1003, 1996.
29. Wald NJ, Rish S, Hackshaw AK. Combining nuchal translucency and serum markers in prenatal screening for Down syndrome in twin pregnancies. *Prenat Diagn* **23**(7):588–592, 2003.
30. Carvalho JS. Early prenatal diagnosis of major congenital heart defects. *Curr Opin Obstet Gynecol* **13**(2):155–159, 2001.
31. Matias A, Montenegro N, Blickstein I. Down syndrome screening in multiple pregnancies. *Obstet Gynecol Clin North Am* **32**(1):81–96, ix, 2005.
32. Sebire NJ, D'Ercole C, Hughes K, Carvalho M, Nicolaides KH. Increased nuchal translucency thickness at 10–14 weeks of gestation as a predictor of severe twin-to-twin transfusion syndrome. *Ultrasound Obstet Gynecol* **10**(2):86–89, 1997.
33. Whitlow BJ, Lazanakis MS, Economides DL. The sonographic identification of fetal gender from 11 to 14 weeks of gestation. *Ultrasound Obstet Gynecol* **13**(5):301–304, 1999.
34. Kagan KO, Gazzoni A, Sepulveda-Gonzalez G, Sotiriadis A, Nicolaides KH. Discordance in nuchal translucency thickness in the prediction of severe twin-to-twin transfusion syndrome. *Ultrasound Obstet Gynecol* **29**(5):527–532, 2007.
35. Maymon R, Dreazen E, Tovbin Y, Bukovsky I, Weinraub Z, Herman A. The feasibility of nuchal translucency measurement in higher order multiple gestations achieved by assisted reproduction. *Hum Reprod* **14**(8): 2102–2105, 1999.
36. Wald NJ, Rodeck C, Hackshaw AK, Walters J, Chitty L, Mackinson AM. First and second trimester antenatal screening for Down's syndrome: the results of the Serum, Urine and Ultrasound Screening Study (SURUSS). *J Med Screen* **10**(2): 56–104, 2003.
37. Cuckle H. Integrating antenatal Down's syndrome screening. *Curr Opin Obstet Gynecol* **13**(2):175–181, 2001.
38. Spencer K. Screening for trisomy 21 in twin pregnancies in the first trimester: does chorionicity impact on maternal serum free beta-hCG or PAPP-A levels? *Prenat Diagn* **21**(9):715–717, 2001.
39. Spencer K, Kagan KO, Nicolaides KH. Screening for trisomy 21 in twin pregnancies in the first trimester: an update of the impact of chorionicity on maternal serum markers. *Prenat Diagn* **28**(1):49–52, 2008.
40. Sebire NJ, Noble PL, Odibo A, Malligiannis P, Nicolaides KH. Single uterine entry for genetic amniocentesis in twin pregnancies. *Ultrasound Obstet Gynecol* **7**(1):26–31, 1996.
41. Yukobowich E, Anteby EY, Cohen SM, Lavy Y, Granat M, Yagel S. Risk of fetal loss in twin pregnancies undergoing second trimester amniocentesis(1). *Obstet Gynecol* **98**(2):231–234, 2001.
42. Millaire M, Bujold E, Morency AM, Gauthier RJ. Mid-trimester genetic amniocentesis in twin pregnancy and the risk of fetal loss. *J Obstet Gynaecol Can* **28**(6):512–518, 2006.
43. Evans MI, Goldberg JD, Horenstein J et al. Selective termination for structural, chromosomal, and mendelian anomalies: international experience. *Am J Obstet Gynecol* **181**(4):893 897, 1999.
44. Taylor MJ, Fisk NM. Prenatal diagnosis in multiple pregnancy. *Baillieres Best Pract Res Clin Obstet Gynaecol* **14**(4):663–675, 2000.
45. Brambati B, Tului L, Guercilena S, Alberti E. Outcome of first-trimester chorionic villus sampling for genetic investigation in multiple pregnancy. *Ultrasound Obstet Gynecol* **17**(3):209–216, 2001.
46. Antsaklis A, Daskalakis G, Souka AP, Kavalakis Y, Michalas S. Fetal blood sampling in twin pregnancies. *Ultrasound Obstet Gynecol* **22**(4):377–379, 2003.
47. Lopriore E, van Wezel-Meijler G, Middeldorp JM, Sueters M, Vandenbussche FP, Walther FJ. Neurodevelopmental outcome after laser therapy for twin-twin transfusion syndrome. *Am J Obstet Gynecol* **196**(1):e20, 2007, author reply e20-21.
48. Quintero RA, Morales WJ, Allen MH, Bornick PW, Johnson PK, Kruger M. Staging of twin-twin transfusion syndrome. *J Perinatol* **19**(8 Pt 1):550–555, 1999.
49. Taylor MJ, Govender L, Jolly M, Wee L, Fisk NM. Validation of the Quintero staging system for twin-twin transfusion syndrome. *Obstet Gynecol* **100**(6):1257–1265, 2002.
50. Yamamoto M, El Murr L, Robyr R, Leleu F, Takahashi Y, Ville Y. Incidence and impact of perioperative complications in 175 fetoscopy-guided laser coagulations of chorionic plate anastomoses in fetofetal transfusion syndrome before 26 weeks of gestation. *Am J Obstet Gynecol* **193**(3 Pt 2): 1110–1116, 2005.
51. Duncombe GJ, Dickinson JE, Evans SF. Perinatal characteristics and outcomes of pregnancies complicated by twin-twin transfusion syndrome. *Obstet Gynecol* **101**(6):1190–1196, 2003.
52. Luks FI, Carr SR, Plevyak M et al. Limited prognostic value of a staging system for twin-to-twin transfusion syndrome. *Fetal Diagn Ther* **19**(3):301–304, 2004.
53. Bajoria R, Wigglesworth J, Fisk NM. Angioarchitecture of monochorionic placentas in relation to the twin-twin transfusion syndrome. *Am J Obstet Gynecol* **172**(3):856–863, 1995.
54. Denbow ML, Cox P, Taylor M, Hammal DM, Fisk NM. Placental angioarchitecture in monochorionic twin pregnancies: relationship to fetal growth, fetofetal transfusion syndrome, and pregnancy outcome. *Am J Obstet Gynecol* **182**(2):417–426, 2000.
55. Taylor MJ, Denbow ML, Tanawattanacharoen S, Gannon C, Cox PM, Fisk NM. Doppler detection of arterio-arterial anastomoses in monochorionic twins: feasibility and clinical application. *Hum Reprod* **15**(7):1632–1636, 2000.
56. Diehl W, Hecher K, Zikulnig L, Vetter M, Hackeloer BJ. Placental vascular anastomoses visualized during fetoscopic laser surgery in severe mid-trimester twin-twin transfusion syndrome. *Placenta* **22**(10):876–881, 2001.
57. Umur A, van Gemert MJ, Nikkels PG, Ross MG. Monochorionic twins and

twin-twin transfusion syndrome: the protective role of arterio-arterial anastomoses. *Placenta* **23**(2-3):201–209, 2002.
58. Fichera A, Mor E, Soregaroli M, Frusca T. Antenatal detection of arterio-arterial anastomoses by Doppler placental assessment in monochorionic twin pregnancies. *Fetal Diagn Ther* **20**(6): 519–523, 2005.
59. Fusi L, McParland P, Fisk N, Nicolini U, Wigglesworth J. Acute twin-twin transfusion: a possible mechanism for brain-damaged survivors after intrauterine death of a monochorionic twin. *Obstet Gynecol* **78**(3 Pt 2):517–520, 1991.
60. Tanawattanacharoen S, Taylor MJ, Letsky EA, Cox PM, Cowan FM, Fisk NM. Intrauterine rescue transfusion in monochorionic multiple pregnancies with recent single intrauterine death. *Prenat Diagn* **21**(4):274–278, 2001.
61. Bajoria R, Ward S, Sooranna SR. Atrial natriuretic peptide mediated polyuria: pathogenesis of polyhydramnios in the recipient twin of twin-twin transfusion syndrome. *Placenta* **22**(8-9):716–724, 2001.
62. De Paepe ME, Stopa E, Huang C, Hansen K, Luks FI. Renal tubular apoptosis in twin-to-twin transfusion syndrome. *Pediatr Dev Pathol* **6**(3):215–225, 2003.
63. Bajoria R, Sullivan M, Fisk NM. Endothelin concentrations in monochorionic twins with severe twin-twin transfusion syndrome. *Hum Reprod* **14**(6):1614–1618, 1999.
64. Mahieu-Caputo D, Muller F, Joly D et al. Pathogenesis of twin-twin transfusion syndrome: the renin-angiotensin system hypothesis. *Fetal Diagn Ther* **16**(4):241–244, 2001.
65. Kilby MD, Platt C, Whittle MJ, Oxley J, Lindop GB. Renin gene expression in fetal kidneys of pregnancies complicated by twin-twin transfusion syndrome. *Pediatr Dev Pathol* **4**(2):175–179, 2001.
66. Wee LY, Sullivan M, Humphries K, Fisk NM. Longitudinal blood flow in shared (arteriovenous anastomoses) and non-shared cotyledons in monochorionic placentae. *Placenta* **28**(5-6):516–522, 2007.
67. Galea P BO, We L, Jain V, Sullivan M, Fisk NM. Discordant placental renin elaboration explains paradoxical renin angiotensin activation in monozygous twin fetuses with twin to twin transfusion syndrome. unpublished 2008.
68. Martinez JM, Bermudez C, Becerra C, Lopez J, Morales WJ, Quintero RA. The role of Doppler studies in predicting individual intrauterine fetal demise after laser therapy for twin-twin transfusion syndrome. *Ultrasound Obstet Gynecol* **22**(3):246–251, 2003.
69. Zikulnig L, Hecher K, Bregenzer T, Baz E, Hackeloer BJ. Prognostic factors in severe twin-twin transfusion syndrome treated by endoscopic laser surgery. *Ultrasound Obstet Gynecol* **14**(6):380–387, 1999.
70. Zosmer N, Bajoria R, Weiner E, Rigby M, Vaughan J, Fisk NM. Clinical and echographic features of in utero cardiac dysfunction in the recipient twin in twin-twin transfusion syndrome. *Br Heart J* **72**(1):74–79, 1994.
71. Karatza AA, Wolfenden JL, Taylor MJ, Wee L, Fisk NM, Gardiner HM. Influence of twin-twin transfusion syndrome on fetal cardiovascular structure and function: prospective case-control study of 136 monochorionic twin pregnancies. *Heart* **88**(3):271–277, 2002.
72. Barrea C, Alkazaleh F, Ryan G et al. Prenatal cardiovascular manifestations in the twin-to-twin transfusion syndrome recipients and the impact of therapeutic amnioreduction. *Am J Obstet Gynecol* **192**(3):892–902, 2005.
73. Lougheed J, Sinclair BG, Fung Kee Fung K et al. Acquired right ventricular outflow tract obstruction in the recipient twin in twin-twin transfusion syndrome. *J Am Coll Cardiol* **38**(5):1533–1538, 2001.
74. Delsing B, Lopriore E, Blom N, Te Pas AB, Vandenbussche FP, Walther FJ. Risk of persistent pulmonary hypertension of the neonate in twin-to-twin transfusion syndrome. *Neonatology* **92**(2):134–138, 2007.
75. Gardiner HM, Taylor MJ, Karatza A et al. Twin-twin transfusion syndrome: the influence of intrauterine laser photocoagulation on arterial distensibility in childhood. *Circulation* **107**(14): 1906–1911, 2003.
76. Senat MV, Deprest J, Boulvain M, Paupe A, Winer N, Ville Y. Endoscopic laser surgery versus serial amnioreduction for severe twin-to-twin transfusion syndrome. *N Engl J Med* **351**(2):136–144, 2004.
77. Ville Y, Hyett J, Hecher K, Nicolaides K. Preliminary experience with endoscopic laser surgery for severe twin-twin transfusion syndrome. *N Engl J Med* **332**(4):224–227, 1995.
78. Quintero RA, Comas C, Bornick PW, Allen MH, Kruger M. Selective versus non-selective laser photocoagulation of placental vessels in twin-to-twin transfusion syndrome. *Ultrasound Obstet Gynecol* **16**(3):230–236, 2000.
79. Quintero RA, Bornick PW, Morales WJ, Allen MH. Selective photocoagulation of communicating vessels in the treatment of monochorionic twins with selective growth retardation. *Am J Obstet Gynecol* **185**(3):689–696, 2001.
80. Stirnemann JJ, Nasr B, Quarello E et al. A definition of selectivity in laser coagulation of chorionic plate anastomoses in twin-to-twin transfusion syndrome and its relationship to perinatal outcome. *Am J Obstet Gynecol* **198**(1):62 e1–6, 2008.
81. Wee LY, Taylor MJ, Vanderheyden T, Wimalasundera R, Gardiner HM, Fisk NM. Reversal of twin-twin transfusion syndrome: frequency, vascular anatomy, associated anomalies and outcome. *Prenat Diagn* **24**(2):104–110, 2004.
82. Lewi L, Jani J, Cannie M et al. Intertwin anastomoses in monochorionic placentas after fetoscopic laser coagulation for twin-to-twin transfusion syndrome: is there more than meets the eye? *Am J Obstet Gynecol* **194**(3):790–795, 2006.
83. Robyr R, Lewi L, Salomon LJ et al. Prevalence and management of late fetal complications following successful selective laser coagulation of chorionic plate anastomoses in twin-to-twin transfusion syndrome. *Am J Obstet Gynecol* **194**(3):796–803, 2006.
84. Hecher K, Diehl W, Zikulnig L, Vetter M, Hackeloer BJ. Endoscopic laser coagulation of placental anastomoses in 200 pregnancies with severe mid-trimester twin-to-twin transfusion syndrome. *Eur J Obstet Gynecol Reprod Biol* **92**(1):135–139, 2000.
85. Cavicchioni O, Yamamoto M, Robyr R, Takahashi Y, Ville Y. Intrauterine fetal demise following laser treatment in twin-to-twin transfusion syndrome. *Br J Obstet Gynaecol* **113**(5):590–594, 2006.
86. Gratacos E, Van Schoubroeck D, Carreras E et al. Impact of laser coagulation in severe twin-twin transfusion syndrome on fetal Doppler indices and venous blood flow volume. *Ultrasound Obstet Gynecol* **20**(2):125–130, 2002.
87. Robyr R, Boulvain M, Lewi L et al. Cervical length as a prognostic factor for preterm delivery in twin-to-twin transfusion syndrome treated by fetoscopic laser coagulation of chorionic plate anastomoses. *Ultrasound Obstet Gynecol* **25**(1):37–41, 2005.
88. Engineer N, O'Donoghue K, Wimalasundera R, Fisk NM. A controlled intervention study of the relationship between cervical length and polyhydramnios in complicated monochorionic twin pregnancies. *Am J Obstet Gynecol* **197**(6):S51, 2007.
89. De Lia JE, Carr MH. Pregnancy loss after successful laser surgery for previable twin-twin transfusion syndrome. *Am J Obstet Gynecol* **187**(2):517–518, 2002, author reply 518.
90. Deprest JA, Van Schoubroeck D, Van Ballaer PP, Flageole H, Van Assche FA, Vandenberghe K. Alternative technique for Nd: YAG laser coagulation in twin-to-twin transfusion syndrome with anterior placenta. *Ultrasound Obstet Gynecol* **11**(5):347–352, 1998.
91. Lopriore E, Hecher K, Vandenbussche FP, van den Wijngaard JP, Klumper FJ, Oepkes D. Fetoscopic laser treatment of twin-to-twin transfusion syndrome followed by severe twin anemia-polycythemia sequence with spontaneous resolution. *Am J Obstet Gynecol* **198**(2): e4–e7, 2008.

92. Bower SJ, Flack NJ, Sepulveda W, Talbert DG, Fisk NM. Uterine artery blood flow response to correction of amniotic fluid volume. *Am J Obstet Gynecol* **173**(2):502–507, 1995.
93. Mahieu-Caputo D, Meulemans A, Martinovic J et al. Paradoxic activation of the renin-angiotensin system in twin-twin transfusion syndrome: an explanation for cardiovascular disturbances in the recipient. *Pediatr Res* **58**(4):685–688, 2005.
94. Fisk NM, Tannirandorn Y, Nicolini U, Talbert DG, Rodeck CH. Amniotic pressure in disorders of amniotic fluid volume. *Obstet Gynecol* **76**(2):210–214, 1990.
95. Fuchs AR, Goeschen K, Husslein P, Rasmussen AB, Fuchs F. Oxytocin and initiation of human parturition. III. Plasma concentrations of oxytocin and 13,14-dihydro-15-keto-prostaglandin F2 alpha in spontaneous and oxytocin-induced labor at term. *Am J Obstet Gynecol* **147**(5):497–502, 1983.
96. Csapo AI, Lloyd-Jacob MA. Effect of uterine volume on parturition. *Am J Obstet Gynecol* **85**:806–812, 1963.
97. Moise KJ Jr, Dorman K, Lamvu G et al. A randomized trial of amnioreduction versus septostomy in the treatment of twin-twin transfusion syndrome. *Am J Obstet Gynecol* **193**(3 Pt 1):701–707, 2005.
98. Dickinson JE, Evans SF. Obstetric and perinatal outcomes from the australian and New Zealand twin-twin transfusion syndrome registry. *Am J Obstet Gynecol* **182**(3):706–712, 2000.
99. Mari G, Roberts A, Detti L et al. Perinatal morbidity and mortality rates in severe twin-twin transfusion syndrome: results of the International Amnioreduction Registry. *Am J Obstet Gynecol* **185**(3): 708–715, 2001.
100. Umur A, Van Gemert MJ, Ross MG. Amniotic fluid and hemodynamic model in monochorionic twin pregnancies and twin-twin transfusion syndrome. *Am J Physiol Regul Integr Comp Physiol* **280**(5):R1499–1509, 2001.
101. Quintero RA, Dickinson JE, Morales WJ et al. Stage-based treatment of twin-twin transfusion syndrome. *Am J Obstet Gynecol* **188**(5):1333–1340, 2003.
102. Frusca T, Soregaroli M, Fichera A et al. Pregnancies complicated by twin-twin transfusion syndrome: outcome and long-term neurological follow-up. *Eur J Obstet Gynecol Reprod Biol* **107**(2):145–150, 2003.
103. Saito M, Pontes AL, Porto Filho FA et al. Septostomy with amniodrainage in the treatment of twin-to-twin transfusion syndrome: a 16-case report. *Arch Gynecol Obstet* **275**(5):341–345, 2007.
104. Lim YK, Tan TY, Zuzarte R, Daniel ML, Yeo GS. Outcomes of twin-twin transfusion syndrome managed by a specialised twin clinic. *Singapore Med J* **46**(8):401–406, 2005.
105. Fox C, Kilby MD, Khan KS. Contemporary treatments for twin-twin transfusion syndrome. *Obstet Gynecol* **105**(6):1469–1477, 2005.
106. Middeldorp JM, Lopriore E, Sueters M et al. Twin-to-twin transfusion syndrome after 26 weeks of gestation: is there a role for fetoscopic laser surgery? *Br J Obstet Gynaecol* **114**(6):694–698, 2007.
107. Middeldorp JM, Sueters M, Lopriore E et al. Fetoscopic laser surgery in 100 pregnancies with severe twin-to-twin transfusion syndrome in the Netherlands. *Fetal Diagn Ther* **22**(3): 190–194, 2007.
108. Fisk NM, Tan TY, Taylor MJ. Stage-based treatment of twin-twin transfusion syndrome. *Am J Obstet Gynecol* **190**(5):1491–1492, 2004.
109. Moise KJ Jr. Neurodevelopmental outcome after laser therapy for twin-twin transfusion syndrome. *Am J Obstet Gynecol* **194**(5):1208–1210, 2006.
110. O'Donoghue K, Cartwright E, Galea P, Fisk NM. Stage I twin-twin transfusion syndrome: rates of progression and regression in relation to outcome. *Ultrasound Obstet Gynecol* **30**(7):958–964, 2007.
111. Roberts D, Neilson J, Kilby M, Gates S. Interventions for the treatment of twin-twin transfusion syndrome. *Cochrane Database Syst Rev* **1**:CD002073, 2008.
112. Lopriore E, Nagel HT, Vandenbussche FP, Walther FJ. Long-term neuro-developmental outcome in twin-to-twin transfusion syndrome. *Am J Obstet Gynecol* **189**(5):1314–1319, 2003.
113. Graef C, Ellenrieder B, Hecher K, Hackeloer BJ, Huber A, Bartmann P. Long-term neurodevelopmental outcome of 167 children after intrauterine laser treatment for severe twin-twin transfusion syndrome. *Am J Obstet Gynecol* **194**(2):303–308, 2006.
114. Banek CS, Hecher K, Hackeloer BJ, Bartmann P. Long-term neurodevelopmental outcome after intrauterine laser treatment for severe twin-twin transfusion syndrome. *Am J Obstet Gynecol* **188**(4):876–880, 2003.
115. Delle Urban LA, Righini A, Rustico M, Triulzi F, Nicolini U. Prenatal ultrasound detection of bilateral focal polymicrogyria. *Prenat Diagn* **24**(10): 808–811, 2004.
116. Denbow ML, Battin MR, Cowan F, Azzopardi D, Edwards AD, Fisk NM. Neonatal cranial ultrasonographic findings in preterm twins complicated by severe fetofetal transfusion syndrome. *Am J Obstet Gynecol* **178**(3):479–483, 1998.
117. Quarello E, Molho M, Ville Y. Incidence, mechanisms, and patterns of fetal cerebral lesions in twin-to-twin transfusion syndrome. *J Matern Fetal Neonatal Med* **20**(8):589–597, 2007.
118. Sutcliffe AG, Sebire NJ, Pigott AJ, Taylor B, Edwards PR, Nicolaides KH. Outcome for children born after in utero laser ablation therapy for severe twin-to-twin transfusion syndrome. *Br J Obstet Gynaecol* **108**(12):1246–1250, 2001.
119. Cincotta RB, Gray PH, Phythian G, Rogers YM, Chan FY. Long term outcome of twin-twin transfusion syndrome. *Arch Dis Child Fetal Neonatal Ed* **83**(3):F171–176, 2000.
120. Sonigo PC, Rypens FF, Carteret M, Delezoide AL, Brunelle FO. MR imaging of fetal cerebral anomalies. *Pediatr Radiol* **28**(4):212–222, 1998.
121. Garel C, Brisse H, Sebag G, Elmaleh M, Oury JF, Hassan M. Magnetic resonance imaging of the fetus. *Pediatr Radiol* **28**(4):201–211, 1998.
122. Righini A, Zirpoli S, Mrakic F, Parazzini C, Pogliani L, Triulzi F. Early prenatal MR imaging diagnosis of polymicrogyria. *Am J Neuroradiol* **25**(2):343–346, 2004.
123. James WH. A note on the epidemiology of acardiac monsters. *Teratology* **16**(2):211–216, 1977.
124. Van Allen MI, Smith DW, Shepard TH. Twin reversed arterial perfusion (TRAP) sequence: a study of 14 twin pregnancies with acardius. *Semin Perinatol* **7**(4): 285–293, 1983.
125. Gembruch U, Viski S, Bagamery K, Berg C, Germer U. Twin reversed arterial perfusion sequence in twin-to-twin transfusion syndrome after the death of the donor co-twin in the second trimester. *Ultrasound Obstet Gynecol* **17**(2):153–156, 2001.
126. Fisk NM, Ware M, Stanier P, Moore G, Bennett P. Molecular genetic etiology of twin reversed arterial perfusion sequence. *Am J Obstet Gynecol* **174**(3):891–894, 1996.
127. Healey MG. Acardia: predictive risk factors for the co-twin's survival. *Teratology* **50**(3):205–213, 1994.
128. Moore TR, Gale S, Benirschke K. Perinatal outcome of forty-nine pregnancies complicated by acardiac twinning. *Am J Obstet Gynecol* **163**(3):907–912, 1990.
129. Tan TY, Sepulveda W. Acardiac twin: a systematic review of minimally invasive treatment modalities. *Ultrasound Obstet Gynecol* **22**(4):409–419, 2003.
130. Weisz B, Peltz R, Chayen B et al. Tailored management of twin reversed arterial perfusion (TRAP) sequence. *Ultrasound Obstet Gynecol* **23**(5):451–455, 2004.
131. Wong AE, Sepulveda W. Acardiac anomaly: current issues in prenatal assessment and treatment. *Prenat Diagn* **25**(9):796–806, 2005.
132. Robyr R, Yamamoto M, Ville Y. Selective feticide in complicated monochorionic

twin pregnancies using ultrasound-guided bipolar cord coagulation. *Br J Obstet Gynaecol* **112**(10):1344–1348, 2005.

133. Hecher K, Lewi L, Gratacos E, Huber A, Ville Y, Deprest J. Twin reversed arterial perfusion: fetoscopic laser coagulation of placental anastomoses or the umbilical cord. *Ultrasound Obstet Gynecol* **28**(5):688–691, 2006.
134. Lee H, Wagner AJ, Sy E et al. Efficacy of radiofrequency ablation for twin-reversed arterial perfusion sequence. *Am J Obstet Gynecol* **196**(5): 459 e1–4, 2007.
135. Rodis JF, McIlveen PF, Egan JF, Borgida AF, Turner GW, Campbell WA. Monoamniotic twins: improved perinatal survival with accurate prenatal diagnosis and antenatal fetal surveillance. *Am J Obstet Gynecol* **177**(5):1046–1049, 1997.
136. Allen VM, Windrim R, Barrett J, Ohlsson A. Management of monoamniotic twin pregnancies: a case series and systematic review of the literature. *Br J Obstet Gynaecol* **108**(9):931–936, 2001.
137. Arabin B, Laurini RN, van Eyck J. Early prenatal diagnosis of cord entanglement in monoamniotic multiple pregnancies. *Ultrasound Obstet Gynecol* **13**(3):181–186, 1999.
138. Overton TG, Denbow ML, Duncan KR, Fisk NM. First-trimester cord entanglement in monoamniotic twins. *Ultrasound Obstet Gynecol* **13**(2):140–142, 1999.
139. Aisenbrey GA, Catanzarite VA, Hurley TJ, Spiegel JH, Schrimmer DB, Mendoza A. Monoamniotic and pseudomonoamniotic twins: sonographic diagnosis, detection of cord entanglement, and obstetric management. *Obstet Gynecol* **86**(2): 218–222, 1995.
140. Abuhamad AZ, Mari G, Copel JA, Cantwell CJ, Evans AT. Umbilical artery flow velocity waveforms in monoamniotic twins with cord entanglement. *Obstet Gynecol* **86**(4 Pt 2): 674–677, 1995.
141. Su LL. Monoamniotic twins: diagnosis and management. *Acta Obstet Gynecol Scand* **81**(11):995–1000, 2002.
142. Roque H, Gillen-Goldstein J, Funai E, Young BK, Lockwood CJ. Perinatal outcomes in monoamniotic gestations. *J Matern Fetal Neonatal Med* **13**(6):414–421, 2003.
143. Hansen LM, Donnenfeld AE. Concordant anencephaly in monoamniotic twins and an analysis of maternal serum markers. *Prenat Diagn* **17**(5):471–473, 1997.
144. van den Wijngaard JP, Umur A, Ross MG, van Gemert MJ. Modelling the influence of amnionicity on the severity of twin-twin transfusion syndrome in monochorionic twin pregnancies. *Phys Med Biol* **49**(6):N57–64, 2004.
145. Dodd JM, Crowther CA. Evidence-based care of women with a multiple pregnancy. *Best Pract Res Clin Obstet Gynaecol* **19**(1):131–153, 2005.
146. Peek MJ, McCarthy A, Kyle P, Sepulveda W, Fisk NM. Medical amnioreduction with sulindac to reduce cord complications in monoamniotic twins. *Am J Obstet Gynecol* **176**(2): 334–336, 1997.
147. Pasquini L, Wimalasundera RC, Fichera A, Barigye O, Chappell L, Fisk NM. High perinatal survival in monoamniotic twins managed by prophylactic sulindac, intensive ultrasound surveillance, and cesarean delivery at 32 weeks' gestation. *Ultrasound Obstet Gynecol* **28**(5):681–687, 2006.
148. Spencer RS. Theoretical and analytical embryology of conjoined twins: part I: embryogenesis. *Clin Anat* **13**(1):36–53, 2000.
149. Machin GA. Heteropagus conjoined twins due to fusion of two embryos. *Am J Med Genet* **78**(4):388–390, 1998.
150. The international clearinghouse for Birth Defects Monitoring Systems. Conjoined twins: an epidemiological study based on 312 cases. *Acta Genet Med Gemellol Roma* **40**:325–335, 1991.
151. Woo JS, Liang ST, Lo R. Characteristic pattern of Doppler umbilical arterial velocity waveform in conjoint twins. *Gynecol Obstet Invest* **23**(1):70–72, 1987.
152. Bonilla-Musoles F, Machado LE, Osborne NG et al. Two-dimensional and three-dimensional sonography of conjoined twins. *J Clin Ultrasound* **30**(2):68–75, 2002.
153. McHugh K, Kiely EM, Spitz L. Imaging of conjoined twins. *Pediatr Radiol* **36**(9):899–910, 2006.
154. Spitz L. Surgery for conjoined twins. *Ann R Coll Surg Engl* **85**(4):230–235, 2003.
155. Spitz L, Kiely EM. Experience in the management of conjoined twins. *Br J Surg* **89**(9):1188–1192, 2002.
156. Li SJ, Ford N, Meister K, Bodurtha J. Increased risk of birth defects among children from multiple births. *Birth Defects Res A Clin Mol Teratol* **67**(10): 879–885, 2003.
157. Chen CJ, Wang CJ, Yu MW, Lee TK. Perinatal mortality and prevalence of major congenital malformations of twins in Taipei city. *Acta Genet Med Gemellol (Roma)* **41**(2-3):197–203, 1992.
158. Hendrix NW, Chauhan SP. Sonographic examination of twins. From first trimester to delivery of second fetus. *Obstet Gynecol Clin North Am* **25**(3):609–621, 1998.
159. Little J, Bryan E. Congenital anomalies in twins. *Semin Perinatol* **10**(1):50–64, 1986.
160. Bahtiyar MO, Dulay AT, Weeks BP, Friedman AH, Copel JA. Prevalence of congenital heart defects in monochorionic/diamniotic twin gestations: a systematic literature review. *J Ultrasound Med* **26**(11):1491–1498, 2007.
161. Manning N, Archer N. A study to determine the incidence of structural congenital heart disease in monochorionic twins. *Prenat Diagn* **26**(11):1062–1064, 2006.
162. Sebire NJ, Sepulveda W, Hughes KS, Noble P, Nicolaides KH. Management of twin pregnancies discordant for anencephaly. *Br J Obstet Gynaecol* **104**(2):216–219, 1997.
163. Sebire NJ, Snijders RJ, Santiago C, Papapanagiotou G, Nicolaides KH. Management of twin pregnancies with fetal trisomies. *Br J Obstet Gynaecol* **104**(2):220–222, 1997.
164. Blickstein I, Kalish RB. Birthweight discordance in multiple pregnancy. *Twin Res* **6**(6):526–531, 2003.
165. Victoria A, Mora G, Arias F. Perinatal outcome, placental pathology, and severity of discordance in monochorionic and dichorionic twins. *Obstet Gynecol* **97**(2):310–315, 2001.
166. Sebire NJ, D'Ercole C, Hughes K, Rennie J, Nicolaides KH. Dichorionic twins discordant for intrauterine growth retardation. *Arch Dis Child Fetal Neonatal Ed* **77**(3):F235–236, 1997.
167. Blickstein I, Jacques DL, Keith LG. A novel approach to intertriplet birth weight discordance. *Am J Obstet Gynecol* **188**(4):1026–1030, 2003.
168. Kalish RB, Chasen ST, Gupta M, Sharma G, Perni SC, Chervenak FA. First trimester prediction of growth discordance in twin gestations. *Am J Obstet Gynecol* **189**(3):706–709, 2003.
169. Sebire NJ. Routine uterine artery Doppler screening in twin pregnancies? *Ultrasound Obstet Gynecol* **20**(6):532–534, 2002.
170. Yu CK, Papageorghiou AT, Boli A, Cacho AM, Nicolaides KH. Screening for pre-eclampsia and fetal growth restriction in twin pregnancies at 23 weeks of gestation by transvaginal uterine artery Doppler. *Ultrasound Obstet Gynecol* **20**(6):535–540, 2002.
171. Hill LM, Guzick D, Chenevey P, Boyles D, Nedzesky P. The sonographic assessment of twin growth discordancy. *Obstet Gynecol* **84**(4):501–504, 1994.
172. Blickstein I, Goldman RD, Mazkereth R. Adaptive growth restriction as a pattern of birth weight discordance in twin gestations. *Obstet Gynecol* **96**(6):986–990, 2000.
173. Vanderheyden TM, Fichera A, Pasquini L et al. Increased latency of absent end-diastolic flow in the umbilical artery of monochorionic twin fetuses. *Ultrasound Obstet Gynecol* **26**(1):44–49, 2005.
174. Hecher K, Jauniaux E, Campbell S, Deane C, Nicolaides K. Artery-to-artery anastomosis in monochorionic twins. *Am J Obstet Gynecol* **171**(2):570–572, 1994.

175. Wee LY, Taylor MJ, Vanderheyden T, Talbert D, Fisk NM. Transmitted arterio-arterial anastomosis waveforms causing cyclically intermittent absent/reversed end-diastolic umbilical artery flow in monochorionic twins. *Placenta* **24**(7): 772–778, 2003.
176. Gratacos E, Lewi L, Carreras E et al. Incidence and characteristics of umbilical artery intermittent absent and/or reversed end-diastolic flow in complicated and uncomplicated monochorionic twin pregnancies. *Ultrasound Obstet Gynecol* **23**(5):456–460, 2004.
177. Huber A, Diehl W, Zikulnig L, Bregenzer T, Hackeloer BJ, Hecher K. Perinatal outcome in monochorionic twin pregnancies complicated by amniotic fluid discordance without severe twin-twin transfusion syndrome. *Ultrasound Obstet Gynecol* **27**(1):48–52, 2006.
178. Gratacos E, Lewi L, Munoz B et al. A classification system for selective intrauterine growth restriction in monochorionic pregnancies according to umbilical artery Doppler flow in the smaller twin. *Ultrasound Obstet Gynecol* **30**(1):28–34, 2007.
179. Mari G, Detti L, Levi-D'Ancona R, Kern L. 'Pseudo' twin-to-twin transfusion syndrome and fetal outcome. *J Perinatol* **18**(5):399–403, 1998.
180. Gratacos E, Carreras E, Becker J et al. Prevalence of neurological damage in monochorionic twins with selective intrauterine growth restriction and intermittent absent or reversed end-diastolic umbilical artery flow. *Ultrasound Obstet Gynecol* **24**(2):159–163, 2004.
181. Sebire NJ, Thornton S, Hughes K, Snijders RJ, Nicolaides KH. The prevalence and consequences of missed abortion in twin pregnancies at 10 to 14 weeks of gestation. *Br J Obstet Gynaecol* **104**(7):847–848, 1997.
182. Burke MS. Single fetal demise in twin gestation. *Clin Obstet Gynecol* **33**(1): 69–78, 1990.
183. Sebire NJ, Snijders RJ, Hughes K, Sepulveda W, Nicolaides KH. The hidden mortality of monochorionic twin pregnancies. *Br J Obstet Gynaecol* **104**(10):1203–1207, 1997.
184. Fusi L, Gordon H. Twin pregnancy complicated by single intrauterine death. Problems and outcome with conservative management. *Br J Obstet Gynaecol* **97**(6):511–516, 1990.
185. Kilby MD, Govind A, O'Brien PM. Outcome of twin pregnancies complicated by a single intrauterine death: a comparison with viable twin pregnancies. *Obstet Gynecol* **84**(1): 107–109, 1994.
186. Gonen R, Heyman E, Asztalos E, Milligan JE. The outcome of triplet gestations complicated by fetal death. *Obstet Gynecol* **75**(2):175–178, 1990.
187. Bajoria R, Wee LY, Anwar S, Ward S. Outcome of twin pregnancies complicated by single intrauterine death in relation to vascular anatomy of the monochorionic placenta. *Hum Reprod* **14**(8):2124–2130, 1999.
188. Benirschke K. Intrauterine death of a twin: mechanisms, implications for surviving twin, and placental pathology. *Semin Diagn Pathol* **10**(3):222–231, 1993.
189. Bulla M, von Lilien T, Goecke H, Roth B, Ortmann M, Heising J. Renal and cerebral necrosis in survivor after in utero death of co-twin. *Arch Gynecol* **240**(2):119–124, 1987.
190. Bejar R, Vigliocco G, Gramajo H et al. Antenatal origin of neurologic damage in newborn infants. II. Multiple gestations. *Am J Obstet Gynecol* **162**(5):1230–1236, 1990.
191. Szymonowicz W, Preston H, Yu VY. The surviving monozygotic twin. *Arch Dis Child* **61**(5):454–458, 1986.
192. Ong SS, Zamora J, Khan KS, Kilby MD. Prognosis for the co-twin following single-twin death: a systematic review. *Br J Obstet Gynaecol* **113**(9):992–998, 2006.
193. Nicolini U, Poblete A. Single intrauterine death in monochorionic twin pregnancies. *Ultrasound Obstet Gynecol* **14**(5):297–301, 1999.
194. Senat MV, Loizeau S, Couderc S, Bernard JP, Ville Y. The value of middle cerebral artery peak systolic velocity in the diagnosis of fetal anemia after intrauterine death of one monochorionic twin. *Am J Obstet Gynecol* **189**(5):1320–1324, 2003.
195. Ozcan T, Thornburg L, Mingione M, Pressman E. Use of middle cerebral artery peak systolic velocity and intrauterine transfusion for management of twin-twin transfusion and single fetal intrauterine demise. *J Matern Fetal Neonatal Med* **19**(12):807–809, 2006.
196. Simonazzi G, Segata M, Ghi T et al. Accurate neurosonographic prediction of brain injury in the surviving fetus after the death of a monochorionic cotwin. *Ultrasound Obstet Gynecol* **27**(5):517–521, 2006.
197. Righini A, Kustermann A, Parazzini C, Fogliani R, Ceriani F, Triulzi F. Diffusion-weighted magnetic resonance imaging of acute hypoxic-ischemic cerebral lesions in the survivor of a monochorionic twin pregnancy: case report. *Ultrasound Obstet Gynecol* **29**(4):453–456, 2007.
198. Glenn OA, Norton ME, Goldstein RB, Barkovich AJ. Prenatal diagnosis of polymicrogyria by fetal magnetic resonance imaging in monochorionic cotwin death. *J Ultrasound Med* **24**(5):711–716, 2005.
199. Eddleman KA, Stone JL, Lynch L, Berkowitz RL. Selective termination of anomalous fetuses in multifetal pregnancies: two hundred cases at a single center. *Am J Obstet Gynecol* **187**(5):1168–1172, 2002.
200. Denbow ML, Overton TG, Duncan KR, Cox PM, Fisk NM. High failure rate of umbilical vessel occlusion by ultrasound-guided injection of absolute alcohol or enbucrilate gel. *Prenat Diagn* **19**(6):527–532, 1999.
201. Lewi L GE, Ortibus E, Van Schoubroeck D, Carreras E, Higueras T, Perapoch J, Deprest J. Pregnancy and infant outcome of 80 consecutive cord coagulations in complicated monochorionic multiple pregnancies. *Am J Obstet Gynecol* **194**(3):782–789, 2006.
202. Ville Y, Hyett JA, Vandenbussche FP, Nicolaides KH. Endoscopic laser coagulation of umbilical cord vessels in twin reversed arterial perfusion sequence. *Ultrasound Obstet Gynecol* **4**(5):396–398, 1994.
203. Lemery DJ, Vanlieferinghen P, Gasq M, Finkeltin F, Beaufrere AM, Beytout M. Fetal umbilical cord ligation under ultrasound guidance. *Ultrasound Obstet Gynecol* **4**(5):399–401, 1994.
204. Quintero RA, Romero R, Reich H et al. In utero percutaneous umbilical cord ligation in the management of complicated monochorionic multiple gestations. *Ultrasound Obstet Gynecol* **8**(1):16–22, 1996.
205. Tsao K, Feldstein VA, Albanese CT et al. Selective reduction of acardiac twin by radiofrequency ablation. *Am J Obstet Gynecol* **187**(3):635–640, 2002.
206. Moise KJ Jr, Johnson A, Moise KY, Nickeleit V. Radiofrequency ablation for selective reduction in the complicated monochorionic gestation. *Am J Obstet Gynecol* **198**(2):198 e1–5, 2008.
207. Spadola AC, Simpson LL. Selective termination procedures in monochorionic pregnancies. *Semin Perinatol* **29**(5):330–337, 2005.
208. Shevell T, Malone FD, Weintraub J, Thaker HM, D'Alton ME. Radiofrequency ablation in a monochorionic twin discordant for fetal anomalies. *Am J Obstet Gynecol* **190**(2):575–576, 2004.
209. Hirose M, Murata A, Kita N, Aotani H, Takebayashi K, Noda Y. Successful intrauterine treatment with radiofrequency ablation in a case of acardiac twin pregnancy complicated with a hydropic pump twin. *Ultrasound Obstet Gynecol* **23**(5):509–512, 2004.
210. Jolly M, Taylor M, Rose G, Govender L, Fisk NM. Interstitial laser: a new surgical technique for twin reversed arterial perfusion sequence in early pregnancy. *Br J Obstet Gynaecol* **108**(10):1098–1102, 2001.
211. O'Donoghue K BO, Pasquini L, Chappell L, Wimalasundera RC,

Fisk NM. Interstitial laser for fetal reduction in monochorionic multiple pregnancy: loss rate and association with aplasia cutis congenita. *Prenat Diagn, in press*, 2008.

212. Rodeck C, Deans A, Jauniaux E. Thermocoagulation for the early treatment of pregnancy with an acardiac twin. *N Engl J Med* **339**(18):1293–1295, 1998.
213. Lam YH, Lee CP, Tang MH, Lau E. Thermocoagulation for selective reduction of conjoined twins at 12 weeks of gestation. *Ultrasound Obstet Gynecol* **16**(3):267–270, 2000.
214. Young BK, Roque H, Abdelhak Y, Timor-Tristch I, Rebarber A, Rosen R. Endoscopic ligation of umbilical cord at 19 week's gestation in monoamniotic monochorionic twins discordant for hypoplastic left heart syndrome. *Fetal Diagn Ther* **16**(1):61–64, 2001.
215. Quintero RA. *Diagnostic and operative fetoscopy*. New York: Parthenon Publishing, p.137, 2002.
216. Middeldorp JM, Klumper FJ, Oepkes D, Lopriore E, Kanhai HH, Vandenbussche FP. Selective feticide in monoamniotic twin pregnancies by umbilical cord occlusion and transection. *Fetal Diagn Ther* **23**(2):113–117, 2007.
217. Petterson B, Nelson KB, Watson L, Stanley F. Twins, triplets, and cerebral palsy in births in Western Australia in the 1980s. *Br Med J* **307**(6914):1239–1243, 1993.
218. Wimalasundera RC, Trew G, Fisk NM. Reducing the incidence of twins and triplets. *Best Pract Res Clin Obstet Gynaecol* **17**(2):309–329, 2003.
219. Skrablin S, Kuvacic I, Simunic V, Bosnjak-Nadj K, Kalafatic D, Banovic V. Long-term neurodevelopmental outcome of triplets. *Eur J Obstet Gynecol Reprod Biol* **132**(1):76–82, 2007.
220. Topp M, Huusom LD, Langhoff-Roos J, Delhumeau C, Hutton JL, Dolk H. Multiple birth and cerebral palsy in Europe: a multicenter study. *Acta Obstet Gynecol Scand* **83**(6):548–553, 2004.
221. Luke B, Brown MB. Contemporary risks of maternal morbidity and adverse outcomes with increasing maternal age and plurality. *Fertil Steril* **88**(2):283–293, 2007.
222. Ellison MA, Hotamisligil S, Lee H, Rich-Edwards JW, Pang SC, Hall JE. Psychosocial risks associated with multiple births resulting from assisted reproduction. *Fertil Steril* **83**(5): 1422–1428, 2005.
223. Berkowitz RL, Lynch L, Chitkara U, Wilkins IA, Mehalek KE, Alvarez E. Selective reduction of multifetal pregnancies in the first trimester. *N Engl J Med* **318**(16):1043–1047, 1988.
224. Evans MI, Fletcher JC, Zador IE, Newton BW, Quigg MH, Struyk CD. Selective first-trimester termination in octuplet and quadruplet pregnancies: clinical and ethical issues. *Obstet Gynecol* **71**(3 Pt 1):289–296, 1988.
225. Dumez Y, Oury JF. Method for first trimester selective abortion in multiple pregnancy. *Contrib Gynecol Obstet* **15**:50–53, 1986.
226. Stone J, Belogolovkin V, Matho A, Berkowitz RL, Moshier E, Eddleman K. Evolving trends in 2000 cases of multifetal pregnancy reduction: a single-center experience. *Am J Obstet Gynecol* **197**(4): 394 e1–4, 2007.
227. Brambati B, Tului L. First trimester fetal reduction: its role in the management of twin and higher order multiple pregnancies. *Hum Reprod Update* **1**(4):397–408, 1995.
228. Evans MI, Ciorica D, Britt DW, Fletcher JC. Update on selective reduction. *Prenat Diagn* **25**(9):807–813, 2005.
229. Evans MI, Berkowitz RL, Wapner RJ et al. Improvement in outcomes of multifetal pregnancy reduction with increased experience. *Am J Obstet Gynecol* **184**(2):97–103, 2001.
230. Antsaklis A, Souka AP, Daskalakis G et al. Pregnancy outcome after multifetal pregnancy reduction. *J Matern Fetal Neonatal Med* **16**(1):27–31, 2004.
231. Evans MI, Britt DW. Fetal reduction. *Semin Perinatol* **29**(5):321–329, 2005.
232. Wimalasundera R. Selective reduction and termination of multiple pregnancies. In *Multiple pregnancy*, MBP Kilby, H Critchley, D Field (eds), pp. 89–108. RCOG Press, 2006.
233. Papageorghiou AT, Liao AW, Skentou C, Sebire NJ, Nicolaides KH. Trichorionic triplet pregnancies at 10-14 weeks: outcome after embryo reduction compared to expectant management. *J Matern Fetal Neonatal Med* **11**(5): 307–312, 2002.
234. Papageorghiou AT, Avgidou K, Bakoulas V, Sebire NJ, Nicolaides KH. Risks of miscarriage and early preterm birth in trichorionic triplet pregnancies with embryo reduction versus expectant management: new data and systematic review. *Hum Reprod* **21**(7):1912–1917, 2006.
235. Evans MI, Kaufman MI, Urban AJ, Britt DW, Fletcher JC. Fetal reduction from twins to a singleton: a reasonable consideration? *Obstet Gynecol* **104**(1): 102–109, 2004.
236. Brambati B, Tului L, Camurri L, Guercilena S. First-trimester fetal reduction to a singleton infant or twins: outcome in relation to the final number and karyotyping before reduction by transabdominal chorionic villus sampling. *Am J Obstet Gynecol* **191**(6):2035–2040, 2004.
237. Child TJ, Henderson AM, Tan SL. The desire for multiple pregnancy in male and female infertility patients. *Hum Reprod* **19**(3):558–561, 2004.
238. Hojgaard A, Ottosen LD, Kesmodel U, Ingerslev HJ. Patient attitudes towards twin pregnancies and single embryo transfer – a questionnaire study. *Hum Reprod* **22**(10):2673–2678, 2007.
239. Britt DW, Risinger ST, Mans M, Evans MI. Anxiety among women who have undergone fertility therapy and who are considering multifetal pregnancy reduction: trends and implications. *J Matern Fetal Neonatal Med* **13**(4): 271–278, 2003.
240. McKinney M, Downey J, Timor-Tritsch I. The psychological effects of multifetal pregnancy reduction. *Fertil Steril* **64**(1):51–61, 1995.
241. McKinney M, Leary K. Integrating quantitative and qualitative methods to study multifetal pregnancy reduction. *J Womens Health* **8**(2): 259–268, 1999.
242. Britt DW, Evans MI. Sometimes doing the right thing sucks: frame combinations and multi-fetal pregnancy reduction decision difficulty. *Soc Sci Med* **65**(11): 2342–2356, 2007.
243. Bryan E. Loss in higher multiple pregnancy and multifetal pregnancy reduction. *Twin Res* **5**(3):169–174, 2002.
244. Chow JS, Benson CB, Racowsky C, Doubilet PM, Ginsburg E. Frequency of a monochorionic pair in multiple gestations: relationship to mode of conception. *J Ultrasound Med* **20**(7):757–760, 2001, quiz 761.
245. De Catte L, Camus M, Foulon W. Monochorionic high-order multiple pregnancies and multifetal pregnancy reduction. *Obstet Gynecol* **100**(3): 561–566, 2002.
246. Geipel A, Berg C, Katalinic A et al. Prenatal diagnosis and obstetric outcomes in triplet pregnancies in relation to chorionicity. *Br J Obstet Gynaecol* **112**(5):554–558, 2005.
247. Pruggmayer MR, Jahoda MG, Van der Pol JG et al. Genetic amniocentesis in twin pregnancies: results of a multicenter study of 529 cases. *Ultrasound Obstet Gynecol* **2**(1):6–10, 1992.
248. Horger EO, 3rd, Finch H, Vincent VA. A single physician's experience with four thousand six hundred genetic amniocenteses. *Am J Obstet Gynecol* **185**(2):279–288, 2001.
249. Antsaklis A, Souka AP, Daskalakis G, Kavalakis Y, Michalas S. Second-trimester amniocentesis vs. chorionic villus sampling for prenatal diagnosis in multiple gestations. *Ultrasound Obstet Gynecol* **20**(5):476–481, 2002.
250. Ghidini A, Lynch L, Hicks C, Alvarez M, Lockwood CJ. The risk of second-trimester amniocentesis in

twin gestations: a case-control study. *Am J Obstet Gynecol* **169**(4):1013–1016, 1993.

251. Toth-Pal E, Papp C, Beke A, Ban Z, Papp Z. Genetic amniocentesis in multiple pregnancy. *Fetal Diagn Ther* **19**(2):138–144, 2004.
252. Pergament E, Schulman JD, Copeland K et al. The risk and efficacy of chorionic villus sampling in multiple gestations. *Prenat Diagn* **12**(5):377–384, 1992.
253. Wapner RJ, Johnson A, Davis G, Urban A, Morgan P, Jackson L. Prenatal diagnosis in twin gestations: a comparison between second-trimester amniocentesis and first-trimester chorionic villus sampling. *Obstet Gynecol* **82**(1):49–56, 1993.
254. van den Berg C, Braat AP, Van Opstal D et al. Amniocentesis or chorionic villus sampling in multiple gestations? Experience with 500 cases. *Prenat Diagn* **19**(3):234–244, 1999.
255. De Catte L, Liebaers I, Foulon W. Outcome of twin gestations after first trimester chorionic villus sampling. *Obstet Gynecol* **96**(5 Pt 1):714–720, 2000.
256. Ville Y, Hecher K, Gagnon A, Sebire N, Hyett J, Nicolaides K. Endoscopic laser coagulation in the management of severe twin-to-twin transfusion syndrome. *Br J Obstet Gynaecol* **105**(4):446–453, 1998.
257. Huber A, Diehl W, Bregenzer T, Hackeloer BJ, Hecher K. Stage-related outcome in twin-twin transfusion syndrome treated by fetoscopic laser coagulation. *Obstet Gynecol* **108**(2): 333–337, 2006.
258. Ierullo AM, Papageorghiou AT, Bhide A, Fratelli N, Thilaganathan B. Severe twin–twin transfusion syndrome: outcome after fetoscopic laser ablation of the placental vascular equator. *Br J Obstet Gynaecol* **114**(6):689–693, 2007.

CHAPTER

47 In utero stem cell transplantation

Sicco Scherjon and Elles in't Anker

KEY POINTS

- This chapter deals with the ontogeny and characteristics of hematopoietic and mesenchymal stem cells and with the possibilities, limitations and future developments of intrauterine stem cell transplantation
- Prenatal intrauterine therapy with stem cells has shown limited success so far. Until now, only low levels of engraftment of donor cells in the recipient have been shown
- Stem cells are characterized by their ability for self-renewal and the possibility to differentiate into different cell lineages
- Fetal liver is an attractive source of hematopoietic stem cells (HSC) because of the high number of HSC, the low number of T cells and the greater proliferation capacity
- Mesenchymal stem cells (MSC) are able to differentiate into different connective tissue lineages
- First-trimester MSC are better candidates for cell based therapy compared to adult sources
- MSC possibly have immunomodulatory properties, which makes them an attractive source for clinical use, especially in graft-versus-host disease and solid organ rejection

INTRODUCTON

Intrauterine fetal therapy (IUTx) with stem cells (SC) is a promising technique for the treatment of a variety of hematological, metabolic and immunological diseases[1]. The background of the technique is that via reconstitution of a missing or defective cell line, correction of a genetic defect becomes possible[2]. Although the diagnostic possibilities of many different congenital diseases have been realized by invasive and non-invasive techniques in the first trimester, prenatal intrauterine therapy with stem cells has shown limited success so far. Postnatal transplantation of hematopoietic stem cells (HSC) is, up till now, the treatment of choice for a broad spectrum of these congenital diseases such as α- and β-thalassemia, severe combined immunodeficiency syndrome (SCID) and different storage diseases[3,4]. However, in those cases where there is already organ damage at birth resulting from an inborn error of metabolism and also when the disorders can be diagnosed and treated early enough in pregnancy, IUTxSC might be an attractive treatment modality in the future.

Furthermore, the limitations of postnatal HSC transplantation are being increasingly realized. First, in many cases, a human leukocyte antigen (HLA)-compatible stem cell donor is not available. Secondly, the presence of T cells with major histocompatiblity (MHC) differences in the graft may lead to activation of donor T cells in the recipient and alloreactivity against the recipient, i.e. graft-versus-host disease (GVHD). Thirdly, transplantation of HSC will be (too) late in cases where the disease has caused organ damage to the fetus, leading to disability or death. This makes the already longstanding interest in intrauterine therapy with stem cells, which was first mentioned in the publication of Davis in 1967[5], more than understandable. Other advantages include the possibility of transplanting a relatively large number of stem cells per kilogram fetal weight, especially if transplanted in early fetal life; the migrational and developmental patterns and supportive environments apparent in fetal stem cell compartments, needed by these stem cells to achieve engraftment[149]; the supposed relative immaturity of the fetal immune system, unable to mount an adequate immune response[23]; the possibility of induction of specific fetal tolerance to donor stem cells; and the avoidance of conditioning in the fetus, such as myeloablation or chemotherapy[6,7].

During the further development of the immune system, these foreign antigens may be included in the 'self' repertoire of the fetus, resulting in immunological tolerance. After having induced tolerance, even after the establishment of very low levels of fetal chimerism, the percentage of donor cells in the recipient can be increased substantially, without inducing GVHD, by having a second late fetal or early neonatal transplant. These strategies have been experimentally tested in various animal models[8,9].

IN UTERO TRANSPLANTATION OF STEM CELLS

Animal studies have included experiments in the mouse, monkey, chicken, dog, pig and goat[8,10–15,147]. However, the majority of experimental work on in utero transplantation of hematopoietic stem cells (IUTxHSC), has been performed in the sheep model[16,17]. IUTxSC with the use of ultrasound-guided transplantation was shown to be feasible already in the first trimester in a fetal sheep model. Although the success of engraftment (18%) and the level of engraftment (0.8% of the total number nucleated cells) remains low, the feasibility for early in utero transplantation was shown with this model[18]. (Fetal) stem cells of many different sources have been used and, especially, the IUTx of human fetal liver derived stem cells into normal fetal sheep have resulted in long-term hematological chimerism, ranging in engraftment percentage from 10 to 15%[19]. Other stem cells types have been used for transplantation, such as umbilical cord blood[20] and adult bone-marrow-derived SC. Lack of success in some studies raises the question of whether the source of stem cells, sample variation in MSC populations derived from different donors[148], or certain host species are more resistant to transplantation. Cross species engraftment with human MSC in previously unexposed immune competent rat is feasible, although rejection of the transplant can occur in a xenogenetic model[21]. However, swine-derived MSC in an acute myocardial infarction non-obese diabetes/SCID mouse model resulted in minimal engraftment, but had a profound effect on post infarction cardiac function[22]. Recently, the induction of tolerance to solid organ transplantations without immunosupression with no signs of rejection has been achieved in the fetal pig model[23]. In mice, IUTxHSC was shown to be effective when the donor cells have some proliferative advantage over host cells. For instance, high levels of engraftment were obtained when normal HSC were transplanted into W-mutant anemic mice. These mice have a congenital defect in the W-gene, which encodes the receptor for stem cell factor (c-kit), resulting in severe macrocytic anemia. IUTxHSC in these mice resulted in complete erythroid reconstitution by donor hematopoiesis and treatment of the anemia[24,25]. Immunodeficient mice provide further examples of permissive recipients due to lineage deficiency. Lymphoid reconstruction after IUTxHSC was observed in SCID mice, in which there is early arrest of T- and B-cell development[26]. Thus, in the presence of a lineage deficiency, IUTxHSC can selectively reconstitute the defective lineage. However, experiments in normal animals, in which there is no competitive advantage for donor cells, have demonstrated that IUTxHSC results in only low levels of engraftment of donor cells in the recipient[27]. In fetal sheep this engraftment ranges between 5 and 14%[28].

Thus far, over 40 cases of IUTx using HSC in human fetuses have been described[29–31]. These transplants have been performed in fetuses affected by immunodeficiencies, white blood cell disorders, hemoglobinopathies, sickle cell anemia, Rhesus disease and metabolic storage disease[30]. The transplantation settings in these cases were different. The gestational age at the time of the transplantation, but also the stem cell source, the stem cell dose and the route of transplantation differed among these IUTx using HSC. Significant engraftment has only been attained in fetuses affected by SCID[31–35]. In immunologically competent fetuses, engraftment of donor cells was very low and had no impact on the clinical course of the disease being treated. In homozygous-thalassemia (2 cases reported) and beta-thalassemia (13 cases reported), although some level of engraftment may have been achieved, all children remained transfusion dependent[36]. Also, in sickle cell disease (n = 3) and in Rhesus-immunization (n = 3) no change in the clinical course could be demonstrated. Adding a mild myeloablative protocol, by giving the mother low-dose dexamethasone before the IUTxHSC, resulted in a higher level of microchimerism, suggesting a different approach[37]. Other strategies, such as the use of CD26 inhibition, shown in animal models to increase homing and engraftment of HSC, might be of interest in modulating the level of chimerism[38].

Most clinical experience and successes of IUTx with HSC have been reported in fetuses affected by immunodeficiencies[31,35]. In at least 8 children, engraftment has been reported, with immunocompetent T-, NK- and (not always) B-cell reconstitution, accounting for the more benign course of the disease. Although the advantages are clear (less expensive, no need for any chemotherapy or radiation, no need for isolation with its profound psychological advantage and theoretically a lower risk of graft versus host disease because maternal chimerism in the fetus is prevented), the nearly 100% success of neonatal bone marrow transplantion, using HLA-identical siblings in these diseases is still preventing the shift from neonatal to fetal treatment. Also the technical risk, with an estimated fetal loss of 1% related to an IUTx, needs to be taken into account. Successful engraftment after IUTx with stem cells in metabolic storage diseases (7 cases reported)[39] has been documented in only one case, with no effect on clinical course. This makes the indication questionable for these diseases, although on scientific and clinical grounds (with possibly already one severely affected child), they are an important group. Success has been reported (5 cases) in osteogenesis imperfecta, although long-term outcome, both considering the functionality of the graft and clinical outcome, and the influence of the IUTx on the phenotype of the disease, is still uncertain[40]. Despite being transplanted relatively late in pregnancy, the success of engraftment might partly be related to the type of stem cell (mesenchymal stem cell: MSCs) which was used. The unique immunological properties (see further) of these cells, being immunosuppressive, could have been a factor in these transplants. The positive effects on engraftment, even across transplantation mismatches, possibly due to the immunomodulatory capacities of MSC, opens up a more general application, by incorporating or co-transplanting these cells in (HSC) transplantation protocols[41–43]. Also the feasibility of these cells for treating storage diseases and others is promising.

As a result of the disappointing outcome of IUTxHSC in humans thus far, relatively few further clinical transplants are being performed today. In particular, it has become uncertain whether the fetal immune incompetent window ('window of opportunity') between prenatal diagnosis and the gestational age for transplantation can be successfully used to induce immune tolerance for donor cells.

Engraftment barriers for in utero transplantation of stem cells

Different barriers are thought to be responsible for the low engraftment of donor cells after IUTxHSC. The first barrier is the lack of space available for homing and engraftment of donor cells in the expanding fetal hematopoietic compartment. The rapid fetal growth suggests an enormous expansion of fetal hematopoietic cells. It has been assumed that, in these rapidly expanding organs, available hematopoietic homing sites are present, allowing donor cells to engraft. However, it is conceivable that due to the high production of hematopoietic cells, limited space is available for donor HSC to engraft. The second barrier is the immune system of the fetus. It was assumed that the human fetus is tolerant to foreign antigens until the 18th week of gestation and transplants are accepted without the need for immune suppression[44]. However, recently it was shown that alloreactive T lymphocytes are present in the fetal liver already in the first trimester of pregnancy[45,46]. Therefore, it is now thought that the 'window of opportunity' for IUTxHSC is rather small.

A third barrier for engraftment is the competition which occurs between donor and recipient cells. Due to the high production of hematopoietic cells in the fetus, donor cells have to compete with endogenous fetal cells. Lack of successful competition will result in low engraftment of donor cells. Theoretically, adding supporting cells to the graft can increase their competitiveness.

STEM CELL BIOLOGY

Stem cells are characterized by their ability for self-renewal and the possibility to differentiate into at least one mature cell type. They are present in many different tissues. Several classes of stem cells are recognized. Fertilized oocytes are totipotent, which means that they are able to differentiate into all cell types resulting in a complete organism. Cells derived from the preimplantation embryo, from the morula or blastocyst stage, are called embryonic stem cells (ESCs). These cells are able to differentiate into most tissues and organs and are therefore called pluripotent. In 1998, it was reported for the first time that human embryonic stem cells (hESCs) were derived from embryos at the blastocyst stage[47]. Stem cells present in later life and also stem cells collected from fetal, neonatal and adult tissue are still multipotent as they are able to differentiate into specific lineages, depending on their origin. Several sources of stem cells such as bone marrow, contain hematopoietic stem cells (HSC) as well as mesenchymal stem cells (MSC). The suggestion that fetal stem cell are more plastic and have a higher replicative potential than adult stem cells, make these fetal cells potentially better candidate cells for transplantation.

Hematopoietic stem cell (HSC)

Ontogeny of HSC

Hematopoiesis is the process whereby HSCs continuously proliferate and differentiate resulting in the renewal of progenitor cells and mature blood cells. This includes, respectively, progenitor cells of the myeloid and lymphoid cell lineages, which further differentiate into lymphocytes, macrophages, platelets and erythrocytes (Fig. 47.1). There is a gradual change during embryonic and fetal life in the site where hematopoiesis takes place. It might be that for hematopoiesis there is the need not only for HSC but also for special supporting microenvironments. Bone marrow stromal cells or mesenchymal stem cells could control and support the proliferation and differentiation of HSC by cellular interactions and the production of certain lineage-specific factors, cytokines and growth factors that stimulate multiple lineages like erythropoietin (EPO), stem cell factor (SCF), macrophage colony-stimulating factor (M-CSF), thrombopoeietin (TPO), Flt3-ligand, interleukins (Il-3, Il-6, Il-11), leukaemia inhibitor factor (LIF) and granulocyte-macrophage colony stimulating factor (GM-CSF)[48,49].

Sites of hematopoiesis

At very early gestational ages – from around 16–20 days of embryonic development – the first signs of hematopoiesis are found outside the fetus, in the mesoderm of the extra embryonic

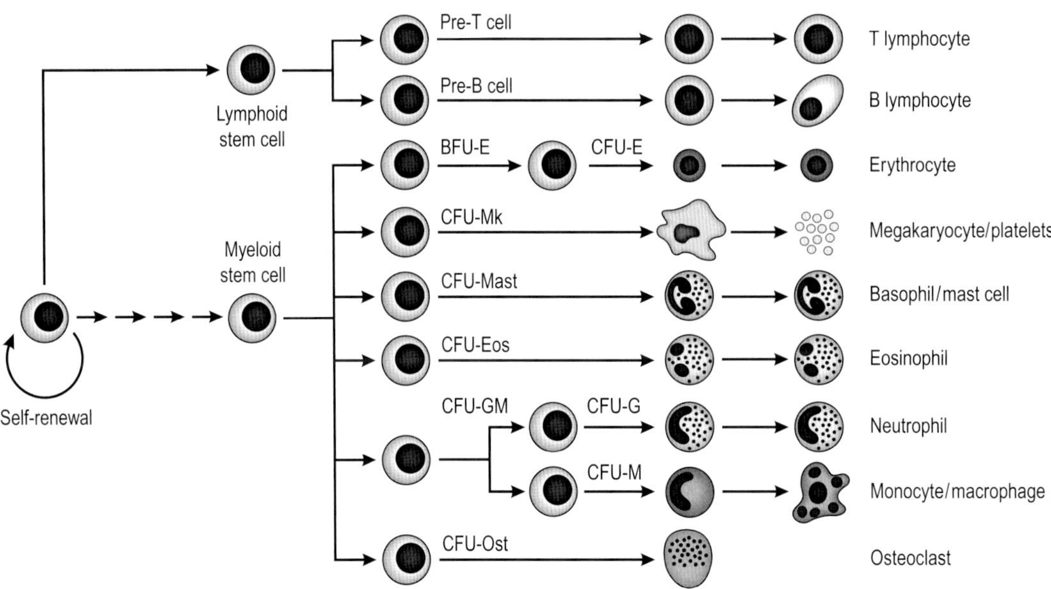

Fig. 47.1 Schematic overview of hematopoietic cell development.

yolk sac[50–52]. Only a primitive erythropoiesis is found in the *blood islands* as only cells from the erythroid cell line are produced and (as there is no expulsion of the nucleus) only nucleated red cells, synthesizing only embryonic hemoglobins, are produced in early embryonic life. There are arguments that circulation of primitive erythrocytes occurs between the yolk sac and the cardiac cavity not earlier than from day 19 or 21. In addition, granulocyte-macrophage progenitors are found in the yolk sac, which disappear together with the erythroid progenitors from the 6th–8th week onwards. Already from the 5th week, an additional, independent pool of hematopoietic progenitor cells, phenotypically characteristic for hematopoietic progenitors ($CD34^+ CD45^+ Lin(eage)^-$), are identified at the ventral endothelium of the dorsal aorta[52–54], also called the aorta-gonad-mesonephros (AGM). These cells are considered to be responsible for further fetal hematopoiesis[50], seeding the fetal liver and later the other hematopoietic tissues[55]. The first organ to be colonized with hematopoietic cells is the fetal liver; this occurs from week 6 concomitant with the start of embryonic cardiac activity. Besides erythropoiesis, which is the major activity found in the liver cells, the granulocytic and magakaryoctic lineages are also found[56]. With the transition from yolk sac to liver there is also a change in the type of hemoglobin produced, now becoming fetal Hb ($\alpha\gamma$), and forming definitive enucleated erythrocytes. In week 8, 88% of the circulating blood cells are still of the primitive type[51]. From week 7 onwards, hematopoietic cells are found in the spleen, with the highest number of $CD34^+$ cells between 14 and 22 weeks. It is still a point of discussion whether the fetal spleen is really a hematopoietic organ or a place were precursor cells are entrapped, making the spleen only part of a recirculation system of stem cells[57]. The final organ for hematopoiesis becomes the fetal bone marrow. Bone marrow stroma appears in the clavicula from the 9–10th week of gestation and somewhat later (from the 11th week) in human medullary cavities. Active hematopoiesis is found at 12–13 weeks and, from 22 weeks onwards, all cell lines can be found in bone marrow, making this compartment in the second trimester of pregnancy the central hematopoietic organ[51,58], from where HSC reside primarily and from where they circulate in the peripheral blood. By that time, fetal bone marrow is similar to adult bone marrow, although in fetal bone marrow no plasma cells and no lymph follicles can be found. From the 22–24th week, it gives rise to all cells of the hematopoietic system including red cells, white cells and platelets. From this gestational age umbilical cord blood is a clearly documented source of HSC[59,60]. Around 30–45% of fetal blood is circulating in the placenta and the umbilical cord. The concentration of HSC in umbilical cord blood is at least 100-fold greater than in adult peripheral blood.

Sources of HSC

Fetal liver is an attractive source for HSC. First, fetal liver has a high number of HSC (especially in early pregnancy). Secondly, the number of T cells (post-thymic) is low. This makes the chances of graft-versus-host disease after transplantation very unlikely. Because these cells have a longer telomere length than HSC derived from umbilical cord blood or adult bone marrow, they have a greater proliferation capacity, resulting in an engraftment advantage[61,62].

Umbilical cord blood (UCB) is a rich source of HSC. First-trimester UCB contains more CD34+ cells than term UCB. However, only 5% of the CD45+ population in UCB are CD34+[63]. The percentage of HSC (of the total number of nucleated cells) is lower compared to adult bone marrow: 1% versus 1–3%. However, the number of the most primitive HSC ($CD34^+ CD38^-$) is probably the same for the two sources[64]. The number of hematopoietic progenitors is highest in second-trimester UCB. Besides the easy availability of UCB HSC, there is a lower risk for GVHD after a cord blood transplantation[65], making it even possible to transplant with one or two mismatches. After the first successful UCB transplantation was performed in 1988[66] with a related donor, the interest in storage of UCB has increased enormously. More than 150 000 UCB have been stored world-wide in cord blood banks. More than 2000 patients have received UCB-derived HSC from related or unrelated cord blood.

Adult bone marrow has been the most frequently used source of stem cells. It is a safe source and a second transplant using the same donor is feasible. Because harvesting of adult bone marrow is an invasive procedure, with drawbacks such as the need for general anesthesia, the collection of stem cells after peripheral stem cell mobilization (with GM-CSF) has become the strategy of choice. Another advantage of peripheral mobilized stem cells is the rapid engraftment of hematopoietic cells and a faster immune reconstitution[67].

Mesenchymal stem cells (MSC)

Friedenstein first showed that isolated progenitor cells from the rat bone marrow were able to differentiate into osteoblasts[68]. These MSC appeared to be an adherent, fibroblast-like population that were able to differentiate into different connective tissue after transplantation[69]. Bone marrow stroma consists of many different cells, including endothelial cells, macrophages, marrow myofibroblasts and adipocytes. Marrow stromal stem cells or mesenchymal stem cells were shown to be multipotent, non-hematopoietic cells, capable of differentiating into cells of the connective lineage such as adipose tissue[70], marrow stroma, cartilage, smooth muscle, cardiomyocytes[71], tendon and bone[72,73] (Fig. 47.2).

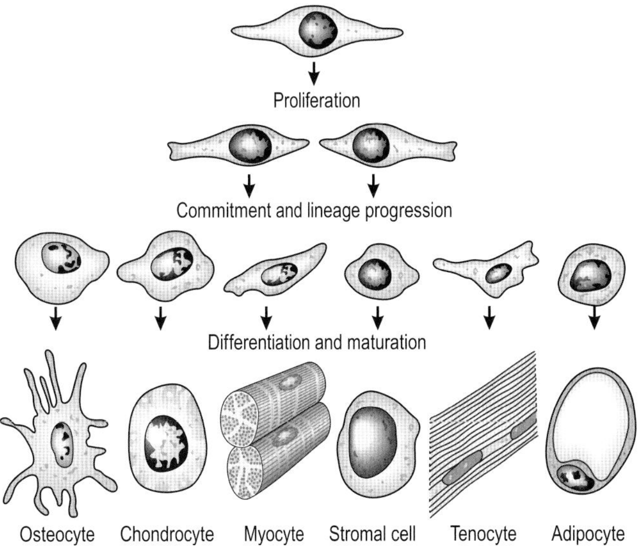

Fig. 47.2 Schematic overview of mesenchymal stem cell differentiation.

Ontogeny of MSC

Hematopoiesis in the bone marrow is preceded by the development of the stromal cell compartment, which regulates hematopoiesis by secreting cytokines and facilitating cell–stromal cell contacts. MSC are characterized by self-renewal, *multi*potentiality and proliferative capacity. Bone marrow also contains an earlier precursor, the multipotent adult progenitor cell (MAPC), which has a *pluri*potent differentiation capacity for not only mesenchymal cells, but also into endothelial and endodermal cell lineages[74]. There is no unique phenotype for MSC. The selection and isolation of MSC relies therefore on the culture of cell suspensions in specific culture media and the subsequent adherence capacity on plastic dishes[75]. Although they are rare in the adult human body, MSC can easily be expanded for more than 30 passages, proliferating into spindle-shaped cells and forming confluent cultures. Although they look by light microscopy more or less the same, they differ by their expansion capacity (also depending on from where the cells were harvested from and how they were cultured). A panel of antibodies can be used to characterize cultured MSC by FACS analysis. They are lineage negative (do not express hematopoietic markers CD34, CD45 and CD14 or endothelial markers CD31, vWF) but stain positive for stromal markers CD73 (SH-4), CD105 (SH-2, endoglin), CD166, and for the adhesion markers CD90 (Thy-1) and CD29[73,76]. Recently, STRO-1 and VCAM-1 (CD106) have been used to enrich the population of MSC before expanding them in culture[77]. In addition, negative selection using CD45, CD34 and CD11b can be effective in isolation and purification protocols. Cultured MSC express HLA- class I and do not express (extracellular) HLA class II and the co-stimulatory molecules[78]. HLA class II expression by MSC can be induced by interferon γ (IFN-γ).

MSC play a role in the formation of the supportive extracellular matrix, which contributes to an appropriate microenvironment for hematopoietic cells. They are able to produce fibronectin, laminin, collagen and proteoglycans. In addition, cytokines and growth factors important for HSC expansion and differentiation are produced by MSC[79]. They also carry receptors able to ligate cells from the hematopoietic lineage, such as ICAM 1 and 2, most probably to be able to give physical support for HSC[80].

Adipogenic differentiation is induced with indomethacin, dexamethasone, bovine insulin and 1-methyl-3-isobutylzantine (IBMX). Within 3 weeks, lipid vacuoles can be visualized using Oil red O staining. Osteogenic differentiation is induced with ascorbic acid, dexamethasone and β-glycerol phosphate. This differentiation can be visualized by staining with alkaline phosphatase or with Alizarin red S solution for the calcium deposition. Chondrogenic differentiation is induced by the use of transforming growth factor-β2 (TGF-β2): visualization is done by an antibody against the type II collagen. Myoblast induction is done with the use of 5-azacytidine and also differentiation into cardiomyocytes has been reported[81].

In vivo, it has been shown that MSC can contribute to the regeneration of many tissues, e.g. liver[82], endometrium, skeletal, neuronal[83] and heart tissue.

Sources of MSC

MSC were first identified in adult bone marrow[84] and later in many other adult tissue such as adipose tissue[85], periosteum[86], muscle[87], connective tissue, skin, nervous system tissue[88], endometrium[89,90] and peripheral blood[91]. Bone marrow is the most common source of MSC and shows a decrease in the number of MSC with age: from 1 in 10^4 nucleated bone marrow cells at birth to 1 in 2×10^6 at the age of 80[92,93], indicating that these cells are rare in the human adult bone marrow[94]. In fetal tissues, MSC have been derived from many different sources: first-trimester bone marrow, blood and liver[95], second-trimester kidney and pancreas[96], lung[97], amniotic fluid[98,99], cord blood[97,100] and placenta[101–103]. First-trimester MSC seem to be a more promising cell type as they express, which adult MSC do not, some pluripotency markers such as Nanog, SSEA-3 and SSEA-4; they have longer telomeres and a greater telomerase activity and are more readily expandable, making them a better candidate for cell-based therapies if compared to adult sources[104]. Although disputed in the beginning of MSC research, it is now clearly demonstrated that UCB contains MSC. UCB is an alternative and attractive source for MSC as it contains much younger cells which are considered to have a much higher proliferation and differentiation capacity[63,93,105,106]. Not only first-trimester UCB contains MSC, but term UCB also[107] with multilineage differentiation capacity for e.g. adipose tissue, neuronal tissue, bone forming capacity[108] and hepatocyte-like cells, neuroglial-like cells, bone and cartilage differentiation[107]. Recently, it was shown that cells isolated from both first-trimester and term placenta have an MSC morphology with both multilineage differentiation potential and cell surface expression characteristic of MSC and embryonic stem (ES) cell markers[103,109,110]. We and others also found that early second-trimester amniotic fluid contains MSC[102,111]. Intrauterine transplantation with MSC in sheep showed engraftment and site-specific differentiation[21,112].

Plasticity

Although the mechanism behind the unique plasticity of stem cells to become another cell type is still debated, it seems most plausible to occur – at least for adult bone marrow – via direct differentiation from several populations of multipotent stem cells. Other mechanisms like cell fusion (as occurring in the placenta) and dedifferentiation (unipotent stem cell becoming multipotent again) seem to be less likely. Via direct differentiation, the stem cells, partly depending on the specific environment, undergo a unidirectional process to become a specific cell type[75]. Certain genes and transcription factors are repressed, while others become activated. As an example of this process, it was recently shown that MSC derived from amnion and chorion were able to differentiate, depending on the culture medium used, to chondrocytes, osteocytes, adipose tissue, with also some neurogenic and myogenic differentiation[103]. The homing process of MSC is, however, poorly understood. It seems that MSC are triggered to specific differentiation in the context of tissue damage, which may be a beneficial mechanism associated with tissue repair. MSC might be dormant in certain niches in the adult e.g. the bone marrow, and after damage has occurred they migrate and home at specific sites of tissue damage[82,113]. MSC chemoattractant molecules like SDF-1, HGF/SF, LIF, VEGF, HIF-1 and CXCR4 are locally upregulated during tissue damage, recruiting MSC to the site of damage.

Immunology

When MSC were shown to engraft even in immunocompetent sheep fetuses, it was realized that they might have immunomodulatory properties. This is partly explained because MSC do not express HLA class II and co-stimulatory molecules (B7-1 and B7-2). In co-culture experiments, human MSC do not induce proliferation of allogenic lymphocytes, neither after the addition of CD28-stimulating antibodies nor after transfection of MSC with the co-stimulatory molecules B7-1 or B7-2[114]. This possibility of reducing immunological rejection was shown in vitro, whereby both autologous and allogenic MSC inhibited the mixed lymphocyte reaction (MLR) resulting in the inhibition of T-cell proliferation[114,115]. This suppression was dose dependent and independent from the sources (rodent, baboon or human) used. The mechanism for suppression is MHC independent and is most probably mediated by a soluble factor, at least in some systems, cell–cell contact is not needed[116,117]. Other mechanisms have been proposed, some of which need cell–cell contact[115,118]. Suppression might rely on the secretion of certain cytokines, e.g. a decrease in the production of TGF-β, HGF, prostaglandin E2, TNF-α or an increase in the production of Il-10. Recently, the possibility was raised that MSC induce regulatory antigen presenting cells (APCs; deletional APCs) or regulatory T cells[119–121] resulting in a dose dependent and contact-dependent inhibition of the T-cell response. The modulatory effect of MSC could also rely on an inhibition of monocyte-derived myeloid dendritic cells (DC) differentiation[120,121], while plasmacytoid DCs increased their production of IL-10[119]. Also the production of 2,3-dioxygenase (IDO) by MSC could have an inhibiting effect on T cells. IDO catalyzes tryptophan to kynurenine and, via the depletion of tryptophan T-cell proliferation, is inhibited[122]. Both undifferentiated and differentiated MSC fail to induce a proliferative response in vitro in allogeneic lymphocytes. Even transduction with the co-stimulatory molecules B7-1 and B7-2 did not stimulate the proliferation of alloreactive T cells[117]. They also escape, in vitro, recognition by alloreactive T cells[123]. The possibility of modifying the immune response because of an anti-proliferative, immunomodulatory effect might make these cells of potential clinical relevance in GVHD[124] and in the prevention of solid organ rejection.

Possible therapeutic applications of MSC (experimental work with MSC)

Studies in animals and various clinical settings have shown a potential role for MSC in different therapeutic applications. Either local implantation or systemic transplantation of specialized cells could be favored by MSC or the transplantation of MSC could be the primary purpose. The possibility of reducing immunological rejection and thereby homing induction has been shown in vivo, whereby the addition of MSC promoted the engraftment of HSC transplantation. MSC have also been used for tissue engineering, whereby both in the antenatal and neonatal period, systemic treatment of osteogenesis imperfecta in immunocompetent fetuses or neonates with fully mismatched MSC showed persistence of donor cells as well as a beneficial effect on the disease process[40,125].

The possible role for fetal and adult human MSC in the enhancement of engraftment and proliferation of HSC has been demonstrated both in animal models, i.e. the fetal sheep[126,127] and the NOD/SCID mouse[128] and in clinical studies. In women treated for breast cancer with myeoloablative therapy and thereafter with myeloreconstitution, co-transplanting HSC with MSC, showed enhancement of engraftment and a rapid hematopoietic recovery[129]. It is still open for discussion if this enhanced engraftment is related to the MSC per se or the cytokines produced by them which promotes homing and/or engraftment. It could also be that MSC are precursors for the bone marrow stroma, thereby providing a supporting tissue structure for the HSC or enhancing HSC engraftment via cytokines produced by the MSC network. The immune suppressive effects of MSC might also have a possible role in the prevention and treatment of GVHD and in the prevention of rejection, both in allogeneic stem cell transplantation[124,130] and in solid organ transplantation[131]. In the future, a possible role in the treatment of severe autoimmune diseases can also be foreseen.

A new line of future applications might be in the field of regenerative medicine. MSC are capable of differentiating into well-defined tissues and might be used to restore e.g. cartilage defects. Cells induced from MSC can generate a cardiomyogeneic phenotype[132]. In humans, the engraftment of these cells in the myocardium and especially their functional properties remain controversial[133,134,146]. In animal models, MSC injected locally around tendon defects show an improvement in function[135]. In human arthritic knees, injection of MSC into the joint stimulated the regeneration of cartilage[136].

In pregnancy, a possible application of MSC would be in healing premature rupture of membranes (PROM). Several treatments for PROM have been suggested, including amnion patch, amnion graft, maternal blood clot patch and fibrin glue, but success has been limited[137]. The presence of MSC in amnion could help in the understanding of healing of ruptured fetal membranes and could represent a first step in the development of tissue engineering strategies in cases of PROM.

Inborn errors of metabolism might also be amenable to IUTxSC. MSC are able to produce certain enzymes which, even after engraftment of low numbers of MSC, are able to have a positive effect on outcome in patients with metabolic diseases, such as lysosomal storage diseases[138]. The possible success of IUTxSC in these diseases relies on the fact that severe tissue damage occurring before birth might be prevented. The best examples for neonatal treatment are MLD (metachromatic leukodystrophy: arylsulfatase A deficiency), infantile Krabbe's disease (globoid cell leukodystrophy: GCL) and Hurler's disease. All these diseases, when treated at a very early stage, might have an impressive improvement in CNS functioning. In Hurler's disease, because of the deficiency of the lysosomal enzyme α-L-iduronidase, there is an accumulation of glycosaminoglycan resulting in progressive mental retardation and fatal cardiac involvement[139]. Good neuropsychological outcome is related to the age at which an MSC transplantation is performed. Mental retardation can be prevented even with very low levels of engraftment. Direct injection of cultured and differentiated MSC into mouse nervous tissue was shown to delay neurological defects (and death) in Niemann-Pick disease, a degenerative central nervous system disease based on a sphingomyelinase deficiency[83]. Also infantile Krabbe's disease, an autosomal recessive disease where there is a deficiency of the lysosomal enzyme galatocerebrosidase, characterized by a failure of central and peripheral myelination resulting in a rapidly progressing neurologic deterioration, might benefit from IUTxSC. Both disease models show the feasibility of this treatment, whereby only minimal engraftment is associated with a delay in the occurrence of detrimental effects on the central nervous system. Neonatal transplantation with UCB-derived stem cells favorably influenced the natural history of the disease[140]. In these cases, neonatal transplantation might be relatively late as already some irreversible central nervous damage has occurred prenatally and, because neonatal transplantation needs cytostatic conditioning, they would be good candidates for IUTxSC. An example, where IUTxSC was not successful was shown in chronic granulomatous disease (CGD). CGD is a genetically heterogeneous disorder where neonates suffer from serious and sometimes fatal infections because of defective activation of cytotoxic immune cells. The defect in the gene coding for the disease is known and located on the X chromosome and can be diagnosed by CVS. As the disease could be cured by the presence of only a small percentage of granulocytes, IUTxSC was chosen as a treatment modality in a pregnancy where the fetus had been diagnosed prenatally to be affected[141]. The fetus was transplanted intraperitoneally at 14 weeks with 1×10^7 paternally derived HSC (CD34+). However, no evidence of engraftment was found at the age of 1 year. It is suggested that this could be related to insufficient space in the bone marrow, but also that the fetus might even at that gestational age be immunocompetent as T cells are present in fetal liver from 7 weeks onward and in fetal blood from 13.5 weeks. Recently, profound differences in engraftment were shown between syngeneic versus allogeneic IUTxHSC in the 14-day-old fetal mouse model, whereby all allogeneic engraftment was lost after birth. All syngeneic animals had a sustained engraftment, suggesting that engraftment space in the bone marrow compartment is not the central issue. Most probably allogeneic cells are eliminated by the adaptive immune response even in the 14-day-old fetal mouse, whereby the elimination occurs neonatally within 2–5 weeks after IUTxHSC[142]. Another case of IUTxSC has been reported where antenatally the diagnosis of globoid cell leukodystrophy was made. Transplantation of 5×10^9 cells/kg fetal weight $CD34^+$ paternally derived cells in a fetus considered to be preimmune (13.5 weeks gestational age) resulted in extensive engraftment[39]. The child died 7 weeks postpartum with the diagnosis of overengraftment resulting in vascular plugging. In two other cases, in which 1 log lower doses were used, no engraftment could be demonstrated[143]. Osteogenesis imperfecta could also benefit substantially from IUTxSC. A mutation in the genes that encode for collagen type I causes insufficient scaffolding for bone formation, resulting in bone fragility and skeletal deformities affecting 1 in 10000 births. Transplantation of allogeneic bone-marrow-derived MSC in children with osteogenesis imperfecta resulted in in the development of donor-derived osteoblast and repair of bone defects and fractures[125,144]. Recently, it was demonstrated that IUTx with MSC in a fetus with an osteogenesis imperfecta phenotype resulted in the homing and engraftment of these cells in the fetus[40]. This study and the neonatal experience give some credence to an effect of MSC transplantation in this otherwise incurable disease.

IUTxSC remains an experimental form of therapy where most successes have been encountered in SCID and BLS. To be successful in other diseases – as shown with the CGD case – greater understanding of barriers preventing SC engraftment are still needed.

CONCLUSIONS

Isolation of MSC from various fetal and adult tissues has resulted in an enormous amplification of biological concepts in regenerative medicine. Fetal stem cells may have a greater potential for expansion and differentiation than adult. In particular, the possibility of isolating and expanding MSC – and perhaps other cell types – from amniotic fluid and placenta promises to be another valuable source of progenitor cells.

Future applications of MSC include the correction of inborn errors of metabolism, tissue engineering and enhancement of engraftment of HSC.

REFERENCES

1. Tiblad E, Westgren M. Fetal stem-cell transplantation.. *Best Pract Res Clin Obstet Gynaec* **22**:189–201, 2008.
2. Surbek DV, Holzgreve W, Nicolaides KH. Haematopoietic stem cell transplantation and gene therapy in the fetus: ready for clinical use? *Hum Reprod Update* **7**:85–91, 2001.
3. Krivit W, Whitley CB. Bone marrow transplantation for genetic diseases. *N Engl J Med* **316**:1085–1087, 1990.
4. Fischer A, Landais P, Friedrich W et al. European experience of bone-marrow transplantation for severe combined immunodeficiency. *Lancet* **336**:850–854, 1990.
5. Davies J. Clinicopathological conference. A case of haemolytic disease with congenital rubella demonstrated at the Royal Postgraduate Medical School. *Br Med J* **2**:819–822, 1967.
6. Brent L, Linch DC, Rodeck CH et al. On the feasibility of inducing tolerance in man: a study in the cynomolgus monkey. *Immunol Lett* **21**:55–61, 1989.
7. Pahal GS, Jauniaux E, Kinnon C, Tracher AJ, Rodeck CH. Normal development of human fetal hematopoiesis between eight and seventeen weeks' gestation. *Am J Obstet Gynecol* **183**:1029–1031, 2000.
8. Hayashi S, Peranteau WH, Shaaban AF, Flake AW. Complete allogeneic hematopoietic chimerism achieved by a combined strategy of in utero hematopoietic stem cell transplantation and postnatal donor lymphocyte infusion. *Blood* **100**:804–812, 2002.
9. Peranteau WH, Hayashi S, Hsieh M, Shaaban AF, Flake AW. High level allogeneic chimerism achieved by prenatal tolerance induction and postnatal nonmyeoloablative bone marrow transplantation. *Blood* **100**:2225–2234, 2002.
10. Kim HB, Shaaban AF, Yang EY, Liechty KW, Flake AW. Microchimerism and tolerance after in utero bone marrow transplantation in mice. *J Surg Res* **77**:1–5, 1998.
11. Harrison MR, Slotnick RN, Crombleholme TM, Golbus MS, Tarantal AF, Zanjani ED. In-utero transplantation of fetal liver haemopoietic stem cells in monkeys. *Lancet* **2**(8677):1425–1427, 1989.
12. Devine SM, Cobbs S, Jenings M, Bartholomew A, Hoffman R. Mesenchymal stem cells distribute to a wide range of tissues following systemic infusion in nonhuman primates. *Blood* **101**:2999–3001, 2003.
13. Shields LE, Bryant EM, Easterling TR, Andrews RG. Fetal liver cell transplantation for the creation of lymphohematopoietic chimerism in fetal baboons. *Am J Obstet Gynecol* **173**:1157–1160, 1995.
14. Blakemore K, Hattenburg C, Stetten G et al. In utero hematopoietic stem cell transplantation with haploidentical donor adult bone marrow in a canine model. *Am J Obstet Gynecol* **190**:960–973, 2004.
15. Pochampally RR, Neville BT, Schwarz EJ, Li MM, Prockop DJ. Rat adult stem cells

(marrow stromal cells) engraft and differentiate in chick embryos without evidence of cell fusion. *Proc Natl Acad Sci USA* **101**:9282–9285, 2004.

16. Flake AW, Harrison MR, Zanjani ED. In utero stem cell transplantation. *Exp Hematol* **19**:1061–1064, 1991.
17. Zanjani ED, Ascensao JL, Flake AW, Harrison MR, Tavassoli M. The fetus as an optiomal donor and recipient of hematopoietic stem cells. *Bone Marrow Transplant* **10**(suppl 1):107–114, 1992.
18. Young AJ, Holzgreven W, Dudler L, Schoeberlein A, Surbek DV. Engraftment of human cord blood-derived stem cells in preimmune ovine fetuses after ultrasound-guided in utero transplantation. *Am J Obstet Gynaecol* **189**:698–701, 2003.
19. Zanjani ED, Pallavacini MG, Ascensao JL, Flake AW, Harrison MR, Tavassoli M. Human-ovine xenogenic transplantation of stem cells in utero. *Bone Marrow Transplant* **9**(Suppl 1):86–89, 1992.
20. Srour EF, Hoffman R, Zanjani D. Animal models for human hematopoiesis. *J Hematother* **1**:143–153, 1992.
21. Grinnemo KH, Mansson A, Dellgren G et al. Xenoreactivity and engraftment of human mesenchymal stem cells transplanted into infarcted rat myocardium. *J Thorac Cardiovasc Surg* **127**:1293–1300, 2004.
22. Nakamura Y, Wang X, Xu C et al. Xenotransplantation of long term cultured swine bone marrow-derived mesenchymal stem cells. *Stem Cells* **25**:612–620, 2007.
23. Lee PW, Cina RA, Randolph MA et al. In utero bone marrow transplantation induces kidney allograft tolerance across a full major histocompatibility complex barrier in swine. *Transplantation* **79**: 1084–1090, 2005.
24. Fleischman RA, Mintz B. Prevention 1996 of genetic anemias in mice by microinjection of normal hematopoietic stem cells into the fetal placenta. *Proc Natl Acad Sci USA* **76**:5736–5740, 1979.
25. Blazar BR, Taylor PA, Vallera DA. Adult bone marrow-derived pluripotent hematopoietic stem cells are engraftable when transferred in utero into moderately anemic fetal recipients. *Blood* **85**:833–841, 1995.
26. Blazar BR, Taylor PA, Vallera DA. In utero transfer of adult bone marrow cells into recipients with severe combined immunodeficiency disorder yields lymphoid progeny with T- and B-cell functional capabilities. *Blood* **86**:4353–4366, 1995.
27. Zanjani ED, Pallavicini MG, Ascensao JL et al. Engraftment and long-term expression of human fetal hemopoietic stem cells in sheep following transplantation in utero. *J Clin Invest* **89**:1178–1188, 1992.
28. Zanjani ED, Almeida-Porada G, Flake AW. Retention and multilineage expression of human hematopoietic stem cells in human-sheep chimeras. *Stem Cells* **13**: 101–111, 1995.
29. Linch DC, Rodeck CH, Nicolaides K, Jones HM, Brent L. Attempted bone-marrow transplantation in a 17-week fetus. *Lancet* **22**(8521):1453, 1986.
30. Shields LE, Lindton B, Andrews RG, Westgren M. Fetal hematopoietic stem cell transplantation: a challenge for the twenty-first century. *J Hematother Stem Cell Res* **11**:617–631, 2002.
31. Westgren M, Ringden O, Bartmann P et al. Prenatal T-cell reconstitution after in utero transplantation with fetal liver cells in a patient with X-linked severe combined immunodeficiency. *Am J Obstet Gynecol* **187**:475–482, 2002.
32. Touraine JL, Raudrant D, Royo C et al. In-utero transplantation of stem cells in bare lymphocyte syndrome. *Lancet* **1**:1382, 1989.
33. Flake AW, Roncarolo MG, Puck JM et al. Treatment of x-linked severe combined immunodeficiency by in utero transplantation of paternal bone marrow. *N Engl J Med* **335**:1806–1810, 1996.
34. Lanfranchi A, Neva A, Tettoni K et al. In utero transplantation (IUT) of parental CD34+ cells in three patients affected by primary immunodeficiencies. *Bone Marrow Transplant* **21**:S127, 1998.
35. Wengler GS, Lanfranchi A, Frusca T et al. In-utero transplantation of parental CD34 haematopoietic progenitor cells in a patient with X-linked severe combined immunodeficiency (SCIDXI). *Lancet* **348**:1484–1487, 1996.
36. Westgren M, Ringdén O, Eik-Nes et al. Lack of evidence of permanent engraftment after in utero fetal stem cell transplantation in congenital hemoglobinopathies. *Transplantation* **61**:1176–1179, 1996.
37. Renda MC, Daimiani G, Fecarotta E et al. In utero stem cell transplantation after a mlld immunosuppression: evidence of paternal ABO cDNA in β-thalassemia affected fetus. *Blood Transfus* **3**:55–65, 2005.
38. Peranteau WH, Endo M, Adibe OO, Merchant A, Zoltick PW, Flake AW. CD26 inhibition enhances allogeneic donor-cell homing and engraftment after in utero hematopoietic-cell transplantation. *Blood* **108**:4268–4274, 2006.
39. Bambach BJ, Moser HW, Blakemore KB et al. Engraftment following in utero bone marrow transplantation for globoid cell leukodystrophy. *Bone Marrow Transplant* **19**:399–402, 1997.
40. Le Blanc K, Gotherstrom C, Ringden O et al. Fetal mesenchymal stem-cell engraftment in bone after in utero transplantation in a patient with severe osteogenesis imperfecta. *Transplantation* **79**:1607–1614, 2005.
41. Shields LE, Gauer L, Delio P, Potter J, Sieverkropp A, Andrews RG. Fetal immune suppression as adjuvant therapy for in utero hematopoietic stem cell transplantation in nonhuman primates. *Stem Cells* **22**:759–769, 2004.
42. Le Blanc K, Ringden O. Immunobiology of human mesenchymal stem cells and future use in hematopoietic stem cell transplantation. *Biol Blood Marrow Transplant* **11**:321–334, 2005.
43. Le Blanc K, Samuelsson H, Gustafsson B et al. Transplantation of mesenchymal stem cell to enhance engraftment of hematopoietic stem cells. *Leukemia* **21**:1733–1738, 2007.
44. Crombleholme TM, Langer JC, Harrison MR, Zanjani ED. Transplantation of fetal cells. *Am J Obstet Gynecol* **164**:218–230, 1991.
45. Renda MC, Fecarotta E, Dieli F et al. Evidence of alloreactive T lymphocytes in fetal liver: implications for fetal hematopoietic stem cell transplantation. *Bone Marrow Transplant* **25**:135–141, 2000.
46. Renda MC, Fecarotta E, Maggio A et al. In utero fetal liver hematopoietic stem cell transplantation: is there a role for alloreactive T lymphocytes? *Blood* **96**:1608–1609, 2000.
47. Thomson JA, Itskovitz-Eldor J, Shapiro SS et al. Embryonic stem cell lines derived from human blastocysts. *Science* **282**: 1145–1147, 1998.
48. Clark BR, Gallagher JT, Dexter TM. Cell adhesion in the stromal regulation of haemopoiesis. *Baillieres Clin Haematol* **5**:619–652, 1992.
49. Metcalf D. Mechanism of human hematopoiesis. In *Haematopoietic Cell Transplantation*, 2nd edn, ED Thomas, KG Blume, SJ Forman (eds), pp. 48–57. Malden: Blackwell Science Inc, 1999.
50. Tavian M, Hallais MF, Péault B. Emergence of intraembryonic hematopoietic precursors in the pre-liver human embryo. *Development* **126**:793–803, 1999.
51. Palis J, Yoder MC. Yolk-sac hematopoiesis: the first blood cells of mouse and man. *Exp Hematol* **29**:927–936, 2001.
52. Tavian M, Péault B. Embryonic development of the human hematopoietic system. *Int J Dev Biol* **49**:243–250, 2005.
53. Tavian M, Coulombel L, Luton D et al. Aorta-associated CD34+ hematopoietic scells in the early human embryo. *Blood* **87**:67, 1996.
54. Peault B, Tavian M. Hematopoietic stem cell emergence in the human embryo and fetus. *Ann NY Acad Sci* **996**:123–140, 2003.
55. Medvinsky A, Dzierzak E. Definitive hematopoiesis is autonomously initiated by the AGM region. *Cell* **86**:897–906, 1996.
56. Migliaccio G, Migliaccio AR, Petti S et al. Human embryonic hemopoiesis. Kinetics of progenitors and precursors underlying

the yolk sac-liver transition. *J Clin Invest* **78**:51–60, 1986.
57. Wolf BC, Luevano E, Neiman RS. Evidence to suggest that the human fetal spleen is not a hematopoietic organ. *Am J Clin Pathol* **80**:40–44, 1983.
58. Tavassoli M, Minguell JJ. Homing of hemopoietic progenitor cells to the marrow. *Proc Soc Exp Biol Med* **196**:367–373, 1991.
59. Broxmeyer HE, Douglas GW, Hangoc G et al. Human umbilical cord blood as a potential source of transplantable hematopoietic stem/progenitor cells. *Proc Natl Acad Sci USA* **86**:3828–3832, 1989.
60. Gluckman E, Rocha V, Boyer-Chammard A et al. Outcome of cord-blood transplantation from related and unrelated donors. Eurocord Transplant Group and the European Blood and Marrow Transplantation Group. *N Engl J Med* **337**:373–381, 1997.
61. Lansdorp PM. Developmental changes in the function of hematopoietic stem cells. *Exp Hematol* **23**:187, 1995.
62. Taylor PA, McElmurry RT, Lees CJ, Harrison DE, Blazar BR. Allogenic fetal liver cells have a distinct competitive engraftment advantage over adult bone marrow cells when infused into fetal as compared with adult severe combined immunodeficient recipients. *Blood* **99**:1870–1872, 2002.
63. Campagnoli C, Roberts IA, Kumar S, Bennet PR, Bellantuono I, Fisk NM. Identification of mesenchymal/stem/progenitor cells in human first-trimester fetal blood, liver and bone marrow. *Blood* **98**:2396–2402, 2001.
64. Hao QL, Shah AJ, Thiemann FT, Smogorzewska EM, Crooks GM. A functional comparison of CD34 + CD38- cells in cord blood and bone marrow. *Blood* **86**:3745–3753, 1995.
65. Rocha V, Wagner JE, Jr,, Sobocinski KA et al. Graft-versus-host disease in children who have received a cord-blood or bone marrow transplant from an HLA-identical sibling. Eurocord and International Bone Marrow Transplant Registry Working Committee on Alternative Donor and Stem Cell Sources. *N Engl J Med* **342**: 1846–1854, 2000.
66. Gluckman E, Broxmeyer HA, Auerbach AD et al. Hematopoietic reconstitution in a patient with Fanconi's anemia by means of umbilical-cord blood from an HLA-identical sibling. *N Engl J Med* **321**: 1174–1178, 1989.
67. Arai S, Klingemann HG. Hematopoietic stem cell transplantation: bone marrow vs. mobilized peripheral blood. *Arch Med Res* **34**:545–553, 2003.
68. Friedenstein AJ, Piatetzky-Shapiro II, Petrakova KV. Osteogenesis in transplants of bone marrow cells. *J Embryol Exp Morphol* **16**:381–390, 1966.
69. Friedenstein AJ, Petrakova KV, Kurolesova AI, Frolova GP. Heterotopic of bone marrow. Analysis of precursor cells for osteogenic and hematopoietic tissues. *Transplantation* **6**:230–247, 1968.
70. Rydén M, Dicker A, Götherström C et al. Functional characterization of human mesenchymal stem cell-derived adipocytes. *Biochem Biophys Res Comm* **311**:391–397, 2003.
71. Fukada K. Reprogramming of bone marrow mesenchymal stem cells into cardiomyocytes. *CR Biol* **325**:1027–1038, 2002.
72. Prockop DJ. Marrow stromal cells as stem cells for nonhematopoietic tissues. *Science* **276**:71–74, 1997.
73. Pittinger MF, MacKay AM, Beck SC et al. Multilineage potentials of adult human mesenchymal stem cells. *Science* **284**: 1740–1747, 1999.
74. Reyes M, Verfaillie CM. Characterization of multipotent adult progenitor cells, a subpopulation of mesenchymal stem cells. *Ann NY Acad Sci* **938**:231–233, 2001.
75. Kemp CK, Hows J, Donaldson C. Bone marrow-derived mesenchymal stem cells. *Leuk Lymph* **46**:1531–1544, 2005.
76. Kucia M, Reca R, Jala VR et al. Bone marrow as a home of heterogeneous population of nonhematopoietic stem cells. *Leukemia* **199**:1118–1127, 2005.
77. Gronthos S, Zannettino AC, Hay SJ et al. Molecular and cellular characterisation of highly purified stromal stem cells derived from human bone marrow. *J Cell Sci* **116**:1827–1835, 2003.
78. Götherström C, Ringdén O, Tammik C, Zetterberg E, Westgren M, Le Blanc K. Immunologic properties of human fetal mesenchymal stem cells. *Am J Obstet Gynecol* **190**:239–245, 2004.
79. Haynesworth SE, Baber MA, Caplan AI. Cytokine expression by human marrow-derived mesenchymal progenitor cells in vitro: effects of dexamethasone and IL-1 alpha. *J Cell Physiol* **166**:585–592, 1996.
80. Majumdar MK, Thiede MA, Mosca JD, Moorman M, Gerson SL. Phenotypic and functional comparison of cultures of marrow derived mesenchymal stem cells (MSCs) and stromal cells. *J Cell Physiol* **176**:57–66, 1998.
81. Fukuda K. Development of regenerative cardiomyocytes from mesenchymal stem cells for cardiovascular tissue engineering. *Artif Organs* **25**:187–193, 2001.
82. Lagase E, Conners H, Al-Dahalimy M et al. Purified hematopoiietic stem cells can differentiate into hepatocytes in vivo. *Nat Med* **6**:1229–1234, 2000.
83. Jin HK, Carter JE, Huntley GW et al. Intracerebral transplantation of mesenchymal stem cells into acid sphingomyelinase-deficient mice delays the onset of neurological abnormalities and extend their life span. *J Clin Invest* **109**:1183–1191, 2002.
84. Jiang Y, Jahagirdar BN, Reinhardt RL et al. Pluripotency of mesenchymal stem cells derived from adult marrow. *Nature* **418**(6893):41–49, 2002.
85. De Ugarte DA, Morizono K, Elbarbary A et al. Comparison of multi-lineage cells from human adipose tissue and bone marrow. *Cells Tissues Organs* **174**:101–109, 2003.
86. Nakahara H, Dennis JE, Bruder SP, Haynesworth SE, Lennon DP, Caplan AI. In vitro differentiation of bone and hypertrophic cartilage from periosteal-derived cells. *Exp Cell Res* **195**:492–503, 1991.
87. Jiang Y, Vaessen B, Lenvik T, Blackstad M, Reyes M, Verfaillie CM. Multipotent progenitor cells can be isolated from postnatal murine bone marrow, muscle, and brain. *Exp Hematol* **30**:896–904, 2002(b).
88. Nunes MC, Roy NS, Keyoung HM et al. Identification and isolation of multipotential neural progenitor cells from the subcortical white matter of the adult human brain. *Nat Med* **9**:439–447, 2003.
89. Chan RWS, Schwab KE, Gargett CE. Clonogenicity of human endometrial epithelial and stromal cells. *Biol Reprod* **70**:1738–1750, 2004.
90. Schwab KE, Chan RW, Gargett CE. Putative stem cell activity of human endometrial epithelial and stromal cells during the menstrual cycle. *Fertil Steril* **84**(Suppl 2):1124–1130, 2005.
91. Zvaifler NJ, Marinova-Mutafchieva L, Adams G et al. Mesenchymal precursor cells in the blood of normal individuals. *Arthritis Res* **2**:477–488, 2000.
92. Caplan AI. The mesengenic process. *Clin Plast Surg* **21**:429–435, 1994.
93. D'Ippolito G, Schiller PC, Ricordi C, Roos BA, Howard GA. Age-related osteogenic potential of mesenchymal stromal stem cells from human vertebral bone marrow. *J Bone Miner Res* **14**:1115–1122, 1999.
94. Castro-Malaspina H, Gay RE, Resnick G et al. Characterization of human bone marrow fibroblast colony forming cells (CFU-F) and their progeny. *Blood* **56**: 289–301, 1980.
95. Campagnoli C, Fisk NM, Bennet PR, Overton TG, Roberts IAG. Circulating multipotent haematopoietic progenitors in first trimester fetal blood. *Blood* **95**:1967–1972, 2000.
96. Hu Y, Liao L, Wang Q et al. Isolation and identification of mesenchymal stem cells from human fetal pancreas. *J Lab Clin Med* **141**:342–349, 2003.
97. Noort WA, Kruisselbrink AB, in't Anker PS et al. Mesenchymal stem cells promote engraftment of human umbilical cord blood-derived CD34(+) cells in NOD/SCID mice. *Exp Hematol* **30**:870–878, 2002.
98. in't Anker PS, Noort WA, Kruisselbrink AB et al. Nonexpanded primary lung and bone marrow-derived mesenchymal cells promote the engraftment of umbilical cord blood-derived CD34+

cell inNOD/SCID mice. *Exp Hematol* **31**:881–889, 2003.

99. De Coppi P, Bartsch G, Siddiqui MM et al. Isolation of amniotic stem cell lines with potential for therapy. *Nat Biotechnol* **25**:100–106, 2007.
100. Erices A, Conget P, Minguell JJ. Mesenchymal progenitor cells in human umbilical cord blood. *Br J Haematol* **109**:235–242, 2000.
101. Kaviani A, Perry TE, Barnes CM et al. The placenta as a cell source in fetal tissue engineering. *J Pediatr Surg* **37**: 995–999, 2002.
102. in 't Anker PS, Scherjon SA, Keur CK et al. Isolation of mesenchymal stem cells of fetal and maternal origin from human placenta. *Stem Cells* **22**:1338–1345, 2004.
103. Portmann-Lanz CB, Schoeberlein A, Huber A et al. Placental mesenchymal stem cells as potential autologous graft for pre- and perinatal neurogeneration. *Am J Obstet Gynecol* :664–673, 2006.
104. Guillot PV, Götherström C, Chan J, Kurata H, Fisk NM. Human first trimester fetal mesenchymal stem cells (MSC) express pluripotency markers, grow faster, and have longer telomeres compared to adult MSC. *Stem Cells* **25**:646–654, 2007.
105. Yu M, Xiao Z, Shen L, Li L. Mid-trimester fetal blood-derived adherent cells share characteristics similar to mesenchymal stem cells but full-term umbilical cord blood does not. *Br J Haematol* **124**:666–675, 2004.
106. Götherström C, Ringdén O, Westgren M, Tammik C, Le Blanc K. Immunomodulatory effects of human fetal liver-derived mesenchymal stem cells. *Bone Marrow Transplant* **32**:265–272, 2003.
107. Lee OK, Kuo TK, Chen WM, Lee KD, Hsieh SL, Chen TH. Isolation of multipotent mesenchymal stem cells from umbilical cord blood. *Blood* **103**:1669–1675, 2004.
108. Goodwin HS, Bicknese AR, Chien SN, Bogucki BD, Quinn CO, Wall DA. Multilineage differentiation activity by cells isolated from umbilical cord blood: expression of bone, fat, and neural markers. *Biol Blood Marrow Transplant* **7**:581–588, 2001.
109. Yen BL, Huang HI, Chien CC et al. Isolation of multipotent cells from human term placenta. *Stem Cells* **23**:3–9, 2005.
110. Miao Z, Jin J, Chen L et al. Isolation of mesenchymal stem cells from human placenta: comparison with human bone marrow mesenchymal stem cells. *Cell Biol Int* **30**:681–687, 2006.
111. Tsai MS, Lee JL, Chang YJ, Hwang SM. Isolation of human multipotent mesenchymal stem cells from second-trimester amniotic fluid using a novel two-stage culture protocol. *Hum Reprod* **19**:1450–1456, 2004.
112. Mackenzie TC, Flake AW. Human mesenchymal stem cells persist, demonstrate site-specific multipotential differentiation, and are present in sites of wound healing and tissue regeneration after transplantation into fetal sheep. *Blood Cells Mol Dis* **27**:601–604, 2001.
113. Lapidot T, Dar A, Kollet O. How the stem cells find their way home? *Blood* **106**:1901–1910, 2005.
114. Bartholomew A, Sturgeon C, Siatskas M et al. Mesenchymal stem cells suppress lymphocyte proliferation in vitro and prolong skin graft survival in vivo. *Exp Hematol* **30**:42–48, 2002.
115. Di Nicola M, Carlo-Stella C, Magni M et al. Human bone marrow stromal cells suppress T-lymphocyte proliferation induced by cellular or nonspecific mitogenic stimulation. *Blood* **99**:3838–3843, 2002.
116. Le Blanc K, Tammik L, Sundberg B, Haynesworth SE, Ringdén O. Mesenchymal stem cells inhibit and stimulate mixed lymphocyte cultures and mitogenic responses independently of the major histocompatibility complex. *Scand J Immunol* **57**:11–20, 2003.
117. Klyushenenkova E, Mosca JD, Zernetkina V et al. T cell responses to allogeneic human mesenchymal stem cells: immunogenicity, tolerance, and suppression. *J Biomed Sci* **12**:47–57, 2005.
118. Puissant B, Barreau C, Bourin P et al. *Br J Haemtol* **129**:118–129, 2005.
119. Aggarwal S, Pittenger MF. Human mesenchymal stem cells modulate allogeneic immune cell responses. *Blood* **105**:1815–1822, 2005.
120. Beyth S, Borovsky Z, Mevorach D et al. Human mesenchymal stem cells alter antigen-presenting cell maturation and induce T cell unresponsiviness. *Blood* **105**:2214–2219, 2005.
121. Maccario R, Podesta M, Moretta A et al. Interaction of human mesenchymal stem cells with cells involved in alloantigen-specific immune response favors the differentiation of $CD4^+$ T-cell subsets expressing a regulatory/suppressive phenotype. *Haematologica* **90**:516–525, 2005.
122. Meissel R, Zibert A, Laryea M, Gobel U, Daubener W, Dilloo D. Human bone marrow stromal cells inhibit allogeneic T-cell responses by indoleamine 2,3-dioxygenase-mediated tryptophan degradation. *Blood* **103**:4619–4621, 2004.
123. Tse WT, Pendleton JD, Beyer WM, Egalka MC, Guinan EC. Suppression of allogeneic T-cell proliferation by human marrow stromal cells: implications in transplantation. *Transplantation* **75**: 389–397, 2003.
124. Le Blanc K, Rasmusson I, Sundberg B et al. Treatment of severe acute graft-versus-host disease with third party haploidentical mesenchymal stem cells. *Lancet* **363**:1439–1441, 2004.
125. Horwitz EM, Gordon PL, Koo WK. Isolated allogenic bone marrow-derived mesenchymal cells engraft and stimulate growth in children with osteogenesis imperfecta: implications for cell therapy of bone. *Proc Natl Acad Sci USA* **99**:8932–8937, 2002.
126. Almeida-Porada G, Flake AW, Glimp HA, Zanjani ED. Cotransplantation of stroma results in enhancement of engraftment and early expression of donor hematoipoeitic stem cells in utero. *Exp Hematol* **27**:1569–1575, 1999.
127. Almeida-Porada G, Porado C, Tran N, Zanjani ED. Contransplantation of human stromal cell progenitors into preimmune fetal sheep results in early appearance of human donor cells in circulation and boosts cell levels in bone marrow at later points after transplantation. *Blood* **95**:3620–3627, 2000.
128. in't Anker PS, Scherjon SA, Klijburg- van de Keur C et al. Amniotic fluid as a novel source of mesenchymal stem cells for therapeutic transplantations. *Blood* **102**:1548–1549, 2003.
129. Koç ON, Gerson SL, Cooper BW et al. Rapid hematopoietic recovery after coinfusion of autologous-blood stem cells and culture-expanded marrow mesenchymnal stem cells in advanced breast cancer patients receiving high-dose chemotherapy. *J Clin Oncol* **18**: 307–316, 2000.
130. Benvenuto F, Ferrari S, Gerdoni E et al. Human mesenchymal stem cells promote survival of T cells in a quiescent state. *Stem Cells* **25**:753–1760, 2007.
131. Wu GD, Nolta JA, Jin YS et al. Migration of mesenchymal stem cells to heart allografts during chronic rejection. *Transplantation* **75**:679–685, 2003.
132. Makino S, Fukuda K, Miyoshi S et al. Cardiomyocytes can be generated from marrow stromal cells in vitro. *J Clin Invest* **103**:697–705, 1999.
133. Toma C, Pittenger MF, Cahill KS, Byrne BJ, Kessler PD. Human mesenchymal stem cells differentiate to a cardiomyocyte phenotype in the adult murine heart. *Circulation* **105**:93–98, 2002.
134. Kang H-J, Kho SH, Jang MK, Lee SH, Shin HY, Ahn HS. Early engraftment kinetics of two units cord blood transplantation. *Bone Marrow Transplant* **38**:197–201, 2006.
135. Young RG, Butler DL, Weber W, Caplan AI, Gordon SL, Fink DJ. Use of mesenchymal stem cells in a collagen matrix for Achilles tendon repair. *J Orthop Res* **16**:406–413, 1998.
136. Wakitani S, Yamamoto T. Response of the donor and recipient cells in mesenchymal cell transplantation to cartilage defect. *Microsc Res Tech* **58**:4–18, 2002.

137. Bilic G, Ochsenbein-Kölble N, Hall H, Huch R, Zimmerman R. In vitro lesion repair by human amnion epithelial and mesenchymal cells. *Am J Obstet Gynecol* **190**:87–92, 2004.
138. Vellodi A. Lysosomal storage disorders. *Br J Haematol* **128**:413–431, 2004.
139. Conway J, Dyack S, Crooks BN, Fernandez CV. Mixed donor chimerism and low level iduronidase expression may be adequate for neurodevelopmental protection in Hurler Syndrome. *J Pediatr* **147**:106–108, 2005.
140. Escolar ML, Poe MD, Provenzale JM et al. Transplantation of umbilical-cord blood in babies with infantile Krabbe's disease. *N Engl J Med* **352**:2069–2081, 2005.
141. Muench MO, Rae J, Bárcena A et al. Transplantation of a fetus with paternal Thy-1^+ $CD34^+$ cells for chronic granulomatous disease. *Bone Marrow Transplant* **27**:355–364, 2001.
142. Peranteau WH, Endo M, Adibe OO, Flake AW. Evidence for an immune barier after in utero hematopoietic cell transplantation. *Blood* **109**:1331–1333, 2007.
143. Blakemore K, Moser HW, Corson VL et al. An update on in utero bone marrow transplantation for Krabbe disease. *J Mol Neurosci* **13**:238–239, 1999.
144. Horwitz EM, Prockop DJ, Fitzpatrick LA et al. Transplantability and therapeutic effects of bone marrow-derived mesenchymal cells in children with osteogenesis imperfecta. *Nat Med* **5**: 309–313, 1999.
145. Kang HJ, Kim HS, Zhang SY et al. Effects of intracoronary infusion of peripheral blood stem-cells mobilised with granulocyte-colony stimulating factor on left ventricular systolic function and restenosis after coronary stenting in myocardial infarction: the MAGIC cell randomised clinical trial. *Lancet* **363**: 751–756, 2004.
146. Lee PW, Cina RA, Randolph MA et al. Stable multilineage chimerism across full MHC bariers without graft-versus-host-disaese following in utero bone marrow transplantation in pigs. *Exp Hematol* **33**:371–379, 2005.
147. Phinney DG, Kopen G, Righter W, Webster S, Tremain N, Prockop DJ. Donor variation in the growth properties and osteogenic potential of human marrow stromal cells. *J Cell Biochem* **75**:424–436, 1999.
148. Shaaban AF, Kim HB, Milner R, Flake AW. A kinetic model for the homing and migration of prenatally transplanted marrow. *Blood* **94**:3251–3257, 1999.

CHAPTER 48

Fetal gene therapy

Anna David and Charles H Rodeck

KEY POINTS

- This chapter discusses why gene therapy in the fetus may be advantageous for treatment or prevention of certain congenital diseases
- Studies of gene therapy in fetal animal models of congenital disease show that long-term therapeutic gene expression at sufficiently high levels can be achieved to provide phenotypic cure and fetal tolerance to the product of the introduced gene develops
- Minimally invasive ultrasound-guided injection techniques can be used to target gene therapy to fetal organs
- Observed risks of fetal gene therapy include insertional mutagenesis, vector toxicity, fetal immune response, maternal and fetal morbidity and mortality; theoretical risks such as germline gene transfer and aberrant fetal development have not yet been seen in preclinical studies
- Currently fetal gene therapy remains at the experimental stage

INTRODUCTION

Gene therapy burst onto the scene in the 1980s and the first human gene therapy trials began over 10 years ago[1]. But, in spite of continuous technological progress, most clinical results have been disappointing. The reasons are many and include difficulty targeting the appropriate organ, a robust immune response to the therapy in adults and low level expression of the therapeutic gene product. Many of these difficulties may be avoidable by applying the therapy to the fetus and recent preclinical work has shown proof-of-principle for phenotypic cure of congenital disease in animal models using fetal gene therapy. This chapter examines the evidence for fetal gene therapy and discusses how it might work in clinical practice.

WHAT IS GENE THERAPY?

Gene therapy delivers genetic material to the cell to generate a therapeutic effect by correcting an existing abnormality or providing cells with a new function. To do this, a vector is used to deliver the genes into the appropriate cell. Genes may be inserted into somatic cells or into germ cells. Somatic gene therapy treats an individual patient by insertion of genes into cells that are either outside the body (ex vivo), for example hematopoietic stem cells (HSCs) grown in culture, or in vivo by, for example intramuscular injection; pluripotential stem cells or differentiated cells may be targeted. Germline gene therapy would target oocytes or spermatocytes and might have the potential to eradicate inherited diseases in future generations. It is, however, currently neither scientifically nor medically justifiable, technically unsafe and unpredictable and is therefore considered to be ethically unacceptable[2].

IS THERE A NEED FOR FETAL GENE THERAPY?

Congenital disease places a huge burden on the community and the health service. A study of pediatric inpatient admissions in 1996 in a USA children's hospital found that wholly genetic conditions accounted for one-third of hospital admissions and for 50% of the total hospital charges for that year[3]. Thus a preventative strategy, such as fetal gene therapy, could have an important social and economic impact.

A criticism leveled at fetal gene therapy is that gene transfer to an individual after birth may be as effective and probably safer than prenatal treatment. Indeed, current conventional treatment of some genetic disease, for example, dietary restriction in phenylketonuria, is highly effective. For many genetic diseases, however, treatment is palliative rather than curative, resulting in patients living longer but with a reduced quality of life. This has been particularly seen in cystic fibrosis, in which life expectancy has risen from school age in 1955 to the mid-thirties today (Cystic Fibrosis Foundation). To achieve this, however, patients require daily chest physiotherapy, antibiotic treatment, dietary supplementation, insulin for diabetes mellitus and, in many cases, lung transplants which require immunosuppressive therapy in addition. Effective treatment in utero could cure genetic disease, or at least provide partial correction that may have a huge impact on disease progression.

What are the advantages of fetal application?

1. Fetal gene therapy may offer particular benefits in certain early onset genetic disorders in which irreversible pathological damage to organs occurs before or shortly after birth[4]. For many such diseases, the organ may be difficult to target after birth, for example the lung in cystic fibrosis, the brain in urea cycle disorders, or the skin in epidermolysis bullosa, and fetal treatment may take advantage of developmental changes to access organs that are inaccessible after birth.
2. Gene transfer to the developing fetus targets rapidly expanding stem cell populations providing a large population of transduced cells to provide a therapeutic effect. For example, after intravascular administration of lentivirus vectors to fetal mice, expression of a marker gene appeared to be distributed in the liver in focal clusters, suggesting they may have arisen from individual progenitors[5,6].
3. The fetus has a size advantage in a number of ways. Delivery of equivalent or even higher doses per kg body mass of factor IX (FIX) adenovirus vectors to dogs and mice resulted in a reduced circulating concentration of FIX clotting factor in the larger animal, making it difficult to scale vector doses from small to large species based on body mass alone[7]. Production of clinical grade vector is time-consuming and expensive and the small size of the fetus could lead to increased vector biodistribution at the same vector dose as an adult.
4. The fetus has a functionally immature immune system compared to an adult which may be to its advantage. World-wide up to 50% of adults have pre-existing humoral immunity to adenovirus and adeno-associated virus serotypes from which commonly used gene therapy vectors are derived[8]. Even in the absence of a pre-existing immune sensitivity, vector administration to adults often results in the development of an immune response that reduces the duration and level of transgene expression. For example, after intramuscular injection of adenovirus vector containing the dystrophin gene into adult Duchenne muscular dystrophy transgenic mice, antibodies to the dystrophin protein were detected[9]. This complication is particularly important when gene therapy is aiming to correct a genetic disease in which complete absence of a gene product is observed.

Immune tolerance to exogenous protein can be induced in the fetus if the protein is introduced before the immune system is competent. Tolerance also requires that the exogenous protein expression is maintained, albeit at low level, and so the ability of the vector to give long-term expression is vital. In newborn mice that are more susceptible to immune tolerization than human neonates, administration of adenovirus vectors achieved long-term correction of type VII mucopolysaccharidosis[10], whereas use of this vector to correct genetic disease in adult mice gives only temporary expression of the transgene in most cases[11]. In a mouse animal model of hemophilia B, one study showed that the functionally immature fetal immune system does not respond to the product of the introduced gene (see later) and, therefore, immune tolerance can be induced[12]. There was a similar finding after intraperitoneal injection of retrovirus vector into first-trimester fetal sheep, when a blunted humoral response and reduced in vitro lymphocyte proliferation was observed after immune challenge with β-galactosidase protein postnatally[13]. This means that treatment could be repeated after birth, if a single fetal treatment was not sufficient to cure the individual of the disease.

WHICH DISEASES COULD FETAL GENE THERAPY BE USED FOR?

Fetal gene therapy has been proposed to be appropriate for life-threatening disorders, in which prenatal gene delivery maintains a clear advantage over cell transplantation or postnatal gene therapy and for which there are currently no satisfactory treatments available[14]. Some of the diseases that may be suitable for fetal treatment are listed in Table 48.1. Preclinical studies are encouraging. Fetal application of gene therapy in mouse models of congenital disease such as hemophilia A[15] and B[12], congenital blindness[16], Crigler-Najjar type 1 syndrome[17] and Pompe disease (glycogen storage disease type II)[18] have shown phenotypic correction of the condition. Progress in the treatment of one condition, hemophilia B, is discussed in detail here to illustrate recent progress.

Deficiency in factor VIII (FVIII) and FIX proteins of the blood coagulation cascade result in hemophilias A and B, respectively, and have a combined incidence of around 1 in 8000 people[19]. Current treatment uses replacement therapy with human FVIII or FIX which is expensive but effective. Beneficial effects occur after achieving only 1% of the normal levels of clotting factor. Unfortunately, a proportion of patients develop antibodies to therapy leading to ineffective treatment and occasional anaphylaxis[20]. Indeed, the complications of hemophilia treatment, which include the major risk of HIV and hepatitis B infections, have, in some cases, been far worse than the diseases themselves, increasing their morbidity and mortality[21]. The clotting proteins are required in the blood and can be secreted functionally from a variety of tissues, thus the actual site of production is not so important as long as therapeutic plasma levels are realized.

Adult gene therapy strategies have concentrated on application to the muscle or the liver, achieving sustained FIX expression in adult hemophiliac dogs or mice after intramuscular or intravascular injection of adeno-associated virus[22–24]. In clinical trials using adeno-associated virus in hemophilia B patients, only short-term and low-level FIX expression has so far been observed, however, which was due to a cell-mediated immune response to transduced hepatocytes[25,26].

In contrast, intravenous injection into fetal hemophiliac mice of an HIV-lentivirus human FIX vector resulted in permanent partial phenotypic correction[12]. Hemophilic mice expressed a mean human FIX plasma concentration of 12% of the normal human level for the duration of the study (up to 14 months). This was one of the first studies to prove the principle that fetal gene therapy could correct the phenotype and effectively cure a congenital disease.

Treatment of genetic disease is a lifelong challenge. Short-term obstetric problems, such as prematurity, prevention of white matter brain injury and, above all, fetal growth restriction,

Table 48.1 **Examples of candidate diseases for fetal gene therapy**

Disease	*Therapeutic gene product*	*Target cells/organ*	*Age at onset*	*Incidence*	*Life expectancy*
Cystic fibrosis (CF)	CF transmembrane conductance regulator	Airway and intestinal epithelial cells	Third trimester of pregnancy	1:4000	Mid-thirties
Duchenne muscular dystrophy	Dystrophin	Myocytes	2 years	1:4500	25 years
Spinal muscular atrophy	Survival motor neuron protein	Motor neurons	6 months (type 1)	1:10 000	2 years
Hemophilia	Human factor VIII or IX clotting factors	Hepatocytes	1 year	1:6000	Adulthood with treatment
β-thalassemia	Globin	Erythrocyte precursors	<1 year	1:2700	<20 years in developing countries
Lysosomal storage disease, e.g. Gaucher	Glucocerebrosidase	Hepatocytes	9.5 years	1:9000 overall 1:59 000	<2 years
Urea cycle defects, e.g. ornithine carbamylase deficiency	Ornithine transcarbamylase	Hepatocytes	2 days	1:30 000 overall 1:105 000	2 days (severe neonatal onset)
Severe combined immunodeficiency	γc cytokine receptor (X-linked SCID)	Hematopoietic precursor cells	Birth	1:1 000 000	<6 months if no bone marrow transplant
Epidermolysis bullosa e.g. dystrophica	Type VII collagen	Keratinocytes	Birth	1:40 000	Adulthood
Hypoxic ischemic encephalopathy	Neurotrophic factors	Cortical neurons	Birth	1:1000	Adulthood
Severe intrauterine growth restriction	Placental growth factors	Trophoblast	Fetus	1:500	Days

may be amenable to gene therapy approaches. Impaired utero-placental perfusion is believed to be an underlying problem in fetal growth restriction (FGR). We have recently shown that injection of adenovirus vectors containing the VEGF-A gene into the uterine artery of mid-gestation fetal sheep increases uterine artery blood flow and causes relaxation of the uterine arteries (see below). Further work is needed to study how long the effect on uterine artery blood flow lasts, but it is likely that even short-term increases for a few weeks may be sufficient to improve the morbidity and mortality associated with severe fetal growth restriction[27].

HOW MIGHT FETAL GENE THERAPY BE APPLIED?

The vectors

Vectors are agents that are used to carry the therapeutic gene into the cell so that it can have its effect. The development of efficient vector systems is crucial for the success of gene therapy in the adult and fetus. The ideal vector for fetal gene therapy of congenital disease would introduce a transcriptionally regulated gene into all organs relevant to the genetic disorder by a single safe application that would achieve efficient and durable gene expression. Although none of the current vector systems meet all these criteria, many have characteristics that are beneficial to the fetal approach.

Non-viral vectors are an attractive option in fetal gene therapy because of their perceived better safety profile and their ability to transfer very large fragments of genetic material. Some fetal studies have shown encouraging results. Intrahepatic injection of the cationic polymer polyethylenimine (PEI) in late gestation fetal mice enhanced gene transfer to the liver as compared with administration of naked DNA. Encouragingly, the marker gene expression was 40-fold higher marker per milligram of protein in fetuses compared with adults[28]. Gene transfer to the fetal sheep airway epithelium was also achieved using guanidium-cholesterol cationic liposomes delivered into the trachea in mid-gestation fetal sheep[29]. Unfortunately, current non-viral systems are hindered by their low transfection efficiency and short expression time. Manipulation of non-viral vector particles can overcome some of their problems. For example, altering the chemical structure of carbon bonds within cationic liposome-DNA complexes improves their transfection efficiency and reduces their toxicity in vivo[30]. Other developments include artificial chromosomes and Epstein-Barr virus-based plasmids.

DNA introduced as plasmid molecules remains episomal and will be lost with cell division which is rapid in the fetus and could be a particular disadvantage. Transient gene transfer may be useful in the management of a developmental condition where therapy is only required for a relatively short time. For instance, short-term transgene expression via injection of a liposome that inhibited fibronectin synthesis into the ductus arteriosis of mid-trimester fetal sheep, maintained a patent ductus arteriosus prior to surgery for congenital heart defects in neonatal sheep[31].

Adenovirus vectors are attractive vectors for proof-of-principle studies in fetal gene therapy since they achieve highly efficient gene transfer in a wide range of fetal tissues depending on the route of administration[32]. Although they do not specifically have a tropism for the liver, these vectors strongly infect liver tissue after intravenous delivery[33]. Gene expression is usually transient[15] as the vector does not integrate into the host genome and is rapidly diluted by the active cellular proliferation taking place in the fetus. Although the vector is highly immunogenic in adults, fetal administration can produce extended gene expression and induction of immune tolerance to the transgene[33] and, in some cases, also to the vector[34], although immune responses to adenovirus are reported after fetal application[35] even in early gestation[32]. To reduce the immunogenicity and toxicity of the vector, all adenoviral coding sequences can be eliminated to generate so called 'gutless vectors'[36,37]. Novel hybrid vectors that take advantage of adenovirus infectivity and the permanent nature of integrative vectors such as retroviruses and lentiviruses may also prove useful in the fetus[38,39].

Adeno-associated virus vectors (AAV) are considered to be less toxic and immunogenic than early generation adenovirus vectors, although an immune response to transgenic protein has been observed after fetal intramuscular injection of AAV[40]. Long-term transgene expression can be achieved after muscular, peritoneal or amniotic injection into the fetal mouse[41–43] and rat[44]. AAV vectors integrate into the genome at only low frequency and therefore they are likely to be diluted rapidly by the increasing tissue mass that occurs in the fetus. Integration of the wild-type virus is predominantly at a specific functionally unimportant location on human chromosome 19 reducing the theoretical risk of insertional mutagenesis. However, certain recombinant vectors integrate preferentially into active genes in mice and may induce chromosomal deletions of up to 2 kb which could have an impact on fetal development[45]. Both wild-type adenovirus and AAV infection have been associated with miscarriage and perinatal morbidity and this will need further investigation before in utero application can be considered in the human[46,47].

Retroviruses and the closely related *lentiviruses* are able to integrate permanently into the genome thus offering the possibility of permanent gene delivery. Moloney leukemia retrovirus (MLV) was the first vector to be applied fetally to investigate the dispersion of neuronal clones across the developing cerebral cortex of fetal mice[48]. Since then, MLV has been used in a number of fetal studies of gene therapy, giving long-term expression in rats[49], sheep[50] and non-human primates[51] after intraperitoneal and intrahepatic delivery. Retroviruses require dividing cells for gene transfer[52] which suggests that they may be better suited for use in fetal, rather than adult tissues, where cells are rapidly dividing. Human serum can almost completely inactivate some retroviral particles[53] which limits their use in vivo, although increased resistance to serum inactivation can be achieved by generating retroviruses from particular human packaging cells[39] or by pseudotyping, which replaces the natural envelope of the retrovirus with an envelope from another virus[54]. A particular problem with in utero application is that amniotic fluid has a mild inhibitory effect on retrovirus infection in vitro[55]. This was probably responsible for the poor gene transfer observed after intra-amniotic application of retroviruses in fetal sheep[56] and non-human primates[57].

Lentiviruses, such as those based on HIV, can also infect non-dividing cells[58], although gene transfer to the liver is improved by cell cycling in some lentiviruses[59]. Pseudotyping improves lentivirus stability and allows vector titers to be improved by ultracentrifugation. Different viral envelopes allow gene transfer to be targeted to specific tissues, for example intramuscular and intrahepatic injection into fetal mice of an HIV vector pseudotyped with vesicular stomatitis virus protein G (VSVG) envelope preferentially transduced the fetal liver, whereas pseudotyping with Mokola or Ebola envelope proteins gave most efficient transduction of the myocytes[6]. Lentivirus vectors integrate into the genome randomly and are therefore theoretically able to cause insertional mutagenesis (see later).

Route and time of application of fetal gene therapy

Developments in vector technology must be accompanied by improvements in minimally invasive methods of delivering vectors to the fetus if fetal gene therapy is to be clinically applicable. Traditionally, invasive surgical techniques such as maternal laparotomy or hysterotomy have been performed to access the fetus in small and even large animal models. It is likely that non-human primates will be the ultimate animal model that will have to be used for safety studies in immediate preparation for a clinical trial of fetal gene therapy. However, their high maintenance costs, difficult breeding conditions and ethical concerns have encouraged investigation of fetal gene therapy in the sheep, which is a well-established animal model of human fetal physiology. Using the pregnant sheep, ultrasound-guided injection techniques from fetal medicine practice have been adapted and new methods developed to deliver gene therapy to specific organs in the fetal sheep (Table 48.2). For example, ultrasound-guided delivery of adenovirus vectors into the fetal sheep trachea results in gene expression in the fetal airways and, into the fetal sheep stomach, targets gene expression to the fetal small bowel[60,61] (Figs 48.1 and 48.2). Maternal mortality in the pregnant sheep is negligible and fetal mortality was between 3 and 15% depending on the route of injection. Over 90% of the fetal mortality was due to iatrogenic infection, usually with known fleece commensals. Invasive procedures, such as tracheal injection, had a complication rate of 6% related to blood vessel damage within the thorax[62]. Intracardiac and umbilical vein injection had an unacceptably high procedure-related fetal mortality in first-trimester fetal sheep[32] and umbilical vein injection was only reliably achieved from 70 days of gestation, equivalent to 20 weeks of gestation in humans[63]. More recently, ultrasound guidance has been used in non-human primates to deliver gene therapy into the amniotic cavity or for direct injection of the lung and liver parenchyma by teams in the USA[51,64,65]. The relevant time windows for the different application routes in man still need to be

Table 48.2 **Application routes for gene delivery to different fetal organs using ultrasound-guided injection of the sheep fetus**

Route of application	*Gestational age of application*		*Target organ (s)*
	Sheep fetus (D: days)	*Equiv. gestational age in human fetus (weeks)*	
Intra-amniotic	From D33 onwards[32]	From W10 onwards	Skin, fetal membranes
Intraperitoneal	From D50 onwards[32]	From W14 onwards[93,94]	Peritoneum, liver, diaphragm
Intrahepatic	From D50 onwards[32]	From W14 onwards	Liver
Intramuscular	From D50 onwards[32]	From W14 onwards	Muscle
Umbilical vein	From D70 onwards[32,63,95]	From W20 onwards[96]	Systemic delivery (predominantly liver, adrenal gland)
Intrapleural	From D60 onwards[97]	From W16 onwards	Intercostal and diaphragm muscles
Intracardiac	From D100 onwards[98]	From W20 onwards[99]	Systemic delivery (predominantly liver, adrenal gland)[100]
Intratracheal	From D80–115[60,62,101]	From W22–32	Airways
Intragastric	From D60 onwards[61]	From W16 onwards	Stomach, small and large bowel, liver
Cerebral ventricles	From D55–65[63]	W15–17	Choroid plexus, lateral ventricle and neurocortex

The equivalent gestational ages in the human fetus are illustrated based on human studies or current fetal medicine practice, or by extrapolation from experiments in the sheep fetus. The sheep gestation period is 145 days

established with respect to technical feasibility, fetal physiology and the development of the fetal immune system. In the human fetus, the immune system develops from 12 to 14 weeks of gestation when profound increases in circulating T lymphocytes can be observed[66]. Thus, it may be necessary to deliver gene therapy before this gestational age, which will limit the routes of application that can be safely used.

Stem cell gene therapy

Stem cell fetal gene therapy uses in utero transplantation of gene corrected stem cells to treat a congenital defect. After isolation and culture of the stem cells, gene transfer would be achieved in vitro using gene therapy vectors. The advantage of such a system is that only the stem cells would be targeted, avoiding transduction of the fetal germline or other tissues, and the maternal tissues. It would also permit assessment of the efficiency and safety of gene transfer to the stem cells prior to transplantation.

There are a number of drawbacks, however, with this type of fetal therapy. The type of stem cell used needs to be tailored to the congenital disease to be treated and isolation and culture of some stem cell types in sufficient numbers, for example neurons, may be difficult. Although stem cells have a large proliferative capacity, in vitro culture and expansion of cell numbers can induce differentiation that depletes the number of long-term repopulating stem cells. In vitro transduction with integrating vectors such as retrovirus requires cycling cells, and transferring quiescent stem cells into the cycling stage with growth factors, for example, may also induce differentiation[67].

The success of fetal stem cell therapy depends critically on the ability to transfer genes into stem cells in vitro. Gene transfer into murine HSCs can be achieved with high efficiency using retroviral vectors[68]. Studies show retroviral gene transfer into large animal[69] and human HSCs[70] is less successful, although transduction of fetal HSCs is more efficient than that of adult cells[71]. Improved gene transfer can be achieved by using retroviral vectors pseudotyped with different envelopes, for example the RD114 envelope from the feline endogenous virus[72] and long-term efficient transduction of CD34+ human HSCs can be attained with lentiviral vectors[73].

Mesenchymal stem cells (MSCs) are becoming increasingly more important for transplantation therapy. Circulating fetal MSCs are present from the first trimester and can be efficiently transduced with retroviral vectors[74]. Fetal MSCs have also been isolated from second-trimester amniotic fluid taken at amniocentesis for prenatal diagnosis and these may provide an excellent source of cells for intrauterine fetal tissue engineering[75].

WHAT ARE THE RISKS OF FETAL GENE THERAPY?

There are various safety issues in relation to in utero gene therapy that need to be addressed before such therapy could be applied clinically[76,77]. There is a theoretical risk that the therapeutic gene product or vector that is required later in life to correct a genetic disease, could interfere with normal fetal development. This has been suggested in the case of cystic fibrosis, where in utero infection of rats at 16–17 days' gestation with a recombinant adenovirus carrying the human cystic

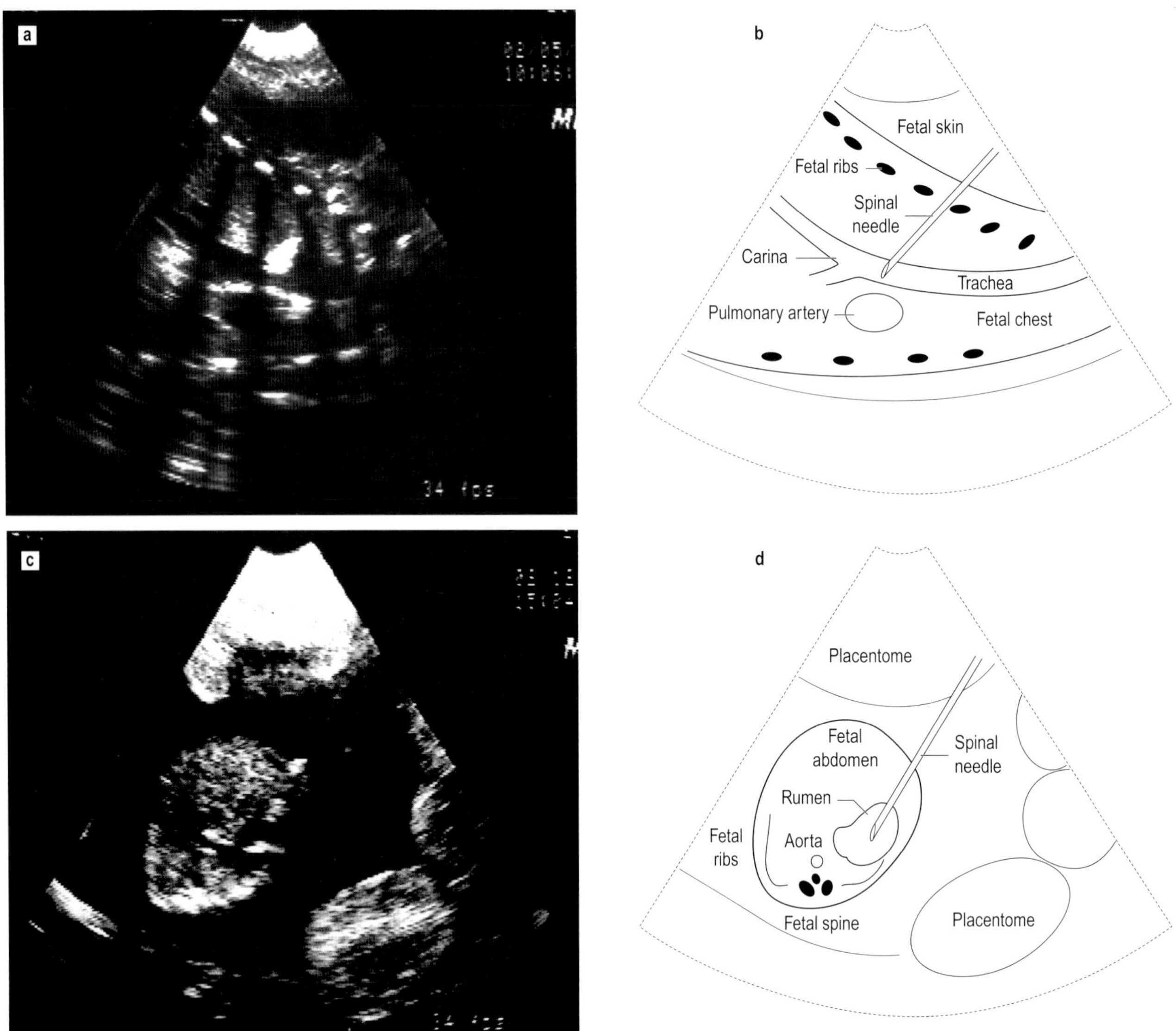

Fig. 48.1 Ultrasound-guided delivery of gene therapy to the fetal sheep trachea and stomach. (a) Ultrasonogram and (b) diagram of sheep fetus at 114 days of gestation in longitudinal section. A 20-gauge spinal needle is inserted into the fetal thorax between the 3rd and 4th rib, penetrates the lung parenchyma and enters the fetal trachea just proximal to the carina. (c) Ultrasonogram and (d) diagram of sheep fetus at 61 days of gestation in transverse section. A 22-gauge spinal needle is inserted into the fetal stomach.

fibrosis transmembrane receptor gene, resulted in altered lung development and morphology[78]. The effects of a transgenic protein on developmental processes will be difficult to predict, depending on the time of gestation and the type of protein introduced, which will require careful long-term monitoring. An established risk factor of integrating viral vectors is insertional mutagenesis. This was recently seen after gene therapy in very young children after transplantation of hematopoietic stem cells that had been transduced ex vivo with a retroviral vector for X-linked severe combined immunodeficiency[79]. Analysis of the lymphocytes showed that the transgene had been inserted adjacent to a potential oncogene, LMO2, the product of which has been implicated in the pathogenesis of leukemias[80]. As well as being related to the type of vector used, the outcome of insertional mutagenesis induced by gene vectors may be influenced by the intrinsic properties of the target cell, and extrinsic factors such as the fetal environment and disease-specific factors influencing clonal competition in vivo.[81] The fetal system may be particularly sensitive to such events since integrating vectors prefer to insert their genomes into chromatin in open configuration. A very high postnatal incidence of liver tumors of prenatally treated mice was observed after application of an early form of third-generation equine infectious anemia virus (EIAV) vectors but not when using a similar vector with an HIV backbone[82]. It is not clear whether insertional mutagenesis has caused this phenomenon, but the observation suggests that the fetus may be particularly sensitive to adverse effects associated with this vector system. Further work is needed to address this issue and to devise strategies to determine and possibly direct integration sites.

While one of the aims of prenatal gene therapy is to achieve immune tolerance to the transgene and delivery system, vectors must be designed to be sufficiently different to the wild type so that the immune system remains able to mount an effective immune response against wildtype virus infection. Germline transmission is another potential concern. Fetal somatic gene

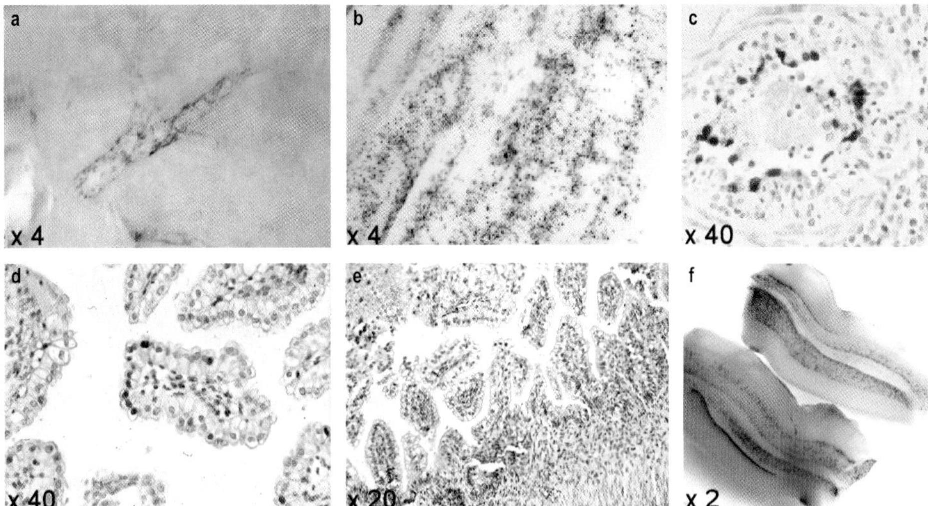

Fig. 48.2 Expression of transgenic lacZ in the fetal sheep airways and gut after application of gene therapy to the fetus. Positive X gal histochemistry (blue cells, a and f) and positive β-galactosidase immunohistochemistry (brown stained nuclei, b–e) of fetal tissues is shown. Fetuses were sampled 2 days after ultrasound-guided injection of an adenovirus vector containing the lacZ gene. (a–c) Positive lacZ expression is seen in the medium sized airways and in the trachea (b) after delivery of the vector into the mid-gestation fetal trachea. (d–f) Positive lacZ expression is seen in the small bowel (d), rectum (e) and (f) stomach after delivery to the early-gestation fetal stomach.

therapy does not aim to modify the genetic content of the germline but inadvertent gene transfer to the germline could occur and prenatal vector administration could carry a higher risk of inadvertent gene delivery to germ cells[83]. In the fetus, compartmentalization of the primordial germ cells in the gonads is complete by 7 weeks of gestation in humans and it is unlikely therefore that any therapy applied after this time would result in germline gene transfer. The chances of germline transduction occurring in the mother are also low, because there is a blood-follicle barrier present in the ovary and the eggs are held in meiotic metaphase arrest until fertilization. Examination of germ cells after delivery of retroviral vectors[50,84] or adenoviral vectors[32] to early gestation fetal sheep, and after intraperitoneal delivery of AAV to fetal mice[43,85], has not shown any detectable transmission. Results from evaluation of maternal tissues in studies of large animals after fetal gene therapy are reassuring and suggest no germline gene transfer to the mother[32,51,64].

Many of these issues are not confined to fetal or even adult gene therapy and concerns regarding germline transmission can be raised in particular for chemotherapy and infertility treatment[86]. Tissue-specific vector targeting is an important and potentially safer strategy that may target vectors to specific tissues[54].

Fetal gene therapy would give a third option to parents following prenatal diagnosis of inherited disease, where currently the only choices are termination of pregnancy or acceptance of an affected child. Many parents when faced with a baby with a genetic disease decide to terminate the pregnancy in a procedure that is very safe for the mother and totally effective. A prenatal gene therapy strategy will have to be extremely safe, reliable and effective at treating the disease[87].

Any fetal therapy or procedure poses risks of infection, immune reactions and the induction of preterm labor for the fetus and the potential to harm the mother. A conflict of interest might potentially arise since treating the fetus may not be in the mother's best interest but, in UK law, a fetus has no rights per se. Currently used fetal treatments, such as fetal blood transfusion for anemia, are effective and carry a low risk for the mother such that the risk-benefit analysis falls heavily on the side of treatment. For experimental fetal procedures, the risk-benefit analysis is uncertain and it is therefore especially important that the mother gives informed consent[88]. This can be difficult since the decision to participate in a fetal gene therapy trial will occur close to the time of prenatal diagnosis of the condition. The professionals involved in counseling the parents must present the information in a non-biased way and ensure that resources are set aside for long-term surveillance of the mother and fetus after birth. The parents must also consider that fetal treatment in this pregnancy may pose risks for a future pregnancy by potentially affecting the mother's health.

For parents who would not have continued with an affected pregnancy, a partial cure of an affected child resulting in a poor quality of life would be the worst case scenario, and we must not forget the first rule of medicine to 'do no harm'. Testing the fetus after gene therapy treatment to evaluate its effectiveness is an option. This presents a risk to the pregnancy but allows termination of pregnancy if no effective gene expression can be detected. Such a strategy was used in a case report of in utero stem cell transplanation for X-linked SCID, in which a couple requested evaluation of stem cell engraftment following transplantation[89]. Following intraperitoneal injection of fetal liver cells at 14 weeks of gestation, analysis of fetal blood at 24 and 33 weeks of gestation showed 10% and 50% chimerism confirming engraftment and the parents continued with the pregnancy.

HOW MIGHT FETAL GENE THERAPY WORK?

Assuming that a safe and effective fetal gene therapy approach was to be possible, how might it work in practice? Figure 48.3 shows a possible scheme for a hypothetical syndrome X, an autosomal recessive condition which results in severe morbidity. Without an effective screening strategy with accurate prenatal diagnosis for syndrome X, many families would not know

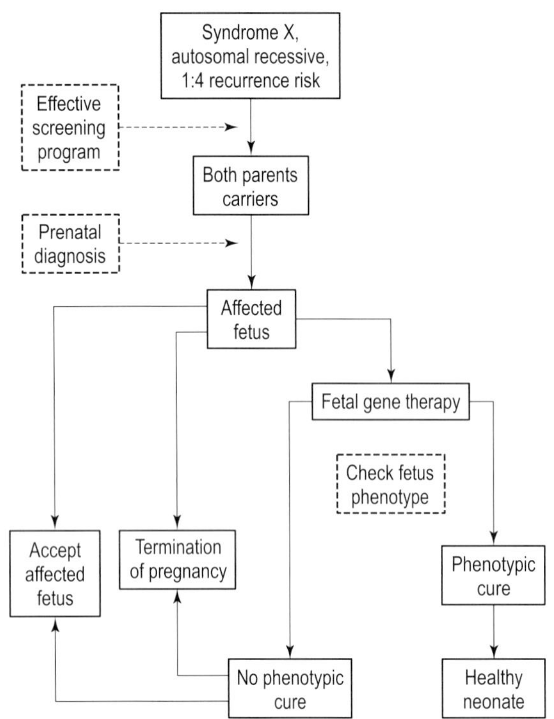

Fig. 48.3 How fetal gene therapy might work in practice: treatment of a hypothetical syndrome X, an autosomal recessive condition that results in severe morbidity.

that they were at risk until an affected child was born. For the next pregnancy, the parents could choose to have prenatal diagnosis of syndrome X in the fetus prior to the gestational age for optimum gene therapy treatment, by non-invasive prenatal diagnosis using cell free fetal DNA if available, or by chorionic villus sampling. The mother would undergo the invasive procedure to treat the fetus at the best time to target the affected organ. The option of further invasive testing to confirm expression of the curative gene product later in the pregnancy could be available. An alternative strategy is preimplantation genetic diagnosis (PGD) which is often proposed as the most sensible option for parents at risk of having an affected fetus. The main limitations of in vitro fertilzation (IVF) and PGD are the ovulation induction and invasive procedures that the woman is required to have, that only 20–30% of couples achieve a pregnancy per cycle[90] and that some embryos will be disposed of, which, for some individuals, is of concern[91].

CHALLENGES FOR THE FUTURE

Application of fetal gene therapy in humans will critically depend on our ability to demonstrate its safety and efficiency in preventing or treating severe genetic disease. Improvements in vector design and safety and in delivery techniques to the fetus are key. A better understanding of the development of the fetal immune response to vector and gene products, as well as improved knowledge of the candidate diseases to be treated is also vital. Animal models of severe genetic diseases in the mouse and generation of large animal transgenic models will be useful to demonstrate proof of principle for in utero treatment, although ultimately it is likely that some safety studies will need to be performed in non-human primates. Regulating the expression of transgenic protein will need to be explored to prevent any adverse effects by over-expression.

One criticism leveled at fetal gene therapy is a belief that couples pregnant with an affected child would be unlikely to proceed with prenatal gene therapy and would opt for a termination instead. The general public remains concerned that ethical discussion about issues such as gene therapy, cloning and the Human Genome Project are falling behind the technology[92]. There is almost no research in this area, and the views of the general public and patient groups need to be solicited as this technology comes closer to the clinic. Research is also needed into how adequate information on the risks and benefits of these novel techniques can best be provided for the general public. This will enable couples to have an educated involvement in the decision-making process alongside health professionals.

SUMMARY

Fetal gene therapy offers the potential for clinicians not only to diagnose but also to treat inherited genetic disease. Fetal application may prove better than application in the adult for treatment, or even prevention of early onset genetic disorders such as cystic fibrosis and Duchenne muscular dystrophy. Gene transfer to the developing fetus targets rapidly expanding stem cell populations that are inaccessible after birth. Integrating vector systems give permanent gene transfer. In animal models of congenital disease, the functionally immature fetal immune system does not respond to the product of the introduced gene and, therefore, immune tolerance can be induced.

For the treatment to be acceptable, it must be safe for both mother and fetus, and preferably avoid germline transmission. Recent developments in the understanding of genetic disease, vector design and minimally invasive delivery techniques have brought fetal gene therapy closer to clinical practice. However, more research needs to be done before it can be introduced as a therapy. Currently, fetal gene therapy remains an experimental procedure. Better understanding of the development of genetic disease in the fetus and improvements in vector design and targeting of fetal tissues should allow this technology to move into clinical practice.

REFERENCES

1. Blaese RM, Culver KW, Miller AD et al. T lymphocyte-directed gene therapy for ADA- SCID: initial trial results after 4 years. *Science* **270**:475–480, 1995.
2. Clothier CM. *Report of the committee on the ethics of gene therapy, CM 1788*. London: HMSO Publications, 1992.
3. McCandless SE, Brunger JW, Cassidy SB. The burden of genetic disease on inpatient care in a children's hospital. *Am J Hum Genet* **74**:121–127, 2004.
4. Coutelle C, Douar A-M, Colledge WH, Froster U. The challenge of fetal gene therapy. *Nat Med* **1**:864–866, 1995.

5. Waddington SN, Mitrophanous KA, Ellard F et al. Long-term transgene expression by administration of a lentivirus-based vector to the fetal circulation of immuno-competent mice. *Gene Ther* **10**:1234–1240, 2003.
6. MacKenzie TC, Kobinger GP, Kootstra NA et al. Efficient transduction of liver and muscle after in utero injection of lentiviral vectors with different pseudotypes. *Molec Ther* **6**:349–358, 2002.
7. Chuah MK, Schiedner G, Thorrez L et al. Therapeutic factor VIII levels and negligible toxicity in mouse and dog models of hemophilia A following gene therapy with high-capacity adenoviral vectors. *Blood* **101**:1734–1743, 2003.
8. Bessis N, GarciaCozar FJ, Boissier MC. Immune responses to gene therapy vectors: influence on vector function and effector mechanisms. *Gene Ther* **11**:S10–sS17, 2004.
9. Gilchrist SC, Ontell MP, Kochanek S, Clemens PR. Immune response to full-length dystrophin delivered to Dmd muscle by a high-capacity adenoviral vector. *Molec Ther* **6**:359–368, 2002.
10. Kamata Y, Tanabe A, Kanaji A et al. Long-term normalization in the central nervous system, ocular manifestations, and skeletal deformities by a single systemic adenovirus injection into neonatal mice with mucopolysaccharidosis VII. *Gene Ther* **10**:406–414, 2003.
11. Cheng SH, Smith AE. Gene therapy progress and prospects: gene therapy of lysosomal storage disorders. *Gene Ther* **10**:1275–1281, 2003.
12. Waddington SN, Nivsarkar MS, Mistry AR et al. Permanent phenotypic correction of Hemophilia B in immunocompetent mice by prenatal gene therapy. *Blood* **104**:2714–2721, 2004.
13. Tran ND, Porada CD, Almeida-Porada G, Glimp HA, Anderson WF, Zanjani ED. Induction of stable prenatal tolerance to b-galactosidase by in utero gene transfer into preimmune sheep fetuses. *Blood* **97**:3417–3423, 2001.
14. Wilson JM, Wivel NA. Report on the potential use of gene therapy in utero. Gene Therapy Advisory Committee. *Hum Gene Ther* **10**:689–692, 1999.
15. Lipshutz GS, Sarkar R, Flebbe-Rehwaldt L, Kazazian H, Gaensler KML. Short-term correction of factor VIII deficiency in a murine model of hemophilia A after delivery of adenovirus murine factor VIII in utero. *Proc Nat Acad Sci USA* **96**:13324–13329, 1999.
16. Dejneka NS, Surace EM, Aleman TS et al. In utero gene therapy rescues vision in a murine model of congenital blindness. *Molec Ther* **9**:182–188, 2004.
17. Seppen J, van der Rijt R, Looije N, van Til NP, Lamers WH, Elferink RPJO. Long-term correction of bilirubin UDPglucuronyltransferase deficiency in rats by in utero lentiviral gene transfer. *Molec Ther* **8**:593–599, 2003.
18. Rucker M, Fraites TJ, Porvasnik SL et al. Rescue of enzyme deficiency in embryonic diaphragm in a mouse model of metabolic myopathy: Pompe disease. *Development* **131**:3007–3019, 2004.
19. Furie B, Limentani SA, Rosenfield CG. A practical guide to the evaluation and treatment of hemophilia. *Blood* **84**:3–9, 1994.
20. Lusher JM. Inhibitors in young boys with haemophilia. *Baillieres Best Pract Res Clin Haematol* **13**:457–468, 2000.
21. Soucie JM, Nuss R, Evatt B et al. Mortality among males with hemophilia: relations with source of medical care. The Hemophilia Surveillance System Project Investigators. *Blood* **96**:437–442, 2000.
22. Chao H, Samulski RJ, Bellinger D, Monahan PE, Nichols T, Walsh CE. Persistent expression of canine factor IX in hemophilia B canines. *Gene Ther* **6**:1695–1704, 1999.
23. Herzog RW, Yang EY, Couto LB et al. Long-term correction of canine hemophilia B by gene transfer of blood coagulation factor IX mediated by adeno-associated viral vector. *Nat Med* **5**:56–63, 1999.
24. Snyder RO, Miao C, Meuse L et al. Correction of hemophilia B in canine and murine models using recombinant adeno-associated viral vectors. *Nat Med* **5**:64–70, 1999.
25. Manno CS, Pierce GF, Arruda VR et al. Successful transduction of liver in hemophilia by AAV-Factor IX and limitations imposed by the host immune response. *Nat Med* **12**:342–347, 2006.
26. Manno CS, Chew AJ, Hutchison S et al. AAV-mediated factor IX gene transfer to skeletal muscle in patients with severe hemophilia B. *Blood* **101**:2963–2972, 2003.
27. David AL, Torondel B, Zachary I, et al. Local delivery of VEGF to the uterine arteries increases vessel relaxation and placental perfusion in the pregnant sheep. SGI Annual Meeting, Washington DC, March 2007. *Reprod Sci* **14**(1Suppl), 2007.
28. Gharwan H, Wightman L, Kircheis R, Wagner E, Zatloukal K. Nonviral gene transfer into fetal mouse livers (a comparison between the cationic polymer PEI and naked DNA). *Gene Ther* **10**:810–817, 2003.
29. Luton D, Oudrhiri N, De Lagausie P et al. Gene transfection into fetal sheep airways in utero using guanidinium-cholesterol cationic lipids. *J Gene Med* **6**:328–336, 2004.
30. Fletcher S, Ahmad A, Perouzel E, Heron A, Miller AD, Jorgensen MR. In vivo studies of dialkynoyl analogues of DOTAP demonstrate improved gene transfer efficiency of cationic liposomes in mouse lung. *J Med Chem* **49**:349–357, 2006.
31. Mason CA, Bigras JL, O'Blenes SB et al. Gene transfer in utero biologically engineers a patent ductus arteriosus in lambs by arresting fibronectin-dependent neointimal formation. *Nat Med* **5**:176–182, 1999.
32. David AL, Cook T, Waddington S et al. Ultrasound guided percutaneous delivery of adenoviral vectors encoding the b-galactosidase and human factor IX genes to early gestation fetal sheep in utero. *Hum Gene Ther* **14**:353–364, 2003.
33. Waddington SN, Buckley SMK, Nivsarkar M et al. In utero gene transfer of human factor IX to fetal mice can induce postnatal tolerance of the exogenous clotting factor. *Blood* **101**:1359–1366, 2003.
34. Lipshutz GS, Flebbe-Rehwaldt L, Gaensler KML. Reexpression following readministration of an adenoviral vector in adult mice after initial in utero adenoviral administration. *Molec Ther* **2**:374–380, 2000.
35. McCray PB, Armstrong K, Zabner J et al. Adenoviral-mediated gene transfer to fetal pulmonary epithelia in vitro and in vivo. *J Clin Invest* **95**:2620–2632, 1995.
36. Chen HH, Mack LM, Kelly R, Ontell M, Kochanek S, Clemens PR. Persistence in muscle of an adenoviral vector that lacks all viral genes. *Proc Natl Acad Sci N Am* **94**:1645–1650, 1997.
37. Schiedner G, Morral N, Parks RJ et al. Genomic DNA transfer with a high-capacity adenovirus vector results in improved in vivo gene expression and decreased toxicity. *Nat Genet* **18**:180–183, 1998.
38. Murphy SJ, Chong H, Bell S, Diaz RM, Vile RG. Novel integrating adenoviral/retroviral hybrid vector for gene therapy. *Hum Gene Ther* **13**:745–760, 2002.
39. Kubo S, Mitani K. A new hybrid system capable of efficient lentiviral vector production and stable gene transfer mediated by a single helper-dependent adenoviral vector. *J Virol* **77**:2964–2971, 2003.
40. Jerebtsova M, Batshaw ML, Ye X. Humoral immune response to recombinant adenovirus and adeno-associated virus after in utero administration of viral vectors in mice. *Pediatr Res* **52**:95–104, 2002.
41. Bouchard S. Prolonged expression of adenovirus and adeno-associated virus following fetal administration in the preimmune period. *Molec Ther* **3**:S393–sS394, 2001.
42. Schneider H, Mühle C, Douar A-M et al. Sustained delivery of therapeutic concentrations of human clotting factor IX–a comparison of adenoviral and AAV vectors administered in utero. *J Gene Med* **4**:46–53, 2002.
43. Lipshutz GS, Titre D, Brindle M, Bisconte AR, Contag CH, Gaensler KM. Comparison of gene expression after intraperitoneal delivery of AAV2 or AAV5 in utero. *Molec Ther* **8**:90–98, 2003.

44. Garrett DJ, Cohen CJ, Larson JE. Long term modification of adult physiology following in utero gene transfer using an AAV vector. *Genet Vaccines Ther* **2**, 2004.
45. Nakai H, Montini E, Fuess S, Storm TA, Grompe M, Kay MA. AAV serotype 2 vectors preferentially integrate into active genes in mice. *Nat Genet* **34**:297–302, 2003.
46. Baschat AA, Towbin J, Bowles NE, Harman CR, Weiner CP. Is adenovirus a fetal pathogen? *Am J Obstet Gynecol* **189**:758–763, 2003.
47. Burguete T, Rabreau M, Fontanges-Darriet M et al. Evidence for infection of the human embryo with adeno-associated virus in pregnancy. *Hum Reprod* **14**:2396–2401, 1999.
48. Walsh C, Cepko CL. Widespread dispersion of neuronal clones across functional regions of the cerebral cortex. *Science* **255**:434–441, 1992.
49. Hatzoglou M, Lamers W, Bosch F, Wynshaw-Boris A, Clapp DW, Hanson RW. Hepatic gene transfer in animals using retroviruses containing the promoter from the gene for phosphoenolpyruvate carboxykinase. *J Biol* **265**:17285–17293, 1990.
50. Porada CD, Tran N, Eglitis M et al. In utero gene therapy: transfer and long-term expression of the bacterial neo^r gene in sheep after direct injection of retroviral vectors into preimmune fetuses. *Hum Gene Ther* **9**:1571–1585, 1998.
51. Tarantal AF, O'Rourke JP, Case SS et al. Rhesus monkey model for fetal gene transfer: studies with retroviral-based vector systems. *Molec Ther* **3**:128–138, 2001.
52. Miller DG, Adam MA, Miller AD. Gene transfer by retrovirus vectors occurs only in cells that are actively replicating at the time of infection. *Molec Cell Biol* **10**:4239–4242, 1990.
53. Welsh RJ, Cooper NR, Jensen FC, Oldstone MB. Human serum lyses RNA tumor viruses. *Nature* **257**:612–614, 1975.
54. Engelstädter M, Buchholz CJ, Bobkova M et al. Targeted gene transfer to lymphocytes using murine leukaemia virus vectors pseudotyped with spleen necrosis virus envelope proteins. *Gene Ther* **8**:1202–1206, 2001.
55. Douar A-M, Themis M, Sandig V, Friedmann T, Coutelle C. Effect of amniotic fluid on cationic lipid mediated transfection and viral infection. *Gene Ther* **3**:789–796, 1996.
56. Galan HL, Bennett ML, Tyson RW et al. Inefficient transduction of sheep in utero after intra-amniotic injection of retroviral producer cells. *Am J Obstet Gynecol* **187**:469–474, 2002.
57. Bennett M, Galan H, Owens G et al. In utero gene delivery by intraamniotic injection of a retroviral vector producer cell line in a nonhuman primate model. *Hum Gene Ther* **12**:1857–1865, 2001.
58. Lewis P, Hensel M, Emerman M. Human immunodeficiency virus infection of cells arrested in the cell cycle. *EMBO* **11**:3053–3058, 1992.
59. Park F, Ohashi K, Chiu W, Naldini L, Kay MA. Efficient lentiviral transduction of liver requires cell cycling in vivo. *Nat Genet* **24**:49–52, 200;.
60. Peebles D, Gregory LG, David A et al. Widespread and efficient marker gene expression in the airway epithelia of fetal sheep after minimally invasive tracheal application of recombinant adenovirus in utero. *Gene Ther* **11**:70–78, 2004.
61. David AL, Peebles DM, Gregory L et al. Clinically applicable procedure for gene delivery to fetal gut by ultrasound-guided gastric injection: toward prenatal prevention of early-onset intestinal diseases. *Hum Gene Ther* **17**:767–779, 2006.
62. David AL, Weisz B, Gregory L et al. Ultrasound-guided injection and occlusion of the trachea in fetal sheep. *Ultrasound Obstet Gynaecol* **28**:82–88, 2006.
63. Coutelle C, Themis M, Waddington SN et al. Gene therapy progress and prospects: fetal gene therapy – first proofs of concept – some adverse effects. *Gene Ther* **12**:1601–1607, 2005.
64. Larson JE, Morrow SL, Delcarpio JB et al. Gene transfer into the fetal primate: evidence for the secretion of transgene product. *Molec Ther* **2**:631–639, 2000.
65. Tarantal AF, Lee CI, Ekert JE et al. Lentiviral vector gene transfer into fetal rhesus monkeys (Macaca mulatta): lung-targeting approaches. *Molec Ther* **4**:614–621, 2001.
66. Pahal GS, Jauniaux E, Kinnon C, Thrasher AJ, Rodeck C. Normal development of human fetal hematopoiesis between eight and seventeen weeks' gestation. *Am J Obstet Gynecol* **183**:1029–1034, 2000.
67. Kittler EL, Peters SO, Crittenden RB et al. Cytokine-facilitated transduction leads to low-level engraftment in nonablated hosts. *Blood* **90**:865–872, 1997.
68. Eglitis MA, Kantoff P, Gilboa E, Anderson WF. Gene expression in mice after high efficiency retroviral-mediated gene transfer. *Science* **230**:1395–1398, 1985.
69. Bodine DM, Moritz T, Donahue RE et al. Long-term in vivo expression of a murine adenosine deaminase gene in rhesus monkey hematopoietic cells of multiple lineages after retroviral mediated transfer into CD34+ bone marrow cells. *Blood* **82**:1975–1980, 1993.
70. Ward M, Richardson C, Pioli P et al. Transfer and expression of the human multiple drug resistance gene in human CD34+ cells. *Blood* **84**:1408, 1994.
71. Ekhterae D, Crumbleholme T, Karson E, Harrison MR, Anderson WF, Zanjani ED. Retroviral vector-mediated transfer of the bacterial neomycin resistance gene into fetal and adult sheep and human hematopoietic progenitors in vitro. *Blood* **75**:365–369, 1990.
72. Ward M, Sattler R, Grossman IR et al. A stable murine-based RD114 retroviral packaging line efficiently transduces human hematopoietic cells. *Molec Ther* **8**:804–812, 2003.
73. Case SS, Price MA, Jordan CT et al. Stable transduction of quiescent CD34(+)CD38(−) human hematopoietic cells by HIV-1-based lentiviral vectors. *Proc Natl Acad Sci N Am* **96**:2988–2993, 1999.
74. Campagnoli C, Bellantuono I, Kumar S, Fairburn LJ, Roberts I, Fisk NM. High transduction efficiency of circulating first trimester fetal mesenchymal stem cells: potential targets for in utero ex vivo gene therapy. *Br J Obstet Gynaecol* **109**:952–954, 2002.
75. Tsai MS, Lee JL, Chang YJ, Hwang SM. Isolation of human multipotent mesenchymal stem cells from second-trimester amniotic fluid using a novel two-stage culture protocol. *Hum Reprod* **19**:1450–1456, 2004.
76. Fletcher JC, Richter G. Human fetal gene therapy: moral and ethical questions. *Hum Gene Ther* **7**:1605–1614, 1996.
77. Recombinant DNA Advisory Committee. Prenatal gene transfer: scientific, medical, and ethical issues. *Hum Gene Ther* **11**:1211–1229, 2000.
78. Morrow SL, Larson JE, Nelson S, Sekhon HS, Ren T, Cohen JC. Modfication of development by the CFTR gene in utero. *Molec Genet Metab* **65**:203–212, 1998.
79. Hacein-Bey-Abina S, von Kalle C, Schmidt M et al. A serious adverse event after successful gene therapy for X-linked severe combined immunodeficiency. *N Engl J Med* **348**:255–256, 2003.
80. Juengst ET. What next for human gene therapy? *Br Med J* **326**:1410–1411, 2003.
81. Baum C, Kustikova O, Modlich U, Li Z, Fehse B. Mutagenesis and oncogenesis by chromosomal insertion of gene transfer vectors. *Hum Gene Ther* **17**:253–263, 2006.
82. Themis M, Waddington SN, Schmidt M et al. Oncogenesis following delivery of a nonprimate lentiviral gene therapy vector to fetal and neonatal mice. *Molec Ther* **12**:763–771, 2005.
83. Billings PR. In utero gene therapy. *Nat Med* **5**:255–261, 1999.
84. Tran ND, Porada CD, Zhao Y, Almeida-Porada G, Anderson WF, Zanjani ED. In utero transfer and expression of exogenous genes in sheep. *Exp Hematol* **28**:17–30, 2000.
85. Lipshutz GS, Gruber CA, Cao Y, Hardy J, Contag CH, Gaensler KML. In utero delivery of adeno-associated viral vectors: intraperitoneal gene transfer produces long-term expression. *Molec Ther* **3**:284–292, 2001.
86. Schneider H, Coutelle C. In utero gene therapy: the case for. *Nat Med* **5**:256–257, 1999.

87. Coutelle C, Rodeck C. On the scientific and ethical issues of fetal somatic gene therapy. *Gene Ther* **9**:670–673, 2002.
88. Burger IM, Wilfond BS. Limitations of informed consent for in utero gene transfer research: implications for investigators and institutional review boards. *Hum Gene Ther* **11**:1057–1063, 2000.
89. Westgren M, Ringden O, Bartmann P et al. Prenatal T-cell reconstitution after in utero transplantation with fetal liver cells in a patient with X-linked severe combined immunodeficiency. *Am J Obstet Gynecol* **187**:475–482, 2002.
90. Wells D, Delhanty JD. Preimplantation genetic diagnosis: applications for molecular medicine. *Trends Molec Med* **7**:23–30, 2001.
91. Snowdon C, Green JM. Preimplantation diagnosis and other reproductive options: attitudes of male and female carriers of recessive disorders. *Hum Reprod* **12**:341–350, 1997.
92. Brown P. Regulations not keeping up with developments in genetics, says poll. *Br Med J* **321**:1369, 2000.
93. Muench MO, Rae J, Barcena A et al. Transplantation of a fetus with paternal Thy-1(+)CD34(+) cells for chronic granulomatous disease. *Bone Marrow Transplant* **27**:355–364, 2001.
94. Touraine JL. Induction of transplantation tolerance in humans using stem cell transplants prenatally or postnatally. *Transplant Proc* **31**:2735–2737, 1999.
95. Themis M, Schneider H, Kiserud T et al. Successful expression of b-galactosidase and factor IX transgenes in fetal and neonatal sheep after ultrasound-guided percutaneous adenovirus vector administration into the umbilical vein. *Gene Ther* **6**:1239–1248, 1999.
96. Nicolini U, Nicolaidis P, Fisk NM, Tannirandorn Y, Rodeck C. Fetal blood sampling from the intrahepatic vein: analysis of safety and clinical experience with 214 procedures. *Obstet Gynaecol* **76**:47–53, 1990.
97. Weisz B, David AL, Gregory LG et al. Targeting the respiratory muscles of fetal sheep for prenatal gene therapy for Duchenne muscular dystrophy. *Am J Obstet Gynecol* **193**:1105–1109, 2005.
98. Newnham JP, Kelly RW, Boyne P, Reid SE. Ultrasound guided blood sampling from fetal sheep. *Aus J Agricult Res* **40**:401–407, 1989.
99. Chinnaiya A, Venkat A, Dawn C et al. Intraheptatic vein fetal blood sampling: current role in prenatal diagnosis. *J Obstet Gynaecol Res* **24**:239–246, 1998.
100. Wang G, Williamson R, Mueller G, Thomas P, Davidson BL, McCray PB, Jr. Ultrasound-guided gene therapy to hepatocytes in utero. *Fetal Diagn Ther* **13**:197–205, 1998.
101. David AL, Peebles DM, Gregory L et al. Percutaneous ultrasound-guided injection of the trachea in fetal sheep: a novel technique to target the fetal airways. *Fetal Diagn Ther* **18**:385–390, 2003.

SECTION 9

The neonate

49 Interface of fetal and neonatal medicine 703
Malcolm Chiswick

CHAPTER 49

Interface of fetal and neonatal medicine

Malcolm Chiswick

KEY POINTS

- Improved survival rates of very preterm infants have been achieved in some cases at the expense of chronic morbidity which may extend for weeks or months beyond the neonatal period
- Bronchopulmonary dysplasia is the most common and serious late in-hospital morbidity among very preterm newborn infants
- Ethical concepts in the management of babies born at the margins of viability are helpful in defining problems but are of limited help providing solutions for clinicians. Problems in delivery room care arise from poor communication between staff, between staff and patients, and lack of awareness of common pitfalls. This is best addressed through agreed protocols
- The use of antenatal steroids is currently the most helpful measure for reducing the risk of intraventricular-periventricular hemorrhage in very preterm infants
- Focal periventricular leukomalacia, diagnosed by neonatal ultrasonography, is now very uncommon. However, in around one-third of very preterm infants magnetic resonance brain imaging at term equivalent shows abnormal signal consistent with diffuse white matter abnormality. Triggering events, including infection and hypoxia-ischemia may occur at a time when the developing brain is vulnerable, before 32 weeks' gestation, but a continuing process of damage to myelin precursor cells is possible. This is relevant to the known risk of learning impairments in very preterm infants
- In term infants, most examples of neonatal encephalopathy associated with clinical features of perinatal asphyxia are associated with acute lesions of the brain suggestive of an intrapartum cause
- Mild hypothermia commencing after birth in infants with encephalopathy appears to be safe. Early results suggest that the combined outcome of death or disability at 18 months is reduced in treated infants. The results are not conclusive and treatment should only be offered in the context of randomized controlled trials, or in connection with an appropriately maintained database accessible to other users

INTRODUCTION

The science of fetal medicine has advanced our understanding of the factors that control fetal health and that generate disease, as exemplified by the preceding chapters. Improved methods of fetal diagnosis and therapies have played an important part in improving outcomes, but the influence of fetal disease on subsequent well-being is complex. The fetal–neonatal interface is just one aspect of a continuum that extends into infancy, childhood and adult life. This chapter focuses on very preterm birth and cerebral hypoxia-ischemia in term infants. These conditions have been selected because they are determinants of long-term outcome and because they illustrate some of the complexities of the fetal–neonatal interface in its influence on disease processes.

VERY PRETERM BIRTH

Around 7–8% of live births in England and Wales occur at less than 37 weeks' gestation. A small minority of these infants, probably amounting to a little over 1% of all live preterm births, are born at less than 32 weeks' gestation and their chances of surviving to be discharged home from the neonatal unit has improved in the past 20 years. However, this has been achieved at the expense of chronic morbidity which may extend many weeks or months beyond the neonatal period. Indeed, for some, the legacy extends into childhood and adult life.

Causal pathways for this morbidity may entail the following concepts:

- Severe in-hospital neonatal morbidity progressing into the early months of life may simply reflect preterm birth before structural and functional maturation of various organ systems. In other words, beyond the margins of viability there are other aspects of functional maturity that profoundly limit adaptation to extrauterine life.
- Treatments that encourage survival may expose morbidity which might have already been determined during fetal life due to maternal disorders, or an adverse intrauterine environment.
- Many relatively common disorders in the perinatal period have been shown to involve processes which reflect the expression of genes.
- Certain treatments may cause or contribute to morbidity.

Bronchopulmonary dysplasia (BPD)

BPD, also known as 'chronic lung disease', is the most common and serious late in-hospital morbidity among very preterm newborn infants. A protracted course of respiratory insufficiency may culminate in death, discharge home on oxygen therapy, multiple rehospitaliztion episodes in the first year of life, and neurodevelopmental disability. The definition of BPD is based on a continuing need for supplemental oxygen at 36 weeks' post-conceptional age (PCA) or 28 days according to a less restrictive definition. Among very preterm infants, the incidence of BPD increases with decreasing gestational age. The EPICure study, conducted in 1995, showed that the incidence of oxygen dependency at 36 weeks' PCA was as high as 86% at ≤23 weeks' gestation, 77%, at 24 weeks and 70% at 25 weeks[1]. In contrast, at 27–30 weeks, the incidence is less than 15%.

The incidence of BPD varies considerably between neonatal units and this is partly due to the definition and how active the neonatal staff are in trying to wean infants from supplemental oxygen. Some infants are nursed in less than 30% supplemental oxygen for several weeks without being challenged by a step-wise reduction in their inspired oxygen concentration, or by a trial of nursing in air while monitoring their oxygen saturation levels. When challenged in this way shortly before 36 weeks' PCA, a proportion of infants have satisfactory oxygen saturation levels in air, and therefore, by definition, do not have BPD[2]. Precision in the diagnosis is important to facilitate the study of large homogeneous populations of affected infants in order to determine antenatal and neonatal influences, treatments and outcomes. A diagnosis based on a prior air-challenge for those receiving minimal oxygen led to less variation in the incidence of BPD between participating centers, and the apparent fall in incidence was comparable with the magnitude to the treatment effects seen in some clinical trials[2].

The clinical pattern of this disorder has changed coincidentally with the improved survival rates of very preterm infants. Earlier descriptions emphasized BPD as a complication of severe respiratory distress syndrome with a continuing need for ventilation and oxygen. A progressive deterioration in the chest X-ray occurred culminating in air trapping, emphysematous bullae and fibrosis. There was also additional histological evidence of small airway damage among those that died. Damage to the immature lung due to the trauma of mechanical ventilation and pulmonary oxygen toxicity played a major etiological role. This pattern of disease, although still seen, is less common, probably due in part to a reduction in the incidence of severe respiratory distress syndrome (RDS) as a result of antenatal steroids and surfactant therapy.

Atypical BPD occurs in extremely preterm infants, most of whom will have received mechanical ventilation and supplemental oxygen during the first week as a general supportive measure. Some of these infants have only mild or no RDS and, by the end of the first week, they no longer require assisted ventilation and are nursed in minimal oxygen (less than 30%). Their course is then characterized by unexpected pulmonary deterioration during the second week of life with an increasing requirement of oxygen culminating in chronic respiratory insufficiency which persists beyond 36 weeks' PCA.

The basis of atypical BPD is impaired development of the immature lung, probably due to disruption of the normal interplay between epithelial and endothelial cells. Pulmonary vascularization is dependent on lung epithelial development and, conversely, the lung epithelium affects capillary morphogenesis. It is likely that the appropriate spatial and temporal expression of angiogenic factors, including vascular endothelial growth factors, have an important role in this interplay[3].

A role for inflammatory mediators originating in utero in the pathogenesis of BPD is supported by elevations of interleukin (IL)-6, TNF-α, IL-1β, and IL-8 in amniotic fluid of mothers delivering preterm in association with increased risk of BPD in the infants[4]. Of particular interest is that chorioamnionitis was one of the most significant risk factors for atypical BPD among infants who had not suffered from RDS[5]. This supports the idea that chorioamnionitis might protect against RDS, perhaps through enhancing pulmonary maturation, while exposing the fetal lung to inflammatory mediators and making it vulnerable to postnatal insults such as ventilatory trauma and hyperoxia.

An interest in the genetic implications of BPD was stimulated by the observation that the BPD status in one twin was a highly significant predictor of the disorder in the other twin, even after allowing for confounding variables[6]. Given the many etiological factors implicated in BPD, there are probably many genes that regulate its occurrence through lung development, pro- and anti-inflammatory mediators, tissue damage and repair[7].

The longer term neurodevelopmental morbidity associated with BPD is confounded to some extent by the preponderance of very preterm survivors of the condition. Nonetheless, there is evidence that BPD is an *additional* risk for global cognitive impairment, especially impaired language development, visual-motor coordination and behavioral problems[8]. The possibility that the use of postnatal steroids for the prevention or treatment of BPD may lead to white matter damage or impaired myelination has provoked caution such that their use has diminished during the past 5 years.

Pulmonary outcomes following BPD have been recently reviewed[9]. Some infants have a significant disturbance in pulmonary mechanics and gas exchange throughout infancy and require nursing at home in supplemental oxygen. Lung function shows a tendency to improve in childhood with growth of the lungs, although residual small airway disease is common with an increased incidence of wheezing. Up to 50% of infants, even if not oxygen dependent, nonetheless have frequent readmissions to hospital with pulmonary infections.

Live birth at the margins of viability

The ethical issues in caring for babies of borderline viability have been widely addressed[10,11] culminating in a land-mark publication by a Working Party of the Nuffield Council on Bioethics[12]. The considerations are well known and focus on the need to act in the *best interests of the infant*, which includes balancing the likely outcome, including the predicted quality of life, with the degree of pain and suffering entailed in on-going intensive care, an awareness of the notion of futility and acknowledgment that parents also have an interest.

Although these ethical concepts are very helpful in *defining the issues*, they are rarely of much help in providing a *clinical solution* to the problem of the delivery room care of such babies. The analytical approach of the bioethicist raises issues which, in order to resolve, demand a level of clinical predictive knowledge which simply does not exist. At its most basic level, the 'best interest' argument is one that defines the infant as a unique individual. In most cases, the neonatologist does not know whether the unique individual born, for example, at 23 weeks' gestation will behave like the majority of such infants or will manifest his or her uniqueness in some other way – perhaps by surviving to be discharged home with a good neurodevelopmental outcome.

The results of the EPICure study of babies born at less than 26 weeks' gestation in the British Isles during a 10-month period in 1995, followed up to the age of 6 years, are summarized in Table 49.1. A further study, 'EPICure 2', will report on outcomes for babies born at less than 27 weeks' gestation during 2006. Preliminary results indicate that survival rates per admission for intensive care have significantly improved at 24 weeks and over but not at 22–23 weeks. However, by the time neurodevelopmental outcomes are available, there may well be shifts in perinatal care, illustrating that in the context of ethical dilemmas surrounding the care of extremely preterm infants, there is a need for accurate *early markers* of neurodevelopmental outcome – clinical, neurophysiological and brain imaging.

The analysis of data from large populations of infants born at the margins of viability may help to determine predictors of survival that operate before birth in a way that will contribute to decision making immediately after delivery. Possible candidates include the fetal growth trajectory, use of antenatal steroids and tocolytics, chorioamnionitis, gender and whether singleton or multiple births. The development of neonatal networks with uniform standards of data collection should, in the future, be able to provide continuous data using computer-aided methodology linking different networks.

The Working Party of the Nuffield Council on Bioethics concluded that the long-term neurodevelopmental outcome data of the EPICure study remain the best available for advising parents in the UK on likely outcomes. However, it was felt that somewhat better survival rates were now being achieved. Their recommendations concerning the resuscitation and on-going intensive care for babies born at 21–25 completed weeks of gestation are summarized in Table 49.2.

When things go wrong in the delivery room and culminate in parental complaints, it is rarely due to misplaced ethical values or serious conflict between what the parents want to happen and how the neonatologist sees things or a failure to act lawfully. Instead, problems commonly result from inadequate communication between professionals and between professionals and parents, and from a lack of awareness of the many clinical pitfalls that can arise following birth at the margins of viability.

Outcome information presented to parents can easily be misunderstood. It is important to clarify the distinction between survival rates per 1000 live births and survival rates expressed in relation to admissions to the neonatal intensive care unit (see Table 49.1). Another source of misunderstanding comes about when survival data are linked with disability rates. For example, at the margins of viability, there is only a small difference between rates of survival with minimal or no disability and

Table 49.1 **Survival and outcome rates of the EPICure study[1,2]**

	Completed weeks of gestation			
	22w	*23w*	*24w*	*25w*
Live births (n)	138	241	382	424
Admitted to NMU (n%)	22 (16)	131 (54)	298 (78)	357 (84)
Survival rates (n%)				
Per live births	2 (1)	26 (11)	100 (26)	186 (44)
Per admission	2 (9)	26 (20)	100 (34)	186 (52)
Assessed at 6 years[3] (n%)	**2 (100)**	**22 (88)**	**73 (74)**	**144 (79)**
Severe disability[4]	1(50)	5 (23)	21 (29)	26 (18)
Moderate[5]	0	9 (41)	16 (22)	32 (22)
Mild/no[6]	1(50)	5 (36)	36 (49)	86 (60)

[1]*Pediatrics* **106**: 659-671, 2000; [2]*N Engl J Med* **352**:9-19, 2005; [3]Only 1–3 patients at each gestation died before assessment; [4]Highly dependent on caregivers, e.g. unable to walk, very low IQ, profound hearing loss, blind; [5]Reasonable level of independence, e.g. able to walk, below average IQ, correctable hearing loss, impaired vision; [6]Mild learning difficulty, squint, (or no disability)

Table 49.2 **Summary of recommendations for the resuscitation at birth of babies born at borderline viability**[1]

Gestation	*Standard*	*Exceptions*
21 weeks	No resuscitation (considered an experimental procedure)	Only as part of research protocol
22 weeks	No resuscitation	At parents' request after prolonged and fully informed discussion of the risks, implications and the likely outcome
23 weeks	Could not be defined	Precedence to parents' wishes. If left to clinicians then the clinical team should 'determine what constitutes appropriate care for that particular baby'
24 weeks	Resuscitation	*Unless* parents and clinicians agree that in the light of the baby's condition that it is not in his or her best interests
25 weeks	Resuscitation	*Unless* severe abnormality incompatible with any significant period of survival

[1]Nuffield Council on Bioethics. Dilemmas in current practice: babies born at the borderline of viability. Critical Care Decisions in Fetal and Neonatal Medicine: Ethical Issues. November 2006, 67-87.

rates of survival with major disability expressed per 1000 live births. This is because of the major impact of *mortality* which numerically outweighs any consideration of disability.

When counseling parents, it is important that they understand the difference between *viability* (the ability to sustain life) and *vitality* (being alive). Confusion may arise when a mother is counseled to the effect that her fetus is too immature to survive and that continuous fetal heart rate monitoring is futile. It is not always appreciated by parents that their baby is likely to be born alive, that the state of the infant at birth is rarely predictable, and that there will still be an issue of the management and care of the infant after birth. This particular problem of poor communication is compounded if only a perfunctory examination of the baby is made and signs of life are missed or ignored. A major delivery room crisis may occur when such an infant unexpectedly shows increasing vigor.

These and other similar problems are best resolved through agreed delivery room policies and management arrangements, which should include care of the dying baby. Having an agreed protocol which is understood and enacted by everyone entails an acknowledgment that, in terms of decisions around resuscitation and on-going intensive care, we may not always get it right and, *with hindsight*, it may be judged that an alternative approach would have been better. Management protocols are aimed at ensuring that parents are appropriately and helpfully informed and that babies born at the margins of viability are not met by confusion and crises in the delivery room.

BRAIN LESIONS IN VERY PRETERM INFANTS

The two most common and significant intracerebral lesions of very preterm infants are intraventricular-periventricular hemorrhage and white matter damage. These lesions may coexist in some infants.

Intraventricular-periventricular hemorrhage (IVH-PVH)

Bleeding in and around the ventricular system of the brain occurs in 15–20% of infants born at 32 weeks' gestation or less, although more mature infants may also be affected. Serial ultrasound brain scans done by the cot-side show that most of these hemorrhages occur on the first day of life and around 80–90% have happened by 72 hours. The most common presentation is by incidental observation on an ultrasound brain scan, and this applies especially to small and moderate hemorrhages. Some of these infants develop subtle signs such as reduced spontaneous movement, hypotonia and a reduced level of arousal. The least common presentation is sudden and rapid deterioration with seizures or decerebrate posturing, stupor and fixed pupils and this is prone to occur with extremely large bleeds.

The origin of bleeding is within the germinal matrix below the subependyma, which consists of a rich and fragile vascular network within a matrix of undifferentiated glial cells and neuronal precursors. Using histochemical markers, autopsy studies recently showed that the coverage of blood vessels by astrocyte end-feet increased consistently in the cerebral cortex and white matter from 19 to 40 weeks' gestation, whereas coverage was less in the germinal matrix especially between 23 and 34 weeks. This may contribute to the fragility of germinal matrix vasculature and propensity to hemorrhage[13].

A major factor contributing to the etiology of bleeding from this fragile vasculature is impaired autoregulation of cerebral blood flow in the preterm infant, especially perturbations of flow which can be precipitated by a wide range of clinical factors. The fall in the incidence of IVH-PVH in the last 20 years is probably attributable to the use of antenatal steroids and surfactant therapy, both treatments reducing the incidence of severe RDS – an important risk factor for hemorrhage. Given that IVH-PVH occurs in the first few days of life, it is important to know whether there are avoidable antenatal risk factors, aside from preterm birth and failure to give antenatal steroids. Retrospective observational studies are often hampered by an array of confounding variables which probably explains the conflicting results between studies. Candidate risk factors requiring more detailed study include intrauterine growth impairment, placental inflammation and intrauterine infection.

Hemorrhage confined to the germinal matrix and small intraventricular bleeds caused by seepage of blood through the floor of the ventricle generally carry a good prognosis. However, there is growing interest in the possibility that destruction of the germinal matrix may lead to subtle impairments as a result of loss of glial cell precursors of oligodendrocytes leading to impaired myelination. Overt neurodevelopmental problems, including cerebral palsy, severe learning disability and epilepsy, are more likely with larger lesions complicated by periventricular hemorrhagic infarction and post-hemorrhagic obstructive hydrocephalus.

White matter damage

Our understanding of white matter damage, which includes a spectrum of injury, has developed considerably in recent years. Earlier concepts based on neonatal cranial ultrasonography emphasized the importance of *focal white matter damage*, commonly referred to as periventricular leukomalacia (PVL) and manifest mainly as periventricular echodensity and cystic change. Histopathologically, the lesion is characterized by necrosis in the periventricular region affecting all cellular elements, progressing to cystic change, gliosis, and culminating in loss of periventricular white matter and secondary ventricular enlargement.

The periventricular region in very preterm infants is a vascular watershed area at the interface of long and short penetrating arteries from the pial surface and basal penetrating arteries. Although direct experimental evidence is lacking, impaired cerebral vascular autoregulation of very preterm infants together with the anatomy of vascular supply probably explain the vulnerability of the periventricular region to hypoxic-ischemic damage. There is a well-established association of maternofetal infection with white matter damage acting through inflammatory mediators. It is possible that intrauterine exposure of the fetus to inflammatory cytokines increases vulnerability to hypoxic-ischemic damage. The mechanisms are not mutually exclusive and cerebral ischemia may result from vasoactive effects of endotoxins and cytokines; furthermore, there is a cytokine response to hypoxia-ischemic injury.

In spite of this, understanding the relationship of PVL to clinical events before or after birth has never been entirely clear. Periventricular echodensities or cystic change may be present at birth on ultrasound scans indicating intrauterine causative factors, yet the antenatal or intrapartum history do not always reveal adverse events. Similarly, infants with normal scans in the first week or two of life may develop periventricular echodensities and cysts in subsequent weeks, yet have a relatively benign neonatal course. Considering the improved survival of very preterm infants and that, unlike IVH-PVH, there is a lack of any preventative measures, one would expect a rising incidence of focal white matter damage. This has not been the case – in fact, focal white matter damage as conventionally diagnosed by neonatal ultrasonography is now very uncommon and affects less than 5% of very preterm infants.

There are pitfalls in the use of neonatal cranial sonography for the diagnosis of PVL. When periventricular cysts are present, they can normally be detected by ultrasound. However, periventricular echodensities can be more difficult to interpret. Echodensities of prognostic significance may be overlooked and, conversely, inexperienced operators may over-interpret periventricular echoes which are normal.

Focal PVL, especially when extensive and cystic, may be associated with *diffuse white matter damage* involving the deep white matter and culminating in time with atrophy and secondary ventricular dilatation. However, MRI examinations made at the equivalent of term in infants born very prematurely have shown a high incidence of diffuse high signal intensity in white matter even in the *absence* of neonatal ultrasound evidence of focal PVL. In a prospective study, the incidence of non-cystic diffuse white matter abnormality diagnosed in this way was reported to be 35% and, in around half of these cases, the neonatal ultrasound scan was normal or showed transient echodensities[14]. Nonetheless, the term PVL is commonly used as a general term applied to diffuse as well as focal damage to the white matter.

The significance of diffuse high signal intensity in the white matter has been clarified by diffusion-weighted brain imaging using a technique which provides a measure of diffusion of water in tissue. This has clearly shown that the high signal intensity in the white matter is truly indicative of white matter *abnormality* rather than a normal biological phenomenon[15]. Although the precise neuropathologic substrate for this injury is unclear, it is likely that preoligodendrocytes, myelin precursors, play a key role and both hypoxic-ischemic injury and infection may be implicated in the pathogenesis. While the triggering events may occur at a time when the developing brain is vulnerable, before 32 weeks' gestation, a continuing process of damage to myelin precursors implicating activated microglia may subsequently occur[16].

Focal PVL, especially with cystic change, is typically associated with cerebral palsy, most commonly spastic diplegia. Many affected children also have a range of impairments of cognitive and behavioral function which are probably related to associated more diffuse white matter damage. Further follow-up studies will probably reveal the extent to which diffuse white matter damage in the absence of focal PVL is responsible for learning impairments in children who have escaped cerebral palsy.

HYPOXIC-ISCHEMIC BRAIN DAMAGE IN TERM INFANTS

Central to our understanding of hypoxic-ischemic injury at term is the notion that, after successful resuscitation at birth, rapid recovery of cerebral energy metabolism occurs but some hours later secondary energy failure intervenes and is associated with many intracerebral biochemical changes which culminate in cell death, mainly by apoptosis[17]. These changes are summarized in Table 49.3. The relevance of this knowledge is that it points the way to possible neural rescue interventions by interruption of some of the pathways concerned.

The *clinical* expression of secondary energy failure is a constellation of non-specific clinical signs known as an encephalopathy and includes, in varying degrees, a disturbance in muscle tone, seizures and an altered level of arousal and poor feeding. Among infants whose encephalopathy is likely attributable to cerebral hypoxia-ischemia, the severity of the encephalopathy is a helpful guide to long-term outcome[18]. Mild encephalopathy has virtually a zero risk of neonatal mortality or severe disability. Moderate encephalopathy, distinguished by the occurrence of seizures, has about a 6% mortality and a 20% incidence of severe disability in survivors; in contrast, severe encephalopathy characterized by stupor or coma has a mortality of around 60% and a 75% incidence of severe disability. The relevance of neonatal encephalopathy is in marked contrast to other potential predictors of outcome such as the results of continuous fetal heart rate monitoring, fetal scalp or umbilical cord pH and the Apgar score, which are unhelpful.

Table 49.3 **Summary of intracerebral events involved in the pathogenesis of hypoxic-ischemic brain damage**

Primary cerebral energy failure[1]
Experimental evidence in animals indicates that a hypoxic-ischemic insult leads to: ▪ cessation of cerebral oxidative metabolism ▪ increase in cerebral lactic acid ▪ a fall in intracellular pH ▪ failure of ionic transport mechanisms ▪ necrotic cell death
Restoration of cerebral energy levels
Resuscitation at birth leads to a rapid restoration of cerebral energy
Secondary cerebral energy failure
Some hours after resuscitation a secondary fall in cerebral energy occurs in association with: ▪ increased excitatory activity ▪ accumulation of intracellular calcium ▪ accumulation of toxic free radicals ▪ enhanced cytokine expression ▪ increase in cerebral lactic acid ▪ *rise* in intracellular pH ▪ mitochondrial dysfunction ▪ apoptosis and necrosis

[1]Chemicals that reflect energy metabolism can be measured in the brain by magnetic resonance spectroscopy. A fall in the ratio of phosphocreatine to inorganic phosphate is an indicator of impaired energy metabolism

Neonatal encephalopathy has itself been used as an outcome to investigate the role of preconception, antepartum and intrapartum characteristics in its etiology[19,20]. These studies have revealed a wide spectrum of risks, including socioeconomic markers, and antepartum factors such as maternal thyroid disease, severe pre-eclampsia, fetal growth retardation and bleeding[19]. This has led to a view that neonatal encephalopathy, even when preceded by signs of 'fetal distress' and a low Apgar score, may reflect dominant antepartum insults, with the fetus responding poorly to relatively mild hypoxia during labor – the already compromised fetus. In these and similar studies, the relative importance of antepartum and intrapartum factors is influenced by the precise criteria used for the definition of neonatal encephalopathy, especially whether it includes a measure of perinatal asphyxia, such as the infant's condition at birth and the umbilical cord pH value, in addition to the neurological signs of encephalopathy.

When brain MRI examinations are made within 2 weeks of birth, it is possible to distinguish acute lesions of recent onset (presumed intrapartum) from established lesions, such as atrophy and porencephaly, which are presumed to have an antepartum cause. Among infants with encephalopathy *and* some features of perinatal asphyxia (such as late decelerations on fetal monitoring, depressed respiration at birth or an arterial cord blood academia), acute evolving lesions compatible with recent hypoxic-ischemic injury were observed in 80% and consisted of bilateral abnormalities in basal ganglia, thalami, cortex or white matter. In contrast, less than 1% had evidence of an established lesion of antepartum origin[21]. In the same study, infants who presented with neonatal seizures alone without features of perinatal asphyxia had an incidence of acute ischemic or hemorrhagic lesions of around 70%, but the spectrum of injury was quite different and consisted mainly of focal infarction. Lesions of presumed antepartum origin were seen in only 3%.

These observations do not rule out the possibility of antepartum predisposition to damage. They do, however, support the notion that the train of hypoxic-ischemic events that culminate in neurodisability occurs at a time when improved methods of intrapartum diagnosis, together with postnatal neuroprotection, may be beneficial for some infants.

Brain MRI examination is used as a research tool in the neonatal period. There is, however, considerable experience of MRI in the investigation of children with cerebral palsy. In a study from eight European centers[22], the MRI brain scans of 351 children with cerebral palsy were classified according to the lesions seen. The most common finding was white matter damage which was observed in 43%, with a quarter of these children being born at term. Basal ganglia lesions and cortical or subcortical lesions, which are consistent with intrapartum perinatal hypoxia-ischemia, together accounted for 22% of lesions.

Bilateral lesions of the basal ganglia and thalamus have special relevance because of the evidence that they are associated with a causal event characterized by acute profound hypoxia-ischemia of relatively brief duration[23,24]. Such lesions have been reported following cord prolapse, abruption, eclampsia, maternal circulatory collapse and the sudden onset of severe fetal bradycardia. Early observations showing that newborns who are resuscitated after severe depression of vital signs at birth including cardiac arrest do not necessarily develop disabilities suggest that there must be some tolerance to this type of insult. Based to a large extent on animal evidence, the notion has grown that human fetuses can withstand a period of 10 minutes or so of profound acute hypoxia before brain damage develops. A degree of precision seems to have been accepted by lawyers who may use the expression 'the 10-minute rule'. This poses a huge challenge for obstetric practice because it implies that to avoid injury delivery needs to be expedited within 10 minutes of the onset of the insult, which itself can rarely be precisely defined.

Hypothermia rescue therapy

Following hypoxic-ischemic injury, mild hypothermia has a neuroprotective effect and this is probably exerted by amelioration of various adverse processes shown in Table 49.3, in addition to reducing the cerebral metabolic rate for glucose and oxygen and the extent of secondary energy failure.

Following diverse animal experiments and preliminary studies in human infants designed to test the safety of hypothermia and the logistics, there have been several randomized controlled trials testing the effect of head cooling or whole body cooling in newborns with suspected hypoxic-ischemic encephalopathy. The longest period of follow-up so far is 18 months which has been achieved in only two reported trials. The 'CoolCap' study[25] used selective head cooling for 72 hours while aiming to maintain the rectal temperature at 34–35°C. The entry criteria were moderate or severe encephalopathy and abnormal amplitude integrated electroencephalography (aEEG). A total of 234 infants were randomized and there was no significant difference in the incidence of the composite outcome of death or severe disability at 18 months (treated 55%, control 66%). However, when adjustment was made for the severity of the aEEG, there was a significant benefit for those infants with less severe aEEG changes.

The study of the National Institute of Child Health and Human Development (NICHD) network[26] employed whole body cooling aiming for an esophageal temperature of 33.5°C for 72 hours. The entry criteria were moderate or severe encephalopathy with either severe acidosis or with perinatal complications and resuscitation at birth. A total of 208 infants were randomized and the composite outcome of death or moderate or severe disability occurred in 44% of the treated group and in 62% of controls ($P = 0.01$). However, when mortality and disability were analyzed individually, there was no significant difference in their incidence between the two study groups.

These and other smaller trials are promising but leave many unanswered questions[27]. Although mild hypothermia appears to be safe, further information is needed so that the appropriate population can be targeted for treatment in a way that may yield long-term benefit with minimal cost. Hypothermia rescue therapy should be used only in the context of randomized controlled trials, or in connection with an appropriately maintained database which is accessible to other users.

REFERENCES

1. Costeloe K, Hennessy E, Gibson AT, Marlow N, Wilkinson AR and for the EPICure Study Group. The EPICure study: outcomes to discharge from hospital for infants born at the threshold of viability. *Pediatrics* **106**:659–671, 2000.
2. Walsh MC, Yao Q, Gettner P et al. National Institute of Child Health and Human Development Neonatal Research Network. Impact of a physiologic definition on bronchopulmonary dysplasia rates. *Pediatrics* **114**:1305–1311, 2004.
3. Chess PR, D'Angio CT, Pryhuber GS, Maniscalco WM. Pathogenesis of bronchopulmonary dysplasia. *Semin Perinatol* **30**:171–178, 2006.
4. Speer CP. Inflammation and bronchopulmonary dysplasia. *Semin Neonatol* **8**:29–38, 2003.
5. Choi CW, Kim BI, Park JD, Koh YY, Choi J-H, Choi Y. Risk factors for the different types of chronic lung diseases of prematurity according to the preceding respiratory distress syndrome. *Pediatr Int* **47**:417–423, 2005.
6. Parker RA, Lindstrom DP, Cotton RB. Evidence from twin study implies possible genetic susceptibility to bronchopulmonary dysplasia. *Semin Perinatol* **20**:206–209, 1996.
7. Bhandari V, Gruen JR. The genetics of bronchopulmonary dysplasia. *Semin Neonatol* **30**:185–191, 2006.
8. Anderson PJ, Doyle LW. Neurodevelopmental outcome of bronchopulmonary dysplasia. *Semin Perinatol* **30**:227–232, 2006.
9. Bhandari A, Panitch HB. Pulmonary outcomes in bronchopulmonary dysplasia. *Semin Perinatol* **30**:219–226, 2006.
10. Ethical issues at the outset of life. In *Contemporary issues in fetal and neonatal medicine*, Weil WB, Benjamin M (eds). Boston: Blackwell Scientific Publications, 1987.
11. Hussain N, Rosenkrantz TS. Ethical considerations in the managements of infants born at extremely low gestational age. *Semin Perinatol* **27**:458–470, 2003.
12. Nuffield Council on Bioethics. Dilemmas in current practice: babies born at the borderline of viability. *Critical Care Decisions in Fetal and Neonatal Medicine: Ethical Issues* (November):67–87, 2006.
13. El-Khoury N, Braun A, Hu F et al. Astrocyte end-feet in germinal matrix, cerebral cortex, and white matter in developing infants. *Pediatr Res* **59**:673–679, 2006.
14. Inder TE, Anderson NJ, Spencer C, Wells S, Volpe JJ. White matter injury in the premature infant: a comparison between serial cranial sonographic and MR findings at term. *Am J Neuroradiol* **24**:805–809, 2003.
15. Counsell SJ, Allsop JM, Harrison C et al. Diffusion-weighted imaging of the brain in preterm infants with focal and diffuse white matter abnormality. *Pediatrics* **112**:1–7, 2003.
16. Volpe JJ. Cerebral white matter injury of the preterm infant – more common than you think (commentary). *Pediatrics* **112**:176–180, 2003.
17. Edwards AD, Azzopardi DV. Perinatal hypoxia-ischemia and brain injury. *Pediatr Res* **47**:431–432, 2000.
18. Peliowski A, Finer NN. Birth asphyxia in the term infant. In *Effective care of the newborn infant*, JC Sinclair, MB Bracken (eds), pp. 249–279. Oxford: Oxford University Press, 1992.
19. Badawi N, Kurinczuk JJ, Keogh JM. Antepartum risk factors for newborn encephalopathy: the Western Australian case-control study. *Br Med J* **317**:1549–1553, 1998.
20. Badawi N, Kurinczuk J, Keogh JM et al. Intrapartum risk factors for newborn encephalopathy: the Western Australian case-control study. *Br Med J* **317**:1554–1558, 1998.
21. Cowan F, Rutherford M, Groenedaal F et al. Origin and timing of brain lesions in term infants with neonatal encephalopathy. *Lancet* **367**:36–42, 2003.
22. Bax M, Tydeman C, Flodmark O. Clinical and MRI correlates of cerebral palsy. The European Cerebral Palsy Study. *J Am Med Assoc* **296**:1602–1608, 2006.
23. Rolan EH, Poskitt K, Rodriguez E, Lupton B, Hill A. Perinatal hypoxic-ischemic thalamic injury: clinical features and neuroimaging. *Ann Neurol* **44**:161–166, 1998.
24. Krageloh-Mann I, Helber A, Mader I et al. Bilateral lesions of the thalamus and basal ganglia: origin and outcome. *Dev Med Child Neurol* **44**:477–484, 2002.
25. Gluckman P, Wyatt JS, Azzopardi D et al. Selective head cooling after neonatal encephalopathy. *Lancet* **365**:1619–1620, 2005.
26. Shankarin S, Laptook AR, Ehrenkranz RA et al. Whole-body hypothermia for neonates with hypoxic-ischaemic encephalopathy. *N Eng J Med* **353**: 1574–1584, 2005.
27. Azzopardi D, Edwards AD. Hypothermia. *Semin Fet Neonat Med* **12**:303–310, 2007.

Self-assessment scenarios

Pranav Pandya

QUESTIONS

Chapter 19 (Image SA-01)

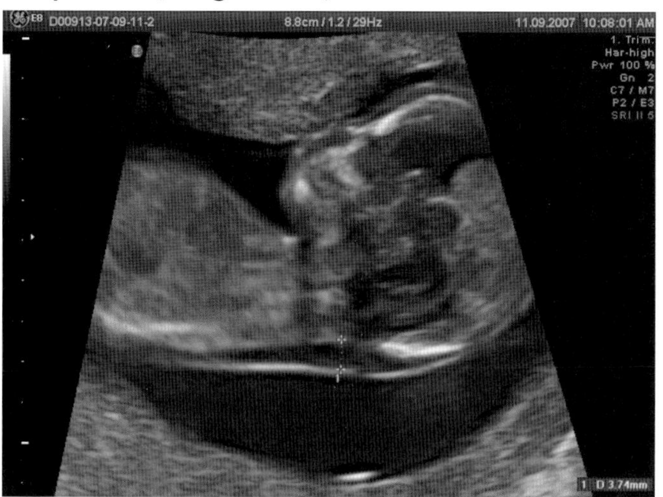

Q1. What does the Image SA-01 show?
Q2. What is the differential diagnosis?
Q3. What is your management?

Chapter 20 (Image SA-02)

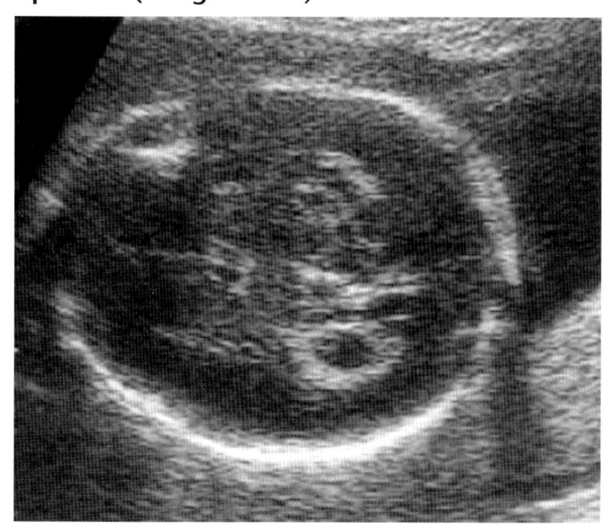

Q1. What does the Image SA-02 show?
Q2. What is your management?

Chapter 28 (Image SA-03)

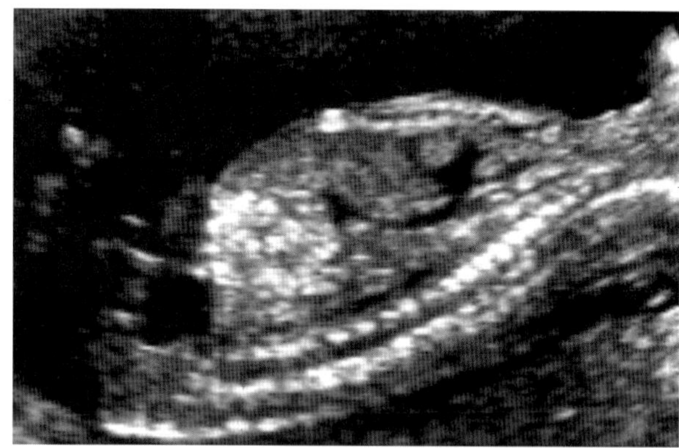

Q1. What does the Image SA-03 show?
Q2. What is the differential diagnosis?
Q3. What is your management?

Chapter 30 (Image SA-04)

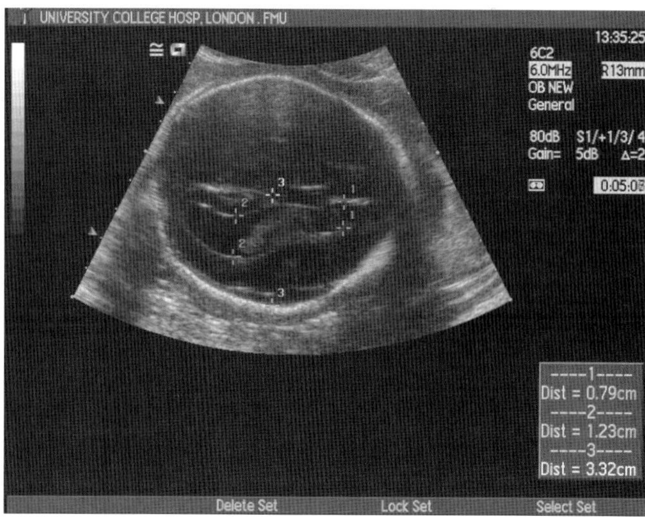

Q1. What does the Image SA-04 show?
Q2. What is it commonly associated with?
Q3. What is your management?
Q4. What is the prognosis if the abnormality remains unchanged?

Chapter 31 (Image SA-05)

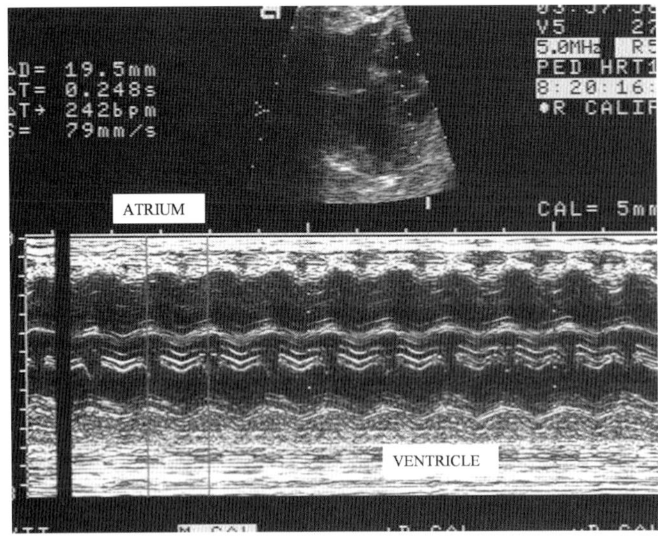

Q1. What is the likely diagnosis?
Q2. What is your management?

Chapter 32

Scenario A (Image SA-06)

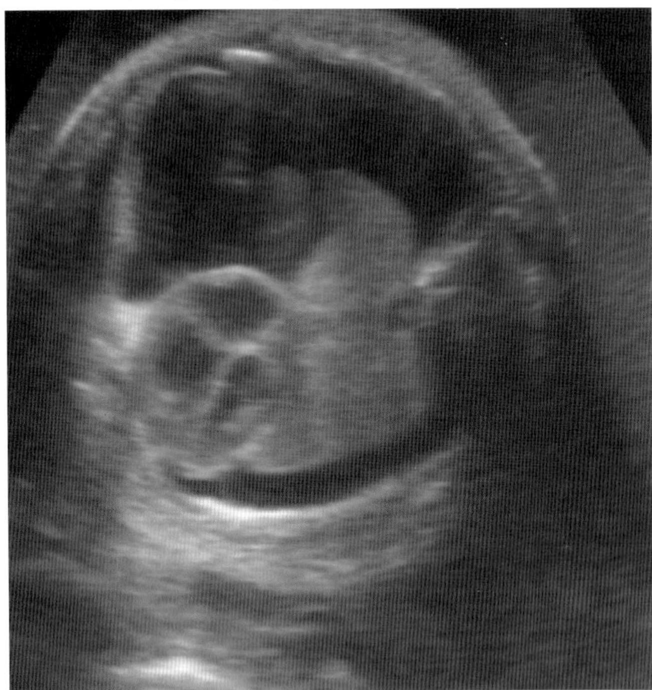

Q1. What does the Image SA-06 show?
Q2. What are the most common possible causes if isolated?
Q3. What is your management?
Q4. What is the prognosis?

Scenario B (Images SA-07 and SA-08)

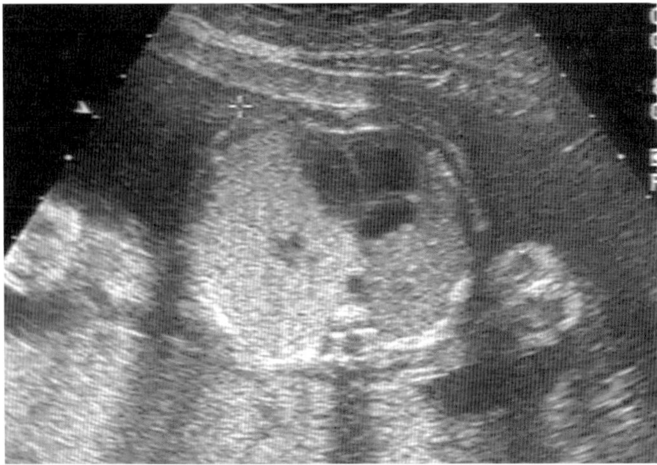

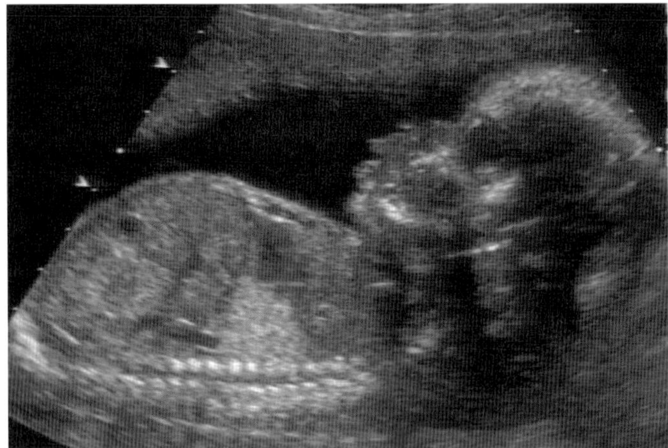

Q1. What do the Images SA-07 and SA-08 show and what is the likely diagnosis?
Q2. What is the differential diagnosis?
Q3. What is your management?
Q4. What is the prognosis of this condition?

Chapter 33 (Images SA-09 and SA-10)

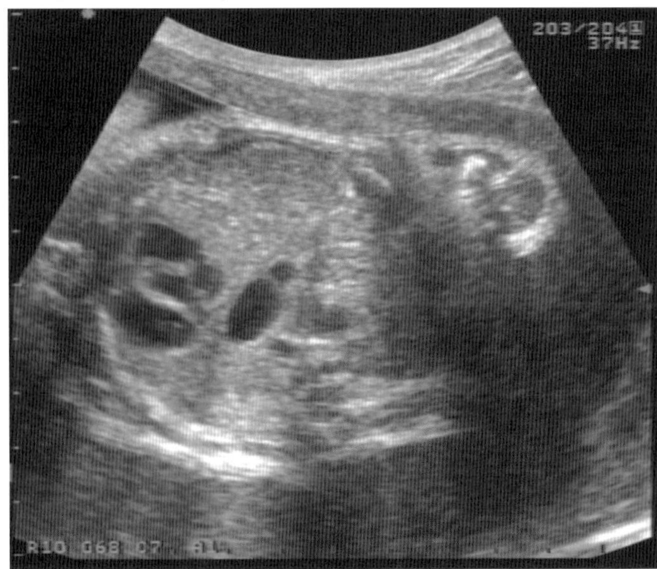

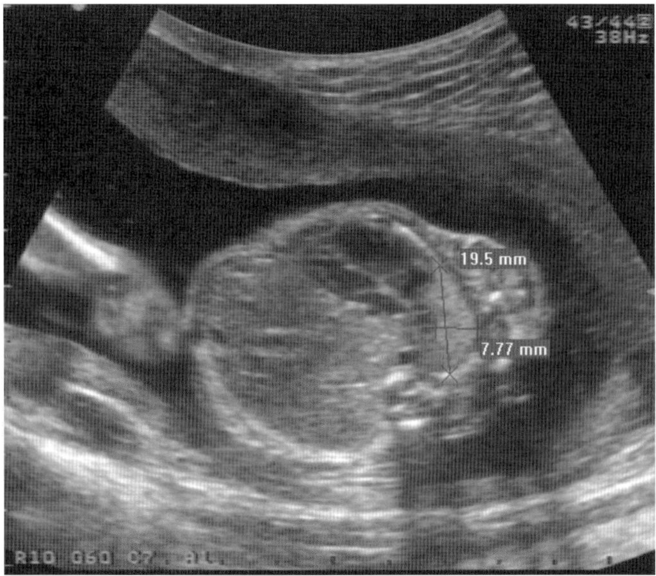

Q1. What do the Images SA-09 and SA-10 show?
Q2. What is the differential diagnosis?
Q3. What is your plan of management?
Q4. What markers are associated with a poor prognosis?
Q5. What is the survival rate?

Chapter 34

Scenario A (Images SA-11 and SA-12)

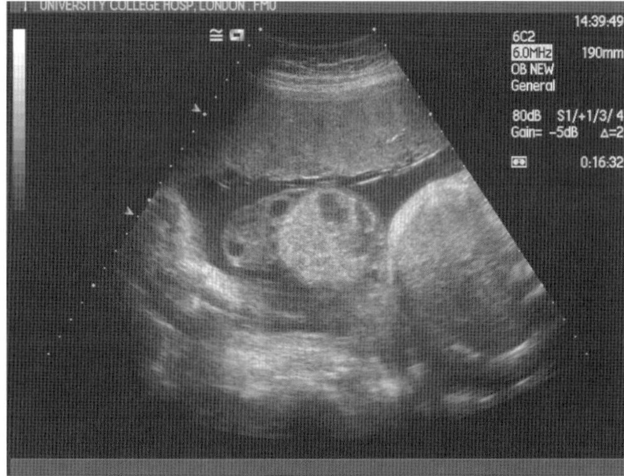

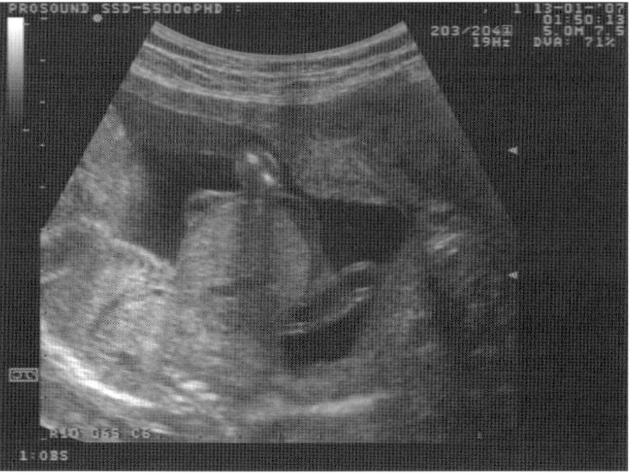

Q1. What is the likely diagnosis in images SA-11 and SA-12?
Q2. What abnormalities is this condition associated with?
Q3. What is the management of this abnormality?
Q4. What is the prognosis?

Scenario B (Images SA-13 and SA-14)

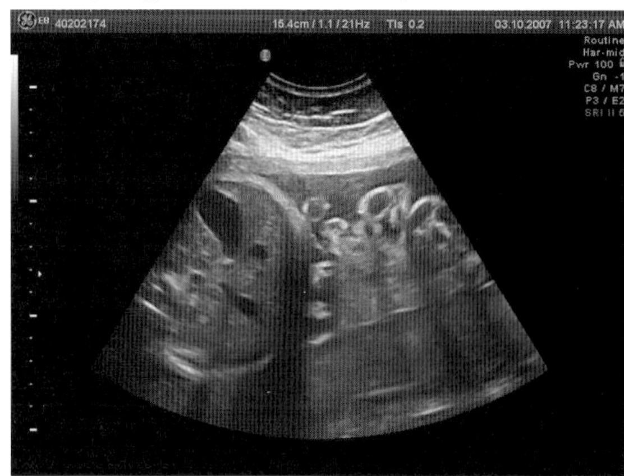

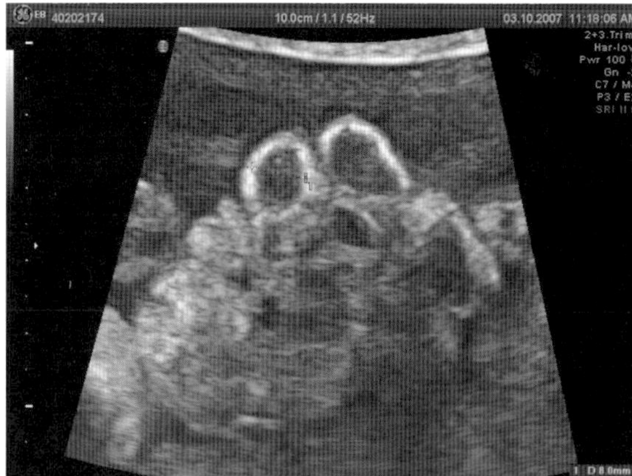

Q1. What is the likely diagnosis in images SA-13 and SA-14?
Q2. How do you distinguish this condition from the main differential?
Q3. What is the management of this abnormality?

Chapter 35

Scenario A (Image SA-15)

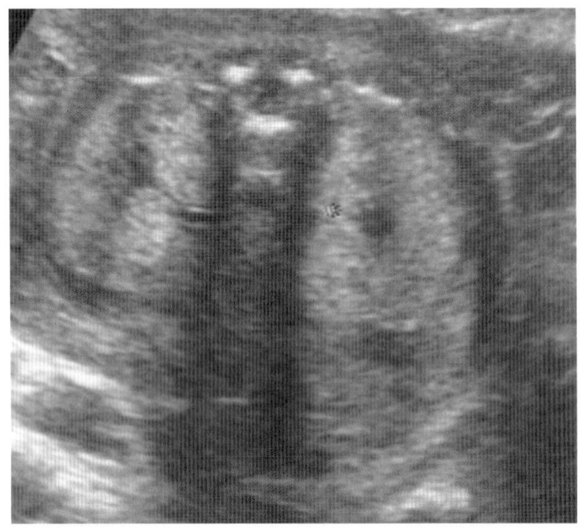

Q1. What does the Image SA-15 show?
Q2. What is the differential diagnosis?
Q3. What is your management?
Q4. What is the prognosis for each of the above differentials?
Q5. What is the recurrence risk for each differential?

Scenario B (Image SA-16)

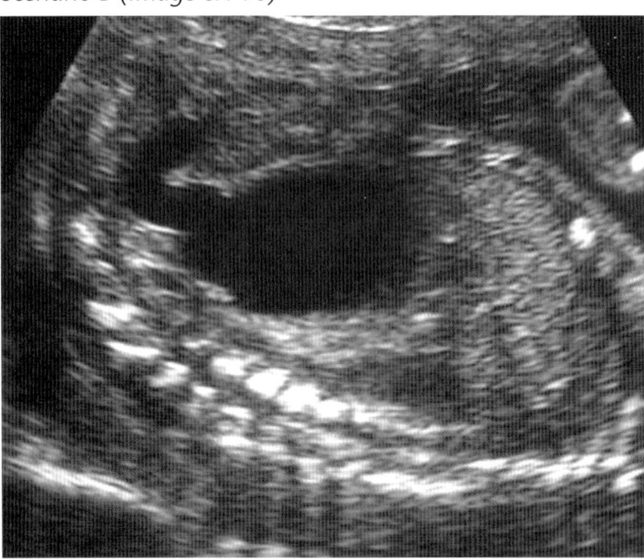

Q1. What does the Image SA-16 show?
Q2. What is the most likely diagnosis?
Q3. What are the other possible ultrasound features of the most likely diagnosis?
Q4. What is the management?
Q5. What is the recurrence risk?

Chapter 36

Q1. A fetus has a femur length below the 3rd centile at 20 weeks of gestation What is the management in this pregnancy?

Chapter 37 (Image SA-17)

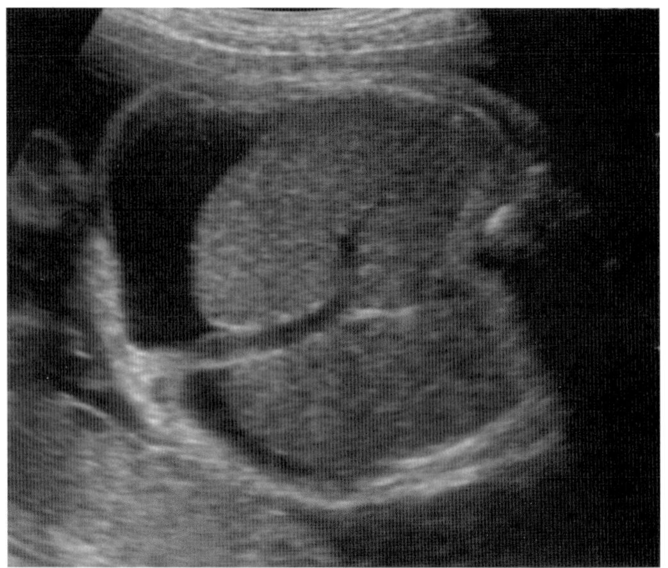

Q1. What does the Image SA-17 show?
Q2. What is the differential diagnosis?
Q3. What is your management?

Chapter 38 (Image SA-18)

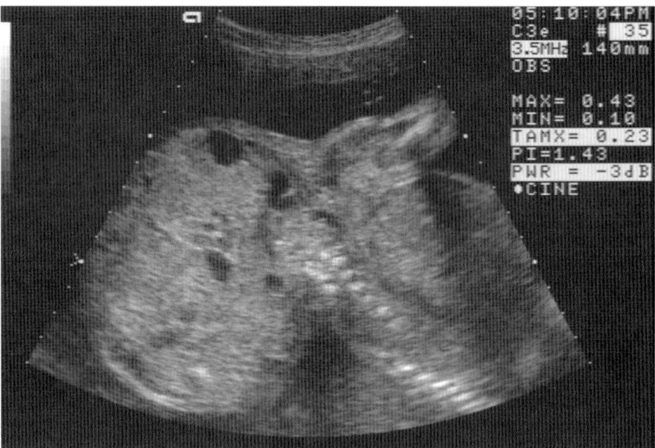

Q1. What does the Image SA-18 show?
Q2. How can this condition be classified?
Q3. What is the incidence?
Q4. What is your antenatal management?

Chapter 39 (Images SA-19)

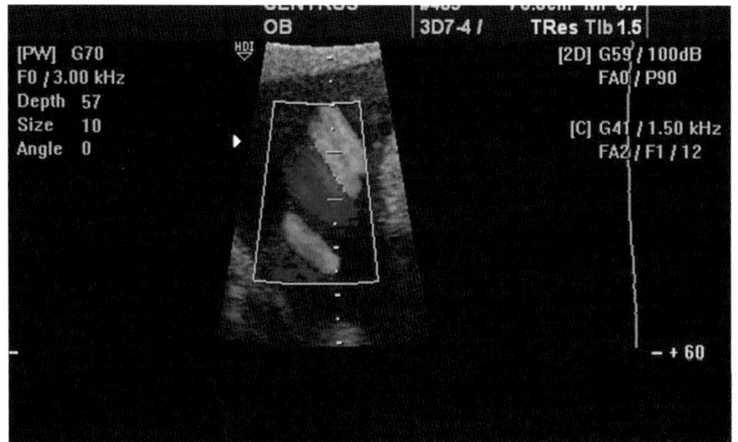

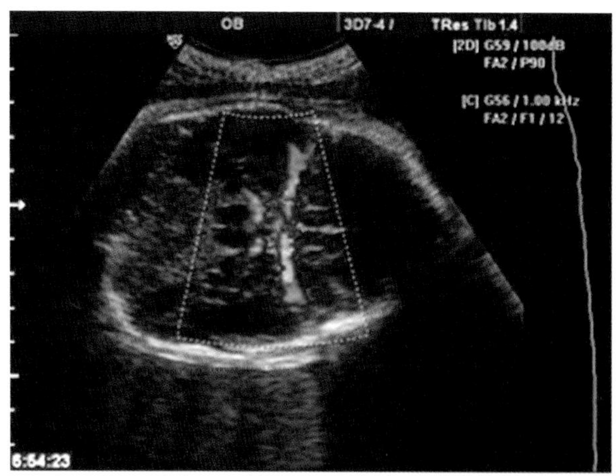

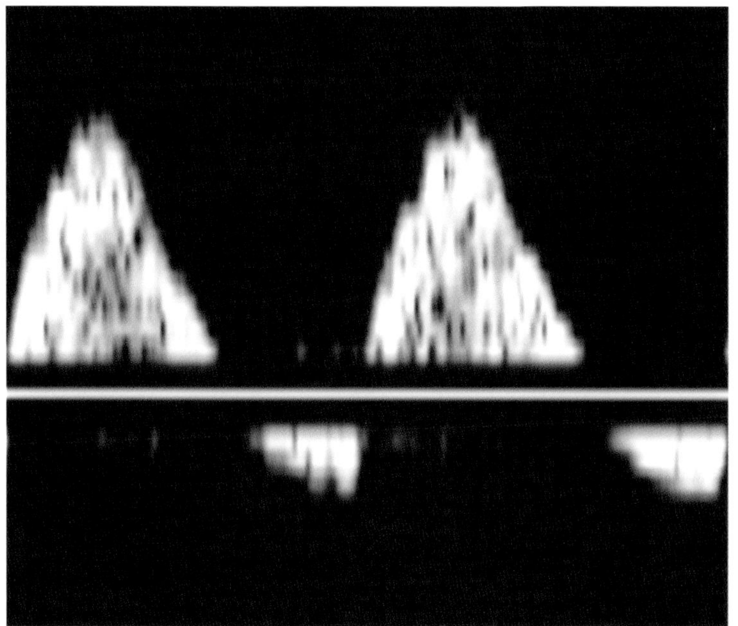

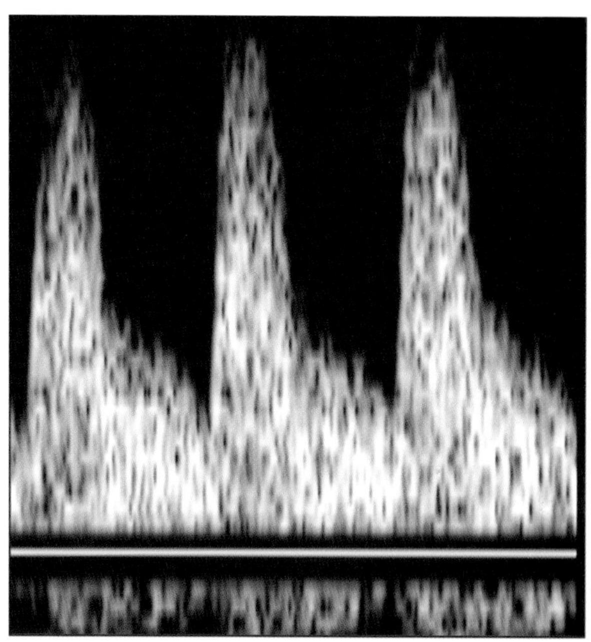

Q1. What do the Images SA-19 show?
Q2. What is your management?

Chapter 40 (Image SA-20)

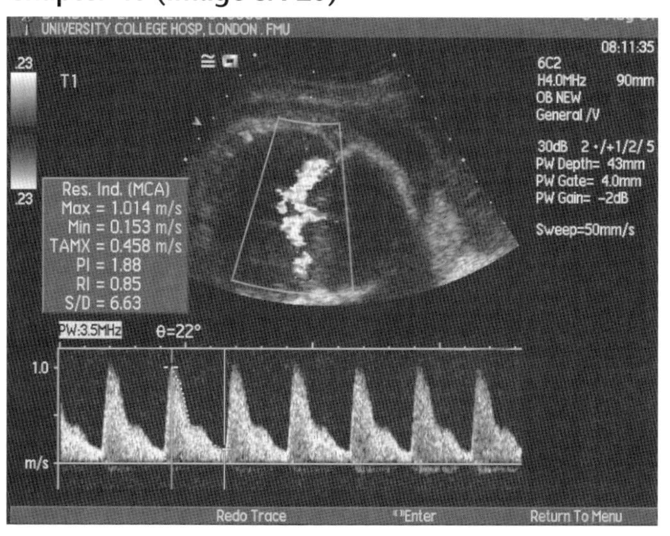

Q1. What does the Image SA-20 show?
Q2. What is your management?

Chapter 41 (Image SA-21)

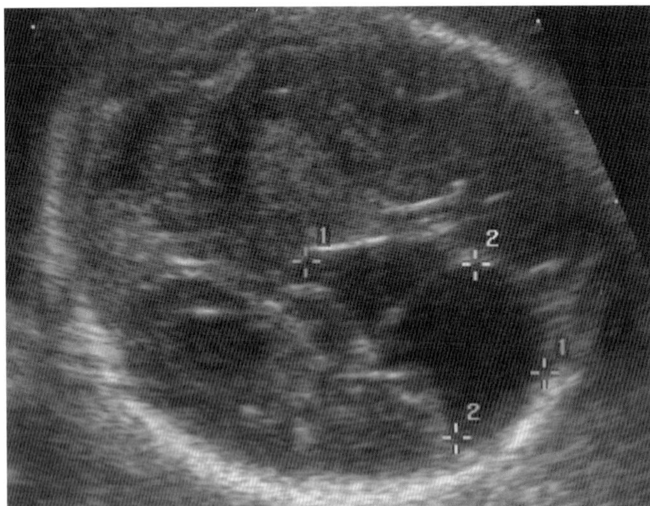

Q1. What does the Image SA-21 show?
Q2. What is the differential diagnosis?
Q3. What is your management?
Q4. What is the prognosis?

Chapter 45

Scenario A (Image SA-22)

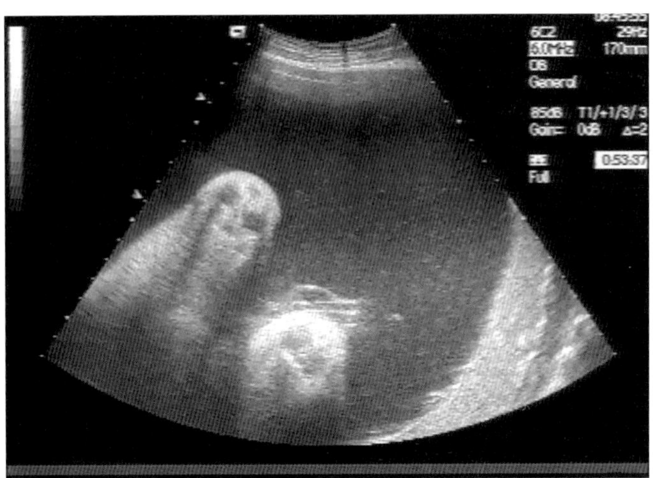

Q1. What does the Image SA-22 show?
Q2. What are the causes of this condition?
Q3. What is your management?

Scenario B (Images SA-23 and SA-24)

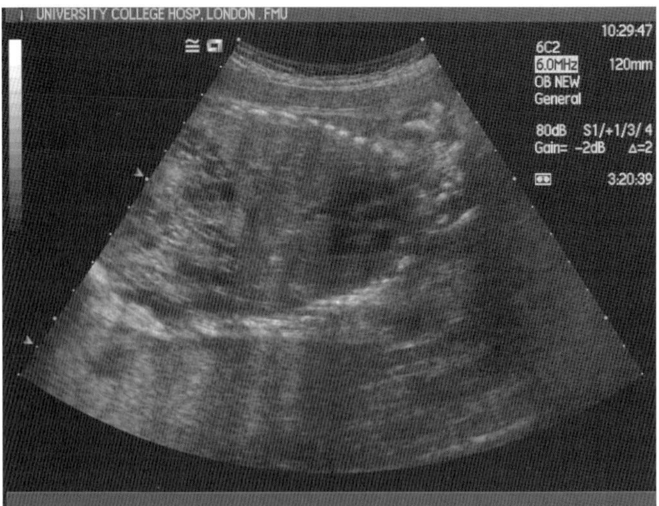

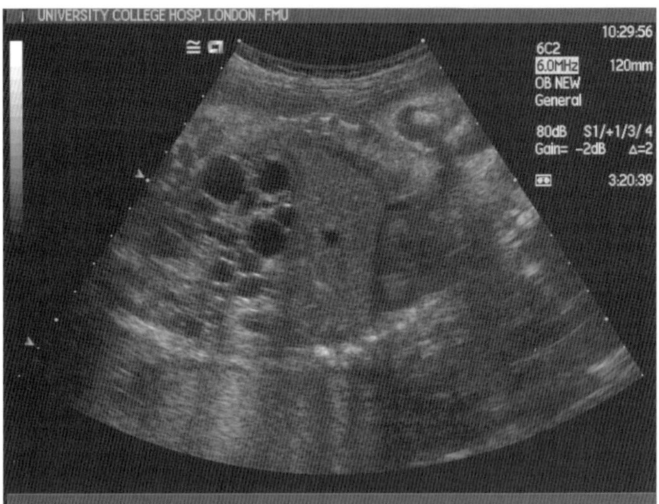

Q1. What do the Images SA-23 and SA-24 show?
Q2. What are the causes of this condition?
Q3. What is your management?

Chapter 46 (Images SA-25 and SA-26)

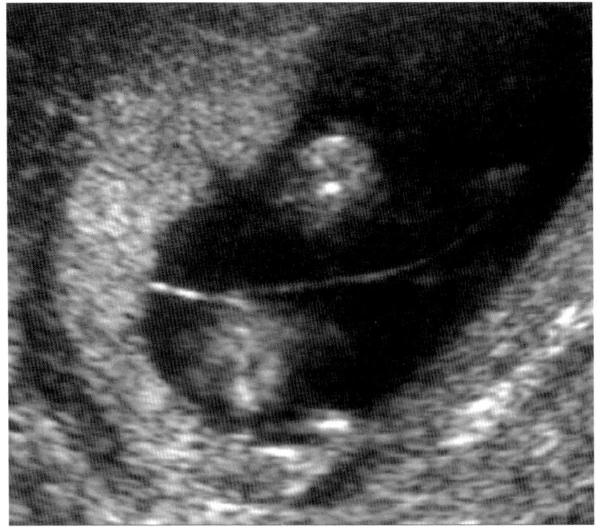

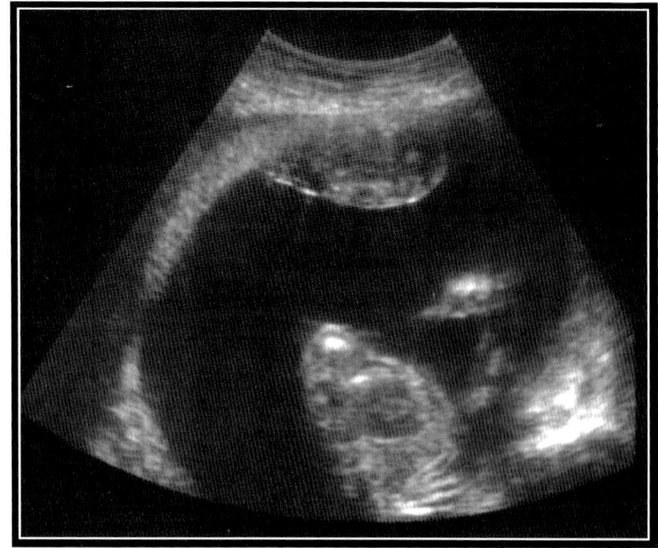

Q1. What do the Images SA-25 and SA-26 show?
Q2. What is the diagnosis?
Q3. What is the management?

ANSWERS

Chapter 19

A1. Increased fetal nuchal translucency

A2. Normal fetus
Chromosomal abnormality, trisomy 21, 18, 13, 45X
Cardiac defect
Congenital diaphragmatic hernia (CDH)
Exomphalos
Skeletal dysplasia
Genetic syndrome, e.g. Noonan's

A3. Detailed scan – look for markers and major structural anomalies, e.g. nasal bone, ductus venosus, tricuspid regurgitation, exomphalos, diaphragmatic hernia, megacystis
Offer fetal karyotyping – chorionic villus sampling (CVS) at 11–14 weeks
If chromosomes normal: detailed and cardiac scan at 15 and 20 weeks
If resolves reassure – good prognosis
Persistent edema {> 6 mm} – TORCH screen (Toxoplasmosis, rubella, cytomegalovirus, herpes simplex), consider genetic syndrome
The bigger the nuchal measurement, the greater the risk of fetal loss and the less likelihood of a normal baby.

Chapter 20

A1. Choroid plexus cysts

A2. Detailed scan
Ask about screening (maternal serum hCG <0.5 MoM increases risk of trisomy 18)
Risk of trisomy 18 is background risk if isolated
Risk of trisomy 21 not increased
No repeat scan required

Chapter 28

A1. Hyperechogenic bowel

A2. Normal
Ingested blood
Chromosomal abnormality
Infection
Intrauterine growth restriction
Cystic fibrosis (CF)

A3. Ask about vaginal bleeding
Detailed scan – evidence of intrauterine bleeding (placental lakes/particles in amniotic fluid) other markers of trisomy 21, dilated bowel
Consider fetal karyotype if other markers seen
TORCH screen (Toxoplasmosis, rubella, cytomegalovirus, herpes simplex)
CF screen
Serial scans for growth including uterine artery Dopplers at 24 weeks

Chapter 30

A1. Mild ventriculomegaly

A2. Chromosomal abnormalities
Congenital infection (TORCH screen, Toxoplasmosis, rubella, cytomegalovirus, herpes simplex)
Other central nervous system (CNS) abnormalities
Extra-CNS abnormalities
Genetic syndromes
Brain hemorrhage e.g. fetal alloimmune thrombocytopenia

A3. Detailed scan
TORCH (Toxoplasmosis, rubella, cytomegalovirus, herpes simplex) serology
Anti-platelet antibody screen
Fetal karyotyping
Repeat scan to look for progression
Consider fetal MRI

A4. Isolated bilateral or unilateral ventriculomegaly with an atrial width of 10–12 mm has an extremely high chance of an entirely normal outcome, especially for male fetuses, whereas with isolated bilateral ventriculomegaly of 12–15 mm or with asymmetrical dilatation of both ventricles the risk of developmental delay in this group is probably of the order of 15% overall, with 8% experiencing moderate to severe neurodevelopmental problems and the remaining 7% having only mild delay.

Chapter 31

A1. A dysrrhythmia – supraventricular tachycardia

A2. Detailed scan
Refer for fetal echocardiography
Consider medical treatment or delivery depending on gestational age and fetal well-being (e.g. Digoxin if non-hydropic or flecainide if hydropic)
Serial scans
If hydropic, admit to hospital and give the drug treatment directly to the fetus by injection into the umbilical vein
May require cesarean section for delivery – difficult to monitor fetal heart rate in labor

Chapter 32

Scenario A

A1. Bilateral pleural effusions

A2. Primary – excessive production or reduced absorption of lymphatic fluid
Secondary –
Chromosomal
Thoracic lesion – congenital cystic adenomatoid malformation (CCAM)/Congenital diaphragmatic hernia (CDH)/sequestration of the lung
Infection – cytomegalovirus (CMV)
Genetic syndrome, e.g. Noonans/Opitz

A3. Detailed scan
Congenital infection screen
Karyotype
Serial scans
Consider shunt/drainage

A4. Depends on associated features and gestation
Good – 70% survival if unilateral (50% if bilateral)

Scenario B

A1. Bright area in lung
Congenital cystic adenomatoid malformation of the lung (CCAM)

A2. Pulmonary sequestration
Congenital diaphragmatic hernia
Tumor

A3. Detailed scan
No karyotype
Serial scans
Refer to pediatric surgeon

A4. Good if unilateral >90% survival. Poor if hydrops develops 15% survival
30% resolve prenatally
All require postnatal follow-up and imaging

Chapter 33

A1. Left-sided congenital diaphragmatic hernia (CDH) (SA-09) with heart deviated to right and stomach bubble in chest behind heart
Measurement of the right lung area to calculate the lung: head ratio (LHR) (SA-10)

A2. CCAM
Pulmonary hypoplasia

A3. Detailed scan
Fetal echocardiography
Offer fetal karyotyping
Refer to pediatric surgeons
Discuss termination of pregnancy (TOP)
Serial scans
Delivery in unit with neonatal intensive care and pediatric surgery
Tracheal occlusion is highly specialised and experimental

A4. Abnormal karyotype
Congenital heart disease
Liver in chest
Polyhydramnios
Reduced lung:head ratio

A5. 60–70% if isolated

Chapter 34

Scenario A

A1. Exomphalos

A2. Trisomy 18 and 13
Congenital heart disease
Cloacal abnormalities/bladder extrophy
Genetic syndromes e.g. Beckwith–Wiedemann

A3. Detailed scan including fetal echocardiography
Karyotype
Refer to pediatric surgeons
Delivery in a unit with pediatric surgery

A4. Good if isolated (95% survival)
Depends on associated abnormalities

Scenario B

A1. Gastroschisis

A2. Defect in the anterior abdominal wall to the right of umbilicus
Normal cord insertion
Free floating bowel/no covering membrane

A3. Detailed scan
Not associated with chromosomal abnormalities – karyotype not offered
Refer to pediatric surgeons
Delivery in a unit with pediatric surgery; plan for vaginal delivery
Serial scans looking for intrauterine growth restriction and bowel dilatation
Consider delivery at 37 weeks or earlier if bowel dilatation

Chapter 35

Scenario A

A1. Big bright kidneys

A2. Infantile polycystic kidney disease (autosomal recessive)
Genetic syndrome e.g. Beckwith–Wiedemann
Normal variant
Adult polycystic kidney disease (autosomal dominant)
Rare metabolic syndromes, e.g. nephrocalcinosis
Trisomy 13

A3. Ask about family history
Detailed scan
Consider karyotype
Consider scanning kidneys of parents

A4. Lethal
Depends on syndrome (likely poor)
Good
Maybe poor if antenatally diagnosed
Depends on syndrome (likely to be poor)
Lethal

A5. 1 in 4
Depends on syndrome
Sporadic
Depends on syndrome
1 in 2
0.75% + maternal age related risk for trisomy 13 (low)

Scenario B

A1. Midline cystic structure in pelvis — likely megacystis and dilated proximal urethra

A2. Posterior urethral valves

A3. 'Keyhole' sign
Thick-walled bladder
Reduced amniotic fluid volume
Hydronephrosis +/− dilated ureter
Echogenic small kidneys
Small chest

A4. Consider karyotype
Determine gender
Offer termination of pregnancy
Consider aspiration to test urinary function – Na/Ca/β2 microglobulin
Consider vesicoamniotic shunt

A5. Sporadic

Chapter 36

A1. Look at the parents' size
Confirm gestational age (wrong dates?)
Look for markers for chromosomal aneuploidy
Fetal growth restriction – measure the fetal biometry, assess amniotic fluid volume and check uterine artery Dopplers and fetal Dopplers (umbilical artery +/− middle cerebral artery)
Measure all the long bones and look for bowing/fractures
Measure thorax/abdominal circumference ratio (<0.8 suggest small thorax)
Skull – look for macrocranium, frontal bossing, clover-leaf
Hands – look for polydactyly, trident hands
Calcification – hypomineralization

Chapter 37

A1. Fetal ascites

A2. Fetal anemia – fetal red cell alloimmunization, parvovirus
Hydrops
Infection
Meconium peritonitis
Urinary ascites
Metabolic syndrome

A3. Detailed scan + fetal echocardiography
Non-invasive assessment for fetal anemia – peak systolic velocity in the middle cerebral artery
TORCH + parvovirus serology
Invasive fetal karyotyping – consider fetal blood sampling +/− intrauterine transfusion

Chapter 38

A1. Sacrococcygeal teratoma

A2. Types I–IV: type I completely external, type IV completely internal

A3. 1 in 40 000 births
F:M = 4:1 {malignant change more common in males}

A4. Refer to tertiary center
Serial scans – monitor size, polyhydramnios and signs of hydrops
Consider amniodrainage
Refer to pediatric surgeons
Consider mode of delivery – may need cesarean section
Fetal surgery may be considered in a few cases

Chapter 39

A1. Reversed end diastolic flow in umbilical artery and increased diastolic velocities in the middle cerebral artery suggestive of redistribution of cardiac output

A2. Measure fetal biometry
Ultrasound scan for anomalies and markers of aneuploidy
Measure amniotic fluid volume
Fetal heart rate monitoring (cardiotocogram)
Assess maternal well-being – blood pressure, proteinuria
Give antenatal prophylactic steroids
Consider delivery

Chapter 40

A1. Increased peak systolic velocity in the middle cerebral artery

A2. Detailed scan looking for signs of fetal anemia (ascites, cardiomegaly, hydrops)
Check maternal blood group and measure antibodies
Maternal serology for parvovirus
Depending on gestation consider fetal blood sampling and intrauterine transfusion. If >34 weeks consider delivery

Chapter 41

A1. Cystic lesion in brain

A2. Intracranial hemorrhage (e.g. alloimmune thrombocytopenia)
Infection
Arachnoid cyst

A3. Detailed scan
Look for maternal antiplatelet antibodies
Maternal TORCH serology
Consider fetal MRI

A4. Depends on etiology, location and size
Can be very poor: brain damage, hydrocephalus, fetal death

Chapter 45

Scenario A

A1. Polyhydramnios

A2. Polyuria (diabetes)
Difficulty swallowing (neuromuscular or obstruction)
Placental tumors
Twin-twin transfusion syndrome

A3. Detailed scan
Exclude diabetes mellitus/gestational diabetes
Treat underlying cause, e.g. diabetes
Consider amniodrainage if mother symptomatic or tense polyhydramnios with risk of preterm rupture of membranes

Scenario B

A1. Anhydramnios and an echogenic cystic mass in the abdomen – possible multicystic dyplastic kidneys

A2. Rupture of membranes
Renal agenesis/severe renal anomalies/outflow obstruction
Severe growth restriction

A3. Detailed scan – use power Doppler to help identify renal arteries
Uterine artery and umbilical artery Dopplers
Speculum examination if considering ruptured membranes

Chapter 46

A1. 'T' sign
Severe amniotic fluid imbalance at the top of picture 'Stuck twin'

A2. Monochorionic diamniotic twin pregnancy
Twin-to-twin transfusion syndrome

A3. Fetoscopic laser ablation of communicating vessels
Amniodrainage

Appendix: Charts of fetal measurements

LS Chitty and Douglas G Altman

INTRODUCTION

There are hundreds of published papers presenting charts (standards) of fetal measurements. Unfortunately, many of these are methodologically unsound and thus of dubious value. The appropriate design and analysis of studies to derive reference centiles for fetal size can be found in the literature[1–3].

In this appendix, we present tables and charts of various measurements of fetal size derived from data collected in a prospective study which was designed expressly for the purpose of developing reference ranges[2,4–8]. In some cases, these differ slightly from those presented previously[4], as a result of improvements to the modelling procedure. We also include charts derived from other data sets. In some cases (e.g. fetal hematological measurements), ideal study design is not possible as samples have to be collected opportunistically when assessment is made for a clinical indication. In these cases, we have tried to include charts from studies with methodology as close as possible to the optimum. Where appropriate, we have added brief comments about methodological problems. For some measurements, because of inadequate documentation in published papers, we have been unable to produce suitable charts and tables although some data exist in the literature.

TABLES AND CHARTS

The tables and charts in the following pages show 5th, 50th and 95th centiles for each measurement by exact gestational age. For those attributed to Chitty et al. (or Chitty and Altman), fractional polynomial regression models were used; details of the methods of analysis are described[1,2]. The dating charts show predicted gestational age (in weeks and days) by fetal size. For these charts only data up to approximately 35 weeks of gestation are included, i.e. biparietal measurement (BPD) <89 mm, head circumference <322 mm and femur length <67 mm[5]. The 5th and 95th centiles tabulated here are slightly narrower than those published before, because the earlier paper[5] included tabulations of 95% rather than 90% ranges.

It is important to note that there are two fetal size and dating charts for the BPD to account for the different methods of making this measurement. In one it was measured from the proximal echo of the fetal skull to the distal side of the border deep to the ultrasound beam (outer–outer) and for the other, it was measured from the proximal edge to the proximal edge of the deep border (outer–inner). The differences in measurement are small, but the user should take care to use the chart appropriate to his/her measurement technique. All circumference measurements[6–8] (and others presented here) were derived from the maximum diameters using the equation $\pi\ (d_1 + d_2)/2$ where d_1 and d_2 were the two diameters. As with the BPD charts, there are two charts for the dating and two size charts for fetal head circumference measurements to take account of the different methods of measuring the BPD, which is d_1 in the equation used to derive the circumference.

REFERENCES

1. Altman DG, Chitty LS. Design and analysis of studies to derive charts of fetal size. *Ultrasound. Obstet Gynaecol* **3**: 378–384, 1993.
2. Altman DG, Chitty LS. Charts of fetal size: 1. Methodology. *Br J Obstet Gynaecol* **101**:29–34, 1994.
3. Royston P, Wright EM. How to construct 'normal ranges' for fetal variables. *Ultrasound Obstet Gynecol* **11**: 30–38, 1998.
4. Chitty LS, Altman DG. Charts of fetal size. In *Ultrasound in obstetrics and gynaecology*, K Dewbury, H Meire, D Cosgrove (eds), pp. 513–567. Edinburgh: Churchill Livingstone, 1993.
5. Altman DG, Chitty LS. New charts for ultrasound dating of pregnancy. *Ultrasound. Obstet Gynecol* **10**:1–18, 1997.
6. Chitty LS, Altman DG, Henderson A, Campbell S. Charts of fetal size: 2. Head measurements. *Br J Obstet Gynaecol* **101**:35–43, 1994.
7. Chitty LS, Altman DG, Henderson A, Campbell S. Charts of fetal size: 3. Abdominal circumference. *Br J Obstet Gynaecol* **101**:125–131, 1994.
8. Chitty LS, Altman DG, Henderson A, Campbell S. Charts of fetal size: 4. Femur length. *Br J Obstet Gynaecol* **101**:132–135, 1994.
9. Aoki S, Hata T, Kitao M. Ultrasonic assessment of fetal and neonatal spleen. *Am J Perinatol* **9**:361–367, 1992.
10. Vintzileos AM, Neckles S, Campbell WA, Andreoli JW, Kaplan BM, Nochimson DJ. Fetal liver ultrasound measurements during normal pregnancy. *Obstet Gynecol* **66**:477–480, 1985.
11. Merz E, Wellek S, Bahlmann F, Weber G. Sonographische Normkurven des fetalen knöchernen Thorax und der fetalen Lunge. *Geburtsh Frauenheilk* **55**:77–82, 1995.
12. Robinson HP, Fleming JEE. A critical evaluation of sonar crown–rump length measurements. *Br J Obstet Gynaecol* **89**:926–930, 1982.

13. Nicolaides KH, Economides DL, Soothill PW. Blood gases, pH, and lactate in appropriate- and small-for-gestational-age fetuses. *Am J Obstet Gynecol* **161**: 996–1001, 1989.
14. Arduini D, Rizzo G. Normal values of pulsatility index from fetal vessels: a cross-sectional study on 1556 healthy fetuses. *J Perinat Med* **18**:165–172, 1990.
15. Bower S, Vyas S, Campbell S, Nicolaides KH. Color Doppler imaging of the uterine artery in pregnancy: normal ranges of impedance to blood flow, mean velocity and volume of flow. *Ultrasound. Obstet Gynecol* **2**:261–265, 1992.
16. Moore TR, Cayle JE. The amniotic fluid index in normal human pregnancy. *Am J Obstet Gynecol* **162**:1168–1173, 1990.
17. Nicolaides KH, Soothill PW, Clewell WH, Rodeck CH, Mibashan RS, Campbell S. Fetal haemoglobin measurement in the assessment of red cell isoimmunisation. *Lancet* i:1073–1075, 1988.
18. Nicolini U, Fisk NM, Rodeck CH, Beacham J. Fetal urine biochemistry: an index of renal maturation and dysfunction. *Br J Obstet Gynaecol* **99**: 46–50, 1992.
19. Hadlock FP, Harrist RB, Sharman RS, Deter RL, Park SK. Estimation of fetal weight with the use of head, body, and femur measurements – a prospective study. *Am J Obstet Gynecol* **151**: 333–337, 1985.
20. Chitty LS, Campbell S, Altman DG. Measurement of the fetal mandible – feasibility and construction of a centile chart. *Prenat Diagn* **13**:749–756, 1993.

LIST OF TABLES AND CHARTS

1. Biparietal diameter (outer–outer)
2. Biparietal diameter (outer–inner)
3. Head circumference (derived from diameters) (a) using biparietal diameter outer–outer
4. Head circumference (derived from diameters) (b) using biparietal diameter outer–inner
5. Abdominal circumference (derived from diameters)
6. Head circumference/abdominal circumference ratio
7. Femur length
8. Humerus length
9. Radius length
10. Ulna length
11. Tibia length
12. Fibula length
13. Foot length
14. Mandible length
15. Transverse cerebellar diameter
16. Internal orbit diameter
17. External orbit diameter
18. Posterior horn/hemisphere ratio
19. Kidney length
20. Spleen length
21. Liver length
22. Thoracic circumference (derived from diameters)
23. Biparietal diameter (outer–outer) – dating chart
24. Biparietal diameter (outer–inner) – dating chart
25. Head circumference (derived from diameters) – dating chart (a) using biparietal diameter outer–outer
26. Head circumference (derived from diameters) – dating chart (b) using biparietal diameter outer–inner
27. Femur length – dating chart
28. Transverse cerebellar diameter – dating chart
29. Crown–rump length – dating chart
30. Umbilical vein Po_2
31. Umbilical vein Pco_2
32. Umbilical vein pH
33. Umbilical artery pulsatility index
34. Descending aorta pulsatility index
35. Renal artery pulsatility index
36. Internal carotid artery pulsatility index
37. Middle cerebral artery pulsatility index
38. Non-placental uterine artery pulsatility index
39. Placental uterine artery pulsatility index
40. Amniotic fluid index
41. Fetal hemoglobin
42. Fetal urinary sodium
43. Fetal weight estimated from abdominal circumference and femur length
44. Fetal weight from abdominal circumference (AC) and femur length (FL) (in mm)

1. **Biparietal diameter (outer–outer)**

Weeks of gestation	*Centiles (mm)*		
	5th	*50th*	*95th*
12	16.0	19.7	23.4
13	19.8	23.5	27.3
14	23.4	27.3	31.2
15	27.1	31.0	35.0
16	30.7	34.7	38.8
17	34.2	38.3	42.5
18	37.7	41.9	46.1
19	41.1	45.4	49.7
20	44.4	48.8	53.3
21	47.6	52.2	56.7
22	50.8	55.5	60.1
23	53.9	58.7	63.4
24	57.0	61.8	66.6
25	59.9	64.8	69.7
26	62.7	67.8	72.8
27	65.5	70.6	75.7
28	68.1	73.4	78.6
29	70.7	76.0	81.3
30	73.1	78.6	84.0
31	75.5	81.0	86.5
32	77.7	83.3	88.9
33	79.8	85.5	91.2
34	81.8	87.6	93.4
35	83.7	89.6	95.5
36	85.5	91.5	97.4
37	87.1	93.2	99.3
38	88.6	94.8	100.9
39	89.9	96.2	102.5
40	91.1	97.5	103.9
41	92.2	98.7	105.2
42	93.1	99.7	106.3

Source: Chitty et al.[6]

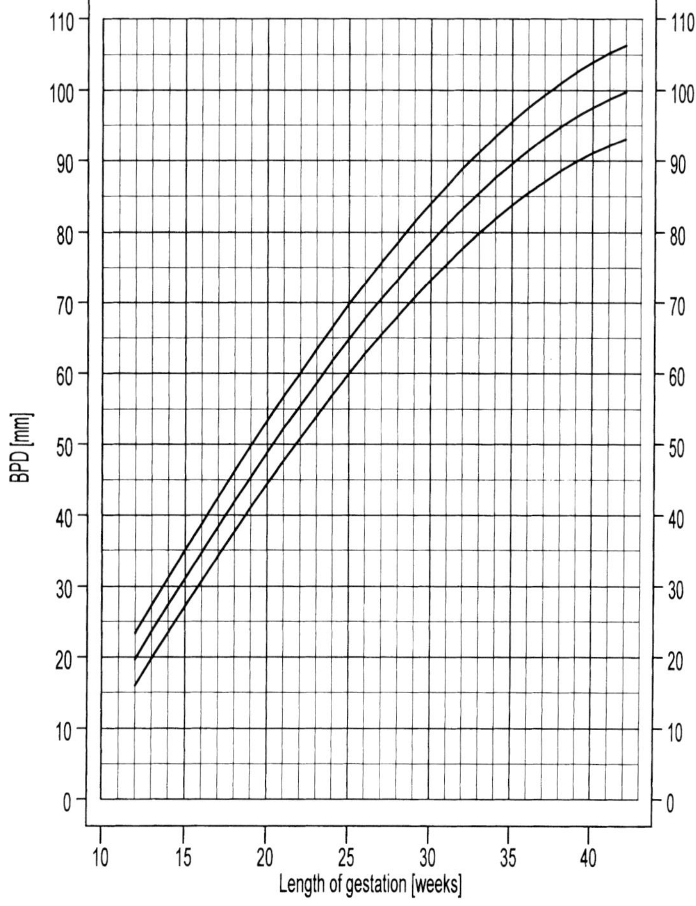

2. **Biparietal diameter (outer–inner)**

Weeks of gestation	Centiles (mm) 5th	50th	95th
12	14.9	18.3	21.7
13	18.5	22.0	25.5
14	22.0	25.6	29.2
15	25.6	29.3	33.0
16	29.0	32.8	36.7
17	32.4	36.3	40.3
18	35.7	39.8	43.9
19	39.0	43.2	47.4
20	42.3	46.5	50.8
21	45.4	49.8	54.2
22	48.5	53.0	57.5
23	51.5	56.1	60.7
24	54.4	59.2	63.9
25	57.3	62.1	67.0
26	60.1	65.0	70.0
27	62.8	67.8	72.9

Weeks of gestation	Centiles (mm) 5th	50th	95th
28	65.3	70.5	75.7
29	67.9	73.1	78.4
30	70.3	75.7	81.1
31	72.6	78.1	83.6
32	74.8	80.4	86.0
33	76.9	82.6	88.4
34	78.9	84.7	90.6
35	80.7	86.7	92.7
36	82.5	88.6	94.7
37	84.1	90.3	96.5
38	85.6	92.0	98.3
39	87.0	93.5	99.9
40	88.3	94.8	101.4
41	89.4	96.1	102.7
42	90.4	97.2	103.9

Source: Chitty et al.[7]

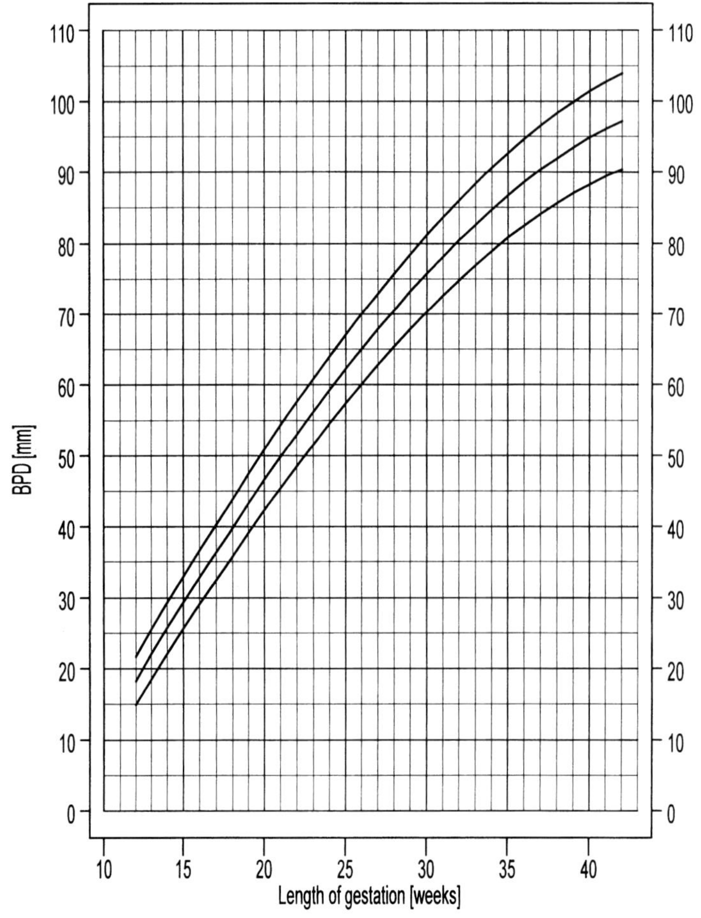

3. **Head circumference (derived from diameters)**

(a) using biparietal diameter outer–outer

Weeks of gestation	Centiles (mm)		
	5th	50th	95th
12	57.1	68.1	79.2
13	70.8	82.2	93.6
14	84.2	96.0	107.8
15	97.5	109.7	121.9
16	110.6	123.1	135.7
17	123.4	136.4	149.3
18	136.0	149.3	162.7
19	148.3	162.0	175.7
20	160.4	174.5	188.6
21	172.1	186.6	201.1
22	183.6	198.5	213.3
23	194.8	210.0	225.3
24	205.6	221.2	236.9
25	216.1	232.1	248.1
26	226.2	242.6	259.0
27	235.9	252.7	269.5
28	245.3	262.5	279.6
29	254.3	271.8	289.4
30	262.8	280.7	298.7
31	270.9	289.2	307.6
32	278.6	297.3	316.0
33	285.8	304.9	324.0
34	292.6	312.0	331.5
35	298.8	318.7	338.5
36	304.6	324.8	345.0
37	309.8	330.4	351.0
38	314.5	335.5	356.5
39	318.7	340.0	361.4
40	322.3	344.0	365.8
41	325.3	347.4	369.6
42	327.7	350.3	372.8

Source: Chitty et al.[6]

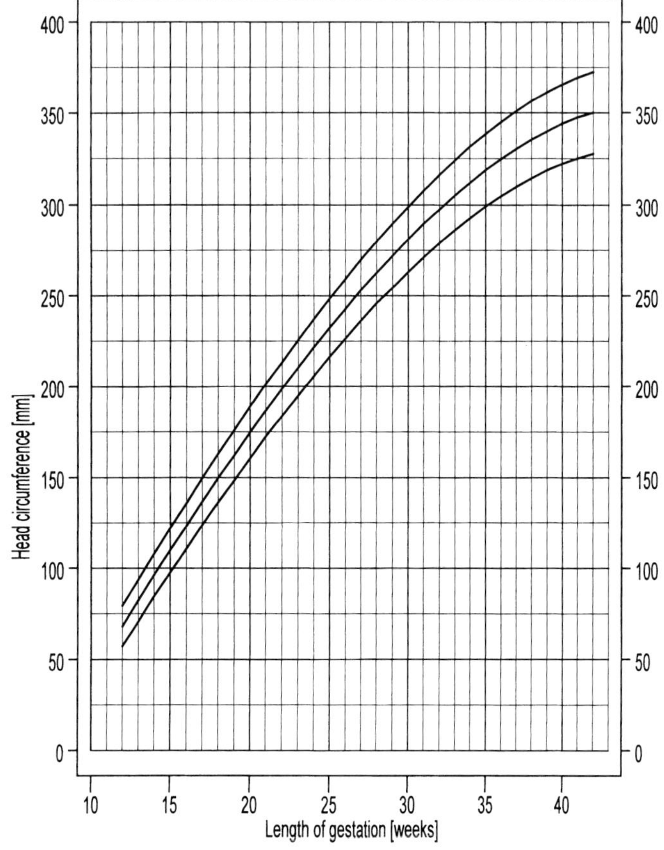

4. **Head circumference (derived from diameters)**
(b) using biparietal diameter outer–inner

Weeks of gestation	Centiles (mm) 5th	50th	95th
12	55.5	65.8	76.1
13	69.0	79.7	90.4
14	82.2	93.4	104.5
15	95.3	106.9	118.4
16	108.1	120.1	132.1
17	120.7	133.2	145.6
18	133.1	146.0	158.9
19	145.2	158.6	171.9
20	157.1	170.9	184.6
21	168.7	182.9	197.0
22	180.0	194.6	209.2
23	191.0	206.0	221.1
24	201.7	217.1	232.6
25	212.0	227.9	243.8
26	222.0	238.3	254.6
27	231.6	248.4	265.1
28	240.9	258.0	275.2
29	249.7	267.3	285.0
30	258.2	276.2	294.3
31	266.2	284.7	303.2
32	273.8	292.7	311.6
33	281.0	300.3	319.7
34	287.7	307.5	327.2
35	293.9	314.1	334.3
36	299.7	320.3	340.9
37	304.9	326.0	347.0
38	309.6	331.1	352.6
39	313.8	335.7	357.7
40	317.5	339.8	362.2
41	320.6	343.4	366.1
42	323.1	346.3	369.5

Source: Chitty and Altman (unpublished)

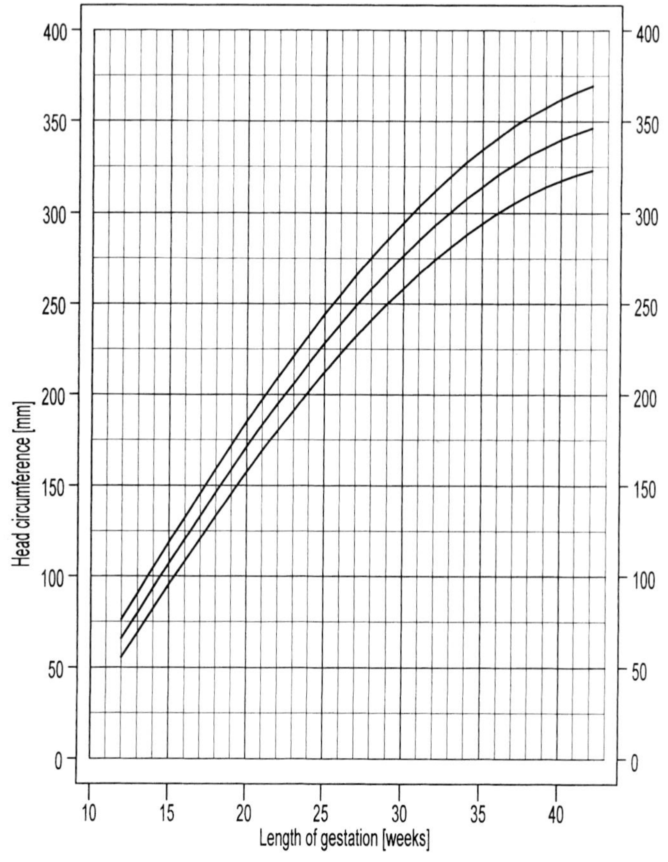

5. Abdominal circumference (derived from diameters)

Weeks of gestation	Centiles (mm)		
	5th	*50th*	*95th*
12	49.0	55.8	62.6
13	59.6	67.4	75.2
14	70.1	78.9	87.7
15	80.5	90.3	100.1
16	90.9	101.6	112.4
17	101.1	112.9	124.7
18	111.3	124.1	136.9
19	121.5	135.2	149.0
20	131.5	146.2	161.0
21	141.4	157.1	172.9
22	151.3	168.0	184.7
23	161.0	178.7	196.4
24	170.6	189.3	208.0
25	180.1	199.8	219.5
26	189.5	210.2	230.8
27	198.8	220.4	242.1
28	207.9	230.6	253.2
29	216.9	240.5	264.2
30	225.8	250.4	275.0
31	234.5	260.1	285.7
32	243.1	269.7	296.3
33	251.5	279.1	306.7
34	259.8	288.4	317.0
35	267.9	297.5	327.0
36	275.8	306.4	337.0
37	283.6	315.1	346.7
38	291.2	323.7	356.3
39	298.6	332.1	365.7
40	305.8	340.4	374.9
41	312.9	348.4	383.9
42	319.7	356.2	392.7

Source: Chitty et al.[7]

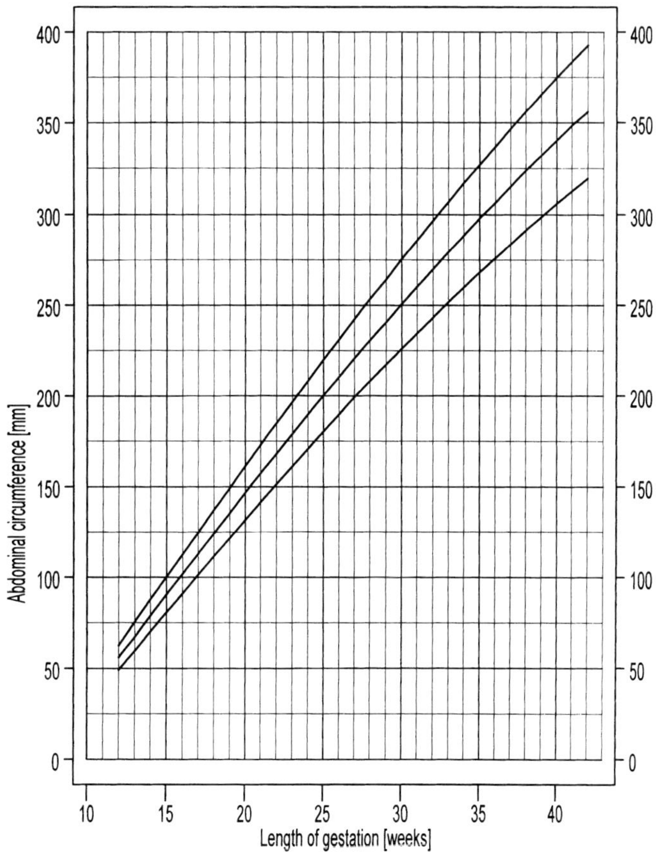

6. **Head circumference/abdominal circumference ratio**

Weeks of gestation	*Centiles*		
	5th	*50th*	*95th*
12	1.13	1.23	1.33
13	1.13	1.23	1.33
14	1.13	1.22	1.32
15	1.12	1.22	1.32
16	1.12	1.21	1.31
17	1.11	1.21	1.31
18	1.11	1.20	1.30
19	1.10	1.20	1.30
20	1.10	1.19	1.29
21	1.09	1.19	1.28
22	1.08	1.18	1.28
23	1.08	1.17	1.27
24	1.07	1.17	1.26
25	1.06	1.16	1.26
26	1.05	1.15	1.25
27	1.05	1.14	1.24

Weeks of gestation	*Centiles*		
	5th	*50th*	*95th*
28	1.04	1.13	1.23
29	1.03	1.13	1.22
30	1.02	1.12	1.21
31	1.01	1.11	1.21
32	1.00	1.10	1.20
33	0.99	1.09	1.19
34	0.98	1.08	1.18
35	0.97	1.07	1.16
36	0.96	1.06	1.15
37	0.95	1.05	1.14
38	0.94	1.03	1.13
39	0.92	1.02	1.12
40	0.91	1.01	1.11
41	0.90	1.00	1.10
42	0.89	0.98	1.08

Source: Chitty and Altman (unpublished)

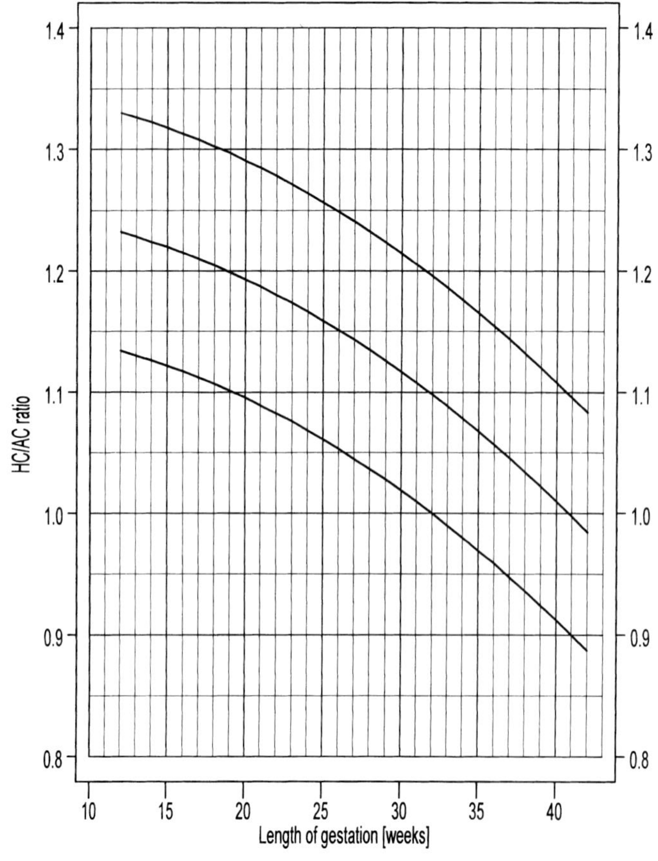

7. **Femur length**

Weeks of gestation	Centiles (mm)		
	5th	*50th*	*95th*
12	4.8	7.7	10.6
13	7.9	10.9	13.9
14	11.0	14.1	17.2
15	14.0	17.2	20.4
16	17.0	20.3	23.6
17	19.9	23.3	26.7
18	22.8	26.3	29.7
19	25.6	29.2	32.8
20	28.4	32.1	35.7
21	31.1	34.9	38.6
22	33.8	37.6	41.5
23	36.4	40.3	44.3
24	38.9	42.9	47.0
25	41.4	45.5	49.6
26	43.7	48.0	52.2
27	46.0	50.4	54.7
28	48.3	52.7	57.1
29	50.4	55.0	59.5
30	52.5	57.1	61.7
31	54.5	59.2	63.9
32	56.4	61.2	66.0
33	58.2	63.1	68.0
34	59.9	64.9	69.9
35	61.5	66.6	71.7
36	63.0	68.2	73.4
37	64.4	69.7	75.0
38	65.7	71.1	76.5
39	66.9	72.4	77.9
40	68.0	73.6	79.1
41	68.9	74.6	80.3
42	69.8	75.6	81.3

Source: Chitty et al.[8]

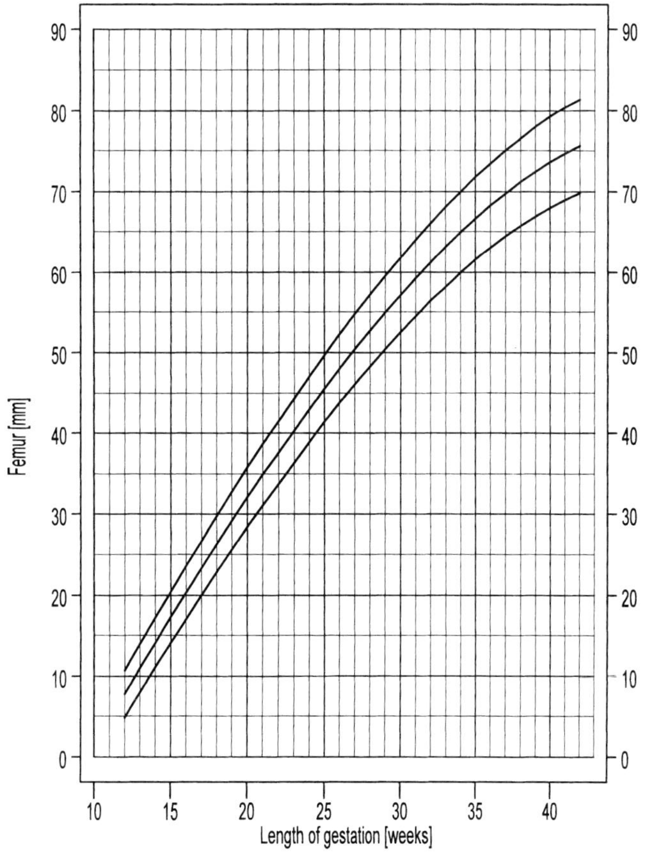

8. **Humerus length**

Weeks of gestation	*Centiles (mm)*		
	5th	***50th***	***95th***
12	4.1	7.1	10.1
13	7.6	10.7	13.8
14	11.0	14.1	17.2
15	14.1	17.3	20.6
16	17.2	20.4	23.7
17	20.1	23.4	26.7
18	22.8	26.2	29.6
19	25.4	28.9	32.4
20	28.0	31.5	35.0
21	30.4	34.0	37.6
22	32.7	36.3	40.0
23	34.8	38.6	42.3
24	36.9	40.7	44.6
25	38.9	42.8	46.7
26	40.9	44.8	48.7
27	42.7	46.7	50.7
28	44.4	48.5	52.6
29	46.1	50.2	54.4
30	47.7	51.9	56.1
31	49.2	53.5	57.7
32	50.6	55.0	59.3
33	52.0	56.4	60.8
34	53.3	57.8	62.3
35	54.6	59.1	63.6
36	55.7	60.3	64.9
37	56.8	61.5	66.2
38	57.9	62.6	67.4
39	58.9	63.7	68.5
40	59.8	64.7	69.6
41	60.7	65.6	70.6
42	61.5	66.5	71.5

Source: Chitty and Altman (unpublished)

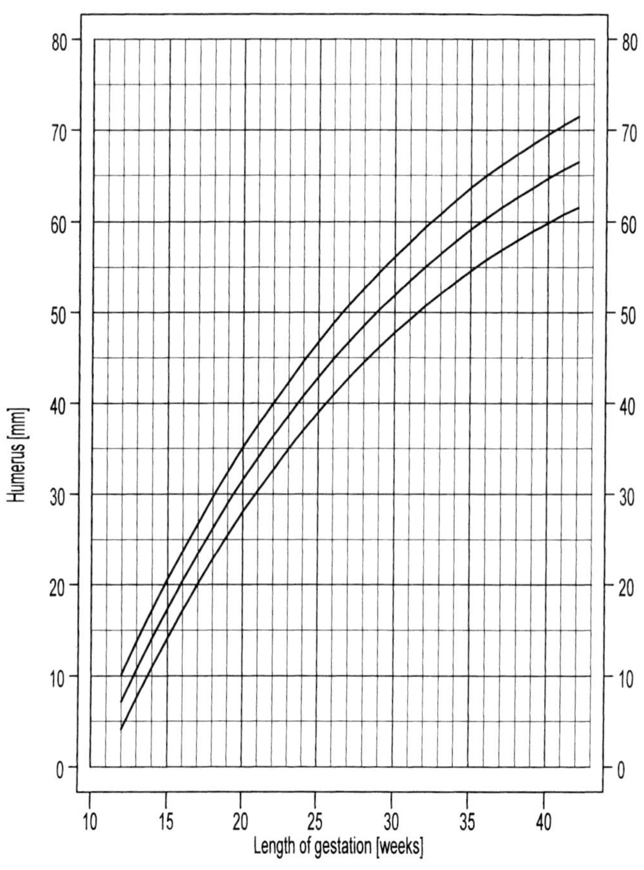

9. **Radius length**

Weeks of gestation	*Centiles (mm)*		
	5th	*50th*	*95th*
12	2.6	5.5	8.4
13	5.3	8.2	11.2
14	8.0	11.0	14.1
15	10.8	13.9	17.0
16	13.5	16.7	19.8
17	16.1	19.3	22.6
18	18.6	21.9	25.2
19	20.9	24.4	27.8
20	23.2	26.7	30.2
21	25.3	28.9	32.4
22	27.3	30.9	34.6
23	29.2	32.9	36.6
24	30.9	34.7	38.5
25	32.6	36.5	40.3
26	34.2	38.1	42.1
27	35.7	39.7	43.7
28	37.1	41.2	45.3
29	38.4	42.6	46.7
30	39.6	43.9	48.1
31	40.8	45.1	49.5
32	41.9	46.4	50.8
33	43.0	47.5	52.0
34	44.0	48.6	53.1
35	45.0	49.6	54.3
36	45.9	50.6	55.3
37	46.8	51.6	56.3
38	47.6	52.5	57.3
39	48.4	53.3	58.3
40	49.1	54.2	59.2
41	49.9	55.0	60.0
42	50.6	55.7	60.9

Source: Chitty and Altman (unpublished)

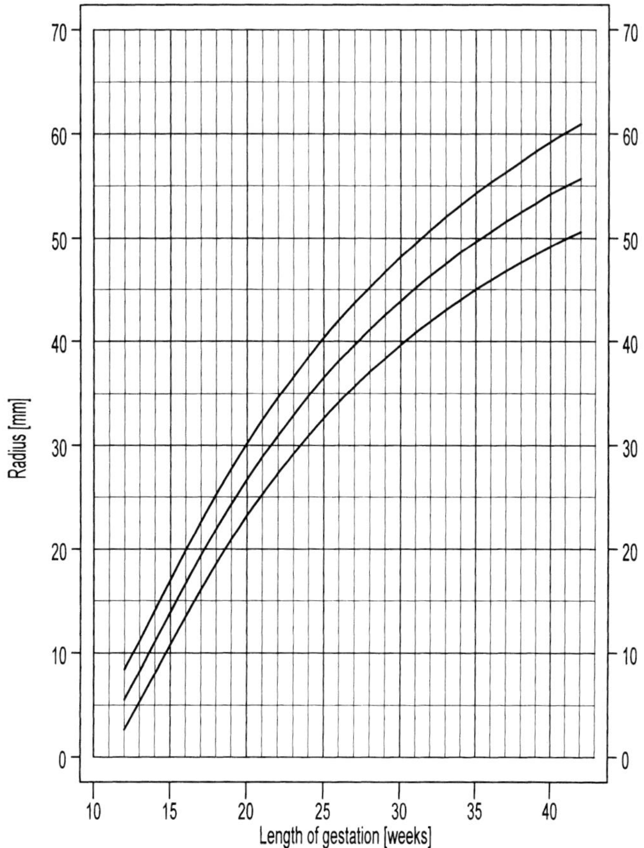

10. **Ulna length**

Weeks of gestation	Centiles (mm)		
	5th	*50th*	*95th*
12	4.4	7.3	10.3
13	6.6	9.6	12.7
14	9.3	12.4	15.5
15	12.1	15.3	18.5
16	15.0	18.2	21.5
17	17.8	21.2	24.5
18	20.6	24.0	27.5
19	23.3	26.8	30.3
20	25.8	29.4	33.0
21	28.3	32.0	35.6
22	30.6	34.4	38.1
23	32.8	36.6	40.5
24	34.9	38.8	42.7
25	36.9	40.9	44.9
26	38.8	42.8	46.9
27	40.5	44.7	48.9
28	42.2	46.5	50.7
29	43.8	48.2	52.5
30	45.3	49.8	54.2
31	46.8	51.3	55.8
32	48.2	52.7	57.3
33	49.5	54.1	58.8
34	50.7	55.4	60.2
35	51.9	56.7	61.5
36	53.0	57.9	62.8
37	54.1	59.1	64.0
38	55.1	60.2	65.2
39	56.1	61.2	66.4
40	57.0	62.2	67.5
41	57.9	63.2	68.5
42	58.8	64.1	69.5

Source: Chitty and Altman (unpublished)

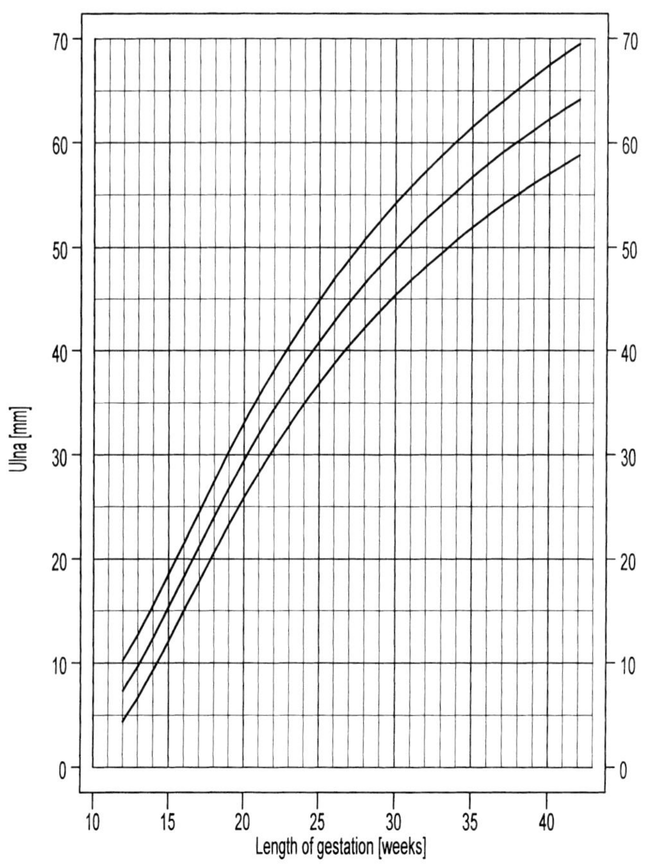

11. Tibia length

Weeks of gestation	Centiles (mm) 5th	50th	95th
12	4.8	7.6	10.4
13	6.3	9.2	12.0
14	8.4	11.4	14.4
15	11.0	14.1	17.1
16	13.8	16.9	20.1
17	16.6	19.9	23.1
18	19.5	22.8	26.1
19	22.3	25.7	29.1
20	25.0	28.5	32.0
21	27.7	31.2	34.8
22	30.2	33.8	37.5
23	32.6	36.4	40.1
24	35.0	38.8	42.6
25	37.2	41.0	44.9
26	39.3	43.2	47.2
27	41.3	45.3	49.4
28	43.2	47.3	51.4
29	45.0	49.2	53.4
30	46.7	51.0	55.3
31	48.3	52.7	57.1
32	49.9	54.4	58.8
33	51.4	55.9	60.5
34	52.8	57.5	62.1
35	54.2	58.9	63.6
36	55.5	60.3	65.1
37	56.7	61.6	66.5
38	57.9	62.9	67.8
39	59.0	64.1	69.1
40	60.1	65.2	70.4
41	61.2	66.4	71.6
42	62.2	67.4	72.7

Source: Chitty and Altman (unpublished)

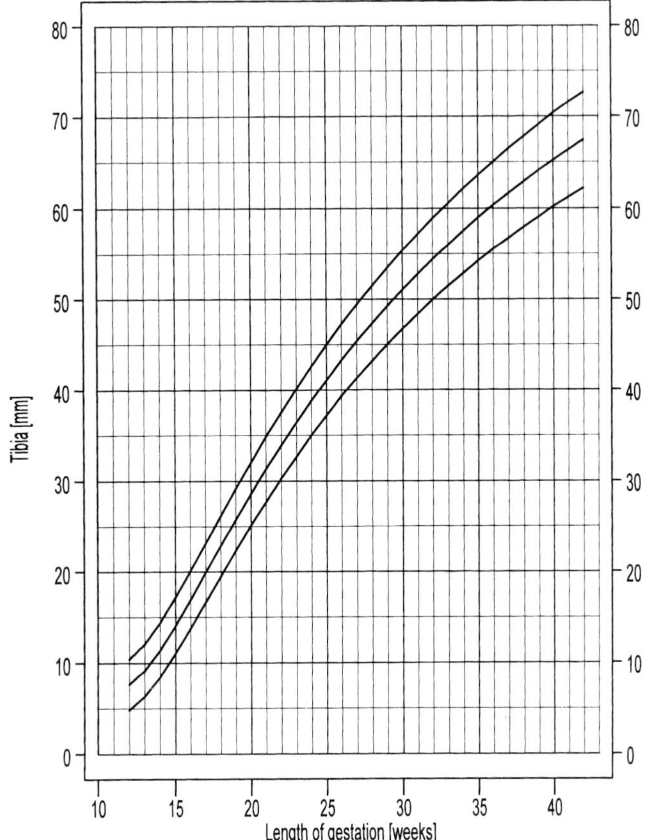

12. **Fibula length**

Weeks of gestation	Centiles (mm) 5th	50th	95th
12	4.0	6.8	9.6
13	5.6	8.5	11.4
14	7.9	10.8	13.8
15	10.5	13.5	16.6
16	13.3	16.4	19.5
17	16.1	19.3	22.5
18	18.9	22.2	25.5
19	21.7	25.1	28.5
20	24.4	27.9	31.3
21	26.9	30.5	34.1
22	29.4	33.1	36.8
23	31.8	35.5	39.3
24	34.0	37.9	41.7
25	36.2	40.1	44.0
26	38.2	42.2	46.3
27	40.2	44.3	48.4
28	42.0	46.2	50.4
29	43.8	48.0	52.3
30	45.4	49.8	54.2
31	47.0	51.5	55.9
32	48.5	53.1	57.6
33	50.0	54.6	59.2
34	51.3	56.1	60.8
35	52.6	57.5	62.3
36	53.9	58.8	63.7
37	55.1	60.1	65.1
38	56.2	61.3	66.4
39	57.3	62.5	67.7
40	58.4	63.6	68.9
41	59.4	64.7	70.1
42	60.3	65.8	71.2

Source: Chitty and Altman (unpublished)

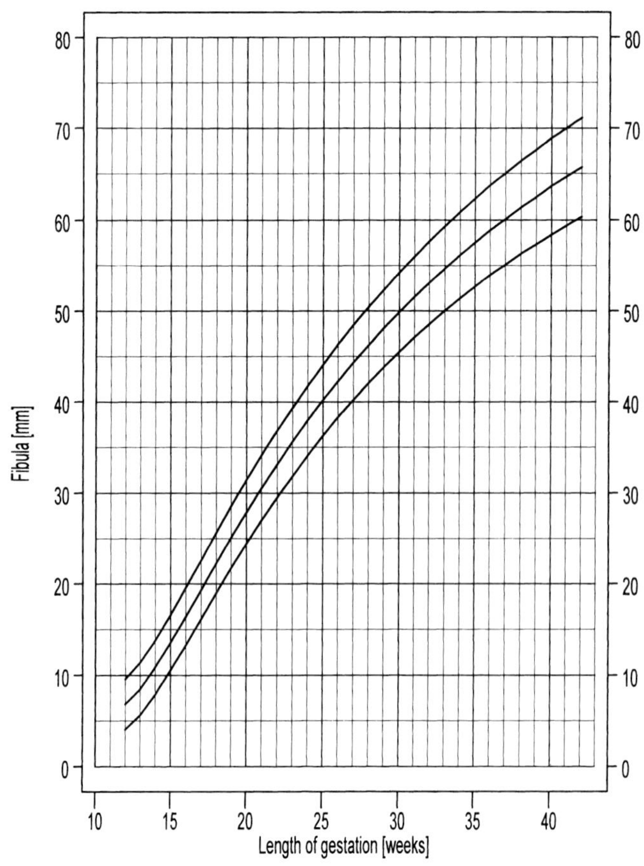

13. Foot length

Weeks of gestation	*Centiles (mm)*		
	5th	*50th*	*95th*
12	6.3	8.9	11.5
13	8.9	11.7	14.5
14	11.7	14.6	17.6
15	14.5	17.6	20.7
16	17.3	20.6	23.9
17	20.1	23.6	27.1
18	22.9	26.6	30.3
19	25.8	29.6	33.5
20	28.6	32.6	36.6
21	31.4	35.6	39.8
22	34.2	38.6	42.9
23	36.9	41.5	46.0
24	39.6	44.4	49.1
25	42.3	47.2	52.1
26	44.8	50.0	55.1
27	47.4	52.7	58.0
28	49.8	55.3	60.8
29	52.2	57.9	63.5
30	54.5	60.4	66.2
31	56.8	62.8	68.8
32	58.9	65.1	71.2
33	60.9	67.3	73.6
34	62.8	69.4	75.9
35	64.7	71.4	78.1
36	66.4	73.3	80.2
37	68.0	75.0	82.1
38	69.4	76.7	83.9
39	70.8	78.2	85.6
40	72.0	79.6	87.2
41	73.0	80.8	88.6
42	74.0	81.9	89.9

Source: Chitty and Altman (unpublished)

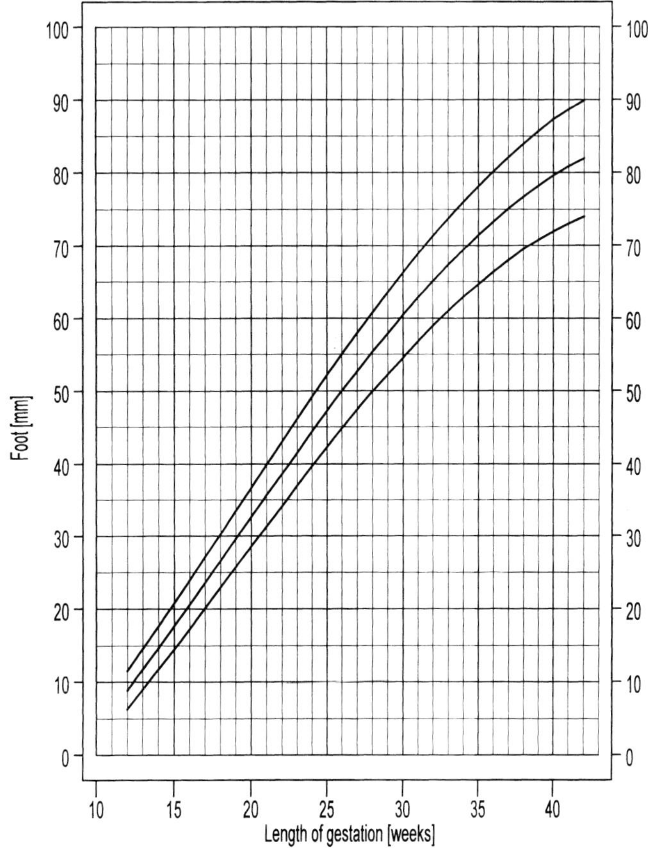

14. **Mandible length**

Weeks of gestation	Centiles (mm) 5th	50th	95th
12	6.3	8.0	9.8
13	8.2	10.3	12.3
14	10.1	12.4	14.6
15	11.9	14.4	16.9
16	13.7	16.4	19.1
17	15.3	18.3	21.3
18	17.0	20.2	23.4
19	18.5	22.0	25.4
20	20.1	23.7	27.4
21	21.5	25.5	29.4
22	23.0	27.1	31.3
23	24.4	28.8	33.2
24	25.7	30.4	35.0
25	27.1	32.0	36.8
26	28.4	33.5	38.6
27	29.7	35.0	40.4
28	30.9	36.5	42.1

Source: Chitty et al.[20]

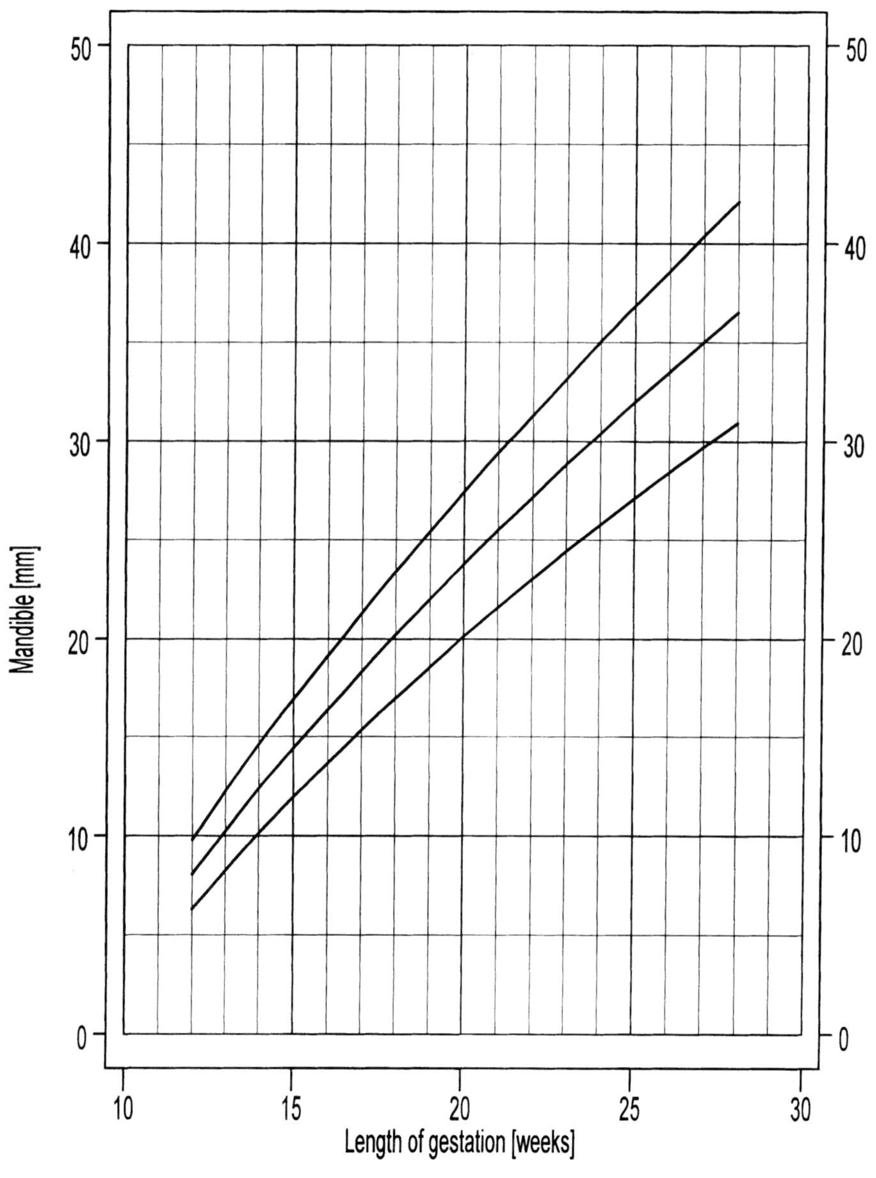

15. **Transverse cerebellar diameter**

Weeks of gestation	Centiles (mm)		
	5th	*50th*	*95th*
12	10.5	11.3	12.1
13	11.2	12.1	13.0
14	12.0	13.0	14.0
15	12.8	13.9	15.0
16	13.7	14.9	16.1
17	14.6	15.9	17.3
18	15.6	17.1	18.6
19	16.7	18.2	20.0
20	17.7	19.5	21.4
21	18.9	20.8	22.9
22	20.0	22.1	24.4
23	21.2	23.5	26.0
24	22.4	24.9	27.7
25	23.6	26.4	29.4
26	24.9	27.8	31.1
27	26.1	29.3	32.8

Weeks of gestation	Centiles (mm)		
	5th	*50th*	*95th*
28	27.3	30.7	34.6
29	28.5	32.1	36.3
30	29.6	33.5	37.9
31	30.7	34.8	39.5
32	31.7	36.1	41.1
33	32.6	37.2	42.5
34	33.4	38.2	43.8
35	34.1	39.2	45.0
36	34.6	39.9	46.0
37	35.0	40.5	46.9
38	35.3	41.0	47.5
39	35.4	41.2	47.9
40	35.4	41.3	48.2
41	35.2	41.2	48.2
42	34.8	40.8	47.9

Source: Chitty and Altman (unpublished)

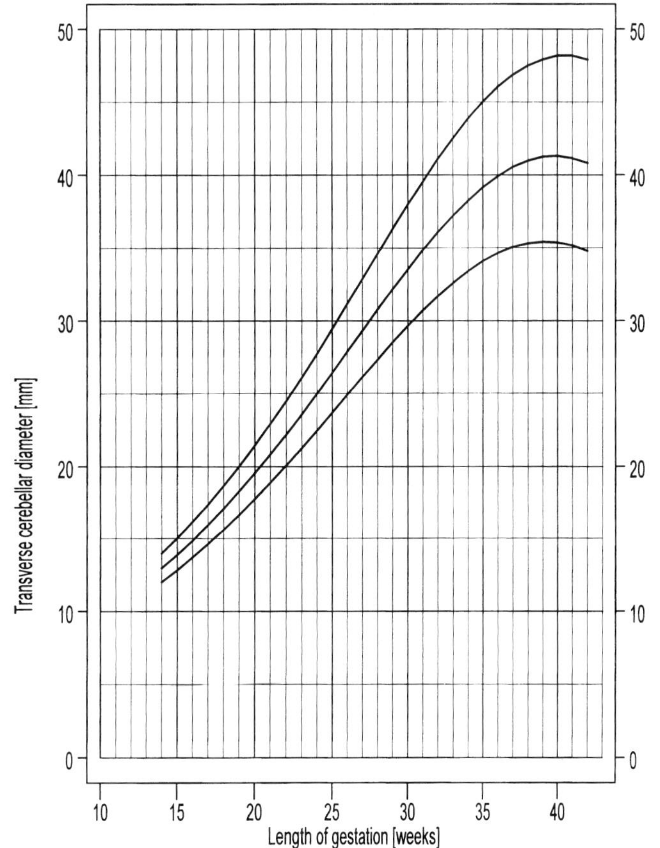

16. **Internal orbit diameter**

Weeks of gestation	Centiles (mm) 5th	50th	95th
12	4.8	5.7	6.9
13	5.6	6.8	8.1
14	6.4	7.7	9.3
15	7.2	8.7	10.5
16	7.9	9.6	11.5
17	8.6	10.4	12.5
18	9.3	11.2	13.5
19	9.9	11.9	14.3
20	10.4	12.6	15.2
21	11.0	13.2	15.9
22	11.4	13.8	16.6
23	11.9	14.3	17.3
24	12.3	14.8	17.9
25	12.7	15.3	18.4
26	13.1	15.7	19.0
27	13.4	16.1	19.4
28	13.7	16.5	19.9
29	14.0	16.9	20.3
30	14.3	17.2	20.7
31	14.5	17.5	21.1
32	14.8	17.8	21.4
33	15.0	18.0	21.7
34	15.2	18.3	22.0
35	15.4	18.5	22.3
36	15.6	18.7	22.6
37	15.7	19.0	22.8
38	15.9	19.1	23.1
39	16.0	19.3	23.3
40	16.2	19.5	23.5
41	16.3	19.7	23.7
42	16.5	19.8	23.9

Source: Chitty and Altman (unpublished)

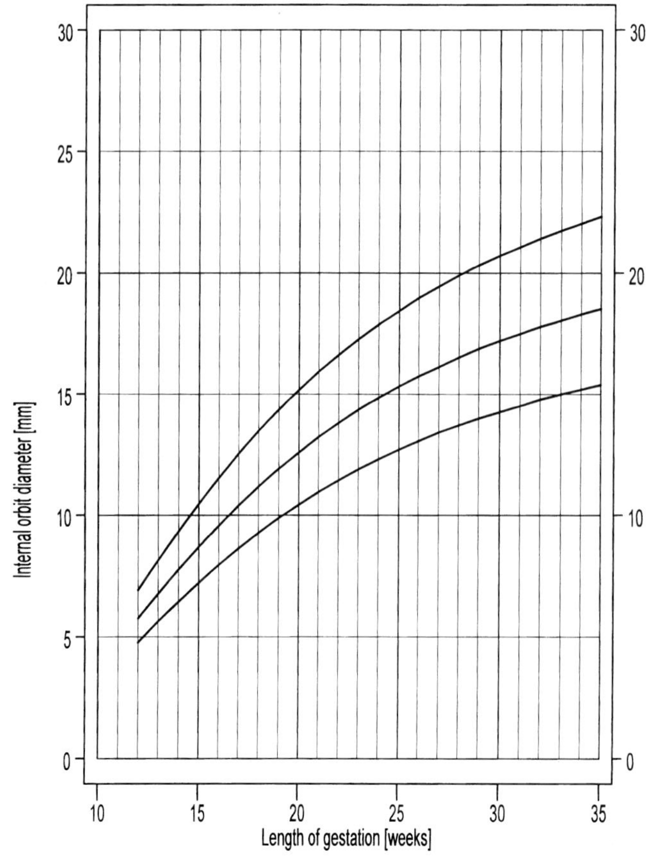

17. External orbit diameter

Weeks of gestation	Centiles (mm) 5th	50th	95th
12	12.0	13.3	14.7
13	14.2	15.6	17.3
14	16.3	18.0	19.9
15	18.4	20.3	22.4
16	20.5	22.6	25.0
17	22.5	24.8	27.4
18	24.5	27.0	29.8
19	26.4	29.1	32.1
20	28.2	31.1	34.4
21	30.0	33.1	36.5
22	31.7	35.0	38.6
23	33.3	36.8	40.6
24	34.9	38.5	42.5
25	36.4	40.2	44.4
26	37.9	41.8	46.1
27	39.3	43.3	47.9
28	40.6	44.8	49.5
29	41.9	46.3	51.1
30	43.2	47.6	52.6
31	44.4	49.0	54.1
32	45.5	50.3	55.5
33	46.6	51.5	56.8
34	47.7	52.7	58.2
35	48.7	53.8	59.4
36	49.7	54.9	60.6
37	50.7	56.0	61.8
38	51.6	57.0	62.9
39	52.5	58.0	64.0
40	53.4	59.0	65.1
41	54.2	59.9	66.1
42	55.0	60.8	67.1

Source: Chitty and Altman (unpublished)

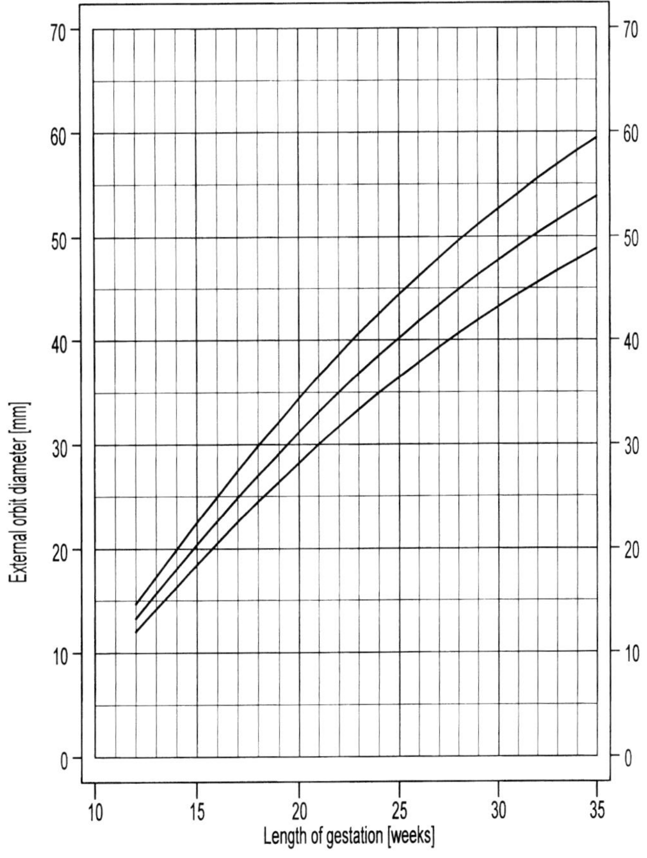

18. **Posterior horn/hemisphere ratio**

Weeks of gestation	Centiles (mm)		
	5th	50th	95th
12	0.50	0.61	0.71
13	0.46	0.56	0.67
14	0.42	0.52	0.63
15	0.39	0.49	0.59
16	0.36	0.45	0.55
17	0.33	0.42	0.52
18	0.30	0.39	0.49
19	0.28	0.37	0.46
20	0.25	0.34	0.43
21	0.23	0.32	0.41
22	0.21	0.30	0.39
23	0.20	0.28	0.37
24	0.18	0.26	0.35
25	0.17	0.25	0.33
26	0.16	0.23	0.31
27	0.15	0.22	0.30
28	0.14	0.21	0.28
29	0.13	0.20	0.27
30	0.12	0.19	0.26
31	0.12	0.18	0.25
32	0.11	0.18	0.24
33	0.11	0.17	0.23
34	0.10	0.16	0.22
35	0.10	0.16	0.22
36	0.10	0.16	0.21
37	0.10	0.15	0.21
38	0.10	0.15	0.20
39	0.10	0.15	0.20
40	0.10	0.15	0.20
41	0.10	0.15	0.20
42	0.11	0.15	0.20

Source: Chitty and Altman (unpublished)

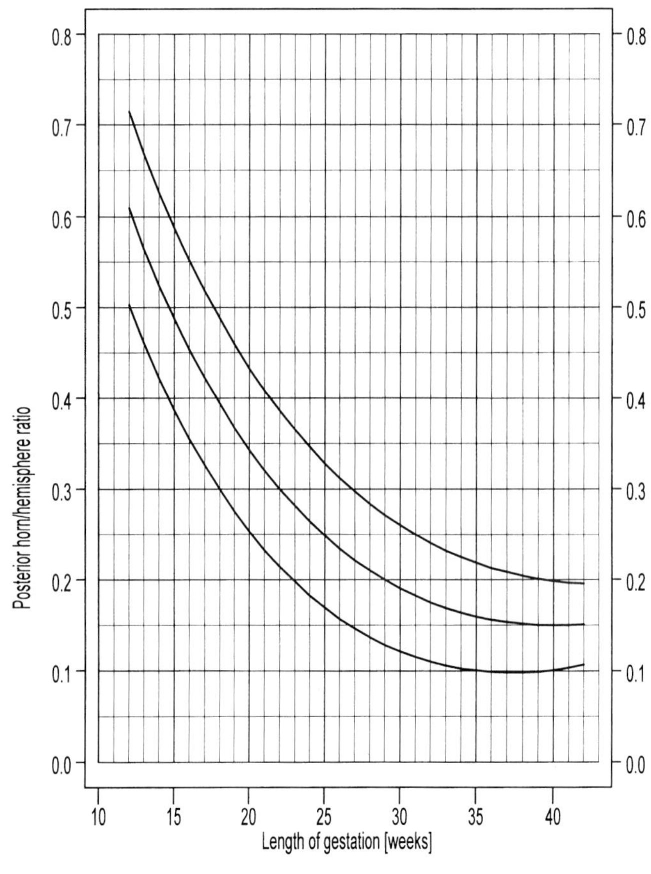

19. Kidney length

Weeks of gestation	Centiles (mm) 5th	50th	95th
12	5.2	6.3	7.7
13	6.4	7.8	9.4
14	7.7	9.3	11.3
15	9.0	11.0	13.3
16	10.5	12.7	15.4
17	11.9	14.5	17.6
18	13.4	16.3	19.8
19	15.0	18.2	22.1
20	16.5	20.0	24.3
21	18.0	21.8	26.5
22	19.5	23.6	28.7
23	20.9	25.4	30.9
24	22.3	27.1	32.9
25	23.7	28.8	35.0
26	25.0	30.4	36.9
27	26.3	31.9	38.8
28	27.5	33.4	40.5
29	28.6	34.7	42.2
30	29.7	36.0	43.8
31	30.7	37.2	45.2
32	31.6	38.3	46.6
33	32.4	39.4	47.8
34	33.2	40.3	48.9
35	33.9	41.1	50.0
36	34.5	41.9	50.9
37	35.1	42.6	51.7
38	35.6	43.2	52.4
39	36.0	43.7	53.1
40	36.3	44.1	53.6
41	36.6	44.5	54.0
42	36.9	44.8	54.4

Source: Chitty and Altman (unpublished)

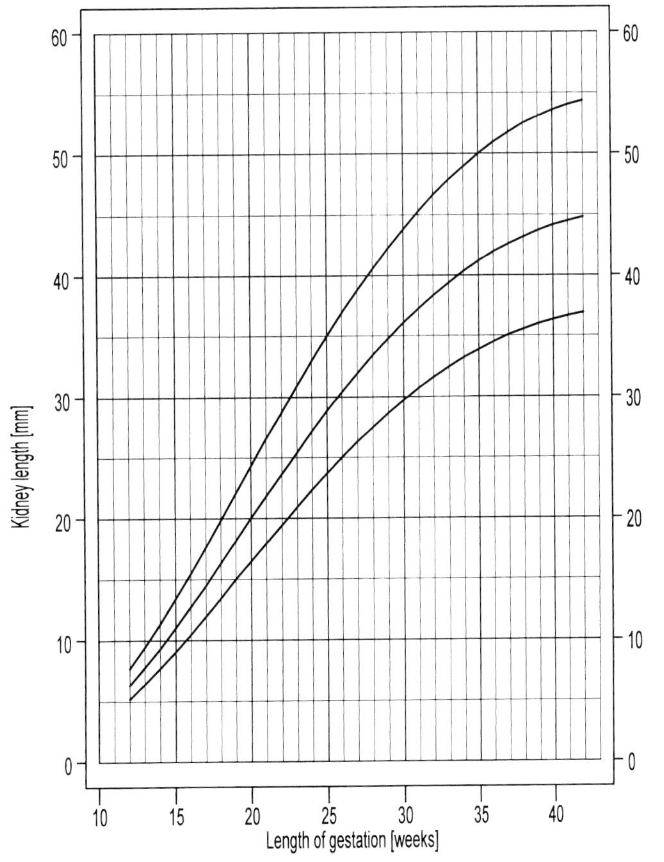

20. **Spleen length**

Weeks of gestation	Centiles (mm) 5th	50th	95th
20	11.1	15.2	19.2
21	13.0	17.0	21.0
22	14.8	18.8	22.8
23	16.6	20.6	24.6
24	18.4	22.4	26.4
25	20.2	24.2	28.2
26	21.9	25.9	30.0
27	23.6	27.6	31.7
28	25.3	29.3	33.3
29	26.9	30.9	34.9
30	28.4	32.5	36.5
31	29.9	33.9	38.0
32	31.3	35.3	39.4
33	32.6	36.6	40.7
34	33.8	37.8	41.9
35	34.9	38.9	43.0
36	35.9	39.9	44.0
37	36.8	40.8	44.8
38	37.5	41.6	45.6
39	38.1	42.2	46.2
40	38.6	42.6	46.7
41	38.9	43.0	47.0

Source: Aoki et al.[9]
Comment: Excluded birthweight <10th or >90th centile; SD taken as constant

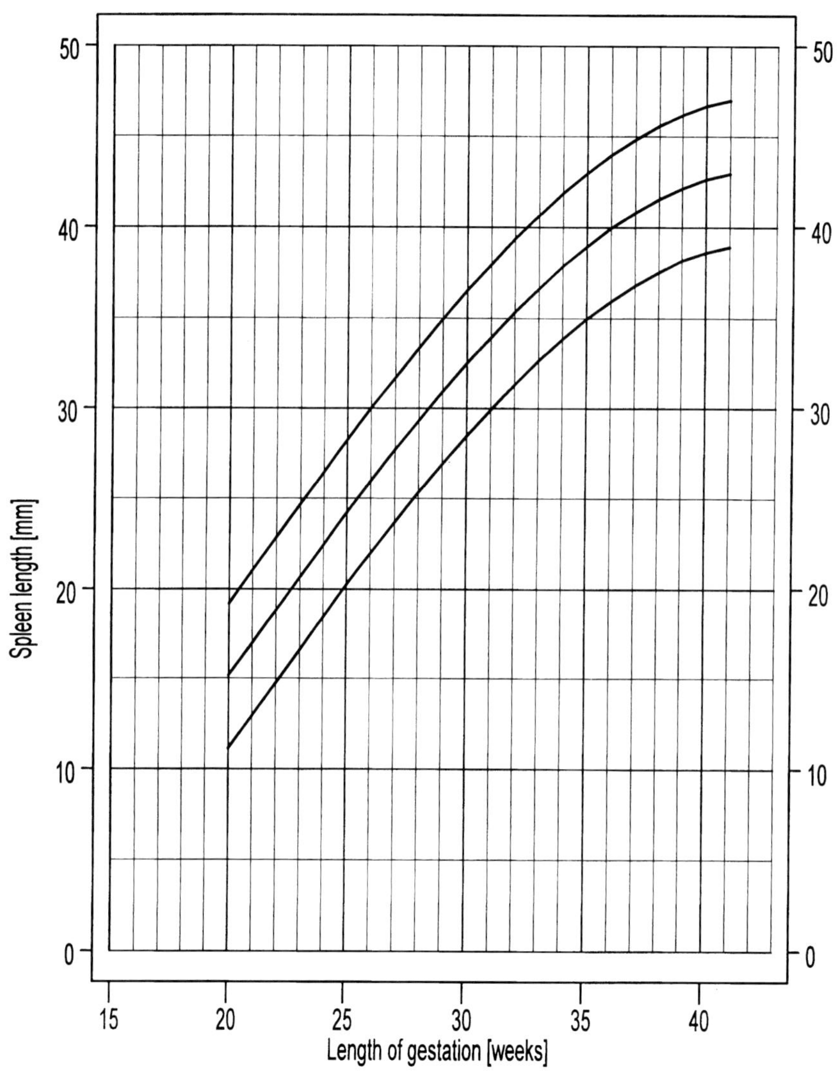

21. Liver length

Weeks of gestation	Centiles (mm)		
	5th	*50th*	*95th*
20	22.9	26.7	30.6
21	24.2	28.1	32.0
22	25.5	29.5	33.5
23	26.8	30.9	35.0
24	28.0	32.2	36.5
25	29.3	33.6	37.9
26	30.6	35.0	39.4
27	31.9	36.4	40.9
28	33.2	37.8	42.3
29	34.5	39.1	43.8
30	35.8	40.5	45.3
31	37.0	41.9	46.8
32	38.3	43.3	48.2
33	39.6	44.7	49.7
34	40.9	46.0	51.2
35	42.2	47.4	52.7
36	43.5	48.8	54.1
37	44.7	50.2	55.6
38	46.0	51.6	57.1
39	47.3	52.9	58.6
40	48.6	54.3	60.0
41	49.9	55.7	61.5

Source: Vintzileos et al.[10]

Comment: Excluded birthweight <10th or >90th centile and IUGR. Fetuses included more than once. Data reanalyzed from tabulated means and SDs

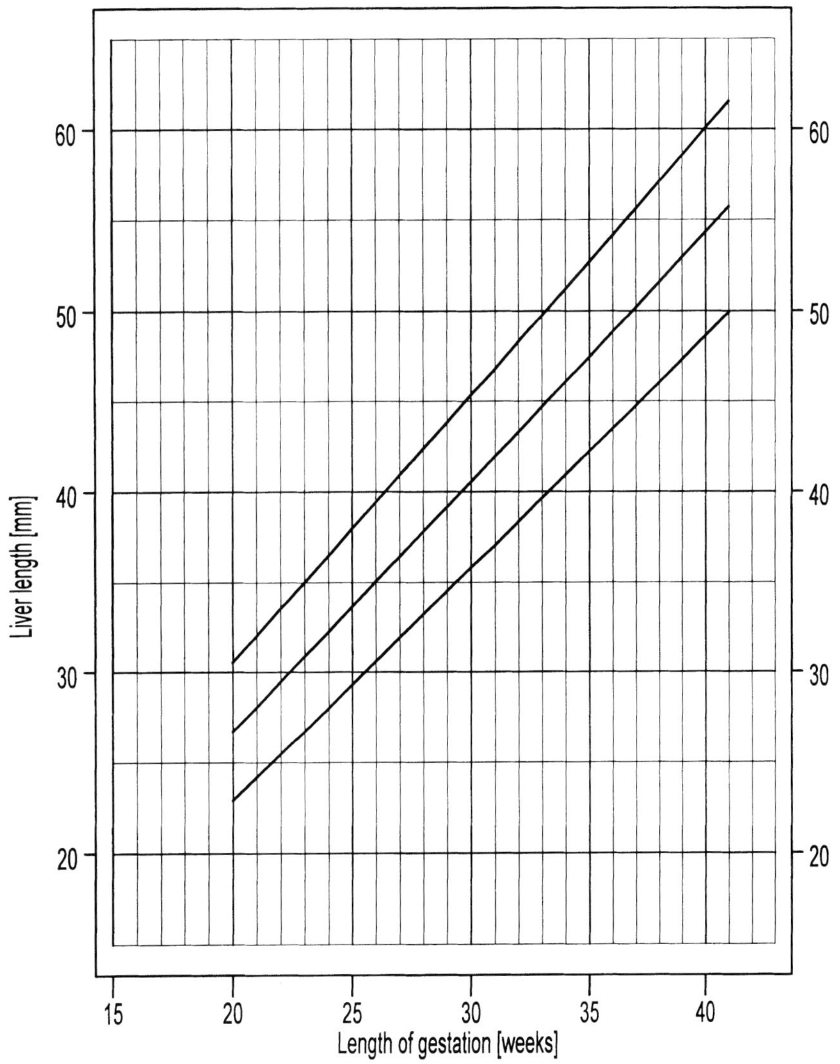

22. **Thoracic circumference (derived from diameters)**

Weeks of gestation	Centiles (mm)		
	5th	50th	95th
12	44	60	77
13	49	66	83
14	56	74	91
15	64	81	99
16	72	89	107
17	80	98	116
18	87	106	124
19	96	114	133
20	103	122	141
21	111	131	150
22	119	139	158
23	127	147	167
24	135	155	175
25	142	163	183
26	150	170	191
27	157	178	199
28	164	185	206
29	171	192	214
30	177	199	221
31	183	206	228
32	189	212	234
33	195	218	240
34	201	223	246
35	205	229	252
36	210	234	257
37	214	238	262
38	218	242	266
39	221	245	270
40	224	248	273
41	226	251	275

Source: Merz et al.[11]
Comment: Excluded IUGR

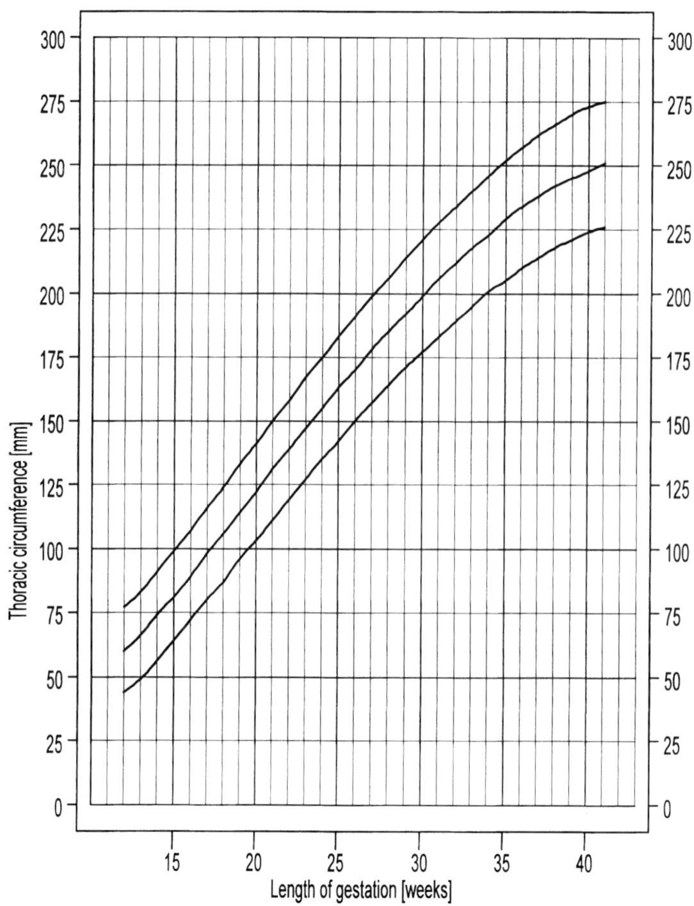

23. **Biparietal diameter (outer–outer) – dating chart**

	Centiles (weeks + days)		
BPD (mm)	***5th***	***50th***	***95th***
22	11 + 6	12 + 4	13 + 3
24	12 + 2	13 + 1	14 + 0
26	12 + 6	13 + 4	14 + 4
28	13 + 2	14 + 1	15 + 1
30	13 + 6	14 + 5	15 + 5
32	14 + 2	15 + 2	16 + 2
34	14 + 6	15 + 5	16 + 6
36	15 + 2	16 + 2	17 + 3
38	15 + 6	16 + 6	18 + 0
40	16 + 2	17 + 3	18 + 5
42	16 + 6	18 + 0	19 + 2
44	17 + 3	18 + 4	20 + 0
46	18 + 0	19 + 2	20 + 4
48	18 + 3	19 + 6	21 + 2
50	19 + 0	20 + 3	22 + 0
52	19 + 4	21 + 1	22 + 5
54	20 + 1	21 + 5	23 + 3
56	20 + 5	22 + 2	24 + 1
58	21 + 2	23 + 0	24 + 6
60	22 + 0	23 + 5	25 + 4
62	22 + 4	24 + 2	26 + 2
64	23 + 1	25 + 0	27 + 0
66	23 + 5	25 + 5	27 + 6
68	24 + 3	26 + 3	28 + 4
70	25 + 0	27 + 1	29 + 3
72	25 + 5	27 + 6	30 + 1
74	26 + 2	28 + 4	31 + 0
76	27 + 0	29 + 2	31 + 6
78	27 + 4	30 + 0	32 + 4
80	28 + 2	30 + 5	33 + 3
82	29 + 0	31 + 4	34 + 2
84	29 + 5	32 + 2	35 + 1
86	30 + 2	33 + 1	36 + 1
88	31 + 0	33 + 6	37 + 0
90	31 + 5	34 + 5	37 + 6

Source: Altman and Chitty[5]

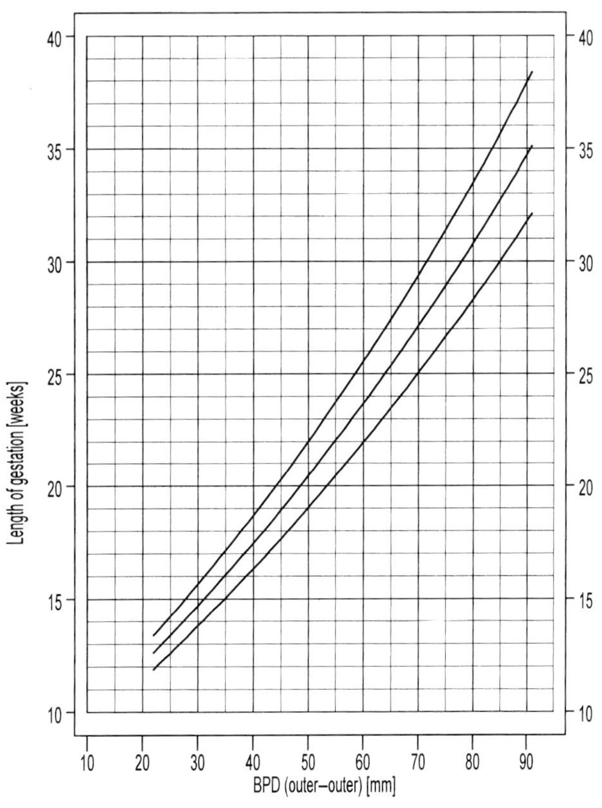

24. **Biparietal diameter (outer–inner) – dating chart**

	Centiles (weeks + days)		
BPD (mm)	*5th*	*50th*	*95th*
22	12 + 2	13 + 0	13 + 6
24	12 + 5	13 + 4	14 + 3
26	13 + 2	14 + 1	15 + 0
28	13 + 5	14 + 5	15 + 4
30	14 + 2	15 + 1	16 + 1
32	14 + 6	15 + 5	16 + 5
34	15 + 2	16 + 2	17 + 3
36	15 + 6	16 + 6	18 + 0
38	16 + 3	17 + 3	18 + 5
40	17 + 0	18 + 1	19 + 2
42	17 + 3	18 + 5	20 + 0
44	18 + 0	19 + 2	20 + 5
46	18 + 4	19 + 6	21 + 2
48	19 + 1	20 + 4	22 + 0
50	19 + 5	21 + 1	22 + 5
52	20 + 2	21 + 6	23 + 3
54	21 + 0	22 + 4	24 + 1
56	21 + 4	23 + 1	24 + 6
58	22 + 1	23 + 6	25 + 5
60	22 + 5	24 + 4	26 + 3
62	23 + 3	25 + 2	27 + 1
64	24 + 0	26 + 0	28 + 0
66	24 + 5	26 + 5	28 + 5
68	25 + 2	27 + 3	29 + 4
70	26 + 0	28 + 1	30 + 3
72	26 + 5	28 + 6	31 + 2
74	27 + 2	29 + 4	32 + 0
76	28 + 0	30 + 2	32 + 6
78	28 + 5	31 + 1	33 + 5
80	29 + 3	31 + 6	34 + 5
82	30 + 1	32 + 5	35 + 4
84	30 + 6	33 + 3	36 + 3
86	31 + 4	34 + 2	37 + 2
88	32 + 2	35 + 1	38 + 2

Source: Altman and Chitty[5]

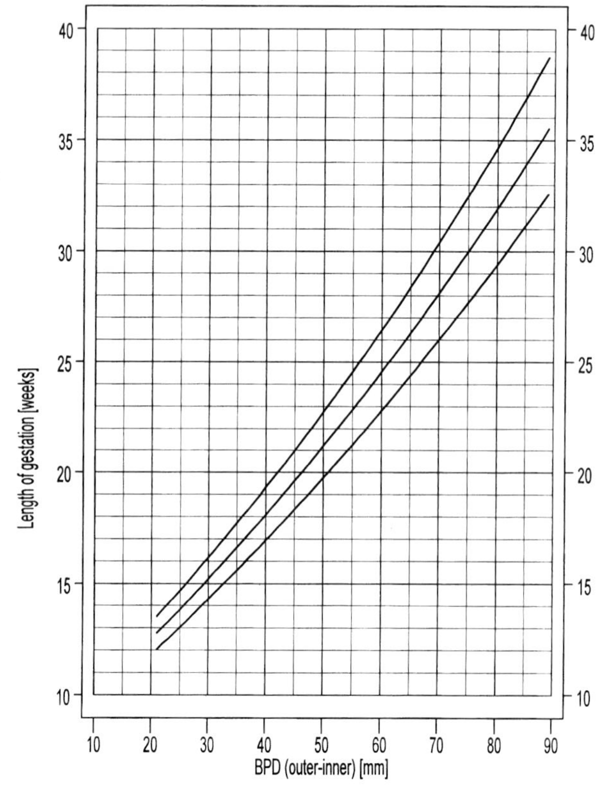

25. **Head circumference (derived from diameters) – dating chart** *(a) using biparietal diameter outer–outer*

Head circ. (mm)	Centiles (weeks + days) 5th	50th	95th
80	11 + 4	12 + 4	13 + 4
90	12 + 3	13 + 2	14 + 2
100	13 + 2	14 + 1	15 + 1
110	14 + 0	15 + 0	16 + 0
120	14 + 6	15 + 6	16 + 6
130	15 + 5	16 + 4	17 + 5
140	16 + 3	17 + 3	18 + 3
150	17 + 2	18 + 2	19 + 2
160	18 + 1	19 + 1	20 + 1
170	18 + 6	19 + 6	21 + 0
180	19 + 5	20 + 5	21 + 6
190	20 + 3	21 + 4	22 + 5
200	21 + 1	22 + 2	23 + 4
210	22 + 0	23 + 1	24 + 3
220	22 + 5	24 + 0	25 + 3
230	23 + 4	24 + 6	26 + 3
240	24 + 2	25 + 6	27 + 3
250	25 + 1	26 + 5	28 + 3
260	26 + 0	27 + 5	29 + 4
270	26 + 6	28 + 6	30 + 6
280	27 + 6	30 + 0	32 + 1
290	28 + 6	31 + 1	33 + 4
300	29 + 6	32 + 3	35 + 2
310	31 + 0	33 + 6	37 + 0
320	32 + 2	35 + 3	38 + 6

Source: Altman and Chitty[5]

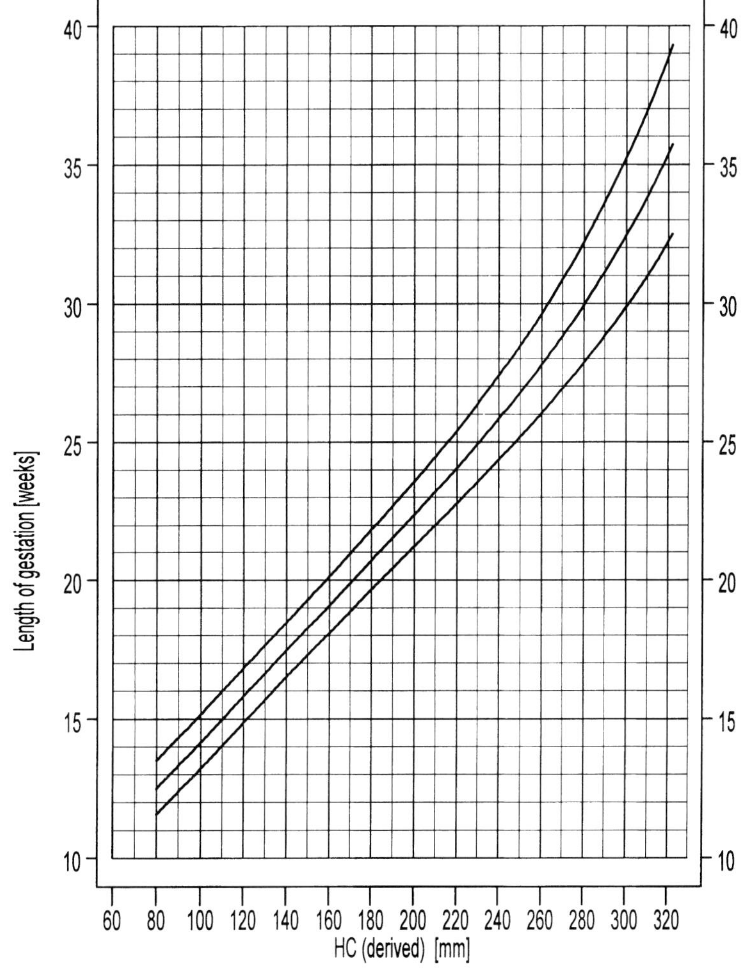

26. **Head circumference (derived from diameters) – dating chart** *(b) using biparietal diameter outer–inner*

Head circ. (mm)	*Centiles (weeks + days)*		
	5th	*50th*	*95th*
80	11 + 6	12 + 5	13 + 5
90	12 + 5	13 + 4	14 + 4
100	13 + 3	14 + 3	15 + 3
110	14 + 2	15 + 2	16 + 1
120	15 + 1	16 + 0	17 + 0
130	16 + 0	16 + 6	17 + 6
140	16 + 5	17 + 5	18 + 5
150	17 + 4	18 + 4	19 + 3
160	18 + 3	19 + 2	20 + 2
170	19 + 1	20 + 1	21 + 1
180	20 + 0	21 + 0	22 + 0
190	20 + 5	21 + 6	22 + 6
200	21 + 4	22 + 4	23 + 6
210	22 + 2	23 + 3	24 + 5
220	23 + 1	24 + 3	25 + 5
230	23 + 6	25 + 2	26 + 5
240	24 + 5	26 + 1	27 + 5
250	25 + 4	27 + 1	28 + 6
260	26 + 3	28 + 1	30 + 1
270	27 + 2	29 + 2	31 + 3
280	28 + 2	30 + 3	32 + 6
290	29 + 1	31 + 5	34 + 2
300	30 + 2	33 + 0	36 + 0
310	31 + 3	34 + 3	37 + 5
320	32 + 4	36 + 0	39 + 5

Source: Chitty and Altman (unpublished)

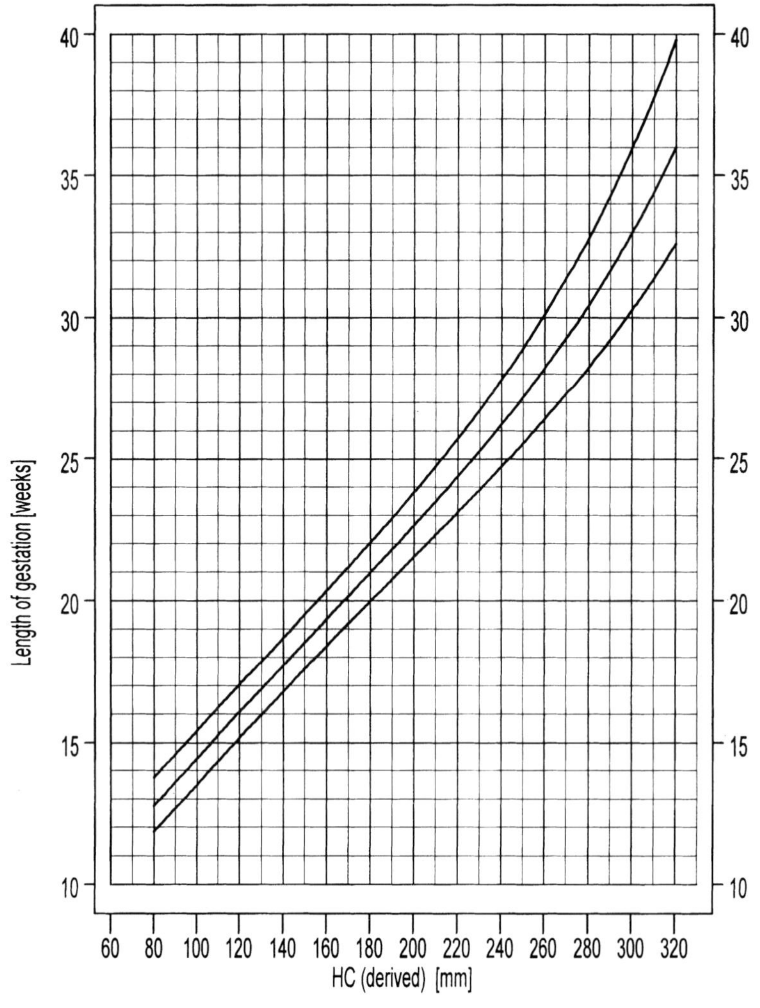

27. **Femur length – dating chart**

Femur (mm)	*Centiles (weeks + days)* 5th	50th	95th
10	12 + 2	13 + 0	13 + 5
12	12 + 6	13 + 4	14 + 2
14	13 + 2	14 + 1	15 + 0
16	13 + 6	14 + 5	15 + 4
18	14 + 3	15 + 2	16 + 2
20	15 + 0	16 + 0	17 + 0
22	15 + 4	16 + 4	17 + 4
24	16 + 1	17 + 2	18 + 2
26	16 + 6	17 + 6	19 + 0
28	17 + 3	18 + 4	19 + 5
30	18 + 0	19 + 2	20 + 4
32	18 + 5	20 + 0	21 + 2
34	19 + 2	20 + 5	22 + 0
36	20 + 0	21 + 3	22 + 6
38	20 + 5	22 + 1	23 + 5
40	21 + 3	22 + 6	24 + 4
42	22 + 1	23 + 5	25 + 3
44	22 + 6	24 + 3	26 + 2
46	23 + 4	25 + 2	27 + 1
48	24 + 2	26 + 1	28 + 1
50	25 + 1	27 + 0	29 + 0
52	25 + 6	27 + 6	30 + 0
54	26 + 5	28 + 5	31 + 0
56	27 + 4	29 + 5	32 + 0
58	28 + 3	30 + 4	33 + 0
60	29 + 2	31 + 4	34 + 1
62	30 + 1	32 + 4	35 + 2
64	31 + 0	33 + 4	36 + 2
66	32 + 0	34 + 4	37 + 3

Source: Altman and Chitty[5]

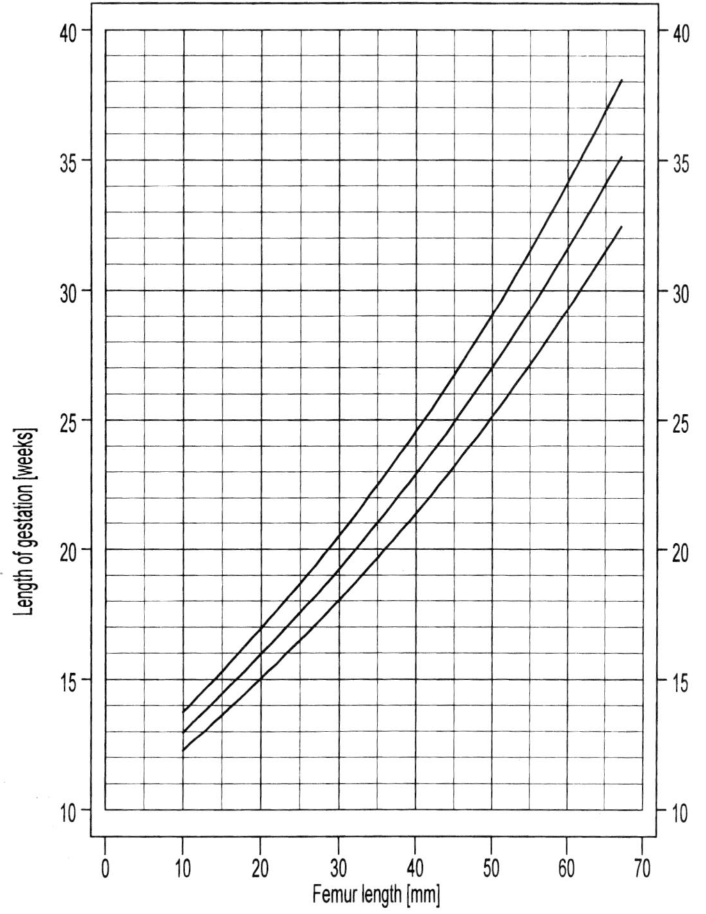

28. **Transverse cerebellar diameter (TCD) – dating chart**

	Centiles (weeks + days)		
TCD (mm)	*5th*	*50th*	*95th*
13	13 + 2	14 + 3	15 + 5
14	14 + 1	15 + 2	16 + 5
15	15 + 0	16 + 2	17 + 4
16	15 + 6	17 + 0	18 + 3
17	16 + 5	17 + 6	19 + 2
18	17 + 3	18 + 5	20 + 0
19	18 + 2	19 + 4	20 + 6
20	19 + 0	20 + 3	21 + 5
21	19 + 6	21 + 1	22 + 4
22	20 + 4	22 + 0	23 + 3
23	21 + 2	22 + 5	24 + 2
24	22 + 0	23 + 4	25 + 1
25	22 + 4	24 + 2	26 + 1
26	23 + 2	25 + 0	27 + 0
27	23 + 6	25 + 6	27 + 6
28	24 + 3	26 + 4	28 + 6
29	25 + 0	27 + 2	29 + 5
30	25 + 4	28 + 0	30 + 5
31	26 + 1	28 + 6	31 + 5
32	26 + 4	29 + 4	32 + 5
33	27 + 1	30 + 2	33 + 6
34	27 + 4	31 + 0	34 + 6
35	27 + 6	31 + 5	36 + 0
36	28 + 2	32 + 3	37 + 1

Source: Altman and Chitty[5]

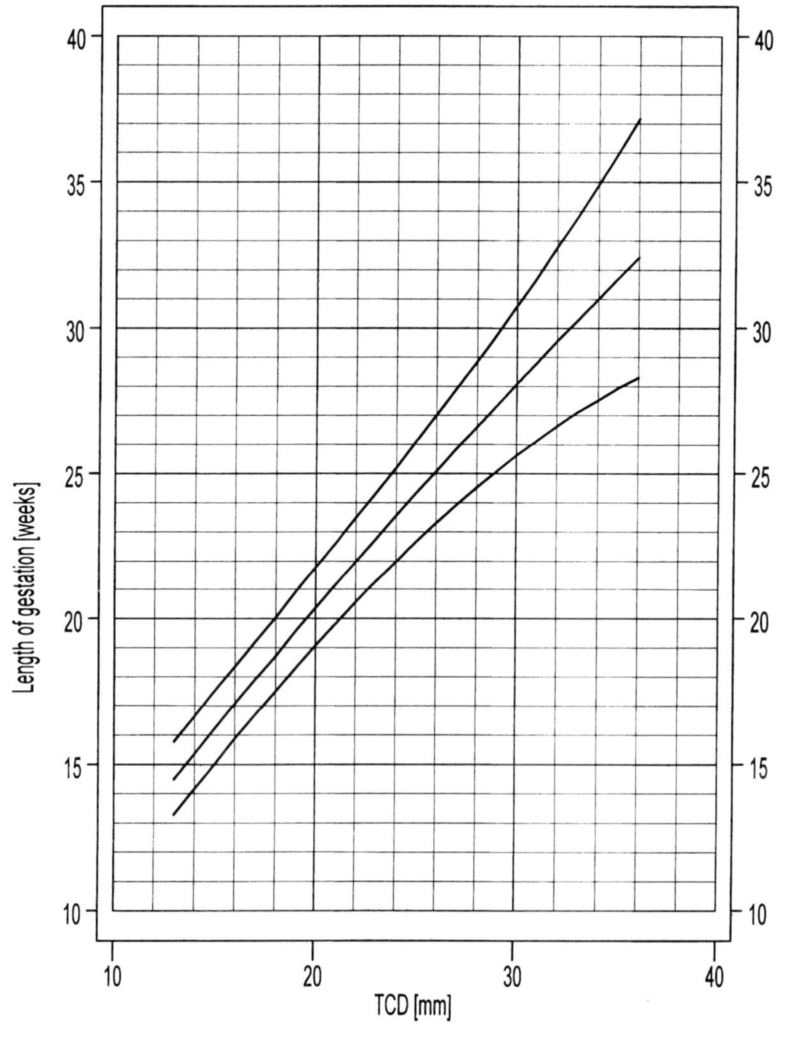

29. Crown–rump length – dating chart

Crown–rump ength (mm)	*Centiles (weeks + days)*		
	5th	*50th*	*95th*
4	5 + 3	6 + 0	6 + 4
6	6 + 0	6 + 3	7 + 0
8	6 + 2	6 + 6	7 + 3
10	6 + 5	7 + 2	7 + 6
12	7 + 0	7 + 4	8 + 1
14	7 + 3	7 + 6	8 + 3
16	7 + 5	8 + 2	8 + 5
18	8 + 0	8 + 3	9 + 0
20	8 + 1	8 + 5	9 + 2
22	8 + 3	9 + 0	9 + 4
24	8 + 5	9 + 2	9 + 6
26	8 + 6	9 + 3	10 + 0
28	9 + 1	9 + 5	10 + 2
30	9 + 3	9 + 6	10 + 3
32	9 + 4	10 + 1	10 + 5
34	9 + 5	10 + 2	10 + 6
36	10 + 0	10 + 4	11 + 0
38	10 + 1	10 + 5	11 + 2
40	10 + 2	10 + 6	11 + 3
42	10 + 4	11 + 0	11 + 4

Crown–rump length (mm)	*Centiles (weeks + days)*		
	5th	*50th*	*95th*
44	10 + 5	11 + 2	11 + 6
46	10 + 6	11 + 3	12 + 0
48	11 + 0	11 + 4	12 + 1
50	11 + 1	11 + 5	12 + 2
52	11 + 3	11 + 6	12 + 3
54	11 + 4	12 + 1	12 + 4
56	11 + 5	12 + 2	12 + 6
58	11 + 6	12 + 3	13 + 0
60	12 + 0	12 + 4	13 + 1
62	12 + 1	12 + 5	13 + 2
64	12 + 2	12 + 6	13 + 3
66	12 + 3	13 + 0	13 + 4
68	12 + 4	13 + 1	13 + 5
70	12 + 5	13 + 2	13 + 6
72	12 + 6	13 + 3	14 + 0
74	13 + 0	13 + 4	14 + 1
76	13 + 1	13 + 5	14 + 2
78	13 + 2	13 + 6	14 + 2
80	13 + 3	14 + 0	14 + 3

Source: Robinson and Fleming[12]

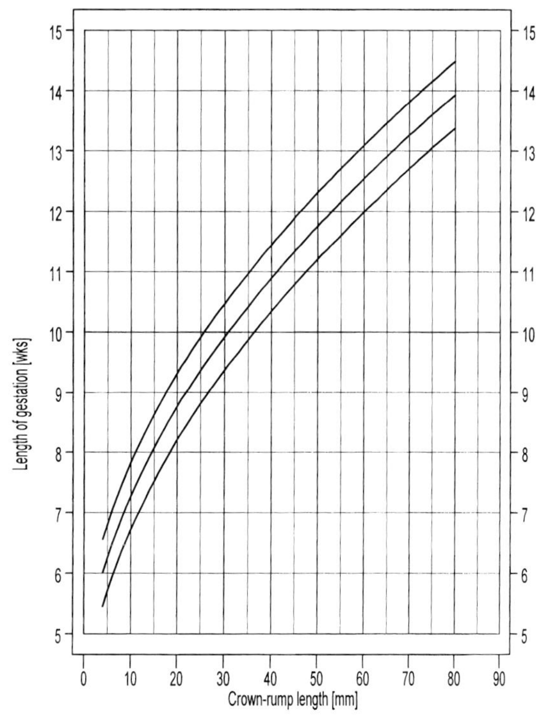

30. **Umbilical vein Po_2**

Weeks of gestation	*Centiles (mmHg)*		
	5th	*50th*	*95th*
18	37.5	49.7	61.9
19	36.5	48.7	60.9
20	35.5	47.7	59.9
21	34.5	46.7	58.9
22	33.5	45.7	57.9
23	32.5	44.7	57.0
24	31.5	43.7	56.0
25	30.5	42.8	55.0
26	29.5	41.8	54.0
27	28.5	40.8	53.0
28	27.6	39.8	52.0
29	26.6	38.8	51.0
30	25.6	37.8	50.0
31	24.6	36.8	49.0
32	23.6	35.8	48.0
33	22.6	34.8	47.1
34	21.6	33.8	46.1
35	20.6	32.8	45.1
36	19.6	31.9	44.1
37	18.6	30.9	43.1
38	17.7	29.9	42.1

Source: Nicolaides et al.[13]
Comment: Model not fully specified; SD taken as constant

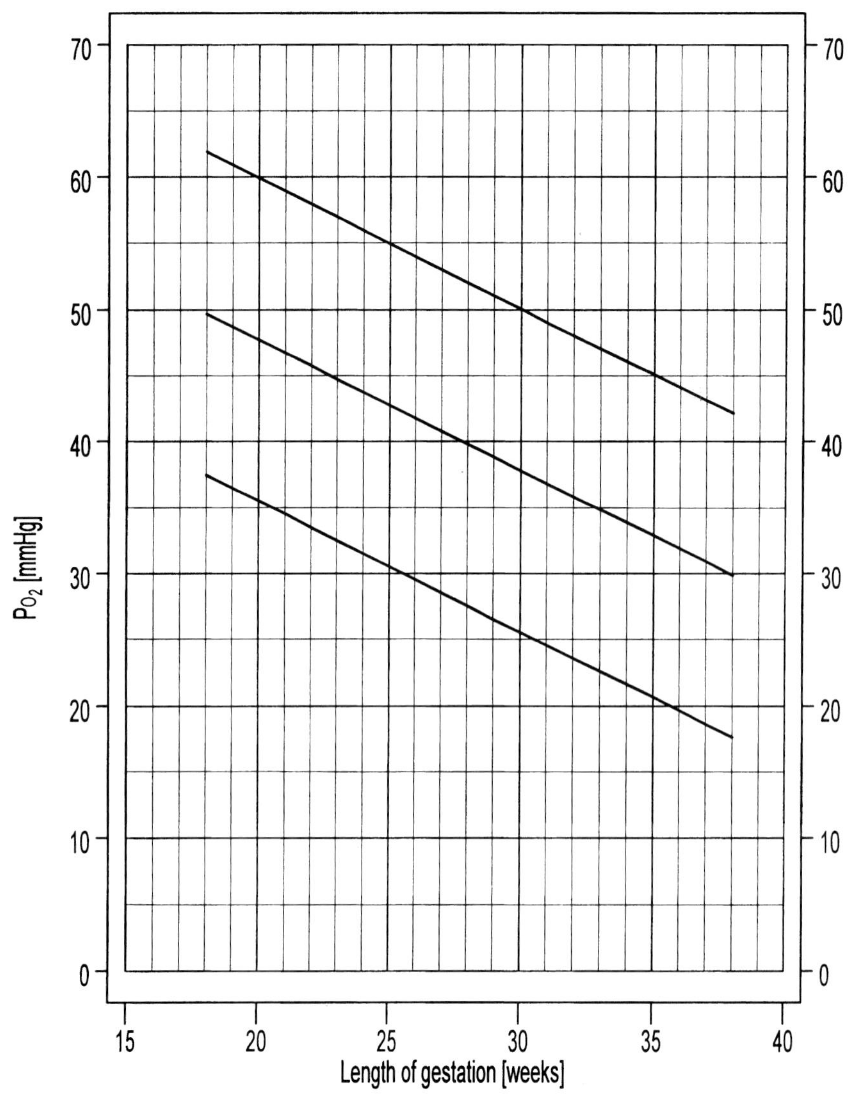

31. **Umbilical vein Pco_2**

Weeks of gestation	Centiles (mmHg)		
	5th	*50th*	*95th*
18	27.1	33.4	39.6
19	27.3	33.6	39.8
20	27.5	33.8	40.1
21	27.8	34.0	40.3
22	28.0	34.2	40.5
23	28.2	34.5	40.7
24	28.4	34.7	40.9
25	28.6	34.9	41.2
26	28.9	35.1	41.4
27	29.1	35.3	41.6
28	29.3	35.6	41.8
29	29.5	35.8	42.0
30	29.7	36.0	42.3
31	30.0	36.2	42.5
32	30.2	36.4	42.7
33	30.4	36.7	42.9
34	30.6	36.9	43.1
35	30.8	37.1	43.4
36	31.1	37.3	43.6
37	31.3	37.5	43.8
38	31.5	37.8	44.0

Source: Nicolaides et al.[13]

Comment: Model not fully specified; SD taken as constant

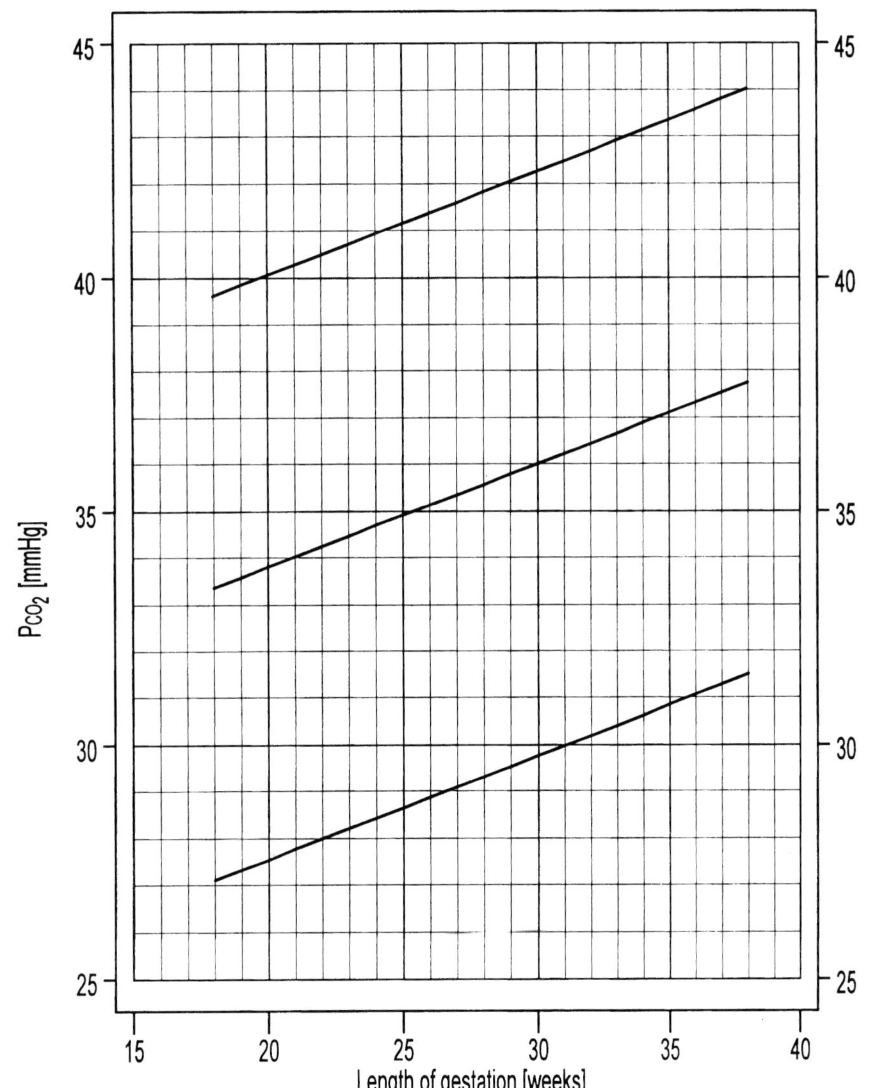

32. **Umbilical vein pH**

Weeks of gestation	Centiles 50th		
	5th	50th	95th
18	7.38	7.42	7.47
19	7.38	7.42	7.47
20	7.37	7.42	7.47
21	7.37	7.42	7.46
22	7.37	7.42	7.46
23	7.37	7.41	7.46
24	7.37	7.41	7.46
25	7.36	7.41	7.46
26	7.36	7.41	7.45
27	7.36	7.41	7.45
28	7.36	7.40	7.45

Weeks of gestation	Centiles		
	5th	50th	95th
29	7.36	7.40	7.45
30	7.35	7.40	7.45
31	7.35	7.40	7.44
32	7.35	7.40	7.44
33	7.35	7.39	7.44
34	7.35	7.39	7.44
35	7.34	7.39	7.44
36	7.34	7.39	7.43
37	7.34	7.39	7.43
38	7.34	7.38	7.43

Source: Nicolaides et al.[13]
Comment: Model not fully specified; SD taken as constant

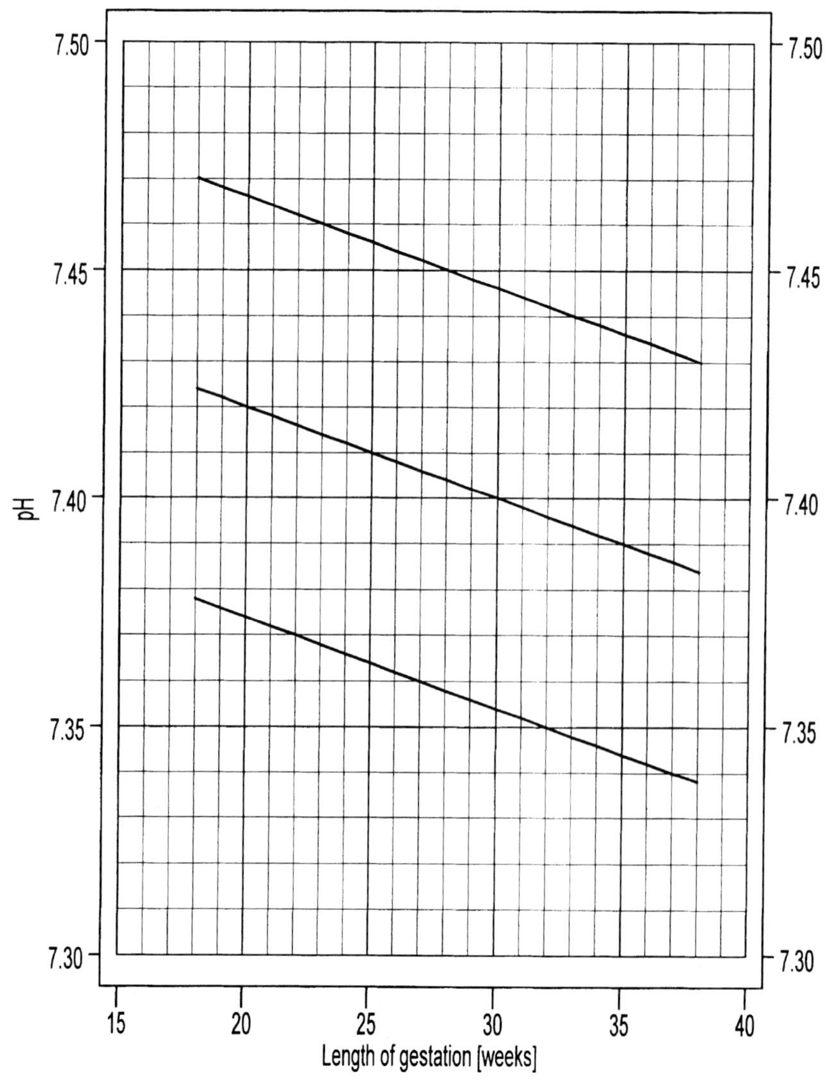

33. **Umbilical artery pulsatility index**

Weeks of gestation	Centiles		
	5th	*50th*	*95th*
20	1.04	1.54	2.03
21	0.98	1.47	1.96
22	0.92	1.41	1.90
23	0.86	1.35	1.85
24	0.81	1.30	1.79
25	0.76	1.25	1.74
26	0.71	1.20	1.69
27	0.67	1.16	1.65
28	0.63	1.12	1.61
29	0.59	1.08	1.57
30	0.56	1.05	1.54
31	0.53	1.02	1.51
32	0.50	0.99	1.48
33	0.48	0.97	1.46
34	0.46	0.95	1.44
35	0.44	0.94	1.43
36	0.43	0.92	1.42
37	0.42	0.92	1.41
38	0.42	0.91	1.40
39	0.42	0.91	1.40
40	0.42	0.91	1.40
41	0.42	0.92	1.41
42	0.43	0.93	1.42

Source: Arduini and Rizzo[14]

Comment: Excluded IUGR; SD taken as constant

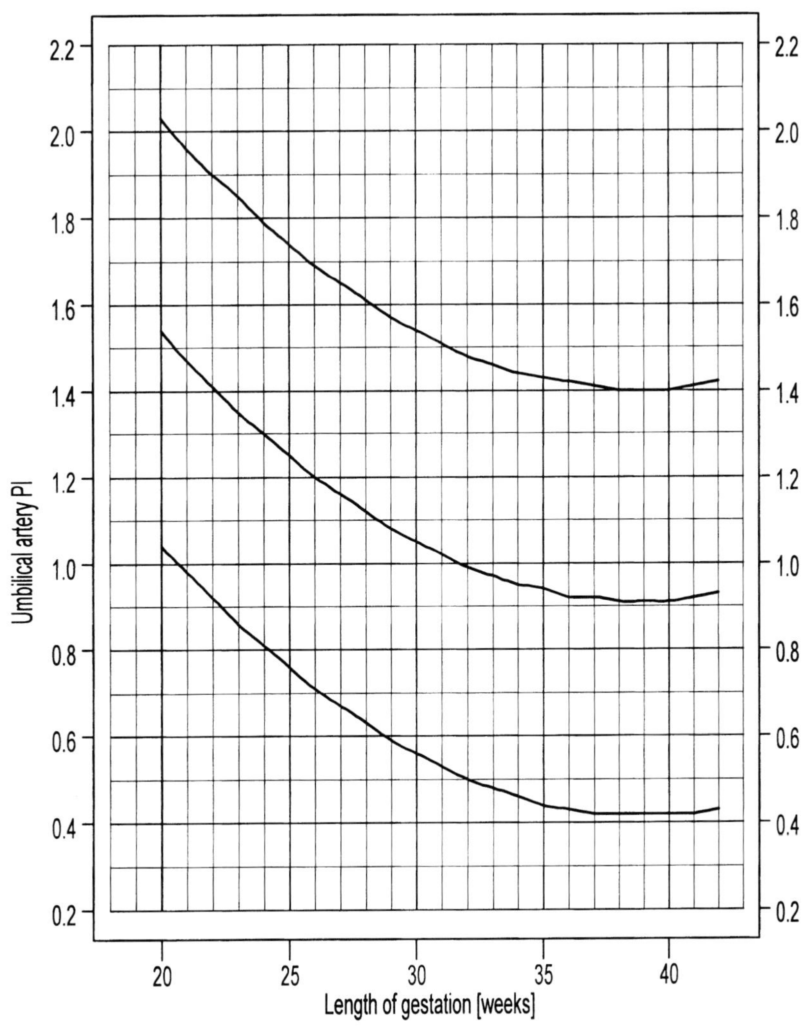

34. Descending aorta pulsatility index

Weeks of gestation	Centiles 5th	50th	95th
20	1.54	1.97	2.39
21	1.54	1.97	2.40
22	1.54	1.97	2.40
23	1.55	1.97	2.40
24	1.55	1.98	2.40
25	1.55	1.98	2.40
26	1.55	1.98	2.41
27	1.56	1.98	2.41
28	1.56	1.99	2.41
29	1.56	1.99	2.41
30	1.56	1.99	2.42
31	1.57	1.99	2.42

Weeks of gestation	Centiles 5th	50th	95th
32	1.57	2.00	2.42
33	1.57	2.00	2.42
34	1.57	2.00	2.43
35	1.58	2.00	2.43
36	1.58	2.00	2.43
37	1.58	2.01	2.43
38	1.58	2.01	2.44
39	1.59	2.01	2.44
40	1.59	2.01	2.44
41	1.59	2.02	2.44
42	1.59	2.02	2.45

Source: Arduini and Rizzo[14]
Comment: Excluded IUGR; SD taken as constant

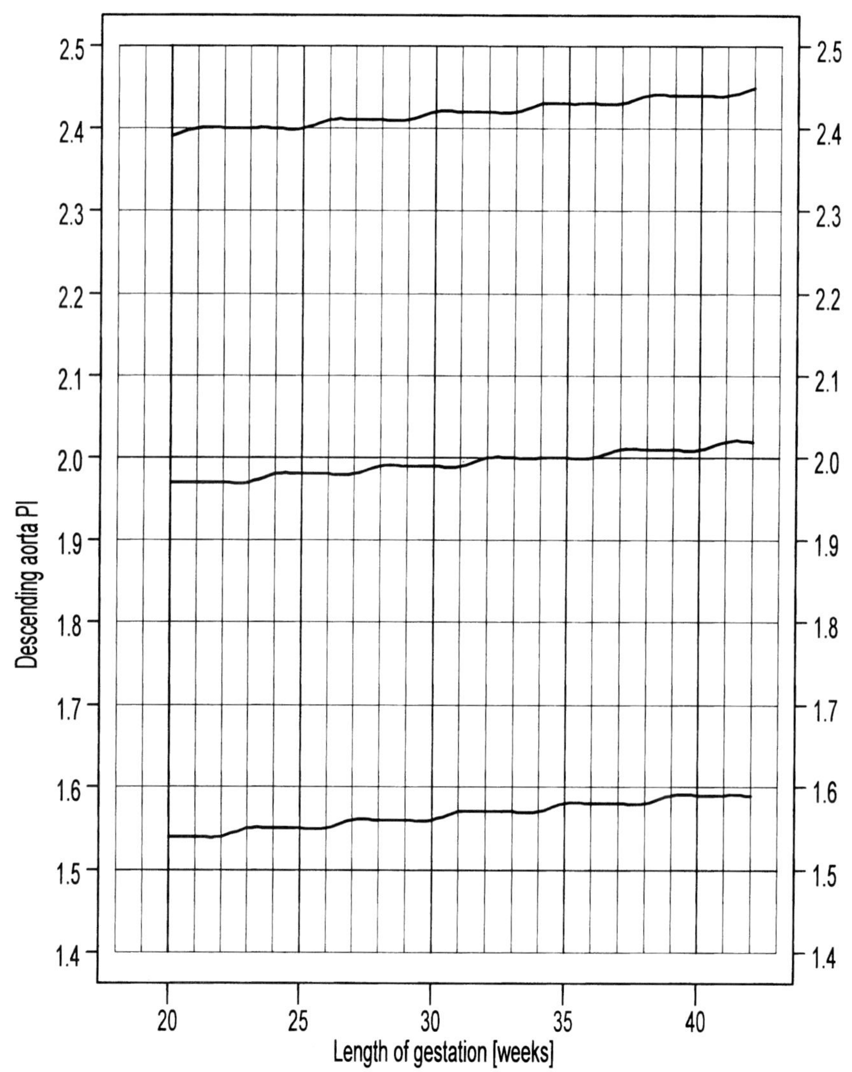

35. Renal artery pulsatility index

Weeks of gestation	Centiles 5th	50th	95th
20	1.61	2.52	3.43
21	1.59	2.50	3.41
22	1.57	2.48	3.39
23	1.55	2.46	3.36
24	1.54	2.44	3.34
25	1.52	2.42	3.32
26	1.50	2.40	3.29
27	1.48	2.38	3.27
28	1.46	2.35	3.25
29	1.44	2.33	3.23
30	1.42	2.31	3.20
31	1.40	2.29	3.18

Weeks of gestation	Centiles 5th	50th	95th
32	1.38	2.27	3.16
33	1.36	2.25	3.14
34	1.34	2.23	3.12
35	1.32	2.21	3.10
36	1.30	2.19	3.08
37	1.28	2.17	3.06
38	1.25	2.15	3.04
39	1.23	2.13	3.02
40	1.21	2.11	3.00
41	1.19	2.08	2.98
42	1.16	2.06	2.96

Source: Arduini and Rizzo[14]
Comment: Excluded IUGR; SD taken as constant

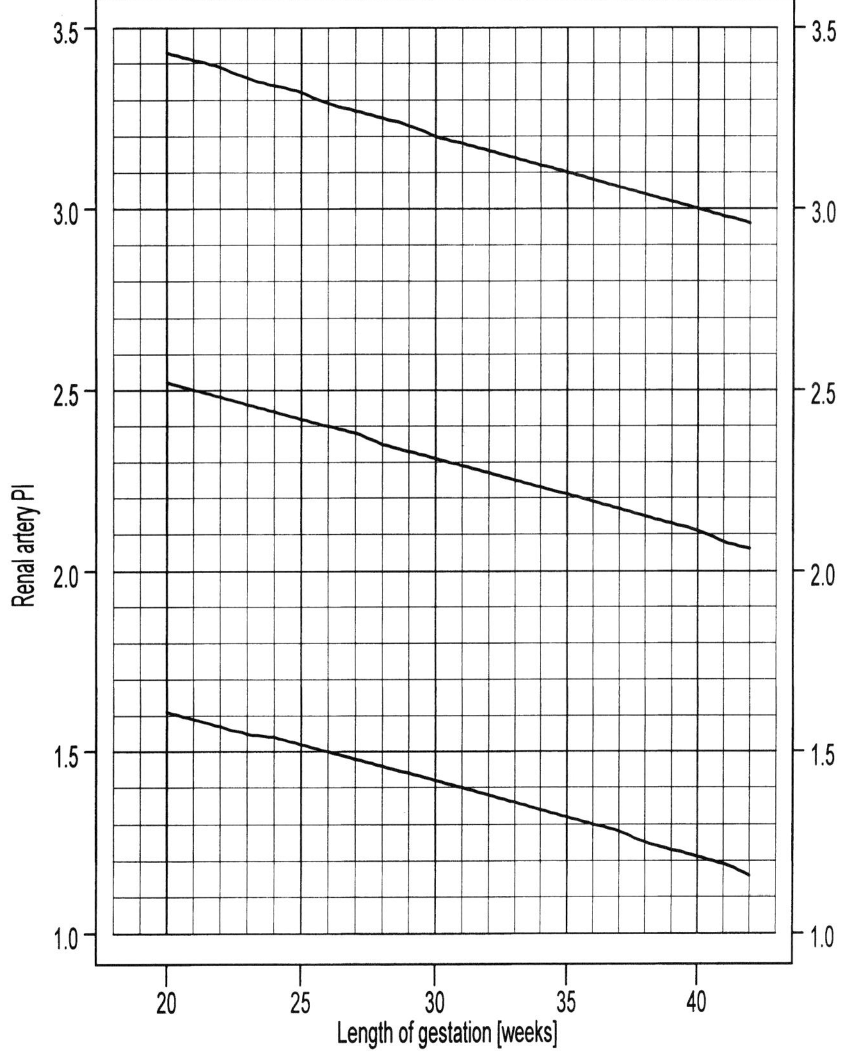

36. Internal carotid artery pulsatility index

Weeks of gestation	Centiles 5th	50th	95th
20	1.19	1.65	2.10
21	1.22	1.68	2.13
22	1.25	1.70	2.15
23	1.28	1.73	2.18
24	1.30	1.75	2.20
25	1.31	1.76	2.21
26	1.33	1.78	2.22
27	1.34	1.79	2.23
28	1.34	1.79	2.24
29	1.35	1.79	2.24
30	1.34	1.79	2.24
31	1.34	1.79	2.23
32	1.33	1.78	2.23
33	1.32	1.77	2.21
34	1.30	1.75	2.20
35	1.28	1.73	2.18
36	1.26	1.71	2.16
37	1.23	1.68	2.13
38	1.20	1.65	2.10
39	1.17	1.62	2.07
40	1.13	1.58	2.03
41	1.09	1.54	1.99
42	1.05	1.50	1.95

Source: Arduini and Rizzo[14]
Comment: Excluded IUGR; SD taken as constant

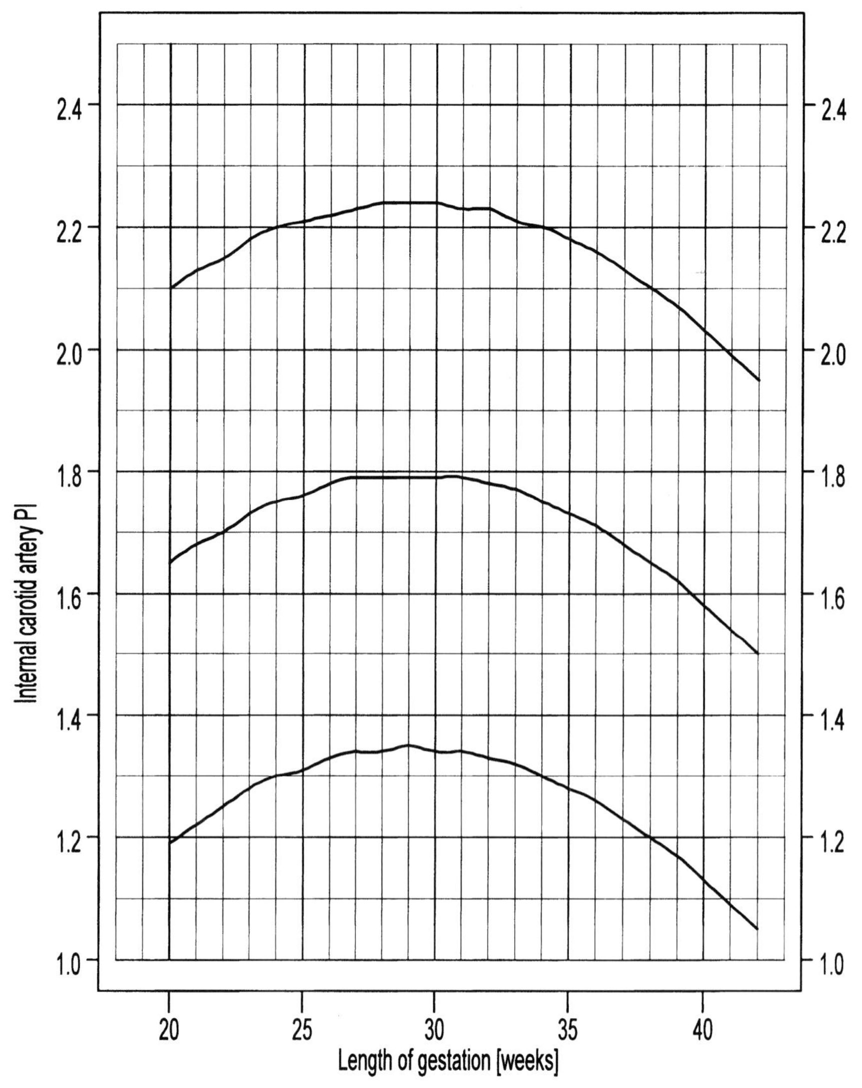

37. **Middle cerebral artery pulsatility index**

Weeks of gestation	*Centiles*		
	5th	*50th*	*95th*
20	1.36	1.83	2.31
21	1.40	1.87	2.34
22	1.44	1.91	2.37
23	1.47	1.93	2.40
24	1.49	1.96	2.42
25	1.51	1.97	2.44
26	1.52	1.98	2.45
27	1.53	1.99	2.45
28	1.53	1.99	2.46
29	1.53	1.99	2.45
30	1.52	1.98	2.44
31	1.51	1.97	2.43
32	1.49	1.95	2.41
33	1.46	1.93	2.39
34	1.43	1.90	2.36
35	1.40	1.86	2.32
36	1.36	1.82	2.28
37	1.32	1.78	2.24
38	1.27	1.73	2.19
39	1.21	1.67	2.14
40	1.15	1.61	2.08
41	1.08	1.55	2.01
42	1.01	1.48	1.94

Source: Arduini and Rizzo[14]
Comment: Excluded IUGR; SD taken as constant

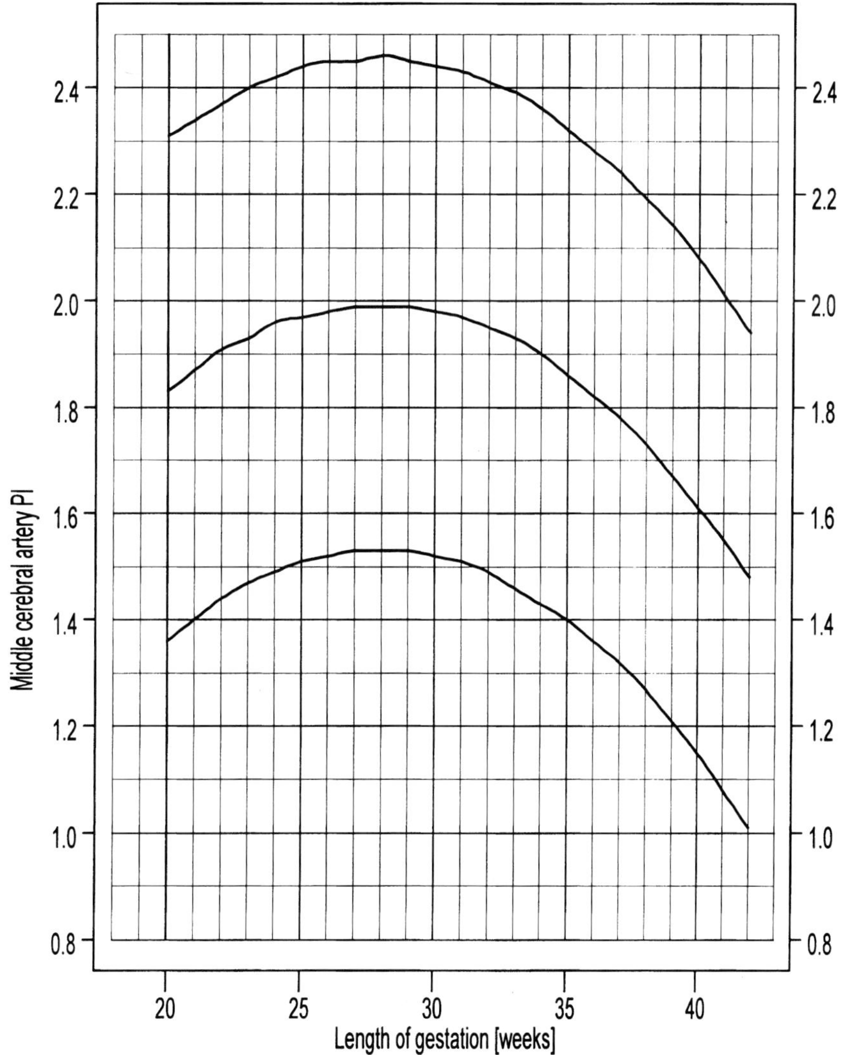

38. Non-placental uterine artery pulsatility index

Weeks of gestation	Centiles 5th	50th	95th
18	0.75	1.23	2.02
19	0.73	1.21	1.98
20	0.72	1.18	1.94
21	0.71	1.16	1.90
22	0.69	1.13	1.86
23	0.68	1.11	1.82
24	0.66	1.09	1.79
25	0.65	1.07	1.75
26	0.64	1.05	1.72
27	0.62	1.02	1.68
28	0.61	1.00	1.65
29	0.60	0.98	1.61
30	0.59	0.96	1.58
31	0.58	0.94	1.55
32	0.56	0.93	1.52
33	0.55	0.91	1.49
34	0.54	0.89	1.46
35	0.53	0.87	1.43
36	0.52	0.85	1.40
37	0.51	0.84	1.37
38	0.50	0.82	1.34
39	0.49	0.80	1.32
40	0.48	0.79	1.29
41	0.47	0.77	1.27
42	0.46	0.76	1.24

Source: Bower et al.[15]
Comment: Model not fully specified

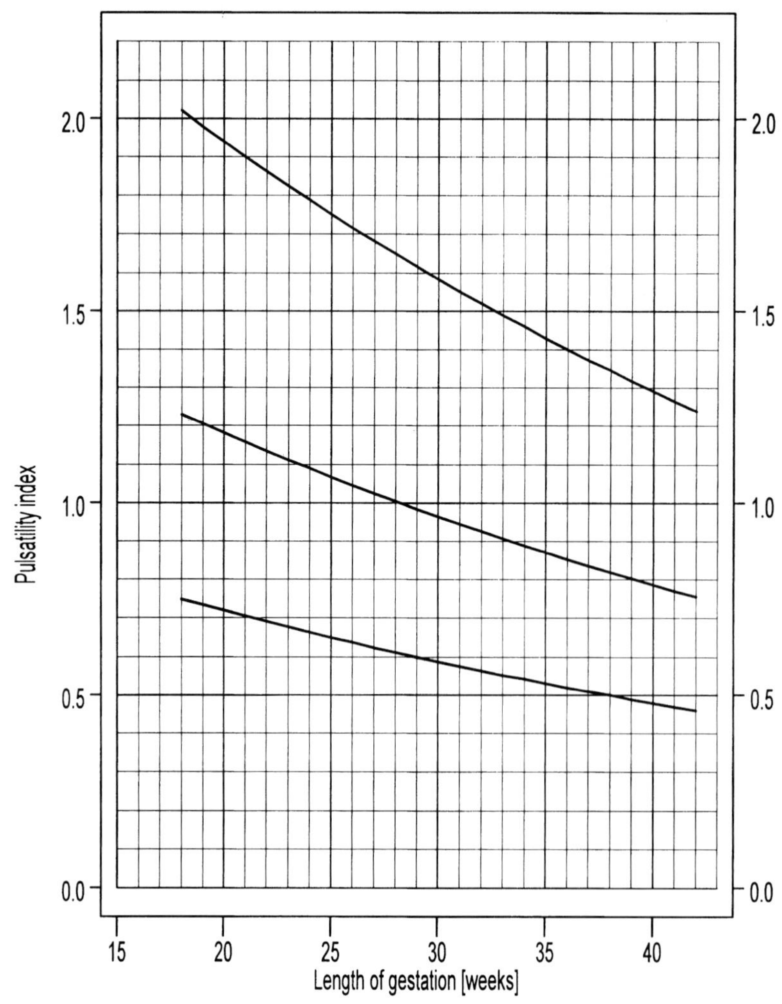

39. **Placental uterine artery pulsatility index**

Weeks of gestation	Centiles 5th	50th	95th
18	0.55	0.90	1.47
19	0.53	0.87	1.43
20	0.52	0.85	1.39
21	0.50	0.82	1.35
22	0.49	0.80	1.31
23	0.47	0.78	1.27
24	0.46	0.75	1.24
25	0.45	0.73	1.20
26	0.43	0.71	1.17
27	0.42	0.69	1.13
28	0.41	0.67	1.10
29	0.40	0.65	1.07
30	0.39	0.63	1.04
31	0.37	0.61	1.01
32	0.36	0.60	0.98
33	0.35	0.58	0.95
34	0.34	0.56	0.92
35	0.33	0.55	0.90
36	0.32	0.53	0.87
37	0.31	0.52	0.85
38	0.31	0.50	0.82
39	0.30	0.49	0.80
40	0.29	0.47	0.78
41	0.28	0.46	0.75
42	0.27	0.45	0.73

Source: Bower et al.[15]
Comment: Model not fully specified

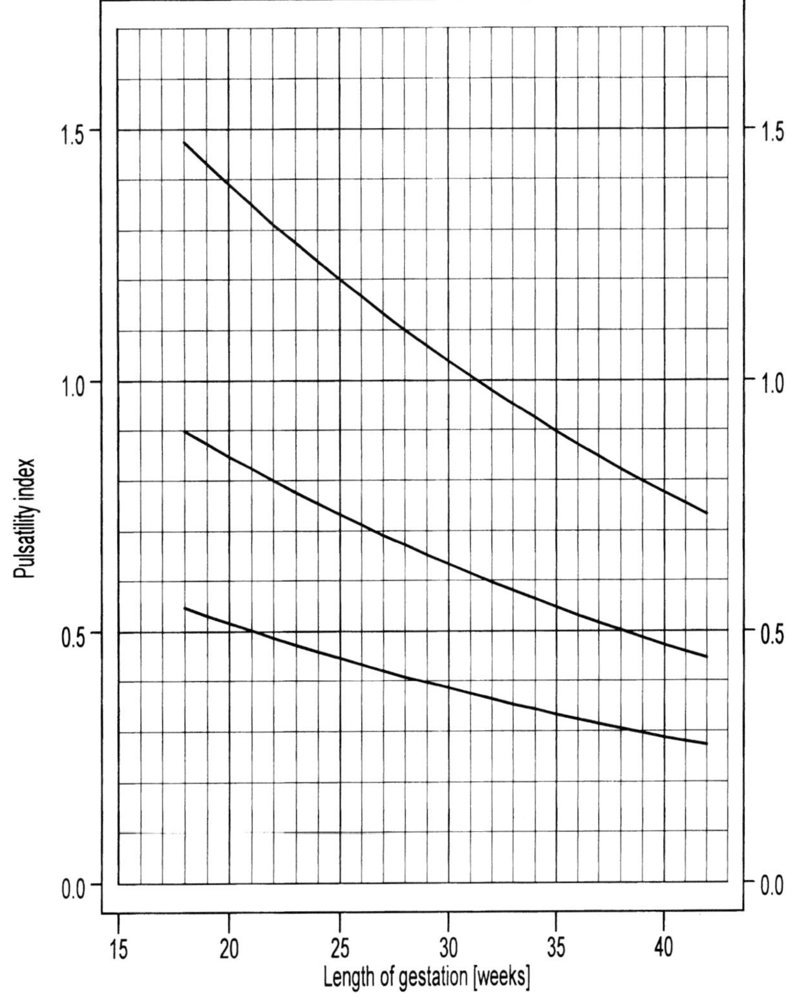

40. **Amniotic fluid index**

Weeks of gestation	*Centiles 50th*		
	5th	*50th*	*95th*
16	79	121	185
17	83	127	194
18	87	133	202
19	90	137	207
20	93	141	212
21	95	143	214
22	97	145	216
23	98	146	218
24	98	147	219
25	97	147	221
26	97	147	223
27	95	146	226
28	94	146	228
29	92	145	231

Weeks of gestation	*Centiles*		
	5th	*50th*	*95th*
30	90	145	234
31	88	144	238
32	86	144	242
33	83	143	245
34	81	142	248
35	79	140	249
36	77	138	249
37	75	135	244
38	73	132	239
39	72	127	226
40	71	123	214
41	70	116	194
42	69	110	175

Source: Moore and Cayle[16]

Comments: Excluded birthweight <10th or >90th centile. Model not fully specified

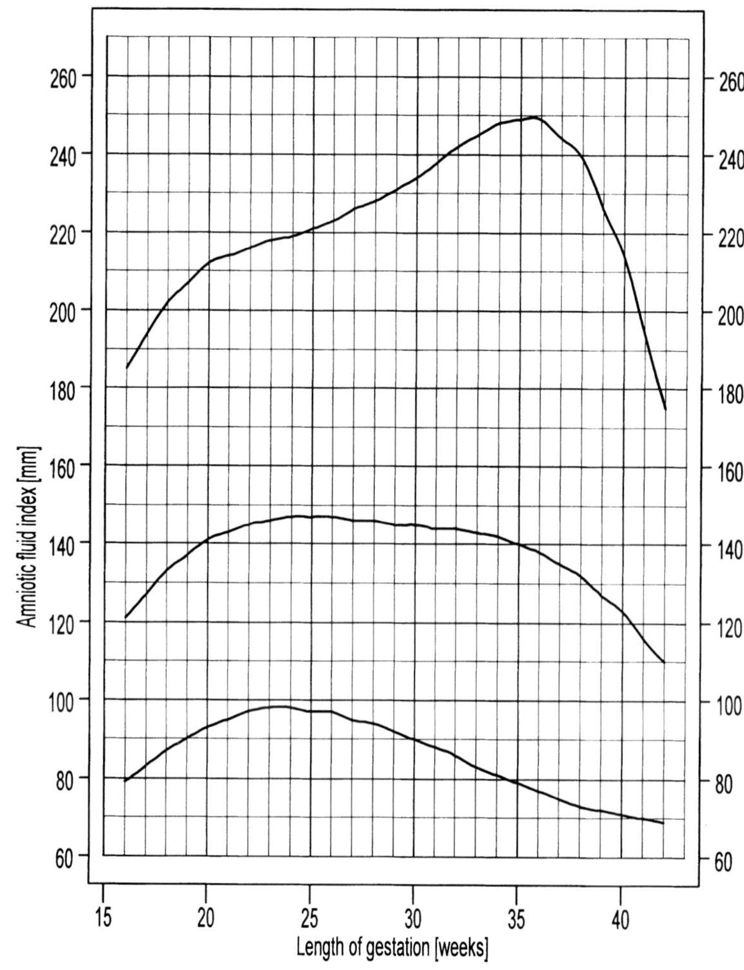

41. **Fetal hemoglobin**

Weeks of gestation	Centiles (g/dl)		
	5th	50th	95th
16	9.1	10.6	12.2
17	9.3	10.8	12.3
18	9.4	11.0	12.5
19	9.6	11.1	12.7
20	9.7	11.3	12.8
21	9.9	11.4	13.0
22	10.0	11.6	13.1
23	10.2	11.7	13.3
24	10.3	11.9	13.4
25	10.5	12.1	13.6
26	10.7	12.2	13.8
27	10.8	12.4	13.9
28	11.0	12.5	14.1
29	11.1	12.7	14.2
30	11.3	12.8	14.4
31	11.4	13.0	14.5
32	11.6	13.1	14.7
33	11.8	13.3	14.8
34	11.9	13.5	15.0
35	12.1	13.6	15.2
36	12.2	13.8	15.3
37	12.4	13.9	15.5
38	12.5	14.1	15.6
39	12.7	14.2	15.8
40	12.8	14.4	15.9

Source: Nicolaides et al.[17], Royston and Wright[3]

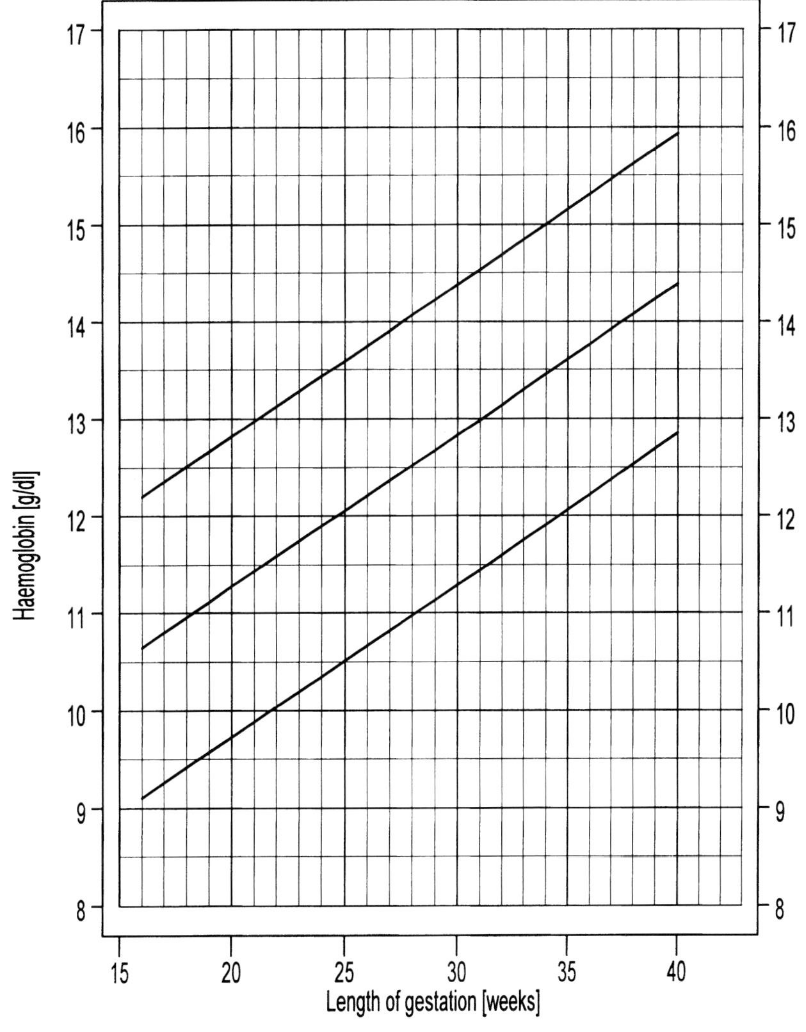

42. **Fetal urinary sodium**

Weeks of gestation	*Centiles (mmol/l)*		
	5th	*50th*	*95th*
18	70.6	87.0	107.1
19	62.8	77.3	95.2
20	56.4	69.5	85.6
21	51.3	63.2	77.8
22	47.2	58.1	71.5
23	43.9	54.0	66.5
24	41.2	50.8	62.5
25	39.2	48.3	59.5
26	37.7	46.4	57.2
27	36.6	45.1	55.6
28	36.0	44.4	54.7
29	35.8	44.1	54.3
30	36.0	44.4	54.6
31	36.6	45.1	55.6
32	37.7	46.4	57.1
33	39.2	48.2	59.4

Source: Nicolini et al.[18]
Comment: Based on sample of 26

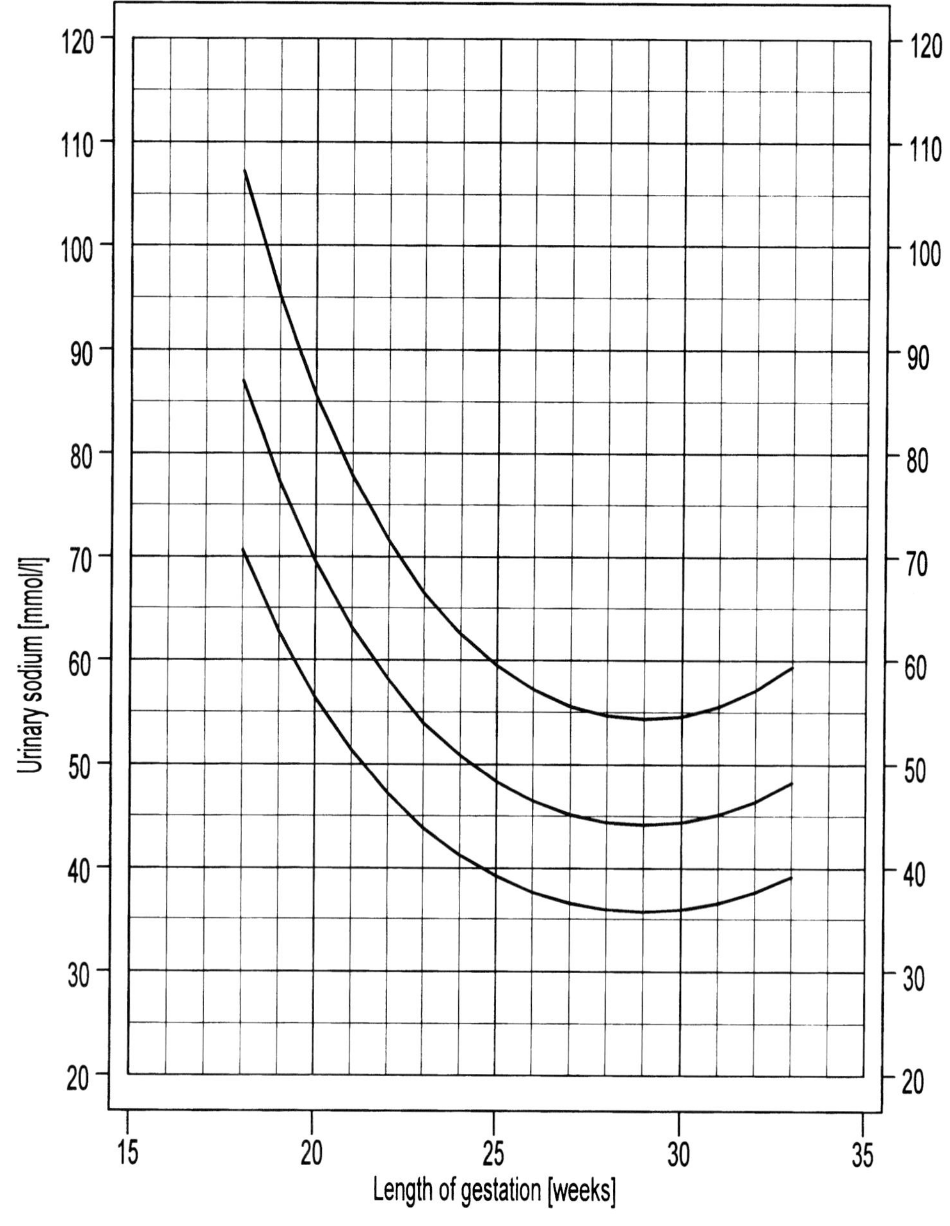

43. Fetal weight estimated from abdominal circumference and femur length

Femur length (mm)	*Abdominal circumference (mm)*										
	200	***220***	***240***	***260***	***280***	***300***	***320***	***340***	***360***	***380***	***400***
40	654	774	918	1087	–	–	–	–	–	–	–
42	689	813	960	1133	–	–	–	–	–	–	–
44	726	854	1004	1181	1389	–	–	–	–	–	–
46	765	896	1050	1231	1442	–	–	–	–	–	–
48	806	941	1099	1283	1497	1748	–	–	–	–	–
50	850	988	1149	1337	1555	1808	–	–	–	–	–
52	895	1037	1202	1393	1615	1871	2168	–	–	–	–
54	943	1089	1258	1452	1676	1936	2235	–	–	–	–
56	994	1144	1316	1513	1741	2003	2304	2650	–	–	–
58	1048	1201	1376	1577	1808	2072	2374	2721	–	–	–
60	1104	1261	1440	1644	1877	2143	2447	2795	–	–	–
62	1163	1324	1506	1713	1949	2217	2523	2870	3265	–	–
64	–	1390	1575	1786	2024	2294	2600	2948	3341	3787	–
66	–	1459	1648	1861	2102	2373	2680	3027	3419	3861	4360
68	–	1532	1724	1940	2182	2456	2763	3109	3498	3936	4428
70	–	–	1803	2021	2266	2540	2848	3193	3579	4012	4498
72	–	–	–	2107	2353	2628	2935	3279	3662	4090	4568
74	–	–	–	2196	2443	2719	3026	3367	3747	4170	4640
76	–	–	–	–	2537	2813	119	3458	3834	4251	713
78	–	–	–	–	2635	2910	215	3551	3923	4333	787
80	–	–	–	–	–	3011	314	3647	4014	4418	862

AC = abdominal circumference
FL = femur le4gth
Source: Hadlock et al.[19]
Equation: Log_{10} weight = 1.304 + 0.005281 × AC + 0.01938 × FL − 0.00004 × AC × FL

44. **Fetal weight From abdominal circumference (AC) and femur length (FL) (in mm)**

Weeks of gestation	Centiles (g)		
	5th	50th	95th
16	120	142	163
17	150	176	203
18	185	218	251
19	226	267	307
20	275	324	373
21	331	390	448
22	395	465	535
23	468	551	634
24	549	647	744
25	640	754	867
26	740	872	1003
27	850	1001	1152
28	968	1140	1312
29	1095	1290	1485
30	1231	1450	1669
31	1374	1618	1863
32	1524	1795	2066
33	1680	1978	2277
34	1840	2168	2495
35	2005	2361	2718
36	2172	2558	2945
37	2341	2757	3174
38	2511	2957	3403
39	2680	3156	3633
40	2848	3354	3860
41	3013	3549	4085
42	3176	3741	4305

Source: Hadlock et al.[19]
Comment: Related to gestation using Chitty et al.[6–8]
Equation: Log_{10} weight = 1.304 + 0.005281 × AC + 0.01938 × FL − 0.00004 × AC × FLSD = 7.7% of weightSD = standard deviation

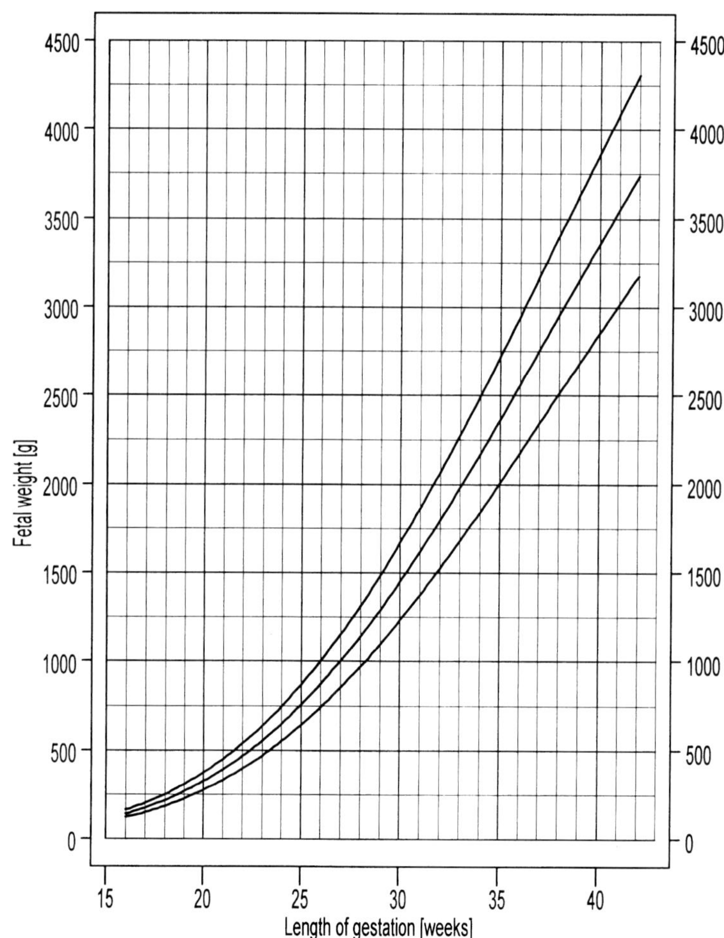

INDEX

NB: Page numbers in **bold** refer to figures and tables

A

Abdomen, 447–456
  biliary tree abnormalities, 452–453
  bowel abnormalities
    functional, 451–452
    structural, 447–451
  intestinal accidents, 453–455
  liver abnormalities, 452–453
  midline herniations, 455–456
  ultrasound appearance, normal, 447
Abdominal circumference (AC), 546–547, 551, 663
Abnormalities, 265–277
  anatomy scan
    first-trimester, 276–277
    mid-trimester, 266–267, **267**
  biliary tree, 452–453
  blood, **83**, 521–522, **521**
  bowel *see* Bowel abnormalities
  cardiovascular, 519–520
  chorionic villus sampling (CVS), 298–299
  chromosome *see* Chromosome abnormalities
  cystic hygroma, septated, 276
  discordant, 662–663
  ductus venosus assessment, 276
  femoral, **486**
  gallbladder, 453
  hemoglobin, 339–340
  intrauterine growth restriction (IUGR), 544
  liver, 452–453
  nasal bone, **271**, 276
  nuchal translucency measurement, 275, **275**
  skeletal *see* Skeletal abnormalities, fetal
  thoracic, 521
  tricuspid regurgitation, 276
  vascular, fetal, 402–403, **404**
  see also Aneuploidy
Absent end-diastolic flow (AEDF), 548, 551, 552, 553, 663
Absent/reversed end-diastolic flow (AREDF)
  cyclical (cyclic AREDF), 663
  velocities, 82, 85
Acetylcholinesterase (AChE) measurements, 245
Achondrogenesis, **490–491**, 491
Achondroplasia, 506, **506**
Acid α-glucosidase (GAA), 365
Acid-base balance, 100–101
Acromesomelic dysplasia, 506–507, **507**
Actin filaments, 6–7, **7**
Activator Ca^{2+}, 123
Adeno-associated virus vectors (AAV), 692, 695
Adenomatous polyposis coli (APC gene), 326
Adenosine, 424
Adenosine deaminase (ADA), 366
Adenovirus vectors, 692
Adenylosuccinase deficiency, 366
Adrenocorticotrophic hormone (ACTH), 141, 142, 592
Advanced maternal age (AMA), 327
Afterload, 126–127, **127**
  sensitivity, 128
Age
  gestational, 664
  maternal, 248–250, **249**, 306, 327, 542, 604
  post-conceptional (PCA), 704
  postovulatory, 25
Age-Adjusted Ultrasound Risk Assessment (AAURA), 273
Aggregate reviews, 201
Akinesia, fetal, 191, **191**
Allele drop-out (ADO), 326, 355
Allele-specific oligonucleotides (ASOs), 338
Alloimmune disease, 111
Alloimmune thrombocytopenia (NAIT)
    see Fetal and neonatal alloimmune thrombocytopenia (FNAIT)
Alpha blockers, 163
Alpha-fetoprotein (AFP), 81, 274
  amniotic fluid, 245
  Down's syndrome, 247–248, 251, 255, 257–261
  levels, 245–246, 535
  as marker, 244–245, **244**
  maternal circulation, 245
  maternal serum (MSAFP), 81, 250, 384, 485, 598
    levels, 245
    maternal weight, **258**
    open spina bifida screening, 245
    overlapping distributions, **248**
    screening, 81, 250–251, **250**, 251–252, **251**, **253**
  measurement, 243–244
Alveolar stage, 134, **135**
Ambystoma, 24
Ameloblasts, 18
Amino acid, 102–103, **102**
  disorder, 367–368, **367**
Aminosalicylates (ASA), 168
Amiodarone, 423
Amniocentesis, 255, 267, 292–295, 341
  complications, 294
  counseling before, 294–295
  indications for, 293
  metabolic disorders, 359
  multiple pregnancy, 652–653, **652**
  red cell alloimmunization, 566, **566**
  technique for, 293–294, **294**
Amniocytes, cultured (CA), 595
Amnioreduction, 657
  medical, 661
Amniotic fluid, 642–647
  alpha-fetoprotein (AFP), 245
  cells, **312**
  DNA, 341
  index (AFI), 551, 643–644, **644**, 645, 657
  kidney/urinary tract disorders, 461–462
  Liley's chart, **566**
  normal, 473
  oligohydramnios, **643**, 644–645, **645**
  polyhydramnios, **643**, 645–647, **646**
  as sample, 306
  volume, 547, 642–644, **643**, **644**, **646**
Amphioxus, 46
Amplification refractory mutation system (ARMS), 339
Amputations, congenital, 508
Analyte values, 246–247, **247**
Anatomical abnormalities
  fetal, 266–267, 276–277
  maternal, 604
Anchoring junctions, 8–9
Anemia, fetal, 521–522, 523
Anencephaly, **246**, 382, **383**, **385**
Aneuploidy, 276
  anomalies, 267–269, **268**, **269**
  autosomal, 307
  biometric markers, 270
  combined screening, 275
  conditions of, 274
  congenital heart disease (CHD), **416**
  intrauterine growth restriction (IUGR), 544
  screening, 327–328
  sex chromosome, 307
  sonographic markers, 267, 269–272, **269**, **270**, **271**
    first-trimester, 274–275, 612–613, **613**
    significance of, 272–273, **272**, **273**
  specific chromosomes, **307**
  zygosity, 650–651
Angelman syndrome, 321
Angiogenesis, 80
Angiogenic mesenchyme, 12, 20, 22
Angiopoietin growth factor, 87–88
Angiotensin I receptor, 152, 153
Angiotensin II receptor, 152
  antagonists, 163
Angiotensin-converting enzyme (ACE) inhibitors, 151, 152, 163, 472
Animals
  disease, 112–113
  model terminology, 5
  nephron studies, 151
Antenatal Results and Choices (ARC), 234, 235, 236–237, 238, 239
Antenatal Screening and Newborns Programmes, 231
Antenatal Screening Web Resource (AnSWeR), 228

Antiarrhythmic drugs, 165–166, **166**
Antibody levels, 564
Antibody-dependent cell-mediated cytotoxicity assay (ADCC), 564
Anticoagulation agents, 164–165
Anticonvulsant syndromes, fetal (FACS), 173, 682
Antidepressants, tricyclic, 174
Anti-epilepsy drugs (AEDs), 172–173
Antigen, human, **580**
  sensitization, 572–573
Antihypertensive drugs, 161–163, **163**
Anti-Kell
  antibody levels, 564
  sensitization, 573
Antimalarial drugs, 169
Antiphospholipid syndrome (APLS), 605
Antiplatelet agents, 164–165
Antiviral treatment, 624–625, 631
Anus, imperforate, 450–451, **450**
Aorta, overriding, 417–418, **417**
Aorta-gonad-mesonephros (AGM), 148, 681
Aortic stenosis/atresia, 421, **421**
Apert syndrome, **489**
Apical ectodermal ridge (AER), 18
Apicomplexa, subclass *Coccidian*, 631
Apoptosis, 13, 74
Arachnoid cysts, 403–404, **405**
Arginine vasopressin (AVP), 139
Argument, ethics and rational, 209
Arnold-Chiari I/II malformation, 45
Arrhythmias, 165
  cardiac, 423–424
  drugs for, 165–166, **166**
Arterial pressure, 127–128, **128**, **130**
Artery-to-artery anastomosis (AAA), 192, 650, 654–655, 658
Artery-to-vein anastomosis (AVA), 654–655, 657
Arthrogryposis multiplex congenita, 191
Arylsulfatase E (ARSE) gene, 504, 506
Ascites
  bowel perforation, **454**
  fetal, 514, **515**
  urinary, 464
Asherman's syndrome, 74
Aspirin, low-dose, 164
  cautions, 164
Assisted reproductive techniques (ART), 649, 668
Association of Clinical Cytogenetecists (ACC), 311
Asymmetric intrauterine growth restriction (IUGR), 542
Asymptomatic states, α-thalassemia, 333
Atenolol, 162
Atria and inflow tract, 49–52
Atrial bigeminy, 423, **423**
Atrial ectopic beats, 424
Atrial isomerism, left/right, 422
Atrial natriuretic factor (ANF), 49, 52
Atrial natriuretic peptide (ANP), 655
Atrial premature beats (APBs), 165
Atrial septal defects, 415
Atrioventricular canal (AVC), 49
Atrioventricular septal defect (AVSD), 268, **268**, 269, 418, **418**
Australian and New Zealand Registry, amnioreduction, 657
Autoimmune diseases, 111–112, 169
Autonomy, patient, 226
Autopsy *see* Perinatal postmortem
Autosomal dominant inheritance, 319
Autosomal dominant polycystic kidney disease, 471–472
Autosomal recessive inheritance, 319
Autosomal recessive polycystic kidney disease, 471, **471**
Autosomal structural rearrangement, 308–309, 309–310
  sex chromosome, 310
  unbalanced, 310
'Avoidability', concept of, 198
Azathioprine (AZA), 167–168

B

B cells, 22, 66
Bacterial vaginosis (BV), 604
Balanced reciprocal translocations, 308–309, **309**
Ballantyne's syndrome, 626
Balloon atrial septostomy, fetal, 425
Bardet-Biedel syndrome (BBS), 322
'Barker Hypothesis', 147, 198
Barrier, placental, 81, 98, **98**
  integrity of, 81
Basal lamina, 8, **9**
Basal plasma membrane (BM), 98, 99, 100
  amino acids, 103
Basal plate, 69–70
Basement membrane, 8, 81, 98
Bauplan, 5
Beckwith-Wiedemann syndrome, 187, 455, 472
Behavioral responses, 545
Beneficence, 217
Bereavement *see* Perinatal postmortem; Prenatal diagnosis
Beta$_2$-agonists, inhaled, 166
Beta-blockers, 162, 165
Betamethasone, 167
Bias, 199
Biliary tree abnormalities, 452–453
Binucleation stage, 123
Biochemical markers, 546
Biometrics, 546, **547**
  markers, 270
Biophysical profile (BPP), 551, 552
Biopsy forceps, curved, 296, **296**
Biparietal diameter (BPD) measurements, 245, 546
Bipolar cord
  diathermy, 666
  occlusion, 666
Birth
  ethical issues, 213
  margins of viability, 705–706, **705**, **706**
  very preterm, 703–706, **705**
    brain lesions, 706–707
Bladder
  dilatation, 464, **464**, **465**
  embryology, 460
  extrophy, 451
  outlet obstruction, 462
Blake's pouch cyst, 400
Blastocysts, 63, 71
  biopsy, 324–325
Blastomeres, **327**
  aspiration, **324**
Blastula, 3
Bleeding *see* Hemorrhage
Bleomycin (BLM), 530
Blood
  donor, 569
  islands, 681
  Kell positive, 573
  red cells (RBC), 168
  umbilical cord (UCB), 681, 682
  vessels, innervation of, 22
  see also Red cell alloimmunization
Blood, fetal, 359
  abnormalities, 521–522, **521**
  ABO group, 567
  transfusion *see* Intrauterine blood transfusion
  see also Fetal blood sampling
Blood flow, 98
  coronary, 129–130, **130**
  fetal organ, 125, **125**, **126**
  fetoplacental, 81–82
  hemochorial, 71
  maternal, intervillous space, 76–77, 76
  patterns, **56**
Blood, maternal, 282–288
  DNA sequences, fetal, 284–285, **284**, 563
  Down's syndrome, 287–288
  fetomaternal traffic, 341
    consequences, 285
    diagnosis, 283–284
  pre-eclampsia, 285–287
Blood pressure (BP), 161, 162
  changes, **122**
Blood-brain barrier, 113
Body plan, 5, 27–31, **29**, **30**, **31**
  stage, 30
Body weight, 188
Bone morphogenetic proteins (BMPs), 23
Bone nomenclature, **478**
Bones, long, 486, **492**
  bowing, 500–503
Bowel abnormalities
  duplication cyst, **452**
  echogenic, 270, **270**, 350, 447–448
  functional, 451–452
  perforation, **454**
  structural, 447–451
Brachycephaly, 271
Bradyarrhythmias, 166
Bradycardias, 165, 166, 423, **423**
Brain
  damage, 658, 706–707
    hypoxic-ischemic, 707–709, **708**
  early fetal, 37, **38**, **380**
    intrauterine infections, 401–402
Brain-derived neurotrophic factor (BDNF), 23
Brain-to-liver ratio (BLR), 188
Branching morphogenesis, 15–16, **15**, 437
Breast feeding
  aminosalicylates (ASA), 168
  antimalarial drugs, 169
  azathioprine (AZA), 167–168
  corticosteroids, 167
  cyclophosphamide, 169
  cyclosporin A, 169
  methotrexate, 168
  mycophenolate mofetil, 168–169
  tacrolimus, 170
  tumour necrosis factor antagonists, 170
  vaccination, 174
'Brenner Hypothesis', 150
Bronchopulmonary dysplasia (BPD), 704
Bronchopulmonary sequestration (BPS), 429, 430, 434
Brucella, 604

C

Cadherins, 9
Caenorhabditis elegans, 13
Calcification, intra-abdominal, **455**
Calcifications, 532
Calcium, 101
  antagonists, 165
  channel blockers, 162
  supplementation, 163
  transport, 99
Calyces, 20
Camptomelic dysplasia, 500–501, **502**

Canadian Early and Mid-trimester Amniocentesis Trial (CEMAT), 293
Canalicular stage, 134, **135**
Capillary endothelium, fetal, 98
Capillary growth, **80**
Carbamazepine, 172, 173
Carbimazole/methimazole (CBZ), 172
Carbohydrate metabolism disorders, 364–366, **365**
Carbon dioxide, 100–101
Carboxylase deficiency, multiple, 596
Cardiac arrhythmias, 423–424
  treatment of, 165
Cardiac contractions, 28
Cardiac function curve (CFC), 127, **127**
Cardiac looping, 48–49, **50**, **51**
Cardiac output, fetal, 125–128
  determinants, 126–128
  distribution of, 125–126
Cardiologists, fetal, 413
Cardiothoracic ratio (CTR), fetal, 344–345
Cardiotocography (CTG), 551, 552, 553, 566, 661, 664, 665
Cardiovascular abnormalities, 519–520
Cardiovascular conditions, hydrops, 517
Cardiovascular disease, renin-angiotensin system (RAS) changes, 153
Cardiovascular system, 119–131
  adult circulation, 123–124
  cardiac development, 119–123, **120**, **121**, **122**, **123**
  fetal circulation, 124, **124**
  fetal hemodynamics, 124–130
  see also Heart, development of
Cardioverters, 165
Carnegie staging system, 25, 26
Case studies, 198–199
Case-controlled studies, 199
Catecholamines, 143
Cat-eye syndrome, 311
Catheter shunt placement, 431–432, **432**
Cell adhesion molecules (CAMs), 9
Cell-cell junctions, 8–10, **10**
Cell-free DNA (cfDNA), 282
Cell-free RNA, 282
Cell-matrix junctions, 12
Cellular interaction, 74
Cellular mechanisms, 6–23
  cycles, 14, **14**
  cytokines/growth factors, 22–23
  embryonic tissue, 8–12
  epithelial/mesenchymal
    interactions, 15–22
    transformation, 12
  general characteristics, 6–8
  induction and division, 12–13
  tissue interactions, 14–15
Celom, 28–29, **29**
Centers for Disease Control and Prevention (USA), 294, 629, 633, 636
Central nervous system, fetal, 35, 379–406
  anatomy, 379–381, **380**, **381**, **382**, **383**
  cerebellar development disorders, 396–400
  intracranial cysts, 403–405
  intrauterine infections, 401–402
  neuronal migration, 396, **397**
  neuronal proliferation disorders, 393–396
  prenatal insults, 400–401
  primary neurulation disorders, 381–386
  prosencephalic development disorders, 388–391
    mid-line, 391–393, **391**, **392**
  secondary neurulation disorders, 386–388
  vascular abnormalities, 402–403, **404**
Cephaloceles, fetal, **384**
Cerebellar development disorders, 396–400
Cerebral artery
  middle (MCA), 293, 549, **550**, 551–553, 565, **565**
    peak systolic velocity (MCA PSV), 565, 567, 572–573, 626–627, 657, 665
Cerebral lesions, 400–401, **400**, **401**
Cerebral palsy, **668**
Cervical teratoma, 530–531, **531**, **532**
Chambers, absent/hypoplastic, 419, **419**
Chest, small, associated dysplasias, 495–500
Chick stage series, 24–25
Chickenpox-zoster virus, 629–631
  congenital varicella syndrome, 630, **630**
Chick-quail chimera experiment, 37
Children's Hospital of Philadelphia (CHOP), 429, 442
Chlamydia trachomatis, 604
Chloridorrhea, congenital, 452
Choledochal cysts, 452, 453, **453**
Chondrodysplasia punctata
  rhizomelic, 503–504, **504**
  X-linked recessive, 504, **505**, 506
Chondroitin sulfate, 10
'Chorion regression syndrome', 77
Chorionic villus cells (CVC), 358–359
  cultured (CCVC), 595
Chorionic villus sampling (CVS), 341
  complications of, 297–299
  confined placental mosaicism, 544, 548
  counseling before, 299–300
  as diagnostic procedure, 292, 293, 295–300
  DNA, 341
  Down's syndrome, 249, 255
  endocrine disorders, 593
  indications for, 295
  laboratory aspects of, 299
  metabolic disorders, 358, 359, 369
  multifetal pregnancy reduction, 668
  multiple pregnancy, 653, **653**
  risk of fetal loss, 606
  techniques of, 295–297, **295**, **296**, **297**
  transabdominal (TA), 296, 297
  transcervical (TC), 296, 297
Chorionicity, 523, 650, 664
Choroid plexus cysts (CPCs), 274, 404–405, **405**
Chromosome abnormalities, 307–311, **307**, 519, 603–604
  embryos, 325, 326–328, **327**
  mosaicism, 308, 325, **328**
  single gene disorder overlap, 320–321
Chromosomes, 305
  analysis, 187
  paints, 312, **313**
Chronic granulomatous disease (CGD), 684
Chronic lung disease (CLD), 143
Chronic renal failure, **467**
Circulation
  adult, 123–124
  embryo-placental, 77
  fetal, 124, **124**, 125
  fetoplacental, 81–82, 548–549, **549**
  maternal, 245
  uteroplacental, 548, **548**
  see also Blood, maternal
CLASP study, 164
Cleavage stage biopsy, 324, **324**
Cleidocranial dysplasia, 45
Clinical information, perinatal postmortem, 183, **184–185**
Clinical and Laboratory Standards Institute, 260
Clinodactyly, **271**
Cloacal anomalies, complex, 462
Cloacal extrophy, 451
Closed spina bifida with lipoma, **388**
Cocaine, 605
Coccidian, 631
Cochrane Collaboration, 201
Cochrane Database of Systematic Reviews, 201
Cochrane meta-analysis, 606
Cochrane review, 296, 658
Codes of conduct, professional, 217
Codes of Practice
  postmortem consent, 183
  for postmortems, 182–183
Cole-Hughes syndrome, 395
Collaborative Eclampsia Trial, 199
Collaborative studies (UK)
  First, 246, 248
  Second, 245
Collagen, 10–11
  type I, 11, 20, 492, 501
  type II, 11, 16
    transient expression of, **17**
  type III, 11, 15–16
  type IV, 8, 12, 20, 22
  type V, 11
  type VII, 12
  type IX, 12
  type XI, 11
  type XII, 12
Collecting ducts, of kidney, 20
College of American Pathologists, 260
Colony-stimulating factors (CSFs), 23
Committed cells, 12
Communicating junctions, 9
Communication, effective, 235
Comparative genomic hybridization (CGH), 187, 293, 313, 324, 325
Competent tissue, 15
Competitive oligonucleotide priming (COP), 339
Complete hydatidiform mole (CHM), 607
Computed tomography (CT), 478, 530, 621, 662
Confidential Enquiry reports, 198
Confined placental mosaicism (CPM), 299, 306, 308, 325
  chorionic villus sampling (CVS) and, 544
  counseling, 300
Congenital abnormalities of the genital and urinary tract (CAKUT), 154
Congenital adrenal hyperplasia (CAH), 592–594, **593**
Congenital bilateral absence of the vas deferens (CBAVD), 353
Congenital cystic adenomatoid malformation (CCAM), 429, 430–431, 439
  fetal lobectomy, 432
  surgery, 432–433, **432**
    exit procedure, 433–434, **434**
Congenital diaphragmatic hernia (CDH), 437–444
  associated anomalies, 440
  embryology, 438
  etiology, 437–438
  genetics, 438
  management, pre-/perinatal, 442–444
  natural history, 438–439
  prenatal diagnosis, 439–442, **440**, **441**
  pulmonary hypoplasia, 438
  severity prediction, 439–440
Congenital Diaphragmatic Hernia Registry, 443
Congenital disorder of glycosylation (CDG) syndrome, 366
Congenital heart disease (CHD), 412–425
  auditing outcomes, 424–425
  classification, 415–423
  delivery, timing, 424
  family history, 413
  fetal cardiologists, 413
  intervention, fetal, 443–444

Congenital heart disease (CHD) (*continued*)
management
perinatal, 424
in pregnancy, 424–425
new technologies/therapies, 425
screening, 412–413
first trimester, 414–415, **414**
training, 413–414
Congenital hypothyroidism (CHT), 354
Congenital myotonic dystrophy (CMD), 482, 485
Connective tissue, 45, 78, 81
Connexon, 9
Conradi Hünermann, 504
CONSORT guidelines, 200
Contamination, misdiagnosis, 326
Contingent screening, 256
Contractility, 127–128
Contraction, cardiac, **123**
'CoolCap' study, 708
Coomb's method, 564
Coomb's test, 567
Copy number variants (CNVs), 310, 311, 313
Cord occlusion, 666
Cordocentesis, 344
Cornelia de Lange syndrome, **488**
Coronal planes, **380**, **383**
Coronary flow, 129–130, **130**
Coroner's jurisdiction, 182
Corpus callosum (CC), agenesis (ACC), 391–393, **391**, **392**
Corticosteroids, 167
oral, 167
systemic, 167
Cortisol, 141
Coumarin embryopathy, 164–165
Counseling
before amniocentesis, 294–295
before chorionic villus sampling (CVS), 299–300
confined placental mosaicism (CPM), 300
congenital heart disease (CHD), 415
screening, 346
skeletal abnormalities, fetal, 511
'Couple testing' for CF carrier status, 352
Cranial meningocele, **384**
Cranial nerves, 37, 530
Craniorachischisis, 382
'Critical titer', 564
Cromolyn, 166
Crown-rump length (CRL), 26, 257, 295, 546, 609–611, **610**, 651
Cultured amniocytes (CA), 595
Cultured chorionic villus cells (CCVC), 595
Cyclo-oxygenase (COX), 153
Cyclophosphamide, 169
Cyclosporin A, 169
Cystic adenomatoid malformation
congenital (CCAM), 429, 430–431, 432–433, **432**, 433–**434**, 434, 439
volume ratio (CVR), 431
Cystic fibrosis (CF), 325–326, 349–355
antenatal screening, 352–354, **353**
'bright gut', **454**
clinical overview, 349
echogenic bowel as marker, 350
family history, 352
newborn screening, 254–255, **354**
preimplantation testing, 355
presymptomatic testing, 350–355
transmembrane conductance regulator (CFTR) gene, 349, 350, **351**, 352–353, 355
Cystic Fibrosis Foundation, 689
Cystic hygroma, 268, **269**
/lymphangioma, 528–530, **529**
septated, 276
Cystic kidneys, 472
Cysts, 631
arachnoid, 403–404, **405**
blastocysts, 63, 71
choledochal, 452, 453, **453**
hepatic, 452
intracranial, 403–405
microcysts, **468**
oocysts, 631
Cytogenetic analysis, 305–315
chromosome abnormalities, 307–311, **307**
future prospects, 315
prenatal samples, 306
referral indications, 306
targeted testing, 315
techniques/applications, 311–315
Cytokines, 22–23
Cytomegalic inclusion disease (CID), 621
Cytomegalovirus (CMV), 189, 293, 401, **401**, 620–625, **624**
congenital, 585, 621–622
fetal anemia, 522
prenatal diagnosis, 622–623
primary, 544, 548
Cytoskeleton, 6–8, **7**
Cytotrophoblast cells, 64, 77, 80, 81
Cytotrophoblast layer, 71

D

Dandy-Walker continuum, 397–398, **397**, **398**, **399**
Data
datasets, routine, 197–198
'dredging', 197
monitoring, 200
Data Monitoring Committees, 200
Death, fetal, 297, 298
co-twin, 664
intrauterine (IUFD), 185, 189–192 *passim*, 626, 649, 656–658, 663–665, 670
see also Perinatal postmortem; Prenatal diagnosis
Decidualization, 64–65
Decision making, 226, **226**
after prenatal diagnosis, 235–237
Deep vein thrombosis, 165
7-Dehydrocholesterol reductase (DHCR7), 596
Delivery
congenital heart disease (CHD), 424
hydrops fetalis (HF), 524
intrauterine growth restriction (IUGR), 552–553
Denaturing gradient gel electrophoresis (DGGE), 339
Dendritic cells (DC), 67
Dental lamina, 16
Dental papilla, 16, 18
Depression, treatment of, 173–174
Deren, O., 271
Dermatan sulfate, 10
Dermatological diseases, 301
Dermomyotome, 39
Detection rates, 247–248, **257**, **259**, **262**
Determined cells, 12–13
Developmental Stages in Human Embryos (O'Rahilly & Müller), 25
Dexamethasone, 167
Diabetes mellitus, 170–171, 413
Diagnostic procedures
deletions by gap-PCR, 334, **334**
differential, 439
invasive, 292–301, 566–567, 651–652
MLPA deletions, 334
molecular, 334, 334–335, 338–339, 340
non-invasive, 282–288, 287–288, 565–566
pitfalls, 342
point mutation, 335
preimplantation, 341–342
strategy, 341–342
tests, 198, **198**
see also Preimplantation genetic diagnosis; Prenatal diagnosis
Diastrophic dysplasia, 507, **508**
sulfate transporter gene (DTDST), 491, 507
Dichorionic (DC) twins, 649–650, 651, 652, 653–654, 662–665
Dichorionic triamniotics (DCTA), 650
Differential diagnosis, 439
Differentiation, 13
cell, 13, **13**
epithelial cells, 141–142, **142**
trophoblast, **64**
Diffusion tensor magnetic resonance imaging (DTMRI), 391
Diffusion-limited transport, blood, 98
Digenic inheritance, 322
DiGeorge's syndrome, 43, 45, 312
Dihydropyrimidine dehydrogenase (DHPDH), 366
Diltiazem, 162
Dipalmitoyl phosphatidylcholine (DPPC), 143
DIPex, 228
DISCERN criteria, 227, **227**
Discordancy
abnormalities, 662–663
double, 420, **420**
fetal growth, 663–664
ventriculoarterial connection, 419–420, **420**
Disease
fetomaternal trafficking, 111–113
animal, 112–113
human, 111–112
pregnancy-associated progenitor cell, 113
gene therapy, 690–691, **691**
life-long, 130
maternal, 482, 485, **485**, 543
'of theories', 287
perinatal, 649–650
pre-existing, 160
Disease modifying antirheumatic drugs (DMARDs), 170
Distinctions, drawing, 210
Diuretics, 162–163
Dizygotic (DZ) twins, 650, 662
DNA
analysis, 359–360
cell-free, 285–287
fetomaternal trafficking, 341, 563
repair, 366-367, **366**
Doppler
color flow, 464
congenital diaphragmatic hernia (CDH), 439, 442
pulsed, 423
surveillance, growth discordancy, 663
time intervals, 425
tissue imaging, 424
Doppler studies, **549**, **550**, 551–552, **552**
abnormal, 553
color, 403
early pregnancy failure (EPF), 612
normal, 552–553
red cell alloimmunization, 565, **565**
Dorsal induction, disorders of, 381
Double discordancy, 420, **420**
Double-needle technique, 297, **297**
Douglas, Gordon, 283
Down's syndrome, 248–261, **307**, 309, 315, 449
echogenic bowel, 448
fetal nuchal translucency (NT), ultrasound, 252, 254, **254**

maternal age, 248–250, **249**, 306
screening
detection rates, **257**, **259**
first trimester, 251–252, **253**, 254
integrated, 254–256, **255**
non-invasive, 287–288
quality control/assessment, 260–261
refinements, 257–260
risk cut-off levels, 259–260, **259**
second trimester, 250–251, **250**, **251**
validation trials, 256–257, **257**
termination rates, 236
in twins, **651**, 668
see also Trisomy 21
Drugs *see* Medicines, maternal
Duchenne muscular dystrophy (DMD), 301, 321, 325–326
Ductus arteriosus, 124, **124**
Ductus venosus (DV), 124, **124**, 545
assessment, 276
Duodenal atresia, 268, **269**, **646**
Duodenal obstruction, 449, **449**
Duplex kidneys, 470, **470**
Dural sinus thrombosis, 403, **404**
Duty-based philosophies, 214, 217
Dysmorphic facial features, 173
Dysplasias, skeletal, 480–491, **481–482**, **483–484**

E

Early pregnancy failure (EPF), 602–614
aneuploidy, first-trimester markers, 612–613, **613**
clinical assessment, 607–608
diagnosis, 606
clinical/ultrasound criteria, 608–612, **608**
early pregnancy units (EPUs), 613, 614
endocrinology, 608
etiology of, 603–606
histopathological analysis, 606–607
incidence, 602–603, **603**
management, 613–614
pathophysiology, 606–607, **607**
terminology, 608, **608**
Ebstein malformation, 420
Echocardiography, 530
Echogenic bowel, Down's syndrome, 448
Echogenic intracardiac focus (EICF), **273**, 274
Echogenic renal parenchyma, **468**
Ectoderm, 4
fly-paper model, skull development, 16
neural/surface interaction, 16, **16**, **17**, 18
surface/somatopleuric mesenchymal interaction, 18, **19**
Ectodermal placodes, 35
Ectomesenchyme, 4
Ectopic kidneys, 470
Edema
musculoskeletal problems, 491
nuchal, 515
scalp, **516**
skin, **516**
Effective Care in Pregnancy and Childbirth, 201
Eicosanoids, 153
Elastin, 10, 12
Electrocardiogram (ECG), 424, 425
Electrocoagulation, 468
Electrophysiological assessment, 425
Ellis van Creveld syndrome, 499, **501**
Embryogenesis, perfusion during, 74–75
Embryonic period, 27, **28**, 133
induction, 12–13
tissue, 8–12
interactions, 14–15
see also Staging embryo development
Embryonic stem cells (ESCs), 680
Emopamil-binding protein (EBP) gene, 504
Enamel organ, 16
Encephalocele, 382, 384, **384**, 472
End-diastolic flow, 82, 85
absent (AED), 548, 551, 552, 553, 663
reversed (RED), 548, 551, 552, 553, 663
End-diastolic pressure (EDP), 126
End-diastolic volume (EDV), 126
Endocrine control, fetal growth, 542
Endocrine disorders, 170–172, 592–595, 604
Endocrinology, 608
Endoderm, 4
splanchnopleuric mesenchyme interactions, 18–20
Endothelial differentiation, 85–86
growth factors, 86–88
Endothelium, fetal, 81
Endovascular migration, trophoblast cells, 66
Engraftment barriers, 679–680
Entactin, 8
Environmental toxins, 606
Enzyme replacement therapy (ERT), 357, 360
Enzyme-linked immunoabsorbent assays (ELISA) techniques, 286, 584, 585, 628, 630
Enzymes, 153
analysis, 359
Epiblast, 4
predictive rates of cell population, **4**
EPICure study, 704, 705, **705**
Epidemiological techniques, 197–202
case studies, 198–199
diagnostic tests, 198, **198**
evidence-based medicine, 201–202
experimental studies, 199–200
monitoring, 260, **260**
perinatal mortality surveys, 198
routine datasets, 197–198
systematic reviews, 201
Epidermal growth factor (EGF), 22, 87, 153
Epigenetic cascades, 14
Epilepsy, drugs for, 172–173, 413
Epiphyses, stippled, 503–506
Epithelium, 8–10
cell differentiation, 141–142, **142**
/mesenchyme
interactions, 15–22
transformation, 12
Equine infectious anemia virus (EIAV), 694
Erythropoietin, 23
Escherichia coli, 294
ESHRE PGD Consortium, 324, 325, 327, **327**
Ethical issues, 207–219
birth, 213
case study, 207–208
components, **211**
descriptive/prescriptive analysis, 208–209
duty/goal/rights based philosophies, 217
examples, **208**, **211**
fetal worth, 212
changes in, 213
'fetus as patient', 215–216
frameworks for analysis, 214–215
human worth, 212
importance of, 208
improving expertise, **219**
law, 217–218
maternal-fetal actors, 211–212, **211**
obligations, 213–214
philosophers, 209–210
principles/algorithms, 217
professional, 217
questions, 210–211
theory and practice, 209
trouble, 218–219, **218**
virtue, 217
Ethnic minorities, information giving, 226
Ethnicity, 259
Ethylenediaminetetraacetic acid (EDTA), 350
Etiquette, 217
Eurofetus trial, 657, 658
European Society for Pediatric Endocrinology, 594
Eustachian valves, 51
Evacuation of retained products of conception (ERPC), 613
Evidence-based medicine, 201–202
clinical practice, 197
Evolution hypothesis, head, 46
Ex utero intrapartum therapy (EXIT), 429, 530, 531–532, **532**
Exocelomic cavity (ECC), 608
Exomphalus, 455–456, **455**
Expectant management, 613
Experimental studies, 199–200
Extra structurally abnormal chromosomes (ESACs), 311
Extracardiac malformations (ECM), **416**
Extracellular matrix (ECM), **11**, 12, 141
degradation by trophoblast, 66
receptors, 9
trophoblast cell interactions, 65–66
Extracorporeal membrane oxygenation (ECMO), 143, 432, 434, 441, 442–443
Extraembryonic celom, 29, **29**
Extraembryonic tissue, 4
Extraocular muscles, 44
Extravillous trophoblast (EVT), 606

F

Face, 486, **488**, **506**
defects, **391**
development of, 43
FAMA test, 630
Family history, 258, 352, 413
Farber disorder, 360
FASTER (first- and second-trimester evaluation of risk), 256, **257**, 275, 276, 294
Fathers, prenatal diagnosis, 239
Federal Aviation Administration, 606
Feet, 488, **488**
Femoral abnormalities, **486**
Femur length (FL), 546, 551
Fetal akinesia deformation sequence (FADS), 191
Fetal akinesia/hypokinesia sequence (FAHS), 191
Fetal alcohol syndrome (FAS), 605–606
Fetal Anomaly Screening programme (NSC), 231
Fetal blood sampling (FBS), 292, 300, **300**
multiple pregnancy, 654
red cell alloimmunization, 567
Fetal breathing movements (FBM), 137, 139
Fetal growth restriction (FGR), 67, 691
Fetal heart rate (FHR), 544, 566, 610
Fetal hydrops *see* Hydrops fetalis (HF)
Fetal infections, 620–636
chickenpox-zoster virus, 629–631
cytomegalovirus (CMV), 401, **401**, 585, 620–625, **624**
intrauterine, 401–402
parvovirus B19, 625–627, **626**
perinatal, 630
rubella, 627–629
syphilis, 634–636, **636**
toxoplasmosis, 631–634, **632**, **633**
Fetal Medicine Foundation, 261
Fetal and neonatal alloimmune thrombocytopenia (FNAIT), 579, 581–584, **583**
natural history, 584
prenatal management, 585–587, **586**

Fetal thrombotic vasculopathy (FTV), 189
Feticide, 238, 665–667
  elective late, 667
  multifetal, 668–669
Fetomaternal trafficking, 341
  consequences, 285
  diagnosis, 283–284
  disease, 111–113
  DNA, 341, 563
  in humans, 111
  in mouse model, 110–111
  stem cells, 113
  see also Maternofetal exchange, placental function; Maternofetal trafficking
Fetoplacental circulation, 81–82, 548–549, **549**
Fetoplacental ratio (FPR), 189, 651
Fetoscopy, 560
Fibrinoid, matrix-type, 73
Fibroblast growth factor (FGF), 23
Fibroblast growth factor receptor gene 3 (FGFR3), 495, 506
Fibronectin, 10, 12
Fibrous proteins, 10
Filaments
  actin, 6–7, **7**
  intermediate, **7**, 8
First UK Collaborative Study, 246, 248
FIX expression, 690
Flecainide, 423
Flow reserve, 130
Flow-limited transport, blood, 98
Fluids, fetal, 359
Fluorescence in situ hybridization (FISH), 187, **312**, 313, **313**
Folic acid supplementation, 246
Food and Drug Administration (FDA), 158, 598, 633
  categories, 160, **161**
Foramen ovale, 124, **124**
Forearm defects, 508, **509**, **510**
Frameworks for analysis, 214–215
Free fatty acids (FFA), 103–104
'Free-hand' technique, 293
Frontonasal dysplasia, 384
Functional assessment, imaging, 425
Functional residual capacity (FRC), 138
Fusion stage, 119, **120**

G

Galactosemia, 597
Gallbladder abnormalities, 453
Gallstones, 453
Galt gene, 365, 597
Ganglia, **35**
Gap junctions, 9–10
Gap-PCR diagnosis, 334, **334**, 339
Gastric mucosa, 20
Gastrointestinal tract (GIT), 447
  splanchnopleuric mesenchyme/endoderm interactions, 20
Gastroschisis, 456, **456**
Gastrula, 3
Gaucher disease, 357
'G-banded' chromosomes, 305
Gene therapy, 689–696
  application routes, 691–693, **693**, **694**, **695**
  defined, 689
  diseases, 690–691, **691**
  future challenges, 696
  need for, 689–690
  risks, 693–695
Generalizability, 200, 218
Genetic factors
  cardiovascular, 121
  control, fetal growth, 542
  hydrops fetalis, 519
  imprinting, 321
  red cell alloimmunization, 562–563, **562**
  single gene disorder overlap, 321–322
  sonogram, 267, **268**
  see also Mendelian genetics; Preimplantation genetic diagnosis
Genitalia, external, 460
Genomic imprinting, 321
  intrauterine growth restriction (IUGR), 544
Germ layers, 3–4
Gestation, multiple, 258
Gestational age, 257, 664
Gestational diabetes mellitus (GD), 170
Gestational sac size, 608–609, **609**
Gestational trophoblastic disorders (GTD), 607
Glial cell line-derived neurotrophic factor (GDNF), 148–149
Glioependymal cysts, 404
Globin genes, 331, 333, **334**
Glomerular filtration rate (GFR), 152
Glucocorticoids, 104, 143
Glucose, 101–102, **102**
  transport, 99
Glucosephosphate isomerase (GPI), 366
Glyburide, 170
Glyceraldehyde-3-phosphate dehydrogenase (GAPDH) gene, 285
Glycerolkinase (GK) deficiency, 366
Glycocalyx, 6
Glycogen storage disease (GSD), 365
Glycoproteinoses, 362–363, **362**
Glycosaminoglycans (GAGs), 10–11
Goal-based philosophies, 214–215, 217
Graft-versus-host disease (GVHD), 678, 681, 683
Granulocyte-macrophage colony-stimulating factor (GM-CSF), 22
Graves' disease, 111, 172, 394
Great arterial disproportion, 421–422, **422**
Green fluorescent protein (GFP)
  cells, 114
  transgene, 110–111, 112
Grieving, 238
GROW software program, 546
Growth, fetal, **13**, 22–23, 541–543
  capillary, **80**
  definitions, 541–542
  discordancy, 663–664
  endocrine control, 542
  genetic control, 542
  maternal constraint, 542–543
  normal, 542
  surveillance, 663
  trophoblast differentiation, 86–88
  see also Intrauterine growth restriction (IUGR)
Growth Restriction Intervention Trial (GRIT), 553
Guillian-Barré syndrome, 170
Guilt, 240

H

Hamartoma, hepatic, 452
Hands, 488, **488–489**
Hashimoto's disease, 111–112, 594
Hassall's corpuscles, 188, **189**
Hb Bart's disease, 522
Hb Bart's hydrops fetalis, 333
Hb C, 340
Hb E, 340
Hb H disease, 333
Hb S, 340
Head circumference (HC), 546–547
Head, development of, 33–46
  axial view, **382**
  connective tissue, 45
  early brain, 37, **38**
  evolution hypothesis, 46
  external features, 45–46
  face, 43
  innervation, 44
  muscles, **34**, 44
  neural crest cells, 35–36, **35**, **36**
    fate maps, predictive, 37–38
  neural tube
    paraxial mesenchyme, 36
    patterning, 37, **39**
  neuromeres, 37, **38**
  neurulation, 36
  notochord formation, 36–37
  palate, 43–44
  pharyngeal arches, 41–43, **42**
    angiogenic mesenchyme in, 45
    innervation of, 44
    paraxial mesenchyme in, **34**, 44
    skeletal elements, 43
  pharynx, **34**, 41
  skull, 39
  somite formation, 39–41, **40**
Heart, development of, 47–57
  atria and inflow tract, 49–52
  cardiac looping and chamber formation, 48–49, **50**, **51**
  early stages, 47–48
  ventricles and outflow tract, 52–57, **54**, **56**
  see also Cardiovascular system; Congenital heart disease (CHD)
Heart rate, 126, 610
Helicobacter pylori, 598
HELLP syndromes, 285–286
Helsinki ultrasound trial, 266
Hemangioma, hepatic, 453
Hematological abnormalities, 521–522, **521**
Hematopoietic stem cells (HSC), 678, 679–680, 680–684, 693
  ontogeny, 680, **680**
  sites of, 680–681
  sources, 681
Hemochorial blood flow, 71
Hemodynamic responses, 544–545
Hemodynamics, fetal, 124–130
Hemoglobin concentration, fetal, **561**
Hemoglobinopathies, 331–342
  abnormal hemoglobins, 339–340
  α-thalassemia, 333–335
  β-thalassemia, 335–339, **336–337**
  δβ-thalassemia, 339
  diagnosis
    pitfalls, 342
    preimplantation, 341–342
    prenatal, **334**, 340–341
  fetomaternal traffic, 341
  globin genes, 331, 333, **334**
  thalassemia/sickle-cell disorders phenotypes, **332**
Hemolytic disease of fetus and newborn (HDFN), 559, 560–561, 564, 572
Hemopoietic colony-stimulating factors (CSFs), 23
Hemorrhage
  intracranial, **400**
  intraventricular-periventricular (IVH-PVH), 706–707
Hensen's node, 35
Heparan sulfate, 10–11
Heparin, 10, 85, 164
Heparin-binding epidermal growth factor, 87
Heparin-induced thrombocytopenia (HIT), 164
Hepatic cyst, 452
Hepatic hamartoma, 452
Hepatic hemangioma, 453

Hepatic teratoma, 452–453
Hepatocyte growth factor (HGF), 86
Hereditary persistence of fetal hemoglobin (HPFH), 339
Herniations, midline, 455–456
Heteroduplex analysis, 339
Heterotaxy syndromes, 422
Hippocratic Oath, 217
Hirschsprung's disease, 22, 454
Historical control studies, 199
Hitch-hiker
great toes, **508**
thumbs, **508**
HLA antigens, 580, 581, 583
Hofbauer cells, 79
Holocarboxilase synthetase gene (HCS), 596
Holoprosencephaly (HPE), 389, **389**, **390**
facial defects, **391**
Homologous gene quantitative PCR (HGQ-PCR), 315
'Horizons', embryos, 25
Horseshoe kidney, 470, 472
Hospital autopsy, 182
'Housekeeping proteins', 13
Hox genes, 37, 43, 46
Human chorionic gonadotropin (HCG), 172
Human embryonic stem cells (hESCs), 680
Human epidermal growth factor receptor (HER) proteins, 87
Human Genetic Variation Society (HGVS), 350
Human Genome Project, 197
Human immunodeficiency virus (HIV), 634, 635, 690, 692, 694
Human leukocyte antigens (HLA), 66, 67, 113–114
platelet disorders, 580, 581, 583
in utero transplantation, 678, 679, 683
Human platelet antigens (HPA), 582–583, 586
antibodies, 585
donor, 585
pheno-/genotyping, 584–585
Human stage series, 25
Human Tissue Act (2004), 182
Human Tissue Authority (HTA), 182–183
Huntington disease, 320
Huntington gene, 315
Hurler syndrome, 360, 361, 363, 683
Hyaline membrane disease, 142
Hyaluronic acid, 10–11
Hydatidiform moles, 307–308, 321
complete, 308
partial, 308
Hydralazine, 162
Hydranencephaly, 400–401
Hydronephrosis, 462, 463, **463**, **464**
bilateral fetal, **645**
Hydropic abortion (HA), 607
Hydrops fetalis (HF), 429, 431–432, 514–524
clinical evaluation, 523–524
immune, 517
infectious causes, 522–523
metabolism errors, 363–364
non-immune, 517, **518**, 519–523, **520**, **521**
obstetrics/delivery, 524
pathophysiology, 515, 517
perinatal postmortem, 190–191, **190**
prenatal diagnosis, 514–515, **515**, **516**, **517**
red cell alloimmunization, 561–562, **561**
Hydroureter, 464
Hydroxychloroquine (HCQ), 169
Hypermineralization dysplasias, 491–495
Hyperoxia, placental, 88
Hyperprolactinemia, 604
Hypertension, **151**, 161–163, **163**
Hyperthyroidism, 594–595
maternal, 172
Hypoblast, 4
Hypophosphatasia, 491–492
Hypoplasia, 140–141, 271, **271**
Hypoplastic valves/chambers, 419, **419**
Hypothermia rescue therapy, 708–709
Hypothyroidism, 594
maternal, 171
Hypoxic-ischemic brain damage, 193, 707–709, **708**
Hysterotomy, 532

I

Iatrogenic causes, early pregnancy failure (EPF), 606
Idiopathic thrombocytopenia (ITP), 579–581, 585, 587
diagnosis, 580–581
management, 581, **582**
natural history, 579–580
Ileal atresia, 450
Imaging, 265, 391, 424
functional assessment, 425
perinatal postmortem, 186
see also Magnetic resonance imaging (MRI)
Immature intermediate villi, 79, **79**
Immune factors
mesenchymal stem cells (MSC), 682–683
pregnancy loss, 605
see also Hydrops fetalis (HF); Platelet disorders, fetal; Thrombocytopenia
Immune response, to implanting placenta, 63–67
abnormal, **65**
decidualization, 64–65
leukocyte cells, 66
nidation, 63
trophoblast cells, 64, **64**, **65**
endovascular migration, 66
extracellular matrix (ECM) interactions, 65–66
major histocompatibility complex (MHC) antigens, 66
uterine NK cell recognition, 67, **67**
Immunization, 174, **174**
Immunoglobulin, 101, 170
Immunoreactive trypsinogen (IRT), 354–355
Immunosuppressants, 167–170, **171**
'Implantation window', 63
In utero stem cell transplantation, 678–684
engraftment barriers, 679–680
stem cell biology, 680–684
In vitro fertilization (IVF), 63, 323–324, 327–328, 370, 563, 696
Indication, counseling, 299–300
Individual patient data (IPD) meta-analyses, 201
Induction, embryonic, 12–13
Infantile Refsum disease, 364, **364**
Infection
congenital, 544, 548, 621–624
early pregnancy failure (EPF), 604
hydrops fetalis (HF), 522–523
intrauterine, 297, 627
maternal, 621, 625–626, 627–628, 629–630, 631–632, 634–635
see also Fetal infections
Inferior vena cava (IVC), 124, 422
Information giving *see under* Screening
Informed choice, 226
measuring, 231
Inner cell mass (ICM), 325
Innervation
blood vessel, 22
head, 44
pharyngeal arches, 44
Installation-free sampling technique, 294
Institute of Medical Genetics (Glasgow), 354
Instructive interactions, 14–15
principles of, **16**
Insulin-like growth factor (IGF), 22, 86, 140, 153, 542
Insults, prenatal, 400–401
Integrin family, 9, 12
'Intention to treat', 200
Interferon (IFN), 22
Interferon-beta 1, 170
Interleukin (IL), 22, 23
Intermediate filaments, **7**
Intermediate risk group, 256
International Birth Defects Information Systems (IBIS), 160
International Blood Group Reference Laboratory, 563
International declarations, 217
International Fetal Medicine and Surgery Society, 533
International Nephrology associations, 150
International Platelet Antigen Working Party, 582
Interstitial laser ablation, 667
Interventricular septum, 120
Intervillous space (IVS), 76–77, 606–607
Intestinal accidents, 453–455
Intestinal duplication, 451, **452**
Intestinal perforation, 454–455, **454**, **455**
Intra-abdominal calcification, **455**
Intracardiac focus, echogenic, 270, **270**
Intrachromosomal insertions, 309
Intracranial cysts, 403–405
Intracranial hemorrhage (ICH), 400, 581, 584, 586–587
Intracytoplasmic sperm injection (ICSI), 326
Intraembryonic celom, 28–29, **29**
Intraembryonic mesoderm/intermediate mesenchyme interactions, 20–22, **21**
Intrafetal ablation, 666, **667**
Intrafunic KCl injection, 665
Intrauterine blood transfusion (IUT), 567–573, 627
intraperitoneal (IPT), 571–572
intravascular (IVT), 560, 567, 568–570, **569**, **571**, 572
Intrauterine fetal death (IUFD), 185, 189–192 *passim*, 626, 649, 656–658, 663–665, 670
Intrauterine fetal therapy (IUTx), 678, 679–680
Intrauterine growth restriction (IUGR), 82–85, 274, 485, 543–554
causes, 543–544
defined, 541–542
delivery, 552–553
management, 549–552
oligohydramnios, 644
pathological diagnosis, 188–190
pediatric consequences, 553–554
perinatal postmortem, 188–190, **189**, **190**
placental basis of, 78, 82, **83**, **84**
placental transport, 100, 105
postnatal management, 553
prenatal diagnosis, 545–549
substrate deprivation, 544–545
symmetrical vs asymmetrical, 190
twins, 664
Intrauterine hematomas (IUH), 612, **612**
Intrauterine infections, 297, 627
fetal, 401–402
Intravascular fetal blood transfusion (IVT), 560, 567, 568–570, **569**, **571**, 572
Intravenous immunoglobulin (IVIG), 572, 586–587
Intraventricular-periventricular hemorrhage (IVH-PVH), 706–707
Intuition, 209
Investing mesenchyme, 18
Iron, 101

J

James Lind Library, 201
Jarisch-Herxheimer reaction, 636
Jejunal atresia, 450, **450**
Jeunes asphyxiating thoracic dystrophy, 498–499, **500**
Joints, 488
Joubert syndrome, 399, **399**

K

Karyotypes
 45, X, 307
 47, XXY, 307
 47, XYY, 307
 analysis, 305–306, **306**, 311–312, **312**, 315
Karyotyping, 187, 305–306
 fetal, 295
 intrauterine growth restriction (IUGR), 547–548
 kidney/urinary tract disorders, 465
 multiple pregnancy, 653–654
Kell positive blood, 573
Keratan sulfate, 10
Keratinocyte growth factor (KGF), 430
Kidneys/urinary tract, development, 147–154
 eicosanoids, 153
 metanephros development, 152
 nephron endowment, 149–152
 normal, sonographic, 460–461, **460**
 renal development, 148–149
  agenesis/malformations, 153
 renin-angiotensin system (RAS), 152–153
Kidneys/urinary tract, disorders, 459–473
 associated anomalies, screening, 465
 classification/pathology, 461
 embryology, 459–460
 kidney anomalies, 469–472
  classification/pathology, 469
  number, 469–470, **470**
  position, 470
  prenatal diagnosis/management, 472–473
 renal function, fetal, 459–460, 465–467, **467**, **468**
  renal hypoplasia, 471
 urinary outflow obstruction, 462
 uropathies, fetal, 461
 prenatal diagnosis, sonographic, 462–464
 prenatal management, 464–469
KIR receptors, 67, **67**
Kleihauer test, 191, 570
Kleihauer-Betke test, 523, 569
Klinefelter's syndrome, 307, **307**
 termination rates, 236
Klippel-Feil disease, 45
Kniest dysplasia, 507–508
Krabbe's disease, 360, 361, 683

L

Labetalol, 162
Laboratory
 diagnosis, 623, 625–626, 627–628, 629–630, 632, 635
 results failure, counseling, 300
Lacunar stage, 71
Lamina densa, 8
Lamina lucida, 8
Laminin, 8, 10, 12
Laplace's law, 126, 129
Large polygonal cells, 73
Laser
 ablation, 468, 656–657, **656**, **659**, **660**, 667
 coagulation, 666
Last menstrual period (LMP), 257, 546
Lateral halves of somites, 4
Lateral plate cells, 4
Laurence-Moon-Bardet-Biedl syndrome, 472
Lecompte maneuver, 420
Legislation, 217–218
 on postmortems, 182
Leiden University Medical Centre (LUMC), 587
Lentiviruses, 692
Lethal multiple pterygium syndrome (LMPS), 191
Leucine catabolism, 368
Leukocyte cells, 66
Leukocyte immunoglobulin-like receptors (LILR), 67
Leukotriene receptor antagonists, 167
Likelihood ratio (LR), 198, 248, 273, 651
Limbs
 defects, lower, 508, 510, **511**
 deficiency, 508, **509**, **510**
 girdles, 488
 reduction defects (LRD), 298–299
 short/straight, 506–508
 surface ectoderm/somatopleuric mesenchymal interactions, 18, **19**
Lipidoses, 360–362
Lipids, 103–104, **104**
Lipoprotein lipase (LPL), 103
Lithium, 174
Liver, 20
 abnormalities, 452–453
 biopsy, fetal, 300–301
 herniation, fetal, 440–441, **440**, **441**
Locus control region (LCR), 339
Logic, use of, 210
London Dysmorphology Database, 508, **509**, **510**
Long chain acyl CoA dehydrogenase (LCHAD) deficiency, 368
Long QT syndrome, 423
Long-chain polyunsaturated fatty acids (LCPUFA), 103–104
Looping stage, 120, **120**
Loss, fetal *see* Death, fetal
Low birth weight, defined, 542
Low molecular weight heparin (LMWH), 164, 165
Lower urinary tract obstruction (LUTO), 461, 462
Lung growth, 133–143
 development stages, 133–134, **134**, **135**
 fetal breathing, 137
 fetal liquid in, 137–139, **138**
  clearance at birth, 139
  control of secretion, 137–138
  control of volume, 138–139, **138**, **139**
 hypoplasia, 140–141
 immaturity treatments, 143
 maturation, 141–142
 pulmonary circulation, 136–137
 pulmonary surfactant, 142–143
 regulation of fetal, 139–140
 stretch mechanisms, 140
Lung lesions, fetal, 429–434
 clinical surgery, 431–434
 prenatal diagnosis, 430–431
Lungs
 splanchnopleuric mesenchyme/endoderm interactions, 18–20
 to head ratio (LHR), 441–442, 443–444
 volume measurements, 441–442
Luteinizing hormone (LH), 604
'Luxury proteins', 13
Lymphangioma, cystic, 528–530, **529**
Lymphocytes, 22
Lysosomal storage diseases, 360–364, **361**, **362**

M

Macrocephaly, 395–396, **395**
Macrophages, 22
Magnetic activator cell sorter (MACS) enrichment, 285
Magnetic resonance imaging (MRI), 430, 478
 central nervous system (CNS), 379, 395, 396, 398, 403
 congenital diaphragmatic hernia (CDH), 439, 440, 442
 multiple pregnancy, 658, 662
 perinatal postmortem, 182, 186
Magpie Trial, 200
Major aortopulmonary collaterals (MAPCAS), 417
Major calyces, 20
Major histocompatibility complex (MHC), 66, 78, 678
Male cells, fetal, **283**
Malformations
 of cortical development (MCD), 396
 pre-existing, 160
 see also Abnormalities
Malnutrition, 543
Markers
 alpha-fetoprotein (AFP), 244–245, **244**
 biochemical, 546
 bowel, echogenic, 350
 maternal weight, 258, **258**
 molecular, 26
 skeletal, 270
 sonographic, 267, 269–272, **269**, **270**, **271**
  first-trimester, 252, **253**, 612–613, **613**
  second trimester, 250–251, **250**, **251**
  significance of, 272–273, **272**, **273**
 urinary analyte, 469
Maroteaux-Lamy syndrome, 360, 363
Mass Array™ system, 287, 346
Maternal cell contamination (MCC), 358
Maternal fetal medicine (MFM), 669
Maternal and Perinatal Health Programme (WHO), 286
Maternal serum (MS), 608
 alpha-fetoprotein (MSAFP) *see under* Alpha-fetoprotein (AFP)
Maternofetal exchange, placental function, 97–105
 acid-base balance/carbon dioxide/protons, 100–101
 amino acids, 102–103, **102**
 barrier, placental, 98, **98**
 clinical implications, 104–105
 diffusion distance, 81
 glucose, 101–102, **102**
 immunoglobulins, 101
 iron, 101
 lipids, 103–104, **104**
 nutrient transporters, 104
 oxygen, 99
 transport
  calcium, 101
  sodium, 100
  types, 98–99
 water, 100
Maternofetal trafficking
 human, 113–114
 mouse, 114
 see also Fetomaternal trafficking
Matrix metalloproteinases (MMP), 66
Mature intermediate villi, 79, **79**
Mean cell/corpuscular hemoglobin (MCH), 333, 335, 339, 346, 347
Mean cell/corpuscular volume (MCV), 333, 335, 339, 346, 347
Measurement charts, fetal, 721, 723–766
 list of, 722

Meckel-Gruber syndrome, 384, 472, 473
Meckel's cartilage, 43
Meconium peritonitis, 455
Medial halves of somites, 4
Medicines and Healthcare Products Regulatory Agency (MHRA), 158
Medicines, maternal, 158–174
 antiarrhythmics, 165–166, **166**
 anticoagulation/antiplatelet agents, 164–165
 anti-epilepsy drugs, 172–173
 asthma, 166–167
 depression, treatment of, 173–174
 drug metabolism, 160
 drug-induced effects, on fetus, 160
 early pregnancy, 482, **485**
  failure (EPF), 605–606
 endocrine disorders, 170–172
 fetal breathing movements (FBM), 137
 Food and Drug Administration (FDA) categories, 160, **161**
 hypertension, 161–163, **163**
 immunosuppressants, 167–170, **171**
 placenta, 160
 pre-existing disease/malformation, 160
 teratogen, defined, 158, **159**, 160
 timing/dosage, 160, **161**
 vaccination, 174, **174**
Medium chain acyl-CoA dehydrogenase (MCAD), 368
Megacystis-microcolon-intestinal-hypoperistalsis syndrome (MMIHS), 452, 465
Megalencephaly, **394**
Megaureter, 462
Mendelian genetics, 318–322
 new, 320–322
 traditional teaching, 319–320
Meningocele, cranial, **384**
Menkes disease, 368
Mesencephalon, 37
Mesenchymal stem cells (MSC), 111, 113, 679–680, 693
 differentiation, 681, **681**
 immunology, 682–683
 ontogeny, 682
 plasticity, 682
 sources, 682
 therapeutic applications, 683–684
Mesenchyme, 4
 angiogenic, 20, 22, 45
 cells, 10–12, **11**
 /epithelium
  interactions, 15–22
  transformation, 12, **21**
 investing, 18
 paraxial, **34**, 36, 39–41, **40**, 44
 prechordal, 37
 somite-derived, 22
 villi, **79**, 80
Mesoblast, 4
Mesoderm, 4
Mesonephros, 148, **148**
Messenger ribonucleic acid (mRNA), 22, 70, 77, 287–288
 lung tissue, 143
Meta-analysis, 201
Metabolic disorders, 357–370, 595–597
 amino/organic acid disorder, 367–368, **367**
 amniocentesis and, 359
 carbohydrate disorders, 364–366, **365**
 chorionic villi (CV), 358–359
 DNA analysis, 359–360
 enzyme analysis, 359
 fetal blood/fluids/tissue, 359
 future developments, 369–370
 hereditary, **520**
 list of, **369**
 lysosomal storage diseases, 360, **361**, **362**
 metabolite analysis, 359
 nucleotide disorder, 366–367, **366**
 peroxisomal disorders, 364, **364**
 prenatal diagnosis, 357–358
  detection, 360
  prerequisites, 358
Metabolism
 drug, 160
 fetal, 545
Metachromatic leukodystrophy (MLD), 683
Metanephric blastema, 20
Metanephric mesenchyme (MM), 148, 149, 154
Metanephros development, 152
 urine production/analysis, fetal, 152
Metformin, 171
Methionine synthase (MTR), 598
Methotrexate (MTX), 168
Methyldopa, 161–162
Methylmalonic acidemia (MMA), 595
Methyltetrahydrofolate reductase (MTHFR), 598, 605
Microarray, 307
 comparative genomic hybridization (CGH), 313
 studies, 187
 testing, theory of, **313**
Microcephaly, 393–395, **394**, **395**
Microchimerism, 110
Microcolon-megacystis-intestinal hypoperistalsis syndrome (MMIHS), 452, 465
Microcysts, **468**
Microdeletions, 320–321
Microduplications, 320
Microglobulins, 466
Microseptostomy, 657
Microtubules, 7–8, **7**
Microvillous plasma membrane (MVM), 98, 99, 100–101
 amino acids, 102–103
 lipids, 103–104
Middle cerebral artery (MCA), 293, 549, **550**, 551–553, 565, **565**
 peak systolic velocity (MCA PSV), 565, 567, 572–573, 626–627, 657, 665
Midline herniations, 455–456
Minor calyces, 20
Minoxidil, 163
'Mirror-hydrops', 626
Miscarriage, 67
 incomplete, 611, **611**
 missed, 611, **611**
 threatened, 610–611
Misdiagnosis, 328
Mitoses, proliferative, 13
Mixed lymphocyte reaction (MLR), 683
M-mode assessment, 425
Molar pregnancy, 308
Molecular defects, 333, 335–338, **336–337**
Molecular diagnosis, 334–335, 338–339, 340
Molecular markers, 26
Moloney leukemia retrovirus (MLV), 692
Molybdenum cofactor deficiency, 366
Monitoring
 prenatal, 550–551
 risk, 563–566
Monoamine oxidase inhibitors (MAOIs), 173
Monoamniotic (MA) twins, 660–661, **661**, 667
Monocarboxylate transporter (MCT), 100
Monochorionic (MC) twins, 649, 651, 652, 654–662, 662–665, 669–670
 diamniotic (MCDA), 649, 656, 661
 perinatal postmortem, 191–192, **192**
 vascular occlusion in, 665–667
Monoclonal antibody immobilization of platelet antigens assay (MAIPA), 581, 585
Monoclonal antibody solid phase platelet antibody test (MASPAT), 584
Monocyte chemiluminescence (CL) test, 564
Monocyte monolayer assay (MMA), 564
Monogenic disorders, 325–326
Monopolar thermocoagulation, 667
Monozygotic twins (MZ), 649, 653, 662
Morbus Werlhoff *see* Idiopathic thrombocytopenia (ITP)
Mosaicism, 299, 300, 306, 308, 328, **328**
 chromosomal, 325
Mucolipidoses, 361–362
Mucopolysaccharidoses (MPS), **362**, 363
Müllerian duct, 25
Multicystic dysplasia, kidney, 471, **471**
Multi-dimensional Measure of Informed Choice (MMIC), 231
Multifactorial disorders, single gene disorder overlap, 321–322
Multifetal pregnancy reduction (MFPR), 651, 653, 666, 668, 670
 ethical dimensions of, 669
Multinucleated giant cells, 74
Multiple displacement amplification (MDA), 326, 355
Multiple sclerosis, 170
Multiples of the median (MoM), 245, 246–247, 247–248, **247**, 259–261
Multiplex ligation-dependent probe amplification (MLPA), 307, 314, 334, 350
Multipotent adult progenitor cells (MAPC), 682
Muscle biopsy, fetal, 300–301
Muscle scaffold model, 45
Mustard procedure, 420
Mutagenetically separated polymerase chain reaction (MS-PCR), 339
Mutation analysis, 360
Myasthenia gravis, 170
Mycophenolate mofetil (MM), 168–169
Mycoplasma hominis, 604
Myelomeningocele (MMC), 384–386, **387**
Myocyte
 mature, 121–122, **121**, **122**, 123, **123**
 size, 123
Myotonic dystrophy, 320, **320**

N

Narrative reviews, 201
Nasal bone, 276
 hypoplasia, 271, **271**
National Asthma Education Prevention Program (NAEPP), 166
National Down's syndrome screening programme (UK), 226
National External Quality Assessment Scheme (NEQAS) (UK), 260
National Health Service (NHS), screening programmes, 229, 230
National Institute of Child Health and Development (NICHD), 284, 709
National Institute for Health and Clinical Excellence (NICE), 469
National Institutes of Health (NIH), 265, 284, 658
National Perinatal Epidemiology Unit (Oxford), 199, 201
National Screening Committee (NSC) (UK), 226, 227, 228, 229, 231, 274, 651
Natriuretic peptide receptor B gene (NPR2), 506
Natural killer (NK) cells, 66, 605
 recognition, uterine, 67, **67**
Neck muscles, **34**, 44
'Negative studies', 200
Neocerebellum malformations, 399–400

Neonatal adrenoleukodystrophy (NALD), 364, **364**
Neonatal alloimmune thrombocytopenia (NAIT) *see* Fetal and neonatal alloimmune thrombocytopenia (FNAIT)
Neonatal medicine, 703
- hypoxic-ischemic brain damage, 707–709, **708**
- very preterm birth, 703–706, **705**
  - brain lesions, 706–707

Nephrectomy
- bilateral, 153
- unilateral, 151–152

Nephroblastomatosis, 472
Nephron endowment, 149–152
- importance of, 150, **150**, **151**
- measuring, 150
- nephrogenesis regulation, 149, **150**
- normal number, 149, **149**, **150**
- unilateral nephrectomy, 151–152
- in utero factors, 150–151
  - animal studies, 151
  - human studies, 151

Nephropathies, fetal, 472
Nerve growth factor (NGF), 22, 23
Neural crest cells, 4–5, 35–36, **35**, 42, 44–46
- contribution to ganglia, **35**
- fate maps, predictive, 37–38
- interactions, 16, **17**, 18
- migration routes, **35**

Neural primordium, fate map, **36**
Neural tube, 36
- defects (NTD), 597–598
  - *see also* Open neural tube defects
- paraxial mesenchyme, 36
- patterning, 37, **39**

Neuroblastoma, 535–536, **535**
Neurocranium, 39
Neurodevelopmental retardation, counseling, 393
Neurological injury, 664
- brain, 658

Neuromeres, 37, **38**
Neuronal ceroid lipofuscinosis (NCL), 363
Neuronal migration, 396, **397**
Neuronal proliferation disorders, 393–396
Neurulation, 36
Neurulation disorders
- primary, 381–386
- secondary, 386–388

Neutrophil extracellular traps (NET), 286
Nicolaides method, 273, **274**
Niemann-Pick disease, 361
Nifedipine, 162
NIFTY study, 284, 288
Nijmegen breakage syndrome, 367
Nitric oxide (NO), 137
Non-competent tissue, 15
Non-immune hydrops fetalis (NIHF), 626
Non-ketotic hyperglycinemia, 368
Non-maleficence, 217
Noonan syndrome, 421
Normality, defining, 26
'Norwood' procedure, 421
Notochord, 4
- formation, 36–37
- process, 35, 36

Nuchal edema, 515
Nuchal fold (NF), 269–270, **269**, 274
Nuchal translucency (NT), 262, 412
- Down's syndrome, 252, 254–255, **254**, 258, 261
- invasive procedures, 295–296
- measurement, accurate, 275, **275**
- metabolic errors, 363–364
- multiple pregnancy, 651, 668
- musculoskeletal problems, 491
- quality review (NTQR) program, 261

Nucleotide metabolism disorder, 366–367, **366**
Nuffield Council on Bioethics, Working Party of, 705
Nutrient transporters, 104
Nyberg method, 273, **274**

O

OAPR (odds of being affected given a positive result), 247
Obligations, 213–214
Obstetrics
- history, 563–564
- management, hydrops fetalis (HF), 524
- multiple pregnancy, 661
- timescales, 26–27, **27**

Oculomotor muscles, 44
Odontoblasts, 16
Oligohydramnios, 140, **643**, 644–645, **645**
- severe, 465, **470**, 472–473

Oocysts, 631
Open neural tube defects (ONTD), 244–246, 257, 258
- alpha-fetoprotein (AFP) as marker, 244–245, **244**
- diagnostic studies, 245
- folic acid supplementation impact, 246
- impact of screening, 246, **246**
- medications, 384

Open spina bifida
- cranial signs, **387**
- screening, 245, **246**

Optic cup, 16, **16**
ORACLE trial, 200
Organ injury, 664
Organic acid disorder, 367–368, **367**
Organisation of Teratology Information Specialists (OTIS), 160
'Ossification model', 41, 45
Osteogenesis imperfecta
- type IIA, IIB, IIC, 492, **492**, **493**, **494–495**, 495
- type III (OI III), 501, **502–503**
- type IV (OI IV), 501, 503, **504**

Ovarian teratomas, 321
Overriding aorta, 417–418, **417**
Oxcarbazepine, 172
Oxford Database of Perinatal Trials, 201
Oxygen
- delivery, fetal organ, **126**
- exchange, 99
- transport, 98–99

P

Pacemakers, 165
Palate, 43–44
Paleocerebellum malformations, 397–399
Paling palette, **229**
Palmitoyl protein thioesterase (PPT), 363
Paracentric inversions, 309
Paralysis, fetal, 568
Paraxial mesenchyme, **34**, 36, 44
- somatogenesis, 39–41, **40**

Parental conflict theory, 542
Parental reaction *see* Prenatal diagnosis
Parietal glomerular cells, 21
Partial hydatidiform mole (PHM), 607
Partners, prenatal diagnosis, 239
Parvovirus B19, 191, 625–627, **626**
- prenatal diagnosis, 626–627

Passive immunization, varicella-zoster virus (VZV) infection, 631
Paternal uniparental disomy for chromosome 14, 499–500
Patients
- fetus as, 215–216
- perinatal postmortem, 181

'Pattern recognition', 209
Peak systolic velocity (PSV), 565, 567, 572–573, 626–627, 657, 665
Pelvic dilatations, 462, 463, **463**
Pena-Shokeir syndrome type 1, 191
Pentalogy of Cantrell, 456
Peptide nucleic acid (PNA) clamping, 285
Percutaneous shunting in lower urinary tract obstruction (PLUTO) RCT, 469
Perfusion during embryogenesis, 74–75
Pericardial effusion, 515, **516**
Pericentric inversions, 309
Perinatal complications, multiple pregnancy, 660, 661
Perinatal disease, 649–650
Perinatal mortality surveys, 198
Perinatal postmortem, 181–183, 524
- authorization for, 182–183
- clinical information, 183, **184–185**
- examination, 183–188
  - delay, 183
  - external, 183, **183**, 186, **186**
  - further tests, 187
  - histology, 186, **186**
  - imaging, 186
  - internal, 186
  - placenta, 187–188, **187**
- fetal akinesia, 191, **191**
- hydrops fetalis (HF), 190–191, **190**
- intrapartum/early neonatal death, 192–193
- intrauterine growth restriction (IUGR), 188–190, **189**, **190**
- monochorionic twins, 191–192, **192**
- reasons for, 181–182
- value of, 182

Peripheral nervous system, 35
Perirenal urinoma, 464
Periventricular leukomalacia (PVL), 401, **401**, 707
Perlecan, 8, 11
Permissive interactions, 14–15
Peroxisomal disorders, 364, **364**
Persistent junctional reciprocating tachycardia (PJRT), 424
Persistent pulmonary hypertension of the newborn (PPHN), 173
Pharyngeal arches, 41–43, **42**
- angiogenic mesenchyme in, 45
- innervation of, 44
- paraxial mesenchyme in, 44
- skeletal elements, 43

Pharynx, **34**, 41
Phenobarbitone, 172
Phenylketonuria (PKU), 354, 368
Phenytoin, 172
Philosophers, 209–210
Phosphomannomutase (PMM), 366
Physicians for Human Rights, 218
'Pinopods', 63
Placenta
- architecture, 654–655, **655**
- bed disease, 82
- ground glass appearance, 515, **517**
- growth factor (PIGF), 87–88, 286
- hyperoxia, 88
- insufficiency, 104
- intrauterine growth restriction (IUGR), 82, 543
- mesenchymal dysplasia, **187**
- perinatal postmortem examination, 187–188, **187**
- primary functions of, 97
- specific 4 gene (PLAC4), 287–288
- thickness, 344
- twin, **192**
- *see also* Immune response, to implanting placenta

Placental development, 69–88
at delivery, 69–70, **70**
barrier, placental, 81
integrity of, 81
blood flow
fetoplacental, 81–82
hemochorial, 71
maternal, intervillous space, 76–77, **76**
early stages, 71–73, **71**
insufficiency, prenatal diagnosis, **84**, 85
intrauterine growth restriction (IUGR)/ pre-eclampsia, 82–85, **83**, **84**
perfusion during embryogenesis, 74–75, **76**
trophoblasts
/endothelial differentiation, 85–88
extravillous phenotypes, 73–74
invasion regulation, 74
uteroplacental arteries transformation, 75–76, **75**
villi, **72**, 77
architecture of trees, 77–78, **78**
villous development, **72**, 77, 78–81, **79**, **80**
see also Maternofetal exchange, placental function
Placental transfer (PT), 160
aminosalicylates (ASA), 168
antimalarial drugs, 169
azathioprine (AZA), 168
cyclosporin A, 169
interferon-beta 1, 170
methotrexate, 168
tacrolimus, 170
Placentome, 70
Placodal cells, contribution to ganglia, **35**
Plasma
maternal, fetal DNA in, 341
membrane, 6
Plasminogen activator (PA) system, 66
Plasticity
developmental, 130
stem cell, 682
Platelet disorders, fetal
alloantibodies, 583–584, **583**
alloantigens, 581–582, **582**, **583**
nomenclatures, **580**, 582–583
diagnosis, 584–587
human antigens, **580**
thrombocytopenia
fetal and neonatal alloimmune (FNAIT), 581–584, **583**, 585–587, **586**
idiopathic (ITP), 579–581, **582**
immune causes, 579, **580**
non-immune causes, 578–579, **579**
Platelet immunofluorescence test (PIFT), 580–581
Platelet-derived growth factor (PDGF), 22, 140, 430
Pleural effusions, 514, **516**
Point mutation diagnosis, 335
Polar body analysis, 323–324
Polycystic kidney disease, 471–472, **471**
Polycystic ovarian syndrome (PCOS), 604
Polygonal cells, large, 73
Polyhydramnios, 430, 448, 472, 532, **643**, 645–647, **646**
Polymorphic eruptions of pregnancy (PEP), 285
Polymorphic nuclear leukocytes (PMNLs), 620, 624
Polyploidization, 74
Pompe disease, 360, 361, 365
Population parameters, 247
Porencephaly, congenital, 400, **401**
Porphyria, acute intermittent, 322
Positive predictive value (PPV), 663
Postaxial polydactyly, 472
Post-conceptional age (PCA), 704
Posterior fossa fluid collection, 400
Postmortem *see* Perinatal postmortem
Postnatal therapy, 468, 553
Postovulatory age, 25
Post-term pregnancies, 644
Potassium chloride (KCl), 665, 670
Potter's syndrome, 153
Practice, theory, 209
Prader-Willi syndrome, 321
Pragmatic trial, 199
Prechordal mesenchyme, 37
Prechordal skull, 46
Predictive adaptive response, 543
Pre-eclampsia, 67, **67**, 82–**83**, **84**, 161, 164
cell-free fetal DNA, 285–287
key observations in, 287
Pre-existing disease/malformation, 160
Pregnancy
-associated progenitor cells, 113
dating, 546
disorders, 64, **65**
outcomes, adverse, 158
see also Early pregnancy failure (EPF)
Pregnancy, multiple, 649–670
dichorionic twin, 653–654, 662–665
higher order, 654, 667–670, **668**
monochorionic twin, 191–192, **192**, 654–662, 662–665, 665–667, 669–670
prenatal diagnosis, 650–654
reduction (feticide), 665–667, 668–669
Pregnancy-associated plasma protein-A (PAPP-A), 274
Pregnancy-induced hypertension (PIH), 161
Preimplantation genetic diagnosis (PGD), 323–329, 341, 370, 696
approach to, 323–325
chromosomal abnormalities, embryos, 325
detection, 326–328, **327**
early pregnancy failure, 602
embryo sexing, 326, **327**
endocrine disorders, 593
future developments, 328–329
monogenic disorders, 325–326
testing, 355
Preimplantation genetic haplotyping (PGH), 326
Prelacunar stage, 71
Preload, 126
Premature rupture of the membranes (PROM), 683
Prenatal diagnosis (PND), 234–240
abnormalities, **622**
bad news, breaking, 235
congenital diaphragmatic hernia (CDH), 439–442, **440**, **441**
congenital varicella syndrome, 630, **630**
cytomegalovirus (CMV), 622–623
decision making after, 235–237
follow-up support, 239–240
hemoglobinopathies, **334**, 340–341, **340**
hydrops fetalis (HF), 514–515, **515**, **516**, **517**
impact of, 235
intrauterine growth restriction (IUGR), 545–549
kidney anomalies, 472–473
lung lesion, 430–431
metabolic disorders, 357–358, 360
multiple pregnancy, 650–654
partners, 239
parvovirus B19, 626–627
placental development deficiency, **84**, 85
pregnancy continuation, 237
rubella, 628–629
skeletal abnormalities, 480, 482, 485
staff issues, 240
syphilis, 635–636
termination, 237–238
psychological effects of, 238–239
thalassemia, 341–342
toxoplasmosis, fetal, 633
uropathies, fetal, 462–464
Pressure-volume curves, 129
Preterm labour (PTL), 612
Preterm premature rupture of the membranes (PPROM), 547, 612, 644, 656–657, 666, 669
Primary biliary cirrhosis (PBC), 111–112
'Primary' proteins, 13
Primer-specific amplification, 338–339
Primidone, 172
Primitive node, 35
Primitive streak, 4
Primordial germ cells, 4
Proficiency testing, external, 260
Progenitor cells, 13, 113
Progress zone, 18
Prolactin, 647
Proliferative mitoses, 13
Promethazine, 572
Pronephros, 148
Propylthiouracil (PTU), 172, 594, 595
Prosencephalic development disorders, 388–391
cleavage, 389, **389**, **390**, 391
formation, 388–389
mid-line, 391–393, **391**, **392**
Prosencephalon, 37
Prostaglandin, 420
Proteins
cell, 13
fatty acid transfer (FATP), 103–104
human epidermal growth factor receptor (HER), 87
receptors, 12
Proteoglycans, 10–11
Proton nuclear magnetic resonance spectroscopy, 466
Protons, 100–101
'Prune-belly' syndrome, 207
'Pseudodeficiency' (PsD), 360
Pseudoglandular stage, 134, **135**
Pseudoporencephaly, 400
'Pseudorisk', 651
Psychological effects, of termination, 238–239
Publication bias, 200
Pulmonary circulation, 136–137
blood flow (PBF), 136, 137
changes at birth, 137
functional development, 136–137
structural development, 136, **136**
Pulmonary embolus, 165
Pulmonary hypoplasia, 438
Pulmonary stenosis/atresia, **420**, 421
Pulmonary surfactant, 142–143
composition of, 142–143
synthesis/release, 143
Pulmonary vascular resistance (PVR), 136, 137, 143
Pulsatility index (PI), 548, 551, 612
Purine nucleoside phosphorylase (PNP) deficiencies, 366
Pyelectasis, 463, **463**, 465
defined, 462
Pyruvate carboxylase (PC), 365
Pyruvate dehydrogenase (PDH), 365–366
Pyruvate kinase (PK) deficiency, 366

Q

QF-PCR (quantitative fluorescence polymerase chain reaction), 187, 307, 308, 311, 313–314, **314**, 315
Quadruplets, 668
Quantal, cell cycle, 13
Quantal mitosis, 13
Quantitative fluorescence polymerase chain reaction (QF-PCR), 187, 307, 308, 311, 313–314, **314**, 315
Queen Mother's Hospital, Glasgow, 265

R

Radiofrequency ablation (RFA), 660, 666, **667**
Radioresistant DNA synthesis (RDS), 367
Randomized controlled trials (RCT), 199–200
 amnioreduction, 657
 data monitoring, 200
 endocrine disorders, 604
 explanatory vs pragmatic, 199–200
 factorial design, 200
 'intention to treat', 200
 NIH multicenter selective laser, 658
 PLUTO, 469
 publication bias, 200
 randomization, 199
 sample size calculations, 200
Rapid Plasma Reagin(RPR), 635
Rara, 8
Rathke's pouch, 36, 38
Receiver operator curves (ROCs), 198
Recurrent miscarriage (RM), 603
Red blood cells (RBC), 168
Red cell alloimmunization, 559–573
 alternative treatment, 572
 antigen sensitization, 572–573
 future trends, 573
 history, 559–560
 hydrops fetalis (HF), 561–562, **561**
 invasive testing, 566–567
 management, 567–573
 mechanism, 560–563
 monitoring risk, 563–566
 pathophysiology, 560–561
Reduction mechanisms, maternofetal diffusion distance, 81
Reflux, 461, 462
Reichert's cartilage, 43
Renal agenesis, 469–470, **470**
Renal factors *see* Kidneys/urinary tract, development; Kidneys/urinary tract, disorders
Renal pyelectasis, 270, **270**
Renal tubular dysgenesis, 472
Renin-angiotensin system (RAS), 152–153, 655
 altered, 152–153
 cardiovascular disease, 153
Repetitive implantation failure (RIF), 327
Respect for autonomy and justice, 217
Respiratory distress syndrome (RDS), 142, 143, 704, 706
Restricted cells, 12
Restriction enzyme analysis (RE-PCR), 339
Resuscitation, **706**
Retroviruses, 692
Reversed end-diastolic flow (RED), 82, 85, 548, 551, 552, 553, 663
Reviews, systematic, 201
RHCD gene, 563
RHCE gene, 562–563
RHD gene, 562–563
RHD genotyping, 284
Rheumatoid arthritis (RA), 169
Rhizomelic chondrodysplasia punctata, 364, **364**, 503–504, **504**
Rhombencephalon, 37
Rhombomeres, 37, **38**
Rights-based philosophies, 214, 217
Risk
 cut-off levels, 259–260, **259**
 fetal loss, counseling, 300
 individual, 247
 information giving, 228–229, **229**
Robertsonian translocations, 309, **310**, 311
Routine Antenatal Diagnostic Imaging with Ultrasound (RADIUS), 265
Royal College of Obstetricians and Gynaecologists (RCOG), 265–266, 412, 613
Royal College of Pathologists, 181
Rubella, 627–629
 congenital, 628, **628**
 prenatal diagnosis, 628–629
 prevention, 629

S

Sacrococcygeal teratoma (SCT), 532–535, **532**, **533**, **534**
Sacrococcygeal tumors, 452
SAFE network, 284
Sagittal planes, **381**, **383**
Salmonella typhi, 604
Sample size calculations, 200
'Sandal gap' toe, 270–271
Sanfilippo disease, 363
Sarcolemma (SL), 121–122, 123
Sarcomeres, 122, **122**
Sarcoplasmic reticulum (SR), 121, 123
Sartans, 163
Scalp edema, **516**
Schizencephaly, 400, **401**
Science, 286
Sclerotome, 39
Screen positive/negative result, 256, 347
Screening, newborn, 254–255, **354**
Screening, prenatal, 225–231
 combined/integrated/contingent, 230, 275
 congenital heart disease (CHD), 412–413, 413–414, 414–415
 cystic fibrosis (CF), 352–354
 first- vs second-trimester, 230
 gestational trophoblastic disorders (GTD), 607
 history/overview, 243–244
 information giving
  DISCERN criteria, 227, **227**
  ethnic minorities, 226
  importance of, 225–226
  resources, 227–228
  risk and, 228–229, **229**
  technology specific, 229–231
 informed choice, 226
  measuring, 231
 integrated, 254–256, **255**
 mathematical principles, 246–248
 for multiple conditions, 231
 non-invasive, 282–288
 quality control/assessment, 260–261
 safety, 255
 for thalassemias, 344–347
 see also Ultrasound
Second UK Collaborative Study, 245
'Secondary' proteins, 13
Selection bias, 199
Selective serotonin reuptake inhibitors (SSRIs), 173
Self-assessment, 711–720
 answers, 717–720
 questions, 711–717
Sensitivity test, 198
Sensorineural hearing loss (SNHL), 621–622
Septal defects, 415, 417, 418
Septation stage, 120, **120**, **121**
 cardiac chamber, **120**
 truncus arteriosus, 120–121, **121**
Septo-optic dysplasia, 393
Septum pellucidum, agenesis (ASP), 393, **393**
Sequential screening, 256
Serum biochemistry, 651
Severe combined immunodeficiency syndrome (SCID), 678, 679, 695
Sex chromosome, 307
 /phenotype discordance, 310–311
 structural rearrangement, 310
Sexing
 embryo, 326, **327**
 fetal, 460
Short ribbed polydactyly syndromes (SRPS), 495, **497**, 498, **498**
SHOX gene, 310
Shunts
 with balanced anatomy, 415
 with unbalanced anatomy, 418, **419**
Sickle Cell and Thalassemia Screening Programme (NHS), 340
Sickle-cell disease (SS), 340
 phenotypes, **332**
Single gene disorders, 318–322
 new teaching, 320–322
 numbers of, 319, 320
 traditional teaching, 319–320
Single needle technique (CVS), 296–297
Single nucleotide polymorphism (SNP), 346
 analysis, 112
Single nucleotide polymorphism (SNP) locus, 288
Single strand conformation polymorphism (SSCP), 326
Single-allele base extension reaction (SABER), 346
Single-operator technique (CVS), **296**
Sinu-atrial foramen, 49
Sinus horns, 49
Sjögren syndrome, 111–112
Skeletal abnormalities, fetal, 478–511
 counseling, 511
 dysplasias, classification, 480–491, **481–482**, **483–484**
 hydrops, 519
 individual conditions, 241–510
 prenatal diagnosis of, 480, 482, 485
 sonographic features, 485–491, **486**
  normal, 480, **480**
 terminology, 478, **479**
Skin
 biopsy, fetal, 300–301
 edema, **516**
Skull, 39, 485–486, **486**
 base, 41
 prechordal, 46
 vault, 41
Sly syndrome, 361, 363
Small for gestational age (SGA), 544, 545, 546, 548, 549, 553
 defined, 541–542
Smith-Lemli-Opitz syndrome (SLOS), 187, 363, 369, **369**, **520**, 596–7
Smoking, 259, 606
 women, 543
Sodium, 100
Sodium valproate, 173
Sodium-proton exchanger (NHE), 100
Somatogenesis, 39–41, **40**
'Somatomedins', 22
Somatopleuric mesenchymal/surface ectoderm interaction, 18, **19**
Somite-derived mesenchyme, 22
Somites, lateral/medial halves, 4
Sonographic diagnosis
 kidney/urinary tract disorders, 462–464, 465
 multiple pregnancy, 660, 661, 662
 see also Central nervous system, fetal; Skeletal abnormalities, fetal
Sonographic marker detection
 first-trimester, 274–275
 risk assessment, 273–274, **274**

'soft', 269–270, **269**, 270–271, **270**, **271**
significance of, 272–273, **272**, **273**
variability, 271–272
see also Ultrasound
Sonographic markers of fetal aneuploidy (SMFAs), 267
Sotolol, 423
Sotos syndrome, 395–396
SOX9 gene, 500–501
'Special relationships', concept of, 213–214
Specialty guidelines, 217
Specificity test, 198
Sphingolipidoses, 360–361, **361**
Spina bifida
fetal, 81
prevalence, **385**
see also Open spina bifida
Spinal cord development, **39**
Spinal dysraphisms, classification, **387**
Spine, 486, **487**
Splanchnopleuric celomic epithelium, 18
Splanchnopleuric mesenchyme, 22
endoderm interactions, 18–20
Spondyloepiphyseal dysplasia congenita (SEDC), 498, **499**
Sprengel's deformity, 45
SRY gene, 285, 310, 563
Staff training, 240
Staging embryo development, 24–31
body plan, 27–31, **29**, **30**, **31**
chick series, 24–25
embryonic period, 27, **28**
human series, 25
molecular markers, 26
normality, 26
obstetric timescales, 26–27, **27**
Standards/guidelines, 261
Stem cells, 13
biology, 680–684
fetomaternal trafficking, 113
gene therapy, 693
Stem villi, 78–79, **79**
Steroidogenic pathway, **593**
Steroids *see* Corticosteroids
Stillbirth, 182
Streptococcus pyogenes, 530
Stroke volume, 126, **128**, **130**
Stromal connective tissue, 78, 81
Substrate deprivation, 544–545
Sulfapyridine, 168
Sulfasalazine, 168
Surfactant *see* Pulmonary surfactant
Surgery
evacuation of retained products of conception (ERPC), 613
fetal, 431–434, 468
heart, 419
mortality, 420
SURUSS (serum, urine, ultrasound study), 256, **257**, 259, 275
Symmetric IUGR, 542
Symphysio-fundal height (SFH), 545–546
Syncytial fusion, 74, 77
Syncytial knots, 77–78, **78**
Syncytiotrophoblast, 81, 98
fetal, 110
Syncytiotrophoblast microvilli (STBM), 286
Syndecans, 12
Syphilis, 634–636, **636**
congenital, 402, **402**, 635–636, **636**
prenatal diagnosis, 635–636
Systematic errors, 199
Systemic lupus erythematosus (SLE), 111–112, 168, 169, 485
Systemic sclerosis, 111

T

T cells, 22, 66
Tachycardias, 423–424
broad complex, 165–166
narrow complex, 165
Tachyzoites, 631
Tacrolimus, 170
Tay-Sachs disease, 358, 360–361
Tei index, 425
Telemedicine, 425
10-minute rule, 708
Tenascin, 20
TenneyParker change, 189
Teratogen, defined, 158, **159**, 160
Teratogenic drugs, 413
Teratoma
cervical, 530–531, **531**, **532**
hepatic, 452–453
sacrococcygeal (SCT), 532–535, **532**, **533**, **534**
Term Breech Trial, 199–200
Terminal differentiation, cell, 13, **13**
Terminal sac stage, 134, **135**
Terminal villi, 79, **79**
abnormal development, **83**
Termination, 236, 237–238, 468, 624
psychological effects of, 238–239
Termination of Pregnancy Act (1967), 413
Terminology, 3–5
animal model, 5
current, 4–5
early pregnancy failure (EPF), 608, **608**
fetal staging, 26
origin of traditional, 3–4
'Tertiary' proteins, 13
Thalassemias
α, 333–335
α major, 344–345
β, 335–339, **336–337**
δβ, 339
β major, 345–346
disorder phenotypes, **332**
prenatal diagnosis, 341–342
screening, 344–345, 346–347
Thanatophoric dysplasia, **396**, 486, 495, **496–497**
Thebesian valves, 51
Theophylline, 166–167
Theory and practice, 209
Therapy, fetal, 468–469
Thoracic abnormalities, 521
Thorax, **440**, 489, 491, **494–495**, **496**
Thought experiments, 210
Thrombocytopenia, 578–579, **579**
heparin-induced (HIT), 164
immune causes, 579, **580**
non-immune causes, 578–579, **579**
see also Fetal and neonatal alloimmune thrombocytopenia (FNAIT); Idiopathic thrombocytopenia (ITP)
Thrombolysis, 165
Thrombophilias, 605
Thrombopoietin plasma (Tpo) levels, 580, 585
Thrombotic vasculopathy, fetal, **190**
Thromboxane A (TAX2), 164
Thyroid disorders, 171–172, 594–595
Thyroid hormones, 143
Thyroid stimulating hormone (TSH), 171, 172, 594, 595, 604
Thyrotropin-releasing hormone (TRH), 143, 200
Thyroxine, 143
Tidal volume, 137
Tight junctions, 8
Tissue
competent/non-competent, 15
embryonic, 8–12, 14–15
fetal, 300–301, 359
Tissue-non-specific alkaline phosphotase gene (TNSALP), 491–492
Toxins, 543, 605–606
Toxoplasma gondii, 402, **402**
Toxoplasmosis, fetal, 293, 631–634, **632**, **633**
anemia, 522
congenital, 632–633
prenatal diagnosis, 633
prevention, 633–634
treatment, 633
Tracheal occlusion (TO), 443–444
Tracheoesophageal atresia, 448–449, **448**
Training
screening, 412–413
staff, 240
Transabdominal (TA)
examination, 379
technique, **295**, 296, **296**
Transabdominal (TA) chorionic villus sampling (CVS), 296, 297
Transcervical (TC) chorionic villus sampling (CVS), 296, 297
Transcervical (TC) technique, **295**, 296, **296**
Transforming growth factor
-α, 87
β (TGFβ), 22–23, 86–87
Transplacental hemorrhage (TPH), 560
Transport
calcium, 101
sodium, 100
types, 98–99
Transvaginal (TVS) examination, 379
TRAP (twin reversed arterial perfusion) sequence, 658, 660
Treponema carateum, 634
Treponema endemicum, 634
Treponema pallidum (TP), 634–635
Treponema pertenue, 634
Trichorionic triamniotic triplets (TCTA), 650
Tricuspid atresia, **419**
Tricuspid regurgitation (TR), 276
Tricuspid valve dysplasia, 420
Tricyclic antidepressants, 174
Trigger gradient, 74
Triiodothyronine, 143
Triplets, 650, 668–669
Triploidy, 307–308, 472
full, 307–308
mosaic, 308
Trisomy 13, **307**
mosaicism, 308
Trisomy 15, 321
Trisomy 16, 324
Trisomy 18, 250, 258, 274, **307**, 472
mosaicism, 308
prenatal testing
first-trimester, 261–262
integrated, 262, **262**
second-trimester, 261, **261**
Trisomy 21, **268**, 268–276 *passim*, **269**, **271–273**, 287, 325, 653
cytogenetics, **307**, 315
mosaicism, 308
see also Down's syndrome
Triturus cristatus, 24
Triturus taeniatus, 24
Trophectoderm (TE), 325
Trophoblast cells, 64, **64**, **65**, 71–72, **73**
endovascular migration, 66
extracellular matrix (ECM) degradation, 65–66
'invasion impairment', 286
invasion regulation, 74
major histocompatibility complex (MHC) antigens, 66

Trophoblast cells (*continued*)
- small spindle-shaped extravillous, 73–74
- uterine NK cell recognition, 67, **67**

Trophoblast differentiation
- growth factors, 86–88
- molecular control, 85–88
- transcription factors, 85–86

Trophoblast plugs, 76–77
TRUFFLE (trial of umbilical and fetal flow in Europe), 553
Truncus arteriosus septation, 120–121, **121**
Tumors, fetal, 528–536
- cervical teratoma, 530–531, **531**, **532**
- cystic hygroma/lymphangioma, 528–530, **529**
- ex utero intrapartum treatment (EXIT), 531–532, **532**
- neck masses, differential diagnosis, **526**
- neuroblastoma, 535–536, **535**
- sacrococcygeal teratoma (SCT), 532–535, **532**, **533**, **534**

Tumour necrosis factor (TNF), 22
- antagonists (anti-TNF), 170

Turner's syndrome, **307**, 472, 519, 529
- termination rates, 236

Twin reversed arterial perfusion (TRAP) sequence, 654, 658, 660, 665, 666–667
Twins, 293, 300
- conjoined, 661–662
- dichorionic (DC), 649–650, 651, 652, 653–654, 662–665
- dizygotic (DZ), 650, 662
- Down's syndrome, **651**, 668
- monoamniotic (MA), 660–661, **661**, 667
- monochorionic *see* Monochorionic (MC) twins
- monozygotic twins (MZ), 649, 653, 662
- surviving, 664

Twin-twin transfusion syndrome (TTTS), 192, 523, 647–651 *passim*, 654–658, 661–670 *passim*
- echocardiograph features, 656
- systemic response, 655–656
- treatment, 656–657, 657–658, **659**

Tyrosinemia type I, 368

U

UKOSS Project, 199
Ultrasound, 182, 230–231, 528
- diagnosis, 622–623, **622**
- early pregnancy failure (EPF), 612
- genetic sonogram, 267, **268**
- real-time, 301
- red cell alloimmunization, 564
- routine, 265–266
- sensitivity, factors affecting, 266–267, **268**
- SURUSS (serum, urine, ultrasound study), 256, **257**
- two dimensional, 344–345, **345**
- three dimensional, 277, 612
- *see also* Sonographic marker detection

Umbilical artery (UA), 548, 552, 553, 612
Umbilical circulation, 124
Umbilical cord
- blood (UCB), 681, 682
- coiling, 188
- ligation, 666

Umbilical vein (UV), **300**, 545
- catheter, 443

'Unexplained IUGR', 549–550
Unfractionated heparin (UFH), 164
Unilateral renal agenesis (URA), 154
Uniparental disomy (UPD), 299, 311, 544
University of California (San Francisco) (UCSF), 429, 441–442, 443–444
University College London Hospital (UCLH), 485, 572
Urachal diverticulum, 462
Urea cycle disorders, 300–301
Ureaplasma urealyticum, 604
Ureteric budding, 20, 148–149
Ureteric ducts, 20
Ureterocele, 462
Ureteropelvic junction (UPJ), 153
- obstruction, 462

Ureters, 459–460
Urethral atresia, 464
Urinary analyte markers, 469
Urinary tract *see* Kidneys/urinary tract, development; Kidneys/urinary tract, disorders
Uroenteric fistula, 465
Uterine NK cell recognition, 67, **67**
Uteroplacental arteries transformation, 75–76, **75**
Uteroplacental circulation, 548, **548**
Uteroplacental insufficiency (UPI), 82, 542, 543
Uteroplacental ischemia, 189

V

Vaccination, 174, **174**, 627, 629, 631
Vaccine In Pregnancy (VIP) registry, 629
VACTERAL sequence, 470
VACTERL sequence, 481
Vagal stimulation, 165
Vaginal bleeding, 297
Validation trials, 256–257, **257**
Valproate, 173
Valves, absent/hypoplastic, 419, **419**
Valvuloplasty, fetal, 425
Varicella syndrome, 293, 630
- prenatal diagnosis, 630, **630**

Varicella-zoster virus (VZV), 629–631
Vascular abnormalities, fetal, 402–403, **404**
Vascular anastomoses, 654–655, **655**
Vascular endothelial growth factor (VEGF), 85, 87–88
Vascular occlusion, 665–667
Vascularization, fetal, **79**
Vasculosyncytial membrane (VSM), 79
Vasodilators, 163
VATER sequence, 448–449, 451, 481, 509–510
Vectors, 691–692
Vein of Galen, 402–403, **403**
Vein-to-vein anastomosis (VVA), 654–655
Venereal Disease Research Laboratory (VDRL), 635
Venous return curve (VRC), **127**
Veno-venous (VV) anastomoses, 192
Ventricles and outflow tract, 52–57, **54**, **56**
Ventricular disproportion, 421–422, **422**
Ventricular fibrillation/flutter, 166
Ventricular geometry, 128–129, **128**, **129**, **130**
Ventricular premature beats (VPB), 166
Ventricular septal defects (VSD), 415, 417, **420**
- large, 417
- multiple, 417

Ventricular tachycardias (VT), 165–166
Ventriculoarterial connections, discordant, 419–420, **420**
Ventriculomegaly, 387–388, **388**
Verapamil, 162, 424
Very long chain acyl dehydrogenase (VLCAD) deficiency, 368
Very long chain fatty acids (VLCFA), 364
Very low birth weight (VLBW) babies, 285
Very low density lipoprotein (VLDL), 103
Vesicoamniotic shunting, **469**
Vesicoureteric junction (VUJ), 153
Vesicoureteric reflex (VUR), 153
Vesicular stomatitis virus protein G (VSVG), 692
Villous development, **72**, 77, 78–81, **80**
- architecture of trees, 77–78, **78**
- capillary growth, **80**
- fetal vascularization of, **79**
- routes of, **80**
- types, **79**
- ultrastructure of, **79**

Virtue ethics, 217
Visceral epithelial podocytes, 21
Viscerocranium, 39
Vitamin deficiency, 151
Vitamin Study Research Group, Medical Research Council (MRC), 598
Vitamin supplementation, 163
Volvulus, congenital, 453–454

W

Walker-Warburg syndrome, 384
Warfarin, 164–165
Water, maternofetal exchange, 100
Weaver syndrome, 395–396
Weight
- estimated fetal(EFW), 546, 549, 551, 663
- maternal, 257–258, **258**

White matter damage, 707
Wilkins Pediatric Endocrine Society, 594
Wilms' tumor (WT-1), 149
Wilson disease, 598
Wolffian duct (WD), 148, 154, 459
Wolman disease, 360, 361
Word analysis, 209–210
World Health Organisation (WHO), 299, 633
World Medical Assembly, 218

X

Xenopus, 5
X-linked adrenoleukodystrophy (ALD), 364, **364**
X-linked diseases, 326, **327**, 358
X-linked dominant inheritance, 319–320
X-linked recessive chondrodysplasia punctata, 504, **505**, 506
X-linked recessive inheritance, 319
X-ray, 186

Y

Yolk sac, secondary (SYS), 610, **610**

Z

Zellweger syndrome, 363, 364, **364**
Zone of polarizing activity (ZPA), 18, **19**

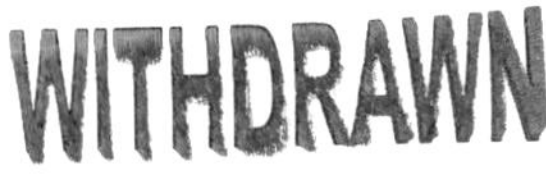

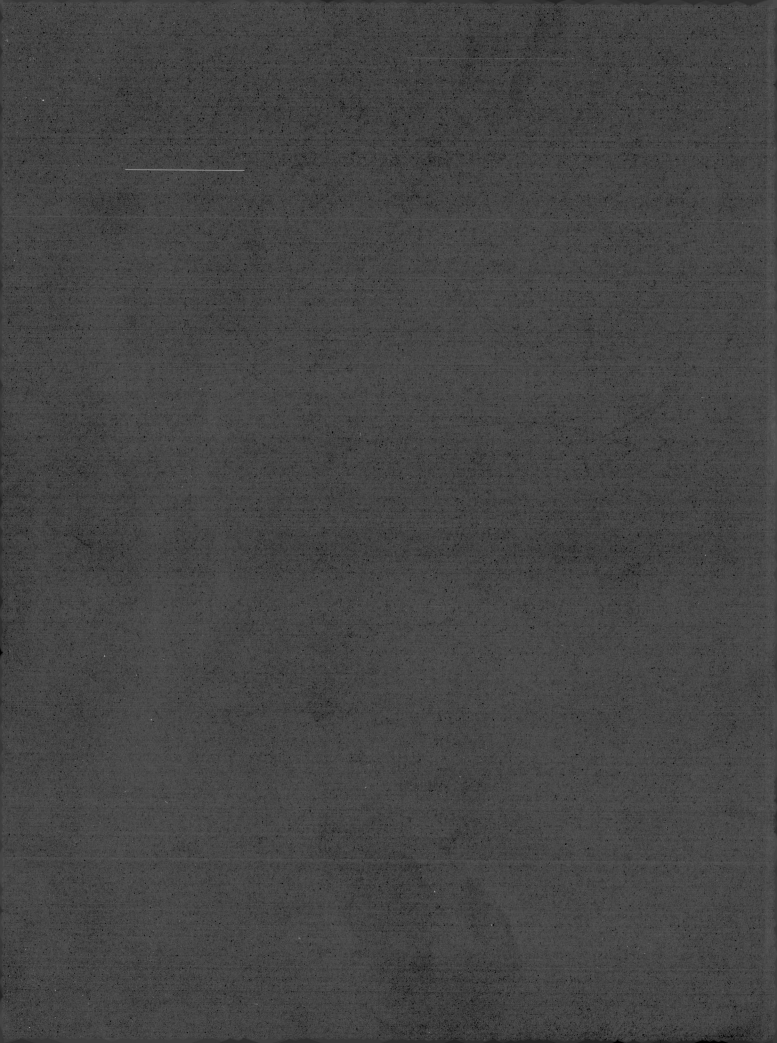